PEARSON'S COMPREHENSIVE MEDICAL CODING

A PATH TO SUCCESS

Second Edition

Lorraine M. Papazian-Boyce, MS, CPC

AHIMA-Approved ICD-10-CM/PCS Trainer

Educator of the Year—Instruction, 2011,
Career Education Corporation

Most Promising New Textbook Excellence Award, 2013, 2016,
Textbook and Academic Authors Association

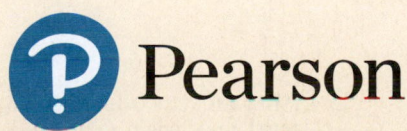

Senior Vice President, Portfolio Management: Adam Jaworski

Director of Portfolio Management: Marlene McHugh Pratt

Portfolio Management Assistant: Emily Edling

Vice President, Content Production and Digital Studio: Paul DeLuca

Managing Producer, Health Science: Melissa Bashe

Content Producer: Faye Gemmellaro

Editorial Project Manager: Pearson CSC, Meghan DeMaio

Full-Service Project Manager: Pearson CSC, Patty Donovan

Operations Specialist: Maura Zaldivar-Garcia

Creative Digital Lead: Mary Siener

Director, Digital Production: Amy Peltier

Digital Studio Producer, REVEL and eText 2.0: Ellen Viagnola

Digital Content Team Lead: Brian Prybella

Digital Content Project Lead: Lisa Rinaldi

Vice President, Product Marketing: Brad Parkins

Product Marketing Manager: Rachele Strober

Senior Field Marketing Manager: Brittany Hammond

Full Service Project Management and Composition: Pearson CSC

Inventory Manager: Vatche Demirdjian

Interior Design: Pearson CSC

Cover Design: Studio Montage

Cover Art: ESB Basic/Shutterstock, Dotshock/Shutterstock, Flamingo Images/Shutterstock, Monkey Business Images/Shutterstock, Billion Photos/Shutterstock, Kekyalyaynen/Shutterstock

Printer/Binder: LSC Communications, Inc.

Cover Printer: LSC Communications, Inc.

Notice: The authors and the publisher of this volume have taken care that the information and technical recommendations contained herein are based on research and expert consultation and are accurate and compatible with the standards generally accepted at the time of publication. Nevertheless, as new information becomes available, changes in clinical and technical practices become necessary. The reader is advised to carefully consult manufacturers' instructions and information material for all supplies and equipment before use, and to consult with a health care professional as necessary. This advice is especially important when using new supplies or equipment for clinical purposes. The authors and publisher disclaim all responsibility for any liability, loss, injury, or damage incurred as a consequence, directly or indirectly, of the use and application of any of the contents of this volume.

Credits and acknowledgments borrowed from other sources and reproduced, with permission, in this textbook. CPT copyright 2018 American Medical Association. All rights reserved. CPT is a registered trademark of the American Medical Association.

Library of Congress Cataloging-in-Publication Data

Names: Papazian-Boyce, Lorraine, author.

Title: Pearson's comprehensive medical coding : a path to success / Lorraine M. Papazian-Boyce.

Other titles: Comprehensive medical coding

Description: Second edition. | Boston : Pearson, 2019. | Includes bibliographical references and index.

Identifiers: LCCN 2018008010 | ISBN 9780134818801 (student edition) | ISBN 0134818806

Subjects: | MESH: International statistical classification of diseases and related health problems. 10th revision. Clinical modification. | International statistical classification of diseases and related health problems. 10th revision. Procedure coding system. | Current procedural terminology (Standard ed.: 1998) | International classification of diseases. 9th revision. Clinical modification. | Healthcare common procedure coding system. | Clinical Coding | Disease--classification | International Classification of Diseases | Problems and Exercises

Classification: LCC R728.8 | NLM W 80 | DDC 616.001/2--dc23

LC record available at https://lccn.loc.gov/2018008010

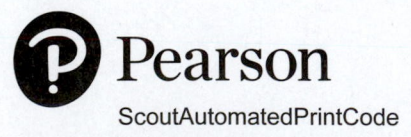

ISBN-10:   0-13-481880-6

ISBN-13:   978-0-13481880-1

Your path to success in life starts with a decision to begin the journey.

Thank you to my family, friends, and colleagues who have supported and guided my path and life adventures.

Brief Table of Contents

SECTION FOUR

ICD-10-PCS Procedure Coding   951

SECTION FIVE

Putting It All Together   1167

Contents

SECTION THREE

CPT/HCPCS Procedure Coding 441

SECTION FOUR

ICD-10-PCS Procedure Coding 951

SECTION FIVE

Putting It All Together   1167

Preface

Pearson's Comprehensive Medical Coding: A Path to Success, 2e is a comprehensive text on the healthcare industry's coding systems: ICD-10-CM/PCS, CPT, and HCPCS. I am honored that the first edition was awarded *Most Promising New Textbook* by the Textbook and Academic Authors Association.

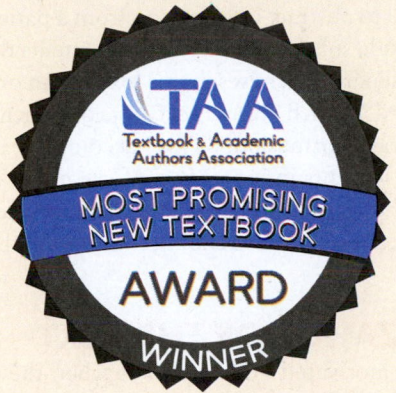

This text is intended for students studying coding at career colleges, community colleges, and universities. Students might be planning to become dedicated coders or be preparing for a related role, such as health information specialist, clinician, or administrator. The book is also useful for professional coders and providers, as well as billers, claims examiners, and medical assistants.

The material is written to be friendly to those with basic exposure to medical terminology and limited or no experience in the medical field. The flexibility of the organization allows the text to be used for a single comprehensive coding course or divided among separate courses on diagnosis coding, physician procedure coding, and inpatient hospital procedure coding. The "Instructor's Resource Manual" provides suggested outlines for various course configurations.

Over 6,200 exercise questions—more than any other coding text—give students ample opportunity to develop and fine-tune their skills. Progressively challenging exercises embedded within the text of each chapter build on one another and guide students through coding principles. End-of-chapter review questions further challenge students and reinforce key concepts.

NEW TO THE SECOND EDITION

My goal in the second edition is to provide updated information, clarify details where needed, and enhance what already works well to make it more useful to students and instructors. Highlights of improvements include:

- Completely updated to 2019 ICD-10 CM/PCS, CPT, HCPCS code sets
- Added a new appendix with all 115 "Key Criteria to Abstracting" tables for easy pull-out reference
- Updated learning objectives to align with the revised Bloom's Taxonomy articulated by AHIMA

- Added two chapters—"Advanced Coding" and "Professionalism and Patient Relations"—to the print text
- Moved most information on hospital reimbursement to Chapter 2, "Coding and Reimbursement"
- Added information on electronic coding tools to Chapter 2, "Coding and Reimbursement"
- Updated and reorganized ICD-10-PCS chapters for easier reference
- Added "Key Criteria to Abstracting" tables for characters 3 through 7 of ICD-10-PCS codes in Chapter 47
- Added multiple-choice coding questions in all coding chapters to mirror certification exam format
- Expanded emphasis on coding guidelines for all code sets
- Created new Professional Profiles to open each section
- Created new anatomic illustrations to enhance challenging concepts, including a new figure depicting the seven PCS surgical approaches and their variations
- Removed first edition chapter, "Transition ICD-10 CM/PCS"
- Removed first edition chapters on ICD-9-CM
- Updated and added tables, charts, and figures
- Updated and added new coding examples
- Updated and reorganized chapter review questions
- Added pertinent new coding information
- Added laterality to pertinent codes
- Expanded modifier coverage
- Updated and added Guided Examples where appropriate
- Updated all SpeedeCoder screenshot figures
- Updated Coder's Index
- Updated Glossary
- Added new "References" section at the end of the book, listing all sources mentioned in the text
- Updated *Success Step* and *Coding Caution* features for new coding guidelines
- Streamlined page layout by integrating selected content from first edition *Success Step* and *Coding Caution* features into the running narrative

CONCEPTUAL APPROACH

The goal of this text is not only to create a comprehensive coding text but to approach coding in a way that gives instructors unique tools to communicate successfully and gives students a unique approach to learn effective coding skills. This approach is applied to all code sets and has proven successful in the classroom over the past eight years of this text and its predecessor, *ICD-10-CM/PCS Coding: A Map for Success*. Four concepts are the focus of each chapter.

Abstracting, Assigning, and Arranging Codes

Students need a simple and methodical approach to the complex coding process. This text organizes coding around the learning mnemonic for an "Ace" coder: *abstract, assign, and arrange (sequence)* codes. Each coding chapter includes a section of the chapter for each concept, complete with a Guided Example and exercises.

The *Abstracting* section of each chapter focuses on how to read and interpret documentation and identify key pieces of information without assigning any codes. A unique and original table, Key Criteria for Abstracting, appears for each body system to guide students through details specific to each body system.

The *Assigning* section of each chapter focuses on the mechanics of navigating the coding manuals and determining the correct code. Annotated and color-coded illustrations of pages from the indices and tabular lists of each coding manual visually guide students through what can sometimes be a dizzying array of Main Terms, subterms, and code options.

The *Arranging* section of each chapter focuses on identifying when multiple codes are required and how to sequence them, as well as how to apply modifiers based on coding guidelines and conventions.

The *Official Guidelines for Coding and Reporting* (OGCR) and CPT guidelines are integrated into each chapter's discussion and highlighted with examples. We do not reprint guidelines in their entirety as is done in many texts. Students should be directed to the current year's guidelines in their coding manuals or online.

Guided Examples walk students through the three steps of coding and reveal the critical thinking process of applying guidelines and negotiating the intricacies of the coding manuals. By consistently and repeatedly focusing on these basic skills, the outcome is students who can tackle a variety of coding scenarios with confidence.

Application of Medical Terminology

Medical terminology skills present one of the greatest challenges to coding students. Unique features in this book help students apply what they learned in medical terminology and anatomy courses to coding. Each chapter begins with a review of medical terminology applicable to the body system being discussed. To support the emphasis on anatomy in ICD-10-CM/PCS, body system diagrams are dually labeled with the English word and the medical combining form, such as *stomach* and *gastr/o*. This helps students make both visual and verbal connections with medical terms. Commonly used prefixes and suffixes, as well as easily confused medical terms, are presented within each body system. Terminology exercises and examples in each chapter show students how to continue building terminology skills and apply them to coding. This section of the chapter reviews medical terminology skills students may have learned in a previous course and introduces basic concepts for students new to medical terminology. Curricula that does not have a medical terminology prerequisite should direct students to online tutorials to familiarize them with basic skills. The outcome is students who understand the terminology they encounter in coding exercises and, as a result, code more accurately.

Relationship of Diagnoses and Procedures

Students need to understand how diagnoses and procedures relate to each other. Every chapter highlights diagnoses and the related treatments together so students learn the relationship between the two. Exercises describe both diagnoses and services, even though the coding focus is on one or the other. End-of-chapter exercises in the procedure coding chapters require both diagnosis and procedure codes. The outcome is students who comprehend the full coding picture and, as a result, make a smooth transition into coding full cases.

Context of the Patient Encounter

Students need to abstract information from a patient encounter rather than code solely from isolated statements that are five to ten words in length. Exercises in this text use an original "mini-medical-record," which presents excerpts of patient, diagnostic, and procedural information. "Tips" accompany difficult exercises to help students interpret the information. The outcome is students who learn abstracting skills in every exercise and are better prepared for advanced coding courses and the workplace.

ORGANIZATION OF THE TEXT

Students are motivated and confident when they understand why they are studying a subject and where they are going before they begin. The organization of this text gives students a context and framework for coding, covers the technical coding topics for each code set in detail, then wraps up the content with a look ahead.

Section One, "Foundations of Coding", establishes the basis of the coding career and the reimbursement process. Students enter coding class with many questions about their future careers, so those questions are addressed up front. Then, by walking students through the claims and reimbursement process, they gain a contextual understanding of how codes are used and how they affect an organization's success.

Section Two, "ICD-10-CM Diagnosis Coding", arranges chapters based on ease of student learning, rather than following the strict order of the coding manual. Four chapters that are used across all body systems appear before the individual body system chapters: symptoms, neoplasms, Z-codes, and external cause codes. The Instructor's Resource Manual provides a cross-walk for those who wish to teach chapters in the traditional order of the coding manual.

Each ICD-10-CM coding manual chapter is covered in one textbook chapter. No coding manual chapters are combined or split, which allows great flexibility to adapt the book to any curriculum format. The chapters can be taught in any order that best suits the curriculum.

Section Three, "CPT/HCPCS Procedure Coding", presents procedure coding for body systems *in the same order as Section Two*, with one body system per chapter. This is convenient for programs that wish to pair diagnosis and procedure coding.

Chapter 27 provides a basic overview of CPT and HCPCS modifiers. Additional details and examples are presented in the section in individual CPT body system chapters. This helps students develop their understanding as they progress through the course rather than isolating all modifier information in a single chapter.

Chapter 28 provides a basic overview of Evaluation and Management (E/M) coding. Subsequent chapters build on this foundation by presenting an E/M case, documentation guidelines, and Guided Example at the end of each CPT body system chapter. This enables students to develop their understanding of E/M throughout the course and to appreciate the total context of a given medical specialty. This approach also allows instructors to be selective about the depth of information covered in class. They can choose to include or exclude the more advanced E/M sections, as applicable to their specific program curriculum.

Section Four, "ICD-10-PCS Coding", provides an introduction to inpatient hospital coding. The emphasis is on helping students understand the purpose of each character of an ICD-10-PCS code and on identifying the characteristics of and differences between ICD-10-PCS root operations. Medical and surgical root operations, which account for 85% of all PCS codes, are covered in greatest detail, in Chapters 46-53, to help students learn the structure and use of ICD-10-PCS. These skills are then applied to the other sections of PCS in Chapters 54-55.

Section Five, "Putting It All Together", consists of two chapters, previously available online. Chapter 56 introduces students to coding from chart notes and operative reports, with hands-on practice. Chapter 57 discusses professionalism in depth to bring students full circle from where they started in Chapter 1 with an introduction to careers.

FEATURES

Consistent pedagogical elements appear in each chapter to facilitate instruction and learning.

Learning Objectives—Each chapter begins with a list of the primary skills students should have after completing the chapter, aligned with Bloom's Taxonomy levels of learning.

Key Terms and Abbreviations—A list of the important terms students need to know but may not have learned in previous classes is provided at the beginning of each chapter. These terms are set in blue boldface type and are defined upon first appearance in the chapter. They are also included in the Glossary at the end of the book.

Chapter Outline—A list of the major topics covered in the chapter appears at the beginning.

Introduction—The text uses analogies at the beginning of chapters to create a "hook" with a common frame of reference and provides a familiar perspective for relating to new information. ICD-10-CM/PCS chapters use travel analogies while CPT chapters use shopping analogies. Instructors can use these analogies as a springboard for student engagement in classroom discussion.

Success Step—Short tips help students abstract, assign, and arrange (sequence) codes.

Coding Caution—Short warnings alert students to coding situations that can be tricky or confusing.

Coding Practice—Coding exercises throughout the chapter consist of three to six patient scenarios related to a specific chapter topic, using the mini-medical-record format. The first exercise in the coding chapters reviews medical terms related to the body system or type of procedure and introduces students to simple coding for the body system. Subsequent exercises walk students through the skills of abstracting, assigning, and sequencing codes. Exercises increase in difficulty as the chapter progresses, while remaining appropriate for an introductory course.

Guided Examples—Step-by-step demonstrations allow students to experience the thinking process of a seasoned coder as they observe a coder abstract, assign, and sequence codes from a mini-medical-record.

Figures—Anatomic illustrations show English names and medical terms for major body parts and organs. Original drawings of disease processes and selected anatomic details clarify difficult coding concepts. Annotated diagrams of sample pages from the coding manuals guide students' understanding of layout and appropriate use. Photographs and graphics portray key points and clarify new information.

Tables—Tables provide definitions of terms, conditions, and treatments, key criteria for abstracting diagnoses, procedures and root operations, and comparative information that highlights key concepts.

Summary—Each chapter ends with a brief restatement of key points in the chapter.

Typefaces and Punctuation

Distinct fonts and color-coding enable students to visually identify various types of information. Typefaces are intermixed in the narrative to highlight information taken directly from a medical record or the coding manual. Three special fonts are used as follows:

- Key terms and abbreviations
- Simulated content in a patient's medical record
- **Codes, code titles, and instructional notes from the coding manuals**

The names of chapters, sections, and selected features in the coding manuals are treated as proper nouns and are therefore capitalized. This use is to be distinguished from the common use of a term. For example, the Digestive System subsection of the CPT manual is treated as a proper noun and capitalized. The organ system known as digestive system is a common noun and not capitalized. In Section Four, ICD-10-PCS, the term *Character* is capitalized when referring to the positions in a PCS code. The term *Table* is capitalized when referring to the reference tables in the PCS coding manual. The names of PCS-identified body systems, body parts, approaches, and devices are treated as proper nouns and thus capitalized when referring to a specific value in the PCS code set. Such terms usually appear in the text's designated font for codes. When a body system, body part, or approach is referenced as a common noun, it is not capitalized. This variation in capitalization is intentional for the sake of clarity and is not a copyediting or proofreading error. Information that appears in **this font** is a direct quote from the coding manuals. Spelling, punctuation, and abbreviations reflect the styles of the respective coding manuals and have not been copyedited to Pearson's style for the text. This practice is intentional for the sake of consistency with the coding manuals and is not a copyediting or proofreading error.

End-of-Chapter Material

The review at the end of each chapter reinforces key concepts, provides opportunity for additional skills practice, and offers resources for additional learning.

Concept Quiz—Definitions and key concepts are reviewed using ten completion and ten multiple-choice questions. Multiple-choice questions include three coding questions formatted similarly to the certification examinations' format.

Keep on Coding—Twenty-five coding exercises in a one-line statement format provide beginning student practice.

Coding Challenge—Ten coding scenarios drawn review beginning and intermediate coding skills with an emphasis on applying the official coding guidelines. The Coding Challenge exercises in procedure coding chapters require both diagnosis and procedure codes for integrative practice. The length of courses and structure of curriculum varies widely among colleges. Based on an individual school's format, instructors may choose to incorporate Coding Challenge exercises into an introductory class or revisit them in a more advanced course.

End-of-Book Material

The following material at the end of the text provides reference information for students.

Glossary—The Glossary defines key terms, supplemental terms, and abbreviations.

Index—An alphabetic cross-walk identifies page references for major topics discussed in this text.

Coders' Index—The Coder's Index lists all codes found in the text and where they are discussed.

Key Criteria to Abstracting Tables—A quick reference pull-out guide provides easy access to all of the Key Criteria to Abstracting tables that appear in the coding chapters.

Resources

- Textbook

The instructor package:

- Instructor's Resource Manual contains detailed lesson plans, homework, discussion topics and teaching tips to help faculty plan and manage the medical coding course
- Answer Key for all exercises in the text
- PowerPoint® slides that align with learning objectives and summarize key learning points
- Testgen® computerized test bank

Interactive Media

Visit our new MyHealthProfessions Lab to accompany *Pearson's Comprehensive Medical Coding: A Path to Success*, 2e. Here you'll find extensive resources, including:

- A pre-/post-test homework engine, which enables students to learn and master concepts as homework, preparing them for classroom work.
- Access your free trial of SpeedeCoder® online medical coding software at **http://sec.pearsonhighered.com**.

ABOUT THE AUTHOR

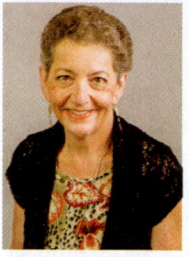

Lorraine M. Papazian-Boyce, MS, CPC
AHIMA-Approved ICD-10-CM/PCS Trainer
Lorraine M. Papazian-Boyce is an award-winning author and instructor. She received the Most Promising New Textbook Award—2016 from the Textbook and Academic Authors Association for this text. She also authored the Pearson text *ICD-10-CM/PCS Coding: A Map for Success*, which received the Most Promising New Textbook Award—2013. She was named Educator of the Year—Instruction in 2011 by Career Education Corporation (CEC).

Lorraine holds an MS in Health Systems Management from Rush University (Chicago) and the Certified Professional Coder (CPC) credential. She is an AHIMA-Approved ICD-10-CM/PCS Trainer. She has taught coding at several ground and online colleges.

Lorraine has over 35 years of experience in healthcare administration as a college instructor, in both traditional and online settings; owner of a medical billing service; office manager; consultant to hospitals, nursing homes, and physicians; and board of directors officer. She is a frequent speaker on billing, coding, and healthcare management. She has taught most aspects of healthcare operations and reimbursement both to practicing professionals and in a formal academic career college setting. She is known as someone who is thorough in covering material and effective in communicating it to learners, in both oral and written formats. She knows exactly where in the curriculum college students struggle, what their questions are, and what techniques best clarify information for them. As a former employer and as an externship coordinator, she also knows what today's students need to succeed in the medical workplace. Her driving passion is taking complex technical subjects and breaking them down into practical, understandable pieces that others can implement.

She is a contributor and/or subject matter expert to several Pearson texts, including *Pearson's Comprehensive Medical Assisting*, 4th ed., by Nina M. Beaman, et al.; *Medical Coding: A Journey*, by Beth A. Rich; *Administrative Medical Assisting: Foundations and Practices*, 2nd ed., by Christine Malone; *Guide to Medical Billing and Coding*, 3rd edition, by Sarah Brown and Lori Tyler; *Comprehensive Health Insurance:*

Billing, Coding, and Reimbursement, by Deborah Vines, Ann Braceland, Elizabeth Rollins, and Susan H. Miller; *A Guided Approach to Intermediate and Advanced Coding,* by Jennifer Lame and Glenna Young; *Mastering Medisoft,* by Bonnie J. Flom; *Medical Assisting: Foundations and Practices,* by Margaret Frazier, et al.; and *Medical Insurance Billing* Course Connect.

ACKNOWLEDGEMENTS

Developing and updating this text has been a long, challenging, exciting, and rewarding experience. I am deeply appreciative to those who walked with me on this journey. Hopefully our healthcare system is a bit better as a result of everyone's efforts on this text.

Marlene Pratt, Director, Portfolio Management, recognized my unique approach to coding and supported my vision to create a comprehensive coding solution. She assembled a development and production team who worked tirelessly throughout the project: Faye Gemmellaro, Content Producer; Joan Gill, Developmental Editor, who has been my publishing mentor and friend for more than 12 years; the production team at SPi; and many others unknown to me who finessed the details of this book.

A special thanks is due to Pearson's marketing team whom I've had the pleasure to work with over the years. Your enthusiasm and support for this text has brought a new coding experience to thousands of students and instructors: Brittany Hammond, Senior Field Marketing Manager; Regina Forbes, Sales Director; and Jeff McIlroy, Sales Director; and the many fun and dedicated inside and field reps.

Subject Matter Experts

A team of subject matter experts wrote exercises, reviewed content for accuracy, and added their expertise to the first edition of the text. Their work continues to help make the second edition the best medical coding text available.

- **Angela R. Campbell, MSHI, RHIA,** *AHIMA Approved ICD-10-CM/PCS Trainer; Medical Insurance Manager, Eastern Illinois University; Instructor, Ultimate Medical Academy*
- **Kate Gabriel-Jones, CPC,** *author, Medical Coding: Evaluation and Management*
- **Mary Lou Hilbert, MBA, RHIT, CCS,** *Subject Matter Expert, Health Information Management Service Center, Parallon*
- **Krystal S. Phillips, RHIA, CHTS-IS,** *Adjunct Instructor, Columbus State Community College*
- **Christine Tufts-Maher, MSHI, MS, RHIA,** *Professor, Seminole State College of Florida*

REVIEWERS

Reviewers from the front lines in the field provided valuable insight and confirmation of this text's approach.

Reviewers of the Second Edition

Angela Campbell, MSHI, RHIA
AHIMA-Approved ICD-10-CM/PCS Trainer
Instructor – Health Information Technology
Ultimate Medical Academy
Tampa, Florida

Nicole Copemann, MSHA, RHIA, CPC
Program Manager, Health Information Technology
Seminole State College of Florida
Sanford, Florida

Mary Lou Hilbert, MBA, RHIT, CCS
Coding Lead, Subject Matter Expert
Health Information Management Service Center, Parallon
San Antonio, Texas

Jennifer Lamé, MPH, RHIT
AHIMA Approved ICD-10-CM/PCS Trainer
Program Director, Health Information Technology
Southwest Wisconsin Technical College
Fennimore, Wisconsin

Donna Maher, RHI, CPC-A
Instructor, Medical Administrative Programs
Renton Technical College
Renton, Washington

Donna Stanley, Ed. S., RHIA, CCS
Director, Health Care Information Programs
Wallace State Community College
Hanceville, Alabama

Christine Tufts-Maher, MSHI, MS, RHIA
Professor
Seminole State College of Florida
Sanford, Florida

Rose Wilkerson, MPA, CPC
Assistant Professor, Medical Coding/Billing
Northwest Florida State College
Niceville, Florida

Reviewers of the First Edition

Geanetta Johnson Agbona, CPC, CPC-I, CBCS
Instructor, Medical Coding
South Piedmont Community College
Charlotte, North Carolina

Felecia Calloway, MBA, CCA, CBCS
Instructional Systems Designer
Virginia College
Montgomery, Alabama

Ora Clark, RHIT, AHIMA, CPC, AAPC
Medical Insurance/Billing & Coding Adjunct Faculty
Oconee Fall Line Technical College
Dublin, Georgia

Michelle Cranney, DHSc, RHIA, CCS-P, CPC
Assistant Professor, Health Information Management
Ashford University
Seattle, Washington

Janet A. Evans, RN, MBA, MS, CCS, CPC-I
Instructor, Introduction to HCPCS (CPT) Coding
Burlington County College
Pemberton, New Jersey

Chemo Faustino, CPC
Program Director, Medical Billing & Coding
Sanford-Brown College
Ft. Lauderdale, Florida

Michelle Griggs, CPC, CPC-I, CPMA
Program Director, Medical Insurance/Billing & Coding
Virginia College
Richmond, Virginia

Wahiyda Harding, RHIA, CCS, CTR
Program Chair, Medical Insurance/Billing & Coding
Westwood College
Atlanta, Georgia

Kerry Heinecke, MS, RHIA
Program Director, HIM
Mid-State Technical College
Marshfield, Wisconsin

Susan Herzberg, RHIA, CCS, CCS-P
Adjunct Professor, Medical Coding
Westchester Community College
Valhalla, New York

Mary Anita Kahler, RHIT, ICD 10-CM Trainer
Instructor, Medical Insurance/Billing & Coding
Coastal Carolina Community College
Jacksonville, North Carolina

Bobbie J. Lautenschlager, CCA, CMRS, CPC
Program Director, Medical Billing & Coding
American School of Technology
Columbus, Ohio

Robin Maddalena, CMT, CEHRS
Adjunct Professor, Medical Insurance/Billing & Coding,
   Electronic Health Records
Tunxis Community College
Farmington, Connecticut

Kim S. Norris, MBA, CPC
Program Director, Medical Billing & Coding
Carrington College
Tucson, Arizona

Lakisha Parker, AAS, CPC, CPC-I, ACPAR
Program Director, Medical Billing & Coding/Healthcare
   Reimbursement
Virginia College
Birmingham, Alabama

Elizabeth Roberts, CPC, CBCS, ICD-10 CM/PCS Trainer
Former Instructor, Medical Billing & Coding at Virginia
   College
Current Independent ICD-10 Consultant
Las Cruces, New Mexico

Gerald Robinson, CPC, ICD-10-CM/PCS Trainer
HIM Director & Adjunct Instructor
Ultimate Medical Academy
Tampa, Florida

Rolando Russell, MBA/HCM, CPC, CPAR
Program Director
Ultimate Medical Academy
Tampa, Florida

Jennifer J. Talbot, RHIA, CCS-P, ICD-10-CM/PCS Trainer
Program Director, HIT
Kirtland Community College
Roscommon, Michigan

Jeanette Thomas, RHIA, RHIT, CPC-H, CPC
Instructor, Health Information Systems
Clayton State University
Morrow, Georgia

Lydia Wikoff
Instructor, Billing & Coding
Southeastern College
Jacksonville, Florida

Guide to Key Features

This Guide to Key Features acquaints users with the text and shows them how to use the pedagogical features to their greatest advantage.

Chapter Opener Features

Learning Objectives—Each chapter begins with a list of the primary skills students should have after completing the chapter, aligned with Bloom's Taxonomy levels of learning.

Learning Objectives

After completing this chapter, you should have the skills to:

16.1 Spell and define the key words, medical terms, and abbreviations related to the nervous system and sense organs. (Remember)

16.2 Summarize the structure, function, and common conditions of the nervous system and sense organs. (Understand)

16.3 Adhere to the Official Guidelines for Coding and Reporting related to the nervous system and sense organs. (Apply)

Key Terms and Abbreviations—A list of the important terms students need to know but may not have learned in previous classes is provided at the beginning of each chapter. These terms are set in blue boldface type and are defined upon first appearance in the chapter. They are also included in the Glossary at the end of the book.

Key Terms and Abbreviations

absence	focal
Alzheimer's disease (AD)	generalized
atonic	grand mal
aura	gustatory
brain	hemiplegia
central nervous system (CNS)	homeostasis
clonic	idiopathic
complex partial	intractable
dementia	late onset
distributed	localized

Chapter Outline—A list of the major topics covered in the chapter appears at the beginning.

Chapter Outline

- **Nervous System Refresher**
- **Coding Guidelines for the Nervous System**
- **Abstracting for Conditions of the Nervous System**
- **Assigning Codes for Conditions of the Nervous System**
- **Arranging Codes for Conditions of the Nervous System**
- **Coding Neoplasms of the Nervous System**

In-Chapter Features

Introduction—The text uses analogies at the beginning of chapters to create a "hook" with a common frame of reference and provides a familiar perspective for relating to new information. ICD-10-CM/PCS chapters use travel analogies while CPT chapters use shopping analogies.

INTRODUCTION

Electrical problems can be one of the most troublesome to solve. A defect in the electrical system located in one part of a car can create a problem in a completely different area. The human nervous system is the electrical system in our bodies, sending and receiving messages that enable us to perform all functions.

A neurologist specializes in diagnosing and treating conditions of the nervous system. Neurosurgeons specialize in performing surgical procedures on the nervous system. Primary care physicians treat uncomplicated conditions of the nervous system and refer more complex cases to a specialist.

Success Step—Short tips help students abstract, assign, and arrange (sequence) codes.

Coding Caution—Short warnings alert students to coding situations that can be tricky or confusing.

SUCCESS STEP

Physicians do not need to use the exact word *intractable* to allow coders to abstract a migraine or epilepsy as intractable. Acceptable terms that mean intractable are *pharmacoresistant*, *pharmacologically resistant*, *treatment resistant*, *refractory*, and *poorly controlled*.

CODING CAUTION

Do not assume that all seizure activity is epilepsy. Seizures may also be caused by high fever, psychological disorders, or other medical conditions such as narcolepsy, Tourette syndrome, or cardiac arrhythmia.

Coding Practice—Coding exercises throughout the chapter consist of three to six patient scenarios related to a specific chapter topic, using the mini-medical-record format. The first exercise in the coding chapters reviews medical terms related to the body system or type of procedure and introduces students to simple coding for the body system.

CODING PRACTICE

Exercise 16.1 Nervous System Refresher

Instructions: Use your medical terminology skills and resources to define the following conditions related to the nervous system, then assign the default diagnosis code.

Follow these steps:

- Use slash marks "/" to break down each term into its root(s) and suffix.
- Define the meaning of the word based on the meaning of each word part.
- Assign the default ICD-10-CM diagnosis code for the condition using the Index and Tabular List.

Example: neuropathy neuro/pathy   Meaning *abnormal condition of a nerve*   ICD-10-CM Code *G62.9*

1. neuroma (benign)   Meaning _____   ICD-10-CM Code _____
2. neuromyelitis   Meaning _____   ICD-10-CM Code _____
3. encephalomyeloradiculitis   Meaning _____   ICD-10-CM Code _____
4. causalgia   Meaning _____   ICD-10-CM Code _____
5. neuromyotonia   Meaning _____   ICD-10-CM Code _____
6. myelinolysis   Meaning _____   ICD-10-CM Code _____
7. hemichorea   Meaning _____   ICD-10-CM Code _____
8. meningoencephalopathy   Meaning _____   ICD-10-CM Code _____
9. myasthenia   Meaning _____   _____

Subsequent exercises walk students through the skills of abstracting, assigning, and sequencing codes. Exercises increase in difficulty as the chapter progresses, while remaining appropriate for an introductory course.

CODING PRACTICE

Exercise 16.5 Coding Neoplasms of the Nervous System

Instructions: Read the mini-medical-record of each patient's encounter, then abstract, assign, and sequence ICD-10-CM diagnosis codes using the Index and Tabular List. Write the code(s) on the line provided.

1. OFFICE Gender: F Age: 6
Reason for encounter: Review CT scan of head
Assessment: Benign hypothalamic astrocytoma (tumor arising from star-shaped cells that form the supportive tissue of the brain)
Plan: Surgery to remove the tumor
1 ICD-10-CM Code _____

2. INPATIENT HOSPITAL Gender: F Age: 62
Reason for admission: Management of pain following pleurectomy of right lung due to non-small-cell carcinoma (NSCLC) of the right lung
Assessment: Chronic post-thoracotomy (incision into the chest) pain
Plan: Discharge to home with fentanyl (a narcotic pain reliever) transdermal patch and home health follow up
Tip: The principal diagnosis is the condition that is the reason for the admission. Refer to OGCR I.C.6.b.5.
2 ICD-10-CM Codes _____

3. INPATIENT HOSPITAL Gender: F Age: 71
Reason for admission: Pain management
Assessment: Nerve root compress d/t stage 4 diffuse large B-cell non-Hodgkin's lymphoma
Tip: Refer to OGCR I.C.6.b.5).
3 ICD-10-CM Codes _____

4. INPATIENT HOSPITAL Gender: M Age: 5
Reason for admission: Craniotomy with tumor resection
Assessment: Primary medulloblastoma of the central cerebellum
Plan: Chemotherapy was provided before discharge, follow up in office to establish chemotherapy and radiotherapy plan
Tip: Refer to OGCR I.C.2.e.
2 ICD-10-CM Codes _____

5. INPATIENT HOSPITAL Gender: F Age: 67
Reason for admission: Anemia due to chemotherapy the brain, also provided IV pain management
Assessment: Left ovarian cancer with metastases to
Plan: Refer to hospice
Tip: Refer to OGCR I.C.2.c.2) and I.C.2.e.
5 ICD-10-CM Codes _____

Guided Examples—Step-by-step demonstrations allow students to experience the thinking process of a seasoned coder as they observe a coder abstract, assign, and sequence codes from a mini-medical-record.

Guided Example of Assigning Codes for Symptoms and Signs

Refer to the following example to learn how to assign codes for symptoms. This case is similar to the earlier example of Chad Wang, who was seen for nausea, vomiting, and diarrhea and was diagnosed with gastroenteritis. However, notice how this example should be coded differently based on the wording of the Assessment.

Date: 6/1/yy   Location: Branton Family Practice
Provider: Kristen Conover, MD
Patient: Charlene Winger   Gender: F   Age: 15
Chief Complaint: Nausea, vomiting, and diarrhea
Assessment: Suspected gastroenteritis
Plan: Stool culture, bedrest, and plenty of fluids

▶ Sherry checks for instructional notes in the Tabular List.

❑ She cross-references the beginning of category **R11** and reads the **Excludes1** instructional note. None of the conditions listed describe the patient, so she may proceed.

❑ She cross-references the beginning of the block **R10-R19** and reads the **Excludes1** instructional note. None of the conditions listed describe the patient, so she may proceed.

❑ She cross-references the beginning of **Chapter 18 (R00-R99)** and reads the detailed instructional notes. She determines that note **(e) cases in which a more precise diagnosis was not available** describes this case and that she is coding correctly.

▶ Next, Sherry searches the Index for the Main Term **Diarrhea**.

Figures—Anatomic illustrations show English names and medical terms for major body parts and organs. Original drawings of disease processes and selected anatomic details clarify difficult coding concepts. Annotated diagrams of sample pages from the coding manuals guide students' understanding of layout and appropriate use. Photographs and graphics portray key points and clarify new information. Screen shots from online coding software introduce students to computerized coding.

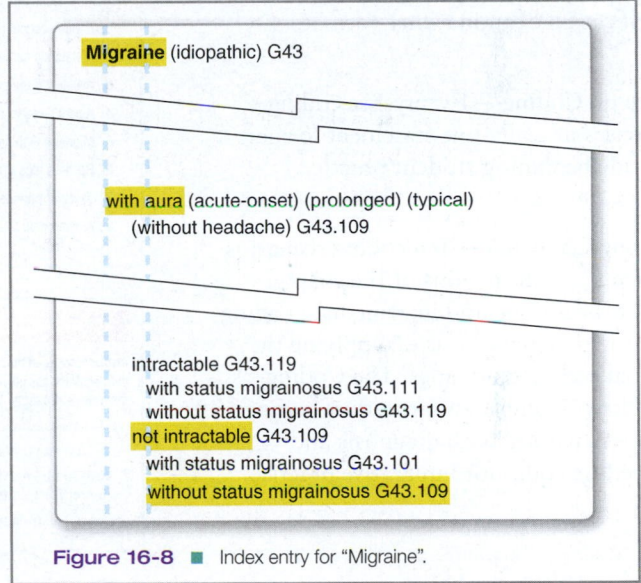

Figure 16-8 ■ Index entry for "Migraine".

Tables—Tables provide definitions of terms, conditions, and treatments, key criteria for abstracting diagnoses, procedures and root operations, and comparative information that highlights key concepts.

Table 16-2   ■   **COMMON DISEASES OF THE NERVOUS SYSTEM**

Condition	Definition
Alzheimer's disease	A progressive degenerative brain disease
Amyotrophic lateral sclerosis (ALS) or Lou Gehrig disease	A chronic, terminal neurological disease characterized by a progressive loss of motor neurons and muscle atrophy
Bell's Palsy	Inflammation of the seventh (VII) cranial nerve, the facial nerve
Cerebral palsy	A functional disorder of the brain manifested by motor impairment
Chronic pain syndrome (CPS)	A collection of pain conditions lasting more than six months and unresponsive to treatment
Cluster headache	Unilateral pain in the eye or temple
Complex regional pain syndrome	A chronic pain syndrome in which an extremity experiences intense burning pain and changes in skin texture and temperature; also called reflex sympathetic dystrophy (RSD)

CHAPTER SUMMARY

In this chapter you learned that:

- The function of the nervous system is to direct the body's response to internal and external stimuli and coordinate the activities of other organ systems.
- ICD-10-CM provides Official Guidelines for Coding and Reporting (OGCR) for the nervous system and sense organs in OGCR section I.C.6, which provides detailed discussion of coding for pain, including general coding information, postoperative pain, chronic pain, neoplasm-related pain, and chronic pain syndrome.
- Because of the variety of conditions addressed under the nervous system, coders need general criteria for abstracting conditions

of the nervous system overall and specific criteria for abstracting pain, headaches, epilepsy, and Parkinson disease.
- OGCR contain specific guidelines for assigning codes for hemi-plegia, monoplegia, and pain.
- When the purpose of the encounter is to manage the pain, sequence the code for pain first; when the purpose of the encounter is to treat the underlying condition, sequence the code for the cond
- Primary mal
brain is a co

Summary—Each chapter ends with a brief restatement of key points in the chapter.

End-of-Chapter Features

The review at the end of each chapter reinforces key concepts and provides opportunity for additional skills practice.

Concept Quiz—Definitions and key concepts are reviewed using ten completion and ten multiple-choice questions. Multiple-choice questions include three coding questions formatted similarly to the certification examinations' format.

Keep on Coding—Twenty-five coding exercises in a one-line statement format provide beginning student practice.

Coding Challenge—Ten coding scenarios drawn from all sections of the chapter review beginning and intermediate coding skills with an emphasis on applying the official coding guidelines. The Coding Challenge exercises in procedure coding chapters require both diagnosis and procedure codes for integrative practice.

CONCEPT QUIZ

Take a moment to look back at the nervous system and sense organs and solidify your skills. Try to answer the questions from memory first, then refer back to the discussion in the chapter if you need a little extra help.

Completion

Instructions: Write the term that completes each statement based on the information you learned in this chapter. Choose from the list below. Some choices may be used more than once and some choices may not be used at all.

30	epilepsy
60	hydrocephalus
72	laterality
brain	meningitis
CNS	PNS
dominance	spina bifida

2. What medical term means "resistant to treatment"?
   A. Vasodilation
   B. Chronic
   C. Refractory
   D. Idiopathic

3. What type of seizures are the result of abnormal activity on both sides of the brain?
   A. Simple partial
   B. Psychomotor
   C. Status epilepticus
   D. Generalized

4. How would you code the following scenario? *A patient with previously diagnosed Parkinson disease is also diagnosed with dementia today.*
   A. G31.83, F02.80
   B. G20, F02.80
   C.

KEEP ON CODING

Instructions: Read the diagnostic statement, then use the Index and Tabular List to assign and sequence ICD-10-CM diagnosis codes. Write the code(s) on the line provided.

1. Pneumococcal meningitis. ICD-10-CM Code(s) _____

2. Metastatic carcinoma of the thalamus from primary cancer of the right breast. ICD-10-CM Code(s) _____

3. Accidental puncture of the meninges during a nervous system operative procedure. ICD-10-CM Code(s) _____

4. Alpers disease. ICD-10-CM Code(s) _____

5. Migraine with an aura. ICD-10-CM Code(s) _____

6. Restless legs syndrome. ICD-10-CM Code(s) _____

7. Vascular parkinsonism. ICD-10-CM Code(s) _____

8. Amyotrophic lateral sclerosis. ICD-10-CM Code(s) _____

CODING CHALLENGE

Instructions: Read the mini-medical-record of each patient's encounter, then abstract, assign, and sequence ICD-10-CM diagnosis codes using the Index and Tabular List. Write the code(s) on the line provided.

1. OUTPATIENT HOSPITAL Gender: M Age: 36

Reason for encounter: Patient presents to the infusion center for treatment of meningitis

Assessment: Staphylococcal meningitis

(continued)

1. (continued)

Plan: FU in 3 days and 1 week after antibiotic infusions are complete

Tip: Read the instructional notes in the Tabular List.

2 ICD-10-CM Codes _____

Foundations of Coding

Welcome to your new career in coding! You are in for the trip of a lifetime, one that is sure to take you to new and unknown places, a few familiar ones, and perhaps some that seem a little scary. This text lays out the path to follow, complete with success steps and caution signs.

Section One: Foundations of Coding acquaints you with the medical coding field, potential career opportunities, and how coding relates to reimbursement and payment. It also introduces the three skills of the "Ace" coder—abstracting, assigning, and arranging (sequencing) codes—skills that are the foundation of working with all medical codes.

PROFESSIONAL PROFILE

Jennifer Holland, RHIT, CPC, CIRCC
Coding Audit Response Specialist
Novant Health, Inc.

I have worked in the health information management (HIM) field for 16 years and in coding for 13 years. My first exposure to coding was as an insurance claims specialist where I would process the insurance claims based on the member's benefits. My first coding job was in the HIM department assisting the preregistration team with CPT codes for preauthorizations and precertifications.

Currently I work as a coding audit response specialist working with the charge description master (CDM), billing, and coding denials. I also perform audits as requested by leadership, research trends and offer solutions, and assist teammates with any questions they may have. I enjoy that coding is always changing and that makes it interesting. No two charts are ever the same.

The most challenging part of the job is getting answers to difficult questions that involve other stakeholders in the organization, such as other departmental supervisors, managers, team leads, and clinical documentation staff. I am able to meet the challenge by researching and providing my information to my own supervisor, who will then communicate with the other stakeholders. Usually if there needs to be further dialogue, my supervisor will set up a meeting for the discussion to take place where we are able to come to an agreement.

I use an encoder in my job for assigning ICD-10-CM and CPT codes. The software also allows me to look up Correct Coding Initiative (CCI) edits and access coding resources like the *CPT Assistant*.

I have two associate degrees, one in health information technology (HIT) and one in medical office administration. Both degrees have aided in my career preparation because they gave me an understanding of billing and coding. My degree in medical office administration taught me the ins and outs of working in a medical office.

I have my registered health information technician (RHIT), certified professional coder (CPC), and certified interventional radiology cardiovascular coder (CIRCC) certifications. I believe these credentials are vital to my career as it shows potential employers that I am not a novice to this field. They show employers my dedication and commitment to the field and how I will pursue opportunities to maintain and continue my education.

I am a member of AAPC and AHIMA, as well as the North Carolina HIMA local chapter. In my local chapter I have served as the education chair and mentorship program coordinator.

My advice to students is to stay focused, work hard, be patient, continually learn, and do not despise small beginnings. Learn as much as you possibly can and explore new opportunities when afforded to you. You never know what may come of the opportunity that is presented to you.

Chapter
1

Your Coding Career

Chapter Outline

- **What Is Coding?**
- **Understanding Patient Encounters**
- **Certification**
- **Coding Careers**

Learning Objectives

After completing this chapter, you should have the skills to:

1.1 Spell and define the key words, medical terms, and abbreviations related to your coding career. (Remember)

1.2 Describe coding, HIPAA-mandated code sets, and coding skills. (Understand)

1.3 Explain how patient encounters relate to coding. (Understand)

1.4 Describe the types of coding certification. (Understand)

1.5 Summarize the career path and performance expectations for a coding career. (Understand)

Key Terms and Abbreviations

AAPC	arrange	code set	inpatient encounter
abstract	assign	coding	midlevel job
admitting privileges	attending physician	covered entities	outpatient encounter
advanced-level job	career path	diagnosis	payers
amend	case production	document	procedure
American Health Information Management Association (AHIMA)	certification	encounter	query
	clinical documentation improvement (CDI)	entry-level job	sequence
ancillary	code	Health Insurance Portability and Accountability Act (HIPAA)	

In addition to the key terms listed here, students should know the terms defined within tables in this chapter.

INTRODUCTION

When starting on a trip, you are more likely to get where you want to go when you have a destination in mind. In this chapter you learn about your ultimate destination: the coding profession. By understanding what coding is, the nature of patient encounters, professional certification, and potential career opportunities, you will formulate ideas on your career goals and the steps needed to reach them.

Many jobs in the healthcare field work with codes even though they may not have a job title of coder. For example, medical assistants, billers, schedulers, and medical secretaries may use codes as part of their jobs. This text uses the term *coder* to refer to those who assigns, reads, or uses codes as part of job responsibilities.

A wide variety of healthcare professionals, in addition to medical doctors (MDs), provides patient services and uses codes to bill for their services. For example, dentists (DDSs or DMDs), osteopaths (DOs), chiropractors (DCs), and nurse practitioners (NPs) also bill their services with the same codes as physicians. This text uses the terms *physician* and *provider* interchangeably to refer to any healthcare professional who provides services that are billed with codes.

WHAT IS CODING?

Coding is the process of accurately assigning codes to verbal descriptions of patients' conditions and the healthcare services provided to treat those conditions. Medical codes are a combination of letters and numbers, three to seven characters in length. Diagnosis codes describe patient illnesses, diseases, conditions, injuries, or other reasons for seeking healthcare services. Procedure codes describe the services healthcare professionals provide to patients, such as evaluation, consultation, testing, treatments, and surgery.

Code Sets

The healthcare system in the United States uses several distinct systems of medical codes, called code sets, for different purposes. The various systems were developed by different organizations and follow different guidelines for their use. The Health Insurance Portability and Accountability Act (HIPAA), a federal law passed in 1996, has numerous provisions relating to consumer health insurance and electronic health transactions. HIPAA defines the code sets that covered entities must use for electronic health transactions and the purpose of each (■ Table 1-1). Covered entities are health plans, healthcare clearinghouses, and healthcare providers who electronically transmit any health information in connection with transactions for which the Department of Health and Human Services (HHS) has adopted standards.

> ### SUCCESS STEP
>
> When speaking of ICD-10-CM/PCS, coding professionals often use the shorthand *CM* to refer to ICD-10-CM and the shorthand *PCS* to refer to ICD-10-PCS.

Three Skills of an "Ace" Coder

Coding is more than looking up numbers in a manual or software program. Accurate coding requires three major skills, which are described next: abstracting, assigning, and arranging

Table 1-1 ■ HIPAA-MANDATED CODE SETS

Code Set Name	Purpose	Developed By	Code Format and Examples
CDT Codes on Dental Procedures and Nomenclature	Dental services (occupies section D of HCPCS codes)	American Dental Association (ADA)	Letter *D* + 4 numbers • D7230
CPT Current Procedural Terminology	Hospital outpatient and physician procedures and services	American Medical Association (AMA)	5 numbers • 99213 • 36415
HCPCS Healthcare Common Procedure Coding System	Supplies, items, and services not covered by CPT, physician and nonphysician services, Medicare services, supplies	Centers for Medicare and Medicaid Services (CMS)	1 letter + 4 numbers • A6461 • G9874
ICD-10-CM International Classification of Diseases, 10th Revision, Clinical Modification	Diagnoses	National Center for Health Statistics (NCHS) based on ICD-10 from the World Health Organization (WHO)	3 to 7 alphanumeric characters • I10 • A52.15 • T50.A11D
ICD-10-PCS International Classification of Diseases, 10th Revision, Procedure Coding System	Hospital inpatient procedures	CMS	7 alphanumeric characters • 0B7B8DZ • 4A04XB1 • F029GCZ
NDC National Drug Codes	Identification of the manufacturer, product, and package size of all drugs and biologics recognized by the Food and Drug Administration (FDA)	Department of Health and Human Services (HHS)	10 numbers divided into 3 segments • 1234-5678-90 • 12345-678-90 • 12345-6789-0

(sequencing). Memorize these definitions and remind yourself of them each time you sit down to code.

Abstracting

Before coders can assign codes, they **abstract** information from the medical record. To abstract, coders read the medical record and determine which elements of the encounter require codes. They identify the reason for the encounter, diagnostic statements from the physician, complications and coexisting conditions, and the services provided. If the medical record is not properly abstracted, it is impossible to assign the correct codes. Each code set has rules for abstracting, and some rules are specific to a particular condition or procedure.

SUCCESS STEP

The term *abstract* also describes a task in health information management in which inpatient coders review the medical record and cull data required for reporting, such as patient demographics and length of stay.

Assigning

Coders must select or **assign** codes to accurately describe both the information documented in the medical record and the patient's condition and services. Each character of the code must be correct. Diagnosis and procedure codes must reflect the highest level of specificity possible and contain the correct number of characters for that code. The official guidelines on how to assign codes vary among code sets because each has slightly different requirements.

Arranging (Sequencing)

When more than one diagnosis or procedure code is required for an encounter, coders must **arrange**, or **sequence**, the codes in a specific order. This coding step requires that you learn the rules for multiple coding (*situations in which more than one code is required*). Sequencing rules are different for each code set. Code sequencing affects how reimbursement is calculated. Official coding guidelines of the various code sets dictate the proper sequencing, based on the codes assigned and the circumstances of the patient encounter. Codes that are not sequenced properly are considered to be incorrect.

CODING PRACTICE

Exercise 1.1   What Is Coding?

Instructions: Write the answers to the following questions in the space provided.

1. Define *coding.* _____
   _____
   _____
   _____

2. What is the difference between diagnosis coding and procedure coding? _____
   _____
   _____

3. List and briefly define the three skills of an "Ace" coder. _____
   _____
   _____
   _____

UNDERSTANDING PATIENT ENCOUNTERS

Coders assign diagnosis and procedure codes to a patient **encounter** (*a specific interaction between a patient and healthcare provider*) after an encounter has been completed. The provider documents the reason(s) for the encounter and the services provided in the patient's medical record. Coders read the medical record and other information the physician provides to identify the main reason for the encounter, any additional reasons for the service, the main service provided, and any additional services provided. The following sections describe an overview of patient encounters with the healthcare system, including the types of encounters and the process of an encounter. This helps coders better understand their role.

Types of Encounters

Patient encounters are generally classified by the location of the encounter because different coding and billing rules apply

to each. The two basic types of locations are outpatient and inpatient, which are described next.

Outpatient Encounters

An **outpatient encounter** is a physician interaction with a patient who receives services and has not been formally admitted to a healthcare institution, such as an acute-care hospital, long-term care facility, or rehabilitation facility. Patients request outpatient encounters when they have particular health problems, need preventive services, or for follow-up or ongoing treatment for known problems. ■ TABLE 1-2 lists examples of outpatient encounters.

Inpatient Encounters

An **inpatient encounter** is a physician interaction with a patient who has been formally admitted to a healthcare facility, such as an acute-care hospital, long-term care facility, or rehabilitation facility. Patients cannot admit themselves to a facility; a

Table 1-2   ■   **EXAMPLES OF OUTPATIENT ENCOUNTERS**

Setting	Purpose	Examples
Ambulatory surgery	Surgical procedure that does not require an overnight stay in the hospital	Tonsillectomy, cataract removal
Cardiology lab	Testing to evaluate a heart problem	EKG, echocardiogram, cardiac catheterization
Diagnostic radiology	Imaging study to evaluate or diagnose a health problem	X-ray, MRI, CT, PET
Emergency department	Treatment of an injury or health problem that cannot be delayed without harm to the patient	Broken leg, chest pain
Laboratory	Specimen collection	Blood draw
Observation	Extended monitoring that may require an overnight stay but does not meet the requirements for a formal inpatient admission	Chest pain
Physical therapy	Treatment of a musculoskeletal problem	Therapeutic exercises, electrical muscle stimulation
Physician office	Evaluation and management of a new or existing health problem; preventive care services	Back pain, diabetes checkup, immunization
Therapeutic radiology	Receive a treatment using radiation	Anticancer radiation therapy

physician must admit a patient for a specific medical reason, which is to either diagnose or treat a health problem. Physicians contract with hospitals for **admitting privileges**, meaning they have authority to admit patients and care for them in a specific hospital. They write admitting orders, conduct an admitting history and physical, and complete paperwork required by the institution. One physician, usually the one who admits the patient, is the **attending physician** who oversees and coordinates all aspects of the patient's care while an inpatient. Other physicians also may be involved in the diagnosis or treatment of the patient. A patient may also receive **ancillary** services—such as laboratory, radiology, or physical therapy—as an inpatient.

The facility codes and bills for the room, board, nursing care, use of the operating room, and most ancillary services. Physicians code and bill for services they personally provide, such as hospital visits, surgical procedures, and interpretation of laboratory or radiology tests. A third-party company may contract with the facility to provide services such as radiology or physical therapy, in which case that company codes and bills its own services to the patient.

Therefore, coders do not code for everything pertaining to a specific patient. They code for the services provided by their employer, such as the hospital, the surgeon, or the physical therapist. They also code for the diagnoses that describe why the patient received these particular services, but they do not code for unrelated diagnoses.

Steps in the Encounter

While each encounter is unique to the patient's situation, it generally involves three steps: diagnosis, treatment, and documentation ■ FIGURE 1-1).

Diagnosis

When a patient presents to a physician with a health problem, the physician needs to establish a diagnosis. If a diagnosis was established in a previous encounter, the physician reviews the patient's progress and updates the diagnosis. Establishing or

updating a diagnosis involves a history, a physical examination, and testing.

History. A physician takes a patient's medical history, which includes questions about current symptoms and past medical problems. Because most symptoms can be caused by several different conditions, the physician asks a series of questions to narrow the possibilities. If a diagnosis was established in a previous encounter, the physician updates the history based on what has happened since the last encounter.

Physical Examination. The physician conducts a physical examination to further identify and evaluate abnormalities. The examination may focus on a specific body system or it may cover the entire body. Examinations include visual inspection, palpation (*physical touching*), and auscultation (*listening to various parts of the body*).

Testing. A physician performs or orders diagnostic tests, including blood tests, imaging, biopsies, and physical function tests, such as EKGs, based on the patient's situation. In some cases, the patient's condition does not require any tests.

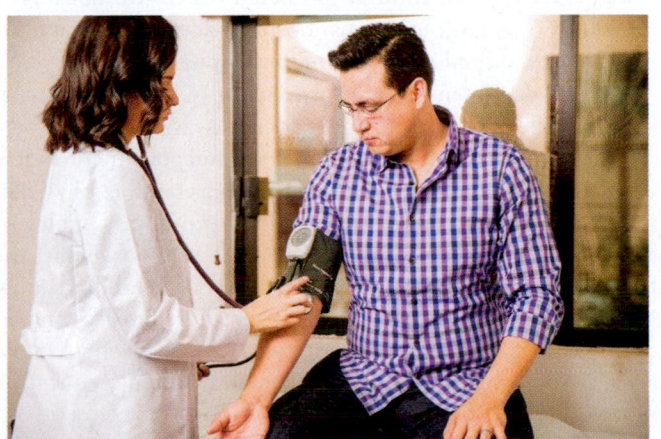

Figure 1-1 ■ Patient encounters include a diagnosis, treatment plan, and documentation.

Antoniodiaz/Shutterstock

Based on the findings from these sources, the physician identifies the most likely diagnosis and the rationale for it. Depending on the complexity of the problem, the physician may determine the diagnosis in a single encounter or it may take multiple patient encounters and multiple rounds of testing to arrive at a conclusion.

Treatment Plan

After establishing the diagnosis, the physician formulates a treatment plan. The treatment plan may include medication, surgery, lifestyle changes, or therapy. For complicated problems that take time to diagnose, the physician may treat symptoms to provide relief to the patient until the underlying cause is determined. Payers do not reimburse for every treatment recommended by physicians. Some treatments require preauthorization by the payer. As codes become more specific and detailed, payers update requirements and often place more restrictions on approvals. If a payer does not offer reimbursement for a recommended service, patients have the option to pay for it themselves. Providers may negotiate a payment plan to make this more manageable for patients. Preauthorization is discussed in greater detail throughout this text.

Coders do not code for services listed in the treatment plan that will be provided at a later date or by a different provider. Code only for services completed on a specific date of service.

Documentation

After each patient encounter, the physician must **document** the encounter, recording the reason for the encounter, the diagnostic techniques used, tests or treatments planned, and the overall assessment of the patient.

Although physicians generally do not assign the final codes, they must ensure that their documentation provides the information required for accurate coding. Physicians need to be knowledgeable of documentation requirements for ICD-10-CM diagnoses and CPT procedures. Those who perform inpatient hospital procedures also must be familiar with ICD-10-PCS requirements. Recall that hospitals use PCS codes to report the facility portion of inpatient procedures that physicians perform. Even though physician offices do not report ICD-10-PCS codes, physicians' hospital documentation must provide the required information for hospital coders.

Clinical documentation improvement (CDI) is an internal process to identify areas in which documentation does not provide all the information needed to code and educate providers regarding the details needed. Hospitals as well as physician practices conduct studies that evaluate random samples of various types of medical records. They determine whether the documentation contains the required level of detail for coding to the greatest level of specificity. Then they develop a priority list of specific diagnoses and procedures that require more detail or other changes and implement a provider education process.

Physician documentation is the basis from which coders assign diagnostic and procedure codes for each encounter. Coders *do not* do the following:

- Determine what is wrong with the patient
- Determine what condition(s) the patient has based on the symptoms
- Code for services provided prior to the current encounter
- Code for services planned but not provided during the current encounter
- Code for services delivered by other providers
- Code for past conditions that are resolved
- Code for current conditions that the physician does not document as relevant to the current encounter

When the documentation is unclear, coders do not make assumptions about missing information. They send a **query** (*a written communication asking for clarification and/or additional details*) to the physician for more information. The physician must **amend** (*add information to*) the medical record, if necessary.

Guided Example of a Patient Encounter

Refer to the following example to learn more about how physicians diagnose a problem, develop a treatment plan, and document patient encounters. Sherry Whittle, CPC, is a fictitious certified coder who guides you through documentation and coding.

▶ Patient Norman Markowitz, age 41, schedules an office appointment to see Dr. Kristen Conover, a family practice physician, on January 5, due to back pain.

❑ Dr. Conover takes a history by asking Mr. Markowitz when the pain started, how severe it is, what makes it better or worse, and if it has occurred before.

❑ She performs a physical examination to see if she can detect abnormalities such as tightness, lumps, knots, or protrusions.

❑ She asks Mr. Markowitz to perform specific maneuvers, such as standing, sitting, and leaning forward or backward, to determine his physical abilities.

❑ She uses a reflex hammer to test his reflexes.

❑ She takes an x-ray in the office, which is negative for a fracture.

▶ Next, Dr. Conover provides a treatment plan.

❑ She prescribes methocarbamol and tramadol to relieve Mr. Markowitz's back pain while waiting for results of blood tests and an MRI. She orders blood tests, which come back negative for arthritis on January 12.

❑ She schedules Mr. Markowitz for an MRI examination on January 17, which reveals a displaced intervertebral disc.

❏ After she receives the MRI results of a displaced disc, she asks Mr. Markowitz to schedule another appointment for follow-up.

▶ Dr. Conover documents the January 5 encounter.

Date: 01/5/yy

Patient: Norman Markowitz   Gender: M   Age: 41

Chief complaint: Low back pain that started about a month ago.

Assessment: Patient was last seen 6 months ago for annual checkup.

History: Detailed history of low back pain problem that started about a month ago. Patient does not recall a specific incident or injury that may have led to the pain.

Examination: Lumbar region is tight to palpation. Patient shows limited range of motion on flexion, extension and rotation. Reflexes are normal. X-ray taken in office is negative for fracture.

Plan: Rx methocarbamol and tramadol. Lab work ordered. MRI scheduled for January 17.

▶ On January 24, Mr. Markowitz returns for a follow-up visit to review next steps.

❏ They discuss treatment options and decide to continue medication and refer Mr. Markowitz for physical therapy.

❏ They also discuss the possibility of surgery if physical therapy does not provide adequate relief.

▶ Dr. Conover documents the January 24 encounter.

Date: 01/24/yy

Patient: Norman Markowitz   Gender: M   Age: 41

Reason for encounter: Follow-up on MRI and lab results

Assessment: Bloodwork is negative for arthritis. MRI shows displacement of L4-5 disc.

Plan: Continue medication. Referral made to physical therapy. Consider surgery if physical therapy does not provide relief. Follow up 6 weeks.

▶ Sherry Whittle, CPC, codes for two outpatient encounters for Mr. Markowitz, January 5 and January 24, because those were the two dates that Dr. Conover saw him in the office.

▶ For the January 5 encounter, Sherry assigns the ICD-10-CM diagnosis code **M54.5 Low back pain** because Dr. Conover had not yet determined the cause of the back pain.

❏ She assigns CPT procedure codes for the office visit and the x-ray that was performed in the office.

❏ She does not assign procedure codes for the blood test or the MRI because Dr. Conover did not provide those services. She does not assign codes for the medications prescribed because the prescription will be filled at the patient's pharmacy. These services will be billed by the organization that provides the service. The physician's service of writing the prescription is included in the office visit code.

▶ Sherry finalizes the codes for January 5:

(1) ICD-10-CM: **M54.5 Low back pain**

(2) CPT: **99214 Office or other outpatient visit for the evaluation and management of an established patient, which requires at least 2 of these 3 key components: A detailed history; A detailed examination; Medical decision making of moderate complexity.**

(3) CPT: **72100 Radiologic examination, spine, lumbosacral; 2 or 3 views**

▶ For the January 24 encounter, Sherry assigns the ICD-10-CM diagnosis code **M51.26 Other intervertebral disc displacement, lumbar region** because Dr. Conover established the diagnosis based on the MRI results.

❏ She also assigns a CPT code for the office visit.

❏ She does not assign procedure codes for physical therapy because Mr. Markowitz will go to a physical therapy clinic for the service. The physical therapy clinic will bill for the services it provides.

❏ She does not assign procedure codes for surgery because surgery was not performed.

▶ Sherry finalizes the codes for January 24:

(1) ICD-10-CM: **M51.26 Other intervertebral disc displacement, lumbar region**

(2) CPT: **99213 Office or other outpatient visit for the evaluation and management of an established patient, which requires at least 2 of these 3 key components: An expanded problem focused history; An expanded problem focused examination; Medical decision making of low complexity.**

▶ Finally, Sherry enters the codes and billing information into the computer and submits the claims to the patient's insurance company for payment.

CODING PRACTICE

Exercise 1.2   **Understanding Patient Encounters**

Instructions: Write the answers to the following questions in the space provided.

1. When do coders assign codes to patient encounters?

_____

_____

_____

2. What are the three steps in a patient encounter?

_____

_____

_____

3. What are the three elements involved in establishing a diagnosis?

_____

_____

_____

CERTIFICATION

Certification is a voluntary achievement that documents that a coder has attained a certain level of proficiency by passing a rigorous examination. Certification is offered by professional organizations and is an additional step beyond a formal educational degree. It does not replace a degree and a degree generally is not required to become certified. Certification began as a form of recognition before there were many educational degrees in this area. Today, certification plus education enhances a coder's professional standing and often results in higher compensation.

Certification is not mandated by federal or state governments and is not a legal requirement. Individual employers determine whether certification is required and which certification is acceptable.

Most large clinics and hospitals require coders to be nationally certified. Two organizations offer coding certifications that are recognized by most employers: **AAPC** (formerly known as the American Academy of Professional Coders) and the **American Health Information Management Association (AHIMA)**. Both organizations offer several certification credentials, each with a unique focus.

AAPC

Founded in 1988, AAPC has historically focused on physician-based and outpatient coders. Current membership is approximately 155,000. AAPC has local chapters in many cities that hold monthly meetings and workshops and provide networking opportunities for members. Members must follow the AAPC Code of Ethics, which outlines ethical principles of professional conduct related to integrity, respect, commitment, competence, fairness, and responsibility. AAPC offers a wide variety of certifications related to the business side of coding, encompassing areas such as professional (physician) coding, billing, medical auditing, clinical documentation, medical compliance, and physician practice management. The primary certification is Certified Professional Coder (CPC), which focuses on coding of services, procedures, and diagnoses for physician offices. The Certified Outpatient Coder (COC) certification focuses on outpatient hospital services,

and the Certified Professional Coder-Payer (CPC-P) focuses on coding and reimbursement skills needed by **payers** (*insurance companies or public programs that pay for healthcare services*). The Certified Professional Coder-Apprentice (CPC-A) is earned by coders with less than two years' professional experience. AAPC also offers specialty coding certifications that enable coders to demonstrate superior levels of expertise in a medical specialty, such as orthopedics, obstetrics, or cardiology. Coders take a separate examination to achieve each type of certification.

AHIMA

Founded in 1928 as the Association of Record Librarians of North America, AHIMA has historically focused on hospital coders and clinical records. Current membership is approximately 103,000. AHIMA's goal is to advance informatics, data analytics, and information governance for healthcare while continuing to lead and support world-class HIM practices and standards. AHIMA has 52 Component State Associations (CSAs) that provide professional education and networking opportunities for members. Members must follow the AHIMA Code of Ethics, which outlines 11 ethical principles related to the coding profession's values and ethical behavior.

The primary certification is Certified Coding Specialist (CCS), which focuses on hospital inpatient and outpatient coding. The Certified Coding Specialist-Physician (CCS-P) certification focuses on physician-based coding. The Certified Coding Associate (CCA) credential is geared toward entry-level coders with little or no job experience. Additional certifications are offered in more specialized functions such as the administration of privacy and security programs in healthcare organizations, data analysis, and medical records administration. Each type of certification requires coders to take a separate examination. When considering which certification to pursue, it is helpful to know if one particular credential is preferred over another in the local geographic area. Research this information by reviewing job postings, talking to the human resources department at area employers, and asking experienced coders in the community. As their careers progress, some coders choose to obtain certification in more than one area of expertise, such as both physician and inpatient, and may become certified by both AAPC and AHIMA. Refer to the organizations' websites, **www.aapc.com** and **www.ahima.org**, to determine the current requirements for earning each certification.

> ### SUCCESS STEP
>
> Joining your local chapter of AAPC or AHIMA will give you the chance to get to know coders in other companies and can potentially lead to future job opportunities. Networking in this manner is an important part of your career path.

CODING PRACTICE

Exercise 1.3   Certification

Instructions: Write the answers to the following questions in the space provided.

1. What is certification?

_____

_____

_____

2. List and define three certifications offered by AAPC.

_____

_____

_____

3. List and define three certifications offered by AHIMA.

_____

_____

_____

CODING CAREERS

Most coding students are seeking a long-term coding career. In addition to learning the mechanics of coding, students are wise to begin learning about their career path and job performance expectations for accuracy and productivity.

Career Path

A career path is the progression of jobs and responsibilities throughout one's working life. In coding, like most careers, new graduates do not start at the top; they start at a basic level and work their way up with greater responsibility and more skills at each level. The career options, compensation, and benefits generally increase at each level of advancement. Advancement may come from within the same organization or it may come by moving to a new organization. In order to plan a possible career path, coding students want to learn about the job market, levels of advancement, and internal and external jobs.

Understanding the Job Market

Coders have many career options regarding where they work and what type of job they perform. While many students imagine themselves working in a hospital, the healthcare field offers many other types of organizations as well. Potential employers include all types of healthcare providers, payers, and third-party service organizations such as medical billing services. Sometimes it is best to start out in a small medical or dental office to get basic experience and then move to a larger organization later in your career. Working for a health insurance company or medical billing service can give coders a broad range of experience that will open up many career options later on. ■ TABLE 1-3 lists examples of various types of healthcare employers.

There are many job titles in the field of medical coding (■ TABLE 1-4). The same job might be called by different titles.

Table 1-3   ■   EXAMPLES OF TYPES OF ORGANIZATIONS THAT MAY REQUIRE CODING SKILLS

❏ Acupuncturist (LAc)	❏ Medical billing service
❏ Ambulance service	❏ Naturopathic office (ND)
❏ Ambulatory surgery center (ASC)	❏ Nursing facility (NF)
❏ Chiropractic office (DC)	❏ Optometrist (OD)
❏ Clearinghouse	❏ Osteopath (DO)
❏ Consulting firm	❏ Pharmacy
❏ Dental office	❏ Physician office (medical, surgical, all specialties) (MD)
❏ Durable medical equipment (DME) supplier	❏ Physical therapy clinic
❏ Health insurance company	❏ Self-insured employer
❏ Home healthcare	❏ Temporary staffing agency
❏ Hospital	❏ Third-party administrator (TPA)
❏ Laboratory	❏ Workers' compensation (WC)

Table 1-4 ■ EXAMPLES OF JOB TITLES THAT MAY REQUIRE CODING SKILLS

❑ Accounts receivable (A/R) specialist	❑ Insurance follow-up specialist
❑ Admitting clerk	❑ Insurance verifier
❑ Billing clerk	❑ Intake specialist
❑ Charge entry specialist	❑ Medical biller
❑ Claims analyst	❑ Medical receptionist
❑ Claims processor	❑ Medical records clerk
❑ Coder I/Coder II	❑ Patient account specialist
❑ Coding assistant	❑ Patient financial services clerk
❑ Electronic claims processor	❑ Patient service representative
❑ Health information analyst	❑ Refund specialist
❑ Insurance biller	❑ Scheduler

in two different organizations, so it is good to be open minded about potential job titles.

Levels of Advancement

Most coders look for an entry-level job upon graduation in order to gain basic skills, become familiar with the healthcare field, and establish excellent work habits. When possible, coders can look for a job in healthcare that builds on previous experience in a call center, bookkeeping, customer service, or patient care. Some companies offer internships (*paid training programs for those new to the field*), but this is not the norm.

After a few years of experience at entry level, coders potentially become eligible for advancement to a midlevel job. A midlevel job allows coders to expand their skills, learn new specialties, assume more independence, and take on more responsibility.

After five or so years of proven experience, coders can progress to an advanced-level job. Advanced-level jobs require

a solid track record of good performance in a related area. Advanced-level jobs often include management of others but may also focus on a specialized area of expertise, such as chart auditing. Technical specialization is an excellent career path for coders who are not interested in supervision or management of others. ■ TABLE 1-5 shows examples of a coding career path in a physician office, a hospital, and an insurance company.

SUCCESS STEP

Some job titles, such as accounts receivable specialist or biller, are also used by nonmedical businesses. Even the job title coder can apply to a computer engineer. When searching job postings, remember to specify a search for the healthcare field.

Table 1-5 ■ EXAMPLES OF A CODING CAREER PATH

	Years of Experience	Physician Office	Hospital	Insurance Company
Entry level	0–2 years	Front office receptionist Medical records file clerk Charge data entry operator	Admissions representative Cashier Billing office data entry clerk Patient account representative	Member services representative Claims representative trainee Sales assistant
Midlevel	3–5 years	Coding specialist Insurance verifier Referral coordinator Billing specialist Home-based coder	Outpatient billing clerk Medical documentation researcher Patient accounts team leader Coding assistant	Claims analyst Provider services representative Member services team leader Hospital claims specialist
Advanced level	More than 5 years	Billing manager Coding manager Chart auditor Collections manager	Chart auditor Medical records manager Inpatient coding specialist Home-based coder Cancer registrar Patient accounts manager	Supervisor, member services Supervisor, claims processing Claims auditor Legal researcher
		Consulting - Freelance coder - Business owner - Trainer - Author - Instructor		

Internal and External Job Openings

When coders are ready to change jobs and advance their careers, they may seek a new job internally within their current organization, or they may choose to look externally for a job with a different company.

Many organizations post their job openings internally, available only to current employees, for a period of time before they are advertised to the public. This means that established employees can apply for a promotion or transfer to another department but stay with the same company and keep their benefits. Companies like to promote from within because they are already familiar with the employee's personality and work ethic. Therefore, one good career strategy for a coder is to identify a desired employer, secure an entry-level job in that company, perform at a high level, and take advantage of opportunities to move to another job in the same company when ready.

Coders can also move between types of organizations, such as from an insurance company to a doctor's office or hospital. When coders start in a small office that has limited advancement opportunities, they can progress by moving to a larger organization or another small one that has an opening at a more advanced level. When they want to gain experience in another aspect of the healthcare industry, they can seek employment with a different type of organization. If an ultimate career goal, such as a hospital coding position, cannot be achieved in the first job, then coders can plan a career path to help get there.

Performance Expectations

Whatever career path coders choose, or even if they are not sure where they want to end up, it is always important to demonstrate excellent job attendance, follow directions, and meet the employer's expectations for quantity and quality of work. Every job task is an opportunity to earn a good reference, and it is those recommendations that help coders get to the next step in their careers.

Performance expectations are the outcomes employers need coders to achieve in order to demonstrate competence in the job. Coding jobs have high expectations because securing payment for services from insurance companies requires a high degree of accuracy and productivity by coders. Most employers have expectations related to coding accuracy and productivity.

Coding Accuracy

Coding accuracy involves the three coding skills discussed earlier in this chapter: abstracting, assigning, and arranging (sequencing). The average expectation for coding accuracy in these three areas is 95–98%. New coders' work is reviewed by a mentor or supervisor until they achieve the required level of accuracy. Samples of all coders' work are reviewed by supervisors and peers on an ongoing basis to ensure that everyone maintains a high level of accuracy. High accuracy is required to be eligible for greater responsibility, advancement, or special benefits such as working from home.

Productivity

Not only is accuracy critical to a coder's job, high productivity (*the amount of work accomplished in a specified time frame*) is also necessary. Productivity skills include keyboarding and case production, which are discussed next.

Keyboarding. Most coders use computers to determine or enter the codes. Therefore, high levels of speed and accuracy in keyboarding are essential. Coders must be proficient in alphanumeric (*a combination of letters and numbers*) keyboarding because most codes contain both letters and numbers. Many employers require that coders pass a keyboarding test before they schedule a job interview. Each employer sets its own speed requirement; 30–40 words per minute (wpm) or 9,000–12,000 keystrokes per hour (ksph) are common minimums. In keyboarding, any errors are deducted from the overall speed, so it is best to work on accuracy first, and then build up speed after the basics are mastered. With daily keyboarding drills, most students can achieve this minimum level in six months or less.

Case Production. Most coders are expected to meet a **case production** standard to code a specific number of cases each day, while maintaining high accuracy. The specific production standard is based on the type of record being coded; whether coders are assigning diagnosis codes, procedure codes, or both; whether coders work from paper or electronic charts; and what other responsibilities, such as billing, coders do at the same time. For example, coders who specialize in radiology coding generally code more encounters per hour than coders who specialize in complex surgical procedures because the records they are coding from are far less complicated. Each employer sets case production standards applicable to specific jobs within the organization.

Professional Skills

In addition to coding skills, coders also need several professional skill sets. These skills supplement your technical coding skills to help you perform all aspects of a job successfully. If you are rusty in one or more of these areas, refer to books and reliable Internet resources to refresh your skills. Important skills include:

- **Medical terminology**—Coders must be able to identify medical terms, a skill that includes breaking down unfamiliar words into a prefix, root, and suffix to define the meaning. It is not possible to code accurately without knowing the definition of medical terms used in clinical documentation.

- **Anatomy and physiology**—Coders must be familiar with the body's organ systems, their purpose, function, and pathology. They must be able to visualize the site where a procedure is performed, identify how the site is accessed, and the steps taken by the physician.

- **Basic arithmetic**—Knowledge of addition, subtraction, multiplication, division, and percentages is necessary to evaluate reimbursement aspects of coding. The ability to read simple statistical tables is needed to understand official publications.

- **Computer and Internet skills**—Coders use several specialized software programs such as electronic health records and encoders, as well as basic word processing and spreadsheet applications. They also must access information on government and payer websites and portals. Coders need to be able to learn new software quickly, often with minimal instruction, and work with multiple applications simultaneously.

- **Professional communication**—Coders need to communicate with each other, physicians, payers, and patients clearly, accurately, and nondefensively. Each method of communication—face-to-face, written, electronic, and telephone—requires unique skills and techniques.

- **Legal and ethical compliance**—Every aspect of healthcare is government by federal, state, and local regulations. Employers and professional associations maintain ethical standards that must be followed. Coders must be knowledgeable of all these requirements and follow them without complaint.

- **Critical thinking**—Many aspects of coding are not spelled out in black and white. Coders often must integrate information from several disciplines and apply it to the situation facing them to decide the appropriate course of action.

- **Team player**—Coders work as part of team and must be able to follow directions and give and accept help, support, and guidance as needed. There is a great deal of pressure in the healthcare environment to complete work accurately and quickly with limited resources. A positive attitude and a willingness to contribute to the organization is important to a successful career.

CODING PRACTICE

Exercise 1.4 Coding Careers

Instructions: Write the answers to the following questions in the space provided.

1. List five types of organizations that may require coding skills.

_____

_____

_____

_____

_____

2. Why do coding jobs have high performance expectations?

_____

_____

_____

_____

3. What keyboarding speed rate is commonly required by employers? _____

4. Why are medical terminology skills important for coders?

_____

CHAPTER SUMMARY

In this chapter you learned that:

- Coding is the process of accurately assigning codes to verbal descriptions of patients' conditions and the healthcare services provided to treat those conditions.

- The three skills of an "Ace" coder are abstracting, assigning, and arranging (sequencing).

- Coders assign diagnosis and procedure codes to patient encounters after an encounter is completed.

- Certification is a voluntary achievement that documents a coder having attained a certain level of proficiency by passing a rigorous examination offered by AAPC or AHIMA.

- A career path is the progression of jobs and responsibilities throughout one's working life.

- Performance expectations are the outcomes employers need coders to achieve in order to demonstrate competence in the job.

CONCEPT QUIZ

Take a moment to look back through this chapter and solidify your skills. This is your opportunity to pull together everything you have learned.

Completion

Instructions: Write the term that completes each statement based on the information you learned in this chapter. Choose from the following list. Some choices may be used more than once, and some choices may not be used at all.

abstract	assume	inpatient
accuracy	attending	outpatient
amend	career path	procedure
ancillary	code	query
arrange	covered entities	testing
assign	diagnosis	treatment

1. _____ codes describe patient illnesses, diseases, conditions, injuries, or other reasons for seeking healthcare services.

2. The three skills of an "Ace" coder are to _____ information from the medical record, _____ the accurate code, and _____ the codes in proper order.

3. A/an _____ encounter is a physician interaction with a patient who has not been formally admitted to a healthcare institution, such as an acute care hospital, long-term care facility, or rehabilitation facility.

4. A/an _____ encounter is a physician interaction with a patient who has been formally admitted to a healthcare facility, such as an acute care hospital, long-term care facility, or rehabilitation facility.

5. _____ services include laboratory, radiology, or physical therapy.

6. The _____ physician oversees and coordinates all aspects of the patient's care.

7. A _____ is the progression of jobs and responsibilities throughout one's working life.

8. The _____ plan may include medication, surgery, lifestyle changes, or therapy.

9. A _____ is a written communication asking for clarification and/or additional details.

10. _____ are health plans, healthcare clearinghouses, and healthcare providers who electronically transmit any health information in connection with transactions for which the Department of Health and Human Services (HHS) has adopted standards.

Multiple Choice

Instructions: Circle the letter of the best answer to each question based on the information you learned in this chapter.

1. What code set is used for diagnosis coding?
   A. HCPCS
   B. CPT
   C. ICD-10-CM
   D. ICD-10-PCS

2. What code set is used for hospital inpatient procedure coding?
   A. CDT
   B. CPT
   C. ICD-10-CM
   D. ICD-10-PCS

3. Which code set is used to report dental procedures?
   A. ICD-10-CM
   B. CDT
   C. DSM-V
   D. NDC

4. What term describes a specific interaction between a patient and healthcare provider?
   A. Admission
   B. Office visit
   C. Observation
   D. Encounter

5. Which service is an example of an inpatient encounter?
   A. Ambulatory surgery
   B. Hospital admission
   C. Emergency department
   D. Observation

6. Which task is the responsibility of coders?
   A. Determine what condition(s) the patient has based on the symptoms.
   B. Assign diagnostic and procedure codes for patient encounters after an encounter is completed.
   C. Code for services planned, but not provided, during the current encounter.
   D. Code for past conditions that are resolved.

7. What or who determines which certification is needed for a specific job?
   A. Employers
   B. HIPAA regulations
   C. CMS
   D. Individual states

8. What kind of job do most coders seek upon graduation in order to gain basic skills, become familiar with the healthcare field, and establish excellent work habits?
   A. Hospital
   B. Entry level
   C. Midlevel
   D. Advanced level

9. Which position is an example of an entry-level job?
   A. Data entry clerk
   B. Insurance verifier
   C. Inpatient coding specialist
   D. Coding assistant

10. Which method of posting job openings makes them available only to current employees for a period of time before they are advertised to the public?
    A. Internally
    B. Externally
    C. Online
    D. Word of mouth

Chapter 2

Coding and Reimbursement

Chapter Outline

- **Healthcare Payers**
- **Documentation**
- **Life Cycle of an Insurance Claim**
- **Reimbursement Methods**
- **Healthcare Claims**
- **Federal Compliance**
- **Health Information Technology**

Learning Objectives

After completing this chapter, you should have the skills to:

2.1 Spell and define the key words, medical terms, and abbreviations relating to reimbursement. (Remember)

2.2 Describe the types of healthcare payers. (Understand)

2.3 Explain the importance and content of documentation. (Understand)

2.4 Describe the life cycle of an insurance claim. (Understand)

2.5 Summarize the most common reimbursement methods for physicians, inpatient hospitals, and outpatient hospitals. (Understand)

2.6 Recognize the major healthcare claims formats. (Understand)

2.7 Explain the federal compliance initiatives. (Understand)

Key Terms and Abbreviations

837I
837P
abuse
ambulatory payment classification (APC)
ANSI ASC X12N Version 5010
audit
automatic adjudication
book-based encoder
beneficiary
capitation
case-based payment
Centers for Medicare and Medicaid Services (CMS)
certified EHR technology (CEHRT)
Children's Health Insurance Program (CHIP)
clean claim
CMS-1500
compliance
computer-assisted coding (CAC)

conversion factor (CF)
denied
Department of Health and Human Services (HHS)
diagnosis-related group (DRG)
discounted fee schedule
documentation
DRG grouper
edit check
electronic health record (EHR)
encoder
entitlement program
explanation of benefits (EOB)
False Claims Act (FCA)
fee schedule
fraud
front-end edit check
geographic practice cost index (GPCI)
group health plan

hierarchical condition category (HCC)
individual health insurance
inpatient prospective payment system (IPPS)
logic-based encoder
managed care plan
manual review
Medicaid
medical necessity
medical payment
medical record
medical review
Medicare
Medicare administrative contractor (MAC)
Medicare Advantage
Medicare Physician Fee Schedule (MPFS)
Medicare Physician Fee Schedule Database (MPFSDB)
Medicare severity-adjusted DRG (MS-DRG)

Medigap
National Uniform Billing Committee (NUBC)
National Uniform Claim Committee (NUCC)
negotiated rate schedule
Office of the Inspector General (OIG)
Original Medicare
outpatient prospective payment system (OPPS)
overcoding
Part A
Part B
Part C
Part D
per diem payment
personal injury protection (PIP)
preferred provider
private health insurance
progress note
promoting interoperability (PI) program

prompt pay
prospective payment system (PPS)
Qui Tam
reconcile
recovery audit contractor (RAC)
rejected claim
relative value unit (RVU)
remittance advice (RA)
resource-based relative value scale (RBRVS)
self-insured health plan
suspended
third-party administrator (TPA)
third-party payer
Tricare (TC)
UB-04
Veterans Health Administration (VHA)
whistleblower
workers' compensation (WC)

In addition to the key terms listed here, students should know the terms defined within tables in this chapter.

INTRODUCTION

When driving, you know that you need to obey the laws and that some laws, such as the speed limit, vary from town to town and state to state. If you miss seeing a speed limit sign, you know the state police will not accept that as an excuse. In healthcare, you also need to understand the rules of different entities, such as different payers. Even if your ultimate job does not directly involve billing, you still want to have a basic understanding of how your work as coder impacts reimbursement so you can become a valuable team member.

HEALTHCARE PAYERS

Third-party payers are entities other than the patient or physician who pay for healthcare services. According to the National Center for Health Statistics, *National Health Expenditures by Type of Service and Source of Funds: Calendar Years 1960 to 2015*, payers reimburse physicians and hospitals for 87% of all healthcare services in the United States. Patients pay the remaining 13% of services directly. Third-party payers include several government programs, private insurance companies, workers' compensation, and automobile medical payments insurance. Coders need to understand the various types of third-party payers because each has separate, and sometimes conflicting, rules about coding and billing.

All healthcare payments to hospitals, physicians, and other providers are based on coding. Procedure codes describe the services provided to patients. Physicians and hospitals assign money charges to each procedure code. Diagnosis codes justify why the services were needed. When the diagnosis code(s) does not adequately explain why the services were provided, payment may be denied or delayed.

Government Programs

Health benefit plans funded by federal or state governments pay for 60% of healthcare services. These are entitlement programs for which beneficiaries (*recipients of services*) qualify based on specific criteria. The various types of government and private insurance programs are summarized in the following sections.

Medicare

Medicare, sometimes abbreviated as MCR, was established in 1965. Medicare is funded by the federal government and is the single largest payer of healthcare services in the United States, accounting for 27% of healthcare payments. Medicare is administered by the Centers for Medicare and Medicaid Services (CMS), which is a division of the Department of Health and Human Services (HHS). Medicare pays for healthcare services for most people age 65 and over, people of any age with end-stage renal disease, and people with disabilities. Because it is so large, Medicare has a tremendous impact on healthcare policy and payment trends and, by extension, on coding. Other government programs and private health insurance are not required to follow Medicare rules, but it is not unusual for them to follow Medicare's lead to a considerable extent. The Medicare program has four parts, each of which also has separate rules and coding guidelines.

Part A. Medicare Part A, also called Original Medicare or traditional Medicare, is hospital insurance that covers a specific list of services for inpatient hospital care, skilled nursing facilities, hospice, and home healthcare. Most Americans who have worked as an adult, or are married to someone who has, are automatically eligible for Part A and do not pay a premium to receive benefits. They do pay deductibles and coinsurance.

Part B. Medicare Part B covers a specific list of physician services, outpatient hospital care, and home healthcare. It was created to provide medical coverage in addition to the hospital coverage of Part A. Part B is optional and most people are required to pay a premium to enroll, as well as deductibles and coinsurance.

Medicare Part A and Part B claims are processed by private companies called Medicare administrative contractors (MACs). Many Medicare coding and billing rules are the same across the country, but MACs have latitude in how certain policies are interpreted and applied. Therefore, coders need to keep up to date on the national rules, as well as the MAC rules.

Part C. Medicare Part C, also called Medicare Advantage, is an optional replacement of Part A and Part B that is offered by private health insurance companies. Many Part C plans are managed care and often have a preferred or required network of providers. Private insurance companies are paid through contracts with Medicare and believe they can provide care more cost effectively than traditional Medicare, thus making a profit. Patients choose Part C when they believe they can receive more benefits for the same or slightly more cost. The amount of premium, deductible, and coinsurance varies with each plan offered by a private company.

Part D. Medicare Part D, also called prescription drug coverage, is offered by private insurance companies through contracts with Medicare and provides limited benefits for prescription drugs. Patients choose from a variety of private plans, each of which may cover different medications, and select the one that covers the majority of their most costly prescriptions. Patients pay premiums, deductibles, and coinsurance. According to Medicare, most Part C plans also include Part D.

Medigap. Medigap is a Medicare supplement insurance policy sold by private insurance companies to fill gaps in Part A and Part B coverage. In most states, patients choose from 10 standardized plans labeled Plan A through Plan J. Medigap policies apply only to Original Medicare, not Part C.

Medicaid

Medicaid, sometimes abbreviated as MCD, also established in 1965, is a program for low-income families that is funded jointly by the federal government and state governments. It accounts for 23% of national healthcare payments. CMS establishes the general plan requirements, but states have considerable latitude in determining eligibility and coverage rules. Billing and coding requirements are also determined and administered by each state.

Other Government Programs

Other government programs include:

- **Tricare (TC)**—Health insurance coverage for family members of active duty personnel and for retired military personnel and their families.
- **Children's Health Insurance Program (CHIP)**—Established in 1997 by the federal government to provide health insurance to children in families with incomes below 200% of the federal poverty level.
- **Veterans Health Administration (VHA)**—An integrated healthcare delivery system with more than 1,400 sites of care, including hospitals, community clinics, community living centers, and various other facilities, to provide health services to veterans with service-connected disabilities.

Private Health Insurance

Private health insurance is coverage for healthcare services offered by private corporations, such as Aetna, Cigna, or United Healthcare, and not-for-profit organizations, such as Blue Cross and Blue Shield. About 35 companies issue the overwhelming majority of private health insurance plans nationwide. Thousands of different plans with different requirements and benefits exist. Private health insurance pays for 40% of national healthcare expenses. The three major sources of private health insurance are group health plans, self-insured plans, and individual insurance. Each insurance company and each plan offered by a company may have different requirements for coding and billing. Typically, the provider's coding and billing departments maintain files on the requirements of each plan. Most laws regarding private health insurance companies are determined by each state's legislature and implemented by the state Department of Insurance.

Group Health Plans

Approximately 56% of Americans are covered by a **group health plan** offered through their employer or union. The employer or union contracts with a private insurance company to provide a specific list of benefits to its employees. Often, they negotiate more than one option, each with a different set of benefits and different costs. The advantage of a group health plan is that the risk, or cost of medical care, is shared by a large number of people, resulting in lower premiums.

Employees choose which plan they want to enroll in based on its benefits and costs. Typically the employer pays the majority of the monthly premium and deducts a smaller portion of the premium, such as 10% or 20%, from employees' paychecks. Usually employees can cover their family members for an additional cost. In addition, employees pay deductibles and coinsurance or copayments for the actual services they receive.

Self-Insured Health Plans

Self-insured health plans are offered by large employers or unions who, rather than purchasing group health insurance, set aside money in a reserve fund and pay for employees' medical expenses from the fund. States regulate how much money employers must set aside in order to ensure that they will have enough money to pay catastrophic (high-cost) medical expenses.

In all other respects, a self-insured plan works similarly to a group health plan in that a specific list of benefits is covered, and, typically, employees pay a small monthly premium, deductibles, coinsurance, and copayments for medical care received. Often claims are processed by a private company called a **third-party administrator (TPA)**.

Individual Health Insurance

Individual health insurance, also called direct purchase, is a plan that people purchase directly from a health insurance company or through a health insurance exchange. Direct purchase is most often done by those who are self-employed or do not have benefits through an employer or government program. Approximately 16% of Americans are covered by individual health insurance.

Workers' Compensation

Workers' compensation (WC) plans pay for medical costs due to employment-related injuries or illnesses. Each state establishes its own requirements for WC insurance, but must comply with federal minimums. WC may be offered by private insurance companies approved by the state, large companies who self-insure, or a statewide insurance pool. Employers pay insurance premiums to cover the costs of care injured employees receive. Federal government employees are covered by federal WC plans.

WC programs are not subject to HIPAA regulations because they do not qualify as a health insurance plan. However, states have separate privacy and security rules that govern WC. WC plans may have unique coding and billing requirements, such as their own private code sets. Coding departments need to maintain a file containing these unique requirements.

Automobile Insurance

Automobile insurance policies often include **medical payments**, also called med pay, coverage, or **personal injury protection (PIP)**, a benefit that pays for medical expenses incurred during an automobile accident. Automobile insurance is regulated by each state's Department of Insurance, not by federal or HIPAA laws that govern health insurance companies. Auto insurance companies often contract with external bill review companies to review medical claims and recommend payment amounts. Coders need to be aware of any special requirements for patients being treated for automobile accident injuries. Typically the coding or billing department maintains a file detailing these requirements for each company.

Managed Care Plans

Managed care plans are companies that attempt to control the cost of healthcare while providing better outcomes. There are many different forms of managed care, but, in general, managed care plans contract with physicians, hospitals, and other providers to offer services for a lower fee than health plans; then they contract with private health insurance companies and self-insured plans to promote an exclusive network of **preferred providers**. When patients use preferred providers, they are responsible for lower out-of-pocket costs for deductibles, coinsurance, and copayments than if they select a provider not on the preferred list. Managed care plans are not a separate type of insurance, but rather a way of offering services to patients who are enrolled in a group health plan, self-insured plan, or individual health plan. Managed care plans also offer services to Medicare Part C programs, Medicaid, and even WC. Managed care companies are regulated primarily by federal laws. Well-known managed care plans include Kaiser Permanente, Anthem, and Humana.

CODING PRACTICE

Exercise 2.1   **Healthcare Payers**

Instructions: Write the answers to the following questions in the space provided.

1. Medicare pays for healthcare services for whom?

_____

2. Medicaid pays for healthcare services for whom?

_____

3. What are the three types of private health insurance plans?

_____

_____

_____

DOCUMENTATION

Payers have freedom to determine what services they will include in an insurance policy within state and federal requirements, but they also have a contractual obligation to pay for these services. To fulfill this obligation they may request information to determine whether the service is covered, including the site (location) of service; the medical need for and appropriateness of the diagnostic and therapeutic services provided; and the accuracy of codes for services billed based on the medical record.

Medical Necessity

The fact that a physician determines a patient needs a particular service or supply item does not mean that the insurance company or payer will agree. **Medical necessity** (*establishing the medical need for services*) is one of several criteria payers use to determine if, and how much, they will pay for a particular service. One of the reasons that payers establish medical necessity rules is to avoid paying unscrupulous providers who might provide a service just so they could receive payments, not because the patient actually needs the service or would benefit

from it. It also helps prevent patients from demanding services they do not need, such as expensive tests or cosmetic surgery.

Each of the payers discussed earlier in this chapter establishes its own definition of medical necessity and writes it into each insurance policy. ■ TABLE 2-1 lists common criteria for medical necessity and examples of each. By law, Medicare can pay only for services that are medically necessary, which is defined as services and supplies that

- Are needed to diagnose or treat a medical condition or improve the functioning of a malformed body member;
- Meet the standards of good medical practice in the local area; and
- Are not mainly for the convenience of the patient or physician.

In addition to a general definition of medical necessity, payers may also establish criteria for specific conditions, such as limiting the number of physical therapy visits for back pain; requiring an x-ray before ordering more expensive magnetic resonance imaging (MRI); or restricting the age and frequency of preventive screening, such as a screening mammogram every

Table 2-1   ■   **EXAMPLES OF MEDICAL NECESSITY CRITERIA**

Criterion	Appropriate Example	Inappropriate Example
Improve a patient's condition	Physical therapy to treat an acute back injury	Ongoing physical therapy to maintain general back comfort
Evidence-based practice	Medications proven to benefit patients based on scientific studies	Experimental drugs or treatments
Rendered by appropriate provider	Patient going to internal medicine or family practice physician to diagnose an initial symptom (e.g., stomach pain)	Patient going directly to gastroenterologist and having many expensive tests performed to diagnose an initial symptom of stomach pain
Least-restrictive setting	Suture removal in physician office; outpatient cataract surgery	Suture removal in the emergency department; inpatient cataract surgery without a medical reason
Not for patient or physician convenience	Liposuction for medical reasons	Liposuction for cosmetic reasons

two years for women over age 50. When providers recommend a treatment that varies from the insurance company's standard list, they may need to obtain preauthorization and provide special reports to justify the service. For some conditions, specific medical necessity criteria are not public information, and patients may learn of them only after a claim is **denied** (*the claim was processed and found to be ineligible for payment*).

Coders should not manipulate codes in a way that distorts or alters the diagnoses and procedures as documented in the medical record. This is unethical and fraudulent. Coders do need to be certain they are accurately describing everything that was done for the patient and the reasons for which the services were provided.

The Medical Record

The **medical record** is the comprehensive collection of all information on a patient at a particular facility. A medical record may be paper-based (Figure 2-1), electronic (Figure 2-2), or hybrid (a combination of both). It provides a written, chronological record of the patient's care, including important facts, findings, and observations about an individual's health history and health status (■ FIGURE 2-1 and ■ FIGURE 2-2). It reports past and present illnesses, examinations, tests, treatments, and outcomes and is a legal document that verifies the care provided. The diagnosis and procedure codes reported on the health insurance claim form or billing statement must be supported by information in the medical record for each encounter. Patients have separate medical records with each physician they see and each facility to which they are admitted. With the growth of electronic health records and the purchase of many provider offices by large healthcare corporations, it is becoming easier for providers to access information from other facilities. Sharing of medical information is regulated by HIPAA.

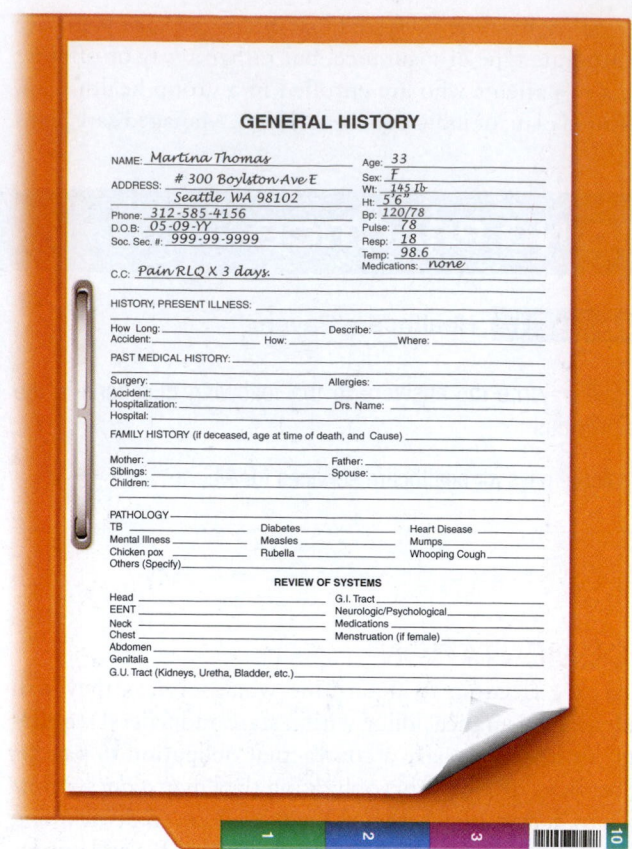

Figure 2-1 ■ Example of a paper-based medical record.

SUCCESS STEP

The medical record is admissible in a court of law as evidence and must be handled with the same care as any legal document.

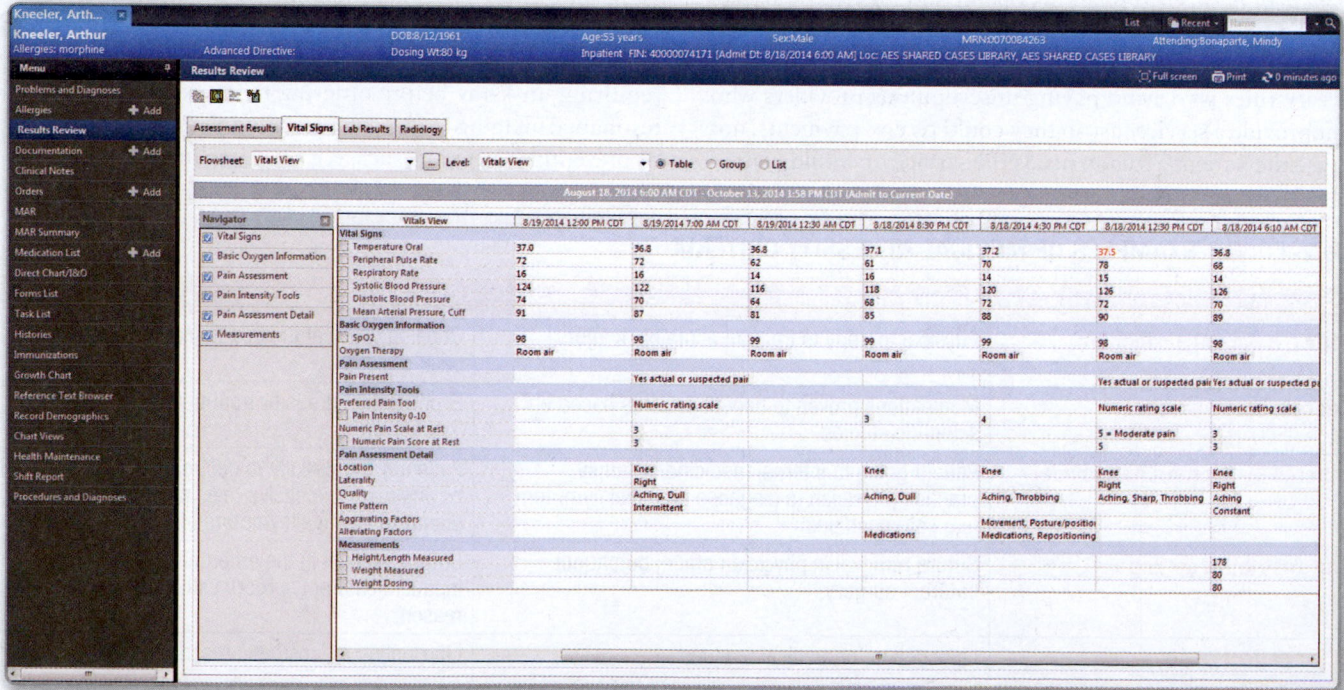

Figure 2-2 ■ Example of an electronic health record. *Source:* © *by Cerner Corporation. Used by permission of Cerner Corporation.*

Documentation is the written or electronic record of medical care and services provided. The word *documentation* is used to refer to the overall medical record as well as to **progress notes** (*the record of a specific patient encounter*). Thorough documentation is necessary, not only because it is the basis for delivering high-quality patient care but also because it helps improve reimbursement. Excellent documentation can reduce the amount of time needed to code a claim, result in more accurate and complete coding, and minimize common problems associated with claims processing. ■ TABLE 2-2 shows major elements of a progress note and how coders use each type of information. ■ TABLE 2-3 shows

major elements of a medical record and how coders use each type of information.

Clinical documentation improvement (CDI) is a program implemented by many hospitals that educates physicians and helps them achieve complete documentation that accurately reflects the care patients receive. CDI specialists review patients' charts concurrently (while the patient is in the hospital) and retrospectively (after the patient is discharged) to identify missing or inadequate documentation and query the physician for clarification when needed. They also provide ongoing education to help physicians better understand and comply with documentation requirements for each code set.

Table 2-2 ■ **ELEMENTS OF A PROGRESS NOTE AND THEIR USE IN CODING**

Element	Description	Coding Application
Chief complaint (CC)	The problem that has brought the patient to see the doctor (nausea, pain) or other reason for the visit (annual checkup)	Code for symptoms if the physician does not make a definitive diagnosis for an outpatient encounter.
History of the present illness (HPI)	An interview of the patient regarding symptoms related to the chief complaint and how the problem has progressed	May add details to the diagnostic statement.
Physical examination (PE)	A hands-on evaluation of the patient's vital signs, physical functions, and organ systems relevant to the chief complaint	May add details to the diagnostic statement.
Assessment	The diagnostic statement; the cause of the patient's current symptoms	This is the starting point for assigning diagnosis codes. Verify the details using other areas of the medical record when necessary.
Plan	The treatment that was or will be provided to address the symptoms	Inpatient hospitals code for procedures performed during the stay. Outpatient hospitals and physicians code for services provided during the encounter. Do not code for future planned treatments.

Table 2-3 ■ **ELEMENTS OF A MEDICAL RECORD AND THEIR USE IN CODING**

Element	Description	Coding Application
Progress notes	Description of specific encounters with the patient	Code each patient encounter based on the progress notes for that visit.
Obstetric history	Prior pregnancies, complications, and their outcomes	Use specific codes for first pregnancy, previous multiple pregnancies, and history of certain complications.
Surgical history	Date and type of past operations, operative reports (a narrative of exactly how the surgeon performed the procedure)	Assign codes for acquired absence (*surgical removal*) of certain organs. When an operation is performed during the current encounter, review the operative report to determine the exact procedure performed and the postoperative diagnosis.
Medications and medical allergies	Current and past medications; allergies to specific medications	Code for long-term use of certain medications.
Family history	The health status of immediate family members, causes of death (if known), diseases common in the family	Assign codes for family history of certain conditions.
Social history	Education, occupation, religious affiliation, natural support network, lifestyle habits (tobacco, alcohol, illicit drug use, sexual activity)	Assign codes for certain lifestyle habits.
Immunization history	Date and type of past vaccinations, titers (blood tests proving immunity to a specific disease)	Do not code for past vaccinations.
Lab test/pathology results	Reports from lab tests; report from pathology regarding specimen testing	Code abnormal test results only when the physician indicates significance and makes no certain diagnosis. Review pathology reports for biopsy results (e.g., malignant neoplasm).
Ancillary reports	Narrative reports or copies of reports from additional services such as EKGs, imaging	Code abnormal results only when the physician indicates significance and makes no certain diagnosis.

CODING PRACTICE

Exercise 2.2 Documentation

Instructions: Write the answers to the following questions in the space provided.

1. What is medical necessity? _____
_____
_____

2. List three examples of medical necessity criteria.
_____
_____
_____

3. What is the difference between the medical record and progress notes? _____
_____

LIFE CYCLE OF AN INSURANCE CLAIM

There are many steps involved in converting a patient encounter into a paid insurance claim. Each step needs to be completed in a timely and accurate manner in order for providers to receive correct payment for their services. The exact procedures are not the same in every office and every hospital, but the general process is similar.

Before the Encounter

The life cycle of an insurance claim begins when the patient calls the physician to make an appointment, a patient arrives at the emergency department, or a physician admits a patient to the hospital. Although providers do not code or bill for scheduling an appointment, the appointment begins when providers begin collecting insurance information. When time allows, patients preregister by completing paperwork regarding their health condition and insurance prior to the appointment. The provider verifies eligibility with the insurance company through a telephone call or secure website in order to determine if the patient is covered by insurance and what services are covered and/or require preauthorization.

During the Encounter

When patients arrive for their appointment or hospital admission, they complete registration forms or confirm the preregistration information, provide a copy of their insurance card, and possibly make a payment, if required by the insurance. They see the physician and/or receive the treatments and procedures needed. The physician documents the patient's problem in a progress note and may check off services and diagnoses on an encounter form or in the electronic health record. Finally, patients check out; schedule the next appointment, if needed; and may make a payment if they did not pay before they saw the physician.

After the Encounter

After the encounter is complete, the specific steps for coding and billing depend on how the encounter is recorded. In a physician's office that uses encounter forms, the physician will have already checked off the services and diagnoses for the visit. The encounter form is given to the billing department for data entry into the computer. If no encounter form is used, the chart is given to the coding department, where a coder reviews the progress note, assigns diagnosis and procedure codes, and enters the codes into the computer. The billing department verifies that all information for the encounter is complete. Usually the computer system automatically inserts the charges for each procedure entered by the coder, so billers also verify that all charges are present and accurate. When they have completed their verifications, billers flag the claim in the computer as ready to be submitted to the insurance company.

Most offices transmit claims electronically, usually daily or weekly depending on the volume of claims. Small offices with 10 or fewer employees may print out claims on paper billing forms and mail them, but this is becoming less common.

At the Clearinghouse

Most electronic claims are submitted to an electronic claims clearinghouse. The clearinghouse accepts the provider's claims, processes them through edit checks to verify that required information is present, then forwards them electronically to the various payers. A front-end edit check is an electronic process that scans the claims for valid data including the policy number, patient name, provider number, diagnosis codes, and procedure codes. The provider receives an electronic report of any missing data, such as a nonexistent code number or a missing policy number. The provider corrects the claim and resubmits it. Clearinghouses allow providers to streamline claims submission by sending all claims to one central recipient, rather than having to establish separate electronic accounts with every payer, which could consist of hundreds of organizations. Government claims can be sent through a clearinghouse or directly to the payer. Clearinghouses charge a fee for their services; claims sent directly to government payers do not incur a processing fee.

At the Insurance Company

Payers also perform front-end edit checks for valid member names, policy numbers, codes, and other information. Claims that contain missing or invalid information are automatically rejected by the computer. A rejected claim is one that is not accepted into the insurance company's computer system for processing due to missing or invalid data. Providers may learn of rejected claims through an electronic or paper report. However, sometimes they may not know the claim was rejected until they notice that payment was never received. When paper claims are submitted, the insurance company either scans them or enters data manually, then runs the front-end edit.

Clean claims are those that pass the front-end edit checks and have no missing or invalid information. Most clean claims are processed using **automatic adjudication,** a process in which the computer automatically determines which procedure codes are covered, calculates how much the insurance company is obligated to pay, then triggers the payment. Medicare is required to pay clean claims within 14 days of receipt. Many private payers also pay clean claims within a few days of receipt.

The payment may be sent to the provider either electronically or by a paper check. The insurance company also sends a **remittance advice (RA)** or **explanation of benefits (EOB),** a statement that lists all the services the provider billed, which ones were accepted for payment, how much the insurance company will pay, how much the patient owes, and how much will not be paid. If there are any services that are not eligible to be paid, the statement lists the reasons. Although the terms *RA* and *EOB* are often used interchangeably, the RA is the statement sent to the provider and the EOB is the statement sent to the patient. The EOB contains information similar to the RA, but it may be formatted differently and contain fewer details, such as no diagnosis or procedure codes.

Some claims are **suspended** from the automatic process for **manual review.** Reasons that claims are suspended include:

- High dollar amounts
- Specific diagnoses and procedures that the payer may wish to monitor
- Medical necessity review
- Illogical information, such as a patient gender or age that does not match the codes
- Questions about the patient's enrollment status
- Any other reason the payer may want to research

A claims analyst reviews the claim, determines if more information is needed from the provider or patient, and sends a letter if needed. Sometimes the claims analyst may have medical questions about the claim, such as if the procedure was appropriate for the diagnosis or if all of the services were medically necessary. These claims are sent to the **medical review** department, where a nurse, physician, or other clinician investigates the situation. They also may send a letter to the provider or patient requesting additional information or copies of documentation.

Clean claims may be processed within a few days of receipt, but claims that require manual review may take several weeks. Most states have **prompt pay** laws that require insurance companies to process claims within a specific period of time, such as 30 or 45 days. If the claim cannot be processed because of missing or incorrect information, insurance companies must issue any inquiry letters to providers or patients within this time frame.

After Insurance Processing

After the payer has processed the claim, the provider receives a check or electronic deposit and an RA. Depending on the sophistication of the provider's computer system, the payment may be automatically posted to the patient's account or a person may need to manually enter it into the computer or manual bookkeeping system. The biller or payment poster **reconciles** the RA. They compare the RA to the original bill to verify that each service billed was paid in the amount expected.

If payment was denied for one service or for the entire claim, an accounts receivable specialist needs to investigate the reason. Usually the reason is stated on the RA, but the specialist may need to call the insurance company for clarification. Solutions may involve obtaining additional information from the patient, asking the coding department to review the documentation and the codes assigned, or providing copies of documentation. ■ TABLE 2-4 gives examples of coding problems that

Table 2-4 ■ **CODING PROBLEMS CAUSING REJECTED OR DENIED CLAIMS**

Problem	Example
Characters in a code are mistyped, creating an invalid code.	Diagnosis code **007.0** instead of **O07.0** (number *zero* instead of letter *O*) PCS code **0J533ZZ** instead of **0J553ZZ**
Codes have too many or too few characters.	Diagnosis code **T20.511** instead of **T20.511A** Diagnosis code **Q68.10** instead of **Q68.1**
Diagnosis does not match the procedure.	Diagnosis code **K28.0 Acute gastrojejunal ulcer with hemorrhage** with a procedure code for removal of gallbladder. This may happen when the code was mistyped and should have been **K82.0 Obstruction of gallbladder**.
Codes are sequenced incorrectly.	Diagnosis codes **M36.1 Arthroplasty in neoplastic disease** and **C91.A0 Mature B-cell leukemia Burkitt type not having achieved remission**. An instructional note with code **M36.1** instructs the coder to "Code first underlying neoplasm."
Additional codes are required.	Diagnosis code **I69.891 Dysphagia following other cerebrovascular disease** instructs coder to "Use additional code to identify the type of dysphagia."
The services described in one code are included (bundled) into another code.	CPT procedure code **58150** includes removal of uterus, ovaries, and fallopian tubes, so these should not be billed separately.
Patient age or gender does not match the diagnosis or procedure.	Diagnosis code **O09.611 Supervision of young primigravida, first trimester** used for 18-year-old, but the code is defined as younger than age 16 at expected date of delivery.
A CPT procedure code requires a modifier in order to be paid.	Two lesions of the same size on the same site are removed. Append CPT modifier **-59** to the second lesion to identify it as a separate lesion and not a duplicate line item.

may cause claim rejections or denials. The provider needs to respond to insurance company inquiries quickly because any delay by the provider adds to the time it takes to receive payment. A new prompt payment period begins when the payer receives the requested information.

After all insurance payments are received and follow-up is complete, the office sends the patient a bill for any deductible, coinsurance, or patient-responsibility amounts that have not been paid.

CODING PRACTICE

Exercise 2.3   Life Cycle of an Insurance Claim

Instructions: Write the answers to the following questions in the space provided.

1. Why does the life cycle of an insurance claim begin when the patient calls the physician to make an appointment?

_____

_____

_____

_____

2. Define *automatic adjudication.*

_____

_____

_____

_____

3. List three coding problems that cause rejected or denied claims.

_____

_____

_____

_____

REIMBURSEMENT METHODS

The healthcare industry uses many different reimbursement, or payment, methods for services. The methods vary by type of payer, the setting—such as physician office, outpatient hospital, or inpatient hospital—and the type of service. Payment methods for the major settings are summarized below. Details of reimbursement methods vary by payer and by region of the country. More information is provided later in this text in the introductory chapters for each code set (Chapter 3, "Introduction to ICD-10-CM Diagnosis Coding"; Chapter 25, "Introduction to CPT Procedure Coding"; and Chapter 46, "Introduction to ICD-10-PCS Procedure Coding").

Reimbursement Terminology

A fee schedule is a list of specific services with charges. Each provider is free to set fees at any level they believe reasonably covers their costs and profit. Payers rarely accept a provider's established fee schedule, but instead issue a **negotiated rate schedule** or a **discounted fee schedule**. In a negotiated rate schedule, the payer specifies the fee it determines to be acceptable, or allowable, for each individual service on the provider's fee schedule. In a discounted fee schedule, the payer specifies the percentage of the provider's fee schedule it considers to be acceptable, such as 80% of the provider's rate. The negotiated or discounted rates function as the maximum amount the payer will allow when processing claims.

A **prospective payment system (PPS)** is a reimbursement method in which payment is made based on a predetermined, fixed amount per case. The payment amount for a particular service is based on a defined classification system of that service. The classification method is unique to each setting or type of services, as described in the next section. Medicare defines prospective payments for most services except physician services. Most other payers who use prospective payment adapt Medicare's system and rates as they determine appropriate. Medicare uses the **inpatient prospective payment system (IPPS)** for inpatient hospital services and the **outpatient prospective payment system (OPPS)** for outpatient hospitals.

Capitation is a prospective payment method in which physicians are paid a fixed amount per month for each member assigned to them, regardless of whether that person requests services. This payment is used primarily by health maintenance organizations (HMOs) for physician services. The rationale is that capitation discourages physicians from ordering unnecessary services because such costs are deducted from their payments. Payer costs and physician income are more predictable. There is concern that capitation creates a negative incentive for physician practices to accept only the healthiest, least costly patients and discourages them from ordering potentially important, but costly, specialty services.

Physician Reimbursement

Physicians are reimbursed based on fee schedules and capitation. Medicare publishes the **Medicare Physician Fee Schedule (MPFS)**, which is updated annually. Each procedure code is assigned a relative weight based on the resources required to provide it, which include work, practice expense, and malpractice. The weight is further adjusted based on the geographic location. The resulting relative value is converted into a fee. Because of the many factors involved, each physician can have a unique payment schedule. Additional incentive payments are made by Medicare based on meeting certain quality and electronic health record criteria.

Medicare uses a **resource-based relative value scale (RBRVS)** to establish physician reimbursement rates, which are published in the MPFS. The MPFS lists the Medicare rates for a specific provider for each CPT code and is updated annually. A **relative value unit (RVU)** identifies the amount of work and expense involved in providing a particular service. Medicare establishes three types of RVU components for each CPT code—physician work, practice expense, and malpractice—that are added together to produce the total RVU. An RVU of 1.0 reflects an average amount of work and expense. RVUs higher than 1.0 reflect a greater-than-average amount of work and expense, whereas RVUs less than 1.0 reflect a lower-than-average amount of work and expense.

The RBRVS also factors in a **geographic practice cost index (GPCI)** for each RVU component that reflects the differences in the cost of doing business in different regions of the country and different zip codes. To establish fees, Medicare multiplies the total RBRVS value for a CPT code by the annual **conversion factor (CF)**. For example, a conversion factor of $35 means that an RBRVS value of 1.0 is worth $35 on the MPFS. A code with an RBRVS value of 0.5 would be worth $17.50. A code with an RBRVS value of 2.0 would be worth $70. A code with an RBRVS value of 10.0 would be worth $3,500. When Medicare adjusts prices each year, it publishes a new conversion factor that is applied to all CPT codes.

Medicare publishes RBRVS information on its website. Many encoder software programs make RBRVS information available to the user. Private payers may adopt Medicare RVUs and RBRVS, modify them, or establish their own.

The **Medicare Physician Fee Schedule Database (MPFSDB)** is the source of all information related to CPT code reimbursement for Medicare. It contains not only the fees, as the MPFS does, but also the RVUs, GPCI, CF, global surgery days (*the number of follow-up days included in a surgical procedure*), accepted modifiers, and other relevant information. A searchable version of the MPFSDB is available on the CMS website.

Physicians provide services in many settings: the medical office, an ambulatory surgery center, outpatient hospital departments such as radiology or cardiac catheterization lab, and inpatient hospitals. Although the services are provided in a location other than the medical office, physicians are still responsible for coding and billing the services they provide in those settings. Services provided at locations other than the medical office often have two billing components: the facility fee and the professional fee. The facility fee covers the cost of the building, equipment, technician, and other staff, as applicable. The professional fee covers the cost of the physician's time. The facility, such as the hospital or ambulatory surgery center, bills the facility fee, and the physician bills the professional fee.

Inpatient Hospital Reimbursement

Inpatient hospitals are reimbursed based on fee schedules, **per diem payment** (*an all-inclusive flat charge per day*), and prospective payment. The most common prospective payment classification method is **diagnosis-related groups (DRGs)**. **Hierarchial condition category (HCC)** coding further fine tunes reimbursement.

Diagnosis-Related Groups

DRGs are a prospective payment method that categorizes patients who are medically related with respect to diagnosis and treatment and statistically have similar lengths of stay. Consequently, they also tend to have similar costs and charges associated with the hospitalization. Several DRG systems have been developed, with the best known being **Medicare severity-adjusted DRGs (MS-DRGs)** used by Medicare. MS-DRGs consist of approximately 800 DRG classifications that aggregate the thousands of diagnoses and procedures available in the coding manuals. DRGs are a case-based prospective payment system. **Case-based payment** means that the rate is determined per case, or per inpatient admission, rather than on a per diem (daily) basis or a fee-for-service basis. A standard payment rate is predetermined based on the average amount of staff, supplies, and other resources typically used and assigned to each DRG. The hospital is paid the same amount for all patients classified to a particular DRG, regardless of the actual costs incurred. Each hospital receives a unique reimbursement rate per DRG based on its geographic location and other factors. This reimbursement method places the risk of cost-effectively managing the patient's stay on the hospital rather than the payer.

Cost outliers are unusual cases in which the cost is above or below a standard threshold amount established for the DRG. High-cost outliers can qualify for additional payment; low-cost outliers can be paid a lower-than-usual rate. Reasons for outliers are unique combinations of diagnoses and surgeries causing high costs, very rare conditions, long lengths of stay, deaths, and cases admitted and discharged on the same day. Examples of comorbidities that may contribute to high-cost outliers are alcoholism, diabetes mellitus, and renal failure. Outlier payments for high-cost outliers help protect the hospital against extraordinary costs incurred from extremely ill patients. Payment reductions for low-cost inliers help protect the insurance company against overpaying.

A **DRG grouper** is software that considers several clinical and demographic characteristics of a patient. After a patient's diagnoses are coded, the case is assigned to a Major Diagnostic Category (MDC) then is classified into a DRG based on seven variables:

- Principal diagnosis
- Secondary diagnoses
- Surgical procedure(s)
- Complications and comorbidities (CC) and major complications and comorbidities (MCC)
- Age and gender
- Discharge status
- Trim points (*the typical high and low length of stay for a diagnosis*)

An example of a MS-DRG is *DRG 375 Digestive Malignancy with Complication or Comorbidity*. The MDC for this DRG is *MDC 06 Diseases and Disorders of the Digestive System*.

DRG payment is increased for cases that are unusually costly or with an unusually high length of stay. In addition, hospitals can receive add-on payments if they treat a high percentage of low-income patients, are a teaching hospital, and a few other factors.

Hierarchical Condition Category Coding

Hierarchical condition category (HCC) coding was developed to estimate future health risks and costs for Medicare Advantage and Medicaid inpatients. The focus is to identify inpatients with chronic, high cost illnesses. To accomplish this, ICD-10-CM diagnosis codes are mapped to approximately 80 HCCs, using software from CMS. Each HCC is assigned a risk adjustment factor (RAF), a numerical score that helps predict the future costs of caring for a patient. These cost estimates are used by insurance companies to establish contracted rates. An example of an HCC is *HCC 11 Colorectal, Bladder, and Other Cancers*.

Most facilities establish a specific job description for an employee who verifies the mapping of HCCs. All of a patient's diagnoses must be documented and coded so that the correct HCC is identified. If key diagnoses are overlooked, the patient will not be classified correctly, thus impacting facility payment.

Outpatient Hospital Reimbursement

Outpatient hospitals are reimbursed based on fee schedules and prospective payment. CMS OPPS assigns individual services to an **ambulatory payment classification (APC)** based on similar clinical characteristics and similar costs. All procedures in an APC are paid at the same rate. Within each APC, payment for ancillary, supportive, and adjunctive items and services is packaged into payment for the primary service. Examples of packaged services include supplies, ancillary services, operating room use, most drugs, laboratory tests, and imaging services. Private payers may adopt Medicare APCs, modify them, establish their own, or pay based on individual CPT codes.

Reimbursement in Other Settings

Each specialized healthcare setting uses a specific and unique reimbursement method. Some of the most common settings are highlighted next.

Ambulatory surgery centers (ASCs) are reimbursed based on negotiated fee schedules and prospective payment. The most common prospective payment classification method is APCs. This is the same overall reimbursement method as used for outpatient hospitals.

Inpatient rehabilitation hospitals and distinct rehabilitation units are reimbursed based on case-mix groups (CMGs). The patient's CMG is determined by a rating of the patient's level of impairment, motor and cognition abilities, and age.

Skilled nursing facilities (SNFs) are reimbursed based on resource utilization groups (RUGs). The patient's RUG is determined by a comprehensive assessment of the patient's caregiving needs using the minimum data set (MDS) evaluation tool. A predetermined per diem (*daily*) amount is paid based on the RUG to which the patient is assigned.

Home health agencies (HHAs) are reimbursed based on home health resource groups (HHRGs). A predetermined payment is made for each 60-day period based on the assessment of the patient. The patient's HHRG is determined by the score on the outcome and assessment information set (OASIS) for each 60-day period. Payment is adjusted if the patient's condition changes significantly.

When working in a new setting, coders must learn specific reimbursement and coding procedures. Coders can research reimbursement information on **www.cms.gov** and other payer websites.

CODING PRACTICE

| Exercise 2.4 | Reimbursement Methods |

Instructions: Write the answers to the following questions in the space provided.

1. Define *negotiated fee schedule*. _____
_____

2. Define *prospective payment system*. _____
_____
_____

3. Define *capitation*. _____
_____
_____

HEALTHCARE CLAIMS

Providers must submit claims for services to payers to receive reimbursement. Specific electronic formats or paper forms are required in each healthcare setting. Electronic standards specify exactly how data is to be submitted, so that payers' computers can read the information submitted by providers and clearinghouses. The standard must be followed by health plans, healthcare clearinghouses, and certain healthcare providers when conducting electronic transactions. The standard includes claims, claims status requests and responses, payment to providers, eligibility requests and responses, referral requests and responses, enrollment and disenrollment in a health plan, coordination of benefits, and premium payments. **ANSI ASC X12N Version 5010** is the name of the approved set of HIPAA standards for electronic transactions. Sometimes you will see it referred to simply as Version 5010. Abbreviations in this designation are:

- ANSI—American National Standards Institute that sets the standards

- ASC—Accredited Standards Committee that is directly responsible

- X12N—The insurance section for the health insurance industry's administrative transactions
- Version 5010A1—The current version of the electronic standards for healthcare transactions

The designation 837 identifies the standard for healthcare claims. Each type of claim has an additional letter such as **837P** for professional claims and **837I** for institutional claims.

Physician Claims

Physicians bill services on the **CMS-1500** form. The electronic format for claims submission of physician services is the 837P (■ FIGURE 2-3). Both formats require the same data elements. The **National Uniform Claim Committee (NUCC)**, chaired by the American Medical Association (AMA), maintains and updates the CMS-1500 form. NUCC also provides specific guidelines for completing a CMS-1500 claim form that are consistent with those for preparing electronic claims and provides a crosswalk between the CMS-1500 and 837P. NUCC guidelines are published in the *1500 Health Insurance Claim Form Reference Instruction Manual*, which is updated each year in July and can be accessed on the Web at **www.nucc.org**. The form contains 33 items, or boxes, that must be completed. The items are grouped into two sections:

- Items 1–13 Patient and insured information
- Items 14–33 Physician or supplier information

The label *ICD ind* in Block 21 identifies the coding system being used on the claim, such **0** for ICD-10-CM.

The patient's primary or first-listed diagnosis is entered in Block 21A, with additional diagnoses in Blocks 21B through 21L.

Procedure information is entered in Block 24, lines 1 through 6. The label *Diagnosis pointer* in block 24E refers to the diagnoses in 21A through 21L that support each procedure.

Inpatient Hospital Claims

Inpatient hospitals bill services on the **UB-04**, also known as the CMS-1450 (■ FIGURE 2-4). The electronic format for claims submission of inpatient services is the 837I. Both formats require the same data elements. The **National Uniform Billing Committee (NUBC)** is chaired by the American Hospital Association (AHA) and consists of representatives from more than 15 healthcare industry groups. NUBC maintains and updates the UB-04 form and provides a crosswalk between the UB-04 and 837I. NUBC also provides specific guidelines for completing a UB-04 claim form that are consistent with those for preparing electronic claims. The form contains 81 form locators, or boxes, that must be completed:

- 1–41 Patient information
- 42–49 Billing information
- 50–65 Payer information
- 66–81 Diagnosis and procedure information

NUBC guidelines are published in the *Official UB-04 Data Specifications Manual*, which is updated each year in July and can be accessed on the Web at **www.nubc.org**.

Some fields require unique two-digit indicators called occurrence codes, condition codes, and value codes to communicate information to the payer. These are informational codes that appear in the instructions for completing the UB-04 form; they are not billing codes and do not appear in the coding manuals. Use of these codes allows flexibility in how certain form locators are used. They make a shorter form than would be possible if every potential data point occupied a dedicated field.

Condition codes identify certain events or circumstances related to a patient. For example, if a condition is employment-related, the biller enters condition code **02** in the first available field of FL 18–28. The code **02** informs the payer that the condition is employment-related.

Occurrence codes and occurrence span codes are used to identify a significant event that could affect payer processing. For example, if an accident or injury caused the condition being treated, the biller enters occurrence code **01** and the date of the accident in the first available field of FL 31–34. The code **01** informs the payer that an accident or injury occurred and the date it happened.

Value codes are entered in FL 39–41 and identify the number and dollar amount of certain services provided. For example, if a patient has physical therapy visits, the biller enters the value code **50** in the Code column on the left side of FL 39a and the actual number of physical therapy visits in the Amount column for FL 39, for example, **5** for five visits. The code **50** informs the payer that physical therapy services were provided, and the number **5** informs the payer that there were five visits.

Revenue codes are entered in FL 42, lines 1–22, with related service and charge information in FL 43–48. This information summarizes charges by department. An itemized bill showing each individual charge item is submitted with the claim.

FL 66 is used to identify the coding system being used on the claim, such as **0** for ICD-10-CM.

The patient's principal diagnosis is entered in FL 67, with additional diagnoses in FL 67A–67Q. The admitting diagnosis appears in FL 69.

The principal procedure is entered in FL 74 and additional procedures in FL 74a–74d.

For detailed instructions on how to complete the UB-04, refer to **www.cms.gov** or **www.nubc.org**.

Outpatient Hospital Claims

Hospitals use the UB-04/837I to bill the facility portion of outpatient services and the CMS-1500/837P to bill any professional services for which they are responsible. The processes are similar to those used by inpatient hospitals and professionals, respectively, except for information related to the location of service.

HEALTH INSURANCE CLAIM FORM

APPROVED BY NATIONAL UNIFORM CLAIM COMMITTEE (NUCC) 02/12

| | PICA | | | | | | | | | | PICA | | |

1. MEDICARE ☐ (Medicare#) MEDICAID ☐ (Medicaid#) TRICARE ☐ (ID#/DoD#) CHAMPVA ☐ (Member ID#) GROUP HEALTH PLAN ☒ (ID#) FECA BLK LUNG ☐ (ID#) OTHER ☐ (ID#)

1a. INSURED'S I.D. NUMBER (For Program in Item 1)
7856321

2. PATIENT'S NAME (Last Name, First Name, Middle Initial)
DOE JOHN A

3. PATIENT'S BIRTH DATE MM 05 DD 15 YY 1980 **SEX** M ☒ F ☐

4. INSURED'S NAME (Last Name, First Name, Middle Initial)
DOE JANE M

5. PATIENT'S ADDRESS (No., Street)

6. PATIENT RELATIONSHIP TO INSURED
Self ☐ Spouse ☒ Child ☐ Other ☐

7. INSURED'S ADDRESS (No., Street)
123 WASHINGTON STREET

CITY | STATE
8. RESERVED FOR NUCC USE
CITY BRANTON | STATE ST

ZIP CODE | TELEPHONE (Include Area Code) ( )

ZIP CODE 11111 | TELEPHONE (Include Area Code) ( )

9. OTHER INSURED'S NAME (Last Name, First Name, Middle Initial)

10. IS PATIENT'S CONDITION RELATED TO:

11. INSURED'S POLICY GROUP OR FECA NUMBER

a. OTHER INSURED'S POLICY OR GROUP NUMBER

a. EMPLOYMENT? (Current or Previous) YES ☐ NO ☒

a. INSURED'S DATE OF BIRTH MM DD YY **SEX** M ☐ F ☐

b. RESERVED FOR NUCC USE

b. AUTO ACCIDENT? YES ☐ NO ☒ PLACE (State)

b. OTHER CLAIM ID (Designated by NUCC)

c. RESERVED FOR NUCC USE

c. OTHER ACCIDENT? YES ☐ NO ☒

c. INSURANCE PLAN NAME OR PROGRAM NAME

d. INSURANCE PLAN NAME OR PROGRAM NAME

10d. CLAIM CODES (Designated by NUCC)

d. IS THERE ANOTHER HEALTH BENEFIT PLAN? YES ☐ NO ☒ If yes, complete items 9, 9a, and 9d.

READ BACK OF FORM BEFORE COMPLETING & SIGNING THIS FORM.
12. PATIENT'S OR AUTHORIZED PERSON'S SIGNATURE I authorize the release of any medical or other information necessary to process this claim. I also request payment of government benefits either to myself or to the party who accepts assignment below.

SIGNED SOF DATE

13. INSURED'S OR AUTHORIZED PERSON'S SIGNATURE I authorize payment of medical benefits to the undersigned physician or supplier for services described below.

SIGNED SOF

14. DATE OF CURRENT ILLNESS, INJURY, or PREGNANCY (LMP) MM DD YY QUAL.

15. OTHER DATE QUAL. MM DD YY

16. DATES PATIENT UNABLE TO WORK IN CURRENT OCCUPATION FROM MM DD YY TO MM DD YY

17. NAME OF REFERRING PROVIDER OR OTHER SOURCE
17a.
17b. NPI

18. HOSPITALIZATION DATES RELATED TO CURRENT SERVICES FROM MM DD YY TO MM DD YY

19. ADDITIONAL CLAIM INFORMATION (Designated by NUCC)

20. OUTSIDE LAB? YES ☐ NO ☐ $ CHARGES

21. DIAGNOSIS OR NATURE OF ILLNESS OR INJURY Relate A-L to service line below (24E) ICD Ind. 0

A. I10 B. I48.91 C. J30.9 D.
E. F. G. H.
I. J. K. L.

22. RESUBMISSION CODE ORIGINAL REF. NO.

23. PRIOR AUTHORIZATION NUMBER

24.

A. DATE(S) OF SERVICE						B. PLACE OF SERVICE	C. EMG	D. PROCEDURES, SERVICES, OR SUPPLIES		E. DIAGNOSIS POINTER	F. $ CHARGES		G. DAYS OR UNITS	H. EPSDT Family Plan	I. ID. QUAL.	J. RENDERING PROVIDER ID. #
From MM	DD	YY	To MM	DD	YY			CPT/HCPCS	MODIFIER							
1	01	15	YY	01	15	YY	11		99205		ABC	205	00	01		NPI	1234567890
2	01	15	YY	01	15	YY	11		95052		C	50	37	10		NPI	1234567890
3	01	15	YY	01	15	YY	11		93000		B	18	25	01		NPI	1234567890
4																NPI	
5																NPI	
6																NPI	

25. FEDERAL TAX I.D. NUMBER SSN ☐ EIN ☒
111222333

26. PATIENT'S ACCOUNT NO.
5831

27. ACCEPT ASSIGNMENT? (For govt. claims, see back) YES ☒ NO ☐

28. TOTAL CHARGE $ 273 62

29. AMOUNT PAID $

30. Rsvd for NUCC Use

31. SIGNATURE OF PHYSICIAN OR SUPPLIER INCLUDING DEGREES OR CREDENTIALS (I certify that the statements on the reverse apply to this bill and are made a part thereof.)
Kristin Conover, MD 1/15/20YY
SIGNED DATE

32. SERVICE FACILITY LOCATION INFORMATION
a. NPI b.

33. BILLING PROVIDER INFO & PH # (555) 555 1111
BRANTON FAMILY PRACTICE
999 MAIN STREET
BRANTON ST 00000
a. 9998887776 b.

NUCC Instruction Manual available at: www.nucc.org **PLEASE PRINT OR TYPE** APPROVED OMB-0938-1197 FORM 1500 (02-12)

CARRIER | PATIENT AND INSURED INFORMATION | PHYSICIAN OR SUPPLIER INFORMATION

Figure 2-3 ■ Example of a completed CMS-1500 claim form.

INPATIENT

1 Any Hospital	2 Any Hospital	3a PAT CNTL # 1234	4 TYPE OF BILL
123 Any Street	456 Any Street	b MED REC # 98765	0111
Philadelphia PA 19103	Philadelphia PA 19103	5 FED. TAX. NO. 221234567	6 STATEMENT COVERS PERIOD FROM 11 03 06 THROUGH 11 04 06	7 RESERVED

8 PATIENT NAME	a Patient ID if different from Sub	9 PATIENT ADDRESS	a 1234 Main Street
b Doe, John		b Philadelphia	c PA d 19111 Country code if other than USA

10 BIRTHDATE	11 SEX	12 DATE	ADMISSION 13 HR	14 TYPE	15 SRC	16 DHR	17 STAT	18 19 20 21 CONDITION CODES 22 23 24 25 26 27 28	29 ACDT STATE	30
03 20 1971	M	11 03 06	08	3	3	12	01	Condition Codes Required identifying Events	PA	RESERVED

31 OCCURRENCE CODE DATE	32 CODE DATE	33 OCCURRENCE CODE DATE	34 OCCURRENCE CODE DATE	35 OCCURRENCE SPAN CODE FROM THROUGH	36 OCCURRENCE SPAN CODE FROM THROUGH	37

a
b Occurrence and Occurrence Span Codes may be used to define a significant event that may affect payer processing — FUTURE USE

38		39 CODE VALUE CODES AMOUNT	40 CODE VALUE CODES AMOUNT	41 CODE VALUE CODES AMOUNT
John Doe 1234 Main Street Philadelphia, PA 19111		a A1 952 00		
		b Value Codes and amounts required when necessary to process claim		
		c		
		d		

42 REV.CD.	43 DESCRIPTION	44 HCPCS/RATE/HPPS CODE	45 SERV. DATE	46 SERV. UNIT	47 TOTAL CHARGES	48 NON-COVERED CHARGES	49
1 0129	Semi-Private	200.00		2	400 00	0 00	Future Use 1
2 0250	Pharmacy			1	50 00	0 00	2
3 0360	OR Services				100 00	0 00	3
4							4
5							5
6							6
7							7
8							8
9							9
10							10
11							11
12							12
13							13
14							14
15							15
16							16
17							17
18							18
19							19
20							20
21							21
22							22
23 PAGE 1 OF 1	CREATION DATE	TOTALS ➤			550 00	0 00	23

50 PAYER NAME	51 HEALTH PLAN ID	52 REL INFO	53 ASG BEN.	54 PRIOR PAYMENTS	55 EST. AMOUNT DUE	56 NPI 2222222222	
A Independence Blue Cross	Report HIPAA National	Y	Y	Required when indicated payer has paid amount to Provider	Amount estimated to be due	57 1234567890	A
B Secondary Payer	Health Plan Identifier					OTHER Secondary	B
C Tertiary Payer	when mendatory					PRV. ID Tertiary	C

58 INSURED'S NAME	59	60 INSURED'S UNIQUE ID	61 GROUP NAME	62 INSURANCE GROUP NO.	
A Doe, John	18	ABC12345678900	Watch Repair, Inc.	1234	A
B Secondary					B
C Tertiary					C

63 TREATMENT AUTHORIZATION CODES	64 DOCUMENT CONTROL NUMBER	65 EMPLOYER NAME	
A 02468	491234	Watch Repair, Inc.	A
B Secondary			B
C Tertiary			C

66 K50114	A Use A through Q to report "Other Diagnosis" if applicable	E	F	G	H	68 Reserved
0	I J K L M N O P Q					

69 ADMIT DX K50114	70 PATIENT REASON DX May be used to report reason for visit	71 PPS CODE 330	72 ECI May be used to report external cause of injury	73 Reserved

74 PRINCIPAL PROCEDURE CODE DATE	a OTHER PROCEDURE CODE DATE	b OTHER PROCEDURE CODE DATE	75	76 ATTENDING NPI 2222222222	QUAL 16 1234569822
0D1B0Z4 08 26 YY			Reserved	LAST Smith FIRST David	
c OTHER PROCEDURE CODE DATE	d OTHER PROCEDURE CODE DATE	e OTHER PROCEDURE CODE DATE		77 OPERATING NPI QUAL	
				LAST FIRST	

80 REMARKS	81CC a B3 292N00000X	78 OTHER NPI QUAL
May be used to report additional	b Secondary	LAST FIRST
information.	c Tertiary	79 OTHER NPI QUAL
	d	LAST FIRST

UB-04 CMS-1450   APPROVED OMB NO.   NUBC™ National Uniform Billing Committee   THE CERTIFICATIONS ON THE REVERSE APPLY TO THIS BILL AND ARE MADE A PART HEREOF.

RED = Required
Black = Situational/Required, if applicable/Reserved

Figure 2-4 ■ Example of a completed UB-04 claim form (with annotations).

CODING PRACTICE

Exercise 2.5 Healthcare Claims

Instructions: Write the answers to the following questions in the space provided.

1. Define *Version 5010A1.* _____

   _____

2. What claim form is used to bill physician services? _____

   _____

3. What is the electronic format used to bill physician services?

   _____

   _____

4. What claim form is used to bill inpatient hospital services? _____

   _____

5. What is the electronic format used to bill inpatient hospital services? _____

FEDERAL COMPLIANCE

Although providers are appropriately concerned about being underpaid or not paid at all, they also need to be concerned about being overpaid. When providers are overpaid they are legally obligated to report the overpayment to Medicare, refund the money, and possibly even pay interest on it.

Using electronically collected data, payers can track patterns of billing, compare a physician to the average or norm, and target providers who deviate from the norm. If an insurance company or Medicare detects a pattern of overpayments due to **overcoding** (*coding for a more complex diagnosis or procedure than is documented*) or improper billing, they can conduct an **audit** (*an investigation of the provider's billing and coding practices*). Going through an audit is time-consuming and costly, but if violations are found, severe financial penalties, loss of Medicare privileges, and even imprisonment are possible.

This should not scare coders but make them aware of the importance of their role and the need for accuracy. Medicare places the responsibility for knowing the rules on providers (and by extension their coders). Medicare's stance is that once they publish a rule, providers should know about it and follow it.

Violating coding and billing rules can be classified as fraud or abuse. **Fraud** is knowingly billing for services that were never given or billing for a service that has a higher reimbursement than the service actually provided. **Abuse** is mistakenly accepting payment for items or services that should not be paid for by Medicare, due to improper coding and billing practices. Examples are billing for a noncovered service, assigning a more costly code to a lesser service, or coding in a way that does not follow national or local coding guidelines.

Compliance simply means following the rules. Healthcare providers must follow rules established by multiple federal, state, and county government agencies. Some rules are specific to healthcare and others pertain to any type of business. Companies and organizations establish compliance programs to actively keep informed about regulations, educate employees, and make sure that everyone in the company is cooperating. Investigation of fraud and abuse is primarily the responsibility of the Office of the Inspector General (OIG) and Recovery audit contractors (RACs).

> ### CODING CAUTION
> You already know that if an officer stops you for speeding, the excuse "I didn't see the sign" will not get you very far. It is the same with Medicare. They expect you to know and follow a multitude of rules, and the rules are usually less clear and less obvious than a speed limit sign on the side of the road.

Office of the Inspector General

Although HIPAA is best known for its privacy rules and healthcare transaction standards, it also created several programs to further control fraud and abuse in healthcare. One of these provisions increased the amount of money the **Office of the Inspector General (OIG)** can spend to investigate fraud and abuse. It also increased the penalties for violations. The OIG is a division of HHS that investigates fraud, abuse, and other noncompliance matters in the Medicare and Medicaid programs. As a result, healthcare fraud and abuse investigations have become a major focus, and a highly profitable one, for the government. The Health Care Fraud and Abuse Control (HCFAC) program's *Annual Report for Fiscal Year 2016* reports a three-year rolling average return on investment of $5.00 recouped for every dollar spent on enforcement activities. Over $3.3 billion was recouped during fiscal year 2016 alone. OIG accomplishes its mission through the False Claims Act (FCA) and compliance programs, which are discussed next.

False Claims Act

OIG uses the **False Claims Act (FCA)** as the basis for much of its investigation and prosecution. The FCA imposes penalties on individuals and companies who defraud government programs. It was passed in 1863, during the Civil War, to combat widespread fraud in which contractors sold the government faulty rifles and ammunition, rotten food, and sick horses. The **Qui Tam** provision of the FCA includes a financial reward to **whistleblowers**, those who turn in violators. The FCA has been updated several times, including 1986, 2009, 2010, and 2016.

Knowingly submitting a bill to a government healthcare program, such as Medicare, that contains incorrect codes is considered to be presenting a false claim for payment because the provider is requesting payment for a service that was not provided. If the same coding or billing error is made repeatedly, it can be considered fraud because the provider is responsible to know all the rules about how services should be billed and coded. The FCA is interpreted in a broad sense to include not only intentional misrepresentation but also errors made from ignorance. Medicare providers and their staff are obligated to know all the Medicare rules.

Compliance Programs

Also as a result of HIPAA, the OIG began promoting voluntary compliance programs for the healthcare industry. The OIG provided guidance to assist healthcare entities in developing effective internal controls to help them be aware of and follow the requirements of federal, state, and private health plans. The OIG believes that healthcare institutions that adopt and implement compliance programs significantly reduce fraud, abuse, and waste. Therefore, investigators tend to be more lenient with organizations that have implemented a voluntary compliance plan. The OIG issued sample compliance programs, which include seven major characteristics:

1. Develop and distribute written standards of conduct, policies, and procedures that address specific areas of potential fraud.
2. Designate a high-level manager to be the chief compliance officer who oversees compliance activities.
3. Develop and implement education and training for employees.
4. Establish a process for reporting exceptions.
5. Develop an internal system to respond to accusations or reports of improper activities and implement disciplinary measures when appropriate.

6. Develop an audit and monitoring system.
7. Investigate and correct system-wide problems and develop policies regarding employment or retention of sanctioned individuals.

The Patient Protection and Affordable Care Act (PPACA), passed in 2010, mandates compliance programs for providers who contract with Medicare, Medicaid, and CHIP. The timeline for defining and implementing compliance programs has not yet been established. This rule places the greatest burden on smaller healthcare providers who never established a voluntary compliance program because now they will have to establish one in order to continue serving Medicare patients.

Recovery Audit Contractor

In the Tax Relief and Health Care Act of 2006, Congress required a permanent and national **Recovery audit contractor (RAC)** program, which was implemented in 2010. The RAC program uses independent contractors to identify improper Medicare payments to healthcare providers and suppliers made on claims of healthcare services provided to Medicare beneficiaries. Improper payments may be overpayments or underpayments. Overpayments can occur when healthcare providers submit claims that do not meet Medicare's coding or medical necessity policies. Underpayments can occur when healthcare providers submit claims for a simple procedure but the medical record reveals that a more complicated procedure was actually performed. Healthcare providers that might be reviewed include hospitals, physician practices, nursing homes, home health agencies, durable medical equipment suppliers, and any other provider or supplier that bills Medicare Parts A and B.

CODING PRACTICE

| Exercise 2.6 | Federal Compliance |

Instructions: Write the answers to the following questions in the space provided.

1. What are the potential consequences of receiving an overpayment from Medicare?

_____

_____

_____

_____

2. Define *overcoding*.

_____

_____

_____

3. What law, passed in 1863, is the basis for much of the OIG's investigation and prosecution?

_____

_____

HEALTH INFORMATION TECHNOLOGY

Hospitals, physicians, and other providers are using health information technology (HIT) advancements to streamline decades-old methods of capturing, storing, and using healthcare data. Proactive coders embrace new technology that increasingly uses computers to perform predictable, repetitive work, positioning themselves to accomplish more complex coding and data analysis tasks and thus adding value to an

organization. Three HIT applications that coders interface with are encoders, EHRs, and computer-assisted coding (CAC).

Encoders

An **encoder** is a computer software program that enables the user to look up medical codes electronically (■ Figure 2-5). A **book-based encoder** is an enhanced electronic coding manual that allows coders to input key words, such as the Main

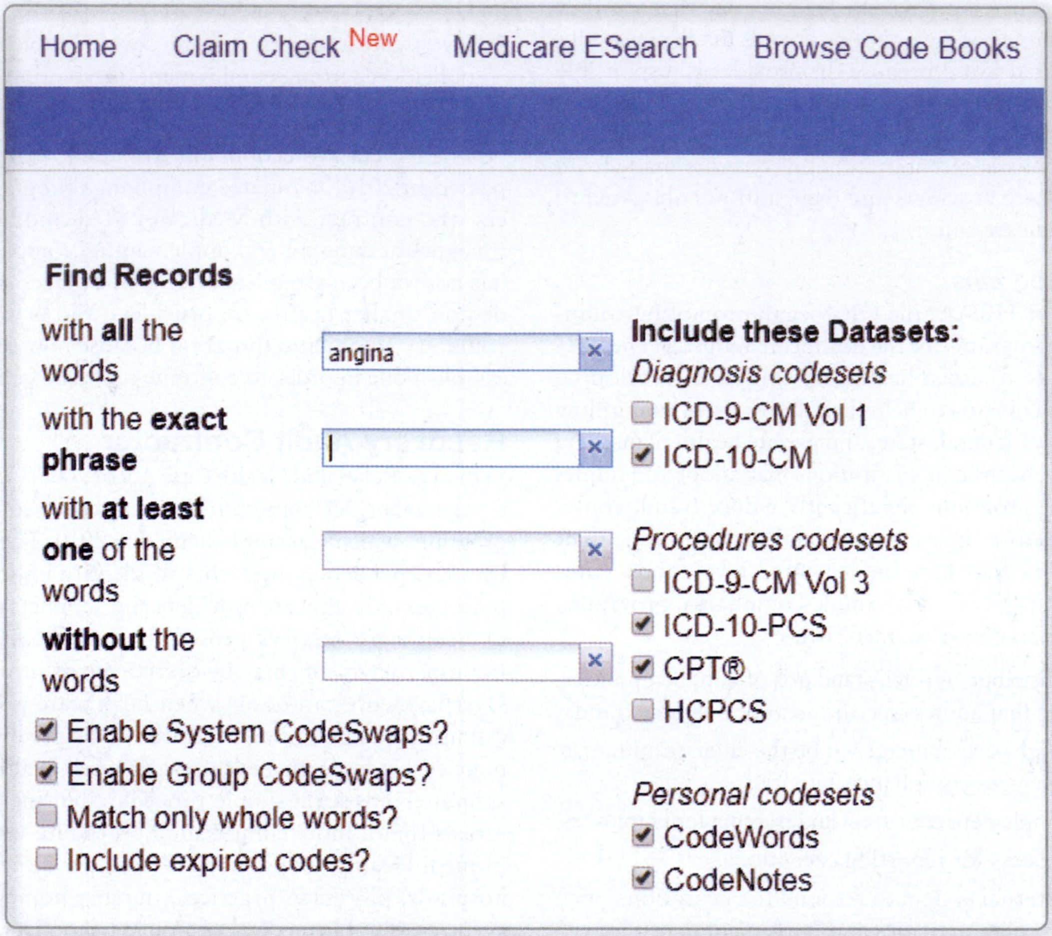

Home	Claim Check New	Medicare ESearch	Browse Code Books

Find Records

with **all** the words: `angina`

with the **exact phrase**: `|`

with **at least one** of the words: ` `

without the words: ` `

☑ Enable System CodeSwaps?
☑ Enable Group CodeSwaps?
☐ Match only whole words?
☐ Include expired codes?

Include these Datasets:

Diagnosis codesets
☐ ICD-9-CM Vol 1
☑ ICD-10-CM

Procedures codesets
☐ ICD-9-CM Vol 3
☑ ICD-10-PCS
☑ CPT®
☐ HCPCS

Personal codesets
☑ CodeWords
☑ CodeNotes

Figure 2-5 ■ Example of an encoder search screen. *Source: SpeedeCoder, Reprinted with permission.*

Term, and access hot links to potential codes. A **logic-based encoder** guides users through a series of questions and menu choices that ultimately lead to code choices. Encoders do not replace physical coding manuals and there are times the physical manuals must be consulted to verify details.

Encoders provide **edit checks** based on the official coding guidelines, instructional notes, and payer rules. An edit check is a feature built into software that alerts users to, or prevents, certain errors based on rules that are programmed into the system (■ TABLE 2-5). An edit check may be as simple as requiring that a patient record have a female gender in order to assign an obstetrics code or as complicated as alerting users when codes are sequenced incorrectly.

An encoder may also cross-reference or hot-link users to reference information, such as the following:

• Official Guidelines for Coding and Reporting (OGCR), ICD-10-CM and ICD-10-PCS
• CPT Guidelines
• *Coding Clinic* newsletter, published by the American Hospital Association
• *CPT Assistant Newsletter*, published by the American Medical Association
• Medical dictionary

Table 2-5 ■ **EXAMPLES OF ENCODER EDIT CHECKS**

❏ Code first
❏ Diagnosis-procedure mismatch
❏ Invalid characters
❏ Manifestation codes
❏ Medicare medical necessity
❏ Mutually exclusive diagnoses
❏ Mutually exclusive procedures
❏ Patient age
❏ Patient gender
❏ Seven characters required
❏ Unacceptable principal diagnosis
❏ Use additional code
❏ Use additional digit(s)

• Anatomic diagrams
• Medicare manual

Encoders are easily updated when quarterly and annual code updates are published. They can create reports that track service utilization and trends, and provide other valuable information to the provider.

Many companies design and sell encoder programs, but the basic functions of all are similar. Menus may be configured differently and the add-on reference tools may vary. Some products interface with other systems in a facility, such as a billing or EHR system; others are standalone programs that can run on any computer. Once coders learn one brand of software, it is usually easy to adapt to others.

An encoder is not a substitute or shortcut to learning how to use the coding manuals. You must still master the basics of abstracting, assigning, and sequencing codes. Coders need to understand what information they must give the software in order for it to provide accurate feedback. An untrained user can make coding errors with an encoder, just as they would using the physical manuals.

Encoders do not always list all the instructional notes and symbols that appear in physical coding manuals. Sometimes logic-based encoders can lead to different and incorrect codes than the coding manual because they do not strictly follow the indexing conventions of the coding manuals. Ultimately, the coding path and guidelines of the official coding manuals must be followed. An encoders is a *work aid* for experienced coders but it is not a substitute for beginning coders to become completely familiar with the official coding manuals.

Electronic Health Records

An electronic health record (EHR) is an electronic version of a patient's medical history and treatments, and is maintained by a provider over time.

Benefits of EHR Systems

At their simplest, EHRs are computerized versions of patients' charts, but when fully implemented, they are real-time, patient-centered records that enable authorized providers to immediately access medical information from remote locations. Key capabilities include the following:

- Contains all of the key administrative clinical data relevant to a person's care under a particular provider, including demographics, progress notes, problem list, medications, vital signs, past medical history, immunizations, laboratory data and radiology reports

- Streamlines the clinician's workflow by sending information to the appropriate parties, such as a pharmacy or a consulting provider, and reducing paperwork and documentation time for providers

- Supports other care-related activities, including evidence-based decision support, quality management, and outcomes reporting

- Improves privacy and security of patient records compared to paper-based systems

One of the key features of an EHR system is that it can be created, managed, and consulted by authorized providers and staff across multiple healthcare organizations (■ Figure 2-6). A single EHR system can bring together information from current and past doctors, emergency facilities, school and workplace clinics, pharmacies, laboratories, and medical imaging facilities. For example:

- A physician can view medications prescribed by other providers to avoid duplication or medication interactions.

- An emergency department can view a patient's medical history to more quickly identify a problem or risk factor.

- A provider can view imaging studies electronically, which may help to understand the progression of a patient's condition.

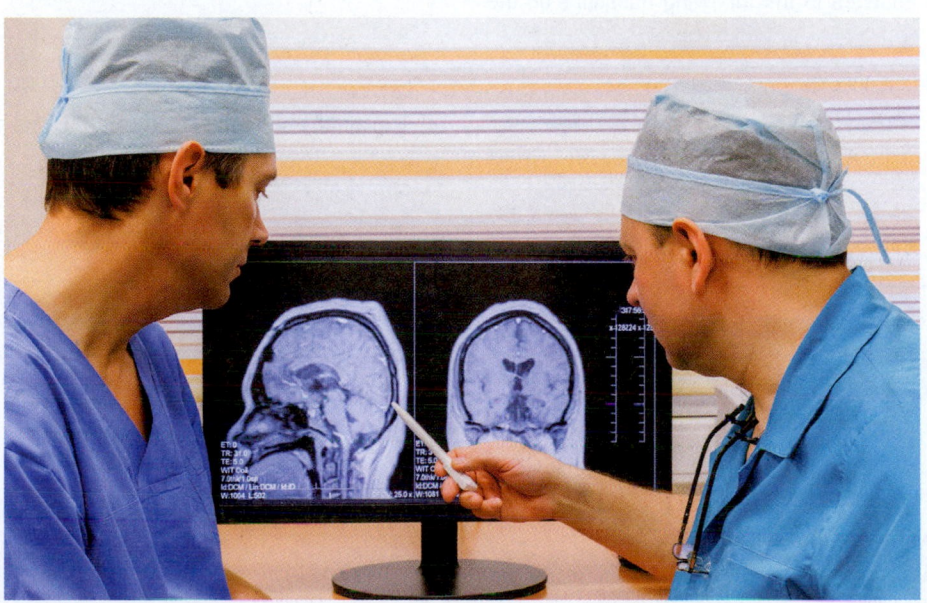

Figure 2-6 ■ EHRs allow doctors to access radiologic images taken by another facility.

Funding Incentives for EHR Systems

The Health Information Technology for Economic and Clinical Health (HITECH) Act, which is part of the American Recovery and Reinvestment Act of 2009 (ARRA), included financial incentives for providers who adopt EHR systems and demonstrate use in ways that can improve quality, safety, and effectiveness of care. The goal behind the funding is to encourage providers to adopt EHR systems sooner than they otherwise would, because Congress believes EHR systems can help improve quality of care and reduce costs.

Under the **promoting interoperability (PI)** program—formerly called meaningful use—eligible Medicare and Medicaid providers can receive payments when they adopt, implement, or upgrade **certified EHR technology (CEHRT)**. The goal is to ensure that the hospitals and providers are equipped to help create a seamless flow of health data information between themselves and the patients. This requires both technological and policy strategies. The primary objectives of PI are to establish standard protocols in four areas:

- Electronic prescribing
- Health information exchange between clinicians
- Exchange of information between providers and patients
- Sharing of clinical data for public health purposes

CEHRT assures purchasers that a specific EHR system provides the necessary features to meet the meaningful use criteria. It also helps providers and patients be confident that the electronic health IT products and systems they use are secure, can maintain data confidentially, and can work with other systems to share information.

A CEHRT system meets the following criteria:

- Includes patient demographic and clinical health information, such as medical history and problem list
- Provides clinical decision support
- Supports physician order entry
- Captures and queries information relevant to healthcare quality
- Exchanges electronic health information with, and integrates such information from, other sources

Computer-Assisted Coding

The move to adopt EHRs and create a national health information infrastructure has created he opportunity for additional technology initiatives, including **computer-assisted coding (CAC)**. CAC is the use of computer software that automatically generates a set of medical codes for review, validation, and use based on clinical documentation provided by healthcare practitioners. It differs from an EHR in that an EHR stores and tracks clinical information but does not convert it into codes. CAC differs from encoders in that encoders require people to conduct an electronic search for each individual code to be assigned, whereas CAC automatically generates codes based on documentation. CAC does not eliminate coders; it transforms their jobs from repetitive, production-oriented tasks into ones of critical thinking, analysis, and auditing.

CODING PRACTICE

Exercise 2.7   Health Information Technology

Instructions: Write your answers to the following questions on the line(s) provided.

1. List five examples of edit checks.

   _____

   _____

   _____

   _____

2. Respond to this scenario: A classmate tells you she does not see the need to look up codes in the physical manual because she will be able to use an encoder in her job. What do you tell her?

   _____

   _____

   _____

3. Describe one example of using an EHR across organizations.

   _____

   _____

   _____

4. Explain the difference between CAC and an encoder.

   _____

   _____

   _____

5. Respond to this scenario: A classmate tells you that she is considering switching majors because all coding will be taken over by computers in the near future. What do you tell her?

   _____

   _____

   _____

CHAPTER SUMMARY

In this chapter you learned that:

- Third-party payers reimburse physicians and hospitals for 87% of all healthcare services in the United States. Coders need to understand the different types of third-party payers because each has separate, and sometimes conflicting, rules about coding and billing.

- To fulfill their contractual obligations, payers may request information to verify whether the service is covered, including the site (location) of service; the medical need for and appropriateness of the diagnostic and therapeutic services provided; and the accuracy of codes for services billed on the claim based on the medical record.

- Each step in the life cycle of an insurance claim must be completed in a timely and accurate manner in order for providers to receive correct payment for their services.

- The healthcare industry uses many different reimbursement, or payment, methods for services. The methods vary by type of payer, the setting—such as physician office, outpatient hospital, or inpatient hospital—and the type of service.

- Providers must submit claims for services to payers to receive reimbursement using specific electronic formats or paper forms in each healthcare setting.

- Providers are legally obligated to report any overpayment to Medicare, to refund the money, and possibly even pay interest on it.

- Proactive coders embrace new technology, such as encoders, electronic health records, and computer-assisted coding that perform predictable, repetitive work, and position themselves to accomplish more complex coding and data analysis tasks, which adds value to an organization.

CONCEPT QUIZ

Take a moment to look back through this chapter and solidify your skills. This is your opportunity to pull together everything you have learned.

Completion

Instructions: Write the term that completes each statement based on the information you learned in this chapter. Choose from the following list. Some choices may be used more than once and some choices may not be used at all.

abuse	medical necessity	Part D
compliance	medical record	progress notes
DRG	Medigap	RA
EOB	OIG	RCA
family history	Part A	social history
FCA	Part B	TC
fraud	Part C	VHA

1. _____ is Medicare's hospital insurance that covers a specific list of services for inpatient hospital care, skilled nursing facilities, hospice, and home healthcare.

2. _____ is a Medicare supplement insurance policy sold by private insurance companies to fill gaps in Part A and Part B coverage.

3. _____ is health insurance coverage for family members of active duty personnel and for retired military personnel and their families.

4. _____ is the health status of immediate family members, causes of death (if known), and diseases common in the family.

5. _____ is the prospective payment method used by Medicare to reimburse inpatient hospitals.

6. The _____ is a statement that lists all the services the provider billed, which ones were accepted for payment, how much the insurance company will pay, how much the patient owes, and how much will not be paid.

7. _____ is knowingly billing for services that were never given or billing for a service that has a higher reimbursement than the service provided.

8. _____ is mistakenly accepting payment for items or services that should not be paid for by Medicare.

9. _____ investigates fraud, abuse, and other noncompliance matters in the Medicare and Medicaid programs.

10. _____ programs include seven major characteristics and are intended to reduce fraud, abuse, and waste.

Multiple Choice

Instructions: Circle the letter of the best answer to each question based on the information you learned in this chapter.

1. Who regulates med pay or personal injury protection from automobile insurance policies?
   A. Each state's Department of Insurance
   B. HIPAA
   C. CMS
   D. Each state's Department of Transportation

2. What program is funded jointly by the federal and state governments?
   A. Medicare
   B. Medicaid
   C. Workers' compensation
   D. Self-insured health plan

3. What is an example of the medical necessity criterion evidence-based practice?
   A. Suture removal in the emergency department
   B. Liposuction for medical reasons
   C. A patient going to an internal medicine or family practice physician to diagnose an initial symptom of stomach pain
   D. Medications proven to benefit patients based on scientific studies

4. When should the provider verify eligibility with the insurance company?
   A. Before the encounter
   B. During the encounter
   C. After the encounter
   D. After insurance company processing

5. What type of software allows coders to input key words, such as the Main Term, and access hot links to potential codes?
   A. Encoder
   B. EHR
   C. CAC
   D. Edit check

6. What method does Medicare use to establish physician reimbursement rates?
   A. GPCI
   B. DRG
   C. RBRVS
   D. CMS-1500

7. What organization maintains and updates the UB-04?
   A. NUBC
   B. CMS
   C. ANSI
   D. NUCC

8. What term means knowingly submitting a bill to a government healthcare program, such as Medicare, that contains incorrect codes?
   A. Medical necessity
   B. Denial
   C. False claim
   D. RA

9. What type of program does the Patient Protection and Affordable Care Act (PPACA) mandate for providers who contract with Medicare, Medicaid, and CHIP?
   A. Edit check
   B. Contractor
   C. Compliance
   D. Fraud and abuse

10. Who does the RAC program use to identify Medicare overpayments and underpayments to healthcare providers and suppliers?
    A. Edit checkers
    B. Independent contractors
    C. Compliance officers
    D. HIPAA officers

SECTION TWO

ICD-10-CM Diagnosis Coding

Section Two: ICD-10-CM Diagnosis Coding discusses how to identify the reasons for a medical encounter. This section guides you through the steps of diagnosis coding for each body system. You learn how to apply the three skills of an "Ace" coder—abstract, assign, and arrange—to report patients' diseases, conditions, injuries, and other diagnostic information for patient encounters in inpatient, outpatient, and physician office settings.

PROFESSIONAL PROFILE

Nicolas A. Joye, MSHI, RHIT, CPMA, CCS
Coding Manager, Coding Solutions
M*Modal

I have been coding for five years within the outpatient vendor environment. I code facility and professional evaluation and management (E/M), observation, outpatient surgery, emergency room, and ancillary services. My educational experiences provided the foundation for my growth as a healthcare professional and have helped me develop a problem-solving mindset.

In my first coding job I was an apprentice coder for M*Modal, which included working for Johns Hopkins University Hospital as an outpatient physician clinic coder. With my certified coding associate (CCA) credential, M*Modal provided an opportunity for me to learn various outpatient chart types. All of my charts were audited until I reached 90% accuracy level. After I successfully learned the outpatient coding environment, I began to develop my career into management.

Now as a coding manager, I coordinate coding services for a large umbrella network. My work involves supporting a team of 30 coders throughout daily workflow processes as well as working with senior management. Outstanding customer communication and customer service is essential in my position. I am also a technical super-user for the integrated revenue cycle and document management systems. I am responsible for training new coders to utilize several different types of software for revenue cycle and document management. I also use in-house software to monitor and support team performance quality and production improvement.

For me, the most enjoyable aspect of coding revolves around the required intellectual challenge. We continually explore pathophysiology and healthcare delivery, while at the same time exceeding quality and productivity standards on a day-to-day basis. There can be a lot of technical constraints that challenge my coding staff to meet quality and productivity standards. As the manager, I must make sure that each coder has a smooth workflow process so they can succeed in a constantly changing environment.

I hold the registered health information technician (RHIT), certified professional medical auditor (CPMA), and certified coding specialist (CCS) certification credentials. These credentials played a pivotal role in my job-hunting process throughout my career because employers have certification requirements to qualify for job consideration.

I am active in several professional organizations, including the Arizona American Health Information Management Association (AZHIMA), Healthcare Information System Society (HIMSS), and AAPC.

My educational background includes master of science in health care informatics, bachelor of science in psychology, and associates of applied science focused on health information technology. Currently, I am participating in a doctorate of business administration program with expected graduation in May 2021.

Entry-level coders should work hard to obtain the RHIA, RHIT, CCS, or CPC credentials. These credentials are often required to obtain a job with healthcare facilities and coding vendors. Coders should join their state chapter AHIMA and AAPC professional associations because this exposure outlines future career pathways and potential mentors. It is important for coders to understanding their current position within a career pathway and identify a future plan to keep progressing.

Chapter 3

Introduction to ICD-10-CM Diagnosis Coding

Chapter Outline

- **Overview of ICD-10-CM**
- **Organization of ICD-10-CM**
- **ICD-10-CM Guidelines and Conventions**
- **Abstracting Diagnoses**
- **Assigning Diagnosis Codes**
- **Arranging Diagnosis Codes**
- **ICD-10-CM Coding and Reimbursement**

Learning Objectives

After completing this chapter, you should have the skills to:

3.1 Spell and define the key words, medical terms, and abbreviations related to ICD-10-CM coding. (Remember)

3.2 Summarize the history and purpose of ICD-10-CM. (Understand)

3.3 Describe the organization of the ICD-10-CM manual. (Understand)

3.4 Adhere to ICD-10-CM Official Guidelines for Coding and Reporting. (Apply)

3.5 Define ICD-10-CM conventions. (Remember)

3.6 Identify how to abstract diagnostic information from the medical record. (Apply)

3.7 Demonstrate how to assign diagnosis codes. (Apply)

3.8 Utilize the guidelines for arranging (sequencing) diagnosis codes. (Apply)

3.9 Articulate the relationship between accurate diagnosis coding and reimbursement. (Apply)

Key Terms and Abbreviations

abstract

arrange

assign

block (ICD-10-CM)

category (ICD-10-CM)

chapter (ICD-10-CM)

circumstances of admission

clinically significant condition

code (ICD-10-CM)

coding path

combination code

complication or comorbidity (CC)

convention

Coordination and Maintenance Committee

default code (ICD-10-CM)

eponym

etiology

first-listed diagnosis

four cooperating parties

hospital-acquired conditions (HACs)

initial encounter (ICD-10-CM)

instructional note

International Classification of Diseases, 10th Revision (ICD-10)

International Classification of Diseases, 10th Revision, Clinical Modification (ICD-10-CM)

late effect

Main Term

major complication or comorbidity (MCC)

manifestation

morbidity

mortality

multiple coding

National Center for Health Statistics (NCHS)

nonessential modifier (ICD-10-CM)

Official Guidelines for Coding and Reporting (OGCR)

present on admission (POA)

principal diagnosis

relevant

sequela (ICD-10-CM)

sequence

subcategory (ICD-10-CM)

subchapter (ICD-10-CM)

subsequent encounter (ICD-10-CM)

subterm

uncertain diagnosis

Uniform Hospital Data Discharge Set (UHDDS)

In addition to the key terms listed here, students should know the terms defined within tables in this chapter.

INTRODUCTION

When you take your vehicle to a mechanic for service, the mechanic needs to figure out what is wrong before the car can be fixed. Similarly, when patients see physicians, physicians must diagnose the condition before they know what services to provide. In this chapter you learn how to code for the conditions that physicians diagnose.

This chapter provides an introduction to ICD-10-CM diagnosis coding and lays the foundation for the remaining chapters in this section. You become acquainted with the history, purpose, and terminology of diagnosis coding; the organization of the ICD-10-CM coding manual, and the official guidelines and conventions. You follow a guided example of the three skills of an "Ace" coder as they relate to diagnosis coding: how to abstract, assign, and arrange diagnosis codes. Finally, you are introduced to the relationship between diagnosis codes and reimbursement.

OVERVIEW OF ICD-10-CM

The *International Classification of Diseases, 10th Revision, Clinical Modification* (ICD-10-CM) is used to code diagnoses that describe patient illnesses, diseases, conditions, injuries, or other reasons for seeking healthcare services. ICD-10-CM is the United States' clinical modification of the World Health Organization's (WHO) International Classification of Diseases, 10th Revision (ICD-10). The inclusion of the term *clinical modification* in the United States' ICD-10-CM emphasizes the intent of the modification to classify and manage data related to the actual examination and treatment of patients. Uses in the United States include tracking morbidity, indexing medical records, reporting ambulatory as well as inpatient care, and reflecting advances in medical care. The Health Insurance Portability and Accountability Act (HIPAA) mandates the use of ICD-10-CM by all covered entities that handle electronic claims. As a result, ICD-10-CM is the standard for communication among healthcare providers, regulators, and payers. ■ TABLE 3-1 summarizes the characteristics of ICD-10-CM.

The History of ICD-10-CM Coding

Diagnosis coding originated in seventeenth-century England when statistical data about deaths was collected through the London Bills of Mortality and assigned numerical codes. The *International Classification of Diseases* was formally organized in the early twentieth century, known simply as ICD. It was periodically updated and expanded, so revision numbers were assigned, such as ICD-1, ICD-2, and so on. ICD-9 was implemented in 1979. The United States developed the first clinical modification, known as ICD-9-CM, which was used from 1979 to 2015.

ICD-10-CM was implemented on October 1, 2015, after nearly 20 years of development, testing, and debate within the healthcare industry. The *International Classification of Diseases, 10th Revision* (ICD-10), without the Clinical Modification (CM) designation, is a worldwide reporting system developed by WHO for classifying epidemiological (*study of diseases in large populations*) and **mortality** (*causes of death*)

Table 3-1 ■ CHARACTERISTICS OF ICD-10-CM

Feature	ICD-10-CM
Name	*International Classification of Diseases, 10th Revision, Clinical Modification*
Developed by	National Center for Health Statistics (NCHS)/Centers for Disease Control and Prevention (CDC), based on World Health Organization (WHO) ICD-10 code set
Used by	All HIPAA entities
Purpose	Diagnosis coding
Number of codes	70,000+
Code length	3–7 characters
Code structure	3-character category
	4th, 5th, 6th characters for etiology, anatomic site, severity
	7th character for additional information
First character	1st character is always alphabetic
Subsequent characters	2nd character is always numeric; all other characters may be alphabetic or numeric
Decimal point	Mandatory after 3rd character on all codes
7th Character	Some codes use a 7th character to provide additional information
Placeholders	Character X is used as a placeholder in certain 6- and 7-character codes

data. After its first full release in 1994, the system was gradually adopted by over 130 countries internationally.

The Purpose of ICD-10-CM Coding

The United States **National Center for Health Statistics (NCHS)** (a division of the Centers for Disease Control and Prevention [CDC]) adapted and expanded ICD-10 to focus on **morbidity** (*causes of disease and illness*) in the United States. This adaptation has the phrase Clinical Modification attached to the name, creating the full name *International Classification of Diseases, 10th Revision, Clinical Modification* (ICD-10-CM). The code set provides diagnoses for tracking and billing patient encounters and uses terminology and details consistent with medical practice in the United States. All modifications in ICD-10-CM must conform to WHO conventions for ICD-10. The United States has used ICD-10-CM for coding and classifying mortality data from death certificates since January 1, 1999, but the code set was not adopted for billing and reimbursement use until 2015.

ICD-10-CM is a HIPAA-mandated code set for all HIPAA-covered entities:

- Providers, such as hospitals, physicians, skilled nursing facilities, rehabilitation facilities, and home health agencies
- Payers, such as private insurance companies and government Medicare and Medicaid programs
- Other HIPAA-covered entities, such as software vendors, clearinghouses, and third-party billing services

Medical Terminology Used in ICD-10-CM Coding

Medical terminology skills are essential to coding. Physicians document using medical terms to identify anatomic sites, diseases, and procedures. The coding manual uses medical terms to classify conditions. Coders must be able to interpret unfamiliar medical terms by breaking them into the components of root, suffix, and prefix. They must be able to identify terms that are synonymous and those that have slightly different meanings. Medical word parts originate primarily from Greek and Latin, as well as other languages, giving rise to multiple medical terms with the same English meaning. For example, both *osse/o*, from Latin, and *oste/o*, from Greek, mean "bone." The anatomic figures in this text display labels in English as well as the most common medical term root(s) or combining form(s). Each body system chapter lists examples of how to build medical terms. Coders should have immediate access to an online and hardcopy medical dictionary and medical terminology text. ■ TABLE 3-2 lists medical term suffixes that describe diagnoses. ■ TABLE 3-3 gives a refresher on how to build medical terms for different diagnoses related to the same anatomic site.

Table 3-2 ■ **MEDICAL TERM SUFFIXES THAT DESCRIBE DIAGNOSES**

Suffix	Meaning	Example
-al	pertaining to	streptococcal (*pertaining to the streptococcus organism*)
-algia	condition of pain	cephalgia (*pain in the head*)
-asthenia	condition of weakness, absence	myasthenia (*muscle weakness*)
-cele	hernia, bulge	enterocele (*bulging or hernia of the small intestine*)
-emia	condition of the blood	uremia (*condition of blood in the urine*)
-ia	condition of	cardia (*condition of the heart*)
-ism	state of	hypothyroidism (*condition of lowered thyroid function*)
-itis	inflammation	gastritis (*inflammation of the stomach*)
-lithiasis	condition of calculus	cystolithiasis (*calculus in the bladder*)
-oma	tumor	sarcoma (*malignant tumor*)
-osis	condition of	endometriosis (*condition of the lining of the uterus*)
-pathy	abnormal condition of	retinopathy (*abnormal condition of the retina*)
-penia	lack of, deficiency of	osteopenia (*deficiency of bone*)
-plasm	growth	neoplasm (*new growth*)
-plegia	condition of lack of, paralysis	hemiplegia (*paralysis of one side*)
-ptosis	drooping	blepharoptosis (*drooping of the eyelid*)
-ptysis	spit, cough	hemoptysis (*spitting or coughing of blood*)
-rrhea	flow	amenorrhea (*lack of monthly flow*)
-uria	condition of the urine	glycosuria (*condition of sugar in the urine*)

Source: © PB Resources, Inc. Used with permission.

Table 3-3 ■ **EXAMPLE OF CONSTRUCTING MEDICAL TERMS FOR DIAGNOSES**

Combining Form	Prefix	Suffix	Complete Medical Term
cardi/o (*heart*)			**cardi + algia** (*pain in or near the heart*)
			card + itis (*inflammation of the heart*)
neur/o (*nerve*)		**-algia** (*pain*)	**neur + algia** (*pain in a nerve*)
	poly- (*many, much*)	**-itis** (*inflammation*)	**neur + itis** (*inflammation of a nerve*)
		-plegia (*paralysis*)	**neuro + plegia** (*paralysis of a nerve*)
			poly + neur + algia (*pain in many nerves*)
			poly + cardia (*rapid heart rate*)

Source: © PB Resources, Inc. Used with permission.

ORGANIZATION OF ICD-10-CM

Accurate coding of diagnoses is necessary in order to explain why services were provided. To code accurately, coders need to be familiar with the overall organization of the manual, the distinct sublevels of organization, and the significance of each, as well as the process for updating ICD-10-CM. Locate the Contents page near the front of the manual and become familiar with the contents and organization of the ICD-10-CM manual listed in ■ TABLE 3-4. The purpose of each of these Contents topics is discussed later in this chapter.

Chapter Structure

The last section of the Contents page, ICD-10-CM Tabular List of Diseases and Injuries, is further subdivided into 21 chapters. Each chapter contains codes for a body system or related conditions. Coders must become acquainted with the chapter topics within ICD-10-CM as well as the internal structure within each chapter in order to locate information and follow instructional notes. Instructional notes are official coding directions throughout the ICD-10-CM manual. Coders are required to follow instructional notes in order to abstract, assign, and arrange codes accurately. The various types of instructional notes are discussed later in this chapter.

The location within the ICD-10-CM chapter structure where instructional notes appear dictates what codes to which they apply. Each chapter is subdivided into blocks, categories, subcategories, and codes (■ FIGURE 3-1) as described below:

- A **block** or **subchapter** is a contiguous range of codes within a chapter.

- A **category** is three characters in length. A three-character category that has no further subdivisions is called a code.

- A **subcategory** is either four or five characters. Each level of subdivision after a category and before a code is a subcategory. A four- or five-character subcategory that has no further subdivisions is called a code.

- A **code** is the final level of subdivision. Codes may be three, four, five, six, or seven characters in length (■ TABLE 3-5, page 40). All codes in the Tabular List of the official version of the ICD-10-CM appear in boldface type. Entries that require a seventh character are referred to as codes, not subcategories, even though they are not complete without the seventh character.

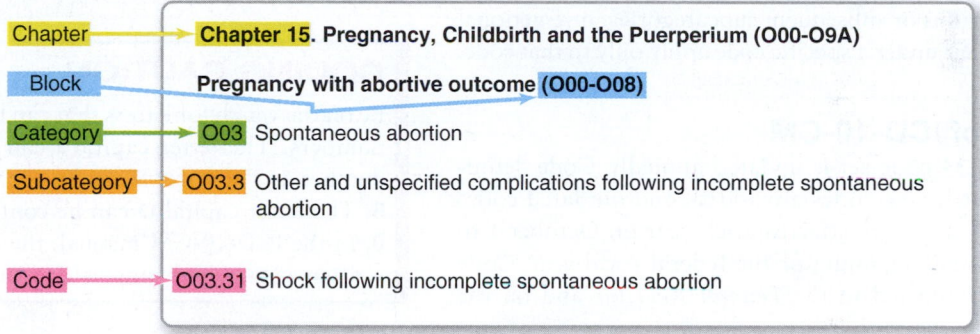

Figure 3-1 ■ Organizational structure of ICD-10-CM chapters.

Table 3-4 ■ OVERVIEW OF THE ICD-10-CM MANUAL

Type of Information	Name of Section	Purpose
Introductory material	Preface	Information and rules on how to use the manual.
	Introduction	
	How to Use the ICD-10-CM	
	ICD-10-CM Official Conventions	
	Additional Conventions	
	ICD-10-CM Official Guidelines for Coding and Reporting	
Index	ICD-10-CM Index to Diseases and Injuries (Index)	Alphabetical list of diseases and injuries, reasons for encounters, and external causes. Two tables provide quick look-ups, one for neoplasms and one for drugs and chemicals causing injury. Coders must always reference one of these indices or tables when searching for a code.
	ICD-10-CM Table of Neoplasms	
	ICD-10-CM Table of Drugs and Chemicals	
	ICD-10-CM Index to External Causes	
Tabular List	ICD-10-CM Tabular List of Diseases and Injuries	Alphanumerical list of diseases and injuries, reasons for encounters, and external causes. Provides additional instruction on how to use, assign, and sequence codes. Coders must always reference the Tabular List to verify a code, after consulting the Index, and before assigning the final code.

Table 3-5 ■ **EXAMPLES OF ICD-10-CM CODES WITH VARYING NUMBER OF CHARACTERS**

Code Length	Example
3-character code	I10 Essential (primary) hypertension
4-character code	G03.1 Chronic meningitis
5-character code	K70.30 Alcoholic cirrhosis of liver without ascites
6-character code	M51.44 Schmorl's nodes, thoracic region
7-character code	T22.761A Corrosion of third degree of right scapular region, initial encounter
7-character code with placeholder X	T51.0X1D Toxic effect of ethanol, accidental (unintentional), subsequent encounter
	V52.0XXS Driver of pick-up truck or van injured in collision with two- or three-wheeled motor vehicle in nontraffic accident, sequela
	O33.4XX1 Maternal care for disproportion of mixed maternal and fetal origin, fetus 1

Instructional notes can appear at the beginning of a chapter, block, category, subcategory, or under a code title. Any instructional notes listed at the beginning of the chapter apply to all codes within that chapter. Instructional notes at the beginning of a block apply to all codes within that block but not to other blocks. Instructional notes at the beginning of the category apply to all codes within that category but not to previous or subsequent categories. Instructional notes at the beginning of the subcategory apply to all codes within that subcategory but not to previous or subsequent subcategories. Instructional notes that appear under a specific code apply only to that code.

Updating of ICD-10-CM

The ICD-10-CM code set is updated annually. Code definitions are revised, new codes are added, and outdated codes are deleted. Updates are effective each year on October 1 to coincide with the beginning of the federal fiscal year. Code changes are published in the *Federal Register* and on the websites for the CMS and the Centers for Disease Control and Prevention (CDC). Each HIPAA-covered entity must update its systems and paperwork to incorporate the changes. The ICD-10-CM Coordination and Maintenance Committee oversees all changes. The Coordination and Maintenance Committee is a federal interdepartmental committee comprised of representatives from the four cooperating parties: CMS, NCHS, the American Hospital Association (AHA), and the American Health Information Management Association (AHIMA).

CODING CAUTION

Be on the watch for letters that can be easily confused with numbers. The letter capital **I** can be confused with the number **1**. The letter **S** can be confused with the number **5**. The letter capital **O** can be confused with the number **0**. In the ICD-10-CM manual, the number zero might be written as to help distinguish it from the capital letter **O**.

CODING PRACTICE

Exercise 3.1   Organization of ICD-10-CM

Instructions: Look up the following entries in the ICD-10-CM manual. Determine if each entry is a block, category, subcategory, or code. Circle the correct description.

Example: F01 Vascular dementia   *category*

1. D56 Thalassemia	Block	Category	Subcategory	Code
2. F20.0 Paranoid schizophrenia	Block	Category	Subcategory	Code
3. Diseases of esophagus, stomach and duodenum (K20–K31)	Block	Category	Subcategory	Code
4. O60.12 Preterm labor second trimester with preterm delivery second trimester	Block	Category	Subcategory	Code
5. O48.1 Prolonged pregnancy	Block	Category	Subcategory	Code
6. S37.0 Injury of kidney	Block	Category	Subcategory	Code
7. S67 Crushing injury of wrists, hand and fingers	Block	Category	Subcategory	Code
8. T28.1XXS Burn of esophagus, sequela	Block	Category	Subcategory	Code
9. Visual disturbances and blindness (H53–H54)	Block	Category	Subcategory	Code
10. F01.5 Vascular dementia	Block	Category	Subcategory	Code

ICD-10-CM GUIDELINES AND CONVENTIONS

ICD-10-CM is accompanied by official guidelines and conventions, both of which direct the coder how to use the manual.

Official Guidelines for Coding and Reporting

The **Official Guidelines for Coding and Reporting (OGCR)** is the official set of rules that provide information and direction in identifying the diagnoses to be reported. Coders are required to apply the OGCR when coding. The OGCR is updated annually and published at the same time as the code set or shortly thereafter. It usually appears in the front of the coding manual and can be downloaded from **www.cms.gov** and **www.cdc.gov**. Refer to the Contents page of the ICD-10-CM manual to locate the ICD-10-CM Official Guidelines for Coding and Reporting (OGCR) and ICD-10-CM Conventions.

- OGCR is a set of rules that complement the conventions and instructional notes to provide additional information and direction in identifying the diagnoses to be reported. HIPAA requires that coders adhere to OGCR when assigning ICD-10-CM diagnosis codes.

- **Conventions** are the use of symbols, typeface, and layout features to succinctly convey interpretive information. Conventions appear in the section ICD-10-CM Official Conventions. Most conventions also appear in OGCR, Section I.A.

Refer to the ICD-10-CM manual and locate the first page of the OGCR, which contains a detailed list of contents. The topics are referenced by an alphanumeric outline numbering system. For example, OGCR I.C.1.a refers to OGCR section I, subsection C, level 1, and sublevel 1. An overview of each OGCR section is provided next.

Section I

OGCR Section I, Conventions, General Coding Guidelines and Chapter Specific Guidelines, contains the following major divisions:

A. Conventions for the ICD-10-CM: The general rules for the use of the coding manual independent of the guidelines. Most, but not all, of the conventions listed here also appear in the separate preceding section, ICD-10-CM Official Conventions.

B. General Coding Guidelines: Overall rules that apply to all chapters in ICD-10-CM.

C. Chapter-Specific Coding Guidelines: Guidelines for specific diagnoses and/or conditions, divided by ICD-10-CM chapter. Unless otherwise indicated within a specific guideline, these apply to all healthcare settings. This is by far the largest section of OGCR.

Section II

Section II, Selection of Principal Diagnosis, describes rules for abstracting the main diagnosis for inpatient settings. The guidelines for inpatient settings are different than for outpatient settings. **Principal diagnosis** applies only to inpatient settings. It is the "condition established after study to be chiefly responsible for occasioning the admission of the patient to the hospital for care," as defined by the **Uniform Hospital Data Discharge Set (UHDDS)**. The UHDDS is a list of data elements and definitions prepared by the Centers for Disease Control and Prevention and used by hospitals for inpatient discharge data collection. Refer to the coding manual to review the topics in this section.

Section III

Section III, Reporting Additional Diagnoses, describes rules for abstracting secondary or extra diagnoses, in addition to the principal diagnosis, for inpatient settings. Refer to the coding manual to review the topics in this section.

Section IV

Section IV, Diagnostic Coding and Reporting Guidelines for Outpatient Services, describes rules for abstracting diagnoses in outpatient settings. Coding guidelines for outpatient diagnoses vary in several ways from those for inpatient diagnoses. The two most notable differences are:

- In the outpatient setting, the **first-listed diagnosis** is the diagnosis, condition, problem, or other reason for the encounter shown in the medical record to be chiefly responsible for the services provided. First-listed diagnosis applies only to outpatient settings; principal diagnosis applies only to inpatient settings. Secondary or additional diagnoses apply to all healthcare settings.

- Coding guidelines for inconclusive or **uncertain diagnoses** (*diagnoses preceded by the words* probable, possible, suspected, questionable, rule out, working diagnosis, *or a similar word*) were developed for inpatient reporting and do not apply to outpatients.

Refer to the coding manual to review the topics in this section.

SUCCESS STEP

The OGCR is updated each year after the coding manual is published. Although the coding manual is updated in October, the OGCR may not be updated until after the physical manual is published. Refer to the websites of CMS at **www.cms.gov** or the CDC at **www.cdc.gov** to download the most current guidelines.

Conventions

Coders' skills to recognize and interpret the conventions are crucial to interpreting ICD-10-CM instructions and assigning the accurate codes. The most commonly used conventions appear in ■ TABLE 3-6 (page 42). The table identifies where each convention is discussed in OGCR. Examples appear later in this chapter as well as throughout this text. Refer to the OGCR for a complete list of conventions.

In addition to the official ICD-10-CM conventions, many publishers include proprietary symbols and color-coding that

Table 3-6 ■ MOST FREQUENTLY USED CONVENTIONS IN ICD-10-CM

Convention	Meaning/Use	OGCR Reference
4th 5th 6th 7th	Tabular: Some publishers place a symbol in front of a code to indicate that an additional character is needed for the code to be complete. This text uses the symbols shown here.	Publisher-specific convention
- Short dash	Tabular and Index: Additional characters should be assigned in place of the -. The additional characters may be number or letters.	This symbol is used but not explained in OGCR or Conventions.
() Parentheses	Index and Tabular: Nonessential modifiers that describe the default variations of a term. These words are not required to appear in the documentation in order to use the code.	I. A.7
: Colon	Tabular: Appears after an incomplete term that requires one or more modifiers following the colon to be classified to that code or category.	I. A.7
[] Square brackets	Index: Indicates sequencing on etiology/manifestation codes or other paired codes. The code in square brackets [ ] should be sequenced second. Tabular: Synonyms, alternative wording, explanatory phrases.	I. A.7
And	Tabular: Means and/or.	I. A.8 I. A.14
Code Also	Tabular: More than one code may be required to fully describe the condition.	I. A.17
Code First/Use Additional Code	Tabular: Provides sequencing instructions for conditions that have both an underlying etiology and multiple body system manifestations and certain other codes that have sequencing requirements.	I. A.13
Excludes1	Tabular: Mutually exclusive codes. None of the codes that appear after it should be used with the original code itself.	I. A.12. a
Excludes2	Tabular: The condition excluded is not part of the condition represented by the code but may be reported together if documented.	I. A.12. b
Includes notes	Tabular: Begin with the word **Includes** and further define, clarify, or give examples.	I. A.10
Inclusion terms	Tabular: A list of synonyms or conditions included within a classification.	I. A.11
NEC	Index and Tabular: Not Elsewhere Classifiable. The medical record contains additional details about the condition, but there is not a more specific code available to use.	I. A.6. a & b
NOS	Tabular: Not Otherwise Specified. Information to assign a more specific code is not available in the medical record.	I. A.6. a & b
See	Index: It is necessary to reference another Main Term or condition to locate the correct code.	I. A.16
See Also	Index: Coder may refer to an alternative or additional Main Term if the desired entry is not found under the original Main Term.	I. A.16
With	Tabular: In a code title, means *with* or *due to*.	I. A.15
With/Without	Tabular: Within a set of alternative codes, describe options for final character.	Conventions
X	Tabular: A placeholder in codes with fewer than six characters that require a seventh character. The **X** itself has no meaning and is not replaced with an actual number or letter. In some codes, the **X** is used to reserve room for future expansion.	I. A.4 I. A.5

alert the user to special rules, warnings, and guidelines. The key to publisher-specific conventions usually appears in the introductory portion of the coding manual as well as at the bottom of each page.

Several of the most important conventions are discussed next. Refer to the ICD-10-CM manual and look up the examples that follow.

Exclusion Notes

ICD-10-CM Tabular List utilizes two exclusion notes: Excludes1 and Excludes2. Exclusion notes may appear at the beginning of a block, category, subcategory, or after a code.

Notes at the category or subcategory level apply to all codes that follow, so it is important to check for these notes not only under the code, but also under the preceding block, category, and subcategory headings.

EXAMPLE: Refer to category **K55 Vascular disorder of intestine** in the Tabular List and notice the note **Excludes1: necrotizing enterocolitis of newborn (P77.-)**. This note applies to all the subsequent codes, **K55.0** through **K55.9**. If coders read only the notes for one code, such as **K55.1**, they would miss the added instruction at the beginning of the category **K55**.

Excludes1 indicates that the condition represented by the code and the condition listed as excluded are mutually exclusive and should not be coded together. When an Excludes1 note appears under a code, none of the codes that appear after it should be used with the code where the note appears.

EXAMPLE: The Excludes1 note under **K55** means that **necrotizing enterocolitis of newborn (P77.-)** should not be reported with any of the codes within the **K55** category.

Excludes2 indicates that the condition excluded is not part of the condition represented by the code, but the patient may have both conditions at the same time. These conditions are not mutually exclusive. When an Excludes2 note appears under a code, it is acceptable to use the main code and the excluded code if the patient is documented to have both conditions.

EXAMPLE: Refer to the Tabular List entry **K86.0 Alcohol induced chronic pancreatitis** and notice the note **Excludes2: alcohol induced acute pancreatitis (K85.2)**. The second condition, alcohol-induced acute

pancreatitis, is not included in code **K86.0** but may be reported together with it if the documentation states that the patient has both conditions.

Some codes may have both Excludes1 and Excludes2 notes.

EXAMPLE: The block **Diseases of liver (K70-K77)** has an Excludes1 note for **Jaundice NOS (R17)**, meaning that **R17** should not be reported with any of the codes from **K70** through **K77**. The same block also has several Excludes2 notes. The conditions listed under Excludes2 are not included in any of the codes **K70** through **K77** but may be reported together with them if the patient is documented to have both conditions. **K77** may appear on a different physical page than the block heading, so the coder who fails to review the beginning of the category will not be aware of these important instructions.

If a code does not have any exclusion notes, then it can be used with any other code that is supported by the medical record and the OGCR.

CODING PRACTICE

| Exercise 3.2 | Conventions: Exclusion Notes |

Instructions: For each pair of codes, indicate whether they can be used together based on the exclusion notes. Look up the first code listed in each question. Read the Excludes1 and Excludes2 note(s) and determine whether the second code can be reported together with the first code. Circle the correct answer.

1. G43.001 and G43.709	OK	Do not use together
2. D56.1 and D57.411	OK	Do not use together
3. H71.00 and H60.410	OK	Do not use together
4. M21.532 and M21.721	OK	Do not use together
5. O07.0 and O04.84	OK	Do not use together
6. R22.2 and R19.01	OK	Do not use together
7. R29.890 and N63	OK	Do not use together
8. M80.012 and M89.712	OK	Do not use together
9. S83.015A and M23.204	OK	Do not use together
10. T38.0X5D and T49.0X5D	OK	Do not use together

Use Additional Characters
ICD-10-CM alerts coders to use additional characters on a code in two ways:

• A short dash (-) at the end of a code number in the Index
• A publisher's symbol in front of a code in the Tabular List

When coders see one of these conventions, it means a subcategory needs additional characters and the coder should look down to the next level for more specificity. When neither

symbol appears, coders should still review the Tabular List closely to ensure that no additional characters are required. In ICD-10-CM the additional values for characters 4 through 6 are listed below the subcategory. ■ FIGURE 3-2, p. 40 illustrates an example of a symbol to use additional characters.

EXAMPLE: OGCR C.12.a.2) for Chapter 12, "Diseases of Skin and Subcutaneous Tissue (L00-L99)," states, **Assignment of the code for unstageable pressure ulcer (L89.--0) should be based on the clinical documentation**.

5th K94.2 Gastrostomy complications
    K94.20 Gastrostomy complication, unspecified
    K94.21 Gastrostomy hemorrhage
    K94.22 Gastrostomy infection
    K94.23 Gastrostomy malfunction

Figure 3-2 ■ Example of a symbol to use additional character.
Source: © PB Resources, Inc. Used with permission.

The use of two short dashes (- -) means that this guideline applies to all codes beginning with **L89** and ending in **0**, such as **L89.000, L89.010, L89.130**, etc. In the earlier example, **Excludes1: necrotizing enterocolitis of newborn (P77.-)**, the designation **P77.-** uses the short dash (-) to indicate all codes beginning with **P77**.

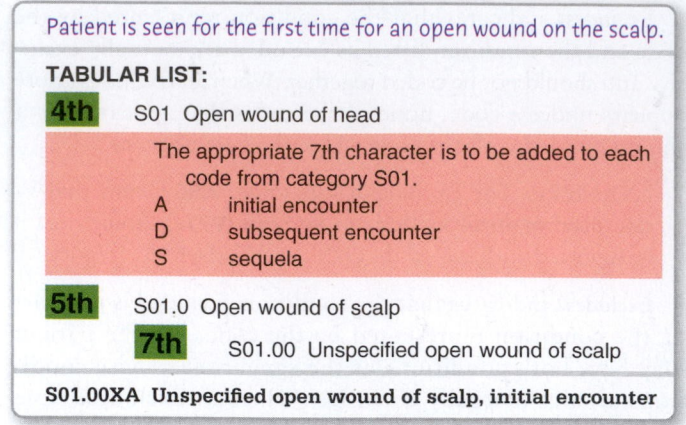

Figure 3-3 ■ Example use of a placeholder (X) and a 7th character (A).

SUCCESS STEP

Many publishing companies print the ICD-10-CM coding manual and each company uses variety of symbols, color-coding, and fonts to alert coders to the need for additional characters. This text uses symbols to indicate that additional characters are required: **4th 5th 6th** and **7th**. If you do not see similar symbols in your edition of the coding manual, check the introductory material at the beginning of the manual to learn what symbols the publisher uses.

Seventh Characters and Placeholders

Some codes require a seventh character that reports special information. The seventh character must appear in the seventh position, regardless of the length of the code. The need for a seventh character may be indicated by a symbol preceding a code. When a three-, four-, or five-character code requires a seventh character, the placeholder **X** must fill any empty positions preceding the seventh position. The **X** itself has no meaning and is not replaced with an actual number or letter. Definitions for the seventh character may appear immediately above the code entry, or at a preceding block, category, or subcategory level.

The range of codes the seventh characters apply to is dictated by where the characters and definitions appear within the organizational hierarchy. Codes that require a seventh character are invalid if the seventh character is omitted; therefore, the claim may be rejected by the payer. ■ FIGURE 3-3 illustrates an example entry in the Tabular List that requires both a seventh character and a placeholder. To assign a code for *unspecified open wound of scalp, initial encounter*, follow these steps in the Tabular List:

- Select code **S01.00**.
- Because the code is only five characters in length, the publisher may list a symbol that reminds you to add the

placeholder **X** for the sixth character, before adding the seventh character.

- Finally, add the seventh character **A** to designate the initial episode of care.
- The final code is **S01.00XA**.

Laterality

ICD-10-CM contains a new OGCR, Section I.B.13, Laterality. For conditions that affect bilateral sites, such as eyes, ears, arms, and legs, the fifth or sixth character indicates whether the condition affects the right or left side. Approximately 30% of ICD-10-CM codes include a designation for laterality. A limited number of these codes also provide an option for bilateral (*both sides affected*). If there is no designation for bilateral, assign separate codes for the right side and the left side. If laterality is unspecified, assign the code for **unspecified** side. The implementation of laterality is one example of why ICD-10-CM has so many codes. ICD-10-CM has four codes plus a subcategory heading (five entries total) for a single condition such as *Marginal corneal ulcer* (■ FIGURE 3-4).

SUCCESS STEP

It is important to notice exactly where a set of seventh character definitions appears within the organizational hierarchy. When the seventh characters and definitions appear at the beginning of a chapter, they are used with all subsequent codes in the chapter; when they appear at the beginning of a block, they are used with all codes in the block; when they appear at the beginning of a category or subcategory, they are used with all codes in the category or subcategory, respectively.

ICD-10-CM code	Description	Level of organization
H16.04	Marginal corneal ulcer	Subcategory
H16.041	Marginal corneal ulcer, right eye	Code
H16.042	Marginal corneal ulcer, left eye	Code
H16.043	Marginal corneal ulcer, bilateral	Code
H16.049	Marginal corneal ulcer, unspecified eye	Code

Figure 3-4 ■ Example of laterality in ICD-10-CM.

CODING PRACTICE

Exercise 3.3 **Conventions: Use Additional Characters, Seventh Characters, and Placeholders**

Instructions: Look up the following codes in the Tabular List and determine whether each is correct, needs additional characters, needs a placeholder, and/or needs a seventh character. Some codes may need more than one of these items. If the code is correct, circle *Correct*. If the code is incorrect, circle *Incorrect* and write the correct code in the space provided.

1. E65 Localized adiposity: Correct Incorrect, should be

   _____

2. E66 Morbid obesity due to excess calories: Correct Incorrect, should be _____

3. G43.1 Migraine with aura, not intractable, with status migrainosus: Correct Incorrect, should be _____

4. I48.9 Unspecified atrial fibrillation: Correct Incorrect, should be

   _____

5. O31.00 Papyraceous fetus, first trimester, fetus 1: Correct Incorrect, should be _____

6. O29.8X2 Other complications of anesthesia during pregnancy, second trimester: Correct Incorrect, should be

   _____

7. S71.151 Bite, right thigh, sequela: Correct Incorrect, should be

   _____

8. S84.22 Injury of cutaneous sensory nerve at lower leg level, left leg, initial encounter: Correct Incorrect, should be

   _____

9. S72.02 Displaced fracture of epiphysis, left femur, subsequent encounter for closed fracture with nonunion: Correct Incorrect, should be _____

10. T59.6X Toxic effect of hydrogen sulfide, accidental, subsequent encounter: Correct Incorrect, should be

   _____

ABSTRACTING DIAGNOSES

Diagnosis coding requires three skills of an "Ace" coder:

- **Abstract**—Read the medical record and determine which elements of the encounter require codes.
- **Assign**—Determine codes that accurately describe the patient's condition, reflect the highest level of specificity possible, and contain the correct number of characters for each code.
- **Arrange (sequence)**—Place codes in the order dictated by the OGCR and instructional notes.

Although coders do not need to memorize specific codes, they do need to memorize the skills and steps of the coding process.

When coders begin the process of assigning diagnosis codes, they do not necessarily know how many codes will be required. In some cases, a **combination code** is available, which describes two or more conditions in a single code. Other times, **multiple coding** is required, which means that two or more codes are needed to fully describe a condition. Coders learn how many codes are needed by following the guidelines, conventions, and instructional notes in the Index, Tabular List, and OGCR.

The first step in coding is to identify the diagnosis(es) to be coded based on the documentation. The OGCR provides guidelines for this task in Section I.B, as well as Section IV for outpatient services and Sections II and III for inpatient services. Chapter-specific guidelines in Section I.C provide more detailed guidance for selected conditions. This section provides an overview of abstracting outpatient and inpatient diagnoses.

SUCCESS STEP

This text uses the term *arrange* as a learning mnemonic for *sequence* in order to remind you of the coding skills of **A**bstract, **A**ssign, and **A**rrange. In the workplace, most professional coders simply use the term *sequence*.

Abstracting Physician and Outpatient Diagnoses

For physician and outpatient coding, the coder needs to identify the main reason for the services provided, which is the first-listed diagnosis. Recall that this is the diagnosis, condition, problem, or other reason for the encounter shown in the medical record to be chiefly responsible for the services provided (OGCR IV.A). Coding conventions and the general (OGCR I.B) and chapter-specific (OCGR I.C) guidelines take precedence over Section IV outpatient guidelines if there is a conflict. Key rules for abstracting outpatient diagnoses are:

- Do *not* code signs or symptoms that are an integral part of the disease process when the diagnosis has been established.

- Do *not* code an uncertain diagnosis, which is indicated in the medical record by words such as *probable, possible, suspected, questionable, rule out,* or *working diagnosis.*

- *Do* code the presenting signs and symptoms when the diagnosis is uncertain. This guideline for outpatient services is different than the guideline for uncertain diagnoses for inpatient services.

- *Do* code additional conditions and signs or symptoms that are not part of the confirmed disease process, in addition to the first-listed diagnosis, when they are managed during the encounter.

- Do *not* code conditions that are resolved, not treated, or have no bearing on the current encounter.

ICD-10-CM also provides codes for encounters due to reasons other than a disease or injury. These may be routine health screenings, preventive care, diagnostic services only, therapeutic services only, preoperative evaluations, prenatal visits, and similar situations. Codes for most of these situations are classified under **Factors Influencing Health Status and Contact with Health Services (Z00-Z99)**. Detailed guidelines appear in OGCR IV and codes are indexed in the Index to Diseases and Injuries.

Abstracting Inpatient Diagnoses

For inpatient coding, the main reason that services were provided is the principal diagnosis. This is "the condition established after study to be chiefly responsible for occasioning the admission of the patient to the hospital for care" (OGCR Section II). Coding conventions and the general (OGCR I.B) and chapter-specific (OGCR I.C) guidelines take precedence over Section II and III inpatient guidelines if there is a conflict. Key rules for abstracting inpatient diagnoses are:

- Do *not* code signs or symptoms that are an integral part of the disease process when the diagnosis has been established.

- *Do* code additional conditions, signs, or symptoms not part of the confirmed disease, in addition to the principal diagnosis, when they are **relevant** to the current admission. Relevant diagnoses, also called **clinically significant conditions,** are defined by UHDDS as "all conditions that coexist at the time of admission, that develop subsequently, or

that affect the treatment received and/or the length of stay. Diagnoses that relate to an earlier episode which have no bearing on the current hospital stay are to be excluded" (OGCR III).

- *Do* code for an uncertain diagnosis if a definitive diagnosis is not available at the time of discharge and/or after all test results are reported. This guideline is different for inpatient services than outpatient. For inpatient, code an uncertain diagnosis as if it exists because it is the reason for the hospital admission and any diagnostic and therapeutic services provided (OGCR II.H).

SUCCESS STEP

You do not always know how many codes you will end up with, or even exactly which conditions require a code, at the time of abstracting. You abstract *potential* conditions and elements to be coded. OGCR and instructional notes in the Tabular List provide further direction about how many and what codes are needed in a specific situation.

Abstracting Using the Mini-Medical-Record

This text uses a mini-medical-record format for examples and exercises, which extracts the most essential information from a patient's medical record. Refer to ■ FIGURE 3-5 to become acquainted with this format and to learn how to interpret it.

Guided Example of Abstracting Diagnoses

■ TABLE 3-7 provides general guidance on how to abstract diagnoses. These abstracting criteria are general questions to ask regarding most conditions. Abstracting questions are a guide, and not every question applies to, or can be answered for, every case. For example, age and gender are not relevant for every diagnosis. Not every case includes signs and symptoms. More detailed abstracting criteria are presented for each body system throughout this text.

Refer to the following example, which begins here and continues throughout the chapter, to learn more about abstracting a diagnosis for an outpatient visit. Follow along with fictitious coder Sherry Whittle, CPC, as she reads the progress notes from patient Eric Beardsley's office visit (refer again to Figure 3-5). Check off each step as you complete it.

▶ First, Sherry reviews the demographic information and reads Mr. Beardsley's chief complaint. Then she refers to TABLE 3-7, Key Criteria for Abstracting Diagnoses, and answers each question from the medical record.

❏ *What are the gender and age of the patient?* Male, age 24

❏ *What is the patient's chief complaint or reason for the encounter?* Pain and swelling in the right ankle

❏ *Is the encounter inpatient or outpatient?* Outpatient (office)

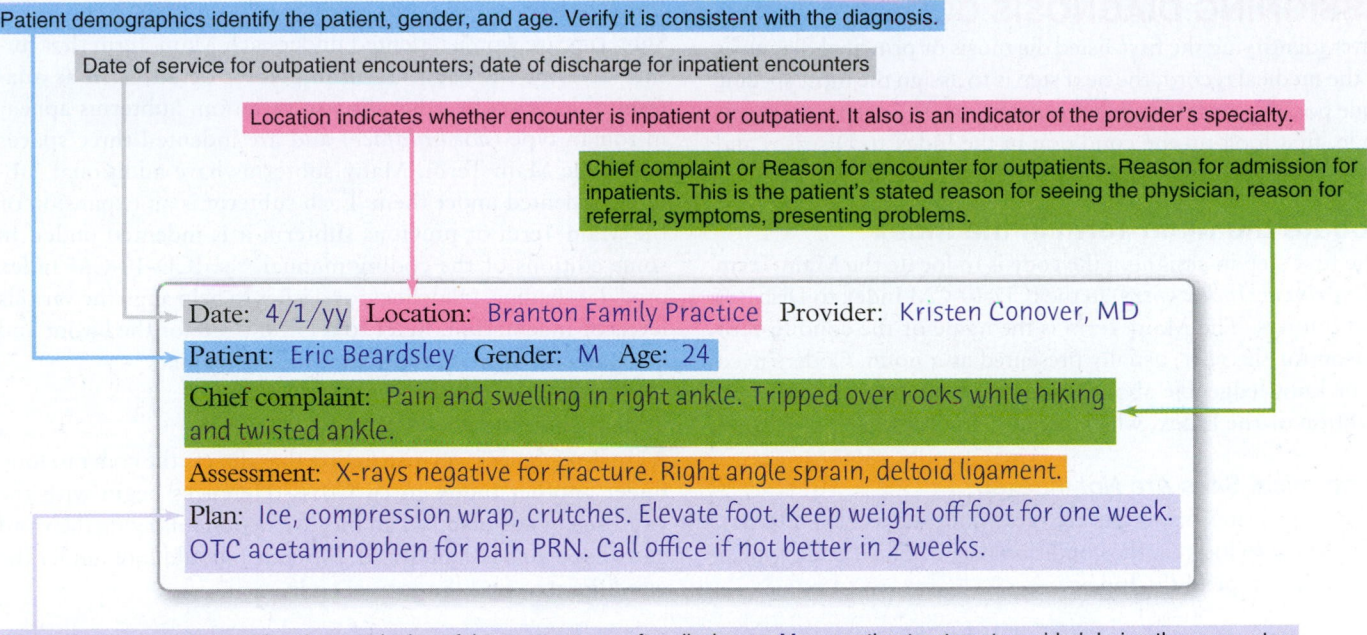

Patient demographics identify the patient, gender, and age. Verify it is consistent with the diagnosis.

Date of service for outpatient encounters; date of discharge for inpatient encounters

Location indicates whether encounter is inpatient or outpatient. It also is an indicator of the provider's specialty.

Chief complaint or Reason for encounter for outpatients. Reason for admission for inpatients. This is the patient's stated reason for seeing the physician, reason for referral, symptoms, presenting problems.

Date: 4/1/yy Location: Branton Family Practice Provider: Kristen Conover, MD

Patient: Eric Beardsley Gender: M Age: 24

Chief complaint: Pain and swelling in right ankle. Tripped over rocks while hiking and twisted ankle.

Assessment: X-rays negative for fracture. Right angle sprain, deltoid ligament.

Plan: Ice, compression wrap, crutches. Elevate foot. Keep weight off foot for one week. OTC acetaminophen for pain PRN. Call office if not better in 2 weeks.

Plan is the treatment plan after the conclusion of the encounter or after-discharge. May mention treatment provided during the encounter.

Figure 3-5 ■ Key to interpreting the mini-medical-record.

Table 3-7 ■ KEY CRITERIA FOR ABSTRACTING DIAGNOSES (GENERAL GUIDELINES)

- ❑ What are the gender and age of the patient?
- ❑ What is the patient's chief complaint or reason for the encounter or inpatient admission?
- ❑ Is the encounter inpatient or outpatient?
- ❑ What symptoms and signs are described?
- ❑ Does the physician provide a definitive diagnosis?
- ❑ Does the physician provide a diagnosis that is uncertain, probable, possible, qualified, or rule out?
- ❑ Which symptoms and signs are integral to the definitive diagnosis?
- ❑ Which symptoms and signs are related, but not integral, to the definitive diagnosis?
- ❑ What unrelated conditions, symptoms, or signs are managed during the encounter?
- ❑ What conditions, symptoms, or signs are not managed during the encounter?
- ❑ What is the laterality, if any, of the condition?
- ❑ What is the treatment plan or procedure? Is it consistent with the diagnosis?
- ❑ Is the condition the result of an injury or external cause?

- ❑ *What symptoms and signs are described?* Pain and swelling

- ❑ *Does the physician provide a definitive diagnosis?* Yes, right ankle sprain, deltoid ligament

- ❑ *Does the physician provide a diagnosis that is uncertain, probable, possible, qualified, or rule out?* No

- ❑ *Which symptoms and signs are integral to the definitive diagnosis?* Pain and swelling

- ❑ *Which symptoms and signs are related, but not integral, to the definitive diagnosis?* None

- ❑ *What unrelated conditions, symptoms, or signs are managed during the encounter?* None

- ❑ *What conditions, symptoms, or signs are not managed during the encounter?* No other conditions, symptoms, or signs were documented

- ❑ *What is the laterality, if any, of the condition?* Right

- ❑ *What is the treatment plan or procedure?* Ice, compression wrap, crutches. *Is it consistent with the diagnosis?* Yes

- ❑ *Is the condition the result of an injury or external cause?* Yes, tripped over rocks while hiking and twisted ankle

▶ Sherry will code the diagnosis *right ankle sprain, deltoid ligament*. Next, she needs to assign the codes.

CODING CAUTION

Coding sounds simple to the casual observer, but as you will learn, it is an extended research process that involves many comparisons and cross-checks. Learning the detailed steps of coding will make you a more accurate coder. Unfortunately, there are no shortcuts.

ASSIGNING DIAGNOSIS CODES

After identifying the first-listed diagnosis or principal diagnosis in the medical record, the next step is to assign the most specific code possible that describes the condition. To assign a diagnosis code, first look up the condition in the Index to Diseases and Injuries (Index), then verify the code in the Tabular List.

Locate the Main Term in the Index

The first step in assigning the code is to locate the **Main Term** (*the primary Index entry*) in the ICD-10-CM Index to Diseases and Injuries. The Main Term is the name of the condition or reason for the visit, usually presented as a noun. Coders need to be knowledgeable about several details regarding the organization of the Index, which are discussed next.

Anatomical Sites Are Not Indexed

Anatomical sites or organs are rarely indexed as Main Terms, so it is best to look up the condition itself. Main Terms appear in boldface type in the Index.

Subterms

Subterms are words indented under each Main Term that further describe the Main Term in greater detail, such as anatomical location or other disease variation. Subterms appear in roman type (*not boldface*) and are indented three spaces under the Main Term. Many subterms have additional subterms indented under them. Each subterm is an expansion of the Main Term or previous subterm it is indented under. In some editions of the coding manual, the ICD-10-CM Index provides shading, guidelines, or dashes to help align the various levels of indentation. Refer to ■ FIGURE 3-6 for the layout and compare the figure to the actual coding manual.

Cross-References

A cross-reference is an instruction that directs the coder to look under another Index entry. Cross-references begin with the word **see** or **see also**. When the instruction following the word **see** or **see also** is capitalized, the coder should look under the word listed to find the correct code.

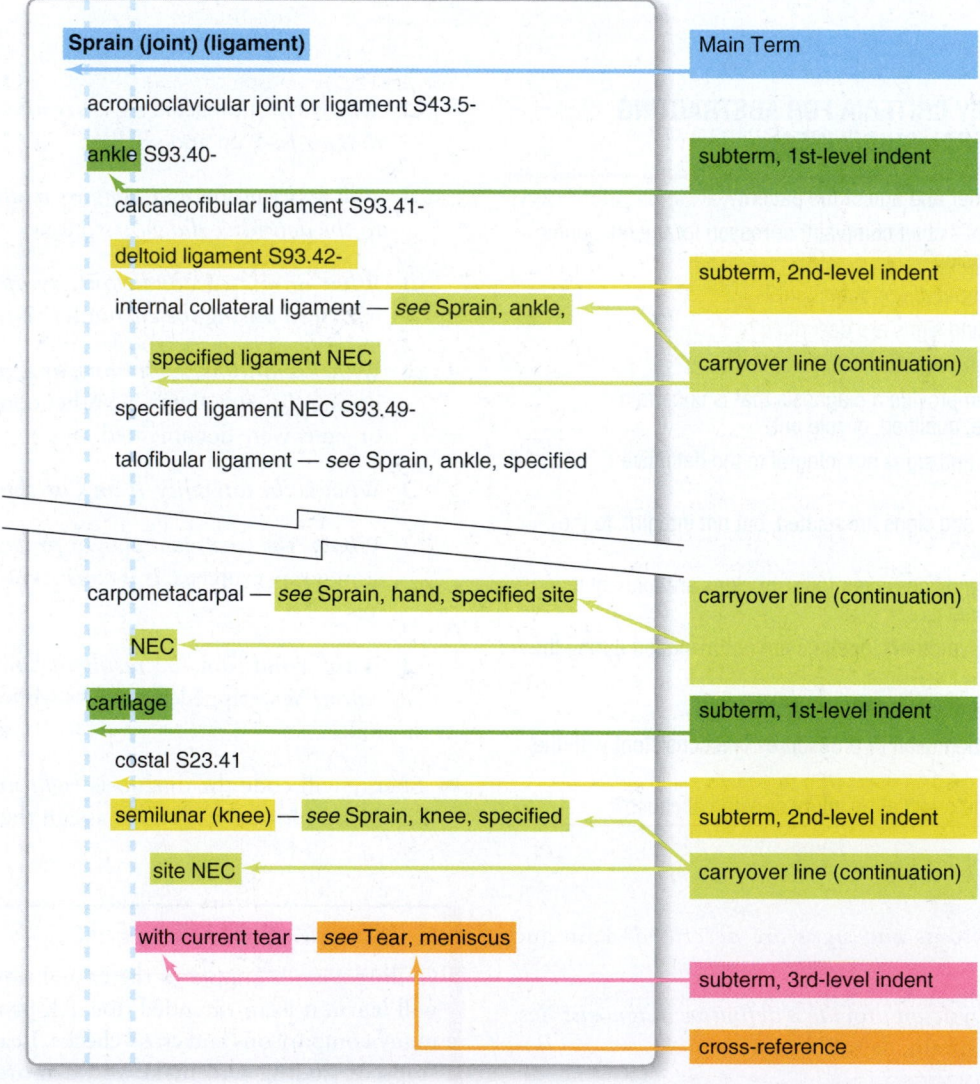

Figure 3-6 ■ Example of Main Term and subterm indents in the Index.

EXAMPLE: Under **Sprain, cartilage, semilunar, with current tear**, the subterm **with current tear** provides cross-referencing instructions to **see Tear, meniscus**. This means the coder should look up the Main Term **Tear** and the subterm **meniscus** in order to locate the code.

Refer to ■ FIGURE 3-7 for an example of a **see also** cross-reference. Notice that the Main Term **Ankyloblepharon** has two subterms. In addition to reviewing these subterms, coders should also cross-reference the Main Term **Blepharophimosis** for additional codes.

Default Codes

A code listed next to a Main Term in the ICD-10-CM Index is referred to as a **default code**. The default code may represent the condition most commonly associated with the Main Term, or it may represent the unspecified code for the condition, which usually ends in **9**. Refer to ■ FIGURE 3-8 for an example of a default code. In this example, if appendicitis is documented in the medical record without any additional information, such as acute or chronic, the default code **K37** should be assigned because it appears next to the Main Term, **Appendicitis**.

Nonessential Modifiers

The words in parentheses ( ) after a Main Term or subterm are **nonessential modifiers**. Nonessential modifiers are included in the default description of the code and do not need to be present in the medical record in order to use the code.

EXAMPLE: Refer again to Figure 3-8. The Main Term **Appendicitis** is followed by the terms **(pneumococcal)** and **(retrocecal)**. These words are nonessential modifiers because they are enclosed in parentheses. This means that pneumococcal and retrocecal appendicitis are automatically included in the default appendicitis code **K37**. However, these words do not need to be present in the medical record in order to assign this code because they are nonessential modifiers. The conditions appendicitis, pneumococcal appendicitis, and retrocecal appendicitis are all classified with the same code, **K37**.

Also notice that in the ICD-10-CM Index, the entry **Appendicitis** has numerous subterms with different codes. Coders must review all the subterms and locate the most specific one before selecting a code to verify. Do not automatically select the default code without reviewing the subterms.

> **Anisocytosis** R71.8
> **Anisometropia (congenital)** H52.31
> <mark>Ankle—*see* condition</mark>
> **Ankyloblepharon (eyelid) (acquired)**—*see also* Blepharophimosis
>   filiforme (adnatum) (congenital) Q10.3
>   total Q10.3

Figure 3-7 ■ Example of a cross-reference in Index.

> **Appendicitis** <mark>(pneumococcal) (retrocecal)</mark> K37

Figure 3-8 ■ Example of Index entry for a default code with nonessential modifiers.

Multiple Coding Paths

Conditions may have multiple **coding paths**, which means they can be indexed under more than one Main Term.

EXAMPLE: Chronic rhinopharyngitis (*inflammation of the nose and throat*) appears under **Rhinopharyngitis, chronic J31.1** and also under **Nasopharyngitis, chronic J31.1**. Both Main Terms lead to the same code because the medical terminology combining forms rhin/o and nas/o both mean "nose." If coders have difficulty locating a Main Term, they can also look under an **eponym** (*named after a person*), a synonym, or other alternative term. In addition, coders can reference broad-ranging Main Terms, such as **Abnormal, Anomaly, Complication, Disease, Findings, Infection, Injury,** or **Syndrome**. In some cases, coders may need to look in several locations under different Main Terms to identify multiple code options before proceeding. This is a normal part of the coding process.

SUCCESS STEP

There are times when you will not be completely sure of which code to look up based on your research in the Index. That is okay. If you locate two or three possible codes in the Index, make note of all of them. After you verify each one in the Tabular List, you will have more information to help determine which code best describes the patient.

Specialized Index Locations

While most conditions and reasons for the encounter are located in the Index to Diseases and Injuries, ICD-10-CM has three additional locations for specialized codes. Some publishers may organize the sections of the coding manual in a different order. Refer to the Table of Contents at the beginning of your coding manual to learn how it is organized.

- *Neoplasms* are indexed in the Table of Neoplasms, located under **N** in the Index to Diseases and Injuries. Some publishers may locate this table immediately after the Index to Diseases and Injuries.

- *Poisonings, adverse effects, and underdosing caused by drugs and chemicals* are indexed in the ICD-10-CM Table of Drugs and Chemicals, which is located following the Index to Diseases and Injuries.

- *External causes of illness and injury* are located in a separate Index, the ICD-10-CM Index to External Causes, which follows the Table of Drugs and Chemicals. External causes are generally reported using codes beginning with the letters **V, W, X,** and **Y** in ICD-10-CM and appear within the Tabular List.

CODING PRACTICE

Exercise 3.4   **Locating the Main Term**

Instructions: Underline the Main Term in each of these diagnoses. Then look up the Main Term and any subterms needed to locate the code in the Index to confirm that you chose the correct term. If the Index cross-references another entry, write the name of the cross-reference in the space provided. Then look up the cross-referenced entry. Do not assign any codes in this exercise.

Example: <u>Short</u> arm: Cross-reference *Deformity, limb, unequal length*

1. Complicated open wound of left ear, initial encounter: Cross-reference _____

2. Deprivation of water, subsequent encounter: Cross-reference _____

3. Urinary tract infection: Cross-reference _____

4. Chickenpox: Cross-reference _____

5. Blackwater fever: Cross-reference _____

6. Gallbladder infection: Cross-reference _____

7. Quartan malaria: Cross-reference _____

8. Cerebrovascular disease: Cross-reference _____

9. Congestive heart failure: Cross-reference _____

10. Type 1 diabetes: Cross-reference _____

Verify Codes in the Tabular List

After identifying the potential code(s) in the Index, the next step in assigning a code is to verify it in the Tabular List. This is an essential step because the Index is not designed to provide the full code or full information about how to use the code. Verifying codes requires cross-referencing information at several points.

A short dash (-) at the end of an Index entry indicates that additional characters are required. Even when a dash is not included at the Index entry, you must refer to the Tabular List to verify that no seventh character is required and to review the instructional notes. Characters for laterality and the seventh character can only be assigned in the Tabular List. The Tabular List also includes instructional notes that must be followed, such as those for sequencing, multiple coding, and inclusion and exclusion notes discussed earlier in the chapter.

To verify a code, look up the code number in the Tabular List and follow these steps:

1. Read the code title to confirm that the code accurately describes the intended condition.

2. Read the instructional notes under the code.

3. Check for symbols preceding the entry indicating that additional characters are required.

4. Cross-reference the titles of the subcategory and the three-character category and read any instructional notes under those titles.

5. Cross-reference the titles of the block and the chapter headings and read any instructional notes under those titles.

6. Compare and contrast any other codes being considered for first-listed or principal diagnosis.

7. Assign all required characters and write down the code, taking time to double check for transcription or typographical errors.

8. Repeat this process for each code required.

Guided Example of Assigning Diagnosis Codes

Continue with the example of Eric Beardsley, who was treated for an ankle sprain, to learn more about assigning codes. Follow along in your ICD-10-CM manual as Sherry Whittle, CPC, locates the code for Mr. Beardsley in the Index. Check off each step as you complete it.

▶ Sherry looks up the entry for **Ankle** and observes a cross-reference note that states **see condition** (refer again to Figure 3-7).

  ❑ She recalls that this is a cross-reference directing her to look up the term that describes the *condition affecting the ankle,* which in this case is a sprain.

  ❑ She does not look up the word *condition.*

  ❑ Sherry will look up the Main Term **Sprain** because that is the condition that affects the ankle.

▶ Sherry locates the Main Term **Sprain** in the Index to Diseases and Injuries.

  ❑ She scans the entire entry for **Sprain**, which continues onto the next several columns on the next page. At the top of each column is a heading **Sprain – continued**, telling her which Main Term is being continued.

  ❑ She notices that all the subterms describe anatomical sites of a sprain.

- ❏ She locates the subterm **ankle**, for the anatomical site.

- ❏ She notices that additional subterms further describe the anatomical site within the ankle, such as **calcaneofibular ligament S93.41-** and **deltoid ligament S93.42-**. These subterms are second-level indents. Both of these entries are part of the overall entry for ankle because they are indented under the subterm **ankle**.

- ❏ Sherry identifies the second-level subterm **deltoid ligament S93.42-** as the best match for Mr. Beardsley's case.

- ❏ The full name of this entry combines the Main Term and each indented subterm: **Sprain + ankle + deltoid ligament** (refer again to Figure 3-6).

- ❏ Sherry notices the Index entry ends with a short dash (-). She knows this means that she will need to assign additional digits when she verifies the code in the Tabular List.

- ▶ Sherry looks up the entry **S93.42** in the Tabular List so she can verify the code.

  - ❏ She notices that this is a subcategory, not a code, because additional characters are required. The symbol **6th** in front of the entry tells her that a sixth character is required.

  - ❏ She confirms the title of the category **Sprain of deltoid ligament** is consistent with the progress note.

- ▶ She reads the code choices listed and notices that the sixth character defines laterality with choices for right ankle, left ankle, and unspecified ankle.

  - ❏ She refers back to the progress note to confirm which ankle was affected.

  - ❏ She selects code **S93.421** for the right ankle.

- ▶ Sherry notices that the symbol **7th** appears in front of the code **S93.421**. This tells her that a seventh character is required to complete the code.

- ❏ The seventh character is not listed under the code, so she knows she needs to review the previous subcategory, category, and block headings to locate the seventh character options. She knows she needs to review these headings anyway in order to locate any possible instructional notes.

- ▶ Sherry confirms the subcategory title **S93.4, Sprain of ankle** is the correct anatomic site because other joints, such as the shoulder, also have a **deltoid** muscle or ligament.

  - ❏ She reads the note **Excludes2: injury of Achilles tendon (S86.0-)** under the subcategory title and verifies that does not apply to her case because the Achilles tendon was not documented.

- ▶ Next, she works back up the organizational hierarchy of the Tabular List until she locates the three-character category heading **S93, Dislocation and sprain of joints and ligaments at ankle, foot and toe level** (■ FIGURE 3-9).

  - ❏ Sherry reads the entries for the **Includes** note under the category heading. She observes that one of the entries is **sprain of cartilage, joint or ligament of ankle, foot and toe**, which is consistent with the Mr. Beardsley's progress note.

  - ❏ Sherry notices the instructional note **Code also any associated open wound** following the Includes list. She understands that if Dr. Conover had documented an open wound in addition to the sprain, she would need an additional code for the wound. Because a wound was not documented, she knows she can bypass this note.

  - ❏ Sherry reads the note **Excludes2: strain of muscle and tendon of ankle and foot (S96.-)** and understands that if Dr. Conover had also documented a muscle or tendon strain, she would need an additional code because **Excludes2** means that **strain of muscle and tendon of ankle and foot (S96.-)** is not included in this category.

  - ❏ Sherry identifies the list of seventh characters for this category.

S93 Dislocation and sprain of joints and ligaments at ankle, foot and toe level
Includes:
avulsion of joint or ligament of ankle, foot and toe
laceration of cartilage, joint or ligament of ankle, foot and toe
sprain of cartilage, joint or ligament of ankle, foot and toe
traumatic hemarthrosis of joint or ligament of ankle, foot and toe
traumatic rupture of joint or ligament of ankle, foot and toe
traumatic subluxation of joint or ligament of ankle, foot and toe
traumatic tear of joint or ligament of ankle, foot and toe
Excludes2: strain of muscle and tendon of ankle and foot (S96.-)
Code also any associated open wound
The appropriate 7th character is to be added to each code from category S93
A - initial encounter
D - subsequent encounter
S - sequela

Figure 3-9 ■ Tabular List entry for category heading S93.

▶ Next, Sherry reviews the seventh character assignments that apply to all codes in category **S93**.

❑ She reviews the progress note to determine if this episode of care was the **initial encounter** (*active treatment*), **subsequent encounter** (*treatment during the healing phase*), or a **sequela** (*late effect or problem after active healing is completed*).

❑ The progress note does not specifically use any of these words, but Sherry determines from the context that this was Mr. Beardsley's first encounter for treatment of the sprain. If this had been a follow-up visit or later problem, Dr. Conover would have explicitly stated that.

❑ The seventh character for initial encounter is **A**, so Sherry assigns **A** at the end of the code, to arrive at **S93.421A**.

▶ Sherry knows she is not quite done. She still needs to check the block and chapter headings for any possible instructional notes.

❑ She is not sure where the block begins, so she refers to the beginning of the entries for codes beginning with **S** in the Tabular List, which coincides with the beginning of the chapter (■ FIGURE 3-10).

❑ She finds an instructional note with the word **NOTE:**, which instructs her to **Use secondary code(s) from**

Chapter 20, External causes of morbidity, to indicate cause of injury. (External cause codes are discussed in Chapter 7, "External Causes of Morbidity (V00–Y99)," in this text.)

❑ She reads the other instructional notes under the chapter heading and finds no other notes that apply to this case.

❑ She scans the list of block headings in this chapter and locates the block for **S90-S99 Injuries to the ankle and foot**.

▶ Sherry turns to the beginning of the block **S90-S99** (■ FIGURE 3-11).

❑ She reads the **Excludes2** notes and determines that they do not apply to this case because none of these conditions are documented.

❑ Sherry is tempted to think it was a waste of time to cross-reference the beginning of the chapter and block for additional instructions because none were found. However, she knows from experience that as soon as she tries to take a shortcut, it backfires on her and causes her to miss important information or instructions.

▶ Sherry assigns diagnosis code **S93.421A** to this encounter. She will also assign external cause codes for tripping while hiking.

ARRANGING DIAGNOSIS CODES

The final step in diagnosis coding is to arrange, or sequence, codes in the correct order when there is more than one diagnosis code. Coders may need to assign more than one diagnosis code when patients have more than one condition that is being treated or managed during an encounter; there is an etiology/manifestation relationship; both acute and chronic conditions are documented; instructional notes in the Tabular List direct the coder to additional codes needed; or multiple coding is required for other reasons. Each of these situations is discussed below.

The OGCR provides direction about how to determine the principal diagnosis for inpatient coding or the first-listed diagnosis for outpatient coding. Sequencing of diagnoses must "tell the story" of the patient encounter or admission. The sequencing of diagnosis codes is essential to proper reimbursement. Payment can be denied or improper payment might be made when diagnosis codes are not sequenced correctly because they will not correctly match up with procedure codes. OGCR references are listed with each topic that follows. In addition,

---

Chapter 19

Injury, poisoning and certain other consequences of external causes (S00-T88)

NOTE: Use secondary code(s) from Chapter 20, External causes of morbidity, to indicate cause of injury. Codes within the T section that include the external cause do not require an additional external cause code.

Use additional code to identify any retained foreign body, if applicable (Z18.-)

Excludes1:
birth trauma (P10-P15)
obstetric trauma (O70-O71)
This chapter contains the following blocks:
S00-09   Injuries to the head
S10-19   Injuries to the neck
S20-29   Injuries to the thorax

S70-79   Injuries to the hip and thigh
S80-89   Injuries to the knee and lower leg
S90-99   Injuries to the ankle and foot
T07   Injuries involving multiple body regions
T14   Injury of unspecified body region

T79   Certain early complications of trauma
T80-88   Complications of surgical and medical care, not elsewhere classified

Figure 3-10 ■ Tabular List entry for Chapter 19.

Injuries to the ankle and foot (S90-S99)

Excludes2:
burns and corrosions (T20-T32)
fracture of ankle and malleolus (S82.-)
frostbite (T33-T34)
insect bite or sting, venomous (T63.4)

Figure 3-11 ■ Tabular List entry for block heading S90–S99.

the OGCR discusses requirements for multiple coding related to specific diseases. Disease-specific sequencing guidelines are discussed throughout this text in the chapters that cover individual body systems.

More Than One Condition Treated

When more than one condition is treated or managed during an encounter, sequence the principal or first-listed diagnosis first. When it is difficult to determine which condition is the principal diagnosis, refer to the following guidelines:

- When two or more interrelated conditions each potentially meet the definition for principal diagnosis, either condition may be sequenced first if the **circumstances of admission** (*facts, signs, and symptoms that require the admission*), the Index, or the Tabular List provide no further guidance (OGCR II.B).

- When two or more distinct conditions equally meet the definition for principal diagnosis, either condition may be sequenced first if the circumstances of admission, the Index, or the Tabular List provide no further guidance (OGCR II.C).

When the principal or first-listed diagnosis is clear, sequence the additional conditions in order of importance to the encounter or in order of severity or risk to the patient's health and well-being.

Etiology/Manifestation

Etiology/manifestation is an ICD-10-CM convention for certain conditions that have both an underlying **etiology** (*cause*) and **manifestations** (*signs and symptoms*) in multiple body systems (OGCR I.A.13). Sequence the etiology first and the manifestation second. Coders may not always know in advance if a particular combination of diseases is an etiology/manifestation relationship, so the ICD-10-CM manual alerts coders with sequencing instructions. Do not apply etiology/manifestation rules if ICD-10-CM does not list instructional notes or other conventions indicating this relationship.

EXAMPLE: Refer to the following example of dementia in Parkinson's disease, where Parkinson's disease is the etiology and dementia is a manifestation. Common sequencing instructions for etiology/manifestation follow with examples:

- The Index lists both conditions and both codes together. The etiology code is first; the manifestation code is second and appears in [brackets]. Always sequence the code in brackets second (■ FIGURE 3-12).

- In the Tabular List entry for the manifestation code, the manual provides an instructional note **Code first** and lists codes for possible etiologies. The condition listed after this note should be sequenced second (■ FIGURE 3-13, p. 54).

- The manifestation code title often includes the phrase **in diseases classified elsewhere**. Code titles with this phrase may be highlighted in the Tabular List as a reminder that manifestation codes may never be the first-listed or principal diagnosis.

- When two codes are listed in the Index, remember to verify both codes in the Tabular List. ■ FIGURE 3-14, page 54 shows the Tabular List entry for the etiology code **G20**.

- Notice that Figure 3-14 has an **Excludes1** note for **dementia with Parkinsonism** and cross-references the coder to **G31.83**. When you cross-reference **G31.83**, you see the code title is **Dementia with Lewy bodies**, which is a specific kind of dementia. Since this condition is not documented in the medical record, use the original code **G20**.

- In some instances, the etiology code in the Tabular List provides the instructional note **Use additional code** and lists common manifestations. Refer to ■ FIGURE 3-15, page 54 to see how this note is used for **Alzheimer's disease, early onset** and **dementia with behavioral disturbance**. Assign and arrange the codes as follows:

(1) **G30.0 Alzheimer's disease with early onset**

(2) **F02.81 Dementia with behavioral disturbance**

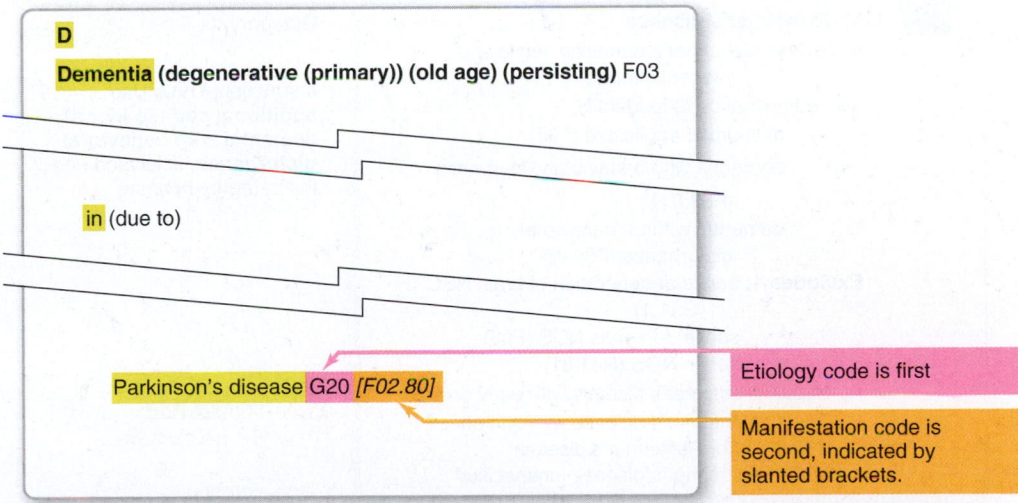

Figure 3-12 ■ Example of Index entry for etiology and manifestation codes.

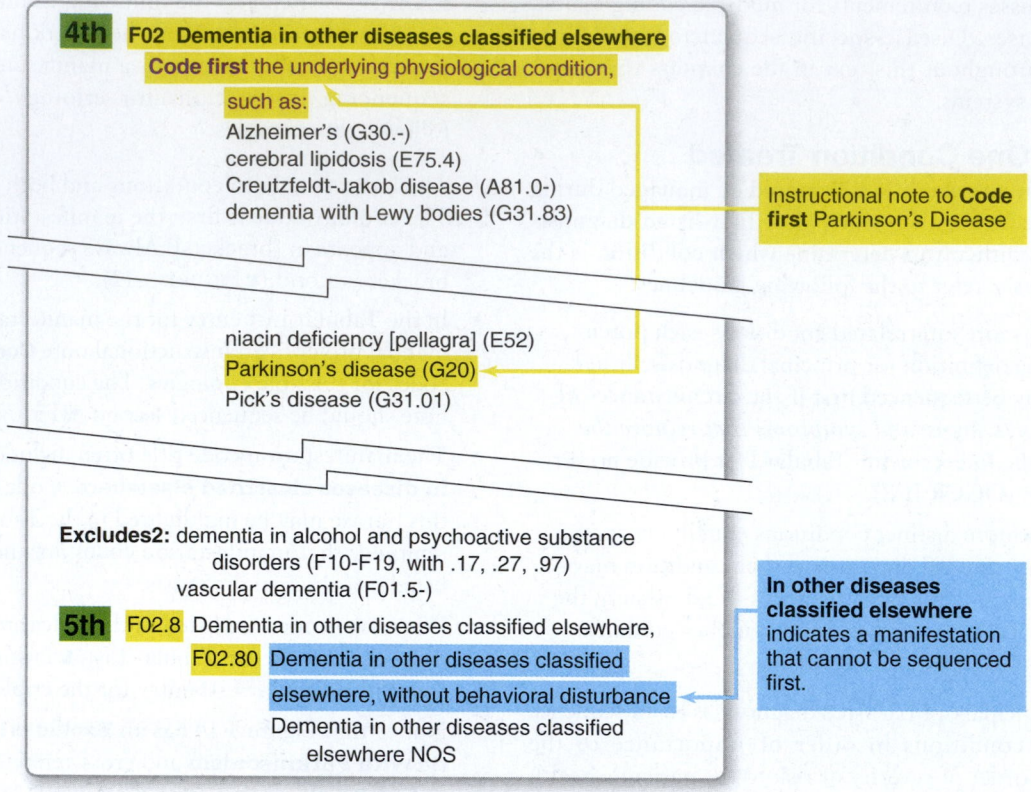

4th **F02 Dementia in other diseases classified elsewhere**
Code first the underlying physiological condition,
such as:
Alzheimer's (G30.-)
cerebral lipidosis (E75.4)
Creutzfeldt-Jakob disease (A81.0-)
dementia with Lewy bodies (G31.83)

Instructional note to **Code first** Parkinson's Disease

niacin deficiency [pellagra] (E52)
Parkinson's disease (G20)
Pick's disease (G31.01)

Excludes2: dementia in alcohol and psychoactive substance
disorders (F10-F19, with .17, .27, .97)
vascular dementia (F01.5-)

5th F02.8 Dementia in other diseases classified elsewhere,
F02.80 Dementia in other diseases classified
elsewhere, without behavioral disturbance
Dementia in other diseases classified
elsewhere NOS

In other diseases classified elsewhere indicates a manifestation that cannot be sequenced first.

Figure 3-13 ■ Example of Tabular List entry with the instructional note "Code first".

G20 Parkinson's disease
Hemiparkinsonism
Idiopathic Parkinsonism or Parkinson's disease
Paralysis agitans
Parkinsonism or Parkinson's disease NOS
Primary Parkinsonism or Parkinson's disease
Excludes1: dementia with Parkinsonism (G31.83)

Figure 3-14 ■ Example of Tabular List entry for an etiology code (G20).

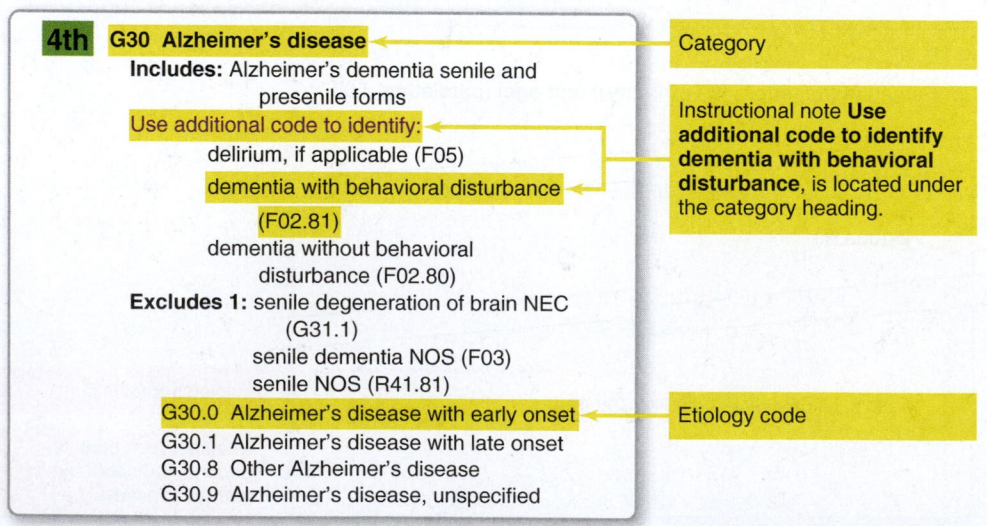

4th **G30 Alzheimer's disease**
Includes: Alzheimer's dementia senile and
presenile forms
Use additional code to identify:
delirium, if applicable (F05)
dementia with behavioral disturbance
(F02.81)
dementia without behavioral
disturbance (F02.80)
Excludes 1: senile degeneration of brain NEC
(G31.1)
senile dementia NOS (F03)
senile NOS (R41.81)
G30.0 Alzheimer's disease with early onset
G30.1 Alzheimer's disease with late onset
G30.8 Other Alzheimer's disease
G30.9 Alzheimer's disease, unspecified

Category

Instructional note **Use additional code to identify dementia with behavioral disturbance**, is located under the category heading.

Etiology code

Figure 3-15 ■ Tabular List entry with the instructional note "Use additional code".

Acute and Chronic Conditions

Providers may document that a patient has both acute and chronic forms of the same condition, such as bronchitis or cholecystitis. The sequencing is determined by how the Index presents the acute and chronic conditions. The Index lists acute and chronic conditions in one of two ways:

- The Index may list subterms for both acute and chronic at the same level of indentation.
- When this occurs, sequence the code for acute first and the code for chronic second (OGCR I.B.8) (■ FIGURE 3-16).
- The Index may list **chronic** as a subterm of **acute**, or vice versa, which leads to a combination code (■ FIGURE 3-17, page 52). When this occurs, assign one code, the combination code, that describes both conditions: **K81.2 Acute cholecystitis with chronic cholecystitis**

Regardless of how the Index lists the entries, always verify the codes in the Tabular List and follow any instructional notes.

Instructional Notes

The Index and Tabular List provide instructional notes and verbal conventions that direct coders how to sequence codes. When these rules are not followed, the coder's computer often provides an informational message reminding the coder of the rule that needs to be applied. If the claim gets submitted with improper code sequencing or missing codes, the edit checks at the clearinghouse or insurance company may cause the claim to be rejected. It is the coder's responsibility to be familiar with these rules, identify when and where they appear in the coding manual or coding software program, and apply the rule correctly.

Use Additional Code

The Tabular List also lists the instructional note **Use additional code** in other situations besides etiology/manifestation. The note may appear under code, subcategory, category, block, or chapter titles, so the coder must always review these headings for instructions. Refer to the ICD-10-CM manual Chapter 10, "Diseases of the Respiratory System (J00-J99)," and locate the note **Use additional code** under the chapter title. This instructional note applies to all codes in the chapter (OGCR I.A.13).

Do not automatically assign a code from the Use additional code list. The condition must be documented in the medical record. If the etiology documented in the medical record does not appear in the list, refer to the Index and locate the code for the specific etiology documented.

Code First

Code first notes also appear under certain codes that are not specifically manifestation codes but may be due to an underlying cause. When there is a **Code first** note and an underlying condition is present, the underlying condition should be sequenced first (OGCR I.A.13 and I.B.7). Do not automatically assign additional codes when you see an instructional note. The condition must be documented in the medical record in order to assign a code.

Code, if Applicable, Any Causal Condition First

Code, if applicable, any causal condition first notes indicate that this code may be assigned as a principal diagnosis when the causal condition is unknown or not applicable. If a causal condition is known, then the code for that condition should be sequenced as the principal or first-listed diagnosis (OGCR I.B.7).

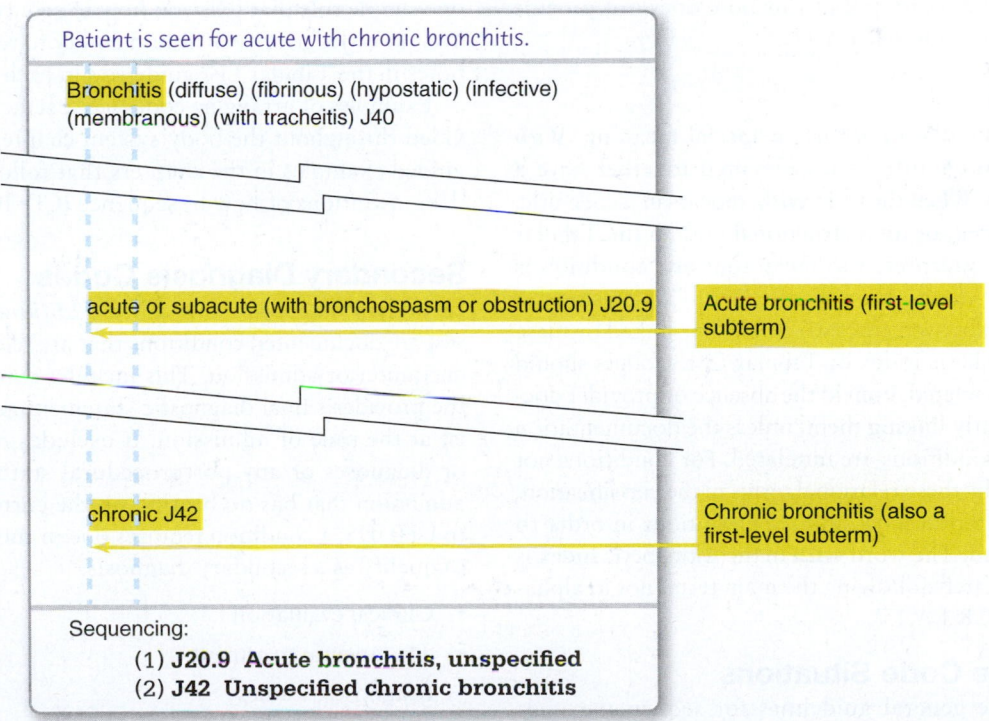

Figure 3-16 ■ Example of multiple coding for an acute and chronic condition.

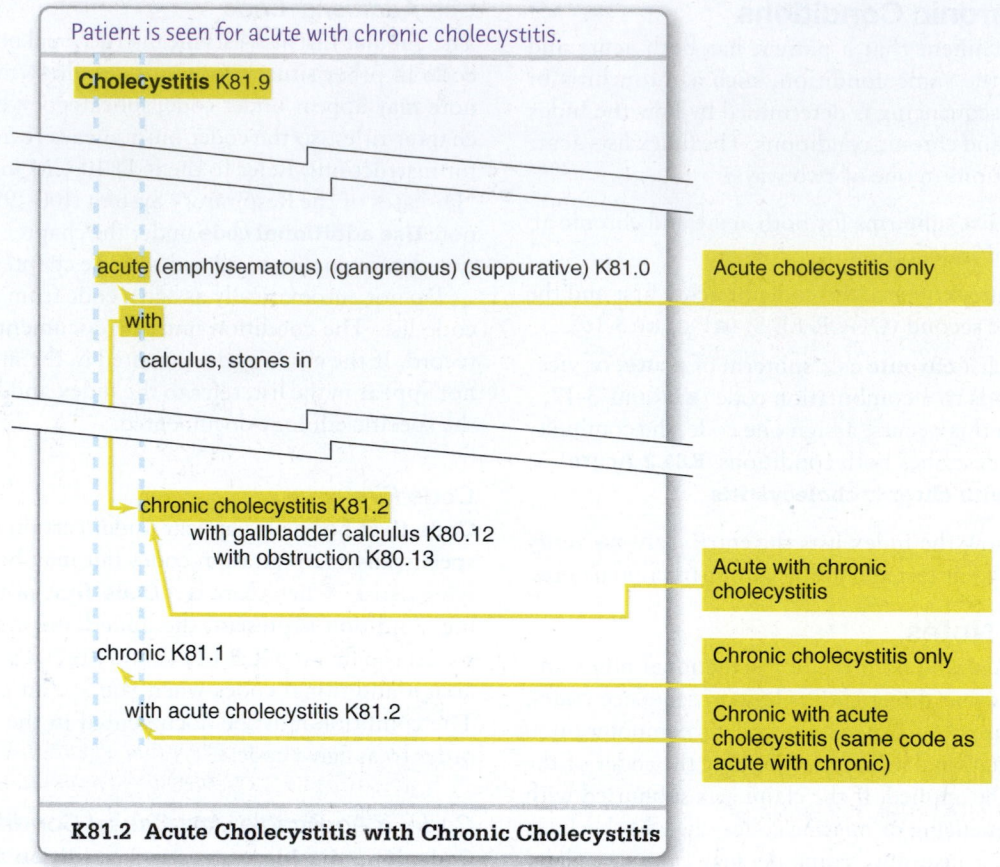

Patient is seen for acute with chronic cholecystitis.

Cholecystitis K81.9

acute (emphysematous) (gangrenous) (suppurative) K81.0 — Acute cholecystitis only

with

calculus, stones in

chronic cholecystitis K81.2
  with gallbladder calculus K80.12
  with obstruction K80.13 — Acute with chronic cholecystitis

chronic K81.1 — Chronic cholecystitis only

with acute cholecystitis K81.2 — Chronic with acute cholecystitis (same code as acute with chronic)

K81.2 Acute Cholecystitis with Chronic Cholecystitis

Figure 3-17 ■ Example of a combination code for an acute with chronic condition.

Code Also

A **Code also** note instructs that two codes may be required to fully describe a condition, but this note does not provide sequencing direction (OGCR I.A.17).

With

In ICD-10-CM, the word *with* has a special meaning. *With* indicates that two conditions documented together have a causal relationship. When the term **with** appears in a code title, the Alphabetic Index, or an instructional note in the Tabular List, it should be interpreted to mean that one condition is *associated with* or *due to* the other. ICD-10-CM presumes a causal relationship between the two conditions linked by these terms in the Alphabetic Index or Tabular List. Coders should code conditions as related, even in the absence of provider documentation explicitly linking them, unless the documentation clearly states the conditions are unrelated. For conditions not specifically linked by these relational terms in the classification, provider documentation must link the conditions in order to code them as related. The word **with** in the Alphabetic Index is sequenced immediately following the main term, not in alphabetical order (OGCR I.A.15).

Other Multiple Code Situations

In addition to the general guidelines for sequencing multiple codes, multiple codes may be needed in many specific situations such as obstetrics, injuries, surgical or procedural

complications, and late effects. OGCR Section I.C, Chapter-Specific Coding Guidelines, defines these rules. There is not one simple rule that tells you how to sequence multiple codes. Your knowledge of OGCR and ability to read all instructional notes in the Tabular List guide you in each situation.

Examples of arranging codes for specific conditions are provided throughout the body system chapters in this text. The guided examples in the chapters that follow provide detailed demonstrations of how to sequence ICD-10-CM codes.

Secondary Diagnosis Codes

Secondary diagnoses, also called *additional* or *other* diagnoses, are documented conditions that are relevant to the current encounter or admission. This includes conditions included in the provider's final diagnostic statement and those that coexist at the time of admission. It excludes resolved conditions or diagnoses or any postprocedural status from a previous admission that has no bearing on the current stay. According to UHDDS, a condition requires one or more of the following to qualify as a secondary diagnosis:

- Clinical evaluation
- Therapeutic treatment
- Diagnostic studies
- Extended length of stay
- Increased nursing care and/or monitoring

ICD-10-CM does not provide definitive sequencing guidelines for secondary diagnoses. Sequencing is usually based on how central the condition is to the encounter/admission, the amount of tests and studies performed or ordered, and the health risk to the patient. Most hospitals establish internal policies that provide additional guidance about when secondary diagnoses should be coded and how they should be sequenced. CMS considers 24 secondary diagnoses (in addition to the principal diagnosis) when determining the MS-DRG, so when patients have more than 24 secondary diagnoses, those affecting DRG assignment must be sequenced within the first 24 on the claim. This includes certain complications, comorbidities, and conditions existing at the time of admission.

More information about coding secondary diagnoses is provided in later chapters of this text that cover individual body systems.

CODING PRACTICE

Exercise 3.5 Abstracting, Assigning, and Arranging Diagnosis Codes

Instructions: Read the diagnostic statement below, then answer the questions that follow to assign the correct codes. Sequence multiple codes in the correct order.

1. Toxic shock syndrome due to *Streptococcus* A

   a. Underline the Main Term, then look it up in the Index.

   b. What is the subterm? _____

   c. Locate the subterm. What code is listed? _____

   d. Locate the code listed in step c in the Tabular List. Is there a symbol indicating that an additional digit is required? _____

   e. What instructional note appears under the code? _____

   f. What is the name of the organism? _____

   g. Cross-reference the block heading A30–A49. Do any instructional notes appear? _____

   h. Cross-reference the title for ICD-10-CM Chapter 1. What does the *Includes* note say? _____

   i. Read the other notes under the Chapter title. Do any of these notes apply to this case? _____

   j. Refer back to the code you looked up in steps c and d. Cross-reference the categories listed in the instructional note. Which category do you need? _____

   k. Which code in this category do you assign for the organism? _____

   l. Cross-reference the block title B95–B97. Is there an instructional note? _____ Read the note.

   m. You have identified two codes for this case. Which code is sequenced first? _____

   n. Which code is sequenced second? _____

ICD-10-CM CODING AND REIMBURSEMENT

ICD-10-CM coding has significant impact on reimbursement because diagnoses identify the reason(s) that services are provided. If a service is not justified by an appropriate diagnosis code, it is not paid. The effect is slightly different for physician and inpatient services.

Physician Reimbursement

Although physicians are paid for procedure codes, each procedure code must be linked with one or more diagnoses that support the reason it is needed. On the CMS-1500 form or the 837P electronic format in a computerized billing program, block 24F requires the letter of the pointer, or cross-reference, of the diagnosis in block 21.

Refer again to Figure 2-3 in Chapter 2 of this text, Figure 2-3, Example of a "Example of a completed CMS-1500 claim form".

The diagnoses are listed in the order of importance for this particular visit, which is based on physician documentation:

- Block 21A: **I10 Essential (primary) hypertension**
- Block 21B: **I48.91 Unspecified atrial fibrillation**
- Block 21C: **J30.9 Allergic rhinitis, unspecified**

The procedure code for the office visit evaluation and management is listed first, then the other procedure codes are listed in descending cost order. Each procedure is matched with one or more diagnoses:

- Block 24D, Line 1: **99205 Office or other outpatient visit for the evaluation and management of a new patient.** This service is supported by all three diagnoses, so the pointers **ABC** are listed in block 24F, line 1.
- Block 24D, Line 2: **95052 × 10 Photo patch test(s) (specify number of tests).** This service is supported by

diagnosis **J30.9**, so the pointer **C** is listed in block 24F, line 2.

- Block 24D, Line 3: **93000 Electrocardiogram, routine ECG with at least 12 leads; with interpretation and report**. This service is supported by diagnosis **I48.91**, so the pointer **B** is listed in block 24F, line 3.

If the diagnosis codes for essential hypertension and atrial fibrillation are missing, it is unlikely that the electrocardiogram procedure would be paid. If the diagnosis code for allergic rhinitis is missing, the procedure for the photo patch tests would not be paid. This is an example. There are several diagnosis codes that could support any of these procedures, based on patient circumstances.

Inpatient Hospital Reimbursement

Inpatient hospitals must determine which diagnosis is the principal diagnosis—"the condition established after study to be chiefly responsible for occasioning the admission of the patient to the hospital for care." Refer to Figure 2-4 in Chapter 2 of this text, Figure 2-4, Example of a completed UB-04 claim form (with annotations). The principal diagnosis is listed in FL 66. The diagnosis is **K50.114 Crohn's disease of large intestine with abscess**. Additional diagnoses, if any, would be listed in FL 66A through 66Q. The principal diagnosis, along with the principal procedure in FL 74, is a key factor in determining the DRG on which reimbursement is based. The principal procedure is **0D1B0Z4 Bypass ileum to cutaneous, Open approach**. The DRG, listed in FL 71, is **330 Major Small & Large Bowel Procedures W CC**.

If the wrong principal diagnosis is listed, the claim could be denied, or the case could be classified into a different DRG that pays an incorrect amount.

The *ICD-10-CM/PCS MS-DRG Definitions Manual*, published by CMS and updated annually, lists certain diagnoses as a **complication or comorbidity (CC)** or a **major complication or comorbidity (MCC)** because they pose a higher risk of mortality. An MCC is more serious than a CC. For example, chronic respiratory failure is classified as an MCC, whereas acute respiratory failure is classified as a CC. Because CC and MCC conditions are more complicated to treat, they can move a patient to a higher-paying DRG.

The *ICD-10-CM/PCS MS-DRG Definitions Manual* also lists certain conditions as **hospital-acquired conditions (HACs)**. HACs are conditions that begin during a patient's hospital stay but are considered reasonably preventable through proper protocols, referred to as evidence-based practices, because they are based on research and clinical evidence. Examples of an HAC are a fractured hip due to a fall while in the hospital and an infection that started during the stay. When such a condition is **present on admission (POA)**, it qualifies the patient for a higher-paying DRG. For example, if a patient is admitted with a fracture due to a fall or an existing infection, these conditions must be identified as POA on the claim.

Various indicator letters identify whether a condition was present at the time of inpatient admission (Y), not present at the time of inpatient admission (N), unknown whether present at the time of admission because of inadequate documentation (U), or clinically undetermined whether present at the time of admission (W). This designation alerts Medicare that the patient qualifies for a higher-paying DRG. On the UB-04, the indicator letter is entered at the eight character of a diagnosis code. On the 837I, the indicator is entered into a designated field on the input screen.

Private payers vary in how they handle CCs, MCCs, HACs, and POA, so each payer's rules must be checked. CCs, MCCs, and HACs are not addressed in detail in this text. Some ICD-10-CM coding manuals provide an appendix with detailed reference information on these criteria.

Refer to Chapter 2, "Coding and Reimbursement," for more information on physician, inpatient hospital, and outpatient hospital reimbursement.

CHAPTER SUMMARY

In this chapter you learned that:

- ICD-10-CM is used to code diagnoses that describe patient illnesses, diseases, conditions, injuries, or other reasons for seeking healthcare services. It is used by all HIPAA-covered entities.

- ICD-10-CM is accompanied by Official Guidelines for Coding and Reporting (OGCR) and Conventions, both of which direct the coder in how to use the manual.

- Diagnosis coding involves the three skills of an "Ace" coder:

  - Abstract—Read the medical record and determine which elements of the encounter require codes

  - Assign—Determine codes that accurately describe the patient's condition, reflect the highest level of specificity possible, and contain the correct number of characters for that code

  - Arrange—Place codes in the order dictated by the guidelines and instructional notes (sequence).

- The OGCR provide guidelines for abstracting the first-listed diagnosis for physician and outpatient encounters and the principal diagnosis for inpatient encounters.

- Assigning diagnosis codes requires coders to locate the Main Term in the Index, then verify the code in the Tabular List. All instructional notes and guidelines must be followed.

- OGCR provides several guidelines to determine when multiple diagnosis codes and how they should be arranged (sequenced).

- ICD-10-CM coding has significant impact on reimbursement because diagnoses identify the reason(s) that services are provided. If a service is not justified by an appropriate diagnosis code, it is not paid. The effect is slightly different for physician and inpatient services.

CONCEPT QUIZ

Take a moment to look back at diagnosis coding and solidify your new skills. This is your opportunity to pull together everything you have learned.

Completion

Instructions: Write the term that completes each statement based on the information you learned in this chapter. Choose from the list below. Some choices may be used more than once and some choices may not be used at all.

-	Code Also
( )	Code First
*	Excludes1
:	Excludes2
[ ]	Includes
	POA
	See
	Use Additional Code
	With
	X

1. The _____ convention identifies nonessential modifiers that describe the default variations of a term.

2. The _____ convention identifies mutually exclusive codes that should not be used together.

3. The _____ convention appears after the code number and tells the coder to assign additional characters.

4. The _____ convention is used in the Index to identify a code that should be sequenced second.

5. The _____ convention means that one condition is associated with or due to the other.

6. The _____ convention is a placeholder in codes with less than six characters that require a seventh character.

7. The _____ convention indicates that the condition excluded is not part of the condition represented by the code, but the patient may have both conditions at the same time.

8. The _____ convention instructs the coder to sequence the etiology first.

9. The _____ convention instructs the coder to sequence the manifestation second.

10. The _____ convention instructs the coder to reference another Main Term or condition to locate the correct code.

Multiple Choice

Instructions: Circle the letter of the best answer to each question based on the information you learned in this chapter.

1. When should signs and symptoms be coded in the inpatient setting?
   A. When they are relevant to the current admission and are not integral to the confirmed diagnosis.
   B. When the diagnosis is uncertain.
   C. When they are an integral part of the confirmed diagnosis.
   D. When they are related to a previous, resolved condition.

2. What is the name for the diagnosis, in the outpatient setting, that describes *the diagnosis, condition, problem, or other reason for the encounter shown in the medical record to be chiefly responsible for the services provided*?
   A. Principal
   B. Uncertain
   C. First-listed
   D. Main Term

3. What type of diagnoses are preceded by the words *probable, possible, suspected, questionable, rule out, working diagnosis,* or a similar word?
   A. Principal
   B. Uncertain
   C. First-listed
   D. Main Term

4. What is the name for the diagnosis, in an inpatient setting, that is *the condition established after study to be chiefly responsible for occasioning the admission of the patient to the hospital for care*?
   A. Principal
   B. Uncertain
   C. First-listed
   D. Main Term

5. What are the rules that complement the conventions and instructional notes to provide additional information and direction in identifying the diagnoses to be reported?
   A. OGCR
   B. Conventions
   C. Exclusions
   D. Instructional notes

6. What is the term for the use of symbols, typeface, and layout features to succinctly convey interpretive information?
   A. OGCR
   B. Conventions
   C. Exclusions
   D. Instructional notes

(continued)

(continued from page 59)

7. Which coding step means to read the medical record and determine which elements of the encounter require codes?
   A. Abstracting
   B. Assigning
   C. Arranging
   D. Cross-referencing

8. What is the name of a contiguous range of codes within a chapter in ICD-10-CM?
   A. Block
   B. Category
   C. Section
   D. Subcategory

9. Which OGCR topic defines separate codes for the right and left sides of the body?
   A. Bilateral
   B. Multiple coding
   C. Arranging
   D. Laterality

10. What type of condition can qualify a patient for a higher-paying DRG?
   A. Etiology
   B. Nonessential modifier
   C. HAC
   D. MCC

KEEP ON CODING

Instructions: Read the diagnostic statement and underline the Main Term. Then use the Index and Tabular List to assign and sequence ICD-10-CM diagnosis codes. Write the code(s) on the line provided.

1. Acquired flat foot, left. ICD-10-CM Code(s) _____

2. Encounter for immunotherapy. ICD-10-CM Code(s) _____

3. Stage 3 pressure ulcer, left buttock. ICD-10-CM Code(s) _____

4. Alcohol dependence. ICD-10-CM Code(s) _____

5. Fistula, left elbow. ICD-10-CM Code(s) _____

6. Family history of alcohol abuse. ICD-10-CM Code(s) _____

7. Body mass index of 38 in an adult. ICD-10-CM Code(s) _____

8. Benign hypertension. ICD-10-CM Code(s) _____

9. Dysphagia following a cerebral infarction with difficulty swallowing. ICD-10-CM Code(s) _____

10. Severe rebound abdominal pain in the left lower quadrant. ICD-10-CM Code(s) _____

11. Repeated falls. ICD-10-CM Code(s) _____

12. Merkel cell carcinoma of the right eyelid. ICD-10-CM Code(s) _____

13. Pain due to malignant neoplasm. ICD-10-CM Code(s) _____

14. Type 2 diabetes mellitus. ICD-10-CM Code(s) _____

15. Insect bite, left ankle, subsequent encounter. ICD-10-CM Code(s) _____

16. Second- and third-degree chemical burns, right ankle, initial encounter. ICD-10-CM Code(s) _____

17. Fused toes, bilateral. ICD-10-CM Code(s) _____

18. Chronic cystitis with hematuria. ICD-10-CM Code(s) _____

19. Pneumocystis pneumonia. ICD-10-CM Code(s) _____

20. Anemia. ICD-10-CM Code(s) _____

21. Encounter for blood typing. ICD-10-CM Code(s) _____

22. Ventilator-associated pneumonia. ICD-10-CM Code(s) _____

23. Head lice. ICD-10-CM Code(s) _____

24. Polyhydramnios, second trimester, fetus 3. ICD-10-CM Code(s) _____

25. Acute otitis externa, right ear. ICD-10-CM Code(s) _____

CODING CHALLENGE

Instructions: Read the mini-medical-record, then answer the questions that follow to abstract, assign, and arrange (sequence) the correct codes.

OFFICE

Gender: M   Age: 75

Chief complaint: Visit to monitor hypertension and congestive heart failure (CHF). Complains of (c/o) increased shortness of breath (SOB).

Assessment: Chronic combined systolic and diastolic heart failure, due to hypertension. Patient is a current and long-term tobacco user. Change diuretic. Use supplemental oxygen (O_2) as needed (PRN).

Part 1: Abstract

1. Read through the mini-medical-record. Observe the patient demographics. Compare the chief complaint to the final assessment.

   a. What symptom did the patient report in the chief complaint?

   _____

   b. What two conditions are stated in the assessment?

   _____
   _____

2. a. Is the symptom integral to one of the conditions stated in the assessment? _____

   b. Should you code for the symptom? _____

   c. Why or why not? _____

   d. What is the first condition due to? _____

   _____

Part 2: Assign

3. You can look up the conditions in any order you wish, as long as you sequence them correctly in the end based on the instructional notes you find during this exercise.

   Today, begin by coding the underlying condition, the condition that the heart failure is *due to*.

   a. Look up the Main Term **Hypertension** in the Index, then the subterm **heart, with, heart failure**. What code is listed? _____

   b. Verify this code in the Tabular List. Is there a symbol in front of this code indicating that you need additional characters?

   _____

4. a. What does the instructional note under the code say?

   _____

   b. Based on this instructional note, should the code for **Hypertension** be sequenced first or second?

   _____

5. a. Locate the beginning of this block for **Hypertensive diseases**. Read the instructional notes. Now refer back to the mini-medical-record. What lifestyle habit is documented? _____

   b. Which instructional note applies to this patient? (*Tip: History* describes a past condition that no longer exists.)

   _____

   You will verify this code later in this exercise.

   c. Review the instructional notes at the beginning of ICD-10-CM Chapter 9. Do any of these notes apply to this patient? _____

6. a. Now determine the code for heart failure. Look again at the instructional note under the code for **Hypertension**. What code is listed in the instructional note? _____

   _____

   b. What does the short dash (-) at the end of the code mean?

   _____

7. a. Verify the code listed in the instructional note. Review the four-character subcategories under this heading and locate the one that describes **Combined systolic and diastolic heart failure**. Write down the subcategory code.

   _____

   b. Now review the five-character codes under this subcategory. What code describes **Chronic combined systolic and diastolic heart failure**? _____

   _____

8. Cross-reference the three-character category heading for **Heart failure**. Read through the instructional notes. What condition should be coded first that applies to this patient?

   _____

   This code should match the one you assigned in step 3a. The instructional note confirms that you assigned the correct first code or alerts you to the fact that the first code was not correct.

9. Now you need to assign a third code for the lifestyle habit you listed in step 5a above. List the code here. _____

   _____

   Verify the code. (This code is sequenced last.)

Part 3: Arrange

10. You have identified three codes for this case. Review your answers in the previous questions to determine the correct sequencing.

    a. What code is sequenced first based on the instructional notes in steps 4b and 8?

    _____

    b. What code is sequenced second? _____

    c. What code is sequenced third? _____

Chapter 4

Symptoms, Signs, and Abnormal Clinical and Laboratory Findings, Not Elsewhere Classified (R00-R99)

Chapter Outline

- **Symptoms and Signs Refresher**
- **Coding Guidelines for Symptoms and Signs**
- **Abstracting Symptoms and Signs**
- **Assigning Codes for Symptoms and Signs**
- **Arranging Codes for Symptoms and Signs**

Learning Objectives

After completing this chapter, you should have the skills to:

4.1 Spell and define the key words, medical terms, and abbreviations in this chapter. (Remember)

4.2 Compare and contrast symptoms, signs, abnormal clinical findings and abnormal laboratory findings, and confirmed diagnoses. (Evaluate)

4.3 Adhere to the Official Guidelines for Coding and Reporting related to symptoms, signs, and abnormal findings. (Apply)

4.4 Examine and abstract symptoms, signs, abnormal findings, and confirmed diagnoses from the medical record. (Analyze)

4.5 Demonstrate how to assign codes for symptoms, signs, abnormal findings, and confirmed diagnoses. (Apply)

4.6 Utilize guidelines for arranging (sequencing) codes for symptoms, signs, abnormal findings, and confirmed diagnoses. (Apply)

Key Terms and Abbreviations

abnormal	modifier	related
confirmed	National Institutes of Health	systemic inflammatory response
Glasgow Coma Scale	Stroke Scale (NIHSS)	syndrome (SIRS)
impression	qualified	unrelated
integral	qualifier	

In addition to the key terms listed here, students should know the terms defined within tables in this chapter.

INTRODUCTION

When you notice an unusual vibration or sound in your car, you know you need to get to the nearest mechanic quickly because these are symptoms and signs of an underlying problem. The mechanic may perform a visual inspection or conduct diagnostic testing to determine the source of the problem and repair it.

Patients experience a symptom or notice a change in their health, so they go to the doctor to have it checked out. The physician interviews the patient, conducts a physical examination, and orders any necessary tests. At times, physicians can make a diagnosis quickly and, at other times, they must order further testing or consult with a specialist.

Coders must learn to distinguish patient symptoms, signs, abnormal findings, and test results from the underlying diagnosis. Physicians of all specialties evaluate symptoms, signs, and abnormal findings.

As you read this chapter, open your medical terminology book and keep a medical dictionary handy to refresh your memory of any unfamiliar terms. Also bookmark reliable Internet sites. These resources are especially important to help you learn what symptoms or signs are common with various conditions.

SYMPTOMS AND SIGNS REFRESHER

To determine a patient's diagnosis, a physician evaluates numerous sources of information: the patient's chief complaint and description of the problem, a visual observation of the patient, a physical examination, and results of laboratory tests, imaging, and other evaluations. The physician's goal is to establish a definitive diagnosis and prescribe a treatment plan to cure the problem and/or alleviate the symptoms. An abnormal test result or clinical finding is one in which the readings are not within the normal reference range established for that particular test. Sometimes a confirmed diagnosis is not possible because the physician needs multiple encounters, extended testing, evaluation by specialists, surgery, or other procedures to arrive at a diagnosis.

Refer to ■ TABLE 4-1 to review the meanings of various types of diagnostic data.

Symptoms and signs are often identified with prefixes or suffixes that are applied to word roots from specific body systems. Refer to ■ TABLE 4-2 for a refresher on how to build medical terms related to symptoms, signs, and abnormal findings.

CODING CAUTION

Be aware of easily confused medical terms that have similar spellings and different meanings, such as:

dysphagia (*difficulty swallowing*) and **dysphasia** (*difficulty speaking*)

hem/e (*blood*) and **hemi-** (*half, side*)

hypo- (*low, below*) and **hyper-** (*high, excessive*)

Table 4-1   ■   DEFINITION AND EXAMPLES OF DIAGNOSTIC DATA SOURCES

Data	Definition	Example
Symptom	Subjective evidence of a disease or condition, usually reported by the patient	Pain, anxiety, fatigue, nausea
Sign	Objective evidence of a disease or condition that can be observed by the physician	Fever, limp, crying, bleeding, vomiting
Abnormal clinical finding	Evidence of a disease or condition discovered through physical examination or testing	Palpation of a lump or mass, irregular EKG, x-ray showing a fracture
Abnormal laboratory test	Result of a chemistry test, blood test, biological culture that is outside of (higher or lower than) the normal numerical range, or microscopic specimen examination that differs from the standard visual features	Elevated or low blood glucose, high or low complete blood count, microscopic dysplasia

Table 4-2   ■   EXAMPLE OF CONSTRUCTING MEDICAL TERMS FOR SYMPTOMS, SIGNS, AND ABNORMAL FINDINGS

Combining Form/Prefix	Suffix	Complete Medical Term
dys- (prefix; *abnormal, painful*)		**dys + uria** (*difficulty urinating*)
		dys + phagia (*difficulty swallowing*)
	-**uria** (*condition of urine*)	**dys + meno + rrhea** (*difficulty or painful menstrual flow*)
hem/e, hemat/o (*blood*)	-**ptysis** (*to spit, cough*)	**hemat + uria** (*blood in urine*)
	meno + rrhea (*menstrual flow*)	**hemo + ptysis** (*coughing up blood*)
poly- (prefix; *many*)		**poly + uria** (*frequent urination*)
		poly + meno + rrhea (*frequent menstrual flow*)

CODING PRACTICE

Exercise 4.1 Symptoms and Signs Refresher

Instructions: Define the following symptoms, signs, and abnormal findings, then assign the diagnosis code.

Follow these steps:

- Use slash marks "/" to break down each term into its root(s) and suffix.
- Define the meaning of the word, based on the meaning of each word part.
- Assign the default ICD-10-CM diagnosis code for the condition using the Index and Tabular List.

Example: dysuria dys/ur/ia   Meaning *condition of painful urination*   ICD-10-CM Code *R30.0*

1. dyspnea   Meaning _____   ICD-10-CM Code _____

2. nocturia   Meaning _____   ICD-10-CM Code _____

3. aphagia   Meaning _____   ICD-10-CM Code _____

4. epistaxis   Meaning _____   ICD-10-CM Code _____

5. lymphadenopathy   Meaning _____   ICD-10-CM Code _____

6. hyperemesis   Meaning _____   ICD-10-CM Code _____

7. hypoxemia   Meaning _____   ICD-10-CM Code _____

8. cyanosis   Meaning _____   ICD-10-CM Code _____

9. glycosuria   Meaning _____   ICD-10-CM Code _____

10. tachycardia   Meaning _____   ICD-10-CM Code _____

CODING GUIDELINES FOR SYMPTOMS AND SIGNS

Coders should understand the organization of this ICD-10-CM chapter, chapter-wide and commonly used instructional notes in Tabular List, and the relevant OGCR. This information is necessary for accurate coding.

ICD-10-CM Chapter 18, "Symptoms, Signs, and Abnormal Clinical and Laboratory Findings, Not Elsewhere Classified (R00-R99)," contains 14 blocks or subchapters that are divided by anatomic site. Review the block names and code ranges listed at the beginning of Chapter 18 in the ICD-10-CM manual to become familiar with the content and organization.

This chapter includes symptoms, signs, and abnormal results of clinical and laboratory procedures. It also includes ill-defined conditions that do not fit anywhere else in ICD-10-CM or that can be indicative of multiple conditions. Signs and symptoms that point to a specific diagnosis appear in other chapters of the classification. For example, fevers of unknown origin or that are drug induced appear in this chapter, but fevers with a known cause, such as a fever due to heat or a specific organism, appear in other chapters. An abnormal blood culture appears in this chapter, but an abnormal white blood cell count is classified to ICD-10-CM Chapter 3, "Diseases of the Blood and Blood Forming Organs."

ICD-10-CM provides Official Guidelines for Coding and Reporting (OGCR) for symptoms, signs, and abnormal clinical and laboratory findings in OGCR section I.C.18. OGCR provides a detailed discussion of when to report and not report codes from this chapter. OGCR also discusses coding of symptoms and signs related to several specific conditions: repeated falls, coma, functional quadriplegia, systemic inflammatory response syndrome (SIRS), the NIH stroke scale (NIHSS), and death not otherwise specified (NOS). Additional OGCR related to symptoms, signs, and abnormal findings appear in OGCR I.B.4, 5, and 6; II.A and II.E; and IV.D and IV.H. Specific OGCR are discussed and cited throughout this chapter.

Review the instructional notes at the beginning of the chapter that discuss how coders should report codes in this chapter. Also review the **Excludes2** note, which lists several conditions not classified to this chapter. Frequent instructional notes throughout the chapter direct coders to use multiple codes to describe related or underlying conditions associated with various symptoms. The subcategory for **Coma (R40.2-)** requires coders to assign a seventh character to identify the Glasgow Coma Scale rating.

ABSTRACTING SYMPTOMS AND SIGNS

Abstracting requires coders to be knowledgeable of disease processes and the related symptoms, signs, abnormal clinical findings, and abnormal laboratory test results so they can distinguish which elements should be coded and which should not. They also must distinguish when a physician makes a confirmed diagnosis, in contrast to when the diagnosis is uncertain, because different coding rules apply to these situations.

■ TABLE 4-3 highlights key questions to answer when reviewing the medical record. Coders use answers to these questions when assigning and sequencing codes. Remember that the

Table 4-3 ■ **KEY CRITERIA FOR ABSTRACTING SYMPTOMS, SIGNS, ABNORMAL FINDINGS, AND CONFIRMED CONDITIONS**

❏ What symptoms does the patient report?

❏ What signs does the physician document?

❏ What abnormal laboratory findings are reviewed?

❏ What confirmed diagnoses are documented?

❏ What diagnoses are identified as uncertain with words such as *possible, probable, rule out, suspected*?

❏ Which symptoms, signs, and abnormal findings are integral to the condition?

❏ Which symptoms, signs, and abnormal findings are related but not integral to the condition?

❏ Which symptoms, signs, and abnormal findings are unrelated to the condition?

abstracting questions are a guide and that not every question applies to, or can be answered for, every case. For example, not all patients have abnormal laboratory findings. Details that will help answer these questions follow in the remainder of this section of the chapter.

Integral, Related, and Unrelated Findings

Coders must distinguish between symptoms, signs, and abnormal findings that are an **integral** (*routine*) part of a disease process, those that are **related** (*a symptom, finding, or sign connected to a disease but not routinely associated with it*) but not integral, and those that are **unrelated** (*a symptom, sign, or abnormal finding not connected to a disease*). They need a solid understanding of common conditions and their symptoms so they can make these distinctions. Refer to ■ TABLE 4-4 to review symptoms, signs, and abnormal findings for commonly diagnosed conditions.

Table 4-4 ■ **SYMPTOMS, SIGNS, AND ABNORMAL FINDINGS FOR COMMONLY DIAGNOSED CONDITIONS**

Condition	Symptoms and Signs	Abnormal Findings
Allergic contact dermatitis	Rash, erythema, pruritus, burning	
Anemia	Fatigue, shortness of breath (SOB), decreased exercise tolerance	Folic acid
Appendicitis	Right lower quadrant (RLQ) pain, fever, nausea, vomiting	
Asthma	Dyspnea, difficulty exhaling, wheezing	
Benign prostatic hyperplasia (BPH)	Nocturia, polyuria, dysuria, oliguria	
Cerebrovascular accident (CVA)	Headache, muscular weakness, speech disturbance, loss of consciousness	Angiography, computerized tomography (CT) scan, magnetic resonance imaging (MRI)
Colorectal cancer	Melena, change in bowel habits, lower abdominal pain	Biopsy, colonoscopy
Congestive heart failure (CHF)	SOB, fatigue, edema	Electrocardiogram (ECG, EKG), echocardiogram (ECC), blood pressure (BP), x-ray
Dementia	Language, memory, and mood deficits	
Depression	Prolonged sadness, sleep and appetite changes, feelings of guilt and anxiety	
Diabetes mellitus (DM)	Polyuria, polydipsia	Hyperglycemia, elevated glucose, elevated HbA1C (*glycated hemoglobin—a blood test to identify 90-day levels of glucose*)
Endometriosis	Pelvic pain, diarrhea, constipation, menorrhagia, fatigue	
Epilepsy	Convulsions, seizures	Electroencephalogram (EEG)
Gastroenteritis	Nausea, vomiting, diarrhea, abdominal pain	Stool culture
Gout	Joint pain, heat, swelling, redness	
Hiatal hernia	Indigestion, heartburn, acid reflux, esophagitis	
Hypercholesterolemia	Asymptomatic (*without symptoms*)	Elevated serum cholesterol
Hypertension (HTN)	Asymptomatic	Elevated blood pressure
Leukemia	Fatigue, weight loss, fever, hemorrhages	Blood tests
Osteoarthritis (OA)	Joint pain and stiffness, muscle weakness, enlarged joints	X-ray
Pneumonia	Chest pain, fluid in lungs, fever, productive cough	X-ray
Rosacea	Flushing, persistent erythema, papules pustules, telangiectasia	
Urinary tract infection (UTI)	Polyuria, dysuria, hematuria	Urinalysis

Integral Symptoms

When a diagnosis is confirmed, assign codes to the named condition, but do *not* assign codes for the symptoms, signs, and abnormal findings that are integral to the condition (OGCR I.B.4 and 5; I.C.18.a). Integral or routine symptoms are those that most patients with the condition experience.

EXAMPLE: The physician documents *fever and RLQ pain due to acute ruptured appendicitis*. Fever and pain are symptoms integral to a ruptured appendix, so the coder assigns a code only for the appendicitis. Do *not* assign codes for fever and pain.

Do not code clinical findings that are integral to the condition.

EXAMPLE: The physician documents *three elevated BP readings over the past three months. Hypertension*. The coder assigns a code for hypertension, but not for elevated blood pressure, because a series of elevated blood pressure readings is the definition of hypertension.

Do not code laboratory test results that are integral to the condition.

EXAMPLE: The physician documents *elevated glucose HbA1C results, type 2 diabetes*. The coder assigns a code for type 2 diabetes, but not for elevated glucose or HbA1C because those tests are used to establish the diagnosis.

Do code for the symptoms, signs, abnormal clinical findings, or abnormal test results when a diagnosis is not stated.

EXAMPLE: The physician documents *three elevated BP readings over the past three months*. The coder assigns a code for elevated blood pressure, but not hypertension, because the physician did not document hypertension as a diagnosis.

EXAMPLE: The physician documents *elevated glucose HbA1C results. Refer to dietician for meal plan*. The coder assigns a code for elevated glucose, but not diabetes, because the physician did not document diabetes as a diagnosis. Coders should not assign a diagnosis that is not documented.

Related Symptoms

Do code for symptoms that are related to the disease process but not integral to it (OGCR I.B.6). Related symptoms are those that patients occasionally experience with the confirmed diagnosis but are not common or routine.

EXAMPLE: The physician documents *RLQ pain, fever, vomiting, dehydration due to acute ruptured appendicitis. Administered IV fluids*. Dehydration is the result of the fever and vomiting associated with appendicitis but is not a routine part of the condition. Additional treatment was provided for the dehydration. Therefore, assign a code for dehydration in addition to ruptured appendicitis.

Unrelated Symptoms

Do code for symptoms that are unrelated to the confirmed diagnosis (OGCR I.C.18.b). Unrelated symptoms are those that are not associated with the confirmed diagnosis and may indicate an additional problem or condition.

EXAMPLE: The physician documents *fever, difficulty breathing, hemoptysis, x-ray positive for pneumonia, sputum culture for hemoptysis*. Fever and difficulty breathing are integral to pneumonia, which the physician confirmed with a chest x-ray. Hemoptysis is not a symptom associated with pneumonia, so it should be coded in addition to pneumonia.

SUCCESS STEP

Be proactive and keep a reference book on diseases on your desk so you can consult it when you are unsure if a symptom is integral, related, or unrelated. Consider creating "tip sheets" with notes on conditions commonly coded in your office to guide you through the learning process. If you are unsure about a symptom, consult a colleague or supervisor; do not guess.

Uncertain Diagnoses

When physicians cannot establish a definite diagnosis, outpatient coders assign codes for the symptoms, signs, and abnormal findings until a diagnosis is established (OGCR IV.H). Coders must interpret the terms physicians use in documentation in order to understand whether a diagnosis is confirmed or uncertain. An uncertain diagnosis is one that the physician is not completely confident of. Particularly in the outpatient setting, physicians may require multiple visits, consultation with a specialist, and test results in order to determine a diagnosis. Coders assign codes for symptoms until the diagnosis is established. After the diagnosis is established, they no longer code the symptoms that are integral to the condition.

By default, interpret any diagnostic statement as **confirmed**, one the physician is confident of, *unless* the physician indicates it is uncertain. A diagnosis may be uncertain when a patient has symptoms and signs that can be attributed to many different conditions or when test results do not provide clear data. An uncertain diagnostic statement contains **qualifiers** or **modifiers** *(word(s) that limit the meaning of another)* before the name of the condition (■ TABLE 4-5).

Table 4-5 ■ **TERMS INDICATING UNCERTAIN DIAGNOSES**

❏ likely	❏ rule out (R/O)
❏ possible	❏ still to be ruled out
❏ probable	❏ suspected
❏ questionable	

An uncertain diagnosis is also called a **qualified** diagnosis. The words *qualified* and *qualifier* have two opposite meanings. One common meaning is *meeting a standard or set of criteria*. An alternative meaning is one of *limiting or restricting*. When coders and physicians use the expression *qualified diagnosis*, they are using the second meaning of the word, a *diagnosis that is limited or uncertain*.

Physicians may use the description **impression** in their progress notes for the diagnostic statement. The word *impression* also carries multiple meanings, which sometimes causes confusion for new coders. One meaning is *an idea or belief that is vague or unclear*. Physicians use an alternate meaning, *an effect produced on the mind by outside stimuli*. Therefore, use of the word *impression* does not describe an uncertain diagnosis.

In the outpatient setting, do not assign a code to an uncertain diagnosis. Instead, code the symptoms, signs, and abnormal test results documented by the physician (OGCR IV.D and H). In the inpatient setting, when the diagnosis documented at the time of discharge is stated as uncertain, code the condition as if it existed (OGCR III.A and IV.H). The rationale for this guideline is that the diagnostic workup, arrangements for further workups, and initial treatments provided must relate to the principal diagnosis.

Abnormal Clinical and Laboratory Findings

When coding inpatient services, abstract abnormal clinical and laboratory findings *only* when the provider documents their clinical significance. Do not automatically abstract and code all findings that are outside the normal range. In rare cases, the provider may order additional tests to further evaluate abnormal findings, or prescribe a treatment, but not document their clinical significance. In this situation, coders should query the provider regarding the possible significance of the findings (OGCR III.B).

Guided Example of Abstracting Symptoms and Signs

Refer to the following example to learn more about abstracting symptoms, signs, and abnormal findings. Sherry Whittle, CPC, is a fictitious coder who guides you through this case.

Date: 6/1/yy Location: Branton Family Practice
Provider: Kristen Conover, MD
Patient: Chad Wang   Gender: M   Age: 6
Chief Complaint: Nausea, vomiting, and diarrhea
Assessment: Gastroenteritis
Plan: Bed rest and plenty of fluids

Follow along as Sherry Whittle, CPC, reviews the medical record and abstracts the diagnosis. Check off each step after you complete it.

▶ Sherry begins by referring to Key Criteria for Abstracting Symptoms, Signs, Abnormal Findings, and Confirmed Conditions (Table 4-3).

❏ *What symptoms does the patient report?* Nausea, vomiting, and diarrhea

❏ *What signs does the physician document?* None

❏ *What abnormal laboratory findings are reviewed?* None

❏ *What confirmed diagnoses are documented?* Gastroenteritis

❏ *What diagnoses are identified as uncertain with words such as* possible, probable, rule out, suspected? None

❏ *Which symptoms, signs, and abnormal findings are integral to the condition?* All

❏ *Which symptoms, signs, and abnormal findings are related but not integral to the condition?* None

❏ *Which symptoms, signs, and abnormal findings are unrelated to the condition?* None

▶ Because the symptoms of nausea, vomiting, and diarrhea are all integral to gastroenteritis, Sherry does not abstract these items to code.

❏ The only diagnosis code to be assigned is gastroenteritis. (You will learn how to do this when you study the digestive system.)

CODING PRACTICE

| Exercise 4.2 | Abstracting Symptoms and Signs |

Instructions: Read the mini-medical-record of each patient's encounter and answer the abstracting questions. Write the answer on the line provided. Do not assign any codes.

1. OFFICE   Gender: M   Age: 61

Reason for encounter: Review result of liver function study

Assessment: Abnormal liver function test *(continued)*

1. (continued)

Plan: Biopsy

a. Does the physician state a confirmed diagnosis?

_____

b. Is this a sign, a symptom, an abnormal clinical finding, or an abnormal laboratory test?

_____

c. What Main Term will you look up in the Index?

_____

(continued)

CODING PRACTICE *(continued)*

2. INPATIENT HOSPITAL   Gender: M **Age:** 74

Reason for admission: Irregular heartbeat, chest pain, and lightheadedness

Assessment: Atrial fibrillation

Plan: Cardiologist evaluation

Tip: Do not code symptoms that are integral to a confirmed condition.

a. What symptoms and signs are mentioned?
_____

b. Does the physician state a confirmed diagnosis?
_____

c. Are all of the symptoms and signs integral to the diagnosis? _____

d. Which symptoms and signs should be coded?
_____

e. What condition will you code? _____
_____

---

3. INPATIENT HOSPITAL   Gender: F **Age:** 16

Reason for admission: Repeated seizures

Assessment: Seizures of unknown cause

Plan: Continued follow-up with neurologist, medication

a. Does the physician state a confirmed diagnosis?
_____

b. What symptom should be coded? _____
_____

c. What is the Main Term? _____

---

4. OFFICE   Gender: F **Age:** 45

Chief complaint: Polydipsia, polyuria, and difficulty sleeping, most recent blood test showed hyperglycemia

Assessment: Type 2 diabetes, possible sleep apnea

Plan: Evaluate for sleep apnea

a. What symptoms and signs are mentioned? _____
_____

b. Does the physician state a confirmed diagnosis?
_____ What is it? _____

c. Does the physician state an uncertain diagnosis?
_____ What is it? _____

(continued)

---

4. (continued)

d. Should you code an uncertain diagnosis for an outpatient encounter? _____ What should you code instead?_____

e. Which symptoms and signs are integral to the confirmed diagnosis? _____

f. Which symptoms and signs relate to the unconfirmed diagnosis? _____

g. What two conditions/symptoms will you code?
_____

---

5. OFFICE   Gender: M **Age:** 29

Chief complaint: Extreme nervousness and irritability

Assessment: R/O hyperthyroidism

Plan: Thyroid workup

a. What symptoms and signs are mentioned?
_____

b. What does R/O (rule out) mean? _____
_____

c. Does the physician state a confirmed diagnosis?
_____

d. Does the physician state an uncertain diagnosis?
_____ What is it? _____

e. What two conditions/symptoms will you code?
_____

---

6. INPATIENT HOSPITAL   Gender: M **Age:** 52

Reason for admission: Abdominal pain

Discharge diagnosis: Epigastric pain due to acute pancreatitis or cholangitis *(inflammation of the common bile duct)*

Plan: Pain medication, antibiotics as precaution, further imaging

Tip: This is a hospital discharge, so inpatient OGCR applies.

a. What symptoms and signs are mentioned? _____
_____

b. Does the physician state a confirmed diagnosis?
_____

c. What alternative or comparative diagnoses does the physician document? _____

ASSIGNING CODES FOR SYMPTOMS AND SIGNS

The most challenging aspect of coding for symptoms, signs, and abnormal findings is distinguishing integral, related, and unrelated symptoms and distinguishing confirmed and uncertain diagnoses. After this is accomplished, assigning codes is relatively straightforward. The Main Term for many symptoms and signs codes is the name of the symptom or sign. Combination codes also exist for definitive diagnoses and certain related symptoms. Coding for abnormal test results can be more challenging and is discussed later in this section.

The physician's diagnosis stands on its own. Coders do not assign codes to symptoms to justify why the physician arrived at the diagnosis. Assign codes for the symptoms only if the diagnosis is not confirmed. When the diagnosis is confirmed, code only the diagnosis, not the symptoms (OGCR I.A.19).

Codes for Symptoms and Signs

Main Term entries for most symptoms and signs in the Index are often the name of the symptom or sign, such as pain, fever, vomiting, or weakness. Review the subterms carefully for anatomic sites or other descriptions of the condition. If none of the specific subterms apply, use the default code immediately following the Main Term.

Refer to the Main Term **Fever** in the ICD-10-CM Index (■ FIGURE 4-1). The default code is **R50.9**. More than 200 subterms describe specific types or causes of fever. When a subterm applies, verify and assign the code listed with the subterm. When no subterm applies, verify and assign the default code.

> ### SUCCESS STEP
>
> When you code for an uncertain diagnosis in an inpatient setting, assign the usual code for the condition. Do not assign any additional codes to indicate it is uncertain.

Combination Codes

Do use combination codes when available. ICD-10-CM contains combination codes that identify both the definitive diagnosis and certain related symptoms. When using this kind of combination code, do not assign an additional code for the related symptom.

EXAMPLE: The physician documents *Type 2 diabetes with gastroparesis*. ICD-10-CM provides an entry in the Index for **Diabetes, with gastroparesis E11.43**. Use the combination code and do not assign a separate code for gastroparesis.

Codes for Abnormal Findings

Physicians may receive test results from the laboratory that are abnormal, but they are still unable to establish a firm diagnosis. In this situation, coders assign codes for the abnormal test result (■ FIGURE 4-2). To locate the Main Term for abnormal clinical and laboratory findings, identify the word in the diagnostic statement that describes how the result differs from normal. Refer to ■ TABLE 4-6, page 70 for commonly used Main Terms and examples of subterm entries. Also be alert for instructional notes and cross-references in the Index that may lead to alternative entries.

Fever (inanition) (of unknown origin) (persistent) (with chills) (with rigor) R50.9
   abortus A23.1
   Aden (dengue) A90
   African tick-borne A68.1
   American
      mountain (tick) A93.2
      spotted A77.0
   aphthous B08.8
   arbovirus, arboviral A94

Figure 4-1 ■ Example of Index entry for a sign ("Fever") with subterms.

Codes for SIRS Due to Noninfectious Process

The **systemic inflammatory response syndrome (SIRS)** (*a complex inflammatory state affecting the whole body*) can develop as a result of both infectious and noninfectious processes. For example, trauma, malignant neoplasm, or pancreatitis can give rise to SIRS even though no infectious process is documented. First assign a code for the underlying condition, followed by code **R65.10 Systemic inflammatory response syndrome (SIRS) of non-infectious origin without acute organ dysfunction** or code **R65.11 Systemic inflammatory response syndrome (SIRS) of non-infectious origin with acute organ dysfunction**. When an associated acute organ dysfunction is documented, assign a code for the specific type of organ dysfunction (OGCR I.C.18.g). Locate codes for SIRS in the Index under the Main Term **Syndrome**, then the subterm **systemic inflammatory response syndrome (SIRS)**.

SIRS due to an infectious process, sepsis, and septic shock are discussed in Chapter 20, "Certain Infectious and Parasitic Diseases (A00–B99)," of this text.

Glasgow Coma Scale Codes

ICD-10-CM provides codes for rating the severity of a coma, a state of unconsciousness from which the patient cannot be aroused. The **Glasgow Coma Scale** is a standardized system for

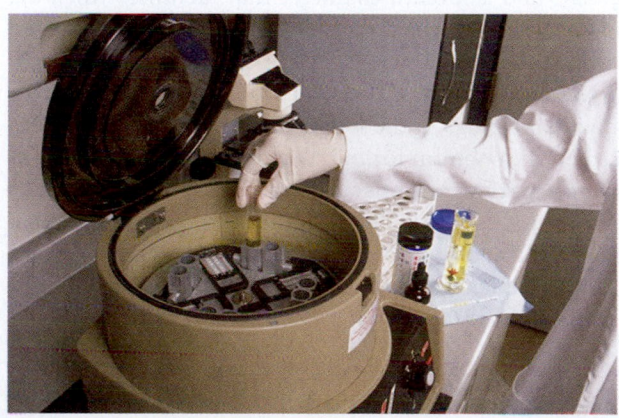

Figure 4-2 ■ Laboratory technician performing a urinalysis test.
Source: Michal Heron/Pearson Education/PH College.

Table 4-6 ■ **MAIN TERMS COMMONLY USED FOR ABNORMAL FINDINGS**

Main Term	Diagnostic Statement Examples	Index Entry Examples
Abnormal	Abnormal liver function test	Abnormal, function studies, liver
	Abnormal hemoglobin in urine	Abnormal, urine, hemoglobin
Anomaly	Heart auricle anomaly	Anomaly, heart, auricle
	Hip anomaly	Anomaly, hip, NEC
Deficiency	Low growth hormone	Deficiency, hormone, growth
	Vitamin D deficiency	Deficiency, vitamin D
Elevated	High fasting glucose	Elevated, fasting glucose
	Elevated blood pressure	Elevated, blood pressure
Findings, abnormal, inconclusive, without diagnosis	Lead in blood	Findings, in blood, lead
	Abnormal urine glucose	Findings, urine, glucose
Loss	Transient loss of consciousness	Loss, consciousness, transient

assessing the level of consciousness of patients with an acute brain injury. Reactions to specific stimuli are reported using a numerical value in three categories: eye opening, verbal responsiveness, and motor responsiveness. The three scores are then added together. The lowest values are the worst clinical scores. (For more information about the Glasgow Coma Scale, refer to www.glasglowcomascale.org.)

Codes in the subcategory **R40.2- Coma** report the level of responsiveness in each category, as well as the total score. These codes are intended primarily for use by trauma registries (*state and national reporting systems that collect data on seriously injured patients*), but can be reported by any setting where this information is collected. OGCR I.C.18.e explains that they can be used in conjunction with traumatic brain injury, acute cerebrovascular disease, and sequelae of cerebrovascular disease, as well to assess the status of the central nervous systems for nontraumatic conditions, such as monitoring in the intensive care unit.

Three codes are required to report the Glasgow Coma Scale assessment:

- **R40.21- Coma scale, eyes open**
- **R40.22- Coma scale, best verbal response**
- **R40.23- Coma scale, best motor response**

Each code requires a sixth character that identifies the level of response and a seventh character that identifies when the assessment was performed. If the total score is documented in the medical record, report it using a code from subcategory **R40.24 Glasgow Coma Scale, total score**. To locate codes for the individual ratings in the Index, search for the Main Term **Coma**, then the subterm for the specific rating, such as **opening of eyes**, **verbal response**, or **motor response**. To locate codes for the total score in the Index, search for the Main Term **Glasgow coma scale**. Codes for the coma scale are secondary codes, to be sequenced after the principal or first-listed diagnosis, such as those for a skull fracture or intracranial injury.

EXAMPLE: An unconscious patient who fell off scaffolding at a construction site is seen in the emergency department. The patient's level of responsiveness is assessed upon arrival:

- Eye opening—None (1 point)
- Verbal response—None (1 point)
- Best motor response—Extension (2 points)
- Total score—4 points

The coder assigns the following codes for the Glasgow Coma Scale:

- **R40.2112 Coma scale, eyes open, never, at arrival to emergency department**
- **R40.2212 Coma scale, best verbal response, none, at arrival to emergency department**
- **R40.2322 Coma scale, best motor response, extension, at arrival to emergency department**
- **R40.2432 Glasgow coma scale score 3-8, at arrival to emergency department**

In addition, the coder assigns codes for the diagnosis, such as traumatic brain injury, any other injuries, and the cause of the fall.

National Institutes of Health Stroke Scale Codes

Patients who have experienced a cerebral infarction (**I63.-**) can be evaluated using the **National Institutes of Health Stroke Scale (NIHSS)**. The NIHSS is a 15-item neurologic examination stroke scale used to evaluate the effect of acute cerebral infarction in several areas: levels of consciousness, language, neglect, visual-field loss, extraocular movement, motor strength, ataxia, dysarthria, and sensory loss. Ratings for each item are scored by a trained observer using 3 to 5 scoring levels, with a score of 0 as normal. There is an allowance for untestable items. For more information on the NIHSS, refer to www.nihstrokescale.org.

ICD-10-CM provides codes in the subcategory **R29.7- National Institutes of Health Stroke Scale** to report the patient's score. Report one code from the range **R29.700** to **R29.742** that identifies the patient's total score. To locate codes in the Index, search for the Main Term **NIHSS**. These are secondary codes, to be reported after the code that identifies the type of cerebral infarction (OGCR I.C.18.i).

Guided Example of Assigning Codes for Symptoms and Signs

Refer to the following example to learn how to assign codes for symptoms. This case is similar to the earlier example of Chad Wang, who was seen for nausea, vomiting, and diarrhea and was diagnosed with gastroenteritis. However, notice how this example should be coded differently based on the wording of the Assessment.

Date: 6/1/yy   Location: Branton Family Practice

Provider: Kristen Conover, MD

Patient: Charlene Winger   Gender: F   Age: 15

Chief Complaint: Nausea, vomiting, and diarrhea

Assessment: Suspected gastroenteritis

Plan: Stool culture, bedrest, and plenty of fluids

Follow along as Sherry Whittle, CPC, assigns codes for nausea, vomiting, and diarrhea. Check off each step as you complete it.

▶ First, Sherry abstracts the case.

❑ She reads the presenting symptoms *nausea, vomiting, and diarrhea*.

❑ She reads the Assessment *suspected gastroenteritis*.

❑ She notes that "suspected" makes gastroenteritis an uncertain diagnosis.

❑ As a result, she identifies the three symptoms—nausea, vomiting, and diarrhea—to code and does not code gastroenteritis.

▶ Sherry searches the Index for the Main Term **Nausea** (■ Figure 4-3).

❑ She reads the nonessential modifier **(without vomiting)**, which is the default for code R11.0.

❑ She locates the subterm **with vomiting, R11.2**, which provides a combination code for two of the symptoms of this patient.

▶ Sherry verifies code **R11.2** in the Tabular List.

❑ She reads the code title for **R11.2 Nausea with vomiting, unspecified** and confirms that this accurately describes the symptoms.

Nausea (without vomiting) R11.0
   with vomiting R11.2
    gravidarum — *see* Hyperemesis, gravidarum
    marina T75.3
    navalis T75.3

Figure 4-3 ■ Index entry for "Nausea, with vomiting."

▶ Sherry checks for instructional notes in the Tabular List.

❑ She cross-references the beginning of category **R11** and reads the **Excludes1** instructional note. None of the conditions listed describe the patient, so she may proceed.

❑ She cross-references the beginning of the block **R10-R19** and reads the **Excludes1** instructional note. None of the conditions listed describe the patient, so she may proceed.

❑ She cross-references the beginning of **Chapter 18 (R00-R99)** and reads the detailed instructional notes. She determines that note **(e) cases in which a more precise diagnosis was not available** describes this case and that she is coding correctly.

▶ Next, Sherry searches the Index for the Main Term **Diarrhea**.

❑ She reads through all of the available subterms but finds none that apply. She checks the documentation to confirm that the diarrhea is not stated as either viral or bacterial. It is not, and that is likely the reason a stool culture was obtained.

❑ She selects the default entry **Diarrhea, diarrheal (disease) (infantile) (inflammatory) R19.7**.

▶ Sherry verifies code **R19.7** in the Tabular List.

❑ She reads the code title for **R19.7 Diarrhea, unspecified** and confirms that this accurately describes the symptom because more detailed information is not provided in the medical record.

❑ She reads the **Excludes1** instructional note under code **R19.7**, which states **Excludes1: functional diarrhea (K59.1), neonatal diarrhea (P78.3), psychogenic diarrhea (F45.8)**. The documentation does not describe any of these types of diarrhea, so she knows her code is correct and can continue.

▶ Sherry checks for instructional notes in the Tabular List.

❑ She cross-references the beginning of category **R19** and identifies the instructional note **Excludes1: acute abdomen (R10.0)**. This does not describe the patient's symptoms so she knows she can proceed.

❑ She cross-references the beginning of the block **R10-R19** and chapter in the previous step and verifies that there are no notes that would change the code she selected.

▶ Sherry reviews the codes she has assigned for this case.

❑ **R11.2 Nausea with vomiting, unspecified**

❑ **R19.7 Diarrhea, unspecified**

▶ Next, Sherry must determine how to sequence the codes.

CODING PRACTICE

Exercise 4.3 Assigning Codes for Symptoms and Signs

Instructions: Read the mini-medical-record of each patient's encounter, review the information abstracted in Exercise 4.2, and assign ICD-10-CM diagnosis codes using the Index and Tabular List. Write the code(s) on the line provided.

1. OFFICE   Gender: M   Age: 61

Reason for encounter: Review result of liver function study

Assessment: Abnormal liver function test

Plan: Biopsy

1 ICD-10-CM Code _____

2. INPATIENT HOSPITAL   Gender: M   Age: 74

Reason for admission: Irregular heartbeat, chest pain, and lightheadedness

Assessment: Atrial fibrillation

Plan: Cardiologist evaluation

Tip: Do not code symptoms that are integral to a confirmed condition.

1 ICD-10-CM Code _____

3. INPATIENT HOSPITAL   Gender: F   Age: 16

Reason for admission: Repeated seizures

Assessment: Seizures of unknown cause

Plan: Continued follow-up with neurologist, medication

1 ICD-10-CM Code _____

ARRANGING CODES FOR SYMPTOMS AND SIGNS

In general, multiple codes for symptoms, signs, and abnormal findings are sequenced using the same guidelines as any other codes. Special situations include coding for a confirmed diagnosis and related symptoms, coding for a confirmed diagnosis and unrelated symptoms, coding symptoms followed by a diagnosis, and coding symptoms with no confirmed diagnosis. These are discussed next.

Confirmed Diagnosis and Related Symptoms

The physician may document a confirmed diagnosis and a symptom, sign, or abnormal finding that is related but not integral. Sequence the confirmed diagnosis first, followed by the related symptom (■ FIGURE 4-4).

Confirmed Diagnosis and Unrelated Symptoms

The physician may document a confirmed diagnosis and an unrelated symptom, sign, or abnormal finding. Sequence the code chiefly responsible for the services provided first. When both the confirmed diagnosis and the unrelated symptom are equally responsible, sequence either code first (■ FIGURE 4-5).

Symptoms with No Confirmed Diagnosis

The physician may document only symptoms, signs, and abnormal findings and no confirmed diagnosis. Assign the main reason for the encounter as the principal or first-listed diagnosis. When more than one symptom is equally responsible for the encounter, sequence either code first.

Patient seen for RLQ pain, fever, vomiting, dehydration due to acute ruptured appendicitis. Administered IV fluids.

(1) **K35.2 Acute ruptured appendicitis with generalized peritonitis**
(2) **E86.0 Dehydration**

Figure 4-4 ■ Example of sequencing for confirmed diagnosis and related symptom.

Patient c/o of fever, difficulty breathing, hemoptysis. X-ray is positive for pneumonia. Sputum culture is ordered for hemoptysis.

(1) **J18.9 Pneumonia**
(2) **R04.2 Hemoptysis**

Figure 4-5 ■ Example of sequencing for a confirmed diagnosis and unrelated symptom.

Guided Example of Arranging Symptoms and Signs Codes

To practice skills for sequencing codes for symptoms and signs, continue with the example from earlier in the chapter about patient Charlene Winger, who was seen for symptoms of nausea, vomiting, and diarrhea, with no confirmed diagnosis.

Follow along in your ICD-10-CM manual as Sherry Whittle, CPC, sequences the codes. Check off each step after you complete it.

▶ First, Sherry confirms the diagnosis codes she assigned.

❑ **R11.2 Nausea with vomiting, unspecified**

❑ **R19.7 Diarrhea, unspecified**

▶ Sherry determines that the physician documented only symptoms but no confirmed diagnosis.

❑ The documentation does not state that one symptom was chiefly responsible for the encounter.

❑ Therefore, either diagnosis may be sequenced first.

▶ Sherry finalizes the codes and sequencing for this case:

(1) **R11.2 Nausea with vomiting, unspecified**

(2) **R19.7 Diarrhea, unspecified**

CODING PRACTICE

Exercise 4.4   Arranging Codes for Symptoms and Signs

Instructions: Read the mini-medical-record of each patient's encounter, review the information abstracted in Exercise 4.2, assign ICD-10-CM diagnosis codes using the Index and Tabular List, and arrange the codes in proper sequence. Write the code(s) on the line provided.

---

1. OFFICE   Gender: F   Age: 45

Chief complaint: Polydipsia, polyuria, and difficulty sleeping, most recent blood test showed hyperglycemia

Assessment: Type 2 diabetes, possible sleep apnea

Plan: Evaluate for sleep apnea

Tip: Determine which symptoms are integral to diabetes and which one is unrelated.

2 ICD-10-CM Codes _____

---

2. OFFICE   Gender: M   Age: 29

Chief complaint: Extreme nervousness and irritability

Assessment: R/O hyperthyroidism

Plan: Thyroid workup

Tip: A condition described as "rule out" means it is uncertain.

2 ICD-10-CM Codes _____

---

3. INPATIENT HOSPITAL   Gender: M   Age: 52

Reason for admission: Abdominal pain

Discharge diagnosis: Epigastric pain due to acute pancreatitis or cholangitis (*inflammation or infection of the common bile duct*)

Plan: Pain medication, antibiotics as precaution, further imaging

Tip: Because this is a hospital discharge, follow inpatient OCGR.

3 ICD-10-CM Codes _____
_____

CHAPTER SUMMARY

In this chapter you learned that:

- Sometimes a confirmed diagnosis is not possible because the physician needs multiple encounters, extended testing, evaluation by specialists, surgery, or other procedures to arrive at a diagnosis.

- ICD-10-CM Chapter 18, "Symptoms, Signs, and Abnormal Clinical and Laboratory Findings, Not Elsewhere Classified (R00-R99)," includes symptoms, signs, and abnormal results of clinical and laboratory procedures. It also includes ill-defined conditions that do not fit anywhere else in ICD-10-CM or that can be indicative of multiple conditions.

- The OGCR provides a detailed discussion of when to report and not report codes from this chapter. It also discusses coding of symptoms and signs related to several specific conditions that coders should be familiar with.

- Abstracting requires coders to be knowledgeable of disease processes and the related symptoms, signs, abnormal clinical findings, and abnormal laboratory test results so they can distinguish which elements should be coded and which should not.

- The Main Term for many symptoms and signs codes is the name of the symptom or sign. Coding for abnormal test results can be more challenging.

- In general, multiple codes for symptoms, signs, and abnormal findings are sequenced using the same guidelines as any other codes, but a few special situations exist.

CONCEPT QUIZ

Take a moment to look back at symptoms, signs, and abnormal findings and solidify your skills. This is your opportunity to pull together everything you have learned.

Completion

Instructions: Write the term that completes each statement based on the information you learned in this chapter. Choose from the following list. Some choices may be used more than once and some choices may not be used at all.

abnormal	outpatient
clinical	related
confirmed	sign
finding	symptom
inpatient	uncertain
integral	unrelated
laboratory	

1. A (an) _____ is the subjective evidence of a disease or condition, usually reported by the patient.

2. A (an) _____ symptom is a routine part of the disease process.

3. A (an) _____ diagnosis is also called a qualified diagnosis.

4. An abnormal _____ finding is evidence of a disease or condition discovered through physical examination.

5. A (an) _____ is objective evidence of a disease or condition that can be observed by the physician.

6. _____ symptoms are those that patients occasionally experience with the confirmed diagnosis but are not common or routine.

7. A (an) _____ diagnosis might be documented as *rule out*, *suspected*, and *likely*.

8. _____ symptoms are those that are not caused by the confirmed diagnosis and may indicate an additional problem or condition.

9. A (an) _____ laboratory test result is outside of the normal reference range.

10. In the _____ setting, if the diagnosis documented at the time of discharge is uncertain, code the condition as if it existed.

Multiple Choice

Instructions: Circle the letter of the best answer to each question based on the information you learned in this chapter.

1. Which of the following is an example of a symptom?
   A. Nausea
   B. Vomiting
   C. Bleeding
   D. Fever

2. Which of the following is an example of an abnormal clinical finding?
   A. Elevated glucose
   B. Bleeding
   C. Irregular EKG
   D. Microscopic dysplasia

3. How would you code the following scenario? *Patient presents with nausea, vomiting, and diarrhea. Suspected gastroenteritis.*
   A. R11.0, R11.1, R19.5
   B. R11.2, R19.7
   C. K29.0
   D. K29.7, R11.2, R19.7

4. Which of the following conditions are asymptomatic?
   A. Osteoarthritis
   B. Hypertension
   C. Gastroenteritis
   D. Anemia

5. What Main Term should be referenced in the Index to locate the code for *best verbal response* on the Glasgow Coma Scale?
   A. Glasgow
   B. coma
   C. verbal
   D. response

6. When should an uncertain diagnosis be coded as though it existed?
   A. Inpatient setting
   B. Outpatient setting
   C. Emergency department
   D. Never

7. How would you code the following scenario? *A patient is seen for RLQ pain, fever, vomiting, dehydration due to acute ruptured appendicitis.*
   A. K35.2, E86.0
   B. K35.2
   C. K35.2, R11.1, R50.9
   D. E86.0, R11.1, R50.9

8. Which term indicates an uncertain diagnosis?
   A. Confirmed
   B. Integral
   C. Verified
   D. Rule out

9. Why might a physician be unable to document a confirmed diagnosis?
   A. Additional testing is necessary
   B. The code is difficult to locate
   C. The patient has multiple symptoms
   D. The OGCR is unclear

10. How would you code the following scenario? *Patient complains of fever, difficulty breathing, hemoptysis. X-ray is positive for pneumonia. Sputum culture is ordered for hemoptysis.*
    A. R06.02, R04.2, J18.9
    B. R50.9, R04.2, R06.02
    C. J18.9
    D. J18.9, R04.2

KEEP ON CODING

Instructions: Read the diagnostic statement, then use the Index and Tabular List to assign and sequence ICD-10-CM diagnosis codes. Write the code(s) on the line provided.

1. Right lower quadrant rebound abdominal tenderness. ICD-10-CM Code(s) _____

2. Nonvisualization of gallbladder. ICD-10-CM Code(s) _____

3. Heartburn. ICD-10-CM Code(s) _____

4. Absent bowel sounds. ICD-10-CM Code(s) _____

5. Slow heartbeat. ICD-10-CM Code(s) _____

6. Overactivity. ICD-10-CM Code(s) _____

7. Auditory hallucinations. ICD-10-CM Code(s) _____

8. Nosebleed. ICD-10-CM Code(s) _____

9. Shortness of breath. ICD-10-CM Code(s) _____

10. SIRS due to pancreatitis. ICD-10-CM Code(s) _____

11. Excessive sweating. ICD-10-CM Code(s) _____

12. Late walker. ICD-10-CM Code(s) _____

13. Change in bowel habits. ICD-10-CM Code(s) _____

14. Heart murmur. ICD-10-CM Code(s) _____

15. Glasgow Coma Scale rating performed at hospital admission with eye opening—to pain; best verbal response—inappropriate words; best motor response—flexion withdrawal; with a total score of 9. ICD-10-CM Code(s) _____

16. Finding of cocaine in blood. ICD-10-CM Code(s) _____

17. Age-related cognitive decline. ICD-10-CM Code(s) _____

18. Intermittent urinary stream. ICD-10-CM Code(s) _____

19. Hoarseness. ICD-10-CM Code(s) _____

20. Abnormal blood-gas level. ICD-10-CM Code(s) _____

21. Respiratory arrest. ICD-10-CM Code(s) _____

22. Unsteadiness on feet. ICD-10-CM Code(s) _____

23. Abnormal liver scan. ICD-10-CM Code(s) _____

24. Failure to gain weight, 2-month-old child. ICD-10-CM Code(s) _____

25. Febrile seizures, simple. ICD-10-CM Code(s) _____

CODING CHALLENGE

Instructions: Read the mini-medical-record of each patient's encounter, then abstract, assign, and sequence ICD-10-CM diagnosis codes using the Index and Tabular List. Write the code(s) on the line provided.

1. OFFICE   Gender: F   **Age:** 41

Reason for visit: Review abnormal mammogram results

Assessment: Microcalcifications in right breast

Plan: Mammogram with magnification to r/o cancer

1 ICD-10-CM Code _____

2. OFFICE   Gender: F   **Age:** 31

Reason for encounter: Review lung x-ray

Assessment: Abnormal shadow, right lung, inferior lobe

Plan: Refer to pulmonologist

Tip: An x-ray is classified as diagnostic imaging.

1 ICD-10-CM Code _____

3. OFFICE   Gender: F   **Age:** 23

Chief complaint: Review results of blood test performed last week because patient was concerned she had been exposed to HIV

Assessment: Nonconclusive HIV test

Plan: Further testing needed

Tip: Search for the Main Term *HIV* or *Test*.

1 ICD-10-CM Code _____

4. OFFICE   Gender: M   **Age:** 24

Chief complaint: Sneezing, scratchy throat, postnasal drip

Assessment: Suspected seasonal allergies

Plan: OTC antihistamine

3 ICD-10-CM Codes _____

_____

5. INPATIENT HOSPITAL   Gender: M   **Age:** 27

Reason for admission: Lumbar pain, weakness in left leg

Discharge diagnosis: Probable herniated intervertebral lumbar disc, sciatica

Plan: Refer to physical therapy

(continued)

5. (continued)

Tip: The description of the admission and discharge indicates that this was an inpatient stay so follow the OCGR for inpatient settings.

1 ICD-10-CM Code _____

6. OFFICE   Gender: F   **Age:** 24

Reason for encounter: Repeat PAP test

Assessment: Abnormal cervical PAP test result, cytologic (*cellular*) evidence of malignancy

Plan: Possible colposcopy based on repeat test results

1 ICD-10-CM Code _____

7. OFFICE   Gender: M   **Age:** 56

Chief complaint: Review bloodwork results

Assessment: Glucose reading of 107, insulin resistant

Plan: HbA1c in 3 months to check long-term glucose levels

1 ICD-10-CM Code _____

8. OFFICE   Gender: F   **Age:** 36

Chief complaint: Daily headaches

Assessment: Likely migraines

Plan: Refer to neurologist for further testing and evaluation

1 ICD-10-CM Code _____

9. INPATIENT HOSPITAL   Gender: F   **Age:** 62

Reason for admission: Shortness of breath

Assessment: Increased edema, congestive heart failure

Discharge instructions: Begin new diuretic, follow up with cardiologist

1 ICD-10-CM Code _____

10. OFFICE   Gender: F   **Age:** 50

Chief complaint: Review recent lab work

Assessment: All results were normal except for low vitamin D.

Plan: Rx 50,000 IU of vitamin D once a week for 8 weeks; recheck in 8 weeks

Tip: A *low* test result is indexed as *Deficiency*.

1 ICD-10-CM Code _____

Chapter 5

Neoplasms (C00-D49)

Learning Objectives

After completing this chapter, you should have the skills to:

5.1 Spell and define the key words, medical terms, and abbreviations related to neoplasms. (Remember)

5.2 Explain the behavior and common types of neoplasms. (Understand)

5.3 Adhere to the Official Guidelines for Coding and Reporting related to neoplasms. (Apply)

5.4 Examine and abstract diagnostic information from the medical record for coding neoplasms. (Analyze)

5.5 Demonstrate how to assign codes for neoplasms and related conditions. (Apply)

5.6 Utilize guidelines for arranging (sequencing) codes for neoplasms and related conditions. (Apply)

Chapter Outline

- **Neoplasm Refresher**
- **Coding Guidelines for Neoplasms**
- **Abstracting for Neoplasms**
- **Assigning Codes for Neoplasms**
- **Arranging Codes for Neoplasms**

Key Terms and Abbreviations

adenocarcinoma
adjuvant therapy
behavior
benign
biopsy
CA in situ
cancer
carcinoma (CA)

carcinoma of unknown primary (CUP)
cell type
external radiotherapy
family history
histology
internal radiotherapy
leukemia

malignant
metastasize
neoplasm
oncologist
overlapping lesion
pathologist
personal history
primary (malignant neoplasm)

prognosis
screening
secondary (malignant neoplasm)
site of origin
staging
topography

In addition to the key terms listed here, students should know the terms defined within tables in this chapter.

INTRODUCTION

Driving into a pothole can be quite a jolt to the system. When potholes are not repaired quickly, they grow bigger and more dangerous each day. The medical field has its own potholes. One of them is cancer, a collection of diseases that affects nearly every person either directly or indirectly.

An oncologist is a physician who specializes in diagnosing and treating tumors. Medical oncologists specialize in medical treatments such as chemotherapy. Surgical oncologists specialize in surgical treatment, such as the surgical excision of malignant tumors (*cancer*). Radiation oncologists specialize in treating malignant tumors with radiation therapy. Physician specialists of a particular body system may also be involved in treating patients with tumors and cancer affecting that body system.

NEOPLASM REFRESHER

Neoplasms are abnormal growth of new tissue, which may be malignant (*life-threatening*) or benign (*not life-threatening*). Malignant neoplasms are commonly referred to as cancer. Neoplasms can occur in any body system and at any anatomic site. Oncologists are physicians who specialize in the diagnosis and treatment of tumors. In order to code neoplasms, coders need to be familiar with neoplasm-related terminology, benign neoplasm behavior, and malignant neoplasm behavior.

Neoplasm-Related Terminology

Neoplasms are classified based on the behavior (*malignant or benign*), topography or site of origin (*anatomic site where the growth begins*), histology (*type of tissue*), and cell type (*characteristics or appearance of the cell*) of the growth. As you learn about different types of neoplasms, remember to put together the root or combining form for body parts you already know with suffixes and prefixes to define new terms for conditions and procedures related to neoplasms.

For example, the suffix *-oma* means "tumor" and *gastr/o* means "stomach," so *gastroma* refers to a neoplasm in the stomach (gastr/oma). Sarc/o refers to connective tissue, so *sarcoma* refers to a neoplasm of connective tissue (sarc/oma) and is nearly always malignant.

Terms for neoplasms frequently contain more than one root to fully describe the tumor. For example, adenocarcinoma (adeno/carcin/oma) has two roots to describe a cancerous (carcin/o) tumor in a gland (aden/o). Refer to ■ TABLE 5-1 for a refresher on how to build medical terms related to neoplasms.

Benign Neoplasm Behavior

A benign neoplasm does not have the ability to invade surrounding tissue or spread to other parts of the body. Types of benign neoplasms are tumors, warts, moles, polyps, and fibroids. In some cases, physicians can determine if a neoplasm is benign or malignant through visual inspection. If they believe the growth could be malignant or are unsure of its behavior, they perform a biopsy (*the scraping, punching, or cutting or removal of a small piece of skin body tissue or fluid sample for laboratory analysis*) to obtain a specimen. They send the specimen to the laboratory where a pathologist (*a physician who studies and identifies diseases through laboratory analysis*) examines it, usually microscopically.

Many benign neoplasms present no health problems and require no treatment. However, a large benign neoplasm can apply pressure to or interfere with surrounding organs or structures, which can create health problems. For example, a benign brain tumor is not cancerous, but it can compress cranial nerves or apply pressure to areas of the brain and may need to be removed to protect brain function. ■ TABLE 5-2 outlines the differences between benign and malignant neoplasms.

Malignant Neoplasm Behavior

The ability of malignant neoplasms to metastasize (*spread and invade organs*) makes them life threatening. When tumors invade vital organs, they cause organ malfunction, leading to death if not treated. It is important to distinguish between the common term cancer and the medical terms *malignant neoplasm* and carcinoma (sometimes abbreviated CA). Refer to the following to review the similarities and differences in these terms:

- Carcinoma is a malignant tumor of epithelial cells, which line body cavities and organs. Not all areas of the body have epithelial cells, so true carcinoma only occurs in structures that contain epithelial cells.

Table 5-1   ■   **EXAMPLE OF CONSTRUCTING MEDICAL TERMS FOR NEOPLASMS**

Combining Form/Prefix	Suffix	Complete Medical Term
sarc/o (*connective tissue*)	**-plasm** (*growth*)	**neo + plasm** (*new growth*)
my/o (*muscle*)	**-oma** (*tumor*)	**sarc + oma** (*tumor of connective tissue*)
carcin/o (*cancerous*)		**aden + oma** (*tumor of a gland*)
aden/o (*gland*)		**myo + sarc + oma** (*tumor of connective tissue and muscle*)
neo- (*prefix; new*)		**adeno + carcin + oma** (*cancerous tumor of a gland*)

Table 5-2 ■ **COMPARISON OF BENIGN AND MALIGNANT NEOPLASM CHARACTERISTICS**

Characteristic	Benign Neoplasm	Malignant Neoplasm
Rate of growth	Grows slowly	Grows rapidly
Encapsulation	Is encapsulated	Is not encapsulated
Differentiation	Well-differentiated (*has cells that resemble the normal cells from which they arose*)	Anaplastic and undifferentiated (*has cells that undergo permanent change, abnormal rapid proliferation*)
Growth pattern	Grows by expansion and causes pressure on surrounding tissue	Has invasive growth and metastasis
Metastasis	Nonmetastatic (*cells remain localized and do not spread*)	Spreads through bloodstream and lymphatic system Causes extensive tissue destruction due to invasiveness
Recurrence	Does not recur when surgically removed	Can recur when surgically removed if invasive growth has occurred
Cachexia	Produces no cachexia (*extreme weakness, fatigue, wasting, and malnutrition*)	Produces cachexia

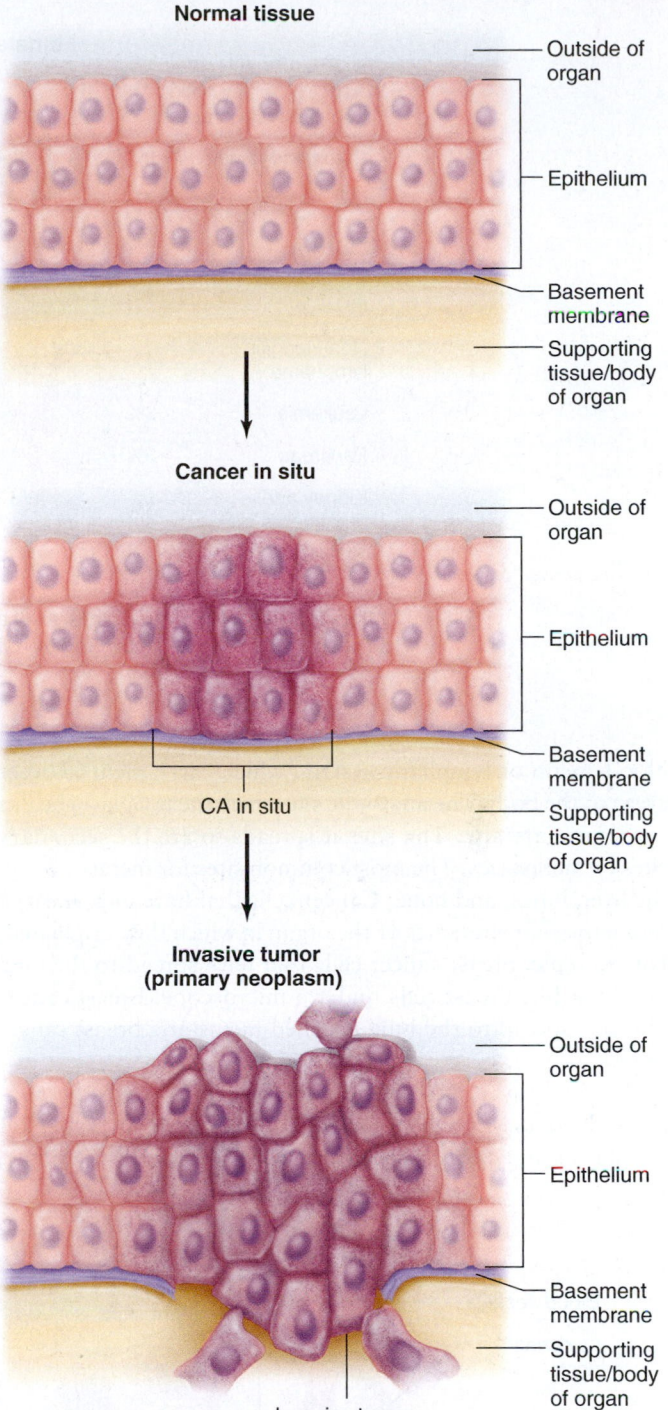

Figure 5-1 ■ Progression of CA in situ to primary neoplasm.

- Carcinoma in situ (**CA in situ**) refers to cells that have begun to change but are contained within the epithelial layer. When malignant cells break through the epithelial membrane into the organ, they become a **primary** malignant neoplasm (■ FIGURE 5-1).

- Malignant neoplasm is a life-threatening new growth of any type of tissue. Although malignant neoplasms are cancerous, not all are classified as carcinoma. Malignant neoplasms can also occur in other types of cells such as bone, muscle, and fat.

- Cancer, in its most limited meaning, is synonymous with carcinoma. However, our language uses cancer loosely to refer to many types of malignancies, including ones that are not tumors. For example, cancer is often used to describe leukemia, which is a malignant disease of the blood-forming organs but does not produce tumors.

- Be aware of different forms of the word *metastasize*, which literally means "beyond control." *Metastasize* (verb) means "to transform or spread diseased cells." *Metastasis* (noun) is the process of spreading or the condition resulting from the spread of diseased cells. *Metastases* (plural) refer to multiple secondary tumors or sites. *Metastatic* (adjective) means "pertaining to having spread."

Cancer is not one disease but, rather, a group of over 100 diseases in which cells in one part of the body begin to mutate and grow out of control. The American Cancer Society (ACS) estimates that one-half of all men and one-third of all women will develop cancer at some point in their lives. The most common sites of cancer are the prostate for men, breast for women, lung, and colon/rectum (■ FIGURE 5-2, page 80). The most common childhood cancers are leukemia and medulloblastoma, a cancer that affects the cerebellum, brain, and spinal cord.

Cells become cancerous due to damaged DNA that is not repaired as it is in normal cells. The damaged cells do not die as they normally should but, rather, replicate and make new damaged cells. Cancer spreads when the damaged cells invade nearby tissues and when damaged cells move into the

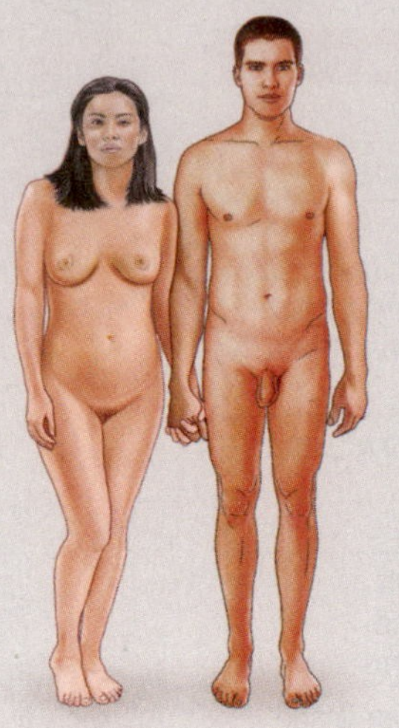

Female		Male	
Breast	30%	Prostate	19%
Lung and bronchus	12%	Lung and bronchus	14%
Colon and rectum	8%	Colon and rectum	9%
Uterine corpus	7%	Urinary bladder	7%
Thyroid	5%	Melanoma of the skin	6%
Melanoma of the skin	4%	Kidney and renal pelvis	5%
Non-Hodgkin's lymphoma	4%	Non-Hodgkin's lymphoma	5%
Leukemia	3%	Leukemia	4%
Pancreas	3%	Oral cavity and pharynx	4%
Kidney and renal pelvis	3%	Liver and intrahepatic bile duct	3%
Other	21%	Other	21%

Figure 5-2 ■ Most frequent sites of new cancer cases.
Data source: American Cancer Society, Cancer Facts and Figures 2017.

bloodstream or lymphatic system, which carry them to other areas of the body. The anatomic site where the neoplasm begins is the primary site. The sites it spreads to are the **secondary** sites or metastases. The most common sites for metastases are the liver, lungs, and bone. Cancer cells that have metastasized retain the characteristics of the organ in which they originated. For example, breast cancer cells that have spread to the lung still look like breast cells under a microscope. Breast cancer that has spread to the lung is called metastatic breast cancer (■ FIGURE 5-3).

Topography refers to the anatomic site where the neoplasm begins. Many histological and cell types of malignant neoplasms and cancers can affect any given site. For example,

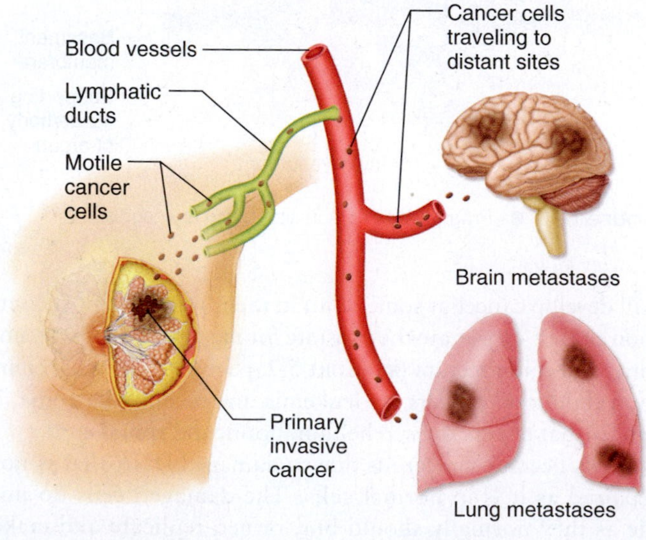

Figure 5-3 ■ Metastasis of breast cancer to the brain and lung.

colorectal cancer includes the following histological types, each of which originates from a different type of tissue:

- Adenocarcinoma, which originates in the glands
- Leiomyosarcoma, which originates in smooth muscle tissue
- Lymphoma, which originates in the lymph nodes
- Malignant melanoma, which originates in pigment cells of the skin
- Neuroendocrine, which originates in hormone-producing cells that are a cross between nerve cells and endocrine cells

Each of these histological types can appear in many different organs. For example, adenocarcinoma may appear in the colon, prostate, lungs, breast, stomach, pancreas, and cervix. Each histological type may have a variety of cell subtypes, which are often named based on their appearance. For example, adenocarcinoma of the colon has a mucinous cell subtype (*comprised of at least 60% mucus*) and a signet ring cell subtype (*looks like a ring when viewed microscopically*). Physicians must identify the specific subtype of cell in order to determine the behavior, the patient's **prognosis** (*expected outcome*), and treatment plan. Hundreds of different cell subtypes are known for various topographical and histological types of cancer.

Coders need to know how malignant neoplasms and other cancers are diagnosed and treated in order to abstract, assign, and sequence codes.

Diagnosis

Physicians diagnose cancer through **screening** (*examination or testing of individuals with no diagnosis or symptoms to identify those at high risk*) examinations or in response to patient symptoms. Screening examinations detect certain types of cancer at an early stage. Cancer that is detected during an early stage is more likely to respond to treatment. Examples of screening tests include:

- Colonoscopy—Colon cancer
- Mammogram—Breast cancer
- Papanicolaou (PAP) test—Cervical cancer
- Prostate-specific antigen (PSA) blood test—Prostate cancer
- Digital rectal examination (DRE)—Prostate cancer

When patients present with symptoms, physicians may diagnose cancer with blood tests, biopsies, and imaging, such as computed tomography (CT), magnetic resonance imaging (MRI), or positron emission tomography (PET) (■ FIGURE 5-4). After making a diagnosis of cancer, physicians determine the stage and grade of the disease in order to help determine the best course of treatment.

Staging. Staging is the process of determining how far the cancer has spread. Several staging systems exist and various systems are used for specific types of cancers. Two common staging systems are TNM and stage grouping. TNM staging assigns numbers to describe how far the primary tumor (T) has grown in its original site; extent of spread to regional (nearby) lymph nodes (N), and whether the cancer has metastasized (M) to other organs of the body. The results of TNM staging are then combined into stage grouping. Stage grouping uses numbers to designate the malignancy from the least advanced (stage 0) to the most advanced (IV). The specific criteria for each stage of TNM and stage grouping are unique to each anatomic site. For example, the definition of stage II colon cancer is different than stage II breast cancer. Physicians state the diagnosis by referencing the stage of cancer at the time it is discovered. However, all cancers will eventually become the highest stage if left untreated. Staging information helps coders confirm whether the disease has metastasized.

Grading. Grading describes how closely the cancer cell type looks like a normal cell when viewed microscopically. A pathologist determines the grade through microscopic inspection of a tissue or fluid specimen. The grade is rated from G1, a low-grade cell that looks much like normal tissue, to G4, a high-grade cell that looks very abnormal. Low-grade cancers tend to grow and spread more slowly than high-grade cells. Several different grades of cancer cells can affect any given anatomic site, so physicians must determine each patient's exact cell type and its grade. The grade of the cell does not change as the disease progresses.

Physicians use the combination of stage and grade to determine a patient's treatment plan and prognosis. Stage and grade are independent of each other. A patient can have a low stage and high grade, a high stage and a low grade, or any combination in between. For example, a patient with a lymphoma type that is stage IV (widespread) and grade G1 (slow growing), such as follicular cell lymphoma, may have a better outcome than a patient with a type of carcinoma of the uterus that is stage I (localized) but grade G4 (rapidly growing and spreading), such as clear cell carcinoma.

Treatment

Physicians recommend treatment plans based on topography, stage, and grade of cancer as well as the patient's age and health condition. The three primary types of treatment are surgery, chemotherapy, and radiotherapy. They may be used alone or in conjunction with each other. When more than one type of treatment is used, the additional treatments are referred to as adjuvant therapies. Some malignancies are more responsive to one type of treatment than another. Which treatments are used, and in what order, is unique to each type of cancer and each patient.

Surgery. Surgery is performed to remove the tumor and a portion of the healthy tissue around the tumor to be certain that all the malignancy is removed. It is most successful when a tumor is small and localized. Surgery is also used to treat some complications of cancer, such as blockage or pain due to a tumor.

Chemotherapy. Chemotherapy is the use of drugs to kill cancer cells. It may be used before surgery, to shrink the size of a large tumor so it is easier to remove, or after surgery, to kill any potentially remaining diseased cells. Chemotherapy is also used to treat widespread metastases that cannot be surgically removed. Drugs may be administered intravenously or orally, or a combination of both. Immense progress has been made in recent years to improve the specificity of chemotherapy drugs, the ability of the drug to target cancerous cells but not damage healthy cells.

Radiotherapy. Radiotherapy can be external or internal. External radiotherapy directs precise doses of x-ray beams at specific sites in order to kill or shrink tumors and cancerous cells. Internal radiotherapy uses radioactive pellets or containers within a body cavity to target the malignant area. Radiotherapy may be used before surgery to shrink the size of a tumor or after surgery to slow potential metastasis.

Each treatment method has its advantages and drawbacks. Unfortunately, treatments aimed at killing cancer cells also kill healthy cells, resulting in side effects for patients. Patients, their families, and their physicians make difficult and personal decisions regarding what is best in any given situation.

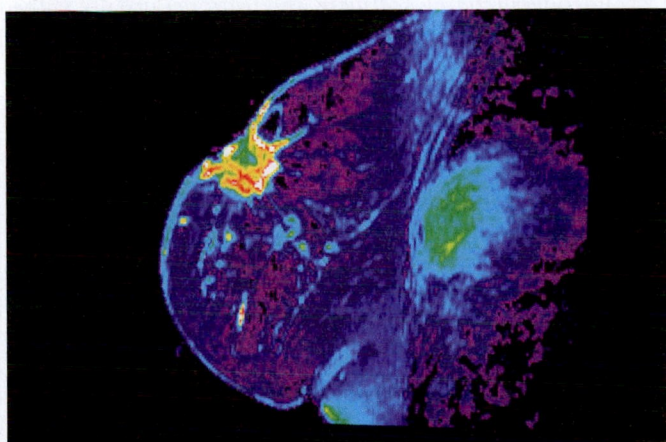

Figure 5-4 ■ MRI image of the breast.
Source: © Dr. Steven Harmes/National Cancer Institute (NCI).

CODING PRACTICE

Exercise 5.1   Neoplasm Refresher

Instructions: Use your medical terminology skills and resources to define the following neoplasms. Do not assign codes. Follow these steps:

- Use slash marks "/" to break down each term into its root(s) and suffix.
- Define the meaning of the word, based on the meaning of each word part.

Example: sarcoma sarc/oma   Meaning *neoplasm of connective tissue*

1. osteosarcoma _____   Meaning _____
2. leiomyoma _____   Meaning _____
3. lipoma _____   Meaning _____
4. liposarcoma _____   Meaning _____
5. adenoma _____   Meaning _____
6. adenocarcinoma _____   Meaning _____
7. osteoma _____   Meaning _____
8. melanoma _____   Meaning _____
9. neuroblastoma _____   Meaning _____
10. lymphoma _____   Meaning _____

CODING GUIDELINES FOR NEOPLASMS

Coders should understand the organization of this ICD-10-CM chapter, chapter-wide and commonly used instructional notes in Tabular List, and the relevant OGCR. This information is necessary for accurate coding.

ICD-10-CM Chapter 2, "Neoplasms (C00-D49)," contains 21 blocks or subchapters that are divided by anatomic site. Review the block names and code ranges listed at the beginning of Chapter 2 in the ICD-10-CM manual to become familiar with the content and organization. This chapter classifies all malignant and most benign neoplasms. Some benign neoplasms are classified in the specific body system chapter. For example, adenomas of the prostate are classified in ICD-10-CM Chapter 14, "Diseases of the Genitourinary System (N00-N99)."

Notice the following characteristics of codes in the neoplasm chapter:

- Codes beginning with C classify malignant neoplasms.
- Codes beginning with D classify neoplasms in situ, benign, and of uncertain or unspecified behavior.
- Some codes contain an alphabetic character in the third position of the code, such as C7A, C7B, and D3A.

ICD-10-CM codes for neoplasm in bilateral anatomic sites usually include specific codes for laterality. Codes for leukemia contain characters to identify whether the disease is in remission or relapse.

ICD-10-CM provides Official Guidelines for Coding and Reporting (OGCR) for neoplasms in OGCR section I.C.2. OGCR provides specific direction for sequencing codes for multiple neoplasms, complications, adjuvant therapies, and other situations. In addition, frequent instructional notes throughout the chapter direct coders to use multiple codes to describe harmful lifestyle habits, such as tobacco use or exposure, that contribute to neoplasms. Coding for harmful lifestyle habits is discussed in Chapter 6, "Factors Influencing Health Status and Contact with Health Services (Z00-Z99)," of this text.

Instructional notes at the beginning of ICD-10-CM Chapter 2 address functional activity, morphology, overlapping sites, and malignant neoplasm of ectopic tissue.

Although it may take a few years of coding experience to memorize every OGCR for neoplasms, new coders can memorize the fact that this ICD-10-CM chapter has many guidelines. Some coding manuals provide the guidelines in the Tabular List. Encoders (*coding software applications*) usually embed links to the guidelines. Specific OGCR guidelines are discussed and cited throughout this chapter of the text.

CODING CAUTION

When diagnosis codes have a letter for other than the first or last character, they can be tricky to locate because they do not appear in a manner consistent with alphanumeric rules. For example, category **C7A** is sequenced after **C75** and before **C76**, but category **D3A** appears after **D36** and before **D37**. Be aware of this inconsistency and know that you may need to take a few moments to locate the code. Look at the beginning of the chapter in the ICD-10-CM manual and read the list of categories to learn where these unique codes appear in the chapter sequence.

ABSTRACTING FOR NEOPLASMS

When abstracting patient cases with neoplasms, coders must look for several pieces of information that will help determine the first-listed or principal diagnosis and the sequencing of any additional diagnoses. Refer to OGCR I.C.2 for detailed guidance on abstracting neoplasms. ■ TABLE 5-3 highlights key questions to answer when reviewing the medical record. Coders use answers to these questions when assigning and sequencing codes. Remember that the abstracting questions are a guide and that not every question applies to, or can be answered for, every case. For example, complications of cancer may not be present in every patient.

Abstracting Metastases

An important task in abstracting is determining the sites of the primary and any secondary neoplasms. Coders must give special attention to the specific wording used to describe various neoplasm sites. In particular, take note of the prepositions *from*, *to*, and *in* because they describe the direction in which the neoplasm has spread. Refer to ■ TABLE 5-4 to better understand how metastases are documented.

Table 5-3 ■ KEY CRITERIA FOR ABSTRACTING NEOPLASMS

- ❏ What is the histologic description of the neoplasm or cancer?
- ❏ What is the anatomic site of the neoplasm?
- ❏ Is the neoplasm stated as malignant or benign?
- ❏ If malignant, is the neoplasm primary, secondary, in situ, or of unknown histologic origin?
- ❏ Has the malignant neoplasm metastasized? If so, to what sites?
- ❏ What complications are documented, such as anemia, dehydration, or a surgical complication?
- ❏ If anemia is present, is it due to the malignancy itself or due to a treatment such as chemotherapy, radiotherapy, or immunotherapy?
- ❏ Is the reason for the encounter or admission the malignancy or an unrelated condition?
- ❏ If the reason for the encounter is the malignancy, what is the specific purpose?
  - Treatment of the primary site
  - Treatment of a metastatic site(s)
  - Treatment of a complication
  - Chemotherapy
  - Radiotherapy
  - Immunotherapy
  - Pain management
  - Determination of the extent of malignancy
  - Aftercare
  - Follow-up care
- ❏ Is the patient in remission from leukemia, multiple myeloma, or malignant plasma neoplasm?
- ❏ If the primary malignancy was previously excised, is there any remaining evidence of primary malignancy, metastasis, or any related treatment?
- ❏ Does the patient have a personal history or family history of malignant neoplasm?

Table 5-4 ■ ALTERNATIVE DESCRIPTIONS OF METASTASES

Statement	Primary Site	Secondary Site(s)
Colon cancer with metastasis *to* the liver	Colon	Liver
Metastatic liver cancer *from* the colon	Colon	Liver
Metastatic colon cancer	Colon	Unknown
Metastatic cancer *in* the lung, liver, and bone	Unknown	Lung, liver, and bone
Liver metastases	Unknown	Liver

Guided Example of Abstracting Neoplasms

Refer to the following example here and throughout the chapter to learn more about coding for neoplasms. Karla Destefano, CPC, is a fictitious certified coder who guides you through the coding process.

Date: 5/1/yy   Location: East Side Oncology

Provider: Richard Blackford, MD

Patient: Anthony Payne   Gender: M   Age: 68

Reason for encounter: Review test results to determine extent of prostate cancer

Assessment: Adenocarcinoma of prostate with metastasis to colon

Plan: Surgery to be followed with radiotherapy

Follow along in your ICD-10-CM manual as Karla abstracts the diagnosis. Check off each step after you complete it.

▶ Karla begins by reviewing the medical record to abstract the diagnosis. She refers to the Key Criteria for Abstracting Neoplasms (Table 5-3).

- ❏ *What is the histologic description of the neoplasm or cancer?* Adenocarcinoma

- ❏ *What is the anatomic site of the neoplasm?* Prostate

- ❏ *Is the neoplasm stated as malignant or benign?* Adenocarcinoma by definition is malignant. In addition, the fact that it has spread indicates it is malignant

- ❏ *If malignant, is the neoplasm primary, secondary, in situ, or of unknown histologic origin?* The prostate is primary because it is not stated as secondary

- ❏ *Has the malignant neoplasm metastasized? If so, to what sites?* She notes that the secondary site is the colon

- ❏ *What complications are documented?* None

- ❏ *Is the reason for the encounter or admission the malignancy or an unrelated condition?* The malignancy

- ❏ *Does the patient have a personal history or family history of malignant neoplasm?* None stated

▶ Next, Karla will assign the codes.

CODING PRACTICE

Exercise 5.2 Abstracting Diagnoses for Neoplasms

Instructions: Read the mini-medical-record of each patient's encounter and answer the abstracting questions. Write the answer on the line provided. Do not assign any codes.

1. OFFICE   Gender: F   Age: 59

Reason for encounter: Chemotherapy

Assessment: Adenocarcinoma of the right breast, lower outer quadrant, with metastasis to the brain

Plan: Return for next treatment in 3 weeks

a. What is the primary site? _____

b. Is metastasis documented? Where? _____

c. Are any complications documented? _____

d. What is the specific purpose of the visit? _____

2. INPATIENT HOSPITAL   Gender: F   Age: 44

Procedure: Embolization of uterine fibroids

Postprocedural diagnosis: Intramural (*within the muscle wall*) leiomyoma, uterus

Plan: FU in office in 4 weeks

a. What is embolization? _____

b. What is a leiomyoma? _____

c. What is the anatomic site? _____

d. Is the neoplasm malignant or benign? _____

3. OFFICE   Gender: M   Age: 43

Reason for encounter: Review results of biopsy and CT scan

Assessment: Gastric adenocarcinoma, fundus

Plan: Surgery to be followed by radiotherapy

a. What is the primary site? _____

b. What part of the stomach is the fundus? _____

3. (continued)

c. Is metastasis documented? Where? _____

d. Are any complications documented? _____

e. What is the specific purpose of the visit? _____

4. INPATIENT HOSPITAL   Gender: F   Age: 15

Reason for admission: Limb-salvage surgery after chemotherapy to shrink tumor

Procedure description: Successfully cut out tumor from left thigh

Postprocedural assessment: Osteosarcoma in the left thigh

Plan: Discharge in 1–2 days

a. What is the primary site? _____

b. Is metastasis documented? _____

c. Are any complications documented? _____

d. What is the specific purpose of the encounter? ____

e. What is the medical term for the bone in the thigh? ____

5. INPATIENT HOSPITAL   Gender: M   Age: 67

Reason for admission: Anemia

Assessment: Anemia due to classical lymphocyte-depleted Hodgkin's lymphoma

Plan: Administer IV iron supplements

a. What is the primary neoplasm? _____

b. Is metastasis documented? _____

c. What complication is documented? _____

d. What is the reason for the admission? _____

(continued)

(continued)

CODING PRACTICE *(continued)*

6. INPATIENT HOSPITAL   Gender: M   Age: 61

Reason for procedure: Brainstem tumor

Procedure description: Used Gamma Knife surgery to destroy tumor

Postprocedural diagnosis: Squamous cell carcinoma of the lung with brainstem metastases

Plan: FU in office 1 week, evaluate for chemotherapy

Tip: Look up unfamiliar terms in a medical dictionary or on the Internet.

(continued)

6. (continued)

a. What is the primary neoplasm? _____
_____

b. Is metastasis documented? What site? _____
_____

c. Which site is the reason for the procedure? _____
_____

d. What is Gamma Knife surgery? _____
_____

ASSIGNING CODES FOR NEOPLASMS

Assigning codes for neoplasms involves three steps:

1. Search for the histological term in the Index to Diseases and Injuries.
2. Locate the anatomic site and behavior in the Table of Neoplasms.
3. Verify the code(s) in the Tabular List.

Search for the Histological Term in the Index

Coders use both the Index to Diseases and Injuries and the Table of Neoplasms to locate codes for neoplasms. Careful abstracting and attention to the terms in the documentation determine how to locate the code.

When the histological type is documented, search for that term in the Index. The histological term identifies the tissue type of a neoplasm, such as carcinoma, melanoma, sarcoma, or leukemia. When the Index lists a code for the histological type, coders may proceed to the Tabular List to verify the code (■ FIGURE 5-5).

In many cases, the Index lists a cross-reference note to the Table of Neoplasms, such as **specified site -** *see* **Neoplasm, malignant**. In this situation, coders need to refer to the Table of Neoplasms, locate the column for Malignant Primary, then locate the anatomic site in the left-hand column (■ FIGURE 5-6). Recall that the Table of Neoplasms appears in the Index to Diseases and Injuries under the letter **N** in most editions of the ICD-10-CM manual. Some publishers place it after the Index to Diseases and Injuries.

SUCCESS STEP

To help remember where the Table of Neoplasms is located and to find it quickly, place an adhesive tab along the top edge of the first page of the Table of Neoplasms. By placing it on the top edge, it will not be obscured by other tabs for the Index to Diseases and Injuries and the Tabular List.

Personal or Family History

When physicians document that patients are at risk due to a personal or family history of malignant neoplasm, assign a code for the history. **Personal history** is a condition the patient had in the past, was removed or resolved, and is no longer being treated, but has the potential for recurrence and therefore may require continued monitoring. To locate codes for personal history, search the Index for the Main Term **History** and subterm **personal**, then the second-level modifying term **malignant neoplasm**. Finally, locate the subterm for the anatomic site.

Family history is a condition that a patient's family member had in the past or currently has that causes the patient to be at higher risk of also contracting or developing the disease. The family member may be alive or deceased. The family member's malignancy may have been removed and/or may still be undergoing treatment. To locate codes for family history, search the Index for the Main Term **History** and subterm **family**, then the second-level subterm **malignant neoplasm**. Finally, locate the subterm for the body system. It is very important to locate the correct subterm—**personal** or **family**—before selecting the anatomic site.

The significance of personal or family history must be documented by the physician as relevant to the current condition or encounter. Patients must have a blood relationship to the family member, such as a parent or sibling. The history of grandparents, aunts, and uncles may be relevant for certain cancers with proven genetic links, such as breast cancer.

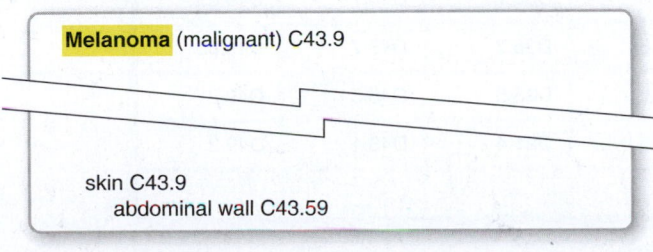

Melanoma (malignant) C43.9

skin C43.9
abdominal wall C43.59

Figure 5-5 ■ Example of Index entry for a histological type of neoplasm.

Carcinoma (malignant) — *see also* Neoplasm, by site, malignant
acidophil
specified site — *see* Neoplasm, malignant, by site

Figure 5-6 ■ Example of a cross-reference to the Table of Neoplasms.

Locate Site and Behavior in the Table of Neoplasms

The Table of Neoplasms lists the codes for neoplasms by anatomic site. Anatomic sites appear in the left column of the table in alphabetical order (■ FIGURE 5-7). Many sites have indented subterms, similar to indentations in the Index to Diseases and Injuries. Subterms in the Table of Neoplasms describe specific locations within a large anatomic site. For example, the anatomic site **abdomen, abdominal** has subterms for **cavity**, **organ**, **viscera**, and **wall**. **Abdomen, wall** has second-level subterms for **connective tissue** and **skin**.

The Table of Neoplasms has six columns, one for each anatomic site, that describe the possible behavior of the neoplasm:

- Malignant Primary
- Malignant Secondary
- CA in situ
- Benign
- Uncertain Behavior (*the physician documents that they have not determined whether the neoplasm is malignant or benign*)
- Unspecified Behavior (*the physician does not document whether the neoplasm is malignant or benign*).

The description of the neoplasm will often indicate which of the six columns to use. For example, benign fibroadenoma of breast is coded using the Benign column; carcinoma in situ of cervix uteri is coded using the CA in situ column. Some sites do not have codes in all six columns because some behaviors do not occur in certain sites. For example, cancer in situ does not occur in bone, muscle, or connective tissue. Cancer in situ occurs only in epithelial cells, and these sites do not have epithelial cells. When a malignant neoplasm is not specified as primary, secondary, or in situ, code it as primary. Secondary malignant neoplasm and CA in situ must be stated in the medical record to assign codes from those columns.

Unknown Anatomic Site

When the anatomic site of the primary or secondary neoplasm is not known, assign a code from the first line of the Table of Neoplasms, which is labeled **Neoplasm, neoplastic**. The same codes also appear under the subterm **Neoplasm, unknown site or unspecified**. There are two common situations when this may occur:

- Carcinoma of unknown primary (CUP) occurs when the neoplasm is diagnosed at a late stage after it has metastasized and the physician is unable to determine the site of origin.
- The secondary site may not be specified when the neoplasm has metastasized to multiple areas throughout the body, and treatment is directed at the overall body rather than one specific site.

The row for **unknown site** provides codes in all six columns, so coders should select the appropriate column. For example, it is possible for the primary site to be specified but not the secondary; for the secondary site to be specified but not the primary; or for neither to be specified. In all cases, coders should query the physician and review all information in the medical record before assigning a code for unspecified site.

Overlapping Lesions

Some anatomic sites provide a listing for overlapping lesions. Overlapping lesions are contiguous sites where the tumor continues from one site to an adjacent one without interruption. Refer to ■ FIGURE 5-8 and review the entries for **lung** in the Table of Neoplasms. Separate entries describe distinct sites within the lung with separate codes. Use the entry for overlapping lesion when the physician documents that two contiguous sites within the lung are affected and the lesions have overlapping boundaries.

Patients may also have multiple tumors in contiguous sites that are not overlapping. For example, distinct tumors in two different lobes of the same lung that do not meet or overlap should be assigned two separate codes for primary malignant

	Malignant Primary	Malignant Secondary	Ca in situ	Benign	Uncertain Behavior	Unspecified Behavior
Neoplasm, neoplastic	C80.1	C79.9	D09.9	D36.9	D48.9	D49.9
abdomen, abdominal	C76.2	C79.8-	D09.8	D36.7	D48.7	D49.89
cavity	C76.2	C79.8-	D09.8	D36.7	D48.7	D49.89
organ	C76.2	C79.8-	D09.8	D36.7	D48.7	D49.89
viscera	C76.2	C79.8-	D09.8	D36.7	D48.7	D49.89
wall	C44.509	C79.2-	D04.5	D23.5	D48.5	D49.2
connective tissue	C49.4	C79.8-	-	D21.4	D48.1	D49.2
skin	C44.509	-	-	-	-	-

Figure 5-7 ■ Example of the Table of Neoplasms.

	Malignant Primary	Malignant Secondary	Ca in situ	Benign	Uncertain Behavior	Unspecified Behavior
lung	C34.9-	C78.0-	D02.2-	D14.3-	D38.1	D49.1
azygos lobe	C34.1-	C78.0-	D02.2-	D14.3-	D38.1	D49.1
carina	C34.0-	C78.0-	D02.2-	D14.3-	D38.1	D49.1
hilus	C34.0-	C78.0-	D02.2-	D14.3-	D38.1	D49.1
lingula	C34.1-	C78.0-	D02.2-	D14.3-	D38.1	D49.1
lobe NEC	C34.9-	C78.0-	D02.2-	D14.3-	D38.1	D49.1
lower lobe	C34.3-	C78.0-	D02.2-	D14.3-	D38.1	D49.1
main bronchus	C34.0-	C78.0-	D02.2-	D14.3-	D38.1	D49.1
mesothelioma-*see* Mesothelioma	-	-	-	-	-	-
middle lobe	C34.2-	C78.0-	D02.21	D14.31	D38.1	D49.1
overlapping lesion	C34.8-	-	-	-	-	-
upper lobe	C34.1-	C78.0-	D02.2-	D14.3-	D38.1	D49.1

Figure 5-8 ■ Example of entry in the Table of Neoplasms for an overlapping lesion.

neoplasm of each lobe. Coders must review the documentation carefully to determine if the sites are overlapping or distinct.

Malignant Neoplasm of the Liver

The liver is a common site for metastasis because it filters the blood, which is a route through which cancer spreads. Primary liver cancer is rare but does occur as the result of cirrhosis and alcoholism. When abstracting and assigning codes for malignant neoplasms of the liver, coders must take extra care to determine if it is primary or secondary.

Verify Codes in the Tabular List

All codes in the Table of Neoplasms must be verified in the Tabular List. Codes listed with a short dash (-) at the end require an additional character for laterality, which must be determined from the Tabular List. The Tabular List also provides instructional notes directing coders when additional codes are required and what sequencing is required. The beginning of ICD-10-CM Chapter 2 (C00-D49) provides several instructional notes that define terms and coding procedures that apply to all codes in the chapter.

Guided Example of Assigning Neoplasm Codes

Continue with the example from earlier in this chapter of Anthony Payne, who saw Dr. Blackford for prostate cancer. Follow along in your ICD-10-CM manual as Karla Destefano, CPC, assigns the codes for the conditions she abstracted. Check off each step after you complete it.

▶ Karla reviews the conditions she abstracted.

❑ Adenocarcinoma of prostate

❑ Metastasis to colon

▶ Karla locates the Main Term for the primary neoplasm in the Index.

❑ She looks up **A, adenocarcinoma**.

❑ The Main Term entry contains a cross-reference note **(see also Neoplasm, malignant, by site)**.

❑ She searches the subterms for **prostate** but cannot find it (■ FIGURE 5-9).

▶ Therefore, she knows she needs to refer to the Table of Neoplasms as directed in the instructional note.

❑ Karla locates the Table of Neoplasms.

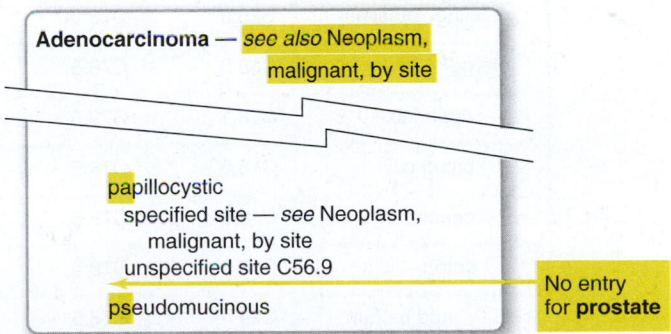

Adenocarcinoma — *see also* Neoplasm, malignant, by site

papillocystic
specified site — *see* Neoplasm, malignant, by site
unspecified site C56.9

pseudomucinous

No entry for **prostate**

Figure 5-9 ■ Index Entry for "Adenocarcinoma" and subterms beginning with "p."

❏ She searches the left column for the subterm **prostate** and locates the entry.

❏ She checks the medical record to confirm that prostate cancer is primary.

❏ She refers to the first code column of the Table of Neoplasms, **Malignant Primary**, and selects the code **C61**.

▶ Next, Karla proceeds to verify the code in the Tabular List.

❏ Karla locates **C61** in the Tabular List and verifies the code title, **Malignant neoplasm of prostate**.

❏ She reviews the **Excludes1** note under the code and sees that **Malignant neoplasm of seminal vesicles** should not be coded here. She double-checks the medical record to be certain that seminal vesicles are not documented.

❏ Karla confirms that the block title **Malignant neoplasms of male genital organs (C60-C63)** contains no additional instructional notes.

❏ Karla reviews the instructional notes at the beginning of **Chapter 2 Neoplasms (C00-D49)**. She determines that they do not apply to this case because she has no functional activity to report (first note); morphology codes are not required for billing (second note); there are no overlapping boundaries (third note); and the neoplasm does not involve ectopic tissue (fourth note).

▶ Karla assigns code **C61 Malignant neoplasm of prostate** for the primary neoplasm.

▶ Karla reviews the medical record and identifies the metastatic site is the colon.

❏ She returns to the Table of Neoplasms and locates the subterm for **intestine**.

❏ Under **intestine** she locates the subterm for **large**, then **colon** (■ Figure 5-10).

❏ She refers to the column **Malignant Secondary** and locates the code **C78.5**.

▶ Karla locates the code in the Tabular List and verifies the title, **C78.5 Secondary malignant neoplasm of large intestine and rectum**.

❏ She reviews the category heading **C78 Secondary malignant neoplasm of respiratory and digestive organs** and confirms this case does not include any of the conditions listed under the **Excludes1** note.

❏ She reviews the block heading **Malignant neoplasms of ill-defined, other secondary and unspecified sites (C76-C80)** and notes that there are no instructional notes.

❏ She already checked the notes at the beginning of **Chapter 2** so she does not need to do so again.

▶ Karla double-checks the medical record one last time to be sure she did not overlook anything. She has assigned the codes:

❏ **C61 Malignant neoplasm of prostate** for the primary neoplasm

❏ **C78.5 Secondary malignant neoplasm of large intestine and rectum** for the metastatic site

▶ Next, Karla needs to sequence the codes.

CODING CAUTION

Although the Table of Neoplasms provides an entry for **C, colon**, it cross-references you to **C79.89 Secondary malignant neoplasm of other specified sites**, which is less specific than **C78.5**. Therefore, it is best to search for colon under the subterms **intestine, large** in order to locate the most specific code.

	Malignant Primary	Malignant Secondary	Ca in situ	Benign	Uncertain Behavior	Unspecified Behavior
intestine, intestinal	C26.0	C78.80	D01.40	D13.9	D37.8	D49.0
large	C18.9	C78.5	D01.0	D12.6	D37.4	D49.0
appendix	C18.1	C78.5	D01.0	D12.1	D37.3	D49.0
caput coli	C18.0	C78.5	D01.0	D12.0	D37.4	D49.0
cecum	C18.0	C78.5	D01.0	D12.0	D37.4	D49.0
colon	C18.9	C78.5	D01.0	D12.6	D37.4	D49.0
and rectum	C19	C78.5	D01.1	D12.7	D37.5	D49.0

Figure 5-10 ■ Table of Neoplasms entry for "Large Intestine, Colon."

CODING PRACTICE

Exercise 5.3	Assigning Codes for Neoplasms

Instructions: Read the mini-medical-record of each patient's encounter, review the information abstracted in Exercise 5.2, and assign ICD-10-CM diagnosis codes using the Index and Tabular List. Write the code(s) on the line provided.

---

1. INPATIENT HOSPITAL   Gender: F   Age: 44

Reason for procedure: Uterine fibroids

Procedure description: Inserted catheter through femoral artery to uterus and injected polyvinyl alcohol (PVA) to block arteries leading to tumor

Postprocedural diagnosis: Intramural (*within the muscle wall*) leiomyoma, uterus

Plan: FU in office in 4 weeks

Tip: The Main Term is the name of the tumor, not its site.

1 ICD-10-CM Code _____

---

2. INPATIENT HOSPITAL   Gender: F   Age: 15

Reason for admission: Limb-salvage surgery after chemotherapy to shrink tumor

Procedure description: Successfully cut out tumor from left thigh

Postprocedural assessment: Osteosarcoma in the left thigh

Plan: Discharge in 1–2 days

Tip: Remember to identify the medical term for the thigh bone.

1 ICD-10-CM Code _____

---

3. OFFICE   Gender: M   Age: 43

Reason for encounter: Review results of biopsy and CT scan

Assessment: Gastric adenocarcinoma, fundus

Plan: Surgery to be followed by radiotherapy

Tip: Under the subterm stomach, search for the specific location within the stomach.

1 ICD-10-CM Code _____

ARRANGING CODES FOR NEOPLASMS

Sequencing of neoplasm codes is determined by the circumstances of the encounter or admission. The findings from abstracting (refer again to Table 5-3) help coders determine how to sequence multiple codes. In particular, be alert for the following circumstances that call for specific sequencing:

- Evaluation or treatment directed at the primary neoplasm
- Evaluation or treatment directed at the metastasis
- Encounter solely for chemotherapy, radiotherapy, or immunotherapy
- Evaluation or treatment for a complication
- Personal or family history of malignant neoplasm

Refer to ■ TABLE 5-5, page 90 for a summary of sequencing rules for neoplasms, then read the more detailed instructions that follow.

Evaluation or Treatment Directed at the Primary Malignancy

When the reason for the encounter is evaluation or treatment of the malignancy, sequence the primary neoplasm first, followed by codes for metastatic sites, complications, or any other relevant conditions (OGCR I.C.2.a and OGCR I.C.2.l.1)). Treatment of the malignancy includes surgical removal of the neoplasm, diagnostic testing to determine the location or extent of the malignancy, and therapies such as paracentesis

(*a surgical puncture of a body cavity to remove ascites*) or thoracentesis (*surgical puncture of the chest wall to remove fluids*).

When *both* the primary and secondary sites are being treated or evaluated, sequence the primary malignancy first, followed by the code(s) for the secondary site(s). Use a code for the primary malignancy as long as the patient is receiving treatment for it, even if the tumor has been surgically removed (OGCR I.C.2.l.1).

Be careful to understand the difference between primary or secondary malignant neoplasm and principal or first-listed diagnosis. The terms *primary* and *secondary neoplasm* refer to the progression of the malignancy: where it started and where it spread to. *Principal* and *first-listed diagnosis* refer to the sequencing of codes. A code for primary neoplasm is not always sequenced first and a code for secondary neoplasm is not always sequenced second. When the metastasis or secondary neoplasm is the main reason for the encounter or admission, it is sequenced first.

Evaluation or Treatment of the Metastasis

When the reason for the encounter is evaluation or treatment of the secondary malignancy or metastasis *only*, sequence the code for the secondary site as the principal or first-listed diagnosis; sequence the code for the primary malignancy as an additional code (OGCR I.C.2.b and OGCR I.C.2.l.2)).

When *both* the primary and secondary sites are evaluated or treated, sequence the primary site first.

Table 5-5 ■ **SUMMARY OF COMMONLY USED SEQUENCING RULES FOR NEOPLASMS**

Reason for Encounter	Sequencing
Evaluation or treatment of primary neoplasm or *both* primary and secondary sites	1. Primary neoplasm 2. Secondary neoplasm
Evaluation or treatment of metastasis	1. Secondary neoplasm 2. Primary neoplasm
Evaluation or treatment *only* for complication of neoplasm (except anemia)	1. Complication 2. Primary neoplasm 3. Secondary neoplasm
Evaluation or treatment of anemia due to neoplasm	1. Neoplasm 2. Anemia
Encounter solely for chemotherapy, radiotherapy, or immunotherapy	1. Encounter for chemotherapy, radiotherapy, or immunotherapy 2. Complications during the therapy, if any 3. Primary neoplasm 4. Secondary neoplasm
Treatment, such as surgery, followed by chemotherapy, radiotherapy, or immunotherapy	1. The neoplasm that was the objective of the treatment 2. Any additional neoplasms
Screening due to family history of malignant neoplasm	1. Screening 2. Family history of malignant neoplasm
Follow-up after completing treatment for a malignant neoplasm that no longer exists	1. Follow-up 2. Personal history of malignant neoplasm
Evaluation or treatment for an unrelated condition	1. Unrelated condition 2. Neoplasm, if documented as relevant

Encounter Solely for Chemo-, Radio-, or Immunotherapy

When the reason for the encounter or admission is *only* for administration of chemotherapy, radiotherapy, or immunotherapy, assign the principal or first-listed diagnosis for **Encounter for**, followed by the name of the therapy (OGCR I.C.2.e.2)). To locate the code in the Index, search for the Main Terms **Chemotherapy**, **Radiotherapy**, or **Immunotherapy**, as appropriate. Sequence codes for the primary and/or secondary neoplasms as additional codes.

When the primary malignancy has been surgically removed but the patient is still receiving treatment, assign the code for **Encounter for** the therapy first, followed by the code for malignant neoplasm. Do not assign a code for personal history of malignant neoplasm while the patient is still receiving treatment, even when it has been surgically removed.

When an episode of care involves surgical removal of the neoplasm followed by chemotherapy or radiation therapy during the *same* episode of care, sequence the neoplasm code first, followed by the **Encounter for** therapy code(s) (OGCR I.C.2.e.1)).

Codes titled **Encounter for** are diagnosis codes that describe the *reason* for the encounter and are referred to as **Z** codes because they begin with the character Z. They are diagnosis codes, not procedure codes. You also must assign procedure codes that describe the service(s) provided using ICD-10-PCS codes for inpatient hospitals or CPT codes for physician office and outpatient services. **Z** codes are discussed in detail in Chapter 6, "Factors Influencing Health Status and Contact with Health Services (Z00-Z99)," of this text.

Evaluation or Treatment for a Complication

When an encounter is for management of a complication associated with a neoplasm, such as dehydration, and the treatment is *only* for the complication, sequence the complication first, followed by the appropriate code(s) for the neoplasm (OGCR I.C.2.l)). However, if treatment is directed at the neoplasm and the complication is *also* treated, sequence the appropriate neoplasm code first, followed by the codes for the complications.

The exception to these sequencing rules is when the complication is anemia. When the encounter is for management of an anemia associated with the malignancy and the treatment is *only* for anemia, sequence the appropriate code for the *malignancy* as the principal or first-listed diagnosis followed by code **D63.0 Anemia in neoplastic disease** (OGCR I.C.2.l.4)).

SUCCESS STEP

To locate the code for anemia due to cancer in the Index, search for the Main Term **Anemia**, then the subterm **in**, then the second-level subterm **neoplastic disease**.

Personal or Family History of Malignant Neoplasm

When a physician documents that family history of malignant neoplasm contributes to a patient's health risk, sequence the diagnosis code for screening first, followed by the history code. For example, a patient with a history of colonic polyps and a family history of colorectal cancer might need a colonoscopy more frequently than the general population. Sequence the codes as follows:

1. Screening for malignant neoplasm of colon
2. Personal history of colon polyps (benign neoplasm)
3. Family history, malignant neoplasm of digestive organs

When a physician sees a patient for follow-up after cancer treatment has been completed and the disease no longer exists at the site treated, assign a code for follow-up first, followed by the appropriate personal history code of the specific site (OGCR I.C.21.c.8)).

The circumstances discussed here are the most common that coders encounter. Refer to the OGCR I.C.2.c for additional detailed guidance on sequencing related to neoplasms.

Guided Example of Arranging Neoplasm Codes

Continue with the example from earlier in this chapter of Anthony Payne, who saw Dr. Blackford for prostate cancer. Follow along in your ICD-10-CM manual as Karla Destefano, CPC, sequences the codes. Check off each step after you complete it.

▶ Karla reviews the codes she assigned.

❑ **C61 Malignant neoplasm of prostate**

❑ **C78.5 Secondary malignant neoplasm of large intestine and rectum**

▶ She reviews the reason for the encounter in the medical record: *review test results to determine extent of prostate cancer*

❑ Therefore, she sequences the primary neoplasm as the first-listed diagnosis, followed by the metastatic site:

(1) **C61 Malignant neoplasm of prostate**

(2) **C78.5 Secondary malignant neoplasm of large intestine and rectum**

CODING PRACTICE

Exercise 5.4 Arranging Codes for Neoplasms

Instructions: Read the mini-medical-record of each patient's encounter, review the information abstracted in Exercise 5.2, assign ICD-10-CM diagnosis codes using the Index and Tabular List, and sequence the codes correctly. Write the code(s) on the line provided.

---

1. OFFICE   Gender: F   Age: 59

Reason for encounter: Chemotherapy

Assessment: Adenocarcinoma of the right breast, lower outer quadrant, which metastasized to multiple overlapping sites in the brain

Plan: Return for next treatment in 3 weeks

Tip: Refer to OGCR I.C.2.e.2) for a reminder on how to sequence these codes. Remember to verify all codes in the Tabular List.

3 ICD-10-CM Codes _____

_____

---

2. INPATIENT HOSPITAL   Gender: M   Age: 61

Reason for procedure: Brainstem tumor

Procedure description: Used Gamma Knife surgery to destroy tumor

Postprocedural diagnosis: Squamous cell carcinoma of the lung with brainstem metastases

Plan: FU in office 1 week, evaluate for chemotherapy

Tip: The site that is the reason for surgery should be sequenced first.

2 ICD-10-CM Codes _____

---

3. INPATIENT HOSPITAL   Gender: M   Age: 67

Reason for admission: Anemia

Assessment: Anemia due to classical lymphocyte-depleted Hodgkin's lymphoma

Plan: Administer IV iron supplements

Tip: Refer to OGCR I.C.2.l.4) for sequencing guidance.

2 ICD-10-CM Codes _____

CHAPTER SUMMARY

In this chapter you learned that:

- Neoplasms are abnormal growth of new tissue, which may be malignant or benign.

- ICD-10-CM Chapter 2, "Neoplasms (C00-D49)," classifies all malignant and most benign neoplasms. Some benign neoplasms are classified in the specific body system chapter.

- ICD-10-CM provides Official Guidelines for Coding and Reporting (OGCR) for neoplasms in OGCR section I.C.2, which provide specific direction for sequencing codes for multiple neoplasms, complications, adjuvant therapies, and other situations.

- When abstracting patient cases with neoplasms, coders must look for several pieces of information that will help determine the first-listed or principal diagnosis and the sequencing of any additional diagnoses.

- Coders use both the Index to Diseases and Injuries and the Table of Neoplasms to locate codes for neoplasms.

- Sequencing of neoplasm codes is determined by the circumstances of the encounter or admission. OGCR provides detailed guidance on sequencing. Coders must determine the main reason for a specific encounter or admission to select the correct first-listed or principal diagnosis.

CONCEPT QUIZ

Take a moment to look back through neoplasms and solidify your skills. This is your opportunity to pull together everything you have learned.

Completion

Instructions: Write the term that completes each statement based on the information you learned in this chapter. Choose from the following list. Some choices may be used more than once and some choices may not be used at all.

adjuvant	malignant
behavior	metastasis
benign	overlapping
CA in situ	primary neoplasm
carcinoma	radiotherapy
chemotherapy	sarcoma
CUP	secondary neoplasm
grading	staging
histology	topography
immunotherapy	

1. _____ describes the anatomic site where the neoplasm begins.

2. _____ describes the tissue type.

3. _____ describes a neoplasm that has spread to other sites.

4. _____ is the process of determining how far the cancer has spread.

5. Examples of _____ therapy include chemotherapy, radiotherapy, and immunotherapy.

6. _____ uses drugs to kill cancer cells.

7. _____ occurs only in epithelial cells.

8. _____ tumors are contiguous sites where the neoplasm continues from one site to the adjacent one without interruption.

9. _____ describes how closely the cancer cell looks like a normal cell when viewed microscopically.

10. _____ means life-threatening.

Multiple Choice

Instructions: Circle the letter of the best answer to each question based on the information you learned in this chapter.

1. Which of the following is a characteristic of characteristics describes benign neoplasms?
   A. Are not encapsulated
   B. Have invasive growth and metastasis
   C. Produce no cachexia
   D. Can recur when surgically removed

2. How do malignant neoplasms metastasize?
   A. Through the exchange of bodily fluids
   B. Through the bloodstream and lymphatic system
   C. Through genetic transmission
   D. Through bacteria

3. What is the personal history of malignant neoplasm?
   A. A condition that a patient's family member had in the past or currently has that causes the patient to be at higher risk of also contracting or developing the disease.
   B. A primary neoplasm that has metastasized.
   C. A condition the patient currently has and is receiving treatment for.
   D. A condition the patient had in the past, was removed or resolved, and is no longer being treated, but has the potential for recurrence.

4. How would you code the following scenario? *A patient is seen for cancer metastases to the left lung.*
   A. C34.92, C79.9
   B. C78.02, C80.1
   C. C34.92, C78.02
   D. D38.1

5. What condition's codes include characters to identify whether the disease is in remission or relapse?
   A. Breast cancer
   B. Leukemia
   C. Benign neoplasms
   D. Adenocarcinoma

6. Where should a coder look to locate a code for personal history of a malignant neoplasm?
   A. Under the Main Term *Personal* and subterm *neoplasm* in the Index
   B. Under the Main Term *History* and subterm *personal* in the Index
   C. In the column titled *Malignant Primary* in the Table of Neoplasms
   D. In the column titled *Personal History* in the Table of Neoplasms

7. How would you code the following scenario? *A patient is seen for dehydration due to colon cancer that has metastasized to multiple sites.*
   A. C18.9, E86.0
   B. E86.0
   C. C18.9
   D. E86.0, C18.9, C79.9

8. How would you code the following scenario? *A patient is admitted for surgery to remove a tumor from the lower inner quadrant of the right breast then receives chemotherapy while still in the hospital.*
   A. Z51.11, C50.311
   B. Z51.11
   C. C50.311
   D. C50.311, Z51.11

9. Which code should be sequenced first when a patient receives a colonoscopy more frequently than normal because of a family history of colon cancer?
   A. Screening
   B. Family history of malignant neoplasm
   C. Personal history of malignant neoplasm
   D. Colon cancer

10. Which code(s) should be assigned when a patient who previously had surgery to remove a malignant neoplasm of the lung has an encounter only for radiotherapy?
    A. Malignant neoplasm only
    B. Encounter for radiotherapy only
    C. Malignant neoplasm first and encounter for radiotherapy second
    D. Encounter for radiotherapy first and malignant neoplasm second

KEEP ON CODING

Instructions: Read the diagnostic statement, then use the Index and Tabular List to assign and sequence ICD-10-CM diagnosis codes. Write the code(s) on the line provided.

1. Carcinoma in situ of false vocal cord. ICD-10-CM Code(s) _____

2. Benign neoplasm of the mouth. ICD-10-CM Code(s) _____

3. Benign carcinoid tumor of the right kidney. ICD-10-CM Code(s) _____

4. Mesothelioma of lung. ICD-10-CM Code(s) _____

5. Metastatic carcinoma of the parietal lobe of the brain. ICD-10-CM Code(s) _____

6. Benign adenomatous polyps of colon. ICD-10-CM Code(s) _____

7. Chief cell adenoma. ICD-10-CM Code(s) _____

8. Kaposi's sarcoma of stomach with HIV. ICD-10-CM Code(s) _____

9. Basal cell carcinoma of right hand. ICD-10-CM Code(s) _____

10. Malignant melanoma of skin of abdominal wall. ICD-10-CM Code(s) _____

11. Malignant neoplasm of nipple of the right breast. ICD-10-CM Code(s) _____

12. Follicular lymphoma, Grade IIIb, inguinal region. ICD-10-CM Code(s) _____

13. Acute leukemia, in relapse. ICD-10-CM Code(s) _____

14. Melanoma of left forearm. ICD-10-CM Code(s) _____

15. Carcinoma in situ, cervical stump. ICD-10-CM Code(s) _____

16. Family history of breast cancer. ICD-10-CM Code(s) _____

17. Personal history of brain cancer. ICD-10-CM Code(s) _____

18. Malignant neoplasm with overlapping lesions in the left upper and lower lobes of the lung, primary. ICD-10-CM Code(s) _____

19. Admission for chemotherapy for ovarian cancer. ICD-10-CM Code(s) _____

20. Malignant primary cancer of the body of the pancreas. ICD-10-CM Code(s) _____

(*continued*)

(continued from page 93)

21. Metastatic cancer to the rib. ICD-10-CM Code(s) _____

22. Anemia due to left intraocular cancer. ICD-10-CM Code(s) _____

23. Metastatic cancer of the liver, with unknown primary site. ICD-10-CM Code(s) _____

24. Invasive (malignant) hydatidiform mole. ICD-10-CM Code(s) _____

25. Adenocarcinoma of the parotid gland with metastasis to the spine. ICD-10-CM Code(s) _____

CODING CHALLENGE

Instructions: Read the mini-medical-record of each patient's encounter, then abstract, assign, and sequence ICD-10-CM diagnosis codes using the Index and Tabular List. Write the code(s) on the line provided.

1. OFFICE   Gender: F   Age: 32

Chief complaint: Management of multiple myeloma

Assessment: Multiple myeloma in remission

Plan: Recheck in 6 months

Tip: The fifth character in the code specifies remission.

1 ICD-10-CM Code _____

2. OUTPATIENT SURGERY   Gender: M   Age: 67

Reason for procedure: Removal of tumor in left cheek

Procedure description: Removed one lesion, 0.5 cm

Postprocedural diagnosis: Basal cell adenoma left parotid salivary gland

Plan: Recheck in 6 months

Tip: The parotid salivary gland is located in the cheek.

1 ICD-10-CM Code _____

3. OFFICE   Gender: F   Age: 57

Chief complaint: Review colon biopsy results

Assessment: Adenocarcinoma in situ in sigmoid colon

Plan: Schedule surgery

Tip: What is another term for the colon? Search for this term to find the code you need.

1 ICD-10-CM Code _____

4. OFFICE   Gender: M   Age: 27

Chief complaint: Evaluate unusual mole on forehead

Assessment: Malignant melanoma

Plan: Schedule removal next week

Tip: Remember to search for the subterm *skin*.

1 ICD-10-CM Code _____

5. OFFICE   Gender: F   Age: 35

Chief complaint: Review pathology results of lesion removed from skin of left breast 1 week ago

Assessment: CA in situ, completely removed

Plan: Self-check entire skin once a month to watch for any additional lesions; schedule a recheck appointment with office in 6 months

1 ICD-10-CM Code _____

6. OUTPATIENT HOSPITAL   Gender: F   Age: 71

Reason for encounter: Radiotherapy to lung

Assessment: Metastatic cancer in the right lung, CUP

Plan: 5 treatments per week for 6 weeks

Tip: The site being treated is the first-listed diagnosis.

3 ICD-10-CM Codes _____

_____

7. OFFICE   Gender: F   Age: 63

Chief complaint: Monitoring of benign neoplasm

Assessment: Benign Islet cell neoplasm of the pancreas

Plan: Return visit if any new problems arise

1 ICD-10-CM Code _____

8. OUTPATIENT HOSPITAL   Gender: F   Age: 66

Reason for encounter: Screening colonoscopy

Assessment: Personal history of carcinoma of the colon which was successfully removed five years ago, no new findings today

Plan: Colonoscopy in 5 years

Tip: Refer to OGCR I.C.21.c.8) for coding and sequencing guidance.

2 ICD-10-CM Codes _____

(continued)

9. INPATIENT HOSPITAL   Gender: M   Age: 48

Reason for admission: Surgery for widespread metastases from pancreatic cancer.

Assessment: Surgery was performed, followed by inpatient chemotherapy.

Plan: Begin weekly regimen of outpatient chemotherapy

Tip: Refer to OGCR I.C.2.e.1).

2 ICD-10-CM Codes _____

10. INPATIENT HOSPITAL   Gender: F   Age: 81

Reason for admission: Admitted from emergency department after collapsing at home, arrived by ambulance

Assessment: Dehydration and hyponatremia (*sodium deficiency*) due to chemotherapy for metastatic bilateral ovarian cancer

Tip: The code for the complication is a combination code. Metastatic ovarian cancer means that the ovary is the primary site and the secondary site is unknown. Refer to OGCR I.B.13 to review rules for coding bilateral conditions. Refer to OGCR I.C.2.e.4) for sequencing guidance.

4 ICD-10-CM Codes _____
_____

Chapter 6

Factors Influencing Health Status and Contact with Health Services (Z00-Z99)

Chapter Outline

- **Purpose of Z Codes**
- **Coding Guidelines for Z Codes**
- **Abstracting for Z Codes**
- **Assigning Z Codes**
- **Arranging Z Codes**

Learning Objectives

After completing this chapter, you should have the skills to:

6.1 Spell and define the key words, medical terms, and abbreviations related to factors influencing health status and contact with health services. (Remember)

6.2 Describe the purpose of codes for factors influencing health status and contact with health services. (Understand)

6.3 Adhere to the Official Guidelines for Coding and Reporting related to factors influencing health status and contact with health services. (Apply)

6.3 Examine and abstract information required for coding factors influencing health status and contact with health services from the medical record. (Analyze)

6.4 Demonstrate how to assign codes for factors influencing health status and contact with health services. (Apply)

6.5 Utilize guidelines for arranging (sequencing) codes for factors influencing health status and contact with health services and related conditions. (Apply)

Key Terms and Abbreviations

ostomy
prophylactic
Z code

In addition to the key terms listed here, students should know the terms defined within tables in this chapter.

INTRODUCTION

Car owners sometimes visit a mechanic even though they have not experienced a breakdown, such as when they seek an oil change or periodic preventive maintenance. In healthcare, patients receive services even though they are not ill or injured. They may seek annual physical examinations, vaccinations, screening examinations, follow-up care, or maternity care. Physicians need to track information about patients' health status, health history, and health risks that do not present current problems but could in the future. In this chapter you learn how to use ICD-10-CM for patient encounters when patients receive healthcare services even though they are not ill or injured.

PURPOSE OF Z CODES

ICD-10-CM Chapter 21 classifies factors influencing health status and contact with health services. For the sake of brevity, this text refers to these codes as **Z codes**. Z codes represent reasons for encounters and may be used in any healthcare setting when the reason for the encounter is not a disease, injury, or external cause that is classified in the preceding ICD-10-CM chapters for body systems (A00 to Y99). Z codes are used in two general types of circumstances:

- A person encounters the health services for some specific purpose that, in itself, is not a disease or injury. Examples are receiving limited care or service for a current condition, donating an organ or tissue, receiving **prophylactic** (*for the prevention of the spread of disease or infection*) vaccination, or discussing a problem.

- A circumstance or problem exists that influences the person's health status, but is not, in itself, a current illness or injury. Examples are being a carrier of a communicable disease, having a family history of certain conditions, and wearing a prosthetic device such as a pacemaker or an artificial limb.

Z codes are classified into 15 categories, which are defined in ■ TABLE 6-1, page 98. Acquaint yourself with these definitions and examples, as they are the foundation for learning to abstract, assign, and sequence Z codes. Refer to the specific Official Guidelines for Coding and Reporting (OGCR) listed for a full discussion of how to use each category.

SUCCESS STEP

Although you do not need to memorize specific codes, it is helpful to memorize the Z code categories and definitions. By knowing the circumstances in which Z codes are required, you will become more accurate when abstracting.

CODING PRACTICE

Exercise 6.1   Introduction to Z Codes

Instructions: Write your answer to each question in the space provided.

1. Give three examples of Z codes that describe the main reason for the encounter. _____
   _____

2. What is the OGCR location of guidelines for each of the following Z code categories?

   Example: History *OGCR I.C.21.c.4)* _____

   a. Contact/Exposure _____

   b. Status _____

   c. Aftercare _____

   d. Routine and Administrative Examinations _____
      _____

Tip: Refer to Table 6-1.

3. Identify the Z code category for each of the following codes:

   Example: Z67.10 Type A blood, Rh positive *Status* _____

   a. Z12.31 Encounter for screening mammogram for malignant neoplasm of breast _____

   b. Z52.4 Kidney donor _____

   c. Z86.59 Personal history of other mental and behavioral disorders _____

   d. Z86.11 Personal history of tuberculosis
      _____

Tip: Refer to Table 6-1.

Table 6-1 ■ **DEFINITIONS AND EXAMPLES OF Z CODE CATEGORIES**

Z Code Category/OGCR	Definition	Example Codes
Contact/Exposure (OGCR I.C.21.c.1))	Patient does not show any sign or symptom of a disease but is suspected to have been exposed to it by close personal contact with an infected individual or is in an area where a disease is epidemic.	Z20.5 Contact with and (suspected) exposure to viral hepatitis Z20.820 Contact with and (suspected) exposure to varicella
Inoculations and vaccinations (OGCR I.C.21.c.2))	A patient receives a prophylactic inoculation or vaccination against a disease. Code first for any routine examination.	Z23 Encounter for immunization
Status (OGCR I.C.21.c.3))	A patient is either a carrier of a disease or has the sequela or residual of a past disease or condition.	Z21 Asymptomatic HIV infection status Z67.10 Type A blood, Rh positive Z68.23 Body mass index (BMI) 23.0-23.9, adult Z94.1 Heart transplant status
History (of) (OGCR I.C.21.c.4))	Personal history codes explain a patient's past medical condition that no longer exists and is not receiving any treatment, but that has the potential for recurrence, and therefore may require continued monitoring. Family history codes are for a patient who has a family member(s) who has had a particular disease, which causes the patient to be at higher risk of also contracting the disease.	Z86.11 Personal history of tuberculosis Z80.3 Family history of malignant neoplasm of breast
Screening (OGCR I.C.21.c.5))	Seemingly well individuals receive testing for disease or disease precursors so that early detection and treatment can be provided for those who test positive for the disease.	Z12.31 Encounter for screening mammogram for malignant neoplasm of breast Z13.1 Encounter for screening for diabetes mellitus
Observation (OGCR I.C.21.c.6))	A person is being observed for a suspected condition that is ruled out. This category is rarely used.	Z03.73 Encounter for suspected fetal anomaly ruled out
Aftercare (OGCR I.C.21.c.7))	The initial treatment of a disease has been performed and the patient requires continued care during the healing or recovery phase or for the long-term consequences of the disease.	Z44.002 Encounter for fitting and adjustment of unspecified left artificial arm Z51.11 Encounter for antineoplastic chemotherapy
Follow-up (OGCR I.C.21.c.8))	Continuing surveillance following completed treatment of a disease, condition, or injury when the condition has been fully treated and no longer exists.	Z08 Encounter for follow-up examination after completed treatment for malignant neoplasm Z39.2 Encounter for routine postpartum follow-up
Donor (OGCR I.C.21.c.9))	Living individuals are donating blood or other body tissue.	Z52.4 Kidney donor
Counseling (OGCR I.C.21.c.10))	A patient or family member receives assistance in the aftermath of an illness or injury, or when support is required in coping with family or social problems.	Z31.5 Encounter for genetic counseling Z69.010 Encounter for mental health services for victim of parental child abuse
Encounters for Obstetrical and Reproductive Services (OGCR I.C.21.c.11))	A patient receives obstetric or reproductive encounters when none of the problems or complications included in the codes from the obstetrics chapter (ICD-10-CM Chapter 15 (O00-O9A)) exist.	Z34.01 Encounter for supervision of normal first pregnancy, first trimester Z37.0 Single live birth Z3A.17 17 weeks gestation of pregnancy
Newborns and Infants (OGCR I.C.21.c.12))	Reports the health supervision and care of foundling, routine child health examination, and classification of birth status of liveborn infants.	Z00.110 Health examination for newborn under 8 days old
Routine and Administrative Examinations (OGCR I.C.21.c.13))	Used for encounters for routine examinations or administrative purposes.	Z00.00 Encounter for general adult medical examination without abnormal findings Z02.1 Encounter for pre-employment examination Z32.01 Encounter for pregnancy test, result positive
Miscellaneous (OGCR I.C.21.c.14))	Additional codes provide useful information on circumstances that may affect a patient's care and treatment.	Z28.01 Immunization not carried out because of acute illness of patient Z53.09 Procedure and treatment not carried out because of other contraindication Z76.0 Encounter for issue of repeat prescription
Nonspecific (OGCR I.C.21.c.15))	Used primarily in inpatient settings when there is no further documentation to permit more precise coding.	Z86.59 Personal history of other mental and behavioral disorders Z92.23 Personal history of estrogen therapy

CODING GUIDELINES FOR Z CODES

Coders should understand the organization of this ICD-10-CM chapter, chapter-wide and commonly used instructional notes in the Tabular List, and the relevant OGCR. This information is necessary for accurate coding.

ICD-10-CM Chapter 21, "Factors Influencing Health Status and Contact with Health Services (Z00-Z99)," contains 15 blocks or subchapters. Review the block names and code ranges listed at the beginning of Chapter 21 in the ICD-10-CM manual to become familiar with the content and organization. This chapter is used to report reasons for encounters that are not due to a current illness or injury or to report health status or risk factors documented as significant by the physician. Instructional notes throughout all ICD-10-CM chapters in the Tabular List alert coders to many circumstances that require Z codes.

ICD-10-CM provides OGCR for Z codes in OGCR section I.C.21. OGCR contains a detailed discussion of the categories of Z codes, when to report them, and which codes may only be sequenced as the principal or first-listed diagnosis. Additional guidelines related to Z codes appear throughout the OGCR, particularly in OGCR I.B.3, I.C.1.a (HIV), I.C.2 (neoplasms), I.C.4 (endocrine), I.C.15 (obstetrics), I.C.19 (injuries), I.C.20 (external causes), and IV.B. Specific OGCR are discussed and cited throughout this chapter of the text.

ABSTRACTING FOR Z CODES

Because Z codes are applicable to a wide variety of situations, there is not one concise rule that guides coders when Z codes are needed. Refer to ■ TABLE 6-2 for guidance on how to abstract for the most commonly used Z codes.

Locate the patient situation in the left column, then refer to the appropriate Main Term in the right column. Remember that the abstracting questions are a guide and that not every encounter requires a Z code. In addition, some situations not in this table also require Z codes, which are discussed later in this chapter.

In addition to using Z codes when they describe the reason for the encounter, coders receive direction to abstract for Z codes from two sources:

- Instructional notes in the Tabular List
- OGCR I.C.21

Identifying the Reason for the Encounter

When a Z code(s) describes the main reason for the encounter, abstracting is fairly straightforward. Coders identify the main reason for the encounter, then search for the Main Term in the Index to Diseases and Injuries (Index) to locate the Z code. Examples of Z codes describing the main reason for the encounter include:

- Aftercare
- Counseling
- Follow-up
- Immunizations
- Observation
- Routine pregnancy
- Routine or administrative examinations (pre-employment, annual checkup)
- Screening examinations (colonoscopy, mammogram)

Table 6-2 ■ **KEY CRITERIA FOR ABSTRACTING Z CODES**

Patient Situation	Main Term
❑ Is the reason for the encounter a routine examination?	Examination
❑ Is the reason for the encounter to receive an inoculation or vaccination against a disease?	Inoculation
❑ Does the physician document a past medical condition that no longer exists and is not receiving any treatment but has the potential for recurrence?	History, personal
❑ Does the physician document that the patient has a family member(s) who has had a particular disease, which causes the patient to be at higher risk of also contracting the disease?	History, family
❑ Is the reason for the encounter testing for disease or disease precursors in seemingly well individuals so that early detection and treatment can be provided?	Screening
❑ Does the physician document a lifestyle habit that poses a risk factor?	Use
❑ Is the reason for the encounter continued care during the healing or recovery phase after initial treatment has been completed?	Aftercare
❑ Is the reason for the encounter continuing surveillance following completed treatment of a disease, condition, or injury when the condition has been fully treated and no longer exists?	Follow-up
❑ Is the reason for the encounter to receive assistance in the aftermath of an illness or injury or for support in coping with family or social problems?	Counseling
❑ Did a woman give birth during the encounter?	Outcome of delivery
❑ Is the patient a newborn who was born during the current admission?	Newborn, born
❑ Was a procedure cancelled or a surgical approach converted?	Procedure
❑ Is a newborn observed for conditions that were suspected but not found to exist?	Observation

Interpreting Instructional Notes

In many circumstances, the Tabular List provides instructional notes directing the coder to assign certain types of Z codes (■ FIGURE 6-1). Examples of Z codes required by instructional notes include:

- Birth status of newborn
- Long-term use of medication
- Occupational risk factors
- Outcome of delivery (following pregnancy)
- Tobacco, alcohol, drug use and dependence

Coders must distinguish between codes for history and current use. As shown in Figure 6-1, instructional notes list a variety of options for Z codes that should be reported. Coders must identify the correct code for the specific situation. Report **history of tobacco dependence (Z87.891)** when tobacco use occurred in the past but the patient is not currently using tobacco. Report **tobacco use (Z72.0)** when the patient currently uses tobacco but is not stated as a smoker and no more specific information about tobacco use is given. Report **tobacco dependence (F17.-)** rather than **tobacco use (Z72.0)** when the medical record documents the dependence or specifically states the patient is a smoker. **Z72.0** is not used frequently because documentation often provides enough information to assign a code from category **F17.- Nicotine dependence** or **Z87.891 Personal history of nicotine dependence**.

CODING CAUTION

Remember that codes in instructional notes should be reported only when they apply to the patient. For example, do not report **Z87.891 Personal history of nicotine dependence** if the patient does not have a history of tobacco use or dependence.

Applying the Official Guidelines

The most challenging situation is when OGCR requires Z codes to describe supplemental information related to the encounter but the Tabular List does not provide instructional notes. The Tabular List cannot anticipate every patient circumstance for every diagnosis in which a Z code is needed. This is when coders' knowledge of OGCR guides them to abstract the

information. Examples of Z codes that may be required by the OGCR and rely on coders' knowledge include:

- Acquired absence of organ or body part
- Artificial opening status
- Blood type
- Body mass index (BMI)
- Carrier
- Do not resuscitate (DNR) status
- Internal or external prosthetics, functional implements, or enabling devices
- Personal or family history
- Postprocedural states
- Problems related to life circumstances such as education, literacy, employment, unemployment, housing, family situation
- Transplant waiting list, recipient, or donor

Guided Example of Abstracting Z Codes

Refer to the following example here and throughout the chapter to learn more about using Z codes. Sherry Whittle, CPC, is a fictitious coder who guides you through coding this case.

Date: 7/1/yy   Location: Branton Medical Center Outpatient Procedure Clinic

Provider: Stanley Garrett, MD

Patient: Angela Holmes   Gender: F   Age: 50

Procedure: Screening colonoscopy

Findings: None

Plan: Next colonoscopy in 10 years

Follow along as Sherry abstracts the Z code. Check off each step as you complete it.

▶ Sherry refers to Key Criteria for Abstracting Z Codes (Table 6-2) and looks for questions that may apply to this patient.

❏ *Is the reason for the encounter a routine examination?* No, although this is a routine colonoscopy, a colonoscopy is not considered to be an examination

❏ *Does the physician document a past medical condition that no longer exists and is not receiving any treatment but that has the potential for recurrence?* No. If the patient were receiving the colonoscopy because of previous colon cancer, then Sherry would answer "yes" and be directed to a different Z code category and a different Main Term.

❏ *Does the physician document that the patient has a family member(s) who has had a particular disease,*

I20 Angina pectoris
Use additional code to identify:
exposure to environmental tobacco smoke (Z77.22)
history of tobacco dependence (Z87.891)
occupational exposure to environmental tobacco smoke
   (Z57.31)
tobacco dependence (F17.-)
tobacco use (Z72.0)

Figure 6-1 ■ Example of instructional notes in Tabular List requiring Z codes (category I20).

which causes the patient to be at higher risk of also contracting the disease? No. If the colonoscopy were being done at a more-frequent-than-normal interval because of having family members with colon cancer, Sherry would answer "yes" and would assign a code for family history of colon cancer.

❑ *Is the reason for the encounter testing for disease or disease precursors in seemingly well individuals so that early detection and treatment can be provided? Yes, this is the definition of a screening*

▶ Next, Sherry will assign the code.

CODING PRACTICE

Exercise 6.2   Abstracting for Z Codes

Instructions: Read the mini-medical-record of each patient's encounter and answer the abstracting questions. Write the answer on the line provided. Do not assign any codes.

1. OFFICE   Gender: M   Age: 52

Reason for encounter: Annual medical examination

Assessment: Comprehensive metabolic panel test results are normal, no new problems

Plan: RTO 1 year

a. What is the reason for the encounter? _____

_____

b. Were there any abnormal findings? _____

If yes, what are they? _____

_____

2. OFFICE   Gender: F   Age: 24

Reason for encounter: Supervision of normal second pregnancy, third trimester, 34 weeks

Assessment: Estimated date of delivery (EDD) 8/3/yy

Plan: RTO 1 week

a. What is the reason for the encounter? _____

_____

b. Were there any abnormal findings? _____

If yes, what are they? _____

_____

3. OFFICE   Gender: M   Age: 76

Reason for encounter: Adjustment of cardiac pacemaker

Assessment: Reprogrammed pacemaker, no problems

Plan: RTO 6 months

a. What is the reason for the encounter? _____

_____

b. Were there any abnormal findings? _____

If yes, what are they? _____

_____

4. OUTPATIENT HOSPITAL   Gender: F   Age: 47

Reason for encounter: Screening mammogram

Assessment: Normal mammogram, both breasts

Plan: Repeat screening 6 months due to personal history of breast cancer

Tip: The National Cancer Institute recommends mammograms every one to two years for women over age 50.

a. What is the reason for the encounter? _____

_____

b. Were there any abnormal findings? _____

If yes, what are they? _____

_____

c. Why is this patient receiving a mammogram more frequently than normal? _____

_____

5. OFFICE   Gender: M   Age: 61

Reason for encounter: 6-month follow-up after removal of prostate due to malignant neoplasm of prostate

Assessment: No new findings, no recurrence of disease, no current treatment

Plan: Next FU 6 months

a. What is the reason for the encounter? _____

_____

b. Were there any abnormal findings? _____

If yes, what are they? _____

_____

c. What past condition is documented? _____

_____

d. A condition that no longer exists but presents potential for recurrence is classified as what? _____

_____

e. What gland was previously removed? _____

_____

(continued)

CODING PRACTICE *(continued)*

6. INPATIENT HOSPITAL Gender: M Age: 48

Reason for admission: Unresolved angina pectoris; current tobacco use

Assessment: EKG negative for AMI, ECC normal, angiogram normal

Discharge Plan: Rx nitroglycerin. Follow-up in office 1 week

(continued)

6. (continued)

a. What is the reason for the encounter? _____
_____

b. Were there any abnormal findings? _____
If yes, what are they? _____
_____

c. What lifestyle habit is documented? _____
_____

ASSIGNING Z CODES

When assigning Z codes, coders need to know what Main Terms to search for in the Index, how to distinguish between diagnosis codes and procedure codes, and when to not use a Z code.

Locating Main Terms

Coders normally search for the name of a condition or disease in the Index in order to locate codes. Because Z codes are not conditions, new coders may be puzzled about what Main Term to search for. Remember to identify the noun that describes the reason or purpose of the encounter. When a surgical procedure is not carried out or the approach is converted, such as conversion of a laparoscopic or thoracoscopic approach to open, search the Index for the Main Term Procedure. Refer to ■ Table 6-3 for commonly used Main Terms.

Distinguishing Diagnoses and Procedures

Recall that the diagnosis is the *reason* a service is provided, whereas the procedure identifies what is actually done. When the reason for the encounter is a screening examination or specific health service, the title of the Z code may look like a procedure code, but it is a diagnosis code—the reason for the encounter. Coders assign a Z code for the diagnosis and an ICD-10-PCS or CPT code for the procedure. (This chapter discusses only Z codes.) Examples of when confusion may occur include:

* Persons encountering health services for examinations. For the diagnosis, assign a Z code (**Z00-Z13**) as the reason for the encounter, then assign a procedure code to identify the complexity of the examination.

* Persons encountering health services in circumstances related to reproduction. For the diagnosis, assign a Z code (**Z30-Z39**) to describe the reason for the encounter, then assign a procedure code to identify the service(s) provided.

* Persons encountering other specific health procedures, such as fitting or adjustment of a prosthetic device, prophylactic or cosmetic surgery, or care of an **ostomy** *(artificial opening between a hollow organ and the skin)*. For the diagnosis, assign a Z code (**Z40-Z53**) to describe the reason for the encounter, then assign a procedure code to identify the service(s) provided.

Identifying When *Not* to Use Z Codes

In some cases, diagnosis codes from body system chapters may include information that coders would otherwise report with a status Z code. When this is the case, do not assign a Z code that repeats the same information as a code from an ICD-10-CM body system chapter. In addition, do not assign aftercare codes when the patient has a current condition that is coded from a body system chapter. Aftercare codes are used only after the initial treatment of a disease has been performed and the patient requires continued care during healing or recovery. Refer to ■ Figure 6-2 to learn more about body system chapter codes that override the need for Z codes.

In the example in Figure 6-2, because the diagnosis code is specific to a colostomy, do not also assign **Z93.3 Colostomy status**. In addition, because the colostomy malfunction is a current condition, do not assign code **Z43.3 Encounter for attention to colostomy**.

Table 6-3 ■ **COMMONLY USED MAIN TERMS FOR Z CODES**

❏ Absence, acquired	❏ History, family
❏ Admission (for)	❏ History, personal
❏ Aftercare	❏ Immunization
❏ Contact	❏ Newborn, born
❏ Counseling	❏ Newborn, twin, triplet, quadruplet
❏ Donor	❏ Outcome of delivery
❏ Encounter (for)	❏ Pregnancy
❏ Examination	❏ Procedure
❏ Exposure	❏ Status
❏ Fitting (and adjustment of)	❏ Supervision (of)
❏ Follow-up	

Patient is seen for a hernia at the site of a colostomy.

CORRECT:
K94.03 Colostomy malfunction
        Mechanical complication of colostomy

INCORRECT:
Z43.3 Encounter for attention to colostomy
Z93.3 Colostomy Status

Figure 6-2 ■ Example of a diagnosis code that overrides the need for a Z code.

Guided Example of Assigning Z Codes

To learn more about assigning Z codes and procedure codes, continue with the example about Angela Holmes, who was seen at Branton Medical Center Outpatient Procedure Clinic for a screening colonoscopy.

Follow along as Sherry Whittle, CPC, assigns the Z code. Check off each step as you complete it.

▶ Sherry searches the Index for the Main Term **Screening** (■ Figure 6-3).

  ❑ She locates the subterm **Colonoscopy, Z12.11**.

  ❑ She reviews the rest of the subterms and also locates **neoplasm (malignant)**, which has a second-level subterm **colon Z12.11**.

  ❑ She determines that both entries point to the same code because the purpose of a screening colonoscopy is to identify any benign polyps or sign of malignant neoplasm.

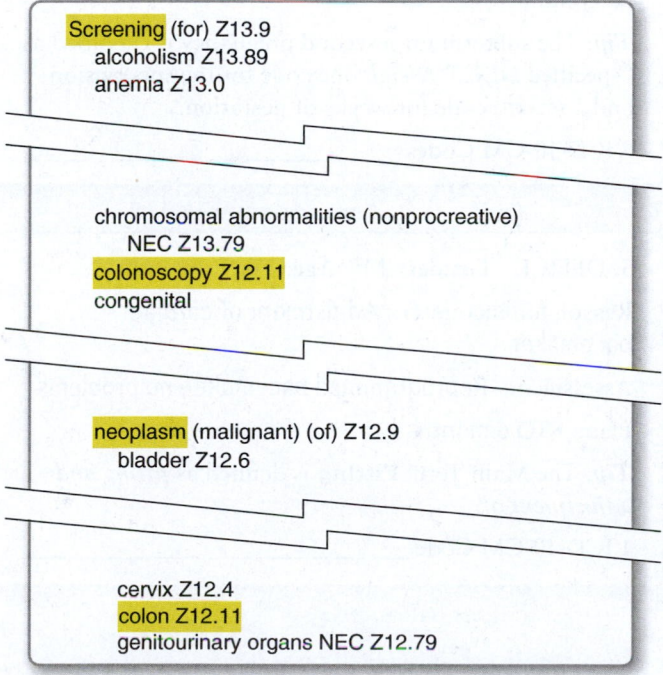

Screening (for) Z13.9
    alcoholism Z13.89
    anemia Z13.0

chromosomal abnormalities (nonprocreative)
    NEC Z13.79
colonoscopy Z12.11
congenital

neoplasm (malignant) (of) Z12.9
    bladder Z12.6

cervix Z12.4
colon Z12.11
genitourinary organs NEC Z12.79

Figure 6-3 ■ Index entry for the Main Term "Screening."

▶ Next, Sherry verifies code **Z12.11** in the Tabular List.

  ❑ She reads the code title for **Z12.11, Encounter for screening for malignant neoplasm of colon** and confirms that this accurately describes the reason for the encounter.

▶ Sherry checks for instructional notes in the Tabular List.

  ❑ She cross-references the beginning of category **Z12, Encounter for screening for malignant neoplasms** and reads the instructional notes (■ Figure 6-4, Page 104).

  ❑ The first instructional note defines what this category is used for. She determines that the patient's encounter meets this definition.

  ❑ The second instructional note states **Use additional code to identify any family history of malignant neoplasm (Z80.-)**. She checks the medical record for documentation of a family history of colon cancer and finds none, so she does not assign a code from **Z80**.

  ❑ The third instructional note is an **Excludes1** note that tells her to *not* use this category for an encounter for diagnostic examination. A diagnostic colonoscopy would be one performed because the patient presented with specific symptoms or signs, such as rectal bleeding, which the physician investigates. This patient did not present with any symptoms, so this note does not change the coding.

▶ Next, Sherry cross-references the beginning of the block **(Z00-Z13)** and reads the instructional notes, which apply to all codes in the block. The **NOTE:** does not apply because there were no abnormal findings of the colonoscopy. The **Excludes1** note does not apply because this encounter was unrelated to pregnancy and reproduction.

▶ She cross-references the beginning of **Chapter 21 (Z00-Z99)** and reads the instructional notes, which describe the use of Z codes.

  ❑ She notices the statement **A corresponding procedure code must accompany a Z code if a procedure is performed**. This confirms her thinking that she should assign a Z code for the diagnosis and a procedure code for the service performed.

▶ Sherry confirms the diagnosis code she has assigned for this case.

  ❑ **Z12.11 Encounter for screening for malignant neoplasm of colon**

▶ Next, Sherry will assign a CPT code to describe the physician's service of performing the colonoscopy. (CPT coding is covered elsewhere in this text.)

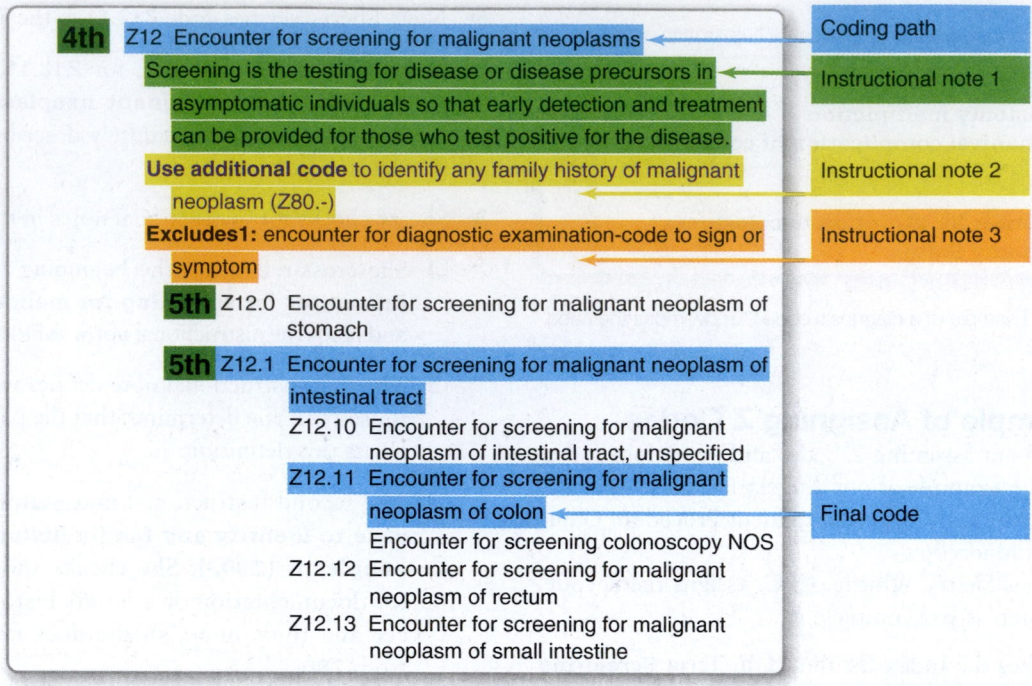

Figure 6-4 ■ Tabular List entry for category Z12 and code Z12.11.

CODING PRACTICE

Exercise 6.3 Assigning Z Codes

Instructions: Read the mini-medical-record of each patient's encounter, review the information abstracted in Exercise 6.2, and assign ICD-10-CM diagnosis codes using the Index and Tabular List. Write the code(s) on the line provided.

---

1. OFFICE   Gender: M   Age: 52

Reason for encounter: Annual medical examination

Assessment: Comprehensive metabolic panel test results are normal, no new problems

Plan: RTO 1 year

1 ICD-10-CM Code _____

---

2. OFFICE   Gender: F   Age: 24

Reason for encounter: Supervision of normal second pregnancy, third trimester, 34 weeks

Assessment: Estimated date of delivery (EDD) 8/3/yy

Plan: RTO 1 week

(continued)

---

2. (continued)

Tip: The subterm for a second pregnancy is classified as "specified NEC." Assign one code for the supervision and a second code for weeks of gestation.

2 ICD-10-CM Codes _____

---

3. OFFICE   Gender: M   Age: 76

Reason for encounter: Adjustment of cardiac pacemaker

Assessment: Reprogrammed pacemaker, no problems

Plan: RTO 6 months

Tip: The Main Term **Fitting** is defined as *fitting and adjustment of.*

1 ICD-10-CM Code _____

ARRANGING Z CODES

Instructional notes in the Tabular List and the OGCR provide sequencing guidance regarding which Z codes are permitted only as the principal or first-listed diagnosis code and which may be the sole diagnosis code or additional (secondary) diagnosis codes.

Determining the Principal or First-Listed Diagnosis

OGCR I.C.21.c.16) lists the Z codes and categories that may be reported *only* as the principal or first-listed diagnosis. This rule does not apply when patients have multiple encounters on the same day and the medical records for the encounters are combined, as sometimes happens for inpatient records.

Instructional notes in the Tabular List and OGCR from other chapters may also provide direction for Z code sequencing. For example, OGCR I.C.21.c.16) lists the following categories as principal or first-listed diagnosis only:

- **Z51.0 Encounter for antineoplastic radiation therapy**
- **Z51.1- Encounter for antineoplastic chemotherapy and immunotherapy**

OGCR I.C.2.e provides additional guidelines, which state:

- When an episode of care involves the surgical removal of a neoplasm, followed by adjunct chemotherapy or radiation therapy during the same episode of care, sequence the *neoplasm* code *first*, then assign any additional diagnoses.
- When more than one type of antineoplastic therapy is provided during the same encounter, either may be sequenced first.

Therefore, coders must review all the OGCR related to an encounter and apply critical thinking skills to compare and contrast the guidelines.

Using a Single Diagnosis Code

Any code listed in OGCR I.C.21.c.16) may be assigned as the sole (only) diagnosis code for an encounter. This is often the case when patients seek specific health services, such as routine and administrative medical examinations or supervision of a normal pregnancy, and have no other problems or conditions.

Status codes and history codes are rarely used as the sole diagnosis code because they do not represent the sole reason for an encounter. For example, codes for family history, BMI, blood type, or DNR describe supplemental information and are used in conjunction with other Z codes or codes from the body system chapters.

CODING CAUTION

Category **Z38 Liveborn infants according to place of birth and type of delivery** must always be sequenced *first* on *newborn* records that include the birth encounter. However, category **Z37 Outcome of delivery** must always be a *secondary* code on records of *mothers* that include the delivery encounter.

Selecting Additional Diagnosis Codes

Any code not listed in OGCR I.C.21.c.16) may be used as a secondary, or additional, diagnosis code. When no specific OGCR exists for sequencing a Z code, follow OGCR that apply to sequencing all diagnosis codes.

CODING PRACTICE

Exercise 6.4 Arranging Z Codes

Instructions: Read the mini-medical-record of each patient's encounter, review the information abstracted in Exercise 6.2, assign ICD-10-CM diagnosis codes using the Index and Tabular List, and sequence them correctly.

---

1. OUTPATIENT HOSPITAL   Gender: F   Age: 47

Reason for encounter: Screening mammogram

Assessment: Normal mammogram, both breasts

Plan: Repeat screening 6 months due to personal history of breast cancer

2 ICD-10-CM Codes _____

---

2. OFFICE   Gender: M   Age: 61

Reason for encounter: 6-month follow-up after removal of prostate due to malignant neoplasm of prostate

Assessment: No new findings, no recurrence of disease, no current treatment

Plan: Next FU 6 months

Tip: Assign codes for the examination, acquired absence of organ, and history of malignant neoplasm.

3 ICD-10-CM Codes _____

_____

(continued)

CODING PRACTICE (continued)

3. INPATIENT HOSPITAL   Gender: M   Age: 48

Reason for admission: Unstable angina pectoris, current tobacco use

Assessment: EKG negative for AMI, ECC normal, angiogram normal

(continued)

3. (continued)

Discharge Plan: Rx nitroglycerin. Follow up in office 1 week

Tip: Remember to read the instructional notes at the beginning of the three-character category.

2 ICD-10-CM Codes _____

CHAPTER SUMMARY

In this chapter you learned that:

- Z codes represent reasons for encounters and may be used in any healthcare setting when the reason for the encounter is not a disease, injury, or external cause that is classified in the preceding ICD-10-CM chapters for body systems (A00 to Y89).

- ICD-10-CM Chapter 21, "Factors Influencing Health Status and Contact with Health Services (Z00-Z99)," reports reasons for encounters that are not due to a current illness or injury or to report health status or risk factors documented as significant by the physician.

- ICD-10-CM provides OGCR for Z codes in OGCR section I.C.21, which contains a detailed discussion of the categories of Z codes, when to report them, and which codes may only be sequenced as the principal or first-listed diagnosis.

- Coders abstract information described by Z codes in three different types of circumstances: Z codes describe the reason for the encounter; instructional notes in the Tabular List direct coders to use Z codes; Z codes are required by the OGCR only.

- When assigning Z codes, coders need to know what Main Terms to search for in the Index, how to distinguish between diagnosis codes and procedure codes, and when not to use a Z code.

- Instructional notes in the Tabular List and the OGCR provide sequencing guidance regarding which Z codes are permitted only as the principal or first-listed diagnosis code and which may be the sole diagnosis code or additional (secondary) diagnosis codes.

CONCEPT QUIZ

Take a moment to look back at health status and health services and solidify your skills. This is your opportunity to pull together everything you have learned.

Completion

Instructions: Write the term that completes each statement based on the information you learned in this chapter. Choose from the following list. Some choices may be used more than once and some choices may not be used at all.

aftercare	newborns and infants
contact/exposure	observation
counseling	obstetrical and reproductive
donor	personal history
family history	routine and administrative examinations
follow-up	
inoculations and vaccinations	screening
miscellaneous	status

1. _____ Z codes describe testing for disease or disease precursors in seemingly well individuals so that early detection and treatment can be provided for those who test positive for the disease.

2. _____ Z codes describe a patient's past medical condition that no longer exists and is not receiving any treatment but that has the potential for recurrence and therefore may require continued monitoring.

3. _____ Z codes describe a person who is being observed for a suspected condition that is ruled out.

4. _____ Z codes describe when a patient or family member receives assistance in the aftermath of an illness or injury.

5. _____ Z codes include codes such as *Z00.00 Encounter for general adult medical examination*.

6. _____ Z codes describe when the initial treatment of a disease has been performed and the patient requires continued care during the healing or recovery phase or for the long-term consequences of the disease.

7. _____ Z codes describe a patient who has a family member(s) who has had a particular disease that causes the patient to be at higher risk of also contracting the disease.

8. *Z53.09 Procedure and treatment not carried out because of other contraindication* is an example of the Z code category for _____.

9. _____ Z codes describe continuing surveillance following completed treatment of a disease, condition, or injury when the condition has been fully treated and no longer exists.

10. _____ services Z codes include codes such as *Z37.0 Single live birth.*

Multiple Choice

Instructions: Circle the letter of the best answer to each question based on the information you learned in this chapter.

1. What is the formal name for Z codes?
   A. Supplemental Reasons for Health Service Encounters
   B. Personal and Family History of Certain Diseases
   C. Factors Influencing Health Status and Health Behavior
   D. Factors Influencing Health Status and Contact with Health Services

2. How would you code the following scenario? *A child is seen for a chickenpox (varicella) vaccination.*
   A. Z20.820
   B. Z23
   C. B01.9
   D. Z28.01

3. What category of Z codes is defined as "A person is being observed for a suspected condition that is ruled out"?
   A. Observation
   B. History
   C. Outcome of delivery
   D. Screening

4. What Z code category is defined as "A patient or family member receives assistance in the aftermath of an illness or injury, or when support is required in coping with family or social problems"?
   A. Aftercare
   B. Follow-up
   C. Counseling
   D. Observation

5. When should you assign a procedure code in addition to a Z code?
   A. Always
   B. When both codes are listed together in the Index
   C. When an instructional note in the Tabular List instructs you to do so
   D. Never

6. How would you code the following scenario? *The patient previously used tobacco, but no longer does.*
   A. Z72.0
   B. Z87.891
   C. Z77.22
   D. F17.201

7. In which healthcare settings(s) should Z codes be used?
   A. Inpatient settings only
   B. Outpatient settings only
   C. Preventive care settings only
   D. Any healthcare setting

8. How would you code the following scenario? *Health examination for newborn 6 days old.*
   A. Z00.110
   B. Z00.111
   C. Z00.121
   D. Z00.11

9. Which code is an example of the Z code category Encounters for Obstetrical and Reproductive Services?
   A. Z32.01 Encounter for pregnancy test, result positive
   B. Z20.4 Contact with and suspected exposure to rubella
   C. Z38.01 Single liveborn infant, delivered by cesarean
   D. Z34.01 Encounter for supervision of normal first pregnancy, first trimester

10. Which code is an example of the Z code category Aftercare?
    A. Z03.73 Encounter for suspected fetal anomaly ruled out
    B. Z08 Encounter for follow-up examination after completed treatment for malignant neoplasm
    C. Z44.002 Encounter for fitting and adjustment of unspecified left artificial arm
    D. Z69.010 Encounter for mental health services for victim of parental child abuse

KEEP ON CODING

Instructions: Read the diagnostic statement, then use the Index and Tabular List to assign and sequence ICD-10-CM diagnosis codes. Write the code(s) on the line provided.

1. Encounter for pregnancy test with a negative result. ICD-10-CM Code(s) _____

2. Blood type AB, Rh positive. ICD-10-CM Code(s) _____

3. Dental examination and cleaning. ICD-10-CM Code(s) _____

4. Surgical procedure canceled per patient decision. ICD-10-CM Code(s) _____

5. Status post heart transplant without complications. ICD-10-CM Code(s) _____

6. Renal dialysis status. ICD-10-CM Code(s) _____

7. Encounter for removal of breast implant. ICD-10-CM Code(s) _____

8. Laparoscopic procedure converted to open. ICD-10-CM Code(s) _____

9. Family history of diabetes mellitus. ICD-10-CM Code(s) _____

10. History of tobacco use. ICD-10-CM Code(s) _____

11. Encounter for paternity testing. ICD-10-CM Code(s) _____

12. Encounter for supervision of high-risk pregnancy in the 20th week (second trimester). ICD-10-CM Code(s) _____

13. Liveborn single female, delivered vaginally in the hospital. ICD-10-CM Code(s) _____

14. Lack of physical exercise. ICD-10-CM Code(s) _____

15. Long-term use of nonsteroidal anti-inflammatory drug (NSAID). ICD-10-CM Code(s) _____

16. Allergy to seafood. ICD-10-CM Code(s) _____

17. Presence of a cerebrospinal shunt. ICD-10-CM Code(s) _____

18. Physical restraint status. ICD-10-CM Code(s) _____

19. Do not resuscitate (DNR) status. ICD-10-CM Code(s) _____

20. Homelessness. ICD-10-CM Code(s) _____

21. Pregnant state incidental to encounter. ICD-10-CM Code(s) _____

22. Personal history of kidney stones. ICD-10-CM Code(s) _____

23. Cystic fibrosis carrier. ICD-10-CM Code(s) _____

24. History of adult neglect. ICD-10-CM Code(s) _____

25. Routine well-child exam, age six months, with abnormal findings. ICD-10-CM Code(s) _____

CODING CHALLENGE

Instructions: Read the mini-medical-record of each patient's encounter, then abstract, assign, and sequence ICD-10-CM diagnosis codes using the Index and Tabular List. Write the code(s) on the line provided.

1. INPATIENT HOSPITAL   Gender: M   Age: 1 day

Assessment: Normal healthy newborn after cesarean delivery here yesterday

Discharge Plan: FU with pediatrician in 2 weeks

Tip: Search under the Main Term *Newborn* and subterm *born*.

1 ICD-10-CM Code _____

2. INPATIENT HOSPITAL   Gender: M   Age: 67

Reason for admission: Initial antineoplastic chemotherapy; risk of tumor lysis syndrome and dehydration

Assessment: Small-cell carcinoma in both lungs; dehydration due to chemotherapy

Discharge Plan: RTO 1 week

Tip: Refer to OGCR I.C.2.e for guidance on code assignment and sequencing. Remember to code for laterality.

4 ICD-10-CM Codes _____

_____

3. OFFICE   Gender: F **Age:** 45

Reason for encounter: Follow-up exam after completing treatment for surgical removal of uterus due to endometrial cancer

Assessment: No new findings

Plan: FU 6 months

Tip: Remember to read all instructional notes in the Tabular List.

3 ICD-10-CM Codes _____

_____

4. INPATIENT HOSPITAL   Gender: F **Age:** 62

Reason for admission: Radical cystectomy followed by inpatient radiotherapy

Assessment: Stage III carcinoma of the bladder, invasive into bladder, no metastasis found

Plan: Continue radiotherapy as outpatient

2 ICD-10-CM Codes _____

5. OFFICE   Gender: M **Age:** 15

Reason for encounter: School sports physical

Assessment: Cleared for football

Plan: Discussed safety precautions and conditioning

1 ICD-10-CM Code _____

6. OFFICE   Gender: M **Age:** 12 months

Reason for encounter: Hepatitis B, MMR, and varicella immunizations

Assessment: Child has a heavy cold today, so immunization was not carried out

Plan: Reschedule when he is healthy

2 ICD-10-CM Codes _____

7. INPATIENT HOSPITAL   Gender: M **Age:** 29

Reason for admission: Patient is a donor match for brother who has end-stage renal disease (ESRD)

Assessment: Removal of kidney for transplantation to brother

Plan: FU in office, 4 weeks

1 ICD-10-CM Code _____

8. OFFICE   Gender: F **Age:** 4

Reason for encounter: Routine 4-year-old exam

Assessment: No new findings. MMR and varicella immunizations administered

Plan: RTO 1 year; call if any new problems

2 ICD-10-CM Codes _____

9. INPATIENT HOSPITAL   Gender: F **Age:** 23

Reason for admission: Normal delivery, 39 weeks' gestation

Outcome: Single liveborn infant

Discharge Plan: FU in office 2 weeks

Tip: Locate the delivery under the Main Term *Delivery* and subterm *normal*. Remember to read the instructional notes in the Tabular List.

3 ICD-10-CM Codes _____

_____

10. OFFICE   Gender: F **Age:** 65

Reason for encounter: Management of coronary artery disease (CAD)

Assessment: Chronic CAD; BP well controlled; smoker

Plan: Renew Rx for the anticoagulant warfarin, which patient has used successfully for 5 years. Discussed eating habits due to borderline cholesterol and the need to quit smoking

Tip: The first code is the disease. Read the instructional notes at the beginning of the category for the second code. The third code is for long-term drug therapy.

3 ICD-10-CM Codes _____

_____

Chapter 7

External Causes of Morbidity (V00-Y99)

Chapter Outline

- **Introduction to External Causes**
- **Coding Guidelines for External Causes**
- **Abstracting for External Causes**
- **Assigning Codes for External Causes**
- **Arranging Codes for External Causes**

Learning Objectives

After completing this chapter, you should have the skills to:

7.1 Spell and define the key words, medical terms, and abbreviations related to external causes of morbidity. (Remember)

7.2 Explain the purpose of external cause codes. (Understand)

7.3 Adhere to the Official Guidelines for Coding and Reporting related to external causes of morbidity. (Apply)

7.4 Examine and abstract information required for coding external causes of morbidity and related conditions from the medical record. (Analyze)

7.5 Demonstrate how to assign codes for external causes of morbidity and related conditions. (Apply)

7.6 Utilize guidelines for arranging (sequencing) codes for external causes of morbidity and related conditions. (Apply)

Key Terms and Abbreviations

activity	complication	misadventure	subsequent encounter
adverse effect	external cause	place of occurrence	terrorism
causal event	initial encounter	sequela encounter	
cause	intent	status	

In addition to the key terms listed here, students should know the terms defined within tables in this chapter.

INTRODUCTION

When your tire fails because the treads are worn down or the retread delaminates, you know the problem is inherent to the tire. When your tire goes flat because you pick up a nail or someone slashes your tires, the cause is external to the tire. In either case, you still need to repair the tire.

In healthcare, some medical problems develop because of the internal failure of an organ system or biological function; other medical problems are due to external causes, such as an accident or assault. These special circumstances require you to identify and code for external causes of illness and injuries.

Physicians of any specialty may use external cause codes, but they are often used in the emergency department, family practice, orthopedics, and ophthalmology because these physicians specialize in circumstances or body systems frequently affected by external causes.

INTRODUCTION TO EXTERNAL CAUSES

External cause codes describe the event or circumstances that caused an injury or medical problem. Diagnosis codes from the body system chapters describe the actual injury or condition that results. External cause codes may be used in any healthcare setting and with any diagnosis code, but they are secondary codes and should *never* be used as a principal or first-listed diagnosis (OGCR I.C.20.a.1) and 6)).

An **external cause** is an event such as an accident, force of nature, assault, or situation that causes an injury or **adverse effect** (*negative physical reaction*), **complication** (*an abnormal medical reaction that results from a medical or surgical procedure*), or **misadventure** (*an error during a medical or surgical procedure*). Examples of external causes include floods, automobile accidents, falls, prescribed or illegal drugs, and medical or surgical procedures.

Many states require the reporting of external cause codes to track statistics. External cause codes assist third-party payers in tracking the liability (*who is at fault*) for medical costs and enable health researchers to collect standardized data for injury research and injury prevention strategies.

CODING GUIDELINES FOR EXTERNAL CAUSES

Coders should understand the organization of this ICD-10-CM chapter, chapter-wide and commonly used instructional notes in the Tabular List, and the relevant OGCR. This information is necessary for accurate coding.

ICD-10-CM Chapter 20, "External Causes of Morbidity (V00-Y99)," contains 34 blocks or subchapters. Review the block names and code ranges listed at the beginning of Chapter 20 in the ICD-10-CM manual to become familiar with the content and organization. Also review the detailed instructional note at the beginning of the chapter that discusses how to use external cause codes. This chapter classifies information about the cause(s) or events external to a patient that give rise to an illness or injury.

ICD-10-CM provides a separate Index to External Causes. Main Terms identify the type of event or action that caused the injury.

Causal event codes identify what happened that caused the injury and almost always require a seventh character: **A** for initial encounter, **D** for subsequent encounter, or **S** for sequela. Diagnosis codes identify the nature of the injury. Place of occurrence codes identify where the injury occurred, including the type of dwelling and room of the house. Activity codes identify what the patient was doing at the time of the injury. Status codes identify the type of employment, military, or unpaid nature of the patient's activity at the time the injury occurred.

ICD-10-CM provides Official Guidelines for Coding and Reporting (OGCR) external causes in OGCR section I.C.20. OGCR provides detailed discussion of when to report codes from this chapter and how they are to be used. Additional OGCR for using external cause codes in conjunction with specific conditions appear throughout the OGCR and as instructional notes throughout the Tabular List. There is no national requirement for mandatory reporting of external cause codes. Providers are encouraged to voluntarily report external cause codes because they provide valuable data for injury research and the evaluation of injury prevention strategies. Specific OGCR are discussed and cited throughout this chapter of the text.

ABSTRACTING FOR EXTERNAL CAUSES

Whenever patients are treated for injuries, adverse effects, or complications from procedures, coders abstract information related to the external cause of the condition. Always abstract before attempting to assign codes. Write down notes with key information to help keep the details organized. Multiple external cause codes are required, each describing a different aspect of the event, if the documentation provides the required information. External cause information that must be abstracted in addition to the clinical diagnosis appears in ■ TABLE 7-1.

Abstracting Intent and Cause

Combination codes report both intent and cause. **Intent** describes whether the event was accidental or intentional. **Cause** or **causal event** describes the event or action that resulted in the injury. Code(s) for intent and cause are reported *every* time the patient receives treatment for the injury (OGCR I.C.20.a.2)).

Table 7-1 ■ **KEY CRITERIA FOR ABSTRACTING EXTERNAL CAUSES**

❏ **Diagnosis:** What physical injury(ies) or health condition did the patient sustain?

❏ **Intent:** What is the purpose or intent of the injury: accidental, self-harm, assault, legal intervention, military operation, or medical procedure?

❏ **Cause/causal event:** How did the injury or health condition happen?

❏ **Place:** Where did the event occur?

❏ **Activity:** What was the patient doing at the time of the event?

❏ **Status:** What was the patient's employment status at the time the event occurred: civilian employment, military, volunteer, or recreational/leisure?

Because intent and cause are described in a combination code, determine the intent first. Doing so helps to locate the Main Term in the Index to External Causes. Options for intent include:

- Accidental
- Self-harm
- Assault
- Result of legal, military, or terrorist activity
- Undetermined

The cause or event code is based on the intent. For example, separate codes exist for an accidental fall, a fall that is a suicide attempt, and a fall that is due to an assault. The vast majority of cause codes are for accidental intent, so accident codes are the most specific. The most common causes of accidents are traffic accidents and falls.

Code the intent as **accidental** when the intent of the cause of an injury or other condition is unknown or unspecified. All transport accident categories assume **accidental** intent (OGCR I.C.20.h)). Abstract the intent as **undetermined** when the documentation specifically states that the intent cannot be determined.

Abstracting the Episode of Care

Coders need to abstract the episode of care, which describes the phase of treatment. Identifying the episode of care is necessary in order to assign the seventh character of an external cause code. Options for the episode of care are:

- **Initial encounter**—Identifies that the patient received active treatment for the injury during the encounter. Initial does not mean *first*, but rather refers to any encounter during *active treatment*, such as initial stabilization of fracture, initial surgery, and cast application.

- **Subsequent encounter**—Identifies that the patient received routine care during the healing phase at the encounter, such as a cast change, an x-ray to monitor healing, or removal of a fixation device.

- **Sequela**—Identifies that the patient was treated for a complication after the healing phase is complete, such as scarring after a burn, dysphagia after a stroke, or arthritis after a fracture.

Abstracting Place of Occurrence, Activity, and Status

Additional details related to the place of occurrence, activity, and status are abstracted when the information is documented.

The **place of occurrence** describes where the injury occurred, such as a public street or a single-family home. Abstract the greatest level of detail possible, such as the type of home—apartment or single-family home—and the specific room.

The **activity** describes what the person was doing when the injury occurred, such as running, playing sports, or preparing food. Be careful to differentiate the activity from the causal event. The causal event, such as a fall, may occur while doing any number of activities, such as running, walking, or working

in the yard. When a person is engaged in an activity, such as walking, an injury could occur as a result of a variety of events, such as falling, tripping, or being struck by an object or vehicle. Every injury should be coded with a causal event, but not every injury requires an activity code. Assign an activity code when it provides additional information.

Status describes the person's employment status in relation to the event that caused the injury (OGCR I.C.20.d and k). The status code indicates whether the event occurred during military activity or whether a civilian was at work or engaged in a volunteer activity.

Guided Example of Abstracting External Causes

Refer to the following example throughout this chapter in order to practice your abstracting, assigning, and arranging external cause code skills. Marcy Elwood, CCS, is a fictitious coder who guides you through coding this case.

Date: 8/1/yy

Location: Branton Medical Center Emergency Department

Provider: Cynthia Hiatt, MD

Patient: Charles Fink Gender: M Age: 24

Reason for encounter: Patient had an accident on his day off. He was painting the outside of his single family home when he fell off a ladder.

Assessment: Fractured left tibia

Plan: Applied long leg cast. Use crutches to keep weight off. Follow-up with orthopedic clinic.

Follow along as Marcy abstracts the diagnosis. Check off each step after you complete it.

▶ Marcy begins by reading the medical record. She refers to the Key Criteria for Abstracting External Causes (refer again to Table 7-1) to abstract the diagnosis. She will abstract all the information first, then assign the actual codes later in this chapter.

❏ *Diagnosis: What physical injury(ies) or health condition did the patient sustain?* She notes that the diagnosis is fractured left tibia because it describes the injury the patient experienced and writes this down.

❏ *Intent: What is the purpose or intent of the injury: accidental, self-harm, assault, legal intervention, military operation, or medical procedure?* She notes that the intent is stated as an accident and writes this down.

❏ *Causal event: How did the injury or health condition happen?* She notes that the causal event is a fall. Specifically, the fall was from a ladder. She writes this down.

❏ *Place of occurrence: Where did the event occur?* She notes that the fall occurred outside of a single-family home. She writes this down.

❏ *Activity: What was the patient doing at the time of the event?* Marcy notes that the patient was painting the outside of his house and writes this down.

❏ *Status: What was the employment status at the time the event occurred: civilian employment, military, volunteer, or recreational/leisure?* Marcy determines the patient was doing the work for personal purposes on his day off. Even though he is employed, the accident was not related to his employment.

▶ Marcy reviews all the data she abstracted for this case and verifies it against the medical record.

❏ Diagnosis: fractured left tibia, initial encounter

❏ Intent and cause: accidental fall from ladder, initial encounter

❏ Place: outside of single-family home

❏ Activity: painting outside of house

❏ Status: personal

▶ Next, Marcy will assign the codes.

CODING PRACTICE

Exercise 7.1   Abstracting for External Causes

Instructions: Read the mini-medical-record of each patient's encounter and answer the abstracting questions. Write the answer on the line provided. Do not assign any codes.

1. INPATIENT HOSPITAL   Gender: F   Age: 85

Chief complaint: Laceration on the forehead. Fell off toilet and hit her head on the sink.

Assessment: 3-cm laceration

Plan: See family physician for suture removal in 10 days

a. What is the diagnosis? _____

_____

b. What event caused the injury? _____

_____

c. Was this an initial, subsequent, or sequela episode of care? _____

_____

2. EMERGENCY DEPT   Gender: F   Age: 5

Reason for encounter: Burn due to accidentally touching hot stove

Assessment: Second-degree burn to the right hand

Plan: Dressed wound. Instructed parent on wound care. Follow up with family physician in 2 weeks. Call if any problems develop.

a. What is the diagnosis? _____

_____

b. What event caused the injury? _____

_____

c. Was this an initial, subsequent, or sequela episode of care? _____

_____

3. INPATIENT HOSPITAL   Gender: M   Age: 25

Reason for admission: Assault by handgun to leg 6 weeks ago. Patient was treated for fracture to femur caused by a bullet. Bullet was removed but fracture has not healed properly so surgery is needed.

Discharge diagnosis: Malunion of nondisplaced comminuted (*bone broken into fragments*) fracture, left femur shaft

Plan: FU in office in 3 weeks

a. What is the diagnosis? _____

_____

b. What event caused the injury? _____

_____

c. Was this an initial, subsequent, or sequela episode of care? _____

_____

4. INPATIENT HOSPITAL   Gender: M   Age: 47

Reason for admission: Heart attack due to overexertion while shoveling snow in driveway of his single-family home.

Discharge diagnosis: Acute myocardial infarction (AMI)

Plan: FU in office in 2 weeks

a. What is the diagnosis? _____

_____

b. What event caused the injury? _____

_____

c. Was this an initial, subsequent, or sequela episode of care? _____

_____

d. Where did the injury occur? _____

_____

(continued)

CODING PRACTICE (continued)

4. (continued)

e. What was the patient doing at the time of the injury?
_____
_____

f. Was the activity done for civilian work, leisure, volunteer service, or military operations? _____
_____

5. (continued)

g. Was she the driver or a passenger? _____
_____

h. What kind of vehicle did she collide with? _____
_____

i. What is the external cause status? _____
_____

---

5. INPATIENT HOSPITAL Gender: **F** Age: **41**

Reason for admission: **Second surgery for fractured scapula, which was the result of a traffic accident. She was driving a van as a volunteer for the swim team and collided with a pickup truck.**

Assessment: **Displaced fracture of body of left scapula, malunion**

a. What is the diagnosis? _____
_____

b. What event caused the injury? _____
_____

c. Was this an initial, subsequent, or sequela episode of care? _____
_____

d. Where did the injury occur? _____
_____

e. What was the patient doing at the time of the injury?
_____
_____

f. What kind of vehicle was the patient in? _____
_____

(continued)

6. EMERGENCY DEPT Gender: **M** Age: **53**

Reason for encounter: **Patient was walking on a public sidewalk while making a delivery as part of his job when he was bit on the leg by a German shepherd dog that was running free in the neighborhood.**

Assessment: **Puncture wound, left calf**

Plan: **Follow up with orthopedic physician in 2 weeks**

a. What is the diagnosis? _____
_____

b. What event caused the injury? _____
_____

c. Was this an initial, subsequent, or sequela episode of care? _____
_____

d. Where did the injury occur? _____
_____

e. What was the patient doing at the time of the injury?
_____
_____

f. Was the activity done for civilian work, leisure, volunteer service, or military operations? _____
_____

ASSIGNING CODES FOR EXTERNAL CAUSES

To assign codes to cases involving external causes, coders use a separate Index to External Causes and verify the codes in the Tabular List. When assigning codes, you may need to refer back to the medical record and abstract additional details based on the specificity of information the code requires. Causal event/intent codes are reported at every encounter related to the injury. Place, Activity, and Status codes are reported only at the first encounter.

Index to External Causes

The Index to External Causes is separate from the Index to Diseases and Injuries (Index) and appears immediately before the Tabular List. When coding cases that involve external causes, use both indices, as follows:

- Use the Index to Diseases and Injuries to locate the diagnosis code(s) for the injury or condition.

- Use the Index to External Causes to locate external cause codes for intent and cause, place of occurrence, activity, and employment status.

In order to use the Index to External Causes successfully, coders must locate Main Terms for each type of external cause code. Coders should also learn how to locate codes specifically for traffic accidents, the most commonly used and largest block in the external cause chapter.

Main Terms

Main Terms for external cause codes for intent and causal event can be located in two ways: search for the intent or search for the event. Regardless of which way coders search for Main Terms, they must be attentive to multiple levels of indented subterms in order to locate the correct code, as follows:

- When searching for intent, the Main Term is the intent, such as **Accident** or **Assault**. Causal events are subterms indented under each Main Term.

- When searching for the causal event, the event is the Main Term, such as **Fall** or **Bite**. Each indent is a subterm under each causal event.

Main Terms for place, activity, and status are located under entries that carry those names: **Place**, **Activity**, and **Status**. Refer to ■ TABLE 7-2 for a list of commonly used Main Terms in the Index to External Causes. As in the Index to Diseases and Injuries, Main Terms have indented subterms that further define the specifics of entry. Remember to carefully review all available subterms in order to locate the most specific code.

Burns are indexed based on the cause of the burn, as follows:

- When burns are caused by contact with a hot object, such as a stove or iron, search under the Main Term **Burn**.

- When burns are caused by a fire with flames, such as a campfire or house fire, search under the Main Term **Exposure (to)** and subterm **fire, flames**.

- Burns from chemical and caustic liquids are classified in the ICD-10-CM Table of Drugs and Chemicals, which is discussed in Chapter 12, "Injury, Poisoning, and Certain Other Consequences of External Causes (S00–T88)," of this text.

Motor Vehicle Accidents

Automobile and other motor vehicle accidents are indexed based on intent, whether they are traffic-related, the mode of transport, and whether the patient was the driver or a passenger. The Index entry for motor vehicle accidents is several pages long and has numerous levels of subterms (■ FIGURE 7-1). It can be challenging to follow. Watch the indentations carefully

Table 7-2 ■ COMMONLY USED MAIN TERMS IN THE INDEX TO EXTERNAL CAUSES

❏ Accident	❏ Incident
❏ Activity	❏ Jump
❏ Assault	❏ Legal
❏ Bite	❏ Military operations
❏ Burn	❏ Misadventure
❏ Complication	❏ Place
❏ Contact	❏ Radiation
❏ Drowning	❏ Status
❏ Explosion	❏ Striking against
❏ Exposure to	❏ Struck by
❏ Failure	❏ Suicide
❏ Fall	❏ War operations
❏ Forces of nature	

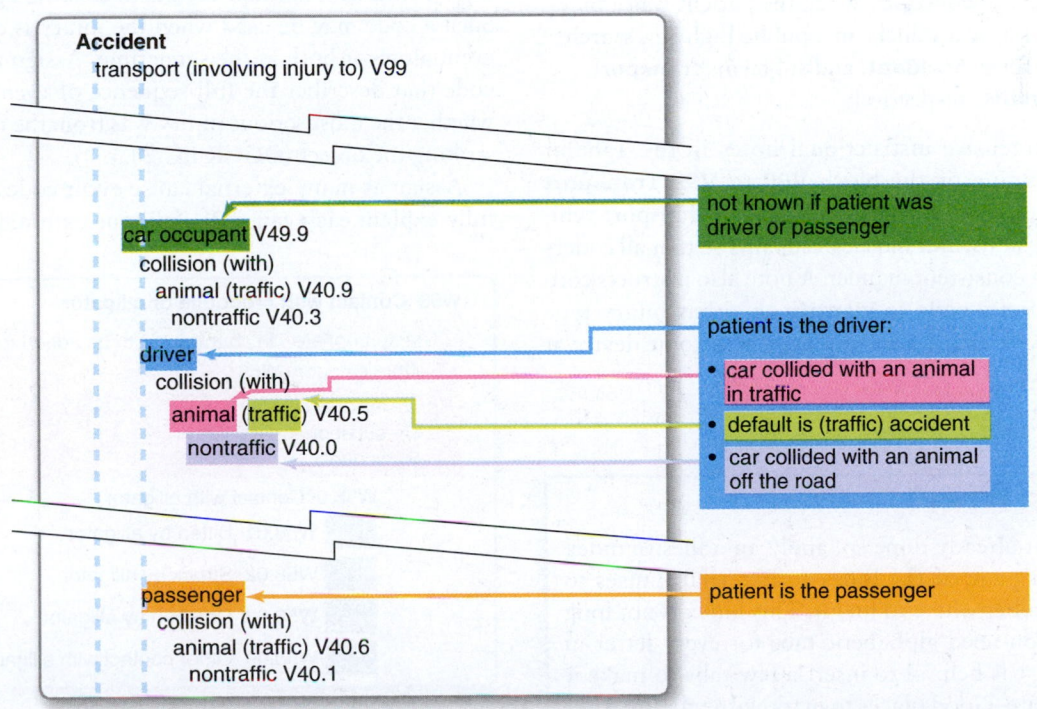

Figure 7-1 ■ Example of the Index to External Causes, Main Term, and subterms for an automobile accident.

to identify each level of subterm. Some codes for motor vehicle accidents require that you navigate as many as seven levels of subterms. Going off track at one level will result in an incorrect code. The most common types of motor vehicle accidents can be located as follows:

1. Locate the Main Term **Accident**.

2. Locate the subterm **transport**, which appears as a left-justified subterm within the first few columns of terms under the Main Term **Accident**. (Highlight the subterm **transport** to make it easier to find later.)

   ▪ Nearly all remaining entries are second-level subterms describing types of transport. These entries and their subterms continue for several pages.

   ▪ The default code for motor vehicle accidents is for a traffic accident, as indicated by the parentheses for a nonessential modifier, **(traffic)**. This refers to an accident that occurs on a public highway.

   ▪ When a vehicle accident occurs anywhere except a public highway, select the subterm **nontraffic** under **Accident**. The Tabular List provides definitions for the various types of accidents.

3. Locate the second-level subterm that identifies the type of vehicle the patient was riding in, such as **bus**, **car**, or **motorcycle**.

4. Locate the third-level subterm to identify the patient as the **driver** or **passenger**.

5. Locate the fourth-level subterm that identifies what object the vehicle collided with, such as **animal**, **car**, or **pedal cycle**.

6. When the patient was a pedestrian who was hit by a vehicle, search under the Main Term **Accident**, and subterms **transport**, then **pedestrian**. When the patient was a bicyclist who was hit by a vehicle on a public highway, search for the Main Term **Accident**, and subterms **transport**, then **pedal cyclist**, respectively.

Review the extensive instructional notes in the Tabular List at the beginning of the block **V00 to V99 Transport Accidents**. These notes provide definitions of transport vehicles, types of collisions, and vehicle occupants so that all coders use the codes in a consistent manner. A note also instructs coders to **Use additional code to identify** an airbag injury, type of street or road, or use of a cell phone or electronic device at time of accident.

Verify in Tabular List

Coders should verify all external cause codes in the Tabular List. Doing so can help catch mistakes that are easily made when navigating multiple levels of indented subterms in the Index to External Causes. In addition, seventh characters can be assigned only from the Tabular List.

Most external cause codes for intent and cause from **V00** to **Y38** require a seventh character to describe the episode of care. Seventh characters for external causes appear under each three-digit category heading in the Tabular List (■ FIGURE 7-2). Some publishers consolidate seventh-character instructions at the beginning of the block, such as **Exposure to animate mechanical forces (W50-W64)**. It is important to become familiar with how your publisher handles these instructions. Refer to ■ TABLE 7-3 to learn when to use each character (OGCR I.C.19.a).

Recall that a publisher's symbol, such as **7th**, means that the final character must be in the seventh position, and coders should assign the placeholder **X** in any unused positions. Because the code **W58.01 Bitten by alligator** is only five characters, add the character **X** in the sixth position before adding the seventh character. For example, **Bitten by alligator, initial encounter** is written as **W58.01XA**.

When the external cause and intent are included in a combination code from another chapter, do not report an additional code from Chapter 20 (OGCR I.C.20.a.8)). For example, **Poisoning by penicillin, accidental** is reported with code **T36.0X1-**. Because the diagnosis code describes both cause and intent, an external cause code is not reported. In addition, do not report place, activity, and status codes with poisonings. Poisonings are discussed in detail in Chapter 12 of this text.

Some external cause codes are combination codes that identify two or more related or sequential events that result in an injury, such as a fall that results in striking against an object. Such a code may be used when the injury is due to either the event alone or both at the same time. Assign the combination code that describes the full sequence of events, regardless of whether the most serious injury was from the fall itself or from striking the object (OGCR I.C.20.a.7).

Assign as many external cause event codes as necessary to fully explain each cause. If only one external cause code can

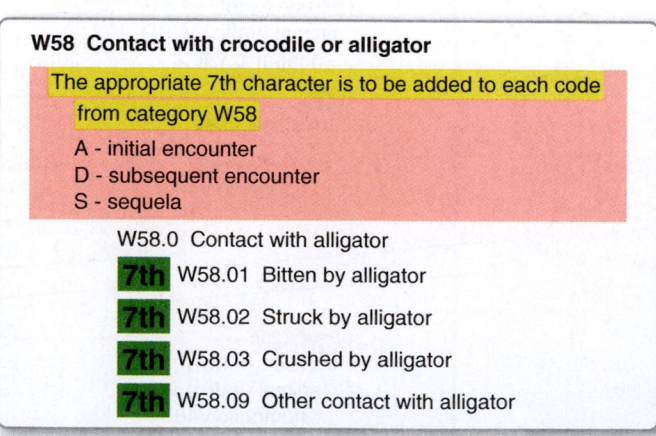

Figure 7-2 ■ Example of the location of seventh characters under category titles in the Index to External Causes.

Table 7-3 ■ **SEVENTH-CHARACTER DEFINITIONS AND EXAMPLES**

7th Character	Definition	Example
A Initial Encounter	Use while the patient is receiving active treatment for the injury.	Surgical treatment Emergency department encounter Evaluation and treatment by a new physician
D Subsequent Encounter	Use for encounters after the patient has received active treatment for the injury and is receiving routine care for the injury during the healing or recovery phase.	Cast change or removal Removal of external or internal fixation device Medication adjustment Visits following injury treatment
S Sequela	Use for complications or conditions that arise as a direct result of an injury after the healing phase is complete.	Scar formation after a burn

be recorded, assign the code most related to the principal diagnosis (OGCR I.C.20.a.4)). However, assign only one code each for place, activity, and status, and report these codes only for the initial encounter.

Assigning Place of Occurrence, Activity, and Status Codes

Place of occurrence, activity, and status codes appear in the block **Supplementary factors related to causes of morbidity classified elsewhere (Y90-Y99)**. An instructional note in the Tabular List instructs coders that these categories may be used to provide supplementary information concerning causes of morbidity. They are not to be used as the only external cause code. The following guidelines apply to all codes for place, activity, and status:

- Assign these codes only once during the patient's course of treatment, at the first visit.
- Do *not* use seventh characters to identify the episode of care.
- Do not report these codes for poisonings, adverse effects, misadventures, or late effects.
- Use these codes only when the *documentation specifically states* that the information is not known or available. When place of occurrence, activity, or status are not documented, omit the code. Do not use place of occurrence code **Y92.9** if the place is not stated or is not applicable (OGCR I.C.20.b). Do not assign **Y93.9 Unspecified activity** if the activity is not stated (OGCR I.C.20.c). Do not assign code **Y99.9 Unspecified external cause status** if the status is not stated (OGCR I.C.20.k).

Place of Occurrence Codes (Y92.-). Report only *one* place per injury and *only* at the initial encounter for treatment (OGCR I.C.20.b and d). Review the category **Y92.-** to familiarize yourself with the various types of settings. Within each setting, such as single-family residence, codes designate the specific room or area where the injury occurred.

Activity Codes (Y93.-). Report *one* activity code per injury when it provides additional information about the event. Report the activity code *only* at the initial encounter for treatment (OGCR I.C.20.c and d). Review the category **Y93.-** to familiarize yourself with the various types of activities. Activity

codes are not applicable to poisonings, adverse effects, medical misadventures, complications, or late effects.

Status Codes (Y99.-). Report *one* status code per injury event and *only* at the initial encounter for treatment. Three specific codes exist for status:

- **Civilian activity done for pay, Y99.0**
- **Military activity, Y99.1**
- **Volunteer activity, Y99.2**

All other status descriptions such as student, hobby, or leisure activity are grouped together under one nonspecific code, **Other external cause status, Y99.8**.

Guided Example of Assigning External Cause Codes

Continue with the example from earlier in the chapter about patient Charles Fink, who fell off a ladder while painting his house, to learn more about using the Index to External Causes.

Follow along in your ICD-10-CM manual as Marcy Elwood, CCS, assigns codes. Check off each step after you complete it.

▶ Marcy reviews the information she abstracted:

- ❑ Diagnosis: fractured left tibia, initial encounter
- ❑ Intent and cause: accidental fall from ladder, initial encounter
- ❑ Place: outside of single-family home
- ❑ Activity: painting outside of house
- ❑ Status: personal

▶ The first code Marcy will assign is the diagnosis code for the injury.

- ❑ She searches the Index to Diseases and Injuries for the diagnosis that she abstracted, fractured left tibia, initial encounter.
- ❑ She locates the Main Term **Fracture, Traumatic** and subterm **tibia S82.20-**.

▶ Marcy verifies the diagnosis code **S82.20-** in the Tabular List.

- ❑ She locates the subcategory title, **S82.20- Unspecified fracture of shaft of tibia**.

❏ The symbol `6th` tells her to assign a sixth character, located below the subcategory title. She assigns the sixth character, **2**, for the left tibia.

❏ The symbol `7th` tells her to assign a seventh character located at the beginning of the category **S82**. She assigns the seventh character, **A**, for the initial encounter for closed fracture.

❏ The diagnosis code is **S82.202A Unspecified fracture of shaft of left tibia, initial encounter for closed fracture**.

▶ Marcy turns her attention to the external cause codes. She locates the Index to External Causes. First, she will code the intent and cause.

▶ Marcy searches the Index to External Causes for the intent and cause of the injury, which she abstracted as accidental fall from ladder.

❏ She locates the Main Term **Fall** and notes that the default intent is **(accidental)**, so she knows she is in the right place.

❏ She locates the subterm **from, off, out of**.

❏ She locates the second-level subterm, **ladder W11**.

▶ Marcy verifies the first external cause code for **accidental fall off ladder**.

❏ She locates the Tabular List entry **W11**. She verifies the external cause code title, **Fall on and from ladder**, which accurately describes the situation.

❏ She cross-references the subchapter title **Other External Causes of Accidental Injury (W00-X58)** to verify that the fall code relates to an accidental intent.

❏ She notices the symbol `7th` in front of the code, which tells her a seventh character is required.

❏ She reviews the seventh character options, which are listed under the code, and identifies that **A** represents **the initial encounter**.

❏ She also notices that because the code is three digits long, she must use the placeholder **X** to fill out the fourth, fifth, and sixth characters of the code.

❏ She assigns the code **W11.XXXA** for **Fall on and from ladder, initial encounter**. Next, she will assign the code for place of occurrence.

▶ Marcy searches the Index to External Causes for the **Place of occurrence**, which she abstracted as outside of single-family home.

❏ She locates the Main Term **Place** and the subterm **residence (non-institutional) (private) Y92.009**. She notices there are more subterms for the type of residence, so she does not assign this code.

❏ She locates the next level of subterm, **house, single family Y92.019**. She notices there are more subterms for the specific location at the house, so she does not assign this code.

❏ She selects the subterm **yard Y92.017** because the accident occurred outside.

▶ Marcy verifies the second external cause code for place of occurrence, **house, single family, yard**.

❏ She locates the Tabular List entry for **Y92.017**.

❏ She verifies the code title, **Garden or yard in single-family (private) house as the place of occurrence of the external cause**, which accurately describes the situation.

❏ She reviews the instructional notes at the beginning of the category **Y92**, which instruct her to report this code only at the initial encounter. Next, she will assign the code for the activity.

▶ Marcy searches the Index to External Causes for the **Activity**, which she abstracted as painting outside of house.

❏ She locates the Main Term **Activity**.

❏ She searches for a subterm that describes painting outside of house, but cannot find anything that specific.

❏ She reviews the subterms again, searching for a broader term that would include painting outside of house.

❏ She locates the subterm **maintenance**, then the subterm **exterior building NEC Y93.H9**.

▶ Marcy verifies the external cause code for activity, **maintenance, exterior building NEC**.

❏ She searches for the Tabular List entry for **Y93.H9**.

❏ She locates the category **Y93** and observes that alphabetic characters for the fourth character of the code begin after **Y93.7** and before **Y93.8**.

❏ She verifies the code title, **Y93.H9 Activity, other involving exterior property and land maintenance, building and construction**, which accurately describes the situation. Next, Marcy will assign a code for the status.

▶ Marcy searches the Index to External Causes for the **Status**, which she abstracted as personal.

❏ She locates the Main Term **Status of external cause** and reviews the subterms.

❏ She notices that there is no entry for personal, but there is an entry for **leisure activity Y99.8**.

▶ Marcy verifies the final external cause code for status, **leisure activity**.

❏ She locates the Tabular List entry for **Y99.8**.

❏ She verifies the code title, **Other external cause status**, which accurately describes the situation.

▶ Marcy reviews the information she located in the Index to External Causes.

❑ Intent and cause: **fall off ladder W11.XXXA**

❑ Place: **house, single family, yard Y92.017**

❑ Activity: **maintenance, exterior building NEC Y93.H9**

❑ Status: **leisure activity Y99.8**

▶ Marcy reviews the diagnosis code, **S82.202A Unspecified fracture of shaft of left tibia, initial encounter**. Next, Marcy needs to determine how to sequence the codes.

CODING PRACTICE

Exercise 7.2   **Assigning Codes for External Causes**

Instructions: Read the mini-medical-record of each patient's encounter, review the information abstracted in Exercise 7.1, and assign ICD-10-CM diagnosis codes using the Index to Diseases and Injuries, the Index to External Causes, and the Tabular List. Write the code(s) on the line provided.

---

1. EMERGENCY DEPT   Gender: F   Age: 85

Chief complaint: Laceration on the forehead. Fell off toilet and hit her head on the sink.

Assessment: 3-cm laceration

Plan: See family physician for suture removal in 10 days

Tip: Code the diagnosis and the external cause event. This medical record does not give you information for place, activity, or status codes.

2 ICD-10-CM Codes _____

---

2. EMERGENCY DEPT   Gender: F   Age: 5

Reason for encounter: Burn due to accidentally touching hot stove

Assessment: Second-degree burn to the right hand

(continued)

---

2. (continued)

Plan: Dressed wound. Instructed parent on wound care. Follow up with family physician in 2 weeks. Call if any problems develop.

Tip: Code the diagnosis and the external cause event. This medical record does not give you information for place, activity, or status codes.

2 ICD-10-CM Codes _____

---

3. INPATIENT HOSPITAL   Gender: M   Age: 25

Reason for admission: Assault by handgun to leg 6 weeks ago. Patient was treated for fracture to femur caused by a bullet. Bullet was removed but fracture has not healed properly so additional surgery is needed.

Discharge diagnosis: Malunion of nondisplaced comminuted (*bone broken into fragments*) fracture, left femur shaft

Plan: FU in office in 3 weeks

Tip: Code the diagnosis and the external cause event. This medical record does not give you information for place, activity, or status codes. On the fracture code, assign the seventh character for *subsequent encounter for closed fracture with malunion.*

2 ICD-10-CM Codes _____

ARRANGING CODES FOR EXTERNAL CAUSES

External cause codes are always secondary codes; they can *never* be the principal or first-listed diagnosis. Sequence external cause codes as follows:

1. The principal or first-listed diagnosis.

2. Secondary diagnosis codes from the body system chapters.

3. External cause combination code for the intent and causal event code that most closely supports the principal or first-listed diagnosis. If more than one intent and causal event code applies, sequence them as follows (OGCR I.C.20.b to f):

1) Child and adult abuse

2) Terrorism events (*events designated by the FBI as terrorism*)

3) Cataclysmic events

4) Transport accidents

4. Place of occurrence code, if required.

5. Activity code, if required.

6. Status code, if required.

If the reporting format on the claim form or computer screen limits the number of external cause codes that can be used in reporting clinical data, report the combination code for the intent and causal event most related to the principal diagnosis. If the format permits capture of additional external cause codes, report intent/cause codes of any additional causal events, including misadventures, before reporting the codes for place, activity, or external status (OGCR I.C.20.b to e)).

Guided Example of Arranging External Cause Codes

Continue with the example about Charles Fink, who fell off a ladder while painting his house, in order to practice skills for arranging external cause codes.

▶ Follow along as Marcy Elwood, CCS, sequences the codes she verified earlier. Check off each step after you complete it.

❏ Marcy sequences the diagnosis code **S82.202A Unspecified fracture of shaft of left tibia, initial encounter for closed fracture** first because it meets the criteria for the first-listed diagnosis.

❏ The second code is the external cause code for intent and causal event, **W11.XXXA Fall on and from ladder, initial encounter**.

❏ The third code is the external cause code for place, **Y92.017 Garden or yard in single-family (private) house as the place of occurrence of the external cause**.

❏ The fourth code is the external cause code for activity, **Y93.H9 Activity, other involving exterior property and land maintenance, building and construction**.

❏ The fifth code is the external cause code for status, **Y99.8 Other external cause status**.

▶ Finally, Marcy cross-references each code against the medical record to be certain that she did not overlook anything.

▶ The final code assignment and sequencing is:

(1) **S82.202A Unspecified fracture of shaft of left tibia, initial encounter for closed fracture**

(2) **W11.XXXA Fall on and from ladder, initial encounter**

(3) **Y92.017 Garden or yard in single-family (private) house as the place of occurrence of the external cause**

(4) **Y93.H9 Activity, other involving exterior property and land maintenance, building and construction**

(5) **Y99.8 Other external cause status**

CODING PRACTICE

Exercise 7.3 **Arranging Codes for External Causes**

Instructions: Read the mini-medical-record of each patient's encounter, review the information abstracted in Exercise 7.1, assign ICD-10-CM diagnosis codes using the Index to Diseases and Injuries, the Index to External Causes, and the Tabular List, and sequence them correctly.

1. INPATIENT HOSPITAL Gender: M Age: 47

Reason for admission: Heart attack due to overexertion while shoveling snow in driveway of his single-family home.

Discharge diagnosis: AMI

Plan: FU in office in 2 weeks

Tip: You need one diagnosis code and three external cause codes.

4 ICD-10-CM Codes _____

_____

2. INPATIENT HOSPITAL Gender: F Age: 41

Reason for admission: Second surgery for fractured scapula, which was the result of a traffic accident. She was driving a van as a volunteer for the swim team and collided with a pickup truck.

(continued)

2. (continued)

Assessment: Displaced fracture of body of left scapula, malunion

Plan: Follow up in office in 3 weeks

Tip: Report place, activity, and status only for the initial encounter.

2 ICD-10-CM Codes _____

3. EMERGENCY DEPT Gender: M Age: 53

Reason for encounter: Patient was walking on a public sidewalk while making a delivery as part of his job when he was bit on the leg by a German shepherd dog that was running free in the neighborhood.

Assessment: Puncture wound, left calf

Plan: Follow up with orthopedic physician in 2 weeks

Tip: This is the initial encounter, so provide the full range of four external cause codes.

5 ICD-10-CM Codes _____

_____

CHAPTER SUMMARY

In this chapter you learned that:

- External cause codes describe the event that created an injury or medical problem.

- ICD-10-CM Chapter 20, "External Causes of Morbidity (V00-Y99)," classifies information about the cause(s) or events external to a patient that give rise to an illness or injury.

- ICD-10-CM provides Official Guidelines for Coding and Reporting (OGCR) in OGCR I.C.20, which discusses when to report codes from ICD-10-CM Chapter 20 and how they are to be used.

- Whenever patients are treated for injuries, adverse effects, or complications from procedures, coders must abstract multiple external cause codes, each describing different aspects of the event.

- Coders use a separate Index to External Causes to locate codes then verify them in the Tabular List. Main Terms for external cause codes for intent and causal event can be located in two ways: search for the intent or search for the event.

- External cause codes are always secondary codes and must be sequenced in a specific order: causal event, place, activity, and status.

CONCEPT QUIZ

Take a moment to look back at external causes and solidify your skills. This is your opportunity to pull together everything you have learned.

Completion

Instructions: Write the term that completes each statement based on the information you learned in this chapter. Choose from the following list. Some choices may be used more than once and some choices may not be used at all.

activity	military operations
adverse effect	misadventure
causal event	place of occurrence
complication	principal
external cause	sequela
falls	subsequent
first-listed	status
initial	suicide
intent	traffic accident

1. _____ codes describe the purpose of the injury as accidental or intentional.

2. _____ is a negative physical reaction.

3. _____ codes describe what the person was doing at the time of the event.

4. _____ codes reporting allows third-party payers to track liability for medical costs.

5. _____ codes describe employment status at the time the event occurred.

6. _____ episode of care identifies that the patient received active treatment for the injury during the encounter.

7. _____ is an error during a medical or surgical procedure.

8. _____ codes are sequenced as the final external cause code.

9. _____ and intent are usually reported with a combination code.

10. _____ is the most commonly used and largest block in the external cause chapter.

Multiple Choice

Instructions: Circle the letter of the best answer to each question based on the information you learned in this chapter.

1. What healthcare setting(s) uses external cause codes?
   A. Outpatient setting only
   B. Emergency department only
   C. Inpatient setting only
   D. All healthcare settings

2. How would you code the following scenario? *A patient is seen in the emergency department after being bitten by an alligator.*
   A. W58.01
   B. W58.01XS
   C. W58.01XD
   D. W58.01XA

3. How should the intent be coded when the intent of the cause of an injury or other condition is unknown or unspecified?
   A. Undetermined
   B. Accidental
   C. Assault
   D. External

4. What type of intent is assumed for all transport accident categories?
   A. Assault
   B. Accidental
   C. Undetermined
   D. External

5. How would you code the following scenario? *A patient is treated for a fractured left tibia after an accidental fall from a ladder while painting the outside of his single-family home.*
   A. S82.202A, W11.XXXA
   B. W11.XXXA, S82.202A, Y92.017, Y93.H9, Y99.8
   C. S82.202A, W11.XXXA, Y92.017, Y93.H9, Y99.8
   D. W11.XXXA, Y92.017, Y93.H9, Y99.8

6. Which type of external cause code is reported at every encounter related to the injury?
   A. Intent and cause
   B. Place
   C. Activity
   D. Status

(continued)

(continued from page 121)

7. Where are external cause codes indexed?
   A. Index to Diseases and Injuries
   B. Index to External Causes
   C. Table of Drugs and Chemicals
   D. Tabular List

8. Which type of code is *running* an example of?
   A. Activity
   B. Injury
   C. Status
   D. Causal event

9. What type of code identifies the person's employment status in relation to the event that caused the injury?
   A. Employment
   B. Activity
   C. Intent
   D. Status

10. How would you code the following scenario? *A patient was a passenger in a car that collided with a deer in the road.*
    A. V40.6XXA
    B. V50.1XXA
    C. V40.1XXA
    D. V50.6XXA

KEEP ON CODING

Instructions: Read the diagnostic statement, then use the Index to External Causes and Tabular List to assign and sequence ICD-10-CM diagnosis codes. Write the code(s) on the line provided.

1. Burn of the hand while onboard a sailboat, initial encounter. ICD-10-CM Code(s) _____

2. Injury occurred while cheerleading (activity code). ICD-10-CM Code(s) _____

3. Injury while using a chainsaw, subsequent encounter. ICD-10-CM Code(s) _____

4. Late effect of being struck by golf ball. ICD-10-CM Code(s) _____

5. Electrocution by a toaster, suicide attempt, initial encounter. ICD-10-CM Code(s) _____

6. Bitten by a raccoon, initial encounter. ICD-10-CM Code(s) _____

7. Overexposure in a tanning bed, sequela. ICD-10-CM Code(s) _____

8. Incorrect procedure performed on correct patient. ICD-10-CM Code(s) _____

9. Pellet gun injury, intent undetermined, initial encounter. ICD-10-CM Code(s) _____

10. Overexposure to sound waves, subsequent encounter. ICD-10-CM Code(s) _____

11. Burned by a hot toaster, initial encounter. ICD-10-CM Code(s) _____

12. Hunting rifle discharge, unknown intent, initial encounter. ICD-10-CM Code(s) _____

13. Excessive fluid administered during a transfusion. ICD-10-CM Code(s) _____

14. Human bite during an assault, initial encounter. ICD-10-CM Code(s) _____

15. Drowning of undetermined intent after a fall in the swimming pool, initial encounter. ICD-10-CM Code(s) _____

16. Blood alcohol level 65 mg/100 mL. ICD-10-CM Code(s) _____

17. Fall into a well, subsequent encounter. ICD-10-CM Code(s) _____

18. Fall from the steps due to ice, initial encounter. ICD-10-CM Code(s) _____

19. Pecked by a macaw, initial encounter. ICD-10-CM Code(s) _____

20. Fall from a motorcycle, driver, in a nontraffic accident, initial encounter. ICD-10-CM Code(s) _____

21. Fall from scaffolding, initial encounter. ICD-10-CM Code(s) _____

22. Subsequent encounter from being stranded in a snow blizzard. ICD-10-CM Code(s) _____

23. Fall from inline roller skates, subsequent encounter. ICD-10-CM Code(s) _____

24. Injured in the garden of a private house (place of occurrence). ICD-10-CM Code(s) _____

25. Failure of sterile precautions during an injection, initial encounter. ICD-10-CM Code(s) _____

CODING CHALLENGE

Instructions: Read the mini-medical-record of each patient's encounter and assign diagnosis codes using the Index to Diseases and Injuries, the Index to External Causes, and Tabular List, and sequence them correctly. Write the code(s) on the line provided.

---

1. INPATIENT HOSPITAL   Gender: F   Age: 20

Reason for admission: Admitted through ED. Patient was on her way home from work and was walking on a local street because there was no sidewalk. It was after dark and a car struck her when the driver did not see her.

Discharge diagnosis: Concussion without loss of consciousness, fracture in the lower end of radius, right arm.

Discharge plan: FU in office 3 weeks. Call if any symptoms such as dizziness or headache.

Tip: Assign a diagnosis code for each injury and assign four external codes. Sequence the concussion as the principal diagnosis.

6 ICD-10-CM Codes _____

---

2. INPATIENT HOSPITAL   Gender: M   Age: 19

Reason for admission: Admitted from ED after fall from canoe and submersion in cold water in Branton Lake. He was instructing a class as part of his job.

Discharge diagnosis: Bradycardia (*slow heart rate*) due to hypothermia, hypoxemia (*oxygen depletion*)

Discharge plan: FU in office 1 week

Tip: Assign three diagnosis codes and five external cause codes. Instructional notes in the Tabular List for hypothermia direct you to one of the external cause codes.

8 ICD-10-CM Codes _____

_____

_____

---

3. INPATIENT HOSPITAL   Gender: M   Age: 20

Reason for admission: Admitted from ED for dislocated shoulder. He was texting his girlfriend while driving on the freeway and ran his motorcycle into a sign post.

Discharge diagnosis: Dislocated right acromioclavicular (*shoulder*) joint, 100% displacement

Discharge plan: Immobilize joint for 2 weeks. FU in office 2 weeks. Recommended course on motorcycle safety.

Tip: The patient's status is not identified.

4 ICD-10-CM Codes _____

_____

---

4. INPATIENT HOSPITAL   Gender: F   Age: 80

Planned procedure: Scheduled for total knee replacement, left knee, due to primary osteoarthritis

Postprocedural diagnosis: Procedure performed in error on right knee, which also had degeneration due to osteoarthritis

Discharge plan: Physical therapy and rehab.

Tip: External cause codes for place, activity, and status are not required because this is a misadventure. In the Index to External Causes, under the entry for *Misadventure, performance of inappropriate operation*, you will see a cross-reference to a different Main Term.

2 ICD-10-CM Codes _____

---

5. INPATIENT HOSPITAL   Gender: M   Age: 21

Reason for admission: Knife stab wounds to the chest after a gang fight in a public park

Discharge diagnosis: Intrathoracic wound with laceration of right lung.

Tip: External cause codes for activity and status are not needed.

3 ICD-10-CM Codes _____

_____

---

6. INPATIENT HOSPITAL   Gender: M   Age: 22

Reason for admission: Admitted from ED. Patient was riding his bicycle for recreation through a parking lot and was hit by a bus. He impacted the handlebar and appears to have internal injuries.

Assessment: Stomach laceration

Tip: The Index to External Causes classifies *bicyclist* using the term *pedal cyclist*.

5 ICD-10-CM Codes _____

_____

---

7. EMERGENCY DEPT   Gender: M   Age: 27

Chief complaint: State police officer arrived by ambulance after being struck in the head by a baton while taking down a suspect. Loss of consciousness for 15 minutes.

Assessment: Concussion to head

Tip: The causal event is legal intervention. Do not assign an activity code because there is none that adds information to the encounter.

3 ICD-10-CM Codes _____

_____

(continued)

(continued from page 123)

8. INPATIENT HOSPITAL   Gender: F   Age: 18

Reason for admission: Stupor, vomiting, muscle cramps, anhidrosis (*lack of sweating*), dyspnea, elevated pulse after being outside in the sun all day at the beach where she was working as a lifeguard, body temperature 104 degrees.

Assessment: Heat stroke with stupor

Tip: Distinguish integral symptoms of heat stroke from complications that the Tabular List instructional notes direct you to code.

5 ICD-10-CM Codes _____

_____

9. OFFICE   Gender: M   Age: 35

Reason for encounter: Second visit for sore back after slipping while playing golf

Assessment: MRI negative for disc damage. Lumbar sprain

Plan: Refer to physical therapy

2 ICD-10-CM Codes _____

10. EMERGENCY DEPT   Gender: M   Age: 28

Chief complaint: Put nail through thumb with nail gun while performing his construction job as a carpenter

Assessment: Puncture wound, right thumb

5 ICD-10-CM Codes _____

_____

Diseases of the Digestive System (K00-K95)

Learning Objectives

After completing this chapter, you should have the skills to:

8.1 Spell and define the key words, medical terms, and abbreviations related to the digestive system. (Remember)

8.2 Summarize the structure, function, and common conditions of the digestive system. (Understand)

8.3 Adhere to the Official Guidelines for Coding and Reporting and instructional notes for the digestive system. (Apply)

8.4 Examine and abstract diagnostic information from the medical record for coding diseases of the digestive system. (Analyze)

8.5 Demonstrate how to assign diagnosis codes for digestive system conditions. (Apply)

8.6 Utilize guidelines for arranging (sequencing) multiple diagnosis codes for digestive system conditions. (Apply)

8.7 Demonstrate how to abstract, assign, and sequence codes for neoplasms of the digestive system. (Apply)

Chapter Outline

- **Digestive System Refresher**
- **Coding Guidelines for the Digestive System**
- **Abstracting for Digestive System Conditions**
- **Assigning Codes for Digestive System Conditions**
- **Arranging Codes for Digestive System Conditions**
- **Coding Neoplasms of the Digestive System**

Key Terms and Abbreviations

accessory organs	colorectal	diverticula	gastrointestinal (GI) system
alimentary canal	comorbidity	diverticulitis	*Helicobacter pylori (H. pylori)*
barium enema	digestive system	diverticulosis	

In addition to the key terms listed here, students should know the terms defined within tables in this chapter.

INTRODUCTION

Your automobile takes in gasoline, utilizes certain components to power the vehicle, and expels the by-products through the exhaust system. A problem at any point in the complicated process affects the way the vehicle functions. The digestive system serves a similar function for your body.

In this chapter you learn more about how the digestive system works, why sometimes it does not work as it should, and how physicians treat these conditions. Gastroenterologists are physicians who specialize in the study, diagnosis, and treatment of digestive system diseases. Dentists specialize in the study,

diagnosis, and treatment of disorders of the oral cavity, which is part of the digestive system. Primary care physicians and internal medicine physicians treat many common digestive system disorders. They refer complex cases to a gastroenterologist or dentist.

DIGESTIVE SYSTEM REFRESHER

The function of the **digestive system**, also called the **gastrointestinal (GI) system**, is to receive nutrients, break them down, absorb them into the blood to be used by the body, and eliminate solid waste products. The digestive system consists of the **alimentary canal** and **accessory organs** (■ FIGURE 8-1).

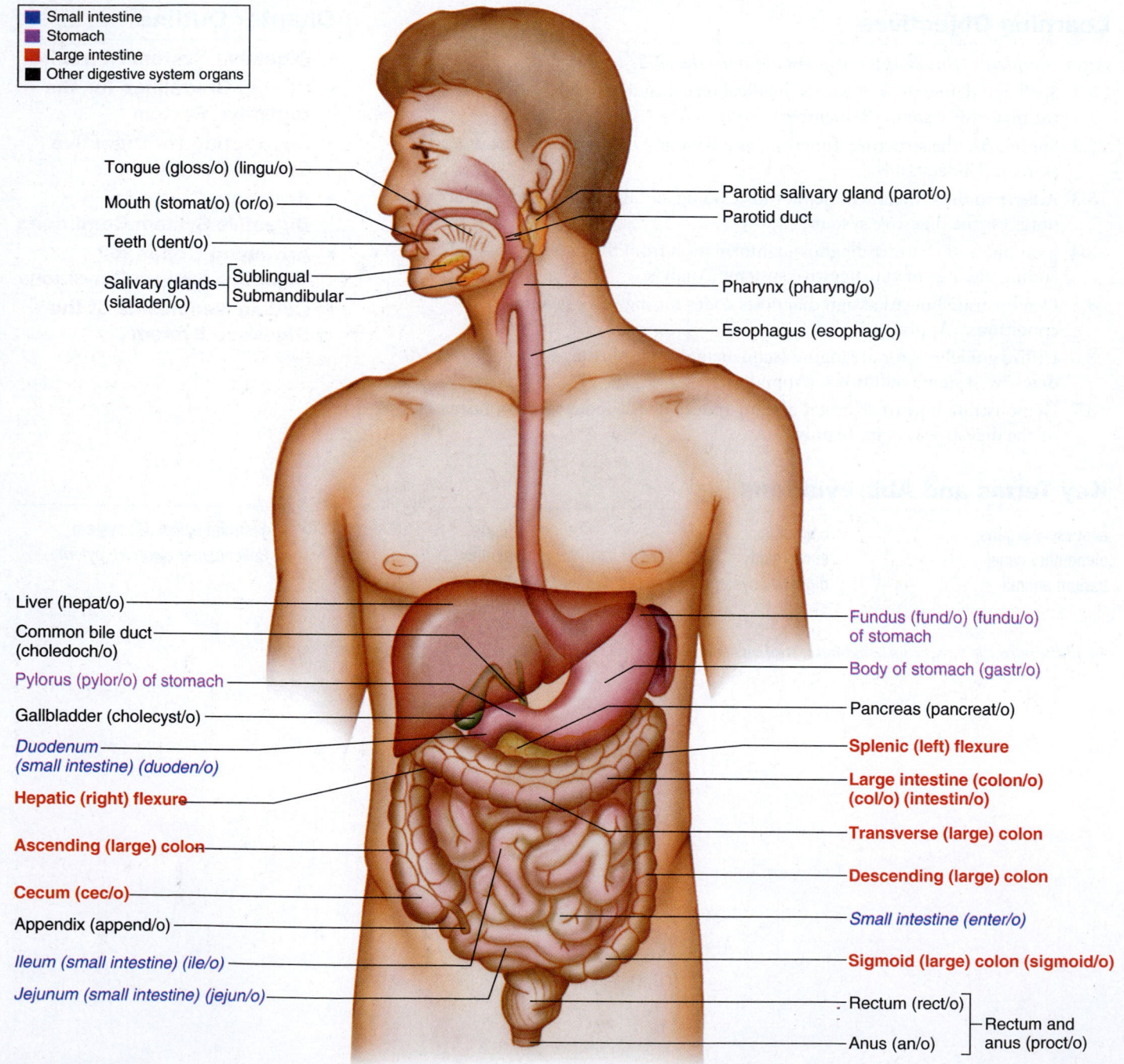

Figure 8-1 ■ The digestive (gastrointestinal) system.

The alimentary canal is a continuous tube, approximately 30 feet in length, which begins at the mouth; continues through the esophagus, stomach, small intestine, and large intestine; and exits the body at the rectum and anus. The accessory organs assist in digestion, but are not directly connected to the alimentary canal. They are the salivary glands, liver, gallbladder, and pancreas. Do not confuse the digestive system (an organ system) with the abdomen (a body region or cavity). Digestive system organs are located in the head, neck, thoracic cavity, abdominal cavity, and pelvic cavity.

Each structure in the digestive system is labeled with its name as well as its medical terminology root/combining form in Figure 8-1. Remember to apply medical terminology skills to combine the root or combining form for the body part with suffixes to define new terms for conditions and procedures, as shown in ■ TABLE 8-1.

CODING CAUTION

Be alert for medical word roots with similar spellings but different meanings:

chole/o (*bile or gall*), **col/o** (*colon*), and **colp/o** (*vagina*)

cholecyst/o (*gallbladder*) and **cyst/o** (*bladder or sac, often used in reference to the urinary bladder*)

ile/o (*ileum, part of the small intestine*) and **ili/o** (*ilium, the pelvic bone*)

ileum (*small intestine*) and **ileus** (*a paralytic condition of the small intestine*)

Conditions of the Digestive System

The functions of the digestive system are:

- Ingestion—Taking in of food (mouth, esophagus; aided by the salivary glands)
- Digestion—Breaking-down of food (stomach, small intestine; aided by the liver, gallbladder, and pancreas)
- Absorption—Transfer of nutrients to the body (small intestine, large intestine)
- Elimination—Removal of solid waste from the body (large intestine, rectum, anus)

Digestive system conditions account for approximately 12% of all inpatient procedures and 20% of all ambulatory procedures, according to the National Institute of Diabetes and Digestive and Kidney Diseases (NIDDK). Treating these conditions costs about $98 billion per year. Over 245,000 people die each year from digestive system conditions. Diseases and conditions of the digestive system can be caused by heredity; the type and amount of food consumed; substance abuse, particularly alcohol and tobacco; or mental health conditions. Diseases are diagnosed through a combination of physical examination, medical history, signs and symptoms, blood tests, imaging, endoscopy, and biopsy. Common treatments include dietary changes, alcohol and tobacco abstinence, medication, and/or surgery.

■ TABLE 8-2 highlights common conditions affecting the digestive system and common diagnostic methods. This table provides a general reference to help understand where a particular diagnosis or procedure fits into the overall picture of the digestive system, but it does not list everything you need to know. Refer to medical resources to learn more about conditions affecting the digestive system.

Table 8-1   ■   **EXAMPLE OF CONSTRUCTING MEDICAL TERMS FOR THE DIGESTIVE SYSTEM**

Combining Form	Suffix	Complete Medical Term
gastr/o (*stomach*) **enter/o** (*intestines*) **colon/o** (*large intestine*)	**-logy** (*study of*)	**gastro + entero + logy** (*the study of the stomach and intestines*)
	-itis (*inflammation*)	**gastr + itis** (*inflammation of the stomach*) **enter + itis** (*inflammation of the intestines*)
	-scopy (*visual examination*)	**gastro + scopy** (*visual examination of the stomach*) **colono + scopy** (*visual examination of the large intestine*)

Table 8-2 ■ **COMMON CONDITIONS AFFECTING THE DIGESTIVE SYSTEM**

Condition	Description	Diagnostic Methods
Appendicitis	Inflammation and possible rupture of the appendix	Blood count, physical examination
Celiac disease	An abnormal immune reaction to gluten and poor absorption of nutrients	Blood tests, intestinal biopsy, presence of dermatitis herpetiformis (DH)
Cholecystitis	Inflammation of the gallbladder	Ultrasound (US), computerized axial tomography (CT), fecal fat test
Choledocholithiasis	Calculi in the common bile duct	US, CT, fecal fat test
Cholelithiasis	Calculi in the gallbladder	US, CT, fecal fat test
Cirrhosis	Scarring of liver tissue that blocks the normal flow of blood through the liver	Blood tests, imaging tests, liver biopsy
Crohn's disease	An inflammatory bowel disease (IBD) with inflammation and ulcers in the alimentary tract characterized by a thickening of the mucous membrane	Blood tests, stool test, endoscopy, biopsy
Diverticular disease	Diverticulosis: The presence of diverticula (*pouches formed when the lining of the intestine pushes through the intestinal muscle layer*) Diverticulitis: A bacterial infection of diverticula	Blood tests, stool sample, digital rectal examination (DRE) colonoscopy, barium enema (*injection of a chalky substance into the colon through the anus and viewing the organs on an x-ray; also called lower GI series*)
Esophagitis	Irritation of the esophagus caused by acid reflux and a weak cardiac sphincter	Physical examination, symptoms of heartburn
Gastritis	Inflammation of the stomach lining	Gastroscopy blood test, stool test, test for *Helicobacter pylori*, or *H. pylori* (*bacteria that causes ulcers*)
Gastroenteritis	Bacterial or viral infection of the stomach and intestines	Stool culture, symptoms of vomiting, nausea, and/or abdominal pain
Gastroesophageal reflux disease (GERD)	Backward flow of stomach contents (food or liquid) into the esophagus	Barium swallow or upper GI series, esophagogastroduodenoscopy (EGD), esophageal manometry
Hepatitis	Inflammation of the liver due to viruses named A, B, or C	Blood tests, liver biopsy
Hernia	Protrusion of an organ through a weakened area in a muscle, such as the diaphragm (hiatal hernia) or groin muscle (inguinal hernia)	X-ray
Intestinal obstruction	A physical blockage of the intestine that prevents waste from passing through	CT, x-ray, barium enema, barium swallow
Irritable bowel syndrome (IBS)	A combination of symptoms such as cramping, abdominal pain, bloating, constipation, diarrhea	Medical history, symptoms, examination, rule out other problems
Pancreatitis	Inflammation of the pancreas	US, CT, endoscopic ultrasound (EUS), magnetic resonance cholangiopancreatography (MRCP)
Stomatitis	Redness, ulcers, and/or bleeding of the mouth due to bacteria, viruses, or fungi	Physical examination, immunological tests, cultures
Ulcer	A sore on the lining of the stomach (gastric ulcer) or duodenum (peptic ulcer)	Blood test for *H. pylori*, urea breath test, stool antigen test, endoscopy, barium swallow
Ulcerative colitis	An IBD with inflammation and sores, called ulcers, in the lining of the rectum and colon	Physical examination, medical history, blood tests, stool sample, colonoscopy, sigmoidoscopy
Volvulus	Twisting of a portion of the small or large intestine or stomach into a loop that obstructs the passage of digestive material	CT, x-ray, barium enema, barium swallow, endoscopy blood tests

CODING PRACTICECODING PRACTICE

Exercise 8.1   Digestive System Refresher

Instructions: Use your medical terminology skills and resources to define the following conditions of the digestive system, then assign the ICD-10-CM diagnosis code.

Follow these steps:

- Use slash marks "/" to break down each term into its root(s) and suffix.
- Define the meaning of the word, based on the meaning of each word part.
- Assign the default diagnosis code for the condition using the Index and Tabular List.

Example: gastritis gastr/itis   Meaning *inflammation of the stomach*   ICD-10-CM Code *K29.70*

1. ileus   Meaning _____   ICD-10-CM Code _____
2. hematemesis   Meaning _____   ICD-10-CM Code _____
3. gingivitis   Meaning _____   ICD-10-CM Code _____
4. volvulus   Meaning _____   ICD-10-CM Code _____
5. stomatitis   Meaning _____   ICD-10-CM Code _____
6. hepatoma   Meaning _____   ICD-10-CM Code _____
7. diverticulitis   Meaning _____   ICD-10-CM Code _____
8. diverticulosis   Meaning _____   ICD-10-CM Code _____
9. proctitis   Meaning _____   ICD-10-CM Code _____
10. cholangitis   Meaning _____   ICD-10-CM Code _____

CODING GUIDELINES FOR THE DIGESTIVE SYSTEM

Coders should understand the organization of this ICD-10-CM chapter, chapter-wide and commonly used instructional notes in the Tabular List, and the relevant OGCR. This information is necessary for accurate coding. Chapter 11 of ICD-10-CM, "Diseases of the Digestive System (K00-K95)," contains 10 blocks or subchapters that are divided by anatomical site. Review the block names and code ranges listed at the beginning of Chapter 11 in the ICD-10-CM manual to become familiar with the content and organization. Review the **Excludes2** note that lists several conditions not classified to this chapter, such as digestive conditions that are perinatal, congenital, pregnancy-related, injuries, symptoms, or neoplasms. Each of these conditions are discussed in the corresponding chapter of ICD-10-CM later in this text. Neoplasms are discussed at the end of this chapter.

Extensive instructional notes direct coders to assign additional codes to identify certain lifestyle habits involving use or exposure to tobacco and alcohol.

ICD-10-CM provides no Official Guidelines for Coding and Reporting (OGCR) for the digestive system. Combination codes that describe complications of digestive system conditions are common. In addition, frequent instructional notes direct coders to use multiple codes to describe the underlying cause or harmful lifestyle habits that contribute to gastrointestinal conditions. Review OGCR sections I.B.7 and I.B.9 of the General Coding Guidelines to review the use of multiple coding and combination codes, respectively. Specific OGCR are discussed and cited throughout this chapter of the text.

ABSTRACTING FOR DIGESTIVE SYSTEM CONDITIONS

When abstracting for the digestive system, coders need to look for manifestations, complications, and lifestyle habits associated with digestive system conditions. Key factors to review for coding cases that involve the digestive system appear in ■ TABLE 8-3. Remember that the abstracting questions are a guide and that not every question applies to, or can be

Table 8-3   ■   **KEY CRITERIA FOR ABSTRACTING DIGESTIVE SYSTEM CONDITIONS**

- ❑ What is the condition?
- ❑ What is the anatomic site?
- ❑ What is the laterality, if any?
- ❑ Is bleeding or hemorrhaging documented?
- ❑ What other manifestations or complications are documented?
- ❑ What comorbidities are documented?
- ❑ What lifestyle habits are documented as current or with a history of, such as alcohol use or abuse and tobacco exposure, use, or abuse?

answered for, every case. For example, lifestyle habits may not be present for every patient.

Manifestations are symptoms and signs that occur as a result of the underlying condition. Certain digestive system diseases can exist alone or as a manifestation of another condition. For example, liver disorders can be a manifestation of congenital syphilis or congenital toxoplasmosis.

Common complications in the digestive system are bleeding, obstruction, and infection. Ulcers, enteritis, colitis, and gastritis may occur with or without bleeding. An obstruction is a blockage of an organ and can be caused by calculi (*stones*), tumors, organic matter, or volvulus. Gallbladder and intestinal diseases may occur with or without an obstruction. When an infection is present, coders need to abstract the infectious agent, such as *Streptococcus, Escherichia coli (E. coli),* or *Staphylococcus.*

Lifestyle habits are patient behaviors that cause or contribute to a condition. Lifestyle habits that contribute to many digestive system conditions include use, history of use, dependence, and exposure to tobacco or tobacco smoke and alcohol.

Many digestive system codes are combination codes that include the complication or **comorbidity** (*two diseases occurring together*). Multiple coding is needed for lifestyle habits and for complications and comorbidities that do not have a combination code. When abstracting, coders do not necessarily know which complications and comorbidities will be assigned a combination code and which will require multiple coding.

Guided Example of Abstracting for Digestive System Conditions

Refer to the following example throughout this chapter to practice skills for abstracting, assigning, and sequencing codes for digestive system conditions. Jill Hynes, CPC, is a fictitious coder who guides you through this case.

Date: 9/1/yy   Location: Branton Gastroenterology

Provider: Stanley Garrett, MD

Patient: Gina Addington   Gender: F   Age: 28

Chief complaint: Rectal bleeding, Crohn's disease since age 10

Assessment: Crohn's disease, colon, new complication of rectal bleeding

Plan: Liquid diet 1 week; FU if not improved

Follow along as Jill Hynes, CPC, abstracts the diagnosis. Check off each step after you complete it.

▶ Jill refers to the Key Criteria for Abstracting Digestive System Conditions (refer again to Table 8-3).

❑ *What is the condition?* Crohn's disease

❑ *What is the anatomic site?* Colon

❑ *Is bleeding or hemorrhaging documented?* Yes, rectal bleeding, which is a new complication

❑ *What other manifestations or complications are documented?* None

❑ *What comorbidities are documented?* None

❑ *What lifestyle habits are documented as current or with a history of?* None

▶ Until Jill researches this condition in the ICD-10-CM manual to assign codes, she does not know if Crohn's disease with rectal bleeding will require one or two codes.

CODING PRACTICE

Exercise 8.2 **Abstracting for Digestive System Conditions**

Instructions: Read the mini-medical-record of each patient's encounter and answer the abstracting questions. Write the answer on the line provided. Do not assign any codes.

---

1. OFFICE   Gender: M   Age: 54

Chief complaint: Indigestion

Assessment: Chronic perforated peptic ulcer in stomach with bleeding

Plan: Change diet, change Rx

a. What symptom is documented? _____

_____

(continued)

---

1. (continued)

b. Where is the ulcer located? _____

_____

c. What signs or complications are present? _____

_____

d. Is the ulcer acute or chronic? _____

_____

e. Will you code for the symptoms? _____

Why or why not? _____

_____

f. What is the diagnosis to be coded? _____

_____

(continued)

CODING PRACTICE *(continued)*

2. OUTPATIENT SURGERY   Gender: **F**   Age: **61**

Procedure: **Repair, right inguinal hernia**

Postprocedural diagnosis: **Recurrent right inguinal hernia**

Plan: **FU in office**

a. Where is an inguinal hernia located? _____
_____

b. Is the hernia unilateral or bilateral? _____
_____

c. Is the hernia documented as recurrent? _____
_____

d. Is an obstruction documented? _____
_____

e. Is gangrene documented? _____
_____

3. OFFICE   Gender: **M**   Age: **67**

Reason for visit: **FU on lower GI series**

Assessment: **Ulcerative colitis with fistula**
(an abnormal connection between an organ, vessel, or intestine and another structure)

Plan: **Begin liquid diet, Rx antibiotics, FU 2 weeks**

a. What test is the follow-up visit for? _____
_____

b. Should you code for the test? _____
Why or why not? _____

c. What type of colitis is documented? _____
_____

d. What complication is documented? _____
_____

e. What diagnosis will you code? _____
_____

4. OFFICE   Gender: **M**   Age: **56**

Chief complaint: **Abdominal pain and bloating, fatigue, vomiting**

Assessment: **Alcoholic liver cirrhosis with ascites due to alcohol addiction**

Plan: **Counseled patient regarding abstinence from alcohol, reduce salt intake**

(continued)

4. (continued)

a. What symptoms are documented? _____
_____

b. What is the anatomic site of the cirrhosis? _____
_____

c. What complication is present? _____

d. What is the cause of the cirrhosis? _____
_____

e. What lifestyle habit is documented? _____
_____

f. Will you code the symptoms? _____

Why or why not? _____
_____

g. What diagnosis will you code? _____
_____

5. OFFICE   Gender: **M**   Age: **59**

Chief complaint: **Hematemesis, history of cirrhosis**

Assessment: **Portal hypertension** *(increase in blood pressure in the portal vein)* **with portal hypertensive gastropathy**

Plan: **Endoscopic therapy, drug therapy, and dietary changes**

a. What symptom(s) are documented? _____
_____

b. Is cirrhosis past or present? _____
Why? _____
_____

c. What is the primary condition diagnosed? _____

d. What is the complication? _____
_____

e. Will you code the symptoms? _____
Why or why not? _____

f. Will you code the cirrhosis? _____
Why? _____

g. What is the first-listed diagnosis? _____

(continued)

CODING PRACTICE (continued)

6. OFFICE Gender: M Age: 33

Chief complaint: Redness and tenderness around colostomy site

Assessment: Colostomy infection, cellulitis of abdominal wall due to methicillin-susceptible Staphylococcus aureus (MSSA)

a. What symptom(s) are documented? _____

_____

(continued)

4. (continued)

b. What two conditions are documented? _____

_____

c. What is the infectious agent? _____

_____

d. Will you code the symptoms? _____

Why or why not? _____

ASSIGNING CODES FOR DIGESTIVE SYSTEM CONDITIONS

Coders frequently assign combination codes to describe common complications or manifestations of digestive system conditions. For example, the category **K50 Crohn's disease** contains more than 25 codes, many of which are combination codes that describe common complications of Crohn's disease. Crohn's is an eponym for Burrill Bernard Crohn, a gastroenterologist who identified the condition in 1932. Most codes in category **K50 Crohn's disease** contain six characters:

- Characters 1–3 classify Crohn's disease in general.
- Character 4 identifies the site as the small intestine, large intestine, both, or unspecified.
- Character 5 indicates whether a complication is present.
- Character 6 describes the specific complication.

Index entries for conditions with combination codes can be rather long and involved, with many subterms and many levels of indentation, in order to identify all the possible combinations of conditions. Be thorough when searching these entries to be certain to locate the correct item. When verifying the code in the Tabular List, read the description carefully to be sure it matches the combination of conditions in the scenario. Many wrong turns can be caught when verifying.

ICD-10-CM uses the term *hemorrhage* when describing a bleeding ulcer but uses the term *bleeding* when describing bleeding in gastritis, enteritis, duodenitis, and diverticular disease.

Guided Example of Assigning Digestive System Diagnosis Codes

Continue with the example from earlier in the chapter about patient Gina Addington, who has Crohn's disease, to practice skills for assigning digestive system codes.

Follow along in your ICD-10-CM manual as Jill Hynes, CPC, assigns codes to the diagnosis. Check off each step after you complete it.

▶ Jill begins by locating the Main Term in the Index.

❏ Jill looks up **C, Crohn's disease**.

❏ She reviews the cross-reference note that states **see Enteritis, regional** (■ FIGURE 8-2).

❏ Under the entry for **E, Enteritis, regional** Jill reviews the subterms that describe the various sites within the intestinal tract.

❏ She locates the subterm for **colon**.

❏ Jill reviews the instruction to cross-reference the subterm **Enteritis, regional, large intestine**.

❏ Under the subterm for **large intestine**, Jill reviews the additional subterms that describe various associated conditions and complications.

❏ She refers back to the medical record and identifies the complication of rectal bleeding.

❏ She locates the subentry for **with**, then **rectal bleeding**.

❏ Jill confirms that there are no further subentries under **rectal bleeding** and identifies the code **K50.111** that she will verify in the Tabular List.

▶ Now Jill verifies the code in the Tabular List. She locates the entry for code **K50.111**.

❏ Jill confirms that the code description **Crohn's disease of large intestine with rectal bleeding** accurately describes the diagnosis (■ FIGURE 8-3).

❏ She notes that a seventh character is not required because there is not a symbol next to it and there are no additional codes under it.

❏ Jill reviews the instructional notes at the beginning of the subclassification **K50.1** that state which sites are included. She sees that Crohn's disease of both the colon and rectum are included in this subcategory. The **Excludes1** note reminds her that this entry *excludes* Crohn's disease that affects *both* the large and small

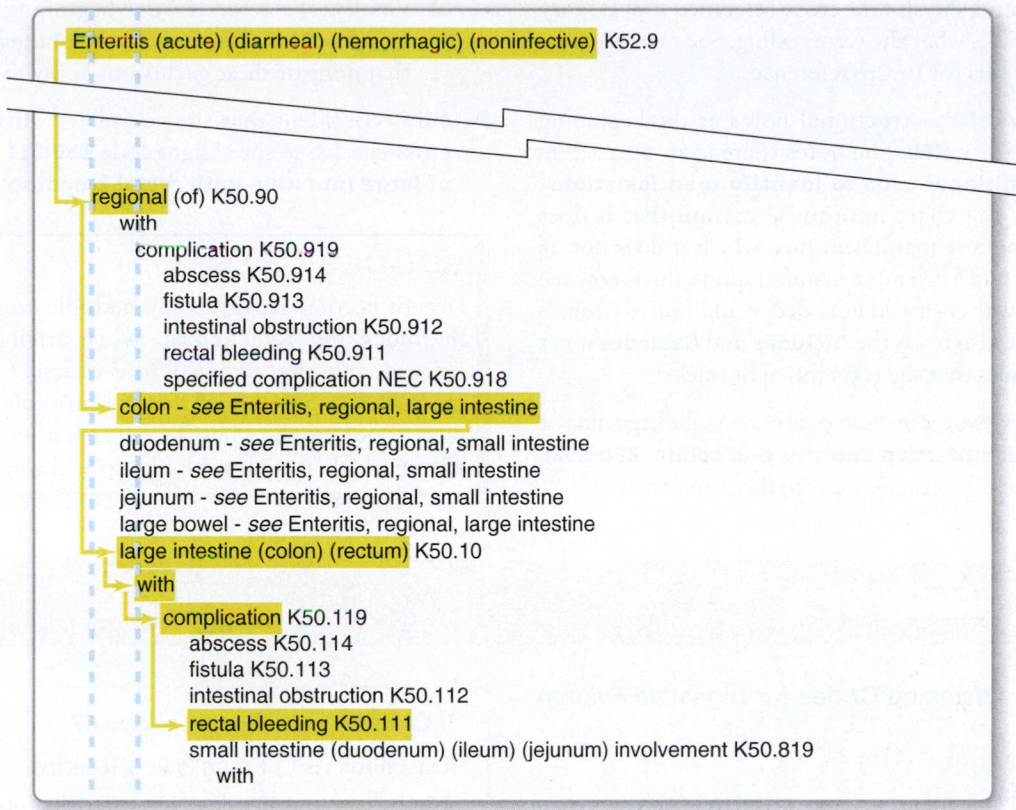

Figure 8-2 ■ Index entry for "Enteritis, regional."

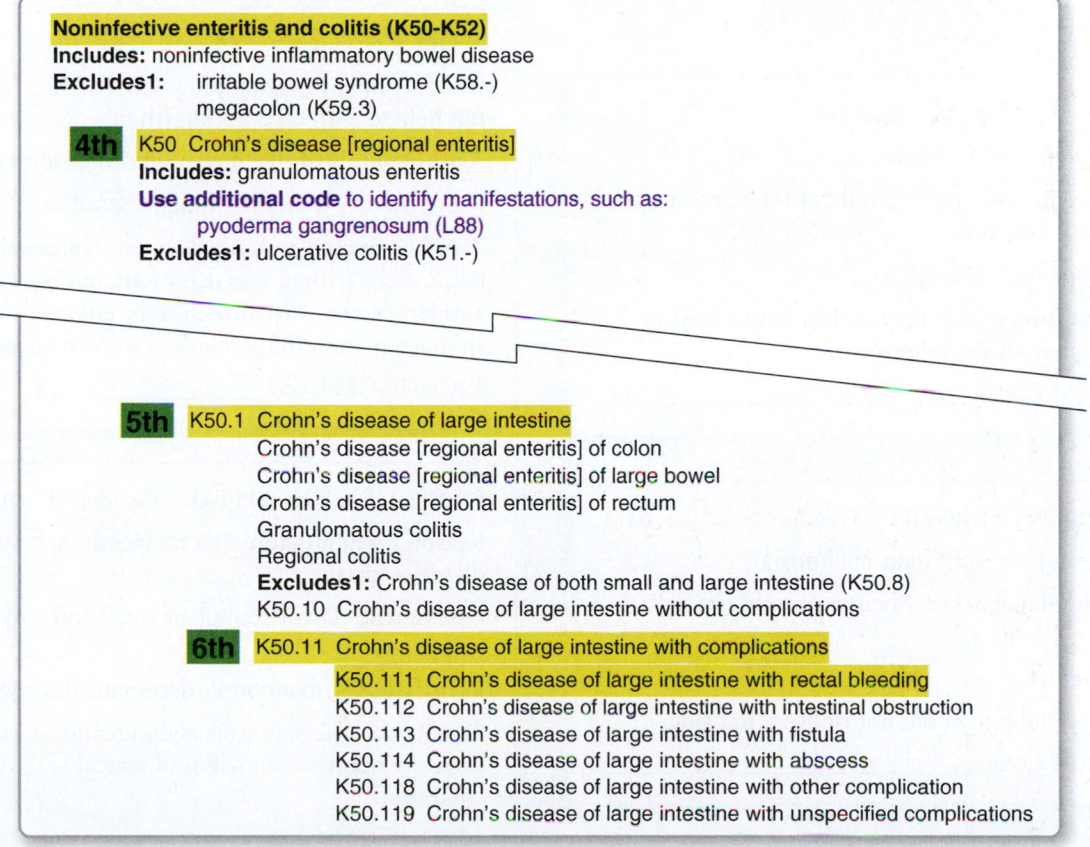

Figure 8-3 ■ Tabular List entry for "Crohn's disease."

intestines and she should cross-reference subcategory **K50.8** if that is what she were coding. She makes a mental note of this for future reference.

❏ She reviews the instructional notes at the beginning of the category **K50**. She notes there is an instruction to **Use additional code to identify manifestations**. Jill checks the chart note to be certain that it does not mention any manifestations, which it does not. If Dr. Garrett had listed more manifestations, this is how she would know they should be coded in addition to Crohn's disease. She also reads the **Includes** and **Excludes** notes and concludes that she is on the right track.

❏ Next, Jill reviews the instructional notes at the beginning of the block **Noninfective enteritis and colitis (K50-K52)**. None of these exclusions apply to the current case.

❏ Finally, she refers to the beginning of ICD-10-CM Chapter 11 and reviews the **Excludes** notes to be sure that none of these exclusions apply to her current case.

▶ Jill is confident that she completed all verifications and cross-checks, so she assigns code **K50.111 Crohn's disease of large intestine with rectal bleeding**.

SUCCESS STEP

Do not become frustrated by multiple cross-references in the Index and Tabular List. When driving, you may see a detour sign that redirects your course. Cross-references are ICD-10-CM's way of making sure you get to the right place. Look up the Main Term listed after the **see** or **see also** note, then continue looking for the needed subterms.

CODING PRACTICE

Exercise 8.3   Assigning Codes for Digestive System Diagnoses

Instructions: Read the mini-medical-record of each patient's encounter, review the information abstracted in Exercise 8.2 for questions 1, 2, and 3, and assign ICD-10-CM diagnosis codes using the Index and Tabular List. For questions 4 and 5, abstract the cases on your own before assigning codes. Write the code(s) on the line provided.

---

1. OFFICE   Gender: M Age: 54

Chief complaint: Indigestion

Assessment: Chronic perforated peptic ulcer in stomach with bleeding

Plan: Change diet, change Rx

Tip: The location of this peptic ulcer is specified, so carefully review all the subterms.

1 ICD-10-CM Code _____

---

2. OUTPATIENT SURGERY   Gender: F Age: 61

Procedure: Repair, right inguinal hernia

Postprocedural diagnosis: Recurrent right inguinal hernia

Plan: FU in office

Tip: Code for unilateral but not right vs. left side.

1 ICD-10-CM Code _____

---

3. OFFICE   Gender: M Age: 67

Reason for visit: FU on lower GI series

Assessment: Ulcerative colitis with fistula

Plan: Begin liquid diet, Rx antibiotics, FU 2 weeks

1 ICD-10-CM Code _____

---

4. OFFICE   Gender: M Age: 31

Chief complaint: Cramping and diarrhea for 3 days, not helped with OTC antidiarrheals

Assessment: Irritable bowel syndrome with diarrhea

Plan: Modify diet, Rx antidepressant

Tip: The doctor prescribed an antidepressant not because the patient was depressed, but because tricyclic antidepressants have proven to be effective in relieving stomach pain in IBS, according to current research.

1 ICD-10-CM Code _____

---

5. INPATIENT HOSPITAL   Gender: F Age: 47

Reason for admission: Rectal bleeding, history of diverticulosis

Assessment: Diverticulitis of small and large intestines with bleeding

Plan: IV fluids, monitoring, determine if surgery is needed

Tip: Review the subterms and indentations in the Index carefully because you will find several variations of this condition.

1 ICD-10-CM Code _____

ARRANGING CODES FOR DIGESTIVE SYSTEM CONDITIONS

To correctly sequence codes for the digestive system, coders need to follow instructional notes in the Tabular List, which direct coders to assign additional codes for associated conditions, underlying causes, and external causes related to digestive system conditions. Instructional notes direct coders whether the cross-referenced codes should be sequenced as additional codes or whether they should be coded first. ■ TABLE 8-4 highlights the most common instructional notes in the digestive system chapter and the categories where they appear. Notice that multiple coding is often required to describe lifestyle habits, such as alcohol or tobacco abuse, that may contribute to digestive system conditions.

Instructional notes may appear at the beginning of the chapter, the beginning of a block or subchapter, the beginning of a three-character category, the beginning of a subcategory, or under the final code. Therefore, it is important to search for information not only directly under the code, but also at the previous levels of the classification hierarchy.

Table 8-4 ■ COMMON INSTRUCTIONAL NOTES FOR THE DIGESTIVE SYSTEM

Content of Instructional Note	Location of Instructional Note
Use additional code to identify: Alcohol abuse and dependence (F10.-)	K20 Esophagitis
	K25 Gastric ulcer
	K26 Duodenal ulcer
	K27 Peptic ulcer
	K28 Gastrojejunal ulcer
	K29.0 Acute gastritis
	K29.2 Alcoholic gastritis
	K70 Alcoholic liver disease
	K86.0 Alcohol-induced chronic pancreatitis
Use additional code to identify: Alcohol abuse and dependence (F10.-) Exposure to environmental tobacco smoke (Z77.22) Exposure to tobacco smoke in the perinatal period (P96.81) History of tobacco dependence (Z87.891) Occupational exposure to environmental tobacco smoke (Z57.31) Tobacco dependence (F17.-) Tobacco use (Z72.0)	K05 Gingivitis and periodontal diseases
	K11 Diseases of salivary glands
	K12 Stomatitis and related lesions
	K13 Other diseases of lip and oral mucosa
	K14 Diseases of tongue
Specify type of infection	K94.02 Colostomy infection
	K94.12 Enterostomy infection
	K94.22 Gastrostomy infection
	K94.32 Esophagostomy infection
	K95.01 Infection due to gastric band procedure
	K95.81 Infection due to other bariatric procedure

Guided Example of Arranging Digestive System Diagnosis Codes

Refer to the following new example to practice skills for sequencing codes for the digestive system. Jill Hynes, CPC, is a fictitious coder who guides you through this case. Jill's abstracting process identified an abscess of the submandibular salivary gland and current heavy tobacco use.

Date: 9/2/yy   Location: Branton Gastroenterology

Provider: Stanley Garrett, MD

Patient: Gary Spates   Gender: M   Age: 52

Chief complaint: "Lump and tenderness in my jaw"

Assessment: Abscess, submandibular salivary gland, heavy current cigarette smoker

Plan: Drain abscess, Rx antibiotics

Follow along in your ICD-10-CM manual as Jill Hynes, CPC, assigns and sequences codes for this case. Check off each step after you complete it.

▶ Jill begins by locating the Main Term in the Index.

❏ Jill looks up **A, Abscess**.

❏ She locates the subterm for **salivary (duct) (gland)**.

❏ Jill confirms that there are no further subentries under **salivary** and identifies the code **K11.3** that she will verify in the Tabular List.

▶ Jill locates code **K11.3** in the Tabular List.

❏ She confirms that the code description **Abscess of salivary gland** accurately describes the diagnosis. She notes that there are no further breakdowns for the specific salivary gland affected.

❏ She reviews the instructional note at the beginning of the category **K11** (■ FIGURE 8-4), which states to **Use additional code**. As she reads the items listed, she observes that they relate to certain lifestyle habits. She knows that an instructional note at the beginning of a category applies to all of the codes in that category, so this instructional note applies to all codes from **K11.0** to **K11.9**. Smoking is

---

K11 Diseases of salivary glands
   Use additional code to identify:
      alcohol abuse and dependence (F10.-)
      exposure to environmental tobacco smoke (Z77.22)
      exposure to tobacco smoke in the perinatal period (P96.81)
      history of tobacco dependence (Z87.891)
      occupational exposure to environmental tobacco smoke (Z57.31)
      tobacco dependence (F17.-)
      tobacco use (Z72.0)

Figure 8-4 ■ Instructional notes for category K11, "Diseases of the salivary glands."

classified as tobacco dependence, per the Index. The fact that tobacco dependence is to be an *additional* code tells her that the abscess should be sequenced first and the tobacco dependence should be sequenced second.

▶ Next, Jill codes for heavy current cigarette smoker.

❑ She notices several possible code options in the instructional note:

- **History of tobacco dependence (Z87.891)**
- **Tobacco dependence (F17.-)**
- **Tobacco use (Z72.0)**

❑ Jill recalls that even though tobacco use is part of Mr. Spates's medical history, OGCR I.C.21.c.4) states she should use **history (of)** codes only to describe a past medical condition that no longer exists. Because Mr. Spates's tobacco use is documented as *current*, she eliminates code **Z87.891, History of tobacco dependence**.

❑ She checks the medical record to see if Dr. Garrett stated tobacco dependence or indicated that he is a smoker. He did, so she chooses **F17.- Tobacco dependence**.

❑ To verify this choice, she searches the Index for the Main Term **Smoker**. The entry lists a cross-reference note, *see* **Dependence, drug, nicotine**.

❑ She searches the Index for the Main Term **Dependence** with the first-level subterm **drug** and the second-level subterm **nicotine**. The entry lists the default code

F17.200. She reviews the third-level subterms and identifies an entry for cigarettes, **F17.210**. No nicotine-induced disorder is documented, so the subterm **with disorder** does not apply.

❑ She verifies **F17.210 Nicotine dependence, cigarettes, uncomplicated** in the Tabular List. She reviews the related code options of **F17.211** through **F17.219**, which identify nicotine dependence in remission or withdrawal. These codes do not apply because the information is not documented.

❑ Next, Jill goes back to the original code and checks for instructional notes at the beginning of the block **Diseases of the oral cavity and salivary glands (K00-K14)**. This block has no further notes.

❑ Finally, she refers to the beginning of ICD-10-CM Chapter 11 and reviews the **Excludes** notes to be sure that none of these exclusions apply to her current case.

▶ Jill is confident that she completed all verifications and cross-checks. She sequences **F17.210** second because the instructional note described it as an additional code.

▶ Jill finalizes the code assignment and sequencing for this case.

(1) **K11.3 Abscess of salivary gland**

(2) **F17.210 Nicotine dependence, cigarettes, uncomplicated**

CODING PRACTICE

Exercise 8.4 Arranging Codes for Digestive System Diagnoses

Instructions: Read the mini-medical-record of each patient's encounter, review the information abstracted in Exercise 8.2 for questions 1, 2, and 3, assign ICD-10-CM diagnosis codes using the Index and Tabular List, and sequence them correctly.

1. OFFICE   Gender: M   Age: 56

Chief complaint: Abdominal pain and bloating, fatigue, vomiting

Assessment: Alcoholic liver cirrhosis with ascites due to alcohol addiction

Plan: Counseled patient regarding abstinence from alcohol, reduce salt intake

Tip: Read the instructional note at the beginning of the category to use an additional code.

2 ICD-10-CM Codes _____

2. OFFICE   Gender: M   Age: 59

Chief complaint: Hematemesis, history of cirrhosis

Assessment: Portal hypertension (*increase in blood pressure in the portal vein*) with portal hypertensive gastropathy

Plan: Endoscopic therapy, drug therapy, and dietary changes

Tip: Code portal hypertension first, then follow the instructional notes to code gastropathy.

3 ICD-10-CM Codes _____
_____

3. OFFICE   Gender: M   Age: 33

Chief complaint: Redness and tenderness around colostomy site

Assessment: Colostomy infection, cellulitis of abdominal wall due to methicillin-susceptible Staphylococcus aureus (MSSA)

(*continued*)

CODING PRACTICE (continued)

3. (continued)

Plan: Rx antibiotics

Tip: Sometimes coding is like a treasure hunt. You never know where it will take you. Read the instructional notes under the code for colostomy infection to identify the second code. Read the instructional notes under the block heading for cellulitis to identify the third code.

3 ICD-10-CM Codes _____

_____

4. OFFICE Gender: M Age: 38

Chief complaint: Fecal incontinence that has not improved

Assessment: Nontraumatic anal sphincter tear

Plan: Sphincteroplasty

(continued)

4. (continued)

Tip: Read the instructional notes under the code for nontraumatic anal sphincter tear to identify the second code.

2 ICD-10-CM Codes _____

5. OFFICE Gender: M Age: 14

Procedure: 2 dental fillings

Postprocedural diagnosis: Caries (*cavities*), tooth 2 pit and fissure surface, enamel only; tooth 3 pit and fissure surface, penetrating dentin

Plan: 6-month check-up

Tip: Assign separate codes for each tooth because the depth of the caries was different on each one. Dentists identify each tooth with a number, beginning at the right rear molar on the top of the mouth.

2 ICD-10-CM Codes _____

CODING NEOPLASMS OF THE DIGESTIVE SYSTEM

Neoplasms of the digestive system do not appear in ICD-10-CM Chapter 11 (K00-K95); they appear in Chapter 2 (C00-D49). Codes for neoplasms of the digestive system appear in two different blocks within the neoplasm chapter:

- Malignant neoplasm of lip, oral cavity and pharynx (C00-C14)
- Malignant neoplasm of digestive organs (C15-C26)

Review these two blocks in the ICD-10-CM manual to become familiar with the content.

According to the Centers for Disease Control and Prevention, the most common sites for cancer in the digestive system are the colon and rectum; cancer of these sites is referred to as colorectal cancer. Colorectal cancer is the third most common cancer in the United States and, in most cases, develops slowly over many years. The number of deaths due to colorectal cancer has declined over the last several decades, largely because cases are being detected early and treatment methods have improved. Colorectal cancer, which most often begins as a polyp, can be detected early through a colonoscopy. Cancer that is detected early is more easily treated. Colorectal cancer can be prevented through removal of polyps during a colonoscopy, before they have time to turn into cancer. Distinguishing statistics for deaths due to colon cancer from those due to

rectal cancer is difficult because the cause of death has been misclassified historically on death certificates, often listed as colon cancer rather than specifying the exact site.

To locate codes for colorectal cancer, search the Table of Neoplasms for the entry **intestine, large, colon**. Identify whether the disease affects only the colon or both the colon and rectum because there are different codes, as shown in ■ FIGURE 8-5, page 138. Specificity of the code will assist in improving data collection for this type of cancer.

The liver is a common site of cancer in the digestive system because many types of cancer metastasize to the liver. The liver filters the blood, which is one of the main ways that cancer cells move throughout the body. Most cancer found in the liver is metastatic. Primary liver cancer occurs most often in patients with cirrhosis and alcoholic liver disease. When coding for cancer in the liver, verify whether it is primary or metastatic.

The incidence rate (*occurrence of new cases*) for cancer of the oral cavity and pharynx is nearly twice as high for men as for women. Approximately 30% of cases are diagnosed at a local stage, leading to a better survival rate than for cancers detected later. Patients with malignant neoplasms of the esophagus, stomach, and pancreas have low survival rates because they have few symptoms and are usually not diagnosed until a late stage, when the neoplasms have already metastasized.

Neoplasm	Malignant Primary	Malignant Secondary	Ca in situ	Benign	Uncertain Behavior	Unspecified Behavior
- intestine, intestinal	C26.0	C78.80	D01.40	D13.9	D37.8	D49.0
- - large	C18.9	C78.5	D01.0	D12.6	D37.4	D49.0
- - - appendix	C18.1	C78.5	D01.0	D12.1	D37.3	D49.0
- - - caput coli	C18.0	C78.5	D01.0	D12.0	D37.4	D49.0
- - - cecum	C18.0	C78.5	D01.0	D12.0	D37.4	D49.0
- - - colon	C18.9	C78.5	D01.0	D12.6	D37.4	D49.0
- - - - and rectum	C19	C78.5	D01.1	D12.7	D37.5	D49.0

Figure 8-5 ■ Table of Neoplasms entry for "Colorectal cancer."

CODING PRACTICE

Exercise 8.5   Coding Neoplasms of the Digestive System

Instructions: Read the mini-medical-record of each patient's encounter, then abstract, assign, and sequence ICD-10-CM diagnosis codes using the Index and Tabular List. Write the code(s) on the line provided.

---

1. OUTPATIENT SURGERY   Gender: F   Age: 57

Procedure: Screening colonoscopy due to finding of polyps 5 years ago and family history of colon cancer

Finding: 3 new adenomatous polyps were found at the sigmoid flexure and removed

Plan: 5-year follow-up

Tip: Identify where the sigmoid flexure is located. Code the patient's personal history as well as the family history because both present risk factors for the patient.

3 ICD-10-CM Codes _____

_____

---

2. OFFICE   Gender: F   Age: 61

Reason for visit: FU on CT scan

Assessment: Adenocarcinoma of overlapping sites (rectum and sigmoid) of the large intestine

Plan: Refer to oncologist

Tip: A tumor in two sites that are adjacent (*immediately next to each other*) is considered to be overlapping.

1 ICD-10-CM Code _____

---

3. OFFICE   Gender: M   Age: 54

Reason for visit: FU on liver biopsy

Assessment: Hepatocellular cancer due to alcohol dependence and chronic hepatitis C

Plan: Refer to oncologist for evaluation of treatment options

Tip: Read the instructional notes in the Tabular List under the first code to identify the additional conditions that need to be coded.

3 ICD-10-CM Codes _____

_____

---

4. OFFICE   Gender: F   Age: 70

Reason for visit: FU on colonoscopy results

Assessment: Cancer in situ, rectum

Plan: Schedule surgery, refer to oncologist for adjuvant therapy

1 ICD-10-CM Code _____

---

5. OFFICE   Gender: M   Age: 68

Reason for visit: FU on biopsy and imaging

Assessment: Adenocarcinoma of the pancreas with liver and lymph gland metastases

Plan: Chemotherapy, palliative care

Tip: Code for the primary cancer and both metastatic sites.

3 ICD-10-CM Codes _____

_____

CHAPTER SUMMARY

In this chapter you learned that:

- The digestive system consists of the alimentary canal and accessory organs, which provide for ingestion, digestion, absorption, and elimination of food.
- Chapter 11 of ICD-10-CM, "Diseases of the Digestive System (K00-K95)," classifies diseases of the digestive system. OGCR provides no specific guidelines for the digestive system, but there are many instructional notes in the Tabular List.
- When abstracting for digestive system conditions, coders need to look for manifestations, complications, and associated lifestyle habits.

- Coders frequently assign combination codes to describe complications of digestive system conditions.
- To sequence codes for the digestive system, follow instructional notes in the Tabular List, which direct coders to assign additional codes for associated conditions, underlying causes, and external causes related to digestive system conditions.
- Colorectal cancer is the third most common cancer in the United States; the liver is a common site of metastases.

CONCEPT QUIZ

Take a moment to look back at the digestive system and solidify your skills. Try to answer the questions from memory first, then refer to the discussion in this chapter and the Glossary at the end of this book if you need a little extra help.

Completion

Instructions: Write the term that completes each statement based on the information you learned in this chapter. Choose from the following list. Some choices may be used more than once and some choices may not be used at all.

calculi	ile/o
cholecyst/o	instructional notes
col/o	large intestine
colon	liver
colp/o	multiple coding
combination coding	pancreas
cysto/o	rect/o
fund/o	small intestine
hepat/o	stomach

1. _____ is the combining form for colon.
2. _____ is the combining form for gallbladder.
3. _____ is the combining form for liver.
4. _____ is a combining form for small intestine.
5. _____ is the combining form for the top portion of the stomach.
6. _____ describes more than one aspect of a condition, or multiple conditions, in a single code.
7. _____ requires that more than one code be assigned to fully describe a patient's condition.
8. _____ may appear at the beginning of the chapter, the beginning of a block or subchapter, the beginning of a three-character category, the beginning of a subcategory, or under the final code.

9. _____ cancer is most often metastatic.
10. _____ is often required to describe lifestyle habits, such as alcohol abuse or tobacco use, which may contribute to digestive system conditions.

Multiple Choice

Instructions: Circle the letter of the best answer to each question based on the information you learned in this chapter.

1. What term means "transfer of nutrients to the body"?
   A. Ingestion
   B. Digestion
   C. Absorption
   D. Elimination

2. What structures assist in digestion but are not directly connected to the alimentary canal?
   A. Large and small intestines
   B. Accessory organs
   C. Rectum and anus
   D. Teeth

3. How would you code the following scenario? *A patient is seen for alcoholic gastritis with bleeding due to alcohol abuse.*
   A. K29.21, F10.188
   B. K29.2, F10.19
   C. F10.188, K29.21
   D. K29.21, F10.10

4. What is a barium enema?
   A. Swallowing a chalky substance and viewing it on an x-ray
   B. A group of disorders in which the intestines become red and swollen
   C. Endoscopic examination of the esophagus, stomach, and duodenum
   D. Injecting a chalky substance into the colon through the anus and viewing the organs on an x-ray

(*continued*)

(continued from page 139)

5. How would you code the following scenario? *A patient is seen for Crohn's disease of both the large and small intestine.*
   A. K50.10, K50.00
   B. K50.00, K50.10
   C. K50.118
   D. K50.80

6. What does the word root *chole/o* mean?
   A. Colon
   B. Gallbladder
   C. Bile
   D. Vagina

7. Where in the Table of Neoplasms should you look for codes for colorectal cancer?
   A. Intestine, large, colon, and rectum
   B. Cancer, colorectal
   C. Colon, rectum, cancer
   D. Colon, large intestine, colorectal

8. What is MRCP?
   A. Endoscopic ultrasound
   B. Magnetic resonance cholangiopancreatography
   C. Esophagogastroduodenoscopy
   D. Magnetic resonance imaging of colon and pancreas

9. How would you code the following scenario? *A patient is seen for a malignant neoplasm of the colon with the rectum.*
   A. C18.0
   B. C19
   C. C18.8
   D. C18.9, C20

10. What is diverticulitis?
    A. Pouches formed when the lining of the intestine pushes through the intestinal muscle layer
    B. Presence of diverticula
    C. Diversion of the colon
    D. Bacterial infection of diverticula

KEEP ON CODING

Instructions: Read the diagnostic statement, then use the Index and Tabular List to assign and sequence ICD-10-CM diagnosis codes. Write the code(s) on the line provided.

1. Carcinoma of the buccal mucosa. ICD-10-CM Code(s) _____

2. Erosion of teeth due to diet. ICD-10-CM Code(s) _____

3. Enterostomy hemorrhage. ICD-10-CM Code(s) _____

4. Cyst of pancreas. ICD-10-CM Code(s) _____

5. Mucous retention cyst of salivary gland. ICD-10-CM Code(s) _____

6. Cardiospasm. ICD-10-CM Code(s) _____

7. Malignant neoplasm of tongue with a past history of tobacco dependence. ICD-10-CM Code(s) _____

8. Hydrops of the gallbladder. ICD-10-CM Code(s) _____

9. Acute gingivitis, plaque induced. ICD-10-CM Code(s) _____

10. Eosinophilic esophagitis. ICD-10-CM Code(s) _____

11. Hairy leukoplakia. ICD-10-CM Code(s) _____

12. Incisional hernia without obstruction or gangrene. ICD-10-CM Code(s) _____

13. Acute appendicitis with localized peritonitis. ICD-10-CM Code(s) _____

14. Ulcerative pancolitis and abscess. ICD-10-CM Code(s) _____

15. Stage 3 hemorrhoids. ICD-10-CM Code(s) _____

16. Slow-transit constipation. ICD-10-CM Code(s) _____

17. Chronic cholecystitis with cholelithiasis without obstruction. ICD-10-CM Code(s) _____

18. Postprocedural liver failure. ICD-10-CM Code(s) _____

19. Cheilosis. ICD-10-CM Code(s) _____

20. Esophageal ulcer with bleeding. ICD-10-CM Code(s) _____

21. Retained dental root. ICD-10-CM Code(s) _____

22. Glossodynia. ICD-10-CM Code(s)) _____

23. Alcoholic cirrhosis of liver with ascites. ICD-10-CM Code(s) _____

24. Malignant neoplasm of overlapping sections of the esophagus due to cigarette smoking. ICD-10-CM Code(s) _____

25. Hemoperitoneum. ICD-10-CM Code(s) _____

CODING CHALLENGE

Instructions: Read the mini-medical-record of each patient's encounter, then abstract, assign, and sequence ICD-10-CM diagnosis codes using the Index and Tabular List. Write the code(s) on the line provided.

---

1. EMERGENCY DEPT   Gender: M   Age: 15

Chief complaint: Vomiting, acute abdominal pain, RLQ tenderness, T 101.8°.

Assessment: Acute appendicitis with rupture

Plan: Laparoscopic appendectomy

1 ICD-10-CM Code _____

---

2. OFFICE   Gender: F   Age: 41

Reason for visit: Referred by her oncologist for mouth ulcers due to chemotherapy for metastatic colon cancer (*primary colon cancer that has spread*)

Assessment: Oral mucositis, side effect from chemotherapy for metastatic colon cancer

Plan: Oral debridement, pain relief

Tip: First, code for the condition being treated. For the second code, read the instructional note in the Tabular List after you verify the first code. Then, code the colon cancer to identify the reason for the chemotherapy. Finally, code for unspecified metastatic sites.

4 ICD-10-CM Codes _____

---

3. OFFICE   Gender: M   Age: 43

Chief complaint: "My hiatal hernia seems worse than usual"

Assessment: Strangulated hiatal hernia

Plan: Schedule hernia repair

Tip: Strangulation is classified as an obstruction.

1 ICD-10-CM Code _____

---

4. OFFICE   Gender: M   Age: 36

Chief complaint: "I've been having problems with my GERD"

Assessment: GERD

Plan: Adjust Rx, call if problems continue

1 ICD-10-CM Code _____

---

5. INPATIENT HOSPITAL   Gender: F   Age: 52

Reason for admission: Pain RUQ, T 102°, vomiting

Procedure: Laparoscopic cholecystectomy

Discharge diagnosis: Acute cholecystitis with calculi in the common bile duct causing obstruction

Tip: When you search for the Main Term *Cholecystitis*, follow the cross-reference listed in the Index.

1 ICD-10-CM Code _____

---

6. OUTPATIENT SURGERY   Gender: M   Age: 56

Chief complaint: Nausea, vomiting, constipation

Assessment: Inflammatory colon polyps, intestinal obstruction

Plan: High-fiber diet and increased liquids, Rx corticosteroid to reduce inflammation, FU 2 weeks

Tip: Main Term is polyps. Thoroughly review all available subterms to locate the correct combination code.

1 ICD-10-CM Code _____

---

7. OFFICE   Gender: M   Age: 26

Chief complaint: Yellow teeth

Assessment: Amelogenesis imperfecta (*a tooth development disorder in which the teeth are covered with thin, abnormally formed enamel and are easily damaged*)

Plan: Apply crowns

1 ICD-10-CM Code _____

---

8. EMERGENCY DEPT   Gender: M   Age: 12

Chief complaint: "My son forgot that he isn't supposed to eat eggs and ate a hardboiled egg at his friend's house. He has had diarrhea and vomiting for 4 hours and I'm getting worried."

Assessment: Allergic gastroenteritis due to eggs

Plan: Rx antiemetic, antidiarrheal

2 ICD-10-CM Codes _____

(continued)

(continued from page 141)

9. INPATIENT HOSPITAL   Gender: F   Age: 30

Reason for admission: LUQ pain and swelling increasing over the past 3 days, indigestion

Treatment: IV fluids, pain control, nasogastric suctioning

Discharge diagnosis: Acute pancreatitis due to opioid dependence and intoxication

2 ICD-10-CM Codes _____

10. INPATIENT HOSPITAL   Gender: F   Age: 41

Reason for admission: Admitted from ED with severe and steady abdominal pain, fever, excessive perspiration, T 101°

Treatment: IV antibiotics, fluids, colectomy

Discharge diagnosis: Generalized peritonitis due to E. coli, irritable bowel syndrome

3 ICD-10-CM Codes _____

_____

Endocrine, Nutritional, and Metabolic Diseases (E00-E89)

Chapter 9

Learning Objectives

After completing this chapter, you should have the skills to:

9.1 Spell and define the key words, medical terms, and abbreviations related to endocrine, nutritional, and metabolic diseases. (Remember)

9.2 Summarize the structure, function, and common conditions of the endocrine system. (Understand)

9.3 Adhere to the Official Guidelines for Coding and Reporting and instructional notes for endocrine, nutritional, and metabolic diseases. (Apply)

9.4 Examine and abstract diagnostic information from the medical record for coding endocrine, nutritional, and metabolic diseases. (Analyze)

9.5 Demonstrate how to assign diagnosis codes for endocrine, nutritional, and metabolic diseases and related conditions. (Apply)

9.6 Utilize guidelines for arranging (sequencing) multiple diagnosis codes for endocrine, nutritional, and metabolic diseases and related conditions. (Apply)

9.7 Demonstrate how to abstract, assign, and sequence codes for neoplasms of the endocrine system. (Apply)

Chapter Outline

- **Endocrine System Refresher**
- **Coding Guidelines for the Endocrine System**
- **Abstracting for Endocrine System Conditions**
- **Assigning Codes for Endocrine System Conditions**
- **Arranging Codes for Endocrine System Conditions**
- **Coding Neoplasms of the Endocrine System**

Key Terms and Abbreviations

causal relationship	hormones	metabolism	target organ
diabetes mellitus (DM)	hyperglycemia	prediabetes	trachea
diabetic ketoacidosis (DKA)	hyperosmolarity hyperglycemic nonketotic syndrome (HHNS)	serum assay	
endocrine system	hypoglycemia		
HbA1c			

In addition to the key terms listed here, students should know the terms defined within tables in this chapter.

INTRODUCTION

When your vehicle gets a little sluggish, you may decide to use a fuel additive to boost its performance. Your body's hormones are, in a sense, like fuel additives for your car. They perform a variety of tasks that keep other organ systems and structures working smoothly. It is the endocrine system's job to produce, store, and release hormones.

An endocrinologist is a physician who specializes in endocrine, nutritional, and metabolic diseases. When primary care physicians (PCPs) are unable to diagnose or manage a complex endocrine, nutritional, or metabolic condition, they refer the patient to an endocrinologist.

As you read this chapter, open up your medical terminology book and keep a medical dictionary handy to refresh your memory of any unfamiliar terms.

ENDOCRINE SYSTEM REFRESHER

The function of the **endocrine system** is to produce, store, and release **hormones**, which are chemical messengers. Hormones regulate many body functions including growth, development, **metabolism** (*the processes of digestion, elimination, breathing, blood circulation, and maintaining body temperature*), sexual function, reproduction, and mood. The endocrine system consists of several ductless glands that are not directly connected to each other. The function of each gland is summarized in ■ TABLE 9-1. The ovaries and testes function as part of the reproductive system in addition to their endocrine function; the pancreas has an exocrine function in the digestive system in addition to its endocrine function.

In ■ FIGURE 9-1, each structure in the endocrine system is labeled with its name, as well as its medical terminology root/combining form. Refer to ■ TABLE 9-2 for a refresher on how to build medical terms related to the endocrine system.

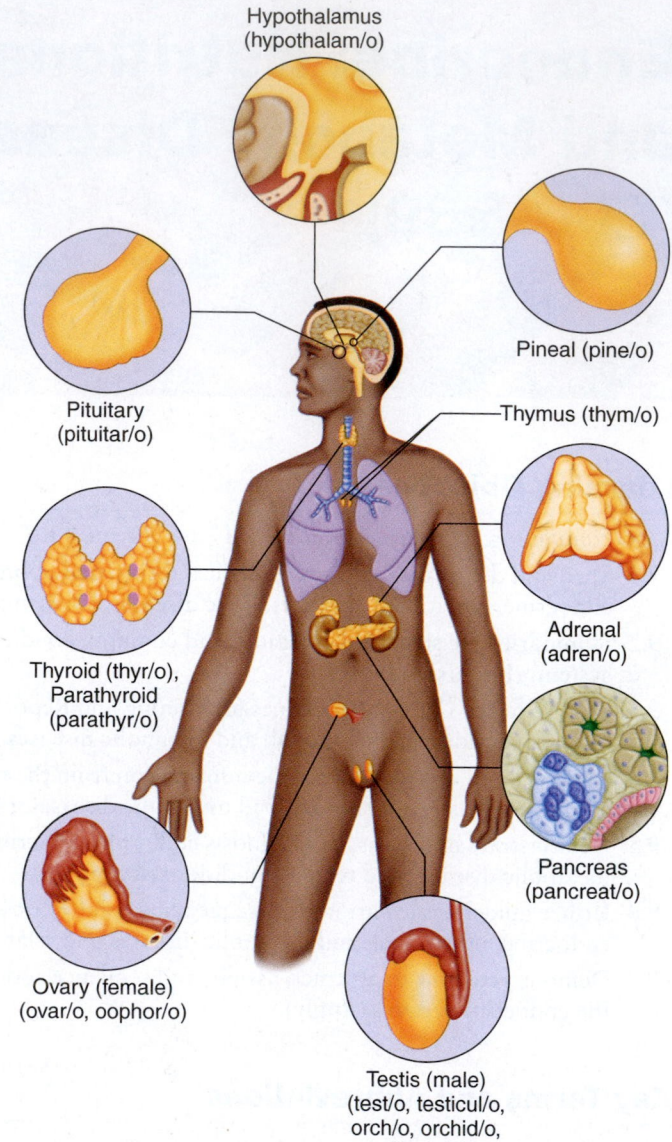

Figure 9-1 ■ The endocrine system.

CODING CAUTION

Be alert for medical terms that are spelled similarly and have different meanings.

ne<u>phr</u>opathy (*kidney disease*) and **ne<u>ur</u>opathy** (*nerve disease*)

hyp<u>o</u>thyroidism (*state of low thyroid function*) and **hyp<u>er</u>thyroidism** (*state of high thyroid function*)

thy<u>r</u>/o (*thyroid*), **thy<u>m</u>/o** (*thymus gland*), and **th<u>alam</u>/o** (*thalamus, a portion of the brain*)

Conditions of the Endocrine System

Endocrine, nutritional, and metabolic disorders tend to have gradual onsets and generalized symptoms such as fatigue, weakness, weight change, hair loss, muscle weakness, nervousness, appetite change, and irritability, making them difficult to diagnose. When a structure in the endocrine system malfunctions, the result is either hypofunction or hyperfunction of a gland, a hormone, or a **target organ** (*the organ receiving hormones*).

Table 9-1 ■ **FUNCTION OF ENDOCRINE GLANDS**

Gland	Endocrine Function
Pituitary	Controls most activity in the endocrine system
Hypothalamus	Controls the pituitary gland
Pineal	Regulates waking/sleeping functions
Thymus	Produces T-cells used by the immune system
Thyroid	Regulates metabolism
Parathyroid	Regulates the level of circulating calcium
Pancreas (Islets of Langerhans)	Synthesis, storage, and release of glucagon and insulin
Adrenal	Secretes steroid hormones
Ovaries/testes (gonads)	Secrete estrogen and testosterone

Table 9-2   ■   **EXAMPLE OF CONSTRUCTING MEDICAL TERMS FOR THE ENDOCRINE SYSTEM**

Combining Form/Prefix	Suffix	Complete Medical Term
glyc/o (*sugar*) **thyr/o** (*thyroid*) **protein/o** (*protein*)	**-emia** (*condition of the blood*) **-uria** (*condition of the urine*) **-ism** (*state of*)	**hypo + glyc + emia** (*low sugar in the blood*) **hyper + glyc + emia** (*excessive sugar in the blood*) **glyco + uria** (*sugar in the urine*)
hypo- (prefix; *below, low*) **hyper-** (prefix; *above, high*)		**hypo + thyroid + ism** (*state of low thyroid function*) **hyper + thyroid + ism** (*state of high thyroid function*)
		protein + emia (*protein in the blood*) **protein + uria** (*protein in the urine*)

Endocrine disorders are best diagnosed through **serum assays** (*lab tests that measure the presence and quantity of a substance in the blood*). Common treatments include injection of hormones, surgical removal of all or part of a gland, and surgical removal of a tumor that is causing the problem.

The most common diseases of the endocrine system are **diabetes mellitus (DM)** and thyroid disorders. These conditions present concepts and terminology that coders must be familiar with.

Diabetes Mellitus

Diabetes mellitus is a condition resulting in elevated glucose levels over an extended period of time and excess excretion of urine, usually due to malfunction of the pancreas. Coders need to be familiar with several types of diabetes, which are highlighted in ■ TABLE 9-3. According to the Centers for Disease Control and Prevention (CDC) *National Diabetes Statistics Report*, diabetes affects more than 9% of the population or 30.3 million people, and an additional 84.1 million people are estimated to have **prediabetes**, a condition in which people have a high blood glucose concentration, but not high enough to be classified as diabetes.

Diabetes causes both acute and chronic complications. Acute complications consist of:

- **Hyperglycemia** is the condition of severely elevated blood glucose levels, usually occurring in type 1 diabetics, due to a lack or deficiency of insulin. Hyperglycemia can cause **diabetic ketoacidosis (DKA)** in which a high level of ketones (*a chemical made when the body breaks down fat into energy*) accumulate in the blood, turning it acidic. Symptoms include nausea and vomiting, abdominal pain, shock, coma, and death if it is not treated immediately.

Table 9-3   ■   **CAUSES OF DIABETES MELLITUS**

Type of Diabetes	Description	Treatment	Frequency
Type 1 diabetes mellitus	Body's immune system attacks pancreatic beta cells so that the pancreas does not produce insulin. (Previously called insulin-dependent diabetes mellitus [IDDM] or juvenile-onset diabetes.)	No prevention or cure known. Patients *must* receive insulin, delivered through injection or pump, to survive.	5% of all diagnosed cases of diabetes
Type 2 diabetes mellitus	Pancreas produces insulin, but the body does not use it properly. In some cases, insulin production is decreased also. (Previously called non-insulin-dependent diabetes mellitus [NIDDM] or adult-onset diabetes.)	Prevent, delay, or reverse the onset of type 2 diabetes with weight loss, increased physical activity, and the medication metformin. Some people *may* need insulin.	90–95% of all diagnosed cases of diabetes
Due to underlying condition (secondary diabetes)	Elevated glucose is caused by medical condition, such as pancreatic disease.	Treat underlying cause if possible. Manage with diet, exercise, medication, and insulin, as needed.	Less than 5% of all diagnosed cases of diabetes
Due to drug or chemical (secondary diabetes)	Elevated glucose is caused by a medication or chemical.	Treat underlying cause if possible. Manage with diet, exercise, medication, and insulin, as needed.	Less than 5% of all diagnosed cases of diabetes
Other specified diabetes (secondary diabetes)	Elevated glucose is caused by another external factor, such as surgery or genetic defect in beta-cell function or insulin action.	Treat underlying cause if possible. Manage with diet, exercise, medication, and insulin, as needed.	Less than 5% of all diagnosed cases of diabetes
Gestational diabetes mellitus (GDM)	Elevated glucose is diagnosed during pregnancy in women with no history of diabetes. (*Note:* Gestational diabetes is coded with pregnancy conditions, rather than the endocrine system.)	Must control the condition quickly to prevent adverse effects on baby. Manage with diet, exercise, and sometimes insulin.	2–10% of pregnant women; using recently updated diagnostic criteria, the rate is expected to increase to 18% of pregnancies

- **Hyperosmolarity hyperglycemic nonketotic syndrome (HHNS)** is elevated glucose without ketoacidosis, usually occurring in elderly type 2 diabetics with other conditions, and can result in hyperosmolar coma and death.
- **Hypoglycemia** is abnormally low blood glucose, often due to excessive use of insulin or other glucose-lowering medications. Symptoms are dizziness, confusion, weakness, tremors, seizures, coma, and brain death.

Chronic complications of diabetes can affect nearly every organ system. The most frequent organ systems affected are:

- Eye (cataracts, blindness)
- Urinary (nephropathy, kidney failure)
- Nervous (neuropathy)
- Circulatory (gangrene, stroke, hypertension, peripheral artery disease [PAD])

SUCCESS STEP

Diabetes mellitus literally means "sweet urine disease." The word *diabetes* is based on the Greek word meaning "siphon." Aretaeus the Cappadocian, a second-century physician, described patients as having polyuria and passing water like a siphon. In 1675, Thomas Willis, the father of modern neuroscience, added *mellitus* because *mel* is the Latin word for "honey" or "sweetness."

Thyroid Disorders

The thyroid is a butterfly-shaped gland in front of the **trachea** (*windpipe*) that produces two hormones, tri-iodothyronine (T3) and thyroxine (T4), that regulate how the body breaks down food and uses or stores energy. ■ TABLE 9-4 summarizes the most common thyroid disorders with which coders need to be familiar.

Table 9-4 ■ COMMON THYROID DISORDERS

Condition	Description	Treatment
Graves' disease (diffuse toxic goiter)	Overproduction by the thyroid gland due to an autoimmune condition in which autoantibodies are directed against the thyroid-stimulating hormone (TSH) receptor.	Disable the thyroid gland's ability to produce hormones through radioactive iodine and/or antithyroid drugs, beta-blockers, thyroidectomy
Hyperthyroidism	Inappropriately elevated thyroid function.	Antithyroid medications (methimazole and propylthiouracil [PTU])
Hypothyroidism	Deficiency of thyroid hormone, usually due to lack of production of the hormone by the thyroid or inadequate secretion of hormones by the pituitary gland or hypothalamus.	Administer supplemental TSH and thyroxine (T4)
Nontoxic goiter	Enlargement of the thyroid that is not associated with overproduction of thyroid hormone or malignancy.	Supplemental thyroid hormone, thyroidectomy
Thyrotoxicosis (thyroid storm)	Excessive quantities of circulating thyroid hormone due to overproduction by the thyroid gland, overproduction originating outside the thyroid, or loss of storage function and leakage from the gland.	Cardiac monitor, supplemental oxygen, aggressive hydration, cooling measures, electrolyte replacement, antithyroid medications

CODING PRACTICE

Exercise 9.1   Endocrine System Refresher

Instructions: Use your medical terminology skills and resources to define the following terms related to the endocrine system, then assign the diagnosis code.

Follow these steps:

- Use slash marks "/" to break down each term into its root(s) and suffix.
- Define the meaning of the word, based on the meaning of each word part.
- Assign the default ICD-10-CM diagnosis code for the condition using the Index and Tabular List.

(continued)

CODING PRACTICE (continued)

Example: hyperthyroidism hyper/thyroid/ism   Meaning _pertaining to excessive thyroid_   ICD-10-CM Code _E05.90_

1. thyrotoxicosis — Meaning _____ — ICD-10-CM Code _____
2. adrenalitis — Meaning _____ — ICD-10-CM Code _____
3. thyromegaly — Meaning _____ — ICD-10-CM Code _____
4. thyroiditis — Meaning _____ — ICD-10-CM Code _____
5. hyperinsulinism — Meaning _____ — ICD-10-CM Code _____
6. hyperlipidemia — Meaning _____ — ICD-10-CM Code _____
7. panhypopituitarism — Meaning _____ — ICD-10-CM Code _____
8. parathyroid tetany — Meaning _____ — ICD-10-CM Code _____
9. hypoparathyroidism — Meaning _____ — ICD-10-CM Code _____
10. acromegaly — Meaning _____ — ICD-10-CM Code _____

CODING GUIDELINES FOR THE ENDOCRINE SYSTEM

Coders should understand the organization of this ICD-10-CM chapter, chapter-wide and commonly used instructional notes in the Tabular List, and the relevant OGCR. This information is necessary for accurate coding. ICD-10-CM Chapter 4, "Endocrine, Nutritional, and Metabolic Diseases (E00-E89)," contains 10 blocks or subchapters that are divided by anatomical site and type of disorder. Review the block names and code ranges listed at the beginning of Chapter 4 in the ICD-10-CM manual to become familiar with the content and organization.

Diabetes mellitus occupies five categories divided by etiology:

- Diabetes due to an underlying condition
- Drug or chemical-induced diabetes
- Type 1 diabetes
- Type 2 diabetes
- Other specified diabetes

Combination codes identify the type of diabetes and manifestations, reducing the need for multiple coding of this common condition.

In addition to the most common conditions of diabetes and thyroid disorders, this ICD-10-CM chapter also classifies other endocrine system conditions, including:

- Dysfunction of other endocrine glands, such as adrenal, pituitary, and parathyroid
- Endocrine-related disorders of glands that serve multiple systems, such as the pancreas, ovaries, and testes
- Nutritional disorders, such as malnutrition and deficiencies of specific vitamins and nutrients
- Obesity
- Disorders of metabolism, such as electrolyte imbalances and the body's inability to properly utilize sugar, fat, or copper

ICD-10-CM provides Official Guidelines for Coding and Reporting (OGCR) for endocrine, nutritional, and metabolic diseases in OGCR section I.C.4. OGCR provides detailed guidance regarding assigning and sequencing codes for diabetes mellitus and secondary diabetes mellitus. Specific OGCR are discussed and cited throughout this chapter.

ABSTRACTING FOR ENDOCRINE SYSTEM CONDITIONS

To abstract diagnoses for endocrine system conditions, coders must distinguish between integral symptoms and signs as opposed to the conditions, complications, and manifestations.

Keep in mind that any diagnosis must be documented by the physician; do not assign a diagnosis based only on test results. Physicians consider a variety of factors, in addition to test results, to establish a diagnosis. They may evaluate a trend of test results over a period of time, order other tests or imaging, or receive an evaluation from a specialist. For example, a patient may have a test result of hyperglycemia but not be diagnosed as diabetic until the result recurs several times over a period of months and additional tests, such as **HbA1c** (_a blood test that measures glucose attached to hemoglobin_) or a glucose tolerance test (GTT), are evaluated. Abstracting for diabetes mellitus (■ TABLE 9-5, page 148) and thyroid disorders (■ TABLE 9-6, page 148) is discussed next.

Abstracting for Diabetes Mellitus

When coders learn how to accurately abstract for diabetes mellitus, they learn detailed skills that serve them well when abstracting many other conditions as well. Diabetes is a commonly coded condition because patients with diabetes tend to have complications necessitating frequent medical care. Table 9-5 (page 148) lists key criteria for abstracting diabetes. Remember that abstracting questions are a general guide and that not all questions apply to every case. For example, not every patient has both acute and chronic complications.

Coders must identify the type of diabetes as type 1, type 2, secondary, or gestational diabetes because each uses different

Table 9-5 ■ KEY CRITERIA FOR ABSTRACTING DIABETES MELLITUS

- ❏ What type of diabetes is documented?
- ❏ Are coexisting conditions documented as related to diabetes?
- ❏ What acute complications are documented?
- ❏ What chronic complications are documented?
- ❏ If secondary DM is documented, what is the cause?
- ❏ If either type 2 or secondary DM is documented, is insulin used on a long-term basis?
- ❏ Is a family history of DM documented?
- ❏ Which problem or complication is the reason for the encounter?

codes. Secondary diabetes must be identified as due to an underlying condition or a drug or chemical. Gestational diabetes is coded from ICD-10-CM Chapter 15, "Pregnancy, Childbirth, and the Puerperium," rather the endocrine system chapter.

Abstracting for Causality

When complications and/or multiple conditions are present, coders must identify whether there is a **causal relationship** (*one disease being caused by another*). The specific words the physician uses in documentation indicate whether and the organization of the Index direct coder. For example, neuropathy may be a complication of diabetes or may be unrelated.

When physicians document *diabetic neuropathy*, where *diabetic* is a modifier of neuropathy, they confirm that the neuropathy is *caused by* diabetes and it is coded as such. Similarly, physicians document a condition with the use of *secondary to*, *due to*, *with*, or *in*, when they are indicating causality. When physicians state that the neuropathy is *unrelated* to diabetes, they are denying a causal relationship and the conditions are coded separately.

If causality is not specifically confirmed or denied by the documentation, the Index provides guidance. OGCR I.A.15 states that when two conditions are linked by the word **with** in the Index, they should be coded as related, unless the physician has specifically documented that they are not related. The entry **with** appears immediately under the Main Term for the condition in the Index rather than in alphabetical order, as shown in the first few rows of ■ FIGURE 9-2. This OGCR applies for all conditions and is especially important when coding diabetes, because this condition causes many complications.

These distinctions are critical when assigning codes. Conditions that arise due to diabetes are usually assigned a combination code describing both conditions. Conditions that are unrelated are assigned separate codes. Refer to ■ TABLE 9-7 (page 150) for examples of how physicians document related and unrelated conditions and how they are coded differently.

Some conditions bear such a strong relationship with diabetes, they are always documented as caused by it, unless explicitly denied by the physician. For example, age-related cataracts occur in most people and are not specifically caused by diabetes. However, research has shown that diabetes causes age-related cataracts to develop earlier and progress faster than in nondiabetic patients, so a causal relationship is always coded unless the physician specifically states they are unrelated (*Coding Clinic* 4Q 2016).

Abstracting for Thyroid Disorders

When abstracting for thyroid disorders, coders must identify the cause of the condition and whether goiter or thyrotoxicosis is documented. The presence of these complications affects code assignment. Some thyroid conditions are congenital, so this information should also be noted. Table 9-7 lists key criteria for abstracting thyroid disorders.

Guided Example of Abstracting Diagnoses for the Endocrine System

Refer to the following example throughout the chapter to practice skills for abstracting and assigning codes for the endocrine system. Tamara Brownlee, CCS-P, is a fictitious coder who guides you through the coding process.

Date: 10/1/yy Location: Branton Medical Center

Provider: Ann Trull, MD

Patient: Justin Kraft Gender: M Age: 12

Reason for admission: Hyperglycemia, ketoacidosis, glycosuria, family history (mother and grandmother) of type 1 diabetes

Tests: Glucose tolerance test (GTT) positive for diabetes. Abdominal x-ray and CT of pancreas are normal.

Discharge diagnosis: New-onset type 1 diabetes

Discharge plan: Insulin injections bid (twice a day), FU office 2 weeks

---

Follow along in your ICD-10-CM manual as Tamara Brownlee, CCS-P, abstracts the diagnosis. Check off each step after you complete it.

▶ Tamara reads the entire medical record and refers to Key Criteria for Abstracting Diabetes Mellitus (Table 9-5).

- ❏ *What type of diabetes is documented?* New-onset type 1 diabetes

- ❏ *Are coexisting conditions documented as related to diabetes?* Tamara notes the symptoms documented under the reason for admission. She identifies that hyperglycemia and glycosuria are integral to type 1 diabetes and should not be coded in addition to the disease (OGCR II.A).

- ❏ *What acute complications are documented?* She identifies that ketoacidosis is an acute complication that should be coded in addition to type 1 diabetes

Table 9-6 ■ KEY CRITERIA FOR ABSTRACTING THYROID DISORDERS

- ❏ Is the condition hyperthyroidism or hypothyroidism?
- ❏ What is the cause of the condition?
- ❏ Is the condition congenital?
- ❏ Is goiter documented?
- ❏ Is thyrotoxicosis crisis documented?

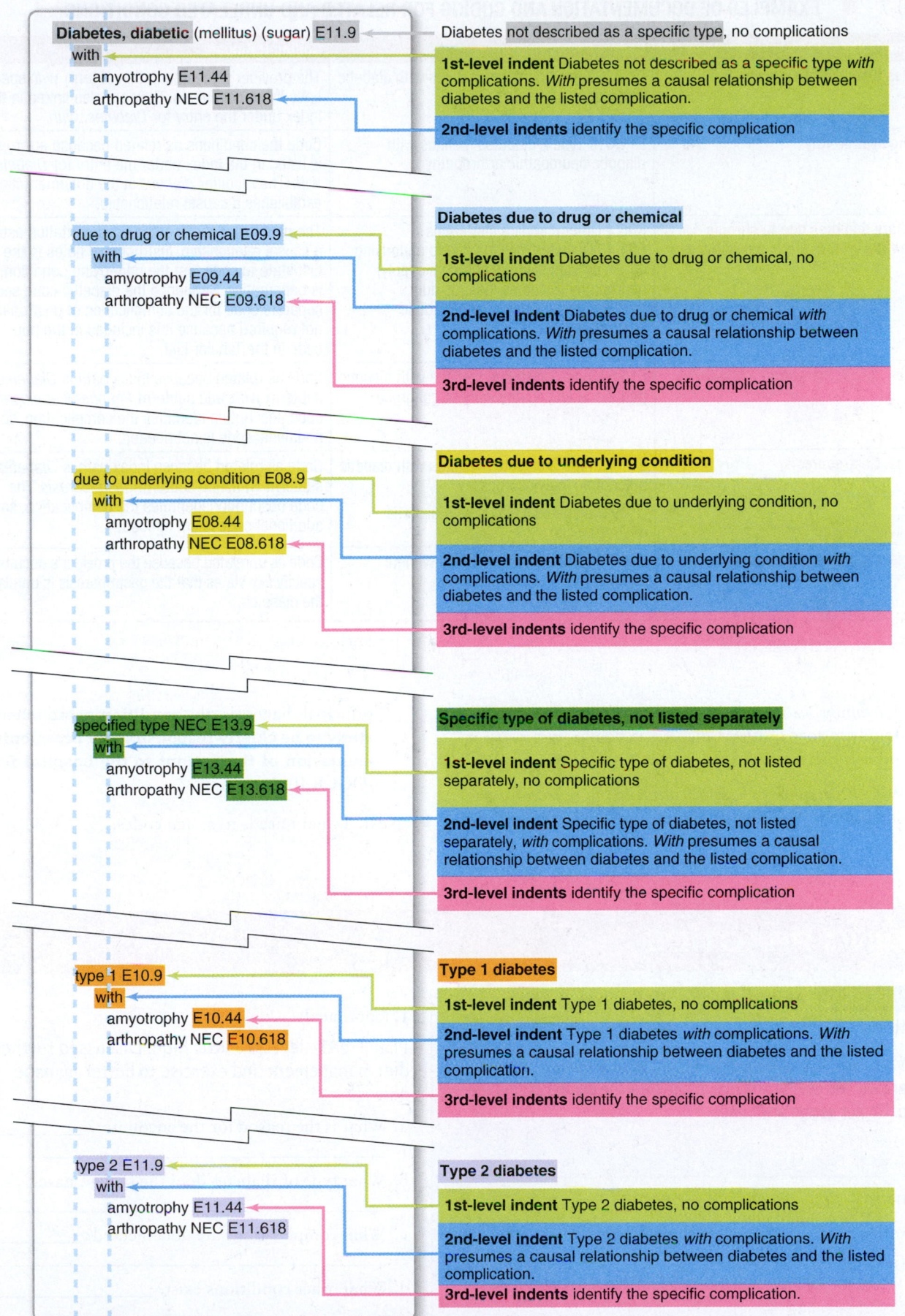

Figure 9-2 ■ Index entry for "Diabetes" showing use of "*with*" and the structure of subterms.

Table 9-7 ■ **EXAMPLES OF DOCUMENTATION AND CODING FOR RELATED AND UNRELATED CONDITIONS**

Documentation	Code	Coding Rationale
Diabetes type 1 with cataract	E10.36 Type 1 diabetes mellitus with diabetic cataract	The provider's documentation of term *with* specifically links these conditions. They are also linked in the Index under the entry for *Diabetes, with.*
Diabetic arthropathy	E11.610 Type 2 diabetes mellitus with diabetic neuropathic arthropathy	Code the conditions as related because arthropathy is listed in the Index under the entry for *Diabetes, with.* The modifier *diabetic* in the documentation also establishes a causal relationship.
Secondary diabetes due to chronic pancreatitis with diabetic gastroparesis	K86.1 Other chronic pancreatitis E08.43 Diabetes mellitus due to underlying condition with diabetic autonomic (poly) neuropathy (Diabetes mellitus due to underlying condition with diabetic gastroparesis)	The modifier *diabetic* in the documentation establishes a causal relationship. Instructional notes in the Tabular List state to code first the underlying condition, which is pancreatitis. Sequence the diabetes code second. A separate code for the complication of gastroparesis is not required because it is included in the notes for the code in the Tabular List.
Diabetes type 1. Peripheral angiopathy.	E10.51 Type 1 diabetes mellitus with diabetic peripheral angiopathy without gangrene	Code as related because Index path is *Diabetes,* subterm *with,* and subterm *Peripheral angiopathy.* The code description identifies the complication, so an additional code is not needed.
Diabetes. Gastroparesis.	E11.43 Type 2 diabetes mellitus with diabetic autonomic (poly)neuropathy. (Type 2 diabetes mellitus with diabetic gastroparesis)	Code as related because Index path is *Diabetes,* subterm *with,* and subterm *gastroparesis.* The code description identifies the complication, so an additional code is not needed.
Diabetes. Unrelated gastroparesis.	E11.9 Type 2 diabetes mellitus without complications K31.84 Gastroparesis	Code as unrelated because the provider's documentation specifically states that the gastroparesis is unrelated to the diabetes.

❏ *Is a family history of DM documented?* She identifies that family history of type 1 diabetes is significant because it poses a risk factor for the patient (OGCR I.C.21.c.4))

❏ *Which problem or complication is the reason for the encounter?* She identifies that type 1 diabetes is the principal diagnosis, the **condition established after study to be chiefly responsible for occasioning the admission of the patient to the hospital for care** (OGCR II)

▶ Next, Tamara needs to assign codes.

CODING PRACTICE

Exercise 9.2   **Abstracting for Endocrine System Conditions**

Instructions: Read the mini-medical-record of each patient's encounter and answer the abstracting questions. Write the answer on the line provided. Do not assign any codes.

1. OFFICE   Gender: M   Age: 56

Reason for encounter: Monitoring of diabetes

Assessment: Type 2 diabetes

(continued)

1. (continued)

Plan: HbA1c level is a little high. Discussed further diet management and exercise to better manage glucose

a. What is the reason for the encounter? _____

_____

b. What type of diabetes does the patient have?

_____

c. What complications are documented? _____

_____

d. What other conditions exist? _____

_____

(continued)

CODING PRACTICE (continued)

2. INPATIENT HOSPITAL   Gender: M   Age: 57

Reason for admission: Cold clammy skin and pallor, rapid breathing & heart rate

Assessment: Hypovolemia

Plan: FU 1 wk

a. What is the reason for the admission? _____
_____

b. What condition(s) is diagnosed? _____
_____

c. What diagnosis(es) should be coded? _____
Why? _____

3. INPATIENT HOSPITAL   Gender: F   Age: 38

Reason for admission: Patient with known hyperthyroidism is admitted for thyroid storm, with fever, tachycardia, hypertension

Assessment: Thyrotoxicosis with thyrotoxic crisis

Plan: Cardiac monitoring, aggressive hydration, electrolyte replacement, antithyroid medications

a. Is the condition hyperthyroidism or hypothyroidism?
_____

b. What is the cause of the condition? _____
_____

c. Is the condition congenital? _____

d. Is goiter documented? _____

e. Is thyrotoxicosis crisis documented? _____
_____

f. Should the symptoms be coded? _____

4. INPATIENT HOSPITAL   Gender: F   Age: 36

Reason for admission: Insulin-induced hypoglycemia

Assessment: Patient has chronic pancreatitis for 2 years with secondary diabetes. Patient has struggled to monitor and self-administer insulin correctly.

Plan: Prescribe insulin pump. FU in office.

a. What is the reason for the encounter? _____
_____

b. What type of diabetes does the patient have?
_____

c. What complications are documented? _____
_____

d. What other conditions exist? _____
_____

(continued)

4. (continued)

e. Should long-term use of insulin be coded? Why or why not? _____

f. What Main Term should you look under in the Index to locate long-term use of insulin? _____
_____

g. What is the principal diagnosis? _____
Why? _____

5. OFFICE   Gender: F   Age: 65

Reason for encounter: Management of longstanding neuropathy

Assessment: Peripheral autonomic neuropathy, unrelated to type 2 diabetes

Plan: FU 6 months

a. What is the reason for the encounter? _____
_____

b. What type of diabetes does the patient have?
_____

c. Is the neuropathy related to the diabetes?
_____
Why or why not? _____

d. What is the first-listed diagnosis? _____

e. What is the additional diagnosis? _____

6. OFFICE   Gender: M   Age: 25

Reason for encounter: Follow up on test results after evaluation of proximal muscle weakness, easy bruising, weight gain

Assessment: Endogenous Cushing's syndrome due to pituitary adenoma

Plan: Evaluate for surgery to remove tumor

a. What is the reason for the encounter? _____
_____

b. What are the symptoms? _____
_____

c. Should the symptoms be coded? _____
Why or why not? _____

d. Is the adenoma malignant or benign? _____
Why? _____

e. What is the first-listed diagnosis? _____

f. What is the cause of the first-listed diagnosis?
_____

g. What is the additional diagnosis? _____

ASSIGNING CODES FOR ENDOCRINE SYSTEM CONDITIONS

When assigning codes for the endocrine system, carefully review the information abstracted from the medical record and determine whether the condition is the primary condition or the result of a disease or condition in another body system. This information will affect what codes to assign and how to sequence them. Special attention to the Index is required. Diabetes is used as an example of assigning codes to endocrine system disorders.

Because diabetes has many variations and complications, coders must be especially careful to follow indented subterms in the Index. The Main Term **Diabetes** has only a few first-level subterm entries, each of which have second- and third-level indented subterms that are used as follows:

- First-level subterms identify the type of diabetes.
- Second-level subterms identify that complications are present through the word **with**.
- Third-level subterms identify the specific complication(s) with each type of diabetes.

The exception is when the type of diabetes is not specified. In this case, the complications are listed directly under the Main Term entry, following the indented subterm **with**. Notice that these are the same codes as **Diabetes, type 2** because OGCR directs coders to assign **type 2 diabetes** when the specific type is not documented in the medical record (OGCR I.C.4.a.2)). When the type of diabetes is specified, search for the corresponding first-level subterm before locating the complication.

Refer again to Figure 9-2 for an abbreviated view of the Index entry **Diabetes**. Selected subterms are shown. Review the first-level subterms and notice that each identifies a different type of diabetes, such as **due to drug or chemical** or **due to underlying condition**. All first-level subterms have the same second- and third-level subterms, such as **amyotrophy** and **arthropathy**. Each instance of **amyotrophy** and **arthropathy** has a different code because it is a combination code of the manifestation *and* the type of diabetes under which it is indented.

Selecting the correct first-level subterm is critical in order to arrive at the correct code because each type of diabetes can have similar complications. Consequently, the same second- and third-level indented terms for complications appear under first-level Index entries for each type of diabetes, but with different codes, because the type of diabetes is different.

Guided Example of Assigning Endocrine System Diagnosis Codes

Continue with the example from earlier in the chapter about patient Justin Kraft, who was admitted to Branton Medical Center due to new onset of type 1 diabetes, to practice skills for assigning codes.

Follow along in your ICD-10-CM manual as Tamara Brownlee, CCS-P, assigns codes. Check off each step after you complete it.

▶ First, Tamara confirms that type 1 diabetes is the principal diagnosis. Diabetic ketoacidosis (DKA) and family history of diabetes are additional diagnoses.

▶ Tamara searches the Index for the Main Term **Diabetes**.

❑ She locates the subterm **type 1**.

❑ She reviews the subterms and locates **ketoacidosis**. She determines that the complication of DKA is a combination code with **type 1 diabetes** and she will not need an additional code for ketoacidosis.

❑ She notes that **ketoacidosis** has a further subterm for **with coma**, and verifies in the medical record that coma is *not* documented.

❑ She makes a note of the code to verify, **E10.10**.

▶ Tamara verifies code **E10.10** in the Tabular List.

❑ She reads the code title for **E10.10, Type 1 diabetes mellitus with ketoacidosis without coma** and confirms that this accurately describes the principal diagnosis.

▶ Tamara checks for instructional notes in the Tabular List.

❑ Tamara cross-references the beginning of category **E10** and verifies that there are no instructional notes.

❑ She cross-references the beginning of the block **Diabetes mellitus (E08-E13)** and verifies that there are no instructional notes that apply to all codes in the block. The instructional notes under **E08** apply only to codes in that category.

❑ She cross-references the beginning of **Chapter 4 (E00-E89)** and reviews the **NOTE:**. She determines that it does not apply to this case because the patient's diabetes is not related to another condition.

▶ Tamara assigns the principal diagnosis **E10.10, Type 1 diabetes mellitus with ketoacidosis without coma**.

▶ Next, Tamara assigns the code for family history of diabetes.

❑ She locates the Main Term **History** in the Index.

❑ She locates the indented subterm **family**.

❑ She locates the second-level indented subterm **diabetes mellitus**, which has the code **Z83.3**.

❑ Tamara verifies the code **Z83.3** in the Tabular List.

❑ She confirms the code title, **Family history of diabetes mellitus**.

❑ She cross-references the beginning of the category, **Z83**; block, **Z77-Z99**; and **Chapter 21 (Z00-Z99)** for instructional notes.

▶ Tamara reviews the codes for this case:

❑ **E10.10 Type 1 diabetes mellitus with ketoacidosis without coma**

❑ **Z83.3 Family history of diabetes mellitus**

▶ Next, Tamara will arrange (sequence) the codes.

CODING PRACTICE

Exercise 9.3 Assigning Codes for Endocrine System Conditions

Instructions: Read the mini-medical-record of each patient's encounter, review the information abstracted in Exercise 9.2, and assign ICD-10-CM diagnosis codes using the Index and Tabular List. Write the code(s) on the line provided.

---

1. OFFICE Gender: M Age: 56

Reason for encounter: Monitoring of diabetes

Assessment: Type 2 diabetes

Plan: HbA1c level is a little high. Discussed further diet management and exercise to better manage glucose.

1 ICD-10-CM Code _____

---

2. INPATIENT HOSPITAL Gender: M Age: 57

Reason for admission: Cold clammy skin and pallor, rapid breathing & heart rate

Assessment: Hypovolemia

Plan: FU 1 wk

1 ICD-10-CM Code _____

---

3. INPATIENT HOSPITAL Gender: F Age: 38

Reason for admission: Patient with known hyperthyroidism is admitted for thyroid storm, with fever, tachycardia, hypertension

Assessment: Thyrotoxicosis with thyrotoxic crisis due to overproduction of thyroid stimulating hormone

Plan: Cardiac monitoring, aggressive hydration, electrolyte replacement, antithyroid medications

1 ICD-10-CM Code _____

ARRANGING CODES FOR ENDOCRINE SYSTEM CONDITIONS

Multiple coding is required throughout the endocrine system as directed by instructional notes in the Tabular List and conventions in the Index to Diseases and Injuries. When multiple coding is required, there is not one simple rule that dictates sequencing. Refer to OGCR and instructional notes in the Tabular List to determine proper sequencing. Diabetes is used for several examples of multiple coding rules because of its complexity, but the guidelines apply to all conditions. Other examples of multiple coding and sequencing are also provided.

Multiple Coding for Diabetes

Multiple coding is required for diabetes to report the following circumstances:

- Patients with unrelated conditions in addition to diabetes
- Patients with more than one diabetic complication
- Additional details about a complication
- Long-term use of insulin with type 2 or secondary diabetes
- Complications due to missing a dose of insulin
- Complications due to the malfunction of an insulin pump
- Any combination of these situations

Examples of coding and sequencing for each of these situations follow.

Multiple Codes Due to Unrelated Conditions

Multiple codes are required when patients have coexisting conditions that are not related to or caused by diabetes, as shown previously in Table 9-6. Sequence the codes according to the documented reason for the encounter. When the encounter is for treatment or management of diabetes, sequence the diabetes code first (■ FIGURE 9-3). When the encounter is for treatment or management of an unrelated condition, sequence that code first (■ FIGURE 9-4, page 154).

Multiple Codes from a Single Diabetes Category

Patients often have more than one complication related to diabetes. Assign as many codes from an ICD-10-CM Chapter 4 category as necessary to describe all documented complications (OGCR I.C.4.a). Sequence the codes according to the reason for the encounter (■ FIGURE 9-5, page 154).

Multiple Coding for Complications

Although all diabetic complications are assigned combination codes from the block **Diabetes mellitus (E00-E13)**, some complications also require codes from other body system chapters to provide additional details. Instructional notes at the beginning of the three-digit category direct the coder and include:

- Code first the underlying condition for secondary diabetes.
- Code first the drug or chemical causing secondary diabetes.
- Use an additional code to identify the stage of chronic kidney disease.

Patient with type 2 diabetes and unrelated peripheral neuropathy sees an endocrinologist for management of diabetes.

(1) **E11.9 Type 2 diabetes mellitus** without complications
(2) **G62.9 Polyneuropathy, unspecified**

Figure 9-3 ■ Example of sequencing when diabetes is the reason for the encounter.

Patient with type 2 diabetes sees a neurologist for management of unrelated peripheral neuropathy.

(1) **G62.9 Polyneuropathy, unspecified**
(2) **E11.9 Type 2 diabetes mellitus without complications**

Figure 9-4 ■ Example of sequencing when an unrelated condition is the reason for the encounter.

Patient sees an ophthalmologist for diabetic cataracts and also has diabetic neuropathic arthropathy.

(1) **E11.36 Type 2 diabetes mellitus with diabetic cataract**
(2) **E11.40 Type 2 diabetes mellitus with diabetic neuropathy, unspecified**

Figure 9-5 ■ Example of sequencing multiple codes from a single diabetes category.

Patient sees an endocrinologist for management of secondary diabetes due to chronic pancreatitis.

Code first the underlying condition
(1) **K86.1 Other chronic pancreatitis**
(2) **E08.9 Diabetes mellitus due to underlying condition without complications**

Figure 9-6 ■ Example of sequencing the underlying condition.

Patient with type 1 diabetes sees wound care for a diabetic foot ulcer with muscle necrosis on the heel of the left foot.

(1) **E10.621 Type 1 diabetes mellitus with foot ulcer**
Use additional code to identify site of ulcer (L97.4-, L97.5-)
(2) **L97.423 Non-pressure chronic ulcer of left heel and midfoot with necrosis of muscle**

Figure 9-7 ■ Example of sequencing details of a complication.

- Use an additional code to identify the site of skin ulcer.
- Use an additional code to identify a complication not listed.

When a patient has secondary diabetes, sequence the underlying cause first, such as the underlying condition or the drug causing the diabetic reaction. Sequence the code for secondary diabetes as an additional code (OGCR I.C.4.a.6)(b)). The instructional note in the Tabular List indicates this with the words **Code first underlying condition** or **Code first drug or chemical** (■ FIGURE 9-6).

When assigning multiple codes to describe additional details about a complication, sequence the code for diabetes first and the additional codes for the details about the complication second. The instructional note in the Tabular List indicates this with the words **Use additional code to identify** (■ FIGURE 9-7).

Multiple Coding for Long-term Use of Insulin

Multiple coding is required to identify long-term insulin use by type 2 diabetics and patients with secondary diabetes. Instructional notes in the Tabular List direct coders to use **Z79.4 Long term (current) use of insulin** to identify long-term insulin use by these patients. Do not assign this code if insulin is given temporarily to bring a type 2 patient's blood glucose under control during an encounter (OGCR I.C.4.a.3)) and (OGCR I.C.4.a.6)(a)). Sequence the diabetes code first and the **Z** code second (■ FIGURE 9-8). **Z79.4** is not required and should not be reported with a diagnosis of type 1 diabetes because all type 1 diabetics must use insulin.

Multiple Coding for Complications Due to Missed Medication Dose

A patient may experience complications if a dose of insulin or oral hypoglycemic drugs is missed. When a diabetic patient has a complication because of missing a dose, multiple codes are needed (OGCR I.C.21.e.5)(c)) (■ FIGURE 9-9):

1. Assign a code to identify the complication (manifestation).
2. Assign a code from the **Underdosing** column of the Table of Drugs and Chemicals to report that an underdoing

occurred. Assign a seventh character to identify the episode of care. Underdosing codes should never be sequenced as the principal or first-listed diagnosis.

3. Assign a code for the reason (intent) for underdosing, if known, such as noncompliance (**Z91.12- Patient's intentional underdosing of medication regimen** or **Z91.13- Patient's unintentional underdosing of medication regimen**) or a complication of care (**Y63.6** through **Y63.9**), which includes the failure of medical personnel to administer the medication. To locate noncompliance Z codes in the Index, search for the Main Term **Noncompliance** or **Underdosing**. When underdosing is an error by medical personnel, search the Index of External Causes for the Main Term **Misadventure to patient during medical or surgical care**, **Nonadministration**, or **Underdosing**.

Be aware that **Underdosing** appears in three places with three different purposes:

- In the Table of Drugs and Chemicals, the **Underdosing** column identifies the drug and nature of the harm done.
- In the alphabetical Index, the Main Term **Underdosing** identifies patient reasons for missing medication dose(s).
- In the Index of External Causes, the Main Term **Underdosing** identifies external events related to the underdosing.

Patient with type 2 diabetes and diabetic nephropathy sees a nephrologist for management of kidney disease. Patient uses insulin to manage the diabetes.

Use additional code to identify control using insulin (Z79.4)
(1) **E11.21 Type 2 diabetes mellitus with diabetic nephropathy**
(2) **Z79.4 Long term (current) use of insulin**

Figure 9-8 ■ Example of sequencing the code for the long-term use of insulin.

Patient with type 2 diabetes is diagnosed with hyperosmolarity without nonketotic hyperglycemic-hyperosmolar coma (NKHHC). Patient has missed several doses of repaglinide because she is low income and is waiting for funds to get the prescription refilled.

(1) **E11.00 Type 2 diabetes mellitus with hyperosmolarity without nonketotic hyperglycemic-hyperosmolar coma (NKHHC)**

(2) **T38.3X6A Underdosing of insulin and oral hypoglycemic [antidiabetic] drugs, Initial encounter**

(3) **Z91.120 Patient's intentional underdosing of medication regimen due to financial hardship**

Figure 9-9 ■ Example of sequencing the code for a missed medication dose.

Multiple Coding for Complications Due to Insulin Pump Malfunction

Diabetic patients may wear an insulin pump to regulate insulin evenly and eliminate self-administering injections. Underdosing or overdosing of insulin due to insulin pump failure is reported with one of two codes from ICD-10-CM Chapter 19, "Injury, Poisoning and Certain Other Consequences of External Causes (S00-T88)," to describe the pump failure and the resulting problem (OGCR I.C.4.a.5)). Also assign codes for the type of diabetes and any related complications (■ FIGURE 9-10).

Multiple Conditions with Multiple Codes

Because diabetes is such a complicated disease, it is not uncommon for coders to encounter cases where several multiple coding situations must be addressed at the same time (■ FIGURE 9-11).

Multiple Coding for Other Endocrine System Conditions

Coders must always be alert for instructional notes in the Tabular List that direct them to assign more than one code. Remember to refer to the beginning of the category and block for instructions when assigning codes from the endocrine system. Common situations in this chapter include the following examples and instructional notes.

1. Assign applicable codes from ICD-10-CM Chapter 4 for complications related to neoplasms or other conditions.
   EXAMPLE: *A patient is treated for functional hyperinsulinism islet cell adenoma of the pancreas.*

   (1) **D13.7 Benign neoplasm of endocrine pancreas**

   (2) **E16.1 Other hypoglycemia**

Patient has diabetes due to pituitary-dependent Cushing's disease and uses insulin to manage her diabetes. Patient is seen today for foot ulcer on right great toe with skin breakdown.

(1) **E24.0 Pituitary-dependent Cushing's disease**

(2) **E08.621 Secondary diabetes mellitus with foot ulcer**

(3) **L97.511 Non-pressure chronic ulcer of other part of right foot limited to breakdown of skin**

(4) **Z79.4 Long term (current) use of insulin**

Figure 9-11 ■ Example of sequencing multiple conditions with multiple codes.

Instructional note at beginning of Chapter 4 E00- E99: All neoplasms, whether functionally active or not, are classified in Chapter 2. Appropriate codes in this chapter (i.e. E05.8, E07.0, E16-E31, E34.-) may be used as additional codes to indicate either functional activity by neoplasms and ectopic endocrine tissue or hyperfunction and hypofunction of endocrine glands associated with neoplasms and other conditions classified elsewhere.

Instructional note under code D13.7: Use additional code to identify any functional activity.

2. Sequence codes from this chapter as additional codes when they are a manifestation of a disease in a different body system.

Patient is seen in the emergency department for ketoacidosis due to the failure of her insulin pump and underdosing. She has type 1 diabetes and moderate bilateral nonproliferative diabetic retinopathy.

(1) **T85.614A Breakdown (mechanical) of insulin pump, initial encounter**
(2) **T38.3X6A Underdosing of insulin and oral hypoglycemic [antidiabetic] drugs, initial encounter**
(3) **E10.10 Type 1 diabetes mellitus with ketoacidosis without coma**
(4) **E10.3393 Type 1 diabetes mellitus with moderate nonproliferative diabetic retinopathy without macular edema, bilateral**

Figure 9-10 ■ Example of sequencing complications from insulin pump failure.

EXAMPLE: *A patient is seen for Dubois thymus due to late congenital syphilis.*

(1) **A50.59 Other late congenital syphilis, symptomatic**

(2) **E35 Disorders of endocrine glands in diseases classified elsewhere**

Instructional note under category E35: Code first underlying disease, such as:

late congenital syphilis of thymus gland [Dubois disease] (A50.5)

3. Assign an additional code to identify the infectious agent in acute infections.

EXAMPLE: *A patient is seen for acute thyroiditis due to Methicillin susceptible Staphylococcus aureus.*

(1) **E06.0 Acute thyroiditis**

(2) **B95.61 Methicillin susceptible Staphylococcus aureus infection as the cause of diseases classified elsewhere**

Instructional note under code E06.0: Use additional code (B95-B97) to identify infectious agent.

4. Assign an additional code to identify intellectual disabilities associated with congenital conditions.

EXAMPLE: *A patient with moderate intellectual disabilities is seen for congenital iodine-deficiency syndrome.*

(1) **E00.2 Congenital iodine-deficiency syndrome, mixed type**

(2) **F71 Moderate intellectual disabilities**

Instructional note under category E00: Use additional code (F70-F79) to identify associated intellectual disabilities.

5. Assign a code for body mass index (BMI), if known, with codes for obesity.

EXAMPLE: *A physician sees a morbidly obese adult patient with a BMI of 43.5 kg/m^2.*

(1) **E66.01 Morbid (severe) obesity due to excess calories**

(2) **Z68.41 Body mass index (BMI) 40.0-44.9, adult**

Instructional note under category E066: Use additional code to identify body mass index (BMI), if known (Z68.-)

6. Assign an additional code for the adverse effect of the drug after the drug-induced endocrine condition that resulted.

EXAMPLE: *A patient is seen for drug-induced thyroiditis due to an adverse effect of lithium.*

(1) **E06.4 Drug-induced thyroiditis**

(2) **T43.8X5A Adverse effect of other psychotropic drugs, initial encounter**

Instructional note under code E06.4: Code for adverse effect, if applicable, to identify drug (T36-T50 with fifth or sixth character 5)

Guided Example of Arranging Endocrine System Diagnosis Codes

To learn more about sequencing codes for the endocrine system, continue with the example about patient Justin Kraft, who was admitted to Branton Medical Center due to new onset of type 1 diabetes. Follow along as Tamara Brownlee, CCS-P, sequences the codes.

▶ Tamara reviews the codes for this case:

❑ **E10.10 Type 1 diabetes mellitus with ketoacidosis without coma**

❑ **Z83.3 Family history of diabetes mellitus**

▶ She identifies that type 1 diabetes is the principal diagnosis, the **condition established after study to be chiefly responsible for occasioning the admission of the patient to the hospital for care** (OGCR II).

❑ A code for family history of a disease is rarely a principal diagnosis.

▶ Tamara finalizes the codes and sequencing for this case.

(1) **E10.10 Type 1 diabetes mellitus with ketoacidosis without coma**

(2) **Z83.3 Family history of diabetes mellitus**

CODING PRACTICE

Exercise 9.4   Arranging Codes for Endocrine System Conditions

Instructions: Read the mini-medical-record of each patient's encounter, review the information abstracted in Exercise 9.2, assign ICD-10-CM diagnosis codes using the Index and Tabular List, and sequence them correctly.

---

1. INPATIENT HOSPITAL   Gender: F   Age: 36

Reason for admission: Insulin-induced hypoglycemia

Assessment: Patient has chronic pancreatitis for 2 years and associated diabetes. Patient has struggled to monitor and self-administer insulin correctly.

Plan: Prescribe insulin pump. FU in office.

Tip: Refer to OGCR for secondary diabetes.

3 ICD-10-CM Codes _____

_____

(continued)

CODING PRACTICE *(continued)*

2. OFFICE   Gender: F Age: 65

Reason for encounter: Management of longstanding neuropathy

Assessment: Peripheral autonomic neuropathy, unrelated type 2 diabetes

Plan: FU 6 months

Tip: The neuropathy is stated as unrelated to the type 2 diabetes.

2 ICD-10-CM Codes _____

3. OFFICE   Gender: M Age: 25

Reason for encounter: Follow up on test results after evaluation of proximal muscle weakness, easy bruising, weight gain

Assessment: Endogenous Cushing's syndrome due to pituitary adenoma

Plan: Evaluate for surgery to remove tumor.

Tip: An adenoma is benign, an adenocarcinoma is malignant.

2 ICD-10-CM Codes _____

CODING NEOPLASMS OF THE ENDOCRINE SYSTEM

Neoplasms of the endocrine system do not appear in ICD-10-CM Chapter 4, "Endocrine, Nutritional, and Metabolic Diseases (E00-E89)"; they appear in Chapter 2 (C00-D49). Codes for neoplasms of the endocrine system appear in the following blocks within the neoplasm chapter:

- C73-C75 Malignant neoplasm of thyroid and other endocrine glands
- C7A Malignant neuroendocrine tumors
- C7B Secondary neuroendocrine tumors
- D3A Benign neuroendocrine tumors

Review these blocks in the ICD-10-CM manual to become familiar with the content.

The most common sites for cancer in the endocrine system are the thyroid and pancreas. Thyroid cancer is the fifth most common cancer in women and accounts for 5% of new cancer cases, according to the American Cancer Society (ACS). Most types of thyroid cancer are treatable, and most patients are cured and have a normal life expectancy. The incidence rates of thyroid cancer in both women and men have been increasing in recent years, which researchers believe is the result of more sensitive detection methods, such as thyroid ultrasound. Pancreatic cancer accounts for 3% of new cancer cases but has a poor survival rate because it is usually not diagnosed until after it has metastasized widely and, therefore, is difficult to treat.

Codes for neoplasms of the ovaries and testes are classified with neoplasms of other reproductive organs.

CODING PRACTICE

Exercise 9.5 Coding Neoplasms of the Endocrine System

Instructions: Read the mini-medical-record of each patient's encounter, then abstract, assign, and sequence ICD-10-CM diagnosis codes using the Index and Tabular List. Write the code(s) on the line provided.

1. INPATIENT HOSPITAL   Gender: F Age: 35

Reason for encounter: Thyroidectomy

Assessment: Serous papillary carcinoma of the thyroid

Plan: Thyroid hormone replacement

1 ICD-10-CM Code _____

2. OFFICE   Gender: M   Age: 7

Reason for encounter: Follow up on a solitary nodule discovered during a routine check-up 10 days ago

Assessment: Follicular adenoma of the thyroid

Plan: Partial thyroidectomy

1 ICD-10-CM Code _____

3. OUTPATIENT HOSPITAL   Gender: M Age: 5

Chief complaint: Review x-ray and CT performed for dyspnea and cough

Assessment: Thymoma

Tip: According to Medscape, the most common location for mediastinal tumors in children is near the trachea, resulting in respiratory symptoms.

1 ICD-10-CM Code _____

(continued)

CODING PRACTICE (continued)

4. INPATIENT HOSPITAL Gender: M Age: 51

Reason for Admission: Surgical removal of carcinoid tumor

Diagnosis: Malignant carcinoid tumor of small intestine with carcinoid syndrome

Plan: FU in office

Tip: In the Index, look up **carcinoid** tumor, not cancer or carcinoma.

2 ICD-10-CM Codes _____

5. INPATIENT HOSPITAL Gender: F Age: 45

Reason for encounter: Chemotherapy

Assessment: Adenocarcinoma of pancreas with metastases to liver, lung, and colon

Tip: Review OGCR I.C.2.e.2) for coding and sequencing reminders.

5 ICD-10-CM Codes _____

_____

CHAPTER SUMMARY

In this chapter you learned the following:

- The function of the endocrine system is to produce, store, and release hormones, which are chemical messengers that regulate body functions including growth, development, metabolism, sexual function, reproduction, and mood.

- ICD-10-CM provides Official Guidelines for Coding and Reporting (OGCR) for endocrine, nutritional, and metabolic diseases in OGCR section I.C.4, which provides detailed guidance regarding assigning and sequencing codes for diabetes mellitus and secondary diabetes mellitus.

- When abstracting diabetes, identify the type of diabetes as type 1, type 2, secondary, or gestational diabetes because each uses different codes.

- When complications and/or multiple conditions are present, coders must identify whether there is a causal relationship.

- When abstracting for thyroid disorders, coders must identify the cause of the condition and whether goiter or thyrotoxicosis is documented.

- When assigning codes for the endocrine system, carefully review the information abstracted from the medical record and determine whether the condition is the primary condition or the result of a disease or condition in another body system.

- Multiple coding is required throughout the endocrine system as directed by instructional notes in the Tabular List and conventions in the Index to Diseases and Injuries.

- The most common sites for cancer in the endocrine system are the thyroid and pancreas.

CONCEPT QUIZ

Take a moment to look back through endocrine, nutritional, and metabolic diseases and solidify your skills. Try to answer the questions from memory first, then refer to the discussion in this chapter and the Glossary at the end of this book if you need a little extra help.

Completion

Instructions: Write the term that completes each statement based on the information you learned in this chapter. Choose from the following list. Some choices may be used more than once and some choices may not be used at all.

body mass index (BMI)

diabetic ketoacidosis (DKA)

Graves' disease

hyperglycemia

hyperosmolarity hyperglycemic nonketotic syndrome (HHNS)

hyperthyroidism

hypoglycemia

hypothalamus

hypothyroidism

metabolism

ovaries

pancreas

pituitary

testes

thyroid

thyrotoxicosis

1. The _____ gland controls most activity in the endocrine system.

2. The _____ and _____ support both the endocrine system and reproductive system.

3. _____ includes the processes of digestion, elimination, breathing, blood circulation, and maintaining body temperature.

4. _____ is elevated glucose without ketoacidosis, usually occurring in elderly type 2 diabetics with other conditions.

5. The _____ is a butterfly-shaped gland in front of the trachea that produces two hormones, tri-iodothyronine (T3) and thyroxine (T4).

6. _____ is excessive quantities of circulating thyroid hormone due to overproduction by the thyroid gland, overproduction originating outside the thyroid, or loss of storage function and leakage from the gland.

7. _____ is a deficiency of thyroid hormone, usually due to lack of production of the hormone by the thyroid or inadequate secretion of hormones.

8. Assign a code for _____, if known, with codes for obesity.

9. _____ is overproduction by the thyroid gland due to an autoimmune condition.

10. Cancer of the _____ accounts for 3% of new cancer cases but has a poor survival rate because it is usually not diagnosed until after it has metastasized widely.

Multiple Choice

Instructions: Circle the letter of the best answer to each question based on the information you learned in this chapter.

1. How would you code the following scenario? *A patient sees an ophthalmologist for moderate nonproliferative diabetic retinopathy in the left eye.*
   A. E11.3392
   B. E11.3322
   C. E10.3392
   D. E11.3312

2. What type of diabetes is one in which elevated glucose is caused by an external factor, such as medication, surgery, pancreatic disease, or other illness?
   A. Type 1 diabetes
   B. Type 2 diabetes
   C. Secondary diabetes
   D. Ketoacidosis

3. What type of diabetes accounts for 90–95% of all diagnosed cases?
   A. Type 1 diabetes
   B. Type 2 diabetes
   C. Secondary diabetes
   D. Gestational diabetes

4. What condition is an accumulation of a high level of ketones in the blood that turns it acidic and becomes life-threatening if not treated immediately?
   A. Hyperglycemia
   B. Diabetic ketoacidosis
   C. Hyperosmolarity hyperglycemic nonketotic syndrome
   D. Hypoglycemia

5. Which of the following disorders is an acute complication?
   A. Cataracts
   B. Hypothyroidism
   C. Diabetes
   D. Ketoacidosis

6. What subterm under a disease entry in the Index, such as Diabetes, directs a coder to code two conditions as related?
   A. Together
   B. In
   C. With
   D. And

7. How would you code the following scenario? *A female patient with type 1 diabetes is seen for routine followup. She reports that she has been taking insulin as directed and her blood glucose level is normal.*
   A. E11.9, Z79.4
   B. E10.9, Z79.4
   C. E10.9
   D. Z79.4

8. What type of code should be sequenced first when a patient has missed a dose of insulin?
   A. An underdosing code from the Table of Drugs and Chemicals
   B. A code to identify the manifestation
   C. A Z code for the long-term use of insulin basis
   D. An external cause code to identify the intent

9. What information do first-level subterms, under the Main Term Diabetes in the Index, identify?
   A. The type of diabetes
   B. That complications are present
   C. The specific complication(s) with each type
   D. Long-term use of insulin.

10. How would you code the following scenario? *A patient has diabetes due to pituitary-dependent Cushing's disease and uses insulin to manage diabetes. The patient is seen today for a foot ulcer on the right great toe with skin breakdown.*
    A. E24.0, E10.621, L97.511, Z79.4
    B. E24.0, E08.621, L97.511, Z79.4
    C. E08.621, E24.0, L97.511, Z79.4
    D. E10.621, L97.511, E24.0, Z79.4

KEEP ON CODING

Instructions: Read the diagnostic statement, then use the Index and Tabular List to assign and sequence ICD-10-CM diagnosis codes. Write the code(s) on the line provided.

1. Type 1 diabetes mellitus with diabetic cataract, right eye. ICD-10-CM Code(s) _____

2. Myxedema coma. ICD-10-CM Code(s) _____

3. Postprocedural hypoparathyroidism. ICD-10-CM Code(s) _____

4. Malignant neoplasm of the thymus gland. ICD-10-CM Code(s) _____

(continued)

(continued from page 159)

5. Argininemia. ICD-10-CM Code(s) _____

6. Diabetes insipidus. ICD-10-CM Code(s) _____

7. Postinfectious hypothyroidism. ICD-10-CM Code(s) _____

8. Drug-induced diabetes mellitus with diabetic neuralgia. ICD-10-CM Code(s) _____

9. Pickwickian syndrome. ICD-10-CM Code(s) _____

10. Type V glycogen storage disease. ICD-10-CM Code(s) _____

11. Thyrotoxicosis factitia. ICD-10-CM Code(s) _____

12. Mixed hyperlipidemia. ICD-10-CM Code(s) _____

13. Type 2 diabetes mellitus with diabetic gangrene. ICD-10-CM Code(s) _____

14. Neonatal adrenoleukodystrophy. ICD-10-CM Code(s) _____

15. Cushing's syndrome. ICD-10-CM Code(s) _____

16. Constitutional gigantism. ICD-10-CM Code(s) _____

17. Long-chain/very-long-chain acyl coenzyme A (CoA) dehydrogenase deficiency. ICD-10-CM Code(s) _____

18. Infantile osteomalacia. ICD-10-CM Code(s) _____

19. Accidental puncture of thyroid during parathyroidectomy procedure. ICD-10-CM Code(s) _____

20. Classical phenylketonuria. ICD-10-CM Code(s) _____

21. Meconium ileus in cystic fibrosis. ICD-10-CM Code(s) _____

22. Hypervitaminosis A. ICD-10-CM Code(s) _____

23. Hypomagnesemia. ICD-10-CM Code(s) _____

24. Infarction of the thyroid gland. ICD-10-CM Code(s) _____

25. Estrogen excess. ICD-10-CM Code(s) _____

CODING CHALLENGE

Instructions: Read the mini-medical-record of each patient's encounter, then abstract, assign, and sequence ICD-10-CM diagnosis codes using the Index and Tabular List. Write the code(s) on the line provided.

1. INPATIENT HOSPITAL   Gender: F   Age: 35

Reason for admission: T 102°F, tachycardia, extreme anxiety, nausea, diarrhea

Assessment: Thyrotoxicosis with goiter and thyroid storm

Plan: Rx PTU (*propylthiouracil*) for thyroid and beta blocker propranolol to control heart rate

1 ICD-10-CM Code _____

2. INvPATIENT HOSPITAL   Gender: M   Age: 42

Reason for admission: Patient found non-responsive. Family reports patient being on a fast.

Assessment: Nondiabetic hypoglycemic coma

Plan: Instructed on diet and glucometer, FU 1 week

1 ICD-10-CM Code _____

3. OFFICE   Gender: F   Age: 25

Chief complaint: Weight loss, decreased appetite, decreased sexual drive, and increased sensitivity to cold

Assessment: Hypopituitarism

Plan: Hormone replacement therapy, FU 4 wk

1 ICD-10-CM Code _____

4. OFFICE   Gender: M   Age: 40

Reason for encounter: FU on lab test results of 24-hour aldosterone excretion rate 18 mcg; 24-h urine sodium above 400 mEq (*milliequivalent*) after presenting with severe hypokalemia, fatigue, muscle weakness, cramping, and hypertension

Assessment: Primary hyperaldosteronism (*Conn's syndrome*) with secondary hypertension

Plan: Medication to normalize BP, Na (*sodium*), electrolytes, and aldosterone

2 ICD-10-CM Codes _____

5. OFFICE   Gender: F   Age: 32

Chief complaint: Irregular and infrequent menstrual periods, recent weight gain, noticeable loss of body hair under arms and pubic area

Assessment: Polycystic ovarian syndrome

Plan: Rx hormones, FU 1 month

1 ICD-10-CM Code _____

6. OFFICE   Gender: F   Age: 51

Reason for encounter: Annual check-up

Assessment: Test results show abnormally low vitamin D level. Patient is obese due to excess calories and has a BMI of 30.5 kg/m^2.

Plan: Rx vitamin D 50,000 IU/week for 8 weeks, then recheck.

Tip: Remember that you need a Z code for the annual checkup.

4 ICD-10-CM Codes _____

_____

7. OFFICE   Gender: M   Age: 48

Chief complaint: Insomnia, hand tremor, hyperactivity, excessive sweating, weight loss

Assessment: Graves' disease with uninodular goiter

Plan: Radioiodine therapy

1 ICD-10-CM Code _____

8. OFFICE   Gender: M   Age: 62

Chief complaint: Open sore on right heel

Assessment: Patient has developed a foot ulcer with skin breakdown due to type 2 diabetes.

Plan: Refer to wound care.

Tip: Read the instructional note to identify the site of the foot ulcer. This is a nonpressure ulcer and it is coded based on the amount of tissue damage.

2 ICD-10-CM Codes _____

9. INPATIENT HOSPITAL   Gender: F   Age: 58

Reason for admission: Admitted from emergency department due to weakness, shortness of breath, and severe abdominal pain with vomiting. Patient forgot to take insulin before going out to dinner.

Assessment: DKA, type 1 DM

Tip: Look up DKA if you're not sure of the meaning. Assign a second code for underdosing of insulin from the Table of Drugs and Chemicals.

3 ICD-10-CM Codes _____

_____

10. INPATIENT HOSPITAL   Gender: F   Age: 71

Reason for admission: Palpitations and muscle weakness

Assessment: Hyperkalemia, hyperosmolality

Plan: Low potassium diet, referred to nutritionist, FU 1 month

2 ICD-10-CM Codes _____

Chapter 10

Diseases of the Skin and Subcutaneous Tissue (L00-L99)

Chapter Outline

- **Integumentary System Refresher**
- **Coding Guidelines for the Skin and Subcutaneous Tissue**
- **Abstracting for Conditions of the Integumentary System**
- **Assigning Codes for Conditions of the Integumentary System**
- **Arranging Codes for Conditions of the Integumentary System**
- **Coding Neoplasms of the Integumentary System**

Learning Objectives

After completing this chapter, you should have the skills to:

10.1 Spell and define the key words, medical terms, and abbreviations related to diseases of the skin and subcutaneous tissue. (Remember)

10.2 Summarize the structure, function, and common conditions of diseases of the skin and subcutaneous tissue. (Understand)

10.3 Adhere to the Official Guidelines for Coding and Reporting related to diseases of the skin and subcutaneous tissue. (Apply)

10.4 Examine and abstract diagnostic information from the medical record for coding diseases of the skin and subcutaneous tissue. (Analyze)

10.5 Demonstrate how to assign diagnosis codes for diseases of the skin and subcutaneous tissue. (Apply)

10.6 Utilize guidelines for arranging (sequencing) multiple diagnosis codes for diseases of the skin and subcutaneous tissue. (Apply)

10.7 Demonstrate how to abstract, assign, and sequence codes for neoplasms of the integumentary system. (Apply)

Key Terms and Abbreviations

actinic keratosis	exfoliation	protection	stage 3 (pressure ulcer)
allograft	folliculitis	psoriasis	stage 4 (pressure ulcer)
alopecia	integumentary	regulation	subcutaneous
autograft	keratosis	sebaceous	sudoriferous
basal cell carcinoma (BCC)	lichen	secretion	synthetic
biopsy	melanoma	sensation	unstageable pressure ulcer
cellulitis	patch testing	squamous cell carcinoma (SCC)	urticaria
culture	pemphigus	stage 1 (pressure ulcer)	vitiligo
erythema multiforme	pityriasis	stage 2 (pressure ulcer)	xenograft

In addition to the key terms listed here, students should know the terms defined within tables in this chapter.

INTRODUCTION

A new car's finish consists of a primer layer that helps the paint adhere to the structure of the car, several layers of paint, and a clear coat on top that serves as a protective finish.

Your skin is the protective covering of your body and also consists of several layers, each with its own function. Repairing damage to the skin can be easy or difficult, depending on how far the damage penetrates.

A dermatologist is a physician who specializes in diagnosing and treating conditions of the skin and subcutaneous tissues. Primary care physicians treat uncomplicated conditions of the skin and subcutaneous tissues. They refer patients with more complex conditions to dermatologists.

INTEGUMENTARY SYSTEM REFRESHER

The **integumentary** (*pertaining to a covering*) system consists of the skin and accessory structures: hair, nails, **sebaceous** (*pertaining to oil*) glands, and **sudoriferous** (*pertaining to sweat*) glands (■ FIGURE 10-1). It is the largest organ in the body, weighing approximately six pounds and covering approximately 20 square feet, which is the size of a

four-by-five-foot rug. The integumentary system has four primary functions:

- **Protection**—Helps prevent invasion by pathogens, mechanical harm, and loss of fluids and electrolytes.
- **Regulation**—Increases and decreases body temperature through constriction and dilation of blood vessels and sweat glands.
- **Sensation**—Contains sensory receptors for pain, touch, heat, cold, and pressure.
- **Secretion**—Gives off perspiration (*water and salt*) to control temperature and sebum (*oil*) to protect from dehydration and penetration by harmful substances.

In Figure 10-1, each structure in the integumentary system is labeled with its name as well as its medical terminology root/combining form. As you learn about conditions and procedures that affect the skin and **subcutaneous** (*under the skin*) structures, remember to apply medical terminology skills to combine word roots, prefixes, and suffixes you already know to define new terms. Refer to ■ TABLE 10-1, (page 164) for a refresher on how to build medical terms related to the integumentary system.

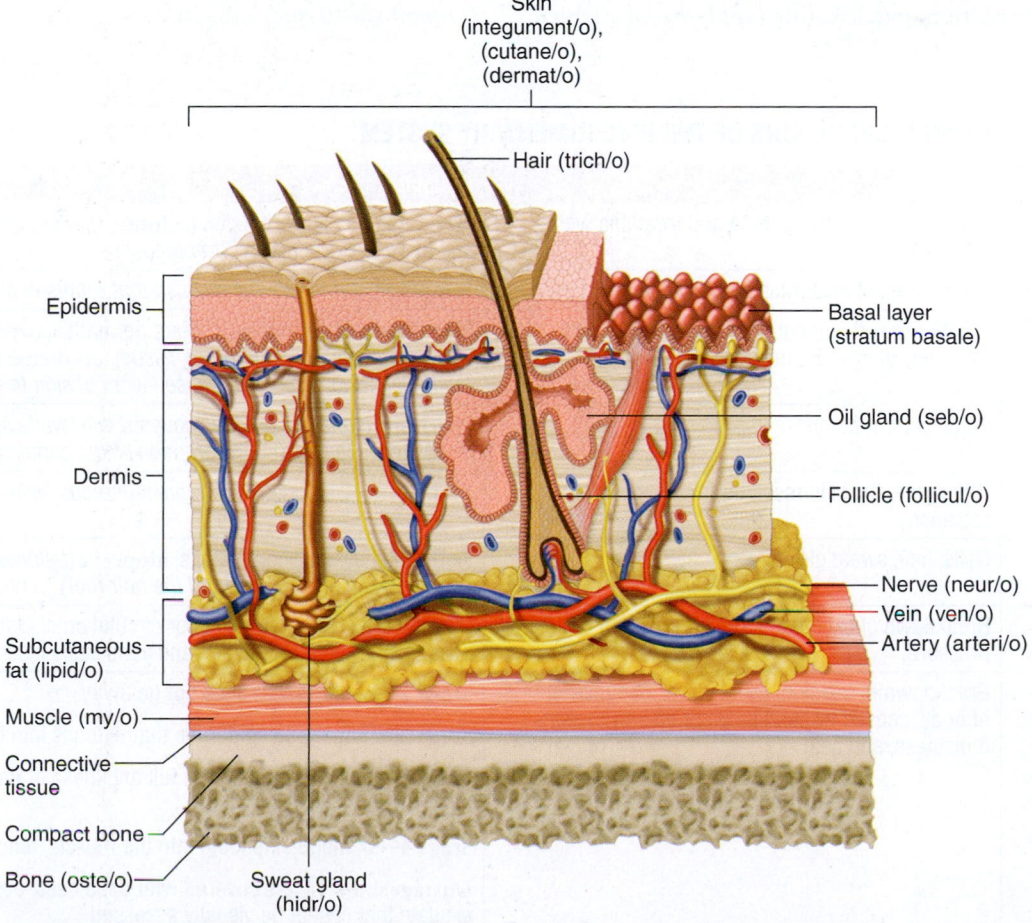

Figure 10-1 ■ The integumentary system.

Table 10-1 ■ **EXAMPLE OF CONSTRUCTING MEDICAL TERMS FOR THE INTEGUMENTARY SYSTEM**

Combining Form/Prefix	Suffix	Complete Medical Term
derm/o, dermat/o (*skin*) cutane/o (*skin*) myc/o (*fungus*) erythr/o (*redness*)	-itis (*inflammation*) -osis (*condition*) -al (*pertaining to*) -plasty (*surgical repair*)	dermat + itis (*inflammation of the skin*) intra + derm + al (*pertaining to within the skin*) erythro + derma (*red skin*) dermo + myc + osis (*skin condition related to fungus*) dermo + plasty (*surgical repair of the skin*)
pachy- (prefix; *thick*) intra- (prefix; *within*) sub- (prefix; *below*)		sub + derm + al (*pertaining to under the skin*) sub + cutane + ous (*pertaining to under the skin*)

CODING CAUTION
Be alert for medical terms that are spelled similarly and have different meanings.

myc/o (*fungus*) and my/o (*muscle*)

urticaria (*hives*) and -uresis (*urination*)

onych/o (*nail*) and onc/o (*tumor*)

Conditions of the Integumentary System
Common conditions of the integumentary system are summarized in ■ TABLE 10-2. Physicians diagnose problems through visual inspection, **patch testing** (*applying an allergen* to the skin to observe the reaction), **biopsy** (*scraping, punching, or cutting a piece of skin and examining it under a microscope*), and **culture** (*performing a test to identify the microorganism that is causing an infection*). Treatments include:

- Medication to treat the underlying condition
- Incision and drainage of fluid
- Surgical removal of the lesion or damaged skin
- Application of replacement tissue using an **autograft** (*tissue from the patient*), **allograft** (*tissue from another person*), **xenograft** (*tissue from an animal*), or a **synthetic** (*manmade tissue*) substitute.

Table 10-2 ■ **COMMON CONDITIONS OF THE INTEGUMENTARY SYSTEM**

Condition	Description	Examples
Bacterial infection	Infection caused by bacteria and treatable with antibiotics	Abscess, furuncle, carbuncle, **cellulitis** (*inflammation under the skin*) due to *Staphylococcus* or *Streptococcus*
Bulla (blister)	Raised area of epidermis filled with fluid	**Pemphigus** (*autoimmune disease that erupts in blisters*)
Dermatitis	A flat or raised eruption that can be caused by irritation, allergy, or infection	Eczema, atopic dermatitis, contact dermatitis, **urticaria** (*hives*), **keratosis** (*overgrowth of horny tissue*), **erythema multiforme** (*red fluid-filled lesions that can cause layers of skin to fall off*)
Papulosquamous disorders	Papules (*firm bumps*) and scales	**Psoriasis** (*round red patches covered with white scales*), **pityriasis** (*rough, dry scales*), **lichen** (*eruption of flat papules*)
Radiation disorders	Damage to the skin resulting from exposure to radiation	Sunburn, **actinic keratosis** (*a precancerous lesion*), radiodermatitis
Skin appendages	Nails, hair, sweat glands	Ingrowing nail, misshaped nails, **alopecia** (*baldness*), **folliculitis** (*inflammation of space around the hair root*), acne, sweat disorders
Nonpressure ulcers	Breakdown of skin that is not the result of prolonged pressure	Diabetic ulcer, ulcers due to poor circulation or clots, such as postphlebitic, postthrombotic, and venostasis ulcers
Decubitus ulcer (pressure ulcer, bed sore)	Breakdown of the skin, usually over bony parts of body, caused by continuous pressure, friction, moistness, and heat	Stage 1—Redness that does not go away Stage 2—Damage to epidermis that extends into the dermis Stage 3—Damage through the full thickness of the dermis and into the subcutaneous tissue (fat) Stage 4—Damage extending into the muscle, tendon, or bone Unstageable—Ulcers covered with dead cells, eschar, or wound exudate that cannot be visually assessed
Pigmentation disorder	Damage to or unhealthy melanin cells that give color to the skin	Age spots, freckles, **vitiligo** (*loss of pigmentation*)

CODING PRACTICE

Exercise 10.1   Integumentary System Refresher

Instructions: Use your medical terminology skills and resources to define the following terms related to the integumentary system, then assign the diagnosis code.

Follow these steps:

- Use slash marks "/" to break down each term into its root(s) and suffix.
- Define the meaning of the word, based on the meaning of each word part.
- Assign the default ICD-10-CM diagnosis code for the condition using the Index and Tabular List.

Example: dermatitis dermat/itis   Meaning *inflammation of the skin*   ICD-10-CM Code *L30.9*

1. pachyderma   Meaning _____   ICD-10-CM Code _____
2. hypertrichosis   Meaning _____   ICD-10-CM Code _____
3. perifolliculitis   Meaning _____   ICD-10-CM Code _____
4. cellulitis   Meaning _____   ICD-10-CM Code _____
5. erythroderma   Meaning _____   ICD-10-CM Code _____
6. pyoderma   Meaning _____   ICD-10-CM Code _____
7. onychocryptosis   Meaning _____   ICD-10-CM Code _____
8. hyperkeratosis   Meaning _____   ICD-10-CM Code _____
9. hidradenitis   Meaning _____   ICD-10-CM Code _____
10. onychodystrophy   Meaning _____   ICD-10-CM Code _____

CODING GUIDELINES FOR THE SKIN AND SUBCUTANEOUS TISSUE

Coders should understand the organization of this ICD-10-CM chapter, chapter-wide and commonly used instructional notes in the Tabular List, and the relevant OGCR. This information is necessary for accurate coding.

ICD-10-CM Chapter 12, "Diseases of the Skin and Subcutaneous Tissue (L00-L99)," contains nine blocks or subchapters that are divided by anatomic site and type of condition. This chapter includes skin disorders and infections other than neoplasms and injuries. Review the block names and code ranges listed at the beginning of Chapter 12 in the ICD-10-CM manual to become familiar with the content and organization.

Take note of the **Excludes2** note at the beginning of the ICD-10-CM chapter, which lists skin conditions not classified in this chapter. The following types of skin disorders are classified in other ICD-10-CM chapters:

- Burns (Chapter 19, "Injury and Poisoning")
- Neoplasms (Chapter 2, "Neoplasms")
- Viral, bacterial, and fungal infections (Chapter 1, "Certain Infectious and Parasitic Diseases")
- Parasites (Chapter 1, "Certain Infectious and Parasitic Diseases")

ICD-10-CM provides Official Guidelines for Coding and Reporting (OGCR) for Diseases of the Skin and Subcutaneous Tissue in OGCR section I.C.12. OGCR provides detailed discussion of assigning codes for both pressure and nonpressure ulcers. Pressure ulcer codes are combination codes that identify the stage, site, and laterality in a single code. Nonpressure ulcers are described based on the depth of tissue involvement. Additional guidelines related to skin infections appear in OGCR I.C.1.b. Guidelines related to burns and other skin injuries appear in OGCR I.C.19.d. Instructional notes throughout the chapter provide information on multiple coding and sequencing. Specific OGCR guidelines are discussed and cited throughout this chapter.

ABSTRACTING FOR CONDITIONS OF THE INTEGUMENTARY SYSTEM

When abstracting for diseases of the integumentary system, coders need to be familiar with the various types of lesions and complications, as well as the systems used to describe the extent of damage to the skin (■ TABLE 10-3, page 166). Remember that the abstracting questions are a guide and that not every question applies to, or can be answered for, every case. For example, not every case has an infectious agent.

Depth of damage is described based on documentation of what layers of tissue are affected. The description varies based on the condition, such as:

- Conditions confined to the epidermis by definition, such as contact dermatitis or superficial lesions, do not require depth descriptions.

- Sunburns are classified by the degree of the burn (■ TABLE 10-4).

- Pressure ulcers are assigned a numerical stage from 1 to 4, based on depth (■ FIGURE 10-2).

- Nonpressure ulcers are classified as:

  - Limited to breakdown of skin
  - Fat layer exposed
  - Muscle involvement without necrosis
  - Necrosis of muscle
  - Bone involvement without necrosis
  - Necrosis of bone

CODING CAUTION

ICD-10-CM uses the Arabic numerals 1, 2, 3, and 4 to identify pressure ulcer stages. The National Pressure Ulcer Advisory Panel, and many physicians, use the Roman numerals I, II, III, and IV. Coders need to be familiar with both ways of writing and reading numbers.

Table 10-3 ■ KEY CRITERIA FOR ABSTRACTING CONDITIONS OF THE INTEGUMENTARY SYSTEM

- ❏ What is the type of lesion (carbuncle, abscess, urticaria, mole, corn)?
- ❏ What is the anatomic site (face, back, hand)?
- ❏ What is the laterality (right or left side)?
- ❏ Is there an underlying cause (another condition, exposure to a drug, or environmental substance)?
- ❏ What is the infectious agent, if any?
- ❏ Are there complications or manifestations (gangrene)?
- ❏ What is the depth or extent of damage?

Table 10-4 ■ CLASSIFICATION OF BURNS

Degree	Name	Description
1st	Superficial	Damage to the epidermis
2nd	Partial thickness	Damage to the epidermis and part of the dermis
3rd	Full thickness	Damage to the entire depth of the dermis

Stage 1: Skin discolored but intact

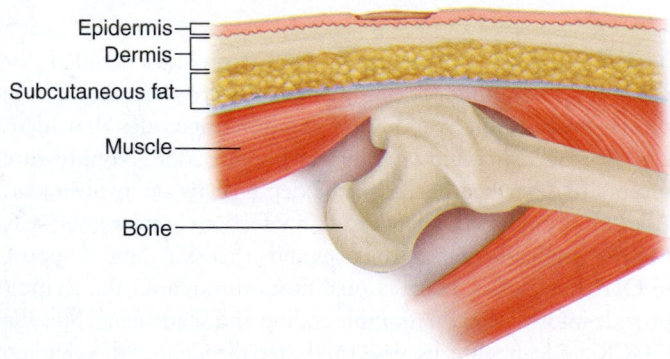

Stage 2: Shallow open ulcer through part of the dermis

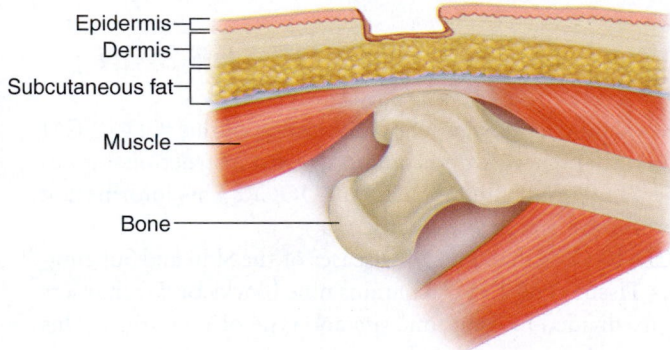

Stage 3: Full-thickness loss of dermis with exposure of subcutaneous fat

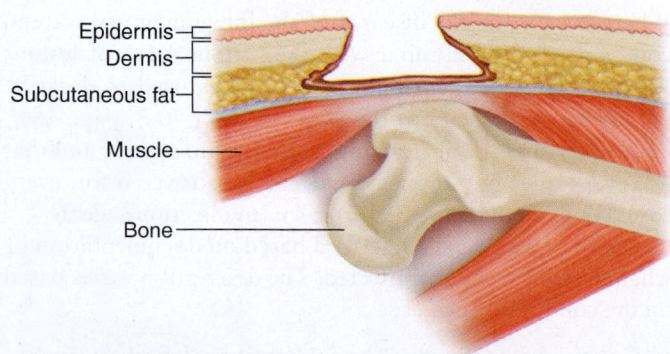

Stage 4: Exposed bone, muscle, or tendon

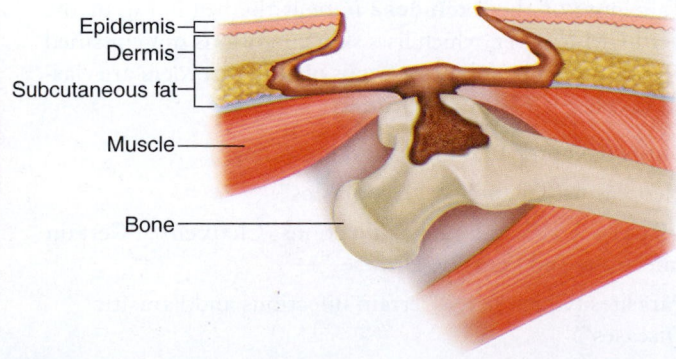

Figure 10-2 ■ Classification of pressure ulcer stages.

Guided Example of Abstracting Diagnoses for the Integumentary System

Refer to the following example throughout this chapter to practice skills for abstracting and assigning codes for the integumentary system. Joshua Grider, CPC, is a fictitious coder who guides you through this case.

Date: 11/1/yy   Location: Dermatology Associates

Provider: Lawrence Staton, MD

Patient: Naomi Vargas   Gender: F   Age: 84

Reason for encounter: Debride and change dressing on pressure ulcer per referral from home health care nurse

Assessment: Damage through the full thickness of the dermis and into the subcutaneous (SC) tissue; stage 3 pressure ulcer, right buttock

Plan: FU visits from home health care

Follow along as Joshua Grider, CPC, abstracts the diagnosis. Check off each step after you complete it.

▶ Joshua reads through the entire record, paying special attention to the reason for the encounter and the final assessment.

❏ He notes that the procedure of debriding the wound is consistent with a stage 3 ulcer. He refers to Key Criteria for Abstracting Conditions of the Integumentary System (Table 10-3).

❏ *What is the type of lesion?* Pressure ulcer

❏ *What is the anatomic site?* Buttock

❏ *What is the laterality?* Right

❏ *Is there an underlying cause?* No

❏ *What is the infectious agent, if any?* None

❏ *Are there complications or manifestations?* No

❏ *What is the depth or extent of damage?* Stage 3

❏ He refers to the definition of pressure ulcer stages and confirms that the description damage through the full thickness of the dermis and into the subcutaneous tissue is consistent with a stage 3 ulcer.

▶ Next, Joshua needs to assign the codes.

CODING PRACTICE

Exercise 10.2   Abstracting for Conditions of the Integumentary System

Instructions: Read the mini-medical-record of each patient's encounter and answer the abstracting questions. Write the answer on the line provided. Do not assign any codes.

1. OFFICE   Gender: F   Age: 5

Chief complaint: Was at the beach all day and did not have sunscreen applied

Assessment: A severe second degree sunburn

a. What is the chief complaint? _____

b. What is the source of the sunburn? _____

c. What degree is the sunburn? _____

d. What is the definition of a second-degree sunburn? _____

2. OFFICE   Gender: F   Age: 17

Chief complaint: Red itchy patches after hiking

Assessment: Contact dermatitis due to poison ivy

a. What is the chief complaint? _____

b. Should you code for the red itchy patches? _____

Why or why not? _____

c. What is the diagnosis? _____

d. What is the Main Term? _____

3. OFFICE   Gender: M   Age: 15

Chief complaint: Red and tender area on the left great toe

Assessment: Ingrown nail

a. What is the reason for the visit? _____

(continued)

CODING PRACTICE *(continued)*

3. (continued)

b. What condition does the physician diagnose?
_____

c. Should you code the redness and tenderness?
_____

Why or why not? _____
_____

---

4. OFFICE   Gender: F   Age: 64

Chief complaint: Evaluation of cellulitis on her right leg

Assessment: Lab results show the cellulitis to be due to Streptococcus A

Plan: Rx oral antibiotics. If it does not improve within 3 days or gets worse, she will need to be admitted for IV antibiotics.

a. What condition is being evaluated? _____
_____

b. What is the anatomic site? _____
_____

c. What is the laterality? _____
_____

d. What is the infectious agent? _____
_____

---

5. OFFICE   Gender: M   Age: 25

Reason for encounter: Follow-up on erythema multiforme minor with stomatitis due to herpes simplex virus

(continued)

---

5. (continued)

Assessment: Stomatitis showing improvement. 15% of his skin is exfoliated.

a. What condition is being treated? _____
_____

b. What is the manifestation? _____
_____

c. What virus caused the condition? _____
_____

d. What does exfoliation mean? _____
_____

e. What is the percentage of exfoliation? _____
_____

---

6. OFFICE   Gender: M   Age: 73

Reason for encounter: Debride and dress chronic ulcer on right calf

Assessment: Chronic ulcer due to postphlebitic syndrome. Healing is progressing. At last visit some muscle necrosis was visible. Today only the fat layer is exposed.

a. What condition is being treated? _____
_____

b. What is the anatomic site? _____
_____

c. What is the laterality? _____
_____

d. Is this a pressure ulcer or a nonpressure ulcer?
_____

e. What is the underlying condition? _____
_____

ASSIGNING CODES FOR CONDITIONS OF THE INTEGUMENTARY SYSTEM

When assigning codes for the integumentary system, coders need to be alert for easily confused Index entries and must use the information abstracted regarding the depth or extent of skin damage, when applicable.

Skin ulcers are classified into separate categories based on whether they are pressure (decubitus) ulcers or nonpressure ulcers. Pressure ulcers are caused by prolonged pressure on an area, usually a bony prominence, such as the heel, elbow, or hip. Pressure ulcers are indexed under the Main Term **Ulcer**, then the subterm **pressure**, then a second-level subterm for the anatomic

site. The most common causes of nonpressure ulcers are diabetes and circulatory problems. Nonpressure skin ulcers are indexed under the Main Term **Ulcer** and a subterm for the anatomic site.

The stage or depth of a pressure ulcer changes as the wound heals or worsens. Assign a code based on the stage documented during the encounter. For an ulcer that worsens during the course of an inpatient admission, two separate codes should be assigned: one code for the site and stage of the ulcer upon admission and a second code for the same ulcer site and the highest stage reported during the stay (OGCR I.C.12.a.6)). When patients have more than one pressure ulcer, assign separate codes for each ulcer (OGCR I.C.12.a.1)).

Some skin conditions cause **exfoliation** (*falling off in scales or layers*) of the skin. These codes provide the instructional note **Use additional code to identify percentage of skin exfoliation (L49-)**.

> ### CODING CAUTION
> Remember to distinguish the *causes* of skin ulcers. A pressure ulcer is caused by continuous pressure on an area, often found in patients with limited mobility. A nonpressure ulcer is due to another cause, such as venous insufficiency or diabetes, not pressure.

Guided Example of Assigning Integumentary System Diagnosis Codes

To practice skills for assigning codes for conditions of the integumentary system, continue with the example from earlier in the chapter about patient Naomi Vargas, who was seen by Dr. Staton due to a stage 3 pressure ulcer on the right buttock.

Follow along in your ICD-10-CM manual as Joshua Grider, CPC, assigns codes. Check off each step after you complete it.

▶ First, Joshua confirms the diagnosis stage 3 pressure ulcer on the right buttock.

▶ Joshua searches the Index for the Main Term **Ulcer**.

❑ He reviews the subterms and notes that many types of ulcers are indexed here, including ulcers in internal organs.

❑ He locates a subterm for **buttock**.

❑ He locates the second-level subterm for **exposed fat layer L98.412**.

▶ Joshua verifies the code in the Tabular List.

❑ He reads the code title **L98.412 Non-pressure chronic ulcer of buttock with fat layer exposed**.

❑ Joshua notices that this code is for a *nonpressure* ulcer, but this is *not* the diagnosis for this patient.

▶ Joshua realizes he selected an incorrect subterm in the Index, so *he returns to the Index* entry for the Main Term **Ulcer** to search for a different subterm.

❑ He locates the subterm **pressure**.

❑ He locates the second-level subterm **buttock L89.3**.

▶ Joshua returns to the Tabular List to verify code **L89.3**.

❑ He reads the category title **L89.3, Pressure ulcer of buttock**.

❑ He notices the convention **5th**, instructing him to assign a fifth character.

❑ He reads the titles of the fifth-character categories and notes that they indicate laterality.

❑ He locates **L89.31 Pressure ulcer of right buttock**.

❑ He notices the convention **6th**, instructing him to assign a sixth character.

❑ He reads the titles of the sixth-character codes and notes that they indicate stage.

❑ He locates **L89.313 Pressure ulcer of right buttock, stage 3**.

❑ He confirms that this accurately describes the diagnosis in the medical record.

▶ Joshua checks for instructional notes in the Tabular List.

❑ He cross-references the beginning of category **L89** and reads the instructional notes.
- The inclusion notes confirm that this category classifies pressure or decubitus ulcers. The **Excludes2** note confirms that other types of ulcers are not coded here.
- He reads the note to **Code first any associated gangrene (I96)**.
- He cross-references the medical record to confirm that gangrene is not documented. He does *not* assign a code for gangrene because gangrene is not documented.

❑ Next, Joshua cross-references the beginning of the block **Other Disorders of the Skin and Subcutaneous Tissue (L80-L99)** and verifies that there are no instructional notes.

❑ Finally, he cross-references the beginning of Chapter 12, "Diseases of the Skin and Subcutaneous Tissue (L00-L99)," and reviews the instructional notes.
- The only instructional note is an **Excludes2** note indicating what conditions are not classified in this chapter.
- He determines that the **Excludes2** does not apply to this case because the patient's condition does not fit the description of any of the listed conditions.

▶ Joshua cross-references the medical record and finalizes the code for this case:

❑ **L89.313 Pressure ulcer of right buttock, stage 3**.

CODING PRACTICE

Exercise 10.3 Assigning Codes for Conditions of the Integumentary System

Instructions: Read the mini-medical-record of each patient's encounter, review the information abstracted in Exercise 10.2, and assign ICD-10-CM diagnosis codes using the Index and Tabular List. Write the code(s) on the line provided.

1. OFFICE   Gender: F   Age: 5

Chief complaint: Was at the beach all day and did not have sunscreen applied

Assessment: A severe second degree sunburn

1 ICD-10-CM Code _____

2. OFFICE   Gender: F   Age: 17

Chief complaint: Red itchy patches after hiking

Assessment: Contact dermatitis due to poison ivy

Tip: Recall that external cause codes for activity are not applicable to poisonings, so you do not need any additional codes.

1 ICD-10-CM Code _____

3. OFFICE   Gender: M   Age: 15

Chief complaint: Red and tender area on the left great toe

Assessment: Ingrown nail

1 ICD-10-CM Code _____

ARRANGING CODES FOR CONDITIONS OF THE INTEGUMENTARY SYSTEM

Sequencing of codes for the integumentary system follows the general coding guidelines OGCR III and IV as well as instructional notes in the Tabular List. In some cases, coders must apply multiple instructional notes for one code. A single category may include notes for **Code first** instructions as well as one or more **Use additional code** instructions. **Code first** means that the code listed should be sequenced before the code from the category in which it appears. **Use additional code** means that the code listed should be sequenced after the code from the category in which it appears.

Guided Example of Arranging Integumentary System Diagnosis Codes

Refer to the following new example of a patient with Stevens-Johnson syndrome to learn how to arrange codes when there are multiple instructional notes. Joshua Grider, CPC, guides you through this case. Review the mini-medical-record in ■ FIGURE 10-3, (page 171) to learn what information Joshua abstracted for each code.

Follow along in your ICD-10-CM manual as Joshua Grider, CPC, assigns and arranges codes. Check off each step after you complete it.

▶ Joshua first assigns the code for Stevens-Johnson syndrome. He locates the Main Term **Stevens-Johnson syndrome**

L51.1 in the Index then refers to the Tabular List to verify the code.

❑ He reads through the instructional notes at the beginning of category **L51** in the Tabular List (■ FIGURE 10-4, page 171).

▶ Joshua reads the first instructional note, which states **Use additional code to identify drug (T36-T50 with fifth or sixth character 5)**.

❑ The documentation states that the condition is the result of taking a prescribed sulfonamide.

❑ Joshua sequences code **T37.0X5A Adverse effect of sulfonamides, initial encounter** as the second code because the instructional note states **Use additional code**, which means the drug code should appear *after* the code from this category (**L51**) for the condition.

▶ Joshua sequences the condition code first, **L51.1 Stevens-Johnson syndrome**.

▶ Joshua reads the second instructional note, which states **Use additional code to identify associated manifestations: stomatitis (K12.-)**.

❑ He refers to the documentation and confirms the manifestation, mouth sores.

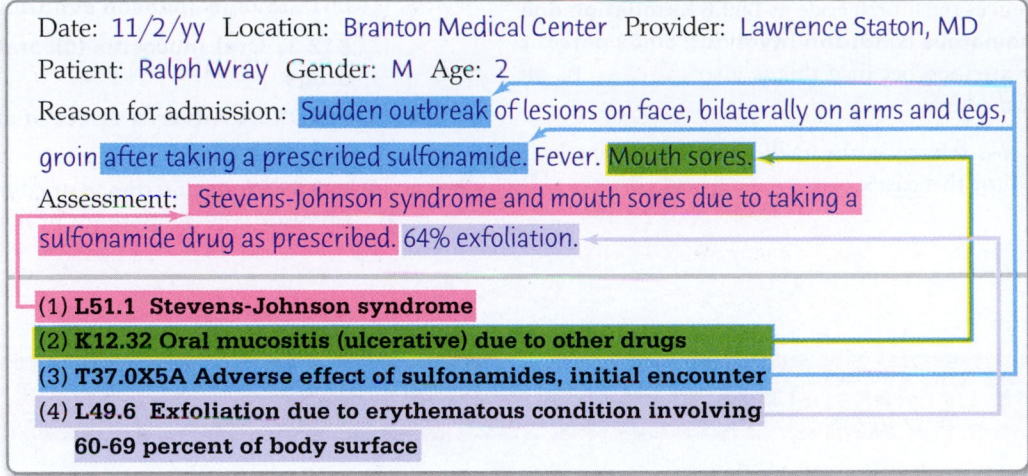

Figure 10-3 ■ Mini-medical-record for arranging integumentary system diagnosis codes.

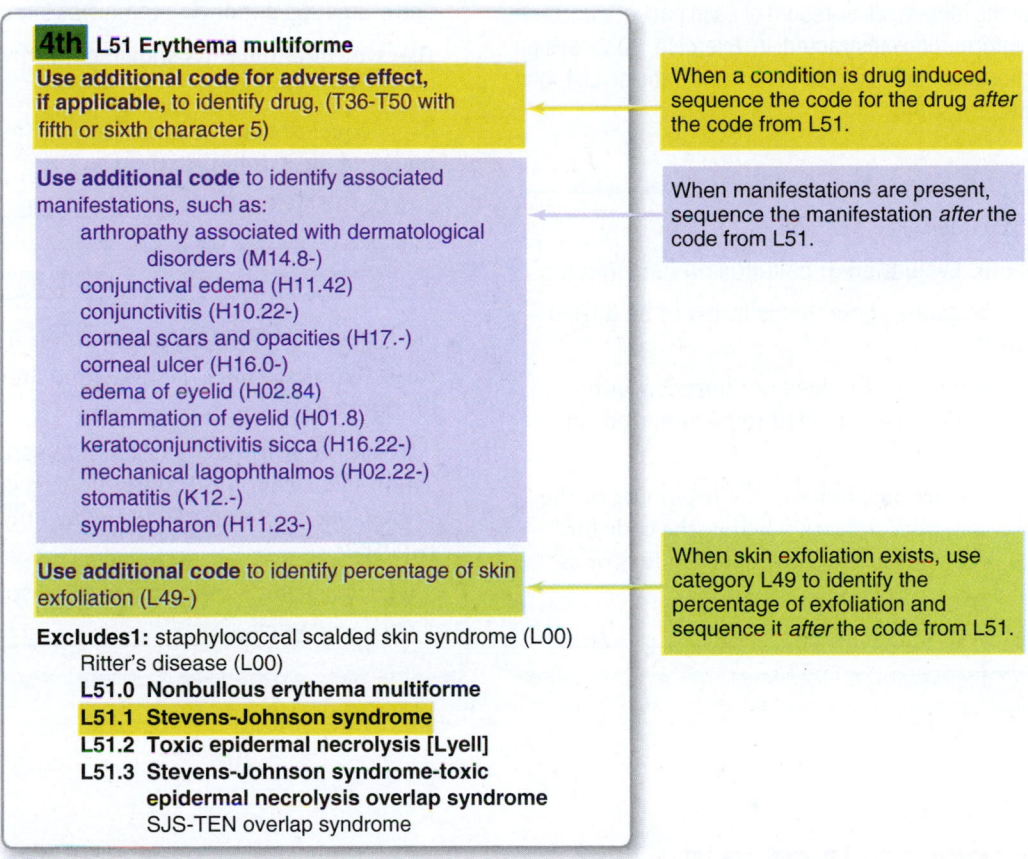

Figure 10-4 ■ Multiple coding and sequencing instructions for all codes within a category.

❑ He sequences the second code as **K12.32 Oral mucositis (ulcerative) due to other drugs** because the instructional note **Use additional code** means the manifestation code should be sequenced *after* the code from this category **(L51)** for the condition. Because it is an adverse effect of the drug, it should be sequenced before the T code for the drug (OGCR I.C.19.e.5)(a)).

▶ Joshua sequences the T code for the drug third, **T37.0X5A Adverse effect of sulfonamides, initial encounter**.

▶ Joshua reads the third instructional note, which states **Use additional code to identify percentage of skin exfoliation (L49-)**.

❑ He refers to the documentation and confirms 64% exfoliation.

❏ He sequences the fourth code as **L49.6 Exfoliation due to erythematous condition involving 60-69 percent of body surface** because this is also stated to be an *additional* code.

❏ Joshua cross-references the medical record and finalizes the codes for this case:

(1) **L51 Stevens-Johnson syndrome**

(2) **K12.32 Oral mucositis (ulcerative) due to other drugs**

(3) **T37.0X5A Adverse effect of sulfonamides, initial encounter**

(4) **L49.6 Exfoliation due to erythematous condition involving 60–69 percent of body surface**

CODING PRACTICE

Exercise 10.4 Arranging Codes for Conditions of the Integumentary System

Instructions: Read the mini-medical-record of each patient's encounter, review the information abstracted in Exercise 10.2, assign ICD-10-CM diagnosis codes using the Index and Tabular List, and arrange them correctly.

---

1. OFFICE Gender: F Age: 64

Chief complaint: Evaluation of cellulitis on her right leg

Assessment: Lab results show the cellulitis to be due to Streptococcus A

Plan: Rx oral antibiotics. If it does not improve within 3 days or gets worse, she will need to be admitted for IV antibiotics.

Tip: Read the instructional notes at the beginning of the three-character category to learn whether the code for the infectious organism should be sequenced first or as an additional code.

2 ICD-10-CM Codes _____

---

2. OFFICE Gender: M Age: 25

Reason for encounter: Follow-up on erythema multiforme and stomatitis minor due to herpes simplex virus

Assessment: Stomatitis showing improvement. 15% of his skin is exfoliated.

Tip: Sequence the condition first, the manifestation second, and the exfoliation third.

3 ICD-10-CM Codes _____
_____

---

3. OFFICE Gender: M Age: 73

Reason for encounter: Debride and dress chronic ulcer on right calf

Assessment: Chronic ulcer due to postphlebitic syndrome. Healing is progressing. At last visit some muscle necrosis was visible. Today only the fat layer is exposed.

Tip: Sequencing is indicated in the instructional notes.

2 ICD-10-CM Codes _____

CODING NEOPLASMS OF THE INTEGUMENTARY SYSTEM

Neoplasms of the integumentary system do not appear in ICD-10-CM Chapter 12, "Diseases of the Skin and Subcutaneous Tissue (L00-L99)." Codes for neoplasms of the integumentary system appear in block C43–C44 in the ICD-10-CM neoplasm chapter.

Skin cancers are named after the type of cell in which they start. The most common cancer in the integumentary system is **basal cell** (*lowest layer of the epidermis*) **carcinoma** (BCC),

according to the Skin Cancer Foundation. **Squamous cell carcinoma (SCC)**, named after the flat squamous cells in which it begins, is also common. BCC and SCC, while malignant, tend to spread slowly and are usually treated with a high degree of success.

The most serious neoplasm of the integumentary system is malignant **melanoma**, a tumor of melanocytes. If found early, melanoma is treatable, but it can metastasize to other areas of the body, in which case it is difficult to treat and usually fatal.

CODING PRACTICE

Exercise 10.5   Coding Neoplasms of the Integumentary System

Instructions: Read the mini-medical-record of each patient's encounter, then abstract, assign, and arrange ICD-10-CM diagnosis codes using the Index and Tabular List. Write the code(s) on the line provided.

---

1. OFFICE   Gender: F   Age: 45

Reason for encounter: Removal of lesions from eyebrow, chin, and lip

Assessment: Removed three lesions, basal cell carcinoma

Plan: Instructed patient to perform skin check monthly

Tip: Remember that you should not report the same diagnosis code twice for the same encounter (OGCR I.B.12).

2 ICD-10-CM Codes _____

---

2. OFFICE   Gender: M   Age: 42

Reason for encounter: Unusual mole on nose

Assessment: Melanoma in situ

Plan: Schedule outpatient surgery to remove

Tip: Remember to look up the Main Term *Melanoma* before deciding whether you should go to the Table of Neoplasms.

1 ICD-10-CM Code _____

---

3. INPATIENT HOSPITAL   Gender: F   Age: 51

Reason for admission: Immunotherapy

Assessment: Metastatic melanoma which started on the back

3 ICD-10-CM Codes _____

_____

---

4. OFFICE   Gender: F   Age: 36

Reason for encounter: Suspicious mole between nose and lip

Assessment: Nevus nasolabial groove

Plan: No treatment necessary

1 ICD-10-CM Code _____

---

5. OFFICE   Gender: M   Age: 68

Reason for encounter: Referred by family physician for areas on left arm where skin is breaking down

Assessment: Merkel cell carcinoma in kidney transplant recipient

Plan: Schedule removal in one week

Tip: Chronic immune suppression is a risk factor for the rare Merkel cell carcinoma. Therefore, code the patient's organ transplant status.

2 IC D-10-CM Codes _____

CHAPTER SUMMARY

In this chapter you learned that:

- The integumentary system consists of the skin and accessory structures: hair, nails, sebaceous glands, and sudoriferous glands.

- ICD-10-CM provides OGCR for Diseases of the Skin and Subcutaneous Tissue in OGCR section I.C.12, which discusses in detail assigning codes for pressure ulcer stages.

- When abstracting for diseases of the integumentary system, coders need to be familiar with the various types of lesions and complications, as well as the systems used to describe the extent of damage to the skin.

- When assigning codes for the integumentary system, coders need to be alert for easily confused Index entries and must use the information abstracted regarding the depth or extent of skin damage for certain conditions.

- Sequencing of codes for the integumentary system follows the general coding guidelines OGCR III and IV as well as instructional notes in the Tabular List.

- Skin cancers are named after the type of cell in which they start, with the most common being basal cell carcinoma (BCC).

CONCEPT QUIZ

Take a moment to look back at diseases of the skin and subcutaneous tissue and solidify your skills. This is your opportunity to pull together everything you have learned.

Completion

Instructions: Write the term that completes each statement based on the information you learned in this chapter. Choose from the following list. Some choices may be used more than once and some choices may not be used at all.

allograft	regulation
autograft	SCC
BCC	secretion
cellulitis	sensation
decubitus	skin
erythema multiforme	stage 1
exfoliation	stage 2
folliculitis	stage 3
hair	stage 4
melanoma	urticaria
nails	xenograft
protection	

1. The skin's _____ function increases and decreases body temperature through constriction and dilation of blood vessels and sweat glands.

2. _____ is an inflammation of space around the hair root.

3. _____ is an inflammation under the skin.

4. A _____ pressure ulcer is a breakdown of the skin, usually over bony parts of the body, caused by continuous pressure, friction, moistness, and heat.

5. _____ is the medical term for hives.

6. _____ is the most common cancer in the integumentary system and accounts for 75% of new skin cancer cases.

7. _____ occurs when skin falls off in layers.

8. *Trich/o* is the combining form for _____.

9. _____ is replacement skin tissue from another person.

10. The skin's _____ function helps prevent invasion by pathogens, mechanical harm, and loss of fluids and electrolytes.

Multiple Choice

Instructions: Circle the letter of the best answer to each question based on the information you learned in this chapter.

1. How would you code the following scenario? *A patient is seen for a stage 2 nonpressure chronic ulcer on the left calf with skin breakdown.*
   A. L89.892
   B. L97.901
   C. L97.221
   D. L97.201

2. What type of disorder are psoriasis, pityriasis, and lichen?
   A. Papulosquamous
   B. Decubitus
   C. Pigmentation
   D. Dermatitis

3. How many stages are pressure ulcers classified into?
   A. Two
   B. Three
   C. Four
   D. Five

4. What is an unstageable pressure ulcer?
   A. One that extends into the muscle, tendon, or bone.
   B. One that has metastasized to other areas of the body.
   C. One that is not documented by a physician.
   D. One that cannot be visually assessed because of dead cells, eschar, or exudate.

5. How would you code the following scenario? *A patient is seen for erythema multiforme with 20% skin exfoliation.*
   A. L51.0, L49.2
   B. L49.2, L51.0
   C. L51.8
   D. L51.9, L49.2

6. What stage of pressure ulcer involves damage through the full thickness of the dermis and into the subcutaneous tissue (fat)?
   A. Stage 1
   B. Stage 2
   C. Stage 3
   D. Stage 4

7. What Main Term and subterm combination is used to locate a code for a pressure ulcer on the right buttock?
   A. Pressure, buttock
   B. Buttock, ulcer
   C. Ulcer, buttock
   D. Ulcer, pressure

8. How would you code the following scenario? *A patient was admitted with a stage 2 pressure ulcer on the sacrum. At discharge, the pressure ulcer was evaluated as having progressed to stage 3.*
   A. L89.152
   B. L89.153
   C. L89.159
   D. L89.152, L89.153

9. What does category L49 identify when skin exfoliation exists?
   A. Percentage of healthy skin
   B. Percentage of lesions
   C. Percentage of exfoliation
   D. Percentage of dermatitis

10. What characteristic are skin cancers are named after?
    A. Anatomic site where they start
    B. Type of cell in which they start
    C. Rate at which they spread
    D. Site they metastasize to

KEEP ON CODING

Instructions: Read the diagnostic statement, then use the Index and Tabular List to assign and sequence ICD-10-CM diagnosis codes. Write the code(s) on the line provided.

1. Infantile eczema. ICD-10-CM Code(s) _____

2. Retiform parapsoriasis. ICD-10-CM Code(s) _____

3. Café au lait spots. ICD-10-CM Code(s) _____

4. Discoid lupus erythematosus. ICD-10-CM Code(s) _____

5. Eosinophilic cellulitis. ICD-10-CM Code(s) _____

6. Stage 3 decubitus ulcer of the right lower back. ICD-10-CM Code(s) _____

7. Trichorrhexis nodusa. ICD-10-CM Code(s) _____

8. Allergic urticaria. ICD-10-CM Code(s) _____

9. Carbuncle of the face. ICD-10-CM Code(s) _____

10. Basal cell carcinoma of skin of right calf. ICD-10-CM Code(s) _____

11. Allergic contact dermatitis due to cosmetics. ICD-10-CM Code(s) _____

12. Solar urticaria. ICD-10-CM Code(s) _____

13. Acne keloid. ICD-10-CM Code(s) _____

14. Nonpressure ulcer of the back with bone involvement without evidence of necrosis. ICD-10-CM Code(s) _____

15. Neurodermatitis. ICD-10-CM Code(s) _____

16. Bockhart's impetigo. ICD-10-CM Code(s) _____

17. Anetoderma of Jadassohn-Pellizzari. ICD-10-CM Code(s) _____

18. Nonbullous erythema multiforme with 45% skin exfoliation. ICD-10-CM Code(s) _____

19. Infantile acne. ICD-10-CM Code(s) _____

20. Vitiligo. ICD-10-CM Code(s) _____

21. Alopecia mucinosa. ICD-10-CM Code(s) _____

22. Onychogryphosis. ICD-10-CM Code(s) _____

23. Malignant melanoma in situ of the right upper eyelid. ICD-10-CM Code(s) _____

24. Postprocedural hemorrhage of skin following dermatologic procedure. ICD-10-CM Code(s) _____

25. Omphalitis in an adult. ICD-10-CM Code(s) _____

CODING CHALLENGE

Instructions: Read the mini-medical-record of each patient's encounter, then abstract, assign, and sequence ICD-10-CM diagnosis codes using the Index and Tabular List. Write the code(s) on the line provided.

1. OFFICE   Gender: F   Age: 27

Reason for encounter: Localized pain in the tail bone area

Assessment: Abscessed pilonidal cyst

Plan: Use depilatory cream and antibiotic, call office if symptoms do not subside

1 ICD-10-CM Code _____

2. OFFICE   Gender: F   Age: 3

Reason for admission: Body covered with blisters, child appears to be in pain

Assessment: Ritter's disease, involving 68 % of body surface

Plan: Rx pain medication, return to burn center for skin debridement

2 ICD-10-CM Codes _____

(continued)

(continued from page 175)

---

3. INPATIENT HOSPITAL   Gender: F   Age: 24

Reason for admission: Painful blisters on the skin and mucous membrane of the mouth

Assessment: Pemphigus vulgaris

Plan: Rx steroids, FU PCP 2 wk

1 ICD-10-CM Code _____

---

4. OFFICE   Gender: M   Age: 47

Reason for encounter: Referred by PCP for red, sore skin lesion

Assessment: Inflamed seborrheic keratosis

Plan: Local anesthetic provided and lesion removed, call office if any redness occurs

1 ICD-10-CM Code _____

---

5. OFFICE   Gender: M   Age: 89

Reason for encounter: Red open skin area in sacral region

Assessment: Pressure ulcer, stage 3, sacral region

Plan: Debrided wound and applied dressing. Refer to wound care clinic for FU.

1 ICD-10-CM Code _____

---

6. OFFICE   Gender: F   Age: 52

Reason for encounter: Redness on the central face across the cheeks, nose, and forehead

Assessment: Rosacea

Plan: Rx oral antibiotics. FU 6 weeks. Advised on diet and lifestyle changes to minimize symptoms.

1 ICD-10-CM Code _____

---

7. OUTPATIENT SURGERY   Gender: M   Age: 44

Reason for encounter: Repair of scar

Assessment: Keloid scar

Plan: Repaired scar, monitor for infection

1 ICD-10-CM Code _____

---

8. OFFICE   Gender: M   Age: 41

Reason for encounter: Swollen lump under skin in right armpit for 2 weeks, fever

Assessment: Carbuncle due to methicillin-susceptible Staphylococcus aureus (MSSA)

Plan: Antibiotic, call if no improvement within 1 week

2 ICD-10-CM Codes _____

---

9. INPATIENT HOSPITAL   Gender: F   Age: 70

Reason for admission: Swelling in left leg with apparent infection

Assessment: Cellulitis, left leg, Streptococcus A

Plan: Rx antibiotics, topical medication, call office if symptoms worsen after discharge

2 ICD-10-CM Codes _____

---

10. OFFICE   Gender: M   Age: 6 months

Reason for encounter: Mother is concerned about severe rash and blistering in child's perinanal area, hips, and buttocks that seems to be getting worse.

Assessment: Diaper dermatitis

Plan: Reviewed diaper hygiene. Rx ointment.

1 ICD-10-CM Code _____

Diseases of the Musculoskeletal System and Connective Tissue (M00-M99)

Chapter 11

Learning Objectives

After completing this chapter, you should have the skills to:

11.1 Spell and define the key words, medical terms, and abbreviations related to diseases of the musculoskeletal system and connective tissue. (Remember)

11.2 Summarize the structure, function, and common conditions of the musculoskeletal system. (Understand)

11.3 Adhere to the Official Guidelines for Coding and Reporting related to diseases of the musculoskeletal system and connective tissue. (Apply)

11.4 Examine and abstract information from the medical record required for coding diseases of the musculoskeletal system and connective tissue. (Analyze)

11.5 Demonstrate how to assign codes for diseases of the musculoskeletal system and connective tissue. (Apply)

11.6 Utilize guidelines for arranging (sequencing) multiple codes for diseases of the musculoskeletal system and connective tissue. (Apply)

11.7 Demonstrate how to abstract, assign, and sequence codes for neoplasms of the musculoskeletal system. (Apply)

Chapter Outline

- **Musculoskeletal System Refresher**
- **Coding Guidelines for the Musculoskeletal System**
- **Abstracting for Conditions of the Musculoskeletal System**
- **Assigning Codes for Conditions of the Musculoskeletal System**
- **Arranging Codes for Conditions of the Musculoskeletal System**
- **Coding Neoplasms of the Musculoskeletal System**

Key Terms and Abbreviations

appendicular skeleton	fatigue fracture	march fracture	pathologic fracture
axial skeleton	femur	metastatic bone disease (MBD)	proximal epiphysis
body	fragility fracture	muscular system	shaft
cartilage	insertion	musculoskeletal (MS) system	skeletal system
delayed	involuntary	neck	tendon
diaphysis	joint	nonunion	traumatic
distal epiphysis	ligament	origin	vertebra
fascia	malunion	osseous	voluntary

In addition to the key terms listed here, students should know the terms defined within tables in this chapter.

INTRODUCTION

Automotive engineers spend thousands of hours designing an amazing chassis that supports and protects you and also allows you to drive in comfort. In the human body, the musculoskeletal system is the chassis that everything else is built on.

Orthopedic physicians specialize in diagnosing and treating conditions of the musculoskeletal system. Orthopedic surgeons may be subspecialists in a particular anatomic site, such as the spine or the knee. Rheumatologists specialize in diagnosing and treating arthritis and other diseases of the joints, muscles, and bones. Physical therapists, or physiotherapists, are non-physician practitioners who hold a master's or doctorate degree and use various physical treatments and exercises to help patients with musculoskeletal conditions or injuries restore function, improve mobility, and reduce pain. Primary care physicians treat uncomplicated conditions of the musculoskeletal system. They refer patients in need of rehabilitation to physical therapists and refer patients with more complex conditions to orthopedic specialists.

As you read this chapter, open up your medical terminology book to the musculoskeletal system and keep a medical dictionary handy to refresh your memory of any unfamiliar terms. The musculoskeletal system has hundreds of structures with scientific names, and no one can remember all of them. Resources ensure that you have the information you need at your fingertips.

MUSCULOSKELETAL SYSTEM REFRESHER

The **musculoskeletal (MS) system** consists of the **skeletal system** and the **muscular system**. The function of the skeletal system is to support the body, protect internal organs, produce blood cells, store minerals, and serve as a point of attachment for the skeletal muscles. The function of the muscular system is to provide for movement of the body as well as the operation of individual organs, maintain body posture, and help produce heat.

Skeletal System

The skeletal system consists of 206 bones, as well as **cartilage** (*fibrous tissue found at the ends of bones*), **ligaments** (*fibrous tissue that connects bones to bones*), **tendons** (*fibrous tissue that connects bones to muscles*), and **fascia** (*fibrous tissue that connects muscle to muscle*). **Joints** are where two or more bones meet. The skeleton has two divisions: the axial skeleton and the appendicular skeleton (■ FIGURE 11-1). The **axial skeleton** contains 80 bones that are basically stationary and make up the skull, sternum, ribs, and **vertebrae** (*bony segments of the spine*). The **appendicular skeleton** contains 126 bones and consists of the arms, shoulders, wrists, hands, legs, hips, ankles, and feet.

Bones are also described by their shapes: long, short, flat, irregular, and sesamoid. Long bones comprise the arms and legs and have three major parts: the **proximal epiphysis**, the rounded end of the bone closest to the trunk; the **diaphysis** or **shaft**, the long narrow part of the bone; and the **distal epiphysis**, the rounded end of the bone furthest from the trunk. The area between the proximal epiphysis and the shaft is the **neck**. The **femur** (*thigh bone*) is an example of a long bone and is the largest bone in the body (■ FIGURE 11-2).

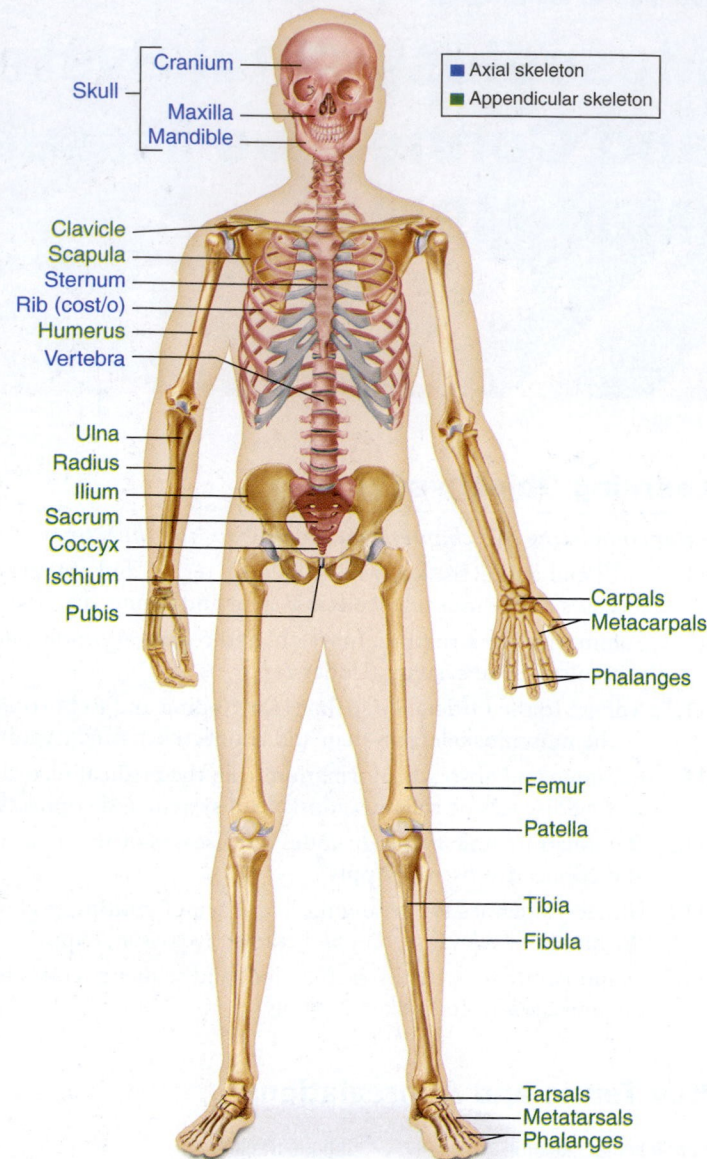

Figure 11-1 ■ The skeletal system.

Short bones are cubical in shape, being of nearly equal length and width. The carpals (*wrist bones*) and tarsals (*ankle bones*) are examples of short bones.

Flat bones are thin, broad, and usually curved. They consist of two parallel layers of compact bone with a layer of spongy bone in between, and they lack the marrow cavity. The ribs, scapulae (*shoulder blades*), and cranium are examples of flat bones.

Irregular bones, such as vertebrae and the ischium (*pelvic bone*), have complex notches and ridges. Sesamoid bones, such as the patella (*kneecap*), develop within a tendon where there is considerable pressure or tension.

Muscular System

The muscular system consists of 600 skeletal muscles that make movement and bodily processes possible (■ FIGURE 11-3). Muscles are classified as **voluntary** (*muscles a person can choose to contract and relax*) and **involuntary** (*muscles that are controlled by a subconscious part of the brain*). Voluntary muscles are attached to the skeleton and enable movement.

Involuntary muscles are in the organs and control bodily functions such as breathing, digestion, and the heartbeat. Muscles are named based on their location and function. Muscles have three distinct parts: the **origin**, where the muscle is fixed; the **body**, or main portion of the muscle; and the **insertion**, where the muscle attaches to a bone that moves.

Remember to apply medical terminology skills to combine word roots, prefixes, and suffixes you already know to define new terms related to the musculoskeletal system. Refer to ■ TABLE 11-1 (page 180) for a refresher on how to build medical terms related to the musculoskeletal system.

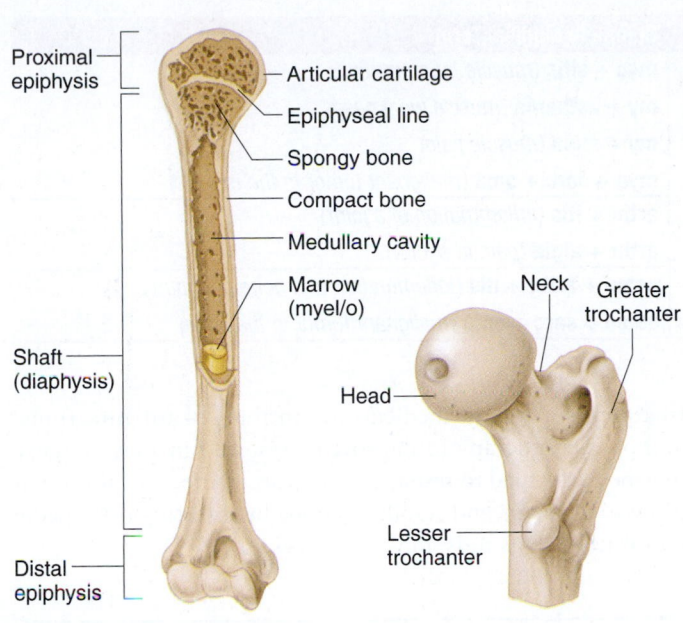

Figure 11-2 ■ The anatomy of a long bone.

> ### CODING CAUTION
> Remember to distinguish between medical terms with similar spellings but different meanings:
>
> **cost/o** (*rib*) and **chondr/o** (*cartilage*)
>
> **ilium** (*pelvic bone*) and **ileum** (*small intestine*)
>
> **my/o** (*muscle*) and **myel/o** (*bone marrow*)
>
> **sacr/o** (*sacrum, lowest part of back*) and **sarc/o** (*flesh, connective tissue*)

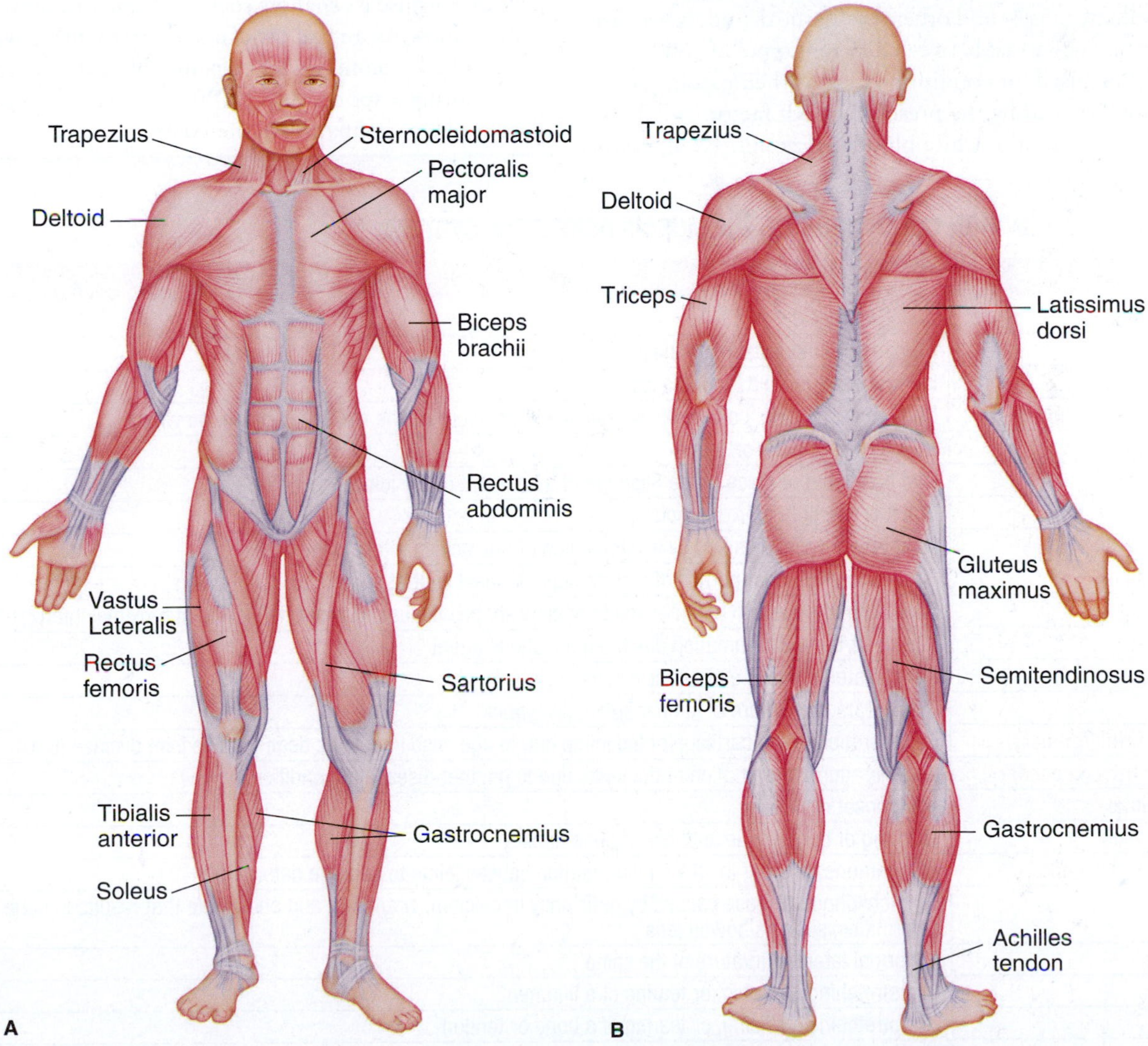

Labels for Figure 11-2:
Proximal epiphysis, Articular cartilage, Epiphyseal line, Spongy bone, Compact bone, Medullary cavity, Marrow (myel/o), Shaft (diaphysis), Distal epiphysis, Neck, Greater trochanter, Head, Lesser trochanter

Labels for Figure 11-3 A (anterior view):
Trapezius, Sternocleidomastoid, Pectoralis major, Deltoid, Biceps brachii, Rectus abdominis, Vastus Lateralis, Rectus femoris, Sartorius, Tibialis anterior, Gastrocnemius, Soleus

Labels for Figure 11-3 B (posterior view):
Trapezius, Deltoid, Triceps, Latissimus dorsi, Gluteus maximus, Biceps femoris, Semitendinosus, Gastrocnemius, Achilles tendon

A   B

Figure 11-3 ■ (A) Selected skeletal muscles (anterior view); (B) selected skeletal muscles and the Achilles tendon (posterior view).

Table 11-1 ■ **EXAMPLE OF CONSTRUCTING MEDICAL TERMS FOR THE MUSCULOSKELETAL SYSTEM**

Combining Form	Suffix	Complete Medical Term
my/o (muscle)		myo + sitis (muscle inflammation)
		my + asthenia (muscle weakness)
	-algia (pain)	my + algia (muscle pain)
	-asthenia (weakness)	myo + sarc + oma (malignant tumor in the muscle)
arthr/o (joint)	-itis (inflammation)	arthr + itis (inflammation of a joint)
	sarc + oma (malignant tumor)	arthr + algia (pain in a joint)
oste/o (bone)		osteo + arthr + itis (inflammation of a bone and joint)
		osteo + sarc + oma (malignant tumor in the bone)

Conditions of the Musculoskeletal System

Coders use medical resources, such as a reference book on diseases, to understand conditions of the musculoskeletal system, diagnostic methods, and common treatments. Common conditions of the musculoskeletal system are highlighted in ■ TABLE 11-2. Conditions are diagnosed through physical examination, imaging, biopsy, and lab tests. X-rays are used to evaluate conditions of the bone because they clearly show the difference between hard tissue and soft tissue. Computerized tomography (CT) and magnetic resonance imaging (MRI) are used to evaluate muscle and other soft-tissue disorders because they show more contrast between different types of soft tissue. Blood tests are used for conditions such as rheumatoid arthritis, which is detected by the presence of Rh factor, and infections, which elevate the white blood cell count. Noninvasive treatments are pain medication, antibiotics for infections, and physical therapy to improve or restore function. Surgery may be performed to reshape a structure, remove an abnormal growth, or repair and stabilize a bone by inserting orthopedic hardware such as rods, pins, or screws.

SUCCESS STEP

The shoulder is the most frequently dislocated joint in the body because its shallow socket allows it to move in many directions. As a result, it can slip out of place when force is applied. You may have seen an athlete dislocate a shoulder during a sporting event, "pop" it back into place, and continue participating in the event.

Table 11-2 ■ **COMMON CONDITIONS OF THE MUSCULOSKELETAL SYSTEM**

Condition	Description
Skeletal System	
Arthritis	Damage or inflammation of the joints
Bursitis	Inflammation of fluid around a joint
Carpal tunnel syndrome	Numbness, tingling, pain, or weakness due to pressure on the median nerve in the wrist
Degeneration	Breakdown of bone or tissue
Dislocation	Two bones out of place at the Slippage of a bone out of the joint
Fracture	Crack or break in a broken bone
Gout, gouty arthritis	Joint inflammation caused by accumulation of uric acid crystals in the joint
Hallux vagas	Enlargement of inner portion of metatarsophalangeal joint at base of big toe; bunion
Hammertoe	Bending of the toe into hammer shape or claw shape because of abnormal flexion of proximal interphalangeal joint
Infection	Muscle or bone inflammation due to an infectious agent
Kyphosis	Exaggerated curvature of thoracic spine
Lordosis	Exaggerated curvature of lumbar spine; swayback
Osteoarthritis (primary)	Degeneration of the cartilage of the joints due to age; also known as degenerative joint disease (DJD)
Osteoarthritis (secondary)	Degeneration/inflammation of the joints due to another disease or condition
Osteomalacia	Adult onset of rickets
Osteoporosis	Thinning of bone tissue and loss of bone density
Rheumatoid arthritis	Autoimmune disorder in which inflammation causes joints to become deformed
Rickets	Early childhood disease caused by deficiency in calcium, vitamin D, and phosphate that results in bone deformities, such as bowed legs
Scoliosis	Abnormal lateral curvature of the spine
Sprain	Overstretching, bruising, or tearing of a ligament
Strain	Overstretching, bruising, or tearing of a bone or tendon
Subluxation	Partial dislocation of bones in a joint

Table 11-2 ■ *(continued)*

Condition	Description
Muscular System	
Fibromyalgia	A collection of symptoms of musculoskeletal pain and fatigue
Ganglion cyst	Benign saclike swelling or cyst that typically develops over a joint or tendon
Muscular dystrophy	A genetic disease that progressively weakens and causes degeneration of skeletal muscles
Myasthenia gravis	A chronic autoimmune neuromuscular disease that causes muscle weakness of the voluntary muscles
Rotator cuff tear	Damage to shoulder muscles and tendons from overuse or traumatic injury
Sprain	Overstretching, bruising, or tearing of a ligament
Strain	Overstretching, bruising, or tearing of a bone or tendon
Tendonitis	Inflammation of a tendon, often caused by overuse
Tetanus	An infectious disease caused by the bacterium *Clostridium tetani* that enters the body through a puncture or open wound and releases a toxin that affects the motor nerves which stimulate the muscles

CODING PRACTICE

Exercise 11.1   Musculoskeletal System Refresher

Instructions: Use your medical terminology skills and resources to define the following conditions related to the musculoskeletal system, then assign the diagnosis code.

Follow these steps:

- Use slash marks "/" to break down each term into its root(s) and suffix.
- Define the meaning of the word, based on the meaning of each word part.
- Assign the default ICD-10-CM diagnosis code for the condition using the Index and Tabular List.

Example: arthritis arthr/itis   Meaning *inflammation of a joint*   ICD-10-CM Code <u>M19.90</u>

1. arthropathy   Meaning _____   ICD-10-CM Code _____

2. osteomyelitis   Meaning _____   ICD-10-CM Code _____

3. fibromyalgia   Meaning _____   ICD-10-CM Code _____

4. lordosis   Meaning _____   ICD-10-CM Code _____

5. chondrocalcinosis   Meaning _____   ICD-10-CM Code _____

6. spondylolisthesis   Meaning _____   ICD-10-CM Code _____

7. chondromalacia   Meaning _____   ICD-10-CM Code _____

8. osteolysis   Meaning _____   ICD-10-CM Code _____

9. tenosynovitis   Meaning _____   ICD-10-CM Code _____

10. fasciitis   Meaning _____   ICD-10-CM Code _____

CODING GUIDELINES FOR THE MUSCULOSKELETAL SYSTEM

Coders should understand the organization of this ICD-10-CM chapter, chapter-wide and commonly used instructional notes in the Tabular List, and the relevant OGCR. This information is necessary for accurate coding.

ICD-10-CM Chapter 13, "Diseases of the Musculoskeletal System and Connective Tissue (M00-M99)," contains 18 blocks or subchapters that are divided by type of condition and type of tissue. Review the block names and code ranges listed at the beginning of Chapter 13 in the ICD-10-CM manual to become familiar with the content and organization.

This chapter includes chronic or recurrent conditions of the joint, bone, and soft tissue, including those of the jaw. It does not include codes for **traumatic** (*acute current injury that results from an accident*) fractures, injuries, congenital and perinatal conditions, neoplasms, or symptoms and signs, which are classified in other ICD-10-CM chapters. Review the **Excludes2** note at the beginning of the chapter to cross-reference the locations of these codes. Most codes require characters for laterality, specificity of site, and/or episode of care. Instructional notes in the ICD-10-CM Tabular List direct coders to assign additional codes for underlying and associated conditions. Osteoporosis codes include options for with and without a current pathological fracture.

ICD-10-CM provides Official Guidelines for Coding and Reporting (OGCR) for the musculoskeletal system in OGCR section I.C.13. OGCR discusses coding for site and laterality, acute traumatic versus chronic or recurrent musculoskeletal conditions, pathologic fractures, and osteoporosis. Additional OGCR related to conditions of the musculoskeletal system appear in OGCR I.C.19 and I.C.20. Specific OGCR guidelines are discussed and cited throughout this chapter of the text.

ABSTRACTING FOR CONDITIONS OF THE MUSCULOSKELETAL SYSTEM

The keys to abstracting diagnoses for the musculoskeletal system are familiarity with the anatomy, knowledge of medical terms, and careful attention to the details of the documented condition. ■ TABLE 11-3 highlights key questions to ask when abstracting musculoskeletal conditions. Pathologic fractures require additional abstracting, shown in ■ TABLE 11-4. Remember that abstracting questions are a general guide and all questions may not apply to every patient. For example, not all conditions have laterality. When there is a traumatic injury, also abstract the external cause.

Guided Example of Abstracting Diagnoses for the Musculoskeletal System

Refer to the following example throughout this chapter to learn skills for abstracting and assigning codes for conditions affecting the musculoskeletal system. Jacob Bates, CCS, is a fictitious coder who guides you through this case.

Follow along as Jacob Bates, CCS, abstracts the diagnosis. Check off each step after you complete it.

▶ Jacob reads through the entire record, paying special attention to the reason for the admission and the discharge plan.

Date: 3/1/yy   Location: Valley Hospital

Provider: Bruce Prentice, MD

Patient: Nadine Tubbs Gender: F Age: 80

Reason for admission: Admitted from physician office where she was seen for hip pain. X-rays showed fracture.

Procedure performed: Repair of fracture with a metal rod

Discharge plan: Pathologic fracture of right femoral neck due to osteoporosis. Referred to rehab for 6 weeks.

He refers to the Key Criteria for Abstracting Pathologic Fractures (Table 11-4).

❑ *Is the fracture traumatic or pathologic?* Pathologic

❑ *What is the underlying disease?* Osteoporosis

❑ *What bone is fractured?* Femur

❑ *What site on the bone is fractured?* Neck

❑ *What is the laterality?* Right

❑ *Is the encounter for active treatment?* Yes, the episode of care is the initial encounter because the fracture was repaired and there is no mention of previous treatment for it

❑ Jacob will not abstract pain because pain is a symptom integral to the condition.

▶ Jacob has completed abstracting. Next, he will assign the codes.

Table 11-3 ■ **KEY CRITERIA FOR ABSTRACTING MUSCULOSKELETAL CONDITIONS**

❑ What type of condition is documented: fracture, dislocation, subluxation, sprain, infection, inflammation, or degeneration?

❑ What type of tissue or structure is affected: bone, joint, cartilage, muscle, tendon, or ligament?

❑ What is the specific subtype of condition (e.g., osteoarthritis vs. rheumatoid arthritis)?

❑ What is the anatomic site?

❑ What is the laterality?

❑ For osteoporosis: Does the patient have a pathologic fracture? Does the patient have a history of healed pathologic fractures?

❑ Is the condition acute, chronic, or a late effect?

❑ Is the encounter for active treatment?

❑ Is the encounter for aftercare during the healing phase?

❑ Is the encounter for follow-up after active healing is complete?

Table 11-4 ■ **KEY CRITERIA FOR ABSTRACTING PATHOLOGIC FRACTURES**

❑ Is the fracture traumatic or pathologic?

❑ What type of pathologic fracture is it?

❑ What is the underlying disease?

❑ What bone is fractured?

❑ What is the laterality?

❑ Were any additional bones fractured?

❑ Is the healing routine, **delayed** (*patient waited to seek care*), **nonunion** (*failure of the ends of the fractured bone segments to reunite*), or **malunion** (*ends of fractured bone segments did not heal with proper alignment*)?

❑ Is the encounter for active treatment?

❑ Is the encounter for aftercare during the healing phase?

❑ Is the encounter for follow-up after active healing is complete?

CODING PRACTICE

Exercise 11.2 Abstracting for Conditions of the Musculoskeletal System

Instructions: Read the mini-medical-record of each patient's encounter and answer the abstracting questions. Write the answer on the line provided. Do not assign any codes.

1. OFFICE Gender: F Age: 48

Chief complaint: Patient came in for management of fibromyalgia which was diagnosed last year. C/o increased pain in lower back and hips.

Assessment: Fibromyalgia

Plan: Refer to physical therapy for modified exercise program and pain relief. Adjusted medication.

a. What are the presenting symptoms? _____

_____

b. What is the underlying condition? _____

_____

c. Should you code the symptoms? _____

Why or why not? _____

_____

d. Should you code an encounter for physical therapy?

_____

Why or why not? _____

_____

2. OFFICE Gender: F Age: 66

Reason for encounter: Management and monitoring of osteoarthritis

Assessment: Degenerative osteoarthritis of the right knee

a. What type of arthritis does the patient have?

_____

b. What is the anatomic site? _____

_____

c. What is the laterality? _____

_____

d. Is the arthritis described as generalized? _____

_____

e. Is the arthritis posttraumatic? _____

_____

3. OFFICE Gender: M Age: 72

Chief complaint: Acute hip pain

Assessment: X-rays show a fracture of the ilium due to age-related osteoporosis

a. What is the presenting symptom? _____

_____

b. What is the diagnosis of the cause of the pain?

_____

c. What is the underlying condition? _____

_____

d. What type of fracture is this? _____

_____

e. Should the symptom be coded? _____

Why or why not? _____

_____

4. OUTPATIENT SURGERY Gender: M Age: 56

Reason for encounter: Vertebroplasty (*injection of acrylic cement into a fractured vertebra to stabilize it*) to correct compression fracture

Assessment: Collapsed vertebrae L3 and L4 due to bone metastasis from prostate cancer

a. What procedure was performed? _____

_____

b. What is the reason for the procedure? _____

_____

c. What is the anatomic site? _____

_____

d. What type of fracture is this? _____

_____

e. What additional diagnoses exist? _____

_____

f. What is the principal diagnosis? _____

_____

g. What is the second diagnosis? _____

_____

h. What is the third diagnosis? _____

_____

CODING PRACTICE (continued)

---

5. OFFICE Gender: M Age: 36

Reason for encounter: Left knee pain

Assessment: Chronic knee derangement due to an old injury of the anterior horn of the medial meniscus. Injury was sustained during a tackle in a college football game 15 years ago.

a. What is the symptom? _____
_____

b. Should you code the symptom? _____
   Why or why not? _____
_____

c. What is the episode of care? _____
_____

d. What is the site within the knee where the original injury occurred? _____
_____

e. What is the laterality? _____
_____

f. What external cause event caused the injury? _____
_____

g. Should you code for the activity? _____
   Why or why not? _____
_____

---

6. OFFICE Gender: F Age: 70

Reason for encounter: Follow-up on test results after complaints of hand pain

Assessment: Elevated WBC count, calcification evident on x-rays. Arthritis in crystal arthropathy (*presence of calcification within soft tissues*) of the right hand due to dicalcium phosphate crystals. Patient previously diagnosed with primary hyperparathyroidism which is associated with this condition.

Plan: Corticosteroid injection, RTO 4 wk

a. What condition is newly diagnosed? _____
_____

b. What is the cause of the condition? _____
_____

c. What is the anatomic site? _____
_____

d. What is the laterality? _____
_____

e. What is the previously existing condition? _____
_____

f. Should the previously existing condition be coded?
_____
   Why or why not? _____

ASSIGNING CODES FOR CONDITIONS OF THE MUSCULOSKELETAL SYSTEM

Assigning codes for musculoskeletal disorders may require coders to cross-reference the medical record multiple times to accurately capture the details of the disorder. This serves as a cross-check for abstracting because it is easy to overlook one or more details. Coders may not know exactly what information is required until they assign the code, review the subterms in the Index, and read the instructional notes in the Tabular List. In addition, careful attention to the spelling of medical terms is necessary to locate the correct term in the Index. Conventions in the Index and Tabular List indicate when multiple coding is required for infections, underlying conditions, and complications. The Tabular List conventions also notify coders when a seventh character is required and what the seventh-character choices are for any given code.

Most of the codes within Chapter 13 have site and laterality designations. The site represents the bone, joint, or muscle involved. For some conditions where more than one bone, joint, or muscle is usually involved in the same type of injury, the Index provides a combination for multiple sites available (OGCR I.C.13.a) (■ FIGURE 11-4).

For some conditions, such as **avascular necrosis of bone** and osteoporosis, the bone may be affected at the upper or lower end. Although the portion of the bone affected may be

at the joint, code the site as the bone, not the joint (OGCR I.C.13.a.1) (■ FIGURE 11-5). Code the joint when the joint capsule itself is affected, as in arthritis.

Recurrent and Chronic Conditions

Some musculoskeletal conditions, such as dislocations and fractures, can result from an acute injury or be a pathological, recurrent, or chronic condition. These various types of conditions are coded differently. Musculoskeletal conditions that are chronic or recurrent are usually assigned a code from this ICD-10-CM chapter (OGCR I.13.b). To locate codes for a pathological, recurrent, or chronic musculoskeletal condition, follow these steps:

1. Search the Index for the Main Term that describes the condition, such as **fracture** or **dislocation**.

2. Locate a subterm for **pathological**, **recurrent**, or **chronic**.

3. Locate a subterm for the anatomic site, such as **hip** or **shoulder**.

4. Verify the code in the Tabular List and assign any additional characters.

When the same type of condition is an acute injury, it should be coded from ICD-10-CM Chapter 19, "Injury, Poisoning and Certain Other Consequences of External Causes (S00-T88)." To locate codes for an acute injury, search the Index for the

Patient has osteochondropathy of ankles, knees, and hip.

Osteochondropathy M93.90
  ankle M93.97-
  elbow M93.92-
  foot M93.97-
  hand M93.94-
  hip M93.95-
  Kienböck's disease of adults M93.1
  knee M93.96-
  multiple joints M93.99

Figure 11-4 ■ Example of a combination code for multiple sites.

Patient has avascular necrosis at the proximal epiphysis of the left radius.

Index:
Necrosis, bone *see also* **Osteonecrosis**
Osteonecrosis, idiopathic aseptic, radius M87.03-
Tabular List:
M87.032 Idiopathic aseptic necrosis of left radius

Figure 11-5 ■ Example of coding the site as bone, not joint.

Main Term that describes the condition, such as **fracture** or **dislocation**, then go directly to the subterm for the anatomic site, such as **hip** or **shoulder**. This leads to the code(s) for the acute injury rather than a chronic condition. Verify the code in the Tabular List and assign any additional characters.

It is essential to verify the code in the Tabular List to ensure that you have located the code for correct type of condition: acute/injury or chronic/recurrent/pathological.

EXAMPLE: *A patient is seen for recurrent dislocation of the left hip.*
This is classified as a recurrent dislocation. Search the Index for the Main Term **Dislocation**. Then locate the subterm **recurrent**. Under recurrent, locate the subterm **hip M24.45-**. Verify the code in the Tabular List and assign the sixth character for laterality: **M24.452 Recurrent dislocation, left hip.**

EXAMPLE: *A patient is seen for dislocation of the left hip due to a fall that happened today.*
This is classified as an acute dislocation. Search the Index for the Main Term **Dislocation**. Then locate the subterm **hip S73.00-**. Verify the code in the Tabular List and assign the sixth character for laterality: **S73.005A Unspecified dislocation of left hip, initial encounter.** Also assign external cause codes for the fall.

SUCCESS STEP

It is common to encounter terms you may be unfamiliar with when coding the musculoskeletal system because there are 206 bones and 600 muscles. A quick check in a medical terminology or anatomy book will help identify the correct site and structure to avoid confusion.

Guided Example of Assigning Musculoskeletal System Diagnosis Codes

Continue with the example from earlier in the chapter about patient Nadine Tubbs, who was admitted to Valley Hospital because of a pathologic fracture, to practice skills for assigning codes for the musculoskeletal system.

Follow along in your ICD-10-CM manual as Jacob Bates, CCS, assigns codes. Check off each step after you complete it.

▶ First, Jacob confirms that the diagnosis is pathologic fracture of the right femoral neck due to osteoporosis.

❏ Jacob searches the Index for the Main Term **Fracture, pathological**. He notes that this is a separate Main Term from **Fracture, traumatic**.

❏ He locates the subterm **due to**.

❏ He locates the second-level subterm **osteoporosis M80.00**.

❏ He notes that there are no further subterms for anatomic site.

❏ However, he does notice a cross-reference for **postmenopausal see Osteoporosis, postmenopausal, with pathological fracture**.

❏ He cross-references the Main Term **Osteoporosis** and the subterm **postmenopausal**.

❏ Now he sees a second-level subterm **with pathological fracture**.

❏ Under this entry he notices no entry for femur, but does see additional subterms for **ilium, ischium**, and **pelvis**, all of which point to **M80.05**. He decides to research this option because these bones are adjacent to the femoral joint and he knows that the ICD-10-CM often classifies them together.

❏ Jacob must follow the cross-reference **Osteoporosis, postmenopausal, with pathological fracture**, or he will select an incorrect code: **M80.00 Age-related osteoporosis with current pathological fracture, unspecified site**. If he does get to code **M80.00**, the words **unspecified site** in the code description should be a red flag and cause him to either return to the Index or review the Tabular List to locate a more specific code for the **femur**.

▶ Jacob verifies code **pelvis M80.05** in the Tabular List.

❏ He reads the code title for **M80.05 Age-related osteoporosis with current pathological fracture, femur** and confirms that this accurately describes the principal diagnosis and identifies the anatomic site of the femur.

❏ Jacob looks for any conventions or instructional notes with the code.

❏ He notices the symbol **6th** that directs him to use a sixth character with **M80.05** for laterality.

❏ He double-checks the medical record to verify the laterality as **right**.

❏ The code for right femur is **M80.051**.

❏ He notices the symbol **7th** that tells him a seventh character is required with **M80.051**.

❏ He refers to the beginning of category **M80** to locate the seventh character.

❏ He selects the seventh character **A, initial encounter** because the episode of care is for active treatment. Even though the patient was previously seen in the physician's office, there active treatment is provided, so seventh character **A** is required.

❏ Jacob verifies that the complete code is **M80.051A**.

▶ Jacob checks for any additional instructional notes in the Tabular List.

❏ Since he is already at the beginning of the three-digit category, he reviews the notes that appear, including the definition of a fragility fracture.

❏ He reviews the note **Use additional code to identify major osseous defect, if applicable** and double-checks the medical record to be certain no defects are documented.

❏ He also double-checks the medical record to see whether there is a personal history of a (healed) osteoporosis fracture, which there is not. If there were, he would need to assign code **Z87.310** for the history.

❏ He cross-references the beginning of the block **M80-M94** and verifies that there are no instructional notes.

❏ He cross-references the beginning of **Chapter 12 (M00-M99)** and reviews the instructional notes. He determines he does not need to assign an external cause code because the patient's fracture was not due to an external cause, but was due to a disease.

▶ Jacob finalizes the code for this case:

❏ **M80.051A Age-related osteoporosis with current pathological fracture, right femur, initial encounter.**

CODING PRACTICE

Exercise 11.3   Assigning Codes for Conditions of the Musculoskeletal System

Instructions: Read the mini-medical-record of each patient's encounter, review the information abstracted in Exercise 11.2, and assign ICD-10-CM diagnosis codes using the Index and Tabular List. Write the code(s) on the line provided.

---

1. OFFICE   Gender: F   Age: 48

Chief complaint: Patient came in for management of fibromyalgia which was diagnosed last year. C/o increased pain in lower back and hips.

Assessment: Fibromyalgia

Plan: Refer to physical therapy for modified exercise program and pain relief. Adjusted medication.

1 ICD-10-CM Code _____

---

2. OFFICE   Gender: F   Age: 66

Reason for encounter: Management and monitoring of osteoarthritis

Assessment: Degenerative osteoarthritis of the right knee

1 ICD-10-CM Code _____

---

3. OFFICE   Gender: M   Age: 72

Chief complaint: Acute hip pain

Assessment: X-rays show a fracture of the ilium due to age-related osteoporosis

Tip: The ilium is classified with the femur in the Tabular List, so both sites are included in the code title, but only one of the sites must be documented to use the code.

1 ICD-10-CM Code _____

ARRANGING CODES FOR CONDITIONS OF THE MUSCULOSKELETAL SYSTEM

When musculoskeletal disorders require multiple coding, coders must be attentive to the sequencing indicated in the instructional notes. Examples of the most commonly encountered situations are discussed next—including pathologic fracture, infectious conditions, osseous defects, and external causes—followed by a new guided example for arranging codes.

Pathologic Fractures

Pathologic fractures, also called fragility fractures, are fractures caused by disease rather than trauma (OGCR I.C.13.d.2). They result from a fall from a standing height or less and would not cause a fracture in a normal healthy bone. ICD-10-CM classifies four types of pathologic fractures and provides instructional notes for sequencing codes (■ TABLE 11-5).

Infectious Conditions

Infectious conditions, such as pyogenic arthritis and myositis, require coders to use an additional code for the infectious agent (■ FIGURE 11-6).

Osseous Defects

Pathologic fractures, osteomyelitis, and osteonecrosis require coders to use an additional code to describe any major bone defects. Pathologic fractures also require an additional code for a history of healed pathologic fractures (■ FIGURE 11-7).

Table 11-5 ■ **DEFINITIONS AND SEQUENCING INSTRUCTIONS FOR PATHOLOGIC FRACTURES**

Type of Fracture	Definition	Instructional Note
Osteoporotic	A fragility fracture in a person with osteoporosis.	Use additional code to identify major osseous (*bone*) defect, if applicable (M89.7-).
		Use additional code to identify personal history of (healed) osteoporosis fracture, if applicable (Z87.310).
Neoplastic	A fragility fracture due to neoplastic disease.	Code also underlying neoplasm.
Stress	Fracture of a bone that has been subjected to repeated use or impact. Also called a **march fracture** or **fatigue fracture**.	Use additional external cause code(s) to identify the cause of the stress fracture.
Other	A fragility fracture caused by a disease other than osteoporosis or neoplasm. Any other type of pathological fracture.	Code also underlying condition.

Patient is seen for pyogenic arthritis in the right elbow due to methicillin-susceptible Staphylococcus aureus.

(1) **M00.021 Staphylococcal arthritis, right elbow**
(2) **B95.61 Methicillin susceptible staphylococcus aureus as the cause of diseases classified elsewhere**

Figure 11-6 ■ Example of sequencing codes for an infectious condition.

Patient is seen for chronic osteomyelitis of left scapula due to methicillin-susceptible Staphylococcus aureus with major osseous defect.

(1) **M86.612 Other chronic osteomyelitis, left shoulder**
(2) **B95.61 Methicillin susceptible staphylococcus aureus as the cause of diseases classified elsewhere**
(3) **M89.712 Major osseous defect, left shoulder region**

Figure 11-7 ■ Example of sequencing codes for osseous defects.

External Cause

Stress fractures and soft-tissue disorders, which are caused by overuse or pressure, require coders to assign and sequence an external cause code as a secondary code. In many cases, the only external cause code will be an activity code because there is not an applicable event code. This is an exception to the general rule that requires that activity codes be assigned only in conjunction with external cause event codes (■ FIGURE 11-8, page 188).

Multiple Sites

Earlier in the chapter, Figure 11-3 demonstrated how to assign a combination code for multiple sites, rather than coding each site separately, when more than one bone, joint, or muscle is involved. Not all categories provide a combination code for multiple sites. When the Index does not provide a code for multiple sites, assign separate codes to indicate each of the sites involved, as shown in ■ FIGURE 11-9, (page 188) (OGCR I.C.13.a). When each site is equally responsible for the encounter, sequence any of the codes first (OGCR II.C and IV).

SUCCESS STEP

When the Index does not provide a subterm for **multiple sites**, also review the Tabular List entries to be certain that no code for multiple sites exists. In some cases, a multiple site code exists in the Tabular List even though it is not listed as a subterm in the Index. The code for **multiple sites** usually appears at the end of a category and ends in the number **8**.

Guided Example of Arranging Codes for the Musculoskeletal System

Refer to the following example to learn skills for arranging codes for conditions affecting the musculoskeletal system. Jacob Bates, CCS, is a fictitious coder who guides you through this case.

Date: 3/1/yy   Location: Valley Hospital

Provider: Bruce Prentice, MD

Patient: Nicholas Taylor   Gender: M   Age: 8

Reason for admission: Chronic recurrent multifocal hematogenous osteomyelitis due to methicillin-resistant Staphylococcus aureus (MRSA) with major osseous defect of the fibula

Procedure performed: Repair of major osseous defect of right fibula

Follow along as Jacob Bates, CCS, abstracts, assigns, and arranges the codes. Check off each step after you complete it.

▶ Jacob follows the abstracting criteria and identifies major osseous defect of the right fibula as the reason for the procedure.

❏ The osseous defect is due to chronic recurrent multifocal hematogenous osteomyelitis, a condition associated with children where it tends to occur in the rapidly growing and highly vascular metaphysis of growing bones.

❏ The associated infectious organism is methicillin-resistant *Staphylococcus aureus*.

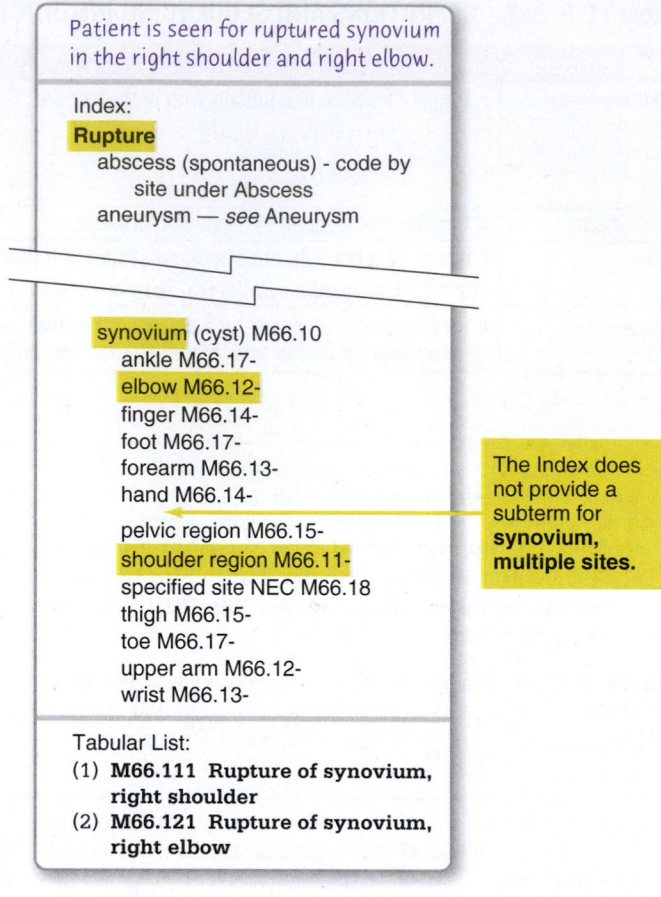

Patient is seen for tendonitis of the left forearm due to overuse in baseball.

Index Entry for Main Term, Tendonitis:
Tendinitis, tendonitis — *see also* Enthesopathy
   Achilles M76.6-

     due to use, overuse, pressure — *see also* Disorder, soft tissue, due to use
      specified NEC — *see* Disorder, soft tissue, due to use, specified NEC

Index Entry for Cross-referenced Main Term, Disorder:
Disorder
  soft tissue M79.9
    ankle M79.9
    due to use, overuse and pressure M70.90
      ankle M70.97-
      bursitis — *see* Bursitis
      foot M70.97-
      forearm M70.93-
      hand M70.94-
      lower leg M70.96-

Tabular List for Category M70:
    Other soft tissue disorders (M70-M79)
M70 Soft tissue disorders related to use, overuse and pressure
    Includes: soft tissue disorders of occupational origin
    Use additional external cause code to identify activity causing disorder (Y93.-)

Final Code Assignment and Sequencing:
(1) **M70.932 Unspecified soft tissue disorder related to use, overuse and pressure, left forearm**
(2) **Y93.64 Activity, baseball**

Figure 11-8 ■ Example of sequencing codes for external causes.

Patient is seen for ruptured synovium in the right shoulder and right elbow.

Index:
Rupture
  abscess (spontaneous) - code by site under Abscess
  aneurysm — *see* Aneurysm

  synovium (cyst) M66.10
    ankle M66.17-
    elbow M66.12-
    finger M66.14-
    foot M66.17-
    forearm M66.13-
    hand M66.14-
    pelvic region M66.15-
    shoulder region M66.11-
    specified site NEC M66.18
    thigh M66.15-
    toe M66.17-
    upper arm M66.12-
    wrist M66.13-

The Index does not provide a subterm for **synovium, multiple sites.**

Tabular List:
(1) **M66.111 Rupture of synovium, right shoulder**
(2) **M66.121 Rupture of synovium, right elbow**

Figure 11-9 ■ Example of assigning separate codes for multiple sites.

► Jacob assigns the following codes:

❑ **M89.761 Major osseous defect, right lower leg**. He locates the code by searching the Index for the Main Term **Defect** and the subterms **osseous, major** and **fibula**. In the Tabular List he assigns the sixth character **1** to identify the right side.

❑ **M86.361 Chronic multifocal osteomyelitis, right tibia and fibula**. He locates the code by searching the Index for the Main Term **Osteomyelitis** and the subterms **chronic, hematogenous,** and **fibula**. In the Tabular List he assigns the sixth character **1** to identify the right side.

❑ **B95.62 Methicillin resistant Staphylococcus aureus infection as the cause of diseases classified elsewhere.**

► Jacob reviews the instructional notes in the Tabular List to determine how to sequence the codes. There are no OGCR that apply to these conditions.

❑ The instructional notes at the beginning of subcategory M89.7 state **Code first underlying disease, if known, such as:...osteomyelitis (M86.-).**

❑ The instructional notes at the beginning of category **M86** state **Use additional code (B95-B97) to identify infectious agent. Use additional code to identify major osseous defect, if applicable (M89.7-).** He reads the **Excludes1** and **Excludes2** notes and determines that they do not list any of the conditions in this case.

❑ Together these notes identify that **M86.361** for osteomyelitis should be sequenced first, even though the immediate reason for the admission was to repair the major osseous defect. Specific direction is not provided regarding the sequencing of the second and third codes, so he lists **M89.761** second since the major osseous defect was the immediate reason for the procedure.

► Jacob finalizes the codes and sequencing for this case:

(1) **M86.361 Chronic multifocal osteomyelitis, right tibia and fibula**

(2) **M89.761 Major osseous defect, right lower leg**

(3) **B95.62 Methicillin resistant Staphylococcus aureus infection as the cause of diseases classified elsewhere**

CODING PRACTICE

Exercise 11.4 Arranging Codes for Conditions of the Musculoskeletal System

Instructions: Read the mini-medical-record of each patient's encounter, review the information abstracted in Exercise 11.2, assign ICD-10-CM diagnosis codes using the Index and Tabular List, and sequence them correctly.

1. OUTPATIENT SURGERY   Gender: M   Age: 56

Reason for encounter: Vertebroplasty *(injection of acrylic cement into a fractured vertebra to stabilize it)* to correct compression fracture

Assessment: Collapsed vertebrae L3 and L4 due to bone metastasis from prostate cancer

Tip: The reason for the vertebroplasty is the principal diagnosis. Sequence metastasis second because it caused the compression fracture. Sequence the primary neoplasm third.

3 ICD-10-CM Codes _____

_____

2. OFFICE   Gender: M   Age: 36

Reason for encounter: Left knee pain

Assessment: Chronic knee derangement due to an old injury of the anterior horn of the medial meniscus. Injury was sustained during a tackle in a college football game 15 years ago.

Tip: An "old injury" is a sequela. Use the Index of External Causes to locate the external cause (event) code.

2 ICD-10-CM Codes _____

3. OFFICE   Gender: F   Age: 70

Reason for encounter: Follow-up on test results after complaints of hand pain

Assessment: Elevated WBC count, calcification evident on x-ray.

Impression: arthritis in crystal arthropathy *(presence of crystal-like deposits in the joints)* of the right hand due to dicalcium phosphate crystals. Patient previously diagnosed with primary hyperparathyroidism which is associated with this condition.

Plan: Corticosteroid injection, RTO 4 wk

Tip: The Main Term can be either *Arthritis* or *Arthropathy*.

2 ICD-10-CM Codes _____

CODING NEOPLASMS OF THE MUSCULOSKELETAL SYSTEM

Neoplasms of the musculoskeletal system do not appear in ICD-10-CM Chapter 12, "Diseases of the Musculoskeletal System and Connective Tissue (M00-M99)." Codes for neoplasms of the musculoskeletal system appear in the block C40-C41 within the neoplasm chapter. Codes for leukemia, which originates in the bone marrow, appear in categories C90-C96.

The most common cancer in the musculoskeletal system is **metastatic bone disease (MBD)** because the bone is a frequent site of metastasis from primary neoplasms in other organs, including the breast, lung, prostate, kidney, and thyroid. According to the American Academy of Orthopaedic Surgeons, approximately 50% of tumors can metastasize to the bone.

Cancer that begins in the bone is called primary bone cancer, or sarcoma, and is named after the specific type of tissue in which it originates, such as osteosarcoma (*sarcoma of bone*) or chondrosarcoma (*sarcoma of cartilage*). Ewing's sarcoma forms in the shaft of long bones, the hip, and ribs. Children and young people are more likely than adults to have bone cancers. Soft-tissue sarcomas are relatively rare but are quite aggressive and dangerous, particularly when they occur in adults.

Leukemia is a cancer that starts in the bone marrow and affects the cells that form new blood cells. About one-third of childhood cancers are leukemias, the most common of which is acute lymphoblastic (lymphocytic) leukemia, according to the American Cancer Society.

All malignant neoplasms in the musculoskeletal system are either primary or secondary. CA in situ does not occur because bone and connective tissue do not have the epithelial cells that give rise to CA in situ.

CODING PRACTICE

Exercise 11.5 Coding Neoplasms of the Musculoskeletal System

Instructions: Read the mini-medical-record of each patient's encounter, then abstract, assign, and sequence ICD-10-CM diagnosis codes using the Index and Tabular List. Write the code(s) on the line provided.

1. INPATIENT HOSPITAL Gender: M Age: 14

Reason for admission: Surgical removal of tumor

Assessment: Osteosarcoma in the right tibia

1 ICD-10-CM Code _____

2. INPATIENT HOSPITAL Gender: F Age: 48

Reason for encounter: Pain management for MBD

Assessment: Left breast cancer with metastasis to bone

Tip: The code for neoplasm-related pain may be assigned as the principal or first-listed code when the stated reason for the admission/encounter is documented as pain control/pain management. The underlying neoplasm should be reported as an additional diagnosis (OGCR I.C.6.b.5).

3 ICD-10-CM Codes _____

_____

3. INPATIENT HOSPITAL Gender: F Age: 13

Reason for admission: Induction chemotherapy with a goal of remission

Assessment: Acute lymphoblastic leukemia

2 ICD-10-CM Codes _____

4. OFFICE Gender: F Age: 63

Reason for encounter: Pain and lump on diaphysis of humerus

Assessment: Possible chondrosarcoma

Plan: CT, MRI

Tip: Remember the guidelines about coding uncertain conditions (OGCR II.H, IV.D, and IV.H). You need to determine whether this is an inpatient or outpatient encounter based on the location stated. You also need to identify where the humerus is.

2 ICD-10-CM Codes _____

5. INPATIENT HOSPITAL Gender: M Age: 16

Reason for admission: Surgical removal of tumor, followed by chemotherapy

Assessment: Ewing's sarcoma, left femur

Tip: Refer to OGCR I.C.2.a and I.C.2.e.1) for sequencing guidance.

2 ICD-10-CM Codes _____

CHAPTER SUMMARY

In this chapter you learned that:

- The musculoskeletal (MS) system consists of the skeletal system, which supports the body, protects internal organs, produces blood cells, stores minerals, and serves as a point of attachment for the skeletal muscles; and the muscular system, which provides for movement of the body, operates individual organs, maintains body posture, and helps produce heat.

- ICD-10-CM provides Official Guidelines for Coding and Reporting (OGCR) for the musculoskeletal system in section I.C.13, which discusses coding for site and laterality, pathologic fractures, and osteoporosis.

- The keys to abstracting for the musculoskeletal system are familiarity with the anatomy, knowledge of medical terms,

and careful attention to the details of the documented condition.

- Assigning codes for musculoskeletal disorders may require coders to cross-reference the medical record multiple times to accurately capture the details of the disorder.

- When codes for musculoskeletal disorders require multiple coding, coders must be attentive to the sequencing indicated in the instructional notes.

- The most common cancer in the musculoskeletal system is metastatic bone disease (MBD) because the bone is a frequent site of metastasis from primary neoplasms in other organs, including the breast, lung, prostate, kidney, and thyroid.

CONCEPT QUIZ

Take a moment to look back at diseases of the musculoskeletal system and connective tissue and solidify your skills. This is your opportunity to pull together everything you have learned.

Completion

Instructions: Write the term that completes each statement based on the information you learned in this chapter. Choose from the following list. Some choices may be used more than once and some choices may not be used at all.

appendicular	malunion
axial	nonunion
cartilage	osteoporosis
delayed	pathologic
diaphysis	proximal epiphysis
distal epiphysis	stress
involuntary	tendons
joints	traumatic
ligaments	voluntary

1. A _____ fracture is an acute current injury that results from an accident.

2. A _____ fracture is a fracture of a bone that has been subjected to repeated use or impact.

3. _____ are fibrous tissue that join muscles to bones.

4. _____ healing occurs when a patient waits to seek care for a fracture.

5. _____ is when the ends of fractured bone segments do not heal with proper alignment.

6. The _____ is the shaft, or long narrow portion of a long bone.

7. The _____ is the rounded end of the bone closest to the trunk.

8. The _____ skeleton consists of the arms, shoulders, wrists, hands, legs, hips, ankles, and feet.

9. _____ are fibrous tissue that connect bones to bones.

10. _____ muscles are controlled by a subconscious part of the brain and control bodily functions such as breathing and digestion.

Multiple Choice

Instructions: Circle the letter of the best answer to each question based on the information you learned in this chapter.

1. What type of fracture occurs as the result of a disease process?
   A. Neoplastic
   B. Traumatic
   C. Pathologic
   D. Stress

2. What is the correct Index path to locate a recurrent dislocation of the hip?
   A. Main Term: Dislocation, Subterm: hip
   B. Main Term: Dislocation, Subterms: Recurrent, hip
   C. Main Term: Recurrent, Subterm: hip, dislocation
   D. Main Term: Hip, Subterms: Recurrent, dislocation

3. How would you code the following scenario? *A patient has osteochondropathy of the right ankle, right knee, and right hip.*
   A. M93.251, M93.261, M93.271
   B. M93.951, M93.961, M93.971
   C. M93.98
   D. M93.99

4. How would you code the following scenario? A *patient is treated for a pathologic fracture of the left femur due to age-related osteoporosis, initial encounter.*
   A. M80.052A
   B. M84.352A
   C. M80.852A
   D. M80.062

5. How would you code the following scenario? *A patient is seen for chronic osteomyelitis of left scapula due to methicillin-susceptible Staphylococcus aureus with major osseous defect.*
   A. B95.61, M86.612, M89.712
   B. M86.612, B95.61, M89.712
   C. M86.612, M89.712, B95.61
   D. M89.712, B95.61, M89.712

6. What structure in the musculoskeletal system are x-rays used to evaluate?
   A. Tendons
   B. Ligaments
   C. Muscles
   D. Bones

7. What condition can be diagnosed based on the presence of Rh factor in the blood?
   A. Infection
   B. Rheumatoid arthritis
   C. Osteoarthritis
   D. Fracture

8. What condition is the failure of the ends of fractured bone segments to reunite?
   A. Delayed healing
   B. Malunion
   C. Nonunion
   D. Pathologic fracture

9. What site in the musculoskeletal system is a frequent site for metastatic cancer?
   A. Muscle
   B. Joints
   C. Tendons
   D. Bone

10. Where does leukemia start?
    A. Blood
    B. Joints
    C. Bone marrow
    D. Tendons

KEEP ON CODING

Instructions: Read the diagnostic statement, then use the Index and Tabular List to assign and sequence ICD-10-CM diagnosis codes. Write the code(s) on the line provided.

1. Pneumococcal arthritis of left ankle. ICD-10-CM Code(s) _____

2. Felty's syndrome, left hip. ICD-10-CM Code(s) _____

3. Dysplastic osteoarthritis of right hip. ICD-10-CM Code(s) _____

4. Lead-induced chronic gout, vertebrae. ICD-10-CM Code(s) _____

5. Panarteritis nodosa. ICD-10-CM Code(s) _____

6. Low-back pain. ICD-10-CM Code(s) _____

7. Rheumatoid nodule, right wrist. ICD-10-CM Code(s) _____

8. Stress fracture, right foot, initial encounter. ICD-10-CM Code(s) _____

9. Plica syndrome, left knee. ICD-10-CM Code(s) _____

10. Psoas tendinitis, right hip. ICD-10-CM Code(s) _____

11. Subacute osteomyelitis, right humerus. ICD-10-CM Code(s) _____

12. Sicca syndrome with myopathy. ICD-10-CM Code(s) _____

13. Rhabdomyosarcoma of the hip, left. ICD-10-CM Code(s) _____

14. Relapsing polychondritis. ICD-10-CM Code(s) _____

15. Spondylolysis, lumbar region. ICD-10-CM Code(s) _____

16. Postsurgical lordosis. ICD-10-CM Code(s) _____

17. Arthralgia of left temporomandibular joint. ICD-10-CM Code(s) _____

18. Rheumatoid bursitis, left hand. ICD-10-CM Code(s) _____

19. Age-related osteoporosis with current pathologic fracture of the right ankle, initial encounter. ICD-10-CM Code(s) _____

20. Achilles tendinitis, right leg. ICD-10-CM Code(s) _____

21. Spinal stenosis, cervical region. ICD-10-CM Code(s) _____

22. Diastasis of muscle of the left shoulder. ICD-10-CM Code(s) _____

23. Spontaneous rupture of the flexor tendon, lower leg. ICD-10-CM Code(s) _____

24. Fibromyalgia. ICD-10-CM Code(s) _____

25. Osteitis deformans of skull. ICD-10-CM Code(s) _____

CODING CHALLENGE

Instructions: Read the mini-medical-record of each patient's encounter, then abstract, assign, and sequence ICD-10-CM diagnosis codes using the Index to Diseases and Injuries, the Index to External Causes, and the Tabular List. Write the code(s) on the line provided.

1. OFFICE   Gender: F   Age: 61

Reason for encounter: Pain, redness, and swelling in left knee

Assessment: Abscess of bursa, left knee, due to Streptococcus A

Plan: Reapply dressing as directed. Take antibiotic as instructed.

2 ICD-10-CM Codes _____

2. INPATIENT HOSPITAL   Gender: F   Age: 32

Reason for admission: Repair of C5 and C6 disc

Assessment: Acute and chronic pain due to herniated cervical disc at C5-C6

Plan: FU with rehab, FU with surgeon 1 wk

1 ICD-10-CM Code _____

3. INPATIENT HOSPITAL   Gender: F   Age: 28

Reason for admission: Admitted for lumbar spinal fusion. She was previously diagnosed with spinal stenosis in her lumbar region. I told her that if the pain could not be controlled, she could opt for surgery. After ongoing efforts to manage the pain unsuccessfully, she decided to have surgery.

Assessment: Osseous stenosis at L3-L4-L5

Plan: FU 1 wk

1 ICD-10-CM Code _____

4. OFFICE   Gender: M   Age: 15

Reason for encounter: Swollen glands and high fever with pain in right shoulder, right elbow, and right hand. Abdominal spasmodic pain and diarrhea

Assessment: Juvenile arthritis with systemic onset (Still's disease), shoulder, elbow, hand, and ulcerative colitis

Plan: Rx anti-inflammatory. RTO 3 wk

2 ICD-10-CM Codes _____

5. INPATIENT HOSPITAL   Gender: F   Age: 21

Reason for admission: Continuing pain in right shoulder after ineffective physical therapy (PT)

Assessment: Frozen right shoulder

Plan: Manipulation under anesthesia for shoulder. Return to PT. FU office 1 wk.

1 ICD-10-CM Code _____

6. OFFICE   Gender: F   Age: 57

Reason for encounter: Pain on left big toe area when walking

Assessment: Hallux valgus, left

Plan: Referred to orthopedic surgeon following unsuccessful treatment with orthotics

1 ICD-10-CM Code _____

7. OFFICE   Gender: M   Age: 47

Reason for encounter: Weakness in the right forefoot

Assessment: Drop foot

Plan: Refer to PT for fitting of lightweight orthoses

1 ICD-10-CM Code _____

8. INPATIENT HOSPITAL   Gender: F   Age: 23

Reason for admission: Rotator cuff repair

Assessment: Recurrent rotator cuff syndrome

Plan: PT, RTO 1 wk

1 ICD-10-CM Code _____

9. INPATIENT HOSPITAL   Gender: M   Age: 1 year

Reason for encounter: Repair of clubfoot

Assessment: Acquired right talipes equinovarus (*clubfoot*)

Plan: PT, RTO 1 wk

1 ICD-10-CM Code _____

10. INPATIENT HOSPITAL   Gender: M   Age: 45

Reason for admission: Sudden onset of pain and swelling in left hip, fever

Testing: Arthrocentesis (*removing fluid from a joint with a needle*), blood culture, x-ray

Assessment: Bacterial pyogenic arthritis due to Pseudomonas aeruginosa, likely due to patient's intravenous drug abuse

3 ICD-10-CM Codes _____

_____

Chapter 12

Injury, Poisoning, and Certain Other Consequences of External Causes (S00-T88)

Chapter Outline

- **Injury and Effects of Drugs Refresher**
- **Coding Guidelines for Injury and Effects of Drugs**
- **Abstracting Diagnoses for Injury and Effects of Drugs**
- **Assigning Diagnosis Codes for Injury and Effects of Drugs**
- **Arranging Diagnosis Codes for Injury and Effects of Drugs**

Learning Objectives

After completing this chapter, you should have the skills to:

12.1 Spell and define the key words, medical terms, and abbreviations related to injury, poisoning, and certain other consequences of external causes. (Remember)

12.2 Describe the common forms of injury and poisoning. (Understand)

12.3 Adhere to the Official Guidelines for Coding and Reporting related to injury, poisoning, and certain other consequences of external causes. (Apply)

12.4 Examine and abstract information from the medical record required for diagnosis coding for injury, poisoning, and certain other consequences of external causes. (Analyze)

12.5 Demonstrate how to assign diagnosis codes for injury, poisoning, and certain other consequences of external causes. (Apply)

12.6 Utilize guidelines for arranging (sequencing) multiple diagnosis codes for injury, poisoning, and certain other consequences of external causes. (Apply)

Key Terms and Abbreviations

burn	contusion	Gustilo classification system	Rule of Nines
circumstances of admission	corrosion	nondisplaced	Salter-Harris classification
clavicle	degree	open (fracture)	total body surface area (TBSA)
closed (fracture)	displaced (fracture)	physis	

In addition to the key terms listed here, students should know the terms defined within tables in this chapter.

INTRODUCTION

As you are driving down the road, you occasionally need to pull over to let an ambulance pass. Your heart may pause for a moment as you wonder, "What happened? Who is in it? Who are their loved ones?" Unfortunately, accidents and injuries are part of life, and coders follow special requirements to code these situations. In this chapter you learn about different types of injuries and undesired effects of drugs, and how physicians treat these conditions.

Any physician may treat injuries and undesired effects of drugs because they can affect any body system. Physician specialties that most commonly treat these conditions are emergency medicine, primary care, orthopedics, and dermatology.

As you read this chapter, refer to anatomic resources on the integumentary system and musculoskeletal systems, both of which are frequently affected by injuries.

INJURY AND EFFECTS OF DRUGS REFRESHER

Injuries and undesired effects of drugs can encompass a wide variety of conditions and a range of definitions, so it is critical that coders understand how ICD-10-CM defines terms, rather than rely on how they might use the words in everyday conversation. Coders use medical resources, such as a reference book on diseases, to understand injuries, diagnostic methods, and common treatments. In particular, coders must be familiar with specific terminology related to burns, traumatic fractures, and poisoning and adverse effects, which are reviewed in detail. Other types of injuries are summarized in ■ TABLE 12-1. Also refer to Table 11-2, Common Conditions of the Musculoskeletal System, for a refresher on dislocations, subluxations, sprains, and strains.

Burns

Burns are damage to skin by heat, electricity, or radiation. In ICD-10-CM, corrosions are damage to skin due to chemicals. Both burns and corrosions are described by the degree (*depth*) of the burn (■ FIGURE 12-1, page 196). Burns of the eye and internal organs are *not* assigned degrees (OGCR I.C.19.d).

Traumatic Fractures

Traumatic fractures result from an accident rather than a disease. The most frequently broken bone in the body is the clavicle (*collar bone*), often caused by a direct blow to the shoulder, such as during a fall, as the result of an automobile collision, or by an outstretched arm that is attempting to break a fall. In babies, clavicle fractures can occur during a difficult delivery. Traumatic fractures are described based on combinations of several criteria:

- Body region
- Specific bone
- Site on the bone
- Line of break (■ FIGURE 12-2, page 196)

  - Open (*the bone breaks through the skin*) or closed (*the bone does not break the skin*)
  - Displaced (*the fragments of bone move out of alignment*) or nondisplaced (*the fragments of bone remain properly aligned*)

Physicians further classify fractures using specially developed classification systems based on the type of fracture. Two such systems that are incorporated into ICD-10-CM are the Gustilo system for open fractures and the Salter-Harris system for epiphysis fractures. Coders must refer to the documentation to determine how the fracture is classified then assign the corresponding diagnosis code.

Gustilo Open Fracture Classification

Open fractures are classified using the Gustilo classification system (■ TABLE 12-2, page 197), which organizes open fractures into three major types depending on the method of injury, extent of soft-tissue damage, and degree of skeletal involvement. Progression from type I to IIIC describes a higher degree of force involved in the injury, increased soft-tissue and bone damage, and greater potential for complications.

Salter-Harris Epiphysis Fracture Classification

Epiphysis fractures are classified using the Salter-Harris classification to identify the involvement of the growth plate (■ FIGURE 12-3, page 197). Fracture of the growth plate is an injury unique to childhood and usually heals without permanent deformity. A small percentage, however, are complicated by growth arrest and subsequent deformity. The Salter-Harris classification aids in estimating both the prognosis and the potential for growth disturbance (■ TABLE 12-3, page 197).

Table 12-1 ■ TYPES OF INJURIES

Injury	Description
Abuse	Physical, emotional, or sexual mistreatment by one person toward another
Complications of care	Unanticipated results of a medical or surgical procedure
Foreign body	An object that does not belong in the body
Laceration	A torn or jagged wound
Open wound	A wound in which underlying tissue is exposed to the air
Penetrating wound Puncture wound	A wound caused by a sharp pointed object passing through the skin into the underlying tissues
Perforation	Cutting or puncturing the wall or membrane of an internal organ or structure
Superficial injury	An injury to the surface of the skin, such as an abrasion, blister, contusion (*bruise*), constriction, insect bite, or superficial foreign body
Traumatic amputation	Severing a body part accidentally
Wound	A cut or opening in the skin or mucous membrane

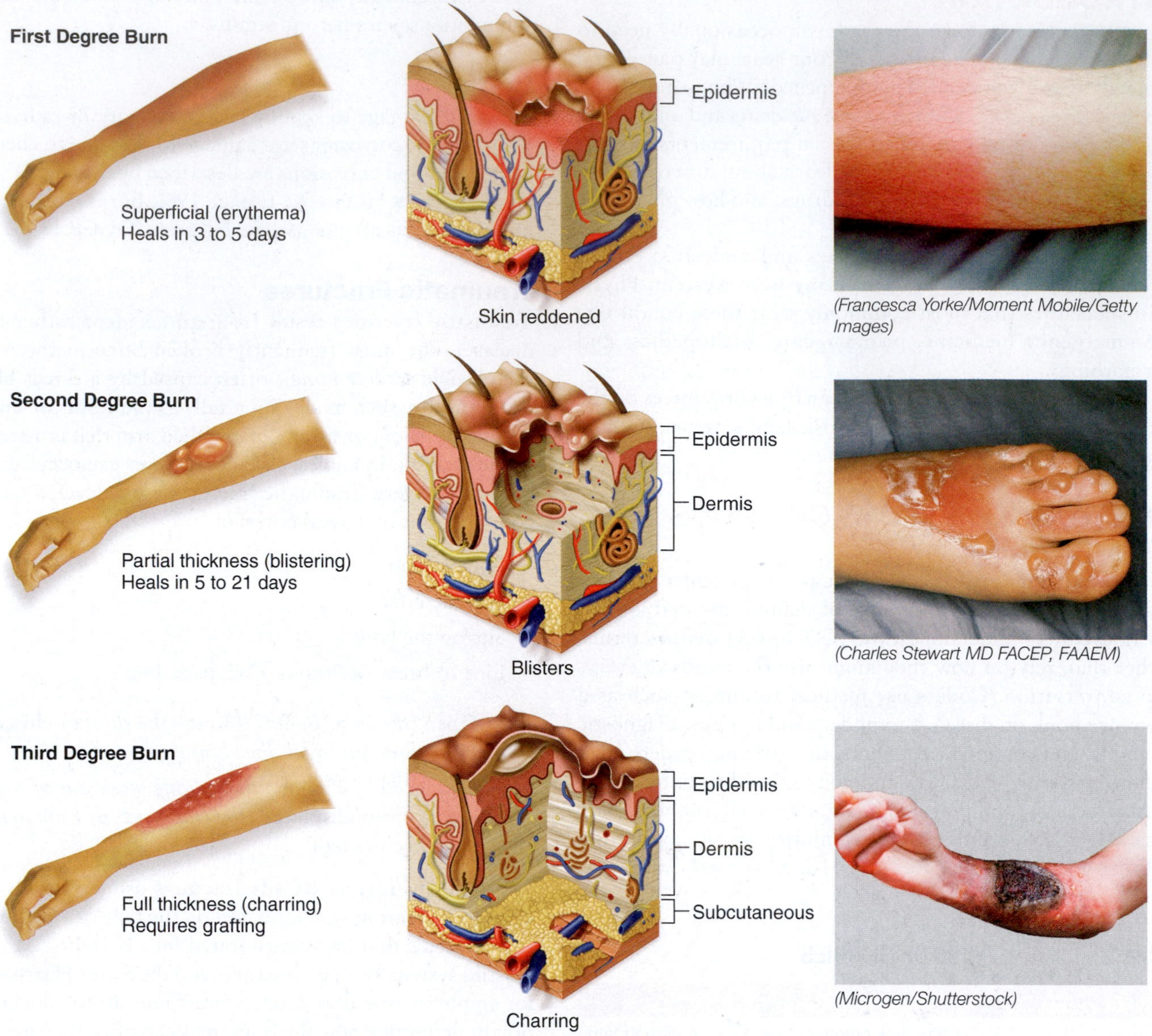

First Degree Burn

Superficial (erythema)
Heals in 3 to 5 days

Epidermis

Skin reddened

(Francesca Yorke/Moment Mobile/Getty Images)

Second Degree Burn

Partial thickness (blistering)
Heals in 5 to 21 days

Epidermis

Dermis

Blisters

(Charles Stewart MD FACEP, FAAEM)

Third Degree Burn

Full thickness (charring)
Requires grafting

Epidermis

Dermis

Subcutaneous

Charring

(Microgen/Shutterstock)

Figure 12-1 ■ Comparison of burn depth. *Source: Pearson Education/PH College.*

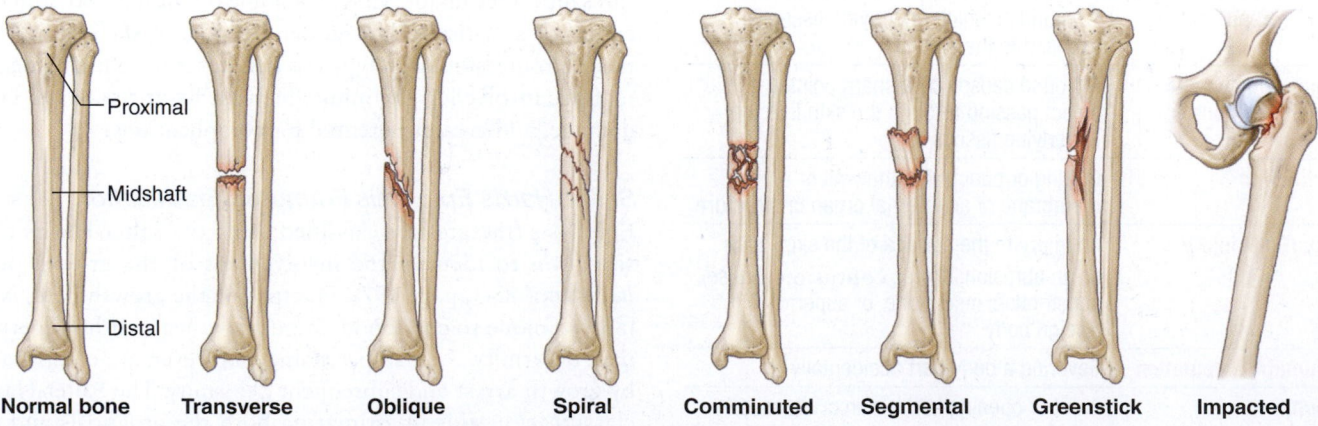

Proximal

Midshaft

Distal

| Normal bone | Transverse | Oblique | Spiral | Comminuted | Segmental | Greenstick | Impacted |

Figure 12-2 ■ Common break lines of fractures.

Table 12-2   ■   **GUSTILO CLASSIFICATION OF OPEN FRACTURES**

Type		Description
I		Wound smaller than 1 cm with minimal soft-tissue injury and clean wound bed. Fracture is usually a simple transverse, short oblique fracture, with minimal comminution (fragmentation).
II		Wound larger than 1 cm with moderate soft-tissue damage, without flaps, avulsions. Fracture is usually a simple transverse, short oblique fracture, with minimal comminution.
III		Fractures that involve extensive damage to the soft tissues, including muscle, skin, and neurovascular structures. The injury is often accompanied by a high-velocity injury or a severe crushing component.
S U B T Y P E	IIIA	Adequate soft-tissue coverage despite soft-tissue laceration regardless of the size of the wound. This includes segmental fractures or severely comminuted fractures.
	IIIB	Extensive soft tissue lost and bony exposure. This is usually associated with massive contamination.
	IIIC	Fracture in which there is a major arterial injury requiring repair for limb salvage.

Table 12-3   ■   **SALTER-HARRIS CLASSIFICATION OF EPIPHYSIS FRACTURES**

Type	Description
I	A transverse fracture through the **physis** (*growth plate*)
II	A fracture through the physis and the metaphysis, sparing the epiphysis
III	A fracture through the physis and epiphysis, sparing the metaphysis
IV	A fracture through all three elements of the bone, the physis, metaphysis, and epiphysis
V	A crush or compression fracture of the physis

Poisoning, Adverse Effects, Toxic Effects, and Underdosing

ICD-10-CM provides specific definitions for injuries from drugs, chemicals, and biological substances (■ TABLE 12-4). Coders need to learn how ICD-10-CM uses these terms and not rely on the common language definition. The use of these definitions when assigning codes is discussed later in this chapter. In this textbook chapter, poisonings, adverse effects, toxic effects, and underdosing are collectively referred to as *effects of drugs.*

Nearly 50% of all exposures to poisoning occur in children under age 6, but this age group accounts for less than 2% of fatalities. Nearly 40% of fatalities occur in persons age 40–59. Intentional poisonings account for nearly 17% of all exposures, with suicidal intent suspected in 12% of cases. The substances most frequently (35%) involved in exposure of adults are analgesics, sedatives/hypnotics/antipsychotics, antidepressants, and cardiovascular drugs. According to the American Association of Poison Control Centers, reported exposures to these classes of drug have increased by two-and-a-half times since 2000.

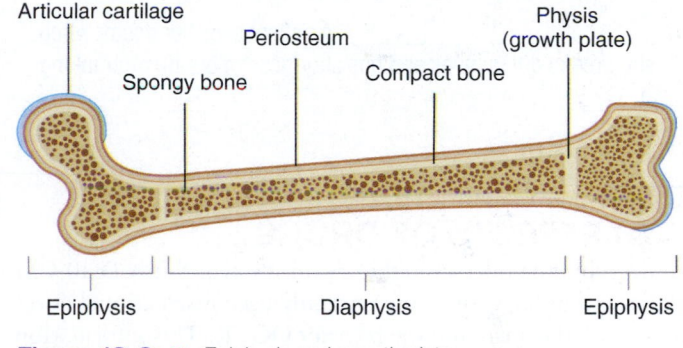

Figure 12-3 ■ Epiphysis and growth plate.
Source: Joshya/Shutterstock.

Table 12-4   ■   **DEFINITIONS FOR INJURIES FROM DRUGS, CHEMICALS, AND BIOLOGICAL SUBSTANCES**

Injury	Definition	Example
Adverse effect	A medication that was correctly prescribed and properly administered causes an undesired physical response.	Allergic reaction to an initial dose of penicillin Interaction between prescribed lithium and Diuril, both taken correctly
Poisoning	The improper use of a medication causes an undesired physical response: • Overdose of any drug, whether intentional or accidental • Error made in prescription, wrong drug given or taken in error • Interaction of drugs and alcohol • Nonprescribed drugs taken with correctly prescribed and administered drug	Administering penicillin to someone known to be allergic Nausea and vomiting and tachycardia from drinking alcohol while taking metformin
Underdosing	Taking less of a medication than is prescribed by a provider or a manufacturer's instruction causes an undesired physical response.	Diabetic ketoacidosis due to taking too little insulin
Toxic effect	A harmful substance is ingested, or comes in contact with a person, and causes an undesired physical response. (Classified as a poisoning on the Table of Drugs and Chemicals.)	Swallowing bleach Rash from wearing latex gloves

CODING PRACTICE

Exercise 12.1 Injury and Poisoning Refresher

Part A

Instructions: Read the following definitions presented in this section. Write the term being defined in the space provided.

1. _____ The fragments of bone move out of alignment

2. _____ Unanticipated results of a medical or surgical procedure

3. _____ Cutting or puncturing the wall or membrane of an internal organ or structure

4. _____ Skin damage due to chemicals

5. _____ A classification system used for open fractures

Part B

Instructions: Read each of the following patient situations and determine whether it is an **adverse effect**, **poisoning**, **underdosing**, or **toxic effect**. Write the answer in the space provided.

6. _____ A patient sees her doctor when she breaks out in hives and has shortness of breath after taking prescribed sulfa for an infection. She has never taken sulfa or had this reaction to any medication before.

7. _____ A diabetic patient who takes prescribed metformin drinks alcohol at a party. He experiences severe nausea and vomiting and tachycardia and is taken to the emergency department.

8. _____ A 2 year old gets into rubbing alcohol while his mother's back is turned. She does not think he drank any of it, but he did rub it in his eyes and is screaming. She calls Poison Control, then rushes him to the emergency department.

9. _____ An elderly woman is seen in the emergency department for an electrolyte imbalance after having taken a newly prescribed diuretic with lithium, which had been prescribed for her last year.

10. _____ A type 1 diabetic is seen in the emergency department for ketoacidosis after getting confused and taking too little insulin.

CODING GUIDELINES FOR INJURY AND EFFECTS OF DRUGS

Coders should understand the organization of this ICD-10-CM chapter, chapter-wide and commonly used instructional notes in the Tabular List, and the relevant OGCR. This information is necessary for accurate coding.

ICD-10-CM Chapter 19, "Injury, Poisoning, and Certain Other Consequences of External Causes (S00-T88)," contains 22 blocks or subchapters that are divided by anatomic site and type of injury. Review the block names and code ranges listed at the beginning of Chapter 19 in the ICD-10-CM manual to become familiar with the content and organization.

This ICD-10-CM chapter includes traumatic injuries to all body systems. The **S** section classifies injuries related to single body regions, such as the head, neck, and hip/thigh. The **T** section classifies injuries to unspecified body regions, effects of foreign bodies, burns, frostbite, poisonings, and other complications and consequences of external causes. The ICD-10-CM chapter is organized to group together all types of injuries for each anatomic region. Codes often require sixth and seventh characters for laterality, episode of care, and other details.

This chapter does not include obstetric trauma, which is classified in categories **O70** and **O71**, or birth trauma, which is classified in categories **P10** through **P15**. It also does not include conditions that arise from a disease process, even though the resulting condition may be similar to a traumatic injury. For example, a pathologic fracture is classified in ICD-10-CM Chapter 13, "Diseases of the Musculoskeletal System and Connective Tissue (M00-M99)," but a traumatic fracture is classified in ICD-10-CM Chapter 19, "Injury, Poisoning, and Certain Other Consequences of External Causes (S00-T88)."

ICD-10-CM Official Guidelines for Coding and Reporting (OGCR) for injury and poisoning appear in section I.C.19, which is divided into the following topics:

a. Application of 7th Characters in Chapter 19

b. Coding of Injuries

c. Coding of Traumatic Fractures

d. Coding of Burns and Corrosions

e. Adverse Effects, Poisoning, Underdosing and Toxic Effects

f. Adult and child abuse, neglect and other maltreatment

g. Complications of care

Instructional notes at the beginning of ICD-10-CM Chapter 19 direct coders to use secondary codes from ICD-10-CM Chapter 20, "External Causes of Morbidity," to indicate the cause of injury. Many codes within section **T** already include the external cause, so those codes do not require an additional external cause code. When a retained foreign body is involved, use an additional code from category **Z18 Retained foreign body fragments** to identify the object. Specific OGCR and instructional notes are discussed and cited throughout this chapter of the text.

ABSTRACTING DIAGNOSES FOR INJURY AND EFFECTS OF DRUGS

Each type of injury has unique criteria for abstracting. Most conditions in ICD-10-CM Chapter 19 also require information on the external cause. Refer to Table 8-1, Key Criteria for Abstracting External Causes, as a refresher on how to abstract data for external causes, and remember to abstract for external causes in addition to the injury. Key criteria for abstracting burns, traumatic fractures, and effects of drugs follow.

Abstracting Burns

Because burns often involve multiple body areas, specific anatomic sites may not be documented. When that is the case, report the percentage of the **total body surface area (TBSA)** affected by second- and third-degree burns. In addition, when a death occurs or more than 20% of the body is affected by third-degree burns, OGCR recommends, but does not require, reporting the percentage of TBSA involved (OGCR I.C.19.d.6)). Physicians estimate the percentage of TBSA using the **Rule of Nines,** which divides the body into areas, each of which comprises 9% of the total body surface area (■ FIGURE 12-4). The percentages vary slightly among adults, children, infants, obese patients, and pregnant women. Key criteria for abstracting burns appear in ■ TABLE 12-5.

Abstracting Traumatic Fractures

Criteria for abstracting traumatic fractures are more detailed than criteria for pathologic fractures. Knowledge of the anatomy of the skeletal system is essential because fractures are identified by their anatomic location. Knowledge of different types of fracture lines is also critical (Figure 12-2). Key criteria for abstracting traumatic fractures appear in ■ TABLE 12-6.

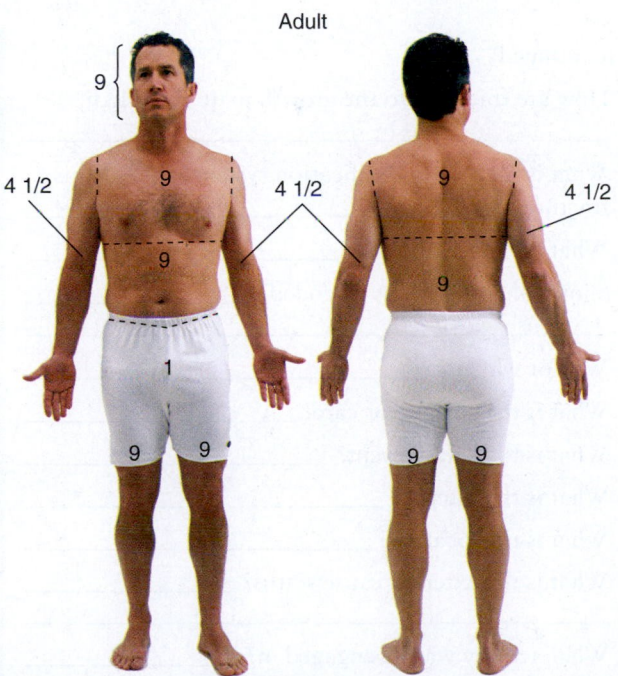

Figure 12-4 ■ "Rule of Nines" for reporting burns (all numbers are percentages of total body surface area.)
Source: Michal Heron/Pearson Education, Inc.

Abstracting Effects of Drugs

When abstracting poisoning, adverse effects, and underdosing, coders must identify the name of the drug or substance involved. Careful attention to spelling is required because drug names may have similar spellings but belong to a different class of drugs. Key criteria for abstracting poisoning and adverse effects appear in ■ TABLE 12-7. Coders must be familiar with the definitions of each type of intent to abstract and code properly. Refer back to Table 12-4 to clarify the terminology.

Table 12-5 ■ KEY CRITERIA FOR ABSTRACTING BURNS

- ❏ Is the burn due to heat or a chemical (corrosion)?
- ❏ What is the anatomic site?
- ❏ What is the laterality?
- ❏ What is the greatest depth (degree) of burn on each site?
- ❏ Are any burns nonhealing?
- ❏ Are any burns infected?
- ❏ What is the episode of care?
- ❏ What percentage of the body surface involves third-degree burns?

Table 12-6 ■ KEY CRITERIA FOR ABSTRACTING TRAUMATIC FRACTURES

- ❏ Is the fracture traumatic or pathologic?
- ❏ Does the patient have osteoporosis?
- ❏ What bone is fractured?
- ❏ What is the laterality?
- ❏ Were any additional bones fractured?
- ❏ Where on the bone is the fracture located?
- ❏ What type of fracture occurred?
- ❏ Is the fracture displaced or nondisplaced? (*Default is displaced.*)
- ❏ Is the fracture open or closed? (*Default is closed.*)
- ❏ For open fractures, what is the Gustilo classification?
- ❏ For epiphysis fractures, what is the Salter-Harris classification?
- ❏ What is the episode of care?
- ❏ Is the healing routine, delayed, nonunion, or malunion?
- ❏ Is the encounter for follow-up after active healing is complete?

Table 12-7 ■ KEY CRITERIA FOR ABSTRACTING POISONING, ADVERSE EFFECTS, AND UNDERDOSING

- ❏ What substance is involved?
- ❏ Is a diagnosis of abuse or dependence on the substance documented?
- ❏ Is the injury a poisoning/toxic effect, adverse effect, or underdosing?
- ❏ Is the injury documented as accidental, intentional self-harm, an assault, or of undetermined intent? (The default intent is *accidental.*)
- ❏ What conditions (manifestations) resulted from the injury?
- ❏ What is the episode of care?

Guided Example of Abstracting Diagnoses for Injury and Adverse Effects

Refer to the following example throughout this chapter to practice skills for abstracting, assigning, and sequencing injury and adverse effects codes. Chelsea Kutcher, CPC-H, is a fictitious coder who guides you through this case.

> Date: 03/1/yy
>
> Location: Branton Medical Center Emergency Department
>
> Provider: Cynthia Hiatt, MD
>
> Patient: Gwen Beene   Gender: F   Age: 23
>
> Reason for encounter: Hives and has shortness of breath
>
> Assessment: Patient has allergic reaction to trimethoprim-sulfamethoxazole prescribed two days ago by her family physician, Dr. Conover, for a urinary tract infection (UTI). She has never taken sulfa or had this reaction to any medication before.
>
> Plan: D/c trimethoprim-sulfamethoxazole, notify PCP

Follow along as Chelsea Kutcher, CPC-H, abstracts the diagnosis. Check off each step after you complete it.

▶ Chelsea reads through the entire record, paying special attention to the reason for the encounter and the final assessment. She notes that the patient has a new allergic reaction to a medication, so she refers to the Key Criteria for Abstracting Poisoning, Adverse Effects, and Underdosing (Table 12-7).

❏ *What substance is involved?* She notes that the substance is trimethoprim-sulfamethoxazole, which is a sulfa-based anti-infective

❏ *Is a diagnosis of abuse or dependence on the substance documented?* No

❏ *Is the injury a poisoning, adverse effect, or underdosing?* She determines that this is an adverse effect because the medication was taken as prescribed and the patient has not had this reaction before

❏ *Is the injury documented as accidental, intentional self-harm, an assault, or of undetermined intent?* Accidental

❏ *What conditions (manifestations) resulted from the injury?* Hives and shortness of breath

❏ *What is the episode of care?* It is the initial encounter because it is a new problem

▶ Next, Chelsea needs to assign the codes.

CODING PRACTICE

Exercise 12.2 Abstracting Diagnoses for Injury and Effects of Drugs

Instructions: Read the mini-medical-record of each patient's encounter and answer the abstracting questions. Write the answer on the line provided. Do not assign any codes.

> 1. EMERGENCY DEPT   Gender: M   Age: 8
>
> Chief complaint: Pain, tenderness, swelling, and distortion on right knee after being tackled while playing football at school
>
> Assessment: X-ray shows type III fracture of growth plate at the upper end of the tibia
>
> Plan: Surgery and internal fixation to ensure proper alignment of the growth plate and the joint surface
>
> a. What bone is fractured? _____
>
>   What is the laterality? _____
>
> b. What site on the bone is injured? _____
>   _____
>
> *(continued)*

1. (continued)

c. How are fractures to the growth plate classified?
   _____

d. What is the type (classification system level) of this fracture? _____

e. What are the symptoms? _____

f. Should the symptoms be coded? _____
   _____

   Why or why not? _____

g. What is the episode of care? _____

h. What is the causal event? _____

i. What is the intent? _____

j. What is the location? _____

k. What is the external cause status? _____
   _____

l. What activity was he engaged in? _____
   _____

CODING PRACTICE (continued)

2. INPATIENT HOSPITAL   Gender: M   Age: 23

Reason for admission: Patient arrived by ambulance after a barn fire that occurred on his own farm which is his job

Assessment: Third degree burns to left forearm, second degree burns to left upper arm and shoulder, smoke inhalation

a. Is the burn due to a controlled flame or an uncontrolled fire? _____

b. What is the degree, site, and laterality of the most serious burn? _____

c. What is the degree, site, and laterality of other burns? _____

d. What does (OGCR I.C.19.d.2) instruct regarding burns of the same local site (three-digit category)? _____

e. What other problems does the patient have? _____ _____

f. What is the episode of care? _____

g. What is the causal event? _____

h. What is the intent? _____

i. What is the location? _____

j. What is the external cause status? _____

k. What activity was he engaged in? _____

3. OFFICE   Gender: F   Age: 35

Reason for encounter: Suture removal from wound to right index finger, sustained when she accidentally cut her finger with a butcher knife while preparing dinner

Assessment: Wound is healed. Removed sutures.

a. What is the injury? _____

b. What is the anatomic site and laterality? _____ _____

c. What is the reason for the encounter? _____

d. What is the episode of care? _____

e. What is the causal event? _____

f. Should you assign an aftercare code for removal of sutures? _____

Why or why not? _____

4. EMERGENCY DEPT   Gender: M   Age: 67

Chief complaint: Irregular pulse, palpitations, confusion

(continued)

4. *(continued)*

Assessment: Cumulative intoxication effect (*a buildup in the body*) from digitalis which had been taken as prescribed for atrial fibrillation. Patient also has stage 2 chronic kidney disease which put him at risk for intoxication.

a. What are the symptoms? _____

Should they be coded? _____

Why or why not? _____

b. Is this an adverse effect or accidental poisoning? _____ _____

Please give the reason for your answer. _____

c. What is the substance? _____

d. What condition was the medication prescribed for? _____

e. What condition raised the patient's risk for intoxication? _____

f. What is the episode of care? _____ _____

5. EMERGENCY DEPT   Gender: F   Age: 19

Chief complaint: Examination after alleged date rape by her boyfriend

Assessment: Conducted physical examination and urine test. Flunitrazepam was found in a urine test. The injury was determined to be sexual assault.

a. What is the substance? _____

b. What is the intent? _____

c. What is the reason for the encounter? _____ _____

d. What event occurred? _____

e. What is the episode of care? _____

f. Who is the perpetrator? _____

g. Should you assign a code to identify the perpetrator? _____

h. Why or why not? _____

6. OFFICE   Gender: M   Age: 31

Chief complaint: Accident in which automobile battery exploded and something got in his eyes while he was working on his car in the driveway at his single family home

Assessment: Sulfuric acid burn on both eyelids and right cornea, second degree sulfuric acid burn to forehead and right cheek

(continued)

CODING PRACTICE (continued)

6. (continued)

a. Is the burn due to heat or a chemical? _____
_____

b. What is the coding term for this type of burn? _____
_____

c. What is the substance? _____

d. What is the anatomic site? _____

e. What is the laterality? _____

f. What is the greatest depth (degree) of burn on each site?
_____

(continued)

6. (continued)

g. What is the episode of care? _____

h. What is the causal event? _____

i. What is the intent? _____

j. What is the location? _____

k. What is the external cause status? _____
_____

l. What is the activity? _____

ASSIGNING DIAGNOSIS CODES FOR INJURY AND EFFECTS OF DRUGS

Each type of injury has unique coding guidelines, so coders need to become familiar with a variety of situations. Because the most severe injuries are often accompanied by less serious injuries, the OGCR instruct coders *not* to assign codes for superficial injuries, such as abrasions or contusions, when more severe injuries, such as an open wound or fracture of the *same* site, are present. Assign codes for the more severe injuries (OGCR I.C.19.b.1)).

Most codes in ICD-10-CM Chapter 19 require a seventh character for the episode of care. In addition to the most common seventh characters for the episode of care—**A Initial encounter**, **D Subsequent encounter**, and **S Sequela**—codes for traumatic fractures often provide additional options within each of these broad categories. Use seventh characters for an **Initial encounter** while the patient is receiving active treatment for the injury. Use seventh characters for a **Subsequent encounter** after the active treatment has been completed and the patient is in the healing phase. Use seventh characters for a **Sequela** for late effects of the injury. A patient may be seen by a new or different provider over the course of treatment for an injury. Assign the seventh character based on whether the patient is undergoing active treatment and *not* whether the provider is seeing the patient for the first time (OGCR I.C.19.a). ■ FIGURE 12-5, (page 203) portrays how the seventh character changes throughout the treatment cycle.

This section of the chapter demonstrates how to assign codes for the three major types of injuries—burns, traumatic fractures, and poisoning—then also discusses two special topics: child or adult abuse and complications of care.

CODING CAUTION

Use character **D Subsequent encounter** for all follow-up and aftercare of injuries. Do not report aftercare **Z** codes with injuries (OGCR I.C.21.c.7) and I.C.19.a).

Assigning Codes for Burns

Burns are classified by anatomic site, depth (degree), extent, and causal event or agent (source). Burns of the eye and internal organs are classified by site and causal event or agent but not by degree. Event and agent codes are external cause codes that are located in the Index to External Causes. The following information summarizes key guidelines to keep in mind when assigning codes for burns (■ FIGURE 12-6, page 204):

- Assign separate codes for each burn site (OGCR I.C.19.d.5)). Search the Index for the Main Term **Burn** and a subterm for the anatomic site.

- When the same local site (three-character category level, **T20-T28**) has multiple burns of different degrees, assign a code only for highest degree recorded in the diagnosis (OGCR I.C.19.d.2)).

- Assign additional codes for any infection of the burn site (OGCR I.C.19.d.4)) and for other related conditions, such as smoke inhalation or respiratory failure (OGCR I.C.19.d.1)c)).

- Assign a code for the percentage of TBSA involved from categories **T31 Burns classified according to extent of body surface involved** or **T32 Corrosions classified according to extent of body surface involved** in the following situations (OGCR I.C.19.d.6)):

  - When the site of the burn is not specified

  - When there is a need for additional data, such as that required by the state health department

  - To provide data for evaluating burn mortality, such as that needed by burn units

  - When a third-degree burn involves 20% or more of TBSA

- Nonhealing burns and necrosis of burned skin are coded in the same way as an acute burn (OGCR I.C.19.d.3)).

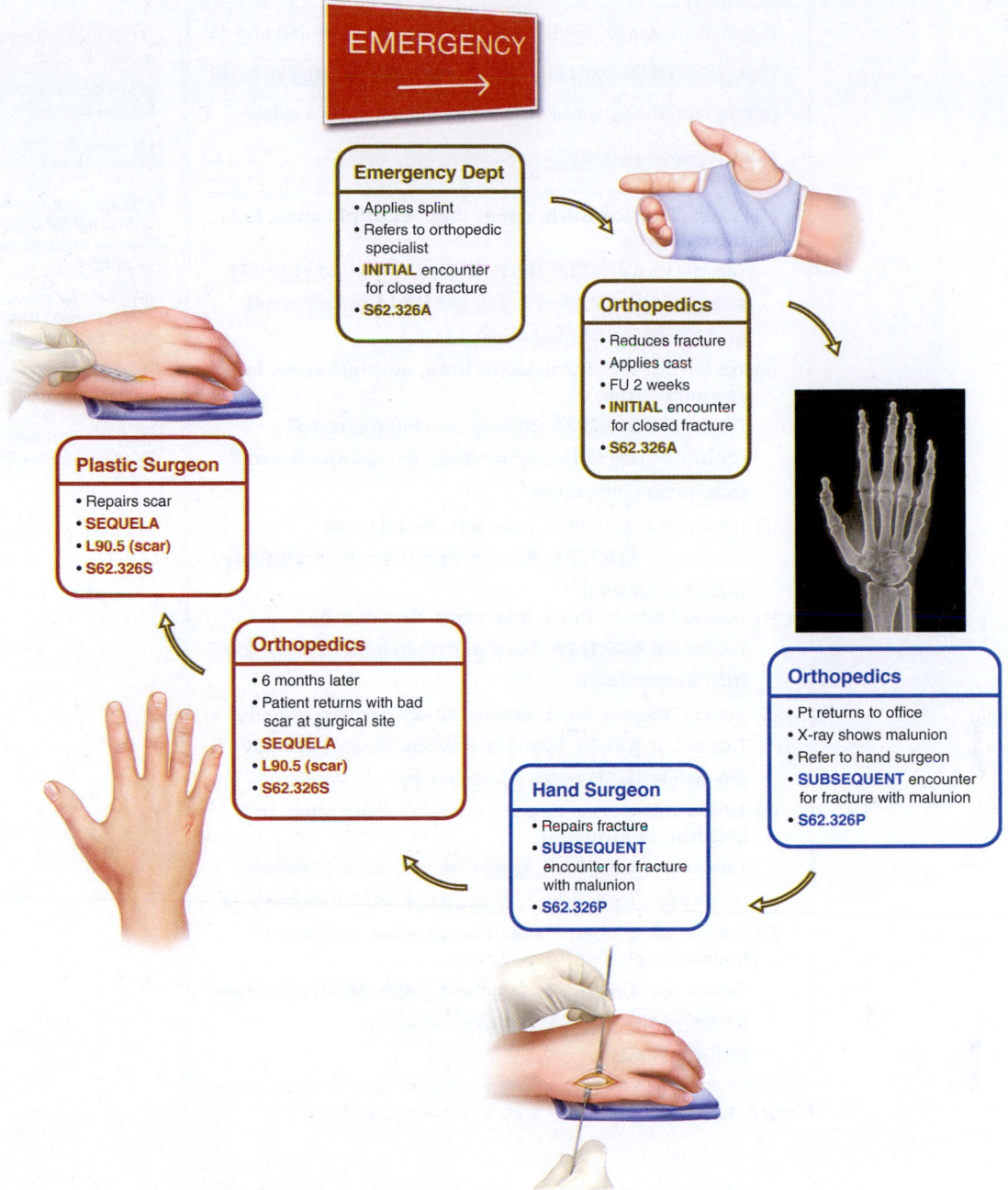

Figure 12-5 ■ Episode of care for code S62.326 "Displaced fracture of shaft of fifth metacarpal bone, right hand".

Assigning Codes for Traumatic Fractures

In addition to the seventh characters **A**, **D**, and **S** used for most injury codes, traumatic fracture codes use several additional seventh characters that describe combinations of the following criteria:

- Open or closed
- Gustilo classification for open fractures (■ FIGURE 12-7, page 204)
- Routine or delayed healing
- Normal union, malunion, or nonunion

Seventh-character options appear at the beginning of each three-digit category and are summarized in ■ TABLE 12-8, (page 205).

The details of code selection vary with the type of fracture. For example, some categories provide separate codes for displaced and nondisplaced fractures. Categories **S49**, **S59**, **S79**, and **S89** classify epiphysis fractures using the Salter-Harris system.

OGCR I.C.19.c provides guidance on the default coding of fractures when certain details are not documented, as follows:

- When a fracture is not documented as open or closed, assign a code for closed.
- When a fracture is not documented as displaced or not displaced, assign a code for displaced.

Patient is treated for multiple third degree burns to her left arm, multiple second degree burns to her left leg, and first degree burns to both feet. She sustained the burns in a house fire of a single family home where she was trapped in a bedroom.

(1) Index to Diseases: **Burn, upper limb, multiple sites, left, third degree**
Tabular List: **T22.392A Burn of third degree of multiple sites of left shoulder and upper limb, except wrist and hand, initial encounter**

(2) Index to Diseases: **Burn, lower limb, multiple sites, left, second degree**
Tabular List: **T24.292A Burn of second degree of multiple sites of left lower limb, except ankle and foot, initial encounter**

(3) Index to Diseases: **Burn, foot, left, first degree**
Tabular List: **T25.122A Burn of first degree of left foot, initial encounter**

(4) Index to Diseases: **Burn, foot, right, first degree**
Tabular List: **T25.121A Burn of first degree of right foot, initial encounter**

(5) Index to Diseases: **Burn, extent, 20–29 percent of body**
Tabular List: **T31.20 Burns involving 20–29% of body surface with 0% to 9% third degree**

(6) External Cause Index: **Exposure, fire, uncontrolled, in building or structure**
Tabular List: **X00.0XXA Exposure to flames in uncontrolled fire in building or structure, initial encounter**

(7) External Cause Index: **Place of occurrence, residence, house, single family, bedroom**
Tabular List: **Y92.013 Bedroom of single-family (private) house as the place of occurrence of the external cause**

(1) Code the third-degree burns

(2) Code the second-degree burns

(3) Code the first-degree burns, left foot

(4) Code the first-degree burns, right foot because there is no code for bilateral

(5) Code for percentage of TBSA burned based on the body areas identified

(6) External cause code for causal event

(7) External cause code for place of occurrence

Figure 12-6 ■ Example of assigning codes for burns.

Patient is seen for follow-up on an open fracture of the right tibia plateau. The fracture occurred at the lateral condyle. The physician classifies the fracture as Type II using the Gustilo scale. X-rays show that the fracture is healing well.

Index: **Fracture, tibia, plateau,** *see* **upper end, bicondylar**
Tabular List:
S82.14 Bicondylar fracture of tibia
        1 sixth digit for **right tibia, displaced**
        E seventh character for **subsequent encounter for open fracture type I or II with routine healing**
Final code: **S82.141E Displaced bicondylar fracture of right tibia, subsequent encounter for open fracture type I or II with routine healing**

Figure 12-7 ■ Example of coding a Gustilo fracture.

Table 12-8 ■ **MATRIX OF SEVENTH CHARACTERS FOR TRAUMATIC FRACTURES OF LONG BONES**

Treatment Phase	Closed	Open Type I or II	Open Type IIIA, B, or C
Initial	A	B	C
Routine healing	D	E	F
Delayed healing	G	H	J
Nonunion healing	K	M	N
Malunion healing	P	Q	R
Sequela	S	S	S

1. Locate the name of the substance in the left-hand column. Some substances have subterms indented below them on the next line.

2. Select the substance code in the column that corresponds to the intent determined during abstracting. A *toxic effect* is coded using the appropriate **Poisoning** columns. When the intent is not stated, code it as accidental.

3. Verify the code in the Tabular List. Do not code directly from the Table of Drugs and Chemicals.

4. Confirm that the code title reflects the intent.

5. Assign the seventh character for the episode of care to the injury code.

6. When more than one substance is involved, repeat the steps for each substance.

7. Assign additional codes to identify the condition(s) or manifestation(s) that resulted. Do not assign a seventh character to the code for the condition/manifestation unless directed to do so by instructional notes in the Tabular List, as occurs with traumatic fractures. Sequencing of codes is discussed later in this chapter.

8. When the intent is underdosing, assign additional codes as follows:

   - When underdosing exacerbates the condition for which the medication was prescribed, assign a code for the condition.

   - Assign a code for noncompliance (**Z91.12-, Z91.13-**) or complication of care (**Y63.6-Y63.9**) to further indicate intent, if known.

> **SUCCESS STEP**
>
> When a patient with known osteoporosis suffers a fracture, remember to assign a code from category **M80 Osteoporosis with current pathological fracture**, rather than a traumatic fracture code. Do this even when the patient has a minor fall or trauma. If the fall or trauma would not usually break a normal, healthy bone, you should assign a code for pathologic fracture due to osteoporosis (OGCR I.C.19.c.1)).

Assigning Codes for Poisoning, Adverse Effects, Toxic Effects, and Underdosing

To assign codes for poisoning/toxic effects, adverse effects, and underdosing, use the Table of Drugs and Chemicals (■ FIGURE 12-8). Assign as many codes as necessary to identify all drugs or medicinal or biological substances (OGCR I.C.19.e.2)). Code each drug or substance separately unless a combination code is listed in the Table of Drugs and Chemicals (OGCR I.C.19.e.4)). Do not assign an additional external cause code because the external cause is included in the injury code.

To use the Table of Drugs and Chemicals, follow these steps:

> **SUCCESS STEP**
>
> The Table of Drugs and Chemicals is located at the end of the Index to Diseases and before the Index to External Causes in most coding manuals. If you haven't already done so, place a red self-adhesive tab along the top edge of the page to make it easier to find.

Substance	Poisoning, Accidental (unintentional)	Poisoning, Intentional self-harm	Poisoning, Assault	Poisoning, Undetermined	Adverse effect	Underdosing
Trimethobenzamide	T45.0X1	T45.0X2	T45.0X3	T45.0X4	T45.0X5	T45.0X6
Trimethoprim	T37.8X1	T37.8X2	T37.8X3	T37.8X4	T37.8X5	T37.8X6
with sulfamethoxazole	T36.8X1	T36.8X2	T36.8X3	T36.8X4	T36.8X5	T36.8X6
Trimethylcarbinol	T51.3X1	T51.3X2	T51.3X3	T51.3X4	-	-
Trimethylpsoralen	T49.3X1	T49.3X2	T49.3X3	T49.3X4	T49.3X5	T49.3X6
Trimeton	T45.0X1	T45.0X2	T45.0X3	T45.0X4	T45.0X5	T45.0X6
Trimetrexate	T45.1X1	T45.1X2	T45.1X3	T45.1X4	T45.1X5	T45.1X6

Figure 12-8 ■ Excerpt from the Table of Drugs and Chemicals.

Special Topics

OGCR provide guidelines for adult and child abuse and complications of care. Coding for these topics is summarized next.

Adult and Child Abuse, Neglect, and Other Maltreatment

Coding of adult and child abuse or neglect is based on whether the medical record documents the abuse as confirmed or suspected (OGCR I.C.19.f)). To learn how to code for abuse, neglect, and other maltreatment, review the following guidelines:

- When the medical record documents abuse or neglect, assign a code for confirmed maltreatment from category **T74.-**.

  1. Search the Index for the Main Term **Maltreatment**.

     - Select a subterm that identifies the victim as **adult** or **child**.

     - Select a second-level subterm for **confirmed**.

  2. Assign an external cause code from the assault section **(X92-Y08)** to identify the cause of any physical injuries.

     - Search the External Cause Index for the Main Term **Assault**, then select the applicable subterm to identify the method of assault.

  3. Assign a perpetrator code **(Y07)** when the perpetrator of the abuse is known.

     - Search the External Cause Index for the Main Term **Perpetrator**, then select the applicable subterm to identify the relationship of the perpetrator to the victim.

- When the medical record documents suspected abuse, assign a code for suspected maltreatment from category **T76.-**.

  1. Search the Index for the Main Term **Maltreatment**.

     - Select a second-level subterm for **suspected**.

  2. For suspected cases of abuse or neglect, *do not* report external cause or perpetrator code.

  3. If a suspected case of abuse, neglect, or mistreatment is ruled out during an encounter, assign code **Z04.71 Encounter for examination and observation following alleged adult physical abuse** or code **Z04.72 Encounter for examination and observation following alleged child physical abuse**, *not* a code from **T76**. The inclusion notes under **Z04.71** and **Z04.72** state **Suspected . . . physical and sexual abuse, ruled out**.

- Sequence the codes as follows (■ FIGURE 12-9):

  1. The code from category **T74.-** or **T76.-** to identify confirmed or suspected abuse, neglect, and other maltreatment.

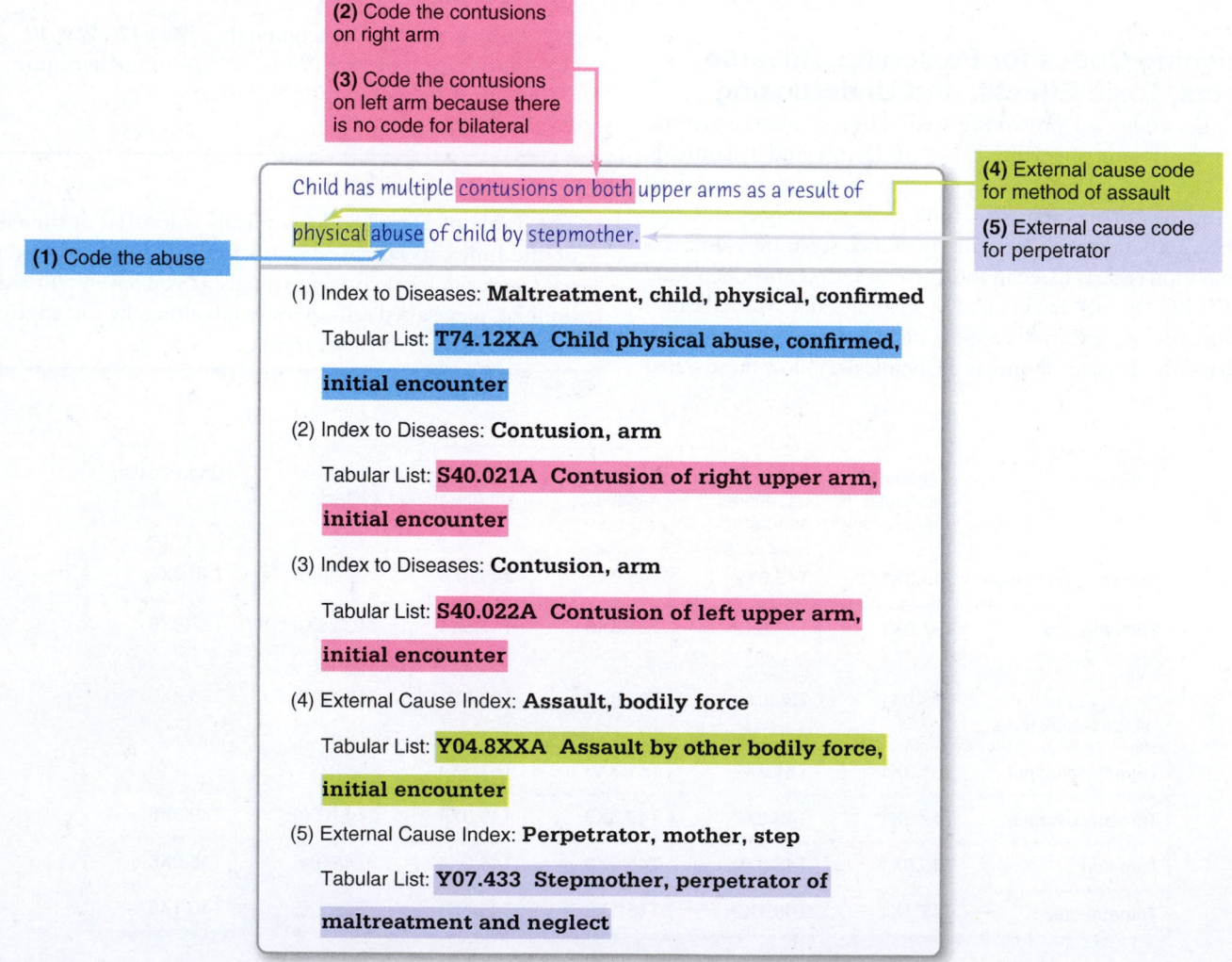

Figure 12-9 ■ Example assigning and sequencing codes for child abuse.

2. Additional codes to identify any associated mental health condition or injury (OGCR I.C.19.f).

3. An external cause code to identify the method of assault.

4. An external cause code to identify the perpetrator (for confirmed abuse only).

Complications of Care

When providers document that a medical or surgical procedure is the cause of a condition, assign a code for the event of a complication (OGCR I.C.19.g.1)(a)) as well as the resulting condition(s) or manifestation(s) as follows:

- Search the Index for the Main Term **Complication**.
  - Locate the first-level subterm that describes the event or procedure that *caused* the problem (■ FIGURE 12-10).
  - Locate the second-level subterm that describes the condition that *resulted*.
  - Locate the third-level subterm that identifies the anatomic site.
- Some complications of care codes are combination codes that describe the nature of the complication as well as the type of procedure that caused the complication.
  - When the external cause is included in a combination code, do not assign an additional external cause code.
- When a complication code is available from a body system chapter, such as those for intraoperative complications, sequence the body system code first, followed by code(s) for the specific complication condition or manifestation, if applicable (OGCR I.C.19.g.5)).

Complications of care include a broad range of conditions that may be due to external causes or may be physical reactions. Complications due to external causes include performing an incorrect procedure, operating on an incorrect site, leaving foreign objects in a patient, perforating a nearby organ or structure during a procedure, malfunction of prosthetic

devices, and certain infections. Complications that are physical reactions include cardiac arrest, respiratory failure, hemorrhaging, or ileus.

Guided Example of Assigning Injury and Adverse Effect Diagnosis Codes

To practice skills for using the Table of Drugs and Chemicals, continue with the example from earlier in the chapter about patient Gwen Beene, who was seen in the Branton Medical Center Emergency Department due to an allergic reaction to trimethoprim-sulfamethoxazole.

Follow along in your ICD-10-CM manual as Chelsea assigns codes. Check off each step after you complete it.

▶ First, Chelsea confirms the diagnosis of hives and shortness of breath due to adverse effect of trimethoprim-sulfamethoxazole.

▶ Chelsea locates the Table of Drugs and Chemicals at the end of the Index to Diseases.

❏ She searches for the Main Term **Trimethoprim** in the left-hand column of the table (Figure 12-8).

❏ She locates the subterm **with Sulfamethoxazole** on the next line.

❏ She locates the column for **Adverse Effects**.

❏ She locates the code where the column for **Adverse Effects** crosses the row for **with Sulfamethoxazole**.

❏ She identifies the code **T36.8X5**.

▶ Chelsea verifies code **T36.8X5** in the Tabular List.

❏ She reads the code title for **T36.8X5 Adverse effect of other systemic antibiotics** and confirms that this accurately describes the diagnosis.

❏ She notes the symbol **7th** that directs her to assign a seventh character.

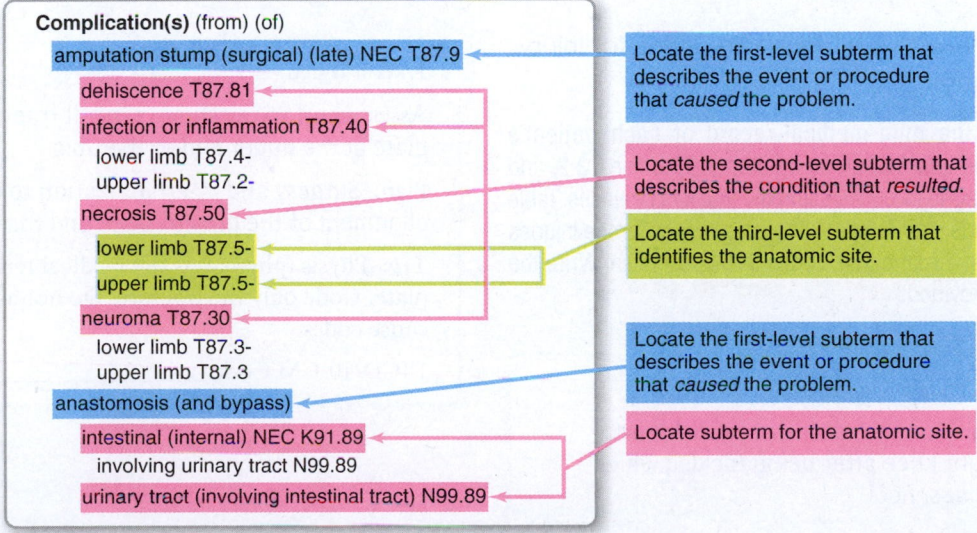

Figure 12-10 ■ Example of Index entry for the Main Term "Complication".

❏ She refers to the beginning of category **T36** to review the seventh characters available for episode of care.

❏ The episode of care is **A, initial encounter** because this is the first encounter for the problem.

❏ She assigns code **T36.8X5A**.

▶ Chelsea checks for instructional notes in the Tabular List.

❏ She cross-references the beginning of the block **Poisoning by, adverse effects of and underdosing of drugs, medicaments and biological substances (T36-T50)** and sees several instructional notes.

❏ She reviews the **Includes** notes that give the definition of poisoning and adverse effect and concludes that she chose the correct category of adverse effect because the medication was properly administered.

❏ She reads another instructional note that says **Code first for adverse effects, the nature of the adverse effect**. Therefore, she knows that she should code for hives and shortness of breath.

❏ She cross-references the beginning of **Chapter 19 (S00-T88)** and reviews the instructional notes. She reads the note that says **Use secondary code(s) from Chapter 20, External causes of morbidity, to indicate cause of injury. Codes within the T section that include the external cause do not require an additional external cause code**. She determines she does not need an additional code for external cause because the code from section **T** includes the cause, which is an adverse effect to a medication.

▶ Chelsea assigns the codes for the manifestations.

❏ She searches the Index for the Main Term **Hives**, which cross-references her to **Urticaria**.

▪ She searches for the Main Term **Urticaria** and the subterm **due to drug**, which directs her to code **L50.0**.

▪ She verifies the code in the Tabular List and confirms the code title **L50.0 Allergic urticaria**.

▪ She cross-references the beginning of the category, block, and chapter for any applicable instructional notes.

❏ She searches the Index for the Main Term **Shortness** and subterm **breath**, which directs her to code **R06.02**.

▪ She verifies the code in the Tabular List and confirms the code title **R06.02 Shortness of breath**.

▪ After cross-referencing the beginning of the category, block, and chapter for any applicable instructional notes, she returns to the Index to locate the code for hives.

▶ Chelsea identifies the codes for this case:

❏ **T36.8X5A Adverse effect of other systemic antibiotics, initial encounter**

❏ **L50.0 Allergic urticaria**

❏ **R06.02 Shortness of breath**

CODING CAUTION

Use the Table of Drugs and Chemicals only for poisoning/toxic effects, adverse effects, and underdosing. Do *not* use this table to report the fact that a patient is taking, or has been prescribed, a medication when no injury is involved.

CODING PRACTICE

Exercise 12.3 Assigning Diagnosis Codes for Injury and Effects of Drugs

Instructions: Read the mini-medical-record of each patient's encounter, review the information abstracted in Exercise 12.2, and assign ICD-10-CM diagnosis codes using the Index to Diseases, Table of Drugs and Chemicals, and Tabular List. Assign codes for the injuries only. Do *not* assign external cause codes in this exercise. Write the code(s) on the line provided.

---

1. EMERGENCY DEPT   Gender: M   Age: 8

Chief complaint: Pain, tenderness, swelling, and distortion on right knee after being tackled while playing football at school

(*continued*)

---

1. (continued)

Assessment: X-ray shows type III fracture of growth plate at the upper end of the tibia

Plan: Surgery and internal fixation to ensure proper alignment of the growth plate and the joint surface

Tip: Physis (physeal) is the medical term for the growth plate. Code only the fracture. Do not assign external cause codes.

1 ICD-10-CM Code _____

CODING PRACTICE (continued)

2. INPATIENT HOSPITAL   Gender: M   Age: 23

Reason for admission: Patient arrived by ambulance after a barn fire that occurred on his own farm which is his job

Assessment: Third degree burns to left forearm, second degree burns to left upper arm and shoulder, smoke inhalation

Tip: Assign a code for the burns and a code for the smoke. Do not code the percentage of body area affected, activity, status, or location external cause codes.

2 ICD-10-CM Codes _____

3. OFFICE   Gender: F   Age: 35

Reason for encounter: Suture removal from wound to right index finger, sustained when she accidentally cut her finger with a butcher knife while preparing dinner

Assessment: Wound is healed. Removed sutures.

Tip: Assign a code for the injury with the appropriate seventh character for care provided during the healing phase. Do not assign external cause codes.

1 ICD-10-CM Code _____

ARRANGING DIAGNOSIS CODES FOR INJURY AND EFFECTS OF DRUGS

Patients with injuries and poisoning often present with multiple problems. The general rule is to sequence the code for the most serious injury first, as determined by the provider and the focus of treatment (OGCR I.C.19.b).

Injuries often involve peripheral nerves or blood vessels. When the primary injury is to the blood vessels or nerves, that injury should be sequenced first. When a primary injury results in minor damage to peripheral nerves or blood vessels, sequence the primary injury first, with additional codes for injuries to nerves, spinal cord, or blood vessels (OGCR I.C.19.b.2)).

Patients may be treated for sequelae or after-effects after the primary injury has healed, such as scars. Sequence first code(s) that describe the after-effect conditions or manifestations. Then report the code that identifies the original injury, with the seventh character **S Sequela** (OGCR I.C.19.a). Refer to ■ FIGURE 12-11 to learn more about sequencing injury codes and sequelae.

Arranging Codes for Burns

When more than one burn is present, the first code should reflect the highest degree of burn (OGCR I.C.19.d.1)). The size of the damaged area is *not* a factor in sequencing burn codes.

The OGCR states that **circumstances of admission** govern the selection of the principal diagnosis or first-listed diagnosis in certain situations. This means that sequencing is based on the specific reason for admission and which injuries are most serious. The circumstances of admission apply when a patient has both internal and external burns (OGCR I.C.19.d.1)(b)) or has other related conditions, such as smoke inhalation and/or respiratory failure (OGCR I.C.19.d.1)(c)).

A patient is treated for a keloid scar that forms following a third degree burn on the right cheek.

(1) **L91.0** Hypertrophic disorders of the skin
(2) **T20.36XS** Burn of third degree of forehead and cheek, sequela

Figure 12-11 ■ Example of coding the sequelae of an injury.

For example, consider a patient with second-degree burns and life-threatening respiratory failure due to smoke inhalation. Sequence respiratory failure first because it is more serious than second-degree burns.

Arranging Codes for Traumatic Fractures

Sequence multiple fractures based on the severity of the fracture (OGCR I.C.19.c.2)). The severity may be determined by either the location of the fracture or the type of fracture. Review the following examples to learn more about sequencing multiple fractures:

- A fracture to the skull is more serious than a fracture to a finger.
- An open fracture is more serious than a closed fracture.
- A fracture that causes damage to another organ, such as a fractured rib that punctures a lung, is more serious than one that does not, such as a fractured arm.

If coders cannot determine the relative severity of multiple fractures based on the documentation, they should consult with their supervisor or query the physician.

Arranging Codes for Effects of Drugs

The OGCR guidelines are different for sequencing poisonings, adverse effects, and underdosings (OGCR I.C.19.e).

Sequence codes for poisonings as follows (OGCR I.C.19.5)(b)):

1. The first code identifies the type and intent of injury (categories **T36** through **T50**). Assign this using the Table of Drugs and Chemicals. Verify the code in the Tabular List and assign a seventh character to identify the episode of care. Assign a code for each drug involved.

2. Subsequent codes identify all resulting conditions or manifestations. Assign these using the Index and Tabular List.

Codes for adverse effects are sequenced in a different order than for poisonings (OGCR I.C.19.5)(a)):

1. The first code(s) identifies the manifestation(s) or resulting condition(s).

2. Subsequent codes identify the **T** code, which is a combination code for the drug and the intent (adverse effect). Assign this using the Table of Drugs and Chemicals. Verify the code in the Tabular List and assign a seventh character to identify the episode of care. Assign a code for each drug involved.

Sequence codes for underdosing encounters as follows (OGCR I.C.19.e. 5)(c)):

1. The first code(s) identifies the manifestation(s) or resulting condition(s).

2. Sequence the underdosing **T** code as an additional code. Assign this using the Table of Drugs and Chemicals. Verify the code in the Tabular List and assign a seventh character to identify the episode of care. Assign a code for each drug involved.

3. Code the medical condition itself when a patient has a relapse or exacerbation of the medical condition for which the drug is prescribed because of the reduction in dose.

4. Sequence a code for complication of care (**Y63.6-Y63.9**) or a **Z** code (**Z91.12-**, **Z91.13**) for noncompliance, as applicable.

Guided Example of Arranging Injury and Adverse Effects Diagnosis Codes

To practice skills for sequencing codes for adverse effects, continue with the example from earlier in the chapter about patient Gwen Beene, who was seen at the Branton Medical Center Emergency Department due to an allergic reaction to trimethoprim-sulfamethoxazole.

Follow along in your ICD-10-CM manual as Chelsea sequences the codes. Check off each step after you complete it.

▶ First, Chelsea confirms the three diagnoses:

- ❏ **T36.8X5A Adverse effect of other systemic antibiotics, initial encounter**
- ❏ **R06.02 Shortness of breath**
- ❏ **L50.0 Allergic urticaria**

▶ Chelsea reviews the instructional notes she found at the beginning of the block T36-T50 that said Code first for adverse effects, the nature of the adverse effect.

- ❏ The words **Code first** mean that the manifestations should be sequenced before the **T** code for the drug that caused the adverse effect.

▶ Chelsea also reviews OGCR I.C.19.e.5)(a) that states:

When coding an adverse effect of a drug that has been correctly prescribed and properly administered, assign the appropriate code for the nature of the adverse effect followed by the appropriate code for the adverse effect of the drug (T36-T50).

- ❏ This confirms that the manifestation codes should be sequenced first, followed by the **T** code.
- ❏ She sequences **R06.02, Shortness of breath** first because it is a more serious condition than hives.

▶ Chelsea finalizes the sequencing for this case:

(1) **R06.02 Shortness of breath**

(2) **L50.0 Allergic urticaria**

(3) **T36.8X5A Adverse effect of other systemic antibiotics, initial encounter**

CODING PRACTICE

Exercise 12.4 Arranging Diagnosis Codes for Injury and Poisoning

Instructions: Read the mini-medical-record of each patient's encounter, review the information abstracted in Exercise 12.2, assign ICD-10-CM diagnosis codes using the Index to Diseases, the Index to External Causes, the Table of Drugs and Chemicals, and the Tabular List, and sequence them correctly. Do assign external cause codes in this exercise.

---

1. EMERGENCY DEPT   Gender: M   Age: 67

Chief complaint: Irregular pulse, palpitations, confusion

Assessment: Cumulative intoxication effect (*a buildup in the body*) from digitalis which had been taken as prescribed for atrial fibrillation. Patient also has stage 2 chronic kidney disease which put him at risk for intoxication.

(continued)

---

1. (continued)

Tip: Sequence codes as follows: 1) the condition that describes the adverse effect, 2) the drug that caused the adverse effect, 3) reason he was at risk.

3 ICD-10-CM Codes _____

_____

---

2. EMERGENCY DEPT   Gender: F   Age: 19

Chief complaint: Examination after alleged date rape by her boyfriend

Assessment: Conducted physical examination and urine test. Flunitrazepam was found in a urine test. The injury was determined to be sexual assault.

Tip: Assign a code for the assault, a code from the Table of Drugs and Chemicals, and one external cause code that identifies the perpetrator.

3 ICD-10-CM Codes _____

_____

CODING PRACTICE (continued)

3. OFFICE   Gender: M   Age: 31

Chief complaint: Accident in which automobile battery exploded and something got in his eyes while he was working on his car in the driveway at his single family home

Assessment: Sulfuric acid burn on both eyelids and right cornea, second degree sulfuric acid burn to forehead and right cheek

Tip: Assign a code from the Table of Drugs and Chemicals, four codes for the injuries, and two external cause

(continued)

3. (continued)

codes for place and status. Read the instructional notes in the Tabular List for help on sequencing. Recall that burns to the eye are not rated by degree. The burn to the cornea is the most serious. The burns to the cheek and forehead are the least serious.

7 ICD-10-CM Codes _____

_____

_____

CHAPTER SUMMARY

In this chapter you learned that:

- Injuries and effects of drugs can encompass a wide variety of conditions and a range of definitions, so it is critical that coders understand how ICD-10-CM defines terms.

- ICD-10-CM Chapter 19, "Injury, Poisoning, and Certain Other Consequences of External Causes (S00-T88)," contains 22 blocks or subchapters that are divided by anatomic site and type of injury.

- ICD-10-CM Official Guidelines for Coding and Reporting (OGCR) for injury and poisoning appear in section I.C.19, which is divided into sections based on the type of injury.

- The most common injuries are burns, fractures, and poisonings, each of which has unique criteria for abstracting.

- Each type of injury has unique coding guidelines, so coders need to become familiar with a variety of situations.

- In general, sequence the code for the most serious injury first, as determined by the provider and the focus of treatment.

- When coding for a poisoning/toxic effect, sequence the T code for the drug and intent first. For adverse effects and underdosings, sequence the codes for the manifestations first.

CONCEPT QUIZ

Take a moment to look back at injury and effects of drugs and solidify your skills. This is your opportunity to pull together everything you have learned.

Completion

Instructions: Refer to category *S72 Fracture of femur* in the ICD-10-CM manual. Read the descriptions of the seventh characters. Write the letter that matches each definition in the space provided. Some choices may be used more than once and some choices may not be used at all.

A	J
B	K
C	M
D	N
E	P
F	Q
G	R
H	S

1. The character _____ describes a subsequent encounter for closed fracture with malunion.

2. The character _____ describes a subsequent encounter for open fracture type IIIA, IIIB, or IIIC with routine healing.

3. The character _____ describes a subsequent encounter for closed fracture with nonunion.

4. The character _____ describes an initial encounter for closed fracture.

5. The character _____ describes an initial encounter for open fracture type IIIA, IIIB, or IIIC.

6. The character _____ describes a subsequent encounter for open fracture type I or II with delayed healing.

7. The character _____ describes sequelae.

8. The character _____ describes an initial encounter for open fracture type I or II.

9. The character _____ describes a subsequent encounter for closed fracture with routine healing.

10. The character _____ describes a subsequent encounter for open fracture type I or II with routine healing.

(continued)

(continued from page 211)

Multiple Choice

Instructions: Circle the letter of the best answer to each question based on the information you learned in this chapter.

1. What condition requires abstracting the depth, anatomic site, and extent?
   A. Poisoning
   B. Fracture
   C. Burn
   D. Abuse

2. What type of fracture is classified by the Gustilo system?
   A. Open fracture
   B. Pathologic fracture
   C. Epiphysis fracture
   D. Comminuted fracture

3. How would you code the following scenario? *A patient is treated for a keloid scar that forms following a third-degree burn on the right cheek.*
   A. L91.0, T20.36XA
   B. L91.0, T20.36XS
   C. L91.0
   D. T20.36XS, L91.0

4. When is a T code that describes the drug and the intent sequenced first?
   A. Poisoning
   B. Adverse effect
   C. Underdosing
   D. All drug-related injuries

5. What Main Term should be located in the Index to assign a code for adult or child abuse?
   A. Abuse
   B. Maltreatment
   C. Child
   D. Confirmed

6. How would you code the following scenario? *A 6-year-old boy is treated for contusions on the right upper arm due to suspected physical abuse by his stepmother.*
   A. T74.12XA, S40.021A, Y04.8XXA, Y07.433
   B. Y04.8XXA, T74.12XA, S40.021A
   C. S40.021A, T76.02XA, Y04.8XXA, Y07.433
   D. T76.02XA, S40.021A, Y04.8XXA, Y07.433

7. When should a code be assigned for complications of care?
   A. Patients have more than one condition.
   B. Providers document that a medical or surgical procedure is the cause of a condition.
   C. Providers perform complicated procedures.
   D. Physician documentation is unclear.

8. How would you code the following scenario? *A patient has an allergic reaction to trimethoprim-sulfamethoxazole prescribed two days ago by her family physician for a urinary tract infection.*
   A. T36.8X5A, N39.0
   B. T36.8X5A, R06.02, L50.0
   C. N39.0, R06.02, L50.0, T36.8X5A
   D. R06.02, L50.0, T36.8X5A

9. How should codes be sequenced when patients are treated for a sequela or after-effects after the primary injury has healed?
   A. Sequence the code that identifies the original injury first and the after-effect second.
   B. Sequence the after-effect condition first and the primary injury second.
   C. Assign codes for the after-effect but not the original injury.
   D. Sequence according to the circumstances of admission.

10. How should codes be sequenced when coding adverse effects?
   A. Sequence according to the circumstances of admission.
   B. Sequence the external cause code first.
   C. Sequence the code for the resulting condition or manifestation first.
   D. Sequence the code for type and intent of injury first.

KEEP ON CODING

Instructions: Read the diagnostic statement, then use the Index and Tabular List to assign and sequence ICD-10-CM diagnosis codes. Write the code(s) on the line provided.

1. Abrasion of the scalp, initial encounter. ICD-10-CM Code(s) _____

2. Fracture of the mandible, subsequent encounter with routine healing. ICD-10-CM Code(s) _____

3. Laceration of the left carotid artery, initial encounter. ICD-10-CM Code(s) _____

4. Muscle strain of the lower back, initial encounter. ICD-10-CM Code(s) _____

5. Accidental ingestion of toxic mushrooms, initial encounter. ICD-10-CM Code(s) _____

6. Bone marrow transplant failure. ICD-10-CM Code(s) _____

7. Crushing injury of the left upper arm, initial encounter. ICD-10-CM Code(s) _____

8. Heat collapse, initial encounter. ICD-10-CM Code(s) _____

9. Fracture of the left sacrum, type 3, subsequent encounter with routine healing. ICD-10-CM Code(s) _____

10. Complete amputation of right breast, traumatic injury, late effect. ICD-10-CM Code(s) _____

11. Late effect of a moderate laceration of the spleen. ICD-10-CM Code(s) _____

12. Nonunion of closed fracture of femoral neck, right. ICD-10-CM Code(s) _____

13. Acute transfusion reaction due to Rh incompatibility, initial encounter. ICD-10-CM Code(s) _____

14. Traumatic compartment syndrome of the left hip, initial encounter. ICD-10-CM Code(s) _____

15. Partial traumatic amputation, left leg, subsequent encounter. ICD-10-CM Code(s) _____

16. Blast injury of right ear, initial encounter. ICD-10-CM Code(s) _____

17. Traumatic hemopneumothorax, subsequent encounter. ICD-10-CM Code(s) _____

18. Foreign body in nostril, initial encounter. ICD-10-CM Code(s) _____

19. Late effect of a third-degree burn of the left ankle. ICD-10-CM Code(s) _____

20. Displaced avulsion fracture of the right ischium, closed, initial encounter. ICD-10-CM Code(s) _____

21. Major contusion of left kidney, traumatic, initial encounter. ICD-10-CM Code(s) _____

22. Displaced longitudinal fracture of right patella, closed, initial encounter. ICD-10-CM Code(s) _____

23. Open bite of the right buttock, subsequent encounter. ICD-10-CM Code(s) _____

24. Sprain of right ankle, initial encounter. ICD-10-CM Code(s) _____

25. Adverse effect of overuse of laxatives, subsequent encounter. ICD-10-CM Code(s) _____

CODING CHALLENGE

Instructions: Read the mini-medical-record of each patient's encounter, then abstract, assign, and sequence ICD-10-CM diagnosis codes using the Index to Diseases, the Index to External Causes, and the Tabular List. Write the code(s) on the line provided.

1. OFFICE   Gender: F   Age: 71

Chief complaint: Swollen and painful right wrist and large bruises on right calf after she tripped and fell in the living room of her apartment yesterday.

Assessment: Colles' fracture. Extensive hematoma on the calf is due to her long term warfarin (*anticoagulant/blood thinner*) therapy. Patient was previously diagnosed with age-related osteoporosis.

Plan: Arm casted, INR (*international normalized ratio blood clotting test*) performed, RTO to access healing of fracture and cast removal.

Tip: Colles' fracture is a fracture to the distal radius. Assign four diagnosis codes and two external cause codes.

6 ICD-10-CM Codes _____

_____

2. OFFICE   Gender: M   Age: 21

Reason for encounter: Follow-up on shoulder dislocation sustained when the motorcycle he was driving collided with an automobile three weeks ago.

Current status: Patient continues to have persistent pain and is unable to work.

Assessment: Dislocated right shoulder, acromioclavicular joint, 150% displacement

(continued)

2. (continued)

Plan: Outpatient surgery scheduled for reducing dislocation. This will be performed under IV sedation. Preop instructions provided to the patient.

Tip: Assign a code for the injury and an external cause code for the accident.

2 ICD-10-CM Codes _____

3. EMERGENCY DEPT   Gender: F   Age: 19

Reason for encounter: Infected wound where she stepped on nail last week

Assessment: Puncture wound left foot

Plan: Continue antibiotic ointment, begin 10 day regime of antibiotics, review status of tetanus immunization. Redress wound. RTO in 3 days.

Tip: Assign a code for the injury and an external cause code. Read the instructional notes for the category.

3 ICD-10-CM Codes _____

_____

4. INPATIENT HOSPITAL   Gender: M   Age: 45

Reason for admission: Admitted from emergency department due to skull fracture. He was unconscious for 90 minutes, but returned to his normal state of consciousness.

Assessment: Open occipital condylar fracture (type I) of base of skull with subarachnoid hemorrhage.

(continued)

(continued)

(continued from page 213)

4. (continued)

Plan: Craniotomy performed based on CT results which showed bleeding. Vessel occlusion performed. Patient in ICU following surg. RTO 4 days post discharge and weekly thereafter for two weeks.

Tip: A combination code describes the injury and the loss of consciousness. The external cause is not documented. Do not assign external cause codes.

2 ICD-10-CM Codes _____

5. EMERGENCY DEPT   Gender: M   Age: 37

Reason for encounter: Ketoacidosis with coma. Admit for observation. Stat blood chemistry and insulin administration.

Assessment: Type 1 diabetic forgot to take insulin. He is here on vacation and got confused due to the time zone change and an erratic schedule.

Plan: FU with endocrinologist when returns home 1 week.

Tip: Follow the guidelines for underdosing. OGCR I.C. 19.e.5)(c).

3 ICD-10-CM Codes _____

_____

6. OFFICE   Gender: M   Age: 34

Reason for encounter: Removal of cast

Assessment: X-rays show full healing of oblique fracture of left radius shaft. Cast removed.

Tip: Do not assign aftercare **Z** codes with injury codes. OGCR I.C.19.a.

1 ICD-10-CM Code _____

7. EMERGENCY DEPT   Gender: F   Age: 28

Chief complaint: Patient was brought in by her neighbor. She was at home stripping wood furniture inside on a rainy day. She got a severe headache and nausea due to the fumes and began vomiting.

Assessment: Acetone toxicity

Plan: OTC medication for headache, restore fluids orally, postpone furniture finishing until it is possible to have better ventilation.

Tip: Assign three diagnosis codes for the poisoning and manifestations and three external cause codes.

6 ICD-10-CM Codes _____

_____

8. OFFICE   Gender: M   Age: 48

Reason for admission: Admitted from emergency department, where he was seen after an accident while riding as a passenger in an off-road recreational vehicle.

Assessment: Transverse fracture right tibia shaft, notified patient's oncologist, who is currently treating him for prostate cancer.

Plan: FU with oncologist and orthopedic surgeon in office.

Tip: Refer to OGCR I.C.2.

3 ICD-10-CM Codes _____

_____

9. INPATIENT HOSPITAL   Gender: M
Age: 18 months

Reason for admission: Child got into some open whiskey and was found unconscious. He had been left alone by his stepfather who ran out to the corner store. Admit for overnight observation.

Assessment: Child neglect and abandonment. Alcohol toxicity. Blood alcohol level (BAC) of .360 (360 mg per 100 ml of blood).

Plan: Stabilize with oxygen and IV fluids. Social service evaluation of home, with mandatory report to Department of Human Services

Tip: Assign three diagnosis codes and three external cause codes for BAC, perpetrator, and place of occurrence. (Do not assign codes for the coma scale.)

6 ICD-10-CM Codes _____

_____

10. INPATIENT HOSPITAL   Gender: F   Age: 22

Chief complaint: Admitted from physician's office after complaining of fast heartbeat

Assessment: Supraventricular tachycardia that is a late effect of a heroin overdose during a suicide attempt 3 months ago

Plan: Stabilized rhythm with vagal maneuvers. Discharged on regime of antiarrhythmic med. Referral for substance addiction.

Tip: Assign codes for the injury and the current manifestation.

2 ICD-10-CM Codes _____

Chapter 13

Diseases of the Circulatory System (I00-I99)

Learning Objectives

After completing this chapter, you should have the skills to:

13.1 Spell and define the key words, medical terms, and abbreviations related to diseases of the circulatory system. (Remember)

13.2 Summarize the structure, function, and common conditions of the circulatory system. (Understand)

13.3 Adhere to the Official Guidelines for Coding and Reporting related to diseases of the circulatory system. (Apply)

13.4 Examine and abstract diagnostic information from the medical record for coding diseases of the circulatory system. (Analyze)

13.5 Demonstrate how to assign codes for diseases of the circulatory system. (Apply)

13.6 Utilize guidelines for arranging (sequencing) multiple diagnosis codes for diseases of the circulatory system. (Apply)

Chapter Outline

- **Circulatory System Refresher**
- **Conditions of the Circulatory System**
- **Coding Guidelines for the Circulatory System**
- **Abstracting for Circulatory System Conditions**
- **Assigning Codes for Circulatory System Conditions**
- **Arranging Codes for Circulatory System Conditions**

Key Terms and Abbreviations

acute myocardial infarction (AMI)
angiography
angioplasty
aorta
aortic valve
arrhythmia
arteriole
artery
atrioventricular bundle (bundle of His)
atrioventricular (AV) node
atrioventricular (AV) valve
atria
autologous
Barlow's syndrome
bundle branch
bypass graft
capillary
cardiac catheterization
cardiac function test
cardiac scan

cardiovascular (CV) system
cerebral
circulatory system
click murmur syndrome
coronary artery bypass graft (CABG)
coronary circulation
current MI
diastole
Doppler ultrasonography
echocardiography
electrocardiography (ECG, EKG)
embolectomy
endarterectomy
endocardium
epicardium
Holter monitor
inferior vena cava
internal mammary artery (IMA)
left atrium
left ventricle

mitral valve
mitral valve prolapse (MVP)
mitral valve stenosis
myocardial infarction (MI)
myocardium
native
nonautologous
nonbiological
non–ST elevation MI (NSTEMI)
nontransmural
occlusion
old (healed) MI
pacemaker
parietal pericardium
pericardium
plaque
precerebral
pulmonary circulation
pulmonary valve
Purkinje fiber
regurgitation

right atrium
right ventricle
sinoatrial (SA) node
ST elevation MI (STEMI)
stent insertion
stress testing
subendocardial
subsequent MI
superior vena cava
systemic circulation
systole
transmural MI
tricuspid valve
valve repair
valve replacement
vein
venography
ventricle
venule
visceral pericardium

In addition to the key terms listed here, students should know the terms defined within tables in this chapter.

INTRODUCTION

When your vehicle's fuel pump is not working correctly, your vehicle may stall when the accelerator is pressed or not start at all. Just as the fuel pump is responsible for circulating gas throughout the engine, the human heart is also a pump with the job of circulating blood. Physicians listen to the heart with a stethoscope and measure blood pressure as part of their diagnostic methods.

In this chapter, you learn more about how the circulatory system works, why it sometimes does not work as it should, and how physicians treat these conditions. Cardiologists are physicians who specialize in diagnosing and treating diseases of the circulatory system. Subspecialities in cardiology include pediatric cardiology and cardiothoracic surgery. Primary care physicians diagnose and treat common conditions of the circulatory systems and refer complex cases to cardiologists.

CIRCULATORY SYSTEM REFRESHER

The function of the **circulatory system**, also called the **cardiovascular (CV) system**, is to distribute blood throughout the body. It consists of the heart, which is the pump, and blood vessels, which are the tubes that carry blood. The distribution or transportation task provides three functions:

- Carries oxygen and nutrients to body tissues for metabolism
- Carries waste products of metabolism to the kidneys and other excretory organs
- Circulates electrolytes and hormones needed to regulate body functions

The circulatory system consists of pulmonary circulation, systemic circulation, and coronary circulation. **Pulmonary circulation**, which occurs between the heart and the lungs, carries deoxygenated blood from the heart to the lungs, where it is replenished with oxygen, then back to the heart. **Systemic circulation**, which occurs between the heart and the rest of the body, carries oxygenated blood away from the heart to the tissues and cells of the body, then carries oxygen-depleted blood back to the heart. **Coronary circulation**, which occurs within the heart, carries blood from the aorta to the tissues of the heart to maintain the function of the heart itself (■ FIGURE 13-1).

According to the Centers for Disease Control and Prevention, heart disease is the leading cause of death in the United States for both men and women, accounting for over 25% of all deaths each year. Every year about 525,000 people have a first heart attack and another 210,000, who previously had a heart attack, have another one. In the United States, health care services, medications, and lost productivity related to heart disease cost more than $207 billion per year.

To understand disorders of the circulatory system, coders need to understand the structure and operation of the heart muscle, the conduction system, and the blood vessels.

The Heart Muscle

The heart is a muscular organ that contains four chambers: two **atria**, which receive blood from the body (**right atrium**) and the lungs (**left atrium**), and two **ventricles**, which eject

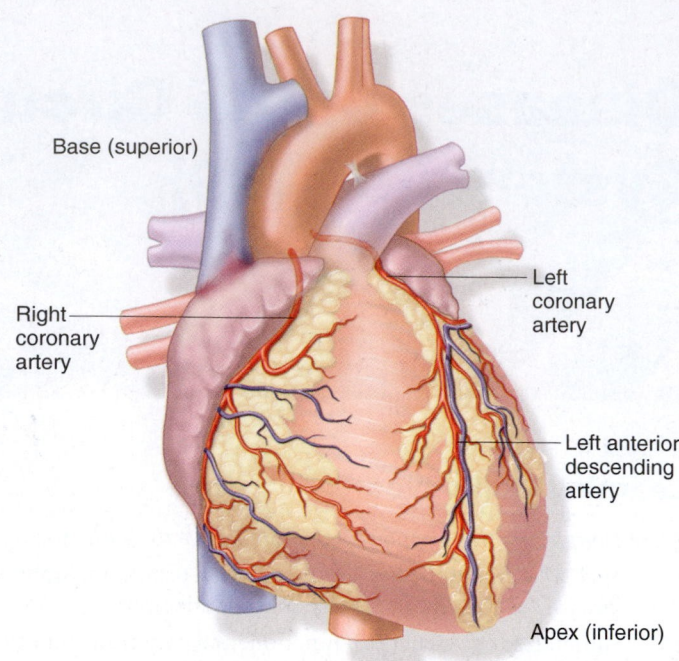

Base (superior)

Right coronary artery

Left coronary artery

Left anterior descending artery

Apex (inferior)

Figure 13-1 ■ The major arteries and vessels of coronary circulation.

blood to the lungs (**right ventricle**) and the body (**left ventricle**) (■ FIGURE 13-2). Four valves control the one-way flow of blood into, through, and out of the heart: the **tricuspid valve** (*right atrium to right ventricle*), **mitral valve** (*left atrium to left ventricle*), **pulmonary valve** (*right ventricle to pulmonary artery*), and **aortic valve** (*left ventricle to aorta*). The mitral and tricuspid valves are **atrioventricular (AV) valves** because they control the flow of blood from atria to ventricles. During every heart cycle, each chamber relaxes as it fills with blood during **diastole** and contracts as it ejects blood during **systole**.

The heart wall is a thick muscle consisting of three layers:

- The **endocardium**, the smooth inner layer that reduces friction as the blood flows through the heart
- The **myocardium**, the thick muscular inner layers that contract to pump blood
- The **pericardium**, a double-walled sac filled with fluid, which is the outer layer

The pericardium consists of the **epicardium** or **visceral pericardium** (*inner layer*) and the **parietal pericardium** (*outer layer*).

Disorders of the Heart Muscle

Myocardial infarction (MI), commonly known as a heart attack, is the death of heart tissue caused by an interruption to the blood supply. The most common cause of MI is **occlusion** (*blockage*) of a coronary artery by **plaque** (*a buildup of cholesterol inside the wall of blood vessels*). MIs are described by the heart wall that is affected: anterior, posterior, or inferior. A **transmural MI** extends through the entire thickness of the heart muscle. A **subendocardial** or **nontransmural** infarction affects only a small portion of the heart wall, usually due to a

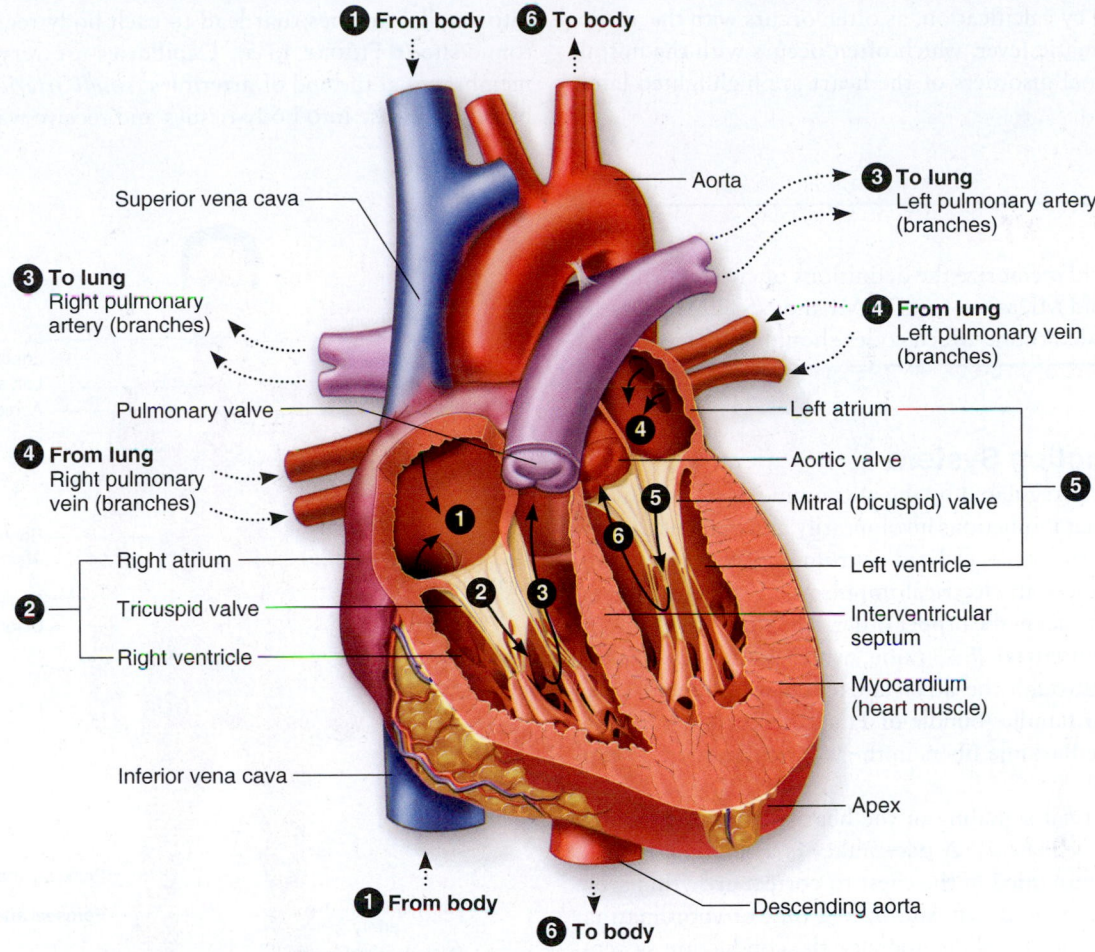

Figure 13-2 ■ The path of blood flow through the heart.

decreased, but not totally occluded, blood supply. Physicians also classify MIs clinically as *type 1* through *type 5* based on the serum (*blood*) level of troponin or creatine kinase–MB mass.

An MI that has occurred within the past four weeks is an **acute myocardial infarction (AMI)**, also referred to as a **current MI**. An MI that occurs within four weeks of a previous AMI is also clinically acute but is referred to as a **subsequent MI** to distinguish it from the original MI. An MI more than four weeks old is an **old (healed) MI**.

MIs are further described based on the results of an electrocardiogram (ECG, EKG) (■ FIGURE 13-3). Each part of the EKG is labeled with a letter denoting a specific phase of the heart's electrical activity. The ST segment is elevated in an MI that completely occludes a vessel, known as **ST elevation MI (STEMI)**. When the vessel is partially blocked, the ST segment is not elevated, resulting in a **non–ST elevation MI (NSTEMI)**.

The valves of the heart can be affected by prolapse, regurgitation, or stenosis. The most common valvular disorder is **mitral valve prolapse (MVP)**, also called **click murmur syndrome** and **Barlow's syndrome**. The two leaflets that comprise the valve fall backward into the left atrium, which results in **regurgitation**, blood leaking backward through the opening. **Mitral valve stenosis** is a narrowing of the valve opening, which

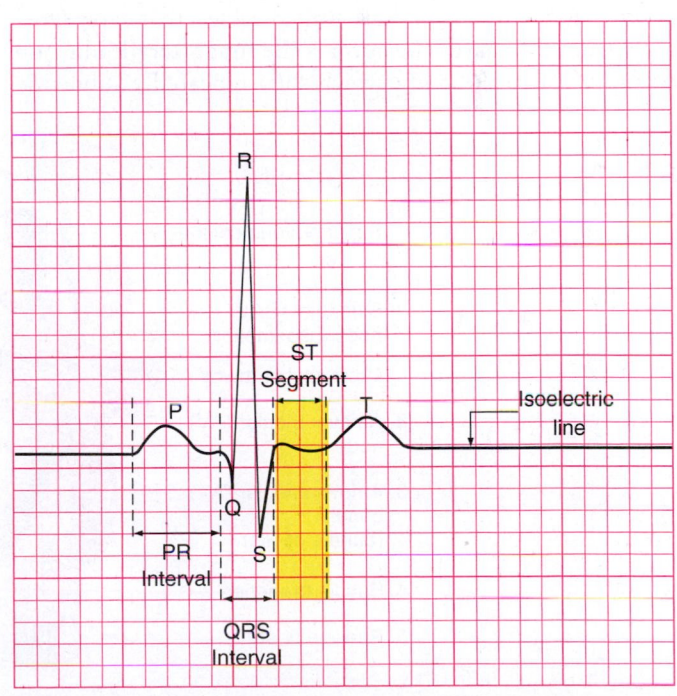

Figure 13-3 ■ Example of an ECG report showing the ST segment.

may be caused by calcification, as often occurs with the aortic valve, or rheumatic fever, which often occurs with the mitral valve. Additional disorders of the heart are highlighted later in this chapter.

into smaller arteries that lead to each body region and anatomic site (■ FIGURE 13-5). **Capillaries** are very thin-walled membranes at the end of **arterioles** (*small arteries*) that allow blood to diffuse into body tissues and receive waste products

---

SUCCESS STEP

Coders should memorize the definitions of current, subsequent, and old MI, as well as STEMI and NSTEMI. These distinctions determine which codes should be assigned.

The Conduction System

The heart rate is regulated by the autonomic nervous system, which means that it functions involuntarily and humans cannot voluntarily control it. Specialized neuromuscular tissue within the heart conducts an electrical impulse that stimulates each chamber to contract in the proper order. The electrical impulses begin in the **sinoatrial (SA) node**, which is the pacemaker of the heart, through the **atrioventricular (AV) node** to the **atrioventricular bundle (bundle of His)**, then through **bundle branches** to the **Purkinje fibers** in the ventricular myocardium (■ FIGURE 13-4).

Faulty electrical signaling in the heart causes **arrhythmia** (*an abnormal heartbeat*). A **pacemaker** is a small electronic device that is implanted in the chest to correct arrhythmia by speeding up, slowing down, smoothing out, or coordinating the heartbeat. Additional disorders of the conduction system are highlighted later in this chapter.

The Blood Vessels

Blood vessels are the pipes that carry the blood through the body. **Arteries** are large, thick-walled vessels that carry blood away from the heart. The **aorta** is the first artery leading out of the heart to the body, which then repeatedly subdivides

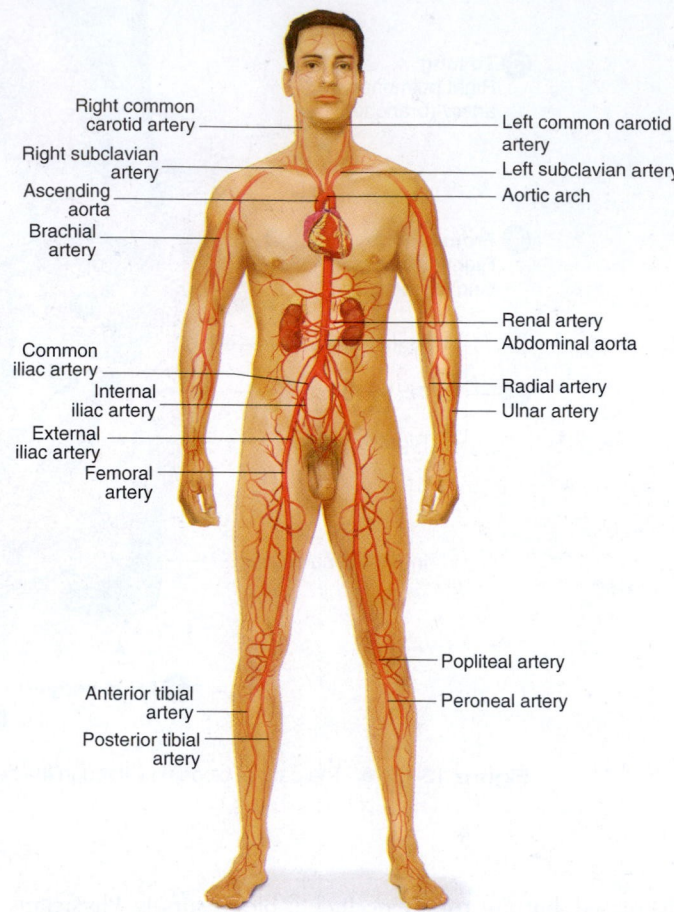

Figure 13-5 ■ The major arteries of systemic circulation.

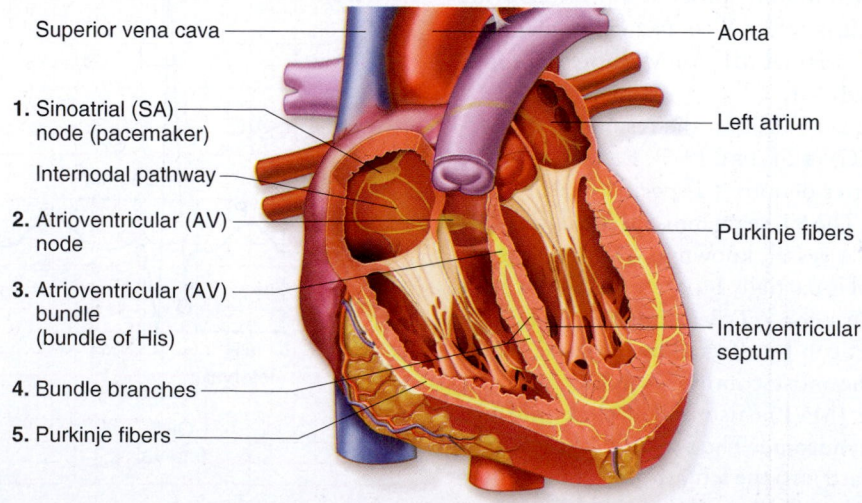

Figure 13-4 ■ The conduction system of the heart.

from the tissues to send back into the bloodstream. **Veins** and **venules** (*small veins*) carry blood from the capillaries back to the heart in successively larger veins leading to the **superior vena cava** and **inferior vena cava**, the largest veins that carry deoxygenated blood back to the right ventricle (■ FIGURE 13-6). Disorders of the blood vessels are highlighted later in this chapter.

In the preceding figures, each structure in the circulatory system is labeled. Arteries and veins are generally named after the anatomic site where they are located. For example, the artery in the femur (*thigh*) is the femoral artery and the vein in the upper leg is the femoral vein. Refer to ■ TABLE 13-1 for a refresher on how to build medical terms related to the circulatory system.

CODING CAUTION

Be alert for medical terms that are spelled similarly and have different meanings.

hemorrhoid (*resembling blood*) and **hemorrhage** (*flow of blood*)

ather/o (*plaque*) and **arteri/o** (*artery*) and **arthr/o** (*joint*)

pericardium (*sack around the heart*) and **perineum** (*the area between the external genitalia and the anus*)

CONDITIONS OF THE CIRCULATORY SYSTEM

Diseases and disorders of the circulatory system can affect the heart muscle, the conduction system of the heart, coronary circulation, or systemic (peripheral) circulation. Diseases of the heart structure are generally caused by a weakness or looseness in one or more components. Diseases of coronary circulation affect the veins and arteries that feed the heart. The most common is the blockage of a coronary artery, which diminishes blood flow to the heart. Diseases of the conduction system result in cardiac arrhythmias, irregularities of the heartbeat. Diseases of systemic circulation include an abnormality in a vein or artery in the arms and legs, such as hardening of the arteries and blockages. Refer to (■ TABLE 13-2, page 220), for a summary of diseases affecting the circulatory system.

This section provides a general reference to help understand the most common diagnoses of the circulatory system but does not list everything you need to know. Use medical terminology skills discussed earlier in this chapter to learn the meaning of unfamiliar words. Remember to keep standard reference books handy in case you get stuck.

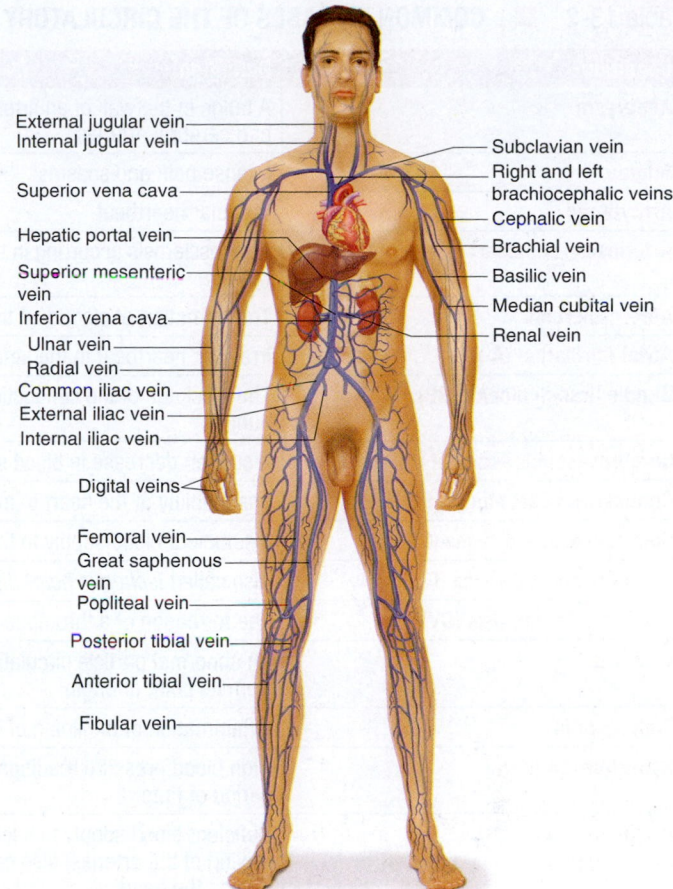

External jugular vein
Internal jugular vein
Superior vena cava
Hepatic portal vein
Superior mesenteric vein
Inferior vena cava
Ulnar vein
Radial vein
Common iliac vein
External iliac vein
Internal iliac vein
Digital veins
Femoral vein
Great saphenous vein
Popliteal vein
Posterior tibial vein
Anterior tibial vein
Fibular vein

Subclavian vein
Right and left brachiocephalic veins
Cephalic vein
Brachial vein
Basilic vein
Median cubital vein
Renal vein

Figure 13-6 ■ The major veins of systemic circulation.

Neoplasms of the Circulatory System

Neoplasms of the cardiovascular system are rare and, when they do occur, most are benign. Secondary or metastatic neoplasms of the heart occur in 1% of the population; primary neoplasms are even more rare.

Diagnostic Methods

Diseases of the circulatory system are diagnosed with laboratory tests, imaging studies, and cardiac function studies, which are described as follows:

- Laboratory tests measure the levels of substances in the blood, such as the following:
  - Cardiac enzymes
    - Creatine phosphokinase (CPK)
    - Lactate dehydrogenase (LDH)
    - Glutamic oxaloacetic transaminase (GOT)

Table 13-1 ■ **EXAMPLE OF CONSTRUCTING MEDICAL TERMS FOR THE CIRCULATORY SYSTEM**

Combining Form	Suffix	Complete Medical Term
my/o (*muscle*)		**endo + cardi + itis** (*inflammation of the lining inside the heart*)
		myo + cardi + itis (*inflammation of the heart muscle*)
angi/o (*vessel*)	**–gram** (*recording*) **–itis** (*inflammation*) **–plasty** (*repair*)	**angio + gram** (*recording of the vessels*)
cardi/o (*heart*)		**electro + cardio + gram** (*electrical recording of the heart*)
		echo + cardio + gram (*recording of the sound of the heart*)
end/o (*within*)		**angio + plasty** (*repair of a blood vessel*)

Table 13-2 ■ **COMMON DISEASES OF THE CIRCULATORY SYSTEM**

Condition	Definition
Aneurysm	A bulge in the wall of an artery due to weakening, most commonly occurring in the abdominal aorta and cerebral arteries
Angina	Intense pain and spasms
Arrhythmia	Irregular heartbeat
Arteriosclerotic heart disease (ASHD)	Atherosclerosis occurring in the coronary arteries; also called *ischemic heart disease* or *coronary heart disease*
Atherosclerosis	The formation of plaque on the inner walls of arteries in the heart
Atrial fibrillation (A-fib)	Irregular heartbeat in the atria characterized by an abnormal quivering of heart fibers
Bundle branch block (BBB)	The blockage of the conduction of electrical impulse through the branches of the atrioventricular bundle
Cerebrovascular accident (CVA)	A sudden decrease in blood supply to the brain; also called *stroke*
Congestive heart failure (CHF)	The inability of the heart to maintain circulation, often resulting in water retention and edema
Coronary artery disease (CAD)	Insufficient blood supply to the heart due to an obstruction of one or more coronary arteries
Coronary heart disease (CHD)	Also called *ischemic heart disease* or *arteriosclerotic heart disease*
Deep vein thrombosis (DVT)	The formation of a thrombus within a deep vein, usually in the leg or pelvis
Embolus	An abnormal particle circulating in the blood, such as an air bubble or thrombus that has broken loose from its point of origin
Endocarditis	Inflammation of the lining of the heart or valves, due to bacteria or another disease
Hypertension (HTN)	High blood pressure readings (exceeding 140/90 mmHg), documented repeatedly over an extended period of time
Ischemia	Deficient blood supply to a local area due to obstruction of the arterial blood flow, usually due to narrowing of the arteries; also called *coronary heart disease* or *arteriosclerotic heart disease* when it affects the heart
Mitral valve prolapse (MVP)	Weakness in the flaps of the mitral valve, which allows blood to flow backward from the right ventricle into the right atrium
Myocardial infarction (MI)	The death of heart tissue due to a blockage of the blood supply
Pericarditis	Inflammation of the pericardial sac that surrounds the heart
Peripheral artery disease (PAD)	Damage to arteries outside the heart resulting in decreased blood flow
Stenosis	A narrowing of a valve or vessel
Thrombus	A clot of blood formed within a blood vessel that remains attached to its point of origin
Transient ischemic attack (TIA)	A brief episode of cerebral ischemia
Ventricular fibrillation (V-fib)	Irregular heartbeat in the ventricles, characterized by an abnormal quivering of heart fibers, which can result in cardiac arrest

- Cholesterol
- Triglycerides
- Imaging studies are visualizations of the circulatory system using x-ray and ultrasound techniques, including:
  - **Angiography** (*x-ray taken after an opaque dye is injected into a blood vessel*)
  - **Cardiac scan** (*a scan of the heart after the patient receives radioactive thallium intravenously*)
  - **Doppler ultrasonography** (*an image created by measuring sound-wave echoes off of tissues and organs*)
  - **Echocardiography** (*noninvasive ultrasound to visualize internal cardiac structures*)
  - **Venography** (*x-ray of the veins by tracing the venous pulse*)

- **Cardiac function tests** measure the capacity of the heart in real time, including:
  - **Cardiac catheterization** (*passage of a thin tube through a blood vessel to the heart to visualize the structure, collect blood samples, and determine the blood pressure of the heart*)
  - **Electrocardiography** (**ECG, EKG**) (*a graphical recording of the electrical activity of the heart*)
  - **Holter monitor** (*a portable EKG worn by the patient for an extended period of hours or days to measure heart activity in a variety of situations*)
  - **Stress testing** (*measuring EKG and oxygen levels as a patient performs an increasing level of exercise on a treadmill or stationary bicycle*)

Treatment Methods

Heart disease is treated with a wide range of medications that regulate circulatory system functions, medical procedures such as a pacemaker or implantable cardioverter-defibrillator to regulate heart activity, and surgery to repair defects. Common procedures include:

- **Angioplasty** (*insertion of an inflatable catheter in a blood vessel that expands to compress plaque against the walls of the vessel*)
- **Bypass graft** (*creation of a new route around a blockage in a blood vessel using a vessel from another part of the body, another person, or a synthetic substitute*)
- **Coronary artery bypass graft (CABG)** (*open-heart surgery to create a bypass around a blocked coronary artery, usually using the* **internal mammary artery [IMA]** *or a vein from the leg*)

- **Embolectomy** (*removal of a clot from a blood vessel*)
- **Endarterectomy** (*removal of the diseased or damaged inner lining of an artery*)
- **Stent insertion** (*placement of a mesh tube in a blood vessel to keep it open; necessary in atherosclerosis*)
- **Valve repair** (*correction of a physical defect*)
- **Valve replacement** (*replacement of a heart valve with an synthetic or porcine [pig] valve*)

Heart transplants, first done in 1967, are the third most common organ transplant in the United States and are performed in extreme cases of heart failure when other treatments have failed. According to the United Network for Organ Sharing (UNOS), approximately 33,000 heart transplants are performed each year in the United States. However, the need is far greater than that but cannot be met, due to a shortage of available donor organs.

CODING PRACTICE

Exercise 13.1 Circulatory System Refresher

Instructions: Use your medical terminology skills and resources to define the following conditions related to the circulatory system, then assign the diagnosis code.

Follow these steps:

- Use slash marks "/" to break down each term into its root(s) and suffix.
- Define the meaning of the word, based on the meaning of each word part.
- Assign the default ICD-10-CM diagnosis code for the condition using the Index and Tabular List.

Example: endocarditis endo/card/itis   Meaning *inflammation of the lining of the heart*   ICD-10-CM Code *I38*

1. hypertension   Meaning _____   ICD-10-CM Code _____
2. myocarditis   Meaning _____   ICD-10-CM Code _____
3. cardiomyopathy   Meaning _____   ICD-10-CM Code _____
4. atheroma   Meaning _____   ICD-10-CM Code _____
5. arteriosclerosis   Meaning _____   ICD-10-CM Code _____
6. arrhythmia   Meaning _____   ICD-10-CM Code _____
7. lymphocele   Meaning _____   ICD-10-CM Code _____
8. thrombophlebitis   Meaning _____   ICD-10-CM Code _____
9. thromboangiitis   Meaning _____   ICD-10-CM Code _____
10. pyopneumopericardium   Meaning _____   ICD-10-CM Code _____

CODING GUIDELINES FOR THE CIRCULATORY SYSTEM

Coders should understand the organization of this ICD-10-CM chapter, chapter-wide and commonly used instructional notes in the Tabular List, and the relevant OGCR. This information is necessary for accurate coding.

ICD-10-CM Chapter 9, "Diseases of the Circulatory System (I00-I99)," contains 11 blocks or subchapters that

are divided by the type of disease. Review the block names and code ranges listed at the beginning of Chapter 9 in the ICD-10-CM manual to become familiar with the content and organization.

This chapter includes disorders that affect the heart and the pulmonary, systemic, and coronary circulatory systems. Conditions may consist of acquired physical dysfunctions or infections.

This chapter does not include congenital diseases of the circulatory system, which are classified in ICD-10-CM Chapter 17, "Congenital Malformations, Deformations, and Chromosomal Abnormalities (Q00-Q99)," or diseases of the blood, which are classified in ICD-10-CM Chapter 3, "Diseases of the Blood and Blood-Forming Organs and Certain Disorders Involving the Immune Mechanism (D50-D89)."

ICD-10-CM provides Official Guidelines for Coding and Reporting (OGCR) for the circulatory system in OGCR section I.C.9. OGCR provides detailed discussion regarding hypertension and its relationship to heart and kidney disease, atherosclerotic coronary artery disease and angina, cerebrovascular accident and disease, acute myocardial infarction, and hypertensive crisis. The Tabular List provides **Excludes2** notes at the beginning of the chapter as well as many instructional notes throughout the chapter regarding additional codes that are required to identify related conditions and lifestyle habits related to tobacco use. Specific OGCR guidelines are discussed and cited throughout this chapter of the text.

ABSTRACTING FOR CIRCULATORY SYSTEM CONDITIONS

Coders need to pay close attention to detail when abstracting for the cardiovascular system because codes must be specific to anatomic site, nature of the disease, and comorbidities. Coders rely on their knowledge of anatomy to identify the exact site of the disorder and their knowledge of diseases to identify the specific form of the disease and coexisting conditions. They also must identify circumstances that require Z codes. Key factors to review when coding cases that involve the circulatory system appear in ■ TABLE 13-3. Remember that the abstracting questions are a guide and that not every question applies to, or can be answered for, every case. For example, the questions about myocardial infarction do not apply to patients who have not had this condition.

Guided Example of Abstracting for Circulatory System Conditions

Refer to the following example throughout this chapter to learn skills for abstracting, assigning, and sequencing circulatory system codes. Tanisha Riemann, CCS-P, is a fictitious coder who guides you through the coding process.

Date: 4/1/yy Location: Branton Medical Center

Provider: Matthew Bunker, MD

Patient: Gordon Rothe Gender: M Age: 76

Reason for admission: Admitted from emergency department due to unstable angina, patient has been on warfarin since a CABG of the left anterior descending coronary artery (LAD) 11 years ago using the left saphenous vein, continues smoke cigarettes, although he states that his usage has decreased

Assessment: Atherosclerosis of grafted vessel

Plan: Balloon angioplasty to clear the partially blocked graft, Rx atorvastatin to address lipid rich plaque

---

Table 13-3 ■ KEY CRITERIA FOR ABSTRACTING CONDITIONS OF THE CIRCULATORY SYSTEM

❏ What part of the circulatory system is affected?
❏ What is the specific anatomic site?
❏ What type of disorder is present?
❏ Is the condition further specified as complete, partial, current, or old (if applicable)?
❏ What is the underlying cause?
❏ What symptoms are documented that are not integral to the condition?
❏ Is the condition acquired or congenital?
❏ Is the condition related to pregnancy?
❏ Does the patient have a current, subsequent, or old MI?
❏ Has the patient had more than one AMI in the past four weeks?
❏ What other cardiovascular conditions coexist?
❏ Does the patient have hypertension with heart or kidney involvement?
❏ What conditions exist in other organ systems?
❏ Which conditions are documented as being related to the cardiovascular condition?
❏ What is the patient's exposure to or use of tobacco?
❏ Does the patient use anticoagulants or antithrombotics on a long-term basis?
❏ Does the patient have a family history of cardiovascular disease?
❏ Does the patient wear a pacemaker?
❏ Has the patient had a CABG?
❏ If a vessel is blocked or diseased, is it an artery or vein? Is it native (*the patient's original vessel*) or a graft?
❏ If a grafted vessel is blocked, is the grafted vessel autologous (*from the patient*), biological nonautologous (*from a source other than the patient, such as a cadaver or animal*), or nonbiological (*synthetic*)?
❏ Is the patient waiting for or a recipient of a heart transplant?

Follow along as Tanisha Riemann, CCS-P, abstracts the diagnosis. Check off each step after you complete it.

▶ Tanisha reads through the entire record, paying special attention to the reason for the encounter and the final assessment. She refers to the Key Criteria for Abstracting Conditions of the Circulatory System (Table 13-3) to guide her review.

❏ She notes the presenting symptom of unstable angina.

❏ *What part of the circulatory system is affected?* Grafted vessel

❏ *What is the specific anatomic site?* The heart, near the left anterior descending coronary artery

❏ *What type of disorder is present?* Blocked graft and atherosclerosis

❏ *Is the condition further specified as complete, partial, current, or old?* Partially blocked

❏ *Does the patient have a current, subsequent, or old MI?* No

❑ *What other cardiovascular conditions coexist?* Lipid-rich plaque

❑ *What is the patient's exposure to or use of tobacco?* The patient continues to smoke cigarettes, although he states that his usage has decreased

❑ *Does the patient use anticoagulants or antithrombotics on a long-term basis?* Yes, the patient has been on warfarin since a CABG 11 years ago

❑ *Has the patient had a CABG?* Yes, 11 years ago

❑ *If a vessel is blocked or diseased, is it an artery or vein?* Vein *Is it native or a graft?* Graft

❑ *If a grafted vessel is blocked, is the grafted vessel autologous, biological nonautologous, or nonbiological?* The graft used the left saphenous vein, so it is autologous

► At this point, Tanisha is not sure of how many codes she will need. She knows that she needs to search the Index and cross-reference any instructional notes in the Tabular List before she knows what her final codes will be.

CODING PRACTICE

Exercise 13.2 **Abstracting for Circulatory System Conditions**

Instructions: Read the mini-medical-record of each patient's encounter and answer the abstracting questions. Write the answer on the line provided. Do not assign any codes.

1. INPATIENT HOSPITAL Gender: F Age: 42

Reason for admission: Admitted from emergency department with subendocardial infarction

Assessment: Nontransmural myocardial infarction

Plan: This is her first event so we will treat it with medication and diet.

a. What is a subendocardial infarction? _____

b. What is a nontransmural infarction? _____

c. What is the Main Term? _____

2. OFFICE Gender: F Age: 68

Reason for encounter: Patient has been taking her BP at home and is concerned about readings that have been increasing over the past 3 months. She claims to be taking the diuretic and beta blocker as directed. Lab results show slightly low potassium.

Assessment: Hypertensive cardiomegaly

Plan: Add spironolactone to the medication regime.

a. What is the cause of the patient's cardiomegaly? _____

b. Should you code for low potassium? _____

c. What is the Main Term? _____

3. INPATIENT HOSPITAL Gender: M Age: 68

Reason for admission: Mitral porcine valvoplasty

Assessment: Mitral valve regurgitation due to prolapse

a. Where is the mitral valve located? _____

b. In your own words, explain what procedure was done. _____

c. In your own words, explain why the procedure was done. _____

4. INPATIENT HOSPITAL Gender: F Age: 71

Reason for admission: Admitted from emergency department with angina. Patient has history of MI 2 years ago, as well as history of TIAs, although the TIAs did not leave any residual deficits.

Assessment: STEMI involving 90% occlusion of the right coronary artery

Procedure: CABG

a. Should you code for angina? _____
   Why or why not? _____

b. What is TIA? _____

c. What is STEMI? _____

d. What is the site of the STEMI? _____

e. Should you code for the old MI? _____

f. In your own words, describe the procedure that was done. _____

(continued)

CODING PRACTICE *(continued)*

---

5. OFFICE   Gender: M   Age: 65

Chief complaint: Increased edema and SOB since last visit

Assessment: HTN and decompensated CHF, A-fib

Plan: We will start by adjusting the diuretic, then evaluate the need for other adjustments based on response after 4 weeks. Continue long-term warfarin and clopidrogel (*an antiplatelet medication*).

a. Define the abbreviations in this scenario. _____
_____

b. Which condition are the edema and SOB most related to? _____

c. What is the causal relationship between HTN and CHF? _____

d. Which condition is the first listed diagnosis? _____
_____

Why? _____

e. What type of medication is warfarin? _____
_____

f. What type of medication is clopidrogel? _____
_____

---

6. INPATIENT HOSPITAL   Gender: M   Age: 57

Reason for admission: Transferred from another hospital where patient was admitted for cerebral infarct 20 hours ago and received tPA (*tissue plasminogen activator*), but now it is evident that a mechanical or surgical embolectomy is needed

Assessment: Cerebral infarction d/t embolus in right middle cerebral artery, cerebral atherosclerosis, HTN, history of tobacco use

Procedure: Surgical embolectomy

a. What is the common term for cerebral infarction? _____

b. What is the cause of the cerebral infarction? _____

c. What is an embolus? _____
_____

d. Is the affected artery **cerebral** (*within the brain*) or **precerebral** (*outside of the brain*)? _____
_____

e. What other medical conditions exist? _____
_____

f. What lifestyle habit is documented? _____

g. In your own words, describe the procedure that was performed. _____
_____

ASSIGNING CODES FOR CIRCULATORY SYSTEM CONDITIONS

Diseases of the circulatory system frequently occur with multiple comorbidities from within the cardiovascular system and/or from other systems. The choice of codes is dependent on the precise wording physicians use in the documentation. The coding of hypertension, a common circulatory system condition, is an example of how documentation affects code choices. Hypertension may occur by itself, in conjunction with chronic kidney disease, heart disease, both kidney and heart disease, or many other conditions. Refer to the following examples to better understand how to interpret physician documentation when assigning codes.

Hypertension

Physicians diagnose hypertension when patients have elevated blood pressure over an extended period of time. Assign a code for hypertension only when the physician has documented for this condition. Do not assign a code for hypertension simply because a patient has an incidental (*random*) high blood pressure reading (■ FIGURE 13-7).

High

　　altitude effects T70.20

　　blood pressure — *see also* Hypertension

　　　　reading (incidental) (isolated) (nonspecific), without diagnosis

　　　　　　of hypertension R03.0

Figure 13-7 ■ Index entry used to located codes for an incidental high blood pressure reading.

When the diagnosis of hypertension is documented, search for the Main Term **Hypertension** in the Index. Assign the default code, **I10 Essential (primary) hypertension**, for hypertension described with the following terms:

- Accelerated
- Benign
- Essential
- Idiopathic
- Malignant
- Systemic

Refer to the Index entry in the ICD-10-CM manual, which identifies these terms as nonessential modifiers by the use of parentheses (■ FIGURE 13-8). Subterms identify codes for use when hypertension occurs with or due to another condition, which is discussed later in this chapter.

In the Tabular List, an instructional note, **Excludes1**, reminds coders that hypertension complicating pregnancy, childbirth, and the puerperium (*postpartum period*) is not coded here. Another instructional note, **Excludes2**, directs coders to look elsewhere for hypertension involving vessels of the brain and eye.

Hypertension with Heart Disease

ICD-10-CM presumes a causal relationship between hypertension and conditions classified to **I50 Heart failure** or **I51.4** through **I51.9**, which includes myocarditis unspecified, myocardial degeneration, cardiomegaly, Takotsubo syndrome, and other ill-defined or unspecified heart disease (■ FIGURE 13-9). Hypertensive heart disease is the leading cause of illness and death due to hypertension. OGCR I.A.9.a.1) provides

guidelines for coding hypertension with heart conditions classified to **I50** or **I51.4** through **I51.9**. Assign codes as follows:

1. Assign a code from category **I11 Hypertensive heart disease**. This category includes any condition in **I51.4** to **I51.9** that is due to hypertension.

2. Also assign a code from category **I50 Heart failure** to identify the type of heart failure as left ventricular, systolic, diastolic, combined, or unspecified. Sequence the code for hypertensive heart disease first and the code for heart failure second (■ FIGURE 13-10).

If the provider has specifically documented a different cause for these same heart conditions (**I50.-, I51.4-I51.9**), assign separate codes. Sequence according to the circumstances of the admission/encounter (■ FIGURE 13-11).

> ### SUCCESS STEP
> To locate CHF in the Index, search for the Main Term **Failure** and the subterm **heart**.

Hypertensive Chronic Kidney Disease

ICD-10-CM presumes a causal relationship between hypertension and chronic kidney disease (CKD) because hypertension is known to cause CKD and CKD is known to cause hypertension. For this reason, the two conditions are linked by the term **with** in the Index. These conditions should be coded as related even in the absence of provider documentation explicitly linking them, unless the documentation clearly states the conditions are unrelated. For hypertension and conditions not specifically linked by relational terms such as **with, associated with**, or **due to** in the classification, provider documentation must link the conditions in order to code them as related (OGCR I.9.a).

OGCR I.C.9.a provides guidelines on coding these conditions when they occur together, unless the physician has

> **Hypertension, hypertensive** (accelerated) (benign) (essential) (idiopathic) (malignant) (systemic) I10

Figure 13-8 ■ Index entry for Main Term "Hypertension" showing nonessential modifiers.

I51.4 Myocarditis, unspecified
Chronic (interstitial) myocarditis
Myocardial fibrosis
Myocarditis NOS
Excludes1: acute or subacute myocarditis (I40.-)
I51.5 Myocardial degeneration
Fatty degeneration of heart or myocardium
Myocardial disease
Senile degeneration of heart or myocardium
I51.7 Cardiomegaly
Cardiac dilatation
Cardiac hypertrophy
Ventricular dilatation
I51.8 Other ill-defined heart diseases
I51.81 Takotsubo syndrome
Reversible left ventricular dysfunction following sudden emotional stress
Stress induced cardiomyopathy
Takotsubo cardiomyopathy
Transient left ventricular apical ballooning syndrome
I51.89 Other ill-defined heart diseases
Carditis (acute)(chronic)
Pancarditis (acute)(chronic)
I51.9 Heart disease, unspecified

Figure 13-9 ■ Tabular List entry for codes I51.4 to I51.9.

> Patient is seen for hypertension and myocarditis with chronic combined congestive heart failure.
>
> (1) **I11.0 Hypertensive heart disease with heart failure**
> (2) **I50.42 Chronic combined systolic (congestive) and diastolic (congestive) heart failure**

Figure 13-10 ■ Example of assigning codes for heart disease and hypertension when a causal relationship is presumed.

> Patient is seen for chronic combined congestive heart failure, and unrelated hypertension.
>
> (1) **I50.42 Chronic combined systolic (congestive) and diastolic (congestive) heartfailure**
> (2) **I10 Essential (primary) hypertension**

Figure 13-11 ■ Example of assigning codes when heart disease and hypertension are documented as unrelated.

> Patient is seen for stage 4 CKD and HTN.
>
> (1) **I12.9 Hypertensive chronic kidney disease with stage 1 through stage 4 chronic kidney disease, or unspecified chronic kidney disease**
> (2) **N18.4 Chronic kidney disease, stage 4 (severe)**

Figure 13-12 ■ Example of assigning codes for hypertensive chronic kidney disease.

specifically documented a different cause for CKD. Assign codes as follows (■ FIGURE 13-12).

1. Assign a code from category **I12 Hypertensive chronic kidney disease** based on the stage of CKD documented. Refer to category **I12** in the ICD-10-CM manual to review the available codes and locate the instructional notes.

2. Assign a code from category **N18 Chronic kidney disease** as an additional code to identify the stage of CKD, as stated in the instructional note (OGCR I.C.9.a.2).

Hypertensive Kidney Disease and Hypertensive Heart Disease

The documentation may state that *both* hypertensive kidney disease and *hypertensive* heart disease exist. Assign codes from combination category **I13, Hypertensive heart and chronic kidney disease**, when there is hypertension with both heart and kidney involvement (OGCR I.A.9.a.3). Assign codes as follows (■ FIGURE 13-13):

1. Assign a code from category **I13 Hypertensive heart and chronic kidney disease**.

2. Also assign a code from category **I50** to identify the type of heart failure, when it is also present.

3. Assign a code from category **N18** to identify the stage of CKD.

Hypertension and Other Conditions

Whenever hypertension exists with another condition, searching Main Terms for both conditions helps ensure that nothing is omitted. Carefully review all available subterms under **Hypertension** to locate any applicable code for the comorbidity. Also locate the Index Main Term entry for the comorbid condition

> Patient is seen for hypertensive myocarditis with chronic combined CHF and stage 4 CKD.
>
> (1) **I13.0 Hypertensive heart and chronic kidney disease with heart failure and stage 1 through stage 4 chronic kidney disease, or unspecified chronic kidney disease**
> (2) **N18.4 Chronic kidney disease, stage 4 (severe)**
> (3) **I50.42 Chronic combined systolic (congestive) and diastolic (congestive) heart failure**

Figure 13-13 ■ Example of assigning codes for hypertensive heart disease and hypertensive chronic kidney disease.

and search for a subterm of hypertension. Refer to OGCR I.C.9.a for additional guidelines on coding hypertension with cerebrovascular disease and retinopathy, as well as secondary, transient, controlled, and uncontrolled hypertension.

Cerebrovascular Accident

When the type or cause of the CVA is documented, search the Index for the Main term **Infarct, Infarction** and first-level subterm **cerebral**. Select the appropriate second-level subterm **due to** to locate the most specific code.

To locate codes for CVA whose cause is not documented, search the Index for one of following Main Terms:

- **Stroke**
- **Accident, cerebral** or **Accident, cerebrovascular**

These Main Terms lead to code **I63.9 Cerebral infarction, unspecified**.

Refer to instructional notes at the beginning of category **I63** for **Includes, Excludes,** and **Use additional code** instructions.

- **Use additional code, if applicable, to identify status post administration of tPA (rtPA) in a different facility within the last 24 hours prior to admission to current facility (Z92.82).** The medication tPA (tissue plasminogen activator) is administered in the case of an ischemic stroke to help dissolve the clot quickly and restore the blood flow to the brain tissue.

- **Use additional code, if known, to indicate National Institutes of Health Stroke Scale (NIHSS) score (R29.7-).** The NIHSS score rates a patient's level of impairment following an ischemic stroke. Refer to Chapter 4, "Symptoms, Signs, and Abnormal Clinical and Laboratory Findings, Not Elsewhere Classified (R00-R99)," of this text for more information on the NIHSS score.

Sequela, or after-effects, of cerebrovascular disease are classified in category **I69 Sequelae of cerebrovascular disease** when conditions in I60-I67 are the original cause of sequelae. Conditions may be specified in the documentation as sequela or residuals and may occur at any time after the onset of the causal condition. Codes are divided by the type of causal event, such as nontraumatic subarachnoid hemorrhage or cerebral infarction, and by the specific sequela, such as memory deficit or monoplegia of an upper limb. Assign as many codes as needed to describe all sequela. Refer to OGCR I.C.9.d. for detailed guidelines.

Guided Example of Assigning Codes for Circulatory System Conditions

To practice skills for assigning codes for the circulatory system, continue with the example from earlier in the chapter about patient Gordon Rothe, who was admitted to Branton Medical Center due to unstable angina.

Follow along in your ICD-10-CM manual as Tanisha assigns codes. Check off each step after you complete it.

▶ First, Tanisha confirms the information she abstracted from the medical record:

❑ Unstable angina

❑ ASHD with occlusion in grafted vein

- ❏ Lipid-rich plaque
- ❏ Anticoagulant use for 11 years
- ❏ Cigarette smoker

▶ Tanisha searches the Index for the Main Term **Angina**.

- ❏ She locates the subterm **unstable I20.0**.

▶ Tanisha verifies code **I20.0** in the Tabular List.

- ❏ She reads the code title for **I20.0 Unstable angina** and confirms that this accurately describes the medical record documentation.

▶ Tanisha checks for instructional notes in the Tabular List.

- ❏ Tamara cross-references the beginning of category **I20** and reads the **Excludes1** note that states **atherosclerosis of coronary artery bypass graft(s) and coronary artery of transplanted heart with angina pectoris (I25.7-)**.

- ❏ The note tells her that **I20.0** cannot be used with a code from **I25.7-** because **Excludes1** means the codes are mutually exclusive.

- ❏ She decides to research the rest of her codes before deciding whether she should include **I20.0**.

▶ Next, Tanisha searches the Index for the Main Term **Atherosclerosis** (■ FIGURE 13-14).

- ❏ She locates the instructional note to cross-reference the Main Term **Arteriosclerosis**.

- ❏ She follows the indented subterms for **coronary (artery), bypass graft, autologous vein, with, angina pectoris, unstable I25.710**.

- ❏ She identifies that she will have a combination code for ASHD and unstable angina.

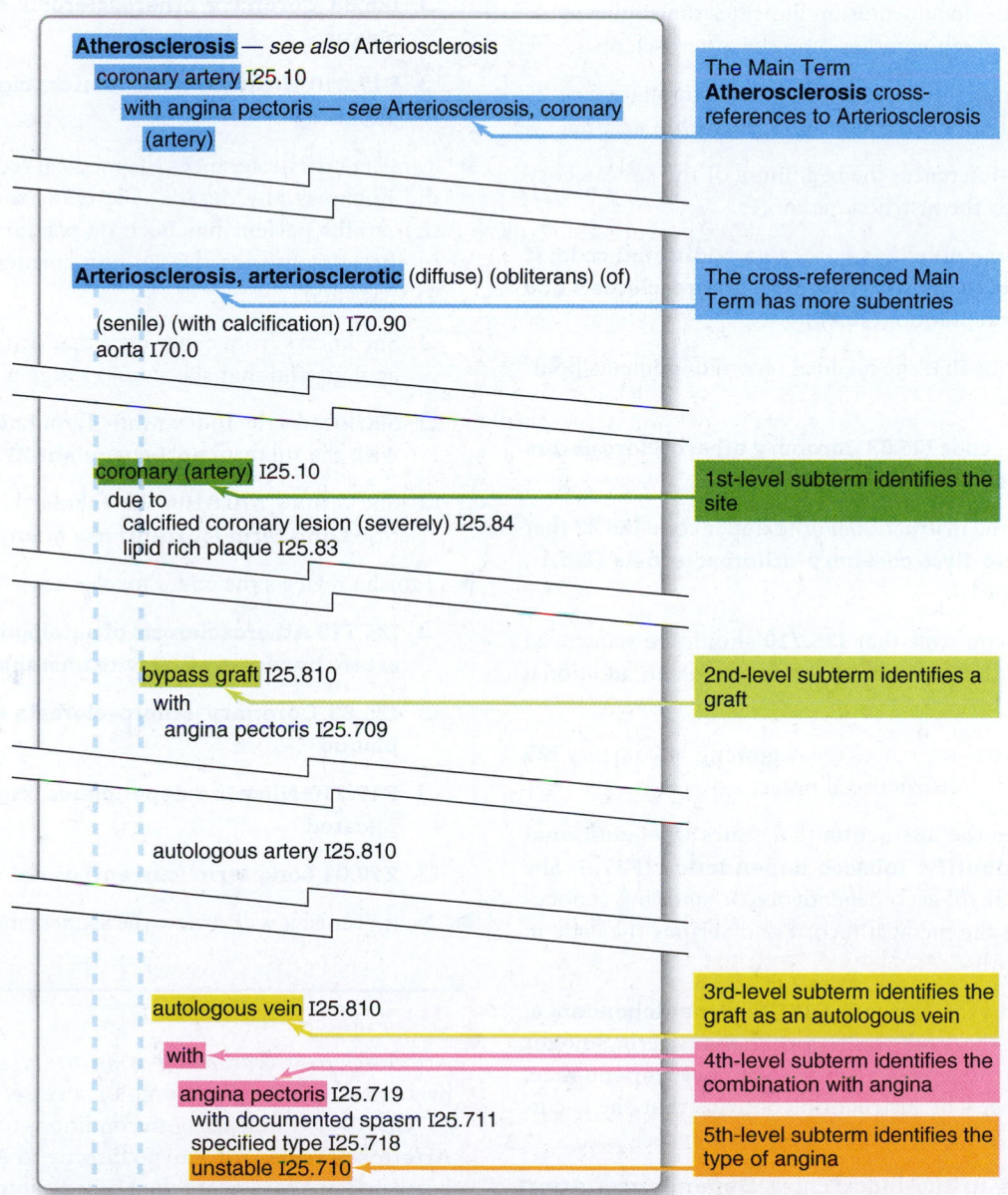

Figure 13-14 ■ Index entry used to locate codes for arteriosclerosis of a grafted autologous vein with unstable angina.

▶ Tanisha verifies code **I25.710** in the Tabular List.

❑ She locates the code title **Atherosclerosis of autologous vein coronary artery bypass graft(s) with unstable angina pectoris** and confirms that all components of the code description are consistent with the documentation.

❑ She reads the note below the code that states **Excludes2: embolism or thrombus of coronary artery bypass graft(s) (T82.8-)**. This instruction does not affect her coding because an embolism or thrombus is not documented.

❑ She also refers to OGCR I.C.9.b, which states:

  ▪ ICD-10-CM has combination codes for atherosclerotic heart disease with angina pectoris. When using one of these combination codes it is not necessary to use an additional code for angina pectoris. A causal relationship can be assumed in a patient with both atherosclerosis and angina pectoris, unless the documentation indicates the angina is due to something other than the atherosclerosis.

❑ She determines that because this is a combination code, she should *not* also assign **I20.0, Unstable angina**.

▶ Tanisha cross-references the beginning of the subcategory **I25.7** and reads the instructional notes.

❑ She reads the note that states **Use additional code, if applicable, to identify coronary atherosclerosis due to lipid rich plaque (I25.83)**.

❑ She confirms that the medical record documents lipid-rich plaque.

❑ She verifies code **I25.83 Coronary atherosclerosis due to lipid rich plaque**.

❑ She reads the instructional note under code **I25.83** that states **Code first coronary atherosclerosis (I25.1-, I25.7-, I25.81-)**.

❑ The note confirms that **I25.710** should be sequenced first and **I25.83** should be sequenced as an additional code.

❑ Tanisha cross-references the beginning of category **I25** and reads the instructional notes.

❑ She notices the instruction that states **Use additional code to identify: tobacco dependence (F17.-)**. She verifies that tobacco dependence or smoking is documented in the medical record and verifies the code in the tabular list.

▶ Tanisha locates the category **F17 Nicotine dependence**. She also cross-checks the Index for the Main Term **Smoker** and reads a cross-reference instruction: *see* **Dependence, drug, nicotine**. The instruction confirms that she is correctly coding smoking as nicotine dependence.

❑ She refers to the Index entry **Dependence, drug, nicotine** and locates the subterm **cigarettes** under **nicotine**.

❑ She verifies the listed code **F17.210** in the Tabular List: **F17.210 Nicotine dependence, cigarettes, uncomplicated**.

▶ Next, Tanisha cross-references the instructional notes for code **I25.710**. She cross-references the beginning of the block **I20-I25** and reads the instructional note that applies to all codes in the block. She determines the note does not apply because it pertains to hypertension, which is not documented in the medical record.

❑ She cross-references the beginning of **Chapter 9 (I00-I99)** for instructional notes that apply to all codes in the chapter. She determines that there are no instructional notes.

▶ Tanisha reviews the codes she has assigned so far:

❑ **I25.710 Atherosclerosis of autologous vein coronary artery bypass graft(s) with unstable angina pectoris**

❑ **I25.83 Coronary atherosclerosis due to lipid rich plaque**

❑ **F17.210 Nicotine dependence, cigarettes, uncomplicated**

▶ Tanisha cross-references the medical record to ensure she did not miss any details. She reads the documentation that states patient has been on warfarin since a CABG of the left anterior descending coronary artery (LAD) 11 years ago.

❑ She knows from experience that warfarin is an anticoagulant and that she should assign a code for it.

❑ She locates the Index Main Term **Long term drug use** with the subterm **anti-coagulant Z79.01**.

❑ She verifies **Z79.01** in the Tabular List and locates the title **Long term (current) use of anticoagulants**.

▶ Tanisha reviews the codes for this case:

❑ **I25.710 Atherosclerosis of autologous vein coronary artery bypass graft(s) with unstable angina pectoris**

❑ **I25.83 Coronary atherosclerosis due to lipid rich plaque**

❑ **F17.210 Nicotine dependence, cigarettes, uncomplicated**

❑ **Z79.01 Long term (current) use of anticoagulants**

▶ Next, Tanisha will review the sequencing of the codes.

SUCCESS STEP

Arteriosclerosis (*hardening of an artery*) is usually caused by atherosclerosis (*hardening of a vessel due to plaque*), so ICD-10-CM indexes both conditions to the Main Term **Arteriosclerosis**. You can go directly to **Arteriosclerosis** in the Index, then locate the needed subterm, rather than searching **Atherosclerosis** first.

CODING PRACTICE

Exercise 13.3 Assigning Codes for Circulatory System Conditions

Instructions: Read the mini-medical-record of each patient's encounter and review the information abstracted in Exercise 13.2 for questions 1–3. For questions 4 and 5, do the abstracting on your own. Assign ICD-10-CM diagnosis codes using the Index and Tabular List. Write the code(s) on the line provided.

1. INPATIENT HOSPITAL Gender: F Age: 42

Reason for admission: Admitted from emergency department with subendocardial infarction

Assessment: Nontransmural myocardial infarction

Plan: This is her first event so we will treat it with medication and diet

1 ICD-10-CM Code _____

2. OFFICE Gender: F Age: 68

Reason for encounter: Patient has been taking her BP at home and is concerned about readings that have been increasing over the past 3 months. She claims to be taking the diuretic and beta blocker as directed. Lab results show slightly low potassium.

Assessment: Hypertensive cardiomegaly

Plan: Add spironolactone to the medication regime.

1 ICD-10-CM Code _____

3. INPATIENT HOSPITAL Gender: M Age: 68

Reason for admission: Mitral porcine valvoplasty

Assessment: Mitral valve regurgitation

Tip: Remember to follow the cross-references in the Index.

1 ICD-10-CM Code _____

4. EMERGENCY DEPT Gender: M Age: 53

Chief complaint: Tachycardia

Assessment: Ventricular flutter

Plan: CPR, external electric shock

Tip: You did not practice abstracting this case earlier, so see how you do on your own.

1 ICD-10-CM Code _____

5. OFFICE Gender: F Age: 38

Chief complaint: Referred by primary care physician for pain in right leg due to varicose veins that have not improved with compression stockings

Assessment: Varicose veins right calf

Plan: Ultrasound to evaluate for thrombus or valve problems. Consider for sclerotherapy.

Tip: You did not practice abstracting this case earlier, so see how you do on your own.

1 ICD-10-CM Code _____

ARRANGING CODES FOR CIRCULATORY SYSTEM CONDITIONS

The circumstances of admission, OGCR, and instructional notes in the Tabular List always determine the selection of the principal or first-listed diagnosis and the sequencing of codes. In some cases sequencing is fairly straightforward and in other cases it can be challenging to sort through multiple sets of instructions. This holds true for patients who have AMI and especially for patients who have had multiple MIs. Refer to the following examples to better understand how to sequence codes for MI.

Myocardial Infarction and Coronary Artery Disease

When a patient with CAD is admitted for an AMI, sequence codes as follows (OGCR I.C.9.b):

1. Sequence the AMI first. To locate MI in the Index, use the Main Term **Infarct, Infarction** and the subterm **myocardium**.

2. Sequence the CAD as an additional code (■ FIGURE 13-15). To locate CAD in the Index, search for the Main Term **Disease**, the first-level subterm **heart**, and the second-level subterm **ischemic**. As an alternative, you can also use the Main Term **Ischemia**.

Patient was admitted for inferior wall STEMI and also has atherosclerotic heart disease.

(1) **I21.19 ST elevation (STEMI) myocardial infarction involving other coronary artery of inferior wall**
(2) **I25.10 Atherosclerotic heart disease of native coronary artery without angina pectoris**

Figure 13-15 ■ Example of sequencing AMI and ASHD.

Acute and Subsequent Myocardial Infarction

An MI is considered to be *acute* or *current* for four weeks after the event. Patients may have two or more MI events within the four-week timeframe. When this occurs, the second and greater MIs are referred to as *subsequent* MIs. An MI is no longer considered acute after four weeks and is then identified as an *old* MI. Code as follows:

- Assign the first MI a code from category **I21.- ST elevation (STEMI) and non-ST elevation (NSTEMI) myocardial infarction**.

- Assign the second event a code for a subsequent AMI from category **I22.- Subsequent ST elevation (STEMI) and non-ST elevation (NSTEMI) myocardial infarction**.

- Sequencing is determined by the AMI that is *chiefly responsible* for the encounter, rather than the order in which the events occurred (OGCR I.C.9.e). Refer to the examples that follow to better understand sequencing rules.

During the course of an admission, STEMI may evolve to NSTEMI and NSTEMI may evolve to STEMI. In both cases, assign the STEMI code (OGCR I.C.9.e.1).

Sequencing in an Admission for AMI Followed by a Subsequent MI

When a patient is admitted for an AMI and has a second AMI during the stay, sequence the codes as follows:

1. Assign a code from category **I21.-** for the original AMI and sequence this condition first because it is the condition chiefly responsible for the admission and services provided.

2. Assign a code from category **I22.-** for subsequent AMI to the second event and sequence it second, as shown in ■ FIGURE 13-16.

SUCCESS STEP

Read the instructional notes at the beginning of categories **I21**, **I22**, and **I23** for definitions and sequencing guidance on MI.

Patient was admitted for STEMI of the anterolateral wall. Two days later, the patient had a separate NSTEMI.

(1) **I21.09 ST elevation (STEMI) myocardial infarction involving other coronary artery of anterior wall**
(2) **I22.2 Subsequent non-ST elevation (NSTEMI) myocardial infarction**

Figure 13-16 ■ Example of sequencing in an admission for AMI followed by a subsequent MI.

Sequencing in an Admission for a Subsequent MI

When a nonhospitalized patient is admitted for a second AMI within four weeks of a previous AMI, assign and sequence codes as follows (■ FIGURE 13-17):

1. Assign a code from category **I22.-** for subsequent MI to the second event. Sequence the subsequent event as the principal diagnosis because it is the reason for the admission and services provided.

2. Assign a code from category **I21.-** for acute MI to the first event. Sequence this code second because it was not the reason for admission.

Sequencing a Current AMI and an Old MI

When more than four weeks elapse between MI events, the first MI is classified as an old or healed MI and only the new AMI is coded as acute. When a nonhospitalized patient is admitted for a second AMI that occurs more than four weeks after a previous AMI, assign and sequence codes as follows (■ FIGURE 13-18):

1. Assign a code for a current AMI from category **I21.-** for the new AMI. Sequence the new event as the principal diagnosis because it is the reason for the admission and services provided.

2. Assign the code **I25.2 Old myocardial infarction** to the first event. Sequence this condition as an additional code because it was not the reason for admission.

Guided Example of Arranging Codes for Circulatory System Conditions

To practice skills for sequencing codes for the circulatory system, continue with the example from earlier in the chapter about patient Gordon Rothe, who was admitted to Branton Medical Center due to unstable angina.

Patient was admitted for a STEMI involving the inferior wall. Three weeks ago, the patient had a transmural MI to the inferoposterior wall.

(1) **I22.1 Subsequent ST elevation (STEMI) myocardial infarction of inferior wall**
(2) **I21.11 ST elevation (STEMI) myocardial infarction involving right coronary artery**

Figure 13-17 ■ Example of sequencing in an admission for a subsequent AMI.

Patient was admitted for AMI involving the LAD coronary artery. Three months ago, the patient had a MI to the anterior wall.

(1) **I21.02 ST elevation (STEMI) myocardial infarction involving left anterior descending coronary artery**
(2) **I25.2 Old myocardial infarction**

Figure 13-18 ■ Example of sequencing a current AMI and an old MI.

Follow along in your ICD-10-CM manual as Tanisha sequences the codes. Check off each step after you complete it.

▶ Tanisha reviews the codes she identified for this case:

❏ **I25.710 Atherosclerosis of autologous vein coronary artery bypass graft(s) with unstable angina pectoris**

❏ **I25.83 Coronary atherosclerosis due to lipid rich plaque**

❏ **F17.210 Nicotine dependence, cigarettes, uncomplicated**

❏ **Z79.01 Long term (current) use of anticoagulants**

▶ Tanisha determines the principal diagnosis.

❏ She reviews the medical record for the reason for admission, which is documented as unstable angina.

❏ She reviews the reason that balloon angioplasty was performed, which is documented as atherosclerosis of grafted vessel.

❏ She confirms that **I25.710 Atherosclerosis of autologous vein coronary artery bypass graft(s) with unstable angina pectoris** meets the definition of principal diagnosis, which is "that condition established after study to be chiefly responsible for occasioning the admission of the patient to the hospital for care" (OGCR II).

❏ She double-checks the instructional note under code **I25.710** in the Tabular List that directs her to use **I25.83 Coronary atherosclerosis due to lipid rich plaque** as an *additional* code, meaning **I25.83** should not be the principal diagnosis.

❏ She double-checks the instructional note under code **I25.83** in the Tabular List that directs her to **Code first** a code from **I25.7-**, meaning that **I25.7.-** should be sequenced *before* **I25.83**.

❏ She also refers to OGCR I.C.9.b, which states:

▪ If a patient with coronary artery disease is admitted due to an acute myocardial infarction (AMI), the AMI should be sequenced before the coronary artery disease.

❏ She determines that the guideline does not affect the sequencing because the patient did not have an AMI.

❏ Therefore, she is confident that **I25.710** is the principal diagnosis and **I25.83** is sequenced second.

❏ She sequences **F17.210 Nicotine dependence, cigarettes, uncomplicated** third because it was specified in an instructional note.

❏ She sequences **Z79.01 Long term (current) use of anticoagulants** as the final code.

▶ Tanisha finalizes the codes and the sequencing for this case:

(1) **I25.710 Atherosclerosis of autologous vein coronary artery bypass graft(s) with unstable angina pectoris**

(2) **I25.83 Coronary atherosclerosis due to lipid rich plaque**

(3) **F17.210 Nicotine dependence, cigarettes, uncomplicated**

(4) **Z79.01 Long term (current) use of anticoagulants**

CODING PRACTICE

Exercise 13.4 Arranging Codes for Circulatory System Conditions

Instructions: Read the mini-medical-record of each patient's encounter, review the information abstracted in Exercise 13.2 for questions 1–3. For questions 4 and 5, do the abstracting on your own. Assign ICD-10-CM diagnosis codes using the Index and Tabular List and sequence them correctly.

---

1. INPATIENT HOSPITAL   Gender: F   Age: 71

Reason for admission: Admitted from emergency department with angina. Patient has history of MI 2 years ago, as well as history of TIAs, although the TIAs did not leave any residual deficits

Assessment: STEMI involving 90% occlusion of the right coronary artery

Procedure: CABG

(continued)

---

1. (continued)

Tip: Assign a Z code for history of TIA.

3 ICD-10-CM Codes _____

_____

---

2. OFFICE   Gender: M   Age: 65

Chief complaint: Increased edema and SOB since last visit

Assessment: HTN and decompensated CHF, A-fib

Plan: We will start by adjusting the diuretic, then evaluate the need for other adjustments based on response after 4 weeks. Continue long-term warfarin and clopidrogel (*an antiplatelet medication*).

Tip: Remember to assign Z codes for the long-term use of the medications.

5 ICD-10-CM Codes _____

_____

CODING PRACTICE (continued)

---

3. INPATIENT HOSPITAL Gender: M Age: 57

Reason for admission: Transferred from another hospital where patient was admitted for cerebral infarct 20 hours ago and received tPA (*tissue plasminogen activator*), but now it is evident that a mechanical or surgical embolectomy is needed

Assessment: Cerebral infarction d/t embolus in right middle cerebral artery, cerebral atherosclerosis, HTN, history of tobacco use

Procedure: Surgical embolectomy

Tip: Remember to read the instructional notes at the beginning of the category and the beginning of the block to identify what you need Z codes for.

5 ICD-10-CM Codes _____

_____

---

4. OFFICE Gender: F Age: 55

Reason for encounter: Management of CHF and A-fib

Assessment: A-fib, chronic diastolic CHF

(continued)

---

4. (continued)

Plan: Refer to wound clinic for a stage 1 venous stasis ulcer on left thigh

Tip: You did not practice abstracting this case earlier, so see how you do on your own.

Use your resources if you need assistance in defining any terms or conditions.

4 ICD-10-CM Codes _____

_____

---

5. INPATIENT HOSPITAL Gender: M Age: 45

Reason for admission: Admitted from emergency department with angina, SOB, tachycardia, hemoptysis. Undergoing treatment for DVT

Assessment: Pulmonary embolism, chronic DVT of left femoral vein

2 ICD-10-CM Codes _____

CHAPTER SUMMARY

In this chapter you learned that:

- The function of the circulatory system, also called the cardiovascular (CV) system, is to distribute blood throughout the body.

- ICD-10-CM provides Official Guidelines for Coding and Reporting (OGCR) for the circulatory system in OGCR section I.C.9 and provides detailed discussion regarding hypertension and its relationship to heart and kidney disease, atherosclerotic coronary artery disease and angina, cerebrovascular accident and disease, and acute myocardial infarction.

- Coders need to pay close attention to detail when abstracting for the cardiovascular system because they assign codes that

  are very specific to anatomic sites, nature of the disease, and comorbidities.

- Diseases of the circulatory system frequently occur with multiple comorbidities from within the cardiovascular system and/or from other systems; consequently, the choice of codes is dependent on the precise wording physicians use in the documentation.

- Sequencing of codes for multiple MIs depends on the circumstances of admission. Carefully determine when each MI occurred and the reason for admission.

CONCEPT QUIZ

Take a moment to look back at the circulatory system and solidify your skills. Try to answer the questions from memory first, then refer back to the discussion in the chapter if you need a little extra help.

Completion

Instructions: Write the term that completes each statement based on the information you learned in this chapter. Choose from the list below. Some choices may be used more than once and some choices may not be used at all.

4	electrocardiography
6	embolectomy
8	embolus
angioplasty	endarterectomy
arrhythmia	endocarditis
atherosclerosis	Holter monitor
bypass graft	ischemia
cardiac catheterization	months
cerebrovascular accident (CVA)	NSTEMI
congestive heart failure (CHF)	STEMI
days	stenosis
deep vein thrombosis (DVT)	weeks

1. Another term for arteriosclerotic heart disease (ASHD) is

   _____.

2. The medical term for stroke is _____.

3. A thrombus that has broken loose from its point of origin and circulates through the bloodstream is a(n)

   _____.

4. The inability of the heart to maintain circulation, often resulting in water retention and edema, is _____.

5. The formation of a thrombus within a deep vein, usually in the leg or pelvis, is _____.

6. Taking a vessel from another part of the body to create a new route around a blockage in a blood vessel is a(n)

   _____.

7. A myocardial infarction is classified as current or acute for _____ weeks.

8. A myocardial infarction that completely occludes a vessel is called _____.

9. Removal of the diseased or damaged inner lining of an artery is a(n) _____.

10. A portable EKG worn by the patient for an extended period of hours or days to measure heart activity in a variety of situations is a(n) _____.

Multiple Choice

Instructions: Circle the letter of the best answer to each question based on the information you learned in this chapter.

1. Which of the following diagnostic statements states or implies a causal relationship?
   A. Chronic kidney disease and congestive heart failure
   B. Hypertensive heart disease
   C. Hypertension and heart disease
   D. STEMI and HTN

2. What Main Term should you locate in the Index to code for acute myocardial infarction?
   A. Heart
   B. Acute
   C. Myocardial
   D. Infarction

3. How would you code the following scenario? *A patient is seen for stage 4 chronic kidney disease and hypertension.*
   A. I12.9, N18.4
   B. N18.4, I10
   C. I12.9
   D. N18.9, I12.9

4. What Main Term should be located in the Index when the cause of CVA is known?
   A. Infarction
   B. Accident
   C. Cerebral
   D. Stroke

5. What Main Term should you locate in the Index to code congestive heart failure?
   A. Congestive
   B. Heart
   C. Failure
   D. Myocardial

6. How would you code the following scenario? *A patient is admitted for a STEMI involving the inferior wall. Three weeks ago, the patient had a transmural MI to the inferoposterior wall.*
   A. I21.19
   B. I22.1, I21.11
   C. I21.A1
   D. I22.1, Z86.79

7. What additional code do the instructional notes at category I63 state is required for a CVA?
   A. A code for the NIHSS score
   B. A code for a previous CVA
   C. A code for the stage of CKD
   D. A code for nicotine dependence

8. What condition has a presumed causal relationship with hypertension?
   A. Cerebrovascular accident
   B. Chronic kidney disease
   C. Acute myocardial infarction
   D. Atherosclerotic heart disease

9. What type of circulation carries blood from the aorta to the tissues of the heart?
   A. Coronary
   B. Endocardial
   C. Pulmonary
   D. Systemic

10. How would you code the following scenario? *A patient is admitted for angina pectoris with documented spasm. A balloon angioplasty is performed to treat atherosclerosis of a partially blocked coronary artery. Patient is a smoker.*
    A. I25.83, Z72.0
    B. I25.710, Z72.0
    C. I25.111, Z72.0
    D. I20.1, I25.83, Z72.0

KEEP ON CODING

Instructions: Read the diagnostic statement, then use the Index and Tabular List to assign and sequence ICD-10-CM diagnosis codes. Write the code(s) on the line provided.

1. Rheumatic myocarditis. ICD-10-CM Code(s) _____

2. Acute cor pulmonale. ICD-10-CM Code(s) _____

3. Floppy nonrheumatic mitral valve syndrome. ICD-10-CM Code(s) _____

4. Nonruptured cerebral aneurysm. ICD-10-CM Code(s) _____

5. Dissection of the iliac artery. ICD-10-CM Code(s) _____

6. Rupture of brachial artery. ICD-10-CM Code(s) _____

7. Postthrombotic syndrome, both legs with inflammation. ICD-10-CM Code(s) _____

8. Intraoperative cardiac arrest during cardiac surgery. ICD-10-CM Code(s) _____

9. Hypertensive heart and stage 3 chronic kidney disease without heart failure. ICD-10-CM Code(s) _____

10. Acute cerebral infarction due to embolism of the posterior cerebral artery, left with tPA administered prior to admission. ICD-10-CM Code(s) _____

11. Variant angina with tobacco use. ICD-10-CM Code(s) _____

12. Intradialytic hypotension. ICD-10-CM Code(s) _____

13. Phlebitis of the right iliac vein. ICD-10-CM Code(s) _____

14. Acute mesenteric lymphadenitis. ICD-10-CM Code(s) _____

15. Portal vein obstruction. ICD-10-CM Code(s) _____

16. Esophageal varices with bleeding. ICD-10-CM Code(s) _____

17. Asymptomatic varicose veins of both legs. ICD-10-CM Code(s) _____

18. Malignant neoplasm of the abdominal aorta. ICD-10-CM Code(s) _____

19. ST elevation myocardial infarction involving the anterior wall. ICD-10-CM Code(s) _____

20. Alcoholic cardiomyopathy with alcohol abuse. ICD-10-CM Code(s) _____

21. Myocardial infarction (STEMI) of left anterior descending coronary artery with old myocardial infarction involving left main coronary artery. ICD-10-CM Code(s) _____

22. Second-degree atrioventricular block, type I. ICD-10-CM Code(s) _____

23. Stuttering following a cerebral infarction, nontraumatic. ICD-10-CM Code(s) _____

24. Premature atrial beats. ICD-10-CM Code(s) _____

25. Chronic venous hypertension, both legs with inflammation. ICD-10-CM Code(s) _____

CODING CHALLENGE

Instructions: Read the mini-medical-record of each patient's encounter, then abstract, assign, and sequence ICD-10-CM diagnosis codes using the Index and Tabular List. Write the code(s) on the line provided.

1. INPATIENT HOSPITAL   Gender: M   Age: 91

Reason for admission: Arrived by ambulance to emergency department for severe abdominal pain

Assessment: Ruptured abdominal aortic aneurysm

Discharge status: Deceased

1 ICD-10-CM Code _____

2. INPATIENT HOSPITAL   Gender: M   Age: 71

Reason for admission: Admitted from emergency department for inferolateral STEMI.

Assessment: On the third day after admission, patient had a second STEMI in the same location.

Procedure: CABG x3

Tip: A CABG was performed to bypass three coronary arteries.

2 ICD-10-CM Codes _____

3. INPATIENT HOSPITAL Gender: F Age: 59

Reason for admission: Spells of dizziness, slow heart rate, and near fainting. Admitted for cardiac work up.

Assessment: EKG showed abnormal waves. Left anterior bundle branch block.

Plan: Patient discharged with FU with cardiologist in 3 weeks

1 ICD-10-CM Code _____

4. INPATIENT HOSPITAL Gender: M Age: 42

Reason for admission: Shortness of breath, generalized weakness, agitation, elevated BP, fever, rapid pulse, history of hyperthyroidism

Assessment: Cardiomyopathy due to thyrotoxicosis with thyroid storm

Plan: Inhibit thyroid hormone synthesis with Methimazole. Beta blockers, body cooling, FU with cardiologist for cardiomyopathy management

2 ICD-10-CM Codes _____

5. INPATIENT HOSPITAL Gender: F Age: 26

Reason for admission: Feet and ankle edema, chest pain, shortness of breath, fever

Assessment: Pericarditis due to Staphylococcus aureus

Plan: Drain fluid from pericardial space, sensitivity testing for suitable antibiotic shows response to methicillin. FU 3 days after discharge

2 ICD-10-CM Codes _____

6. INPATIENT HOSPITAL Gender: F Age: 66

Reason for admission: Painful sore on left calf area, nausea, vomiting

Assessment: Atherosclerosis of nonautologous biological bypass graft with ulceration of left calf with muscle necrosis

Plan: Intravenous fluids, CBC, surgical debridement, wound care. Visiting nurse scheduled daily upon discharge

2 ICD-10-CM Codes _____

7. INPATIENT HOSPITAL Gender: M Age: 75

Reason for admission: Angina pectoris with documented spasm

Assessment: CAD of grafted autologous artery following CABG 8 years ago, hypertensive chronic systolic with diastolic CHF

Plan: Oxygen, vasodilators, beta and calcium channel blockers, angioplasty with stent

3 ICD-10-CM Codes _____

_____

8. OFFICE Gender: F Age: 52

Chief complaint: Dizziness upon sudden standing, temporary visual dimming, numbness and tingling in arms and hands

Assessment: Orthostatic hypotension

Plan: BP to be checked daily and follow instructions related to lifestyle changes (i.e., improve diet and exercise)

1 ICD-10-CM Code _____

9. INPATIENT HOSPITAL Gender: M Age: 82

Reason for admission: Left sided paralysis, inability to walk, inability to formulate words

Assessment: Cerebral infarction due to embolism in right common carotid artery with pharyngeal dysphagia and left non-dominant hemiplegia

Plan: Rehab for mobility and speech, medication to address blood pressure issues. FU with primary care physician

Tip: The carotid artery is located in the neck.

4 ICD-10-CM Codes _____

_____

10. INPATIENT HOSPITAL Gender: M Age: 47

Reason for admission: Chest pain

Assessment: Post-infarctional angina following LAD STEMI 2 weeks ago

Plan: FU 1 week

2 ICD-10-CM Codes _____

Chapter 14

Diseases of the Blood and Blood-Forming Organs and Certain Disorders Involving the Immune Mechanism (D50-D89)

Chapter Outline

- **Blood Refresher**
- **Coding Guidelines for the Blood**
- **Abstracting for Conditions of the Blood**
- **Assigning Codes for Conditions of the Blood**
- **Arranging Codes for Conditions of the Blood**
- **Coding Malignancies of the Blood**

Learning Objectives

After completing this chapter, you should have the skills to:

14.1 Spell and define the key words, medical terms, and abbreviations related to diseases of the blood and blood-forming organs. (Remember)

14.2 Summarize the structure, function, and common conditions of the blood and blood-forming organs. (Understand)

14.3 Adhere to the Official Guidelines for Coding and Reporting related to diseases of the blood and blood-forming organs. (Apply)

14.4 Examine and abstract diagnostic information from the medical record for coding diseases of the blood and blood-forming organs. (Analyze)

14.5 Demonstrate how to assign codes for diseases of the blood and blood-forming organs. (Apply)

14.6 Utilize guidelines for arranging (sequencing) multiple diagnosis codes for diseases of the blood and blood-forming organs. (Apply)

14.7 Demonstrate how to abstract, assign, and sequence codes for malignancies of the blood and blood-forming organs. (Apply)

Key Terms and Abbreviations

anemia	formed element	leukocyte	thrombocyte
aplastic anemia	hemic system	nutritional anemia	vasoocclusive crisis
blood	hemoglobin (Hb)	plasma	white blood cell disorder
bone marrow	hemolytic anemia	relapse	
erythrocyte	hemostasis	remission	

In addition to the key terms listed here, students should know the terms defined within tables in this chapter.

INTRODUCTION

You need to determine if your vehicle runs best on regular grade, premium, or super premium fuel because each has different components. The blood in the human body is comprised of several distinct components and, sometimes, they become out of balance and require medical attention.

A hematologist specializes in diagnosing and treating conditions of the blood and blood-forming organs. Hematologists may specialize in oncology and treat malignancies of the blood. Primary care physicians treat uncomplicated conditions of the blood and refer complex cases to a hematologist.

BLOOD REFRESHER

The function of the **blood**, also called the **hemic system**, is to transport and pass nutrients, oxygen, carbon dioxide, water, proteins, and hormones to cells and to transport waste products to excretory organs. Blood consists of **plasma** (*clear fluid*) and **formed elements**, or blood cells. There are three types of blood cells, which are created in the **bone marrow** (*connective tissue in the cavities of bones*): **erythrocytes** (*red blood cells [RBCs]*), **leukocytes** (*white blood cells [WBCs]*), and **thrombocytes** (*platelets*) (■ FIGURE 14-1). Blood cells are named based on their appearance and ability to accept stain during lab testing (■ FIGURE 14-2). **Hemoglobin (Hb)** is the oxygen-carrying component of erythrocytes. The spleen destroys old erythrocytes, filters microorganisms from the blood, and serves as a reservoir for blood. The spleen functions as part of both the hemic and digestive systems.

In Figure 14-1, each component of blood is labeled with its name, which is based on the medical terminology root. Refer to ■ TABLE 14-1, (page 238) for a refresher on how to build medical terms related to the blood and lymphatic systems.

Refer to ■ TABLE 14-1, (page 238)

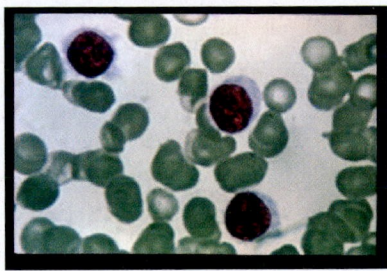

Figure 14-2 ■ Microscopic image of a stained blood cell. *Source:* © *National Institutes of Health.*

Conditions of the Blood

Diseases and disorders of the blood include anemias, hemostasis disorders, and white blood cell disorders. Coders use medical resources, such as a reference book on diseases, to understand conditions of the blood, diagnostic methods, and common treatments.

Anemia is a blood disorder characterized by a reduction in the number of red blood cells, which results in less oxygen reaching the tissues. Although there are more than 400 different

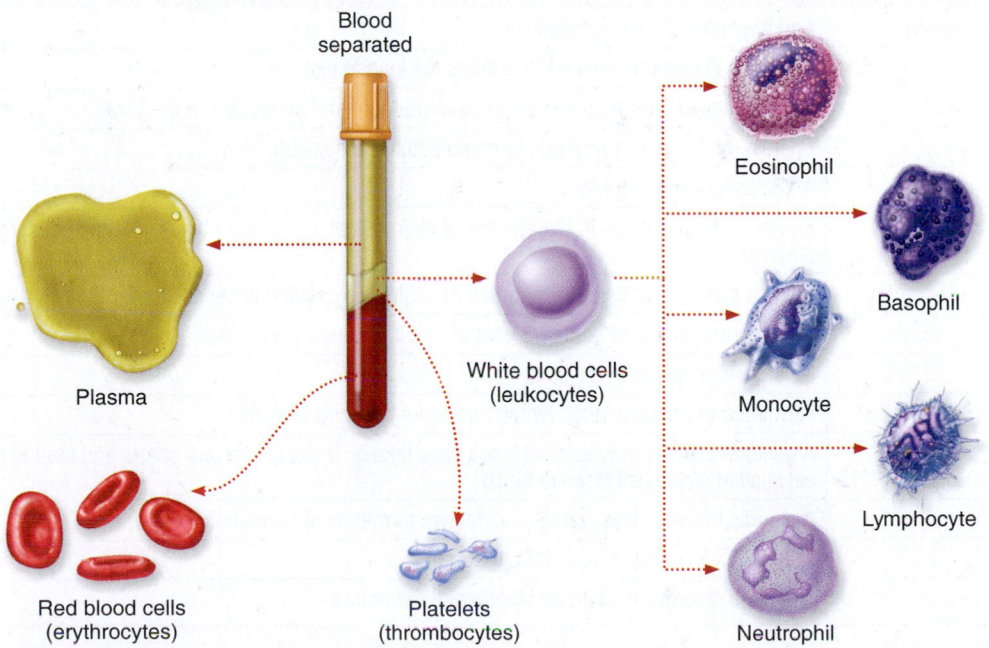

Blood separated

Plasma

White blood cells (leukocytes)

Red blood cells (erythrocytes)

Platelets (thrombocytes)

Eosinophil

Basophil

Monocyte

Lymphocyte

Neutrophil

Figure 14-1 ■ Formed elements of the blood (hemic system).

Table 14-1   ■   **EXAMPLE OF CONSTRUCTING MEDICAL TERMS FOR THE HEMIC SYSTEM**

Combining Form	Suffix	Complete Medical Term
hem/e, hemat/o (*blood*)	**-emia** (*blood condition*) **-penia** (*lack of*) **-cyte** (*cell*) **-phil** (*attraction*) **-poiesis** (*formation*)	**hemato + poiesis** (*formation of blood*) **an + emia** (*lack of blood condition*)
erythr/o- (*red*)		**erythro + cyte** (*red blood cell*) **erythro + cyto + penia** (*lack of red blood cells*) **erythro + poiesis** (*formation of red blood cells*)
leuk/o (*white*)		**leuko + cyte** (*white blood cell*) **leuko + penia** (*lack of white blood cells*) **leuk + emia** (*condition of white blood cells*)

types of anemia, they are classified into the following three groups, based on common etiology (*cause*):

- **Nutritional anemia**—Anemia due to malabsorption or poor dietary intake of iron, folate, and/or vitamin B_{12}

- **Hemolytic anemia**—Anemia due to excessive loss of erythrocytes

- **Aplastic anemia**—Anemia due to loss of red bone marrow

Anemia can result as a complication of other diseases and treatments, including chronic kidney disease (CKD), malignant neoplasms, and antineoplastic therapy such as chemotherapy, radiotherapy, and immunotherapy.

Hemostasis disorders include a range of medical problems that lead to poor clotting and continuous bleeding. Causes include platelet dysfunction, vitamin K deficiency, and clotting factor deficiencies.

White blood cell disorders diminish the body's immune response and increase the risk of infection.

Common blood conditions are summarized in ■ TABLE 14-2. Physicians diagnose blood disorders using blood tests, microscopic examination of blood cells, and bone marrow biopsy. Treatments include correction of nutritional deficiencies and other lifestyle changes, medication to correct the symptom or underlying problem, and transfusion of whole blood or a particular component of the blood.

Remember to keep standard reference books handy to learn more about conditions affecting the blood and blood-forming organs.

Table 14-2   ■   **COMMON BLOOD CONDITIONS**

Condition	Description
Folic acid-deficiency anemia	Anemia due to a lack of folic acid
Hemophilia	A genetic disorder in which blood takes too long to clot
Hypogammaglobulinemia	A deficiency of gamma globulins (protein fraction) and antibodies in the blood
Iron-deficiency anemia	Anemia due to insufficient iron to manufacture hemoglobin
Neutropenia	A decrease in neutrophils
Pancytopenia	An abnormal reduction in the number of all (medical prefix *pan-*) types of blood cells: red, white, and platelets
Pernicious anemia	Anemia due to insufficient absorption of vitamin B_{12}, which is necessary for erythrocyte production
Polycythemia	An abnormal increase in the number of circulating red blood cells
Purpura	Small hemorrhages in the skin
Sarcoidosis	Formation of nodules in the lymph nodes, lungs, bone, and skin
Sickle cell anemia	A genetic disorder in which red blood cells take on a sickle (curved) shape and lead to hemolytic anemia; also called sickle cell disease (SCD)
Thalassemia	A genetic disorder that results in defective formation of hemoglobin
Thrombophilia	A tendency to create blood clots (thrombi)
Von Willebrand's disease	A genetic disorder marked by bleeding of the mucosa

CODING PRACTICE

Exercise 14.1   Refresher on the Blood

Instructions: Use your medical terminology skills and resources to define the following conditions related to the blood and blood-forming organs, then assign the diagnosis code. Follow these steps:

- Use slash marks "/" to break down each term into its root(s) and suffix.
- Define the meaning of the word based on the meaning of each word part.
- Assign the default ICD-10-CM diagnosis code for the condition using the Index and Tabular List.

Example: leukemia leuk/emia   Meaning *disorder of white blood cells*   ICD-10-CM Code *C95.90*

1. hemophilia   Meaning _____   ICD-10-CM Code _____
2. neutropenia   Meaning _____   ICD-10-CM Code _____
3. thrombocytopenia   Meaning _____   ICD-10-CM Code _____
4. leukocytosis   Meaning _____   ICD-10-CM Code _____
5. eosinophilia   Meaning _____   ICD-10-CM Code _____
6. hemoglobinemia   Meaning _____   ICD-10-CM Code _____
7. panhematopenia   Meaning _____   ICD-10-CM Code _____
8. hemolymphangioma   Meaning _____   ICD-10-CM Code _____
9. erythroblastophthisis Meaning _____   ICD-10-CM Code _____
10. leukoerythroblastosis Meaning _____   ICD-10-CM Code _____

CODING GUIDELINES FOR THE BLOOD

Coders should understand the organization of this ICD-10-CM chapter, chapter-wide and commonly used instructional notes in the Tabular List, and the relevant OGCR. This information is necessary for accurate coding.

ICD-10-CM Chapter 3, "Diseases of the Blood and Blood-Forming Organs and Certain Disorders Involving the Immune Mechanism (D50-D89)," contains seven blocks or subchapters that are divided by type of condition. This chapter begins at D50, in the middle of a letter division, rather than at the beginning. Review the block names and code ranges listed at the beginning of Chapter 3 in the ICD-10-CM manual to become familiar with the content and organization.

This ICD-10-CM chapter includes anemia due to nutritional deficiencies, hemolytic anemia, aplastic anemia, coagulation disorders, and disorders of blood-forming organs. It does not include infectious diseases, most diseases of the lymphatic system, or disorders of the circulatory system, all of which are classified in other ICD-10-CM chapters.

ICD-10-CM does not provide Official Guidelines for Coding and Reporting (OGCR) for this chapter. OGCR I.C.2.c.1) and 2) in ICD-10-CM Chapter 2, "Neoplasms," discuss the coding of anemia associated with malignancy, chemotherapy, radiotherapy, and immunotherapy. The Tabular List contains frequent instructional notes to use an additional code for associated conditions and to code first underlying diseases. Specific OGCR guidelines are discussed and cited throughout this chapter of the text.

ABSTRACTING FOR THE BLOOD

Many of the conditions in this ICD-10-CM chapter can have multiple underlying causes and multiple manifestations. Therefore, coders should thoroughly abstract the symptoms, manifestations, and underlying causes documented in the medical record.

Some of these situations use combination codes, some require multiple coding, and others do not need to be coded because they are integral to the condition. For example, approximately 75 ICD-10-CM codes identify various types of anemia. Closely related anemias are classified to the same code. Refer to ■ TABLE 14-3 for guidance on how to abstract

Table 14-3   ■   **KEY CRITERIA FOR ABSTRACTING CONDITIONS OF THE BLOOD**

- ❏ What is the condition?
- ❏ What part of the hemic system does the condition involve?
- ❏ Does the condition have an underlying cause?
- ❏ Is the condition acquired or congenital?
- ❏ If anemia exists, is it due to a neoplasm or chronic disease?
- ❏ If sickle cell disease exists, what is the specific type?
- ❏ If sickle cell disease exists, is the patient in crisis?
- ❏ If sickle cell disease exists, does the patient have a fever?
- ❏ What symptoms are integral to the condition?
- ❏ What manifestations require an additional code?
- ❏ Is the condition drug induced?

conditions of the blood and blood-forming organs, then work through the detailed example that follows. Remember that the abstracting questions are a guide and that not every question applies to, or can be answered for, every case.

Guided Example of Abstracting for Conditions of the Blood

Refer to the following example throughout this chapter to learn skills for abstracting, assigning, and sequencing codes for disorders of the blood and blood-forming organs. Scott Hood, CPC, is a fictitious coder who guides you through the coding process.

Date: 05/11/yy

Location: Branton Medical Center Emergency Department

Provider: Robyn Akin, MD

Patient: Douglas Ketron　Gender: M　Age: 10 months

Reason for encounter: Fever, cough, SOB, bilateral dactylitis (*painful and swollen hands and/or feet*)

Assessment: Vasoocclusive crisis and acute chest syndrome due to HbSS sickle cell disease (SCD)

Plan: Administer oxygen and IV antibiotics, then admit as inpatient

---

Follow along as Scott Hood, CPC, abstracts the diagnosis. Check off each step after you complete it.

▶ Scott reads through the entire record, paying special attention to the reason for the encounter and the final assessment. Scott reviews all the medical terms in the documentation to be sure he understands the case.

❑ He knows from his experience working at a hematology clinic and medical reference books that **vasoocclusive crisis** is a form of sickle cell crisis in which the patient experiences severe pain due to infarctions and that the pain may occur in nearly any location (■ Figure 14-3, page 241).

❑ He is also aware that acute chest syndrome (ACS) is a group of symptoms, often due to a bacterial infection or lung infarction, seen in patients with SCD and can bring on a vasoocclusive crisis.

❑ He notes the presenting symptoms of fever, cough, SOB, and bilateral dactylitis.

▶ Scott refers to the Key Criteria for Abstracting Conditions of the Blood (Table 14-3).

❑ *What is the condition?* Vasoocclusive crisis and acute chest syndrome

❑ *What part of the hemic system does the condition involve?* Circulation

❑ *Does the condition have an underlying cause?* Sickle cell disease

❑ *Is the condition acquired or congenital?* Sickle cell is congenital

❑ *If anemia exists, is it due to a neoplasm or chronic disease?* Not applicable

❑ *If sickle cell disease exists, what is the specific type?* HbSS

❑ *If sickle cell disease exists, is the patient in crisis?* Yes, vasoocclusive crisis

❑ *If sickle cell disease exists, does the patient have a fever?* Yes

❑ *What symptoms are integral to the condition?* Fever, cough, SOB are symptoms of ACS. Dactylitis is a manifestation of SCD

❑ *What manifestations require an additional code?* Fever

❑ *Is the condition drug induced?* No

▶ Scott double-checks the medical record to be certain that he has identified all of the symptoms, conditions, and manifestations.

▶ At this point, Scott has abstracted the information he needs, but he is still unsure of how many codes he will need for this case. He knows that he will need to research the Index and Tabular List to learn what combination codes are available for this case.

SUCCESS STEP

It may not be clear whether a separate code for fever is required at the time of initial abstracting for sickle cell crisis. It becomes clear later when assigning codes in the Tabular List. The abstracting questions specifically ask about fever with sickle cell crisis to help identify the possible need for a code.

Hemoglobin S and Red Blood Cell Sickling

Sickle cell anemia is caused by an inherited autosomal recessive defect in Hb synthesis. Sickle cell hemoglobin (HbS) differs from normal hemoglobin only in the substitution of the amino acid valine for glutamine in both beta chains of the hemoglobin molecule.

When HbS is oxygenated, it has the same globular shape as normal hemoglobin. However, when HbS loses its oxygen, it becomes insoluble in intracellular fluid and crystallizes into rodlike structures. Clusters of rods form polymers (long chains) that bend the erythrocyte into the characteristic crescent shape of the sickle cell.

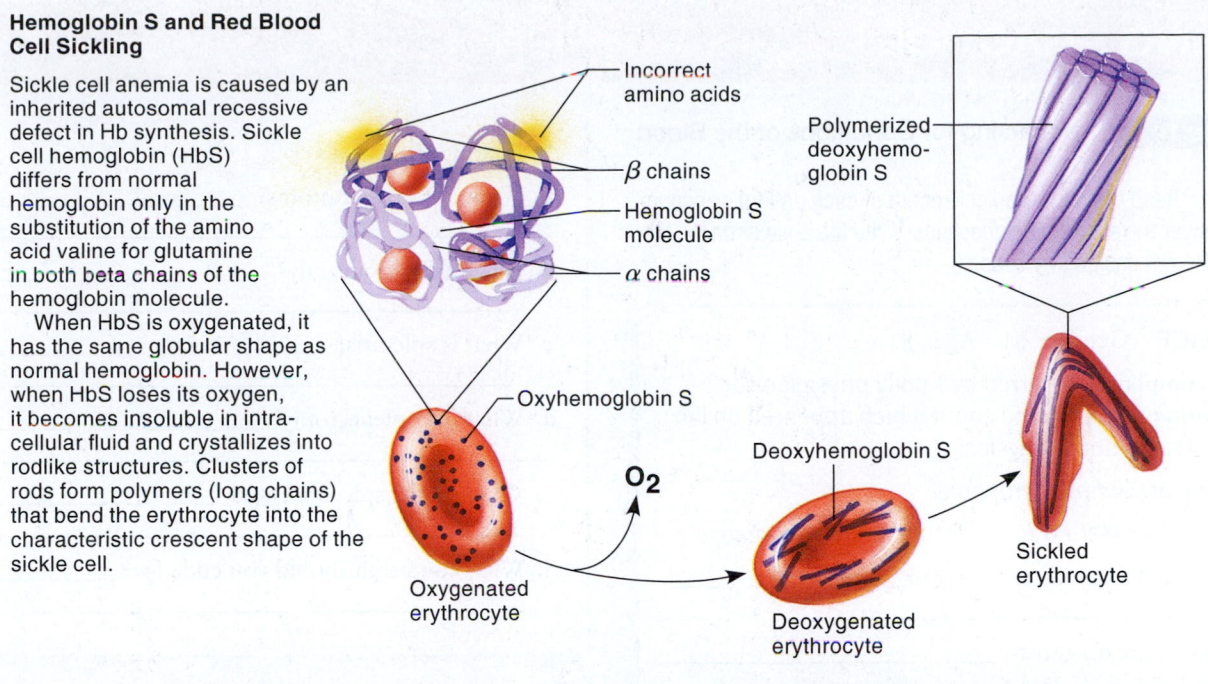

Incorrect amino acids

β chains

Hemoglobin S molecule

α chains

Polymerized deoxyhemoglobin S

Oxyhemoglobin S

Deoxyhemoglobin S

O_2

Oxygenated erythrocyte

Deoxygenated erythrocyte

Sickled erythrocyte

The Sickle Cell Disease Process

Sickle cell disease is characterized by episodes of acute painful crises. Sickling crises are triggered by conditions causing high tissue oxygen demands or that affect cellular pH. As the crisis begins, sickled erythrocytes adhere to capillary walls and to each other, obstructing blood flow and causing cellular hypoxia. The crisis accelerates as tissue hypoxia and acidic metabolic waste products cause further sickling and cell damage.

Sickle cell crises cause microinfarcts in joints and organs, and repeated crises slowly destroy organs and tissues. The spleen and kidneys are especially prone to sickling damage.

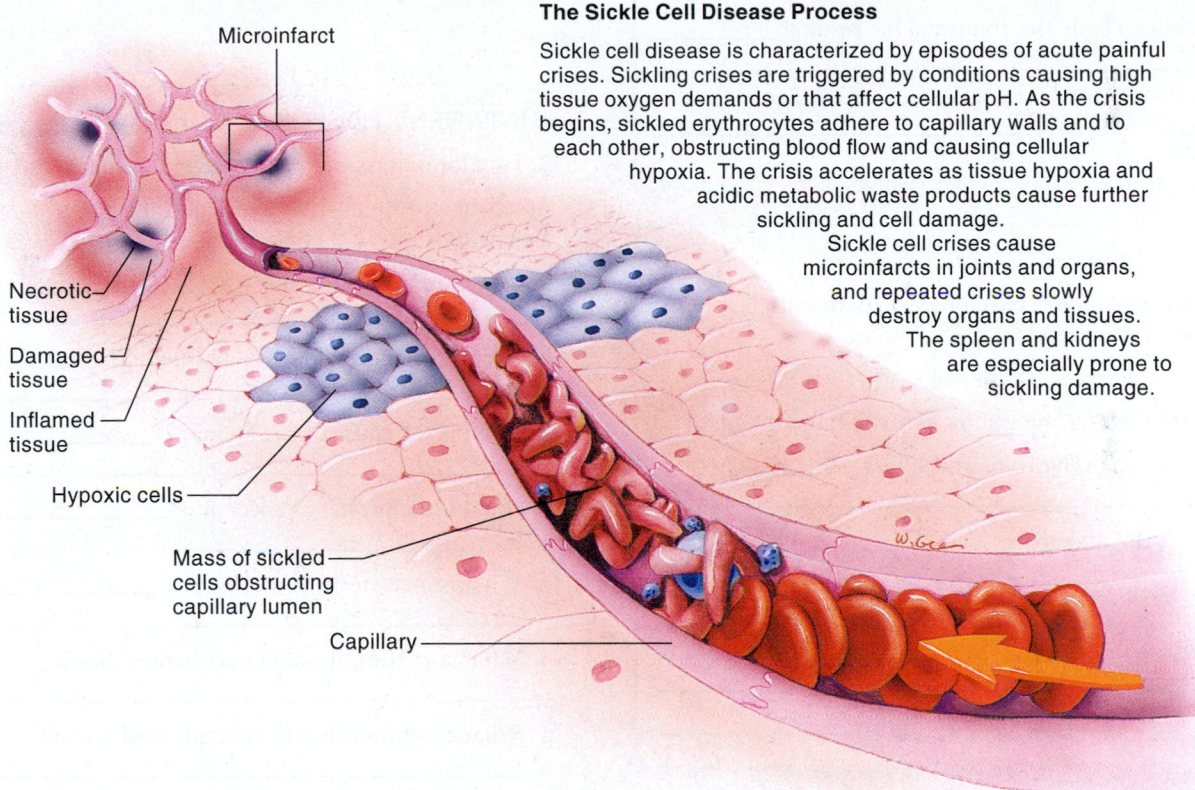

Microinfarct

Necrotic tissue

Damaged tissue

Inflamed tissue

Hypoxic cells

Mass of sickled cells obstructing capillary lumen

Capillary

Figure 14-3 ■ How sickle cell disease affects the patient. *Source: Pearson Education/PH College.*

CODING PRACTICE

Exercise 14.2 **Abstracting for Conditions of the Blood**

Instructions: Read the mini-medical-record of each patient's encounter and answer the abstracting questions. Write the answer on the line provided. Do not assign any codes.

1. OFFICE   Gender: M   Age: 81

Chief complaint: Referred by family physician for reduction in lymphocyte count which appeared on lab results from annual physical

Assessment: Lymphocytopenia

Plan: Further testing to determine underlying cause

a. What is the reason for referral? _____
_____

b. What is the diagnosis? _____
_____

c. Should you code the abnormal lab results? _____
_____

Why or why not? _____
_____

2. OFFICE   Gender: F   Age: 35

Reason for encounter: Numbness in extremities, nausea and vomiting

Assessment: Pernicious anemia

Plan: Vitamin B-12 injections, refer to hematologist

a. What are the symptoms and signs? _____
_____

b. What is the diagnosis? _____
_____

c. Are the symptoms and signs integral to the diagnosis? _____
_____

d. Should you code for the symptoms? _____

3. OFFICE   Gender: M   Age: 52

Reason for encounter: Referred by family physician for pain and swelling in LUQ

Assessment: Splenomegaly due to splenitis

Plan: Schedule splenectomy ASAP

(continued)

3. (continued)

a. What are the symptoms? _____
_____

b. What is splenomegaly? _____

c. What is splenitis? _____
_____

d. What is a splenectomy? _____
_____

e. Where is the spleen located? _____
_____

f. What condition should you code for? _____
_____

4. INPATIENT HOSPITAL   Gender: F   Age: 59

Reason for admission: Weakness, fatigue, confusion

Assessment: Anemia due to chemotherapy for metastatic colon cancer

a. What are the symptoms? _____
_____

b. Are the symptoms integral to anemia? _____
_____

c. What is the cause of the anemia? _____

d. What is the primary cancer site? _____
_____

e. What is metastatic cancer? _____
_____

f. What condition should be sequenced first? _____
_____

g. What condition should be sequenced second? _____
_____

h. What condition should be sequenced third? _____
_____

i. What adverse effect has occurred? _____
_____

CODING PRACTICE (continued)

5. INPATIENT HOSPITAL   Gender: M   Age: 61

Reason for admission: Tachycardia, headaches, fatigue

Assessment: Anemia due to stage 3 chronic kidney disease

Plan: Erythropoiesis stimulating agents (ESAs), supplemental iron

a. What are the symptoms? _____
_____

b. What is the diagnosis? _____
_____

c. Are the symptoms integral to the diagnosis? _____
_____

d. What is the underlying condition? _____
_____

e. Which condition is the principal diagnosis? _____
_____

f. What is the additional diagnosis? _____
_____

6. INPATIENT HOSPITAL   Gender: F   Age: 50

Reason for encounter: Follow up on glucose tolerance test (GTT) and complete chemistry analysis

Assessment: Hyperglycemia due to prediabetes, lab results also indicate iron (Fe)-deficiency anemia

Plan: Manage prediabetes with 1,500 calorie diabetic diet, Rx Fe supplements

a. What is hyperglycemia? _____
_____

b. Should both hyperglycemia and prediabetes be coded? _____
Why or why not? _____

c. Should anemia be coded? _____
Why or why not? _____

d. What type of anemia is present? _____

e. What should be the first-listed diagnosis? _____
_____

f. What is the additional diagnosis? _____
_____

ASSIGNING CODES FOR CONDITIONS OF THE BLOOD

When an ICD-10-CM chapter does not have any OGCR, as is the case with diseases of the blood and blood-forming organs, coders apply the general OGCR (I.A, I.B, II, and III) and follow instructional notes in the Tabular List. When coders thoroughly abstract information, they are poised to assign codes correctly.

Most types of anemia are indexed under the Main Term **Anemia**, followed by subterms that identify the specific type. Because the Index contains over 350 subterms for **Anemia**, remember to search them carefully to locate the most specific code. Refer to ■ FIGURE 14-4 for a sample Index entry showing how to locate aplastic anemia due to drugs.

Anemia is often associated with cancer and may be caused by the disease itself or by adjunct therapy such as chemotherapy, radiotherapy, or immunotherapy. Review the documentation carefully to clearly identify the cause. Chemotherapy may cause anemia or aplastic anemia, which is a result of bone marrow not producing erythrocytes, and each has separate codes (■ TABLE 14-4, page 244). Information about multiple coding for anemia in cancer patients is discussed later in this chapter.

Anemia (essential) (general) (hemoglobin deficiency) (infantile)
  (primary) (profound) D64.9
with (due to) (in)
  disorder of
    anaerobic glycolysis D55.2
    pentose phosphate pathway D55.1
  koilonychia D50.9
achlorhydric D50.8
achrestic D53.1
Addison(-Biermer) (pernicious) D51.0
agranulocytic — *see* Agranulocytosis
amino-acid-deficiency D53.0
aplastic D61.9
  congenital D61.09
  drug-induced D61.1
  due to
    drugs D61.1
    external agents NEC D61.2
    infection D61.2
    radiation D61.2

Figure 14-4 ■ Index entry for "Anemia, aplastic" used to located codes for aplastic anemia due to drugs.

Table 14-4 ■ **ANEMIA CODES FOR CANCER PATIENTS**

Cause of Anemia	Code Assignment
Anemia due to the cancer itself	D63.0 Anemia in neoplastic disease
Aplastic anemia due to chemotherapy	D61.1 Drug-induced aplastic anemia
Other anemia due to chemotherapy	D64.81 Anemia due to antineoplastic chemotherapy

Anemia may be caused by other drugs, in addition to chemotherapy. Drugs such as nonsteroidal anti-inflammatory drugs (NSAIDs) can cause bleeding, which in turn causes anemia. Drugs that suppress the immune system can cause anemia because the hematopoietic function of the bone marrow is suppressed. Other drugs, such as certain antibiotics, antihypertensives, and antiarrythmics, can occasionally destroy erythrocytes prematurely, causing hemolytic anemia. When anemia is drug-induced, the Tabular List instructs coders to assign an external cause code for the substance. Use the Table of Drugs and Chemicals to locate the substance and intent. Refer to OGCR I.C.19.e to review the definitions of each intent column in the Table of Drugs and Poisonings. Anemia also may be caused by CKD, in which case an additional code to identify the stage of kidney disease is required.

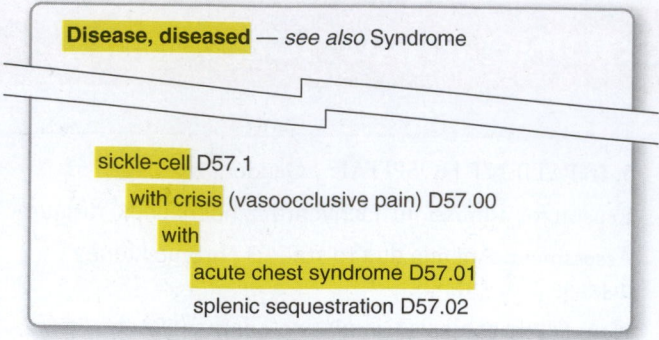

Figure 14-5 ■ Index entry showing a combination code for sickle cell disease with crisis and acute chest syndrome.

SUCCESS STEP

Anemia of newborns and anemia related to pregnancy are not classified in this chapter. ICD-10-CM has separate chapters for conditions of the newborn and pregnancy-related conditions. To locate the codes for anemia of the newborn, search the Main Term **Anemia** and subterm **newborn**. To locate codes for anemia in pregnancy, search the Main Term, **Pregnancy** and subterm **complicated by anemia**.

Guided Example of Assigning Codes for Conditions of the Blood

To practice skills for assigning codes for disorders of the blood and blood-forming organs, continue with the example from earlier in the chapter about patient Douglas Ketron, age 10 months, who was seen in the Branton Medical Center Emergency Department with HbSS sickle cell disease, vasoocclusive crisis, and acute chest syndrome.

Follow along in your ICD-10-CM manual as Scott Hood, CPC, assigns codes. Check off each step after you complete it.

▶ First, Scott confirms the diagnosis in the medical record: HbSS sickle cell with vasoocclusive crisis and acute chest syndrome; and the symptoms and manifestations: fever, cough, SOB, and bilateral dactylitis.

❑ He does not know how many codes he will need, so he begins by coding the main condition, HbSS sickle cell disease.

▶ Scott searches the Index for the Main Term **Disease**.

❑ He locates the subterm **sickle-cell** (■ FIGURE 14-5).

❑ He reviews the second-level subterms and notices that there are subterms for several types of SCD, but not HbSS.

❑ He determines that he will need to use either the default entry under **sickle-cell** or the entry for **specified NEC**, but he will not know for sure until he gets to the Tabular List.

❑ Scott reviews the subterms under **sickle-cell** and locates a third-level subterm **with crisis (vasoocclusive pain)**.

❑ He locates an additional fourth-level subterm **with** that provides a combination code for **acute chest syndrome D57.01**.

▶ Scott verifies code **D57.01** in the Tabular List.

❑ He verifies the code title **D57.01 Hb-SS disease with acute chest syndrome** and confirms that this accurately describes the diagnosis.

❑ He notes that the Tabular List specifies the **D57.0-** category includes HbSS, so he is in the right place and does not need to locate the code for **Other specified sickle cell, NEC** that he had considered in the Index.

❑ He also verifies that this is a combination code for SCD, vasoocclusive crisis, and acute chest syndrome, so he does not need to assign additional codes for vasoocclusive crisis or ACS.

▶ Scott checks for instructional notes in the Tabular List.

❑ He cross-references the beginning of category **D57** and reads the instructional note that states **Use additional code for any associated fever (R50.81)** (■ FIGURE 14-6, page 245).

❑ Before looking up the code for fever, Scott completes the verification of **D57.01**. He cross-references the beginning of the block **Hemolytic anemias (D55-D59)** and verifies that there are no instructional notes.

❑ He then cross-references the beginning of **Chapter 3 (D50-D89)** and verifies that there are no instructional notes.

▶ Now Scott verifies the code for fever contained in the first instructional note, **R50.81**.

❑ He verifies the code title **R50.81 Fever presenting with conditions classified elsewhere** and confirms that this accurately describes the fever.

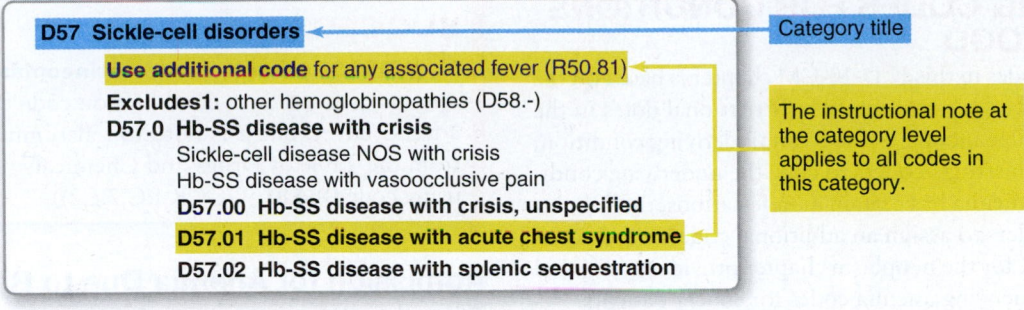

Figure 14-6 ■ Instructional note at the category level in the Tabular List to "Use additional code".

❏ He recognizes that the code is from ICD-10-CM Chapter 18, "Symptoms, Signs and Abnormal Clinical and Laboratory Findings, Not Elsewhere Classified (R00-R99)." He normally would hesitate to assign a code for a sign with a confirmed diagnosis that includes the three main conditions. However, because the instructional note directs him to assign a code for fever, if present, he knows he should assign it. He knows that fever is a sign of infection and that infection is a life-threatening event for a patient with SCD.

▶ Scott is unsure whether he needs to assign a code for bilateral dactylitis, so he researches this condition in the Index and Tabular List.

❏ He locates the Index Main Term **Dactylitis**.

❏ The subterms **sickle-cell** then **Hb-SS** lead him to **D57.00**.

❏ He instantly recognizes that **D57.00** is from the same category as his previous code, **D57.01**.

❏ He verifies **D57.00** in the Tabular List and reads the code title **Hb-SS disease with crisis, unspecified**.

❏ This confirms his thinking that dactylitis is a manifestation of SCD crisis. Because he has already identified **D57.01**, which is a more specific code for SCD crisis, he does not also assign **D57.00**. **D57.00** is a code with unspecified manifestations, so it adds no further information (OGCR I.A.9.b).

▶ Scott reviews the codes he has assigned for this case:

❏ **R50.81 Fever presenting with conditions classified elsewhere**

❏ **D57.01 Hb-SS disease with acute chest syndrome**

▶ Next, Scott needs to confirm the sequencing.

CODING PRACTICE

Exercise 14.3   **Assigning Codes for Conditions of the Blood**

Instructions: Read the mini-medical-record of each patient's encounter, review the information abstracted in Exercise 14.2, and assign ICD-10-CM diagnosis codes using the Index and Tabular List. Write the code(s) on the line provided.

---

1. OFFICE   Gender: M   Age: 81

Chief complaint: Referred by family physician for reduction in lymphocyte count which appeared on lab results from annual physical

Assessment: Lymphocytopenia

Plan: Further testing to determine underlying cause

Tip: The name of the condition is the Main Term.

1 ICD-10-CM Code _____

---

2. OFFICE   Gender: F   Age: 35

Reason for encounter: Numbness in extremities, nausea and vomiting

Assessment: Pernicious anemia

Plan: Vitamin B-12 injections, refer to hematologist

Tip: Look for the Main Term anemia, then look for the subterm that identifies the type of anemia.

1 ICD-10-CM Code _____

---

3. OFFICE   Gender: M   Age: 52

Reason for encounter: Referred by family physician for pain and swelling in LUQ

Assessment: Splenomegaly due to splenitis

Plan: Schedule splenectomy ASAP

1 ICD-10-CM Code _____

ARRANGING CODES FOR CONDITIONS OF THE BLOOD

Sequencing of codes in this ICD-10-CM chapter is based on the circumstances of admission and the instructional notes in the Tabular List. When anemia is due to an underlying condition, the Tabular List instructs coders to code the underlying condition first. When anemia has certain manifestations, the Tabular List instructs coders to assign an additional code for the manifestation. OGCR for the neoplasm chapter provides additional guidance for sequencing anemia codes for cancer patients.

Admission for Anemia Due to Neoplastic Disease

Patients with a malignancy and anemia may be admitted to treat the neoplasm or to treat the anemia. Assign and sequence codes in the same way for both situations. Assign and sequence codes as follows (OGCR I.C.2.c.1)):

1. Assign a code for the neoplasm.
2. Assign code **D63.0 Anemia in neoplastic disease for the anemia**.

Depending on the conventions used by a particular publisher, the Tabular List entry for **D63.0 Anemia in neoplastic disease** may be highlighted or appear in an italic typeface, indicating that it is a manifestation code and should not be sequenced as the first-listed or principal diagnosis (OGCR I.A.13) (■ FIGURE 14-7).

Admission for Anemia Due to Chemotherapy or Immunotherapy

When the admission or encounter is for management of an anemia associated with an adverse effect of chemotherapy or immunotherapy and the *only* treatment is for the anemia, assign and sequence codes as follows (OGCR I.C.2.c.2)):

1. Assign a code for the anemia.
2. Assign a code for the neoplasm.
3. Assign a code for the adverse effect from the Table of Drugs and Chemicals.

> **D63 Anemia in chronic diseases classified elsewhere**
>
> **_D63.0 Anemia in neoplastic disease_**
>
> Code first neoplasm (C00-D49)
> **Excludes1:** aplastic anemia due to antineoplastic chemotherapy (D61.1)
> **Excludes2:** anemia due to antineoplastic chemotherapy (D64.81)
>
> **_D63.1 Anemia in chronic kidney disease_**
>
> Erythropoietin resistant anemia (EPO resistant anemia)
> Code first underlying chronic kidney disease (CKD) (N18.-)
>
> _Manifestation Code_

Figure 14-7 ■ Example of a Tabular List convention for a manifestation code.

Admission for Anemia Due to Radiotherapy

When the admission or encounter is for management of an anemia associated with an adverse effect of radiotherapy, assign and sequence codes as follows (OGCR I.C.2.c.2)):

1. Assign a code for the anemia.
2. Assign a code for the neoplasm.
3. Assign an external cause code for the complication, **Y84.2 Radiological procedure and radiotherapy as the cause of abnormal reaction of the patient, or of later complication, without mention of misadventure at the time of the procedure**.

Admission for Adjunct Therapy

When the admission or encounter is for the purpose of administering adjunct therapy and the patient develops anemia *during* the encounter, assign, and sequence codes as follows (OGCR I.C.2.e.3)):

1. First, assign the appropriate **Z** code for the therapy encounter:
   a. **Z51.11 Encounter for antineoplastic chemotherapy**
   b. **Z51.12 Encounter for antineoplastic immunotherapy**
   c. **Z51.0 Antineoplastic radiation therapy**
4. Assign a second code from the Table of Drugs and Chemicals for the adverse effect when the encounter is for chemotherapy or immunotherapy.
5. Assign a code for the anemia (see Table 14-4).
6. Assign a code for the neoplasm.
7. If the encounter was for radiotherapy, assign code **Y84.2**.

Guided Example of Arranging Codes for Conditions of the Blood

To practice skills for sequencing codes for disorders of the blood and blood-forming organs, continue with the example from earlier in the chapter about patient Douglas Ketron, age 10 months, who was seen in Branton Medical Center Emergency Department with HbSS sickle cell disease, vasoocclusive crisis, and acute chest syndrome.

Follow along in your ICD-10-CM manual as Scott Hood, CPC, sequences the codes. Check off each step after you complete it.

▶ First, Scott confirms the diagnosis codes he believes should be assigned:

❏ **R50.81 Fever presenting with conditions classified elsewhere**

❏ **D57.01 Hb-SS disease with acute chest syndrome**

▶ Scott needs to cross-reference back to the Tabular List to read the sequencing instructions.

❏ Scott reads the instructional note that appears in the Tabular List under code **R50.81**. The note states **Code first underlying condition when associated fever is present, such as with: sickle cell disease (D57.-)** (■ FIGURE 14-8).

　▪ This instruction tells him that SCD should be sequenced first.

❏ Scott double-checks the Tabular List entry for code **D57.01**.

　▪ He is reminded of the instructional note at the beginning of category **D57**, which states **Use**

R50.8 Other specified fever

　R50.81 Fever presenting with conditions classified elsewhere

　　Code first underlying condition when associated fever is present, such as with:
　　　leukemia (C91-C95)
　　　neutropenia (D70.-)
　　　sickle-cell disease (D57.-)

Figure 14-8 ■ Instructional note in the Tabular List to "Code first".

additional code for any associated fever (R50.81).

▪ This note confirms that the code for the fever should be sequenced as an additional, or second, code after the code for SCD.

▶ Scott finalizes the codes and sequencing for this case:

(1) **D57.01 Hb-SS disease with acute chest syndrome**

(2) **R50.81 Fever presenting with conditions classified elsewhere**

CODING PRACTICE

Exercise 14.4　Arranging Codes for Conditions of the Blood

Instructions: Read the mini-medical-record of each patient's encounter, review the information abstracted in Exercise 14.2, assign ICD-10-CM diagnosis codes using the Index and Tabular List, and sequence them correctly.

1. INPATIENT HOSPITAL　Gender: F　Age: 59

Reason for admission: Weakness, fatigue, confusion

Assessment: New anemia due to chemotherapy for metastatic colon cancer

Tip: Read the instructional notes in the Tabular List and refer to OGCR I.C.2c.2) to identify all codes needed and the sequencing.

4 ICD-10-CM Codes _____

_____

2. INPATIENT HOSPITAL　Gender: M　Age: 61

Reason for admission: Tachycardia, headaches, fatigue

Assessment: Anemia due to stage 3 chronic kidney disease

Plan: Erythropoiesis stimulating agents (ESAs), supplemental iron

Tip: Read the instructional notes in the Tabular List for sequencing guidance.

2 ICD-10-CM Codes _____

3. OFFICE　Gender: F　Age: 50

Reason for encounter: Follow up on glucose tolerance test (GTT) and complete chemistry analysis

Assessment: Hyperglycemia due to prediabetes, lab results also indicate iron (Fe)-deficiency anemia

Plan: Manage prediabetes with 1,500 calorie diabetic diet, Rx Fe supplements

Tip: The main focus of the visit is prediabetes.

2 ICD-10-CM Codes _____

CODING MALIGNANCIES OF THE BLOOD

Malignancies of the blood and blood-forming organs do not appear in ICD-10-CM Chapter 3, "Diseases of the Blood and Blood-Forming Organs and Certain Disorders Involving the Immune Mechanism (D50-D89)." Codes for malignancies of the blood and blood-forming organs appear in block C81 to C96 within the neoplasm chapter.

Neoplasms, which are solid tumors, do not form in the blood, so there is no entry for *blood* in the Table of Neoplasms. However, hematological malignancies do affect blood, bone marrow, and lymph nodes. Leukemia and myeloma, which begin in the bone marrow, and lymphoma, which begins in the lymphatic system, are the most common types of blood cancer. The blood is also one of the primary vehicles for metastasis of malignant neoplasms in any organ because it circulates through all organs and body tissues.

Lymphomas, leukemias, and myelomas are named based on the type of cell affected and whether the disease begins in mature or immature cells, so coders must be attentive to the exact name of the malignancy. Examples include:

- Anaplastic large cell lymphoma
- ALK-negative or acute myeloid leukemia with 11q23-abnormality
- Multiple myeloma

New cases of leukemia, lymphoma, and myeloma account for approximately 10% of new cancer cases each year, according to the Leukemia and Lymphoma Society. Leukemia is the most common type of cancer in children, accounting for over 27% of childhood cancer, with acute lymphoblastic leukemia (ALL) being the most common.

To locate codes, search the Index for the Main Term that describes the condition, such as **Lymphoma**, **Leukemia**, or **Myeloma**. Then search for subterms that describe the type and location. Do not search the Table of Neoplasms unless the Index directs you to do so.

Each type of leukemia has three separate codes based on the status of the disease, as follows (OGCR I.C.2.n):

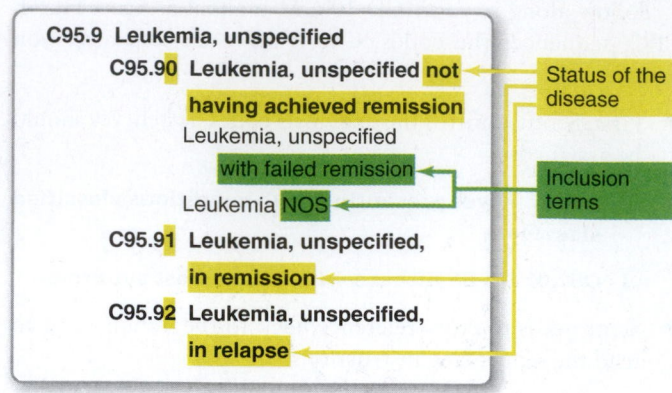

Figure 14-9 ■ Tabular List entry for leukemia showing separate codes for the status of the disease.

- Not having achieved **remission** (*blood counts return to normal and bone marrow samples show no sign of disease*), final digit of **0**
- In remission, final digit of **1**
- In **relapse** (*the return of the disease after remission*), final digit of **2**

When the medical record does not specifically document the status of the disease, assign a code for **not having achieved remission** because the Tabular List classifies **leukemia NOS** under the codes for **leukemia, not having achieved remission** (■ FIGURE 14-9). Also assign a code for **not having achieved remission** when leukemia is documented as *failed remission*.

CODING CAUTION

Remember to distinguish between remission and a personal history of the disease. Personal history defines a condition that no longer exists and is not receiving treatment but has the potential for recurrence and therefore may require continued monitoring (OGCR I.C.21.c.4)). If the documentation is unclear whether the patient is in remission, query the provider (OGCR I.C.2.n).

CODING PRACTICE

Exercise 14.5 Coding Malignancies of the Blood

Instructions: Read the mini-medical-record of each patient's encounter, then abstract, assign, and sequence ICD-10-CM diagnosis codes using the Index and Tabular List. Write the code(s) on the line provided.

1. INPATIENT HOSPITAL Gender: M Age: 78

Reason for admission: Induction chemotherapy

Assessment: Acute myeloid leukemia M7

Tip: Acute myeloid leukemia has eight subtypes. The goal of induction chemotherapy is to achieve remission.

2 ICD-10-CM Codes _____

CODING PRACTICE *(continued)*

2. INPATIENT HOSPITAL   Gender: F   Age: 65

Reason for admission: Chemotherapy

Assessment: Early stage chronic lymphocytic leukemia, B-cell type

Plan: FU in office 1 week. Repeat treatment 3 weeks.

Tip: Refer to OGCR I.C.2.e.

2 ICD-10-CM Codes _____

---

3. OFFICE   Gender: M   Age: 9

Reason for encounter: Monitoring of acute lympho-blastic leukemia (ALL)

Assessment: ALL, in remission

Plan: RTO 3 months

1 ICD-10-CM Code _____

---

4. OFFICE   Gender: F   Age: 22

Reason for encounter: Follow up biopsy of lump in neck

Assessment: Classical Hodgkin's lymphoma with mixed cellularity

Plan: Radiation therapy to neck

1 ICD-10-CM Code _____

---

5. OFFICE   Gender: F   Age: 36

Reason for encounter: Radiation therapy

Assessment: Non-Hodgkin's follicular lymphoma, grade II, stage 3, in neck, abdomen, and pelvic nodes

Plan: Treatment 5x/week for 6 weeks

Tip: Remember to distinguish between grade (how aggressive it is) and stage (how far it has spread).

2 ICD-10-CM Codes _____

CHAPTER SUMMARY

In this chapter you learned that:

- The function of the blood, also called the hemic system, is to transport and pass nutrients, oxygen, carbon dioxide, water, proteins, and hormones to cells and to transport waste products to excretory organs.

- ICD-10-CM does not provide Official Guidelines for Coding and Reporting (OGCR) for this chapter, but the Tabular List contains frequent instructional notes to use an additional code for associated conditions and to code underlying diseases first.

- Many of the conditions in this ICD-10-CM chapter can have multiple underlying causes and multiple manifestations, so coders should thoroughly abstract the symptoms, manifestations, and underlying causes documented in the medical record.

- When an ICD-10-CM chapter does not have any OGCR, as is the case with diseases of the blood and blood-forming organs, coders apply the general OGCR (I.A, I.B, II, and III) and follow instructional notes in the Tabular List.

- Sequencing of codes in this ICD-10-CM chapter is based on the circumstances of admission and the instructional notes in the Tabular List.

- Neoplasms, which are solid tumors, do not form in the blood, but leukemia and myeloma—which begin in the bone marrow—and lymphoma, which begins in the lymphatic system, are the most common types of blood cancer.

CONCEPT QUIZ

Take a moment to look back at diseases of the blood and blood-forming organs and solidify your skills. Try to answer the questions from memory first, then refer back to the chapter if you need a little extra help.

Completion

Instructions: Write the term that completes each statement based on the information you learned in this chapter. Choose from the list below. Some choices may be used more than once and some choices may not be used at all.

aplastic	nutritional
bone marrow	plasma
erythrocytes	polycythemia
formed elements	sarcoidosis
hemic	sickle cell disease
hemoglobin	spleen
hemolytic	thrombocytes
leukocytes	thrombophilia

1. _____ is the oxygen-carrying component of erythrocytes.

2. Blood cells are created in the _____.

3. _____ anemia is due to excessive loss of erythrocytes.

4. _____ are white blood cells.

5. The blood is referred to as the _____ system.

6. _____ is the formation of nodules in the lymph nodes, lungs, bone, and skin.

7. Erythrocytes, leukocytes, and thrombocytes are blood cells, or the _____ of the blood.

8. The spleen destroys old _____ and filters the blood.

9. _____ is an abnormal increase in the number of circulating red blood cells.

10. HbSS is a type of _____.

Multiple Choice

Instructions: Circle the letter of the best answer to each question based on the information you learned in this chapter.

1. Which of the following disorders is classified in ICD-10-CM Chapter 3, "Diseases of the Blood and Blood-Forming Organs"?
   A. Aplastic anemia
   B. Congestive heart failure
   C. Leukemia
   D. High blood pressure

2. What medical term means "formation of blood"?
   A. Hematopoiesis
   B. Hematologist
   C. Hemoglobin
   D. Hemophilia

3. What type of anemia is described by code *D63.0 Anemia in neoplastic disease*?
   A. Aplastic anemia due to chemotherapy
   B. Anemia due to radiotherapy
   C. Anemia due to the cancer itself
   D. Anemia due to antineoplastic chemotherapy

4. What type of disorders include a range of medical problems that lead to poor clotting and continuous bleeding?
   A. Hemostasis
   B. Hemoglobin
   C. Anemia
   D. Purpura

5. How does the coder know how to assign and sequence codes when an ICD-10-CM chapter does not have OGCR?
   A. Use common sense.
   B. Assign the default code listed in the Index.
   C. Ask the supervisor.
   D. Follow instructional notes in the Tabular List.

6. How would you code the following scenario? *A patient with sickle cell thalassemia with crisis is seen for an acute fever.*
   A. R50.81, D57. 419
   B. D57.419, R50.81
   C. D57.40, D56.9, R50.9
   D. R50.9, D57.40

7. What type of external cause code should be assigned when anemia is drug-induced, according to instructions in the Tabular List?
   A. The neoplasm
   B. The injury
   C. The substance
   D. The anemia

8. How would you code the following scenario? *A patient is admitted for aplastic anemia due to chemotherapy for primary lung cancer, overlapping sites of the right lung.*
   A. C34.81, D61.1, T45.1X5A
   B. D61.1, C34.81, T45.1X5A
   C. T45.1X5A, D61.1, C34.81
   D. D61.1, C34.81

9. What is the most common type of childhood leukemia?
   A. Acute myeloid leukemia
   B. Acute lymphoblastic leukemia
   C. Chronic lymphocytic leukemia
   D. Lymphoma

10. How would you code the following scenario? *A patient is seen for lymphoid leukemia, not having achieved remission.*
   A. C91.90
   B. C91.91
   C. C91.92
   D. C91.Z0

KEEP ON CODING

Instructions: Read the diagnostic statement, then use the Index and Tabular List to assign and sequence ICD-10-CM diagnosis codes. Write the code(s) on the line provided.

1. Sideropenic dysphagia. ICD-10-CM Code(s)_____

2. Alpha thalassemia. ICD-10-CM Code(s)_____

3. Sickle cell disease without crisis. ICD-10-CM Code(s)_____

4. Hereditary factor IX deficiency. ICD-10-CM Code(s)_____

5. Bandemia. ICD-10-CM Code(s)_____

6. Cyst of the spleen. ICD-10-CM Code(s)_____

7. Diffuse large B-cell lymphoma, of axilla. ICD-10-CM Code(s)_____

8. Megaloblastic anemia. ICD-10-CM Code(s)_____

9. Pancytopenia due to chemotherapy for metastatic pancreatic cancer. ICD-10-CM Code(s)_____

10. Encounter for chemotherapy for acute monocytic leukemia. ICD-10-CM Code(s)_____

11. Sarcoid arthropathy. ICD-10-CM Code(s)_____

12. Postprocedural hematoma of the spleen following gastric surgery. ICD-10-CM Code(s)_____

13. Cyclic neutropenia. ICD-10-CM Code(s)_____

14. Histiocytic sarcoma. ICD-10-CM Code(s)_____

15. Pyruvate kinase (PK) deficiency anemia. ICD-10-CM Code(s)_____

16. Hemolytic-uremic syndrome. ICD-10-CM Code(s)_____

17. Infantile pseudoleukemia. ICD-10-CM Code(s)_____

18. Heparin-induced thrombocytopenia. ICD-10-CM Code(s)_____

19. Leukopenia. ICD-10-CM Code(s)_____

20. Di George's syndrome. ICD-10-CM Code(s)_____

21. Essential cryoglobulinemia. ICD-10-CM Code(s)_____

22. Protein-deficiency anemia. ICD-10-CM Code(s)_____

23. Evans syndrome. ICD-10-CM Code(s)_____

24. Acquired pure red cell aplasia. ICD-10-CM Code(s)_____

25. Polycythemia due to stress. ICD-10-CM Code(s)_____

CODING CHALLENGE

Instructions: Read the mini-medical-record of each patient's encounter, then abstract, assign, and sequence ICD-10-CM diagnosis codes using the Index and Tabular List. Write the code(s) on the line provided.

1. OFFICE   Gender: M Age: 61

Reason for encounter: Bruising and petechiae, SOB, rapid heart rate, pelvic pain

Assessment: Aplastic anemia due to chemotherapy for prostate cancer with metastasis to the pelvic bones

Plan: Admitted and started on immunosuppressant drugs, received blood transfusion and pain management.

Referral to interventional radiologist to deliver targeted ablation (RFA) to bone metastasis. Pain management at weaker opioid level, RTO weekly for CBC

Tip: Refer to OGCR I.C.2.c.2) for sequencing rules.

4 ICD-10-CM Codes _____

_____

2. INPATIENT HOSPITAL   Gender: M Age: 47

Reason for admission: Severe anemia

Assessment: Anemia due to lung cancer in right lower lobe with metastasis to the bone.

Plan: He received blood transfusions and was discharged home.

Tip: Refer to OGCR I.C.2.c.1) for sequencing rules.

3 ICD-10-CM Codes _____

(continued)

(continued from page 251)

3. OFFICE   Gender: F   Age: 12

Reason for encounter: Management and monitoring of thrombophilia

Assessment: Congenital antithrombin III deficiency

Plan: INR protocol, anticoagulation medication

1 ICD-10-CM Code _____

---

4. INPATIENT HOSPITAL   Gender: F   Age: 53

Chief complaint: Patient states she ran out of the anticoagulant warfarin 5 days ago and now "feels funny."

Assessment: Lupus anticoagulant syndrome, systemic lupus erythematosus

Plan: Restart warfarin, FU in office

Tip: Remember to assign an external cause code for the medication.

3 ICD-10-CM Codes _____

_____

---

5. INPATIENT HOSPITAL   Gender: M   Age: 74

Reason for admission: Bruising, petechiae, hemorrhages, nosebleeds, bleeding gums, extreme fatigue

Assessment: Leukemia, anemia, and thrombocytopenia

Plan: Pt received platelet transfusion. Schedule chemotherapy, Rx anemia support medications

Tip: Pancytopenia is a deficiency of WBCs, RBCs, and platelets.

1 ICD-10-CM Code _____

---

6. OFFICE   Gender: F   Age: 32

Reason for encounter: FU on lab results from daily renal dialysis showing Hb in urine

Assessment: Hemoglobinuria due to dialysis, end stage renal failure

Plan: Erythropoietin protocol, place on kidney replacement list, investigate possibility of family kidney donor. FU for test results in five days

Tip: Remember to assign an external cause code for complication from dialysis.

3 ICD-10-CM Codes _____

_____

---

7. INPATIENT HOSPITAL   Gender: M   Age: 64

Reason for admission: Fever, oral cavity lesions. CBC shows absolute neutrophil count (ANC) is below 500/microliter

Assessment: Neutropenia with fever

Plan: At discharge patient provided guidelines to avoid infections, including use of saline mouth rinses. antibiotic and/or antifungal meds as directed. RTO weekly for CBC.

Tip: Remember to read the instructional notes in the Tabular List.

2 ICD-10-CM Codes _____

---

8. INPATIENT HOSPITAL   Gender: F   Age: 28

Reason for Admission: Palpitations, rapid heartbeat, long bone pain, enlarged, painful spleen. Admit patient for transfusion, IV therapy, pain management, and splenectomy.

Assessment: Sickle cell crisis with splenic sequestration

Plan: RTO in one week for CBC and postoperative check

1 ICD-10-CM Code _____

---

9. INPATIENT HOSPITAL   Gender: F   Age: 45

Reason for Admission: Bone marrow transplant

Assessment: Secondary myelofibrosis due to right breast cancer

Tip: Remember that "due to" means secondary.

2 ICD-10-CM Codes _____

---

10. INPATIENT HOSPITAL   Gender: M   Age: 36

Chief complaint: Unexplained loss of weight, fever, weakness, night sweats, itching, tingling in legs, SOB, elevated red cell count

Assessment: Leukocytosis with polycythemia vera

Plan: FU with clinic one week

2 ICD-10-CM Codes _____

Diseases of the Respiratory System (J00-J99)

Learning Objectives

After completing this chapter, you should have the skills to:

15.1 Spell and define the key words, medical terms, and abbreviations related to the respiratory system. (Remember)

15.2 Summarize the structure, function, and common conditions of the respiratory system. (Understand)

15.3 Adhere to the Official Guidelines for Coding and Reporting related to the respiratory system. (Apply)

15.4 Examine and abstract diagnostic information from the medical record for coding diseases of the respiratory system. (Analyze)

15.5 Demonstrate how to assign codes for diseases of the respiratory system. (Apply)

15.6 Utilize guidelines for arranging (sequencing) multiple diagnosis codes for diseases of the respiratory system. (Apply)

15.7 Demonstrate how to abstract, assign, and sequence codes for neoplasms of the respiratory system. (Apply)

Chapter Outline

- **Respiratory System Refresher**
- **Coding Guidelines for of the Respiratory System**
- **Abstracting for Respiratory System Conditions**
- **Assigning Codes for Respiratory System Conditions**
- **Arranging Codes for Respiratory System Conditions**
- **Coding Neoplasms of the Respiratory System**

Key Terms and Abbreviations

acute exacerbation	chronic bronchitis	laryngitis	status asthmaticus
acute rhinitis	chronic obstructive pulmonary disease (COPD)	larynx	thoracentesis
aerosol therapy	culture and sensitivity	lobe	trachea
airway obstruction	emphysema	lower respiratory tract	tracheal cartilage
allergic rhinitis	endotracheal intubation	lung	tracheostomy tube
alveolus	exchange	nonatopic	upper respiratory tract
atopic	extrinsic	pharyngitis	ventilation-perfusion scan
bronchodilator	hospital-acquired condition (HAC)	pharynx	ventilator
bronchogenic	hypercapnia	productive cough	ventilator-associated pneumonia (VAP)
bronchial tree	hypoxemia	pulmonary function test	
bronchiole	intrinsic	respiratory system	
bronchus		sinusitis	

In addition to the key terms listed here, students should know the terms defined within tables in this chapter.

INTRODUCTION

As you travel to a higher elevation than what you're accustomed to, breathing becomes more difficult. This is not because there is less oxygen in the air but because a decrease in air pressure causes us to inhale less air with each breath.

A pulmonologist specializes in diagnosing and treating conditions of the lungs and lower respiratory system. An otolaryngologist specializes in diagnosing and treating conditions of the upper respiratory system. Primary care physicians treat uncomplicated conditions of the respiratory system and refer more complicated cases to specialists.

RESPIRATORY SYSTEM REFRESHER

The function of the **respiratory system** is to obtain oxygen (O_2) from the air and deliver it to the lungs and blood for distribution to tissue cells and to remove the gaseous waste product carbon dioxide (CO_2) from the blood and lungs and expel it. This process is called **exchange**. The respiratory system also makes it possible to cough, sneeze, and talk.

The respiratory system is divided into the **upper respiratory tract**, which consists of the nose, **pharynx** (*throat*), and **larynx** (*voice box*); and the **lower respiratory tract**, which consists of the **trachea** (*windpipe*), bronchi, and **lungs**

(■ FIGURE 15-1). As air enters the nasal cavity or oral cavity, it is warmed and moistened, then passes through the pharynx, larynx, and trachea. The trachea divides into two **bronchi** (*bronchial tubes*) that lead to the two lungs. Rings of **tracheal cartilage** keep the trachea and bronchi open. In the **bronchial tree**, the bronchi subdivide into smaller and smaller branches, with the smallest being the **bronchioles**, which do not contain rings of cartilage. Bronchioles end in small air sacs in the lungs, **alveoli**.

The lungs consist of spongy tissue with interlacing networks of bronchioles, alveoli, alveolar sacs, blood vessels, and capillaries. The lungs are divided into **lobes** (*segments*). The right lung has three lobes: the superior, middle, and inferior. The left lung has two lobes: the superior and inferior. The lungs receive deoxygenated blood from the heart through the pulmonary artery, reoxygenate it, and send it back to the heart through the pulmonary vein so the heart can pump the blood out to the rest of the body.

In Figure 15-1, each structure in the respiratory system is labeled with its name as well as its medical terminology root/combining form, where applicable. Refer to ■ TABLE 15-1 for a refresher on how to build medical terms related to the respiratory system.

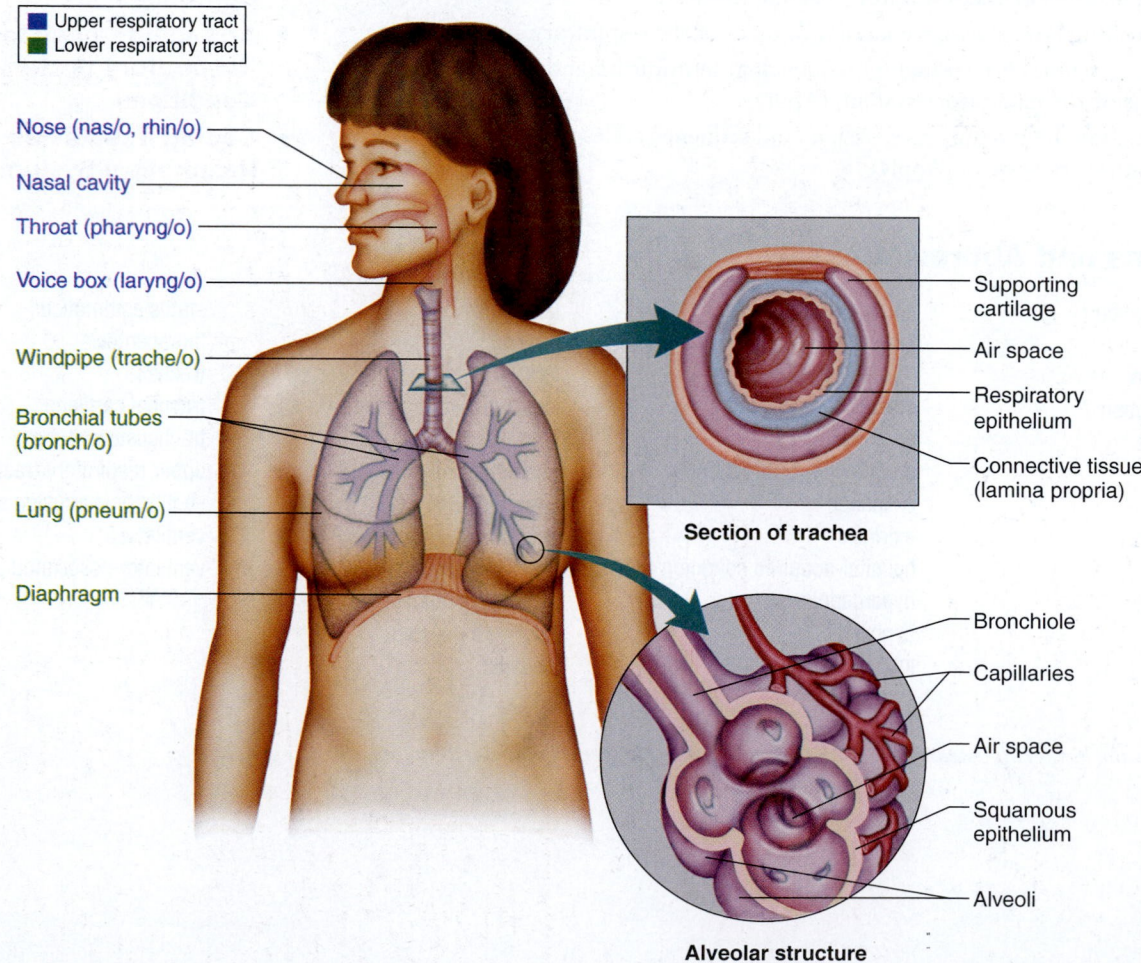

Figure 15-1 ■ The respiratory system.

Table 15-1   ■   **EXAMPLE OF CONSTRUCTING MEDICAL TERMS FOR THE RESPIRATORY SYSTEM**

Prefix/Combining Form	Suffix	Complete Medical Term
dys- (prefix; *abnormal, painful*)	**-scope** (*instrument to view the inside*)	**dys + phonia** (*difficulty speaking*)
	-ectasis (*dilation*)	**dys + pnea** (*difficulty breathing*)
bronch/o (*bronchus*)	**-pnea** (*breathing*)	**broncho + scope** (*instrument to view the bronchus*)
	-phonia (*voice*)	**bronchi + ectasis** (*dilated bronchus*)

SUCCESS STEP

To form the plural of most medical terms, you need to drop the last one or two letters and substitute new letters. For example, one bronch**us** becomes two bronch**i**.

CODING CAUTION

Be alert for medical terms that are spelled similarly and have different meanings.

bronchitis (*inflammation of the bronchus*) and **bronchiol-itis** (*inflammation of the bronchiole*)

pyothorax (*pus in the chest*) and **pneumothorax** (*air in the chest*)

emphysema (*abnormal accumulation of air in body tissue*) and **empyema** (*pus in a body cavity*)

Conditions of the Respiratory System

Respiratory conditions are divided based on whether they affect the upper or lower respiratory tract. Conditions affecting the upper respiratory tract, frequently caused by viruses, include **acute rhinitis** (*common cold*), **allergic rhinitis** (*hay fever*), **sinusitis** (*sinus infection*), **pharyngitis** (*sore throat*), and **laryngitis** (*irritated vocal cords*). Conditions affecting the lower respiratory tract include obstructive diseases (narrowing of the air passages), infection and inflammatory diseases (viral and bacterial infections), and mechanical damage (nontraumatic structural damage to the lung). Refer to ■ TABLE 15-2, (page 252) for a summary of respiratory system conditions.

Coders should have an understanding of asthma, COPD, and ventilator-associated pneumonia because they pose special coding challenges. These are discussed next, followed by an overview of diagnostic and treatment methods.

Asthma

Asthma is a chronic lung disease that affects the bronchi and is characterized by inflammation and narrowing of the airway. A common symptom is wheezing due to bronchospasms. Asthma may be **extrinsic** or **atopic** (*due to allergens*) or **intrinsic** or **nonatopic** (*not due to allergens*). According to the American College of Allergy, Asthma, and Immunology (ACAAI), about one in 12 people in the United States have asthma, with over half experiencing an asthma attack each year.

Physicians diagnose asthma based on the frequency and type of symptoms, forced expiratory volume (FEV), and peak expiratory flow (PEF), which are measurements of lung function. Based on this information, patients' asthma is rated as intermittent or persistent and is classified into one of four severity levels:

1. Mild intermittent
2. Mild persistent
3. Moderate persistent
4. Severe persistent

An **acute exacerbation**, commonly called an asthma attack, is a sudden increase in the intensity or type of symptoms, such as shortness of breath, wheezing, and chest tightness. **Status asthmaticus** is an acute exacerbation that does not respond to the standard medical treatments of bronchodilators and steroids.

Chronic Obstructive Pulmonary Disease

Chronic obstructive pulmonary disease (COPD), one of the most common lung diseases, is the combination of **chronic bronchitis** and **emphysema** as comorbidities. An **airway obstruction** is a reduction in the amount of air inhaled during each breath, most commonly caused by a reduction in the diameter of the bronchioles due to inflammation.

According to the Centers for Disease Control and Prevention, approximately 11% of nursing home residents have COPD and over 5% of noninstitutionalized adults suffer from either chronic bronchitis or emphysema. COPD accounts for over 174,000 emergency department visits per year.

Physicians diagnose chronic bronchitis when patients present with a **productive cough** (*cough with sputum*) on most days for three months in two consecutive years. The most common cause is long-term inhalation of irritants. Emphysema is an enlargement and rupture of alveolar sacs at the end of the bronchioles, causing an abnormal accumulation of air in the tissue. The damage it causes is irreversible, unlike asthma, in which the obstruction is reversible.

Ventilator-Associated Pneumonia

Ventilator-associated pneumonia (VAP) is pneumonia that develops 48 hours or more after mechanical ventilation is initiated. Mechanical ventilation is the administration of oxygen using an endotracheal tube or **tracheostomy tube** (*a surgical opening in the neck leading to the trachea*). Intubation allows

Table 15-2 ■ **CONDITIONS OF THE RESPIRATORY SYSTEM**

Condition	Definition
Acute respiratory distress syndrome (ARDS)	Acute respiratory failure that results in widespread injury to the endothelium in the lung, caused by sepsis, massive blood transfusion, aspiration of gastric contents, or pneumonia
Acute respiratory failure (ARF)	Insufficient oxygen passing from the lungs to the blood, due to hypercapnia (*high carbon dioxide level*), hypoxemia (*low oxygen level*), or both
Asthma	A chronic lung disease that affects the bronchi and is characterized by inflammation of the airway, a reversible obstruction, and reshaping of the airway
Atelectasis	Collapse of a lung, preventing the exchange of oxygen and carbon dioxide
Chronic bronchitis	Inflammation of the bronchi with a productive cough for three months in two consecutive years
Chronic obstructive pulmonary disease (COPD)	The combination of chronic bronchitis and emphysema as comorbidities
Emphysema	An enlargement and rupture of alveolar sacs at the end of the bronchioles, causing an abnormal accumulation of air in the tissue
Influenza	An acute respiratory infection with sudden onset caused by a virus and characterized by fever, chills, headache, muscle aches, cough, and sore throat
Laryngitis	Inflammation of the larynx, resulting in hoarseness
Lobar pneumonia	Bacterial pneumonia that primarily affects one lobe of the lung
Lobular pneumonia	Pneumonia that primarily affects the bronchi and lobules (*clusters of alveoli that surround each bronchial branch*); also called *bronchopneumonia*
Pharyngitis	Inflammation of the throat
Pleurisy	Inflammation of the lining of the lungs and thoracic cavity with oozing of fluid or fibrinous material into the pleural cavity
Pneumoconiosis	Abnormal condition of the lung caused by inhalation of dust particles, such as coal dust (anthracosis), asbestos (asbestosis), iron dust (siderosis), or quartz (silicosis)
Pneumonia	Inflammatory condition of the lung in which the alveoli and air spaces fill with fluid; caused by bacterial, virus, fungi, or chemical irritants (■ FIGURE 15-2)
Pneumothorax	A collection of air between the chest wall and lungs, which may cause the lung to collapse
Pulmonary edema	An abnormal accumulation of fluid in the lungs, especially the alveoli, resulting in dyspnea
Tonsillitis	Inflammation of the tonsils

microorganisms from oral and gastric secretions to invade the tissues of the lower respiratory tract and lung. VAP is more serious than other types of pneumonia because patients who acquire it are in poorer health than the average person. In addition, the types of germs present in a hospital are often more dangerous and more resistant to treatment than those found in the community at large.

SUCCESS STEP

VAP is an example of a **hospital-acquired condition (HAC)**, a serious condition that develops after admission. Medicare does not pay hospitals for the costs incurred to care for HACs and hospitals cannot bill patients for them.

Diagnosis and Treatment of Respiratory Conditions

Diseases of the respiratory system are diagnosed with a wide variety of techniques, including:

- Arterial blood gasses to determine O_2 and CO_2 concentrations
- Biopsy
- Chest x-ray
- Computed tomography scan
- **Culture and sensitivity**—A lab test of secretions, such as sputum, to observe bacterial growth and determine antibiotic effectiveness
- Endoscopy (laryngoscopy, bronchoscopy)

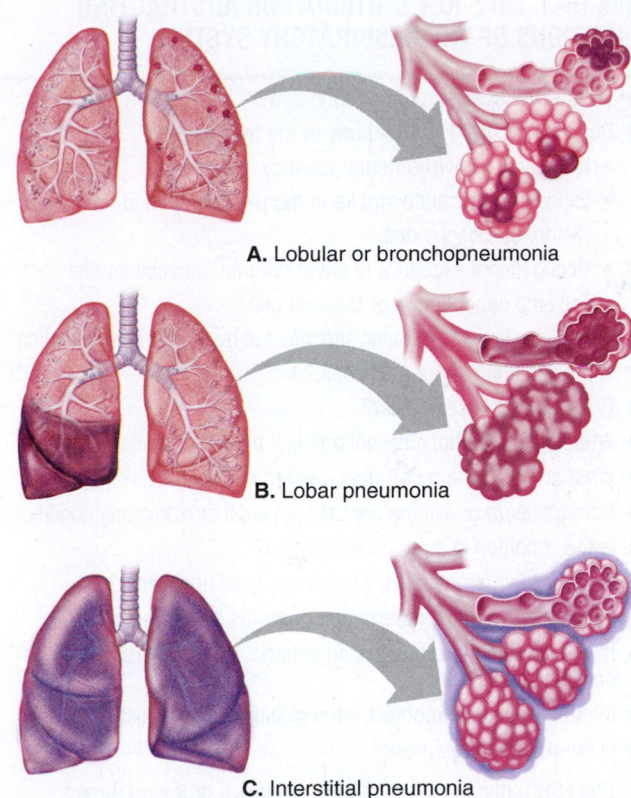

A. Lobular or bronchopneumonia

B. Lobar pneumonia

C. Interstitial pneumonia

Figure 15-2 ■ Types of pneumonia. (**A**) Lobular or bronchopneumonia has a localized pattern. (**B**) Lobar pneumonia has a diffuse pattern within a lung lobe. (**C**) Interstitial pneumonia is typically diffuse and bilateral.

- **Pulmonary function tests**—Diagnostic tests that measure air flow in and out of the lungs, lung volumes, and gas exchange between the lungs and blood
- Ultrasound scanning
- **Ventilation-perfusion scan**—A nuclear medicine test useful in identifying pulmonary emboli by showing whether blood is flowing to all parts of the lung

Respiratory diseases are treated by medications, surgery, and respiratory therapy, including:

- **Aerosol therapy**—Medication suspended in a mist that is inhaled
- **Bronchodilator**—A medication that relaxes muscle spasms in bronchial tubes
- **Endotracheal intubation**—Placement of a tube through the mouth and glottis into the trachea to create a viable airway
- Pulmonectomy or lobectomy
- **Thoracentesis**—Surgical puncture of the chest wall to remove fluids
- Tracheostomy

CODING PRACTICE

Exercise 15.1   **Respiratory System Refresher**

Instructions: Use your medical terminology skills and resources to define the following conditions related to the respiratory system, then assign the diagnosis code. Follow these steps:

- Use slash marks "/" to break down each term into its root(s) and suffix.
- Define the meaning of the word, based on the meaning of each word part.
- Assign the default ICD-10-CM diagnosis code for the condition using the Index and Tabular List.

Example: tonsillitis tonsil/itis   Meaning *inflammation of the tonsil*   ICD-10-CM Code *J03.90*

1. pneumatocel   Meaning _____   ICD-10-CM Code _____
2. bronchiolitis   Meaning _____   ICD-10-CM Code _____
3. pneumohemothorax   Meaning _____   ICD-10-CM Code _____
4. rhinorrhea   Meaning _____   ICD-10-CM Code _____
5. nasopharyngitis   Meaning _____   ICD-10-CM Code _____
6. bronchoalveolitis   Meaning _____   ICD-10-CM Code _____
7. laryngoplegia   Meaning _____   ICD-10-CM Code _____
8. pyothorax   Meaning _____   ICD-10-CM Code _____
9. tracheostenosis   Meaning _____   ICD-10-CM Code _____
10. hydropneumothorax   Meaning _____   ICD-10-CM Code _____

CODING GUIDELINES FOR THE RESPIRATORY SYSTEM

Coders should understand the organization of this ICD-10-CM chapter, chapter-wide and commonly used instructional notes in the Tabular List, and the relevant OGCR. This information is necessary for accurate coding.

ICD-10-CM Chapter 10, "Diseases of the Respiratory System (J00-J99)," contains 11 blocks or subchapters that are divided by type of disorder and anatomic site. Review the block names and code ranges listed at the beginning of Chapter 10 in the ICD-10-CM manual to become familiar with the content and organization.

This chapter includes infections of the upper and lower respiratory tracts, acute and chronic obstructive diseases, lung diseases due to external agents, and respiratory failure. It does not include infectious diseases, smoke inhalation, symptoms and signs, perinatal conditions, or obstetric-related conditions. These conditions are classified in other ICD-10-CM chapters.

ICD-10-CM provides Official Guidelines for Coding and Reporting (OGCR) for the respiratory system in OGCR section I.C.10. OGCR provides a detailed discussion of chronic obstructive pulmonary disease and asthma, acute respiratory failure, influenza, and ventilator-associated pneumonia.

An instructional note at the beginning of ICD-10-CM Chapter 10 in the Tabular List directs coders when they should use an additional code to identify circumstances and lifestyle habits related to tobacco use, tobacco dependence, and tobacco smoke exposure. An additional instructional note directs coders how to assign codes when more than one site in the respiratory system is affected. Instructional notes appear throughout the Tabular List directing coders when additional codes are required for certain categories, including coding the type of asthma and any infection. Review the instructional notes carefully to ensure accurate and complete coding. Specific OGCR and instructional notes are discussed and cited throughout this chapter of the text.

ABSTRACTING FOR RESPIRATORY SYSTEM CONDITIONS

Abstracting diagnoses for the respiratory system requires knowledge of the disease processes because multiple comorbidities are common. Coders need to distinguish between diseases to ensure they abstract all of the required details. In addition to identifying the conditions, coders must also identify the infectious organism and lifestyle habits related to tobacco.
■ TABLE 15-3 lists important questions to ask when abstracting respiratory system conditions.

Guided Example of Abstracting for Respiratory System Conditions

Refer to the following example throughout this chapter to practice skills for abstracting, assigning, and sequencing respiratory system codes. Leanne Riehl, CCS, is a fictional coder who guides you through the coding process.

Table 15-3 ■ **KEY CRITERIA FOR ABSTRACTING CONDITIONS OF THE RESPIRATORY SYSTEM**

- ❏ What is the specific type of condition?
- ❏ Does the record document any of the following?
  - Exposure to environmental tobacco smoke
  - Exposure to tobacco smoke in the perinatal period
  - History of tobacco use
  - Occupational exposure to environmental tobacco smoke
  - Tobacco dependence or tobacco use
- ❏ What is the lowest anatomic site affected by a respiratory infection?
- ❏ Is the condition acute or chronic?
- ❏ Does a lung abscess exist?
- ❏ What is the infectious organism? Is it a virus or bacteria?
- ❏ What are all of the respiratory-related comorbidities?
- ❏ Does influenza or asthma coexist with another respiratory condition?
- ❏ Is the condition in acute exacerbation?
- ❏ If asthma is documented, what is the level of severity?
- ❏ Is asthma in acute exacerbation or status asthmaticus?
- ❏ Is the condition the result of an external cause or procedural complication?
- ❏ If influenza is documented, what manifestations exist?
- ❏ Is the condition recurrent?
- ❏ Does the patient use supplemental oxygen or a **ventilator** (*a machine that assists in breathing*)?

Date: 6/16/yy   Location: Branton Medical Center

Provider: Gilbert Stagg, MD

Patient: Jared Hershman   Gender: M   Age: 73

Reason for admission: Dehydration, started IV fluids

Assessment: Patient who previously smoked cigarettes for 50 years (nicotine dependence) was placed on ventilator due to COPD exacerbation. Patient acquired ventilator associated pneumonia (VAP) due to Pseudomonas. Hospital stay was prolonged due to the VAP.

Plan: Discharged home after 10 days, continue antibiotics, start supplemental O_2

Follow along as Leanne Riehl, CCS, abstracts the diagnosis. Check off each step after you complete it.

▶ Leanne reads through the entire record, paying special attention to the reason for the encounter and the final assessment.

❏ She sees that there are quite a few things going on with this patient, so she needs to break it down step by step. She refers to the Key Criteria for Abstracting Conditions of the Respiratory System (Table 15-3). Because there are several coexisting conditions, she must review all the abstracting questions for each condition.

❏ *What is the specific type of condition?* The reason for the admission is dehydration. She notes that this condition was treated with IV fluids

❏ *What are all of the respiratory-related comorbidities?* After he was admitted, the patient developed VAP

❏ *Does the patient use supplemental oxygen or a ventilator?* Yes, patient was placed on ventilator

❏ *What is the infectious organism?* Pseudomonas *Is it a virus or bacteria?* Bacteria

❏ *Is the condition the result of an external cause or procedural complication?* Yes, the pneumonia is ventilator associated

❏ *Does the record document any current or past tobacco use?* Previously smoked cigarettes for 50 years (nicotine dependence)

▶ Leanne reviews all the information she has gathered about this case.

❏ The patient was admitted for dehydration.

❏ He has COPD.

❏ He experienced an acute exacerbation of COPD.

❏ He has a history of cigarette smoking.

❏ He acquired VAP due to *Pseudomonas*.

▶ At this time, Leanne does not know which of these conditions may need to be coded nor how many codes she will end up with. She will learn about this when she moves on to assigning codes.

CODING PRACTICE

Exercise 15.2 Abstracting for Respiratory System Conditions

Instructions: Read the mini-medical-record of each patient's encounter and answer the abstracting questions. Write the answer on the line provided. Do not assign any codes.

1. OFFICE   Gender: M   Age: 31

Reason for encounter: Patient with previously diagnosed extrinsic asthma presents with increased symptoms of coughing, wheezing, and SOB

Assessment: Symptoms are due to acute exacerbation of mild intermittent asthma.

Plan: Oral steroids and quick relief bronchodilator inhaler

a. What condition was previously diagnosed? _____

b. What are the presenting symptoms? _____

c. What is the cause of the symptoms? _____

d. Which symptoms should you code? _____

e. What is the severity of the patient's asthma? _____

2. OFFICE   Gender: F   Age: 69

Reason for encounter: Productive cough and fever, patient is concerned that she may need medication for COPD which she has not needed for several years

Assessment: Viral pneumonia unrelated to patient's history of COPD

Plan: Rx cough medicine with expectorant, take aspirin for fever, drink plenty of fluids to prevent dehydration

a. What are the patient's symptoms? _____

b. Why was the patient concerned about the symptoms? _____

c. What condition did the physician diagnose?_____

d. What is the difference between viral pneumonia and bacterial pneumonia? _____

e. Is the pneumonia related to the past COPD?_____

f. Should you code the symptoms? _____
   Why or why not? _____

g. Should you code the COPD? _____
   Why or why not? _____

(continued)

CODING PRACTICE (continued)

2. (continued)

Tip: If you are unsure about this, refer to OGCR IV.J.

h. Should you code the pneumonia? _____

   Why or why not? _____

---

3. INPATIENT HOSPITAL Gender: M Age: 72

Reason for encounter: Management of chronic obstructive pulmonary disease, recent self-administered spirometry results have been declining, increased SOB

Assessment: COPD with chronic bronchitis and emphysema

Plan: Nebulizer treatment to administer bronchodilators

a. What chronic disease was previously diagnosed? _____
_____

b. What symptoms does the patient report at this encounter? _____

c. Do these symptoms lead to a new diagnosis?_____
_____

d. Should you code the symptoms? _____

   Why or why not? _____

e. Should you code the COPD? _____

   Why or why not? _____

f. Should you code chronic bronchitis and/or emphysema? _____

   Why or why not? _____

---

4. INPATIENT HOSPITAL Gender: M Age: 80

Reason for admission: Patient with congestive heart failure and on supplemental O₂ admitted from physician's office after presenting with low fever, chills, cough. CHF increases patient risk for complications.

Assessment: Lobular pneumonia and acute bronchitis, both due to Mycoplasma pneumoniae

a. What are the symptoms? _____

b. Should the symptoms be coded? _____

   Why or why not? _____

c. What is the role of CHF in this case? _____
_____

(*continued*)

---

4. (continued)

d. What two conditions were diagnosed? _____
_____

e. Is the bronchitis acute or chronic? _____
_____

f. What is the infectious organism? _____
_____

g. Does the patient have COPD? _____
_____

h. What is the principal diagnosis? _____
_____

Tip: Refer to OGCR II.B.

i. What is the second diagnosis? _____
_____

j. What is the third diagnosis? _____
_____

k. What ongoing medical treatment does the patient use? _____

---

5. INPATIENT HOSPITAL Gender: F Age: 76

Reason for admission: Acute bronchitis

Assessment: COPD with acute bronchitis exacerbation and chronic bronchitis

Plan: Begin oxygen therapy, patient must cease cigarette smoking as it continues to impact her respiratory conditions, counseled her regarding treatment options for tobacco dependence

a. What is the reason for admission? _____
_____

b. What other conditions are documented? _____
_____

c. What is the relationship between COPD and the acute bronchitis? _____

d. Should the acute bronchitis be coded? _____

   Why or why not? _____

e. Should chronic bronchitis be coded? _____

   Why or why not? _____

f. What lifestyle habit should be coded? _____
_____

Tip: You will learn the sequencing when you begin assigning the codes in Exercise 15.4.

CODING PRACTICE (continued)

6. INPATIENT HOSPITAL Gender: F Age: 78

Reason for admission: Asbestosis which is thought to be due to exposure to asbestos particles brought home by her late husband who worked in the fireproofing industry for many years and died of mesothelioma

Assessment: Asbestosis, clubbing of fingers due to the asbestosis, mild persistent asthma

Plan: O_2, thoracentesis, medication, respiratory therapy

a. What is the reason for admission? _____
_____

b. What is clubbing of the fingers due to? _____
_____

(continued)

6. (continued)

c. Should clubbing of the fingers be coded? _____
_____

Why or why not? _____

d. What other diagnosis exists? _____
_____

e. What is the severity of the asthma? _____

f. Should asthma be coded? _____

Why or why not? _____

g. What is the principal diagnosis? _____
_____

ASSIGNING CODES FOR RESPIRATORY SYSTEM CONDITIONS

Coders must be attentive to the details of the case, instructional notes in the Tabular List, and the OGCR to accurately assign codes for respiratory system conditions. They should become familiar with chapter-wide coding considerations as well as information specifically for asthma, COPD, and influenza.

Chapter-Wide Coding

ICD-10-CM Chapter 10, "Diseases of the Respiratory System (J00-J99)," begins with two instructional notes that apply to all codes in the chapter. One instruction pertains to assigning additional codes for lifestyle habits; the other instruction describes how to code when multiple sites within the respiratory system are affected. Coders should also assign status **Z** codes when needed.

Lifestyle Habits

ICD-10-CM Chapter 10 provides an instructional note at the beginning of the chapter that instructs coders to use an additional code, when applicable, to identify various situations related to tobacco use, dependence, and exposure to tobacco smoke (■ FIGURE 15-3). Exposure may include environmental tobacco smoke, occupational exposure to tobacco smoke, and exposure to tobacco smoke during the perinatal period (*before birth through the first 28 days after birth*).

SUCCESS STEP

The Tabular List provides an instructional note to assign an additional code to identify the infectious organism when there is no combination code to describe the condition and the organism.

Use additional code, where applicable, to identify:
 exposure to environmental tobacco smoke (Z77.22)
 exposure to tobacco smoke in the perinatal period (P96.81)
 history of tobacco dependence (Z87.891)
 occupational exposure to environmental tobacco smoke (Z57.31)
 tobacco dependence (F17.-)
 tobacco use (Z72.0)

Figure 15-3 ■ Tabular List instructional notes that apply to all codes in ICD-10-CM chapter 10.

Multiple Sites Affected

Respiratory conditions may affect more than one site within the respiratory system, such as the tonsils and adenoids, trachea and bronchi, or bronchi and lung. When the site is not specifically indexed, assign a code for the lowest anatomical site. This requires coders to follow conventions in the Index carefully and to have knowledge of respiratory system anatomy.

For example, consider a patient seen for tracheobronchitis, an inflammation (-*itis*) of the trachea (trache/o) and bronchi (bronch/o). The Index entry for the Main Term **Tracheobronchitis** cross-references coders to the Main Term **Bronchitis** because the bronchi are located lower than the trachea. The Index entry for the Main Term **Bronchitis** directs coders to **J40** (■ FIGURE 15-4, page 258). In the Tabular List, **Tracheobronchitis** appears as an inclusion term under the code **J40 Bronchitis, not specified as acute or chronic.**

Z Codes

Certain treatments for respiratory conditions require status **Z** codes. The most common are the existence of a tracheostomy, an encounter for tracheostomy care, long-term use of oxygen, and/or ventilator assistance in breathing. If there are

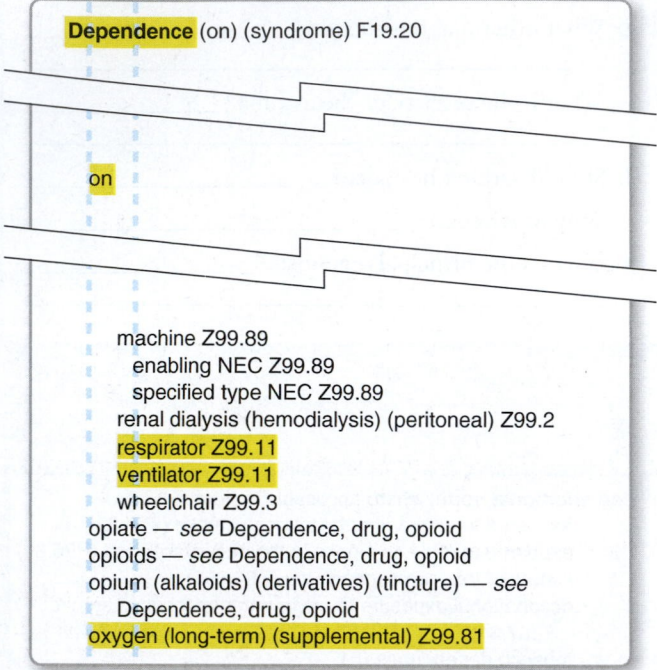

> **J40 Bronchitis, not specified as acute or chronic**
> Bronchitis NOS
> Bronchitis with tracheitis NOS
> Catarrhal bronchitis
> Tracheobronchitis NOS

Figure 15-4 ■ Tabular List entry for bronchitis, with tracheobronchitis as an inclusion term.

> **Dependence** (on) (syndrome) F19.20
>
> on
>
> machine Z99.89
>   enabling NEC Z99.89
>   specified type NEC Z99.89
> renal dialysis (hemodialysis) (peritoneal) Z99.2
> respirator Z99.11
> ventilator Z99.11
> wheelchair Z99.3
> opiate — *see* Dependence, drug, opioid
> opioids — *see* Dependence, drug, opioid
> opium (alkaloids) (derivatives) (tincture) — *see*
>   Dependence, drug, opioid
> oxygen (long-term) (supplemental) Z99.81

Figure 15-5 ■ Index entries for dependence on ventilator or oxygen.

complications from any of these devices, code the complication and do not assign a **Z** code.

Locate codes for tracheostomy status and tracheostomy care under the Main Term **Tracheostomy** in the Index. Locate the **Z** codes for oxygen and ventilator use under the Main Term **Dependence** in the Index (■ FIGURE 15-5).

Assigning Codes for Asthma

Assigning codes for asthma has new requirements in ICD-10-CM. To assign codes for asthma, coders need to identify how the physician has documented the severity of the patient's condition. Be attentive when navigating the Main Term for **Asthma** in the Index because the second-level subterms **with exacerbation** and **with status asthmaticus** appear under multiple first-level subterms, and it is easy to become confused.

By searching the Index for the Main Term **Asthma**, then locating a subterm for either **intermittent** or **persistent**, coders can locate most of the codes they need. The subterm **intermittent** contains only one level of severity, **mild**, then provides choices for **with exacerbation** or **with status asthmaticus**. The subterm **persistent** provides additional subterms for **mild**, **moderate**, or **severe**, then provides choices under each for **with exacerbation** or **with status asthmaticus** (■ FIGURE 15-6).

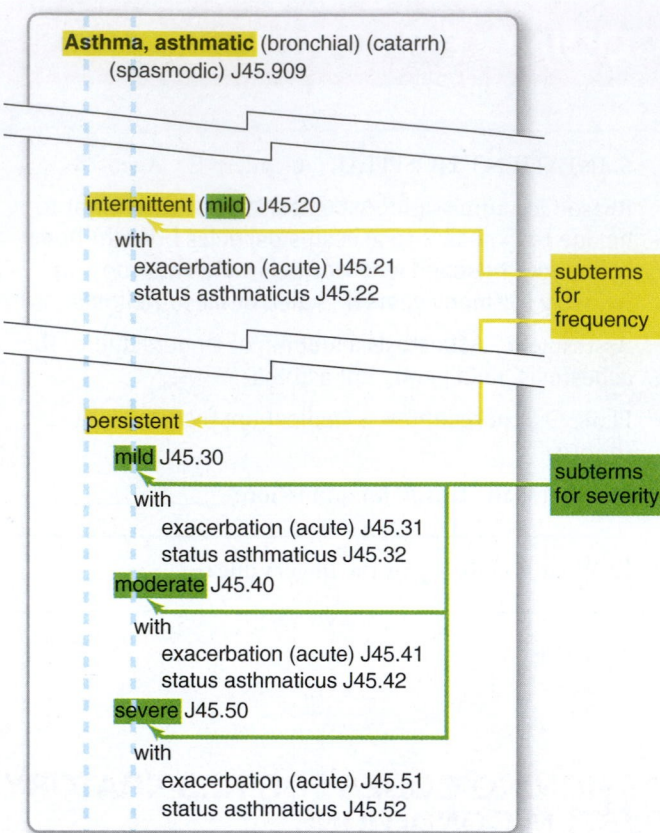

> **Asthma, asthmatic** (bronchial) (catarrh)
>   (spasmodic) J45.909
>
> intermittent (mild) J45.20
>   with
>   exacerbation (acute) J45.21   *subterms for frequency*
>   status asthmaticus J45.22
>
> persistent
>   mild J45.30   *subterms for severity*
>   with
>   exacerbation (acute) J45.31
>   status asthmaticus J45.32
>   moderate J45.40
>   with
>   exacerbation (acute) J45.41
>   status asthmaticus J45.42
>   severe J45.50
>   with
>   exacerbation (acute) J45.51
>   status asthmaticus J45.52

Figure 15-6 ■ Example of the Index entry for "Asthma".

Assigning Codes for COPD and Asthma

The codes in categories **J44 Other chronic obstructive pulmonary disease** and **J45 Asthma** distinguish between uncomplicated cases and those in acute exacerbation. An acute exacerbation is a worsening of a chronic condition. An acute exacerbation is not the same as an infection superimposed on a chronic condition, although an exacerbation may be triggered by an infection.

When asthma occurs with COPD, the Index leads to the entry **Asthma, with chronic obstructive pulmonary disease J44.9**, which appears to be a combination code. However, the Tabular List instructs coders to assign an additional code for the type of asthma. The same holds true for chronic obstructive bronchitis with asthma. Sequencing depends on the circumstances of admission. (OGCR I.C.10.a.1)) (■ FIGURE 15-7).

> Patient with COPD is admitted for severe persistent asthma with status asthmaticus.
>
> (1) **J45.52 Severe persistent asthma with status asthmaticus**
> (2) **J44.9 Chronic obstructive pulmonary disease, unspecified**

Figure 15-7 ■ Example of assigning codes for COPD and asthma.

Assigning Codes for Influenza

When assigning codes for influenza, coders must identify the type of influenza and the manifestations. Influenza codes are divided based on whether the disease is identified as *novel influenza A virus*, other virus, or the virus is unidentified. Novel influenza A, which includes avian influenza and H1N1, has a specific subcategory in the Tabular List (■ FIGURE 15-8). Coders should assign codes from subcategory **J09.X** and **J10** only when the virus is confirmed as one of those listed in the inclusion notes. Confirmation requires a definitive diagnostic statement from the physician but does not require a positive laboratory test. However, if the provider documents *suspected or possible or probable avian influenza*, do not assign a code from **J09.- Influenza due to certain identified influenza viruses**. Instead, assign a code from category **J11.- Influenza due to unspecified influenza virus** (OGCR I.C.10.c).

For all types of influenza, assign a combination code that describes the manifestation(s). The choices include:

- Pneumonia
- Other respiratory
- Gastrointestinal
- Encephalopathy
- Myocarditis
- Otitis media
- Other

Instructional notes in the Tabular List also instruct coders to assign additional codes for lung abscess, pleural effusion, perforated tympanic membrane, sinusitis, the type of pneumonia, and any additional manifestations.

CODING CAUTION

OGCR I.C.10.c, which prohibits coding unconfirmed cases of avian or H1N1 influenza, is an exception to the hospital inpatient guideline OGCR II.H, which says to code uncertain conditions as though they exist. When there is a difference between a general coding guideline and a chapter-specific guideline, you should follow the chapter-specific guideline.

Guided Example of Assigning Codes for Respiratory System Conditions

To practice skills for sequencing codes for the respiratory system, continue with the example from earlier in the chapter about patient Jared Hershman, who was admitted to Branton Medical Center due to dehydration.

Follow along in your ICD-10-CM manual as Leanne Riehl, CCS, assigns codes. Check off each step after you complete it.

▶ First, Leanne reviews all the information she abstracted about the patient. She will tackle each condition, one at a time.

❏ The patient was admitted for dehydration.

❏ He has COPD.

❏ He experienced an acute exacerbation of COPD.

❏ He has a history of cigarette smoking.

❏ He acquired VAP due to *Pseudomonas*.

▶ Leanne searches the Index for the Main Term **Dehydration**.

❏ She identifies the default code **E86.0**.

❏ She reviews the three subterms and verifies that none of them are documented.

▶ Leanne verifies code **E86.0** in the Tabular List.

❏ She reads the code title for **E86.0, Dehydration** and confirms that this accurately describes the documentation.

▶ Leanne checks for instructional notes in the Tabular List.

❏ She cross-references the beginning of category **E86**, reads the **Excludes1** notes, and verifies that they do not apply to this case.

❏ She then cross-references the beginning of the block **E70-E88** and the beginning of the chapter, reads the **Excludes1** notes, and verifies that they do not apply to this case.

❏ Leanne finalizes the code **E86.0 Dehydration**.

4th	**J09**	**Influenza due to certain identified influenza viruses**
	Excludes1:	influenza due to other identified influenza virus (J10.-)
		influenza due to unidentified influenza virus (J11.-)
		seasonal influenza due to other identified influenza virus (J10.-)
		seasonal influenza due to unidentified influenza virus (J11.-)
5th	**J09.X**	Influenza due to identified novel influenza A virus
		Avian influenza
		Bird influenza
		Influenza A/H5N1
		Influenza of other animal origin, not bird or swine
		Swine influenza virus (viruses that normally cause infections in pigs)

Figure 15-8 ■ Tabular List inclusion and exclusion notes for "Influenza due to certain identified influenza viruses".

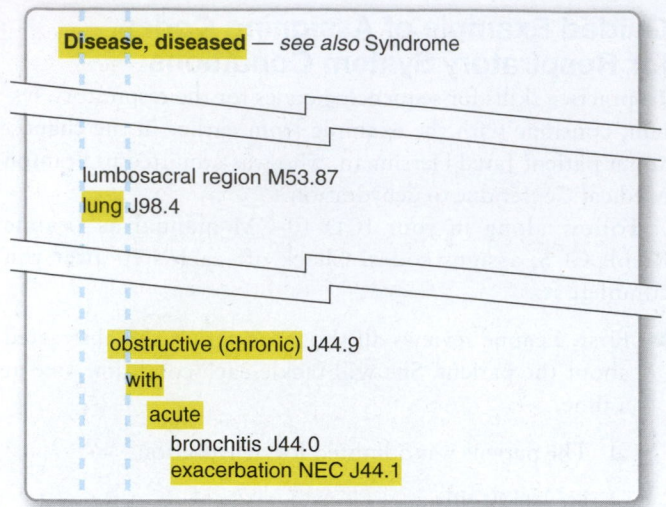

Disease, diseased — *see also* Syndrome

lumbosacral region M53.87
lung J98.4

obstructive (chronic) J44.9
with
acute
bronchitis J44.0
exacerbation NEC J44.1

Figure 15-9 ■ Index entry for chronic obstructive pulmonary disease with acute exacerbation.

▶ Leanne proceeds to assign a code for COPD.

❑ She searches the Index for the Main Term **Disease** and subterm **lung**.

❑ She locates a second-level subterm **obstructive**.

❑ She locates additional subterm levels **with**, **acute**, and **exacerbation** (■ FIGURE 15-9).

❑ Now she knows she will have a combination code for COPD and the acute exacerbation. She identifies the code **J44.1**.

▶ Leanne verifies code **J44.1** in the Tabular List.

❑ She reads the code title for **J44.1 Chronic obstructive pulmonary disease with acute exacerbation** and confirms that this accurately describes the documentation.

❑ She double-checks to be sure that additional characters are not required.

▶ Leanne checks for instructional notes in the Tabular List.

❑ She reads the **Excludes2** notes under code **J44.1** and determines that neither note apples to this case because the patient does not have acute bronchitis and the COPD is not due to an external agent.

❑ She cross-references the beginning of category **J44** and reads the instructional notes.

▪ She determines that the **Excludes1** note does not apply to this case because none of these conditions are documented.

▪ She determines that the note **Code also type of asthma, if applicable (J45.-)** does not apply because asthma is not documented.

❑ She reads the **Use additional code** notes and determines that **history of tobacco dependence (Z87.891)** applies to this case because the patient smoked cigarettes for 50 years. This answers her question as to whether she should code the past nicotine dependence. She verifies this code in the Tabular List. **Z87.891, Personal history of nicotine dependence**.

❑ Leanne continues with cross-referencing and turns the page to the beginning of the block **Chronic lower respiratory diseases (J40-J47)**.

▪ She reads the **Excludes1** and **Excludes2** notes and determines they do not apply to this case because none of these conditions are documented.

❑ She turns to the beginning of **Chapter 10 (J00-J99)** and reads the instructional notes. She locates the same note that appeared under the category heading, **Use additional code for history of tobacco dependence (Z87.891)**. This confirms that she was correct in assigning the **Z** code.

❑ Leanne reviews her working list of diagnoses and notices that she still needs to assign a code for VAP.

▶ Leanne searches the Index for the Main Term **Pneumonia**.

❑ She locates two possible subterms for ventilator-associated pneumonia due to *Pseudomonas*:

▪ **Pseudomonas J15.1**

▪ **ventilator associated J95.851**

❑ To determine whether she needs both of the codes or only one, she knows she needs to verify the codes in the Tabular List.

❑ She verifies the title for code **J15.1 Pneumonia due to Pseudomonas**, which is classified under the category **J15 Bacterial pneumonia, not elsewhere classified**.

❑ She verifies the title for code **J95.851 Ventilator associated pneumonia**, which is classified under the category **J95 Intraoperative and postprocedural complications and disorders of respiratory system, not elsewhere classified**.

❑ Leanne refers to OGCR I.C.10.d, which provides guidelines on coding VAP.

▪ OGCR I.C.10.d.1) states that the code should be used only when the provider has documented VAP. She double-checks the medical record to be certain it is documented.

▪ The guideline also states that she should assign an additional code to identify the infectious organism.

▪ The guideline also states that a code from **J12** to **J18** should not be assigned to identify the type of pneumonia.

❑ Leanne now understands that **J15.1** is for pneumonia due to *Pseudomonas* that patients acquire in the normal course of events and that **J95.851** is specifically for VAP.

❑ She returns to the Tabular List for code **J95.851** and reads the instructional note **Use additional code to identify the organism, if known (B95.-, B96.-, B97.-)**.

This note is consistent with OGCR I.C.10.d, which she consulted. These codes are located in **Chapter 1, Certain Infectious and Parasitic Diseases (A00-B99)** and are used to identify infectious organisms in diseases classified in other ICD-10-CM chapters.

❏ She cross-references the block heading **J95** and sees that it is the same as the category. She sees no further instructional notes.

▶ Leanne cross-references the codes **B95.-, B96.-,** and **B97.-** to locate the code for *Pseudomonas*, **B96.5**, which has the title **Pseudomonas (aeruginosa) (mallei) (pseudomallei) as the cause of diseases classified elsewhere**.

❏ She notices that the terms **(aeruginosa) (mallei) (pseudomallei)** are nonessential modifiers because they are enclosed in parentheses. They describe various species of *Pseudomonas* and do not need to be present in the documentation in order to use the code.

▶ Leanne reviews the codes she has assigned for this case.

❏ **J95.851 Ventilator associated pneumonia**

❏ **Z87.891 Personal history of nicotine dependence**

❏ **J44.1 Chronic obstructive pulmonary disease with acute exacerbation**

❏ **E86.0 Dehydration**

❏ **B96.5 Pseudomonas (aeruginosa) (mallei) (pseudomallei) as the cause of diseases classified elsewhere**

▶ Next, Leanne must determine how to sequence the codes.

CODING PRACTICE

Exercise 15.3 Assigning Codes for Respiratory System Conditions

Instructions: Read the mini-medical-record of each patient's encounter, review the information abstracted in Exercise 15.2, and assign ICD-10-CM diagnosis codes using the Index and Tabular List. Write the code(s) on the line provided.

---

1. OFFICE   Gender: M   **Age:** 31

Reason for encounter: Patient with previously diagnosed extrinsic asthma presents with increased symptoms of coughing, wheezing, and SOB

Assessment: Symptoms are due to acute exacerbation of mild intermittent asthma.

Plan: Oral steroids and quick relief bronchodilator inhaler

Tip: Assign a code for the severity, not extrinsic versus intrinsic.

1 ICD-10-CM Code _____

---

2. OFFICE   Gender: F   **Age:** 69

Reason for encounter: Productive cough and fever, patient is concerned that she may need medication for COPD which she has not needed for several years

(continued)

---

2. (continued)

Assessment: Viral pneumonia unrelated to patient's past history of COPD

Plan: Rx cough medicine with expectorant, take aspirin for fever, drink plenty of fluids to prevent dehydration

1 ICD-10-CM Code _____

---

3. INPATIENT HOSPITAL   Gender: M   **Age:** 72

Reason for encounter: Management of chronic obstructive pulmonary disease, recent self-administered spirometry results have been declining, increased SOB

Assessment: COPD with chronic bronchitis and emphysema

Plan: Nebulizer treatment to administer bronchodilators

Tip: Compare the codes for COPD, COPD with bronchitis, and COPD with emphysema.

1 ICD-10-CM Code _____

ARRANGING CODES FOR RESPIRATORY SYSTEM CONDITIONS

OGCR provides specific instructions regarding sequencing codes for ventilator associated pneumonia and acute respiratory failure (ARF).

Arranging Codes for Ventilator-Associated Pneumonia

VAP is pneumonia that patients acquire as a result of being on a ventilator (■ FIGURE 15-10). The relationship between ventilator use and the pneumonia must be documented by the physician. VAP is a complication of care and is classified separately from other types of pneumonia by ICD-10-CM. OGCR I.C.10.d provides instructions for how to assign codes for VAP as follows:

1. Confirm that the provider has documented the relationship between the ventilator use and the pneumonia.

2. Assign code **J95.851 Ventilator associated pneumonia**. To locate VAP in the Index, search for the Main Term **Pneumonia** and the subterm **ventilator associated**.

3. Assign an additional code from **B95.-, B96.-,** or **B97.-** to identify the infectious organism.

4. Do not assign a code from categories **J12** to **J18** to identify the type of pneumonia.

Patients may be admitted with one type of pneumonia, then be put on a ventilator and also develop VAP. When this happens, assign and sequence codes as follows:

1. Assign a code from categories **J12** to **J18** to identify the pneumonia the patient had at admission. Sequence this as the principal diagnosis.

2. Assign code **J95.851 Ventilator associated pneumonia** for VAP.

3. Assign an additional code from **B95.-, B96.-,** or **B97.-** to identify the infectious organism.

When patients are on a ventilator and do not have VAP or other ventilator-associated complications, assign code **Z99.11 Dependence on respirator [ventilator] status**.

Arranging Codes for Acute Respiratory Failure

Acute respiratory failure (ARF) may be sequenced as either the principal diagnosis or a secondary diagnosis. OGCR I.C.10.b. provides the following guidance:

- When ARF meets the definition of a principal diagnosis, coders should sequence it first, unless another chapter-specific guideline, such as obstetrics, poisoning, HIV, or newborn, provides sequencing direction that takes priority.

- When ARF does not meet the criteria for the principal diagnosis, or arises after admission, coders should sequence it as an additional diagnosis.

- When ARF and another acute condition—such as myocardial infarction, cerebrovascular accident, or aspiration pneumonia—coexist, the circumstances of admission should determine the principal diagnosis.

Guided Example of Arranging Codes for Respiratory System Conditions

To practice skills for sequencing codes for the respiratory system, continue with the example from earlier in the chapter about patient Jared Hershman, who was admitted to Branton Medical Center due to dehydration.

Follow along in your ICD-10-CM manual as Leanne Riehl, CCS, sequences the codes. Check off each step after you complete it.

▶ Leanne confirms the codes she has assigned.

- ❏ **J95.851 Ventilator associated pneumonia**

- ❏ **Z87.891 Personal history of nicotine dependence**

- ❏ **J44.1 Chronic obstructive pulmonary disease with acute exacerbation**

- ❏ **E86.0 Dehydration**

- ❏ **B96.5 Pseudomonas (aeruginosa) (mallei) (pseudomallei) as the cause of diseases classified elsewhere**

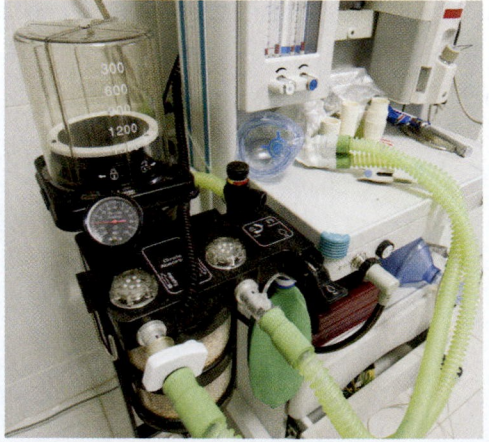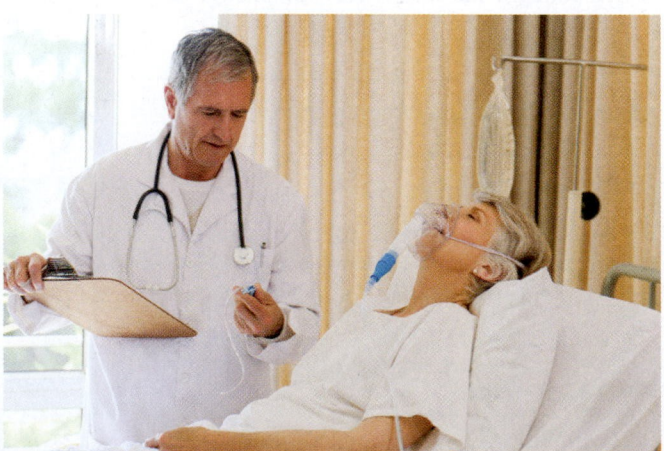

Figure 15-10 ■ Ventilators assist patients with breathing, but can also create an opportunity for pneumonia.
Sources: Paul Vinten/Shutterstock (left) and Wavebreakmedia/Shutterstock (right).

► First, she must determine the principal diagnosis, which the Uniform Hospital Data Discharge Set (UHDDS) defines as "that condition established after study to be chiefly responsible for occasioning the admission of the patient to the hospital for care" (OGCR II).

❏ Leanne checks the medical record and confirms that dehydration was the reason for admission. The COPD exacerbation and VAP developed after admission. Although these conditions were responsible for additional services and prolonged the length of stay, they do not meet the criteria for the reason for admission. She sequences **E86.0 Dehydration** as the principal diagnosis.

❏ Leanne determines that **J44.1 Chronic obstructive pulmonary disease with acute exacerbation** should be the second code because it was the reason the patient was placed on a ventilator.

❏ She sequences **J95.851 Ventilator associated pneumonia** as the third code and **B96.5, Pseudomonas** as

the fourth code. The instructional notes and OGCR indicate that the organism is sequenced in addition to or after the code for VAP.

❏ The final code is **Z87.891 Personal history of nicotine dependence** because it is required by instructional notes and provides supplementary information.

► Leanne finalizes the code assignment and sequencing for this case:

(1) **E86.0 Dehydration**

(2) **J44.1 Chronic obstructive pulmonary disease with acute exacerbation**

(3) **J95.851 Ventilator associated pneumonia**

(4) **B96.5 Pseudomonas (aeruginosa) (mallei) (pseudomallei) as the cause of diseases classified elsewhere**

(5) **Z87.891 Personal history of nicotine dependence**

CODING PRACTICE

Exercise 15.4 Arranging Codes for Respiratory System Conditions

Instructions: Read the mini-medical-record of each patient's encounter, review the information abstracted in Exercise 15.2, assign ICD-10-CM diagnosis codes using the Index and Tabular List, and sequence them correctly.

---

1. INPATIENT HOSPITAL Gender: M Age: 80

Reason for admission: Patient with congestive heart failure on supplemental O₂ admitted from physician's office after presenting with low fever, chills, cough. CHF increases patient risk for complications.

Assessment: Lobular pneumonia and acute bronchitis, both due to Mycoplasma pneumoniae

Tip: Be sure to distinguish between lobar pneumonia and lobular pneumonia. Remember to assign a **Z** code for the supplemental oxygen use.

4 ICD-10-CM Codes _____

_____

---

2. INPATIENT HOSPITAL Gender: F Age: 76

Reason for admission: COPD with exacerbation

Assessment: COPD with acute bronchitis exacerbation and chronic bronchitis

(continued)

---

2. (continued)

Plan: Antibiotics for the infection, begin oxygen therapy, patient must cease cigarette smoking as it continues to impact her respiratory conditions, counseled her regarding treatment options for tobacco dependence

Tip: Read the instructional notes in the Tabular List for sequencing instructions.

3 ICD-10-CM Codes _____

_____

---

3. INPATIENT HOSPITAL Gender: F Age: 78

Reason for admission: Asbestosis which is thought to be due to exposure to asbestos particles brought home by her late husband who worked in the fireproofing industry for many years and died of mesothelioma

Assessment: Asbestosis, clubbing of fingers due to the asbestosis, mild persistent asthma

Plan: O₂, thoracentesis, medication, respiratory therapy

3 ICD-10-CM Codes _____

_____

CODING NEOPLASMS OF THE RESPIRATORY SYSTEM

Neoplasms of the respiratory system do not appear in ICD-10-CM Chapter 10, "Diseases of the Respiratory System (J00-J99)." Codes for neoplasms of the respiratory system appear in the block C30 to C39 within the neoplasm chapter.

The most common site for cancer in the respiratory system is the lung. Lung cancer, rare in people under age 45, is the deadliest type of cancer for both men and women, causing more deaths each year than breast, colon, and prostate cancers combined. Most lung cancer is **bronchogenic**, beginning in the cells that line the bronchi. Cigarette smoking is the leading cause of lung cancer; risk increases with how long people have smoked and the number of cigarettes smoked per day (■ FIGURE 15-11). However, lung cancer occurs in people who have never smoked. According to the American Cancer Society (ACS), an estimated 7,300 nonsmoking adults die each year from lung cancer related to breathing secondhand smoke. Mesothelioma is lung cancer that is usually caused by exposure to asbestos dust.

Primary lung cancer is divided into non-small-cell lung cancer (NSCLC), the most common type; small-cell lung cancer (SCLC), which is aggressive and metastasizes quickly; and mixed small cell/large cell, which includes both NSCLC and SCLC. Lung cancer commonly spreads to the liver, adrenal glands, bone, and brain. According to ACS, five-year survival rates depend on the type of lung cancer and stage when discovered but are lower (16%) compared to other cancers because it is usually not detected until metastasis has occurred. However, NSCLC found in Stage 1 and removed with surgery has a five-year survival rate of 60–70%.

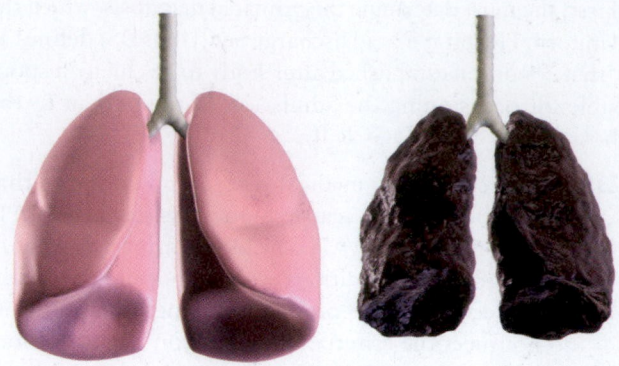

Figure 15-11 ■ Comparison of a healthy lung and the lung of a smoker. *Source: Sebastian Kaulitzki/Shutterstock.*

The lung is also a common site of metastasis from other types of cancer, the most common being bladder, breast, colon, and kidney cancer. If only a small area of the lung is infiltrated and the original tumor has been cured, then surgery to remove the diseased portion of the lung can be beneficial. However, this is rare, and metastasis in the lung usually indicates that the original cancer has spread widely throughout the body and has a poor prognosis.

Although most types of lung cancer are classified in the Table of Neoplasms, coders should always search the Index first for the specific type of malignancy. Mesothelioma is classified in the Index, not the Table of Neoplasms. Codes are divided based on the site within the lung where the tumor is found and also contain laterality.

CODING PRACTICE

Exercise 15.5 Coding Neoplasms of the Respiratory System

Instructions: Read the mini-medical-record of each patient's encounter, then abstract, assign, and sequence ICD-10-CM diagnosis codes using the Index and Tabular List. Write the code(s) on the line provided.

1. INPATIENT HOSPITAL Gender: F Age: 51

Reason for encounter: Radiotherapy for lung cancer due to cigarette smoking

Assessment: NSCLC, upper left lobe

Plan: Return for daily treatments

3 ICD-10-CM Codes _____

_____

2. INPATIENT HOSPITAL Gender: F Age: 56

Reason for encounter: Lung biopsy of mass found on x-ray when patient was treated for pneumonia, CT scan was inconclusive

Assessment: Benign neoplasm in right inferior lobe

Plan: Patient has been asymptomatic so there is no need to do a resection at this time.

1 ICD-10-CM Code _____

3. INPATIENT HOSPITAL Gender: M Age: 55

Reason for encounter: Bilateral cervical lymphadenectomy

(continued)

CODING PRACTICE (continued)

3. (continued)

Assessment: Pharyngeal cancer that has spread to lymph nodes, patient is dependent on alcohol and has a past history of nicotine (cigarette) dependence

Plan: Radiation therapy

Tip: Lymphadenectomy is the surgical removal of a lymph node.

4 ICD-10-CM Codes _____

_____

4. INPATIENT HOSPITAL   Gender: M   Age: 68

Reason for encounter: Right pulmonectomy

Assessment: Bilateral pleural malignant mesothelioma, occupational exposure to asbestos

(continued)

4. (continued)

Plan: Radiotherapy

Tip: Remember to use an external cause code for accidental asbestos poisoning.

2 ICD-10-CM Codes _____

5. OFFICE   Gender: M   Age: 46

Reason for encounter: Sinus pain, facial numbness

Assessment: Squamous cell carcinoma (SCCA), maxillary sinus

Plan: Surgical removal of tumor, to be followed with radiotherapy and chemotherapy

1 ICD-10-CM Code _____

CHAPTER SUMMARY

In this chapter you learned that:

- The function of the respiratory system is to obtain oxygen from the air and deliver it to the lungs and blood for distribution to tissue cells and to remove the gaseous waste product carbon dioxide from the blood and lungs and expel it.

- ICD-10-CM Official Guidelines for Coding and Reporting (OGCR) for the respiratory system, in OGCR section I.C.10, provide detailed discussion of chronic obstructive pulmonary disease and asthma, acute respiratory failure, influenza, and ventilator-associated pneumonia.

- Coders should become familiar with chapter-wide coding considerations as well as information specifically for asthma, COPD, and influenza.

- OGCR provides specific instructions regarding sequencing codes for ventilator-associated pneumonia and acute respiratory failure.

- Codes for neoplasms of the respiratory system appear in the block C30 to C39 in the neoplasm chapter; the most common site of neoplasms is the lung.

CONCEPT QUIZ

Take a moment to look back at the respiratory system and solidify your skills. Try to answer the questions from memory first, then refer back to the discussion in the chapter if you need a little extra help.

Completion

Instructions: Write the term that completes each statement based on the information you learned in this chapter. Choose from the list below. Some choices may be used more than once and some choices may not be used at all.

acute exacerbation	lobar
acute respiratory failure	lobular
alveoli	lower
asthma	novel influenza A
atelectasis	pharyngitis
avian	pleura
bronchi	status asthmaticus
chronic bronchitis	tonsillitis
emphysema	tracheostomy
laryngitis	upper

(continued from page 265)

1. The _____ respiratory tract consists of the nose, pharynx, and larynx.

2. Bronchioles end in small air sacs in the lungs called _____.

3. _____ is the collapse of a lung.

4. _____ is inflammation of the bronchi with a productive cough for three months in two consecutive years.

5. _____ is a chronic lung disease that affects the bronchi and is characterized by reversible obstruction and reshaping of the airway.

6. _____ pneumonia affects the alveoli and is also called bronchopneumonia.

7. _____ is an asthma exacerbation that does not respond to standard treatments.

8. A _____ is a surgical opening in the neck leading to the trachea.

9. _____ includes H1N1 and avian influenza.

10. _____ is inflammation of the throat.

Multiple Choice

Instructions: Circle the letter of the best answer to each question based on the information you learned in this chapter.

1. What is the medical term for a collection of air between the chest wall and lungs, which may cause the lung to collapse?
   A. Atelectasis
   B. Pneumonia
   C. Pneumothorax
   D. Pulmonary edema

2. What term identifies an "asthma attack," or a sudden increase in the intensity or type of symptoms, such as shortness of breath, wheezing, and chest tightness?
   A. Acute exacerbation
   B. Status asthmaticus
   C. Rapid-onset asthma
   D. Severe persistent

3. What is the medical term for a reduction in the amount of air inhaled during each breath, most commonly caused by a reduction in the diameter of the bronchioles due to inflammation?
   A. Airway obstruction
   B. Asthma
   C. COPD
   D. Status asthmaticus

4. When should ventilator-associated pneumonia be coded?
   A. Whenever a patient on mechanical ventilation has pneumonia
   B. When a hospitalized patient acquires pneumonia after admission
   C. When the physician documents that ventilation was required due to pneumonia
   D. When the physician documents the relationship between mechanical ventilation and pneumonia

5. How would you code the following scenario? *A patient with COPD is admitted for severe persistent asthma with status asthmaticus.*
   A. J44.9
   B. J45.52
   C. J44.9, J45.52
   D. J45.52, J44.9

6. How would you code the following scenario? *A 23-year old patient is seen for acute inflammation of the trachea and bronchi.*
   A. J04.10
   B. J20.9
   C. J04.10, J20.9
   D. J20.9, J04.10

7. In what anatomic site does most lung cancer begin?
   A. Bronchi
   B. Right upper lobe of lung
   C. Breast
   D. Trachea

8. How would you code the following scenario? *A patient is seen for ventilator-associated pneumonia due to* Pseudomonas.
   A. J15.1
   B. J95.851
   C. J95.851, J15.1
   D. J95.851, B96.5

9. What disease is the combination of chronic bronchitis and emphysema as comorbidities?
   A. ARDS
   B. COPD
   C. VAP
   D. ARF

10. Which codes does the instructional note *Use additional code, where applicable, to identify exposure to environmental tobacco smoke (Z77.22)* apply to?
    A. Only codes for asthma
    B. Only codes for asthma and COPD
    C. Only codes for asthma, COPD, and pneumonia
    D. All codes in ICD-10-CM Chapter 10

KEEP ON CODING

Instructions: Read the diagnostic statement, then use the Index and Tabular List to assign and sequence ICD-10-CM diagnosis codes. Write the code(s) on the line provided.

1. Acute pharyngitis. ICD-10-CM Code(s) _____
2. Atelectasis. ICD-10-CM Code(s) _____
3. Chylous effusion of the pleura. ICD-10-CM Code(s) _____
4. Allergic rhinitis due to pollen. ICD-10-CM Code(s) _____
5. Malignant neoplasm of the ethmoid sinus, right. ICD-10-CM Code(s) _____
6. Stenosis of the larynx. ICD-10-CM Code(s) _____
7. Chlamydial pneumonia. ICD-10-CM Code(s) _____
8. Acute streptococcal tonsillitis. ICD-10-CM Code(s) _____
9. Avian flu. ICD-10-CM Code(s) _____
10. Acute bronchiolitis due to respiratory syncytial virus. ICD-10-CM Code(s) _____
11. Chronic tonsillitis. ICD-10-CM Code(s) _____
12. Exercised-induced bronchospasm. ICD-10-CM Code(s) _____
13. Postprocedural respiratory failure. ICD-10-CM Code(s) _____
14. Hernia of the mediastinum. ICD-10-CM Code(s) _____
15. Mixed simple and mucopurulent chronic bronchitis. ICD-10-CM Code(s) _____
16. COPD (chronic obstructive pulmonary disease) with acute exacerbation. ICD-10-CM Code(s) _____
17. Carcinoma of the trachea. ICD-10-CM Code(s) _____
18. Acute respiratory failure with hypoxia. ICD-10-CM Code(s) _____
19. Maltworker's lung. ICD-10-CM Code(s) _____
20. Personal history of carcinoma of the lung. ICD-10-CM Code(s) _____
21. Vocal cord paralysis, bilateral. ICD-10-CM Code(s) _____
22. Tracheoesophageal fistula following tracheostomy. ICD-10-CM Code(s) _____
23. Ulcer of the left bronchus. ICD-10-CM Code(s) _____
24. Chronic maxillary sinusitis with exposure to environmental tobacco smoke. ICD-10-CM Code(s) _____
25. Pharyngeal abscess. ICD-10-CM Code(s) _____

CODING CHALLENGE

Instructions: Read the mini-medical-record of each patient's encounter and answer the abstracting questions. Write the answer on the line provided using the Index and Tabular List. Write the code(s) on the line provided.

1. OFFICE   Gender: F   Age: 1

Reason for encounter: Productive cough, SOB, fever

Assessment: Chest x-ray and sputum culture positive for acute bronchitis due to Streptococcus pneumonia. Child exposed to cigarette smoke prenatally and currently because her mother smoked during pregnancy and still does.

Plan: OTC expectorant, acetaminophen to reduce fever, FU one week or sooner if necessary.

(continued)

1. (continued)

Tip: Assign one code for the bronchitis and two codes for smoke exposure.

3 ICD-10-CM Codes _____

_____

2. OFFICE   Gender: F   Age: 9

Reason for encounter: Coughing, wheezing, SOB, and chest tightness during and 10 to 15 minutes after exercising during gym at school

Assessment: Acute exacerbation of mild persistent asthma, intrinsic

(continued)

(continued)

(continued from page 271)

2. (continued)

Plan: Rx bronchodilator, use prior to exercise. FU office visit in one month.

Tip: Remember to code the severity of the asthma.

1 ICD-10-CM Code _____

---

3. INPATIENT HOSPITAL Gender: M Age: 82

Reason for admission: Pneumococcal pneumonia

Assessment: COPD with acute exacerbation required ventilation

Plan: Discharged to skilled nursing facility with oxygen

2 ICD-10-CM Codes _____

---

4. OFFICE Gender: F Age: 84

Reason for encounter: Cracked tracheostomy tube

Assessment: Patient also has sarcoidosis with lung involvement.

Plan: Replaced tracheostomy tube

Tip: A cracked tracheostomy tube is a mechanical complication of a tracheostomy.

2 ICD-10-CM Codes _____

---

5. INPATIENT HOSPITAL Gender: M Age: 33

Reason for encounter: Ethmoidectomy and nasal reconstruction

Assessment: Ethmoidal polyps and hypertrophy of nasal turbinates due to deviated nasal septum

Plan: Excised polyps and repaired deviated nasal septum

3 ICD-10-CM Codes _____

_____

---

6. INPATIENT HOSPITAL Gender: F Age: 23

Reason for encounter: Acute sinus pain, toothache, headache

Assessment: Acute recurrent sinusitis, right maxillary sinus

Plan: Schedule CT scan of sinuses, analgesic, antihistamine, and antibiotic therapy. FU office visit 10 days.

1 ICD-10-CM Code _____

---

7. INPATIENT HOSPITAL Gender: M Age: 89

Reason for admission: Admitted from emergency department due to acute respiratory failure

Assessment: ARF is due to aspiration pneumonia due to gastric secretions, lung abscess, diabetes type 2 with gastroparesis

Plan: Discharged to a skilled nursing facility.

4 ICD-10-CM Codes _____

_____

---

8. INPATIENT HOSPITAL Gender: M Age: 72

Reason for admission: Gram-negative pneumonia

Assessment: Patient's left-sided congestive heart failure and pulmonary edema were managed in addition to the pneumonia. Patient also has chronic back pain with an unknown etiology but it was not a factor during this admission.

Plan: FU with pulmonary clinic and cardiologist in one week

2 ICD-10-CM Codes _____

---

9. INPATIENT HOSPITAL Gender: M Age: 36

Reason for admission: Difficulty breathing

Assessment: Spontaneous pneumothorax secondary to a ruptured bulla

Plan: X-ray confirmed reexpansion of lung, pulmonary clinic FU 1 week

2 ICD-10-CM Codes _____

---

10. INPATIENT HOSPITAL Gender: F Age: 6

Reason for encounter: T&A

Assessment: Chronic tonsillitis with adenoiditis

Plan: FU in office 1 week

1 ICD-10-CM Code _____

Chapter 16

Diseases of the Nervous System and Sense Organs (G00-G99)

Learning Objectives

After completing this chapter, you should have the skills to:

16.1 Spell and define the key words, medical terms, and abbreviations related to the nervous system and sense organs. (Remember)

16.2 Summarize the structure, function, and common conditions of the nervous system and sense organs. (Understand)

16.3 Adhere to the Official Guidelines for Coding and Reporting related to the nervous system and sense organs. (Apply)

16.4 Examine and abstract information from the medical record required for coding conditions of the nervous system and sense organs. (Analyze)

16.5 Demonstrate how to assign codes for conditions of the nervous system and sense organs. (Apply)

16.6 Utilize guidelines for arranging (sequencing) multiple diagnosis codes for conditions of the nervous system and sense organs. (Apply)

16.7 Demonstrate how to abstract, assign, sequence arrange codes for neoplasms of the nervous system and sense organs. (Apply)

Chapter Outline

- **Nervous System Refresher**
- **Coding Guidelines for the Nervous System**
- **Abstracting for Conditions of the Nervous System**
- **Assigning Codes for Conditions of the Nervous System**
- **Arranging Codes for Conditions of the Nervous System**
- **Coding Neoplasms of the Nervous System**

Key Terms and Abbreviations

absence	focal	nervous system	quadriplegia
Alzheimer's disease (AD)	generalized	neurons	reflex sympathetic dystrophy (RSD)
atonic	grand mal	olfactory	refractory
aura	gustatory	Parkinson's disease (PD)	secondary parkinsonism
brain	hemiplegia	parkinsonian	simple partial
central nervous system (CNS)	homeostasis	parkinsonism	spinal cord
clonic	idiopathic	partial	status epilepticus
complex partial	intractable	peripheral nervous system (PNS)	status migrainosus
dementia	late onset	petit mal	tonic
distributed	localized	pharmacoresistant	tonic-clonic
dominance	monoplegia	psychomotor	vasodilation
early onset	myoclonic		

In addition to the key terms listed here, students should know the terms defined within tables in this chapter.

INTRODUCTION

Electrical problems can be one of the most troublesome to solve. A defect in the electrical system located in one part of a car can create a problem in a completely different area. The human nervous system is the electrical system in our bodies, sending and receiving messages that enable us to perform all functions.

A neurologist specializes in diagnosing and treating conditions of the nervous system. Neurosurgeons specialize in performing surgical procedures on the nervous system. Primary care physicians treat uncomplicated conditions of the nervous system and refer more complex cases to a specialist.

NERVOUS SYSTEM REFRESHER

The function of the **nervous system** is to direct the body's response to internal and external stimuli and coordinate the activities of other organ systems. It works with the endocrine system to maintain **homeostasis** (*maintenance of a stable internal physical state*). The nervous system consists of the **central nervous system (CNS)** and **peripheral nervous system (PNS)**. The CNS acts as the control center for the nervous system by processing information and providing short-term control over other organ systems. The CNS consists of the **brain** and **spinal cord**. The brain governs perception of the senses, emotions, consciousness, memory, and voluntary movements (■ FIGURE 16-1). The spinal cord relays information to and from the brain. The PNS consists of the 12 nerves that radiate out from the brain and the 31 pairs of nerves that radiate from the spinal cord to all other areas of the body (■ FIGURE 16-2). The PNS links the CNS with other systems and the sense organs.

In Figures 16-1 and 16-2, each structure in the nervous system is labeled with its name as well as its medical terminology root/combining form where applicable. As you learn about conditions and procedures that affect the nervous system, remember to apply medical terminology skills to use word roots, prefixes, and suffixes you already know to define new terms related to the nervous system. Refer to ■ TABLE 16-1 for a refresher on how to build medical terms related to the nervous system.

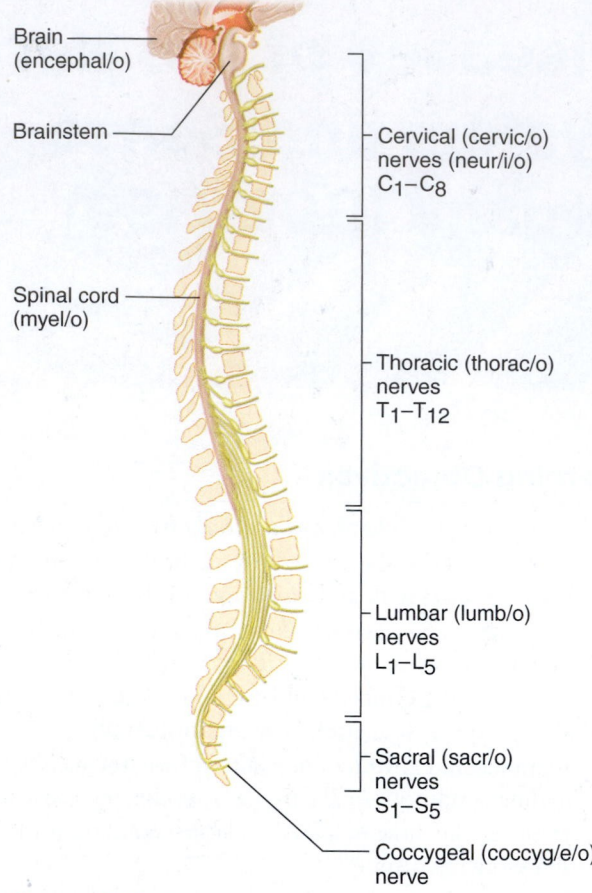

Figure 16-2 ■ The spinal cord and spinal nerves.

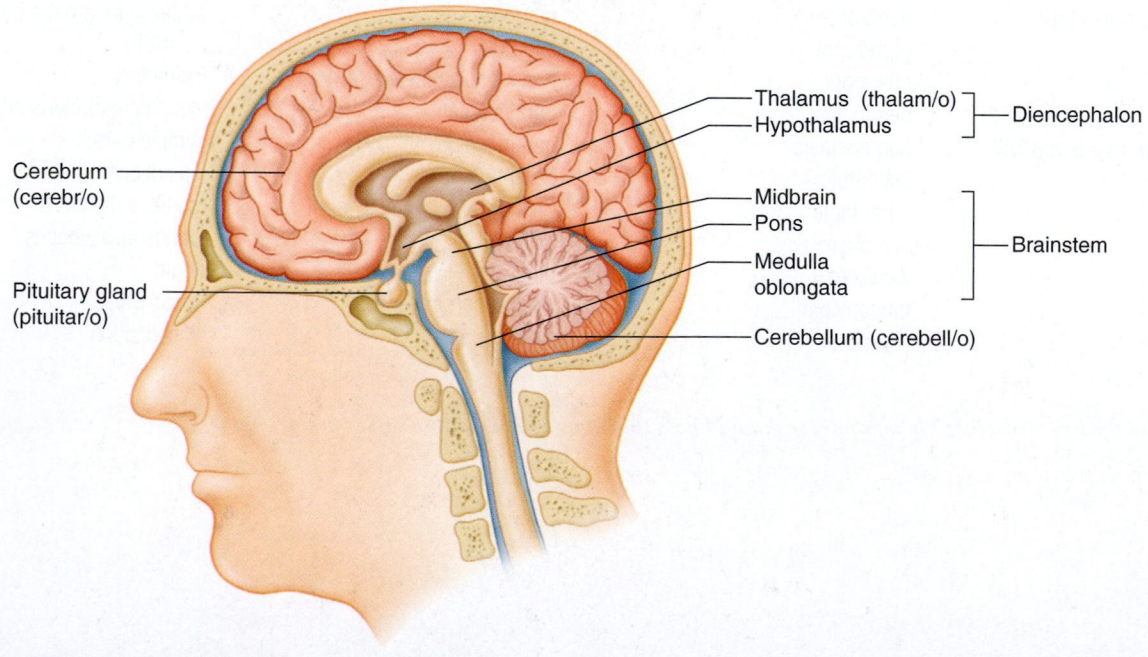

Figure 16-1 ■ The brain.

Table 16-1 ■ **EXAMPLE OF CONSTRUCTING MEDICAL TERMS FOR THE NERVOUS SYSTEM**

Prefix/Combining Form	Suffix	Complete Medical Term
dys- (prefix; *abnormal, painful*)	**-tonia** (*contraction*)	**dys + tonia** (*abnormal contraction*)
hemi- (prefix; *one side*)	**-plegia** (*paralysis*)	**hemi + plegia** (*paralysis on one side of the body*)
neur/i/o (*nerve*)	**-al** (*pertaining to*)	**neuro + plegia** (*paralysis of a nerve*)
		neur + al (*pertaining to nerves*)

CODING CAUTION

Be alert for medical terms with similar spellings but different meanings:

he<u>me</u> (*word root meaning blood*) and he<u>mi</u> (*prefix meaning half*)

<u>cerebro</u>vascular (*pertaining to vessels of the brain*) and <u>cardio</u>vascular (*pertaining to vessels of the heart*)

<u>electroen</u>cephalogram (**EEG**) (*recording of the electrical activity of the brain*) and **electro<u>cardio</u>gram** (**EKG, ECG**) (*recording of the electrical activity of the heart*)

cere<u>brum</u> (*the largest structure of the brain that controls sensory and motor activity*) and cere<u>bellum</u> (*the portion of the brain located below and behind the cerebrum*)

Conditions of the Nervous System

Diseases and disorders of the nervous system include headaches, infectious diseases, CNS disorders, and seizure disorders. Coders use medical resources, such as a reference book on diseases, to understand conditions of the nervous system, diagnostic methods, and common treatments. Refer to ■ TABLE 16-2, (page 276) for a summary of diseases affecting the nervous system.

In particular, coders must be familiar with specific concepts and terminology related to migraine headaches, epilepsy, Alzheimer's disease, and Parkinson's disease, which are highlighted next.

Migraine Headaches

Migraine headaches are severe, debilitating headaches caused by **vasodilation** (*enlargement of the blood vessels*). They may be accompanied by symptoms of nausea and vomiting and sensitivity to light and sound. Before the onset of a migraine, patients may experience an **aura**, such as a sensation of voices or colored light. An **intractable** migraine is one that is resistant to treatment and can also be called **pharmacoresistant** (*resistant to medication*) or **refractory** (*resistant to treatment*). A migraine that lasts more than 72 hours is considered to be **status migrainosus**.

CODING CAUTION

Do not assume that any severe headache is a migraine.

Epilepsy

Epilepsy is a brain disorder in which **neurons** (*clusters of nerve cells*) signal abnormally, causing seizures and/or unconsciousness. Epilepsy may be due to a medical condition or an injury or may be **idiopathic** (*of unknown cause*). Known causes include:

- Alcoholism
- Birth trauma
- Depressed skull fracture
- Penetrating wound
- Infections of the brain
- Dementia
- Stroke or transient ischemic attack (TIA)
- Other traumatic brain injury
- Brain tumor

Seizures are classified as **localized** or **generalized** based on the source of the seizure within the brain. Localized, **partial**, or **focal** seizures occur in one part of the brain. Localized seizures are further classified based on whether consciousness is affected, as follows:

- A **simple partial** seizure affects only a small region of the brain and does not cause loss of consciousness.
- A **complex partial**, or **psychomotor**, seizure is associated with both sides of the cerebrum and causes a change in or loss of consciousness.

Generalized or **distributed** seizures are the result of abnormal activity on both sides of the brain and include the following types:

- **Absence** or **petit mal**—Characterized by muscle twitching or jerking for several seconds
- **Myoclonic**—Jerking and twitching in the upper body, arms, or legs
- **Tonic**—Characterized by prolonged muscle contractions or stiffening
- **Clonic**—Characterized by a series of muscle contractions and relaxations on both sides of the body
- **Tonic-clonic** or **grand mal**—Characterized by a sudden loss of consciousness and falling to the floor; affects the entire brain
- **Atonic**—Characterized by a brief loss of muscle tone

Table 16-2 ■ **COMMON DISEASES OF THE NERVOUS SYSTEM**

Condition	Definition
Alzheimer's disease	A progressive degenerative brain disease
Amyotrophic lateral sclerosis (ALS) or Lou Gehrig disease	A chronic, terminal neurological disease characterized by a progressive loss of motor neurons and muscle atrophy
Bell's Palsy	Inflammation of the seventh (VII) cranial nerve, the facial nerve
Cerebral palsy	A functional disorder of the brain manifested by motor impairment
Chronic pain syndrome (CPS)	A collection of pain conditions lasting more than six months and unresponsive to treatment
Cluster headache	Unilateral pain in the eye or temple
Complex regional pain syndrome	A chronic pain syndrome in which an extremity experiences intense burning pain and changes in skin texture and temperature; also called reflex sympathetic dystrophy (RSD)
Degenerative neural disease	A class of diseases marked by degeneration of nerves and brain tissue, resulting in abnormalities in muscle and sensory functions
Dementia	A loss of brain function that affects memory, thinking, language, judgment, and behavior
Dystonia	Erratic jerky movements due to improperly functioning muscle tension
Encephalitis	A viral inflammation of the brain and meninges
Epilepsy	A brain disorder in which neurons signal abnormally, causing seizures and/or unconsciousness
Huntington's chorea	An inherited progressive, degenerative disease involving loss of muscle control and personality changes
Hydrocephalus	Excess cerebrospinal fluid trapped in the brain
Meningitis	A contagious, acute inflammation of the pia mater and the arachnoid mater in the brain
Migraine headache	A severe, debilitating headache caused by vasodilation
Multiple sclerosis	A chronic, progressive disorder of the CNS characterized by muscle impairment due to patches of hardened tissue in the brain or spinal cord
Narcolepsy	A condition characterized by brief sudden attacks of deep sleep
Parkinson's disease	A degenerative disease that affects muscle control and coordination
Spina bifida	A congenital neural tube defect in which vertebrae do not fuse

Epilepsy is classified as to whether it is intractable. According to the Centers for Disease Control and Prevention, approximately 70% of epilepsy is responsive to medication and 30% is intractable. **Status epilepticus** is an epileptic seizure that lasts more than 30 minutes or is a near-constant state of seizures and is a medical emergency.

CODING CAUTION

Do not assume that all seizure activity is epilepsy. Seizures may also be caused by high fever, psychological disorders, or other medical conditions such as narcolepsy, Tourette syndrome, or cardiac arrhythmia.

Alzheimer's Disease

Alzheimer's disease (AD) is a progressive degenerative brain disease that doubles in prevalence with every five years of age. Early onset and late onset are types of AD defined by age at onset. **Early-onset** AD is diagnosed before age 65 and accounts for approximately 5% of all AD cases, according to the Alzheimer's Association. **Late-onset** AD is diagnosed after age 65 and accounts for the vast majority of AD cases. However, AD is not a normal part of aging.

AD is a progressive disease that worsens over time. The progression is classified as early, middle, and late stage. Do not confuse early- and late-stage progression of AD with early-onset and late-onset, which describe the age of onset.

AD is the most common cause of **dementia** (*a progressive loss of brain function that affects memory, thinking, language, judgment, and behavior*), which is classified in ICD-10-CM Chapter 5, "Mental and Behavioral Disorders."

Parkinson's Disease

Parkinson's disease (PD) is a degenerative disease that affects muscle control and coordination, usually occurring in midlife. Symptoms include tremor, rigid muscles, and loss of normal reflexes. Dementia may be caused by PD or it may occur independently of PD. When *dementia* is diagnosed first, followed at a later time with an additional diagnosis of *Parkinson's disease*, the combined condition is referred to as **parkinsonian** dementia or dementia with **parkinsonism** and assumes the existence of Lewy body disease. When PD is diagnosed first, followed at a later time with an additional diagnosis of dementia, the combined condition is referred to as *Parkinson's disease with dementia*, and the existence of Lewy body disease is not assumed. **Secondary parkinsonism** is Parkinson-type abnormal movements that are caused by medication or another condition.

CODING PRACTICE

Exercise 16.1   Nervous System Refresher

Instructions: Use your medical terminology skills and resources to define the following conditions related to the nervous system, then assign the default diagnosis code.

Follow these steps:

- Use slash marks "/" to break down each term into its root(s) and suffix.
- Define the meaning of the word based on the meaning of each word part.
- Assign the default ICD-10-CM diagnosis code for the condition using the Index and Tabular List.

Example: neuropathy neuro/pathy   Meaning *abnormal condition of a nerve* _____   ICD-10-CM Code *G62.9* _____

1. neuroma (benign)   Meaning _____   ICD-10-CM Code _____
2. neuromyelitis   Meaning _____   ICD-10-CM Code _____
3. encephalomyeloradiculitis   Meaning _____   ICD-10-CM Code _____
4. causalgia   Meaning _____   ICD-10-CM Code _____
5. neuromyotonia   Meaning _____   ICD-10-CM Code _____
6. myelinolysis   Meaning _____   ICD-10-CM Code _____
7. hemichorea   Meaning _____   ICD-10-CM Code _____
8. meningoencephalopathy   Meaning _____   ICD-10-CM Code _____
9. myasthenia   Meaning _____   ICD-10-CM Code _____
10. hemiplegia   Meaning _____   ICD-10-CM Code _____

CODING GUIDELINES FOR THE NERVOUS SYSTEM

Coders should understand the organization of this ICD-10-CM chapter, chapter-wide and commonly used instructional notes in the Tabular List, and the relevant OGCR. This information is necessary for accurate coding.

ICD-10-CM Chapter 6, "Diseases of the Nervous System and Sense Organs (G00-G99)," contains 11 blocks or subchapters that are divided by the type of structure affected. Review the block names and code ranges listed at the beginning of Chapter 6 in the ICD-10-CM manual to become familiar with the content and organization.

This chapter includes disorders of the central and peripheral nervous systems as well as paralytic syndromes. It also includes the **gustatory** (*taste*) and **olfactory** (*smell*) sense organs. The eye and the ear each has its own chapter in ICD-10-CM. This chapter does not include congenital disorders or injuries, which are classified in other ICD-10-CM chapters. This chapter also does not include cerebrovascular disease, which is classified with the circulatory system in block I60-I69. However, it does include transient ischemic attacks and related syndromes that were classified with the circulatory system in ICD-9-CM.

ICD-10-CM provides Official Guidelines for Coding and Reporting (OGCR) for the nervous system and sense organs in OGCR section I.C.6. OGCR provides detailed discussion of coding for pain, including general coding information, postoperative pain, chronic pain, neoplasm-related pain, and chronic pain syndrome. OGCR also discusses the definitions of dominant and nondominant side when coding hemiplegia. OGCR

I.C.19.g.2) discusses pain due to devices, implants, and grafts. OGCR I.C.5.a discusses pain disorders related to psychological factors. Instructional notes throughout the chapter direct coders to use an external cause code, code first the underlying disease, and code first the underlying neoplasm. Specific OGCR guidelines and instructional notes are discussed and cited throughout this chapter of the text.

ABSTRACTING FOR CONDITIONS OF THE NERVOUS SYSTEM

When abstracting, coders analyze the medical record to highlight the key facts of the case and to identify details that will be important when assigning and sequencing codes. As coders gain experience in assigning and sequencing codes, they are able to abstract more quickly and more accurately. Review the questions in ■ TABLE 16-3 to learn key questions

Table 16-3   ■   **KEY CRITERIA FOR ABSTRACTING CONDITIONS OF THE NERVOUS SYSTEM**

- ❏ What is the condition?
- ❏ What is the subtype of the condition?
- ❏ What is the anatomic site?
- ❏ What is the underlying disease, if any?
- ❏ What is the external cause, if any?
- ❏ What is the infectious organism, if any?
- ❏ What laterality is documented?
- ❏ Is paralysis documented?

to ask when analyzing cases related to the nervous system. Remember that the abstracting questions are a guide and that not every question applies to, or can be answered for, every case. Because of the variety of conditions addressed under the nervous system, coders need general criteria for abstracting conditions of the nervous system overall (Table 16-3), as well as specific criteria to abstract pain (■ TABLE 16-4), headaches (■ TABLE 16-5), epilepsy (■ TABLE 16-6), and PD (■ TABLE 16-7).

Table 16-4 ■ KEY CRITERIA FOR ABSTRACTING PAIN

- ❏ What is the site of the pain?
- ❏ What is the underlying cause of the pain?
- ❏ Is the pain due to a device, implant, graft, or trauma?
- ❏ Is the pain postoperative?
- ❏ Is it related to a specific postoperative complication?
- ❏ Is the pain related to a neoplasm?
- ❏ Is pain management the reason for the encounter?
- ❏ Is treatment of the underlying condition the reason for the encounter?
- ❏ Is the pain documented as chronic?
- ❏ Is chronic pain syndrome documented?
- ❏ Is complex regional pain syndrome documented?
- ❏ What psychological factors are associated with the pain?

Table 16-5 ■ KEY CRITERIA FOR ABSTRACTING HEADACHES

- ❏ What specific type of headache is documented?
- ❏ Is it documented as intractable?
- ❏ Is the headache documented as episodic or chronic?
- ❏ Does it affect the entire head or only one side?
- ❏ Is the headache accompanied with aura?
- ❏ Is status migrainosus or duration of 72 hours or more documented?
- ❏ Is the headache associated with another condition such as trauma, menstruation, cerebral infarction, or drug use?

Table 16-6 ■ KEY CRITERIA FOR ABSTRACTING EPILEPSY

- ❏ Is the seizure documented as epilepsy?
- ❏ Is it localized or generalized?
- ❏ Is it documented as intractable?
- ❏ Is status epilepticus or duration of 30 minutes or more documented?
- ❏ Are partial seizures documented as simple or complex?

Table 16-7 ■ KEY CRITERIA FOR ABSTRACTING PARKINSON'S DISEASE

- ❏ Is parkinsonism primary or secondary?
- ❏ Is dementia documented?
- ❏ Is dementia documented as parkinsonian dementia or Parkinson's disease with dementia?
- ❏ Is secondary parkinsonism documented?
- ❏ What is the cause?

SUCCESS STEP

Physicians do not need to use the exact word *intractable* to allow coders to abstract a migraine or epilepsy as intractable. Acceptable terms that mean intractable are *pharmacoresistant*, *pharmacologically resistant*, *treatment resistant*, *refractory*, and *poorly controlled*.

Guided Example of Abstracting for Nervous System Conditions

Refer to the following example throughout this chapter to practice skills for abstracting, assigning, and sequencing nervous system codes. Angelia Harkey, CPC, is a fictitious coder who guides you through the coding process.

Date: 7/11/yy   Location: Branton Medical Center

Provider: Lorene Garman, MD

Patient: Catalina Piatt   Gender: F   Age: 57

Reason for encounter: Patient was admitted from the emergency department where she presented with left sided hemiparesis

Assessment: Imaging studies were negative for CVA, symptoms mitigated within 24 hours, leading to a diagnosis of TIA. Patient received Duradrin (*a vasoconstrictor combination medication*) for classical migraine which responded to treatment. She received routine insulin for type 1 diabetes.

Plan: She was discharged to home with no residual weakness. FU in office 1 week.

Follow along as Angelia Harkey, CPC, abstracts the diagnosis. Check off each step after you complete it.

▶ Angelia reads through the entire record, paying special attention to the reason for the encounter and the final assessment.

- ❏ She notes that the presenting symptoms, left-sided hemiparesis, were temporary and that imaging studies were negative for CVA, which she knows is a cerebrovascular accident, or a stroke.

❑ She reviews Key Criteria for Abstracting Conditions of the Nervous System (Table 16-3, page 277).

❑ *What is the condition?* She notes there is a definitive diagnosis of TIA, which is a transient ischemic attack; a TIA is a brief episode of ischemia that has temporary symptoms but causes no permanent damage

❑ *What is the subtype of the condition?* None was listed

❑ *What is the anatomic site?* A TIA by definition occurs in the brain

❑ *What is the underlying disease, if any?* None

❑ *What is the external cause, if any?* None

❑ *What is the infectious organism, if any?* None

❑ *What laterality is documented?* Temporary left-sided hemiparesis

❑ *Is paralysis documented?* Temporary weakness is documented, but no paralysis

❑ Because the left-sided hemiparesis was temporary and the underlying cause was diagnosed as TIA, she knows she should not code for the presenting symptom.

❑ She identifies that two additional conditions were treated during the admission: classical migraine and type 1 diabetes.

▶ At this time, Angelia has a good idea that she will have three diagnoses, but she will not know for certain until she completes the next step of assigning codes.

CODING PRACTICE

Exercise 16.2   Abstracting Diagnoses for the Nervous System

Instructions: Read the mini-medical-record of each patient's encounter and answer the abstracting questions. Write the answer on the line provided. Do not assign any codes.

---

1. OUTPATIENT HOSPITAL   Gender: F   Age: 31

Reason for encounter: Patient comes in today for a migraine which started 2 days ago with aura

Assessment: Pharmacoresistant migraine

Plan: Administered injection of sumatriptan and discussed potential side effects and how to manage. Rx oral sumatriptan. Patient to call nurse tomorrow to discuss progress.

a. What condition is documented? _____
_____

b. Is it documented as intractable? _____
_____

c. Is it documented as affecting only one side? _____
_____

d. Is the migraine accompanied with aura? _____
_____

e. Is status migrainosus or duration of 72 hours or more documented? _____

f. Is the headache associated with another condition: trauma, menstruation, cerebral infarction, or drug use? _____

---

2. OUTPATIENT HOSPITAL   Gender: M   Age: 9

Reason for encounter: Video EEG (*video to monitor brain activity in real time*) as part of ongoing epilepsy evaluation

Assessment: Benign childhood epilepsy with EEG spikes, poorly controlled at this time

Plan: We are going to start with Rx gabapentin monotherapy (*single-drug therapy*) and reevaluate in 4 weeks, consult with nutritionist re: diet modifications

a. What condition is documented? _____
_____

b. What is the type of epilepsy? _____
_____

c. Is it documented as intractable? _____
_____

d. Is status epilepticus or duration of 30 minutes or more documented? _____

---

3. OFFICE   Gender: M   Age: 51

Reason for encounter: Management of PD, patient reports increased tremor activity and difficulty walking since last visit

Assessment: PD has progressed

Plan: Adjusted medications, referred to physical therapy

a. What symptoms are reported? _____
_____

b. What condition is documented? _____
_____

(continued)

CODING PRACTICE (continued)

3. (continued)

c. Should you code the symptoms? _____
_____

Why or why not? _____
_____

d. Is the condition primary or secondary? _____
_____

e. Is dementia documented? _____
_____

---

4. INPATIENT HOSPITAL Gender: F Age: 33

Reason for admission: Implant neurostimulator (*a device placed under the skin that stimulates the spinal cord by tiny electrical impulses*) for pain control

Assessment: Chronic lumbar pain due to displaced disc at L3-L4, which resulted from a back injury two years ago

Plan: FU 2 weeks

a. What is the reason for admission? _____
_____

b. What is the site of the pain? _____

c. What is the underlying cause of the pain? _____
_____

d. Is the pain due to a device, implant, graft, or trauma? _____

e. Is pain management the reason for the encounter? _____

f. Is treatment of the underlying condition the reason for the encounter? _____
_____

g. Is the pain documented as chronic? _____
_____

h. Is chronic pain syndrome documented? _____

---

5. INPATIENT HOSPITAL Gender: M Age: 86

Reason for encounter: Admitted from nursing facility due to generalized weakness

Assessment: Weakness is due to hyponatremia, patient presents an elopement risk due to late onset AD, dementia with hallucinations, and wandering

(*continued*)

---

5. (continued)

Plan: Discharged to nursing facility

a. What symptom is documented? _____
_____

b. What is the cause of the symptom? _____

c. What type of AD is documented? _____
_____

d. What is an elopement risk? _____
_____

e. Is the dementia accompanied with behavioral disturbances? _____
_____

f. What is the principal diagnosis? _____
_____

g. What additional diagnosis(es) should be coded? _____
_____

Why? _____

---

6. INPATIENT HOSPITAL Gender: F Age: 42

Reason for admission: Admitted from emergency department where patient presented with migraine of 4 days' duration which has not responded to the usual medication

Assessment: Persistent migraine with cerebrovascular infarction, cerebral stenosis of right cerebellar artery, hypertension

a. What specific type of migraine is documented? _____
_____

b. Is it documented as intractable? _____
_____

c. Is the migraine accompanied with aura? _____
_____

d. Is status migrainosus or duration of 72 hours or more documented? _____
_____

e. What other conditions are documented? _____
_____

f. What is the location of the cerebral stenosis? _____
_____

g. What is the principal diagnosis? _____
_____

ASSIGNING CODES FOR CONDITIONS OF THE NERVOUS SYSTEM

OGCR contain specific guidelines for assigning codes for hemiplegia and monoplegia and pain.

Assigning Codes for Hemiplegia and Monoplegia

According to the instructional note at the beginning of categories **G81**, **G82**, and **G83**, codes for hemiplegia (*paralysis of one side of the body*), quadriplegia (*paralysis of all limbs*), and monoplegia (*paralysis of one limb*) from this ICD-10-CM chapter should be assigned when the paralysis is reported without further specification or is stated to be old or longstanding but of unspecified cause. Also use these categories in multiple coding to identify these conditions resulting from any cause. When these conditions result from cerebrovascular disease, assign codes from category **I69 Sequelae of cerebrovascular disease**.

Codes for hemiplegia and monoplegia require coders to assign a fifth character to identify a combination of laterality and dominance. Dominance refers to the side of the body an individual favors, such as being left-handed or right-handed (■ FIGURE 16-3).

For *right-handed* persons, assign the fifth character as follows:

- **1** identifies that the right side (dominant) of a right-handed person is affected.
- **4** identifies that the left side (nondominant) of a right-handed person is affected.

For *left-handed* persons, assign the fifth character as follows:

- **2** identifies that the left side (dominant) of a left-handed person is affected (■ FIGURE 16-4).
- **3** identifies that the right side (nondominant) of a left-handed person is affected.

Assign the fifth character **0** when laterality is not documented.

When laterality is documented but dominance is not, OGCR I.C.6.a instructs coders to code the right side as

Patient, who is left-handed, is seen for left side flaccid hemiplegia.

G81.02   Flaccid hemiplegia affecting left dominant side

Figure 16-4 ■ Example of hemiplegia affecting left dominant side.

dominant and the left side as nondominant (■ FIGURE 16-5). For ambidextrous patients, the default is to code the affected side as dominant.

Assigning Codes for Pain

OGCR I.C.6.b provides detailed guidance for assigning and sequencing codes from category **G89 Pain not elsewhere classified**. Use this category *only* when pain is specified as acute or chronic, postthoracotomy, postprocedural, or neoplasm related. These codes may be used with codes from other categories and other chapters, including site-specific pain codes from ICD-10-CM Chapter 18, "Symptoms, Signs and Abnormal Clinical and Laboratory Findings," when they provide additional information about the condition, such as whether the pain is acute or chronic.

Coders must determine whether the underlying cause of the pain is known. If it is, assign codes from category **G89** *only* when the purpose of the encounter is to provide pain management (■ FIGURE 16-6), but not when the purpose of the encounter is to treat the underlying condition (■ FIGURE 16-7) (OGCR I.C.6.b.1 (a) and (b)).

Patient is seen for monoplegia of the left arm.

G83.24   Monoplegia of upper limb affecting left nondominant side

Figure 16-5 ■ Example of monoplegia with unspecified dominance.

Patient with a displaced C4-C5 disk due to trauma and associated severe chronic neck pain presents for a steroid injection in the spinal canal to relieve pain.

(1) **G89.21   Chronic pain due to trauma**
(2) **M50.221   Other cervical disc displacement at C4-C5 level**

Figure 16-6 ■ Example of an encounter to treat pain.

Patient with low-back pain due to a wedge compression fracture of lumbar vertebra L4 is seen for balloon kyphoplasty (*a procedure to stabilize the vertebral segments*).

S32.040A   Wedge compression fracture of fourth lumbar vertebra, initial encounter for closed fracture

Figure 16-7 ■ Example of an encounter to treat the underlying condition.

5th   G81.0 Flaccid hemiplegia

G81.00   Flaccid hemiplegia affecting unspecified side

G81.01   Flaccid hemiplegia affecting right dominant side

G81.02   Flaccid hemiplegia affecting left dominant side

G81.03   Flaccid hemiplegia affecting right nondominant side

G81.04   Flaccid hemiplegia affecting left nondominant side

Figure 16-3 ■ Tabular List Entry showing dominance and nondominance.

ICD-10-CM provides a specific code and specific OGCR for neoplasm-related pain (OGCR I.C.6.b.5)). Assign code **G89.3 Neoplasm related pain (acute) (chronic)** when pain is documented as either acute or chronic for any of the following:

- Neoplasm related
- Cancer associated
- Due to malignancy
- Tumor associated

Also assign a code(s) for the neoplasm and/or metastases.

Code pain as acute or chronic based on the physician's documentation. There is no specific time frame that defines acute or chronic.

Refer to OGCR I.C.6.b.3) for instructions on coding postoperative pain.

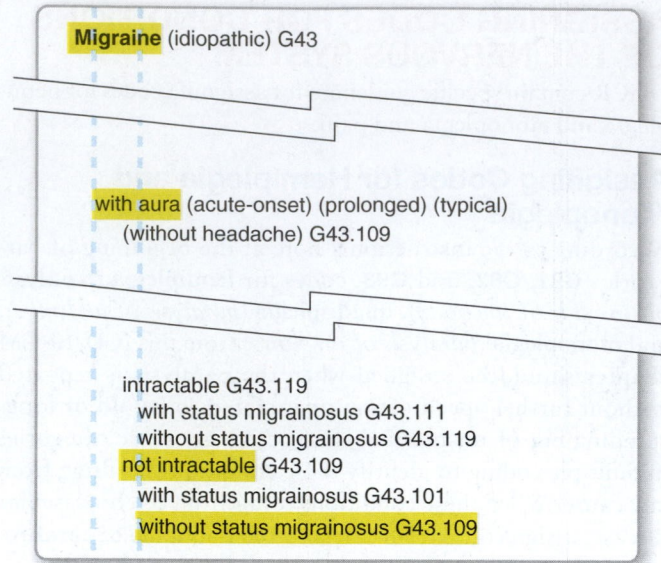

Figure 16-8 ■ Index entry for "Migraine".

> ### CODING CAUTION
>
> Be careful to distinguish codes for chronic pain **(G89.2-)**, chronic pain syndrome **(G89.4)**, and complex regional pain syndrome (CRPS) **(G90.5-)** based on the physician's documentation.

Guided Example of Assigning Codes for Nervous System Conditions

To practice assigning codes for diseases of the nervous system, continue with the example from earlier in the chapter about patient Catalina Piatt, who was admitted to Branton Medical Center due to left-sided hemiparesis.

Follow along in your ICD-10-CM manual as Angelia Harkey, CPC, assigns codes. Check off each step after you complete it.

▶ First, Angelia reviews the conditions she identified during abstracting:

- ❏ TIA
- ❏ Classical migraine
- ❏ Type 1 diabetes

▶ Angelia is most concerned about assigning a code for the migraine, so she begins with this diagnosis. She searches the Index for the Main Term **Migraine**.

- ❏ She locates the subterm **classical** and reads the cross-referencing note in the Index, **see Migraine, with aura**.

- ❏ Staying under the Main Term **Migraine**, she locates the subterm **with aura** (■ FIGURE 16-8).

- ❏ She notices that there are indented third-level subterms for **intractable**, **not intractable**, and **persistent**.

- ❏ She double-checks the medical record and notes that the physician documented classical migraine that

responded to treatment. Because intractable means "not responsive to treatment," she determines that she should select a code for not intractable. Although the physician did not use the exact statement "not intractable," she is confident of the meaning of the term and proceeds.

- ❏ Under the entry for **not intractable**, she reads two additional indented subterms for **with** or **without status migrainosus**.

- ❏ She again double-checks the documentation and confirms that status migrainosus is not documented, so she selects the entry for **without status migrainosus, G43.109**.

- ❏ Angelia verifies code **G43.109** in the Tabular List (■ FIGURE 16-9).

- ❏ She reads the code title **G43.109 Migraine with aura, not intractable, without status migrainosus** and is concerned because the documentation did not state that the migraine was accompanied with aura.

- ❏ She reads the inclusion terms under the category heading **G43.1 Migraine with aura** and sees the term **Classical migraine**. The inclusion term confirms that this is the correct category to classify a classical migraine.

▶ Angelia checks for instructional notes in the Tabular List.

- ❏ Angelia cross-references the beginning of subcategory **G43.1 Migraine with aura** and reads the instructional notes. The note **Code also any associated seizure** does not apply because no seizure was documented.

> **5th** G43.1 Migraine with aura
>   Basilar migraine
>   Classical migraine
>   Migraine equivalents
>   Migraine preceded or accompanied by transient focal
>   neurological phenomena
>   Migraine triggered seizures
>   Migraine with acute-onset aura
>   Migraine with aura without headache
>   (migraine equivalents)
>   Migraine with prolonged aura
>   Migraine with typical aura
>   Retinal migraine
>   **Code also** any associated seizure (G40.-, R56.9)
>   **Excludes1:** persistent migraine aura (G43.5-, G43.6-)
> **6th** G43.10 Migraine with aura, not intractable
>   G43.101 Migraine with aura, not intractable,
>   with status migrainosus
>   G43.109 Migraine with aura, not intractable,
>   without status migrainosus
>   Migraine with aura NOS
> **6th** G43.11 Migraine with aura, intractable
>   G43.111 Migraine with aura, intractable, with
>   status migrainosus
>   G43.119 Migraine with aura, intractable,
>   without status migrainosus

Figure 16-9 ■ Tabular List entry for code G43.1 "Migraine with aura".

❏ She cross-references the beginning of category **G43, Migraine** and reads the **NOTE** that defines intractable. She confirms that this case is not intractable.

❏ Angelia cross-references the beginning of the block **G40-G47 Episodic and paroxysmal disorders** and verifies that there are no instructional notes that apply to all codes in the block.

❏ She cross-references the beginning of Chapter 6 (G00-G99) and reviews the **Excludes2** note. She determines that it does not apply to this case because the patient does not have any of the conditions listed.

❏ Angelia finalizes the code assignment for the migraine, **G43.109, Migraine with aura, not intractable, without status migrainosus.**

▶ Next, Angelia assigns a code for the TIA. She searches the Index for the Main Term **Transient**.

❏ She reads the nonessential modifier **(meaning homeless)** and determines this is not the correct Main Term to use because the condition is not homelessness. The noun *transient* is used to refer to a homeless person. The adjective *transient* means temporary or short-lived and describes the type of ischemia.

❏ She searches the Index for the Main Term **Attack**.

❏ She locates the subterm **transient ischemic (TIA) G45.9** and determines that this is an appropriate entry.

▶ Angelia verifies code **G45.9** in the Tabular List.

❏ She reads the code title **G45.9 Transient cerebral ischemic attack, unspecified** and confirms that this describes the documentation.

❏ She confirms that this is the accurate code by reading the inclusion term **TIA** listed under code **G45.9**.

❏ She quickly rechecks the beginning of the category, block, and chapter for instructional notes and finds no notes that apply to this case.

❏ Angelia finalizes the code assignment **G45.9 Transient cerebral ischemic attack, unspecified**.

▶ Angelia checks her abstracting notes and identifies that she needs to assign a code for type 1 diabetes because it was treated during this admission.

❏ She searches the Index for the Main Term **Diabetes** and the subterm **type 1 E10.9**. No additional complications are documented, so none of the second-level subterms apply.

❏ She turns to the Tabular List to verify the code **E10.9 Type 1 diabetes mellitus without complications**.

❏ She cross-references the beginning of the category **E10**, the block **E08-E13**, and the chapter to identify that there are no further instructional notes that apply.

▶ Angelia reviews the codes for this case:

❏ **E10.9 Type 1 diabetes mellitus without complications**

❏ **G45.9 Transient cerebral ischemic attack, unspecified**

❏ **G43.109 Migraine with aura, not intractable, without status migrainosus**

▶ Next, Angelia must determine how to sequence the codes.

CODING PRACTICE

Exercise 16.3   Assigning Codes for Conditions of the Nervous System

Instructions: Read the mini-medical-record of each patient's encounter, review the information abstracted in Exercise 16.2, and assign ICD-10-CM diagnosis codes using the Index and Tabular List. Write the code(s) on the line provided.

---

1. OFFICE   Gender: F   Age: 31

Reason for encounter: Patient comes in today for a migraine which started 2 days ago with aura

Assessment: Pharmacoresistant migraine

Plan: Administered injection of sumatriptan (*a medication used to treat migraines*) and discussed potential side effects and how to manage. Rx oral sumatriptan. Patient to call nurse tomorrow to discuss progress.

Tip: Be sure to review the meaning of intractable.

1 ICD-10-CM Code _____

---

2. OUTPATIENT HOSPITAL   Gender: M   Age: 9

Reason for encounter: Video EEG as part of ongoing epilepsy evaluation

Assessment: Benign childhood epilepsy with EEG spikes, poorly controlled at this time

Plan: We are going to start with Rx gabapentin monotherapy (*single-drug therapy*) and reevaluate in 4 weeks, consult with nutritionist re: diet modifications

Tip: Read and follow the cross-referencing instruction in the Index.

1 ICD-10-CM Code _____

---

3. OFFICE   Gender: M   Age: 51

Reason for encounter: Management of PD, patient reports increased tremor activity and difficulty walking since last visit

Assessment: PD has progressed

Plan: Adjusted medications, referred to physical therapy

1 ICD-10-CM Code _____

ARRANGING CODES FOR CONDITIONS OF THE NERVOUS SYSTEM

Sequencing codes that include codes for pain is determined by the circumstances of the encounter. When the purpose of the encounter is to manage the pain, sequence the code for pain first. When the purpose of the encounter is to treat the underlying condition, sequence the code for the condition first. Follow the same procedure when coding neoplasm-related pain. Refer to the examples in ■ FIGURE 16-10 and ■ FIGURE 16-11 to learn more about sequencing codes for neoplasm-related pain.

Guided Example of Arranging Codes for Nervous System Conditions

To practice skills for sequencing codes for diseases of the nervous system, continue with the example from earlier in the chapter about patient Catalina Piatt, who was admitted to Branton Medical Center due to left-sided hemiparesis.

Follow along in your ICD-10-CM manual as Angelia Harkey, CPC, sequences the codes. Check off each step after you complete it.

▶ Angelia reviews the codes she assigned for this case:

❑ **E10.9 Type 1 diabetes mellitus without complications**

❑ **G45.9 Transient cerebral ischemic attack, unspecified**

❑ **G43.109 Migraine with aura, not intractable, without status migrainosus**

▶ First, Angelia needs to determine the principal diagnosis.

❑ She refers back to the medical record and confirms that the reason established after study for the admission and the services provided is TIA.

❑ She sequences **G45.9 Transient cerebral ischemic attack, unspecified** first as the principal diagnosis.

Patient is admitted for IV pain control related to metastatic pancreatic cancer.

(1) **G89.3** Neoplasm related pain (acute) (chronic)
(2) **C25.9** Malignant neoplasm of pancreas, unspecified
(3) **C79.9** Secondary malignant neoplasm of unspecified site

Figure 16-10 ■ Example of an encounter to treat neoplasm-related pain.

Patient is admitted for left upper lobectomy for lung cancer and also reports severe neoplasm-related pain.

(1) **C34.12** Malignant neoplasm of upper lobe, left bronchus or lung
(2) **G89.3** Neoplasm related pain (acute) (chronic)

Figure 16-11 ■ Example of an encounter to treat the neoplasm, with pain as an additional diagnosis.

❏ She refers to the OGCR I.C.4 and 6 to determine whether any sequencing guidelines apply for the migraine and diabetes but finds none.

❏ She refers to OGCR Section III, "Reporting Additional Diagnoses," and verifies that because the migraine and the diabetes required therapeutic treatment during the admission, she should assign them as additional diagnoses.

❏ She determines that the migraine required specific treatment and sequences it as the second code.

❏ She determines that the diabetes is a chronic condition and, although routine insulin was administered, there were no diabetic complications requiring attention. She sequences diabetes as the third and final code.

▶ Angelia finalizes the codes and sequencing for this case:

(1) **G45.9 Transient cerebral ischemic attack, unspecified**

(2) **G43.109 Migraine with aura, not intractable, without status migrainosus**

(3) **E10.9 Type 1 diabetes mellitus without complications**

CODING PRACTICE

Exercise 16.4   Arranging Codes for Conditions of the Nervous System

Instructions: Read the mini-medical-record of each patient's encounter, review the information abstracted in Exercise 16.2, assign ICD-10-CM diagnosis codes using the Index and Tabular List, and sequence them correctly.

---

1. INPATIENT HOSPITAL   Gender: F   Age: 29

Reason for admission: Implant neurostimulator (*a device placed under the skin that stimulates the spinal cord by tiny electrical impulses*) for pain control

Assessment: Chronic lumbar pain due to displaced disc at L3-L4 which resulted from a back injury two years ago

Plan: FU 2 weeks

Tip: Review OGCR I.C.6.b.1)(a) and (b)(ii) for sequencing instructions.

2 ICD-10-CM Codes _____

---

2. INPATIENT HOSPITAL   Gender: M   Age: 86

Reason for admission: Admitted from nursing facility due to generalized weakness

Assessment: Weakness is due to hyponatremia, patient presents an elopement risk due to late onset AD, dementia with hallucinations, and wandering

Plan: Discharged to nursing facility

Tip: Sequencing of the additional diagnoses is indicated in the Index and Tabular List.

5 ICD-10-CM Codes _____

_____

---

3. INPATIENT HOSPITAL   Gender: F   Age: 42

Reason for admission: Admitted from emergency department where patient presented with migraine of 4 days' duration which has not responded to the usual medication

Assessment: Persistent migraine with cerebrovascular infarction, cerebral stenosis of right cerebellar artery, hypertension

Tip: Review the subterms in the Index carefully.

3 ICD-10-CM Codes _____

_____

CODING NEOPLASMS OF THE NERVOUS SYSTEM

Neoplasms of the nervous system do not appear in ICD-10-CM Chapter 6, "Diseases of the Nervous System and Sense Organs (G00-G99)." Codes for neoplasms of the nervous system appear in categories C70 to C72 within the neoplasm chapter. Primary malignancies of the nervous system are rare, with the most common being medulloblastoma, an aggressive malignant brain tumor. Benign tumors can cause serious problems not because they are invasive, but because benign tumors in the brain can apply pressure to the cranial nerves. Benign peripheral tumors can cause nerve damage and loss of muscle control in the extremities.

The brain is a common site of metastases from cancers in other organs, most notably lung cancer, breast cancer, and melanoma. Brain metastases affect up to 45% of all cancer patients (Medscape). Chemotherapy can have a negative "double effect" on the brain because the treatment itself may not penetrate the brain well, but can weaken the blood–brain barrier (BBB). This weakness allows cancer cells to infiltrate the CNS, enter the brain, and grow in an environment that is removed from the treatment.

CODING PRACTICE

Exercise 16.5 Coding Neoplasms of the Nervous System

Instructions: Read the mini-medical-record of each patient's encounter, then abstract, assign, and sequence ICD-10-CM diagnosis codes using the Index and Tabular List. Write the code(s) on the line provided.

---

1. OFFICE   Gender: F   Age: 6

Reason for encounter: Review CT scan of head

Assessment: Benign hypothalamic astrocytoma (*tumor arising from star-shaped cells that form the supportive tissue of the brain*)

Plan: Surgery to remove the tumor

1 ICD-10-CM Code _____

---

2. INPATIENT HOSPITAL   Gender: F   Age: 62

Reason for admission: Management of pain following pleurectomy of right lung due to non-small-cell carcinoma (NSCLC) of the right lung

Assessment: Chronic post-thoracotomy (*incision into the chest*) pain

Plan: Discharge to home with fentanyl (*a narcotic pain reliever*) transdermal patch and home health follow up

Tip: The principal diagnosis is the condition that is the reason for the admission. Refer to OGCR I.C.6.b.5).

2 ICD-10-CM Codes _____

---

3. INPATIENT HOSPITAL   Gender: F   Age: 71

Reason for admission: Pain management

Assessment: Nerve root compress d/t stage 4 diffuse large B-cell non-Hodgkin's lymphoma

Tip: Refer to OGCR I.C.6.b.5).

3 ICD-10-CM Codes _____

_____

---

4. INPATIENT HOSPITAL   Gender: M   Age: 5

Reason for admission: Craniotomy with tumor resection

Assessment: Primary medulloblastoma of the central cerebellum

Plan: Chemotherapy was provided before discharge, follow up in office to establish chemotherapy and radiotherapy plan

Tip: Refer to OGCR I.C.2.e.

2 ICD-10-CM Codes _____

---

5. INPATIENT HOSPITAL   Gender: F   Age: 67

Reason for admission: Anemia due to chemotherapy

Assessment: Left ovarian cancer with metastases to the brain, also provided IV pain management

Plan: Refer to hospice

Tip: Refer to OGCR I.C.2.c.2) and I.C.2.e.

5 ICD-10-CM Codes _____

_____

CHAPTER SUMMARY

In this chapter you learned that:

- The function of the nervous system is to direct the body's response to internal and external stimuli and coordinate the activities of other organ systems.

- ICD-10-CM provides Official Guidelines for Coding and Reporting (OGCR) for the nervous system and sense organs in OGCR section I.C.6, which provides detailed discussion of coding for pain, including general coding information, postoperative pain, chronic pain, neoplasm-related pain, and chronic pain syndrome.

- Because of the variety of conditions addressed under the nervous system, coders need general criteria for abstracting conditions

- of the nervous system overall and specific criteria for abstracting pain, headaches, epilepsy, and Parkinson's disease.

- OGCR contain specific guidelines for assigning codes for hemiplegia, monoplegia, and pain.

- When the purpose of the encounter is to manage the pain, sequence the code for pain first; when the purpose of the encounter is to treat the underlying condition, sequence the code for the condition first.

- Primary malignancies of the nervous system are rare, but the brain is a common site of metastases from other cancers.

CONCEPT QUIZ

Take a moment to look back at the nervous system and sense organs and solidify your skills. Try to answer the questions from memory first, then refer back to the discussion in the chapter if you need a little extra help.

Completion

Instructions: Write the term that completes each statement based on the information you learned in this chapter. Choose from the list below. Some choices may be used more than once and some choices may not be used at all.

30	epilepsy
60	hydrocephalus
72	laterality
brain	meningitis
CNS	PNS
dominance	spina bifida
electrocardiogram	spinal cord
electroencephalogram	status epilepticus
encephalitis	status migrainosus

1. The _____ acts as the control center for the nervous system by processing information and providing short-term control over other organ systems.

2. _____ is a viral inflammation of the brain and meninges.

3. _____ is a brain disorder in which neurons signal abnormally, causing seizures and/or unconsciousness.

4. The _____ is a common site of metastases from cancers in other organs.

5. The _____ consists of the 12 nerves that radiate out from the brain and the 31 pairs of nerves that radiate from the spinal cord to all other areas of the body.

6. _____ means a condition is resistant to treatment.

7. _____ refers to the side of the body an individual favors, such as being left-handed or right-handed.

8. _____ is a recording of the electrical activity of the brain.

9. _____ is a congenital neural tube defect in which vertebrae do not fuse.

10. Status epilepticus is an epileptic seizure lasting more than _____ minutes.

Multiple Choice

Instructions: Circle the letter of the best answer to each question based on the information you learned in this chapter.

1. What is the medical term for maintenance of a stable internal physical state of the body?
   A. Hemostasis
   B. Equilibrium
   C. Homeostasis
   D. Intractable

2. What medical term means "resistant to treatment"?
   A. Vasodilation
   B. Chronic
   C. Refractory
   D. Idiopathic

3. What type of seizures are the result of abnormal activity on both sides of the brain?
   A. Simple partial
   B. Psychomotor
   C. Status epilepticus
   D. Generalized

4. How would you code the following scenario? *A patient with previously diagnosed Parkinson's disease is also diagnosed with dementia today.*
   A. G31.83, F02.80
   B. G20, F02.80
   C. F02.80
   D. G31.83

5. Which of the following is a key criterion for abstracting headaches?
   A. Is it localized or generalized?
   B. What is the infectious organism?
   C. Is a duration of 30 minutes or more documented?
   D. Is it accompanied with aura?

6. How would you code the following scenario? *A left-handed patient is seen for flaccid hemiplegia of the right arm.*
   A. G81.01
   B. G81.02
   C. G81.03
   D. G81.04

7. What code category does OGCR I.C.6.b provide detailed guidance for?
   A. G00 Bacterial meningitis, not elsewhere classified
   B. G20 Parkinson's disease
   C. G81 Hemiplegia and hemiparesis
   D. G89 Pain, not elsewhere classified

8. What is another term for classical migraine?
   A. Migraine with aura
   B. Intractable migraine
   C. Cluster headache
   D. Status migrainosus

9. Which of the following is a key criterion for abstracting pain?
   A. Is it due to a device, implant, graft, or trauma?
   B. Is it documented as intractable?
   C. Is paralysis documented?
   D. Is a duration of 72 hours or more documented?

10. How would you code the following scenario? *A patient with a displaced C4-C5 disk due to trauma and associated severe chronic neck pain presents for a steroid injection in the spinal canal to relieve pain.*
    A. M50.221, G89.21
    B. G89.21, M50.221
    C. M50.221, G89.11
    D. G89.11, M50.221

KEEP ON CODING

Instructions: Read the diagnostic statement, then use the Index and Tabular List to assign and sequence ICD-10-CM diagnosis codes. Write the code(s) on the line provided.

1. Pneumococcal meningitis. ICD-10-CM Code(s) _____

2. Metastatic carcinoma of the thalamus from primary cancer of the right breast. ICD-10-CM Code(s) _____

3. Accidental puncture of the meninges during a nervous system operative procedure. ICD-10-CM Code(s) _____

4. Alpers' disease. ICD-10-CM Code(s) _____

5. Migraine with an aura. ICD-10-CM Code(s) _____

6. Restless legs syndrome. ICD-10-CM Code(s) _____

7. Vascular parkinsonism. ICD-10-CM Code(s) _____

8. Amyotrophic lateral sclerosis. ICD-10-CM Code(s) _____

9. Blepharospasm. ICD-10-CM Code(s) _____

10. Childhood absence epilepsy, intractable with status epilepticus. ICD-10-CM Code(s) _____

11. Menstrual migraine, intractable without status migrainosus. ICD-10-CM Code(s) _____

12. Narcolepsy with cataplexy. ICD-10-CM Code(s) _____

13. Huntington's chorea. ICD-10-CM Code(s) _____

14. Headache due to lumbar puncture. ICD-10-CM Code(s) _____

15. Ataxic cerebral palsy. ICD-10-CM Code(s) _____

16. Guillain-Barré syndrome. ICD-10-CM Code(s) _____

17. Myasthenia gravis without exacerbation. ICD-10-CM Code(s) _____

18. Intractable epilepsy with status epilepticus. ICD-10-CM Code(s) _____

19. Primary central sleep apnea. ICD-10-CM Code(s) _____

20. Spasmodic torticollis. ICD-10-CM Code(s) _____

21. Postpoliomyelitis syndrome. ICD-10-CM Code(s) _____

22. Tropical spastic paraplegia. ICD-10-CM Code(s) _____

23. Medulloblastoma. ICD-10-CM Code(s) _____

24. Alzheimer's disease. ICD-10-CM Code(s) _____

25. Episodic tension-type headache. ICD-10-CM Code(s) _____

CODING CHALLENGE

Instructions: Read the mini-medical-record of each patient's encounter, then abstract, assign, and sequence ICD-10-CM diagnosis codes using the Index and Tabular List. Write the code(s) on the line provided.

1. OUTPATIENT HOSPITAL   Gender: M   Age: 36

Reason for encounter: Patient presents to the infusion center for treatment of meningitis

Assessment: Staphylococcal meningitis

(continued)

1. (continued)

Plan: FU in 3 days and 1 week after antibiotic infusions are complete

Tip: Read the instructional notes in the Tabular List.

2 ICD-10-CM Codes _____

2. INPATIENT HOSPITAL   Gender: M   Age: 60

Reason for admission: Acute respiratory distress

Assessment: Myasthenia gravis crisis, chronic inflammatory demyelinating polyneuropathy (CIDP) (*an inflammatory disorder of PNS due to abnormal immune activity*)

Plan: Rx cholinesterase inhibitor and immunosuppressant drugs. FU 1 week

2 ICD-10-CM Codes _____

---

3. OFFICE   Gender: F   Age: 13

Reason for encounter: Increase in number and intensity of myoclonic seizures.

Assessment: Poorly controlled juvenile myoclonic epilepsy (JME)

Plan: Valproic acid dosage changes

Tip: Read the cross-reference instruction in the Index.

1 ICD-10-CM Code _____

---

4. OFFICE   Gender: M   Age: 18

Reason for encounter: EEG

Assessment: Focal seizures

Plan: Rx Dilantin

Tip: Read the cross-reference instruction in the Index.

1 ICD-10-CM Code _____

---

5. OFFICE   Gender: M   Age: 44

Reason for encounter: Continuing lower back pain with radiating pain in left hip. Patient has had surgical repair of several ruptured discs and is overweight and sedentary.

Assessment: Chronic pain syndrome

Plan: Acetaminophen, consult with dietician for weight loss plan, 12 session physical therapy followed by regular exercise, RTO in 4 weeks

2 ICD-10-CM Codes _____

---

6. INPATIENT HOSPITAL   Gender: F   Age: 12

Reason for admission: Recurring headaches, problems with balance, poor coordination, gait disturbances

Assessment: Normal-pressure hydrocephalus

Plan: Placement of ventriculoperitoneal shunt (*a tube that drains fluid from the brain into the peritoneal cavity*)

1 ICD-10-CM Code _____

---

7. OFFICE   Gender: M   Age: 55

Reason for encounter: Sleep study

Assessment: Obstructive sleep apnea, nutritional obesity with BMI 33.0

Plan: Rx continuous positive airway pressure (CPAP) device, refer to dietician for weight loss

3 ICD-10-CM Codes _____
_____

---

8. OFFICE   Gender: F   Age: 68

Reason for encounter: Carpal tunnel release, right hand, endoscopic

Assessment: Carpal tunnel syndrome and diabetes type 2 with polyneuropathy

Plan: FU 3 weeks

2 ICD-10-CM Codes _____

---

9. OFFICE   Gender: F   Age: 58

Reason for encounter: Pain in the calf muscle, muscle weakness and cramping in thighs and upper arms

Assessment: Alcohol dependence with alcoholic myopathy

Plan: Referral to alcohol counseling and nutritionist, RTO 1 week

2 ICD-10-CM Codes _____

---

10. OFFICE   Gender: F   Age: 43

Reason for encounter: Physical therapy

Assessment: Long-standing left-sided hemiplegia due to encephalitis 20 years ago

Plan: return 1 week

Tip: Refer to OGCR I.C.6.a for coding of hemiplegia. The statement "20 years ago" means that the hemiplegia is a sequela of encephalitis.

Chapter 17

Mental, Behavioral, and Neurodevelopmental Disorders (F01-F99)

Chapter Outline

- **Psychiatry Refresher**
- **Coding Guidelines for Psychiatry**
- **Abstracting Diagnoses for Psychiatry**
- **Assigning Diagnosis Codes for Psychiatry**
- **Arranging Diagnosis Codes for Psychiatry**

Learning Objectives

After completing this chapter, you should have the skills to:

17.1 Spell and define the key words, medical terms, and abbreviations related to mental, behavioral, and neurodevelopmental disorders. (Remember)

17.2 Summarize the common types of mental, behavioral, and neurodevelopmental disorders. (Understand)

17.3 Adhere to the Official Guidelines for Coding and Reporting related to mental, behavioral, and neurodevelopmental disorders. (Apply)

17.4 Examine and abstract diagnostic information from the medical record for coding mental, behavioral, and neurodevelopmental disorders. (Analyze)

17.5 Demonstrate how to assign codes for mental, behavioral, and neurodevelopmental disorders. (Apply)

17.6 Utilize guidelines for arranging (sequencing) multiple codes for mental, behavioral, and neurodevelopmental disorders. (Apply)

Key Terms and Abbreviations

abuse (substance)	delusion	Lewy body disease	psychotherapy
addiction	dependence (substance)	mental disorder	schizophrenia
behavioral disorder	hallucination	neurodevelopmental disorder	schizothymia
behavioral disturbance	in remission	paranoia	tolerate
blood alcohol level (BAL)	intellectual disability	perceptual disturbance	use (substance)
delirium	intoxication	psychoactive substance	vascular dementia

In addition to the key terms listed here, students should know the terms defined within tables in this chapter.

INTRODUCTION

According to the National Highway Traffic Safety Administration (NHTSA), on any given day there are 28 deaths due to drunk driving, or one every 51 minutes. Substance abuse is just one of many topics in the ICD-10-CM chapter on mental, behavioral, and neurodevelopmental disorders, but it occupies a significant portion of the codes.

A psychiatrist specializes in diagnosing and treating mental, behavioral, and neurodevelopmental disorders and also prescribes medications to treat those disorders. Other providers who also may treat mental, behavioral, and neurodevelopmental disorders are clinical psychologists, social workers, and therapists. However, these nonphysician providers cannot prescribe medication. Primary care physicians screen for mental, behavioral, and neurodevelopmental disorders and usually refer patients who need treatment to one of these specialists. For the sake of brevity, this chapter refers to mental, behavioral, and neurodevelopmental disorders as *psychiatry*.

As you read this chapter, open up your medical terminology book and keep a medical dictionary handy to refresh your memory of any unfamiliar terms. Many psychiatric conditions are part of your daily vocabulary, so a reference book will help you understand the medical meaning of these terms.

PSYCHIATRY REFRESHER

Mental, behavioral, and neurodevelopmental disorders are real—not imagined—disorders that have diagnostic criteria and are proven to respond to treatment. **Mental disorders** are psychological or physical conditions that disrupt an individual's personality, mind, and emotions in such a way that they affect the ability to function and interact with others. **Behavioral disorders** are manifestations of mental disturbances that result in extreme or disruptive conduct, such as rage, withdrawal, or substance abuse. **Neurodevelopmental disorders** are conditions that result from impaired development of the nervous system during infancy or childhood. Although mental, behavioral, and neurodevelopmental disorders are not fully understood by scientists, they are believed to be caused by a combination of psychological, environmental, biological, and social factors (■ FIGURE 17-1).

As you learn about conditions and procedures related to mental, behavioral, and neurodevelopmental disorders, remember to apply medical terminology skills to use word roots, prefixes, and suffixes you already know to define new terms. Refer to ■ TABLE 17-1, (page 292) for a refresher on how to build medical terms related to mental, behavioral, and neurodevelopmental disorders.

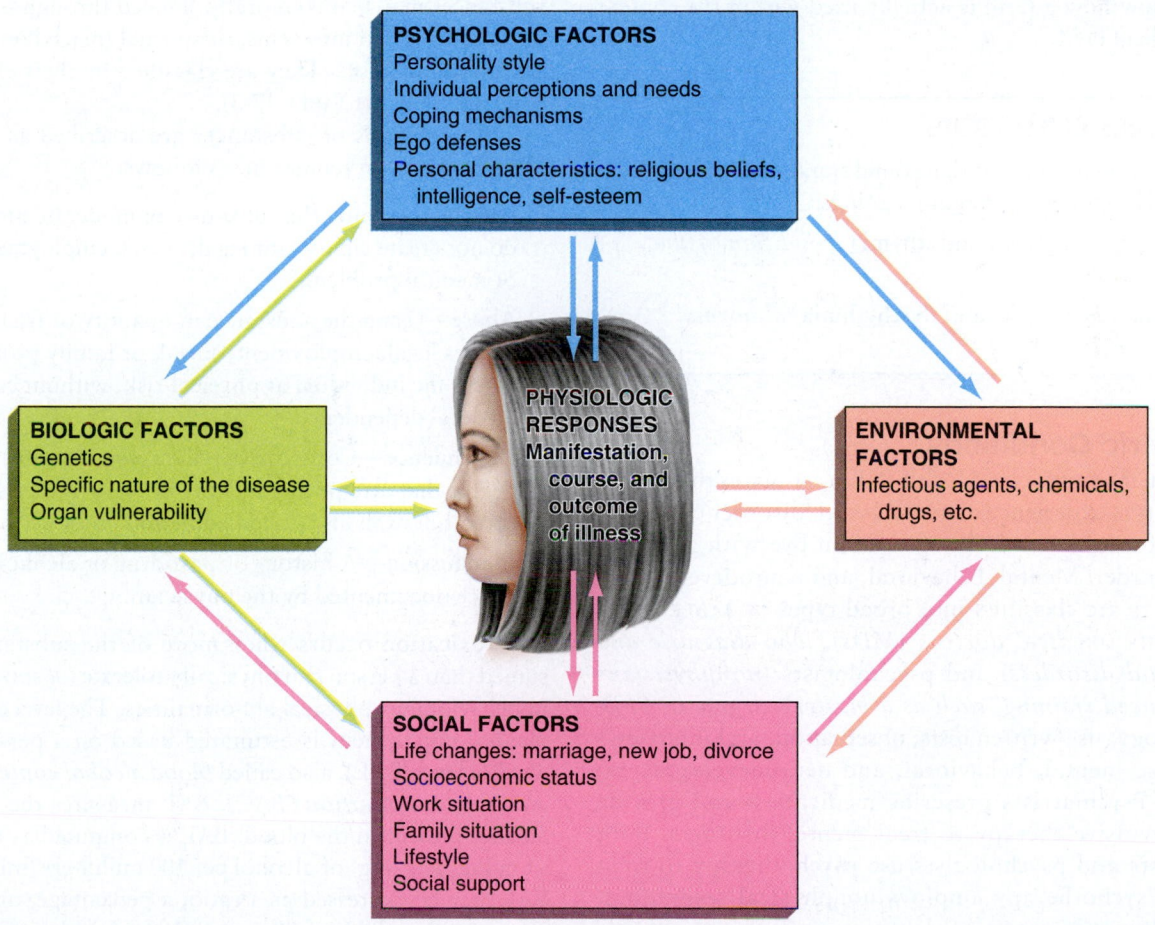

PSYCHOLOGIC FACTORS
Personality style
Individual perceptions and needs
Coping mechanisms
Ego defenses
Personal characteristics: religious beliefs, intelligence, self-esteem

BIOLOGIC FACTORS
Genetics
Specific nature of the disease
Organ vulnerability

PHYSIOLOGIC RESPONSES
Manifestation, course, and outcome of illness

ENVIRONMENTAL FACTORS
Infectious agents, chemicals, drugs, etc.

SOCIAL FACTORS
Life changes: marriage, new job, divorce
Socioeconomic status
Work situation
Family situation
Lifestyle
Social support

Figure 17-1 ■ Factors contributing to mental health and mental illness.

Table 17-1 ■ **EXAMPLE OF CONSTRUCTING MEDICAL TERMS FOR PSYCHIATRIC DISORDERS**

Prefix/Combining Form	Suffix	Complete Medical Term
dys- (prefix; *abnormal, painful*) para- (prefix; *beside*)	-thymia (*condition of the mind or emotion*) -phrenia (*condition of the mind*) -asthenia (*lack of strength*)	dys + thymia (*abnormal condition of the mind*) schizo + thymia (*condition of a split mind*)
schiz/o (*split*)		schizo + phrenia (*condition of a split mind*) para + phrenia (*condition beside the mind*)
psych/o (*mind*)		psycho + genic (*originating in the mind*) psycho + asthenia (*lack of strength in the mind*)

Medical terms may seem confusing because the literal meaning of the word parts may not fully describe how the word is used, particularly in the area of mental, behavioral, and neurodevelopmental disorders. For example, *para-* means "beside" or "beyond" and *-noia* means "mind." The literal meaning of paranoia is beside or beyond the mind, but the word is used to mean a mental condition of delusions of persecution. The suffixes *-thymia* and *-phrenia* both mean "mind," but schizothymia (*tendency toward being severely introverted*) is a different and less serious condition than schizophrenia (*a condition characterized by the inability to distinguish between thoughts and reality*). Coders understand that they use medical terminology skills to gain a basic understanding; they also need to know how a term is actually used within the context of the medical field.

CODING CAUTION

Be alert for medical terms that sound similar but are spelled differently and have different meanings.

thym/o (*thymus gland*) and **-thymia** (*condition of the mind*)

dysthymia (*depression*) and **dysrhythmia** (*abnormal heartbeat*)

Psychiatric Conditions

The National Institutes of Health (NIH) estimates that nearly 18% of adults experience a mental health disorder each year, and 4% of adults and 21% of children live with a serious mental disorder. Mental, behavioral, and neurodevelopmental disorders are classified into broad types (■ TABLE 17-2). Psychiatrists (*medical doctors [MDs], who diagnose and treat mental disorders*) and psychologists (*nonphysicians with advanced training, such as a master's degree or PhD, in psychology*) use written tests, observation, and interviews to diagnose mental, behavioral, and neurodevelopmental disorders. Psychiatrists prescribe medication and provide electroconvulsive therapy to treat mental disorders. Both psychiatrists and psychologists use psychotherapy to treat patients. Psychotherapy employs nonphysical techniques, such as talking, interpreting, listening, rewarding, and role playing, to treat disorders.

In particular, coders must be familiar with the terminology related to psychoactive substance use and dementia in order to code accurately.

Psychoactive Substance Disorders

Psychoactive substances have the ability to alter behavior, impair judgment, or create medical problems. Inappropriate use of such products can create legal, social, employment, family, and medical problems. Psychoactive substance disorders may involve legal substances, such as tobacco, alcohol, and, in some states, cannabis; illegal substances, such as heroin, cocaine, or cannabis; or prescribed medications—such as pain relievers or tranquilizers—that are used inappropriately. Substances may be taken orally, inhaled through breathing or smoking, injected into veins, or snorted (placed on mucosa of the mouth or nose). They are classified by their effect on the mind and body (■ TABLE 17-3).

Usage patterns of substances are described as use, abuse, dependence, or in remission, as follows:

- Use—Consuming the substance in moderate amounts that do not create significant legal, social, employment, family, or medical problems.

- Abuse—Using the substance in quantity or frequency that creates legal, employment, social, or family problems or places the individual at physical risk, without causing physical dependence.

- Dependence—Compulsive reliance on the substance to a degree that attempting to stop creates physical symptoms of withdrawal; also called addiction.

- In remission—A history of past drug or alcohol dependence documented by the physician.

Intoxication occurs when more of the substance is consumed than a person can physically tolerate (*absorb*), resulting in behavioral or physical abnormalities. The level of potential alcohol impairment is estimated based on a person's blood alcohol level (BAL), also called *blood alcohol content* or *blood alcohol concentration (BAC)*. BAL measures the amount of alcohol present in the blood. BAL is computed as the number of milligrams (mg) of alcohol per 100 milliliters (mL) of blood. BAL may be expressed as a ratio, a percentage, or a number. For example, a BAL of *80 mg per 100 mL* is the same as a BAL of *0.08%*, which may also be written without the percent sign

Table 17-2   ■   **COMMON MENTAL, BEHAVIORAL, AND NEURODEVELOPMENTAL DISORDERS**

Type of Disorder	Definition	Examples
Adjustment	Abnormal difficulty in responding to life changes	Adjustment disorder with anxiety, adjustment disorder with depressed mood
Anxiety	Abnormal anxiety that interferes with normal activities	Panic disorder, social phobia, obsessive–compulsive disorder (OCD), posttraumatic stress disorder (PTSD)
Cognitive	Failure to develop or deterioration of mental comprehension	Autism, dementia, intellectual disability
Dissociative	Disruption in consciousness, memory, identity, or perception	Multiple personality amnesia
Eating	Serious disturbance in eating behavior	Anorexia nervosa, bulimia nervosa
Impulse control	Extreme difficulty in controlling impulses, despite the negative consequences	Intermittent explosive disorder, kleptomania, pyromania, pathological gambling
Mood (affective)	Instability of mood	Major depression, mania, bipolar disorder
Personality	Persistent inflexible patterns of behavior that affect interpersonal relationships	Cluster A: Paranoid and schizoid Cluster B: Antisocial, borderline, histrionic, and narcissistic Cluster C: Avoidant, dependent, obsessive–compulsive
Psychotic	Delusions (*false beliefs that hinder the ability to function*) and hallucinations (*false visual, auditory, olfactory, or tactile perceptions*)	Schizophrenia (catatonic type, disorganized type, paranoid type, undifferentiated type, residual type); delusional disorder; brief psychotic disorder
Sexual	Repetitive and prolonged sexual activity and sexual dysfunction that interferes with normal relationships or daily activities	Gender identity disorder, pedophilia, voyeurism
Sleeping	Abnormal sleep problems	Insomnia, sleepwalking
Somatoform	Physical symptoms that are not explained by medical conditions	Hypochondriasis, body dysmorphic disorder (BDD), pain disorder
Substance	Drug and alcohol use, abuse, and addiction	Alcoholism, tobacco dependence, illicit drug use

Table 17-3   ■   **COMMONLY ABUSED SUBSTANCES**

Classification	Effect	Examples
Alcohol (ethanol)	Reduces tension, promotes relaxation	Beer, wine, liquor (scotch, gin, vodka, rum)
Barbiturate (sedative)	Reduces tension, promotes relaxation	Phenobarbital, Tuinal, secobarbital, "downers"
Hallucinogen	Promotes relaxation, changes mood, thoughts, and behavior	Cannabis (marijuana), hashish, LSD, PCP
Narcotic (opiate)	Reduces physical pain and anxiety	Opium, cocaine, heroin, morphine, codeine, meperidine (Demerol), fentanyl, hydrocodone (Vicodin), oxycodone (OxyContin)
Nicotine	Stimulant; increases feelings of confidence and elevates mood	Cigarettes, cigars, pipes, smokeless tobacco, chewing tobacco
Stimulant	Increases feelings of confidence, alertness, and well-being	Amphetamine, "meth" (methamphetamine), dextroamphetamine (Dexedrine), speed, crank
Tranquilizer	Reduces anxiety, induces sleep	Diazepam (Valium), lorazepam (Ativan), alprazolam (Xanax)

as .08. To convert a percentage, such as *0.08%*, to a ratio, simply add a *0* to the end of the percentage and drop the leading decimal point to arrive at *80 mg per 100 mL*.

Dementia

Dementia is a progressive loss of brain function that affects memory, thinking, language, judgment, and behavior. A leading cause is **Lewy body disease** in which patients have abnormal protein structures in certain areas of the brain. **Vascular dementia** is caused by many small strokes. Dementia may be a manifestation of substance abuse disorders or other nervous system diseases such as Parkinson's disease, multiple sclerosis, and Alzheimer disease. Most dementia is accompanied by **behavioral disturbances** such as aggression, wandering, depression, delusion or hallucinations, sleep disturbances, or poor eating habits.

CODING PRACTICE

Exercise 17.1 **Psychiatry Refresher**

Instructions: Use your medical terminology skills and resources to define the following conditions related to mental, behavioral, and neurodevelopmental disorders, then assign the diagnosis code.

Follow these steps:

• Use slash marks "/" to break down each term into its root(s) and suffix.

• Define the meaning of the word, based on the meaning of each word part.

• Assign the default ICD-10-CM diagnosis code for the condition using the Index and Tabular List.

Example: arachnophobia arachno/phobia   Meaning *fear of spiders*   ICD-10-CM Code *F40.210*

1. agoraphobia   Meaning _____   ICD-10-CM Code _____

2. psychasthenia   Meaning _____   ICD-10-CM Code _____

3. trichotillomania   Meaning _____   ICD-10-CM Code _____

4. hypomania   Meaning _____   ICD-10-CM Code _____

5. pedophilia   Meaning _____   ICD-10-CM Code _____

6. hematophobia   Meaning _____   ICD-10-CM Code _____

7. dysmorphophobia   Meaning _____   ICD-10-CM Code _____

8. somnambulism   Meaning _____   ICD-10-CM Code _____

9. paraphilia   Meaning _____   ICD-10-CM Code _____

10. pseudocyesis   Meaning _____   ICD-10-CM Code _____

CODING GUIDELINES FOR PSYCHIATRY

Coders should understand the organization of this ICD-10-CM chapter, chapter-wide and commonly used instructional notes in the Tabular List, and the relevant OGCR. This information is necessary for accurate coding.

ICD-10-CM Chapter 5, "Mental, Behavioral, and Neurodevelopmental Disorders (F01-F99)," contains 11 blocks or subchapters that are divided by the type of disorder. Review the block names and code ranges listed at the beginning of Chapter 5 in the ICD-10-CM manual to become familiar with the content and organization.

This chapter includes mental, behavioral, and neurodevelopmental disorders with physiological causes; personality, mood, and schizophrenic disorders; substance disorders; intellectual disabilities; and developmental disorders. It does not include symptoms and signs, neurological disorders, or congenital conditions.

Categories for mental, behavioral, and neurodevelopmental disorders due to psychoactive substance use, F10 through F19, are detailed. Codes differentiate between abuse, dependence, and unspecified use and also identify complications, such as delusions, hallucinations, or sleep disturbances. Categories for intellectual disabilities, F70 through F79, provide instructional notes to code first any associated physical or developmental disorder.

ICD-10-CM provides Official Guidelines for Coding and Reporting (OGCR) for mental, behavioral, and neurodevelopmental disorders in OGCR section I.C.5. The OGCR provides detailed discussion of pain disorders related to psychological factors and mental, behavioral, and neurodevelopmental disorders due to substance abuse. Additional guidelines related to pain appear in OGCR I.C.6.b. Specific OGCR and instructional notes are discussed and cited throughout this chapter of the text.

The American Psychiatric Association (APA) uses the *Diagnostic and Statistical Manual of Mental Disorders, Fifth Edition* (DSM-5) to diagnose and classify mental disorders. In addition to codes, the manual also lists known causes of disorders, statistics regarding gender, age at onset, prognosis, and research concerning optimal approaches. DSM-5 uses a numbering system different than ICD-10-CM. Users must refer to a crosswalk between DSM-5 and ICD-10-CM to find the equivalent code. DSM is not a HIPAA-approved code set and cannot be used for insurance billing.

ABSTRACTING DIAGNOSES FOR PSYCHIATRY

Many mental, behavioral, and neurodevelopmental disorders have multiple subtypes, so coders must be particularly attentive to the documented wording of the condition. For example, a substance disorder may be stated as *use*, *abuse*, or *dependence*, each of which has a specific meaning and different codes. Some disorders, such as dementia, may have underlying physiological conditions that must be identified and abstracted as well. Diseases and conditions classified in other ICD-10-CM body system chapters—such as the digestive, circulatory, and nervous systems—contain frequent instructional notes to assign an additional code for use, abuse, or dependence on alcohol or nicotine.

The table that follows provides general criteria for abstracting mental, behavioral, and neurodevelopmental disorders (■ TABLE 17-4). Remember that the abstracting questions are a guide and that not every question applies to, or can be answered for, every case. For example, not every disorder is described based on whether it is in remission. Some conditions do have this criterion, so coders should always check the documentation to see if such information is present. Additional tables provide specific criteria for abstracting mood disorders (■ TABLE 17-5) and substance disorders (■ TABLE 17-6).

Guided Example of Abstracting Diagnoses for Psychiatry

Refer to the following example throughout this chapter to learn about abstracting, assigning, and sequencing mental, behavioral,

and neurodevelopmental disorder codes. Ladonna Shuck, CPC, is a fictitious coder who will guide you through the coding process.

Date: 8/11/yy Location: Valley Hospital

Provider: Brett Camden, MD

Patient: Cody Locust Gender: M Age: 58

Reason for admission: Admitted from the emergency department with coma

Assessment: Alcoholic liver failure with coma for 4 hours, alcohol dependent abuse for 15 years with intoxication at admission, BAL .23%. Early onset Alzheimer's dementia with behavioral disturbance was managed as well.

Plan: Discharge to rehab program

Table 17-4 ■ KEY CRITERIA FOR ABSTRACTING GENERAL PSYCHIATRIC DISORDERS

- ❏ What is the disorder?
- ❏ What is the specific subtype of the disorder?
- ❏ Is the disorder due to an underlying physiological condition?
- ❏ Does the patient report symptoms that have no medical cause?
- ❏ What is the severity?
- ❏ Is the condition in remission?

Table 17-5 ■ KEY CRITERIA FOR ABSTRACTING MOOD DISORDERS

- ❏ What is the disorder?
- ❏ Does it have psychotic features?
- ❏ Is the condition current or in remission?
- ❏ Is the current or most recent episode manic, depressed, or mixed?
- ❏ Is the severity mild, moderate, or severe?
- ❏ Is remission partial or full?

Table 17-6 ■ KEY CRITERIA FOR ABSTRACTING PSYCHOACTIVE SUBSTANCE DISORDERS

- ❏ What is the specific substance?
- ❏ What is the class of substance (opioid, sedative, stimulant, hallucinogen, inhalant)?
- ❏ Is the disorder one of use, abuse, or dependence?
- ❏ Does the provider clearly document the relationship between the mental or behavioral disorder and the substance use?
- ❏ What is the blood alcohol level?
- ❏ Is intoxication present?
- ❏ Is withdrawal present?
- ❏ Is delirium (*state of confusion, restlessness, and incoherence*) or perceptual disturbance (*misinterpretation of surroundings or events*) present?
- ❏ Are any associated hallucinations, delusions, or other psychotic conditions present?
- ❏ Is the condition in remission?

Follow along as Ladonna Shuck, CPC, abstracts the diagnosis. Check off each step after you complete it.

▶ Ladonna reads through the entire record, paying special attention to the reason for the encounter and the final assessment. She notes that the patient was admitted with a coma that lasted for four hours and was later diagnosed with alcoholic liver disease.

▶ Ladonna refers to the Key Criteria for Abstracting Psychoactive Substance Disorders (Table 17-6).

- ❏ *What is the specific substance?* Alcohol
- ❏ *Is the disorder one of use, abuse, or dependence?* Dependence
- ❏ *Does the provider clearly document the relationship between the mental or behavioral disorder and the substance use?* Yes, alcoholic liver failure
- ❏ *What is the blood alcohol level?* BAL .23%
- ❏ *Is intoxication present?* Yes, with intoxication at admission
- ❏ *Is withdrawal present?* No
- ❏ *Is delirium or perceptual disturbance present?* No
- ❏ *Are any associated hallucinations, delusions, or other psychotic conditions present?* Early-onset Alzheimer's dementia with behavioral disturbance
- ❏ *Is the condition in remission?* No

▶ Patients with a coma are often rated using the Glasgow Coma Scale. The Glasgow Coma Scale is discussed in Chapter 4, "Symptoms, Signs, and Abnormal Clinical and Laboratory Findings, Not Elsewhere Classified (R00–R99)," of this text. The Glasgow Coma Scale is not applied in this guided example for the sake of brevity.

▶ At this time, Ladonna does not know which of these conditions may need to be coded nor how many codes she will end up with. She will learn about this when she moves on to assigning codes.

CODING PRACTICE

Exercise 17.2   Abstracting Diagnoses for Psychiatry

Instructions: Read the mini-medical-record of each patient's encounter and answer the abstracting questions. Write the answer on the line provided. Do not assign any codes.

---

1. OFFICE   Gender: F   Age: 9

Reason for encounter: Referred by pediatrician for hyperactivity, short attention span, and irritability

Assessment: After testing, symptoms are due to attention deficit hyperactive disorder, predominately hyperactive type

Plan: Start medication and behavior therapy

a. What symptoms are reported? _____

b. What is the disorder?_____

c. What is the specific subtype of the disorder?_____
_____

d. What symptoms should you report? _____
Why? _____

---

2. INPATIENT HOSPITAL   Gender: M   Age: 31

Reason for encounter: Extreme delusions of paranoia

Assessment: Dependent continual user of coke, psychosis with delusions due to dependence and long-term use of cocaine

Plan: Rx to help manage delusions, transfer to rehab

a. What is the specific substance? _____

b. Is the disorder one of use, abuse, or dependence?
_____

c. Does the provider clearly document the relationship between the mental or behavioral disorder and the substance use? _____
_____

d. Is withdrawal present? _____

e. Is delirium or perceptual disturbance present?_____
_____

f. Are any associated hallucinations, delusions, or other psychotic conditions present? _____
_____

---

3. OFFICE   Gender: F   Age: 21

Reason for encounter: Ongoing medical management (*evaluation and renewal of prescription*) of schizophrenia

Assessment: Paranoid schizophrenia

Plan: Medication is managing the condition well and patient is interested in getting a job. Referred to a supported employment service (*a program that assists in locating community-based employment*)

a. What is the reason for the encounter? _____
_____

b. What condition does the medication treat? _____
_____

c. What is the specific subtype of disorder? _____
_____

d. Is the disorder due to an underlying physiological condition? _____

---

4. OFFICE   Gender: M   Age: 10

Reason for encounter: I have been seeing this child for autism, but today his mother is concerned about continuing "fussing and worry about his private parts" that has been going on for quite awhile and his "desire to be like his sister."

Assessment: Gender identity disorder

Plan: Adjusted medications for current autism.

a. What concerns did the mother express? _____
_____

b. What is the disorder? _____

c. What other conditions were managed? _____
_____

d. What condition is the main reason for the encounter? _____

---

5. INPATIENT HOSPITAL   Gender: M   Age: 48

Reason for encounter: Admitted from emergency department for alcohol-induced gastritis with hemorrhaging and intoxication with BAL of .09%

Assessment: Patient has long-term alcohol use with dependence, prior cocaine abuser but states he no longer uses

(continued)

CODING PRACTICE (continued)

5. (continued)

Plan: Patient agreed to counseling after discharge

a. What is the medical condition? _____
_____

b. What substance is the cause? _____

c. Does the provider clearly document the relationship between the mental or behavioral disorder and the substance use? _____
_____

d. Is the disorder one of use, abuse, or dependence? _____

e. Is intoxication present? _____

f. What is the blood alcohol level? _____
How do you write this number as a ratio?_____
_____ mg per 100 mL

g. Is delirium or perceptual disturbance present?_____
_____

h. What substance abuse is in remission? _____
_____

6. INPATIENT HOSPITAL   Gender: M   Age: 56

Reason for encounter: Severe depression due to bipolar disorder

Assessment: Patient is also being treated for liver cirrhosis with ascites due to chronic continuous alcoholism

Plan: Patient has stable living situation so we are going to discharge him to a partial hospitalization program (*a treatment program that participants attend during the day, and return home at night*)

a. What is the mood disorder? _____

b. Is the current or most recent episode manic, depressed, or mixed? _____

c. Does it have psychotic features? _____

d. Is the severity mild, moderate, or severe? _____
_____

e. What physical condition exists? _____

f. What substance disorder is documented?_____
_____

g. Is the disorder one of use, abuse, or dependence?
_____

h. Are any associated hallucinations, delusions, or other psychotic conditions present? _____

i. What condition was chiefly responsible for the admission and services? _____

ASSIGNING DIAGNOSIS CODES FOR PSYCHIATRY

Three types of conditions in this ICD-10-CM chapter present challenges in assigning codes because of the level of detail that must be reported: bipolar disorder, schizophrenic disorders, and substance disorders.

Assigning Codes for Bipolar Disorder

Bipolar disorder has numerous variations based on the episode, severity, and psychotic disturbances that may accompany it. Follow these steps to assign codes for bipolar disorder (■ FIGURES 17-2 and 17-3):

1. Locate the Main Term **Disorder** in the Index.
2. Locate the subterm **bipolar (I)**.
   - For bipolar II disorder, locate the subterm **bipolar II**, which follows the subterm entry for **bipolar (I)**.

> Dr. Camden saw a patient for medication management of bipolar I disorder. After questioning, Dr. Camden documented that the patient reported experiencing severe manic episodes during the past several days.
>
> **F31.13 Bipolar disorder, current episode manic without psychotic features, severe**

Figure 17-2 ■ Example of assigning codes for bipolar disorder.

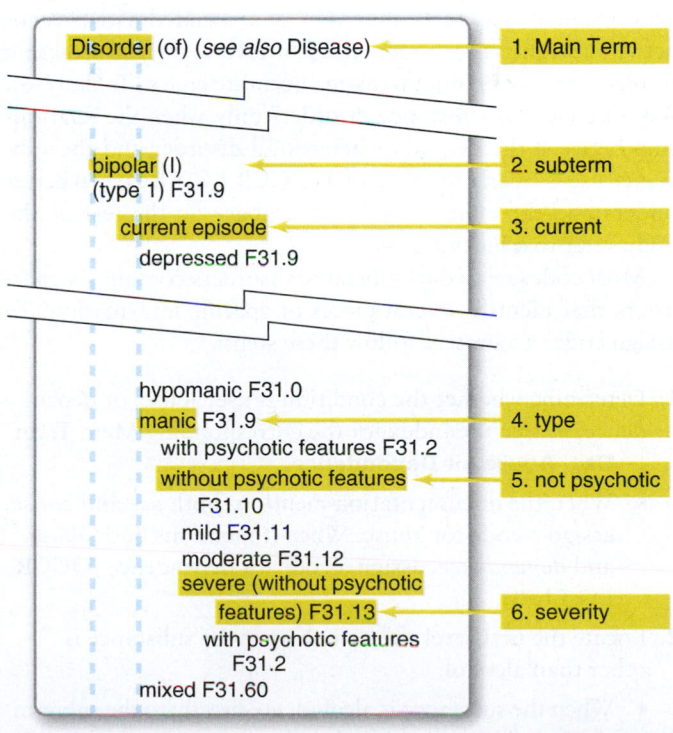

Figure 17-3 ■ Index entry for "Disorder, biopolar" used to locate codes for bipolar disorder.

3. Determine whether the disorder is documented as **current** or **in remission** and locate the corresponding second-level subterm.

4. For current bipolar disorder, identify whether the current episode is **depressed**, **hypomanic**, **manic**, or **mixed** and locate the corresponding third-level subterm.

5. Identify whether the disorder is **with psychotic features** or **without psychotic features** and locate the corresponding fourth-level subterm.

6. For cases **without psychotic features**, select the fifth-level subterm that describes the severity as **mild**, **moderate**, or **severe**. Verify the code in the Tabular List.

7. For bipolar **in remission**, locate the corresponding second-level subterm, then identify whether the remission is **full** or **partial**. Under the corresponding third-level subterm, select the additional subterm that describes the severity. Verify the code in the Tabular List.

8. To code for a *single manic episode*, locate the Main Term **Disorder**, subterm **bipolar**, then the additional subterm **single manic episode**.

Assigning Codes for Schizophrenic Spectrum Disorders

Schizophrenic spectrum disorders (SSDs) include several different disorders, each with different characteristics and diagnostic criteria. Coders must be careful to identify the specific terminology documented in order to assign the correct code. Refer to ■ TABLE 17-7 for a summary of SSDs and associated codes.

Assigning Codes for Psychoactive Substance Disorders

When mental, behavioral, and neurodevelopmental disorders are documented as being caused by or associated with psychoactive substance use, coders need to review their abstracting results carefully in order to assign accurate codes (Table 17-6). Assign codes for substance disorders only when the relationship between the mental or behavioral disorder and the substance use is clearly documented (OGCR I.C.5.b.1)). To better understand the effect of substance abuse on the rest of the body, refer to ■ FIGURE 17-4.

Most codes related to substance disorders contain six characters that identify several pieces of specific information. To assign codes accurately, follow these steps:

1. Determine whether the condition is use, abuse, or dependence. Search the Index for the corresponding Main Term — **Use**, **Abuse**, or **Dependence**.

   - When the documentation mentions both *use* and *abuse*, assign a code for abuse. When it mentions both *abuse* and *dependence*, assign a code for dependence (OGCR I.C.5.b.2)).

2. Locate the first-level subterm **drug** if the substance is other than alcohol.

   - When the substance is alcohol, go directly to the subterm **alcohol**. *Alcoholism* is indexed as **Dependence, alcohol**.

Table 17-7 ■ **ASSIGNING CODES FOR SCHIZOPHRENIC SPECTRUM DISORDERS**

Condition	Description	Code(s)
Schizoaffective disorder	Characterized by an extended period in which schizophrenia is accompanied by major depressive, manic, or mixed episodes	F25.-
Schizoid of childhood (Asperger's syndrome)	Severe and sustained impairment in social interactions and restricted, repetitive patterns of behaviors, interests, and activities	F84.5
Schizoid personality disorder, schizothymia	Persistent withdrawal from social relationships and lack of emotional responsiveness in most situations	F60.1
Schizophrenia	Inability to distinguish between thoughts and reality, think logically, and have normal emotional and social relationships	F20.0 through F20.5
Schizophreniform disorder	Identical to schizophrenia except that the total duration is greater than one month but less than six months; impaired social or occupational functioning may not be apparent	F20.81
Schizotypal personality disorder	Trouble with relationships and disturbances in thought patterns, appearance, and behavior	F21

3. Locate a second-level subterm for the specific substance or class of substance.

   - **Cannabis**, **cocaine**, and **nicotine** are separate subterms.

   - Other substances are classified under subterms for the class of substance: **hallucinogen**, **inhalant**, **opioid**, **sedative**, **stimulant**, or **psychoactive substance NEC** (Table 17-3).

   - When *smoker* is documented, the Index entry **Smoker** directs you to the Main Term **Dependence** and the first- and second-level subterms **drug** then **nicotine**. Select a third-level subterm for the type of nicotine, such as chewing **tobacco** or **cigarettes**, if known.

4. Review the entries under the third-level subterm **with** to locate a combination code for the substance and any manifestations.

5. When the condition is stated as in remission, select the subterm **in remission**.

6. Verify the code in the Tabular List, being certain that all aspects of code title correctly describe the documented diagnosis.

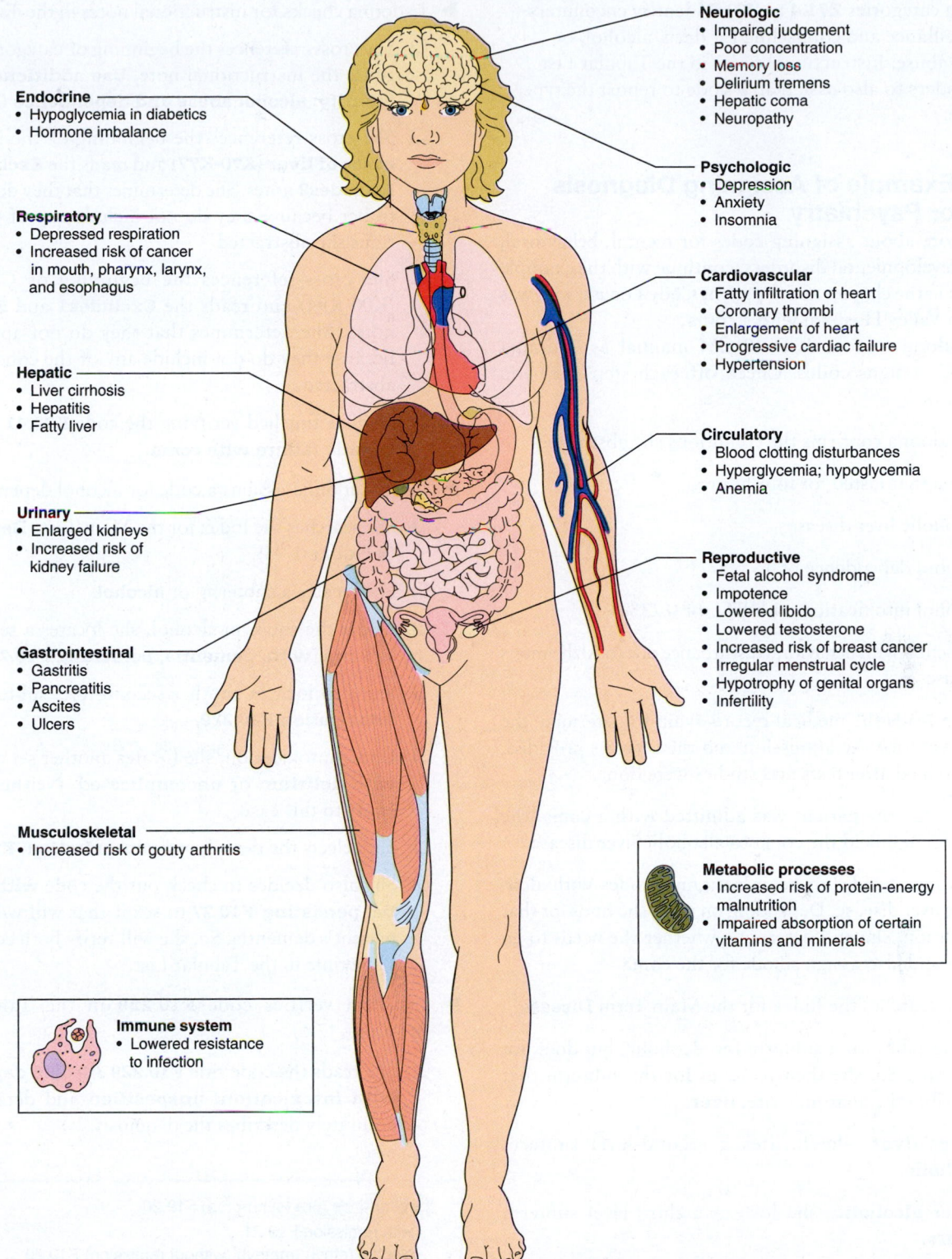

Neurologic
• Impaired judgement
• Poor concentration
• Memory loss
• Delirium tremens
• Hepatic coma
• Neuropathy

Psychologic
• Depression
• Anxiety
• Insomnia

Endocrine
• Hypoglycemia in diabetics
• Hormone imbalance

Respiratory
• Depressed respiration
• Increased risk of cancer
  in mouth, pharynx, larynx,
  and esophagus

Hepatic
• Liver cirrhosis
• Hepatitis
• Fatty liver

Urinary
• Enlarged kidneys
• Increased risk of
  kidney failure

Gastrointestinal
• Gastritis
• Pancreatitis
• Ascites
• Ulcers

Musculoskeletal
• Increased risk of gouty arthritis

Cardiovascular
• Fatty infiltration of heart
• Coronary thrombi
• Enlargement of heart
• Progressive cardiac failure
• Hypertension

Circulatory
• Blood clotting disturbances
• Hyperglycemia; hypoglycemia
• Anemia

Reproductive
• Fetal alcohol syndrome
• Impotence
• Lowered libido
• Lowered testosterone
• Increased risk of breast cancer
• Irregular menstrual cycle
• Hypotrophy of genital organs
• Infertility

Metabolic processes
• Increased risk of protein-energy
  malnutrition
• Impaired absorption of certain
  vitamins and minerals

Immune system
• Lowered resistance
  to infection

Figure 17-4 ■ The multisystem effects of alcohol use, abuse, and dependence.

Z codes related to substance use are needed in some situations:

• Code **Z87.891 Personal history of nicotine dependence** identifies that a person previously was dependent on nicotine but no longer is. This information must be documented by the physician. Patients are considered to be dependent on nicotine but in remission (**F17.201, F17.211,** **F17.221,** or **F17.291**) if they continue to crave nicotine for support, to maintain function, or to survive.

• Code **Z72.0 Tobacco use** reports that the patient has problems related to tobacco use but no further information is documented. This code should be used infrequently.

- Codes in categories **Z71.4** to **Z71.6** identify encounters for surveillance and counseling for drug, alcohol, or tobacco abuse. Instructional notes in the Tabular List direct coders to also assign an **F** code to report the type of abuse.

Guided Example of Assigning Diagnosis Codes for Psychiatry

To learn more about assigning codes for mental, behavioral, and neurodevelopmental disorders, continue with the example from earlier in the chapter about patient Cody Locust, who was admitted to Valley Hospital with a coma.

Follow along in your ICD-10-CM manual as Ladonna Shuck, CPC, assigns codes. Check off each step after you complete it.

▶ First, Ladonna confirms the conditions she abstracted:

❑ Coma that lasted for four hours

❑ Alcoholic liver disease

❑ Alcohol dependence of 15 years

❑ Alcohol intoxication with BAL of 0.23%

❑ Dementia with behavioral disturbance due to Alzheimer's disease

▶ Ladonna reads the medical record again to determine the main reason for the admission and the services provided, as determined after tests and studies were done.

❑ Although the patient was admitted with a coma, the physician linked the coma to alcoholic liver disease.

❑ Ladonna decides to begin assigning codes with alcoholic liver disease. Depending on what she finds for that condition, she will determine whether she needs to go back and also assign a code for the coma.

▶ Ladonna searches the Index for the Main Term **Disease**.

❑ She searches for a subterm for alcoholic, but does not find one. So, she then searches for the subterm that describes the anatomic site, **liver**.

❑ Under **liver**, she locates a second-level subterm **alcoholic**.

❑ Under **alcoholic**, she locates a third-level subterm **failure**.

❑ Under **failure**, she locates a fourth-level subterm **with coma K70.41**.

❑ This code appears to be a combination code that includes both alcoholic liver failure and the coma.

▶ Ladonna verifies code **K70.41** in the Tabular List.

❑ She reads the code title for **K70.41 Alcoholic hepatic failure with coma**. She knows that *hepatic* means "liver" and confirms that this accurately describes the diagnosis.

▶ Ladonna checks for instructional notes in the Tabular List.

❑ She cross-references the beginning of category **K70** and reads the instructional note, **Use additional code to identify: alcohol abuse and dependence (F10.-)**.

❑ She cross-references the beginning of the block **Diseases of liver (K70-K77)** and reads the **Excludes1** and **Excludes2** notes. She determines that they do not apply to her because they do not include any of the conditions she abstracted.

❑ She cross-references the beginning of Chapter 11 (K00-K94) and reads the **Excludes1** and **Excludes2** notes. She determines that they do not apply to her because they do not include any of the conditions she abstracted.

❑ She has finished verifying the code **K70.41 Alcoholic hepatic failure with coma**.

▶ Next, Ladonna assigns a code for alcohol dependence.

❑ She searches the Index for the Main Term **Dependence** (■ FIGURE 17-5).

❑ She locates a subterm for **alcohol**.

❑ Under the subterm alcohol, she locates a second-level subterm, **with, dementia, persisting F10.27**.

❑ She also locates another second-level subterm, **with, intoxication F10.229**.

❑ Under intoxication, she locates another set of choices: **with delirium** or **uncomplicated**. Neither of these apply to this case.

❑ She selects the default entry **intoxication, F10.229**.

❑ She also decides to check out the code **with, dementia, persisting F10.27** to see if that will work for the patient's dementia. So, she will verify both codes at the same time in the Tabular List.

▶ Ladonna verifies code **F10.229** in the Tabular List (■ FIGURE 17-6).

❑ She reads the code title **F10.229 Alcohol dependence with intoxication, unspecified** and determines it accurately describes the diagnosis.

Dependence (on) (syndrome) F19.20
  with remission F19.21
  alcohol (ethyl) (methyl) (without remission) F10.20
    with
      amnestic disorder, persisting F10.26
      anxiety disorder F10.280
      dementia, persisting F10.27
      intoxication F10.229
        with delirium F10.221
        uncomplicated F10.220
      mood disorder F10.24
      psychotic disorder F10.259

Figure 17-5 ■ Index entry for "Dependence, alcohol" used to located codes for alcohol dependence.

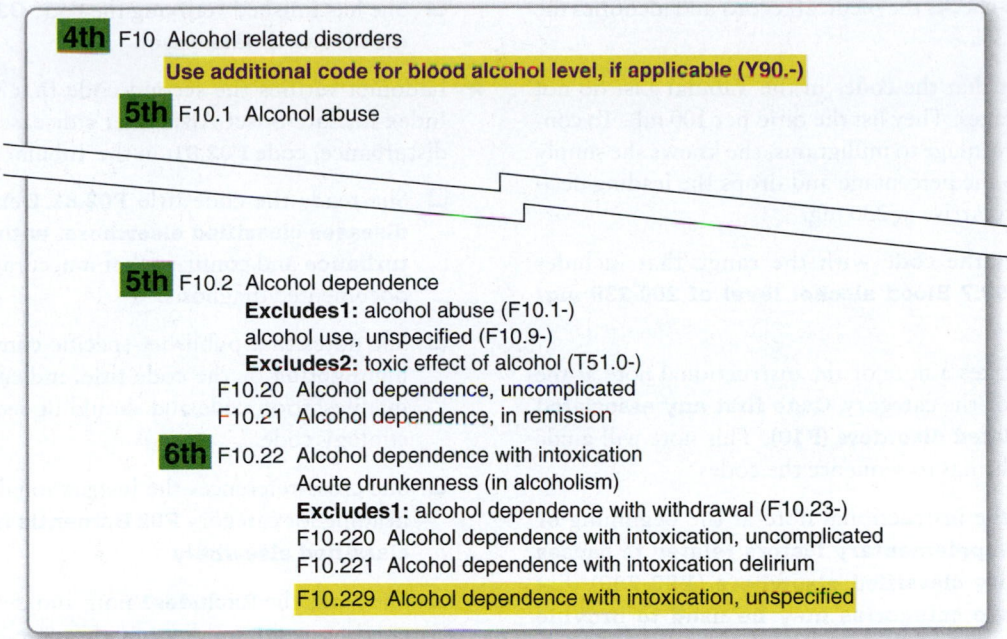

Figure 17-6 ■ Tabular List entry for category F10 "Alcohol related disorders".

❏ Next, she verifies the code **F10.27** and reads the code title: **Alcohol dependence with alcohol-induced persisting dementia**.

- She determines that this code does *not* accurately describe the dementia diagnosis.
- This code describes alcohol-induced dementia, but the medical record documents Alzheimer's dementia.
- She eliminates code **F10.27** from consideration.

❏ Ladonna still needs to check the instructional notes that apply to code **F10.229, Alcohol dependence with intoxication, unspecified**.

❏ She cross-references the beginning of the category **F10 Alcohol related disorders** and reads the instructional note that states, **Use additional code for blood alcohol level, if applicable (Y90.-)**.

- This instructional note applies to this case because the patient was intoxicated and the BAL is documented.

❏ She cross-references the beginning of the block **Mental and behavioral disorders due to psychoactive substance use (F10-F19)** and does not see any instructional notes.

❏ She cross-references the beginning of Chapter 5 (F01-F99). The only notes are an **Includes** note and an **Excludes2** note, neither of which applies to this case.

❏ She has finished verifying the code **F10.229, Alcohol dependence with intoxication, unspecified**.

▶ Next, Ladonna assigns the code for BAL, which the instructional note lists as **Y90.-**.

❏ She locates the entry for **Y90** and reads the category title: **Y90 Evidence of alcohol involvement determined by blood alcohol level** (■ FIGURE 17-7).

❏ She notices the symbol 4th next to the entry, so she knows she must assign an additional character.

Supplementary factors related to causes of morbidity classified elsewhere (Y90-Y99)

NOTE: These categories may be used to provide supplementary information concerning causes of morbidity. They are not to be used for single-condition coding.

4th Y90 Evidence of alcohol involvement determined by blood alcohol level

Code first any associated alcohol related disorders (F10)

Y90.0 Blood alcohol level of less than 20 mg/100 ml
Y90.1 Blood alcohol level of 20–39 mg/100 ml
Y90.2 Blood alcohol level of 40–59 mg/100 ml
Y90.3 Blood alcohol level of 60–79 mg/100 ml
Y90.4 Blood alcohol level of 80–99 mg/100 ml
Y90.5 Blood alcohol level of 100–119 mg/100 ml
Y90.6 Blood alcohol level of 120–199 mg/100 ml
Y90.7 Blood alcohol level of 200–239 mg/100 ml
Y90.8 Blood alcohol level of 240 mg/100 ml or more
Y90.9 Presence of alcohol in blood, level not specified

Figure 17-7 ■ Tabular List entry for category Y90 "Evidence of alcohol involvement determined by blood alcohol level".

❏ She double-checks the medical record and identifies the BAL as 0.23%.

❏ She notices that the codes in the Tabular List do not list percentages. They list the ratio per 100 mL. To convert the percentage to milligrams, she knows she simply adds a 0 to the percentage and drops the leading decimal point to arrive at 230 mg.

❏ She locates the code with the range that includes 230 mg, **Y90.7 Blood alcohol level of 200-239 mg/100 ml**.

❏ She also makes a note of the instructional note at the beginning of the category, **Code first any associated alcohol related disorders (F10).** This note will guide her when she has to sequence the codes.

❏ She reads the instructional note at the beginning of the block **Supplementary factors related to causes of morbidity classified elsewhere (Y90-Y99)** that states: **These categories may be used to provide supplementary information concerning causes of morbidity. They are not to be used for single-condition coding.** This note confirms that BAL is *not* a diagnosis that can stand alone; it must always be assigned in conjunction with other codes that describe the condition.

❏ She has finished verifying the code **Y90.7 Blood alcohol level of 200-239 mg/100 ml.**

▶ Next, Ladonna must determine the code for Alzheimer's with dementia.

▶ Ladonna searches the Index for the Main Term **Disease**.

❏ She locates the subterm **Alzheimer's**.

❏ She checks the medical record for details, then locates the second-level subterm **late onset**.

❏ Under **late onset**, she locates the third-level subterm **with behavioral disturbance G30.1 [F02.81].**

❏ She notices that two codes are provided. She knows that the *[slanted brackets]* are a coding manual convention that identifies the second code as a manifestation that must be sequenced second.

▶ Ladonna verifies code **G30.1** in the Tabular List.

❏ She reads the code title **G30.1 Alzheimer's disease with late onset** and confirms that it accurately describes the documented diagnosis.

❏ She cross-references the instructional notes under the heading for category **G30 Alzheimer's disease**.

❏ She reads the **Includes** and **Excludes1** notes. The conditions listed under **Excludes1** do not describe this case, so this note does not apply.

❏ She checks the beginning of the block and chapter for instructional notes but does not find any that apply to this case.

❏ She has finished verifying the code **G30.1 Alzheimer's disease with late onset**.

▶ Ladonna verifies the second code that was listed in the Index for late-onset Alzheimer's disease with behavioral disturbance, code **F02.81**, in the Tabular List.

❏ She reads the code title **F02.81 Dementia in other diseases classified elsewhere, with behavioral disturbance** and confirms that it accurately describes the documented diagnosis.

❏ She notes that publisher-specific conventions, such as highlighting of the code title, indicates that this is a manifestation code and should be sequenced after the etiology code.

❏ She cross-references the instructional notes under the heading for category **F02 Dementia in other diseases classified elsewhere**.

❏ She reads the **Excludes1** note and determines that the conditions do not describe this case, so this note does not apply.

❏ She reads the note **Code first the underlying physiological condition, such as:** and locates the entry for **Alzheimer's (G30.-).** This instruction confirms the sequencing order. The code for Alzheimer's should be sequenced before the code for dementia because it is the etiology.

❏ She reads the instructional note at the beginning of the block **Mental disorders due to known physiological conditions (F01-F09)** that describes the purpose of this category, but the note does not change the code assigned.

❏ She cross-references the beginning of Chapter 5 (F01-F99) for instructional notes, but does not find any that relate to this case.

❏ She has finished verifying the code **F02 Dementia in other diseases classified elsewhere**.

▶ Ladonna reviews the codes she has assigned for this case.

❏ **K70.41 Alcoholic hepatic failure with coma**

❏ **F10.229 Alcohol dependence with intoxication, unspecified**

❏ **Y90.7 Blood alcohol level, 200-239 mg/100 ml**

❏ **G30.1 Late onset Alzheimer's**

❏ **F02.81 Dementia in diseases classified elsewhere, with behavioral disturbance**

▶ Next, Ladonna must determine how to sequence the codes.

SUCCESS STEP

BAL is indexed in the Index to External Causes under the Main Term **Blood alcohol level**.

CODING PRACTICE

Exercise 17.3   Assigning Codes for Psychiatry

Instructions: Read the mini-medical-record of each patient's encounter, review the information abstracted in Exercise 17.2, and assign ICD-10-CM diagnosis codes using the Index and Tabular List. Write the code(s) on the line provided.

1. OFFICE   Gender: **F**   Age: **9**

Reason for encounter: Referred by pediatrician for hyperactivity, short attention span, and irritability

Assessment: After testing, symptoms are due to attention deficit hyperactive disorder, predominately hyperactive type

Plan: Start medication and behavior therapy

1 ICD-10-CM Code _____

2. INPATIENT HOSPITAL   Gender: **M**   Age: **31**

Reason for encounter: Extreme delusions of paranoia

Assessment: Dependent continual user of coke, psychosis with delusions due to dependence and long-term use of cocaine

Plan: Rx to help manage delusions, transfer to rehab

1 ICD-10-CM Code _____

3. OFFICE   Gender: **F**   Age: **21**

Reason for encounter: Ongoing medical management of schizophrenia

Assessment: Paranoid schizophrenia

Plan: Medication is managing the condition well. Renewed Rx. Patient is interested in getting a job. Referred to a supported employment service

Tip: The first code is a Z code to issue a repeat prescription.

2 ICD-10-CM Codes _____

ARRANGING DIAGNOSIS CODES FOR PSYCHIATRY

Sequencing of codes for mental, behavioral, and neurodevelopmental disorders is determined by instructional notes in the Tabular List. When mental disorders are associated with underlying physical conditions, the Tabular List provides an instructional note, **Code first the underlying physiological condition**. Coders must read the documentation carefully to identify when the physician documents a relationship between a mental disorder and a physiological condition.

Arranging Codes for Pain

ICD-10-CM provides codes to use when pain is documented as exclusively or partially psychological. The guidelines for coding pain are summarized next.

When pain is exclusively psychological with no identifiable medical condition and no documentation of acute or chronic pain, assign **F45.41 Pain disorder exclusively related to psychological factors**.

When pain is exclusively psychological and there is also documentation of acute or chronic pain, assign only code **F45.41** (OGCR I.C.5.a).

When the documentation reports pain with related psychological factors, assign and sequence codes as follows:

1. Assign the appropriate code from category **G89.- Pain, not elsewhere classified**.
2. Assign code **F45.42 Pain disorder with related psychological factors**.

Arranging Codes for Intellectual Disabilities

An instructional note in the Tabular List for intellectual disabilities (F70 through F79) directs coders to **Code first any associated physical or developmental disorders**. Following the lead of mental health advocates, the Social Security Administration adopted the term **intellectual disabilities** to replace the outdated and stigmatized term *mental retardation*. According to DSM-5, the following criteria must be met for a diagnosis of intellectual disabilities:

- An IQ below 70
- Significant limitations in two or more areas of adaptive behavior
- Evidence that the limitations became apparent before the age of 18

Refer to ■ FIGURE 17-8, (page 304) to learn more about sequencing codes for intellectual disabilities.

Guided Example of Arranging Diagnosis Codes for Psychiatry

To learn more about sequencing codes for mental, behavioral, and neurodevelopmental disorders, continue with the example from earlier in the chapter about patient Cody Locust, who was admitted to Valley Hospital with a coma.

Follow along in your ICD-10-CM manual as Ladonna Shuck, CPC, sequences the codes. Check off each step after you complete it.

Patient with moderate intellectual disabilities is seen for neurological endemic cretinism. Patient also has associated overactive disorder and difficulty with verbal expression. Patient is dependent on assistance with personal care.

(1) **E00.0 Congenital iodine-deficiency syndrome, neurological type**
(2) **F80.1 Expressive language disorder**
(3) **F84.8 Other pervasive developmental disorders**
(4) **Z74.1 Need for assistance with personal care**
(5) **F70 Mild intellectual disabilities**

Figure 17-8 ■ Example of sequencing codes for intellectual disabilities.

▶ First, Ladonna confirms the codes she assigned for this case.

❑ **K70.41 Alcoholic hepatic failure with coma**

❑ **F10.229 Alcohol dependence with intoxication, unspecified**

❑ **Y90.7 Blood alcohol level, 200-239 mg/100 ml**

❑ **G30.1 Late onset Alzheimer's**

❑ **F02.81 Dementia in diseases classified elsewhere, with behavioral disturbance**

▶ Ladonna takes a moment to read the medical record to review the details of the case.

❑ She confirms that the principal diagnosis is **K70.41 Alcoholic hepatic failure with coma** because it meets the definition of principal diagnosis defined by the Uniform Hospital Data Discharge Set (UHDDS) (OGCR II).

❑ She determines that the second code should be **F10.229 Alcohol dependence with intoxication, unspecified** because it further describes the principal diagnosis.

❑ Although the code for BAL relates to code **F10.229**, she decides to sequence it as the last code because it is a supplemental code.

❑ She determines that the third code should be **G30.1 Late onset Alzheimer's** because the documentation states that the condition was managed during the admission but does not qualify as the principal diagnosis.

❑ She sequences **F02.81 Dementia in diseases classified elsewhere, with behavioral disturbance** as the fourth code because it is a manifestation code for Alzheimer's and must be sequenced after **G30.1**. During the process of assigning codes, she found four instructional codes directing her to sequence the dementia code after the Alzheimer's code:

- The *[slanted brackets]* convention in the Index
- The instructional note in the Tabular List under category **G30** to **Use additional code** to identify the dementia
- A publisher's convention for the code **F02.81** in the Tabular List that identified it as a manifestation
- The instructional note in the Tabular List under category **F02** to **Code first the underlying condition**, Alzheimer's

❑ She sequences the final code as **Y90.7 Blood alcohol level, 200-239 mg/100 ml** because it is a supplemental code that provides added information but is not a diagnosis code on its own.

▶ Ladonna finalizes the codes and sequencing for this case:

(1) **K70.41 Alcoholic hepatic failure with coma**
(2) **F10.229 Alcohol dependence with intoxication, unspecified**
(3) **G30.1 Late onset Alzheimer's**
(4) **F02.81 Dementia in diseases classified elsewhere, with behavioral disturbance**
(5) **Y90.7 Blood alcohol level, 200–239 mg/100 ml**

CODING CAUTION

When the Tabular List provides the instructional note for Alzheimer's disease to **Code first the underlying condition**, it does not mean that Alzheimer's disease should always be the principal diagnosis. The note describes the relationship between Alzheimer's disease (the etiology) and dementia (the manifestation) (OGCR I.A.13). The principal diagnosis is determined based on the criteria in OGCR II.

CODING PRACTICE

Exercise 17.4 Arranging Diagnosis Codes
for Psychiatry

Instructions: Read the mini-medical-record of each patient's encounter, review the information abstracted in Exercise 17.2, assign ICD-10-CM diagnosis codes using the Index and Tabular List, and sequence them correctly.

1. OFFICE   Gender: M   Age: 10

Reason for encounter: I have been seeing this child for autism, but today his mother is concerned about continuing "fussing and worry about his private parts" that has been going on for quite awhile and his "desire to be like his sister."

Assessment: Gender identity disorder

Plan: Adjusted medications for current autism

2 ICD-10-CM Codes _____

CODING PRACTICE (continued)

2. **INPATIENT HOSPITAL**   Gender: M   Age: 48

Reason for encounter: Admitted from emergency department for alcohol-induced gastritis with hemorrhaging and intoxication with BAL of .09

Assessment: Patient has long-term alcohol use with dependence, prior cocaine abuser but states he no longer uses

Plan: Patient agreed to counseling after discharge

Tip: Follow instructional notes in the Tabular List to help determine sequencing.

4 ICD-10-CM Codes _____
_____

3. **INPATIENT HOSPITAL**   Gender: M   Age: 56

Reason for encounter: Severe depression due to bipolar disorder

Assessment: Patient is also being treated for liver cirrhosis with ascites due to chronic continuous alcoholism

Plan: Patient has stable living situation so we are going to discharge him to a partial hospitalization program

3 ICD-10-CM Codes _____
_____

CHAPTER SUMMARY

In this chapter you learned that:

- Mental, behavioral, and neurodevelopmental disorders are real, not imagined, disorders that have diagnostic criteria and are proven to respond to treatment.

- ICD-10-CM Official Guidelines for Coding and Reporting (OGCR) section I.C.5 provides detailed discussion of pain disorders related to psychological factors and mental, behavioral, and neurodevelopmental disorders due to substance abuse.

- Many mental, behavioral, and neurodevelopmental disorders have multiple subtypes, so coders must be particularly attentive to the documented wording of the condition.

- Three types of conditions in this ICD-10-CM chapter present challenges in assigning codes because of the level of detail that must be reported: bipolar disorder, schizophrenic disorders, and substance disorders.

- When mental disorders are associated with underlying physical conditions, the Tabular List provides an instructional note to code the underlying physiological condition first.

CONCEPT QUIZ

Take a moment to look back at mental, behavioral, and neurodevelopmental disorders and solidify your skills. Try to answer the questions from memory, first, then look back at the discussion in this chapter if you need a little extra help.

Completion

Instructions: Write the term that completes each statement based on the information you learned in this chapter. Choose from the list below. Some choices may be used more than once and some choices may not be used at all.

abuse	intoxication
barbiturate	mood
cognitive	narcotic
dependence	personality
dissociative	psychotic
hallucinogen	sexual
impulse-control	use
in remission	

1. Dementia is an example of a(n) _____ disorder.

2. Voyeurism is an example of a(n) _____ disorder.

3. Kleptomania is an example of a(n) _____ disorder.

4. Bipolar is an example of a(n) _____ disorder.

5. Phenobarbital is an example of the _____ class of drugs.

6. Fentanyl is an example of the _____ class of drugs.

7. LSD is an example of the _____ class of drugs.

8. _____ occurs when more of a substance is consumed than a person can physically tolerate, resulting in behavioral or physical abnormalities.

9. _____ is a past history of a substance disorder.

10. _____ of a substance is consuming it in moderate amounts that do not create significant legal, social, employment, family, or medical problems.

(continued from page 305)

Multiple Choice

Instructions: Circle the letter of the best answer to each question based on the information you learned in this chapter.

1. What type of disorders consist of delusions and hallucinations?
   A. Cognitive disorders
   B. Psychotic disorders
   C. Anxiety disorders
   D. Dissociative disorders

2. What type of disorders are physical symptoms that are not explained by medical conditions?
   A. Affective disorders
   B. Dissociative disorders
   C. Adjustment disorders
   D. Somatoform disorders

3. Which of the following substances is a narcotic?
   A. Secobarbital
   B. PCP
   C. Heroin
   D. Amphetamine

4. What is the term for a progressive loss of brain function that affects memory, thinking, language, judgment, and behavior?
   A. Dementia
   B. Alzheimer's disease
   C. Parkinson's disease
   D. Lewy body disease

5. What Main Term and subterms should be located in the Index to code for *cigarette smoker*?
   A. Main Term: Tobacco use, Subterm: cigarettes
   B. Main Term: Dependence, Subterms: drug, nicotine, cigarettes
   C. Main Term: Cigarette, Subterm: smoker
   D. Main Term: Smoker, Subterm: cigarettes

6. How many mg per 100 mL is a BAL of 0.08%?
   A. 0.8 mg per 100 mL
   B. 8 mg per 100 mL
   C. 80 mg per 100 mL
   D. 800 mg per 100 mL

7. How would you code the following scenario? *A patient is seen for alcohol abuse and dependence.*
   A. F10.10
   B. F10.20
   C. F10.10, F20.20
   D. F20.20, F10.10

8. How would you code the following scenario? *A patient is seen for paranoid schizophrenia.*
   A. F20.0
   B. F21
   C. F23
   D. F25.9

9. How would you code the following scenario? *A 10-year-old patient is seen for attention-deficit hyperactivity disorder, predominantly hyperactive type.*
   A. F94.8
   B. F90.0
   C. F84.3
   D. F90.1

10. What information is stated in the instructional note in the Tabular List for intellectual disabilities (F70 through F79)?
    A. Code first any associated physical or developmental disorders.
    B. Use additional codes for any associated physical or developmental disorders.
    C. Assign combination codes for the intellectual disability and any associated physical or developmental disorders.
    D. Do not code any associated physical or developmental disorders.

KEEP ON CODING

Instructions: Read the diagnostic statement, then use the Index and Tabular List to assign and sequence ICD-10-CM diagnosis codes. Write the code(s) on the line provided.

1. Acute brain syndrome. ICD-10-CM Code(s) _____

2. Catatonic schizophrenia. ICD-10-CM Code(s) _____

3. Thumb-sucking. ICD-10-CM Code(s) _____

4. Bulimia nervosa. ICD-10-CM Code(s) _____

5. Fear of flying. ICD-10-CM Code(s) _____

6. Nicotine dependence with withdrawal. ICD-10-CM Code(s) _____

7. Alcohol abuse with alcohol-induced sleep disorder. ICD-10-CM Code(s) _____

8. Bipolar II disorder. ICD-10-CM Code(s) _____

9. Adjustment disorder with anxiety. ICD-10-CM Code(s) _____

10. Primary hypersomnia. ICD-10-CM Code(s) _____

11. Voyeurism. ICD-10-CM Code(s) _____

12. Autistic disorder. ICD-10-CM Code(s) _____

13. Intellectual disability with IQ level 19. ICD-10-CM Code(s) _____

14. Psychogenic encopresis. ICD-10-CM Code(s) _____

15. Trichotillomania. ICD-10-CM Code(s) _____

16. Abuse of antacids. ICD-10-CM Code(s) _____

17. Dissociative stupor. ICD-10-CM Code(s) _____

18. Sleepwalking. ICD-10-CM Code(s) _____

19. Selective mutism. ICD-10-CM Code(s) _____

20. Psychogenic torticollis. ICD-10-CM Code(s) _____

21. Dysthymic disorder. ICD-10-CM Code(s) _____

22. Hypochondria. ICD-10-CM Code(s) _____

23. Clumsy child syndrome. ICD-10-CM Code(s) _____

24. Cigarette smoker. ICD-10-CM Code(s) _____

25. Cocaine dependence in remission. ICD-10-CM Code(s) _____

CODING CHALLENGE

Instructions: Read the mini-medical-record of each patient's encounter, then abstract, assign, and sequence ICD-10-CM diagnosis codes using the Index and Tabular List. Write the code(s) on the line provided.

1. OFFICE   Gender: M   Age: 19

Reason for encounter: Pattern of exacerbation of asthma attacks on the weekends

Assessment: Psychogenic moderate persistent asthma

Plan: Allergy studies are scheduled in addition to follow-up with a family systems therapist to address the psychogenic component

Tip: Read the instructional notes in the Tabular List to determine the codes and sequencing.

2 ICD-10-CM Codes _____

2. OFFICE   Gender: F   Age: 20

Reason for encounter: Veteran experiencing flashbacks accompanied by nightmares, angry outbursts, hypervigilance, and anxiousness

Assessment: Chronic posttraumatic stress disorder

Plan: Trauma-focused cognitive-behavioral treatment (TFCBT) 12 weeks

1 ICD-10-CM Code _____

3. OFFICE   Gender: M   Age: 52

Reason for encounter: Review results of brain MRI ordered after he complained at a previous visit of episodes of sleepwalking

Assessment: MRI shows brain metastasis from pancreatic cancer; patient has secondary diabetes d/t pancreatic cancer and is on long-term insulin

Plan: Refer to neurologist for further workup on sleepwalking

Tip: Review OGCR I.C.2.a and b for sequencing of neoplasm codes. Review OGCR I.C.4.a.6) regarding secondary diabetes.

5 ICD-10-CM Codes _____

_____

4. OFFICE   Gender: M   Age: 26

Reason for encounter: Patient reports feeling extremely irritable, having cold sweats, and headaches. He went cold turkey for 4 days to try and get off heroin.

Assessment: Symptoms are due to drug withdrawal with heroin dependence

Plan: The patient met with a drug counselor to discuss a more appropriate way to address his addiction, started patient on methadone (*opiate substitute*) treatment

1 ICD-10-CM Code _____

5. INPATIENT HOSPITAL   Gender: F   Age: 36

Reason for encounter: Severe depression, has considered suicide

Assessment: Depression and suicide ideation due to persistent anxiety regarding being unemployed for the past year

Plan: Psychotherapy with no-suicide contract, antidepressant medication, refer to unemployment support group

3 ICD-10-CM Codes _____

_____

6. OFFICE   Gender: M   Age: 43

Reason for encounter: Depressed mood (3-week duration), excessive sleep, fatigue

Assessment: Depressive episode due to bipolar disorder which is in partial remission

Plan: Dosage change of present mood stabilizer, psychotherapy

1 ICD-10-CM Code _____

7. OFFICE   Gender: F   Age: 22

Reason for encounter: Excessive sadness, crying, sleeping, lethargy, feeling emotionally numb. Gave birth 3 weeks ago

Assessment: Postpartum depression

Plan: Interpersonal relationship counseling, Rx SSRI (*selective serotonin reuptake inhibitor*) antidepressant meds, obtain part time mother's helper

1 ICD-10-CM Code _____

8. OFFICE   Gender: F   Age: 10

Reason for encounter: Struggling in school with reading and spelling

Assessment: Developmental dyslexia, spelling disorder

Plan: Special ed schooling, teach compensating and coping skills

2 ICD-10-CM Codes _____

9. INPATIENT HOSPITAL   Gender: F   Age: 16

Reason for admission: Admitted from psychiatrist's office for multiple personality disorder

Assessment: Multiple personality disorder and mild intellectual disability. Patient presents with learning deficiencies (IQ 65) and with physical disability of anemia due to poor nutrition.

Plan: Psychotherapy weekly, transfer patient into special education program at school, home visit by social services to address nutritional issues

Tip: Assign codes for the personality disorder, the cognitive disorder, and the physical disability.

3 ICD-10-CM Codes _____

_____

10. OFFICE   Gender: F   Age: 25

Reason for encounter: Chewing tobacco since age 13 and wants to quit

Assessment: Counseling to address dependence on tobacco

Plan: RTO 1 week

Tip: Read the instructional note in the Tabular List that indicates sequencing.

2 ICD-10-CM Codes _____

Diseases of the Eye and Adnexa (H00–H59)

Learning Objectives

After completing this chapter, you should have the skills to:

18.1 Spell and define the key words, medical terms, and abbreviations related to diseases of the eye and ocular adnexa. (Remember)

18.2 Summarize the structure, function, and common conditions of the eye and ocular adnexa. (Understand)

18.3 Adhere to the Official Guidelines for Coding and Reporting related to diseases of the eye and ocular adnexa. (Apply)

18.4 Examine and abstract diagnostic information from the medical record for conditions of the eye and ocular adnexa. (Analyze)

18.5 Demonstrate how to assign codes for diseases of the eye and ocular adnexa. (Apply)

18.6 Utilize guidelines for arranging (sequencing) multiple diagnosis codes for diseases of the eye and ocular adnexa. (Apply)

18.7 Demonstrate how to abstract, assign, and sequence codes for neoplasms of the eye and ocular adnexa. (Apply)

Chapter Outline

- **Eye Refresher**
- **Coding Guidelines for the Eye**
- **Abstracting for Eye Conditions**
- **Assigning Codes for Eye Conditions**
- **Arranging Codes for Eye Conditions**
- **Coding Neoplasms of the Eye**

Key Terms and Abbreviations

adnexa	cornea	orbital cavity	sclera
choroid	lens	pupil	vitreous body
cone	ocular globe	retina	
conjunctiva	optic nerve	rod	

In addition to the key terms listed here, students should know the terms defined within tables in this chapter.

INTRODUCTION

A camera, particularly a traditional film camera, collects and focuses light in a manner very similar to the human eye. In this chapter you learn more about how the eye and ocular adnexa works, why sometimes they do not work as they should, and how physicians treat these conditions.

An ophthalmologist is a physician (MD) who specializes in diagnosing and treating diseases of the eye. Ophthalmologists may specialize in a specific part of the eye, such as the cornea or the retina. An optometrist is a doctor of optometry (OD) who specializes in examining the eyes and prescribing corrective lenses. Optometrists screen patients for certain eye diseases, such as glaucoma, and refer patients to an ophthalmologist if there are any concerns. Opticians are technical specialists who design, fit, and dispense corrective lenses and other ophthalmic appliances. Dermatologists might treat conditions affecting the eyelid and skin around the eye.

EYE REFRESHER

The eye and ocular **adnexa** (*associated anatomic structures*) make vision possible by receiving light from the external world and converting it into impulses that are transmitted to the brain through the **optic nerve**, which is cranial nerve II. The **ocular globe** refers to the eyeball itself. The eyeball consists of three layers: the **sclera** (*tough, white outer layer*), the **choroid** (*opaque middle layer that supplies blood to the eye*), and the **retina** (*the innermost layer that contains sensory receptor cells*). The **orbital cavity** is the bony structure around the eye, commonly known as the eye socket. The adnexa are the surrounding ocular muscles, eyelids, and **conjunctiva** (*membrane that lines the eyelids*) (■ FIGURE 18-1).

Light rays pass through the **cornea** (*the clear hard portion of the sclera that protects the lens*), **pupil** (*the black central part of the eye that constricts and dilates in response to light*), **lens** (*the clear part of the front of the eye that focuses light rays on the retina*), and **vitreous body** (*the transparent jelly that fills the eyeball and is surrounded by a membrane*) to focus on the retina. **Rods** and **cones** (*light-sensitive receptor cells*) in the retina are stimulated and transmit sensory impulses to the brain, which interprets the impulses as a visual image.

In Figure 18-1, each structure in the eye is labeled with its name as well as its medical terminology root/combining form where applicable. Refer to ■ TABLE 18-1 for a refresher on how to build medical terms related to the eye and ocular adnexa.

Conditions of the Eye

Refer to ■ TABLE 18-2 for a summary of diseases affecting the eye and ocular adnexa. It is important to identify where a condition occurs, such as the eyelid or eyeball, as well as the specific site within the eyeball. Ophthalmologists often specialize in either the front of the eye—the sclera, cornea, pupil, iris, and lens—or the back of the eye—the vitreous gel, macular, optic nerve, and retina.

Common symptoms of eye conditions include blurriness, burning and/or redness; distortion, reduction, or loss of vision;

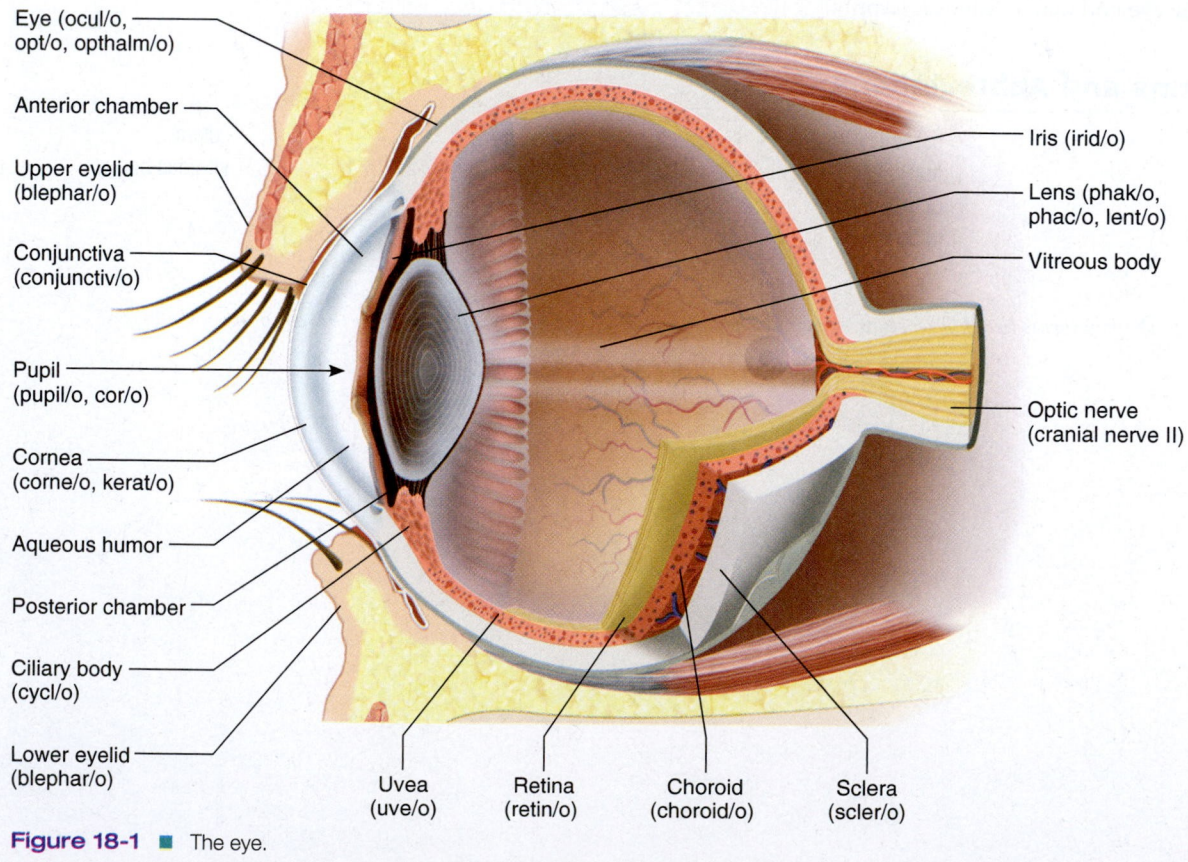

Figure 18-1 ■ The eye.

Table 18-1 ■ **EXAMPLE OF CONSTRUCTING MEDICAL TERMS FOR THE EYE AND OCULAR ADNEXA**

Combining Form	Suffix	Complete Medical Term
retin/o (*retina*)		retin + itis (*inflammation of the retina*)
	-itis (*inflammation*)	retino + pathy (*abnormal condition of the retina*)
blephar/o (*eyelid*)	-ptosis (*drooping*)	blephar + itis (*inflammation of the eyelid*)
	-pathy (*abnormal condition*)	blephar + optosis (*drooping eyelid*)
choroid/o (*vascular coat of the eye*)		choroid + itis (*inflammation of the vascular coat of the eye*)

Table 18-2 ■ **COMMON DISEASES OF THE EYE AND OCULAR ADNEXA**

Condition	Definition
Astigmatism	Blurred vision at all distances, caused by an irregularly shaped cornea
Blepharitis	An inflammation and infection of hair follicles and glands at the margins of the eyelids due to virus, bacteria, allergic response, or exposure to irritants
Cataract	A cloudiness of the lens that usually develops slowly over time due to aging
Chalazion	A small hard cyst on the eyelid caused by blockage of a gland on the eyelid
Conjunctivitis	A viral or bacterial inflammation and infection of the conjunctiva
Diabetic retinopathy	The abnormal expansion of blood vessels and hemorrhaging in the vessels of the retina, caused by diabetes
Glaucoma	An increased fluid pressure within the eye that damages the optic nerve and can cause blindness
Hordeolum	A bacterial inflammation of a sebaceous gland on the edge or lining of the eyelid; also called a *stye*
Hyperopia	Farsightedness, poor near vision
Keratitis	An inflammation and ulceration of the surface of the cornea
Macular degeneration	The gradual loss of central vision due to aging, with no cure (■ Figure 18-2 and ■ Figure 18-3)
Myopia	Nearsightedness, poor distance vision
Presbyopia	Normal age-related loss of focusing ability after age 40
Retinal detachment	The separation of the retina from the choroid layer of the eye

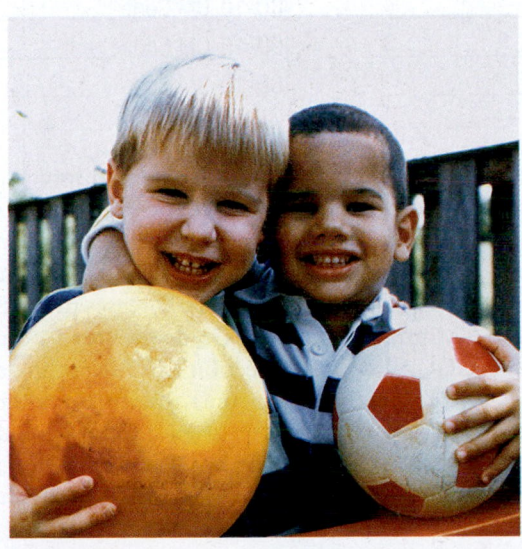

Figure 18-2 ■ Clear image as seen by a person with normal vision. *Source: National Eye Institute, National Institutes of Health.*

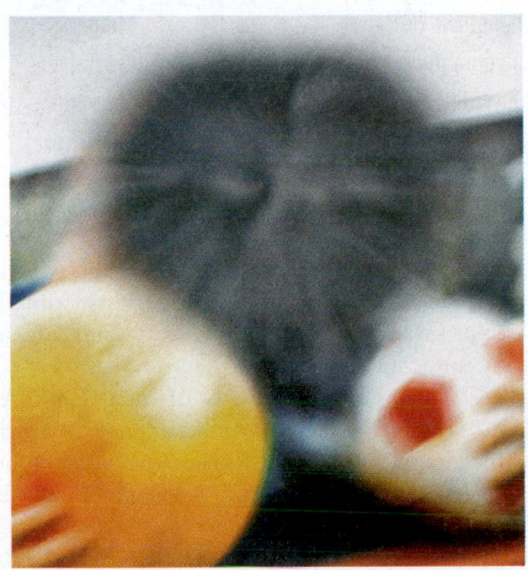

Figure 18-3 ■ Image with darkened central area as seen by a person with macular degeneration and related loss of central vision *Source: National Eye Institute, National Institutes of Health.*

limited movement of the eye or eyelid, pain; and sensations such as spots, floaters, flashes, halos, and starbursts. As with any body system, symptoms and signs can be related to a variety of conditions. Eye conditions are diagnosed through a visual examination using a variety of specialized equipment that allows a physician to see or digitally map the structures of the eye.

Refractive errors are conditions such as myopia, hyperopia, astigmatism, and presbyopia that affect vision due to how the eye collects and focuses light. Refractive errors are diagnosed with a vision test and can be corrected with lenses or surgery. Other methods are used for more complex cases.

CODING CAUTION

Be alert for medical words that sound and are spelled similarly but have different meanings.

uvea (*the middle layer of the eye consisting of the iris, ciliary body, and choroid*) and **uvula** (*a pendant fleshy lobe, most commonly referred to as the one in the back of the mouth*)

keratitis (*inflammation of the cornea*) and **keratin** (*horny tissues found in the epidermis, hair, and nails*)

choroid (*the middle layer of the eye*) and **colloid** (*gelatin-like or mucous substance found in tissues*)

CODING PRACTICE

Exercise 18.1   Eye Refresher

Instructions: Use your medical terminology skills and resources to define the following conditions related to the eye and ocular adnexa, then assign the default diagnosis code.

Follow these steps:

- Use slash marks "/" to break down each term into its root(s) and suffix.
- Define the meaning of the word, based on the meaning of each word part.
- Assign the default ICD-10-CM diagnosis code for the condition, including laterality, using the Index and Tabular List.

Example: conjunctivitis (right eye, acute)   Meaning *inflammation of the lining of the eye*   ICD-10-CM Code *H10.31*
conjunctiv/itis

1. photokeratitis (right eye)	Meaning _____	ICD-10-CM Code _____
2. retinoblastoma (left eye)	Meaning _____	ICD-10-CM Code _____
3. lagophthalmos	Meaning _____	ICD-10-CM Code _____
4. blepharoptosis (bilateral)	Meaning _____	ICD-10-CM Code _____
5. dacryoadenitis (right eye)	Meaning _____	ICD-10-CM Code _____
6. keratomalacia (bilateral)	Meaning _____	ICD-10-CM Code _____
7. retinoschisis (left eye)	Meaning _____	ICD-10-CM Code _____
8. amblyopia (bilateral)	Meaning _____	ICD-10-CM Code _____
9. iridocyclitis	Meaning _____	ICD-10-CM Code _____
10. aphakia (right eye)	Meaning _____	ICD-10-CM Code _____

CODING GUIDELINES FOR THE EYE

Coders should understand the organization of this ICD-10-CM chapter, chapter-wide and commonly used instructional notes in the Tabular List, and the relevant OGCR. This information is necessary for accurate coding.

ICD-10-CM Chapter 7, "Diseases of the Eye and Adnexa (H00–H59)," contains 12 blocks or subchapters that are divided by anatomic site within the eye. Review the block names and code ranges listed at the beginning of Chapter 7 in the ICD-10-CM manual to become familiar with the content and organization. This chapter is one of two in which codes begin with the letter H; codes for the ear and mastoid process occupy codes H60 through H95.

This chapter includes disorders affecting each structure within the eye, glaucoma, and visual disturbances and blindness. It does not include injuries to the eye, congenital conditions,

or infectious, parasitic, or syphilis-related eye disorders, which are classified in other ICD-10-CM chapters. It also does not include diabetic or many other endocrine eye disorders, which are reported with combination codes in ICD-10-CM Chapter 4, "Endocrine, Nutritional, and Metabolic Diseases (E00–E89)."

ICD-10-CM provides Official Guidelines for Coding and Reporting (OGCR) in OGCR section I.C.7 regarding assigning codes for the stages of glaucoma. Instructional notes in the Tabular List guide the coder when additional codes are required. An instructional note at the beginning of the chapter directs coders to use an external cause code following the code for the eye condition when an external cause is involved in creating the eye condition. This note applies to all codes in ICD-10-CM Chapter 7. Most codes include specificity of anatomic site and laterality. Specific OGCR and instructional notes are discussed and cited throughout this chapter of the text.

ABSTRACTING FOR EYE CONDITIONS

The main concerns when abstracting eye conditions are identifying laterality and the presence of underlying conditions, particularly diabetes. The majority of eye conditions require that the laterality be identified. Laterality is expressed at the following levels:

- Right, left, or unspecified eye
- Bilateral, for applicable conditions
- Upper, lower, or unspecified lid of each eye, for applicable conditions

Refer to ■ TABLE 18-3 for guidance on how to abstract conditions of the eye and ocular adnexa. Remember that the abstracting questions are a guide and that not every question applies to, or can be answered for, every case. For example, some conditions, such as glaucoma and conjunctivitis, are designated as acute or chronic, while other conditions, such as cataract(s), are not.

Abstracting Diabetic Eye Conditions

Retinopathy and cataract(s) are common diabetic manifestations. Even though diabetic eye conditions are not classified to ICD-10-CM Chapter 7, coders must know how to abstract them. Laterality is required for most diabetic manifestations. Refer to ■ TABLE 18-4 to learn key criteria for abstracting ophthalmic manifestations of diabetes.

ICD-10-CM presumes a causal relationship between diabetes and most ophthalmic manifestations, unless documented otherwise. This rule is based on clinical standards, OCGR I.A.15, and guidance in the *Coding Clinic* newsletter published by the American Hospital Association. Age-related cataracts are coded as a diabetic manifestation because diabetes accelerates the condition. Refer to Chapter 9, "Endocrine, Nutritional, and Metabolic Diseases (E00-E89)," of this text for more information.

Guided Example of Abstracting for Eye Conditions

Refer to the following example throughout this chapter to learn about abstracting, assigning, and sequencing eye and ocular adnexa codes. Megan Scheidler, CCS-P, is a fictitious coder who guides you through the coding process.

Date: 9/1/yy   Location: Branton Eye Care

Provider: Margo Bittinger, MD

Patient: Jaclyn Vandeventer   Gender: F   Age: 71

Reason for encounter: Referred by optometrist after abnormal findings on a routine vision exam

Assessment: Right normal tension glaucoma, mild stage (*damage to the optic nerve despite normal pressure in the eye*), age related nuclear (*centrally located*) cataracts bilaterally that are interfering with vision

Plan: Drops and medication for glaucoma, we will see how that does, then see if surgery is needed, we will wait on cataract removal until the glaucoma is controlled

---

Follow along as Megan Scheidler, CCS-P, abstracts the diagnosis. Check off each step after you complete it.

▶ Megan reads through the entire record, paying special attention to the reason for the encounter and the final assessment.

❑ She notes that the patient was seen at a clinic by an optometrist who identified some concerns that required the attention of an ophthalmologist.

▶ Megan refers to Key Criteria for Abstracting Conditions of the Eye and Ocular Adnexa (Table 18-3) and begins with glaucoma.

❑ *What is the condition?* Glaucoma (■ FIGURE 18-4).

❑ *What is the subtype of the condition?* Normal-tension glaucoma

Table 18-3   ■   KEY CRITERIA FOR ABSTRACTING CONDITIONS OF THE EYE AND OCULAR ADNEXA

- ❑ What is the condition?
- ❑ What is the subtype of the condition?
- ❑ Is a more specific subtype documented?
- ❑ What is the stage (certain types of glaucoma and macular degeneration)?
- ❑ Is laterality right, left, bilateral, or unspecified?
- ❑ For conditions affecting the eyelid, is the upper or lower lid involved?
- ❑ Is the condition acute or chronic?
- ❑ Is the eye condition secondary to diabetes or a condition from another body system?
- ❑ Do any additional eye conditions exist?
- ❑ Is the condition due to an external cause?

Table 18-4   ■   KEY CRITERIA FOR ABSTRACTING OPHTHALMIC MANIFESTATIONS OF DIABETES

- ❑ Is the diabetes type 1 or type 2?
- ❑ Is the eye condition related to diabetes (per the documentation or ICD-10-CM Index)?
- ❑ Is the condition retinopathy, cataract(s), or other?
- ❑ What is the laterality?

Retinopathy

- ❑ Is retinopathy proliferative or nonproliferative?
- ❑ Is nonproliferative retinopathy mild, moderate, or severe?
- ❑ Is retinopathy accompanied by macular edema?

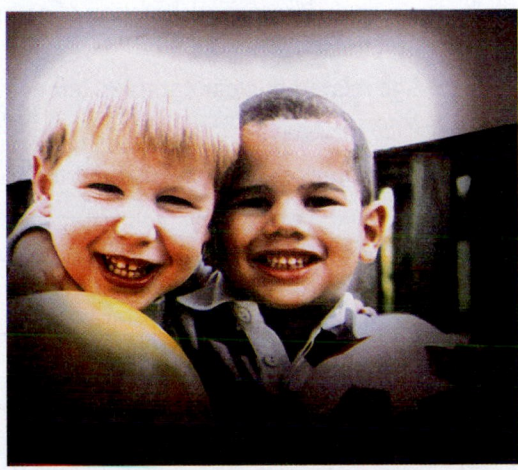

Figure 18-4 ■ Image with darkened edges as seen by a person with glaucoma and related tunnel vision.
Source: National Eye Institute, National Institutes of Health

❑ *Is laterality right, left, bilateral, or unspecified?* Right eye

❑ *What is the stage?* Mild

❑ *Is the condition acute or chronic?* She notes that acute or chronic does not apply to glaucoma

❑ *Is the eye condition secondary to diabetes or a condition from another body system?* No

❑ *Do any additional eye conditions exist?* Yes, cataracts are documented

❑ *Is the condition due to an external cause?* No

▶ Next, Megan abstracts for cataracts (■ FIGURE 18-5).

❑ *What is the condition?* Cataracts

❑ *What is the subtype of the condition?* Age related

❑ *Is a more specific subtype documented?* Nuclear

❑ *Is laterality right, left, bilateral, or unspecified?* The laterality is both eyes; she notes that although the glaucoma affects only the right eye, the cataracts are bilateral

❑ *Is the condition acute or chronic?* Acute or chronic is not applicable to cataracts

❑ *Is the eye condition secondary to diabetes or a condition from another body system?* No

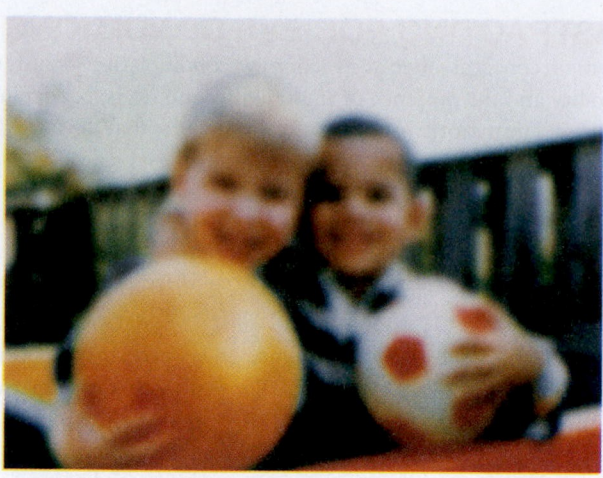

Figure 18-5 ■ Blurry image as seen by a person with cataracts *Source: National Eye Institute, National Institutes of Health.*

❑ *Do any additional eye conditions exist?* No

❑ *Is the condition due to an external cause?* No

▶ At this time, Megan thinks she will need a code for glaucoma and a code for cataracts, but she will not know for certain until she moves on to assigning codes.

CODING PRACTICE

Exercise 18.2 Abstracting for Eye Conditions

Instructions: Read the mini-medical-record of each patient's encounter and answer the abstracting questions. Write the answer on the line provided. Do not assign any codes.

1. OFFICE   Gender: M   Age: 76

Reason for encounter: Phacoemulsification of cataract and intraocular lens (IOL) implant

Assessment: Age related nuclear cataract, left eye

Plan: FU in office in, 2 days

a. Define the procedures that are the reason for the encounter. _____

b. What is the condition? _____

c. What is the subtype of the condition? _____

d. What is the laterality? _____

2. OFFICE   Gender: F   Age: 84

Reason for encounter: Monthly retinal injections

Assessment: Stage 2 wet macular degeneration, in both eyes

Plan: Return 1 month

a. Define the procedure that is the reason for the encounter. _____

b. What is the condition? _____

c. What is the subtype of the condition? _____

d. What is the laterality? _____

3. OFFICE   Gender: F   Age: 69

Reason for encounter: Crusty eyelids

Assessment: Nonulcerative blepharitis on both upper lids

(continued)

CODING PRACTICE (continued)

3. (continued)

Plan: Keep clean, Rx topical antibiotic

a. What is the condition? _____

b. What is the subtype of the condition? _____
_____

c. What is the laterality? _____

d. Is the upper or lower lid involved on the right side?
_____

   On the left side? _____

4. OFFICE   Gender: M   Age: 61

Reason for encounter: Routine eye exam as part of diabetic monitoring

Assessment: Moderate diabetic nonproliferative retinopathy with no macular edema, bilateral

Plan: Be diligent about keeping sugar and BP well controlled, to slow progression of condition

a. What is the reason for the encounter? _____
_____

b. Are there abnormal findings? _____
_____

c. What eye condition is diagnosed? _____
_____

d. Is it proliferative or nonproliferative? _____
_____

e. Is it mild, moderate, or severe? _____
_____

f. Is it accompanied by macular edema? _____
_____

g. What is the underlying condition? _____
_____

h. What is the type? _____
_____

5. OFFICE   Gender: F   Age: 53

Reason for encounter: Blurred vision, eye pain, floaters in both eyes

Assessment: Bilateral anterior uveitis due to juvenile rheumatoid arthritis, associated cataract with neovascularization in left eye also noted

Plan: Eye drops, dark glasses

a. What is the condition? _____

b. What is the laterality? _____

c. What additional eye condition exists? _____
_____

d. What is the subtype of the additional condition?
_____

e. What is the laterality of the additional condition?

f. Is the eye condition secondary to a condition from another body system? _____
_____

6. OFFICE   Gender: F   Age: 54

Reason for encounter: Difficulty seeing, gritty feeling in eyes, ocular hyperemia (*bloodshot eye*)

Assessment: Bilateral grade 2 corneal and conjunctival deposits, likely due to end-stage renal failure, patient has been on dialysis for about 18 months

Plan: Schedule cornea scraping to remove deposits

a. What are the symptoms and signs? _____

b. What two eye conditions are diagnosed? _____
_____

c. What is the laterality? _____

d. Are the symptoms integral to the condition(s)?
_____

e. What is the underlying condition? _____
_____

   What stage?_____

f. How is the underlying condition being treated?
_____

ASSIGNING CODES FOR EYE CONDITIONS

Coders need to be attentive when assigning codes that involve laterality. The fifth or sixth character of the code identifies laterality. Always verify the character for laterality in the Tabular List. Although often the right side is **1**, the left side is **2**, and bilateral is **3**, this is not always the case. In some categories, laterality designations use characters other than **1**, **2**, or **3**. Some codes that have laterality do not provide an option for bilateral because the condition is commonly unilateral.

When a condition affects both eyes, but no code is provided for bilateral, assign two codes: one for the right eye and a second one for the left eye (OGCR I.B.13). For example, disorders of the eyelid have codes for right and left laterality as well as upper and lower but do not usually have codes for bilateral (■ FIGURE 18-6, page 316).

When coding glaucoma, assign a seventh character to identify the stage of glaucoma as **unspecified, mild, moderate, severe, or indeterminate**. Assign as many codes as necessary from category **H40 Glaucoma** to fully describe the type of glaucoma, the affected eye, and the stage (OGCR I.C.7.a).

Patient is seen for senile entropion (*turning inward*) of both upper eyelids.

H02.031	Senile entropion of **right** upper eyelid
H02.034	Senile entropion of **left** upper eyelid

Figure 18-6 ■ Example of assigning codes for a bilateral condition when no code option for bilaterality exists.

Assigning Codes for Diabetic Eye Conditions

Codes for diabetic ophthalmic manifestations are not indexed under the Main Term for the eye condition, such as retinopathy. They are indexed under the Main Term **Diabetes**, then a subterm for the type of diabetes, then a second-level subterm for the specific manifestation, such as retinopathy or cataract(s). In the Tabular List, diabetes is classified in block **E08-E13**. Each three-digit category describes a different form of diabetes. Each category has a specific subcategory for ophthalmic manifestations, which are identified with the fourth character of **3** (■ FIGURE 18-7).

The fifth and sixth characters describe the type of ophthalmic condition. Refer to ■ FIGURE 18-8 to learn more about locating codes for diabetic eye manifestations.

Guided Example of Assigning Codes for Eye Conditions

To learn more about assigning codes for diseases of the eye and ocular adnexa, continue with the example from earlier in the chapter about patient Jaclyn Vandeventer, who was seen at Branton Eye Care due to glaucoma and cataracts.

Follow along in your ICD-10-CM manual as Megan Scheidler, CCS-P, assigns codes. Check off each step after you complete it.

▶ First, Megan confirms the conditions she abstracted.

❏ Right normal tension glaucoma, mild stage

❏ Bilateral age-related nuclear cataracts

▶ Megan searches the Index for the Main Term **Glaucoma** (■ FIGURE 18-9).

❏ She locates the subterm **low tension**.

❏ She reads the cross-reference instruction that states **—see Glaucoma, open angle, low-tension.**

❏ She locates the subterm **open angle, low-tension H40.12-.**

▶ Megan verifies code **H40.12-** in the Tabular List (■ FIGURE 18-10).

❏ She reads the code title for H40.12 Low-tension glaucoma and confirms that this accurately describes the diagnosis.

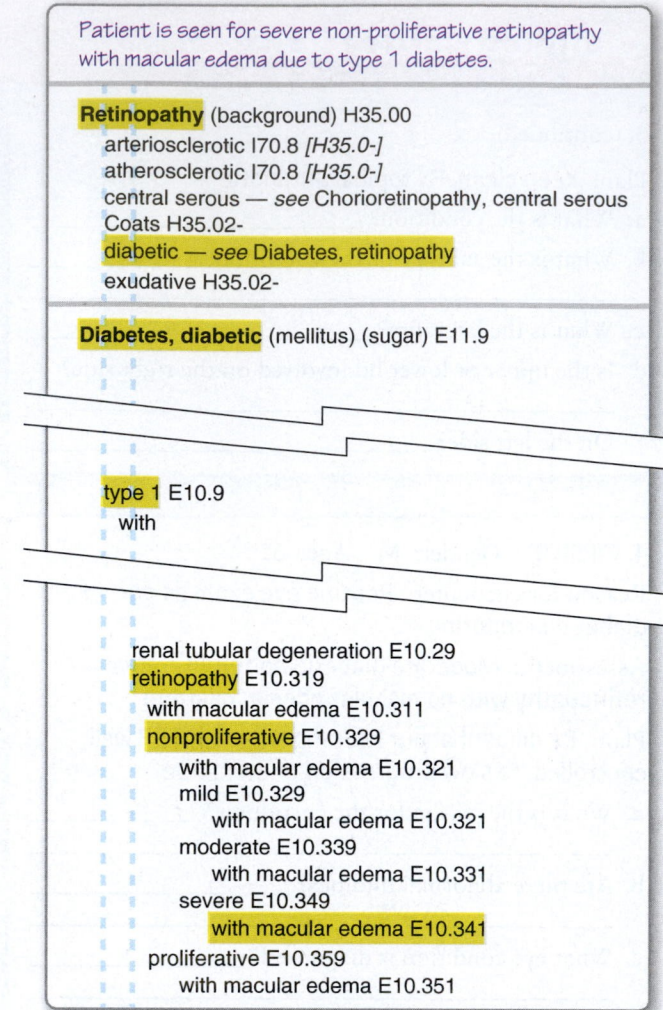

Patient is seen for severe non-proliferative retinopathy with macular edema due to type 1 diabetes.

Retinopathy (background) H35.00
 arteriosclerotic I70.8 *[H35.0-]*
 atherosclerotic I70.8 *[H35.0-]*
 central serous — *see* Chorioretinopathy, central serous
 Coats H35.02-
 diabetic — *see* Diabetes, retinopathy
 exudative H35.02-

Diabetes, diabetic (mellitus) (sugar) E11.9

 type 1 E10.9
  with

 renal tubular degeneration E10.29
 retinopathy E10.319
  with macular edema E10.311
  nonproliferative E10.329
   with macular edema E10.321
   mild E10.329
    with macular edema E10.321
   moderate E10.339
    with macular edema E10.331
   severe E10.349
    with macular edema E10.341
  proliferative E10.359
   with macular edema E10.351

Figure 18-8 ■ Example of Index entry for diabetic retinopathy.

❏ She observes the symbol **6th**, indicating that a sixth digit is required for laterality.

❏ She reviews the choices for laterality and selects **H40.121 Low-tension glaucoma, right eye**.

❏ She notices the **7th** symbol and reads the instructional note under the subcategory **H40.12** to assign a seventh character to identify the stage.

❏ She checks the medical record to verify the stage as mild and selects **H40.1211 Low-tension glaucoma, right eye, mild stage**.

▶ Megan checks for instructional notes in the Tabular List.

❏ She cross-references the beginning of category **H40** and verifies that the only instructional note is an **Excludes1** note that does not apply to the low-tension glaucoma.

E08.3-	Diabetes mellitus due to underlying condition with ophthalmic complications
E09.3-	Drug or chemical induced diabetes mellitus with ophthalmic complications
E10.3-	Type 1 diabetes mellitus with ophthalmic complications
E11.3-	Type 2 diabetes mellitus with ophthalmic complications
E13.3-	Other specified diabetes mellitus with ophthalmic complications

Figure 18-7 ■ Tabular List subcategories for diabetes with ophthalmic manifestations.

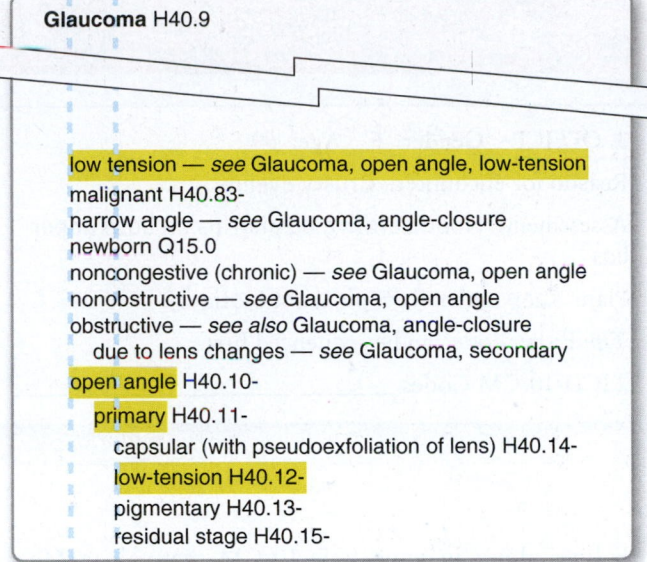

Figure 18-9 ■ Index Entry for "Glaucoma".

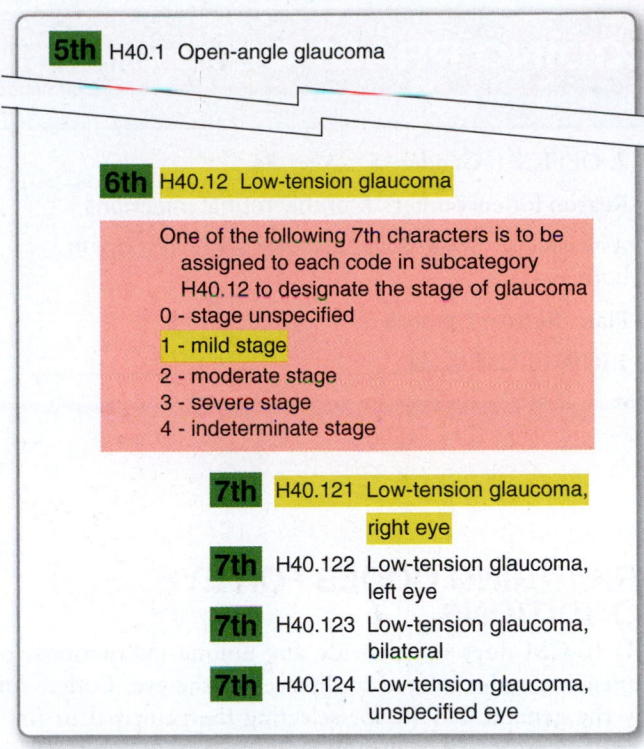

Figure 18-10 ■ Tabular List entry for code H40.12 "Low-tension glaucoma".

❑ She cross-references the beginning of the block **H40-H42** and verifies that there are no instructional notes.

❑ She cross-references the beginning of Chapter 7 (H00-H89) and reviews the instructional note. She determines that it does not apply to this case because the patient's glaucoma is not related to an external cause.

▶ Megan searches the Index for the Main Term **Cataract**.

❑ She locates the subterm **age-related**.

❑ She reads the cross-reference instruction that states —*see* Cataract, senile.

❑ She locates the subterm **senile**.

❑ She locates the second-level subterm **nuclear H25.1**.

▶ Megan verifies code **H25.1** in the Tabular List.

❑ She reads the code title for **H25.1, Age-related nuclear cataract** and confirms that this accurately describes the diagnosis.

❑ She observes the symbol **5th**, indicating that a fifth digit is required for laterality.

❑ She reviews the choices for laterality and selects **H25.13 Age-related nuclear cataract, bilateral**.

▶ Megan checks for instructional notes in the Tabular List.

❑ She cross-references the beginning of category **H25** and verifies that the only instructional note is an **Excludes1** note that does not apply to the low-tension glaucoma.

❑ She cross-references the beginning of the block **H25-H28** and verifies that there are no instructional notes.

❑ She previously checked the beginning of Chapter 7 (H00-H89) and knows that the note does not apply because the cataract is not related to an external cause.

▶ Megan reviews the codes she has assigned for this case.

❑ **H40.1211 Low-tension glaucoma, right eye, mild stage**

❑ **H25.13 Age-related nuclear cataract, bilateral**

▶ Next, Megan must determine how to sequence the codes.

CODING PRACTICE

Exercise 18.3 **Assigning Codes for Eye Conditions**

Instructions: Read the mini-medical-record of each patient's encounter, review the information abstracted in Exercise 18.2, and assign ICD-10-CM diagnosis codes using the Index and Tabular List. Write the code(s) on the line provided.

1. OFFICE   Gender: M Age: 76
Reason for encounter: Phacoemulsification of cataract and intraocular lens (IOL) implant
Assessment: Age related nuclear cataract, left eye
Plan: FU in office 2 days

Tip: Follow cross-referencing instructions in the Index.

1 ICD-10-CM Code _____

(continued)

CODING PRACTICE *(continued)*

2. OFFICE   Gender: F   Age: 84

Reason for encounter: Monthly retinal injections

Assessment: Stage 2 wet macular degeneration, in both eyes

Plan: Return 1 month

1 ICD-10-CM Code _____

3. OFFICE   Gender: F   Age: 69

Reason for encounter: Crusty eyelids

Assessment: Nonulcerative blepharitis on both upper lids

Plan: Keep clean, Rx topical antibiotic

Tip: Either code can be sequenced first.

2 ICD-10-CM Codes _____

ARRANGING CODES FOR EYE CONDITIONS

ICD-10-CM does not provide any unique instructions for sequencing codes related to diseases of the eye. Coders follow the general OGCR for selecting the principal or first-listed diagnosis. They also follow instructional notes within the Tabular List. The most common situations when coders will see instructional notes in this ICD-10-CM chapter are the following:

- When the eye condition is secondary to another condition, sequence the underlying condition first.
- When another associated condition is documented, such as hypertension or glaucoma, assign codes for both conditions and sequence them according to the circumstances of the encounter.
- When the condition is due to a poisoning from a drug, sequence a combination code for the drug and intent first, followed by the code(s) for the eye condition. Use the Table of Drugs and Chemicals to identify the drug and intent.
- When the eye condition results from an adverse effect to a drug, sequence the eye condition first and the drug second. Use the Table of Drugs and Chemicals to identify the drug and intent.
- When the eye condition results from an external cause, sequence the eye condition first, then the external cause codes.

Guided Example of Arranging Codes for Eye Conditions

To learn more about sequencing codes for diseases of the eye and ocular adnexa, continue with the example from earlier in the chapter about patient Jaclyn Vandeventer, who was seen at Branton Eye Care due to glaucoma and cataracts.

Follow along in your ICD-10-CM manual as Megan Scheidler, CCS-P, sequences the codes. Check off each step after you complete it.

▶ First, Megan confirms the codes she assigned.

❑ **H40.1211 Low-tension glaucoma, right eye, mild stage**

❑ **H25.13 Age-related nuclear cataract, bilateral**

▶ Megan reviews the medical record to determine which condition was the main reason for the visit.

❑ The encounter was due to a referral from the optometrist.

❑ Both conditions were evaluated during the visit.

❑ The Tabular List provides no instructional notes regarding sequencing.

▶ Megan evaluates the relative severity of the glaucoma compared to the cataracts.

❑ Glaucoma has already damaged the optic nerve and has the potential to cause permanent damage to vision.

❑ Cataracts, while annoying, do not present a risk of permanent damage.

❑ The physician documents that glaucoma will be treated first, followed by cataract surgery at a later time.

❑ Based on these considerations, Megan sequences the glaucoma first.

▶ Megan finalizes the codes and sequencing for this case:

(1) **H40.1211 Low-tension glaucoma, right eye, mild stage**

(2) **H25.13 Age-related nuclear cataract, bilateral**

CODING PRACTICE

Exercise 18.4   Arranging Codes for Eye Conditions

Instructions: Read the mini-medical-record of each patient's encounter, review the information abstracted in Exercise 18.2, assign ICD-10-CM diagnosis codes using the Index and Tabular List, and sequence them correctly.

---

1. OFFICE   Gender: M   Age: 61

Reason for encounter: Routine eye exam as part of diabetic monitoring

Assessment: Moderate diabetic nonproliferative retinopathy with no macular edema, bilateral

Plan: Be diligent about keeping sugar and BP well controlled, to slow progression of condition

Tip: Assign a Z code for the reason for the encounter. Follow sequencing instructions in the Tabular List.

2 ICD-10-CM Codes _____

---

2. OFFICE   Gender: F   Age: 53

Reason for encounter: Blurred vision, eye pain, floaters in both eyes

(continued)

---

2. (continued)

Assessment: Chronic bilateral anterior uveitis due to juvenile rheumatoid arthritis, associated cataract with neovascularization in left eye also noted

Plan: Eye drops, dark glasses

Tip: Follow cross-referencing instructions in the Index.

3 ICD-10-CM Codes _____

_____

---

3. OFFICE   Gender: F   Age: 54

Reason for encounter: Difficulty seeing, gritty feeling in eyes, ocular hyperemia (*bloodshot eyes*)

Assessment: Bilateral grade 2 corneal and conjunctival deposits, likely due to end-stage renal failure, patient has been on dialysis for about 18 months

Plan: Schedule cornea scraping to remove deposits

Tip: Instructional notes in the Tabular List guide you to the additional codes and sequencing.

4 ICD-10-CM Codes _____

_____

CODING NEOPLASMS OF THE EYE

Neoplasms of the eye and ocular adnexa do not appear in ICD-10-CM Chapter 7, "Diseases of the Eye and Adnexa (H00–H59)." Codes for neoplasms of the eye and ocular adnexa appear in category **C69 Malignant Neoplasm of eye and adnexa** within the neoplasm chapter.

According to the American Society of Clinical Oncology (ASCO), the most common primary malignant neoplasm in the eye among adults is intraocular melanoma, followed by intraocular lymphoma, although both are relatively rare. In children, the most common eye cancer is retinoblastoma (*cancer arising from cells in the retina*).

Metastatic neoplasms are more common than primary neoplasms of the eye. The most common cancers that spread to the eye are breast and lung cancers. Most often, these cancers spread to the uvea. Metastatic breast cancer usually appears in the eye several years after breast cancer treatment has been completed. Metastatic lung cancer to the eye is often the first sign that lung cancer exists. Patients may be surprised to learn that a vision problem is a manifestation of breast or lung cancer.

Cancers of the orbit and ocular adnexa develop from tissues such as muscle, nerve, and skin around the eyeball and are classified as neoplasms of the type of tissue in which they arise. For example, cancers of the eyelid are usually skin cancers and cancers of the eye muscles are usually rhabdomyosarcoma.

When eye cancer needs specific treatment, physicians use targeted radiation therapy to the eye or eye injections of chemotherapeutic drugs. Unfortunately, by the time cancer has metastasized to the eye, patients often have more serious problems to address, and the eye metastasis may not be a high treatment priority.

CODING PRACTICE

Exercise 18.5   Coding Neoplasms of the Eye

Instructions: Read the mini-medical-record of each patient's encounter, then abstract, assign, and sequence ICD-10-CM diagnosis codes using the Index and Tabular List. Write the code(s) on the line provided.

---

1. OFFICE   Gender: M   Age: 8

Reason for encounter: Mother is concerned about a white spot in her son's right eye and says he seems to be cross-eyed

(continued)

CODING PRACTICE (continued)

1. (continued)

Assessment: Retinoblastoma

Plan: Schedule a consultation with ophthalmologic oncologist, pediatric oncologist, and radiation oncologist to determine treatment options

1 ICD-10-CM Code _____

---

2. OFFICE   Gender: F   Age: 58

Reason for encounter: Patient is concerned because she can see a dark spot on the left iris and has been having headaches

Assessment: Melanocytoma with secondary glaucoma

Plan: This is benign and does not require treatment at this time, but we need to monitor the glaucoma

2 ICD-10-CM Codes _____

---

3. OFFICE   Gender: F   Age: 49

Reason for encounter: Blurry vision

Assessment: Metastatic cancer to choroid in both eyes, history of right breast cancer 5 years ago which is no longer under treatment, status post right mastectomy

(continued)

---

3. (continued)

Plan: Targeted radiotherapy, referred back to her oncologist for detection of other possible metastases

3 ICD-10-CM Codes _____

_____

---

4. OFFICE   Gender: F   Age: 56

Reason for encounter: Removal of lesion from right upper eyelid

Assessment: Basal cell carcinoma

1 ICD-10-CM Code _____

---

5. OFFICE   Gender: F   Age: 54

Reason for encounter: Review biopsy and consultation results for salmon colored patch on right conjunctiva

Assessment: Malignant conjunctival lymphoma mucosa associated lymphoid tissue (MALT)

Plan: Refer to oncologist for evaluation for possible systemic lymphoma, then determine course of treatment

1 ICD-10-CM Code _____

CHAPTER SUMMARY

In this chapter you learned that:

- The eye and ocular adnexa make vision possible by receiving light from the external world and converting it into impulses that are transmitted to the brain through the optic nerve.

- ICD-10-CM provides Official Guidelines for Coding and Reporting (OGCR) in OGCR section I.C.7 regarding assigning codes for the stages of glaucoma. An instructional note in the Tabular List at the beginning of the chapter directs coders to use an external cause code following the code for the eye condition when an external cause is involved.

- The majority of conditions in this chapter require that the laterality be identified. When a condition affects both eyes but there is no option for bilateral, assign two codes, one for the right eye and a second one for the left eye.

- ICD-10-CM does not provide any unique instructions for arranging codes related to diseases of the eye, so coders follow the general OGCR for selecting the principal or first-listed diagnosis.

- Metastatic neoplasms are more common than primary neoplasms of the eye, with the most common being metastatic breast and lung cancers.

CONCEPT QUIZ

Take a moment to look back at the eye and ocular adnexa and solidify your skills. Try to answer the questions from memory first, then look back at the discussion in this chapter if you need a little extra help.

Completion

Instructions: Write the term that completes each statement based on the information you learned in this chapter. Choose from the list below. Some choices may be used more than once and some choices may not be used at all.

adnexa	keratitis
cataract	macular degeneration
chalazion	ocular globe
conjunctivitis	optic nerve
diabetic retinopathy	orbital cavity
glaucoma	uvea
hordeolum	uvula
keratin	vitreous body

1. The ocular muscles, eyelids, and conjunctiva make up the
   _____.

2. A(an) _____ is a small hard cyst on the eyelid caused by blockage of a gland on the eyelid.

3. The transparent jelly that fills the eyeball and is surrounded by a membrane is the _____.

4. The condition _____ may be proliferative or nonproliferative.

5. The _____ is the middle layer of the eye consisting of the iris, ciliary body, and choroid.

6. _____ is the gradual loss of central vision due to aging with no cure.

7. A(an) _____ is a bacterial inflammation of a sebaceous gland on the edge or lining of the eyelid.

8. The eye socket is also called the _____.

9. _____ is a viral or bacterial inflammation and infection of the lining of the eyelid.

10. _____ is an inflammation and ulceration of the surface of the cornea.

Multiple Choice

Instructions: Circle the letter of the best answer to each question based on the information you learned in this chapter.

1. What is the separation of the retina from the choroid layer of the eye?
   A. Choroiditis
   B. Macular degeneration
   C. Diabetic retinopathy
   D. Retinal detachment

2. How would you code the following scenario? *A patient is seen for moderate stage low-tension open-angle glaucoma of the left eye.*
   A. H40.1122
   B. H40.112
   C. H40.1222
   D. H40.122

3. What type of conditions affect vision due to how the eye collects and focuses light?
   A. Refractive errors
   B. Retinopathy
   C. Macular degeneration
   D. Glaucoma

4. Which character(s) of a code indicates laterality?
   A. First
   B. Second or third
   C. Fifth or sixth
   D. Seventh

5. How would you code the following scenario? *A 79-year old patient is seen for senile entropion of both upper eyelids.*
   A. H02.032, H02.035
   B. H02.031, H02.034
   C. H02.033, H02.036
   D. H02.039

6. What Main Term are the codes for *diabetic retinopathy* indexed under?
   A. Diabetes
   B. Retinopathy
   C. Either Diabetes or Retinopathy
   D. Manifestation, diabetic

7. What subterm under *Cataracts* should be used to locate *age-related cataracts* in the Index?
   A. Age
   B. Old
   C. Nuclear
   D. Senile

8. How would you code the following scenario? *A patient is seen for follow up of intraoperative floppy iris syndrome attributed to having taken tamsulosin 6 months ago for urinary retention.*
   A. H21.81, R33.0
   B. T44.6X5D, H21.81
   C. H21.81, T44.6X5D
   D. T44.6X5D, H21.81, R33.9

9. What is nuclear cataract?
   A. Located in the center of the eye
   B. The result of exposure to radiation
   C. Beginning to become apparent
   D. Caused by diabetes

10. What is the most common neoplasm that affects the eye?
    A. Intraocular melanoma
    B. Retinoblastoma
    C. Metastasis
    D. Rhabdomyosarcoma

KEEP ON CODING

Instructions: Read the diagnostic statement, then use the Index and Tabular List to assign and sequence ICD-10-CM diagnosis codes. Write the code(s) on the line provided.

1. Abscess of both upper eyelids. ICD-10-CM Code(s) _____

2. Acute atopic conjunctivitis, both eyes. ICD-10-CM Code(s) _____

3. Kayser-Fleischer ring, left eye. ICD-10-CM Code(s) _____

4. Stable keratoconus, right eye. ICD-10-CM Code(s) _____

5. Anterior subcapsular polar age-related cataract, both eyes. ICD-10-CM Code(s) _____

6. Retinopathy of prematurity, stage 1, right eye. ICD-10-CM Code(s) _____

7. Low-tension glaucoma. ICD-10-CM Code(s) _____

8. Malignant melanoma of choroid, right eye. ICD-10-CM Code(s) _____

9. Optic nerve hypoplasia, left eye. ICD-10-CM Code(s) _____

10. Vertical strabismus, right eye. ICD-10-CM Code(s) _____

11. Sebaceous cyst of right lower eyelid. ICD-10-CM Code(s) _____

12. Low vision, both eyes. ICD-10-CM Code(s) _____

13. Cystoid macular edema post cataract surgery, left eye. ICD-10-CM Code(s) _____

14. Convergence insufficiency. ICD-10-CM Code(s) _____

15. Epiphora due to excessive discharge of tears, bilateral. ICD-10-CM Code(s) _____

16. Progressive external ophthalmoplegia, right eye. ICD-10-CM Code(s) _____

17. Horseshoe tear of retina without detachment, left eye. ICD-10-CM Code(s) _____

18. Harada's disease, both eyes. ICD-10-CM Code(s) _____

19. Cortical age-related cataract, right eye. ICD-10-CM Code(s) _____

20. Staphyloma posticum, bilateral. ICD-10-CM Code(s) _____

21. Pseudotumor of the left orbit. ICD-10-CM Code(s) _____

22. Ptosis of both eyelids. ICD-10-CM Code(s) _____

23. Diplopia. ICD-10-CM Code(s) _____

24. Ghost vessels in the cornea of the left eye. ICD-10-CM Code(s) _____

25. Postprocedural blebitis, stage 2. ICD-10-CM Code(s) _____

CODING CHALLENGE

Instructions: Read the mini-medical-record of each patient's encounter, then abstract, assign, and sequence ICD-10-CM diagnosis codes using the Index and Tabular List. Write the code(s) on the line provided.

1. OFFICE   Gender: F   Age: 28

Reason for encounter: Routine vision examination

Assessment: Latent nystagmus, right eye

Plan: Prescription contact lenses

Tip: Assign one code for the eye exam and a second code for the finding.

2 ICD-10-CM Codes _____

2. OFFICE   Gender: M   Age: 48

Reason for encounter: Light flashes for 2 months, dense shadow/curtain progressing toward central vision this morning

Assessment: Detachment of retina with one break, right eye

Plan: Scleral buckle surgery

1 ICD-10-CM Code _____

3. OFFICE   Gender: F   Age: 42

Reason for encounter: Pain and redness in R eye

Assessment: R eye marginal corneal ulcer due to dry eye syndrome which is bilateral, so we will keep watch on the other eye as well

Plan: Pain medication, tear substitute drops, discontinue contact use, RTO tomorrow

2 ICD-10-CM Codes _____

4. OFFICE   Gender: M   Age: 57

Reason for encounter: Noticing mild impairment of vision, redness of eyes, foreign body sensation in eyes

Assessment: Recurrent pterygium, bilateral

Plan: Artificial tears, anti-inflammatory drops, RTO one month

1 ICD-10-CM Code _____

5. OFFICE   Gender: F   Age: 2

Reason for encounter: Scheduled cataract removal

Assessment: Subcapsular posterior juvenile cataract left eye, cerebrotendinous xanthomatosis (*a metabolic disorder related to fat storage*)

Plan: RTO tomorrow, genetic counseling for family, referral to pediatric endocrinologist for FU

2 ICD-10-CM Codes _____

6. OFFICE   Gender: M   Age: 66

Reason for encounter: Sudden painless loss of vision

Assessment: Occlusion of left central retinal artery. Pt has hypertension and CAD which place her at risk for embolism

Plan: Aspirin and Plavix, ocular-digital massage, admit for angiogram to evaluate carotid circulation

3 ICD-10-CM Codes _____

7. OFFICE   Gender: M   Age: 9

Reason for encounter: Child referred to clinic by schoolteacher. Child unable to distinguish the color red from green.

Assessment: Acquired color blindness

Plan: Teach coping skills to distinguish colors

1 ICD-10-CM Code _____

8. OFFICE   Gender: F   Age: 31

Reason for encounter: Cloudy blurred vision

Assessment: Idiopathic corneal edema, bilateral

Plan: Hypertonic eye drops and ointment

1 ICD-10-CM Code _____

9. OFFICE   Gender: F   Age: 68

Reason for encounter: Swelling of lower right eyelid, tenderness, increased tearing

Assessment: Chalazion on right lower eyelid

Plan: Topical antibiotic eye drops for initial infection. RTO 2 months to inject with a corticosteroid if chalazion has not disappeared

1 ICD-10-CM Code _____

10. OFFICE   Gender: F   Age: 16

Reason for encounter: Pink eye, ocular itching, tearing, photophobia, watery discharge, painful socialized swelling on lid

Assessment: Bilateral chronic conjunctivitis due to allergies and a stye on the edge of the right upper lid

Plan: Cold compresses, NSAIDs, mast cell stabilizers, antihistamine, RTO 1 week

2 ICD-10-CM Codes _____

Chapter 19

Diseases of the Ear and Mastoid Process (H60-H95)

Chapter Outline

- **Ear Refresher**
- **Coding Guidelines for the Ear**
- **Abstracting for Ear Conditions**
- **Assigning Codes for Ear Conditions**
- **Arranging Codes for Ear Conditions**

Learning Objectives

After completing this chapter, you should have the skills to:

19.1 Spell and define the key words, medical terms, and abbreviations related to the ear and mastoid process. (Remember)

19.2 Summarize the structure, function, and common conditions of the ear and mastoid process. (Understand)

19.3 Adhere to the Official Guidelines for Coding and Reporting related to diseases of the ear and mastoid process. (Apply)

19.4 Examine and abstract diagnostic information from the medical record for conditions of the ear and mastoid process. (Analyze)

19.5 Demonstrate how to assign codes for diseases of the ear and mastoid process. (Apply)

19.6 Utilize guidelines for arranging (sequencing) multiple diagnosis codes for diseases of the ear and mastoid process. (Apply)

19.7 Demonstrate how to abstract, assign, and sequence codes for neoplasms of the ear and mastoid process. (Apply)

Key Terms and Abbreviations

auditory canal	incus	otitis media (OM)	tympanic membrane
auricle	inner ear	oval window	tympanic membrane perforation (TMP)
cerumen	labyrinth	pinna	
cochlea	malleus	purulent otitis media	tympanum
eardrum	mastoid process	saccule	utricle
equilibrium	middle ear	semicircular canal	vestibulocochlear nerve
external ear	ossicles	stapes	

In addition to the key terms listed here, students should know the terms defined within tables in this chapter.

INTRODUCTION

Many of our memories relate to sounds—a trickling brook, a thundering waterfall, or the music of a concert. Whatever sounds are imbedded in your memory, you have your ears to thank.

An otolaryngologist is a physician who specializes in diagnosing and treating conditions of the ear, nose, and throat (ENT). Primary care physicians treat uncomplicated conditions of the ear, nose, and throat. They refer patients with more complex conditions to otolaryngologists.

Keep your medical reference resources handy as you study this chapter. The ear contains some of the smallest structures in the human body, and it is important to understand the function of each. Experienced coders keep the information they need at their fingertips.

EAR REFRESHER

The ear makes hearing possible by collecting sound waves from the external world and converting them into impulses that are transmitted to the brain through the **vestibulocochlear nerve**, cranial nerve VIII. The ear also maintains **equilibrium**, the sense of balance. The **mastoid process** is the portion of the temporal bone of the skull that juts forward behind the ear.

The ear is divided into three sections: the **external ear**, **middle ear**, and **inner ear** (■ FIGURE 19-1). The external ear consists of the **auricle** or **pinna**, the visible part of the ear, which collects sound waves; the **auditory canal**, which funnels the sound waves; and the **tympanic membrane**, also called the **tympanum** or **eardrum**, which separates the external ear from the middle ear. Glands in the auditory canal produce **cerumen** (*ear wax*) that protects and lubricates the ear.

The middle ear is a small air-filled cavity in the temporal bone that contains the **ossicles**, three small bones that are critical to the hearing process. The ossicles amplify vibrations in the middle ear and transmit them to the inner ear, from the **malleus** (*hammer*) to the **incus** (*anvil*) to the **stapes** (*stirrup*). The stapes is attached to the **oval window**, a thin membrane that covers the opening to the inner ear and passes vibrations to the cochlea.

The inner ear, or **labyrinth**, is a fluid-filled cavity in the temporal bone that contains the **cochlea**, a snail-shaped organ that makes hearing possible, and the sensors for equilibrium, which are the **semicircular canals**, **utricle**, and **saccule**.

In Figure 19-1, each structure in the ear and mastoid process is labeled with its name as well as its medical terminology root/combining form where applicable. Refer to ■ TABLE 19-1, (page 326) for a refresher on how to build medical terms related to the ear and mastoid process.

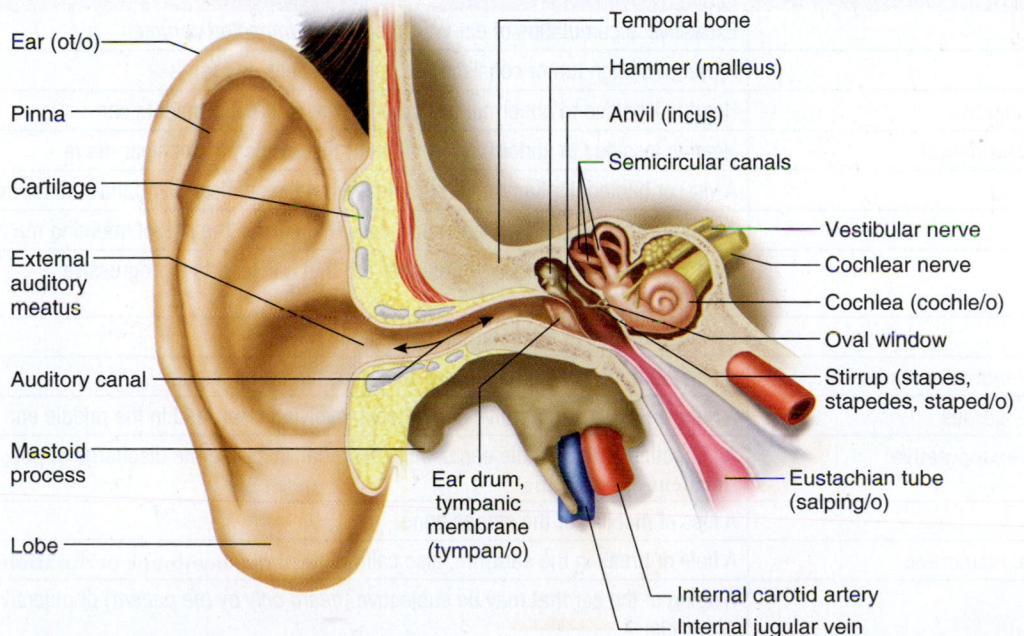

Figure 19-1 ■ The ear and mastoid process.

Table 19-1 ■ **EXAMPLE OF CONSTRUCTING MEDICAL TERMS FOR THE EAR AND MASTOID PROCESS**

Combining Form	Suffix	Complete Medical Term
ot/o (*ear*)		**ot + itis** (*inflammation of the ear*) **oto + plasty** (*surgical repair of the ear*)
myring/o (*eardrum*) **tympan/o** (*eardrum, tympanic membrane*)	**-itis** (*inflammation*) **-plasty** (*surgical repair*) **-tomy** (*make an incision into*)	**myring + itis** (*inflammation of the eardrum*) **myringo + tomy** (*making an incision in the eardrum*) **tympano + plasty** (*surgical repair of the tympanic membrane*)
staped/o (*stapes bone*)		**stapedo + tomy** (*make an incision in the stapes bone*)
mastoid/o (*mastoid process bone, breast shaped*)		**mastoid + itis** (*inflammation of the mastoid process bone*)

Conditions of the Ear

Coders must be familiar with the most common conditions of the ear: hearing loss, or deafness, and otitis media (OM) (*infection of the middle ear*). Approximately 15% of American adults report some degree of hearing loss, and 50% of adults age 75 or older have a hearing impairment, according to the National Institute on Deafness and Other Communication Disorders (NIDCD).

Five of six children experience OM by the time they are three years old, according to NIDCD. Ear infections are the second most common reason for trips to the pediatrician, after wellness visits; almost half of all antibiotic prescriptions

written for children are for ear infections. Untreated OM can lead to complications, such as mastoiditis, hearing loss, perforation of the tympanum, meningitis, facial nerve paralysis, and Ménière's disease. Refer to ■ TABLE 19-2 for a summary of diseases affecting the ear and mastoid process.

Neoplasms of the Ear

Neoplasms of the ear are rare. Basal cell carcinoma and malignant melanoma may occur on the skin of the external ear; these are classified under malignant neoplasms of the skin. Squamous cell carcinoma may occur in the ear canal; adenoid cystic carcinoma may occur in the ear glands.

Table 19-2 ■ **COMMON DISEASES OF THE EAR AND MASTOID PROCESS**

Condition	Definition
Ceruminoma	Excessive accumulation of ear wax, also called *impacted cerumen*
Cholesteatoma	A cyst or benign tumor consisting of epithelial cells and fat
Hearing loss—conductive	Hearing loss due to abnormal formation of the external or middle ear
Hearing loss—sensorineural	Hearing loss due to abnormal formation of the cochlea or cochlear nerve
Labyrinthitis	A viral or bacterial inflammation or infection of the semicircular canals of the inner ear
Mastoiditis	A serious infection of the mastoid process that carries the risk of infecting the brain
Ménière's disease	An abnormality of the fluid of the inner ear that can lead to a progressive hearing loss
Otitis externa	An inflammation of the external ear (pinna)
Otitis media (OM)—nonsuppurative	An inflammation of the middle ear that does not produce pus
Otitis media (OM)—serous	A subtype of nonsuppurative otitis media involving clear fluid in the middle ear
Otitis media (OM)—suppurative	An infection of the middle ear, usually bacterial, involving the discharge of pus, also called purulent otitis media
Otosclerosis	A loss of mobility of the stapes bone
Ruptured tympanic membrane	A hole or break in the eardrum, also called tympanic membrane perforation (TMP)
Tinnitus	Ringing of the ear that may be subjective (*heard only by the patient*) or objective (*audible to the physician*)
Vertigo	A sensation of motion or dizziness

Acoustic neuroma, also called vestibular schwannoma, is a benign tumor of the vestibular cochlear nerve, which connects the ear to the brain. It grows slowly, and people with this condition usually do not show symptoms until after age 30.

This section provides a general reference to help understand the most common diagnoses of the ear and mastoid process. Refer to medical resources to learn more about conditions affecting the ear and mastoid process.

CODING PRACTICE

Exercise 19.1   **Ear Refresher**

Instructions: Use your medical terminology skills and resources to define the following conditions related to the ear and mastoid process, then assign the default diagnosis code.

Follow these steps:

- Use slash marks "/" to break down each term into its root(s) and suffix.
- Define the meaning of the word, based on the meaning of each word part.
- Assign the default ICD-10-CM diagnosis code and laterality for the condition using the Index and Tabular List.

Example: otitis (right) ot/itis   Meaning *inflammation of the right ear*   ICD-10-CM Code <u>H66.91</u>

1. labyrinthitis (bilateral)   Meaning _____   ICD-10-CM Code _____

2. otosclerosis (right)   Meaning _____   ICD-10-CM Code _____

3. cholesteatoma (left)   Meaning _____   ICD-10-CM Code _____

4. mastoiditis   Meaning _____   ICD-10-CM Code _____

5. presbycusis (bilateral)   Meaning _____   ICD-10-CM Code _____

6. otolith (left)   Meaning _____   ICD-10-CM Code _____

7. otorrhagia (left)   Meaning _____   ICD-10-CM Code _____

8. otorrhea   Meaning _____   ICD-10-CM Code _____

9. mastoidalgia (right)   Meaning _____   ICD-10-CM Code _____

10. tympanosclerosis (bilateral)   Meaning _____   ICD-10-CM Code _____

CODING GUIDELINES FOR THE EAR

Coders should understand the organization of this ICD-10-CM chapter, chapter-wide and commonly used instructional notes in the Tabular List, and the relevant OGCR. This information is necessary for accurate coding.

ICD-10-CM Chapter 8, "Diseases of the Ear and Mastoid Process (H60-H95)," contains five blocks or subchapters that are divided by external, middle, and internal ear. Review the block names and code ranges listed at the beginning of Chapter 8 in the ICD-10-CM manual to become familiar with the content and organization.

This chapter is the second of two ICD-10-CM chapters in which codes begin with the letter H; codes for the eye and adnexa occupy codes H00 through H59.

This chapter includes disorders affecting the external, middle, and inner ear, as well as the mastoid process. It does not include injuries to the ear, which are classified in ICD-10-CM Chapter 19.

ICD-10-CM does not provide any Official Guidelines for Coding and Reporting (OGCR) specific to this chapter.

General OGCR in sections I.A, I.B, II, III, and IV direct the coder. Instructional notes in the Tabular List guide coders when additional codes are required. An instructional note at the beginning of the chapter directs coders to use an external cause code following the code for the ear condition when an external cause created the ear condition. This note applies to all codes in ICD-10-CM Chapter 8. Codes identify laterality and detailed anatomic specificity. Instructional notes to **code first the underlying condition** appear throughout the chapter. Specific OGCR and instructional notes are discussed and cited throughout this chapter of the text.

ABSTRACTING FOR EAR CONDITIONS

The primary concerns in abstracting for diagnoses of the ear and mastoid process are laterality, external causes, and tobacco use or exposure. In addition, coders should be aware of the many variations of OM so they can abstract all the needed details.

Table 19-3 ■ **KEY CRITERIA FOR ABSTRACTING CONDITIONS OF THE EAR AND MASTOID PROCESS**

❑ What is the condition?
❑ What is the subtype of the condition?
❑ Is a more specific subtype documented?
❑ What part of the ear is affected?
❑ What is the laterality?
❑ What other conditions coexist?
❑ Is there an underlying disease?
❑ Is the condition due to a drug or external cause?
❑ Is there documentation of current or past use of tobacco or exposure to tobacco smoke?

Abstracting Laterality

The majority of ear conditions require that the laterality be identified. Laterality is expressed at the following levels:

• Right, left, or unspecified ear

• Bilateral, for applicable conditions

• Unilateral, with additional status of contralateral ear, for selected conditions

When a patient has more than one ear condition, the laterality for *each* condition must be identified separately. For example, a patient may have bilateral OM but unilateral TMP in the right or left ear only.

Refer to ■ TABLE 19-3 for guidance on how to abstract conditions of the ear and mastoid process. Remember that abstracting questions are a guide and that not every question applies to, or can be answered for, every case. For example, tinnitus does not have subtype conditions.

Abstracting for Otitis Media

Otitis media requires that coders abstract the basic information required for all ear conditions, plus additional details unique to OM. Coders need to abstract the specific subtype of OM. The two most common are suppurative and serous. Serous is one form of nonsuppurative OM, but coders may occasionally encounter other nonsuppurative types, such as mucoid, allergic, secretory, and seromucinous.

OM is classified as acute, acute recurrent, and chronic. Although there are no universal definitions of these stages, a common practice is to classify recurrent acute otitis media as chronic when it persists for longer than three months and is accompanied by changes in the lining of the middle ear. Coders abstract this information based on how physicians describe the condition in the documentation. When in doubt, query the physician for clarification. Refer to ■ TABLE 19-4 for guidance on how to abstract for otitis media, then work through the detailed example that follows.

CODING CAUTION

Do not assume that all conditions named *otitis* are otitis media. *Otitis* is inflammation of the ear. You need to distinguish between otitis *media*, inflammation of the middle ear, and otitis *externa*, inflammation of the external ear. These are separate conditions with different codes.

Guided Example of Abstracting for the Ear

Refer to the following example throughout this chapter to learn about abstracting, assigning, and sequencing codes for the ear and mastoid process. Gabrielle Javiera, CPC, is a fictitious coder who guides you through the coding process.

> Date: 10/21/yy Location: Ear, Nose, and Throat Specialists
>
> Provider: Shauna Rotz, MD
>
> Patient: Estela Nuno Gender: F Age: 4
>
> Reason for encounter: Ear pain, fever
>
> Assessment: Bilateral acute serous otitis media with total rupture of tympanic membrane of the right ear, no one in the household smokes
>
> Plan: Antibiotics, fat-plug tympanoplasty

Follow along as Gabrielle Javiera, CPC, abstracts the diagnosis. Check off each step after you complete it.

▶ Gabrielle reads through the entire record, with special attention to the reason for the encounter and the final assessment. She refers to the Key Criteria for Abstracting Otitis Media (Table 19-4).

❑ She notes the presenting symptoms: ear pain, fever

❑ *What is the condition?* Otitis media

❑ *What is the subtype of the condition?* Acute serous

❑ *Is it suppurative/purulent, nonsuppurative/serous, or another subtype?* Serous, which is a type of nonsuppurative OM

❑ *What is the laterality?* Bilateral

❑ *Is it acute, acute recurrent, or chronic?* Acute

Table 19-4 ■ **KEY CRITERIA FOR ABSTRACTING OTITIS MEDIA**

❑ What is the subtype of otitis media?
❑ Is it suppurative/purulent, nonsuppurative/serous, or another subtype?
❑ Is it acute, acute recurrent, or chronic?
❑ What is the laterality?
❑ Is there associated rupture of the tympanic membrane?
❑ What is the type or extent of the rupture?
❑ What is the laterality of the rupture?
❑ Is it a manifestation of another disease?
❑ Is there documentation of current or past use of tobacco or exposure to tobacco smoke?

❏ *Is there associated rupture of the tympanic membrane?* Yes

❏ *What is the type or extent of the rupture?* Total

❏ *What is the laterality of the rupture?* She notes that laterality of the rupture is right, although the otitis media is bilateral

❏ *Is it a manifestation of another disease?* No

❏ *Is there documentation of current or past use of tobacco or exposure to tobacco smoke?* No one in the household smokes

❏ Now that she has identified the conditions, she reviews the symptoms again. She determines that ear pain and fever are integral to otitis media and should not be coded (■ FIGURE 19-2).

❏ She reviews the planned treatments and concludes that they are consistent with the condition she abstracted.

▶ At this time, Gabrielle does not know how many codes she will need. She will learn about this when she moves on to assigning codes.

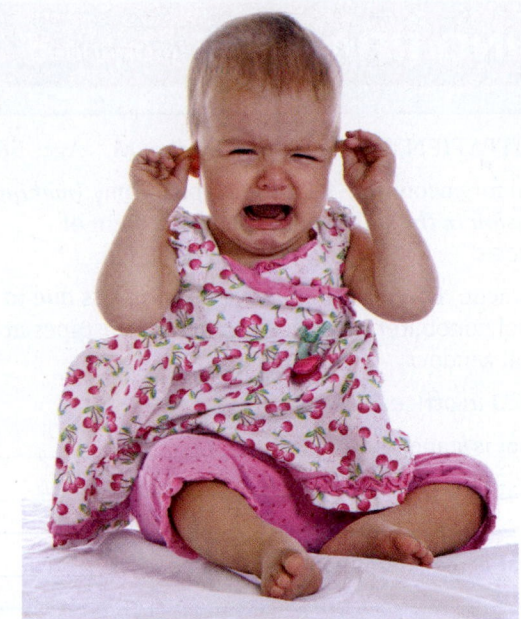

Figure 19-2 ■ Common signs of otitis media are fussiness and pulling at the ear. *Source: John Wollwerth/Shutterstock.*

CODING PRACTICE

Exercise 19.2   Abstracting for Ear Conditions

Instructions: Read the mini-medical-record of each patient's encounter and answer the abstracting questions. Write the answer on the line provided. Do not assign any codes.

---

1. OUTPATIENT HOSPITAL   Gender: M   Age: 7

Reason for encounter: Bilateral tympanoplasty

Assessment: Bilateral chronic serous otitis media

Plan: FU in office 2 weeks

a. What is tympanoplasty? _____

b. What is the condition? _____

c. Is it suppurative or nonsuppurative? _____
_____

d. What is the laterality? _____

e. Is the condition acute or chronic? _____
_____

---

2. OFFICE   Gender: F   Age: 23

Chief complaint: Severe nausea, vomiting, sweating, vertigo

Assessment: Symptoms are due to Ménière's disease, left ear

(continued)

---

2. (continued)

Plan: Diazepam (*a sedative*) for vertigo, it may get better on its own or it may not, will consider surgery if necessary, but we want to follow it for awhile

a. What are the symptoms? _____

b. Will you code the symptoms? _____
Why or why not? _____

c. What condition is diagnosed? _____

d. What is the laterality? _____

---

3. OFFICE   Gender: F   Age: 32

Chief complaint: Ringing and buzzing in right ear, difficulty hearing in right ear

Assessment: Objective tinnitus

Plan: We will try electrical stimulation treatments and see how the condition responds before considering surgery.

a. What are the symptoms? _____

b. Will you code the symptoms? _____
Why or why not? _____

c. What condition is diagnosed? _____
What does *objective* mean? _____

d. What is the laterality? _____

(continued)

CODING PRACTICE (continued)

4. OUTPATIENT SURGERY Gender: M Age: 58

Reason for encounter: Bilateral stapedotomy (*making an incision in the stapes bone*) and placement of prosthesis

Assessment: Bilateral conductive hearing loss due to bilateral nonobliterative otosclerosis of the stapes at the oval window

Plan: FU in office 2 weeks

a. What is stapedotomy? _____

b. What type of hearing loss is documented? _____
_____

c. What is the laterality of the hearing loss? _____
_____

d. What is otosclerosis? _____

e. What is the type of otosclerosis? _____

f. What bone is affected by the otosclerosis? _____
_____

g. What is the laterality of the otosclerosis? _____
_____

5. OFFICE Gender: F Age: 12

Reason for encounter: Left earache, fever, head congestion

Assessment: Acute recurrent suppurative otitis media and acute recurrent sinusitis, mother is a heavy cigarette smoker

Plan: Antibiotics for OM, decongestant, and fluids

a. What are the symptoms? _____

b. What condition is the first condition diagnosed?
_____

c. Is it suppurative or nonsuppurative? _____
_____

d. Is it acute or chronic? _____

e. Is it recurrent? _____

(continued)

5. (continued)

f. Which symptoms relate to the first condition?
_____

g. What is the laterality of the first condition?
_____

h. What condition is the second condition diagnosed?
_____

i. Is it acute or chronic? _____

j. Is it recurrent? _____

k. Which symptoms relate to the second condition?
_____

l. Which condition should you sequence first? _____
_____

Why? _____

m. Is tobacco use or exposure documented? _____

6. OFFICE Gender: M Age: 19

Reason for encounter: Dizziness, nausea, low back pain, headache on right side

Assessment: Dizziness, nausea, and headache due to labyrinthitis, right

Plan: Refer to physical therapy for balance and for LBP

a. What are the symptoms? _____

b. What is labyrinthitis? _____
_____

c. What is the laterality? _____
_____

d. Which symptoms relate to the labyrinthitis? _____
_____

e. What symptom does not relate to labyrinthitis? _____
_____

Should it be coded? _____

Why or why not? _____

ASSIGNING CODES FOR EAR CONDITIONS

The Index provides cross-referencing instructions that redirect coders to alternative Main Terms for many ear conditions. When a condition cannot be located under a Main Term, remember to refer to any alternative Main Terms provided in the cross-reference notes. This is especially helpful when assigning codes for hearing loss and OM.

Assigning Codes for Hearing Loss

Coders may use the Main Term **Deafness** for any condition described as hearing loss or deafness. Hearing **loss** is indexed under the Main Term Loss and the subterm **hearing**. A cross-reference note states **see also Deafness**.

The Index entry for **Deafness** includes a wide range of deaf conditions and causes, whereas **Loss, hearing** indexes conductive and sensorineural hearing loss. It is a good idea to check the entries under both of these Main Terms to ensure you have selected the most appropriate code. In particular, it is important to identify several characteristics:

- What type of deafness or hearing loss is identified, such as conductive, sensorineural, or mixed? Sensorineural incudes conductive, perceptive, and sensory loss. Identify the corresponding subterm.

- On which side does the deafness occur? Identify the subterm that identifies laterality.

- If deafness occurs in only one ear, does the contralateral (*opposite*) side ear experience *restricted* hearing? Identify the subterm that describes the contralateral ear.

- Is the hearing loss caused by an injury? Traumatic hearing loss is indexed under **Injury, nerve, acoustic, specified type NEC.**

- Is the hearing loss psychogenic, hysterical, or emotional in nature? These conditions are coded to **F44.6 Conversion disorder with sensory symptom or deficit.**

EXAMPLE: *A patient is seen who has conductive hearing loss in the right ear and restricted hearing in the left ear.* Index: Loss, hearing, conductive, unilateral, with, restricted hearing on the contralateral side Tabular List: H90.A11 Conductive hearing loss, unilateral, right ear with restricted hearing on the contralateral side

Assigning Codes for Otitis Media

The Index entry **Otitis, media** contains numerous cross-references between second-level subterms, which may seem confusing. Nearly all types of OM can be located under the two second-level subterms **nonsuppurative** and **suppurative.** Third- and fourth-level subterms further identify the specific subtype of OM.

SUCCESS STEP

To make navigating the Index entry for **Otitis, media** easier, highlight the subterm entries for **nonsuppurative** and **suppurative** in your coding manual.

Guided Example of Assigning Codes for Ear Conditions

To learn more about assigning codes for the ear and mastoid process, continue with the example from earlier in the chapter about a patient who was seen due to ear pain and fever.

Follow along in your ICD-10-CM manual and check off each step after you complete it.

▶ First, Gabrielle confirms the diagnoses.

❏ Bilateral acute serous otitis media

❏ Total rupture of tympanic membrane of the right ear

▶ Gabrielle searches the Index for the Main Term **Otitis** (■ Figure 19-3).

❏ She locates the subterm **media.**

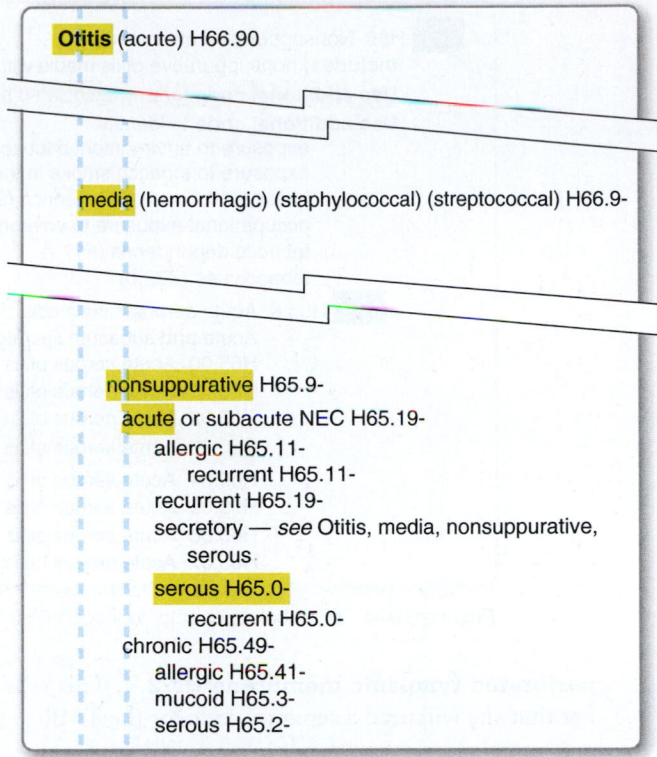

Otitis (acute) H66.90

media (hemorrhagic) (staphylococcal) (streptococcal) H66.9-

nonsuppurative H65.9-
   acute or subacute NEC H65.19-
      allergic H65.11-
         recurrent H65.11-
      recurrent H65.19-
      secretory — *see* Otitis, media, nonsuppurative, serous
      serous H65.0-
         recurrent H65.0-
   chronic H65.49-
      allergic H65.41-
      mucoid H65.3-
      serous H65.2-

Figure 19-3 ■ Index entry for "Otitis, medica, nonsuppurative" used to locate codes for nonsuppurative otitis media.

❏ She knows that serous otitis media is a type of nonsuppurative otitis media, so she locates the second-level subterm, **nonsuppurative.**

❏ She locates the third-level subterm **acute.**

❏ She locates the fourth-level subterm **serous H65.0-.**

▶ Gabrielle verifies **H65.0-** in the Tabular List (■ Figure 19-4, page 332).

❏ She reads the subcategory title for **H65.0 Acute serous otitis media** and confirms that this accurately describes the condition.

❏ She identifies the symbol **5th** in front of the subcategory number, telling her that a fifth digit is required to identify the laterality.

❏ She notices that there are eight codes in this category: four for **acute serous otitis media** and four for **acute serous otitis media, recurrent.**

❏ She verifies that the documentation does not state recurrent, so she selects the code **H65.03 Acute serous otitis media, bilateral.**

▶ Gabrielle checks for instructional notes in the Tabular List.

❏ She cross-references the beginning of subcategory **H65.0** and verifies that there are no instructional notes.

❏ She cross-references the beginning of category **H65** and identifies several instructional notes. The first note states **Use additional code for any associated**

4th H65 Nonsuppurative otitis media
  Includes: nonsuppurative otitis media with myringitis
  Use additional code for any associated perforated tympanic membrane (H72.-)
  Use additional code to identify:
        exposure to environmental tobacco smoke (Z77.22)
        exposure to tobacco smoke in the perinatal period (P96.81)
        history of tobacco dependence (Z87.891)
        occupational exposure to environmental tobacco smoke (Z57.31)
        tobacco dependence (F17.-)
        tobacco use (Z72.0)
  5th H65.0 Acute serous otitis media
        Acute and subacute secretory otitis
        H65.00 Acute serous otitis media, unspecified ear
        H65.01 Acute serous otitis media, right ear
        H65.02 Acute serous otitis media, left ear
        H65.03 Acute serous otitis media, bilateral
        H65.04 Acute serous otitis media, recurrent, right ear
        H65.05 Acute serous otitis media, recurrent, left ear
        H65.06 Acute serous otitis media, recurrent, bilateral
        H65.07 Acute serous otitis media, recurrent, unspecified ear

Figure 19-4 ■ Tabular List entry for code H65.0 "Acute serous otitis media".

perforated tympanic membrane (H72.-). This tells her that she will need a separate code for the TMP.

❏ She reads the other instructional notes that direct her to use an additional code for various circumstances of tobacco use and exposure. She double-checks the medical record and determines that none of these circumstances are documented.

❏ She cross-references the beginning of the block **H65-H75** and verifies that there are no instructional notes.

❏ She cross-references the beginning of Chapter 8 (H60-H95) and reviews the instructional note. She determines that it does not apply to this case because the condition is not due to an external cause.

► Gabrielle proceeds to code the total rupture of the tympanic membrane.

❏ She cross-references the Tabular List entry for **H72.-** that is listed in the instructional note.

❏ She notices there are a lot of codes under category **H72.**

❏ She reviews the subcategory headings until she locates subcategory **H72.82 Total perforations of tympanic membrane.**

❏ She identifies the symbol **6th** in front of the subcategory number, telling her that a sixth digit is required to identify the laterality.

❏ She double-checks the medical record to confirm that laterality for the TMP is right.

❏ She reviews the available code options and selects the code **H72.821 Total perforations of tympanic membrane, right ear.**

► Gabrielle checks for instructional notes in the Tabular List.

❏ She cross-references the beginning of category **H72** and identifies the instructional note that states **Code first any associated otitis media.**

❏ She already checked the instructional notes for the block and chapter, so she does not check them again because she knows they do not apply to this case.

► Gabrielle reviews the codes she has assigned for this case.

❏ **H72.821 Total perforations of tympanic membrane, right ear**

❏ **H65.03 Acute serous otitis media, bilateral**

► Next, Gabrielle must decide how to sequence the codes.

CODING PRACTICE

Exercise 19.3 Assigning Codes for Ear Conditions

Instructions: Read the mini-medical-record of each patient's encounter, review the information abstracted in Exercise 19.2, and assign ICD-10-CM diagnosis codes using the Index and Tabular List. Write the code(s) on the line provided.

1. OUTPATIENT SURGERY   Gender: M   Age: 7

Reason for encounter: Bilateral tympanoplasty

Assessment: Bilateral chronic serous otitis media

Plan: FU in office 2 weeks

1 ICD-10-CM Code _____

CODING PRACTICE (continued)

2. OFFICE   Gender: F   Age: 23

Chief complaint: Severe nausea, vomiting, sweating, vertigo

Assessment: Symptoms are due to Ménière's disease, left ear

Plan: Diazepam for vertigo, it may get better on its own or it may not, will consider surgery if necessary, but we want to follow it for awhile

1 ICD-10-CM Code _____

3. OFFICE   Gender: F   Age: 32

Chief complaint: Ringing and buzzing in right ear, difficulty hearing in right ear

Assessment: Objective tinnitus

Plan: We will try electrical stimulation treatments and see how the condition responds before considering surgery.

1 ICD-10-CM Code _____

ARRANGING CODES FOR EAR CONDITIONS

ICD-10-CM does not provide any unique instructions for sequencing codes related to diseases of the ear. Coders follow the general OGCR for selecting the principal or first-listed diagnosis. They also follow instructional notes within the Tabular List. The most common situations in which coders will see instructional notes in this ICD-10-CM chapter are the following:

- When the ear condition is secondary to another condition, sequence the underlying condition first.
- When the ear condition results from an adverse effect of a drug, sequence the condition first and the drug second. Use the Table of Drugs and Chemicals to identify the drug and intent.
- When OM is accompanied by a perforated tympanic membrane, sequence the OM first and the perforated membrane second.
- When the ear condition is due to an external cause, sequence the ear condition first, followed by the external cause codes.
- Sequence codes describing tobacco use or exposure as secondary codes.

Guided Example of Arranging Codes for Ear Conditions

To learn more about sequencing codes for the ear and mastoid process, continue with the example from earlier in the chapter about a patient who was seen due to ear pain and fever.

Follow along in your ICD-10-CM manual and check off each step after you complete it.

▶ First, Gabrielle confirms the codes she assigned.

❏ **H72.821 Total perforations of tympanic membrane, right ear**

❏ **H65.03 Acute serous otitis media, bilateral**

▶ Gabrielle reviews the instructional notes in the Tabular List to determine how to sequence the codes.

❏ The instructional note for code **H72.821** directs her to **Code first any associated otitis media**. This tells her that the code for otitis media, **H65.03**, should be sequenced first.

❏ The instructional note for code **H65.03** directs her to **Use additional code for any associated perforated tympanic membrane**. This confirms that the code for TMP, **H72.821**, should be sequenced second.

▶ Gabrielle finalizes the codes and sequencing for this case:

(1) **H65.03 Acute serous otitis media, bilateral**

(2) **H72.821 Total perforations of tympanic membrane, right ear**

CODING PRACTICE

Exercise 19.4   Arranging Codes for Ear Conditions

Instructions: Read the mini-medical-record of each patient's encounter, review the information abstracted in Exercise 19.2, assign ICD-10-CM diagnosis codes using the Index and Tabular List, and sequence them correctly.

1. OUTPATIENT SURGERY   Gender: M   Age: 58

Reason for encounter: Bilateral stapedotomy and placement of prosthesis

Assessment: Bilateral conductive hearing loss due to bilateral nonobliterative otosclerosis of the stapes at the oval window

(continued)

(continued)

CODING PRACTICE (continued)

1. (continued)

Plan: FU in office 2 weeks

Tip: *Nonobliterative* means nonblocking. Sequence the underlying condition first because it is the reason for the procedure.

2 ICD-10-CM Codes _____

2. OFFICE   Gender: F   Age: 12

Reason for encounter: Left earache, fever, head congestion

Assessment: Acute recurrent suppurative otitis media and acute recurrent sinusitis, mother is a heavy cigarette smoker in the home

(continued)

2. (continued)

Plan: Antibiotics for OM, decongestant, and fluids

3 ICD-10-CM Codes _____

_____

3. OFFICE   Gender: M   Age: 19

Reason for encounter: Dizziness, nausea, low back pain, headache on right side

Assessment: Dizziness, nausea, and headache due to labyrinthitis, right

Plan: Refer to physical therapy for balance and for LBP

2 ICD-10-CM Codes _____

CHAPTER SUMMARY

In this chapter you learned that:

- The ear makes hearing possible by collecting sound waves from the external world and converting them into impulses that are transmitted to the brain through the vestibulocochlear nerve, cranial nerve VIII.
- ICD-10-CM provides no Official Guidelines for Coding and Reporting (OGCR) for Chapter 8.
- The primary concerns in abstracting for diagnoses of the ear and mastoid process are laterality, external causes, tobacco use or exposure, and the many variations of otitis media.

- The Index provides cross-references that redirect coders to alternative Main Terms for many ear conditions.
- ICD-10-CM does not provide any unique instructions for sequencing codes related to diseases of the ear.

CONCEPT QUIZ

Take a moment to look back at the ear and mastoid process and solidify your skills. Try to answer the questions from memory first, then look back at the discussion in this chapter if you need a little extra help.

Completion

Instructions: Write the term that completes each statement based on the information you learned in this chapter. Choose from the list below. Some choices may be used more than once and some choices may not be used at all.

ceruminoma	mastoid	serous
cholesteatoma	Ménière's disease	suppurative
conductive	middle	tinnitus
external	nonsuppurative	vertigo
inner	recurrent	vestibulocochlear
labyrinthitis	sensorineural	

1. The tympanic membrane is part of the _____ ear.
2. _____ is excessive accumulation of ear wax.
3. _____ hearing loss is due to abnormal formation of the cochlea or cochlear nerve.
4. Otitis media is an infection of the _____ ear.
5. The ossicles are part of the _____ ear.
6. _____ OM involves the discharge of pus.
7. The cochlea is part of the _____ ear.
8. _____ is a viral or bacterial inflammation or infection of the semicircular canals of the inner ear.

9. _____ is a sensation of motion or dizziness.

10. The _____ nerve is also called cranial nerve VIII.

Multiple Choice

Instructions: Circle the letter of the best answer to each question based on the information you learned in this chapter.

1. How would you code the following scenario? *A 7-year-old girl is brought in by her mother and is diagnosed with bilateral recurrent acute serous otitis media and total perforation of the left ear tympanic membrane.*
   A. H65.06, H72.822
   B. H72.822, H65.06
   C. H65.03, H72.823
   D. H72.823, H65.03

2. What term means a loss of mobility of the stapes bone?
   A. Tinnitus
   B. Cholesteatoma
   C. Ménière's disease
   D. Otosclerosis

3. What circumstance does an instructional note at the beginning of Chapter 8 directs coders to assign an additional code for?
   A. External cause
   B. Alcohol use
   C. Tobacco use
   D. Exposure to loud music

4. Which is a subtype of otitis media?
   A. Sensorineural
   B. Supportive
   C. Suppurative
   D. Conductive

5. How would you code the following scenario? *A patient is seen for recurrent acute otitis media that has persisted for four months and is accompanied by changes in the lining of the middle ear. Physician updates the diagnosis to chronic suppurative otitis media, bilateral.*
   A. H66.23
   B. H66.3X3
   C. H66.003
   D. H65.493

6. What is the focus of OGCR for Chapter 8?
   A. Otitis media
   B. Laterality
   C. Hearing loss
   D. There are no OGCR for Chapter 8.

7. What are the most common types OM?
   A. Nonsuppurative and secretory
   B. Suppurative and serous
   C. Chronic and mucoid
   D. Allergic and seromucinous

8. What Main Term does the Index entry for *Loss, hearing* cross-reference coders to?
   A. Sensorineural
   B. Conductive
   C. Deafness
   D. Hearing

9. What second-level subterms are nearly all types of OM indexed under?
   A. Nonsuppurative and suppurative
   B. Acute and chronic
   C. Otitis and media
   D. Serous and recurrent

10. How would you code the following scenario? *A patient is seen for bilateral congenital sensorineural deafness.*
    A. H90.41, H90.42
    B. H90.3
    C. H90.6
    D. H90.5

KEEP ON CODING

Instructions: Read the diagnostic statement, then use the Index and Tabular List to assign and sequence ICD-10-CM diagnosis codes. Write the code(s) on the line provided.

1. Diffuse cholesteatosis, right ear. ICD-10-CM Code(s) _____

2. Noise-induced hearing loss of bilateral inner ears. ICD-10-CM Code(s) _____

3. Mucosal cyst of postmastoidectomy cavity, both ears. ICD-10-CM Code(s) _____

4. Swimmer's ear, left. ICD-10-CM Code(s) _____

5. Exostosis, right external ear canal. ICD-10-CM Code(s) _____

6. Postauricular fistula, both ears. ICD-10-CM Code(s) _____

7. Aural vertigo. ICD-10-CM Code(s) _____

8. Conductive deafness. ICD-10-CM Code(s) _____

9. Cochlear otosclerosis, right ear. ICD-10-CM Code(s) _____

10. Partial loss of ear ossicles, left ear. ICD-10-CM Code(s) _____

(continued)

(continued from page 335)

11. Acute petrositis, both ears. ICD-10-CM Code(s) _____

12. Postoperative stenosis of right external ear canal. ICD-10-CM Code(s) _____

13. Otorrhea, left ear. ICD-10-CM Code(s) _____

14. Basal cell carcinoma of pinna of right ear. ICD-10-CM Code(s) _____

15. Chronic allergic otitis media. ICD-10-CM Code(s) _____

16. Hyperacusis, right ear. ICD-10-CM Code(s) _____

17. Adhesive otitis, left middle ear. ICD-10-CM Code(s) _____

18. Patulous Eustachian tube, both ears. ICD-10-CM Code(s) _____

19. Acute reactive otitis externa, left ear. ICD-10-CM Code(s) _____

20. Acute myringitis, bilateral. ICD-10-CM Code(s) _____

21. Labyrinthine hydrops. ICD-10-CM Code(s) _____

22. Perforation of tympanic membrane, left. ICD-10-CM Code(s) _____

23. Transient ischemic deafness, left. ICD-10-CM Code(s) _____

24. Plasminogen deficiency with otitis media, right ear. ICD-10-CM Code(s) _____

25. Hematoma of pinna, right ear. ICD-10-CM Code(s) _____

CODING CHALLENGE

Instructions: Read the mini-medical-record of each patient's encounter, then abstract, assign, and sequence ICD-10-CM diagnosis codes using the Index and Tabular List. Write the code(s) on the line provided.

1. OFFICE   Gender: M   Age: 6

Reason for encounter: Earache in left ear and fever

Assessment: Acute bullous myringitis, left ear

Plan: Antipyrine and benzocaine ear drops for pain, amoxicillin, RTO 1 week

1 ICD-10-CM Code _____

2. OFFICE   Gender: F   Age: 41

Reason for encounter: Sudden loss of hearing after taking tobramycin as prescribed for an infection

Assessment: Ototoxic bilateral sensorineural hearing loss

Plan: Hearing workup for hearing aids

Tip: Follow any cross-reference notes you find in the Index. Remember to code for the drug using the Table of Drugs and Chemicals.

2 ICD-10-CM Codes _____

3. OFFICE   Gender: M   Age: 21

Reason for encounter: Right ear pain and otorrhagia

Assessment: Polyp of right middle ear and associated cholesteatoma in middle ear

Plan: Removed cholesteatoma, Rx antibiotics, RTO 3 weeks

2 ICD-10-CM Codes _____

4. OFFICE   Gender: M   Age: 11

Reason for encounter: Frequent ear aches

Assessment: Chronic serous otitis media (CSOM), bilateral, with attic rupture of left eardrum

Plan: Rx antibiotics

1 ICD-10-CM Code _____

5. OFFICE   Gender: M   Age: 58

Reason for encounter: Patient had upper respiratory infection (URI) followed by feeling of fullness, popping ears, intermittent sharp ear pain and mild disequilibrium

Assessment: Acute Eustachian salpingitis, left ear, URI

Plan: 10 day course of amoxillin, nasal decongestant limited to short term and only 3–4 times daily

2 ICD-10-CM Codes _____

6. OFFICE   Gender: F   Age: 16

Reason for encounter: Ear pain, recurrent URIs

Assessment: Acute and subacute allergic serous otitis media, bilateral, recurrent; the patient smokes cigarettes and both parents smoke at home

Plan: Ear drops to control pain, refer patient and parents to stop smoking clinic

3 ICD-10-CM Codes _____
_____

7. OFFICE   Gender: M   Age: 17

Reason for encounter: Mild hearing impairment, R ear; has been using q-tips to clean ears

Assessment: Impacted cerumen, right ear

Plan: Removed cerumen with curette, call if any further problems

1 ICD-10-CM Code _____

8. OFFICE   Gender: F   Age: 22

Reason for encounter: Pain, swelling, discharge, and itchiness of outer ear

Assessment: Malignant bilateral otitis externa due to Pseudomonas aeruginosa, diabetes type 1

Plan: Schedule for surgical debridement of necrotic tissue, antipseudomonal antibiotic course of 4–6 weeks, RTO in one week

3 ICD-10-CM Codes _____
_____

9. OFFICE   Gender: F   Age: 9

Reason for encounter: Yellow discharge, redness, and some swelling on left ear lobe after getting her ears pierced

Assessment: Abscess of external ear

Plan: Instruct patient on cleaning area with saline, warm salt water compresses to be performed 4x daily, RTO in 2 days if infection has not mitigated

Tip: Code for the condition only. Do not assign external cause codes.

1 ICD-10-CM Codes _____

10. OFFICE   Gender: M   Age: 4

Reason for encounter: Admitted for intravenous antibiotics and mastoidectomy d/t fever, mastoid swelling, deep ear pain at physician's office

Assessment: Left subperiosteal mastoiditis

Plan: Oral antibiotic, RTO in 1 week

1 ICD-10-CM Code _____

Chapter 20

Certain Infectious and Parasitic Diseases (A00-B99)

Chapter Outline

- **Infectious Disease Refresher**
- **Coding Guidelines for Infectious Diseases**
- **Abstracting for Infectious Diseases**
- **Assigning Codes for Infectious Diseases**
- **Arranging Codes for Infectious Diseases**

Learning Objectives

After completing this chapter, you should have the skills to:

20.1 Spell and define the key words, medical terms, and abbreviations related to infectious and parasitic diseases. (Remember)

20.2 Summarize the types of infectious and parasitic diseases. (Understand)

20.3 Adhere to the Official Guidelines for Coding and Reporting related to infectious and parasitic diseases. (Apply)

20.4 Examine and abstract diagnostic information from the medical record for coding infectious and parasitic diseases. (Analyze)

20.5 Demonstrate how to assign codes for infectious and parasitic diseases. (Apply)

20.6 Utilize guidelines for arranging (sequencing) multiple codes for infectious and parasitic diseases. (Apply)

Key Terms and Abbreviations

acquired immunodeficiency syndrome (AIDS)
asymptomatic
bacteria
Candida
Escherichia coli (E. coli)

fungus
Giardia
helminth
herpes
human immunodeficiency virus (HIV)
inconclusive HIV

indeterminate HIV
localized
multiple organ dysfunction
opportunistic infection
pandemic
parasite
protozoa

Pseudomonas aeruginosa (P. aeruginosa)
serology
smallpox
systemic
varicella
virus

In addition to the key terms listed here, students should know the terms defined within tables in this chapter.

INTRODUCTION

When you travel out of the United States or Canada, you will most likely be required to get some vaccinations. These "travel shots" help protect you from contracting an infectious disease and, as importantly, prevent you from spreading it to others. Most such infectious diseases are classified in ICD-10-CM Chapter 1.

An infectious disease physician specializes in diagnosing and treating infectious diseases. Primary care physicians treat common infectious diseases but refer patients with more complex conditions to an infectious disease specialist.

INFECTIOUS DISEASE REFRESHER

Infectious and parasitic diseases are not a body system; they are a class of diseases that affect the entire body, called systemic diseases. This is in contrast to localized infections, which primarily affect a single organ or body system, such as pneumonia or pharyngitis. Infectious organisms (germs) live in the environment, in the air, on the skin, and inside the body. When the body's immune defenses are weaker than the organism, the organism multiplies to the extent that it causes illness. Infectious organisms are classified by scientists based on the type of cell, shape, and behavior (■ Figure 20-1). Coding infectious diseases requires working with the scientific names of microorganisms that you might not be familiar with. Rely on your medical resources so you have the information you need at your fingertips.

There are four main types of infectious organisms:

- **Bacteria**—One-celled germs that multiply quickly and may release toxins that create illness. Examples are *Escherichia coli (E.coli)* and *Pseudomonas aeruginosa (P. aeruginosa)*.
- **Viruses**—Capsules that contain genetic material and use the body's own cells to multiply. Examples are **varicella** (*chickenpox*) and **herpes** (*shingles*).
- **Protozoa**—One-celled beings, more complex than bacteria, that use other living things as a source of food and a place to live. Examples are *Trichomonas vaginalis* (the cause of trichomoniasis, a sexually transmitted disease) and *Giardia* (*the cause of giardiasis, an intestinal tract infection*).
- **Fungi**—Primitive vegetables that reproduce through spores. Examples include *Candida* (*yeast*) and *Trichophyton rubrum* (the cause of athlete's foot).

The type of infectious organism also determines how physicians treat it. For example, antibiotics treat many bacterial infections but are useless against viruses.

Parasites, also called **helminths**, are plants or animals that live in or on another living organism, or host, and often cause damage to the host. Examples are tapeworm and head lice.

Medical terms related to infectious diseases are built on the word root for the causal organism, which is often named after its shape. As you learn about infectious and parasitic diseases,

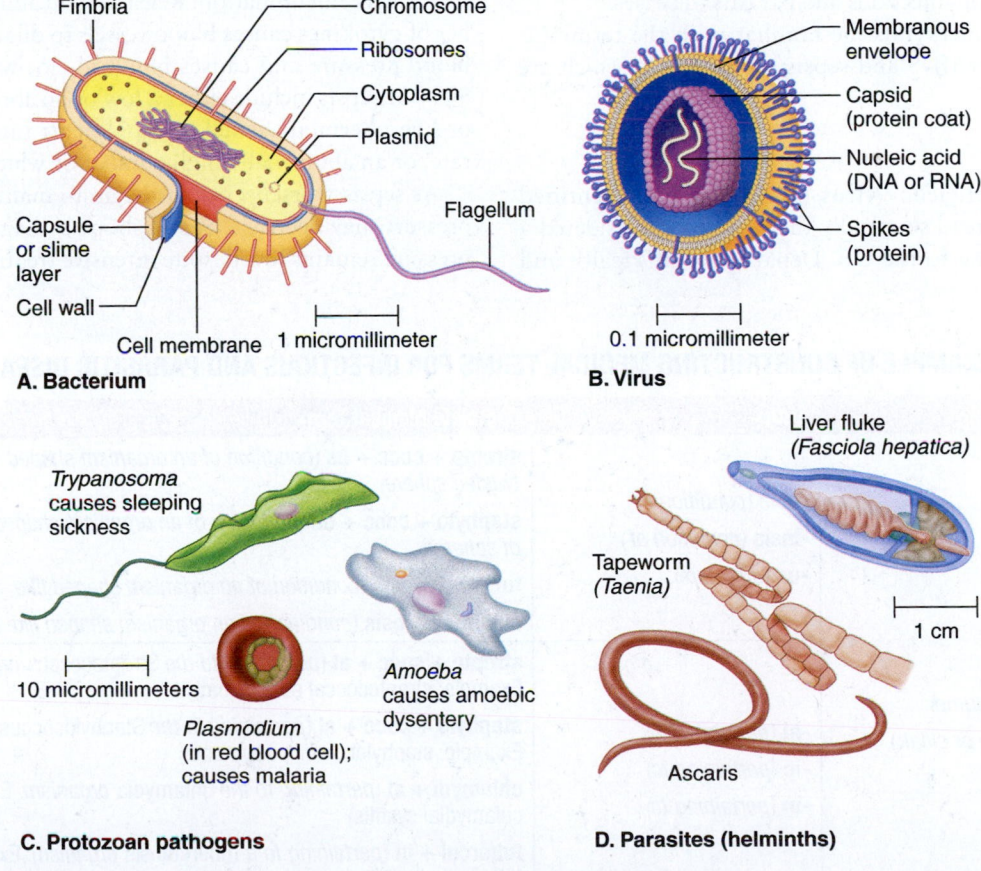

A. Bacterium — Fimbria, Chromosome, Ribosomes, Cytoplasm, Plasmid, Flagellum, Capsule or slime layer, Cell wall, Cell membrane, 1 micromillimeter

B. Virus — Membranous envelope, Capsid (protein coat), Nucleic acid (DNA or RNA), Spikes (protein), 0.1 micromillimeter

C. Protozoan pathogens — *Trypanosoma* causes sleeping sickness, *Plasmodium* (in red blood cell); causes malaria, *Amoeba* causes amoebic dysentery, 10 micromillimeters

D. Parasites (helminths) — Liver fluke (*Fasciola hepatica*), Tapeworm (*Taenia*), Ascaris, 1 cm

Figure 20-1 ■ Pathogens causing infectious and parasitic diseases.

remember to use medical terminology skills to distinguish between word roots for organisms, nouns that describe conditions, and adjectives that mean "pertaining to." When the organism causes a condition, a suffix is added to create a noun or adjective. Refer to ■ TABLE 20-1 for a refresher on how to build medical terms related to infectious and parasitic diseases.

> ### CODING CAUTION
> Be alert for medical word roots that are spelled similarly but have different meanings.
>
> **HIV** (*human immunodeficiency virus*) and **HPV** (*human papilloma virus*, which causes cervical cancer)
>
> **candidiasis** (*a yeast infection*) and **chlamydia** (*a sexually transmitted disease*)
>
> **trichomoniasis** (*a sexually transmitted disease*) and **trichinosis** (*a roundworm infection caused by eating raw pork or certain other meats*)

Common Infectious Diseases

Smallpox is the only infectious disease of humans that the World Health Organization (WHO) has declared to have been eradicated, with the last known case in 1977. Other types of pox (*a disease manifested through eruptions or pustules*), such as chickenpox and Rickettsialpox, still exist. Some infectious diseases that once were common, such as poliomyelitis, are now quite rare in the United States. However, new diseases, such as HIV and Lyme disease, have taken their place. Refer to ■ TABLE 20-2 for a summary of common infectious and parasitic diseases.

In particular, coders must be familiar with the terminology related to HIV/AIDS and sepsis/septic shock, which are highlighted next.

HIV and AIDS

Human immunodeficiency virus (HIV) was first identified in 1983 and has spread so rapidly that it is now considered a pandemic, according to the U.S. Department of Health and Human Services (HHS). HIV is the virus that causes acquired immunodeficiency syndrome (AIDS). It is transmitted through unsafe sex, contaminated needles, blood products, breast milk, and perinatal means, such as the birth process. Screening of blood products for HIV has nearly eliminated the transmission of HIV through blood transfusions in developed countries.

HIV invades T4 lymphocytes and eventually paralyzes the body's immune system. People can be infected with the HIV virus and be asymptomatic (*have no symptoms*) for many years. During this time serology (*blood tests*) will be positive for the virus.

An indeterminate or inconclusive HIV test result means that the antibody test was neither positive nor negative. This may be due to a variety of causes, and the test should be repeated.

AIDS is the final stage of the HIV infection and is diagnosed based on blood cell counts. The symptoms of AIDS are opportunistic infections, diseases that attack those with weakened immune systems but do not develop in those with healthy immune systems (■ TABLE 20-3). Patients with AIDS usually die from an opportunistic infection, such as Kaposi's sarcoma or pneumonia. There is no cure for HIV or AIDS, although researchers have made immense progress in developing drugs that slow the rate at which the disease progresses.

Sepsis, Severe Sepsis, and Septic Shock

Sepsis is the presence of bacteria or their toxins in the blood. Usually, the body's response to infection is limited to the specific area infected. In sepsis, the body has a systemic response, in which all body systems try to fight the infection. The invasive bacteria cause cells in the body to release cytokines, substances that trigger inflammation. Release of an abnormally high number of cytokines causes blood vessels to dilate, which decreases blood pressure and causes blood to clot within vital organs. Signs of sepsis include either a low or an abnormally high fever or hypothermia, as well as rapid heart rate, rapid breathing rate, or an abnormally high number of white blood cells.

As sepsis worsens, organs begin to malfunction and blood pressure may decrease. Septic shock is diagnosed when blood pressure remains low despite intensive treatment. Severe sepsis

Table 20-1 ■ EXAMPLE OF CONSTRUCTING MEDICAL TERMS FOR INFECTIOUS AND PARASITIC DISEASES

Combining Form	Suffix	Complete Medical Term
cocc/o (sphere) strept/o (twisted) staphyl/o (cluster) tubercul/o (knob or bump) chlamyd/o (envelope or cloak)	-osis (condition of) -iasis (condition of) -us (structure)	**strepto + cocc + us** (*condition of an organism shaped like a twisted sphere*) **staphylo + cocc + us** (*condition of an organism shaped like a cluster of spheres*) **tubercul + osis** (*condition of an organism shaped like a knob*) **chlamydi + osis** (*condition of an organism shaped like a cloak*)
	-al (pertaining to) -ic (pertaining to) -in (pertaining to)	**strepto + cocc + al** (*pertaining to the Streptococcus organism. Example: streptococcal sore throat*) **staphylo + cocc + al** (*pertaining to the Staphylococcus organism. Example: staphylococcal pneumonia*) **chlamydi + al** (*pertaining to the Chlamydia organism. Example: chlamydial cystitis*) **tubercul + in** (*pertaining to a Tuberculosis organism. Example: tuberculin test*)

Table 20-2 ■ **COMMON INFECTIOUS AND PARASITIC DISEASES**

Condition	Definition
Acquired immunodeficiency syndrome (AIDS)	A disease caused by the HIV virus that weakens and paralyzes the immune system
Hepatitis	A viral inflammation of the liver
Herpes zoster	A painful, blistering skin rash due to the varicella-zoster virus that causes chickenpox; also called *shingles*
Human immunodeficiency virus (HIV)	A virus that infects and destroys helper T-cells of the immune system and causes AIDS
Human papillomavirus (HPV)	A virus that causes cervical cancer
Leprosy	A chronic bacterial disease characterized by the formation of nodules on the surface of the body
Malaria	An acute or chronic disease caused by parasites and characterized by high fever, shaking chills, flu-like symptoms, and anemia
Methicillin-resistant *Staphylococcus aureus* (MRSA) infection	A type of staph infection that does not respond to commonly used antibiotics
Methicillin-susceptible *Staphylococcus aureus* (MSSA) infection	A type of staph infection that responds to commonly used antibiotics
Mononucleosis	A viral infection causing fever, sore throat, and swollen lymph glands
Multiple drug-resistant organism (MDRO)	A bacteria that survives exposure to many different antibiotics
Nosocomial	Any hospital-acquired infection
Sepsis	A severe, life-threatening, system-wide reaction to infection caused by disease-causing organisms, especially bacteria, in the blood or tissues
Septic shock	Life-threatening low blood pressure due to sepsis
Septicemia	A systemic disease associated with the presence and persistence of bacteria, viruses, fungi, or other organisms or toxins in the blood
Severe sepsis	Acute or multiple organ dysfunction (MOD) due to sepsis
Syphilis	A sexually transmitted disease (STD) caused by bacteria that produces chancres, rashes, and systemic lesions
Systemic inflammatory response syndrome (SIRS)	An acute, system-wide inflammatory reaction with at least two manifestations: fever, tachycardia, tachypnea, leukocytosis, and/or leukopenia
Tuberculosis (TB)	A contagious bacterial infection that involves the lungs but may spread to other organs

is organ malfunction, which results from a blockage of blood flow to vital organs due to blood clots.

Infants, the elderly, and those with weakened immune systems are most likely to get sepsis. Physicians treat sepsis with antibiotics to kill the bacteria, fluids to maintain adequate blood pressure, and mechanical ventilation to aid breathing. Sepsis progresses rapidly, causing death in one-third of those who get it, according to the Centers for Disease Control and Prevention (CDC).

CODING CAUTION

Medicare does not reimburse inpatient hospitals for costs associated with hospital-acquired conditions (HACs; *a preventable condition acquired during a hospital stay*). Inpatient hospitals must report whether conditions are present on admission (POA). Because sepsis and septicemia are common HACs, it is important to correctly identify the POA status. OGCR Appendix I provides detailed guidelines on POA reporting.

Table 20-3 ■ **CONDITIONS COMMON TO AIDS**

Type of Complication	Conditions
Malignancies	Kaposi's sarcoma (*malignant neoplasm of the connective tissue*) lymphoma
Infections	Candidiasis
	Herpes simplex
	Herpes zoster (shingles)
	Pneumonia (*Pneumocystis carinii* pneumonia [PCP])
	Toxoplasmosis
	Tuberculosis
Gastrointestinal symptoms	Diarrhea
	Lack of appetite
	Nausea and vomiting
Neurological symptoms	Confusion and memory loss
	Headaches and visual changes

CODING PRACTICE

Exercise 20.1 Infectious Disease Refresher

Instructions: Use your medical terminology skills and resources to define the following conditions related to infectious and parasitic diseases, then assign the default diagnosis code.

Follow these steps:

- Identify the infectious organism.
- Define the meaning of the condition.
- Assign the diagnosis code for the condition using the Index and Tabular List.

Example: chlamydial cervicitis   Organism *Chlamydia*   Meaning *Inflammation of the cervix due to Chlamydia*   ICD-10-CM Code *A56.09*

1. candidiasis bronchitis   Organism _____   Meaning _____   ICD-10-CM Code _____
2. syphilitic endocarditis   Organism _____   Meaning _____   ICD-10-CM Code _____
3. herpetic eyelid   Organism _____   Meaning _____   ICD-10-CM Code _____
4. typhoid meningitis   Organism _____   Meaning _____   ICD-10-CM Code _____
5. amebiasis cutaneous   Organism _____   Meaning _____   ICD-10-CM Code _____
6. parasitic stomatitis   Organism _____   Meaning _____   ICD-10-CM Code _____
7. Rickettsialpox   Organism _____   Meaning _____   ICD-10-CM Code _____
8. trichomoniasis prostate   Organism _____   Meaning _____   ICD-10-CM Code _____
9. tubercular anus   Organism _____   Meaning _____   ICD-10-CM Code _____
10. gonococcal pharyngitis   Organism _____   Meaning _____   ICD-10-CM Code _____

CODING GUIDELINES FOR INFECTIOUS DISEASES

Coders should understand the organization of this ICD-10-CM chapter, chapter-wide and commonly used instructional notes in the Tabular List, and the relevant OGCR. This information is necessary for accurate coding.

ICD-10-CM Chapter 1, "Certain Infectious and Parasitic Diseases (A00-B99)," contains 22 blocks or subchapters that are divided by the type of infection. Review the block names and code ranges listed at the beginning of Chapter 1 in the ICD-10-CM manual to become familiar with the content and organization. Two letters of the alphabet, *A* or *B*, are used as the first letter of the codes.

This chapter includes parasitic infestations and systemic infections due to viruses, bacteria, protozoa, and fungi. It also includes the named organisms that cause localized infections. This chapter does not include localized infections, which are classified in the body system chapter. Localized infections may be assigned a combination code that identifies the condition and the causal organism, or they may require one code for the condition and a second code from Chapter 1 to identify the causal organism. Instructional notes in the Tabular List, under the code for the localized infection, identify when to assign an additional code for the infectious organism. This chapter also does not include obstetric- or newborn-related conditions, which are classified in ICD-10-CM Chapters 15 and 16, respectively.

ICD-10-CM provides Official Guidelines for Coding and Reporting (OGCR) infectious and parasitic diseases in OGCR section I.C.1. OGCR provides a detailed discussion of assigning and sequencing codes for HIV, sepsis, septic shock, and Zika virus infections. An instructional note at the beginning of Chapter 1 in the Tabular List instructs coders to assign an additional code when an infection is drug resistant. This instruction applies to all codes in Chapter 1. Specific OGCR and instructional notes are discussed and cited throughout this chapter of the text.

ABSTRACTING FOR INFECTIOUS DISEASES

Coders always need to identify the scientific name of the infectious organism and subtype, as well as associated complications or manifestations. Additional details are needed when abstracting HIV/AIDS and sepsis. Refer to ■ TABLE 20-4 for

Table 20-4 ■ **KEY CRITERIA FOR ABSTRACTING INFECTIOUS AND PARASITIC DISEASES**

- ❏ What is the named organism responsible for the patient's condition?
- ❏ What type of organism is it (bacteria, virus, etc.)?
- ❏ What is the subtype of the condition?
- ❏ Is a more specific subtype documented?
- ❏ Does the patient have a condition that is due to *Streptococcus, Staphylococcus,* or *Enterococcus*?
- ❏ Is the infection systemic or localized (organ specific)?
- ❏ Is the organism the cause of a condition that exists in a specific body system?
- ❏ Does the documentation state that the infection is resistant to antibiotics?

guidance on how to abstract infectious and parasitic diseases. Remember that the abstracting questions are a guide and that not every question applies to, or can be answered for, every case. For example, the hepatitis virus has subtypes A, B, or C, but not every organism does. Also remember to abstract for symptoms and determine whether they are integral to the confirmed diagnoses.

Abstracting HIV and AIDS

When abstracting cases involving HIV and AIDS, coders must determine whether physician documentation confirms an HIV infection. In addition, coders must determine whether HIV is asymptomatic or if it manifests itself in AIDS-related conditions. For any encounter with an HIV or AIDS patient, coders must also determine whether the reason for the encounter is related to HIV or AIDS or is an unrelated condition, such as an accident that causes a fracture. Refer to ■ TABLE 20-5 for guidance in abstracting HIV and AIDS cases, then refer to the example that follows (■ FIGURE 20-2).

Abstracting Sepsis, Severe Sepsis, and Septic Shock

When abstracting sepsis, severe sepsis, and septic shock, coders must have a clear understanding of the definitions of these conditions. For example, patients with sepsis and associated acute organ dysfunction are classified as having severe sepsis even if the documentation does not contain

the precise word *severe* (OGCR I.C.1.d.1)(a)). When the documentation is unclear regarding the status of the patient, query the physician for clarification. Coders also abstract the underlying systemic infection, such as *Pseudomonas aeruginosa* or *Escherichia coli*. Refer to ■ TABLE 20-6 for guidance in abstracting these cases, then work through the detailed example that follows.

Guided Example of Abstracting for Infectious Diseases

Refer to the following example throughout this chapter to practice skills for abstracting, assigning, and sequencing infectious and parasitic disease codes. Susanna Vannote, CPC, is a fictitious coder who guides you through the coding process.

Date: 02/11/yy Location: Branton Medical Center

Provider: James Cruickshank, MD

Patient: Faye Gillis   Gender: F   Age: 81

Reason for admission: Admitted to ICU from the emergency department due to acute respiratory failure

Assessment: Gram-negative (E. coli) sepsis with organ failure (POA)

Plan: Discharged to skilled nursing facility

Table 20-5 ■ KEY CRITERIA FOR ABSTRACTING HIV AND AIDS

- ❏ Does the physician clearly document a confirmed diagnosis of HIV positive?
- ❏ Does the patient have symptoms or complications?
- ❏ Is the patient being seen (or admitted) for an HIV-related condition?
- ❏ Is the patient being seen (or admitted) for a condition *un*related to HIV?
- ❏ Has the patient been previously diagnosed with an HIV-related illness?
- ❏ Is the purpose of the encounter HIV testing?
- ❏ Did the patient receive HIV counseling?
- ❏ Is HIV serology inconclusive?

Table 20-6 ■ KEY CRITERIA FOR ABSTRACTING SEPSIS AND SEPTIC SHOCK

- ❏ What is the systemic infection underlying the sepsis?
- ❏ Is a more specific subtype documented?
- ❏ Is the sepsis documented as severe?
- ❏ Is an *associated* acute organ dysfunction documented?
- ❏ Is septic shock documented?
- ❏ Was the severe sepsis present on admission or did it develop after admission?
- ❏ Does a localized (organ-specific) infection exist in addition to sepsis?
- ❏ Is the sepsis the complication of a procedure that was performed?
- ❏ Is the sepsis associated with a wound?
- ❏ Is the sepsis associated with a noninfectious condition (such as trauma)?

Patient with known AIDS is admitted for AIDS-related pneumocystis carinii pneumonia (PCP).

- Does the physician clearly document a confirmed diagnosis of HIV positive? **Yes, a diagnosis of AIDS presumes HIV positive.**
- Does the patient have symptoms or complications? **Yes, pneumonia.**
- Is the patient being seen (or admitted) for an HIV-related condition? **Yes, PCP.**
- Is the patient being seen (or admitted) for a condition unrelated to HIV? **No.**
- Has the patient been previously diagnosed with an HIV-related illness? **Yes, patient is known to have AIDS at the time of admission.**
- Is the purpose of the encounter HIV testing? **No.**
- Did the patient receive HIV counseling? **No.**
- Is HIV serology inconclusive? **No.**

Figure 20-2 ■ Example of abstracting HIV/AIDS.

Follow along as Susanna Vannote, CPC, abstracts the diagnosis. Check off each step after you complete it.

▶ Susanna reads through the entire record, paying special attention to the reason for the encounter and the final assessment. She refers to the Key Criteria for Abstracting Sepsis and Septic Shock (Table 20-6).

❏ *What is the systemic infection underlying the sepsis?* E. coli

❏ *Is the sepsis documented as severe?* No

❏ *Is an associated acute organ dysfunction documented?* Yes, respiratory

❏ *Is septic shock documented?* No

❏ *Was the severe sepsis present on admission or did it develop after admission?* Sepsis was present on admission

❏ *Does a localized (organ-specific) infection exist in addition to sepsis?* No

❏ *Is the sepsis the complication of a procedure that was performed?* No

❏ *Is the sepsis associated with a wound?* No

❏ *Is the sepsis associated with a noninfectious condition (such as trauma)?* No

▶ At this time, Susanna does not know which of these conditions may need to be coded, nor how many codes she will end up with. She will learn about this when she moves on to assigning codes.

CODING PRACTICE

Exercise 20.2   Abstracting for Infectious Diseases

Instructions: Read the mini-medical-record of each patient's encounter and answer the abstracting questions. Write the answer on the line provided. Do not assign any codes.

---

1. OFFICE   Gender: M   Age: 18

Chief complaint: General lack of energy, fatigue, loss of appetite, fever, and chills

Assessment: Suspected Epstein-Barr mononucleosis, which was confirmed by a blood test

Plan: Drink fluids, get rest, acetaminophen or ibuprofen for pain and fever, recovery can take several weeks, call if abdominal pain, difficulty breathing, severe weakness, or persistent high fever

a. What are the symptoms? _____
_____

b. Is the condition uncertain or confirmed? _____
_____

c. What is the named organism? _____
_____

d. Should the symptoms be coded? _____
   Why or why not? _____

---

2. OFFICE   Gender: F   Age: 46

Reason for encounter: Annual work related PPD (*purified protein derivative*) tuberculin test

Assessment: PPD positive for TB, x-ray of lung positive for nodules in lung

(continued)

---

2. (continued)

Plan: Order sputum culture, begin pharmacotherapy

a. What is the named organism responsible for the patient's condition? _____
_____

b. Does the documentation state that the infection is resistant to antibiotics? _____
_____

c. What anatomic site is involved? _____
_____

---

3. INPATIENT HOSPITAL   Gender: F   Age: 70

Reason for admission: Called in for a consult on Staphylococcus aureus pneumonia

Assessment: Culture result shows MSSA

Plan: IV teicoplanin (*an antibiotic*) was successful and patient was discharged with instructions to help prevent recurrence

a. What is the named organism responsible for the patient's condition? _____
_____

b. Does the patient have a condition that is due to *Streptococcus, Staphylococcus,* or *Enterococcus*? _____
_____

c. Does the documentation state that the infection is resistant to antibiotics? _____
_____

CODING PRACTICE (continued)

4. OFFICE   Gender: M   Age: 27

Reason for encounter: Genital chancre (*a firm, nonitchy skin ulcer*)

Assessment: Primary syphilis

Plan: Antibiotics

a. What is the named organism responsible for the patient's condition? _____
_____

b. What is the subtype of the condition? _____
_____

c. Does the patient have a condition that is due to *Streptococcus*, *Staphylococcus*, or *Enterococcus*? _____

d. Does the documentation state that the infection is resistant to antibiotics? _____
_____

5. INPATIENT HOSPITAL   Gender: F   Age: 35

Reason for admission: Admitted from emergency department due to sepsis

Assessment: Staphylococcus aureus sepsis, cause unknown, responsive to antibiotics

Plan: After O$_2$ and IV fluids and antibiotics, patient was discharged home in good condition

a. What is the systemic infection underlying the sepsis? _____

b. Does the documentation state that the infection is resistant to antibiotics? _____
_____

c. Is the sepsis documented as severe? _____
_____

d. Is an associated acute organ dysfunction documented? _____
_____

e. Is the sepsis the complication of a procedure or a wound? _____
_____

6. OFFICE   Gender: M   Age: 26

Reason for encounter: Lesions on the skin of this HIV positive patient

Assessment: Kaposi's sarcoma of the skin

Plan: Refer to oncologist to evaluate extent of the cancer and determine treatment plan

(continued)

6. (continued)

a. Does the physician clearly document a confirmed diagnosis of HIV positive? _____

b. Does the patient have symptoms or complications?
_____

c. Is the patient being seen (or admitted) for an HIV-related condition? _____
_____

7. EMERGENCY DEPARTMENT   Gender: M   Age: 26

Reason for encounter: Toe pain after a horse stepped on his foot

Assessment: Fractured distal phalanx of great toe on the right foot, AIDS patient with Kaposi's sarcoma of the lymph nodes which was not treated at this encounter

Plan: Reduced fracture and applied cast, crutches, FU office 2 weeks

a. What is the reason for the encounter? _____
_____

b. What bone was fractured? _____
_____

c. What is the laterality? _____
_____

d. What is the episode of care? _____
_____

e. Does the physician clearly document a confirmed diagnosis of HIV positive? _____
_____

f. Does the patient have symptoms or complications? _____

g. Is the patient being seen (or admitted) for an HIV-related condition? _____
_____

8. OFFICE   Gender: F   Age: 31

Reason for encounter: Follow up on HIV test results

Assessment: Positive for HIV, asymptomatic, counseled patient on managing the infection

Plan: Refer to HIV support group

a. Did the physician clearly document a confirmed diagnosis of HIV positive? _____
_____

b. Does the patient have symptoms or complications?
_____

(continued)

CODING PRACTICE *(continued)*

---

8. (continued)

c. Is the purpose of the encounter HIV testing? _____
_____

d. Did the patient receive HIV counseling? _____
_____

---

9. (continued)

f. Is the urosepsis documented as HIV related? _____
_____

g. What condition is the reason for the encounter?
_____

---

9. OFFICE   Gender: M   Age: 45

Reason for encounter: HIV positive patient with no related conditions presents with dysuria, weakness, and fever

Assessment: Urosepsis (UTI) d/t E. coli (non-Shiga toxin-producing)

Plan: Antibiotics

a. What are the symptoms? _____
_____

b. What condition is diagnosed? _____
_____

c. What is the infectious organism? _____
_____

   What is the subtype? _____

d. Does the documentation state that the infection is resistant to antibiotics? _____
_____

e. Does the physician clearly document a confirmed diagnosis of HIV positive? _____
_____

(continued)

---

10. INPATIENT HOSPITAL   Gender: F   Age: 77

Reason for admission: Admitted from SNF 1 day post-hospital-discharge with 102°F fever, dyspnea, heart rate 100 per minute, low BP

Assessment: Severe sepsis d/t nosocomial MRSA and associated heart failure, septic shock

Plan: Deceased

a. What is the systemic infection underlying the sepsis?
_____

b. Does the documentation state that the infection is resistant to antibiotics? _____
_____

c. Is the sepsis documented as severe? _____
_____

d. Is septic shock present? _____
   Why or why not? _____
_____

e. Is an associated acute organ dysfunction documented? _____
_____

ASSIGNING CODES FOR INFECTIOUS DISEASES

OGCR provides many detailed guidelines for coding infectious organisms; HIV and AIDS; and sepsis, severe sepsis, and septic shock. Although coders do not need to memorize every guideline, they should memorize the *fact* that OGCR exists for these conditions and refer to OGCR every time they code these conditions.

Assigning Codes for Infectious Organisms

Guidelines describe how to code infectious organisms that are the cause of localized infections and organisms that are resistant to drugs.

Infectious Organisms in Diseases Classified Elsewhere

As discussed earlier in this chapter, localized infections are classified in body system chapters. In some cases, a combination code describes the condition and the infectious organism. In other cases, the body system chapter provides a code for the condition with an instructional note to assign an additional code for the causal agent. Assign a code from one of the following categories:

- **B95 Streptococcus, Staphylococcus, and Enterococcus as the cause of diseases classified to other chapters**

- **B96 Other bacterial agents as the cause of diseases classified to other chapters**

- **B97 Viral agents as the cause of diseases classified to other chapters**

These are causal agent codes and should be assigned only as a secondary code, in conjunction with a principal or first-listed diagnosis code for the localized infection (OGCR I.C.1.b). When an infectious organism causes a systemic infection, assign a code from elsewhere in ICD-10-CM Chapter 1 based on guidance from the Index and OGCR.

E. coli is classified by its strain. O157 is a strain that produces potentially harmful Shiga toxins. Shiga toxins can also be produced by other strains of *E. coli*. Review the code selections under category **B96.2** to identify codes for the various strains of *E. coli*.

Drug-Resistant Organisms

When an organism is stated as resistant to antibiotics or other drugs, report the resistance with a combination code that identifies the organism and its resistance, if one is available. *Staphylococcus aureus* is classified as either susceptible (responsive) to methicillin, described as methicillin-susceptible *Staphylococcus aureus* (MSSA), or resistant to methicillin, described as methicillin-resistant *Staphylococcus aureus* (MRSA). Combination codes for both MSSA and MRSA are located in the Index under the Main Term **MSSA** and **MRSA**, respectively, and also under the Main Term **Staphylococcus**. Read the documentation carefully to identify the correct type of *Staphylococcus aureus*.

When a combination code is not available, report the resistance with two codes: (1) the infection code and (2) a code from category **Z16 Resistance to antimicrobial drugs** (OGCR I.C.1.c). Locate the code for resistance in the Index under the Main Term **Resistance** and subterms **organism, to, drug**, with a final subterm for the class of drug. When an organism is resistance to multiple drugs, select the subterm **multiple drugs (MDRO)** (■ FIGURE 20-3).

Identify nosocomial infections with the external cause code **Y95 Nosocomial condition**, in addition to any other codes for the infection or organism.

Assigning Codes for HIV and AIDS

ICD-10-CM provides detailed guidelines for assigning codes related to HIV and AIDS. Coders must be careful to use the terminology for HIV and AIDS correctly and precisely, as discussed earlier in this chapter. The codes for a patient with HIV or AIDS change as the disease progresses (■ FIGURE 20-4, page 348).

Asymptomatic HIV

Assign code **Z21 Asymptomatic human immunodeficiency virus [HIV] infection status** when the documentation describes the following circumstances (OGCR I.C.1.a.2)(d)):

- HIV positive
- Known HIV

- HIV test positive
- Asymptomatic HIV

To locate the code, search the Index for the Main Term **HIV** and the subterm **positive, seropositive** (■ FIGURE 20-5, page 348). Do not assign code **Z21** when the test results are documented as inconclusive or when the terms *AIDS* or *HIV disease* are documented. These situations are discussed next.

AIDS

Assign code **B20 Human immunodeficiency virus [HIV] disease** in the following documented circumstances:

- Documentation uses the terms *AIDS* or *HIV disease*
- The patient is treated for any HIV-related illness
- The patient is described as having any condition resulting from HIV-positive status
- The patient has been previously diagnosed with AIDS (OGCR I.C.1.a.2)(f))

To locate the code, search the Index for the Main Term **HIV** and use the default code (Figure 20-5) or search for the Main Term **AIDS** and use the default code (■ FIGURE 20-6, page 348).

The ICD-10-CM code description for AIDS is **HIV disease**. Remember to distinguish between the term *HIV disease* and the terms *HIV virus*, *HIV positive*, or *asymptomatic HIV*, each of which describes a different aspect of the HIV/AIDS cycle.

Inconclusive HIV Test Results

Assign code **R75 Inconclusive laboratory evidence of human immunodeficiency virus [HIV]** for patients with inconclusive HIV serology but no definitive diagnosis or manifestations of the illness (OGCR I.C.1.a.2)(e)). Locate this code under the Main Term **HIV** and the subterm **nonconclusive** (Figure 20-5).

Other HIV-Related Encounters

OGCR I.C.1.a.2)(h) provides additional guidelines for coding encounters for testing for HIV, exposure to HIV, HIV counseling, and high-risk behavior. These and other HIV-related codes can be located in the Index under the Main Term **Human** and subterm **immunodeficiency**. The codes for asymptomatic HIV, inconclusive HIV results, and HIV infection are also located under this entry (■ FIGURE 20-7, page 349).

Once a patient has developed an HIV-related illness, you should assign code **B20** for *every* encounter. Patients previously diagnosed with any HIV illness (**B20**) should *never* be assigned to **R75** or **Z21**.

Refer to ■ FIGURE 20-8 (page 349) to learn more about assigning codes for HIV and AIDS. Sequencing of codes for AIDS patients is discussed later in this chapter.

Assigning Codes for Sepsis and Severe Sepsis

ICD-10-CM provides separate OGCR for sepsis and severe sepsis, which are discussed next.

Sepsis

For a diagnosis of sepsis, assign the appropriate code for the underlying systemic infection, which corresponds to the scientific

---

Patient is treated for Klebsiella pneumoniae pneumonia which is not responding to multiple antibiotics.

(1) **J15.0 Pneumonia due to Klebsiella pneumoniae**
(2) **Z16.24 Resistance to multiple antibiotics**

Figure 20-3 ■ Example of coding multiple drug-resistant organisms.

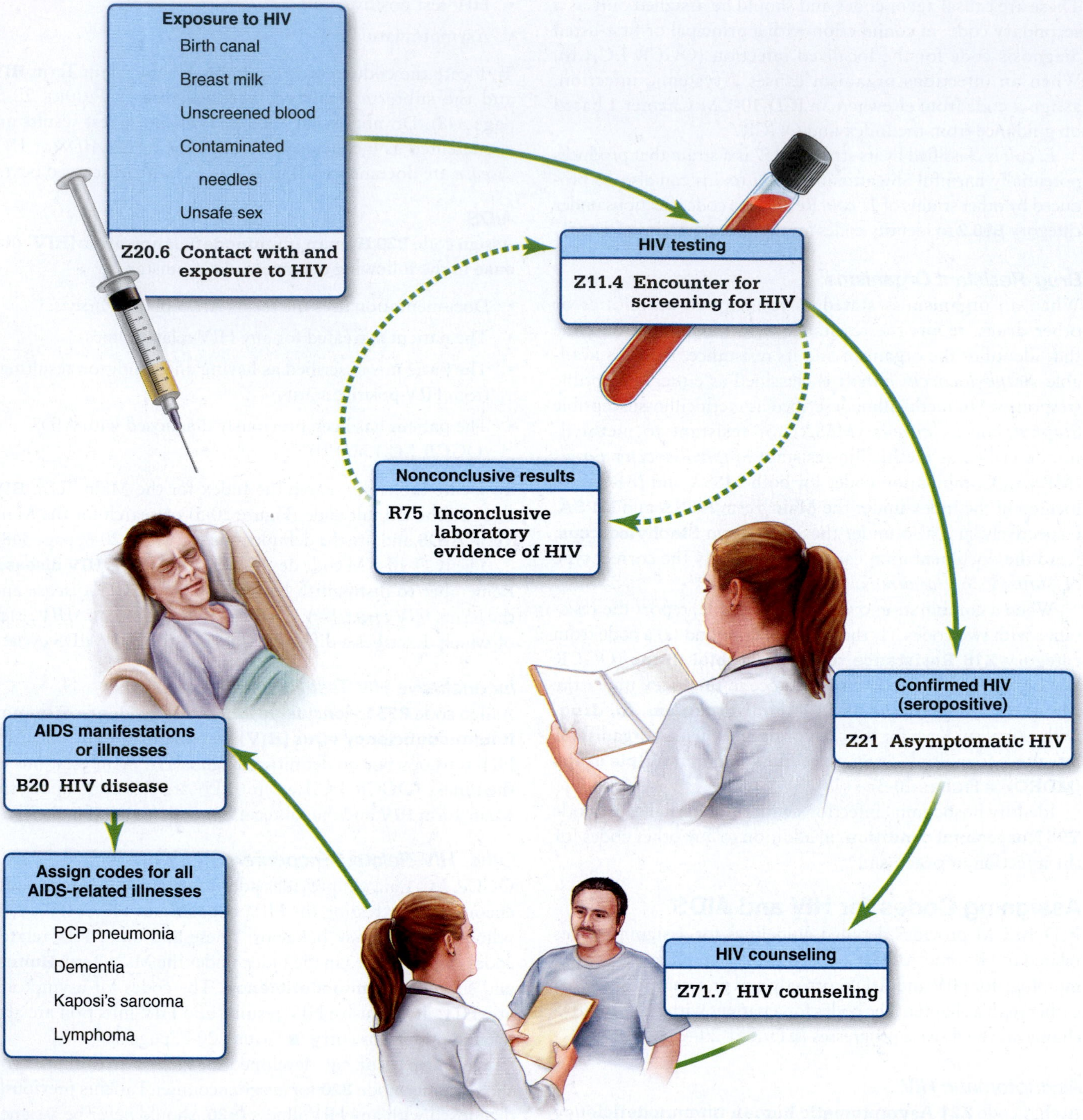

Exposure to HIV

Birth canal

Breast milk

Unscreened blood

Contaminated

needles

Unsafe sex

Z20.6 Contact with and exposure to HIV

HIV testing

Z11.4 Encounter for screening for HIV

Nonconclusive results

R75 Inconclusive laboratory evidence of HIV

Confirmed HIV (seropositive)

Z21 Asymptomatic HIV

AIDS manifestations or illnesses

B20 HIV disease

Assign codes for all AIDS-related illnesses

PCP pneumonia

Dementia

Kaposi's sarcoma

Lymphoma

HIV counseling

Z71.7 HIV counseling

Figure 20-4 ■ Each stage of HIV and AIDS requires unique codes.

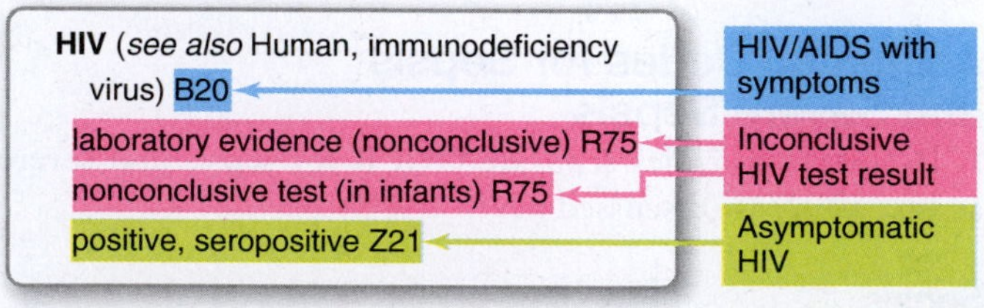

HIV (*see also* Human, immunodeficiency virus) B20

   laboratory evidence (nonconclusive) R75

   nonconclusive test (in infants) R75

   positive, seropositive Z21

HIV/AIDS with symptoms

Inconclusive HIV test result

Asymptomatic HIV

Figure 20-5 ■ Index entry for "HIV".

AIDS (related complex) B20

Figure 20-6 ■ Index entry for "AIDS".

> **Human**
>   bite (open wound) — *see also* Bite
>   intact skin surface — *see* Bite, superficial
>   herpesvirus — *see* Herpes
>   immunodeficiency virus (HIV) disease (infection) B20
>   asymptomatic status Z21
>   contact Z20.6
>   counseling Z71.7
>   dementia B20 *[F02.80]*
>   with behavioral disturbance B20 *[F02.81]*
>   exposure to Z20.6
>   laboratory evidence R75
>   type-2 (HIV 2) as cause of disease classified
>   elsewhere B97.35

Figure 20-7 ■ Index entry for Main Term "Human" with subterm "Immunodeficiency virus".

> Patient with known AIDS is admitted for AIDS-related pneumocystis carinii pneumonia (PCP).
>
> (1) **B20 Human immunodeficiency virus [HIV] disease**
> (2) **B59 Pneumocystosis**

Figure 20-8 ■ Example of assigning codes for HIV/AIDS.

name of the causal organism. If the type of infection or causal organism is not specified, assign code **A41.9 Sepsis, unspecified** (OGCR I.C.1.d.1)(a)). Do not assign a code from subcategory **R65.2 Severe sepsis** unless severe sepsis or an associated acute organ dysfunction is documented. The Index entry for **Septicemia** directs coders to category **A41 Other sepsis**.

Severe Sepsis

When severe sepsis or sepsis *with* organ dysfunction are specifically documented, assign a code from category **R65.2 Severe sepsis** in addition to codes for the infection and organ dysfunction. Assign the fifth character **0** for **without septic shock** or the fifth character **1** for **with septic shock**. When patients have sepsis and *associated* acute organ dysfunction or **multiple organ dysfunction**, follow these instructions for coding severe sepsis (OGCR I.C.1.d.1)(a)(iii)). Documentation must state the association between sepsis and the organ dysfunction. If the medical record documents that the acute organ dysfunction is related to another medical condition, do not assign a code from **R65.2** (OGCR I.C.1.d.1)(a)(iv)). Sequencing of the codes is discussed later in this chapter.

Review the OGCR for additional guidelines regarding:

- Sepsis and severe sepsis with a localized infection (OGCR I.C.1.d.4)).
- Sepsis due to a postprocedural infection (OGCR I.C.1.d.5)).
- Sepsis and severe sepsis associated with a noninfectious process (OGCR I.C.1.d.6)).

Septic Shock

Septic shock, by definition, includes severe sepsis. Therefore, whenever septic shock is documented, assign a code for the systemic infection and also code **R65.21 Severe sepsis with septic shock**.

Assigning Codes for Zika Virus

Zika virus should be coded only when the diagnosis is confirmed by the provider in the documentation (OGCR I.C.1.f). The type of test performed does not need to be stated; the physician's statement of the diagnosis is sufficient. If the provider documents *suspected*, *possible*, or *probable* Zika, do not assign code **A92.5**. Assign a code(s) explaining the reason for the encounter (such as fever, rash, or joint pain) or **Z20.828 Contact with and (suspected) exposure to other viral communicable diseases**. This is an exception to OGCR II.H. that directs coders to code uncertain diagnoses as confirmed for inpatient cases.

Guided Example of Assigning Infectious Disease Codes

To practice skills for assigning codes for infectious and parasitic diseases, continue with the example from earlier in the chapter about patient Faye Gillis, who was admitted to Branton Medical Center due to acute respiratory failure.

Follow along in your ICD-10-CM manual as Susanna Vannote, CPC, assigns codes. Check off each step after you complete it.

▶ First, Susanna confirms the diagnoses.

- ❏ Gram-negative (*E. coli*) sepsis
- ❏ Acute respiratory failure

▶ Susanna searches the Index for the Main Term **Sepsis** (■ FIGURE 20-9).

- ❏ She locates the subterm for the type of sepsis, **Escherichia coli A41.5**.
- ❏ As Susanna continues to review all the subterms under **Sepsis**, she notes an additional subterm that may apply.
  - Immediately under **Sepsis**, she sees the subterm, **with, acute organ dysfunction R65.2**.

▶ Susanna feels confused with so many choices. She remembers that the OGCR contains several guidelines regarding sepsis, so she turns to OGCR I.C.1 near the front of her ICD-10-CM manual for more information.

- ❏ OGCR I.C.1.d.1)(a) states **For a diagnosis of sepsis, assign the appropriate code for the underlying systemic infection**.
  - This tells her she needs a code for Gram-negative sepsis because it is the underlying systemic infection.

> **Sepsis** (generalized) (unspecified organism) A41.9
>   **with**
>   organ dysfunction (acute) (multiple) R65.2
>   with septic shock R65.21
>   actinomycotic A42.7
>
>   Enterococcus A41.81
>   Erysipelothrix (rhusiopathiae) (erysipeloid) A26.7
>   Escherichia coli (E. coli) A41.5
>   extraintestinal yersiniosis A28.2

Figure 20-9 ■ Index entry for "Sepsis".

❑ OGCR I.C.1.d.1)(a)(iii) states **If a patient has sepsis and associated acute organ dysfunction or multiple organ dysfunction (MOD), follow the instructions for coding severe sepsis.**

- This tells her that **acute organ dysfunction** follows the same guidelines as **severe sepsis**, even though the word *severe* was not specifically documented.

❑ OGCR I.C.1.d.1)(b) states **The coding of severe sepsis requires a minimum of 2 codes: first a code for the underlying systemic infection, followed by a code from subcategory R65.2.**

- This confirms that she needs a code for Gram-negative sepsis.

- This tells her that she also needs a code from subcategory **R65.2.**

▶ Susanna verifies subcategory **R65.2, Severe sepsis** in the Tabular List.

❑ She observes that there are many instructional notes under the subcategory title.

❑ She identifies the symbol **5th** in front of the subcategory title, which tells her that a fifth character is required to complete the code.

❑ She locates the fifth-character codes below the instructional notes and determines that code **R65.20 Severe sepsis without septic shock** describes this case because septic shock was not documented.

▶ Susanna reviews the instructional notes in the Tabular List for **R65.20** (■ FIGURE 20-10).

❑ She cross-references the notes at the beginning of subcategory **R65.2.**

❑ The inclusion notes state **Sepsis with acute organ dysfunction.** This accurately describes the case.

❑ She reviews the note **Code first underlying infection, such as:**

❑ None of the conditions listed include the code she assigned for Gram-negative sepsis. However, she recalls that OGCR I.C.1.d.1)(b) already gave her sequencing instructions, which she will review later.

❑ She reviews the note **Use additional code to identify specific acute organ dysfunction, such as:.**

❑ She determines that this note applies because the patient had acute respiratory failure, which is listed in the instruction as **acute respiratory failure (J96.0-).** She will finish verifying the instructional notes for **R65.20,** then assign and verify code for acute respiratory failure.

❑ She cross-references the beginning of category **R65** and verifies that there are no instructional notes that apply to all codes in the category.

❑ She cross-references the beginning of block **R50-R69** and verifies that there are no instructional notes that apply to all codes in the block.

5th R65.2 Severe sepsis
Infection with associated acute organ dysfunction
Sepsis with acute organ dysfunction
Sepsis with multiple organ dysfunction
Systemic inflammatory response syndrome due to infectious process with acute organ dysfunction
Code first underlying infection, such as:
    Infection following a procedure (T81.4)
    Infections following infusion, transfusion and therapeutic injection (T80.2-)
    Puerperal sepsis (O85)
    Sepsis following complete or unspecified spontaneous abortion (O03.87)
    Sepsis following ectopic and molar pregnancy (O08.82)
    Sepsis following incomplete spontaneous abortion (O03.37)
    Sepsis following (induced) termination of pregnancy (O04.87)
    Sepsis NOS A41.9
Use additional code to identify specific acute organ dysfunction, such as:
    acute kidney failure (N17.-)
    acute respiratory failure (J96.0-)
    critical illness myopathy (G72.81)
    critical illness polyneuropathy (G62.81)
    disseminated intravascular coagulopathy [DIC] (D65)
    encephalopathy (metabolic) (septic) (G93.41)
    hepatic failure (K72.0-)
R65.20 **Severe sepsis without septic shock**
    Severe sepsis NOS
R65.21 **Severe sepsis with septic shock**

Figure 20-10 ■ Tabular List entry for code R65.2 "Severe sepsis".

❑ She cross-references the beginning of Chapter 18 (R00-R99) and reviews the instructional notes. These notes apply to assigning codes for symptoms and signs when a more specific diagnosis cannot be established. She determines that she should assign **R65.20** from this chapter, although a more specific diagnosis code is available, because the OGCR specifically directs her to assign a code from category **R65.2.**

▶ Next, Susanna wants to assign a code for acute respiratory failure. She locates the cross-referenced subcategory **J96.0 Acute respiratory failure** in the Tabular List.

❑ She identifies the symbol **5th** in front of the subcategory title, which tells her that a fifth character is required to complete the code.

❑ She reviews the fifth-digit options and determines that the code that best describes the case is **J96.00 Acute respiratory failure, unspecified whether with hypoxia or hypercapnia** because neither hypoxia or hypercapnia were documented.

❑ Susanna cross-references the beginning of category **J96,** the beginning of block **J96-J99,** and the beginning of Chapter 10 (J00-J99) for additional instructional notes and finds none that apply to this case.

▶ Susanna checks her notes and realizes she still needs to verify the code she located in the Index for the underlying infection, **Sepsis, Escherichia coli A41.5**.

❏ She locates the subcategory **A41.5** in the Tabular List, which has the title **Sepsis due to other Gram-negative organisms.** She notices that it requires a fifth character.

❏ She reads the codes listed, which identify various strains of Gram-negative sepsis, and selects code **A41.51 Sepsis due to Escherichia coli [E. coli].**

❏ She confirms that this accurately describes the documented organism.

❏ She cross-references the instructional notes at the beginning of category **A41, Other sepsis.** She determines that the conditions listed do not apply to this case.

❏ She cross-references the beginning of the block **A30-A49** and verifies that there are no instructional notes for this block.

❏ She cross-references the beginning of **Chapter 1 (A00-B99)** and reviews the instructional note that applies to all codes in this chapter. She determines that it does not apply to this case because the infection is not due to an external cause.

▶ Susanna reviews the codes she has assigned for this case.

❏ **R65.20 Severe sepsis without septic shock**

❏ **J96.00 Acute respiratory failure, unspecified whether with hypoxia or hypercapnia**

❏ **A41.51 Sepsis due to Escherichia coli [E. coli]**

▶ Next, Susanna must determine how to sequence the codes.

CODING PRACTICE

Exercise 20.3   Assigning Codes for Infectious Diseases

Instructions: Read the mini-medical-record of each patient's encounter, review the information abstracted in Exercise 20.2, and assign ICD-10-CM diagnosis codes using the Index and Tabular List. Write the code(s) on the line provided.

---

1. OFFICE   Gender: M   Age: 18

Chief complaint: General lack of energy, fatigue, loss of appetite, fever, and chills

Assessment: Suspected Epstein-Barr mononucleosis, which was confirmed by a blood test

Plan: Drink fluids, get rest, acetaminophen or ibuprofen for pain and fever, recovery can take several weeks, call if abdominal pain, difficulty breathing, severe weakness, or persistent high fever

1 ICD-10-CM Code _____

---

2. OFFICE   Gender: F   Age: 46

Reason for encounter: Annual work related PPD tuberculin test

Assessment: PPD positive for TB, x-ray of lung positive for nodules in lung

Plan: Order sputum culture, begin pharmacotherapy

1 ICD-10-CM Code _____

---

3. OFFICE   Gender: F   Age: 31

Reason for encounter: Follow up on HIV test results

Assessment: Positive for HIV, asymptomatic, counseled patient on managing the infection

Plan: Refer to HIV support group

Tip: Refer to OGCR I.C.1.a.2)(d). The second code is for HIV counseling.

2 ICD-10-CM Codes _____

---

4. OFFICE   Gender: M   Age: 27

Reason for encounter: Genital chancre

Assessment: Primary syphilis

Plan: Antibiotics

1 ICD-10-CM Code _____

---

5. INPATIENT HOSPITAL   Gender: F   Age: 35

Reason for encounter: Admitted from emergency department due to sepsis

Assessment: Staphylococcus aureus sepsis, cause unknown, responsive to antibiotics

Plan: After O_2 and IV fluids and antibiotics, patient was discharged home in good condition

Tip: Refer to OGCR I.C.1.d.1)(a).

1 ICD-10-CM Code _____

ARRANGING CODES FOR INFECTIOUS DISEASES

Codes from this ICD-10-CM chapter are sequenced first when the systemic infection qualifies as the principal or first-listed diagnosis. Manifestations or conditions associated with the infection are sequenced after the systemic infection code. This order is indicated in the Tabular List through the use of the instructional notes **Code first** for the systemic infection and **Use additional code** for the associated condition (■ FIGURE 20-11).

CODING CAUTION

Do not confuse the guidelines for sequencing of codes for causal organisms with the sequencing guidelines for etiology and manifestation. When an etiology/manifestation relationship exists, sequencing is specifically designated in ICD-10-CM through the use of conventions, such as brackets in the Index and highlighting in the Tabular List. These conventions direct coders to sequence the etiology first and the manifestation second.

The exception to this guideline is when a localized infection is described with a code from a body system chapter but the causal organism is *not* identified with a combination code. Assign the localized infection from the body system chapter as the first code. Assign a secondary code from the block **Bacterial and viral infectious agents (B95-B97)**, which contains codes to identify the infectious agent in diseases classified elsewhere. This order is indicated in the Tabular List through the use of the instructional notes **Code first** for the primary disease and **Use additional code** for the infectious organism (■ FIGURE 20-12).

Patient is seen for Q fever and associated endocarditis.

(1) **A78 Q fever**
(2) **I39 Endocarditis and heart valve disorders in diseases classified elsewhere**

Figure 20-11 ■ Example of body system disease associated with an infection.

Patient is seen for infective myocarditis due to methicillin-resistant staphylococcal aureus.

(1) **I40.0 Infective myocarditis**
(2) **B95.62 Methicillin resistant Staphylococcal aureus as the cause of diseases classified elsewhere**

Figure 20-12 ■ Example of sequencing for a body system disease due to an infectious organism.

OGCR provides specific guidelines for sequencing codes related to HIV/AIDS and sepsis, severe sepsis, and septic shock. These are discussed next.

Arranging Codes for HIV and AIDS

Sequencing of codes for HIV and AIDS depends on the circumstances of admission. Review the documentation and abstracting notes carefully to determine whether the patient was seen or admitted for treatment related directly to HIV or if the reason for the encounter was an unrelated condition, such as a traumatic injury.

Admission for HIV

When a patient is admitted for an HIV-related condition, assign and sequence codes as follows (OGCR I.C.1.a.2)(a)) (see Figure 20-8):

1. Assign code **B20 Human immunodeficiency virus [HIV] disease**.
2. Assign code(s) for all reported HIV-related condition(s).

Admission for a Condition Not Related to HIV

When a patient with HIV disease is admitted for an unrelated condition, assign and sequence codes as follows (OGCR I.C.1.a.2)(b)) (■ FIGURE 20-13):

1. Assign code(s) for the unrelated condition(s).
2. Assign code **B20 Human immunodeficiency virus [HIV] disease**.
3. Assign code(s) for all reported HIV-related condition(s).

Arranging Codes for Severe Sepsis and Septic Shock

Sequencing of codes for severe sepsis and septic shock is dependent on the circumstances of admission and when the condition develops.

Severe Sepsis

OGCR provides specific sequencing guidelines based on whether severe sepsis is the reason for admission or develops after admission.

Patient is admitted for repair of a partial right rotator cuff tear. Patient also has AIDS with Kaposi's sarcoma of the skin.

(1) **M75.111 Incomplete rotator cuff tear or rupture of right shoulder, not specified as traumatic**
(2) **B20 Human immunodeficiency virus [HIV] disease**
(3) **C46.0 Kaposi's sarcoma of skin**

Figure 20-13 ■ Example of sequencing for an AIDS patient admitted with a nonrelated condition.

Severe Sepsis Present at Admission. When severe sepsis meets the requirements of principal diagnosis, assign and sequence codes as follows (OGCR I.C.1.d.1)(b) and OGCR I.C.1.d.3)):

1. Assign a code for the underlying systemic infection or assign **A41.9 Sepsis, unspecified** if the infection is not specified.

2. Assign either **R65.20 Severe sepsis without septic shock** or **R65.21 Severe sepsis with septic shock**, as appropriate.

3. Assign code(s) for acute organ dysfunction.

Severe Sepsis That Develops after Admission. When severe sepsis develops after admission, assign and sequence codes as follows:

1. Assign code(s) for the condition(s) that meet the requirements of the principal diagnosis.

2. Assign a code for the underlying systemic infection or assign **A41.9 Sepsis, unspecified** if the infection is not specified.

3. Assign either **R65.20 Severe sepsis without septic shock** or **R65.21 Severe sepsis with septic shock**, as appropriate.

4. Assign code(s) for acute organ dysfunction.

Septic Shock

OGCR provide specific sequencing guidelines based on whether septic shock is the reason for admission or develops after admission.

Septic Shock Present at Admission. When septic shock meets the requirements of principal diagnosis, assign and sequence codes as follows (OGCR I.C.1.d.2)):

1. Assign a code for the underlying systemic infection or assign **A41.9 Sepsis, unspecified** if the infection is not specified.

2. Assign code **R65.21 Severe sepsis with septic shock**.

3. Assign code(s) for acute organ dysfunction, when applicable.

Septic Shock That Develops after Admission. When septic shock develops after admission, assign and sequence codes as follows (OGCR I.C.1.d.3)) (■ FIGURE 20-14):

1. Assign code(s) for the condition(s) that meet the requirements of principal diagnosis.

2. Assign a code for the underlying systemic infection or assign **A41.9 Sepsis, unspecified** if the infection is not specified.

3. Assign code **R65.21 Severe sepsis with septic shock**.

4. Assign code(s) for acute organ dysfunction, when applicable.

Patient is admitted for repair of mitral valve stenosis. Two days after the procedure, the patient experiences septic shock due to a deep incisional surgical site infection due to methicillin-resistant staphylococcus aureus.

(1) **I05.0 Rheumatic mitral stenosis**
(2) **T81.42XA Infection following a procedure, deep incisional surgical site, initial encounter**
(3) **A41.02 Sepsis due to methicillin resistant Staphylococcus aureus**
(4) **R65.21 Severe sepsis with septic shock**

Figure 20-14 ■ Example of sequencing for a patient who develops septic shock following a procedure.

Guided Example of Arranging Infectious Disease Codes

To practice skills for sequencing codes for infectious and parasitic diseases, continue with the example from earlier in the chapter about patient Faye Gillis, who was admitted to Branton Medical Center due to acute respiratory failure. Follow along in your ICD-10-CM manual as Susanna Vannote, CPC, sequences the codes. Check off each step after you complete it.

▶ First, Susanna confirms the codes she has assigned.

❏ **R65.20 Severe sepsis without septic shock**

❏ **J96.00 Acute respiratory failure, unspecified whether with hypoxia or hypercapnia**

❏ **A41.51 Sepsis due to Escherichia coli [E. coli]**

▶ Susanna refers back to the OGCR and instructional notes she read earlier.

❏ OGCR I.C.1.d.1)(b) states **The coding of severe sepsis requires a minimum of 2 codes: first a code for the underlying systemic infection, followed by a code from subcategory R65.2.**

❏ This tells her that the code **A41.51** for the systemic infection should be sequenced before **R65.20**.

❏ She is still unsure whether **R65.20** should be sequenced before or after **J96.00**.

❏ She refers back to the instructional note under subcategory **R65.2** that states **Use additional code to identify specific acute organ dysfunction, such as: acute respiratory failure (J96.0-).** This tells her that **J96.00** should be sequenced after **R65.20** because it says that **J96.00-** is an additional code.

▶ Susanna finalizes the codes and sequencing for this case:

(1) **A41.51 Sepsis due to Escherichia coli [E. coli]**

(2) **R65.20 Severe sepsis without septic shock**

(3) **J96.00 Acute respiratory failure, unspecified whether with hypoxia or hypercapnia**

CODING PRACTICE

Exercise 20.4   **Arranging Codes for Infectious Diseases**

Instructions: Read the mini-medical-record of each patient's encounter, review the information abstracted in Exercise 20.2, assign ICD-10-CM diagnosis codes using the Index and Tabular List, and sequence them correctly.

---

1. OFFICE   Gender: M   Age: 26

Reason for encounter: Lesions on the skin of this HIV positive patient

Assessment: Kaposi's sarcoma of the skin

Plan: Refer to oncologist to evaluate extent of the cancer and determine treatment plan

Tip: Refer to OGCR I.C.1.a.2)(a) for sequencing instructions.

2 ICD-10-CM Codes _____

---

2. EMERGENCY DEPT   Gender: M   Age: 26

Reason for encounter: Toe pain after a horse stepped on his foot

Assessment: Fractured distal phalanx of great toe on the right foot. AIDS patient with Kaposi's sarcoma of the lymph nodes which was not treated at this encounter.

Plan: Reduced fracture and applied cast, crutches, FU office 2 weeks

Tip: Refer to OGCR I.C.1.a.2)(b) and (f) for coding and sequencing instructions. Also, remember to assign an external cause code.

4 ICD-10-CM Codes _____

_____

---

3. INPATIENT HOSPITAL   Gender: F   Age: 70

Reason for encounter: Called in for a consult on Staphylococcus aureus pneumonia

Assessment: Culture result shows MSSA

Plan: IV teicoplanin was successful and patient was discharged with instructions to help prevent recurrence

Tip: Refer to OGCR I.C.1.c for coding and sequencing instructions.

1 ICD-10-CM Code _____

---

4. OFFICE   Gender: M   Age: 45

Reason for encounter: HIV positive patient with no related conditions presents with dysuria, weakness, and fever

Assessment: Urosepsis (UTI) d/t E. coli (non-Shiga toxin-producing)

Plan: Antibiotics

Tip: Urosepsis is not sepsis or septicemia. Refer to OGCR I.C.1.a.2)(d) and I.C.1.b.

3 ICD-10-CM Codes _____

_____

---

5. INPATIENT HOSPITAL   Gender: F   Age: 77

Reason for admission: Admitted from SNF 1 day post-hospital-discharge with 102° F fever, dyspnea, heart rate 100 per minute, low BP

Assessment: Severe sepsis d/t nosocomial MRSA and has associated heart failure

Plan: Deceased

Tip: Refer to OGCR I.C.1.d.1) and 2). Assign an external cause code for nosocomial infection.

4 ICD-10-CM Codes _____

_____

CHAPTER SUMMARY

In this chapter you learned that:

- Infectious and parasitic diseases are not a body system; they are systemic diseases that affect the entire body.

- OGCR I.C.1 provides detailed discussion of assigning and sequencing codes for HIV, sepsis, septic shock, and Zika virus infections.

- Coders always need to identify the scientific name of the infectious organism and subtype, as well as associated complications or manifestations.

- Although coders do not need to memorize every guideline, they should memorize the *fact* that OGCR exists for HIV and AIDS and sepsis, severe sepsis, and septic shock; they should refer to OGCR every time they code these conditions.

- Codes from this ICD-10-CM chapter are sequenced first when the systemic infection qualifies as the principal or first-listed diagnosis, followed by codes for associated conditions.

CONCEPT QUIZ

Take a moment to look back through infectious and parasitic diseases and solidify your skills. Try to answer the questions from memory first, then look back at the discussion in this chapter if you need a little extra help.

Completion

Instructions: Write the term that completes each statement based on the information you learned in this chapter. Choose from the list below. Some choices may be used more than once and some choices may not be used at all.

asymptomatic	parasites
bacteria	septic shock
herpes zoster	severe sepsis
HIV	smallpox
HPV	trichinosis
inconclusive	tuberculosis
leprosy	viruses
opportunistic	

1. _____ is a virus that causes cervical cancer.

2. _____ is a roundworm infestation caused by eating raw pork.

3. _____ is a chronic bacterial disease characterized by the formation of nodules on the surface of the body.

4. _____ is organ malfunction due to sepsis.

5. _____ is a virus that causes AIDS.

6. A(an) _____ infection is a disease that attacks people with weakened immune systems but does not develop in those with healthy immune systems.

7. _____ is a painful, blistering skin rash due to the varicella-zoster virus that causes chickenpox.

8. _____ is HIV serology that is neither positive or negative.

9. *Escherichia coli* is an example of _____.

10. _____ is diagnosed when blood pressure remains low despite intensive treatment.

Multiple Choice

Instructions: Circle the letter of the best answer to each question based on the information you learned in this chapter.

1. Which of the following are examples of protozoa?
   A. *Trichomonas vaginalis* and *Giardia*
   B. Varicella and herpes
   C. HIV and AIDS
   D. *Escherichia coli* and *Pseudomonas aeruginosa*

2. What type of conditions are pneumonia and pharyngitis?
   A. Systemic diseases
   B. Infectious agents
   C. Localized infections
   D. Bacteria

3. What characteristic do word roots for causal organisms often describe?
   A. Frequency
   B. Shape
   C. Toxicity
   D. Immunity

4. What is the relationship between AIDS and HIV?
   A. AIDS is the cause of HIV.
   B. AIDS is asymptomatic HIV.
   C. AIDS is an opportunistic infection.
   D. AIDS is the final stage of HIV.

5. When should code Y95 be assigned?
   A. When Zika virus is confirmed
   B. When there is a nosocomial infection
   C. When both sepsis and septic shock are documented
   D. When an AIDS-related condition exists

6. How would you code the following scenario? *An asymptomatic HIV-positive patient is seen.*
   A. B20
   B. Z11.4
   C. Z71.7
   D. Z21

(continued)

(continued from page 355)

7. How would you code the following scenario? *A patient with known AIDS is admitted for AIDS-related pneumocystis carinii pneumonia.*
   - A. B59, B20
   - B. B20, B59
   - C. Z21, B59
   - D. B20, J17

8. What code should be assigned when a patient is treated for any HIV-related illness?
   - A. B20, HIV disease
   - B. B97.35, HIV 2 as the cause of diseases classified elsewhere
   - C. Z0.6, Exposure to HIV
   - D. Z71.7, HIV counseling

9. How would you code the following scenario? *A patient is admitted for right heart failure. Septic shock develops the next day.*
   - A. I50.810, R65.21
   - B. R65.21, I50.810
   - C. I50.810, A41.9
   - D. A41.9, I50.810

10. What condition is the principal diagnosis in this scenario? *A patient with AIDS and associated Kaposi's sarcoma is admitted for repair of a torn rotator cuff.*
   - A. HIV disease
   - B. Kaposi's sarcoma
   - C. HIV as the cause of diseases classified elsewhere
   - D. Rotator cuff tear

KEEP ON CODING

Instructions: Read the diagnostic statement, then use the Index and Tabular List to assign and sequence ICD-10-CM diagnosis codes. Write the code(s) on the line provided.

1. *Salmonella* pyelonephritis. ICD-10-CM Code(s) _____

2. Glanders. ICD-10-CM Code(s) _____

3. Infant botulism. ICD-10-CM Code(s) _____

4. Gonococcal orchitis. ICD-10-CM Code(s) _____

5. Fatal familial insomnia. ICD-10-CM Code(s) _____

6. Postmeasles otitis media. ICD-10-CM Code(s) _____

7. Thrush. ICD-10-CM Code(s) _____

8. Meningococcal meningitis. ICD-10-CM Code(s) _____

9. Acute military tuberculosis. ICD-10-CM Code(s) _____

10. Monkeypox. ICD-10-CM Code(s) _____

11. Cat scratch fever. ICD-10-CM Code(s) _____

12. Postherpetic trigeminal neuralgia. ICD-10-CM Code(s) _____

13. Eczema herpeticum. ICD-10-CM Code(s) _____

14. Viral pericarditis, coxsackie. ICD-10-CM Code(s) _____

15. Toxoplasma myositis. ICD-10-CM Code(s) _____

16. *Rhodesiense* trypanosomiasis. ICD-10-CM Code(s) _____

17. Whooping cough due to *Bordetella pertussis* with pneumonia. ICD-10-CM Code(s) _____

18. Acute hepatitis E. ICD-10-CM Code(s) _____

19. Sepsis due to *Escherichia coli*. ICD-10-CM Code(s) _____

20. Jungle yellow fever. ICD-10-CM Code(s) _____

21. African histoplasmosis. ICD-10-CM Code(s) _____

22. Sequelae of leprosy. ICD-10-CM Code(s) _____

23. Rabies. ICD-10-CM Code(s) _____

24. Chlamydial conjunctivitis. ICD-10-CM Code(s) _____

25. West Nile fever. ICD-10-CM Code(s) _____

CODING CHALLENGE

Instructions: Read the mini-medical-record of each patient's encounter, then abstract, assign, and sequence ICD-10-CM diagnosis codes using the Index and Tabular List. Write the code(s) on the line provided.

1. OFFICE   Gender: F   Age: 52

Reason for encounter: Bloody diarrhea, patient states she is worried she might have cancer

Assessment: Symptoms started a few days after eating hamburgers at a cookout. Hemorrhagic colitis (*inflammation and bleeding of the colon*) due to E. coli.

Plan: Call back if it does not improve within 1 week

Tip: Follow the cross-references in the Index.

1 ICD-10-CM Code _____

2. OFFICE   Gender: M   Age: 44

Reason for encounter: Blisters and scabs on face and left side of body, unexplained pain

Assessment: Disseminated herpes zoster

Plan: Rx pain management medication, Calamine lotion applied topically to blisters and rash, RTO 1 week.

1 ICD-10-CM Code _____

3. OFFICE   Gender: M   Age: 23

Reason for encounter: HIV testing (screening) after unprotected sex with an infected partner

Assessment: Exposure to HIV

Plan: FU in 1 week for results

Tip: You need two Z codes, one for the reason for the encounter and a second for the exposure.

2 ICD-10-CM Codes _____

4. INPATIENT HOSPITAL   Gender: F   Age: 43

Reason for encounter: Antiviral therapy

Assessment: Chronic hepatitis due to hepatitis B

Plan: RTO as protocol for antiviral therapy stipulates, FU liver function tests at next office visit

1 ICD-10-CM Code _____

5. INPATIENT HOSPITAL   Gender: F   Age: 22

Reason for admission: Diarrhea and vomiting, fever

Assessment: Gastroenteritis d/t salmonella food poisoning

Plan: Rx antibiotics. RTO 1 week following discharge

1 ICD-10-CM Code _____

6. INPATIENT HOSPITAL   Gender: M   Age: 84

Reason for encounter: Redness on neck is spreading

Assessment: Cellulitis due to group F streptococcus infection of tracheostomy tube

Plan: Discharge to skilled nursing facility. Rx oral antibiotics and antibiotic cream.

3 ICD-10-CM Codes _____

_____

7. INPATIENT HOSPITAL   Gender: F   Age: 58

Reason for encounter: Recent trip to Sumatra without malaria prophylaxis, 4 day history of fever, sudden onset (SO) left upper quadrant (LUQ) pain and tenderness

Assessment: Plasmodium vivax malaria with splenic rupture

Plan: Post ICU discharge: 14 day course of chloroquine to be taken with food, RTO in 1 week

Tip: Plasmodium vivax is a type of malaria.

1 ICD-10-CM Code _____

8. OFFICE   Gender: M   Age: 7

Reason for encounter: Itchy scalp and rash on the child's neck. Parent suspects that they have identified nits in the patient's hair.

Assessment: Head lice infestation

Plan: Advise head lice shampoo (Rid, Nix).

Tip: Read and follow the cross-reference in the Index.

1 ICD-10-CM Code _____

(continued)

(continued from page 357)

9. OFFICE Gender: M Age: 29

Reason for encounter: Numbness (temperature sensations), multiple pale, diffuse cutaneous lesions

Assessment: BL leprosy (borderline lepromatous leprosy)

Plan: Multidrug therapy (Dapsone, rifampin, and clofazimine) regime initiated, RTO in 3 months

1 ICD-10-CM Code _____

10. INPATIENT HOSPITAL Gender: M Age: 30

Reason for encounter: Admitted from emergency department due to septic shock

Assessment: Sepsis is due to an infected tooth that patient has had for six months

Plan: Rx antibiotic, FU with dentist for extraction when patient is organism free.

Tip: Because the infectious organism is not identified, you need to assign a default NOS code for sepsis. Refer also to OGCR I.C.1.d.1) and 2).

3 ICD-10-CM Codes _____

_____

Learning Objectives

After completing this chapter, you should have the skills to:

21.1 Spell and define the key words, medical terms, and abbreviations related to the urinary system and male and female reproductive systems. (Remember)

21.2 Summarize the structure, function, and common conditions of the urinary system and male and female reproductive systems. (Understand)

21.3 Adhere to the Official Guidelines for Coding and Reporting related to diseases of the genitourinary system. (Apply)

21.4 Examine and abstract diagnostic information from the medical record for conditions of the urinary system and male and female reproductive systems. (Analyze)

21.5 Demonstrate how to assign codes for diseases of the urinary system and male and female reproductive systems. (Apply)

21.6 Utilize guidelines for arranging (sequencing) multiple diagnosis codes for diseases of the urinary system and male and female reproductive systems.

21.7 Demonstrate how to abstract, assign, and arrange codes for neoplasms of the urinary system and male and female reproductive systems. (Apply)

Chapter Outline

- **Genitourinary System Refresher**
- **Coding Guidelines for the Genitourinary System**
- **Abstracting for Genitourinary System Conditions**
- **Assigning Codes for Genitourinary System Conditions**
- **Arranging Codes for Genitourinary System Conditions**
- **Coding Neoplasms of the Genitourinary System**

Key Terms and Abbreviations

Bartholin's gland	fallopian tube	lower urinary tract symptom (LUTS)	reflux nephropathy
benign prostatic hypertrophy	genitourinary (GU) system	nephron	renal pelvis
blood creatinine	glomerular filtration rate (GFR)	ovary	reproductive duct
bulbo-urethral gland	glomerulus	penis	testis
clitoris	hematuria	peritoneal dialysis (PD)	ureter
dialysis	hemodialysis (HD)	peritoneal membrane	urethra
dialysis-related amyloidosis (DRA)	impotence	polycystic kidney disease	urinary bladder
ductal	kidney	polynephritis	urinary tract infection (UTI)
electrolyte	labia major	prostate	uterus
enlarged prostate (EP)	labia minor	prostate-specific antigen (PSA)	vagina
	lobular		

In addition to the key terms listed here, students should know the terms defined within tables in this chapter.

INTRODUCTION

All travelers have their own strategies for managing restroom needs, but everyone driving on an interstate highway looks forward to the next rest area. The genitourinary system consists of three systems: urinary, male reproductive, and female reproductive; each is discussed separately within this chapter.

A urologist specializes in diagnosing and treating conditions of the urinary tract and male reproductive organs, and a nephrologist specializes in diagnosing and treating conditions of the kidney. A gynecologist specializes in diagnosing and treating conditions of the female reproductive organs. Primary care physicians treat common conditions affecting the genitourinary system and refer more complex cases to a specialist.

GENITOURINARY SYSTEM REFRESHER

The **genitourinary (GU) system** includes the urinary system and the male and female genital, or reproductive, systems. The function of the urinary system is to filter, store, and remove waste products from the blood and maintain homeostasis. The function of the genital system is sexual reproduction. The urinary and reproductive systems are grouped together in the coding manual because they arise from the same embryonic tissue, use common structures, and are in close physical proximity. Each major section of this textbook chapter is divided into subsections on the urinary, male reproductive, and female reproductive systems.

Urinary System Refresher

The urinary system consists of two kidneys, two ureters, the urinary bladder, and the urethra (■ FIGURE 21-1). The **kidneys** produce urine and regulate the level of **electrolytes** and body fluid (■ FIGURE 21-2). The **nephrons** are the functioning part of each kidney and filter waste from the blood, beginning with the **glomerulus**, a cluster of capillaries that separates the urinary

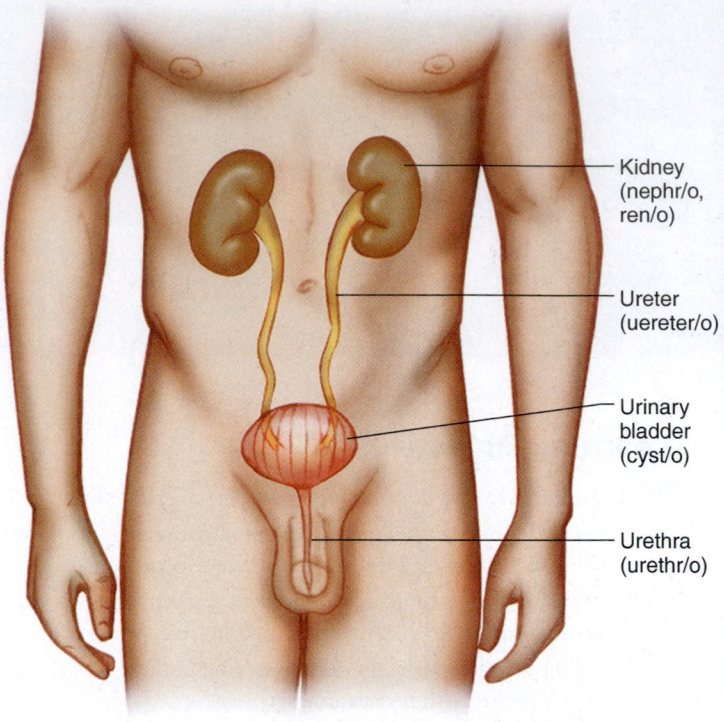

Figure 21-1 ■ The urinary system.

space from the blood. The **renal pelvis** of each kidney collects urine, which then passes through the **ureter** (*a tube that drains each kidney*) to the **urinary bladder**, a muscular sac that holds urine until it is expelled through the **urethra** (*a tube that carries urine out of the body*).

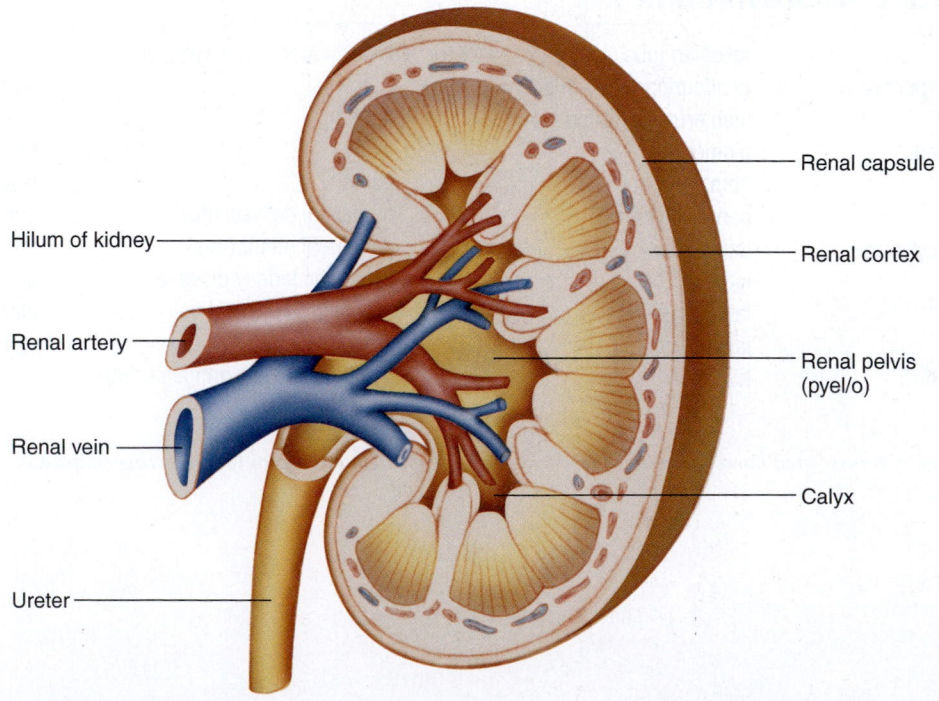

Figure 21-2 ■ The kidney.

Male Reproductive System Refresher

The male reproductive system consists of the external genital organ, internal genital organs, and associated glands (■ FIGURE 21-3). The **penis**, the external male sex organ, is a conduit for the urethra, which carries urine and semen out of the body. The male urethra is approximately eight inches long. Internal genital organs are the **testes** and the **reproductive ducts**. Associated glands are the **prostate** and **bulbo-urethral glands**. The testes also function as part of the endocrine system.

Female Reproductive System Refresher

The female reproductive system also consists of external and internal genital organs (■ FIGURE 21-4, page 362). The external genital organs are the **labia major** and **labia minor** (*folds of flesh that surround and protect the opening to the vagina and urethra*), **Bartholin's gland** (*a gland that secretes mucus*), and the **clitoris** (*a small, sensitive protrusion*). The internal genital organs consist of two **ovaries**, which produce eggs; two **fallopian tubes**, which transport eggs for fertilization and implantation in the uterus; the **uterus**, which is the womb for development of the fetus; and the **vagina**, which is the birth canal. The female urethra, which is one to two inches long and exits the body in front of the vagina, does not function in reproduction.

The female breasts are also part of the reproductive system. The ovaries also function as part of the endocrine system.

In the previous figures, each structure in the genitourinary system is labeled with its name as well as its medical terminology root/combining form, where applicable. Refer to ■ TABLE 21-1 (page 362) for a refresher on how to build medical terms related to the genitourinary system.

> ### CODING CAUTION
>
> Be alert for medical word terms that are spelled similarly but have different meanings.
>
> **prostat/o** (*prostate*) and **proct/o** (*anus and rectum*)
>
> **salpingitis** of the <u>fallopian</u> tube (*part of the female reproductive system*) and salpingitis of the <u>Eustachian</u> tube (*located between the ear and the nasopharynx*)
>
> **ureter** (*two tubes that drain the kidneys into the bladder*) and **urethra** (*a single tube that carries urine from the bladder to the outside of the body*)
>
> **colp/o** (*vagina*) and **col/o** or **col<u>on</u>/o** (*colon or large intestine*)

■ Reproductive system

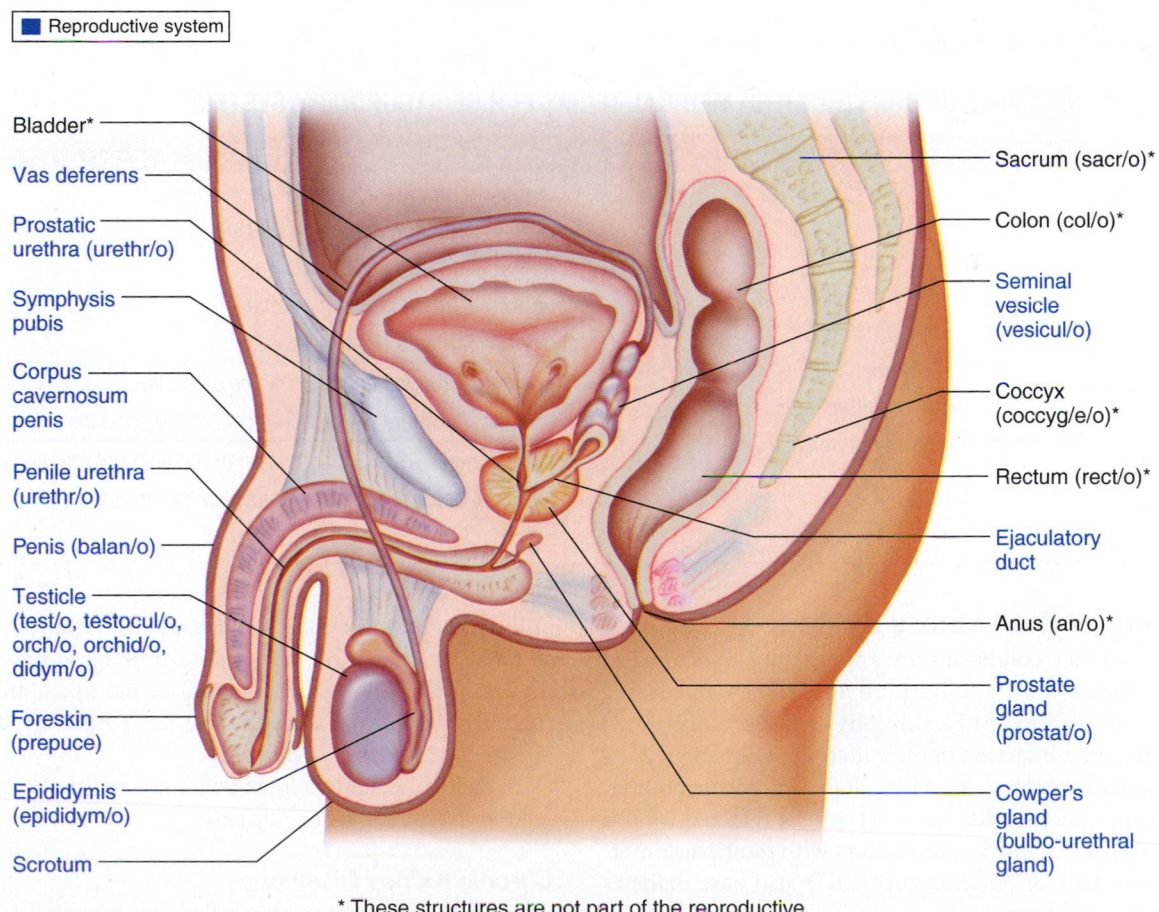

Bladder*

Vas deferens

Prostatic urethra (urethr/o)

Symphysis pubis

Corpus cavernosum penis

Penile urethra (urethr/o)

Penis (balan/o)

Testicle (test/o, testocul/o, orch/o, orchid/o, didym/o)

Foreskin (prepuce)

Epididymis (epididym/o)

Scrotum

Sacrum (sacr/o)*

Colon (col/o)*

Seminal vesicle (vesicul/o)

Coccyx (coccyg/e/o)*

Rectum (rect/o)*

Ejaculatory duct

Anus (an/o)*

Prostate gland (prostat/o)

Cowper's gland (bulbo-urethral gland)

* These structures are not part of the reproductive system and are shown for reference.

Figure 21-3 ■ The male reproductive system.

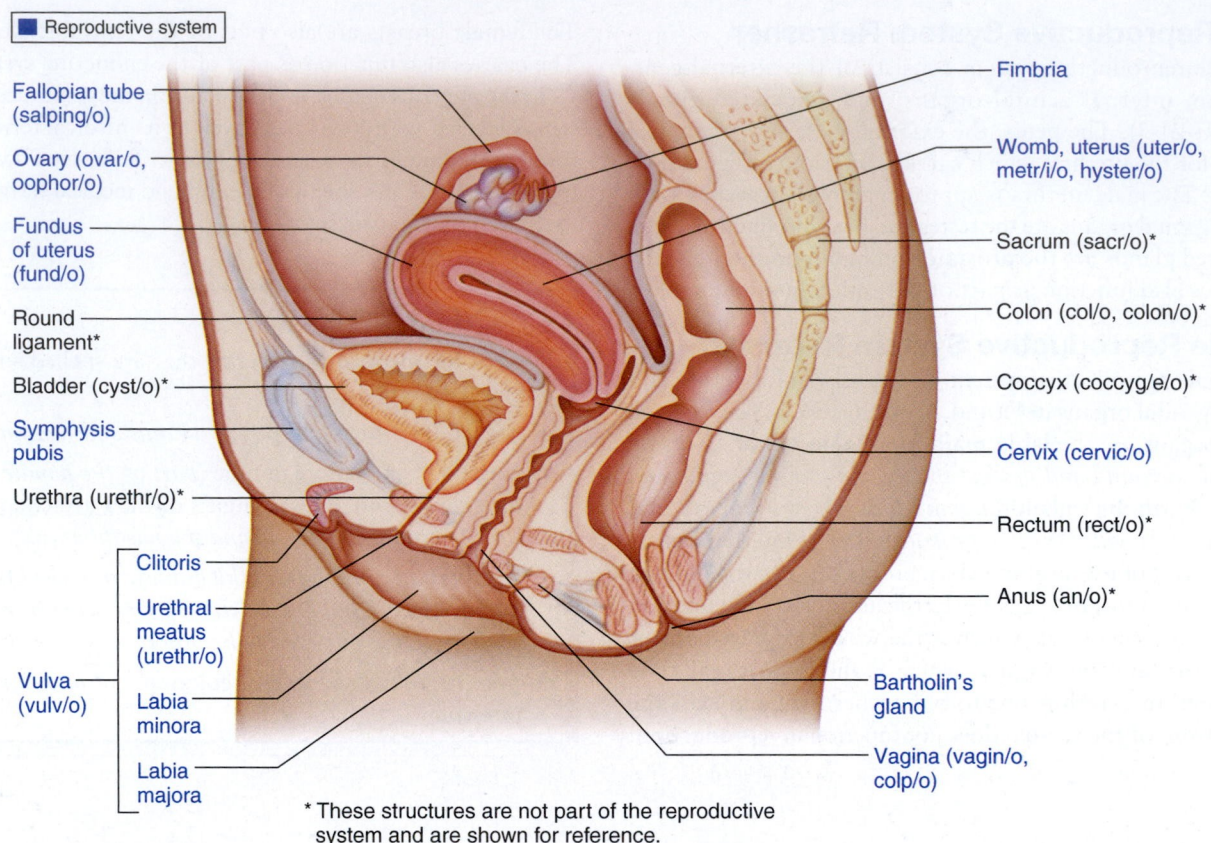

■ Reproductive system

Figure 21-4 ■ The female reproductive system.

* These structures are not part of the reproductive system and are shown for reference.

Table 21-1 ■ **EXAMPLE OF CONSTRUCTING MEDICAL TERMS FOR GENITOURINARY SYSTEM**

Combining Form	Suffix	Complete Medical Term
nephr/o (*kidney*)		**nephro + ptosis** (*drooping of the kidney*)
hemat/o (*blood*)		**cyst + ptosis** (*drooping of the bladder*)
cyst/o (*bladder*)		**hemat + uria** (*blood in urine*)
	-uria (*condition of urine*)	**nephro + lithiasis** (*kidney stones*)
	-ptosis (*to droop*)	**cysto + lithiasis** (*bladder stones*)
	-lithiasis (*condition of stones*)	
prostat/o (*prostate*)	**-itis** (*inflammation*)	**prostat + itis** (*inflammation of the prostate*)
	-ectomy (*surgical excision*)	**prostat + ectomy** (*surgical removal of the prostate*)
end/o (*within*)		**endo + metr + itis** (*inflammation of the lining of the uterus*)
metr/i (*uterus*)		**hyster + ectomy** (*surgical removal of the uterus*)
hyster/o (*uterus*)		

Conditions of the Urinary System

Urologic and kidney conditions are among the most common reasons for doctor visits and hospital admissions. According to the National Institutes of Health (NIH), 40–60% of women have a urinary tract infection in their lifetime, with about 25% experiencing repeat infections. More than 14% of the population has chronic kidney disease (CKD). It is referred to as a disease multiplier because it often occurs with multiple comorbidities. About half of patients with CKD also have diabetes and cardiovascular disease.

Diseases and disorders of the urinary system include infections and inflammations of nearly any anatomic site, glomerular diseases that attack the kidneys' filtering ability, kidney failure, and obstructions. Coders use medical resources, such as reference books on diseases, to understand conditions of the genitourinary system, diagnostic methods, and common treatments. Refer to ■ TABLE 21-2 for a summary of diseases affecting the urinary system.

In particular, coders must be familiar with the terminology related to chronic kidney disease.

Chronic Kidney Disease

Chronic kidney disease, also called *chronic renal failure*, is the slow loss of kidney function over a period of months or years. People are able to live long periods of time with decreased kidney function; symptoms of the disease may not appear until

Table 21-2 ■ **COMMON DISEASES OF THE URINARY SYSTEM**

Condition	Definition
Acute kidney failure	The rapid loss of kidney function over a period of days or weeks
Acute tubular necrosis	Damage to the renal tubules due to reduced blood flow or toxins in the urine
Calculi	Stones that may accumulate in the kidneys, bladder, or ureters
Chronic kidney disease (CKD)	The slow loss of kidney function over a period of months or years
Cystitis	Bacterial infection of the urinary bladder; also called **urinary tract infection (UTI)**
Diabetic nephropathy	Accumulated damage to the glomerulus capillaries due to chronic high blood glucose
Glomerulonephritis	Inflammation of the glomerulus of the kidney, allowing protein and blood into the urine
Hydronephrosis	Distention of the renal pelvis due to excessive urine collection in the kidney, often due to ureteral obstruction (■ Figure 21-5)
Incontinence	The inability to control bladder muscles
Nephritic syndrome	A collection of disorders affecting the kidneys, characterized by nonpurulent inflammatory glomerular disorders that allow proteins and red blood cells to pass into the urine, resulting in proteinuria and **hematuria** (*blood in the urine*)
Nephroptosis	Downward placement of the kidney from its normal location
Nephrotic syndrome	A collection of disorders affecting the kidneys, characterized by proteinuria but not hematuria
Pyelonephritis	Acute or chronic infection of the renal medulla and upper urinary tract as a result of untreated cystitis; also called **polynephritis**
Uremia	Toxic blood condition due to the inability of the kidneys to remove nitrogenous substances from the blood

as little as 10% of kidney function remains. However, the loss of kidney function results in the buildup of toxins in the body, which can have serious effects on most body functions, especially red blood cell production, blood pressure control, vitamin D absorption, and bone health (■ FIGURE 21-6, page 364).

Diabetes and high blood pressure account for two-thirds of the cases of CKD, according to the National Kidney Foundation. Other conditions that cause CKD include **polycystic kidney disease**, glomerulonephritis, medications, autoimmune disorders such as lupus erythematosus and scleroderma, kidney stones, recurrent UTIs, and **reflux nephropathy**. CKD typically has no symptoms in the initial stages, earning its name the "silent killer."

Kidney health is monitored through a wide range of blood tests that are included as part of most routine physical examinations. Persistent protein in the urine is an early sign of

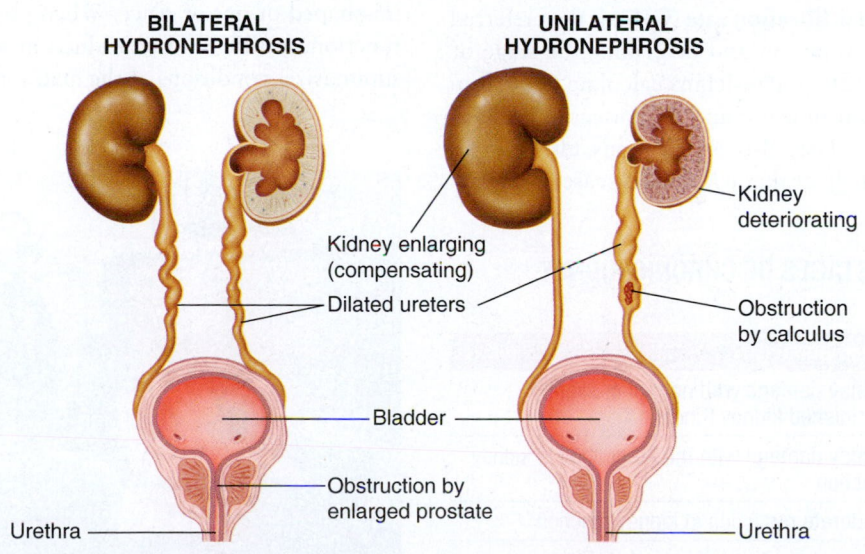

BILATERAL HYDRONEPHROSIS   UNILATERAL HYDRONEPHROSIS

Kidney enlarging (compensating)
Dilated ureters
Kidney deteriorating
Obstruction by calculus
Bladder
Obstruction by enlarged prostate
Urethra
Urethra

Figure 21-5 ■ Hydronephrosis: bilateral and unilateral.

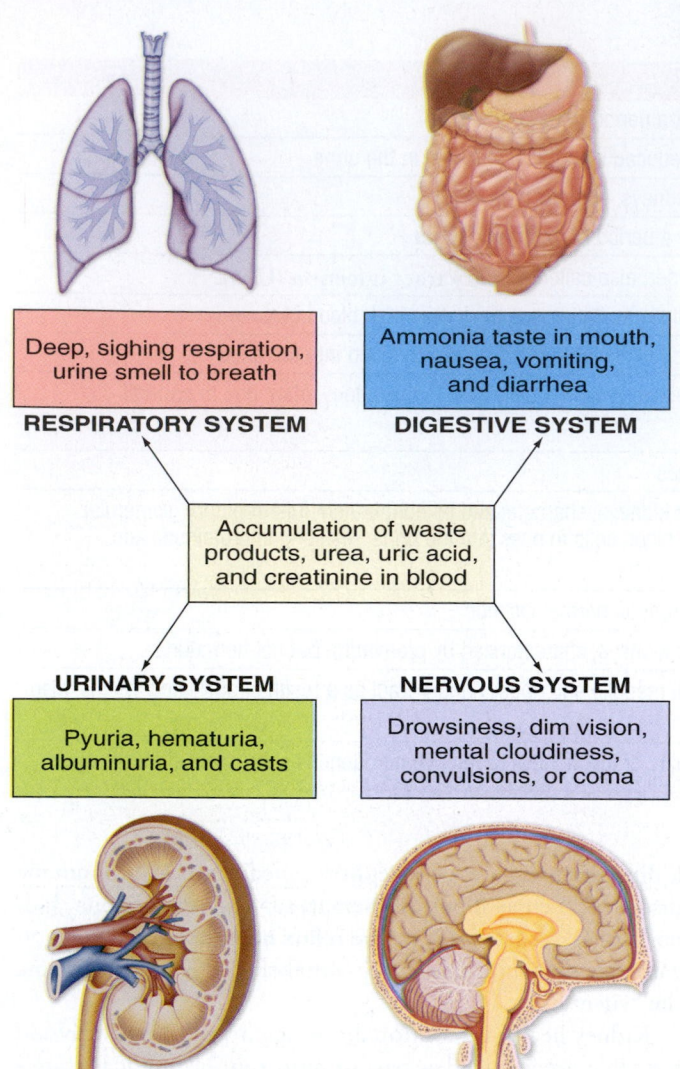

Deep, sighing respiration, urine smell to breath
RESPIRATORY SYSTEM

Ammonia taste in mouth, nausea, vomiting, and diarrhea
DIGESTIVE SYSTEM

Accumulation of waste products, urea, uric acid, and creatinine in blood

URINARY SYSTEM
Pyuria, hematuria, albuminuria, and casts

NERVOUS SYSTEM
Drowsiness, dim vision, mental cloudiness, convulsions, or coma

Figure 21-6 ■ Manifestations of chronic kidney disease.

possible CKD. **Glomerular filtration rate (GFR)** is the preferred way to measure kidney function and determine the stage of kidney disease (■ TABLE 21-3). Physicians calculate GFR from the results of a **blood creatinine** test and the patient's age, race, gender, and other factors. They also use CT scans, ultrasounds, and kidney biopsies to help evaluate kidney disease.

Table 21-3 ■ **THE STAGES OF CHRONIC KIDNEY DISEASE**

Stage	GFR	Description
1	≥90	Kidney damage with normal or slightly diminished kidney function
2	89–60	Kidney damage with mild reduction in kidney function
3a-3b	59–30	Moderate reduction in kidney function
4	29–15	Severe reduction in kidney function
5	<15	Kidney failure; end-stage renal disease (ESRD)

CKD is not curable, but its progress can be slowed through diet, lifestyle, and medication. When CKD reaches stage 5, the kidneys cease to function, and patients must receive **dialysis** or a kidney transplant in order to survive.

Dialysis is a treatment that filters the blood to remove waste, excess salt, and water. Nearly a half-million Americans are on dialysis, according to the National Kidney Foundation. In **hemodialysis (HD)**, the blood is processed through a machine (■ FIGURE 21-7). In **peritoneal dialysis (PD)**, the **peritoneal membrane** (*the lining of the abdomen*) is used to filter the blood. Although the overwhelming majority of dialysis is performed at centralized dialysis centers, it can be done at home with proper training and support. Medicare requires that all patients be offered all dialysis options. Dialysis brings on its own complications as well, including infections and hemorrhaging through the dialysis port access site, electrolyte abnormalities, anemia, cardiac dysfunction, and **dialysis-related amyloidosis (DRA)** (*deposits of the starchy substance amyloid in the joints*) in long-term dialysis patients. Kidney transplants are an option to treat ESRD, making the kidney one of the most frequently transplanted organs.

SUCCESS STEP

ESRD is the only specific disease that Medicare covers for the entire population, regardless of age. Individuals, their guardians, or spouses must meet the Medicare eligibility requirement of 40 quarters of employment and are responsible for the usual Medicare deductibles and coinsurance. Medicare covers dialysis services and transplants.

Conditions of the Male Reproductive System

Conditions of the male reproductive system relate to both the structure and function of the organs. Components may be misshaped or out of place. When portions of the system malfunction, fertility and reproduction are affected. ■ TABLE 21-4 summarizes conditions of the male reproductive system covered

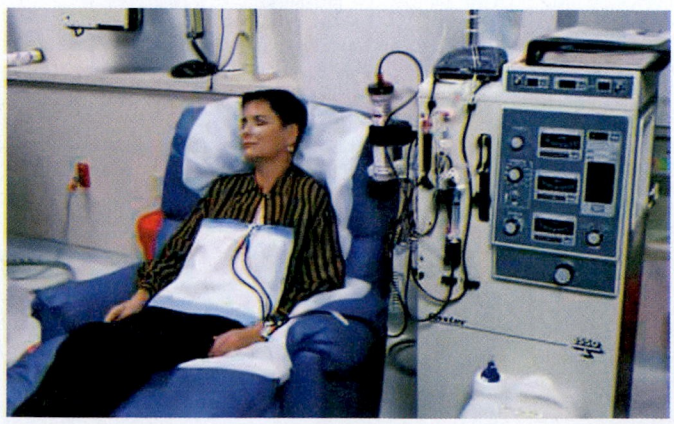

Figure 21-7 ■ A patient undergoing hemodialysis. *Source: Michal Heron.*

Table 21-4 ■ **COMMON DISEASES OF THE MALE REPRODUCTIVE SYSTEM**

Condition	Definition
Benign prostatic hyperplasia (BPH)	The abnormal growth of epithelial cells of the prostate, causing compression or obstruction of the urethra; also called benign prostatic hypertrophy or enlarged prostate (EP)
Erectile dysfunction (ED)	The chronic inability to achieve or maintain a penile erection until ejaculation; also called impotence
Hydrocele	A fluid-filled sack in the scrotum caused by abnormal fetal development, injury, hernia, or blockages
Male factor infertility	A problem in the male genital system that diminishes reproduction, such as inability to ejaculate, lack of sperm production, or lack of live sperm
Prostatic intraepithelial neoplasia (PIN)	Neoplastic changes in the epithelial cells of the prostate ducts showing some features of cancer, but not invasive; a potential precursor of carcinoma or adenocarcinoma
Spermatocele	Benign cystic swelling of sperm in the ducts of the epididymis

Table 21-5 ■ **COMMON DISEASES OF THE FEMALE REPRODUCTIVE SYSTEM**

Condition	Definition
Cervical dysplasia	Abnormal changes in the cells on the surface of the cervix that may lead to cancer if not treated
Cervical intraepithelial neoplasia (CIN)	Cervical dysplasia seen on a cervical biopsy, classified as mild dysplasia (CIN I), moderate to marked dysplasia (CIN II), and severe dysplasia to cancer in situ (CIN III)
Endometriosis	The growth of endometrial tissue in any area other than the uterus
Female factor infertility	A problem in the female genital system that diminishes reproduction, such as scarring or obstruction of the fallopian tubes or abnormal interaction between sperm and the mucous membrane in the cervix
Fibrocystic breast disease	Lumps of benign fibrous tissue in the breast
Genital prolapse	Downward displacement of the uterus or vagina to an abnormal position
Pelvic inflammatory disease (PID)	Inflammation of the female reproductive tract above the cervix
Squamous intraepithelial lesion (SIL)	Cervical dysplasia seen on a PAP test, graded as low grade (LSIL), high grade (HSIL), and possibly cancerous or malignant
Vulvovaginitis	Inflammation of the vulva and vagina due to yeast, bacteria, viruses, parasites, or skin care products

in ICD-10-CM Chapter 14. Sexually transmitted diseases are classified in ICD-10-CM Chapter 1, "Certain Infections and Parasitic Diseases (A00-B99)."

Conditions of the Female Reproductive System

Conditions of the female reproductive system are related to organ position, fertility, and reproduction; they include disorders of the breast in addition to the reproductive organs located in the pelvic region (■ TABLE 21-5). Sexually transmitted diseases are classified in ICD-10-CM Chapter 1, "Certain Infections and Parasitic Diseases (A00-B99)."

This section provides a general reference to help understand the most common diagnoses of the genitourinary system but does not list everything you need to know. Use medical terminology skills discussed earlier in this chapter to learn the meaning of unfamiliar words. Remember to keep standard reference books handy in case you get stuck.

CODING PRACTICE

Exercise 21.1 Genitourinary System Refresher

Instructions: Use your medical terminology skills and resources to define the following conditions related to the genitourinary system, then assign the default diagnosis code. Follow these steps:

- Use slash marks "/" to break down each term into its root(s) and suffix.
- Define the meaning of the word, based on the meaning of each word part.
- Assign the default ICD-10-CM diagnosis code for the condition using the Index and Tabular List.

Example: cystitis cyst/itis   Meaning *inflammation of the bladder*   ICD-10-CM Code <u>N30.90</u>

1. amenorrhea   Meaning _____   ICD-10-CM Code _____

2. cystolithiasis   Meaning _____   ICD-10-CM Code _____

3. dyspareunia   Meaning _____   ICD-10-CM Code _____

(continued)

CODING PRACTICE (continued)

4. hydrocele   Meaning _____   ICD-10-CM Code _____

5. cystoptosis   Meaning _____   ICD-10-CM Code _____

6. nephralgia   Meaning _____   ICD-10-CM Code _____

7. urethrorrhagia   Meaning _____   ICD-10-CM Code _____

8. nephrosis   Meaning _____   ICD-10-CM Code _____

9. ureterocele   Meaning _____   ICD-10-CM Code _____

10. pyelonephrosis   Meaning _____   ICD-10-CM Code _____

CODING GUIDELINES FOR THE GENITOURINARY SYSTEM

Coders should understand the organization of this ICD-10-CM chapter, chapter-wide and commonly used instructional notes in the Tabular List, and the relevant OGCR. This information is necessary for accurate coding.

ICD-10-CM Chapter 14, "Diseases of the Genitourinary System (N00-N99)," contains 11 blocks or subchapters that are divided by anatomic site. Review the block names and code ranges listed at the beginning of Chapter 14 in the ICD-10-CM manual to become familiar with the content and organization.

This chapter includes conditions of the male and female urinary system, the male reproductive system, the female breast, and disorders of the female genital tract. It does not include disorders related to pregnancy, which are classified in Chapter 15, "Pregnancy, Childbirth and the Puerperium (O00-O9A)." It also does not include injuries or congenital conditions of the genitourinary system.

ICD-10-CM provides Official Guidelines for Coding and Reporting (OGCR) diseases of the genitourinary system in OGCR section I.C.14. OGCR provides detailed discussion of chronic kidney disease. Additional OGCR related to hypertensive chronic kidney disease appear in OGCR I.C.9.a.2) and 3). Specific OGCR and instructional notes are discussed and cited throughout this chapter of the text.

ABSTRACTING FOR GENITOURINARY SYSTEM CONDITIONS

Disorders in this chapter have a wide range of abstracting criteria because there is a wide range of organs and types of disorders. Most conditions can be adequately abstracted by being attentive to the specific type and subtype of condition. Certain conditions require additional specific criteria, such as CKD and BPH. Refer to the following tables for guidance on how to abstract conditions of the urinary system (■ TABLE 21-6), male reproductive system (■ TABLE 21-7), and female reproductive system (■ TABLE 21-8), then work through the detailed example that follows. Remember that the abstracting questions are a guide and that not every question applies to, or can be answered for, every case. For example, laterality applies

Table 21-6 ■ KEY CRITERIA FOR ABSTRACTING CONDITIONS OF THE URINARY SYSTEM

❑ What is the condition?
❑ What is the subtype or anatomic site?
❑ What is the laterality, if any?
❑ Is the condition acute or chronic?
❑ Is an obstruction documented?
❑ What is the infectious organism?
❑ Is there a history of recurrent UTIs?
❑ What stage is the chronic kidney disease?
❑ Does the patient receive dialysis?
❑ Is the patient on a transplant waiting list or the recipient of a transplant?
❑ Do any additional conditions coexist?

Table 21-7 ■ KEY CRITERIA FOR ABSTRACTING CONDITIONS OF THE MALE REPRODUCTIVE SYSTEM

❑ Verify the patient's gender.
❑ What is the condition?
❑ What is the subtype or anatomic site?
❑ What is the laterality, if any?
❑ Is the condition acute or chronic?
❑ Is an obstruction documented?
❑ What is the infectious organism?
❑ What symptoms are associated with prostatic hypertrophy?
❑ Do any additional conditions coexist?

Table 21-8 ■ KEY CRITERIA FOR ABSTRACTING CONDITIONS OF THE FEMALE REPRODUCTIVE SYSTEM

- ❏ Verify the patient's gender.
- ❏ What is the condition?
- ❏ What is the subtype or anatomic site?
- ❏ What is the laterality, if any?
- ❏ Is the condition acute or chronic?
- ❏ What is the infectious organism?
- ❏ Do any additional conditions coexist?

to many, but not all, disorders of the breast, but not to most disorders of the kidneys, ureters, ovaries, or fallopian tubes, all of which are paired organs. Also remember to abstract for symptoms and determine if they are integral to the confirmed diagnoses.

Guided Example of Abstracting for Urinary System Conditions

Refer to the following example throughout this chapter to learn skills for abstracting, assigning, and sequencing urinary system codes. Chrystal Crago, CCA, is a fictitious coder who guides you through the coding process.

Follow along as Chrystal Crago, CCA, abstracts the diagnosis. Check off each step after you complete it.

CODING CAUTION

Checking patients' gender helps prevent coding errors, such as picking up a code for the wrong gender, and also helps identify potential keying errors. Never assume a patient's gender based on the name because many common names are androgynous, such as Terry, Taylor, Lynn, or Pat. In addition, if ethnic names are unfamiliar, it is impossible to "guess." Examples are Shing, which is Chinese (male); Iffat, which is Muslim (female); or Gwandoya, which is African (male).

Date: 02/21/yy   Location: Branton Professional Group   Provider: Ann Colyer, MD

Patient: Ronald Coffield   Gender: M   Age: 53

Reason for encounter: ESRD patient presents with ongoing complaints of extreme joint pain

Assessment: Joint pain is due to dialysis-related amyloidosis (DRA), ESRD, HD, on kidney transplant waiting list

Plan: Begin medication regimen despite side effects, and consider surgical intervention

---

▶ Chrystal reads through the entire record, paying special attention to the reason for the encounter and the final assessment. She refers to the Key Criteria for Abstracting Conditions of the Urinary System (Table 21-6).

- ❏ *What is the condition?* Ongoing complaints of extreme joint pain for an ESRD patient

- ❏ *Which system does this case relate to: urinary, male reproductive, or female reproductive?* Urinary

- ❏ *What are the presenting symptom(s)?* Ongoing extreme joint pain

- ❏ *What is the condition?* Amyloidosis

- ❏ *What is the subtype?* ESRD dialysis-related (DRA)

- ❏ *What stage is the chronic kidney disease?* By definition, ESRD is stage 5

- ❏ *Does the patient receive dialysis?* Yes, HD is documented

- ❏ *Is the patient on a transplant waiting list or the recipient of a transplant?* Yes

▶ At this time, Chrystal does not how many codes she will end up with. She will learn about this when she moves on to assigning codes.

CODING PRACTICE

Exercise 21.2   Abstracting for Genitourinary System Conditions

Instructions: Read the mini-medical-record of each patient's encounter and answer the abstracting questions. Write the answer on the line provided. Do not assign any codes.

1. OFFICE   Gender: F   Age: 42

Reason for encounter: Surgery for endometriosis

Assessment: Endometriosis of the uterus

Plan: FU in office 2 weeks

a. Which system does this case relate to: urinary, male reproductive, or female reproductive? _____

_____

(continued)

CODING PRACTICE (continued)

1. (continued)

b. What is the condition? _____
_____

c. What is the subtype or anatomic site? _____
_____

d. Is an infectious organism named? _____
_____

2. OFFICE   Gender: F   Age: 46

Reason for encounter: Painful lumps in both breasts

Assessment: Fibrocystic breast changes

Plan: OTC acetaminophen, heat and ice as needed to relieve local pain

Tip: Physicians use the term *changes* rather than the more traditional *disease* to avoid alarming patients.

a. Which system does this case relate to: urinary, male reproductive, or female reproductive?_____
_____

b. What is the condition? _____
_____

c. What is the anatomic site? _____
_____

d. What is the laterality, if any? _____
_____

e. Is an obstruction documented? _____
_____

f. Do any additional conditions coexist? _____
_____

3. OFFICE   Gender: M   Age: 61

Reason for encounter: Occasional excruciating low back pain

Assessment: Renal and ureteral calculi

Plan: Medical expulsive therapy (MET) *(treatment with drugs to expel the calculi)* with tamsulosin *(an alpha blocker)*

a. Which system does this case relate to: urinary, male reproductive, or female reproductive?_____
_____

b. What are the symptoms? _____
_____

c. What is the condition? _____
_____

(continued)

3. (continued)

d. Does the condition account for the symptom? _____
_____

e. What is the anatomic site? _____
_____

f. What is the laterality, if any? _____
_____

g. Is an obstruction documented? _____
_____

4. OFFICE   Gender: M   Age: 81

Reason for encounter: FU on BPH with obstruction and urinary retention

Assessment: Little improvement seen despite multiple medication adjustments

Plan: Schedule transurethral resection of the prostate (TURP)

a. Which system does this case relate to: urinary, male reproductive, or female reproductive?_____
_____

b. What is the condition? _____
_____

c. Is an obstruction documented? _____
_____

d. What symptoms are associated with prostatic hypertrophy? _____
_____

5. OFFICE   Gender: F   Age: 37

Reason for encounter: Vaginal discharge, burning, redness in perineal area

Assessment: Lab results show bacterial vaginitis due to staphylococcus, which is treatable

Plan: Antibiotics

a. Which system does this case relate to: urinary, male reproductive, or female reproductive?_____
_____

b. What are the symptoms? _____
_____

c. What is the condition? _____
_____

d. What is the subtype of the condition? _____
_____

(continued)

CODING PRACTICE (continued)

5. (continued)

e. What is the infectious organism? _____
_____

f. Is the organism resistant to antibiotic treatment?
_____

---

6. INPATIENT HOSPITAL Gender: F Age: 83

Reason for admission: Nursing facility (NF) patient brought to emergency department with suspected UTI because of signs of confusion and lack of cooperation; history of UTI over the past 2 years

Assessment: UTI due to E. coli, (non-Shiga toxin-producing)

(continued)

---

6. (continued)

Plan: Administered IV antibiotics, discharged after 2 days to NF with Rx

a. Which system does this case relate to: urinary, male reproductive, or female reproductive? _____
_____

b. What is the condition? _____

c. Is an obstruction documented? _____
_____

d. What is the infectious organism? _____
_____

What is the subtype? _____

e. Is there a history of recurrent UTIs? _____
_____

ASSIGNING CODES FOR GENITOURINARY SYSTEM CONDITIONS

Two similar urinary system conditions, nephritic syndrome and nephrotic syndrome, demonstrate the importance of checking cross-referencing instructions in the Index to assign the most specific code available.

Assigning Codes for Nephritic Syndrome and Nephrotic Syndrome

An analysis of word roots and suffixes leads to similar descriptions of nephritis (*inflammation of the kidney*) and nephrosis (*abnormal condition of the kidney*), but, clinically, they are distinct conditions with distinct diagnostic criteria (Table 21-2).

Nephritic syndrome is a collection of disorders affecting the kidneys, characterized by nonpurulent inflammatory glomerular disorders that allow proteins and red blood cells to pass into the urine, resulting in proteinuria and hematuria. The Index entry for the Main Term **Syndrome** and the subterm **nephritic** provides a cross-referencing instruction, *see also* **Nephritis**. It provides additional subterms for **acute**, **chronic**, and **rapidly progressive** (■ FIGURE 21-8). The subterm **with edema**

provides a cross-reference **see Nephrosis** because edema is characteristic of nephrosis.

Coders may feel confused whether they should assign one of the codes listed under **Syndrome, nephritic**, or whether they must follow the cross-reference. Remember the following tips:

- When the condition is *not specified any further* in the documentation, assign the code that follows the appropriate subterm.

- When documentation *provides more details than appear in the Index entry*, follow the cross-referenced Main Term to search for a more specific code.

Whenever you are in doubt if you have the correct code, follow the cross-reference. It only takes a moment and either confirms your initial choice or leads you to a more specific code. Either way, cross-referencing gives you confidence in your coding skills.

Nephrotic syndrome is a collection of disorders affecting the kidneys, characterized by proteinuria and edema but *not* hematuria. The Index entry for the Main Term **Syndrome** and the subterm **nephrotic** provides a cross-referencing instruction, *see also* **Nephrosis**. It provides additional subterms for certain subtypes of the condition.

Refer to ■ FIGURE 21-9 (page 370) to learn more about when to follow the cross-referencing instructions in the Index.

When coders search only under **Syndrome, nephritic, acute**, they identify the code **N00.9 Acute nephritic syndrome with unspecified morphologic changes** (■ FIGURE 21-10, page 370). When they follow the cross-reference to **Nephritis**, then follow the subterms that describe the specific subtype, they identify code **N00.3 Acute nephritic syndrome with diffuse mesangial proliferative glomerulonephritis** (Figure 21-10). Because **N00.3** is a specific code, it is the correct code for this example.

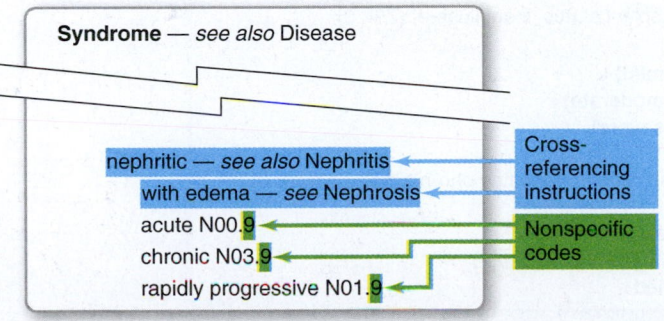

Figure 21-8 ■ Index entry for the Main Term "Syndrome, nephritic" used to locate nephritic syndrome codes.

A mother presents with her 6 year old daughter who has blood in her urine. Urinalysis testing shows albuminuria, hematuria, and proteinuria. A kidney biopsy is also done and after results come back, the physician diagnoses her with acute nephritic syndrome with mesangial proliferative glomerulonephritis.

Index: **Nephritis, acute, diffuse, mesangial proliferative glomerulonephritis**
Tabular List: **N00.3 Acute nephritic syndrome with diffuse mesangial proliferative glomerulonephritis**

Figure 21-9 ■ Example of assigning codes for nephritic syndrome.

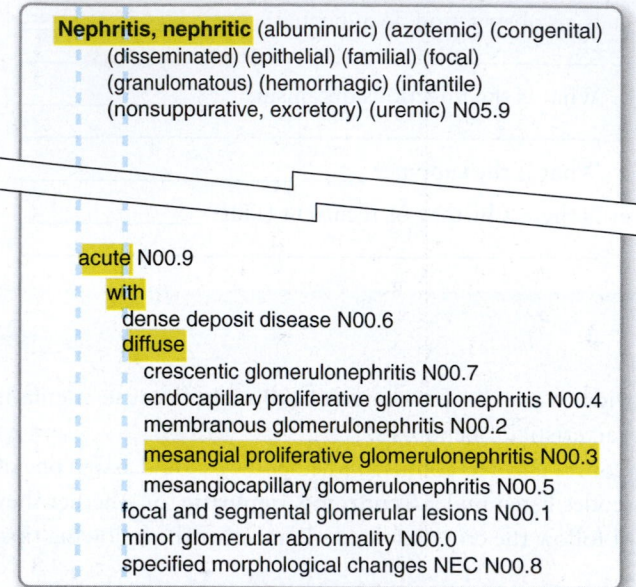

Figure 21-10 ■ Index entry for the Main Term "Nephritis".

Guided Example of Assigning Codes for Urinary System Conditions

To practice skills for assigning codes for diseases of the urinary system, continue with the example from earlier in the chapter about patient Ronald Coffield, who was seen at Branton Professional Group for ESRD and joint pain.

Follow along in your ICD-10-CM manual as Chrystal Crago, CCA, assigns codes. Check off each step after you complete it.

▶ First, Chrystal confirms the information she abstracted:

❏ ESRD

❏ HD

❏ DRA

❏ On transplant waiting list

▶ Chrystal begins with ESRD and searches the Index for the Main Term **Disease**.

❏ She locates the subterm **renal**.

❏ She locates the second-level subterm **end stage (failure) N18.6**.

❏ She notes an additional level subterm **due to hypertension**, but concludes it does not describe this case because the patient's ESRD is not documented as due to hypertension.

▶ Chrystal verifies code **N18.6** in the Tabular List (■ FIGURE 21-11).

❏ She reads the code title for **N18.6 End stage renal disease** and confirms that this accurately describes the diagnosis.

❏ She reads the inclusion note under the code title that states **Chronic kidney disease requiring chronic dialysis**.

❏ She reads the instructional note under the code title that states **Use additional code to identify dialysis status (Z99.2)**.

❏ This tells her to assign a code for dialysis and that it should be a secondary code.

4th **N18 Chronic kidney disease (CKD)**
   Code first any associated:
       diabetic chronic kidney disease (E08.22, E09.22, E10.22, E11.22, E13.22)
       hypertensive chronic kidney disease (I12.-, I13.-)
   Use additional code to identify kidney transplant status, if applicable, (Z94.0)
   N18.1 Chronic kidney disease, stage 1
   N18.2 Chronic kidney disease, stage 2 (mild)
   N18.3 Chronic kidney disease, stage 3 (moderate)
   N18.4 Chronic kidney disease, stage 4 (severe)
   N18.5 Chronic kidney disease, stage 5
       Excludes1: chronic kidney disease, stage 5 requiring chronic dialysis (N18.6)
   N18.6 End stage renal disease
       Chronic kidney disease requiring chronic dialysis
       Use additional code to identify dialysis status (Z99.2)
   N18.9 Chronic kidney disease, unspecified

Figure 21-11 ■ Tabular List entry for category H19 "Chronic kidney disease".

▶ Chrystal checks for other instructional notes in the Tabular List.

❏ She cross-references the beginning of category **N18** and reads the instructional notes.

❏ This patient does not have diabetes or hypertension, so the first two notes do not apply.

❏ The third note that states **Use additional code to identify kidney transplant status, if applicable, (Z94.0)** also does not apply because the patient has not yet received a transplant.

❏ She cross-references the beginning of the block **(N17–N19)** and reviews the **Excludes2** notes. None of them apply because they do not describe ESRD.

❏ She cross-references the beginning of Chapter 14 (N00–N99) and reviews the **Excludes2** notes. None of them apply.

▶ Chrystal moves on to HD and searches the Index for the Main Term **Dialysis**.

❏ She locates the subterm **renal Z99.2**.

❏ This code is the same as the one cross-referenced by the Tabular List under code **N18.6**.

❏ She reviews the rest of the subterms and does not see any others that apply.

▶ Chrystal verifies code **Z99.2** in the Tabular List.

❏ She reads the code title for **Z99.2 Dependence on renal dialysis** and confirms that this accurately describes the diagnosis.

❏ She reads the inclusion items under the code title and learns that this code describes both hemodialysis and peritoneal dialysis.

❏ She reads the **Excludes1** notes, which do not apply.

▶ Chrystal checks for instructional notes in the Tabular List.

❏ She cross-references the beginning of category **Z99.2** and verifies that there are no instructional notes.

❏ She cross-references the beginning of the block **Z77–Z99** and reads the instructional note. It does not apply because there was no follow-up examination.

❏ She cross-references the beginning of Chapter 21 (Z00–Z99) and reviews the instructional notes, which describe the general use and purpose of Z codes. Nothing she reads changes the code assigned.

▶ Next, Chrystal codes for DRA, dialysis-related amyloidosis, and searches the Index for the Main Term **Amyloidosis**.

❏ She locates the subterm **hemodialysis-associated E85.3**.

❏ She reviews the rest of the subterms and does not see any others that apply.

▶ Chrystal verifies code **E85.3** in the Tabular List.

❏ She reads the code title for **E85.3 Secondary systemic amyloidosis** and confirms that this accurately describes the diagnosis.

❏ She reads the inclusion item under the code title and confirms that this code describes **Hemodialysis-associated amyloidosis**.

▶ Chrystal checks for instructional notes in the Tabular List.

❏ She cross-references the beginning of category **E85** and verifies that the **Excludes1** note regarding Alzheimer's disease does not apply.

❏ She cross-references the beginning of the block **E70–E88** and verifies that the **Excludes1** notes do not apply.

❏ She cross-references the beginning of Chapter 14 (E00–E89) and determines that the notes do not apply to this case because the patient does not have any of the conditions listed.

▶ Chrystal finishes by coding *on kidney transplant waiting list* and searches the Index for the Main Term **Waiting**.

❏ She locates the subterm **for organ transplant Z76.82**.

▶ Chrystal verifies code **Z76.82** in the Tabular List.

❏ She reads the code title for **Z76.82 Awaiting organ transplant status** and confirms that this accurately describes the diagnosis. She searches for, but does not find, a code specifically for kidney transplant waiting list.

▶ Chrystal checks for instructional notes in the Tabular List.

❏ She cross-references the beginning of category **Z76** and verifies that there are no instructional notes.

❏ She cross-references the beginning of the block **Z69–Z76** and verifies that there are no instructional notes.

❏ She previously cross-referenced the beginning of **Chapter 21 (Z00–Z99)** and remembers that there are no chapter-wide instructional notes that apply to this case.

▶ Chrystal reviews the codes she has assigned for this case.

❏ **N18.6   End stage renal disease**

❏ **Z99.2   Dependence on renal dialysis**

❏ **E85.3   Secondary systemic amyloidosis**

❏ **Z76.82   Awaiting organ transplant status**

▶ Next, Chrystal must determine how to sequence the codes.

CODING PRACTICE

Exercise 21.3 Assigning Codes for Genitourinary System Conditions

Instructions: Read the mini-medical-record of each patient's encounter, review the information abstracted in Exercise 21.2, and assign ICD-10-CM diagnosis codes using the Index and Tabular List. Write the code(s) on the line provided.

---

1. OFFICE Gender: F Age: 42

Reason for encounter: Surgery for endometriosis

Assessment: Endometriosis of the uterus

Plan: FU in office 2 weeks

1 ICD-10-CM Code _____

---

2. OFFICE Gender: F Age: 46

Reason for encounter: Painful lumps in both breasts

Assessment: Fibrocystic breast changes

Plan: OTC acetaminophen, heat and ice as needed to relieve local pain

Tip: Physicians use the term *changes* rather than the more traditional *disease* to avoid alarming patients.

2 ICD-10-CM Codes _____

---

3. OFFICE Gender: M Age: 61

Reason for encounter: Occasional excruciating low back pain

Assessment: Ureteral calculi

Plan: Medical expulsive therapy (MET) with tamsulosin

Tip: The presence of calculi accounts for the low back pain.

1 ICD-10-CM Code _____

ARRANGING CODES FOR GENITOURINARY SYSTEM CONDITIONS

Coders should be attentive to instructional notes in the Tabular List regarding how to sequence codes for genitourinary conditions due to infections and codes for benign prostatic hyperplasia (BPH) and associated symptoms.

Arranging Codes for Genitourinary Conditions Due to Infections

Because many disorders of the genitourinary system are infections, the Tabular List provides frequent instructional notes directing coders to assign an additional code to identify the infectious organism or underlying condition. Sequence the genitourinary condition first and the infectious organism second (■ FIGURE 21-12).

Patient is seen for acute vaginitis due to Candida.

(1) **N76.0 Acute vaginitis**
(2) **B37.3 Candidiasis of vulva and vagina**

Figure 21-12 ■ Example of arranging codes for a genitourinary condition due to an infectious organism.

Arranging Codes for Benign Prostatic Hyperplasia

Benign prostatic hyperplasia (BPH), or enlarged prostate (EP), is the abnormal growth of epithelial cells of the prostate, causing compression or obstruction of the urethra. Do not confuse the abbreviation EP, which is an enlarged prostate, with the abbreviation ED, which is erectile dysfunction. The condition is common among men over age 50 and may be accompanied by a variety of **lower urinary tract symptoms (LUTS)** (*symptoms relating to urine storage and voiding disturbances*). ICD-10-CM provides separate codes for BPH based on whether LUTS exist. When BPH is accompanied with LUTS, coders must assign codes for LUTS and sequence them after the code for the BPH (■ FIGURE 21-13).

Refer to ■ FIGURE 21-14 to learn more about assigning and sequencing codes for BPH with LUTS. The code for BPH must be sequenced first, followed by the two symptoms. The order of the symptoms does not matter, unless the physician indicates that one is of greater importance.

Guided Example of Arranging Codes for Urinary System Conditions

To practice skills for sequencing codes for diseases of the urinary system, continue with the example from earlier in the chapter about patient Ronald Coffield, who was seen at Branton Professional Group for ESRD and joint pain.

4th N40 Benign prostatic hyperplasia
Includes: adenofibromatous hypertrophy of prostate
benign hypertrophy of the prostate
benign prostatic hypertrophy
BPH
enlarged prostate
nodular prostate
polyp of prostate
Excludes1: benign neoplasms of prostate (adenoma, benign) (fibroadenoma) (fibroma) (myoma) (D29.1)
Excludes2: malignant neoplasm of prostate (C61)
N40.0 Benign prostatic hyperplasia without lower urinary tract symptoms
Enlarged prostate without LUTS
Enlarged prostate NOS
N40.1 Benign prostatic hyperplasia with lower urinary tract symptoms
Enlarged prostate with LUTS
Use additional code for associated symptoms, when specified:
incomplete bladder emptying (R39.14)
nocturia (R35.1)
straining on urination (R39.16)
urinary frequency (R35.0)
urinary hesitancy (R39.11)
urinary incontinence (N39.4-)
urinary obstruction (N13.8)
urinary retention (R33.8)
urinary urgency (R39.15)
weak urinary stream (R39.12)

Figure 21-13 ■ Tabular List entry for code H40.1 "Benign prostatic hyperplasia with lower urinary tract symptoms".

Patient is seen due to complaints of a weak urine stream and straining to urinate. The physician determines these symptoms are due to benign prostatic hyperplasia.

(1) **N40.1 Benign prostatic hyperplasia with lower urinary tract symptoms**
(2) **R39.16 Straining to void**
(3) **R39.12 Poor urinary stream**

Figure 21-14 ■ Example of arranging codes for benign prostatic hyperplasia with lower urinary tract symptoms.

Follow along in your ICD-10-CM manual as Chrystal Crago, CCA, sequences the codes. Check off each step after you complete it.

▶ First, Chrystal confirms the codes she assigned.

❏ **N18.6 End stage renal disease**

❏ **Z99.2 Dependence on renal dialysis**

❏ **E85.3 Secondary systemic amyloidosis**

❏ **Z76.82 Awaiting organ transplant status**

▶ Chrystal must determine the first-listed diagnosis because this was an outpatient office visit.

❏ She reviews OGCR IV.G, which states: **List first the ICD-10-CM code for the diagnosis, condition, problem, or other reason for encounter/visit shown in the medical record to be chiefly responsible for the services provided. List additional codes that describe any coexisting conditions.**

❏ She reviews the medical record and determines that the diagnosis that best meets this definition is DRA. The patient's ongoing complaints of severe joint pain were the main reason for the visit and the services.

❏ She assigns DRA as the first-listed diagnosis.

- Although the DRA is secondary to the ESRD, she did not see any instructional notes that directed her to sequence ESRD first. The word *secondary* in the code title means that DRA is secondary to ESRD, or caused by it. It does not mean that DRA must be sequenced as the second code.

▶ Chrystal determines that ESRD should be the second sequenced diagnosis because it is responsible for the DRA. It takes priority over the **Z** codes, which describe the status of the patient but not specific conditions.

▶ Chrystal sequences HD status as the third code because it is required by the instructional note under code **N18.6**. The instructional note also indicates that HD should be sequenced secondary to ESRD.

▶ Chrystal sequences the code for awaiting organ transplant as the final code.

▶ Chrystal reviews the medical record one final time to ensure that she has captured all the details and that the final codes are consistent with the medical record.

▶ Chrystal finalizes the codes and sequencing for this case:

(1) **E85.3 Secondary systemic amyloidosis**
(2) **N18.6 End stage renal disease**
(3) **Z99.2 Dependence on renal dialysis**
(4) **Z76.82 Awaiting organ transplant status**

CODING PRACTICE

Exercise 21.4 Arranging Codes for Genitourinary System Conditions

Instructions: Read the mini-medical-record of each patient's encounter, review the information abstracted in Exercise 21.2, assign ICD-10-CM diagnosis codes using the Index and Tabular List, and sequence them correctly.

1. OFFICE   Gender: M   Age: 81

Reason for encounter: FU on BPH with obstruction and urinary retention

Assessment: Little improvement seen despite multiple medication adjustments

(continued)

CODING PRACTICE (continued)

1. (continued)

Plan: Schedule transurethral resection of the prostate (TURP)

Tip: Follow instructional notes in the Tabular List for additional codes and sequencing.

3 ICD-10-CM Codes _____

_____

2. OFFICE   Gender: F   Age: 37

Reason for encounter: Vaginal discharge, burning, redness in perineal area

Assessment: Lab results show bacterial vaginitis due to staphylococcus, which is treatable

Plan: Antibiotics

Tip: The type of *Staphylococcus* is not specified.

2 ICD-10-CM Codes _____

3. INPATIENT HOSPITAL   Gender: F   Age: 83

Reason for admission: Nursing facility (NF) patient brought to emergency department with suspected UTI because of signs of confusion and lack of cooperation; history of UTI over the past 2 years

Assessment: UTI due to E. coli (non-Shiga toxin-producing)

Plan: Administered IV antibiotics, discharged after 2 days to NF with Rx

Tip: In the elderly, confusion and lack of cooperation may be the only symptoms of UTI.

3 ICD-10-CM Codes _____

CODING NEOPLASMS OF THE GENITOURINARY SYSTEM

Neoplasms of the genitourinary system do not appear in ICD-10-CM Chapter 14, "Diseases of the Genitourinary System (N00-N99)." Codes for neoplasms of the genitourinary system appear in the following blocks within the neoplasm chapter:

- **C50 Malignant neoplasm of breast**
- **C51-C58 Malignant neoplasm of female genital organs**
- **C60-C63 Malignant neoplasms of male genital organs**
- **C64-C68 Malignant neoplasm of urinary tract**

The most common cancer of the urinary system is bladder cancer, which is the fourth most common cancer among males in the United States, according to the American Cancer Society. Most bladder cancer is transitional cell carcinoma, which starts from the cells lining the bladder. The tumors are classified based on the way they grow. Papillary tumors have a wart-like appearance and are attached to a stalk. Nonpapillary tumors are less common but more invasive, with a poorer outcome. Smoking is a major risk factor for bladder cancer. Other risk factors are a family history of bladder cancer, advanced age, Caucasian race, and male gender.

The most common sites for cancer in the reproductive system are the prostate in males and the breast and ovaries in females, according to NIH.

Prostate cancer is the most common cancer in men and the third most common cause of death from cancer in men of all ages. It is the most common cause of death from cancer in men over age 75. Prostate cancer is rarely found in men younger than 40. The **prostate-specific antigen (PSA)** blood test is performed to screen for prostate cancer, enabling physicians to detect prostate cancer before it causes symptoms. At an early stage, prostate cancer is very treatable through surgery and radiation.

Breast cancer is the most common cancer in women, and the second-leading cause of cancer death in women, according to the American Cancer Society. Most occurrences of breast cancer are **ductal**, starting in the milk ducts. **Lobular** breast cancer starts in the lobules that produce milk. Screening mammograms are proven to be effective at identifying breast cancer in early stages. Treatment of breast cancer in the early stages, through surgery and radiation, has a high success rate.

Ovarian cancer is the fifth most common cause of cancer deaths among women. It causes more deaths than any other type of female genital cancer, largely because its symptoms of bloating, pain, and the feeling of fullness are often attributed to other causes. Ovarian cancer is usually not diagnosed until after it has metastasized, making it difficult to treat.

Genetic testing for mutations in the genes *BRCA1* and *BRCA2* can be helpful in identifying women who are at greater risk of breast or ovarian cancer and men who are at greater risk of breast cancer, prostate cancer, and several other cancers.

CODING PRACTICE

Exercise 21.5 Coding Neoplasms of the Genitourinary System

Instructions: Read the mini-medical-record of each patient's encounter, then abstract, assign, and sequence ICD-10-CM diagnosis codes using the Index and Tabular List. Write the code(s) on the line provided.

1. OFFICE Gender: M Age: 62

Reason for encounter: Review results of needle biopsy which was performed due to elevated PSA

Assessment: Stage 1 adenocarcinoma of the prostate which affects less than 5% of the prostate

Plan: Brachytherapy (*placing radioactive seeds inside the prostate gland*)

1 ICD-10-CM Code _____

2. OUTPATIENT HOSPITAL Gender: M Age: 64

Reason for encounter: Radiation therapy

Assessment: Transitional cell carcinoma bladder cancer with overlapping lesions of the orifice and metastasis to the prostate

Plan: Daily treatments for 3 more weeks

3 ICD-10-CM Codes _____
_____

3. OFFICE Gender: F Age: 60

Reason for encounter: Painful and frequent urination, blood in urine

Assessment: Radiation cystitis as a result of external beam radiotherapy for metastatic ovarian cancer

Tip: The fourth code is an external cause code for a complication of radiotherapy.

4 ICD-10-CM Codes _____
_____

4. OFFICE Gender: F Age: 44

Reason for encounter: FU on imaging for pain and hematuria

Assessment: Angiomyolipoma, right kidney

Plan: Embolization to reduce risk of hemorrhage and shrink the tumor

1 ICD-10-CM Code _____

5. OUTPATIENT HOSPITAL Gender: F Age: 58

Reason for encounter: Lumpectomy

Assessment: Ductal cancer in situ (DCIS) of the left breast, upper inner quadrant

1 ICD-10-CM Code _____

CHAPTER SUMMARY

In this chapter you learned that:

- The genitourinary (GU) system includes the urinary system and the male and female genital, or reproductive, systems. The function of the urinary system is to filter, store, and remove waste products from the blood and maintain homeostasis. The function of the genital system is sexual reproduction.

- ICD-10-CM Official Guidelines for Coding and Reporting (OGCR) I.C.14 provides detailed discussion of chronic kidney disease.

- Disorders in this chapter have a wide range of abstracting criteria because there is a wide range of organs and types of disorders.

- Two similar genitourinary conditions, nephritic syndrome and nephrotic syndrome, demonstrate the importance of checking cross-referencing instructions in the Index in order to assign the most specific code available.

- Coders should be attentive to instructional notes in the Tabular List regarding how to sequence codes for genitourinary conditions due to infections and codes for benign prostatic hyperplasia (BPH) and associated symptoms.

- The most common sites for cancer in the genital system are the prostate in males and the breast and ovaries in females, according to NIH.

CONCEPT QUIZ

Take a moment to look back through diseases of the genitourinary system and solidify your skills. Try to answer the questions from memory first, then look back at the discussion in this chapter if you need a little extra help.

Completion

Instructions: Write the term that completes each statement based on the information you learned in this chapter. Choose from the list below. Some choices may be used more than once and some choices may not be used at all.

calculi	glomerulonephritis
cervical dysplasia	glomerulus
cervical intraepithelial neoplasia	nephritic
CKD	nephron
diabetic nephropathy	nephroptosis
dialysis	nephrotic
ED	renal pelvis
endometriosis	transplant
EP	ureter
ESRD	urethra

1. Urine passes from the renal pelvis through the _____ to the urinary bladder.

2. _____ syndrome is a collection of disorders affecting the kidneys, characterized by nonpurulent inflammatory glomerular disorders that allow proteins and red blood cells to pass into the urine, resulting in proteinuria and hematuria.

3. The _____ is a cluster of capillaries in the kidney that separates the urinary space from the blood.

4. _____ is accumulated damage to the glomerulus capillaries due to chronic high blood glucose.

5. BPH is also called _____.

6. Diseases of the _____ attack the kidneys' filtering ability.

7. _____ is abnormal changes in the cells on the surface of the cervix that may lead to cancer if not treated.

8. _____ is stage 5 chronic kidney disease.

9. _____ are stones that may accumulate in the kidneys, bladder, or ureters.

10. _____ is a treatment that filters the blood to remove waste, excess salt, and water.

Multiple Choice

Instructions: Circle the letter of the best answer to each question based on the information you learned in this chapter.

1. What stage of CKD occurs when the kidneys cease to function, requiring that patients receive dialysis or a kidney transplant to survive?
   A. 1
   B. 3
   C. 4
   D. 5

2. What condition is the accumulation of deposits of the starchy substance amyloid in the joints, seen in long-term dialysis patients?
   A. Dialysis-related amyloidosis
   B. End-stage renal disease
   C. Nephritic syndrome
   D. Nephrolithiasis

3. What is the only specific disease that Medicare covers for the entire population, regardless of age?
   A. BPH
   B. ED
   C. CKD
   D. ESRD

4. What kidney condition is a collection of nonpurulent inflammatory glomerular disorders that allow proteins and red blood cells to pass into the urine, resulting in proteinuria and hematuria?
   A. Nephroptosis
   B. Hydronephrosis
   C. Nephritic syndrome
   D. Nephrotic syndrome

5. What condition does OGCR I.C.14 discuss in detail?
   A. Hypertensive kidney disease
   B. Chronic kidney disease
   C. Nephritic and nephrotic syndrome
   D. Benign prostatic hyperplasia

6. What Main Term and subterm should be located in the Index to locate codes for ESRD?
   A. Main Term: *ESRD*
   B. Main Term: *End*, Subterm: *stage*
   C. Main Term: *Disease*, Subterm: *renal*
   D. Main Term: *Disease*, Subterm: *kidney*

7. How would you code the following scenario? *A patient with ESRD is receiving dialysis.*
   A. Z99.2, N18.6
   B. N18.6, Z99.2
   C. N18.6
   D. Z99.2

8. How would you code the following scenario? *A patient is seen due to complaints of a weak urine stream and straining to urinate. The physician determines these symptoms are due to an enlarged prostate.*
   A. N40.1, R39.16, R39.12
   B. R39.16, R39.12, N40.1
   C. N40.1
   D. R39.16, R39.12

9. How would you code the following scenario? *A patient is seen for acute vaginitis due to Candida.*
   A. B37.3, N76.0
   B. N76.0, B37.3
   C. B37.3
   D. N76.0

10. What condition does the PSA blood test screen for?
    A. Cervical cancer
    B. Benign prostatic hyperplasia
    C. Prostate cancer
    D. Pyelonephritis

KEEP ON CODING

Instructions: Read the diagnostic statement, then use the Index and Tabular List to assign and sequence ICD-10-CM diagnosis codes. Write the code(s) on the line provided.

Urinary System

1. Hydroureter. ICD-10-CM Code(s) _____

2. Cystostomy malfunction. ICD-10-CM Code(s) _____

3. Carcinoma of the left kidney pelvis. ICD-10-CM Code(s) _____

4. Urethrolithiasis. ICD-10-CM Code(s) _____

5. Urethrocele. ICD-10-CM Code(s) _____

6. Interstitial nephritis. ICD-10-CM Code(s) _____

7. Trigonitis. ICD-10-CM Code(s) _____

8. End-stage renal disease, currently receiving dialysis. ICD-10-CM Code(s) _____

9. Terminal atrophy of the kidney. ICD-10-CM Code(s) _____

10. Hypermobility of urethra with urinary stress incontinence. ICD-10-CM Code(s) _____

11. Urinary bladder stone. ICD-10-CM Code(s) _____

12. Ureteritis cystica. ICD-10-CM Code(s) _____

Male Reproductive System

13. Benign prostatic hyperplasia with nighttime urination. ICD-10-CM Code(s) _____

14. Oligospermia. ICD-10-CM Code(s) _____

15. Priapism due to trauma. ICD-10-CM Code(s) _____

16. Infected hydrocele due to *E. coli.* ICD-10-CM Code(s) _____

17. Cyst of tunica albuginea testes. ICD-10-CM Code(s) _____

18. Erectile dysfunction due to type 2 diabetes. ICD-10-CM Code(s) _____

19. Gynecomastia. ICD-10-CM Code(s) _____

Female Reproductive System

20. Torsion of fallopian tube. ICD-10-CM Code(s) _____

21. Decubitus ulcer of cervix. ICD-10-CM Code(s) _____

22. Secondary amenorrhea. ICD-10-CM Code(s) _____

23. Anteversion of uterus. ICD-10-CM Code(s) _____

24. Endometriosis of the intestines. ICD-10-CM Code(s) _____

25. Bartholin's gland cyst. ICD-10-CM Code(s) _____

CODING CHALLENGE

Instructions: Read the mini-medical-record of each patient's encounter, then abstract, assign, and arrange ICD-10-CM diagnosis codes using the Index and Tabular List. Write the code(s) on the line provided.

Urinary System

1. INPATIENT HOSPITAL Gender: M Age: 46

Reason for encounter: Oliguria, drowsy and lethargic, edema

Assessment: Acute renal failure with tubular necrosis and hypertension

Plan: Fluid restriction, diuretics, restrict mineral intake, dialysis if serum potassium remains high

Tip: Chronic renal failure is assumed to be related to hypertension, but acute renal failure is not.

2 ICD-10-CM Codes _____

---

2. INPATIENT HOSPITAL Gender: M Age: 37

Reason for encounter: Bloody urine, edema of feet, ankles, and legs, uncontrolled high BP, upper abdominal pain, general malaise

Assessment: Glomerulonephrosis due to secondary DM which is a result of alcohol dependent chronic pancreatitis, 2 years on insulin

Plan: Adjust BP meds, diuretics, angiotensin-converting enzyme inhibitors

4 ICD-10-CM Codes _____

_____

---

3. OFFICE Gender: F Age: 56

Reason for encounter: Renal dialysis

Assessment: Stage 5 CKD due to autosomal recessive polycystic kidney disease

Plan: Return in 2 days

Tip: Patients typically receive dialysis three times per week.

3 ICD-10-CM Codes _____

_____

Male Reproductive System

4. OFFICE Gender: M Age: 63

Reason for encounter: Painful urination

Assessment: Acute enterococcal prostatitis

Plan: IV antibacterial gram-positive therapy

2 ICD-10-CM Codes _____

---

5. OFFICE Gender: M Age: 16

Reason for encounter: Red and painful foreskin and penis with foul smelling discharge, uncircumcised

Assessment: Balanitis due to E. coli

Plan: Rx antibiotics, hygiene instructions

2 ICD-10-CM Codes _____

Female Reproductive System

6. OFFICE Gender: F Age: 38

Reason for encounter: Urinary incontinence (UI), difficulty with sexual encounters, feeling of pelvic heaviness

Assessment: Cystocele and uterine prolapse, grade 3

Plan: Schedule surgical rectocele and cystocele repair in 3 wk

Tip: Follow the cross-references in the Index.

1 ICD-10-CM Code _____

---

7. OFFICE Gender: F Age: 20

Reason for encounter: Severe pelvic pain and cramps on the first day or two of her monthly period

Assessment: No specific problems except an incidental finding of retroverted uterus, which I do not believe is the cause of the menstrual pain

Plan: Patient advised to begin a daily walking program, ibuprofen or other NSAIDs to be taken 1–2 days prior to her period

2 ICD-10-CM Codes _____

8. OFFICE   Gender: F   Age: 22

Reason for encounter: FU on routine pap smear showing CIN II (unvaccinated for HPV)

Assessment: CIN II

Plan: Schedule for colposcopy in 2 weeks

Tip: If you are unsure whether the CIN is mild, moderate, or severe, review the inclusion notes in the Tabular List for the possible codes.

1 ICD-10-CM Code _____

9. OFFICE   Gender: F   Age: 81

Reason for encounter: Urge incontinence, bladder droops to the vaginal opening

Assessment: Urge incontinence due to grade 2 cystocele on the right side

Plan: Kegel exercises, pessary, RTO in 2 months to schedule surgery if no relief

1 ICD-10-CM Code _____

10. OUTPATIENT HOSPITAL   Gender: F   Age: 41

Reason for encounter: Screening mammogram

Assessment: Suspicious mass, right breast, and bilateral microcalcifications

Plan: Schedule biopsy next week

3 ICD-10-CM Codes _____

_____

Chapter 22

Pregnancy, Childbirth, and the Puerperium (O00-O9A)

Chapter Outline

- **Obstetrics Refresher**
- **Coding Guidelines for Obstetrics**
- **Abstracting Diagnoses for Obstetrics**
- **Assigning Diagnosis Codes for Obstetrics**
- **Arranging Diagnosis Codes for Obstetrics**

Learning Objectives

After completing this chapter, you should have the skills to:

22.1 Spell and define the key words, medical terms, and abbreviations related to pregnancy, childbirth, and the puerperium. (Remember)

22.2 Summarize the structures, processes, and common conditions of pregnancy, childbirth, and the puerperium. (Understand)

22.3 Adhere to the Official Guidelines for Coding and Reporting related to pregnancy, childbirth, and the puerperium. (Apply)

22.4 Examine and abstract diagnostic information from the medical record for coding conditions of pregnancy, childbirth, and the puerperium. (Analyze)

22.5 Demonstrate how to assign diagnosis codes for pregnancy, childbirth, and the puerperium. (Apply)

22.6 Utilize guidelines for arranging (sequencing) multiple diagnosis codes for pregnancy, childbirth, and the puerperium. (Apply)

Key Terms and Abbreviations

amnion	estimated date of delivery (EDD)	multiple gestation	prenatal
amniotic sac	estimated gestational age (EGA)	occipitoanterior (OA)	prepartum
antenatal	fetopelvic disproportion	para (P)	puerperal
antepartum	first trimester	parturition	puerperium
childbirth	gestational condition	peripartum	second trimester
chorion	grand multipara	placenta	singleton
conception	gravida (G)	postpartum	third trimester
delivery	last menstrual period (LMP)	pregnancy	TPAL
dichorionic-diamniotic (DiDi)	monoamniotic	pregnancy-induced hypertension (PIH)	true labor
ectopic	monochorionic		zygote

In addition to the key terms listed here, students should know the terms defined within tables in this chapter.

INTRODUCTION

Pregnancy possesses unique terminology, presents unique complications, and requires unique coding skills. Physicians who specialize in pregnancy and delivery are obstetrician/gynecologists (OB/GYNs). It is common for several OB/GYNs to join together in the same medical practice to provide 24/7 coverage for one another. Obstetric practices may also include a certified nurse midwife (CNM), an advanced practice nurse with specialized education in nursing and obstetrics. A CNM provides care for relatively healthy women with uncomplicated pregnancies.

For the sake of brevity, this chapter refers to pregnancy, childbirth, and the puerperium as obstetrics.

OBSTETRICS REFRESHER

Pregnancy is a normal, temporary condition that occurs within the female body, which begins at the time of **conception** (*fertilization of the female ova by the male sperm*) and ends with the birth of the fetus. The **prenatal** period is the time period from conception to the beginning of labor. It is also called the **prepartum, antepartum,** or **antenatal** period. **Childbirth**, also called **parturition**, is the period of **true labor** (*uterine contractions and dilation of the cervix*) and active **delivery** (*the expulsion of the fetus and placenta from the uterus*). The **puerperium, puerperal** period, or **postpartum** period is the six-week period following childbirth, during which time the female reproductive organs return to the pre-pregnant state. The **peripartum** period is the last month of pregnancy to five months postpartum.

The term (length) of a normal pregnancy is 38–40 weeks. The **estimated date of delivery (EDD)** is determined as 40 weeks from the **last menstrual period (LMP). Estimated gestational age (EGA)** is the number of weeks and days since the LMP. The pregnancy is divided into three trimesters, defined based on gestational age as follows:

- **First trimester**—Less than 14 weeks, 0 days
- **Second trimester**—14 weeks, 0 days to less than 28 weeks, 0 days
- **Third trimester**—28 weeks, 0 days until delivery

A woman's childbearing history is described in terms of **gravida (G)** (*the number of pregnancies*) and **para (P)** (*the number of pregnancies resulting in a fetus of viable gestational age [20 weeks] regardless of whether the fetus was alive at birth*). **Grand multipara** identifies a woman who has had five or more previous pregnancies resulting in a viable fetus. Pregnancies that consist of multiples, such as twins or triplets, count as *one* when describing parity. For example, a woman currently pregnant, who has had one previous pregnancy and gave birth to twins, is gravida 2 (two pregnancies including the current one) and para 1 (has had one pregnancy resulting in a viable fetus). Parity may be further described using **TPAL**, which identifies the number of term births (T), preterm births (P), spontaneous or induced abortions (A), and living children (L). TPAL is written as a four-digit number. Refer to ■ FIGURE 22-1 to learn more about the various ways that childbearing history may be written. The specific format and abbreviations used in obstetrics records can vary by institution. It is important to become acquainted with the format used by the institution(s) you work with.

Each structure in the pregnant uterus is labeled with its name as well as its medical terminology root/combining form in ■ FIGURE 22-2 (page 382). As you learn about conditions and procedures of pregnancy, childbirth, and the puerperium, remember to apply medical terminology skills to combine word roots, prefixes, and suffixes you already know to define new terms. Refer to ■ TABLE 22-1 (page 382) for a refresher on how to build medical terms related to pregnancy, childbirth, and the puerperium.

In particular, coders must be familiar with the terminology related to each aspect of pregnancy, childbirth, and the puerperium.

SUCCESS STEP

If physician documentation of EDD or gestational age differs from the date calculated by the method shown here or another calculation method, coders should utilize the date documented by the physician.

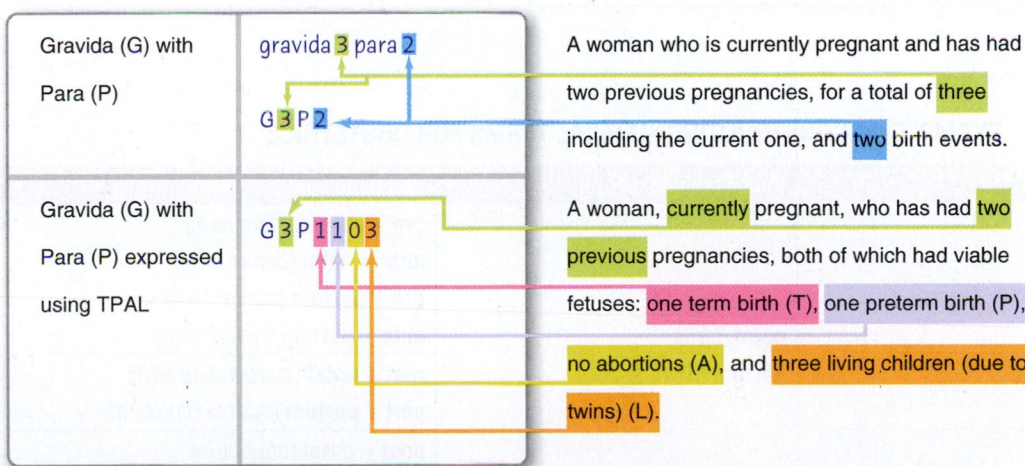

| Gravida (G) with Para (P) | gravida **3** para **2**

G **3** P **2** | A woman who is currently pregnant and has had two previous pregnancies, for a total of three including the current one, and two birth events. |
| Gravida (G) with Para (P) expressed using TPAL | G **3** P **1 1 0 3** | A woman, currently pregnant, who has had two previous pregnancies, both of which had viable fetuses: one term birth (T), one preterm birth (P), no abortions (A), and three living children (due to twins) (L). |

Figure 22-1 ■ Methods of describing childbearing history.

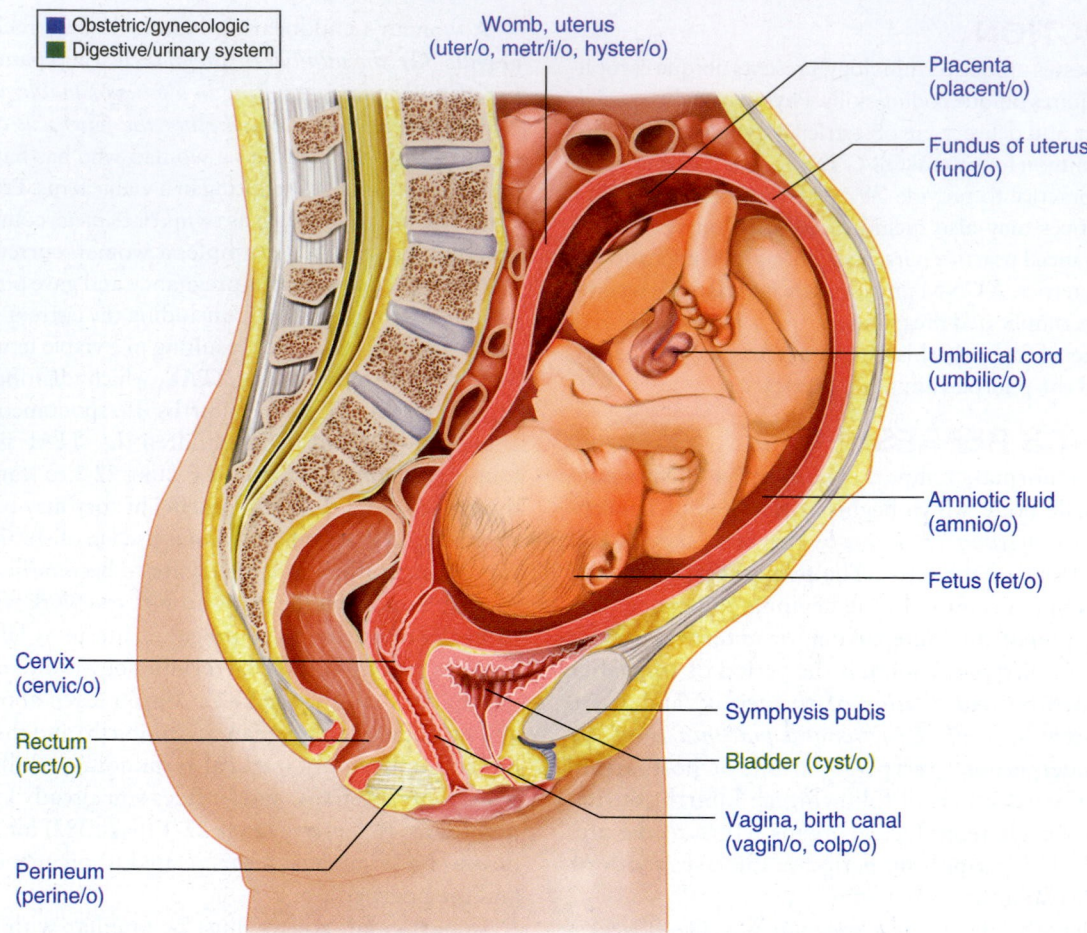

■ Obstetric/gynecologic
■ Digestive/urinary system

Womb, uterus
(uter/o, metr/i/o, hyster/o)

Placenta
(placent/o)

Fundus of uterus
(fund/o)

Umbilical cord
(umbilic/o)

Amniotic fluid
(amnio/o)

Fetus (fet/o)

Symphysis pubis

Bladder (cyst/o)

Vagina, birth canal
(vagin/o, colp/o)

Cervix
(cervic/o)

Rectum
(rect/o)

Perineum
(perine/o)

Figure 22-2 ■ Pregnant uterus in a full-term pregnancy.

CODING CAUTION

Be alert for medical word terms that are spelled similarly but have different meanings.

anti- (*against*) and **ante-** (*before*)

dystocia (*difficult labor*) and **dyspnea** (*difficulty breathing*)

mastalgia (*breast pain*) and **mastitis** (*inflammation of the breast*)

Conditions of Pregnancy

The Centers for Disease Control and Prevention (CDC) reports that there are nearly 4 million live births per year in the United States. Most of these (94%) carry some type of complication that needs to be coded, according to the Agency for Healthcare Research and Quality (AHQR). Hospital stays with pregnancy-related complications tend to be longer and cost more than those without complications.

Table 22-1 ■ **EXAMPLE OF CONSTRUCTING MEDICAL TERMS FOR OBSTETRICS**

Prefix	Root/Combining Form	Complete Medical Term
pre- (*before*)		**pre + natal** (*before birth*)
ante- (*before*)		**ante + natal** (*before birth*)
		pre + partum (*before birth*)
	natal (*birth*)	**ante + partum** (*before birth*)
peri- (*surrounding*)	**partum** (*birth*)	**peri + natal** (*surrounding birth*)
		peri + partum (*surrounding birth*)
post- (*after*)		**post + natal** (*after birth*)
		post + partum (*after birth*)

A normal pregnancy is defined as follows:

- No preexisting conditions
- No new conditions that develop during pregnancy
- Single gestation
- Mother will be over age 16 and under age 35 at EDD

Disorders of the pregnancy may be due to preexisting conditions of the mother, conditions that arise during pregnancy, or conditions of the fetus or amniotic cavity. Refer to ■ TABLE 22-2 for a summary of conditions affecting pregnancy. Coders use medical resources, such as reference books on diseases; to understand conditions of pregnancy, childbirth, and the puerperium; diagnostic methods; and common treatments.

Conditions Due to Pregnancy Compared to Preexisting Conditions

Some conditions, such as Rh incompatibility and pre-eclampsia, occur only during pregnancy. Other conditions, such as diabetes and hypertension, may affect people at any time during their lifetime but also have a pregnancy-related variation. When a condition has been diagnosed before a woman becomes pregnant, it is a preexisting condition. When the condition is first diagnosed during pregnancy, it is a **gestational condition**.

Characteristics of a gestational condition, such as gestational diabetes or gestational hypertension, include:

- The gestational disease has the same symptoms and signs as its nongestational counterpart.
- The condition is not present prior to pregnancy.
- The condition usually begins after the 20th week of pregnancy.
- The condition returns to normal when the pregnancy is over.

When diabetes or hypertension is present, coders must review the documentation carefully to determine whether it is gestational or preexisting to assign the correct codes.

Multiple Gestation

Multiple gestation is a pregnancy with more than one fetus, as in twins, triplets, or sextuplets, and carries greater risk for complications than **singletons** (*pregnancies with one fetus*). The rate of twin births increased over 76% from 1980 to 2009, according to the CDC, and leveled off in subsequent years. The increase in multiple-gestation pregnancies is due to delayed childbearing and expanding use of reproductive technology.

Coders need to be familiar with the terminology used to describe multiple gestation because it affects code assignment. Physicians describe multiple-gestation pregnancies based on the number of **amnions** or **amniotic sacs, chorions,** and **placentas.** This is important because it directly affects the mortality risk of the fetuses. The amniotic sac is a membrane that surrounds the embryo. The chorion is an outer membrane that surrounds the amnion. The space inside the chorion and the amnion is called the amniotic cavity and is filled with amniotic fluid. The amniotic cavity prevents the embryo from drying out and protects it against vibration and shocks. The placenta is the organ that allows for the exchange of oxygen, nutrients, and waste between the fetus and the mother. It attaches to the chorion and consists of chorionic material from the fetus and uterine material from the mother.

When multiple embryos each develop from separate **zygotes** (*fertilized eggs*)—as happens with fraternal twins—each embryo always has its own amnion and chorion, making the pregnancy **dichorionic-diamniotic (DiDi)**.

Identical twins are created when a zygote divides to create two or more identical embryos. Normally, identical embryos are DiDi, with each embryo enclosed in its own amnion and chorion and having its own placenta. However, it is possible for more than one embryo to share a chorion or an amniotic sac. When the chorion is shared, the placenta is also shared. The sharing of the chorion and amnion is determined by how soon after fertilization the egg divides. Refer to ■ TABLE 22-3 (page 384) to learn the possible combinations of twins and ■ FIGURE 22-3 (page 384) to visualize the differences. **Monochorionic** (*sharing the chorion*) twins are at risk for more complications than DiDi twins; **monoamniotic** (*sharing the same amnion*) twins have the greatest risk of mortality.

Table 22-2 ■ COMMON CONDITIONS OF PREGNANCY

Condition	Definition
Chromosomal abnormality	Any of a wide range of disorders in which a fetus has an abnormal number of chromosomes or a structural abnormality in one or more chromosomes
Eclampsia	Convulsions occurring during pregnancy or the puerperium associated with pre-eclampsia
Gestational diabetes	Diabetes that develops during pregnancy in a woman who did not previously have diabetes
Gestational hypertension	Development of hypertension after 20 weeks of gestation in a woman who previously was not diagnosed with hypertension; also called **pregnancy-induced hypertension (PIH)**
HELLP syndrome	Severe pre-eclampsia with **h**emolysis, **e**levated **l**iver enzymes, and **l**ow **p**latelet count
In vitro fertilization (IVF)	Fertilization of an ova in a laboratory dish, followed by introduction into the uterus
Pre-eclampsia	A metabolic disorder of pregnancy that develops after the 20th week and involves gestational hypertension and proteinuria
Preexisting diabetes	Diabetes diagnosed in a woman before she becomes pregnant
Preexisting hypertension	Hypertension diagnosed in a woman before she becomes pregnant
Rhesus (Rh) incompatibility	A condition in which the mother is Rh negative and develops antibodies against a fetus that is Rh positive

Table 22-3 ■ **CONFIGURATIONS OF CHORION, AMNION, AND PLACENTA OF TWINS**

Description	Number of Chorions	Number of Amnions	Number of Placentas	Division of Zygote
Monochorionic-monoamniotic (MoMo)	1	1	1	8–13 days after fertilization
Monochorionic-diamniotic (MoDi)	1	2	1	3–8 days after fertilization
Dichorionic-diamniotic (DiDi)	2	2	2	Less than 3–4 days after fertilization

Monochorionic-Monoamniotic (MoMo)

Monochorionic-Diamniotic (MoDi)

Dichorionic-Diamniotic (DiDi)

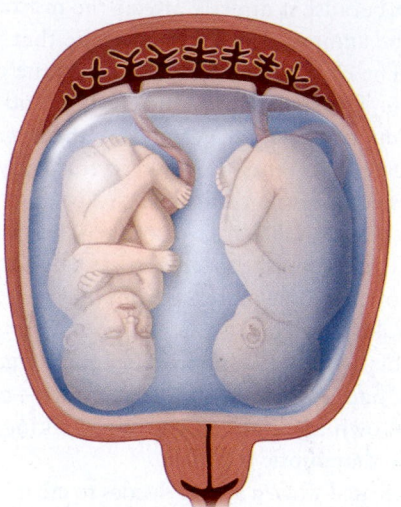 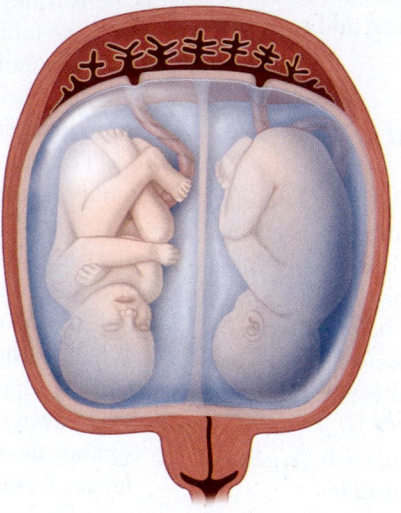 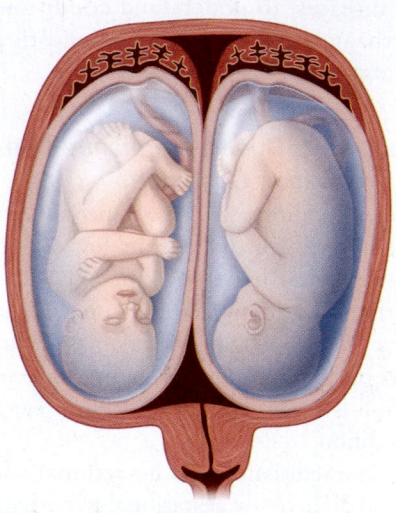

Figure 22-3 ■ Twin configurations of the chorion and amnion.

Conditions of Childbirth

A normal delivery is defined as follows:

- Single liveborn infant
- Full-term pregnancy
- Vaginal delivery with cephalic presentation
- No induction, manipulation, or instrumentation
- No complications

Any labor and delivery that does not meet these criteria is complicated. Complications can occur during any phase of labor and delivery (■ FIGURE 22-4) and multiple complications may affect one mother. Refer to ■ TABLE 22-4 for a summary of conditions affecting labor and delivery.

Conditions of the Puerperium

Postpartum and puerperal conditions arise after delivery and are due to the postpregnancy state. Because some conditions, such as depression, can be preexisting, look for the physician's documentation that describes a condition as puerperal. Refer to ■ TABLE 22-5 for a summary of conditions affecting the puerperium.

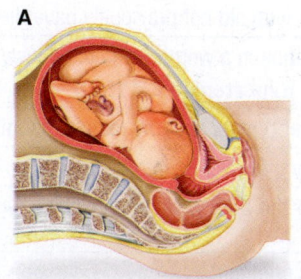 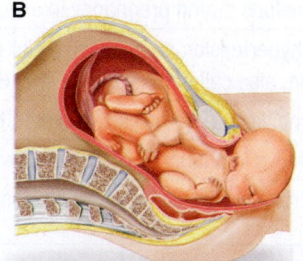 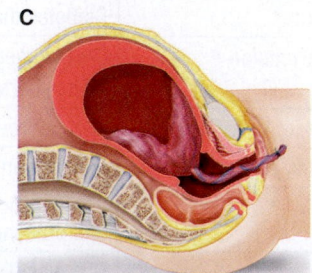

A **DILATION STAGE:** Uterine contractions dilate cervix

B **EXPULSION STAGE:** Birth of baby or expulsion

C **PLACENTAL STAGE:** Delivery of placenta

Figure 22-4 ■ Three stages of labor and delivery.

Table 22-4   ■   **COMMON CONDITIONS OF CHILDBIRTH**

Condition	Definition
Assisted delivery	A delivery of the fetus using mechanical assistance, such as forceps or vacuum extractor; pharmacologic assistance, such as drugs to induce labor; or medical assistance, such as manual rotation of the fetal position
Cephalopelvic disproportion (CPD)	A cause of obstructed labor due to a mismatch between the size of the fetal head and the mother's pelvic brim; also called fetopelvic disproportion
Cesarean delivery	Delivery of the fetus by making a surgical incision into the abdominal wall and uterus; also called *abdominal delivery*
Forceps delivery	Extraction of a fetus from the birth canal by grasping the head with forceps (tongs)
Malposition of fetus	Any presentation of the fetus other than occipitoanterior (OA) (the back of the baby's head is slightly off center in the pelvis with the back of the head toward the mother's left thigh)
Normal spontaneous vaginal birth (NSVB)	Vaginal delivery without mechanical, pharmacologic, or medical assistance
Nuchal cord	The condition of the umbilical cord becoming wrapped around the neck of the fetus
Obstructed labor	Labor in which the fetus cannot progress into the birth canal, despite adequate uterine contractions, due to a physical blockage
Pelvic girdle pain (PGP)	Pain at the back of the pelvis
Placenta previa	A condition in which the placenta partially or fully covers the cervix, posing a risk that it may separate from the wall of the uterus during labor (■ FIGURE 22-5)
Placental infarction	A scarring of the placenta due to inadequate blood supply
Premature rupture of membranes (PROM)	The rupture of the amniotic sac and chorion before the onset of labor. May also be called *prelabor rupture of membranes*
Unstable lie	Repeated changes in the fetal position during or after the 36th week of pregnancy
Vaginal birth	Delivery of the fetus from the uterus through the cervix to the vagina (birth canal)
Vaginal birth after cesarean (VBAC)	Delivery through the vagina after having a cesarean delivery in a previous pregnancy

Table 22-5   ■   **COMMON CONDITIONS OF THE PUERPERIUM**

Condition	Definition
Postpartum depression	Moderate to severe depression after giving birth
Postpartum hemorrhage (PPH)	Excessive bleeding following delivery
Postpartum psychosis	Sudden dramatic onset of psychotic symptoms after giving birth, often occurring in patients with bipolar disorder
Postpartum wound infection	Bacterial infection of a cesarean delivery wound
Puerperal mastitis	Inflammation or infection of the mammary gland in the breast during the postpartum period

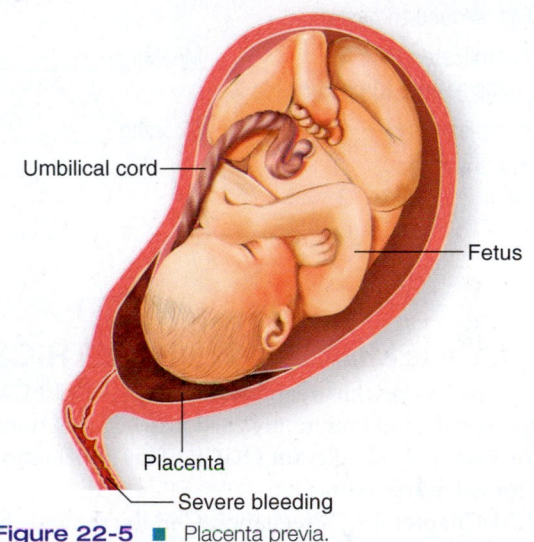

Figure 22-5   ■   Placenta previa.

CODING PRACTICE

Exercise 22.1   Obstetrics Refresher

Instructions: Use your medical terminology skills and resources to define the conditions, then assign the diagnosis code.

Follow these steps:

• Use slash marks "/" to break down the underlined term into its root(s) and suffix.

• Define the meaning of the word, based on the meaning of each word part.

• Assign the default diagnosis code for the condition using the Index and Tabular List.

(continued)

CODING PRACTICE (continued)

Example: Pregnancy, complicated by, endometritis endo/metr/itis   Meaning _inflammation of the lining of the uterus_   ICD-10-CM Code _O86.12_

1. Pregnancy, complicated by, hyperemesis   Meaning _____   ICD-10-CM Code _____

2. Pregnancy, complicated by, antepartum hemorrhage, second trimester   Meaning _____   ICD-10-CM Code _____

3. Pregnancy, complicated by, amnionitis, first trimester   Meaning _____   ICD-10-CM Code _____

4. Pregnancy, complicated by, isoimmunization Rh, second trimester   Meaning _____   ICD-10-CM Code _____

5. Pregnancy, complicated by, oligohydramnios, second trimester   Meaning _____   ICD-10-CM Code _____

6. Pregnancy, complicated by, salpingo-oophoritis, first trimester   Meaning _____   ICD-10-CM Code _____

7. Pregnancy, intraperitoneal   Meaning _____   ICD-10-CM Code _____

8. Pregnancy, supervision of, high risk, older mother, primigravida, second trimester   Meaning _____   ICD-10-CM Code _____

9. Delivery, complicated by, cervical dystocia, third trimester   Meaning _____   ICD-10-CM Code _____

10. Delivery, complicated by, abruptio placentae, third trimester   Meaning _____   ICD-10-CM Code _____

CODING GUIDELINES FOR OBSTETRICS

Coders should understand the organization of this ICD-10-CM chapter, chapter-wide and commonly used instructional notes in the Tabular List, and the relevant OGCR. This information is necessary for accurate coding.

ICD-10-CM Chapter 15, "Pregnancy, Childbirth, and the Puerperium (O00-O9A)," contains nine blocks or subchapters that are divided by the phase of pregnancy and the type of condition. Review the block names and code ranges listed at the beginning of Chapter 15 in the ICD-10-CM manual to become familiar with the content and organization.

This chapter includes pregnancy with abortive outcome, complications of pregnancy, delivery and complications of delivery, and disorders arising during the postpartum period. It does not include reproductive or fertility disorders, which are classified in ICD-10-CM Chapter 14, "Diseases of the Genitourinary System." An instructional note at the beginning of the chapter requires that codes in this chapter are to be used only on the mother's record, never on the newborn's record.

Conditions are classified based on the trimester in which the condition occurs. An instructional note at the beginning of the chapter directs coders to assign an additional code from category **Z3A** to identify the weeks of gestation. Some codes require a seventh character to identify which fetus in a multiple gestation is affected. Examples of how to assign trimester, week, and fetus identifiers are provided later in this chapter.

ICD-10-CM provides Official Guidelines for Coding and Reporting (OGCR) pregnancy, childbirth, and the puerperium in OGCR section I.C.15. OGCR provides detailed discussion of general rules for obstetric cases, selection of OB principal or first-listed diagnosis, supervision of high-risk pregnancies, preexisting conditions, and several specific conditions, including hypertension, diabetes, HIV, alcohol and tobacco use, normal delivery, postpartum, and abortions. OGCR regarding the use of Z codes related to pregnancy, childbirth, and the puerperium appear in OGCR I.C.21.c.11). Specific OGCR and instructional notes are discussed and cited throughout this chapter of the text.

ABSTRACTING DIAGNOSES FOR OBSTETRICS

Because multiple complications are common during pregnancy, childbirth, and the puerperium, coders must be attentive to which complication is the reason for the encounter or admission.

Abstracting Conditions of Pregnancy

It is important to identify all the conditions affecting a pregnant woman, but coders also must identify the main reason for the specific encounter or admission because this will determine the first-listed or principal diagnosis. Refer to ■ TABLE 22-6 for guidance on how to abstract conditions of pregnancy. In particular, coders must be attentive to distinguish between preexisting conditions and pregnancy-related conditions. In particular, become familiar with the criteria for abstracting multiple gestations.

Abstracting Preexisting Conditions and Conditions Due to Pregnancy

Pregnant women can have a medical condition that must be treated in addition to caring for the pregnancy itself. Coders must determine, based on the documentation, if the condition is preexisting (*existed prior to the pregnancy*) or if it developed as a direct result of the pregnancy. Although the symptoms, manifestations, and complications are similar for preexisting and pregnancy-related variations of a disease, different codes are often required (OGCR I.C.15.c.). Two common conditions that fall into this category are diabetes and hypertension.

Preexisting and Gestational Diabetes. Preexisting diabetes should be clearly documented in the medical record and identified as type 1 or type 2. Coders should also identify any additional manifestations of diabetes and whether a type 2 diabetic is on long-term use of insulin or oral hypoglycemic medications. Preexisting diabetes that is treated during pregnancy is *not* gestational diabetes. Gestational diabetes mellitus (GDM)

is first diagnosed during pregnancy, usually during the second or third trimester, and usually resolves after delivery. GDM should be identified as diet-controlled or insulin-controlled. For a refresher on abstracting diabetes, refer to OGCR I.C.4.a and Chapter 10 of this text.

> ### CODING CAUTION
> A patient cannot have *both* preexisting diabetes and gestational diabetes. You need to identify the condition as one or the other. If the documentation is not clear, query the physician.

Preexisting and Gestational Hypertension. Preexisting hypertension should also be clearly documented in the medical record. The type of hypertension and whether the condition involves the heart and/or kidney should also be identified. When a patient with preexisting hypertension develops pre-eclampsia, this combination should be noted. Gestational hypertension is first diagnosed during pregnancy and usually resolves after delivery. Coders must carefully review the documentation for gestational hypertension to determine whether it exists with significant proteinuria, which constitutes pre-eclampsia. Pre-eclampsia should be further identified as mild, moderate, severe, or HELLP syndrome. Finally, coders should note when symptoms of edema and proteinuria are documented without hypertension.

Abstracting Multiple Gestations

Multiple gestation is a complication of pregnancy that places both the mother and the fetuses at higher risk of developing problems. Coders must identify the number of amnions and chorions in all multiple-gestation pregnancies. If the physician has documented that the number of placenta or amniotic sacs cannot be determined, this should also be noted.

Physicians identify each fetus in a multiple gestation by number, such as fetus 1, fetus 2, or fetus 3. There are no rules that determine how to number each fetus; identification is determined by the physician. When a fetus is affected by a prenatal or delivery complication, or the mother is affected by a condition of a fetus, coders must identify which fetus is affected (■ FIGURE 22-6).

Table 22-6   ■   **KEY CRITERIA FOR ABSTRACTING CONDITIONS OF PREGNANCY**

- ❏ Will the patient be under age 16 or age 35 and older at EDD?
- ❏ How many fetuses are there?
- ❏ What trimester is the pregnancy?
- ❏ How many weeks of gestation are completed?
- ❏ How many pregnancies has the patient had, including the current one?
- ❏ How many births has the patient had?
- ❏ What preexisting medical conditions exist?
- ❏ What complications exist?
- ❏ What is the current gestational age?
- ❏ For multiple gestations, how many chorions and amniotic sacs are present?
- ❏ For multiple gestations, which fetus is affected by the complication?
- ❏ What is the main reason for the encounter or the primary complication treated?

Patient is seen in the office in week 36 with mild preeclampsia. She is pregnant with twins, DiDi, and wants to attempt vaginal delivery. Reports sporadic contractions that appear to be false labor. Fetus 2 is currently in breech position. The physician decides to admit her to the hospital for observation.

What is the current gestational age? **36 weeks**
What trimester is the pregnancy? **third**
How many fetuses exist? **two**
How many chorions are present? **two**
How many amnions are present? **two**
What complications exist? **mild preeclampsia**
What other complications exist? **breech presentation**
What fetus is affected? **fetus 2**

Figure 22-6   ■   Example of abstracting for multiple gestation.

Abstracting Conditions of Childbirth

Any delivery that varies from the definition of a normal delivery is complicated and requires that coders identify all the complications that occurred. The definition of a normal delivery is very narrow and specific, so most deliveries do require coding for complications. First, identify the main circumstance or complication of the delivery. Then, identify any additional complications. When a cesarean delivery is performed, identify the main circumstance or complication that establishes the need for the cesarean delivery.

Keep in mind that certain circumstances always qualify as complications, even though they may not seem to be a specific "problem." Circumstantial complications include (■ Figure 22-7):

- Age at EDD under 16 or age 35 and older
- Multiple gestation
- Previous cesarean delivery
- Delivery before 37 or after 40 completed weeks of gestation

Refer to ■ Table 22-7 for guidance in abstracting conditions related to labor, delivery, and childbirth.

Abstracting Conditions of the Puerperium

Some conditions, such as depression or psychosis, may be pre-existing, so coders need to distinguish between conditions that originate in the postpartum period and those that are preexisting. Refer to ■ Table 22-8 for guidance in abstracting conditions related to the puerperium.

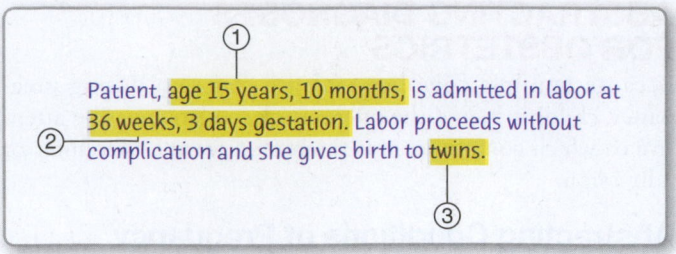

Figure 22-7 ■ Example of a delivery with three complications.

Table 22-7 ■ **KEY CRITERIA FOR ABSTRACTING CONDITIONS OF CHILDBIRTH**

- ❏ What is the reason for the admission?
- ❏ In what week of pregnancy did delivery occur?
- ❏ Is the delivery vaginal or cesarean?
- ❏ What is the reason a cesarean delivery was performed?
- ❏ Has the mother had a previous cesarean delivery?
- ❏ Is there a classical (vertical) or low transverse scar from any previous cesarean delivery?
- ❏ Was there a malposition of the fetus or obstructed labor?
- ❏ What other complications are present?
- ❏ How many fetuses were delivered? Were there any stillbirths?

Abstracting from Obstetric Records

Obstetric records contain unique information and abbreviations not found in other medical records. Refer to ■ Figure 22-8 to learn how to interpret the mini-medical-record used for obstetric cases in this text.

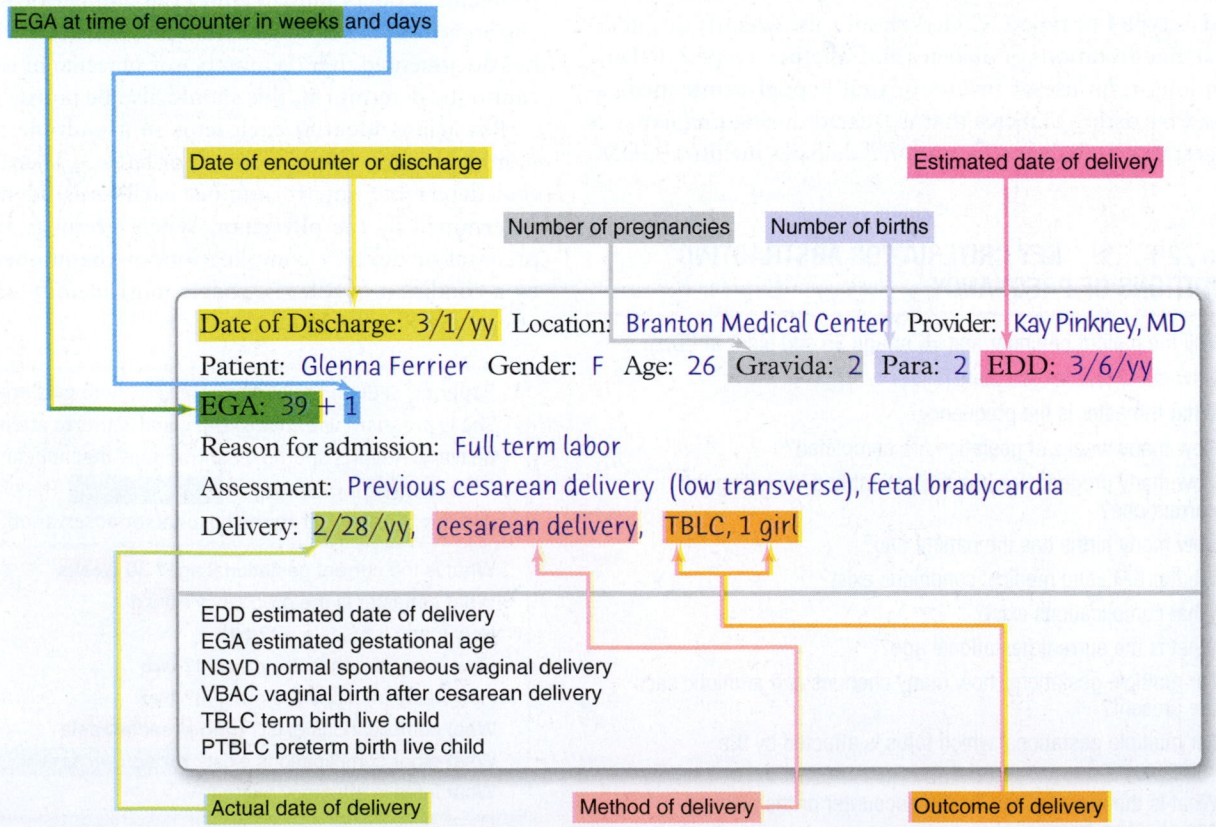

Figure 22-8 ■ Key to interpreting the obstetrics mini-medical-record.

Table 22-8 ■ **KEY CRITERIA FOR ABSTRACTING CONDITIONS OF THE PUERPERIUM**

❑ Is the encounter less than six weeks after delivery?

❑ What complication or condition is treated during the encounter?

❑ Is the condition preexisting or does it originate during the postpartum/puerperal period?

Guided Example of Abstracting Diagnoses for Obstetrics

Refer to the following example throughout this chapter to practice skills for abstracting, assigning, and sequencing pregnancy, childbirth, and the puerperium codes. Daphne Wittman, CCS-P, is a fictitious coder who guides you through the coding process.

Date of discharge: 3/1/yy   Location: Branton Medical Center   Provider: Kay Pinkney, MD

Patient: Glenna Ferrier   Gender: F   Age: 26

Gravida: 2   Para: 2   EDD: 3/6/yy

EGA: 39+1

Reason for admission: Full term labor

Assessment: Attempted vaginal delivery. Labor started off well then slowed. I was concerned that prolonged labor would place the scar from the previous cesarean delivery at risk. In addition, the stress affected the fetal heart rate causing tachycardia so I proceeded with a cesarean delivery.

Delivery: 2/28/yy, cesarean delivery, TBLC, 1 girl, transferred to NICU for monitoring and management of heart rate

Follow along as Daphne Wittman, CCS-P, abstracts the diagnosis. Check off each step after you complete it.

▶ Daphne reads through the entire record, paying special attention to the reason for the admission and the final delivery data. She refers to Key Criteria for Abstracting Conditions of Childbirth (Table 22-7).

❑ *What is the reason for the admission?* Full-term labor

❑ *In what week of pregnancy did delivery occur?* 39+1

❑ *Is the delivery vaginal or cesarean?* Cesarean

❑ *What is the reason a cesarean delivery was performed?* Previous cesarean delivery

❑ *Has the mother had a previous cesarean delivery?* Yes

❑ *Is there a classical (vertical) or low transverse scar from any previous cesarean delivery?* Low transverse

❑ *How many fetuses were delivered?* One female

❑ *Were there any stillbirths?* No, TBLC

❑ *What other complications are present?* Fetal tachycardia

▶ At this time, Daphne does not know how many codes she will end up with. She will learn about this when she moves on to assigning codes.

CODING PRACTICE

Exercise 22.2 Abstracting Diagnoses for Obstetrics

Instructions: Read the mini-medical-record of each patient's encounter and answer the abstracting questions. Write the answer on the line provided. Do not assign any codes.

1. OFFICE   Gender: F   Age: 33

Gravida: 3   Para: 2   EDD: 6/30/yy

EGA: 26+2

Reason for encounter: Vaginal bleeding

Assessment: Placenta previa, hemorrhage

Plan: Bed confinement, RTO 2 weeks, cesarean delivery may be required

(continued)

1. (continued)

a. Will the patient be under age 16 or age 35 and older at EDD? _____

b. What trimester is the pregnancy? _____

How many weeks of gestation are completed?

_____

c. How many pregnancies has the patient had, including the current one? _____

_____

d. How many births has the patient had? _____

_____

e. What preexisting medical conditions exist?

_____

f. What complications exist? _____

_____

(continued)

2. OFFICE Gender: **F** Age: **24**

Gravida: **1** Para: **0** EDD: **3/23/yy**

EGA: **40+2**

Reason for encounter: **Prenatal visit**

Assessment: **Unstable lie**

Plan: **Cesarean delivery today at 1500**

a. Will the patient be under age 16 or age 35 and older at EDD? _____

b. What trimester is the pregnancy? _____

   How many weeks of gestation are completed? _____

c. How many pregnancies has the patient had, including the current one? _____

d. How many births has the patient had? _____

e. What preexisting medical conditions exist? _____

f. What is the current gestational age? _____

g. What complications exist? _____

h. Did the patient deliver at this encounter? _____

i. What is the main reason for the encounter or the primary complication treated? _____

3. OFFICE Gender: **F** Age: **35**

Gravida: **1** Para: **0** EDD: **10/19/yy**

EGA: **10+4**

Reason for encounter: **Establish prenatal care**

Assessment: **Discussed the risks of pregnancy at this age, need for BP and DM monitoring, no problems at this time**

Plan: **Schedule amniocentesis and chorionic villi sampling (CVS)**

a. Will the patient be under age 16 or age 35 and older at EDD? _____

b. What trimester is the pregnancy? _____

   How many weeks of gestation are completed? _____

_____

(continued)

3. (continued)

c. How many pregnancies has the patient had, including the current one? _____

d. How many births has the patient had? _____

_____

e. What preexisting medical conditions exist? _____

f. What is the current gestational age? _____

g. What complications exist? _____

h. What is the main reason for the encounter or the primary complication treated? _____

4. OFFICE Gender: **F** Age: **26**

Gravida: **3** Para: **2** EDD: **7/6/yy** EGA: **24+6**

Reason for encounter: **Prenatal visit, FU on gestational DM diagnosed at last visit**

Assessment: **GTT shows that the diabetes is being adequately controlled through diet**

Plan: **Continue with nutritional plan and good eating habits**

a. Will the patient be under age 16 or age 35 and older at EDD? _____

b. What trimester is the pregnancy? _____

   How many weeks of gestation are completed? _____

_____

c. How many pregnancies has the patient had, including the current one? _____

d. How many births has the patient had? _____

e. What preexisting medical conditions exist? _____

f. What is the current gestational age? _____

g. What complications exist? _____

h. What is the main reason for the encounter or the primary complication treated? _____

CODING PRACTICE *(continued)*

5. OFFICE Gender: F Age: 25

Gravida: 2 Para: 1 EDD: 6/15/yy

EGA: 28+3

Reason for encounter: Routine prenatal visit

Assessment: Rhesus incompatibility

Plan: Rho(D) immune globulin treatment on Monday

a. Will the patient be under age 16 or age 35 and older at EDD? _____

b. What trimester is the pregnancy? _____

   How many weeks of gestation are completed? _____
   _____

c. How many pregnancies has the patient had, including the current one? _____
   _____

d. How many births has the patient had? _____
   _____

e. What preexisting medical conditions exist? _____
   _____

f. What is the current gestational age? _____
   _____

g. What complications exist? _____
   _____

h. What is the main reason for the encounter or the primary complication treated? _____
   _____

6. INPATIENT HOSPITAL Gender: F Age: 18

Gravida: 1 Para: 0 EDD: 4/6/yy EGA: 37+5

Reason for admission: Full term labor

Assessment: Placental infarction

Delivery: 3/22/yy, NSVD, stillborn, 1 girl

a. What is the reason for the admission? _____
   _____

b. In what week of pregnancy did delivery occur?
   _____

c. Is the delivery vaginal or cesarean? _____
   _____

d. Has the mother had a previous cesarean delivery?
   _____

e. Was there a malposition of the fetus or obstructed labor? _____

f. What other complications are present? _____
   _____

6. (continued)

g. How many fetuses were delivered? _____

   Were there any stillbirths? _____
   _____

7. OFFICE Gender: F Age: 30

Gravida: 2 Para: 1 EDD: 10/5/yy

EGA: 12+0

Reason for encounter: Prenatal care, pernicious anemia

Assessment: Blood work has improved, but still not where it should be

Plan: B12 injection

a. Will the patient be under age 16 or age 35 and older at EDD? _____

b. What trimester is the pregnancy? _____

   How many weeks of gestation are completed? _____
   _____

c. How many pregnancies has the patient had, including the current one? _____
   _____

d. How many births has the patient had? _____
   _____

e. What preexisting medical conditions exist? _____
   _____

f. What is the current gestational age? _____
   _____

g. What complications exist? _____
   _____

h. What is the main reason for the encounter or the primary complication treated? _____
   _____

8. INPATIENT HOSPITAL Gender: F Age: 32

Gravida: 2 Para: 2 EDD: 5/18/yy

EGA: 32+2

Reason for admission: Premature rupture of membranes

Assessment: Severe preeclampsia requires cesarean delivery

Delivery: 3/22/yy, classical cesarean, PTBLC, 1 girl

a. What is the reason for the admission? _____
   _____

(continued)

CODING PRACTICE (continued)

8. (continued)

b. In what week of pregnancy did delivery occur? _____
_____

c. Is the delivery vaginal or cesarean? _____
_____

d. What is the reason a cesarean delivery was performed?
_____

e. Was there a malposition of the fetus or obstructed
labor? _____
_____

f. What other complications are present? _____
_____

g. How many fetuses were delivered? _____
_____

Were there any stillbirths? _____
_____

---

9. OFFICE   Gender: F   Age: 15

Birthday: 7/15   Gravida: 1   Para: 0

EDD: 6/1/yy   EGA: 30+4

Reason for encounter: Prenatal care, twins, MoDi

Assessment: Dipstick shows new isolated gestational
proteinuria

Plan: At risk for pre-eclampsia, RTO 4 days for repeat
test.

a. Will the patient be under age 16 or age 35 and older
at EDD? _____

b. What trimester is the pregnancy? _____
How many weeks of gestation are completed? _____
_____

c. How many pregnancies has the patient had, including
the current one? _____
_____

d. How many births has the patient had? _____
_____

(*continued*)

---

9. (continued)

e. What preexisting medical conditions exist? _____
_____

f. What is the current gestational age? _____
_____

For multiple gestations, how many chorions are present?

How many amniotic sacs are present? _____
_____

g. What complications exist? _____
_____

---

10. INPATIENT HOSPITAL   Gender: F   Age: 22

Gravida: 2   Para: 2   EDD: 3/16/yy

EGA: 41+3

Reason for admission: Post term labor

Assessment: Obstructed labor due to CPD, severe
obesity, mother, BMI 41

Delivery: 3/23/yy, cesarean delivery, TBLC, 1 boy

a. What is the reason for the admission? _____
_____

b. In what week of pregnancy did delivery occur? _____
_____

c. Is the delivery vaginal or cesarean? _____
_____

d. Was there a malposition of the fetus or obstructed
labor? _____

e. What other complications are present? _____
_____

f. What is the reason a cesarean delivery was performed?
_____

g. How many fetuses were delivered? _____
Were there any stillbirths? _____

ASSIGNING DIAGNOSIS CODES FOR OBSTETRICS

Coders should acquaint themselves with the organization of obstetrical terms in the Index and must be attentive to distinguish between codes that apply to the mother and those that apply to the infant. In addition, become familiar with how to assign codes to identify the term, the pregnancy, the trimester, and the fetus. Different rules also apply for assigning codes to prenatal visits for normal and high-risk pregnancies.

Locating Obstetrical Main Terms in the Index

The Index groups codes for pregnancy under the Main Term **Pregnancy**. The first-level subterm **complicated by** occupies most of the entry and provides second- and third-level subterms for conditions that complicate pregnancy, such as **abscess** or **placenta previa**. Other first-level subterms describe the type of pregnancy, such as **normal**, **ectopic**, or **multiple gestation**.

The Index groups codes for labor and delivery under the Main Term **Delivery**. The first-level subterms **cesarean for** and **complicated by** occupy most of the entry and provide second- and third-level subterms for conditions that complicate labor and delivery, such as **cord, around neck, with compression** or **obstruction**. A limited number of other first-level subterms describe the type of delivery, such as **normal** or **forceps**.

As with any condition, most obstetrical conditions have multiple coding paths. For example, some complications of labor and delivery are also located under the Main Term **Pregnancy, complicated by**. Some conditions are also indexed under the Main Term for the name of the condition, with a subterm for pregnancy, such as **Diabetes, gestational** or **Rh, incompatibility**.

SUCCESS STEP

Take a few minutes to review the Index entries for **Pregnancy** and **Delivery** in your ICD-10-CM manual. Highlight the beginning and end of the subterm **complicated by**.

Assigning Codes for the Mother's Condition

When both the mother and the newborn are affected by the same condition, assign separate codes for each. Codes in ICD-10-CM Chapter 15 are used *only* on the mother's bill (OGCR I.C.15.a.2)). This is easy to remember because the mother's codes begin with the letter **O**.

When delivery occurs and the newborn receives medical care or occupies a bed, the baby has a separate medical record, separate bills, and separate codes. Codes for the infant begin with **P** and are assigned from ICD-10-CM Chapter 16, "Certain Conditions Originating in the Perinatal Period (P00–P96)." Coding for the infant is discussed in Chapter 23 of this text.

Careful use of the Index is required in order to identify the Main Term and subterms that distinguish between the mother and the infant. A Main Term for the condition will have separate subterms for the mother and the infant. Select the subterm that corresponds to the record being coded. For example, when a mother is treated for Rh incompatibility, the code will be different than the one used when the infant is treated for the same condition (■ FIGURE 22-9).

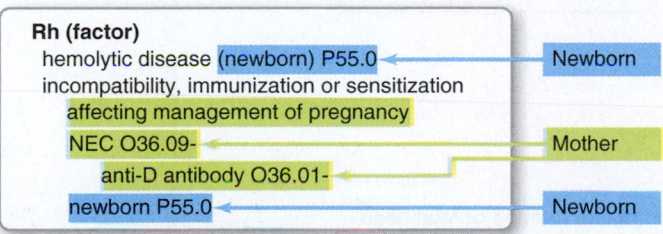

Rh (factor)
 hemolytic disease (newborn) P55.0 ← Newborn
 incompatibility, immunization or sensitization
  affecting management of pregnancy
  NEC O36.09- ← Mother
   anti-D antibody O36.01- ← Mother
  newborn P55.0 ← Newborn

Figure 22-9 ■ Index Entry for "Rh (factor)" showing separate codes for mother and newborn.

Table 22-9 ■ DEFINITION OF PREGNANCY TERMS, WITH CODES

Term	Weeks of Gestation	Code
Preterm pregnancy, delivery, or labor	Less than 37 completed weeks of gestation	O60.0-, O60.1-, O60.2-
Full-term pregnancy	37 completed weeks to less than 40 completed weeks of gestation	No code
Postterm pregnancy	40 completed weeks to 42 completed weeks of gestation	O48.0
Prolonged pregnancy	More than 42 completed weeks of gestation	O48.1

CODING CAUTION

Codes beginning with **P** should *never* be assigned to the mother (OGCR I.C.16.a.1)).

Assigning Codes to Identify the Term of Pregnancy

Preterm labor and delivery, as well as postterm pregnancy, constitute complications and require a code. Term lengths are defined by the gestational age at the time of the encounter (■ TABLE 22-9). Codes are indexed under the Main Term **Pregnancy**, the subterm **complicated by**, and a second-level subterm for **preterm** or **postmaturity**. Alternatively, search for the Main Term **Preterm**, **Postterm**, or **Prolonged**, then locate the appropriate subterm for **pregnancy, labor, or delivery**.

SUCCESS STEP

Be careful to distinguish between the letter **O** (oh) that begins each code, and the number **0** (zero) that occupies other positions. When making handwritten notes, use a cursive O (with a loop at the top) for the letter and write the number zero with a slash through it: **Ø**. By clearly distinguishing handwritten notes, you make it easier to key them in correctly. On the keyboard, use the alphabetic keys for the letter and the numeric keypad or the top row of numbers for zero. If you mix up these two similar characters, the computer in your workplace may not accept your code or, worse, the insurance company may reject your claim as unprocessable (*incapable of being processed*) due to an invalid code.

Assigning Codes to Identify the Trimester and Weeks

Many obstetrics codes require coders to identify the trimester and weeks of gestation. The time frame for each trimester is defined in an instructional note at the beginning of the chapter. Trimesters are identified by the fourth, fifth, or sixth character, depending on the length of the code. The symbol **4th**, **5th**, **6th** or in front of the subcategory entry in the Tabular List indicates that an additional character is needed. The codes for each trimester are listed immediately below the subcategory heading (■ FIGURE 22-10, page 394). Conditions that only occur

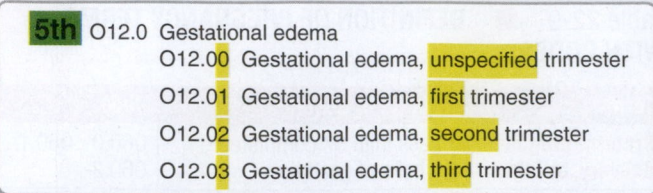

5th O12.0 Gestational edema
O12.00 Gestational edema, unspecified trimester
O12.01 Gestational edema, first trimester
O12.02 Gestational edema, second trimester
O12.03 Gestational edema, third trimester

Figure 22-10 ■ Tabular List entry for "Gestational edema" requiring a trimester designation.

in one trimester, or to which the concept of trimesters does not apply, do not have a character to identify the trimester (OGCR 15.a3), 4), and 5)). For example, codes for ectopic (*located away from the normal site*) pregnancy do not require a trimester designation. **Z3A** codes should not be assigned for pregnancies with abortive outcomes (categories **O00-O08**), elective termination of pregnancy (code **Z33.32**), or for postpartum conditions, as category **Z3A** is not applicable to these conditions (OGCR I.C.21.c.11)).

Assign a code from category **Z3A Weeks of gestation** to identify the number of weeks of gestation completed in the pregnancy. Count only the *completed* weeks of pregnancy. Do not count partial weeks. Locate the code in the Index under the Main Term **Pregnancy** and subterm **weeks**. Category **Z3A** appears after category **Z36** in the Tabular List.

Assigning Codes to Identify the Fetus

Assign a seventh character to identify the fetus involved (OGCR 15.a.6)) when maternal conditions affect the fetus or fetal conditions create maternal complications. Identification of the fetus is based on physician documentation. The applicable codes are designated in the Tabular List by the symbol **7th** or similar designation by most publishers. Seventh-character options are listed in a box at the category or subcategory level

(■ Figure 22-11 and ■ Figure 22-12). Assign the seventh character of **0** in the following situations:

- For singletons
- When it is not possible for the physician to determine which fetus is affected
- When documentation does not identify the affected fetus and the coder cannot obtain clarification from the physician

SUCCESS STEP

Common sense may suggest that when there is only one fetus, you would assign the seventh character of **1**. However, the instructional note directs you to assign the seventh character **0** for a singleton. The character **1** identifies *fetus number one* in a multiple-gestation pregnancy.

Assigning Codes for Prenatal Visits

ICD-10-CM provides codes for routine outpatient prenatal visits, which are classified as **Supervision of pregnancy**. Different rules apply for a normal pregnancy than for high-risk patients.

For routine outpatient visits with no complications present, assign a code from category **Z34 Encounter for supervision of normal pregnancy** as the only diagnosis code. Codes are divided based on whether it is the first pregnancy and also by trimester. If any complication from ICD-10-CM Chapter 15 (O00-O99) exists, the pregnancy is not classified as normal and coders should not assign a code from **Z34**. Locate the code in the Index by searching for the Main Term **Pregnancy**, the subterm **supervision of**, then the second-level subterm **normal**. Select the third-level subterm that identifies the pregnancy as the **first** or **specified NEC** (meaning "not the first"). Verify the code in the Tabular List in order to assign the correct character for the trimester.

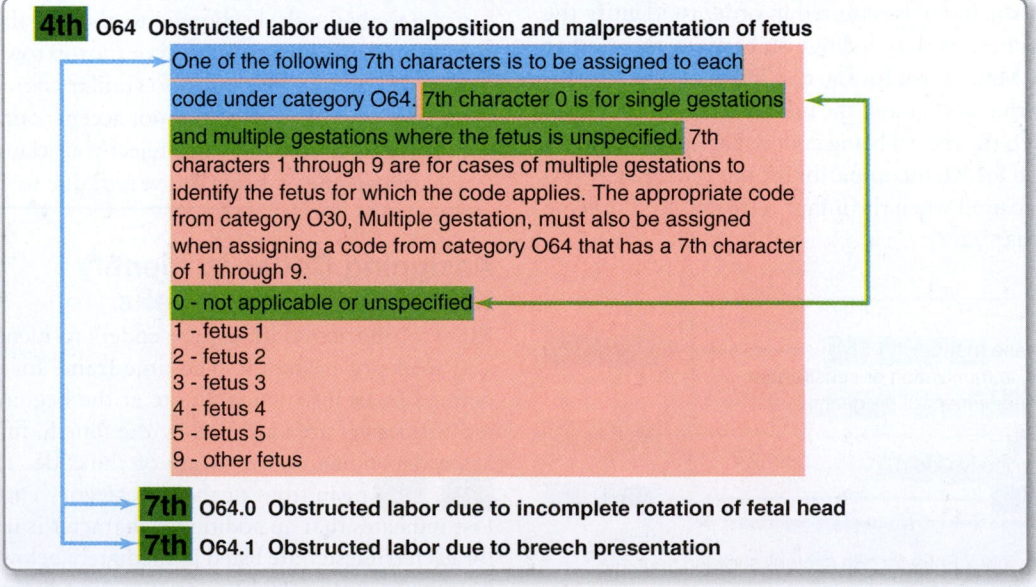

4th O64 Obstructed labor due to malposition and malpresentation of fetus

One of the following 7th characters is to be assigned to each code under category O64. 7th character 0 is for single gestations and multiple gestations where the fetus is unspecified. 7th characters 1 through 9 are for cases of multiple gestations to identify the fetus for which the code applies. The appropriate code from category O30, Multiple gestation, must also be assigned when assigning a code from category O64 that has a 7th character of 1 through 9.

0 - not applicable or unspecified
1 - fetus 1
2 - fetus 2
3 - fetus 3
4 - fetus 4
5 - fetus 5
9 - other fetus

7th O64.0 Obstructed labor due to incomplete rotation of fetal head

7th O64.1 Obstructed labor due to breech presentation

Figure 22-11 ■ Tabular List entry for seventh character identification of fetus.

Fetus 2 presents in the breech position. Physician performs a cesarean delivery due to obstructed labor.

O64.1XX2   Obstructed labor due to breech presentation
(Note: This example only illustrates how to identify the fetus with the seventh character and does not represent complete coding for the case.)

Figure 22-12 ■ Example of assigning a seventh character to identify the fetus.

For all other routine outpatient visits, assign a code from category **O09 Supervision of high-risk pregnancy** as the first-listed code. Assign additional codes from

ICD-10-CM Chapter 15, or other chapters as needed, to describe any complications. Women who are very young—under age 16 at EDD—or older—age 35 and older at EDD—are classified as high-risk pregnancies and should be assigned a corresponding code from category **O09**. Locate the code in the Index by searching for the Main Term **Pregnancy**, the subterm **supervision of**, then the second-level subterm **high risk**. Select the third-level subterm that describes the reason the pregnancy is high risk. Verify the code in the Tabular List in order to assign the correct character for the trimester (■ FIGURE 22-13). Assign codes from **O09 Supervision of high-risk pregnancy** only during the prenatal period. For complications during delivery that result from a high-risk pregnancy, assign codes that identify the complication(s) (OGCR I.C.15.b.4)).

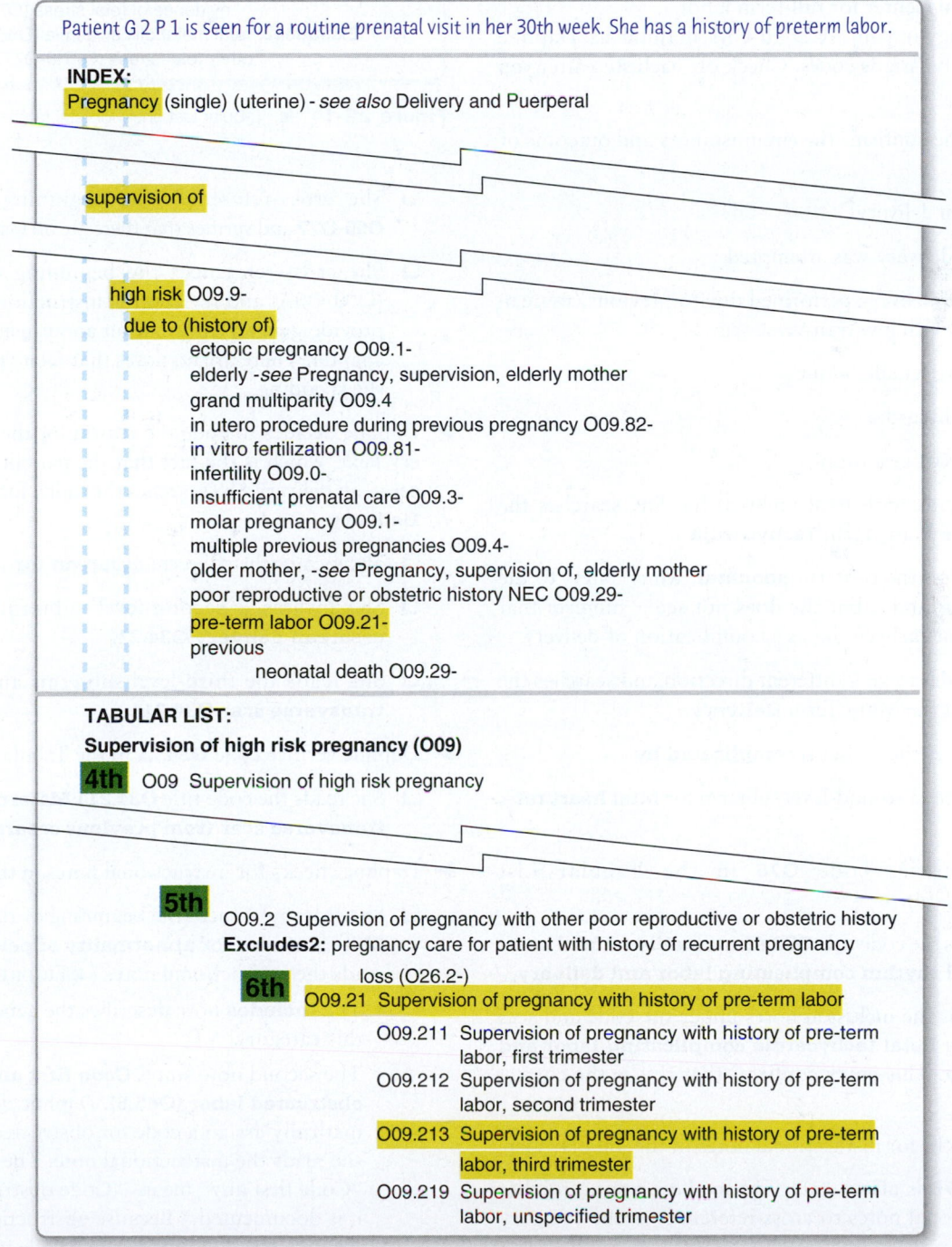

Figure 22-13 ■ Example of selecting the first-listed diagnosis for supervision of a high-risk pregnancy.

SUCCESS STEP

Assign a code from category **Z32** for an encounter for pregnancy testing, childbirth instruction, and childcare instruction. Search under the Main Term **Encounter** and the subterms **pregnancy**, then **test**, then **result** or the subterm **instruction**.

Guided Example of Assigning Obstetrics Diagnosis Codes

To practice skills for assigning codes for pregnancy, childbirth, and the puerperium, continue with the example from earlier in the chapter about patient Glenna Ferrier, who was admitted to Branton Medical Center for full-term labor.

Follow along in your ICD-10-CM manual as Daphne Wittman, CCS-P, assigns codes. Check off each step after you complete it.

▶ First, Daphne confirms the circumstances and outcome of delivery:

❏ Full-term delivery

❏ Vaginal delivery was attempted

❏ Cesarean delivery performed due to previous cesarean delivery, with low transverse scar

❏ Single live female infant

❏ Fetal tachycardia

❏ 39 weeks of gestation

▶ Daphne begins with fetal tachycardia. She searches the Index for the Main Term **Tachycardia**.

❏ She locates the subterm **neonatal**, which refers to the newborn infant, but she does not see a subterm that relates the tachycardia as a complication of delivery.

❏ She decides to go a different direction and searches the Index for the Main Term **Delivery**.

❏ She locates the subterm **complicated by**.

❏ She locates a second-level subterm for **fetal heart rate, O76**.

▶ Daphne verifies code **O76** in the Tabular List (■ FIGURE 22-14).

❏ She reads the code title **O76 Abnormality in fetal heart rate and rhythm complicating labor and delivery**.

❏ She reads the inclusion notes under the code and sees the entry **Fetal tachycardia complicating labor and delivery**. This entry confirms that this is the correct code.

▶ Daphne checks for instructional notes in the Tabular List.

❏ Code **O76** is also a category, so there are no further instructional notes to cross-references at the category level.

O76 Abnormality in fetal heart rate and rhythm complicating labor and delivery
   Depressed fetal heart rate tones complicating labor and delivery
   Fetal bradycardia complicating labor and delivery
   Fetal heart rate decelerations complicating labor and delivery
   Fetal heart rate irregularity complicating labor and delivery
   Fetal heart rate abnormal variability complicating labor and delivery
   Fetal tachycardia complicating labor and delivery
   Non-reassuring fetal heart rate or rhythm complicating labor and delivery
   Excludes1: fetal stress NOS (O77.9)
                 labor and delivery complicated by electrocardiographic evidence of fetal stress (O77.8)
                 labor and delivery complicated by ultrasonic evidence of fetal stress (O77.8)
   Excludes2: fetal metabolic acidemia (O68)
                 other fetal stress (O77.0-O77.1)

Figure 22-14 ■ Tabular List entry for fetal tachycardia.

❏ She cross-references the beginning of the block **O60-O77** and verifies that there are no instructional notes.

❏ She cross-references the beginning of Chapter 15 (O00-O9A) and reviews the instructional notes, which provide general information about using codes in this chapter. There are no notes that relate to the condition she is coding.

▶ Daphne decides to code the reason for the cesarean delivery next, which is the fact that the patient had a previous cesarean delivery. She searches the Index for the Main Term **Delivery**.

❏ She locates the subterm **cesarean for**.

❏ She locates a second-level subterm for **previous cesarean delivery O34.21**.

❏ She reads the third-level subterms and chooses **low transverse scar O34.211**.

▶ Daphne verifies code **O34.21** in the Tabular List.

❏ She reads the code title **O34.211 Maternal care for low transverse scar from previous cesarean delivery**.

▶ Daphne checks for instructional notes in the Tabular List.

❏ She cross-references the beginning of the category **O34 Maternal care for abnormality of pelvic organs** and reads the instructional notes (■ FIGURE 22-15).

▪ The **Includes** note describes the general purpose of this category.

▪ The second note states **Code first any associated obstructed labor (O65.5)**. Daphne does not automatically assign a code for obstructed labor when she reads the instructional note. The expression "Code first any" means "Code obstructed labor, if it is documented." Because obstruction is not documented, she does not assign a code for it.

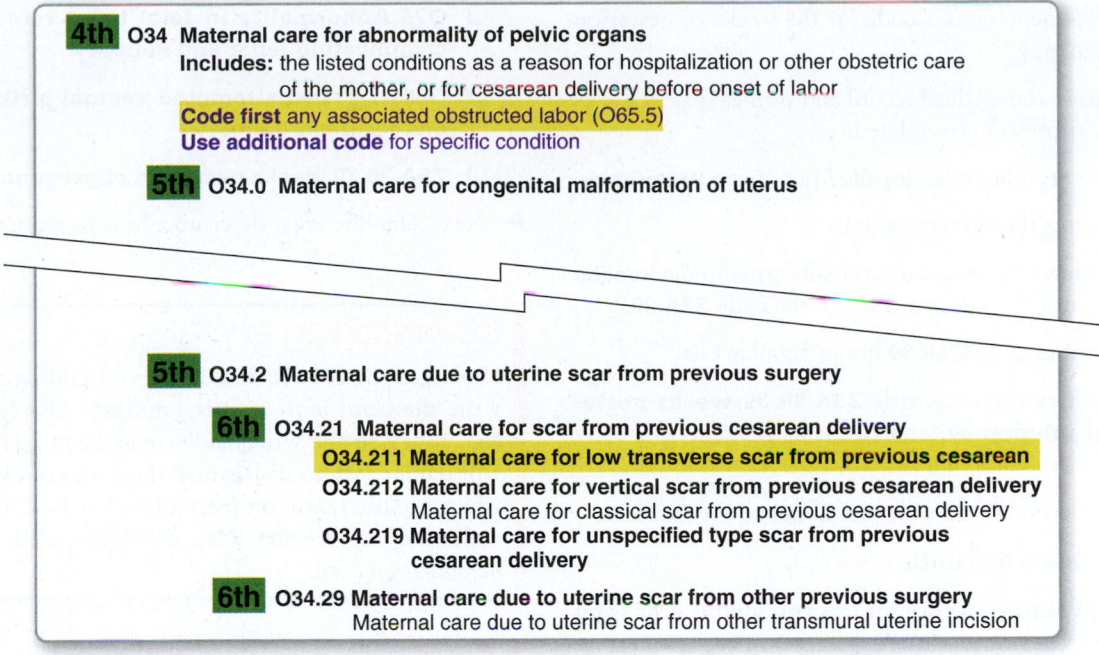

Figure 22-15 ■ Tabular List entry showing instructional notes for category O34 "Maternal care for abnormality of pelvic organs."

- She double-checks the medical record and confirms that obstructed labor is not documented; therefore, this note does not apply.
- The third note states **Use additional code for specific condition**.
- The specific condition is fetal tachycardia, which she has already coded. This note will also provide direction when it is time to sequence the codes.

❑ She cross-references the beginning of the block **O30-O48** and verifies that there are no instructional notes.

❑ She is already familiar with the instructional notes at the beginning of Chapter 15 (O00-O9A) and remembers that there are no notes that relate to the condition she is coding.

▶ Daphne recalls that for every encounter in which a birth occurs, OGCR require coders to assign a **Z** code for outcome of the delivery (OGCR I.C.15.b.5)).

❑ She searches the Index for the Main Term **Outcome of delivery**.

❑ She locates the subterm **single**.

❑ She reviews the second-level subterms under **single** and locates **liveborn Z37.0**.

▶ Daphne verifies the code **Z37.0** in the Tabular List.

❑ She verifies the code title **Z37.0 Single live birth** and confirms that this correctly describes the outcome.

❑ She cross-references the **NOTE:** under the category heading **Z37**, which states **This category is intended for use as an additional code to identify the outcome of delivery on the mother's record. It is not for use on the newborn record.**

❑ This note confirms that she has the correct code for the mother's record.

❑ Daphne quickly checks the beginning of the category **Z30-Z39** for instructional notes and finds none.

❑ She also checks the beginning of Chapter 21 (Z00-Z99) and reviews the instructional notes.

▶ Daphne reviews the medical record to be certain she has captured all the elements that need to be coded for this patient.

❑ She reads that a vaginal delivery was attempted first and this complicated the delivery. She determines that she needs to assign a code for a failed attempt at vaginal delivery after a previous cesarean delivery.

▶ Daphne searches the Index for the Main Term **Delivery** and the subterm **complicated by**.

❑ She locates a second-level subterm **failed**.

❑ She locates a third-level subterm **attempted vaginal birth after previous cesarean delivery O66.41**.

▶ Daphne verifies code **O66.41** in the Tabular List.

❑ She reads the code title **O66.41 Failed attempted vaginal birth after previous cesarean delivery** and confirms that this describes the case.

❑ She reads the instructional note under the code that states **Code first rupture of uterus, if applicable (O71.0-, O71.1).** She determines that the note does not apply because a uterine rupture is not documented.

❑ She has already cross-referenced the beginning of block **O60-O77** and Chapter 15 (O00-O9A) for instructional notes and remembers that there are no instructions that apply to this case.

▶ Finally, Daphne assigns a code for the weeks of gestation of the pregnancy.

❏ She checks the medical record and verifies that 39 weeks of gestation were completed.

❏ She searches the Index for the Main Term **Pregnancy**.

❏ She locates the subterm **weeks**.

❏ She reviews the second-level subterms under **weeks** and locates the subterm **39** with the code **Z3A.39**.

▶ Daphne verifies code **Z3A.39** in the Tabular List.

❏ She verifies the code title **Z3A.39 39 weeks gestation of pregnancy**, and confirms that this correctly describes the outcome.

▶ Daphne reviews the codes she has assigned for this case.

❏ **Z37.0 Single live birth**

❏ **O34.211 Maternal care for low transverse scar from previous cesarean delivery**

❏ **O76 Abnormality in fetal heart rate and rhythm complicating labor and delivery**

❏ **O66.41 Failed attempted vaginal birth after previous cesarean delivery**

❏ **Z3A.39 39 weeks gestation of pregnancy**

▶ Next, Daphne must determine how to sequence the codes.

SUCCESS STEP

Highlight the **NOTE:** at **Z37** in your coding manual and write the word *mother* in the margin. Also highlight the **NOTE:** at **Z38** and write *newborn* in the margin. These tips will remind you to distinguish the codes in category **Z37**, which are used only on the *mother's* record, from similar code titles in category **Z38**, which are used only on the *newborn's* record.

CODING PRACTICE

Exercise 22.3 Assigning Diagnosis Codes for Obstetrics

Instructions: Read the mini-medical-record of each patient's encounter, review the information abstracted in Exercise 22.2, and assign ICD-10-CM diagnosis codes using the Index and Tabular List. All exercises require a code to be from category Z3A to identify the weeks of gestation. Write the code(s) on the line provided.

1. OFFICE   Gender: F   Age: 33

Gravida: 3   Para: 2   EDD: 6/30/yy

EGA: 26+2

Reason for encounter: Vaginal bleeding

Assessment: Placenta previa, hemorrhage

Plan: Bed confinement, RTO 2 weeks, cesarean delivery may be required

2 ICD-10-CM Codes _____

2. OFFICE   Gender: F   Age: 24

Gravida: 1   Para: 0   EDD: 3/23/yy

EGA: 40+2

Reason for encounter: Prenatal visit

Assessment: Unstable lie

Plan: Cesarean delivery today at 1500

3 ICD-10-CM Codes _____

_____

3. OFFICE   Gender: F   Age: 35

Gravida: 1   Para: 0   EDD: 10/19/yy

EGA: 10+4

Reason for encounter: Establish prenatal care

Assessment: Discussed the risks of pregnancy at this age, need for BP and DM monitoring, no problems at this time

Plan: Schedule amniocentesis and chorionic villi sampling (CVS)

Tip: Primigravida means first pregnancy.

2 ICD-10-CM Codes _____

4. OFFICE   Gender: F   Age: 26

Gravida: 3   Para: 2   EDD: 7/6/yy   EGA: 24+6

Reason for encounter: FU on gestational DM diagnosed at last visit

Assessment: GTT shows that the diabetes is being adequately controlled through diet

Plan: Continue with nutritional plan and good eating habits

2 ICD-10-CM Codes _____

CODING PRACTICE *(continued)*

5. OFFICE   Gender: F   Age: 25

Gravida: 2   Para: 1 EDD: 6/15/yy

EGA: 28+3

Reason for encounter: Routine prenatal visit

Assessment: Rhesus incompatibility

Plan: Rho(D) immune globulin treatment on Monday

(continued)

5. *(continued)*

Tip: Select the code for the condition as it affects the mother, not the infant. Refer to OGCR I.C.15.b.2) for sequencing information.

3 ICD-10-CM Codes _____

_____

ARRANGING DIAGNOSIS CODES FOR OBSTETRICS

Coders must be attentive to selecting the principal diagnosis when a delivery occurs and to sequencing codes from Chapter 15 with codes from body system chapters. As in all coding, the principal or first-listed diagnosis is determined by the reason for the admission or encounter, OGCR, and instructional notes in the Tabular List. ■ TABLE 22-10 summarizes key coding and sequencing rules for obstetrics.

Arranging Codes for When a Delivery Occurs

When a delivery occurs, a minimum of two codes are required—one for the delivery diagnosis and one for the outcome of delivery (■ Table 22-10). The principal diagnosis should be the condition that prompted the admission. If multiple conditions prompted the admission, sequence the one most related to delivery as the principal diagnosis. Refer to OGCR I.C.15.b.4) for detailed guidance on selecting the principal diagnosis from the following:

- The code for normal delivery, **O80** (■ TABLE 22-11)
- The main complication of labor and delivery, if that was the reason for admission
- The main reason a cesarean delivery was required, if that was the reason for admission
- The reason for admission if unrelated to any of the above

Search the Main Term **Delivery** and subterm **complicated by** to locate the codes for complications.

The additional code is a code from category **Z37.-**, which describes the outcome of delivery in terms of the number of live infants and/or the number of stillbirths (OGCR I.C.15.b.5)). Search for the Main Term **Outcome of Delivery** for the **Z37.-** code (■ FIGURE 22-16, page 400).

SUCCESS STEP

Assign a code from **Z37.-** only during the admission in which delivery occurs. Do not assign it for subsequent admissions, even if they are for complications of delivery or for postpartum office visits. **Z37.-** is *never* the principal or first-listed code.

Table 22-10 ■ **SUMMARY OF CODE SEQUENCING FOR OBSTETRICS**

Type of Encounter	Index Main Term and Subterms
Routine prenatal visit	1. Pregnancy, supervision 2. Pregnancy, weeks of gestation (Z3A.-)
Complications of pregnancy	1. Pregnancy, complicated by
Normal delivery	1. Delivery, normal (O80) 2. Outcome of delivery, single live birth (Z37.0)
Delivery with complications	1. Delivery, complicated by 2. Outcome of delivery (Z37.-)
Cesarean delivery	1. Delivery, cesarean 2. Outcome of delivery (Z37.-)
Birth encounter for the newborn	1. Newborn + appropriate subterm: born in hospital/born outside of hospital/twin/triplet/quadruplet/multiple born (Z38.-) 2. Newborn, affected by

Table 22-11 ■ **DEFINITION OF A NORMAL DELIVERY, ICD-10-CM CODE O80**

Includes	Excludes
Minimal or no assistance	Fetal manipulation
Episiotomy	Rotation version
Spontaneous	Instrumentation/forceps
Cephalic presentation	Induced labor
Vaginal	Noncephalic presentation
Full-term	Cesarean delivery
Single gestation	Preterm delivery
Live-born infant	Postterm delivery
Resolved antepartum conditions	Prolonged delivery
No other complications	Multiple gestation
	Stillbirth
	Any complication

> Patient gives birth to a baby boy who makes a cephalic presentation. Aside from requesting an epidural and having an episiotomy, the patient has no problems.
>
> (1) Index: **Delivery, normal**
> Tabular List: **O80   Encounter for full-term uncomplicated delivery**
> (2) Index: **Outcome of delivery, single, liveborn**
> Tabular List: **Z37.0   Single live birth**

Figure 22-16 ■ Example of sequencing codes for a delivery.

Arranging Chapter 15 Codes with Codes from Other Chapters

Many complications require a code from Chapter 15 to identify the obstetric complication and an additional code from a body system chapter to describe the details of the condition. Always sequence the Chapter 15 code first (OGCR 15.a.1)). Follow this guideline regardless of whether the condition is preexisting, as in diabetes, or is specific for the postpartum period, as in postpartum thrombophlebitis (■ FIGURE 22-17). The terms *thrombophlebitis* and *phlebothrombosis* are interchangeable in ICD-10-CM. Notice that both terms contain two roots, **phleb-** (*vein*) and **thromb-** (*clot*). Refer to the Tabular List for instructional notes to assign additional codes (■ FIGURE 22-18).

Guided Example of Arranging Obstetrics Diagnosis Codes

To practice skills for sequencing codes for pregnancy, childbirth, and the puerperium, continue with the example from earlier in the chapter about patient Glenna Ferrier, who was admitted to Branton Medical Center for full-term labor.

Follow along in your ICD-10-CM manual as Daphne Wittman, CCS-P, sequences the codes. Check off each step after you complete it.

▶ First, Daphne reviews the codes she has assigned for this case:

❑ **Z37.0 Single live birth**

❑ **O34.211 Maternal care for low transverse scar from previous cesarean delivery**

❑ **O76 Abnormality in fetal heart rate and rhythm complicating labor and delivery**

❑ **O66.41 Failed attempted vaginal birth after previous cesarean delivery**

❑ **Z3A.39 39 weeks gestation of pregnancy**

▶ To better determine the sequencing rules, Daphne reads OGCR I.C.15.b.4, which states the following:

❑ "In cases of cesarean delivery, the selection of the principal diagnosis should be the condition established after study that was responsible for the patient's admission. If the patient was admitted with a condition that resulted in the performance of a cesarean procedure, that condition should be selected as the principal diagnosis."

> Patient is seen for postpartum deep venous phlebothrombosis in the tibial vein of the left leg.
>
> (1) Index: **Phlebothrombosis, puerperal, - see Thrombophlebitis, puerperal**
> Index: **Thrombophlebitis, puerperal, deep**
> Tabular List: **O87.1 Deep phlebothrombosis in the puerperium**
> (2) Tabular List: **Use additional code to identify the deep vein thrombosis (I82.4-, I85.5-, I82.62-, I82.72-)**
> **I82.442 Acute embolism and thrombosis of left tibial vein**

Figure 22-17 ■ Example of sequencing obstetric complications with codes from a body system chapter.

> **O87.1 Deep phlebothrombosis in the puerperium**
> Deep vein thrombosis, postpartum
> Pelvic thrombophlebitis, postpartum
> **Use additional code** to identify the deep vein thrombosis (I82.4-, I82.5-, I82.62-. I82.72-)
> **Use additional code**, if applicable, for associated long-term (current) use of anticoagulants (Z79.01)

Figure 22-18 ■ Tabular List Entry for an obstetric complication requiring additional codes from a body system chapter.

❑ Daphne reviews the medical record and the codes she assigned. The main reason a cesarean delivery was performed was because of the scar from the previous cesarean delivery.

❑ Therefore, the principal diagnosis is **O34.211 Maternal care for low transverse scar from previous cesarean delivery**.

❑ The second code should be the next most important complication, which is the fetal tachycardia.

❑ The third code is failed vaginal delivery.

❑ The fourth code is the outcome of delivery.

❑ The final code is the weeks of gestation.

▶ Daphne finalizes the codes and sequencing for this case:

(1)   **O34.211 Maternal care for low transverse scar from previous cesarean delivery**

(2)   **O76 Abnormality in fetal heart rate and rhythm complicating labor and delivery**

(3)   **O66.41 Failed attempted vaginal birth after previous cesarean delivery**

(4)   **Z37.0 Single live birth**

(5)   **Z3A.39 39 weeks gestation of pregnancy**

CODING PRACTICE

Exercise 22.4   Arranging Diagnosis Codes for Obstetrics

Instructions: Read the mini-medical-record of each patient's encounter, review the information abstracted in Exercise 22.2, assign ICD-10-CM diagnosis codes using the Index and Tabular List, and sequence them correctly.

---

1. **INPATIENT HOSPITAL**   Gender: **F**   Age: **18**

Gravida: **1**   Para: **0**   EDD: **4/6/yy**   EGA: **37+5**

Reason for admission: **Full term labor**

Assessment: **Placental infarction**

Delivery: **3/22/yy, NSVD, stillborn, 1 girl**

Tip: Assign a code for the placental infarction, a code for the fetal death, a code for outcome of delivery, and a code for the weeks of gestation.

4 ICD-10-CM Codes _____

_____

---

2. **OFFICE**   Gender: **F**   Age: **30**

Gravida: **2**   Para: **1**   EDD: **10/5/yy**

EGA: **12+0**

Reason for encounter: **Prenatal care, pernicious anemia**

Assessment: **Blood work has improved, but still not where it should be**

Plan: **B12 injection**

Tip: Read the instructional notes in the Tabular List. Assign a code for the weeks of gestation.

3 ICD-10-CM Codes _____

_____

---

3. **INPATIENT HOSPITAL**   Gender: **F**   Age: **32**

Gravida: **2**   Para: **2**   EDD: **5/18/yy**

EGA: **32+2**

Reason for admission: **Premature rupture of membranes**

Assessment: **Severe preeclampsia requires cesarean delivery**

(continued)

---

3. (continued)

Delivery: **3/22/yy, classical cesarean, PTBLC, 1 girl**

Tip: Assign a code for the reason for the cesarean delivery, a code for PROM, a code for preterm delivery, a code for the outcome of delivery, and a code for the weeks of gestation.

5 ICD-10-CM Codes _____

_____

---

4. **OFFICE**   Gender: **F**   Age: **15**

Birthday: **7/15**   Gravida: **1**   Para: **0**

EDD: **6/1/yy**   EGA: **30+4**

Reason for encounter: **Prenatal care, twins, MoDi**

Assessment: **Dipstick shows new isolated gestational proteinuria**

Plan: **At risk for pre-eclampsia, RTO 4 days for repeat test**

Tip: Assign a code for the diagnosis, a code for the mother's age, a code for the twin pregnancy, and a code for the weeks of gestation.

4 ICD-10-CM Codes _____

_____

---

5. **INPATIENT HOSPITAL**   Gender: **F**   Age: **22**

Gravida: **2**   Para: **2**   EDD: **3/16/yy**

EGA: **41+3**

Reason for admission: **Post term labor**

Assessment: **Obstructed labor due to CPD, severe obesity, mother, BMI 41**

Delivery: **3/23/yy, cesarean delivery, TBLC, 1 boy**

Tip: Assign a delivery code for the obstruction, a code for postterm pregnancy, and a delivery code for the obesity complication, then follow instructional notes in the Tabular List. Also assign a code for the weeks of gestation.

7 ICD-10-CM Codes _____

_____

_____

CHAPTER SUMMARY

In this chapter you learned that:

- Pregnancy is a normal, temporary condition that occurs within the female body, which begins at the time of conception and ends with the birth of the fetus.

- ICD-10-CM provides Official Guidelines for Coding and Reporting (OGCR) in section I.C.15 that cover the general rules for obstetric cases, selection of OB principal or first-listed diagnosis, preexisting conditions, and several specific conditions, including hypertension, diabetes, HIV, alcohol and tobacco use, normal delivery, postpartum, and abortions.

- Because multiple complications are common during pregnancy, childbirth, and the puerperium, coders must be attentive to which complication is the reason for the encounter or admission.

- Coders should acquaint themselves with the organization of obstetrical terms in the Index and must be attentive to distinguish between codes that apply to the mother and those that apply to the infant.

- Coders must be attentive to selecting the principal diagnosis when a delivery occurs and to sequencing codes from ICD-10-CM Chapter 15 with codes from body system chapters.

CONCEPT QUIZ

Take a moment to look back at pregnancy, childbirth, and the puerperium and solidify your skills. Try to answer the questions from memory first, then look back at the discussion in this chapter if you need a little extra help.

Completion

Instructions: Write the term that completes each statement based on the information you learned in this chapter. Choose from the list below. Some choices may be used more than once and some choices may not be used at all.

cephalic	occipitoanterior
conception	para
DiDi	parturition
DiMo	peripartum
fetopelvic	placenta previa
first trimester	pre-eclampsia
gestational hypertension	prenatal
gravida	PROM
HELLP syndrome	puerperium
last menstrual period	Rhesus incompatibility
MoDi	second trimester
MoMo	third trimester
nuchal cord	

1. The _____ period is the last month of pregnancy to five months postpartum.

2. _____ is the period of true labor.

3. The estimated date of delivery is determined as 40 weeks from the _____.

4. _____ is the period from 28 weeks, 0 days until delivery.

5. _____ is the condition of the umbilical cord becoming wrapped around the neck of the fetus.

6. _____ is a condition in which a mother is Rh negative and develops antibodies against a fetus that is Rh positive.

7. _____ is a metabolic disorder of pregnancy that develops after the 20th week and involves gestational hypertension and proteinuria.

8. _____ identifies twin fetuses with one chorion and two amnions.

9. _____ disproportion is also known as cephalopelvic disproportion.

10. _____ is the rupture of the amniotic sac and chorion before the onset of labor.

Multiple Choice

Instructions: Circle the letter of the best answer to each question based on the information you learned in this chapter.

1. How many months after delivery are included in the *peripartum* period?
   A. 0
   B. 1
   C. 5
   D. 6

2. How many *gravida* and *para* describe a woman currently pregnant, who has had one previous pregnancy and gave birth to twins?
   A. Gravida 1 para 2
   B. Gravida 2 para 1
   C. Gravida 2 para 2
   D. Grand multipara

3. How would you code the following scenario? *A patient at 39 weeks gestation gives birth to a baby boy who makes a cephalic presentation*
   A. O80, Z37.0, Z3A.30
   B. Z3A.30, O80, Z37.0
   C. O80, Z37.0
   D. O80

4. What is the length of a full-term pregnancy?
   A. More than 37 completed weeks of gestation
   B. 37 weeks, 0 days of gestation to 39 weeks, 6 days of gestation
   C. 40 completed weeks to 42 completed weeks of gestation
   D. More than 42 completed weeks of gestation

5. How would you code the following scenario? *A patient G 2 P 1 is seen for a routine prenatal visit in her 30th week. She has a history of preterm labor.*
   A. O09.299
   B. Z34.83, Z87.51
   C. O09.213, Z3A.30
   D. Z87.51, Z3A.30

6. Which of the following is a normal delivery?
   A. Induction of labor with vaginal delivery
   B. Vaginal delivery with cephalic presentation
   C. Vaginal delivery of twins
   D. Vaginal delivery at 36 weeks of gestation

7. When is a multiple-gestation pregnancy coded as high risk?
   A. Only when the physician documents it as high risk
   B. Only when a cesarean delivery is required
   C. When there are more than two fetuses
   D. Always

8. How would you code the following scenario? *A patient is seen for postpartum deep venous phlebothrombosis in the popliteal vein of the right leg.*
   A. O87.1
   B. I82.431
   C. I82.431, O87.1
   D. O87.1, I82.431

9. What information about pregnancy does the seventh character of 1 identify in the obstetrics chapter?
   A. The first trimester
   B. A single gestation pregnancy
   C. Fetus 1 in a multiple-gestation pregnancy
   D. Gravida 1

10. How many complications are documented in this case? *A patient age 15 years, 10 months, is admitted in labor at 36 weeks, 3 days gestation. Labor proceeds uneventfully and she gives birth to twins.*
    A. None
    B. One
    C. Two
    D. Three

KEEP ON CODING

Instructions: Read the diagnostic statement, then use the Index and Tabular List to assign and sequence ICD-10-CM diagnosis codes. Write the code(s) on the line provided.

1. Tubal pregnancy, right. ICD-10-CM Code(s) _____

2. Supervision of elderly primigravida, 35-week pregnancy. ICD-10-CM Code(s) _____

3. Threatened abortion. ICD-10-CM Code(s) _____

4. Complication of childbirth due to bariatric surgery status, 36 weeks. ICD-10-CM Code(s) _____

5. Excessive weight gain during first 12 weeks of pregnancy. ICD-10-CM Code(s) _____

6. Pregnancy with preexisting diabetes mellitus, type 1, in puerperium. ICD-10-CM Code(s) _____

7. Pregnancy complicated by breech presentation, 39 weeks' gestation. ICD-10-CM Code(s) _____

8. Galactorrhea. ICD-10-CM Code(s) _____

9. Postpartum thyroiditis. ICD-10-CM Code(s) _____

10. Aspiration pneumonia due to anesthesia during 27th week of pregnancy (26 weeks completed). ICD-10-CM Code(s) _____

11. Acute lymphoblastic leukemia complicating the pregnancy in 31st week (30 weeks completed). ICD-10-CM Code(s) _____

12. Acute renal failure after an incomplete spontaneous abortion. ICD-10-CM Code(s) _____

13. Herpes gestationis, 10 weeks pregnant. ICD-10-CM Code(s) _____

14. Fetal anemia. ICD-10-CM Code(s) _____

15. Failed induction of labor by oxytocin, 40 weeks. ICD-10-CM Code(s) _____

16. Triplet pregnancy delivered at 38 weeks of gestation by cesarean delivery, all liveborn. ICD-10-CM Code(s) _____

17. Preterm labor without delivery, 33 weeks of pregnancy. ICD-10-CM Code(s) _____

18. Alcohol abuse complicating pregnancy at 37 weeks. ICD-10-CM Code(s) _____

19. Normal delivery at 38 weeks' gestation with single liveborn infant. ICD-10-CM Code(s) _____

(continued)

(continued from page 403)

20. Puerperal abscess of nipple. ICD-10-CM Code(s) _____

21. Abnormal glucose level complicating pregnancy, 22 weeks. ICD-10-CM Code(s) _____

22. Hemorrhoids complicating pregnancy at 26 weeks. ICD-10-CM Code(s) _____

23. Maternal care for incompetent cervix, 25 weeks. ICD-10-CM Code(s) _____

24. Kidney infection, in 13th week of pregnancy (12 weeks completed). ICD-10-CM Code(s) _____

25. Physical abuse complicating pregnancy in the 8th week (7 weeks completed). ICD-10-CM Code(s) _____

CODING CHALLENGE

Instructions: Read the mini-medical-record of each patient's encounter, then abstract, assign, and sequence ICD-10-CM diagnosis codes using the Index and Tabular List. Write the code(s) on the line provided.

---

1. EMERGENCY DEPT Gender: F Age: 24

Gravida: 2 Para: 1 EDD: 9/27/yy EGA: 14+2

Reason for encounter: Hurt her shoulder while lifting bags of gravel she was spreading on a walking path in the yard of her single family home, leisure status

Assessment: Sprained right shoulder, does not affect pregnancy

Plan: Ice and sling, FU 1 week

Tip: Remember to assign external cause codes for activity, place of occurrence, and status.

5 ICD-10-CM Codes _____

_____

---

2. OFFICE Gender: F Age: 19

Gravida: 1 Para: 0 EDD: 8/16/yy EGA: 19+6

Reason for encounter: Prenatal care

Assessment: HIV positive

Plan: Anti-HIV drugs beginning in second trimester, newborn to be treated within 8 hrs and for 6 months

Tip: Refer to OGCR I.C.15.f.

3 ICD-10-CM Codes _____

_____

---

3. OFFICE Gender: F Age: 35

Gravida: 2 Para: 0 EDD: 10/25/yy

EGA: 10+0

Reason for encounter: Patient presents for prenatal care after successful IVF

(continued)

---

3. (continued)

Assessment: Previous miscarriage

Plan: Schedule prenatal visits

Tip: Assign a separate code for each risk factor.

4 ICD-10-CM Codes _____

_____

---

4. INPATIENT HOSPITAL Gender: F Age: 28

Gravida: 2 Para: 2 EDD: 4/5/yy EGA: 39+1

Reason for admission: Labor

Assessment: Cord entanglement and compression of fetus 1

Delivery: 3/28/yy, vaginal delivery converted to cesarean delivery, TBLC, 1 girl, 1 boy

Tip: By definition, twins of the opposite sex are DiDi.

4 ICD-10-CM Codes _____

_____

---

5. INPATIENT HOSPITAL Gender: F Age: 31

Gravida: 2 Para: 2 Date of delivery: 3/8/yy

Reason for encounter: Admitted from physician office with fever of 103 degrees F and purulent discharge from operative wound

Assessment: Infected cesarean delivery wound, superficial incisional site, staphylococcus

Plan: Antibiotics, FU 2 weeks

2 ICD-10-CM Codes _____

6. INPATIENT HOSPITAL Gender: F Age: 23

Gravida: 1 Para: 1 EDD: 3/27/yy EGA: 39+4

Reason for admission: Full term labor

Assessment: Obstructed labor due to prolapsed arm presentation, successfully converted to cephalic, with first degree perineal laceration

Delivery: 3/28/yy, NSVD, TBLC, 1 girl

4 ICD-10-CM Codes _____

_____

---

7. INPATIENT HOSPITAL Gender: F Age: 31

Gravida: 3 Para: 2 EDD: 10/11/yy

EGA: 12+5

Reason for admission: Observation for signs of labor or other complications after failed legal abortion due to fetal chromosome abnormality

Assessment: No labor or other complications were noted

Plan: RTO FU in 2 days, supportive and genetic counseling

Tip: Assign codes for the attempted abortion and the underlying reason for the attempt. See OGCR 15.b.3).

3 ICD-10-CM Codes _____

_____

---

8. OFFICE Gender: F Age: 34

Gravida: 2 Para: 2 Date of Delivery: 3/15/yy

Reason for encounter: Postpartum care

Assessment: Abscess of right breast

Plan: Rx antibiotic, RTO 2 weeks

1 ICD-10-CM Code _____

---

9. OFFICE Gender: F Age: 30

Gravida: 1 Para: 0 EDD: 10/18/yy

EGA: 11+3

Reason for encounter: Prenatal visit

Assessment: Long standing essential hypertension

Plan: Antihypertensive therapy, monitor for preeclampsia

2 ICD-10-CM Codes _____

---

10. INPATIENT HOSPITAL Gender: F Age: 21

Gravida: 2 Para: 2 EDD: 5/31/yy

EGA: 31+4

Reason for admission: Premature rupture of membranes

Assessment: Labor started 30 hours post admission, vertical scar from previous cesarean delivery

Delivery: 3/28/yy, VBAC, TBLC, 1 girl

5 ICD-10-CM Codes _____

_____

Chapter 23

Certain Conditions Originating in the Perinatal Period (P00-P96)

Chapter Outline

- **Perinatal Refresher**
- **Coding Guidelines for Perinatal Conditions**
- **Abstracting for Perinatal Conditions**
- **Assigning Codes for Perinatal Conditions**
- **Arranging Codes for Perinatal Conditions**

Learning Objectives

After completing this chapter, you should have the skills to:

23.1 Spell and define the key words, medical terms, and abbreviations related to conditions originating in the perinatal period. (Remember)

23.2 Summarize common conditions originating in the perinatal period. (Understand)

23.3 Adhere to the Official Guidelines for Coding and Reporting related to conditions originating in the perinatal period. (Apply)

23.4 Examine and abstract diagnostic information from the medical record for coding conditions originating in the perinatal period. (Analyze)

23.5 Demonstrate how to assign codes for conditions originating in the perinatal period. (Apply)

23.6 Utilize guidelines for arranging (sequencing) multiple diagnosis codes for conditions originating in the perinatal period. (Apply)

Key Terms and Abbreviations

chromosomal abnormality
deformation
erythroblastosis fetalis
malformation

neonatal mortality
neonate
newborn
newborn birth status

newborn clinically significant condition
perinatal condition

perinatal period
transitory

In addition to the key terms listed here, students should know the terms defined within tables in this chapter.

INTRODUCTION

Newborn babies win over everyone's heart but, unfortunately, some experience medical conditions during the first few weeks of life. This chapter introduces you to some of those conditions.

A pediatrician is a physician who specializes in diagnosing and treating conditions of children, including perinatal conditions. A neonatologist is a pediatric subspecialist who diagnoses and treats complex conditions of newborns. Other medical specialties also have subspecialists in pediatrics and neonatology. For example, a neonatal cardiologist specializes in diagnosing and treating heart conditions of newborns.

PERINATAL REFRESHER

The **perinatal period** begins before birth and continues through the 28th day following birth. An infant is referred to as a **neonate** or **newborn** during the first 28 days of life (■ FIGURE 23-1). After day 28 they are classified as infants or children. **Perinatal conditions** are those that develop before birth or in the first 28 days after birth, but exclude physical **malformations** (*permanent abnormal shape of an organ or body region, resulting from arrested, delayed, or abnormal development of the embryo*), **deformations** (*a change in the size or shape of a normal structure due to physical forces*), and **chromosomal abnormalities** (*the abnormal number or structure of chromosomes*). Perinatal conditions are often **transitory** (*temporary*), but may be long term or permanent as well.

Refer to ■ TABLE 23-1 for a refresher on how to build medical terms related to conditions originating in the perinatal period.

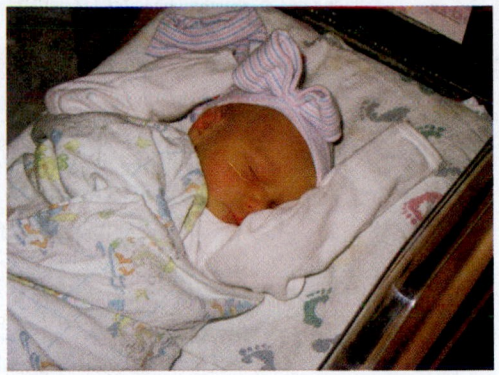

Figure 23-1 ■ A neonate or newborn is 1 to 28 days old. *Source: Bronwen Schulman.*

until after the perinatal period, but because they originated during the perinatal period they are still considered perinatal conditions and are assigned codes from this ICD-10-CM chapter (■ FIGURE 23-2).

Some perinatal conditions, such as retinopathy, apnea, or tachycardia, use similar medical terms as conditions that affect adults. The condition is identified as perinatal by the use of a descriptive term, such as prematurity or newborn, in conjunction with the name of the condition. For example, retinopathy of prematurity, newborn apnea, or newborn tachycardia are perinatal conditions, whereas retinopathy, apnea, and tachycardia can originate at any age. Other perinatal conditions only occur in newborns, such as amnionitis or meconium aspiration syndrome. Refer to ■ TABLE 23-2, page 408 for a summary of conditions originating in the perinatal period.

In particular, coders must be aware of conditions related to neonatal birth weight.

Patient, age 15, is seen for Erb's palsy (*paralysis of the upper arm*), which resulted from damage during birth.

Patient, age 60, is seen for blindness in the left eye, which he has had since birth, as a result of retinopathy of prematurity (ROP).

Patient, age 35, is diagnosed with carcinoma of the vagina, due to exposure to diethylstilbestrol (DES) which her mother took during pregnancy.

Figure 23-2 ■ Examples of perinatal conditions affecting patients later in life.

CODING CAUTION

Be alert for medical word roots that are spelled similarly and have different meanings.

omphal/o (*umbilicus or navel*) and **oophor/o** (*ovary*)

amni/o (*amniotic sac*), **ammon/o** (*ammonium*), and **amin/o** (*amino acid*)

Conditions Originating in the Perinatal Period

Perinatal conditions are defined by the fact that they *originated* during the perinatal period, regardless of when they are diagnosed or treated. Some conditions may not be diagnosed

Table 23-1 ■ **EXAMPLE OF CONSTRUCTING MEDICAL TERMS FOR CONDITIONS ORIGINATING IN THE PERINATAL PERIOD**

Prefix	Root/Suffix	Complete Medical Term
dys- (prefix; *abnormal, painful*)		**dys + pnea** (*difficulty breathing*)
		dys + rhythmia (*abnormal heartbeat*)
tachy- (prefix; *rapid*)	**-pnea** (*breathing*) **-cardi/o** (*heart, heart rate*) **-rhythm/o** (*rhythm, beat*)	**tachy + pnea** (*rapid breathing*)
		tachy + cardia (*rapid heart rate*)
brady- (prefix; *slow*)		**brady + pnea** (*slow breathing*)
		brady + cardia (*slow heart rate*)

Table 23-2   ■   **COMMON CONDITIONS ORIGINATING IN THE PERINATAL PERIOD**

Condition	Definition
Amnionitis	Infection or inflammation of the amniotic sac
Apgar score	An evaluation of a newborn's physical condition, performed 1 and 5 minutes after birth, to determine any immediate need for extra medical or emergency care (named after the physician who designed it, Dr. Virginia Apgar)
Appropriate for gestational age (AGA)	A fetus or newborn infant whose size is within the normal range for his or her gestational age
Birth trauma	Any physical injury to the infant during delivery
Breast engorgement	The temporary enlargement of breasts on female or male newborns, due to high levels of maternal hormones in the infant's blood
Drug withdrawal syndrome	A collection of symptoms of drug withdrawal in an infant who was exposed to narcotics in the uterus; also called *neonatal abstinence syndrome (NAS)*
Exceptionally large newborn	Birth weight more than 4,500 grams (9 pounds, 15 ounces)
Extremely low birth weight (ELBW)	Birth weight of less than 1,000 grams (2 pounds, 3 ounces)
Failure to thrive (FTT)	Inadequate physical growth marked by child's weight for age below the fifth percentile of the standard growth chart
Hemolytic disease of the newborn (HDN)	A blood disorder that occurs when the blood types of a mother and baby are incompatible, also called **erythroblastosis fetalis**
High birth weight (HBW)	Birth weight greater than 4,000 grams (8 pounds, 13 ounces)
Hyperbilirubinemia	High concentrations of bilirubin in the blood, which causes the infant's skin and sclera to turn yellow
Infant of diabetic mother (IDM)	An infant born to a woman who is diabetic
Intrauterine growth restriction (IUGR)	Poor growth of a baby while in the mother's womb during pregnancy. Specifically, it means the developing baby weighs less than 90% of other babies at the same gestational age.
Intraventricular hemorrhage (IVH)	Bleeding in the brain in very low birth weight premature babies, which usually resolves within a few days
Jaundice	A condition due to high bilirubin that causes the skin and parts of the eyes to turn a yellow color
Large for gestational age (LGA)	A fetus or newborn infant who is larger in size than normal for the baby's sex and gestational age, most commonly defined as a weight, length, or head circumference above the 90th percentile at gestational age
Low birth weight (LBW)	Birth weight less than 2,500 grams (5 pounds, 8 ounces)
Meconium aspiration syndrome (MAS)	Condition in which the newborn breathes a mixture of meconium and amniotic fluid into the lungs prior to or during delivery
Meconium peritonitis	Infection of the peritoneal cavity due to perforation of the bowel and leakage of meconium
Newborn ABO incompatibility	An infant with blood type A or B affected by comingling of type O blood from mother with blood type O
Newborn apnea	A condition in which the infant stops breathing
Newborn Rh incompatibility	Rh-positive infant affected by comingling of blood with an Rh-negative mother
Normal birth weight	Birth weight of 2,500 to 4,000 grams (5 pounds, 8 ounces to 8 pounds, 13 ounces)
Omphalitis	Infection of the umbilical stump in a newborn, usually presenting as superficial cellulitis
Respiratory distress syndrome (RDS)	A condition in which the alveolar sacs collapse due to lack of surfactant
Retinopathy of prematurity (ROP)	The abnormal growth of blood vessels in the eye that can lead to vision loss
Small for gestational age (SGA)	A fetus or newborn infant who is smaller in size than normal for the baby's sex and gestational age, most commonly defined as a weight, length, or head circumference below the 10th percentile for the gestational age
Transient tachypnea of the newborn (TTN)	Short-term condition (less than 24 hours) of rapid breathing due to retained lung fluid that occurs shortly after birth in full-term or near-term newborns
Very low birth weight (VLBW)	Birth weight of less than 1,500 grams (3 pounds, 4 ounces)

Birth Weight

Newborn birth weight is a major indicator of newborn health and nutritional status. Both low birth weight (LBW), under 2,500 grams, and high birth weight (HBW), over 4,000 grams, are associated with health problems. Birth weight is directly tied to the estimated gestational age (EGA) at birth. The earlier infants are born, before 37 weeks' gestation, the less they weigh. The longer a pregnancy continues, beyond 40 weeks, the more newborns weigh. Newborns of any EGA can be lighter or heavier in weight or smaller or larger in size compared to other infants of the same EGA. This condition is referred to by a variety of names such as *small for gestational age*, *light for date*, *light for age*, *large for age*, and similar.

LBW is a leading cause of **neonatal mortality** (*death before 29 days of age*). Although it is largely preventable in a developed country such as the United States, over 8% of infants each year are born with LBW, according to the Centers for Disease Control and Prevention (CDC), and nearly six of every 1,000 children die before one year of age. LBW is associated with failure to thrive, dehydration, and feeding disorders, as well as many chronic conditions of the digestive, pulmonary, and cardiovascular systems. Premature infants are weighed daily in the neonatal intensive care unit (NICU) and generally must weigh at least 1,800 grams (four pounds) before being removed from the incubator (■ Figure 23-3). Each hospital sets its own weight standards for discharge, but the infant must be out of the incubator and steadily gaining weight before discharge.

High birth weight is associated with diabetes and certain adult cancers, such as breast, prostate, endometrial, and colon cancer, according to journal articles published by the National Institutes of Health (NIH).

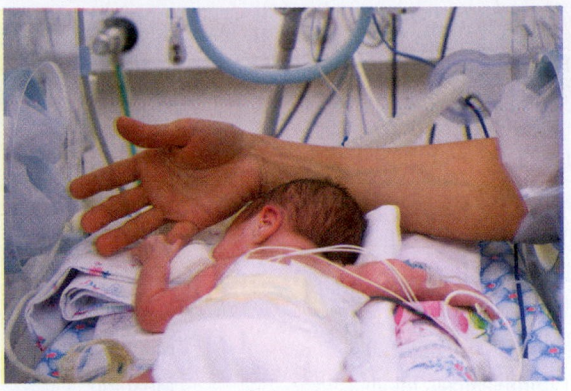

Figure 23-3 ■ Premature babies must weigh 1,800 grams before being released from an incubator. *Source: Fanfo/Fotolia.*

This section provides a general reference to help understand the most common conditions originating in the perinatal period but does not list everything you need to know. Use medical terminology skills discussed earlier in this chapter to learn the meaning of unfamiliar words. Remember to keep standard reference books handy in case you get stuck.

SUCCESS STEP

Newborn birth weight is reported in grams using the metric system. A weight of 2,500 grams is equal to 5 pounds, 8 ounces.

CODING PRACTICE

Exercise 23.1   Perinatal Refresher

Instructions: Use your medical terminology skills and resources to define the following conditions related to conditions originating in the perinatal period, then assign the default diagnosis code.

Follow these steps:

- Use slash marks "/" to break down each underlined term into its root(s) and suffix.
- Define the meaning of the underlined term, based on the meaning of each word part.
- Assign the default ICD-10-CM diagnosis code for the condition using the Index and Tabular List. Locate the Main Term Newborn, then locate the subterms in the order shown.

Example: newborn apnea a/pnea   Meaning *lack of breathing*   ICD-10-CM Code *P28.3*

1. Newborn, affected by, heart rate, tachycardia   Meaning _____   ICD-10-CM Code _____

2. Newborn, affected by, intrauterine blood loss   Meaning _____   ICD-10-CM Code _____

3. Newborn, hyperbilirubinemia   Meaning _____   ICD-10-CM Code _____

4. Newborn, affected by, maternal polyhydramnios   Meaning _____   ICD-10-CM Code _____

5. Newborn, infective mastitis   Meaning _____   ICD-10-CM Code _____

(continued)

CODING PRACTICE *(continued)*

6. Newborn, <u>omphalitis</u>   Meaning _____   ICD-10-CM Code _____

7. Newborn, affected by,   Meaning _____   ICD-10-CM Code _____
   hypoxic ischemic <u>encephalopathy</u>

8. Newborn, affected by,   Meaning _____   ICD-10-CM Code _____
   <u>chorioamnionitis</u>

9. Newborn, <u>hyponatremia</u>   Meaning _____   ICD-10-CM Code _____

10. <u>Erythroblastosis</u> fetalis   Meaning _____   ICD-10-CM Code _____

CODING GUIDELINES FOR PERINATAL CONDITIONS

Coders should understand the organization of this ICD-10-CM chapter, chapter-wide and commonly used instructional notes in the Tabular List, and the relevant OGCR. This information is necessary for accurate coding.

ICD-10-CM Chapter 16, "Certain Conditions Originating in the Perinatal Period (P00-P96)," contains 12 blocks or subchapters that are divided by anatomical site. Review the block names and code ranges listed at the beginning of Chapter 16 in the ICD-10-CM manual to become familiar with the content and organization.

This chapter includes newborn conditions that originate before birth or during the first 28 days of life and result from maternal conditions that are both related and unrelated to pregnancy, birth trauma, and underdevelopment during gestation. They also include respiratory, cardiovascular, metabolic, digestive, and hematological disorders. This chapter does not include fetal conditions that affect the mother or congenital abnormalities, both of which are classified in separate chapters. An instructional note at the beginning of the chapter requires that codes in this chapter are to be used *only* on the newborn's record, never on the mother's record.

The sequencing of chapters in ICD-10-CM is different than in ICD-9-CM. In ICD-10-CM, this chapter, "Certain Conditions Originating in the Perinatal Period (P00-P96)," appears immediately after the obstetrics chapter, "Pregnancy, Childbirth, and the Puerperium (O00-O9A)," and is followed by Chapter 17, "Congenital Malformations, Deformations, and Chromosomal Abnormalities (Q00-Q99)."

ICD-10-CM provides Official Guidelines for Coding and Reporting (OGCR) for conditions originating in the perinatal period in OGCR section I.C.16. OGCR provides detailed discussion of selecting the principal and additional diagnoses and how to report codes from this chapter with those from other chapters. OGCR also discusses specific coding for prematurity, low birth weight, bacterial sepsis of the newborn, stillbirth, and observation and evaluation of newborns for suspected conditions not found. Additional guidelines related to assigning Z codes for newborns and infants appear in OGCR I.C.21.c.12). Specific OGCR and instructional notes are discussed and cited throughout this chapter of the text.

ABSTRACTING FOR PERINATAL CONDITIONS

Coders must take note whether a hospitalization of a newborn includes the birth itself or whether the admission takes place after the birth episode. Abstract all **newborn clinically significant conditions,** defined as any newborn condition that meets the following criteria (OGCR I.C.16.a.6):

- Requires clinical evaluation
- Requires therapeutic treatment
- Requires diagnostic procedures
- Extends length of hospital stay (LOS)
- Increases nursing care or monitoring
- Presents implications for future healthcare needs

The final criterion, conditions that present implications for future healthcare needs, is unique to newborns. When the provider documents newborn conditions that are not treated, but may have implications for future needs, coders should abstract and code this information. This type of information is *not* coded for adults.

Abstracting the birth encounter (■ TABLE 23-3) requires different criteria than abstracting encounters after birth (■ TABLE 23-4). Remember that the abstracting questions are a guide and that not every question applies to, or can be answered for, every case. For example, not all newborns are affected by a maternal condition. Also remember to abstract for symptoms and determine if they are integral to the confirmed diagnoses. After reviewing the abstracting criteria, work through the guided example that follows.

Abstracting from Newborn Records

Newborn records contain unique information and abbreviations not found in other medical records. Refer to ■ FIGURE 23-4 to

Table 23-3 ■ KEY CRITERIA FOR ABSTRACTING BIRTH ENCOUNTERS

❏ Was the infant born in this hospital during this admission?

❏ Was the infant born outside the hospital, then hospitalized?

❏ Was the delivery vaginal or cesarean?

❏ What is the birth weight?

❏ What is the estimated gestational age at time of delivery?

❏ Are any conditions documented as due to prematurity?

❏ Did the infant suffer any birth trauma?

❏ What conditions of the newborn required evaluation, treatment, extended LOS, or increased care or present implications for future healthcare needs?

❏ Was the newborn observed or evaluated for any suspected conditions not found?

❏ What maternal conditions affected the infant?

Table 23-4 ■ KEY CRITERIA FOR ABSTRACTING ENCOUNTERS AFTER THE BIRTH EPISODE

❏ What is the age of the patient?

❏ What is the reason for the encounter?

❏ What condition is documented?

❏ What is the subtype of the condition?

❏ What complications and comorbidities exist?

❏ Is the condition documented as originating in the perinatal period?

learn how to interpret the mini-medical-record used for newborn cases in this text.

Guided Example of Abstracting for Perinatal Conditions

Refer to the following example throughout this chapter to practice skills for abstracting, assigning, and sequencing codes for conditions originating in the perinatal period. Aaron Randell, CCS, is a fictitious coder who guides you through the process.

> Date of discharge: 4/21/yy   Location: Valley Hospital (VH)   Provider: Joann Gwinn, MD
>
> Patient: Derek Leverette   Gender: M   DOB: 4/18/yy
>
> Birth Weight: 1990g   EGA: 34+1
> Method: Cesarean   Location: VH
>
> Assessment: Cesarean performed due to maternal preeclampsia. Infant presented with transient tachypnea (TTN) due to prematurity and was admitted to NICU. O₂ and CPAP therapy were provided, which restored breathing to normal within 48 hours. Patient was discharged with no symptoms.
>
> Plan: FU in office 2 weeks

Follow along as Aaron Randell, CCS, abstracts the diagnosis. Check off each step after you complete it.

▶ Aaron reads through the entire record, paying special attention to the birth data and the final assessment.

❏ He notes that this record is for the birth encounter so he refers to the Key Criteria for Abstracting Birth Encounters (Table 23-3).

❏ *Was the infant born in this hospital during this admission?* Yes

❏ *Was the delivery vaginal or cesarean?* Cesarean

❏ *What is the birth weight?* 1990 grams

❏ *What is the gestational age at time of delivery?* 34 weeks, 1 day

❏ *Are any conditions documented as due to prematurity?* Transient tachypnea

❏ *Did the infant suffer any birth trauma?* No

❏ *What conditions of the newborn required evaluation, treatment, extended LOS, increased care, or present implications for future healthcare needs?* Transient tachypnea

❏ *Was the newborn observed for any suspected conditions not found?* No

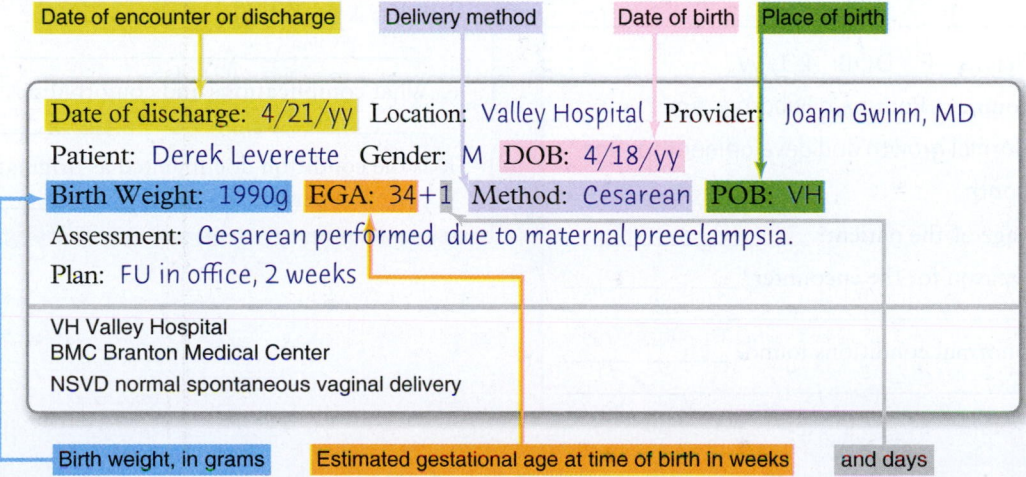

Figure 23-4 ■ Key to interpreting the newborn mini-medical-record.

❏ *What maternal conditions affected the infant?* None. The mother had preeclampsia, but documentation does not state that it affected the infant

▶ At this time, Aaron does not know how many codes he will end up with. He will learn about this when he moves on to assigning codes.

CODING PRACTICE

Exercise 23.2   Abstracting for Perinatal Conditions

Instructions: Read the mini-medical-record of each patient's encounter and answer the abstracting questions. Write the answer on the line provided. Do not assign any codes.

1. INPATIENT HOSPITAL   Gender: F   DOB: 4/22/yy

Birth Weight: 3521g   EGA: 38+2   Type: NSVD

POB: Hospital

Assessment: APGARS 6, 8

Plan: Discharged 1 day after birth. FU in office, 2 weeks

a. Was the infant born in this hospital during this admission? _____

b. Was the delivery vaginal or cesarean? _____ _____

c. What is the birth weight? _____

d. What is the estimated gestational age at time of delivery? _____

e. Are any conditions documented as due to prematurity? _____

f. Did the infant suffer any birth trauma? _____ _____

g. What conditions of the newborn required evaluation, treatment, extended LOS, or increased care or present implications for future healthcare needs? _____ _____

2. OFFICE   Gender: F   DOB: 4/1/yy

Reason for encounter: Routine newborn exam

Assessment: Normal growth and development for age

Plan: RTO 1 month

a. What is the age of the patient? _____

b. What is the reason for the encounter? _____ _____

c. Were any abnormal conditions found? _____ _____

3. OFFICE   Gender: F   DOB: 4/10/yy

Reason for encounter: Neonatal checkup, 13 days old

Assessment: Neonatal diabetes

Plan: Start on sulfonylurea therapy and see how she does. Insulin may not be required. RTO 2 weeks.

a. What is the age of the patient? _____

b. What is the reason for the encounter? _____ _____

c. Were any abnormal conditions found? _____ _____

4. INPATIENT HOSPITAL   Gender: M   DOB: 4/5/yy

Reason for encounter: Admitted for observation from Emergency Department where mother stated she found the baby not breathing

Assessment: No respiratory effort for 15 seconds, resulting in slight cyanosis and bradycardia times one at home and the first hour of observation. After 6 hours of observation determined to be d/t central sleep apnea

Plan: Discharged 18 days after birth. Use sleep apnea monitor and alarm

a. What is the age of the patient? _____

b. What is the reason for the encounter? _____ _____

c. What condition is documented? _____

d. What is the subtype of the condition? _____ _____

e. What complications and comorbidities exist? _____ _____

f. Is the condition documented as originating in the perinatal period? _____

(continued)

CODING PRACTICE (continued)

5. INPATIENT HOSPITAL Gender: M DOB: 4/20/yy

Birth Weight: 3200g EGA: 39+6

Type: Forceps delivery POB: Hospital

Assessment: Admitted to NICU for observation due to fetal bradycardia during labor

Plan: D/c in excellent condition, RTO 2 weeks

a. Was the infant born in this hospital during this admission? _____

b. Was the delivery vaginal or cesarean? _____

c. What is the birth weight? _____

d. What is the estimated gestational age at time of delivery? _____

e. Are any conditions documented as due to prematurity? _____

f. Did the infant suffer any birth trauma? _____

g. What conditions of the newborn required evaluation, treatment, extended LOS, or increased care or present implications for future healthcare needs? _____

h. What maternal conditions affected the infant? _____

6. INPATIENT HOSPITAL Gender: F DOB: 4/21/yy

Birth Weight: 3756g EGA: 43+3 Type: NSVD

Location: Born in car on way to hospital, then admitted, mother reports discolored amniotic fluid

Assessment: Meconium aspiration d/t late delivery with dyspnea and tachypnea, orotracheal intubation x 1 day, O_2 x 2 days, Rx antibiotics prophylactically

Plan: D/c in good condition, RTO 2 weeks

a. Was the infant born in this hospital during this admission? _____

b. Was the infant born outside the hospital then hospitalized? _____

c. Was the delivery vaginal or cesarean? _____

d. What is the birth weight? _____

e. What is the estimated gestational age at time of delivery? _____

(continued)

6. (continued)

f. Are any conditions documented as due to prematurity? _____

g. Did the infant suffer any birth trauma? _____

h. What maternal conditions affected the infant? _____

i. What conditions of the newborn required evaluation, treatment, extended LOS, increased care, or present implications for future healthcare needs? _____

j. What is the subtype of the condition? _____

7. INPATIENT HOSPITAL Gender: F DOB: 4/12/yy

Birth Weight: 2016g EGA: 35+5

Type: NSVD POB: Hospital

Reason for admission: Infant was readmitted 2 days post-discharge from physician office d/t hyperbilirubinemia of prematurity

Assessment: Jaundice d/t preterm delivery, resolved with phototherapy

Plan: Discharged 12 days after birth. FU in office 2 days

a. Was the infant born in this hospital during this admission? _____

b. Was the delivery vaginal or cesarean? _____

c. What is the birth weight? _____

d. What is the estimated gestational age at time of delivery? _____

e. Are any conditions documented as due to prematurity? _____

f. Did the infant suffer any birth trauma? _____

g. What conditions of the newborn required evaluation, treatment, extended LOS, or increased care or present implications for future healthcare needs? _____

(continued)

8. INPATIENT HOSPITAL   Gender: F   DOB: 4/2/yy

Birth Weight: 1923g   EGA: 37+2   Type: cesarean

POB: Hospital

Reason for admission: Transferred from another hospital on 4/3/yy for supervision of weight gain

Assessment: SGA and fetal growth restriction due to maternal preeclampsia and smoking during pregnancy

a. Was the infant born in this hospital during this admission? _____

b. Was the delivery vaginal or cesarean? _____

c. What is the birth weight? _____

d. What is the estimated gestational age at time of delivery? _____

e. Are any conditions documented as due to prematurity? _____

f. Did the infant suffer any birth trauma? _____

g. What maternal conditions affected the infant? _____

h. What conditions of the newborn required evaluation, treatment, extended LOS, or increased care or present implications for future healthcare needs? _____

9. OFFICE   Gender: M   DOB: 4/2/yy

Reason for encounter: Foul smelling urine

Assessment: UTI d/t E. coli (NSTEC)

Plan: Admit to hospital for IV antibiotics

(continued)

9. (continued)

a. What is the age of the patient? _____

b. What is the reason for the encounter? _____

c. What condition is documented? _____

d. What is the subtype of the condition? _____

e. What complications and comorbidities exist? _____

f. Is the condition documented as originating in the perinatal period? _____

10. OFFICE   Gender: F   DOB: 4/20/yy

Reason for encounter: First newborn check at 4 days old, baby was born at home with CNM in attendance

Assessment: Breast engorgement d/t maternal hormones which will resolve on its own. No problems with jaundice.

Plan: RTO 2 weeks

a. What is the age of the patient? _____

b. What is the reason for the encounter? _____

c. What condition is documented? _____

d. What is the subtype of the condition? _____

e. What complications and comorbidities exist? _____

f. Is the condition documented as originating in the perinatal period? _____

ASSIGNING CODES FOR PERINATAL CONDITIONS

To assign codes for newborns, coders must learn how to assign codes for birth status and for specific medical conditions. ICD-10-CM also provides separate codes for newborn medical examinations.

Assigning Codes for Newborn Birth Status

The **newborn birth status** code identifies the location of the birth, the delivery method, and the number of multiples. Assign this code to each infant only once and only when the hospital stay includes the birth episode. The exception is when an infant is born outside the hospital then hospitalized; in that instance, a birth status code should also be assigned. When a discharge includes the birth episode, assign a code from category **Z38.- Liveborn infants according to place of birth and type of delivery**. When a newborn is transferred from another hospital, the hospital where the infant was born reports a code from **Z38.-**. A birth status code should not be reported by the receiving hospital (OGCR I.C.16.a.2)).

Locate the newborn birth status code for singletons in the Index under the Main Term **Newborn**, subterm **born** (■ FIGURE 23-5). For multiple births, locate the Main Term **Newborn**, then the subterm for **twin**, **triplet**, **quadruplet**, or

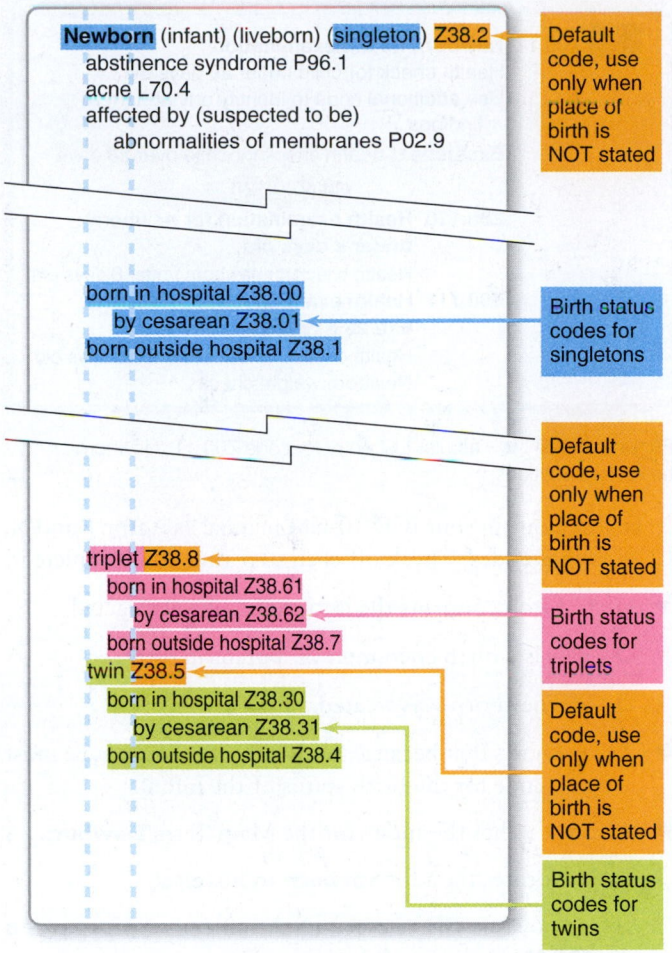

Figure 23-5 ■ Index entries for newborn birth status codes.

quintuplet. Each of these subterms has additional subterms for **born in hospital** and **by cesarean**. Always verify the code in the Tabular List.

Do not confuse category **Z38**, which is for use on the newborn record, with category **Z37 Outcome of delivery**, which is for use on the **mother's** record. Even though both categories have similar code titles, they exist for different purposes. An instructional note at the beginning of each category in the Tabular List clearly defines the respective use and intended purpose.

SUCCESS STEP

Highlight, flag, or draw an icon in your coding manual to remind yourself that **Z37.-** is for the mother and **Z38.-** is for the newborn. Mixing up these two code categories is a common mistake of new coders.

Assigning Codes for Newborn Conditions

Most codes for medical conditions of the newborn are indexed under the Main Term **Newborn**. The subterm **affected by** means to report the code *only* when the newborn is specifically affected by a condition. For example, when an infant is delivered with forceps assistance, assign a code only if the delivery method *affected* the infant. Do not automatically assign a code for forceps delivery to report the *fact* that forceps were used.

The subterm **maternal** describes the effect on the newborn of a condition the mother had during pregnancy, labor, or delivery. For example, when a newborn is affected by the mother's gestational diabetes (GDM), assign a code for **Newborn, affected by, maternal diabetes**. Be aware of the following distinctions among maternal and newborn codes:

- Do *not* assign code **O24.419 Gestational diabetes** to the newborn. This code is for use only with the mother.

- Assign code **P70.0 Syndrome of infant of mother with gestational diabetes** (■ FIGURE 23-6) when the newborn is affected by maternal GDM.

- When the mother has GDM but the newborn is *not* affected by it, do not assign code **P70.0** because the newborn is not affected.

When a code cannot be located under the Main Term **Newborn**, search under the name of the condition itself. Many conditions have a subterm specifically for the newborn, so be certain to review the subterms carefully to locate the appropriate entry (■ FIGURE 23-7). The subterm **transitory** under a newborn condition means that the condition was temporary, as many newborn conditions are.

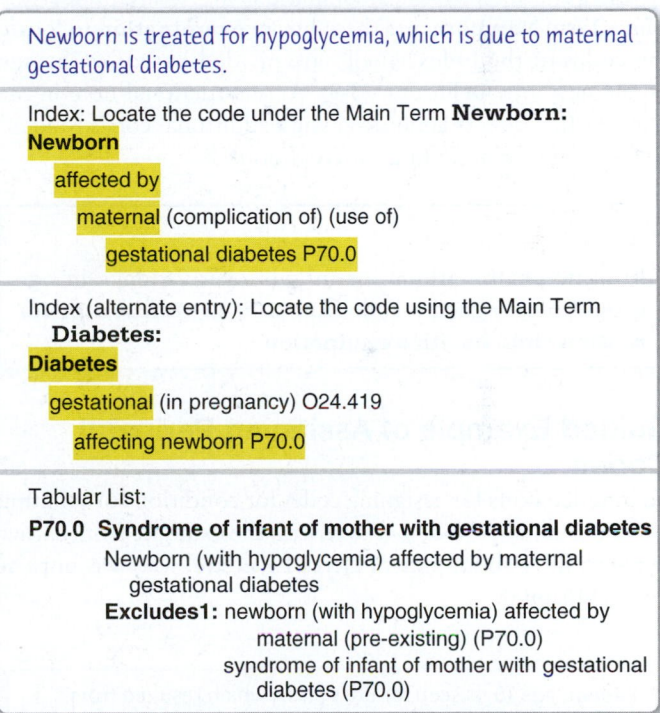

Figure 23-6 ■ Example of assigning codes for an infant affected by a maternal condition.

Newborn is treated for respiratory distress syndrome II.

Respiratory — *see also* condition
   distress syndrome (newborn) (type I) P22.0
      type II P22.1
   syncytial virus, as cause of disease classified elsewhere B97.4

Figure 23-7 ■ Example of locating a newborn code under the main term for the condition.

When a condition that originated during the perinatal period is diagnosed or treated later in life, assign a perinatal code to identify the perinatal origin (OGCR I.C.16.a.4)) (■ FIGURE 23-8).

Some conditions of newborns either can be due to the birth process or be a community-acquired disease. When the documentation does not specify the cause of the condition, the default is to code it as perinatal and to assign a code from ICD-10-CM Chapter 16. When the condition is documented as community acquired, do not assign a code from Chapter 16 (OGCR I.C.16.a.5)).

When a newborn is evaluated for a suspected condition not found after study, assign a **Z** code from category **Z05 Encounter for observation and evaluation of newborn for suspected diseases and conditions ruled out.** Codes from this category can be assigned as a principal or first-listed diagnosis code for readmissions or encounters after the birth episode. Do not assign codes from **Z05** when the patient shows signs and symptoms or a condition has been confirmed. Use codes for the signs, symptoms, or condition for such patients (OGCR I.C.16.b).

Assigning Codes for Neonatal Examinations

Routine neonatal examinations are reported with **Z** codes, just as other routine physical examinations are. Search under the Main Term **Newborn** and the subterm **examination** to locate the codes in the Index. Codes are divided based on the age of the newborn (■ FIGURE 23-9). An instructional note in the Tabular List directs coders to assign additional codes to identify any abnormal findings or conditions.

SUCCESS STEP

Routine examinations for infants over 28 days in age should be assigned a code from **Z00.12- Encounter for routine child health examination.**

Guided Example of Assigning Perinatal Codes

To practice skills for assigning codes for conditions originating in the perinatal period, continue with the example from earlier in the chapter about patient Derek Leverette, who was born at Valley Hospital.

Patient, age 15, is seen for Erb's palsy, which resulted from damage during birth.

Index:
Erb's
    disease G71.02
    palsy, paralysis (brachial) (birth) (newborn) P14.0
       spinal (spastic) syphilitic A52.17
    pseudohypertrophic muscular dystrophy G71.0

Tabular List:
P14.0 Erb's paralysis due to birth injury

Figure 23-8 ■ Example of assigning a code for a perinatal condition later in life.

6th Z00.11 **Newborn health examination**
Health check for child under 29 days old
Use additional code to identify any abnormal findings
Excludes1: health check for child over 28 days old (Z00.12-)
    Z00.110 **Health examination for newborn under 8 days old**
       Health check for newborn under 8 days old
    Z00.111 **Health examination for newborn 8 to 28 days old**
       Health check for newborn 8 to 28 days old
       Newborn weight check

Figure 23-9 ■ Tabular List entry for code Z00.11 "Newborn health examination".

Follow along in your ICD-10-CM manual as Aaron Randell, CCS, assigns codes. Check off each step after you complete it.

▶ First, Aaron confirms the information he abstracted.

❏ This is a birth encounter of a preterm birth.

❏ The newborn was treated for TTN.

▶ Aaron knows that because this is a birth encounter, he must assign a code for the birth status of the infant.

▶ Aaron searches the Index for the Main Term **Newborn**.

❏ He locates the subterm **born in hospital**.

❏ He locates the second-level subterm **by cesarean Z38.01**.

▶ Aaron verifies code **Z38.01** in the Tabular List.

❏ He reads the code title for **Z38.01 Single liveborn infant, delivered by cesarean** and confirms that this accurately describes the birth.

▶ Aaron checks for instructional notes in the Tabular List.

❏ He cross-references the beginning of category **Z38** and reads the instructional note that tells him that this is the correct code for a newborn and it should never be assigned to the mother (■ FIGURE 23-10).

4th Z38 **Liveborn infants according to place of birth and type of delivery**
    NOTE: This category is for use as the principal code on the initial record of a newborn baby. It is to be used for the initial birth record only. It is not to be used on the mother's record.

5th Z38.0 **Single liveborn infant, born in hospital**
    Single liveborn infant, born in birthing center or other health care facility
    Z38.00 **Single liveborn infant, delivered vaginally**
    Z38.01 **Single liveborn infant, delivered by cesarean**

Figure 23-10 ■ Tabular List instructional note for category Z38 "Liveborn infants according to place of birth and type of delivery".

❏ He cross-references the beginning of block **Z30-Z39** and verifies that there are no instructional notes.

❏ He cross-references the beginning of Chapter 21 (Z00-Z99) and reviews the instructional notes, which provide a general description about the use of Z codes. He determines there is no information that applies specifically to this code.

▶ Next, Aaron decides to assign a code for TTN.

▶ Aaron searches the Index for the Main Term **Tachypnea**.

❏ He locates the subterm **newborn P22.1**.

▶ Aaron verifies code **P22.1** in the Tabular List.

❏ He reads the code title for **P22.1 Transient tachypnea of newborn** and confirms that this accurately describes the diagnosis.

▶ Aaron checks for instructional notes in the Tabular List.

❏ He cross-references the beginning of category **P22** and reads the **Excludes1** note. He determines that it does not apply because neither of the conditions excluded are documented for this patient.

❏ He cross-references the beginning of block **P19-P29** and verifies that there are no instructional notes.

❏ He cross-references the beginning of Chapter 16 (P00-P99) and reads the instructional notes. They confirm that codes in this chapter should be used on the newborn's record.

▶ The next code Aaron decides to assign is for the preterm birth.

▶ Aaron searches the Index for the Main Term **Preterm** (■ Figure 23-11).

❏ He locates a subterm **delivery O60.10**.

❏ He reviews the remaining subterm and also locates subterm **newborn P07.30**.

❏ He notices that the codes are from different chapters because they begin with different letters. He decides to check the Tabular List for each code.

❏ He verifies the code title for **O60.10 Preterm labor with preterm delivery, unspecified trimester**.

❏ When he cross-references the beginning of the chapter, he learns that this code is from Chapter 15 "Pregnancy, Childbirth, and the Puerperium (O00-O9A)."

❏ He reads the instructional note in capital letters under the chapter title that states **CODES FROM THIS CHAPTER ARE FOR USE ONLY ON MATERNAL RECORDS, NEVER ON NEWBORN RECORDS**.

❏ This instruction tells him that he should *not* use **O60.10** because he is coding for the newborn, not the mother.

❏ Aaron returns to the Index to review the entries for the Main Term **Preterm** and subterm **newborn**.

❏ He locates a second-level subterm **gestational age**.

❏ He locates the third-level subterm **34 completed weeks (34 weeks, 0 days through 34 weeks, 6 days) P07.37**. He believes this code describes the preterm newborn of gestational age 34 weeks, which is documented in the medical record.

▶ Aaron verifies code **P07.37** in the Tabular List.

❏ He reads the code title for **P07.37, Preterm newborn, gestational age 34 completed weeks**, and confirms that this accurately describes the length of gestation.

▶ Aaron checks for instructional notes in the Tabular List.

❏ He cross-references the beginning of category **P07** and reads the instructional notes, which direct him to assign a code for birth weight in addition to gestational age. The note also provides sequencing instructions (■ Figure 23-12, page 418).

❏ He reads the code selections for low birth weight under subcategories **P07.0** and **P07.1**. He locates the code **P07.17, Other low birth weight newborn, 1750-1999 grams**, which includes the birth weight of this baby, 1790 grams.

❏ He continues cross-referencing and checks the beginning of the block **P05-P08**. He verifies that there are no instructional notes for this block.

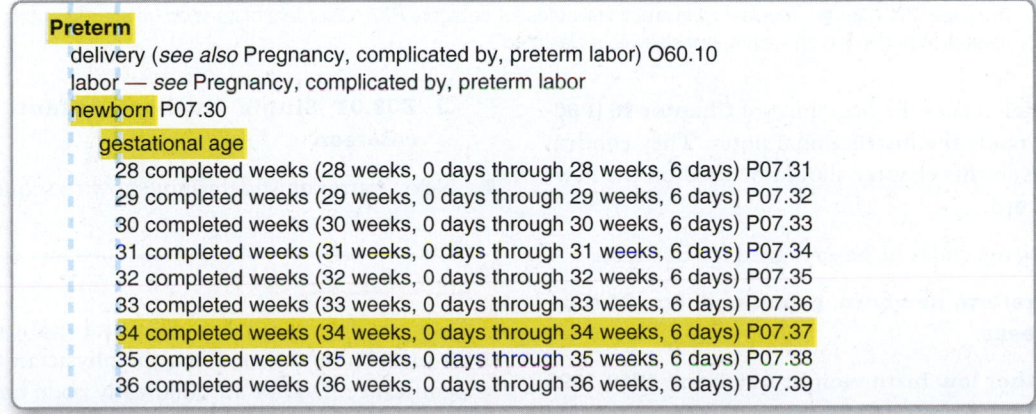

Preterm
delivery (*see also* Pregnancy, complicated by, preterm labor) O60.10
labor — *see* Pregnancy, complicated by, preterm labor
newborn P07.30
gestational age
28 completed weeks (28 weeks, 0 days through 28 weeks, 6 days) P07.31
29 completed weeks (29 weeks, 0 days through 29 weeks, 6 days) P07.32
30 completed weeks (30 weeks, 0 days through 30 weeks, 6 days) P07.33
31 completed weeks (31 weeks, 0 days through 31 weeks, 6 days) P07.34
32 completed weeks (32 weeks, 0 days through 32 weeks, 6 days) P07.35
33 completed weeks (33 weeks, 0 days through 33 weeks, 6 days) P07.36
34 completed weeks (34 weeks, 0 days through 34 weeks, 6 days) P07.37
35 completed weeks (35 weeks, 0 days through 35 weeks, 6 days) P07.38
36 completed weeks (36 weeks, 0 days through 36 weeks, 6 days) P07.39

Figure 23-11 ■ Index entry for "Preterm".

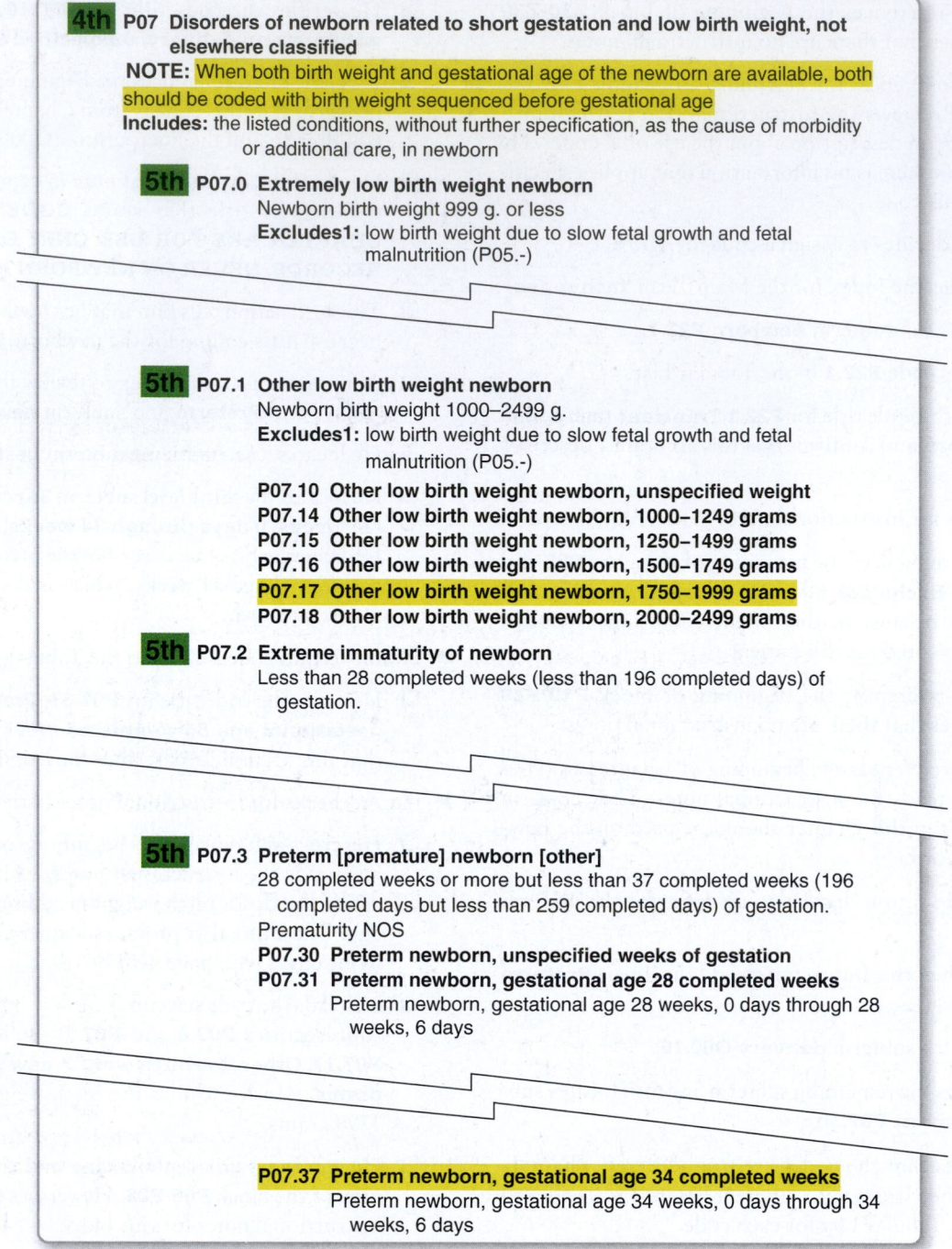

4th P07 **Disorders of newborn related to short gestation and low birth weight, not elsewhere classified**
NOTE: When both birth weight and gestational age of the newborn are available, both should be coded with birth weight sequenced before gestational age
Includes: the listed conditions, without further specification, as the cause of morbidity or additional care, in newborn

5th P07.0 **Extremely low birth weight newborn**
Newborn birth weight 999 g. or less
Excludes1: low birth weight due to slow fetal growth and fetal malnutrition (P05.-)

5th P07.1 **Other low birth weight newborn**
Newborn birth weight 1000–2499 g.
Excludes1: low birth weight due to slow fetal growth and fetal malnutrition (P05.-)
P07.10 **Other low birth weight newborn, unspecified weight**
P07.14 **Other low birth weight newborn, 1000–1249 grams**
P07.15 **Other low birth weight newborn, 1250–1499 grams**
P07.16 **Other low birth weight newborn, 1500–1749 grams**
P07.17 **Other low birth weight newborn, 1750–1999 grams**
P07.18 **Other low birth weight newborn, 2000–2499 grams**

5th P07.2 **Extreme immaturity of newborn**
Less than 28 completed weeks (less than 196 completed days) of gestation.

5th P07.3 **Preterm [premature] newborn [other]**
28 completed weeks or more but less than 37 completed weeks (196 completed days but less than 259 completed days) of gestation.
Prematurity NOS
P07.30 **Preterm newborn, unspecified weeks of gestation**
P07.31 **Preterm newborn, gestational age 28 completed weeks**
Preterm newborn, gestational age 28 weeks, 0 days through 28 weeks, 6 days

P07.37 **Preterm newborn, gestational age 34 completed weeks**
Preterm newborn, gestational age 34 weeks, 0 days through 34 weeks, 6 days

Figure 23-12 ■ Tabular List instructional notes for category P07 "Disorders of newborn related to short gestation and low birth weight, not elsewhere classified".

❑ He cross-references the beginning of **Chapter 16 (P00-P99)** and reads the instructional notes. They confirm that codes in this chapter should be used on the newborn's record.

▶ Aaron reviews the codes he has assigned for this case.

❑ **P07.37 Preterm newborn, gestational age 34 completed weeks**

❑ **P07.17 Other low birth weight newborn, 1750-1999 grams**

❑ **P22.1 Transient tachypnea of newborn**

❑ **Z38.01 Single liveborn infant, delivered by cesarean**

▶ Next, Aaron must determine how to sequence the codes.

SUCCESS STEP

Assign codes for birth weight and gestational age *only* for preterm infants or when the physician documents the significance. Do not automatically code birth weight and gestational age for every baby.

CODING PRACTICE

Exercise 23.3   Assigning Codes for Perinatal Conditions

Instructions: Read the mini-medical-record of each patient's encounter, review the information abstracted in Exercise 23.2, and assign ICD-10-CM diagnosis codes using the Index and Tabular List. Write the code(s) on the line provided.

---

1. INPATIENT HOSPITAL   Gender: F   DOB: 4/22/yy

Birth Weight: 3521g   EGA: 38+2   Type: NSVD

POB: Hospital

Assessment: APGARS 6, 8

Plan: Discharged 1 day after birth. FU in office 2 weeks

Tip: Apgar scores of 6 (one minute after delivery) and 8 (five minutes after delivery) are considered normal.

1 ICD-10-CM Code _____

---

2. OFFICE   Gender: F   DOB: 4/1/yy

Reason for encounter: Routine newborn exam, 4 days

Assessment: Normal growth and development for age

Plan: RTO 1 month

1 ICD-10-CM Code _____

---

3. OFFICE   Gender: F   DOB: 4/10/yy

Reason for encounter: Neonatal checkup, 13 days old

Assessment: Neonatal diabetes

(continued)

---

3. (continued)

Plan: Start on sulfonylurea therapy and see how she does. Insulin may not be required. RTO 2 weeks.

Tip: A checkup is the same as an examination.

2 ICD-10-CM Codes _____

---

4. INPATIENT HOSPITAL   Gender: M   DOB: 4/5/yy

Reason for encounter: Admitted for observation from Emergency Department where mother stated she found the baby not breathing

Assessment: No respiratory effort for 15 seconds, resulting in slight cyanosis and bradycardia times one at home and the first hour of observation. After 6 hours of observation determined to be d/t central sleep apnea.

Plan: Discharged 18 days after birth. Use sleep apnea monitor and alarm at home.

1 ICD-10-CM Code _____

---

5. INPATIENT HOSPITAL   Gender: M   DOB: 4/20/yy

Birth Weight: 3200g   EGA: 39+6

Type: Forceps delivery   POB: Hospital

Assessment: Admitted to NICU for observation due to fetal bradycardia during labor

Plan: D/c in excellent condition, RTO 2 weeks

Tip: Forceps are used only in a vaginal delivery.

2 ICD-10-CM Codes _____

ARRANGING CODES FOR PERINATAL CONDITIONS

Significant perinatal sequencing guidelines relate to selecting the principal diagnosis for the birth episode, assigning codes for the weight and EGA of preterm infants, and sequencing codes for bacterial newborn sepsis.

Selecting the Principal Diagnosis for Birth Encounters

The previous section of this chapter discussed assigning a code from category **Z38** to identify the birth status on a newborn's record. This code is assigned only for hospital admissions that

include the delivery or occur immediately after a birth outside the hospital. Sequence codes as follows:

1. **Z38.-** is *always* sequenced as the principal diagnosis on a newborn's record (OGCR I.C.16.a.2)). This is true regardless of any other conditions or complications that accompany the birth.

2. Sequence additional codes for any conditions that require observation (OGCR I.C.21.c.6)) treatment, further workup, or prolong length of stay or require resource utilization (OGCR I.C.16.c.1)). Conditions that require

current treatment or workup should be sequenced based on their significance according to the provider.

3. Finally, sequence conditions documented as having implications for future healthcare needs (OGCR I.C.16.c.2)).

> ### CODING CAUTION
>
> Conditions not treated but documented as having implications for future healthcare needs should be coded only for newborns, never for adults.

Arranging Codes for Birth Weight and Estimated Gestational Age

A preterm infant may have difficulties due to short gestation or low birth weight. A postterm infant may be at risk for diabetes or other conditions. Assign codes that identify the birth weight and the EGA of the infant when these factors are documented to affect the infant's health status. Also assign codes for any specified conditions. For admissions that include the birth encounter, sequence the codes as follows (OGCR I.C.16.d and e):

1. **Z38.-** Birth status of infant, if the admission includes the birth episode

2. **P07.0-** or **P07.1-** Birth weight (Search the Index for the Main Term **Low**, subterm **birth weight**.) Birth weight should always be sequenced before EGA, but weight is never the principal diagnosis.

3. **P07.2-** or **P07.3-** Weeks of gestation (Search the Index for the Main Term **Preterm**, subterm **newborn**, second-level subterm **gestational age** for 28–36 completed weeks of gestation, or the Main Term **Immaturity**, subterm **extreme of newborn**, second-level subterm **gestational age** for 17–27 completed weeks of gestation.)

4. Other specified conditions

For admissions that do not include the birth encounter, select the principal diagnosis based on the standard criteria in OGCR II.

A full-term or preterm infant may be small for its age due to slow fetal growth or malnutrition. Assign a code from **P05.- Disorders of newborn related to slow fetal growth and fetal malnutrition** in these situations. When you assign a code from **P05**, do *not* assign codes from **P07** for birth weight and EGA.

A postterm infant may be at risk due to being large for its age. Assign a code from **P08 Disorders of newborn related to long gestation and high birth weight** in these situations.

Arranging Codes for Bacterial Newborn Sepsis

Coding bacterial sepsis of a newborn is similar to coding any patient with sepsis, as discussed in Chapter 20 of this text and ICD-10-CM Chapter 1, "Certain Infectious and Parasitic Diseases (A00-B49)." One difference is that perinatal sepsis may be congenital or community acquired. When the source is not documented, the default is congenital and a newborn sepsis code should be assigned (OGCR I.C.16.f). Category **P36 Bacterial sepsis of newborn** provides combination codes that include the most common causal organisms (■ FIGURE 23-13). If the appropriate causal organism is not included in the **P36.-** code,

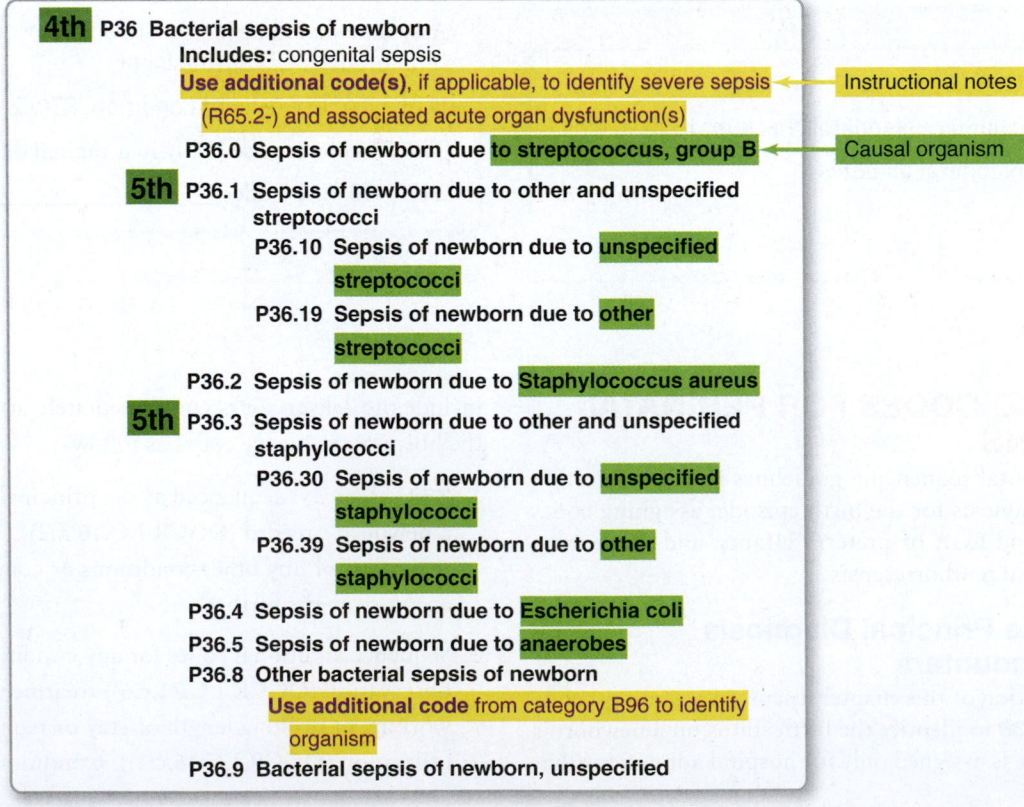

Figure 23-13 ■ Tabular List entry for category P36 "Bacterial sepsis of newborn".

then assign an additional code from category **B96**. Assign and sequence codes as follows:

1. Assign a code from **P36.- Bacterial sepsis of newborn**.

2. If the causal organism is *not* provided in a combination code, assign a code from **B96 Other bacterial agents as the cause of diseases classified elsewhere**.

3. When severe sepsis or septic shock is documented, assign a code from **R65.2- Severe sepsis**.

4. Assign codes for associated acute organ dysfunction(s).

Guided Example of Arranging Perinatal Codes

To practice skills for sequencing codes for diseases of the conditions originating in the perinatal period, continue with the example from earlier in the chapter about patient Derek Leverette, who was born at Valley Hospital.

Follow along in your ICD-10-CM manual as Aaron Randell, CCS, sequences the codes. Check off each step after you complete it.

▶ First, Aaron reviews the codes he assigned.

❏ **P07.37 Preterm newborn, gestational age 34 completed weeks**

❏ **P07.17 Other low birth weight newborn, 1750-1999 grams**

❏ **P22.1 Transient tachypnea of newborn**

❏ **Z38.01 Single liveborn infant, delivered by cesarean**

▶ Aaron refers to OGCR I.C.16.a.2), Principal Diagnosis for the Birth Record.

❏ The OGCR states that a code from **Z38** should be the principal diagnosis for the birth episode. This enables Aaron to determine that the first code should be **Z38.01**.

▶ Aaron refers to OGCR I.C.16.d, Prematurity and Fetal Growth Retardation.

❏ This OGCR states that codes should be assigned based on the documented birth weight and gestational age. It also states that the code for birth weight should be sequenced before the code for gestational age. He also recalls that he read an instructional note under category **P07** with the same information.

❏ Based on this information, Aaron determines that **P07.17** should be the second code and **P07.37** should be the third code.

❏ This leaves **P22.1** as the final code. Aaron checks the notes he wrote earlier to be certain that there are no instructional notes that affect the sequencing of this code.

▶ Aaron finalizes the codes and sequencing for this case:

(1) **Z38.01 Single liveborn infant, delivered by cesarean**

(2) **P07.17 Other low birth weight newborn, 1750-1999 grams**

(3) **P07.37 Preterm newborn, gestational age 34 completed weeks**

(4) **P22.1 Transient tachypnea of newborn**

CODING PRACTICE

Exercise 23.4   Arranging Codes for Perinatal Conditions

Instructions: Read the mini-medical-record of each patient's encounter, review the information abstracted in Exercise 23.2, assign ICD-10-CM diagnosis codes using the Index and Tabular List, and sequence them correctly.

---

1. INPATIENT HOSPITAL   Gender: F   DOB: 4/21/yy

Birth Weight: 3756g   EGA: 43+3   Type: NSVD

Location: Born in car on way to hospital, then admitted, mother reports discolored amniotic fluid

Assessment: Meconium aspiration d/t late delivery with dyspnea and tachypnea, orotracheal intubation x 1 day, O₂ x 2 days, Rx antibiotics prophylactically

Plan: D/c in good condition, RTO 2 weeks

Tip: Meconium-related problems are most common with prolonged gestations.

3 ICD-10-CM Codes _____

_____

---

2. INPATIENT HOSPITAL   Gender: F   DOB: 4/12/yy

Birth Weight: 2016g   EGA: 35+5   Type: NSVD

POB: Hospital

Reason for admission: Infant was readmitted 2 days post-discharge from physician office d/t hyperbilirubinemia of prematurity

Assessment: Jaundice d/t preterm delivery, resolved with phototherapy

Plan: Discharged 12 days after birth. FU in office 2 days

3 ICD-10-CM Codes _____

_____

(continued)

CODING PRACTICE (continued)

3. INPATIENT HOSPITAL Gender: F DOB: 4/2/yy

Birth Weight: 1923g EGA: 37+2 Type: Cesarean

POB: Hospital

Reason for admission: Transferred from another hospital on 4/3/yy for supervision of weight gain

Assessment: SGA and fetal growth restriction due to maternal preeclampsia and smoking during pregnancy

Tip: The term *intrauterine growth restriction* has largely replaced the older term *intrauterine growth retardation*. You also need to determine what type of condition preeclampsia is.

4 ICD-10-CM Codes _____

_____

4. OFFICE Gender: M DOB: 4/2/yy

Reason for encounter: Foul-smelling urine

Assessment: UTI d/t E. coli (NSTEC)

Plan: Admit to hospital for IV antibiotics

2 ICD-10-CM Codes _____

5. OFFICE Gender: F DOB: 4/20/yy

Reason for encounter: First newborn check at 4 days old, baby was born at home with CNM in attendance

Assessment: Breast engorgement d/t maternal hormones, which will resolve on its own. No problems with jaundice.

Plan: RTO 2 weeks

2 ICD-10-CM Codes _____

CHAPTER SUMMARY

In this chapter you learned that:

- The perinatal period begins before birth and continues through the 28th day following birth.

- ICD-10-CM provides Official Guidelines for Coding and Reporting (OGCR) in OGCR I.C.16 regarding selecting the principal and additional diagnoses and how to report codes from this chapter with those from other chapters; also discusses prematurity, low birth weight, bacterial sepsis of the newborn, stillbirth, and observation and evaluation of newborns for suspected conditions not found.

- Coders must take note whether a hospitalization of a newborn includes the birth itself or whether the admission takes place after the birth episode.

- To assign codes for newborns, coders must learn how to assign codes for birth status, for specific medical conditions, and for newborn examinations.

- Significant sequencing guidelines relate to selecting the principal diagnosis for the birth episode, assigning codes for the weight and EGA of preterm infants, and sequencing codes for bacterial newborn sepsis.

CONCEPT QUIZ

Take a moment to look back at conditions originating in the perinatal period and solidify your skills. Try to answer the questions from memory first, then look back at the discussion in this chapter if you need a little extra help.

Completion

Instructions: Write the term that completes each statement based on the information you learned in this chapter. Choose from the list below. Some choices may be used more than once and some choices may not be used at all.

1,000	Erb's palsy
1,500	LBW
2,000	LGA
2,500	MAS
4,000	meconium peritonitis
amin/o	neonate
ammon/o	omphalitis
amni/o	perinatal
amnionitis	transitory
birth trauma	VLBW

1. A newborn with a birth weight of 2,200 grams is classified as _____.

2. Normal birth weight is defined as _____ to _____ grams.

3. _____ is a condition in which the newborn breathes a mixture of meconium and amniotic fluid into the lungs prior to or during delivery.

4. A fetus or newborn infant who is larger in size than normal for the baby's sex and gestational age is classified as _____.

5. _____ is any physical injury to the infant during delivery.

6. _____ is infection of the umbilical stump in a newborn.

7. A _____ perinatal condition is temporary.

8. _____ describes an infant during the first 28 days of life.

9. _____ is the combining form for amniotic sac.

10. _____ grams equals 5 pounds, 8 ounces.

Multiple Choice

Instructions: Circle the letter of the best answer to each question based on the information you learned in this chapter.

1. What is the time frame for the perinatal period?
   A. It begins 28 days before birth and continues through the 28th day after birth
   B. It begins 28 days before birth and continues through birth
   C. It begins before birth and continues through the 28th day after birth
   D. It begins at birth and continues through the 28th day after birth

2. Which of the criteria for "clinically significant conditions" is used *only* for newborns?
   A. A condition that requires clinical evaluation
   B. A condition that increases nursing care or monitoring
   C. A condition that extends length of hospital stay
   D. A condition that presents implications for future healthcare needs

3. How would you code the newborn's birth record in the following scenario? *A full-term infant is born in the hospital with normal vaginal delivery and no complications.*
   A. O80
   B. Z34.03
   C. Z37.0
   D. Z38.00

4. What are perinatal conditions?
   A. Conditions diagnosed during the first 28 days
   B. Conditions that originated before birth or during the first 28 days
   C. Conditions that were treated during the first 28 days
   D. Conditions in the infant that result from a condition of the mother

5. Which of the following conditions is a perinatal condition of the infant?
   A. Meconium aspiration syndrome
   B. Missed abortion
   C. Preeclampsia
   D. Gestational diabetes

6. What term describes the permanent abnormal shape of an organ or body region, resulting from arrested, delayed, or abnormal development of the embryo?
   A. Deformation
   B. Malformation
   C. Chromosomal abnormality
   D. Erb's palsy

7. How would you code the newborn's birth record in the following scenario? *A newborn is treated for bacterial sepsis due to Staphylococcus aureus with septic shock and acute respiratory dysfunction with hypoxia.*
   A. J96.01, P36.2
   B. R65.21, P36.2, J96.01
   C. P36.2, R65.21, J96.01
   D. P36.2, B95.61, R65.21

8. When should a birth status code from Z38 be reported?
   A. A hospital receives a newborn from another hospital
   B. The hospital stay includes the birth episode
   C. A fetus is stillborn
   D. A newborn is readmitted within 28 days of birth

9. How would you code the newborn's birth record in the following scenario? *A newborn is treated for hypoglycemia, which is due to maternal gestational diabetes that was controlled with diet.*
   A. O24.410
   B. E08.9, P70.0
   C. P70.0, O24.410
   D. P70.0

10. What information does a birth status code from Z38 describe?
    A. Weight
    B. Gender
    C. Delivery method
    D. Gestational age

KEEP ON CODING

Instructions: Read the diagnostic statement, then use the Index and Tabular List to assign and sequence ICD-10-CM diagnosis codes. Write the code(s) on the line provided.

1. Transient neonatal myasthenia gravis. ICD-10-CM Code(s) _____

2. Subdural hematoma due to birth injury. ICD-10-CM Code(s) _____

3. Newborn small for date, 1,150 grams. ICD-10-CM Code(s) _____

4. Newborn melena. ICD-10-CM Code(s) _____

5. Congenital pneumonia due to *Pseudomonas*. ICD-10-CM Code(s) _____

6. Postterm newborn, 42 weeks' gestation. ICD-10-CM Code(s) _____

7. Overfeeding of newborn. ICD-10-CM Code(s) _____

8. Neonatal jaundice due to polycythemia. ICD-10-CM Code(s) _____

9. Neonatal craniotabes. ICD-10-CM Code(s) _____

10. Atelectasis of newborn. ICD-10-CM Code(s) _____

11. Transitory ileus of newborn. ICD-10-CM Code(s) _____

12. Neonatal aspiration of blood. ICD-10-CM Code(s) _____

13. Phrenic nerve paralysis due to birth injury. ICD-10-CM Code(s) _____

14. Newborn affected by Cesarean delivery. ICD-10-CM Code(s) _____

15. Preterm newborn, 28 completed weeks. ICD-10-CM Code(s) _____

16. Noninfective neonatal diarrhea. ICD-10-CM Code(s) _____

17. Newborn affected by mother's type 1 diabetes during pregnancy. ICD-10-CM Code(s) _____

18. Neonatal goiter. ICD-10-CM Code(s) _____

19. Anemia of prematurity. ICD-10-CM Code(s) _____

20. Congenital hydrocele. ICD-10-CM Code(s) _____

21. Rh isoimmunization of newborn. ICD-10-CM Code(s) _____

22. Neonatal coma. ICD-10-CM Code(s) _____

23. Cardiac arrest of newborn. ICD-10-CM Code(s) _____

24. Massive umbilical hemorrhage of newborn. ICD-10-CM Code(s) _____

25. Transitory neonatal neutropenia. ICD-10-CM Code(s) _____

CODING CHALLENGE

Instructions: Read the mini-medical-record of each patient's encounter, then abstract, assign, and sequence ICD-10-CM diagnosis codes using the Index and Tabular List. Write the code(s) on the line provided.

1. INPATIENT HOSPITAL   Gender: F   DOB: 4/27/yy

Birth Weight: 4555g   EGA: 40+4   Type: Cesarean

POB: Hospital

Assessment: LGA, watch for diabetes, otherwise healthy

Plan: Discharged 1 day after birth. FU office 2 weeks

2 ICD-10-CM Codes _____

2. INPATIENT HOSPITAL   Gender: M   DOB: 4/28/yy

Birth Weight: 3010g   EGA: 42+0   Type: NSVD

POB: Hospital

Assessment: Postterm, otherwise healthy

Plan: Discharged 1 day after birth. FU office 2 weeks

2 ICD-10-CM Codes _____

3. INPATIENT HOSPITAL   Gender: F   DOB: 4/22/yy

Birth Weight: 1293g   EGA: 30+3   Type: Cesarean

POB: Hospital

Reason for admission: Transferred from another hospital on DOB due to heroin baby

(continued)

3. (continued)

Assessment: Drug withdrawal syndrome complicated by prematurity with underdeveloped lungs

Plan: Discharged 7 days after birth. Weaned off heroin. RTO 3 days post discharge.

Tip: Follow the sequencing rules for poisonings.

4 ICD-10-CM Codes _____

_____

---

4. INPATIENT HOSPITAL   Gender: F   DOB: 4/20/yy

Birth Weight: 3621g   EGA: 39+1   Type: Cesarean

POB: Hospital

Assessment: Hypoglycemia due to GDM, respiratory distress

Plan: Discharged 9 days after birth. FU weekly for first month

4 ICD-10-CM Codes _____

_____

---

5. INPATIENT HOSPITAL   Gender: F   DOB: 4/22/yy

Birth Weight: 3489g   EGA: 38+0   Type: NSVD

POB: Hospital

Assessment: Fractured clavicle during delivery d/t prolapsed arm presentation

Plan: Pin long-sleeved garment to the clothes to immobilize arm if discomfort observed, lift child with care, RTO 1 week

Tip: Discharged 7 days after birth. A prolapsed arm is a malpresentation.

3 ICD-10-CM Codes _____

_____

---

6. INPATIENT HOSPITAL   Gender: M   DOB: 4/15/yy

Reason for encounter: Redness, mild bleeding, and swelling of umbilical stump

Assessment: Omphalitis with hemorrhage

Plan: Begin 2 week regimen of antimicrobial therapy, RTO in one day for reevaluation of condition

1 ICD-10-CM Code _____

---

7. INPATIENT HOSPITAL   Gender: M   DOB: 3/29/yy

Birth Weight: 762g   EGA: 28   Type: NSVD

POB: Hospital

(continued)

---

7. (continued)

Assessment: This infant is the first born of triplets with cardiomyopathy. The second sibling was liveborn with respiratory distress syndrome and jaundice. Fetus 3 stillborn

Plan: Discharged 31 days after birth. RTO 3 days post discharge.

Tip: Each infant has its own record. Code only for the infant who is named on this record.

4 ICD-10-CM Codes _____

_____

---

8. INPATIENT HOSPITAL   Gender: M   DOB: 4/22/yy

Birth Weight: 3256g   EGA: 40+2   Type: NSVD

POB: Hospital

Assessment: Injury to brachial plexus and cannot move arm

Plan: Discharged 7 days after birth. Refer to physical therapist for three months. Reevaluate for reconstructive surgery if no improvement in three months.

2 ICD-10-CM Codes _____

---

9. INPATIENT HOSPITAL   Gender: M   DOB: 4/12/yy

Reason for admission: Admitted on 4/15/yy, 2 days post discharge, with acute respiratory failure d/t severe sepsis

Assessment: Severe sepsis d/t Staphylococcus aureus caused by amnionitis, ARF

Plan: Antibiotic therapy, careful post discharge monitoring, aggressive fluid restoration. RTO 1 week

Tip: Refer to OGCR I.C.16.f.

4 ICD-10-CM Codes _____

_____

---

10. INPATIENT HOSPITAL   Gender: M   DOB: 4/25/yy

Birth Weight: 3185g   EGA: 38+3   Type: NSVD

POB: Hospital

Reason for admission: Transferred from another hospital 6 hours after birth d/t hemolytic disease

Assessment: Transfusion required for hemolytic disease due to ABO isoimmunization

Plan: Discharged 4 days after admission. FU 1 week

1 ICD-10-CM Code _____

Chapter 24

Congenital Malformations, Deformations, and Chromosomal Abnormalities (Q00-Q99)

Chapter Outline

- **Congenital Abnormalities Refresher**
- **Coding Guidelines for Congenital Abnormalities**
- **Abstracting for Congenital Abnormalities**
- **Assigning Codes for Congenital Abnormalities**
- **Arranging Codes for Congenital Abnormalities**

Learning Objectives

After completing this chapter, you should have the skills to:

24.1 Spell and define the key words, medical terms, and abbreviations related to congenital malformations, deformations, and chromosomal abnormalities. (Remember)

24.2 Summarize common congenital malformations, deformations, and chromosomal abnormalities. (Understand)

24.3 Adhere to the Official Guidelines for Coding and Reporting related to congenital malformations, deformations, and chromosomal abnormalities. (Apply)

24.4 Examine and abstract diagnostic information from the medical record for coding congenital malformations, deformations, and chromosomal abnormalities. (Analyze)

24.5 Demonstrate how to assign diagnosis codes for congenital malformations, deformations, and chromosomal abnormalities. (Apply)

24.6 Utilize guidelines for arranging (sequencing) multiple diagnosis codes for congenital malformations, deformations, and chromosomal abnormalities. (Apply)

Key Terms and Abbreviations

abnormal development
anomaly (congenital)
arrested development

chromosomal abnormality
congenital abnormality
deformation

delayed development
malformation (congenital)

In addition to the key terms listed here, students should know the terms defined within tables in this chapter.

INTRODUCTION

Two types of problems with a new vehicle are those due to faulty manufacturing materials and those due to poor workmanship or assembly. Some may be correctable and some may not. Congenital conditions can be thought of in a similar way. Conditions can result from abnormal development of the embryo or physical damage to an anatomical part that developed normally.

In your tour of the congenital malformations, deformations, and chromosomal abnormalities in this chapter you learn more about the types of congenital malformations, deformations, and chromosomal abnormalities, why they arise, and how physicians treat these conditions. For the sake of brevity, this text refers to *congenital malformations*, *deformations*, and *chromosomal abnormalities* as congenital abnormalities. Coders must know the specific differences among these terms. Physicians of any specialty may treat congenital conditions, based on the body system affected.

CONGENITAL ABNORMALITIES REFRESHER

Congenital abnormalities are specific types of perinatal conditions. Both congenital and perinatal conditions originate during pregnancy or the first 28 days of life. Both types of conditions may be diagnosed and treated in utero, during the first 28 days, or at any time later in life. In common usage, the terms are frequently used interchangeably.

In ICD-10-CM, congenital abnormalities include physical malformations, deformations, and chromosomal abnormalities. Conditions that do not meet these definitions are classified as perinatal conditions. A congenital malformation or congenital anomaly is a permanent abnormal shape of an organ or body region, which is due to problems of embryonic development. Malformations may be the result of arrested development, in which embryonic development of a structure stopped before it should have; delayed development, in which embryonic development of a structure started late or progressed slowly; or abnormal development, in which embryonic development of a structure occurred on schedule but took an uncommon physical variation in the womb. Examples of malformations are transposition of the great vessels (aorta and pulmonary artery) and spina bifida.

A deformation or deformity is a change in the size or shape of a normal structure due to extrinsic physical forces, such as intrauterine compression. Examples of deformities are dislocation of the hip and rotational deformities.

A chromosomal abnormality is the abnormal number or structure of chromosomes. Examples are Down syndrome and Prader-Willi syndrome.

As you learn about congenital abnormalities, remember to apply medical terminology skills to combine word roots, prefixes, and suffixes you already know to define new terms. Refer to ■ TABLE 24-1 for a refresher on how to build medical terms related to congenital malformations, deformations, and chromosomal abnormalities.

CODING CAUTION

Be alert for medical terms that are spelled similarly and have different meanings.

hydrocele (*bulge of fluid*) and hydrocephalus (*water or fluid in the head/brain*)

polydactyly (*many fingers or toes*) and syndactyly (*webbed fingers or toes*)

Conditions Related to Congenital Abnormalities

Congenital abnormalities are the leading cause of infant mortality, accounting for 20% of all infant deaths, according to the Centers for Disease Control and Prevention (CDC). Thousands of congenital abnormalities have been identified by physicians. The most common congenital abnormalities are heart defects, cleft lip or cleft palate, and Down syndrome. Certain conditions reflect multiple abnormalities that occur together. For example, tetralogy of Fallot and Shone's syndrome are each a combination of four specific heart abnormalities, but the specific abnormalities are different for each. Although certain congenital abnormalities are known to be caused by genetics, environment, or a combination of both, the cause of more than 70% is unknown, according to the Physicians Committee for Responsible Medicine. Refer to ■ TABLE 24-2, page 428 for a summary of congenital abnormalities.

Table 24-1   ■   **EXAMPLE OF CONSTRUCTING MEDICAL TERMS FOR CONGENITAL ABNORMALITIES**

Prefix/Suffix	Combining Form	Complete Medical Term
a/an- (prefix; *lacking*)		**an + en + cephaly** (*lack of part of the brain*)
en- (prefix; *within*)		**a + tresia** (*lack of an opening*)
micro- (prefix; *small*)	**cephal/o** (*head/brain*)	**micro + cephaly** (*small head*)
	hydr/o (*water*)	**hydro + cephaly** (*water or fluid in the head/brain*)
-cele (suffix; *hernia, bulge*)		**hydro + cele** (*bulge of fluid*)
-tresia (suffix; *opening*)		**en + cephalo + cele** (*hernia in the brain*)

Table 24-2 ■ **COMMON CONGENITAL ABNORMALITIES**

Condition	Definition
Aortic coarctation	A narrowing of the aorta
Cleft lip or palate	A notch or division of the upper lip or roof of the mouth
Developmental dysplasia of the hip (DDH)	Disruption in the normal relationship between the head of the femur and the acetabulum (hip socket)
Down syndrome	A genetic condition in which a person has 47 chromosomes instead of the usual 46; also called *trisomy 21*
Esophageal ring	An abnormal ring of tissue around the esophagus
Hydrocephalus	A buildup of fluid inside the skull
Hydronephrosis	Excessive collection of urine in the kidneys
Hypospadias	A congenital condition in which the opening of the urethra is on the underside, rather than the end, of the penile shaft, and may be located as far down as in the scrotum or perineum
Marfan's syndrome	A genetic disorder of connective tissue characterized by elongated bones and ocular and circulatory defects
Meckel's diverticulum	A congenital bulge in the intestine caused by a remnant of the embryonic yolk stalk
Nonmosaic Down syndrome	The predominant type of Down syndrome, which occurs when there is an extra copy of chromosome 21 in every cell of the body.
Patent foramen ovale	An opening in the septum between the two atria of the heart
Prader-Willi syndrome	A genetic disorder due to a deletion of paternal chromosome 15 and characterized by short stature, intellectual disability, muscle weakness, abnormally small hands and feet, nonfunctioning gonads, and uncontrolled appetite leading to extreme obesity
Rotational deformities	Abnormal position of the femur or tibia
Spina bifida	A birth defect in which the backbone and spinal canal do not close before birth
Tetralogy of Fallot	A congenital heart defect consisting of four malformations: pulmonary stenosis (*obstructed outflow of blood from the right ventricle to the lungs*), ventricle septal defect (VSD) (*an opening between the ventricles*), dextroposition or overriding aorta (*blood from the aorta flowing into both the left and right ventricles*), and hypertrophy (*enlargement*) of the right ventricle
Tongue tie	A condition in which the bottom of the tongue is attached to the floor of the mouth by a band of tissue called the *lingual frenulum*
Transposition of the great vessels	A congenital heart defect in which the aorta and pulmonary artery are switched, preventing pulmonary circulation
Trisomy	A genetic disorder in which a person has three copies, rather than two, of genetic material
Shone's syndrome	A set of four congenital heart defects: a supravalvular mitral membrane (SVMM), parachute mitral valve, subaortic stenosis, and coarctation of the aorta

CODING PRACTICE

Exercise 24.1   Congenital Abnormalities Refresher

Instructions: Use your medical terminology skills and resources to define the following conditions related to congenital malformations, deformations, and chromosomal abnormalities, then assign the default diagnosis code.

Follow these steps:

- Use slash marks "/" to break down each term into its root(s) and suffix.
- Define the meaning of the word, based on the meaning of each word part. When multiple words are listed, define the meaning of the underlined word.
- Assign the default ICD-10-CM diagnosis code for the condition using the Index and Tabular List.

CODING PRACTICE (continued)

Example: microgastria micro/gastr/ia   Meaning _condition of a very small stomach_   ICD-10-CM Code _Q40.2_

1. ichthyosis   Meaning _____   ICD-10-CM Code _____
2. left renal <u>agenesis</u>   Meaning _____   ICD-10-CM Code _____
3. frontal <u>encephalocele</u>   Meaning _____   ICD-10-CM Code _____
4. macrotia   Meaning _____   ICD-10-CM Code _____
5. vaginal <u>atresia</u>   Meaning _____   ICD-10-CM Code _____
6. cryptorchism   Meaning _____   ICD-10-CM Code _____
7. polydactyl   Meaning _____   ICD-10-CM Code _____
8. <u>polycystic</u> kidney disease   Meaning _____   ICD-10-CM Code _____
9. <u>bicornate</u> uterus   Meaning _____   ICD-10-CM Code _____
10. pseudohermaphroditism   Meaning _____   ICD-10-CM Code _____

CODING GUIDELINES FOR CONGENITAL ABNORMALITIES

Coders should understand the organization of this ICD-10-CM chapter, chapter-wide and commonly used instructional notes in the Tabular List, and the relevant OGCR. This information is necessary for accurate coding.

ICD-10-CM Chapter 17, "Congenital Malformations, Deformations, and Chromosomal Abnormalities (Q00-Q99)," contains 11 blocks or subchapters that are divided by organ system. Review the block names and code ranges listed at the beginning of Chapter 17 in the ICD-10-CM manual to become familiar with the content and organization.

This chapter includes congenital physical and chromosomal abnormalities. It does not include acquired variations of conditions that may be either congenital or acquired, which are classified in the corresponding body system chapter. It also does not include conditions originating during the birth process, which are classified in ICD-10-CM Chapter 16, "Certain Conditions Originating in the Perinatal Period (P00-P96)." Codes for cleft palate are divided by anatomic site. Codes for chromosomal abnormalities identify the specific genetic abnormality.

ICD-10-CM provides Official Guidelines for Coding and Reporting (OGCR) for congenital malformations, deformations, and chromosomal abnormalities in OGCR section I.C.17. OGCR provides discussion of sequencing codes from this chapter, multiple coding, and use of these codes throughout the patient lifespan. An instructional note at the beginning of Chapter 17 in the Tabular List states that codes from this chapter should not be used on records of mothers or unborn fetuses. Specific OGCR and instructional notes are discussed and cited throughout this chapter of the text.

ABSTRACTING FOR CONGENITAL ABNORMALITIES

Coders must identify whether a condition is congenital and what manifestations exist. In addition, coders should follow abstracting guidelines for the body system(s) affected.

Many conditions may be either congenital or acquired. Therefore, the coder must identify the documentation regarding when the condition originated. Chromosomal abnormalities and other conditions that are, by definition, congenital, do not require explicit documentation regarding the congenital nature.

Coders should review all manifestations of the congenital condition and identify those that are integral to the condition and those that are not. When a specific code exists for a condition, coders should report only the manifestations that are _related but not integral_ to the condition. When congenital conditions do not have a unique code, assign a nonspecific code and report all manifestations.

Age is not a factor when reporting congenital conditions. Unless a congenital defect can be repaired, congenital conditions exist throughout a patient's life and may be reported at any time.

Refer to ■ TABLE 24-3 for guidance on how to abstract conditions related to congenital malformations, deformations, and chromosomal abnormalities, then work through the detailed example that follows. Remember that the abstracting questions are a guide and that not every question applies to, or can be answered for, every case. Also remember to consult key criteria for abstracting specific body system conditions. For example, to code for a congenital condition documented during the birth encounter, follow the key criteria listed here as well as key criteria for abstracting birth encounters.

Table 24-3 ■ KEY CRITERIA FOR ABSTRACTING CONDITIONS RELATED TO CONGENITAL ABNORMALITIES

- ❏ What is the specific condition?
- ❏ What is the subtype?
- ❏ Is the condition clearly congenital?
- ❏ What manifestations are present?
- ❏ What manifestations are integral to the condition?
- ❏ What complications or comorbidities exist?
- ❏ Which condition or manifestation is the main reason for the encounter?

Guided Example of Abstracting Congenital Abnormalities

Refer to the following example throughout this chapter to practice skills for abstracting, assigning, and sequencing codes related to congenital malformations, deformations, and chromosomal abnormalities. Geneva Deckard, CPC, is a fictitious coder who guides you through the coding process.

Date: 5/21/yy   Location: Branton Medical Center

Provider: Matthew Bunker, MD

Patient: Lucia Ovalle   Gender: F   Age: 9 months

Reason for encounter: Cyanosis, tachypnea, difficulty feeding, and failure to thrive

Assessment: Blood work and imaging studies reveal tetralogy of Fallot (TOF); congenital atrial septal defect (ASD) is also present and can be corrected at the same time as TOF surgery, if parents consent

Plan: Corrective surgery

Follow along as Geneva Deckard, CPC, abstracts the diagnosis. Check off each step after you complete it.

▶ Geneva reads through the entire record, paying special attention to the reason for the encounter and the final assessment. She refers to the Key Criteria for Abstracting Conditions Related to Congenital Abnormalities (Table 24-3).

❏ *What is the specific condition?* Tetralogy of Fallot

❏ *What is the subtype?* Not applicable

❏ *Is the condition clearly congenital?* Yes, the condition is congenital by definition

❏ *What manifestations are present?* Cyanosis, tachypnea, difficulty feeding, and failure to thrive

❏ *What manifestations are integral to the condition?* All manifestations listed are common with TOF

❏ *What complications or comorbidities exist?* Congenital atrial septal defect

❏ *Which condition or manifestation is the main reason for the encounter?* Tetralogy of Fallot

▶ At this time, Geneva does not know which of these conditions may need to be coded, nor how many codes she will end up with. She will learn about this when she moves on to assigning codes.

CODING PRACTICE

Exercise 24.2   **Abstracting for Congenital Abnormalities**

Instructions: Read the mini-medical-record of each patient's encounter and answer the abstracting questions. Write the answer on the line provided. Do not assign any codes.

1. INPATIENT HOSPITAL   Gender: M   Age: 32

Reason for admission: Mitral valve replacement

Assessment: Mitral valve prolapse d/t congenital Marfan's syndrome

Plan: Valve replacement was successful, FU office 2 weeks

a. What is the specific condition? _____

b. What is the subtype? _____

c. Is the condition clearly congenital? _____
_____

d. What manifestations are present? _____

e. What manifestations are integral to the condition?
_____

f. What complications or comorbidities exist? _____
_____

g. Which condition or manifestation is the main reason for the encounter? _____

2. INPATIENT HOSPITAL   Gender: M   Age: 23 days

Reason for admission: Removal of a renal cyst

Assessment: Congenital renal cyst, congenital hydronephrosis

Plan: RTO 2 weeks

a. What is the specific condition? _____

b. What is the subtype? _____

c. Is the condition clearly congenital? _____
_____

d. What manifestations are present? _____
_____

e. What manifestations are integral to the condition?
_____

f. What complications or comorbidities exist? _____
_____

g. Which condition or manifestation is the main reason for the encounter? _____

CODING PRACTICE *(continued)*

3. OFFICE Gender: F Age: 16

Reason for encounter: Referred by family physician for gynecological consult on amenorrhea

Assessment: Ultrasound reveals missing uterus, which has not been surgically removed

a. What is the specific condition? _____

b. What is the subtype? _____

c. Is the condition clearly congenital? _____

_____

d. What manifestations are present? _____

e. What manifestations are integral to the condition?

_____

f. What complications or comorbidities exist? _____

_____

g. Which condition or manifestation is the main reason for the encounter? _____

4. OFFICE Gender: F Age: 30 days

Reason for encounter: FU on endoscopy after referral from pediatrician because infant is constantly spitting up

Assessment: Congenital Schatzki's esophageal ring

Plan: We attempted to dilate the ring and will evaluate for surgery if that is unsuccessful

a. What is the specific condition? _____

b. What is the subtype? _____

c. Is the condition clearly congenital? _____

_____

d. What manifestations are present? _____

e. What manifestations are integral to the condition?

_____

f. What complications or comorbidities exist? _____

_____

g. Which condition or manifestation is the main reason for the encounter? _____

5. OUTPATIENT HOSPITAL Gender: F Age: 1 year

Reason for encounter: Surgical correction of polydactyly

Assessment: Accessory thumb of right hand

Plan: FU office 1 week

a. What is the specific condition? _____

b. What is the subtype? _____

c. Is the condition clearly congenital? _____

5. (continued)

d. What manifestations are present? _____

e. What manifestations are integral to the condition?

_____

f. What complications or comorbidities exist? _____

_____

g. Which condition or manifestation is the main reason for the encounter? _____

6. OFFICE Gender: F Age: 23 days

Reason for encounter: Management of Down syndrome and FU on genetic testing

Assessment: Down syndrome, nonmosaic type, hypotonia, obstructive sleep apnea d/t Down-related hypertrophy of tonsils and adenoids, ASD, also Down related

Plan: FU with cardiologist and neurologist

a. What is the specific condition? _____

b. What is the subtype? _____

c. Is the condition clearly congenital? _____

_____

d. What manifestations are present? _____

e. What manifestations are integral to the condition?

_____

f. Which conditions are related, but not integral, to Down syndrome? _____

g. Which condition or manifestation is the main reason for the encounter? _____

7. INPATIENT HOSPITAL Gender: M Age: 6 days

Birth Weight: 2169g EGA: 38+4 Type: NSVD

POB: Hospital

Assessment: SGA, the blood test FISH (*fluorescent in situ hybridization*) is positive for Prader-Willi syndrome. Hypotonia and abnormally small (*hypoplasia*) testes, which cannot be detected within the scrotal sac, secondary to Prader-Willi.

Plan: Follow feeding plan, evaluate for supplemental growth hormone in 1 month

a. What is the specific condition? _____

b. What is the subtype? _____

c. Is the condition clearly congenital? _____

_____

d. What manifestations are present? _____

(continued)

CODING PRACTICE *(continued)*

7. (continued)

e. What manifestations are integral to the condition?
_____

f. What complications or comorbidities exist? _____
_____

g. Which condition or manifestation is the main reason
for the encounter? _____
_____

---

8. OFFICE Gender: M Age: 30 days

Reason for encounter: Routine examination

Assessment: Infant was born with microgastria and now has failure to thrive

Plan: Refer to nutritionist for feeding guidance, WU for vitamin, mineral, and hormone deficiencies

a. What is the specific condition? _____
_____

b. What is the subtype? _____

c. Is the condition clearly congenital? _____
_____

d. What manifestations are present? _____
_____

e. What manifestations are integral to the condition?
_____

f. What complications or comorbidities exist? _____
_____

g. Which condition or manifestation is the main reason
for the encounter? _____
_____

---

9. INPATIENT HOSPITAL Gender: M Age: 10 days

Birth Weight: 3216g EGA: 38+2 Type: Cesarean

POB: Hospital

Assessment: Meckel's diverticulum and congenital pyloric stenosis with vomiting

Plan: Evaluate effectiveness of pyloric balloon dilation that was performed. If unsuccessful, consider surgery to correct stenosis. Surgery is not needed for Meckel's unless bleeding occurs.

(continued)

---

9. (continued)

a. What is the specific condition? _____
_____

b. What is the subtype? _____

c. Is the condition clearly congenital? _____
_____

d. What manifestations are present? _____

e. What manifestations are integral to the condition?
_____

f. What complications or comorbidities exist? _____
_____

g. Which condition or manifestation is the main reason
for the encounter? _____
_____

---

10. OFFICE Gender: F Age: 3 months

Reason for encounter: Referred by pediatrician due to heart murmur

Assessment: Patent foramen ovale and congenital VSD

Plan: Treat VSD medically, postpone surgery if symptoms increase, no treatment needed for patent foramen ovale at this time, RTO 3 months

a. What is the specific condition? _____

b. What is the subtype? _____
_____

c. Is the condition clearly congenital? _____
_____

d. What manifestations are present? _____
_____

e. What manifestations are integral to the condition?
_____

f. What complications or comorbidities exist? _____
_____

g. Which condition or manifestation is the main reason
for the encounter? _____

ASSIGNING CODES FOR CONGENITAL ABNORMALITIES

ICD-10-CM distinguishes between conditions that can be either congenital in origin or acquired. For some conditions, the default code in the Index is for congenital origin, with the acquired version appearing as a subterm. For other conditions, the default code is for the acquired version, with the congenital origin appearing as a subterm. Coders can determine which variation is identified by the default code in the Index by reading the nonessential modifiers that appear in parentheses after the Main Term. When either of these terms, congenital or acquired, appears as a nonessential modifier, the other term usually appears as a subterm. Refer to ■ FIGURE 24-1 for the Main Term **Deformity** to compare the difference between the subterm **bone**, for which the default is **(acquired)**, and the subterm **brain**, for which the default code is **(congenital)**. Notice that the code for the congenital variation is from ICD-10-CM Chapter 17 and begins with **Q**, while the code for the acquired version does not begin with **Q** but, rather, the letter from the corresponding body system chapter.

When the documentation does not specify either congenital or acquired, assign the default code. Remember that the nonessential modifier in parentheses does *not* have to be present in the documentation in order to assign the code. Some conditions are congenital by definition and do not have an acquired form. When this is the case, the Index does not provide an alternative subterm for acquired and all code options begin with **Q** (■ FIGURE 24-2). Subterms describe variations of the congenital condition.

When a congenital abnormality has been corrected, assign a personal history code to identify the history of the condition (OGCR I.C.17). Search under the Main Term **History**, subterm **personal**, and the second-level subterm for the name of the condition. When the specific condition does not appear as a subterm, search under the Main Term **History**, subterm **personal**, the second-level subterm **congenital malformation**, and a third-level subterm for the body system involved (■ FIGURE 24-3, page 434).

Guided Example of Assigning Congenital Abnormalities Codes

To practice skills for assigning codes for congenital malformations, deformations, and chromosomal abnormalities, continue with the example from earlier in the chapter about patient

> **Hypospadias** Q54.9
> balanic Q54.0
> coronal Q54.0
> glandular Q54.0
> penile Q54.1
> penoscrotal Q54.2
> perineal Q54.3
> specified NEC Q54.8

Figure 24-2 ■ Index Main Term for "Hypospadias," a condition that is only congenital in origin.

Lucia Ovalle, who was diagnosed at Branton Medical Center with tetralogy of Fallot and atrial septal defect.

Follow along in your ICD-10-CM manual as Geneva Deckard, CPC, assigns codes. Check off each step after you complete it.

▶ First, Geneva confirms the conditions she abstracted:

❑ Tetralogy of Fallot

❑ Congenital atrial septal defect

▶ Geneva searches the Index for the Main Term **Tetralogy**.

❑ She locates the entry **Tetralogy of Fallot Q21.3**.

❑ There are no subterms.

▶ Geneva verifies code **Q21.3** in the Tabular List.

❑ She reads the code title for **Q21.3 Tetralogy of Fallot** and confirms that this accurately describes the diagnosis.

▶ Geneva checks for instructional notes in the Tabular List.

❑ She cross-references the beginning of category **Q21** and reads the **Excludes1** instructional note that directs her to *not* use this code if the cardiac septal defect is *acquired*.

❑ She determines that this note does not apply because her patient's condition is congenital.

❑ She cross-references the beginning of the block **Q20-Q28** and verifies that there are no instructional notes.

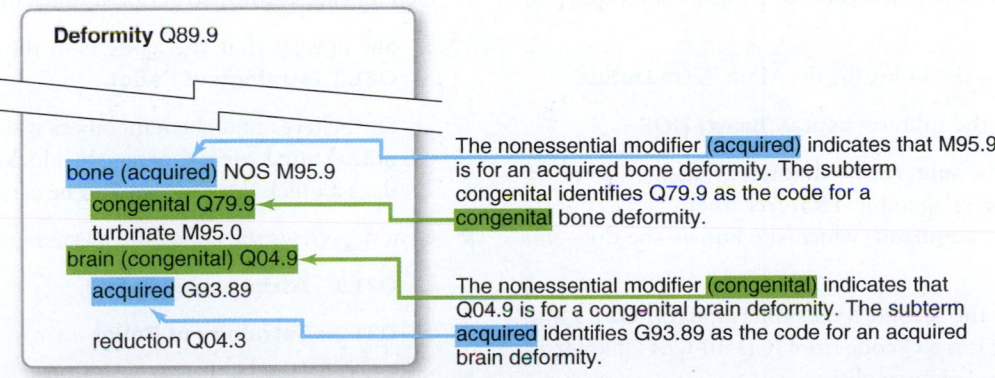

Figure 24-1 ■ Index entry showing "acquired" and "congenital" as nonessential modifiers for subterms.

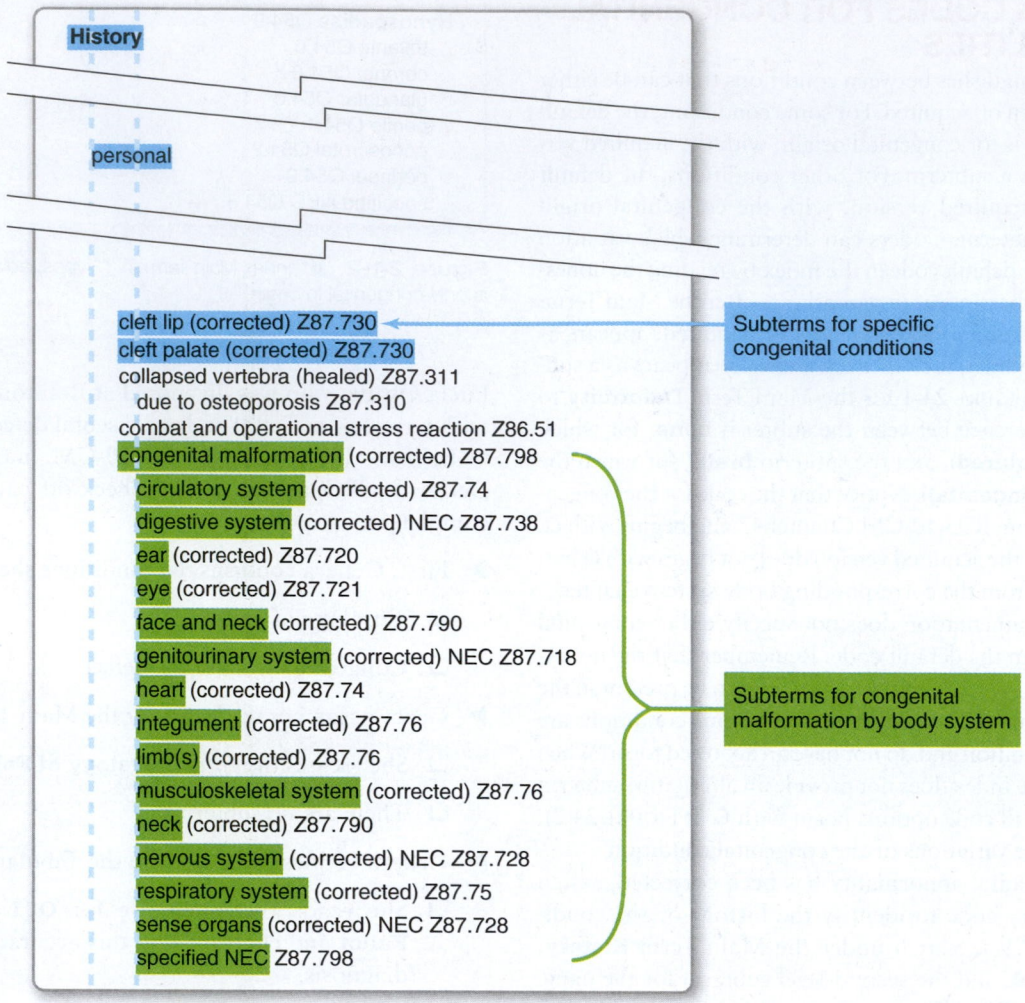

History

personal

cleft lip (corrected) Z87.730
cleft palate (corrected) Z87.730
collapsed vertebra (healed) Z87.311
   due to osteoporosis Z87.310
combat and operational stress reaction Z86.51
congenital malformation (corrected) Z87.798
  circulatory system (corrected) Z87.74
  digestive system (corrected) NEC Z87.738
  ear (corrected) Z87.720
  eye (corrected) Z87.721
  face and neck (corrected) Z87.790
  genitourinary system (corrected) NEC Z87.718
  heart (corrected) Z87.74
  integument (corrected) Z87.76
  limb(s) (corrected) Z87.76
  musculoskeletal system (corrected) Z87.76
  neck (corrected) Z87.790
  nervous system (corrected) NEC Z87.728
  respiratory system (corrected) Z87.75
  sense organs (corrected) NEC Z87.728
  specified NEC Z87.798

Subterms for specific congenital conditions

Subterms for congenital malformation by body system

Figure 24-3 ■ Index entry used to locate personal history of congenital conditions.

❏ She cross-references the beginning of Chapter 17 (Q00-Q99) and reviews the instructional notes. She determines that the **NOTE:** does not apply to this case because the patient is not a mother or a fetus. She determines that the **Excludes1** note does not apply because the condition is not an inborn error of metabolism.

▶ Next, Geneva works on the code for congenital atrial septal defect.

▶ Geneva searches the Index for the Main Term **Defect**.

❏ She locates the subterm **septal (heart) NOS**.

❏ She reads the subterms and notices that there is not a subterm for congenital. However, there is a separate subterm for **acquired**, which she knows she does *not* want.

❏ She locates the second-level subterm **atrial Q21.1** and notices that it is a Q code from ICD-10-CM Chapter 17 on congenital abnormalities.

❏ The third-level subterms under **atrial** relate to myocardial infarction, which does not apply to this patient.

▶ Geneva verifies the code **Q21.1** in the Tabular List.

❏ She reads the code title for **Q21.1 Atrial septal defect** and confirms that this accurately describes the diagnosis.

▶ Geneva checks for instructional notes in the Tabular List.

❏ She notices that this code is in the same category as **Q21.3 Tetralogy of Fallot**.

❏ She believes that she remembers what the instructional notes stated for the category, block, and chapter, but does a quick double-check to be certain.

▶ Geneva reviews the codes she has assigned for this case.

❏ **Q21.1**   **Atrial septal defect**

❏ **Q21.3**   **Tetralogy of Fallot**

▶ Next, Geneva must determine how to sequence the codes.

CODING PRACTICE

Exercise 24.3 **Assigning Codes for Congenital Abnormalities**

Instructions: Read the mini-medical-record of each patient's encounter, review the information abstracted in Exercise 24.2, and assign ICD-10-CM diagnosis codes using the Index and Tabular List. Write the code(s) on the line provided.

1. INPATIENT HOSPITAL   Gender: M   Age: 32

Reason for admission: Mitral valve replacement

Assessment: Mitral valve prolapse d/t congenital Marfan's syndrome

Plan: Valve replacement was successful, FU office 2 weeks

1 ICD-10-CM Code _____

2. INPATIENT HOSPITAL   Gender: M   Age: 23 days

Reason for admission: Removal of a renal cyst

Assessment: Congenital renal cyst, congenital hydronephrosis

Plan: RTO 2 weeks

2 ICD-10-CM Codes _____

3. OFFICE   Gender: F   Age: 16

Reason for encounter: Referred by family physician for gynecological consult on amenorrhea

Assessment: Ultrasound reveals missing uterus, which has not been surgically removed

1 ICD-10-CM Code _____

4. OFFICE   Gender: F   Age: 30 days

Reason for encounter: FU on endoscopy after referral from pediatrician because infant is constantly spitting up

Assessment: Congenital Schatzki's esophageal ring

Plan: We attempted to dilate the ring and will evaluate for surgery if that is unsuccessful

1 ICD-10-CM Code _____

5. OUTPATIENT HOSPITAL   Gender: F   Age: 1 year

Reason for encounter: Surgical correction of polydactyly

Assessment: Accessory thumb of right hand successfully removed

Plan: FU office 1 week

1 ICD-10-CM Code _____

ARRANGING CODES FOR CONGENITAL ABNORMALITIES

Codes for congenital abnormalities may be either a principal/first-listed diagnosis or a secondary diagnosis, based on the circumstances of the encounter and the definition of principal diagnosis in OGCR II (OGCR I.C.17). When a patient has multiple congenital abnormalities, which is not unusual, sequence the codes based on the circumstances of the encounter. Although this chapter does not have many instructional notes in the Tabular List, remember to always look for them and follow their direction for multiple coding and sequencing.

When coding for Down syndrome (**Q90.-**), an instructional note in the Tabular List states **Use additional code(s) to identify any associated physical conditions and the degree of intellectual disabilities (F70-F79)** (■ FIGURE 24-4, page 436).

SUCCESS STEP

When congenital abnormalities are diagnosed as part of the birth episode, assign a code from category **Z38.-** to describe the birth status of the infant. Always sequence the **Z38** code first, followed by codes for congenital or any other conditions.

Guided Example of Arranging Congenital Abnormalities Codes

To practice skills for sequencing codes for congenital malformations, deformations, and chromosomal abnormalities, continue with the example from earlier in the chapter about patient Lucia Ovalle, who was diagnosed at Branton Medical Center with tetralogy of Fallot and atrial septal defect.

Patient who has moderate intellectual disabilities is seen for nonmosaicism Down syndrome. Patient also has associated hypothyroidism and celiac disease.

(1) **Q90.0 Trisomy 21, nonmosaicism (meiotic nondisjunction)**
(2) **F71 Moderate intellectual disabilities**
(3) **E03.9 Hypothyroidism, unspecified**
(4) **K90.0 Celiac disease**

Figure 24-4 ■ Example of arranging codes for Down syndrome.

Follow along in your ICD-10-CM manual as Geneva Deckard, CPC, sequences the codes. Check off each step after you complete it.

▶ First, Geneva confirms the codes she assigned:

❑ **Q21.1 Atrial septal defect**

❑ **Q21.3 Tetralogy of Fallot**

▶ Geneva reviews the medical record to determine which code is the principal diagnosis.

❑ The workup and studies found both conditions, and TOF is the more serious condition because it consists of four malformations. ASD is secondary to TOF.

▶ Geneva finalizes the codes and sequencing for this case:

(1) **Q21.3 Tetralogy of Fallot**
(2) **Q21.1 Atrial septal defect**

CODING PRACTICE

Exercise 24.4 Arranging Codes for Congenital Abnormalities

Instructions: Read the mini-medical-record of each patient's encounter, review the information abstracted in Exercise 24.2, and assign ICD-10-CM diagnosis codes using the Index and Tabular List. Write the code(s) on the line provided.

1. OFFICE Gender: F Age: 23 days

Reason for encounter: Management of Down syndrome and FU on genetic testing

Assessment: Down syndrome, nonmosaic type, hypotonia, obstructive sleep apnea due to Down-related hypertrophy of tonsils and adenoids, ASD, also Down-related

Plan: FU with cardiologist and neurologist

Tip: Nonmosaicism is also called *meiotic nondisjunction*. Be careful to read any *Excludes1* notes you encounter.

3 ICD-10-CM Codes _____

_____

2. INPATIENT HOSPITAL Gender: M Age: 6 days

Birth Weight: 2169g EGA: 38+4

Type: NSVD POB: Hospital

Assessment: SGA, the blood test FISH (*fluorescent in situ hybridization*) is positive for Prader-Willi syndrome. Hypotonia and abnormally small (*hypoplasia*) testes, which cannot be detected within the scrotal sac, secondary to Prader-Willi

4 ICD-10-CM Codes _____

_____

3. OFFICE Gender: M Age: 30 days

Reason for encounter: Routine examination

Assessment: Infant was born with microgastria and now has failure to thrive

Plan: Refer to nutritionist for feeding guidance, WU for vitamin, mineral, and hormone deficiencies

Tip: Be sure to check the age of the patient.

3 ICD-10-CM Codes _____

_____

4. INPATIENT HOSPITAL Gender: M Age: 10 days

Birth Weight: 3216g EGA: 38+2

Type: Cesarean POB: Hospital

Assessment: Meckel's diverticulum and congenital pyloric stenosis with vomiting

Plan: Evaluate effectiveness of pyloric balloon dilation that was performed. If unsuccessful, consider surgery to correct stenosis. Surgery is not needed for Meckel's unless bleeding occurs.

3 ICD-10-CM Codes _____

_____

5. OFFICE Gender: F Age: 3 months

Reason for encounter: Referred by pediatrician due to heart murmur

Assessment: Patent foramen ovale and congenital VSD

Plan: Treat VSD medically, postpone surgery if symptoms increase, no treatment needed for patent foramen ovale at this time, RTO 3 months

2 ICD-10-CM Codes _____

CHAPTER SUMMARY

In this chapter you learned that:

- Congenital abnormalities are specific types of perinatal conditions, which include physical malformations, deformations, and chromosomal abnormalities.

- ICD-10-CM provides Official Guidelines for Coding and Reporting (OGCR) in OGCR section I.C.17, which discuss sequencing codes from this chapter, multiple coding, and use of these codes throughout the patient lifespan.

- Coders must identify whether a condition is congenital and what manifestations exist.

- Coders can determine whether a condition identified by the default code in the Index is the congenital variation or the acquired variation by reading the nonessential modifiers that appear in parentheses after the Main Term.

- Codes for congenital abnormalities may be either a principal/first-listed diagnosis or a secondary diagnosis, based on the circumstances of the encounter.

CONCEPT QUIZ

Take a moment to look back at congenital malformations, deformations, and chromosomal abnormalities and solidify your skills. Try to answer the questions from memory first, then look back at the discussion in this chapter if you need a little extra help.

Completion

Instructions: Write the term that completes each statement based on the information you learned in this chapter. Choose from the list below. Some choices may be used more than once and some choices may not be used at all.

adults	Marfan's syndrome
aortic coarctation	mothers
chromosomal abnormality	newborns
cleft palate	patent foramen ovale
deformity	Prader-Willi syndrome
Down syndrome	spina bifida
hydrocephalus	transposition of the great vessels
hydronephrosis	
hypospadias	Turner's syndrome
malformation	

1. Down syndrome is an example of a
   _____.

2. Dislocation of the hip is an example of a
   _____.

3. _____ is a notch or division of the roof of the mouth.

4. _____ is the excessive collection of urine in the kidneys.

5. _____ is a congenital heart defect in which the aorta and pulmonary artery are switched, preventing pulmonary circulation.

6. An instructional note at the beginning of Chapter 17 in the Tabular List states that codes from this chapter should not be used on records of _____.

7. _____ is a congenital condition in which the opening of the urethra is on the underside of the penile shaft.

8. _____ is a genetic disorder of connective tissue characterized by elongated bones and ocular and circulatory defects.

9. _____ is a genetic condition in which a person has 47 chromosomes instead of the usual 46.

10. _____ is a chromosomal defect in females in which they are missing all or part of one X chromosome.

Multiple Choice

Instructions: Circle the letter of the best answer to each question based on the information you learned in this chapter.

1. Which condition consists of pulmonary stenosis, overriding aorta, ventricle septal defect, and hypertrophy of the right ventricle?
   A. Trisomy
   B. Tetralogy of Fallot
   C. Marfan's syndrome
   D. Patent foramen ovale

2. What condition is a genetic disorder due to a deletion of paternal chromosome 15?
   A. Prader-Willi syndrome
   B. Marfan's syndrome
   C. Shone's syndrome
   D. Down syndrome

3. How would you code the following scenario? *A 9-month-old girl is seen for tetralogy of Fallot and a congenital atrial septal defect with manifestations of cyanosis and failure to thrive.*
   A. Q21.3, Q21.1, R23.0, R62.51
   B. Q24.9, P92.6
   C. Q21.3, Q21.1
   D. Q21.1, Q21.3

4. What additional codes should be assigned with codes for Down syndrome (Q90.-)?
   A. The degree of intellectual disabilities
   B. Identification of whether the condition is congenital or acquired
   C. The age of the patient
   D. The type of Down syndrome

(continued from page 437)

5. What medical term describes that part of the brain is missing?
   A. Microcephaly
   B. Hydrocephaly
   C. Anencephaly
   D. Encephalopathy

6. How would you code the following scenario? *A patient is seen for a congenital bone deformity.*
   A. M95.9
   B. Q79.9
   C. Q04.9
   D. M95.0

7. What type of code should be assigned when the documentation does not specify whether a condition is congenital or acquired?
   A. Assign a code for congenital.
   B. Assign a code for acquired.
   C. Assign a code for NOS.
   D. Assign the default code listed in the Index.

8. What code should you assign after a congenital abnormality has been corrected?
   A. Assign a code for the congenital condition.
   B. Assign a code for personal history of the condition.
   C. Assign the default code.
   D. Do not assign any code.

9. What should the principal diagnosis be when congenital abnormalities are diagnosed as part of the birth episode?
   A. Determine principal diagnosis according to the circumstances of admission.
   B. Principal diagnosis should be the most serious congenital condition.
   C. Principal diagnosis should be any birth trauma.
   D. Principal diagnosis should be the birth status of the infant.

10. How would you code the following scenario? *A patient who has moderate intellectual disabilities is seen for nonmosaicism Down syndrome. Patient also has associated hypothyroidism and celiac disease.*
    A. F71, Q90.0, E03.9, K90.0
    B. Q90.0, F71, E03.9, K90.0
    C. E03.9, K90.0, Q90.0, F71
    D. K90.0, F71, Q90.0, E03.9

KEEP ON CODING

Instructions: Read the diagnostic statement, then use the Index and Tabular List to assign and sequence ICD-10-CM diagnosis codes. Write the code(s) on the line provided.

1. Congenital glaucoma. ICD-10-CM Code(s) _____

2. Accessory ovary. ICD-10-CM Code(s) _____

3. Karyotype 45, X. ICD-10-CM Code(s) _____

4. Schwannomatosis. ICD-10-CM Code(s) _____

5. Lobster-claw, left hand. ICD-10-CM Code(s) _____

6. Congenital clawfoot. ICD-10-CM Code(s) _____

7. Congenital cyst of the pancreas. ICD-10-CM Code(s) _____

8. Anomaly of the aqueduct of Sylvius. ICD-10-CM Code(s) _____

9. Ectopic kidney. ICD-10-CM Code(s) _____

10. Supernumerary nipple. ICD-10-CM Code(s) _____

11. Laryngocele. ICD-10-CM Code(s) _____

12. Cleft lip, median. ICD-10-CM Code(s) _____

13. Low-set ears. ICD-10-CM Code(s) _____

14. Anencephaly. ICD-10-CM Code(s) _____

15. Arnold-Chiari syndrome with hydrocephalus. ICD-10-CM Code(s) _____

16. Plagiocephaly. ICD-10-CM Code(s) _____

17. Marfan's syndrome. ICD-10-CM Code(s) _____

18. Blue sclera. ICD-10-CM Code(s) _____

19. Ebstein's anomaly. ICD-10-CM Code(s) _____

20. Atresia of the aorta. ICD-10-CM Code(s) _____

21. Short rib syndrome. ICD-10-CM Code(s) _____

22. Congenital spondylolysis. ICD-10-CM Code(s) _____

23. Strawberry nevus. ICD-10-CM Code(s) _____

24. Epidermolysis bullosa letalis. ICD-10-CM Code(s) _____

25. Congenital hiatal hernia. ICD-10-CM Code(s) _____

CODING CHALLENGE

Instructions: Read the mini-medical-record of each patient's encounter, then abstract, assign, and sequence ICD-10-CM diagnosis codes using the Index and Tabular List. Write the code(s) on the line provided.

1. INPATIENT HOSPITAL   Gender: M   Age: 15 days

Birth Weight: 3421g   EGA: 39+0   Type: NSVD

POB: Hospital

Assessment: Unilateral cleft lip on left side, with cleft palate, hard

Plan: Detailed review of estimated repair protocol with parents. Visiting nurse to supervise feeding for 2 days. RTO 3 days.

Tip: Infant was discharged 15 days after birth.

2 ICD-10-CM Codes _____

2. INPATIENT HOSPITAL   Gender: F   Age: 50

Reason for encounter: Patient was attempting to adjust her office chair when the mechanism gave and caught and crushed her finger

Assessment: Finger crush injury of right hand, congenital deficiency of the development of hands and fingers, bilaterally, complicates the repair

Plan: Arm and hand loosely wrapped in splint, elevate hand above elbow. RTO in one day, schedule reconstruction after swelling has abated.

Tip: There is not a specific external cause code for this accident. Code as exposure to inanimate mechanical forces.

4 ICD-10-CM Codes _____
_____

3. INPATIENT HOSPITAL   Gender: F   Age: 2

Reason for encounter: Reconstructive heart surgery

Assessment: Congenital Shone's syndrome with aortic stenosis, subaortic stenosis, aortic coarctation, bicuspid aortic valve

Plan: FU in office 3 days

4 ICD-10-CM Codes _____
_____

4. INPATIENT HOSPITAL   Gender: M   Age: 1 day

Birth Weight: 2421g   EGA: 36+0   Type: Cesarean

POB: Hospital

Reason for encounter: Spina bifida suspected at second trimester screening and confirmed by ultrasound and at birth; infant was born yesterday

Assessment: Spina bifida of the thoracic region

Plan: Surgical repair recommended

Tip: This is an inpatient consultation with a pediatric neurologist. When coding for the physician, do not report the birth status of the infant, which is reported only on the inpatient record.

1 ICD-10-CM Code _____

5. OFFICE   Gender: M   Age: 2

Reason for encounter: Referral from neurologist

Assessment: Lingual frenum extending toward the tip of tongue, which is fused to mouth floor and affects speech

Plan: Refer for speech therapy

1 ICD-10-CM Code _____

6. OFFICE   Gender: M   Age: 5

Reason for encounter: Referred by pediatrician for dysphagia

Assessment: Congenital esophageal web with esophageal spasm and reflux esophagitis

Plan: Schedule balloon dilatation and electrocauterization

3 ICD-10-CM Codes _____
_____

(continued)

(continued from page 439)

---

7. OFFICE Gender: **M** Age: **1 year**

Reason for encounter: **Preoperative exam for cryptorchism repair tomorrow**

Assessment: **Cleared for surgery, bilateral perineal cryptorchism**

Plan: **Surgery tomorrow at 11:00 a.m.**

Tip: Assign a Z code for the preoperative exam.

2 ICD-10-CM Codes _____

---

8. OFFICE Gender: **M** Age: **1 month**

Reason for encounter: **Fitting of knee braces, bilateral**

Assessment: **Congenital genu recurvatum**

Plan: **Instruct parents on daily passive physical therapy, schedule pt treatments x 12 on weekly basis**

Tip: Assign a Z code for the fitting of the braces. Genu recurvatum is a minor backward curving of knee joints, causing bowed legs.

2 ICD-10-CM Codes _____

---

9. INPATIENT HOSPITAL Gender: **M** Age: **1 day**

Birth Weight: **3011g** EGA: **38+0** Type: **NSVD**

POB: **Hospital**

Assessment: **Penoscrotal hypospadias**

Plan: **Discharged 1 day after birth. We will keep an eye on the hypospadias to see if treatment is necessary or if it will correct independently, FU in office 2 days for jaundice check**

2 ICD-10-CM Codes _____

---

10. INPATIENT HOSPITAL Gender: **F** Age: **9 days**

Birth Weight: **3011g** EGA: **38+0** Type: **Cesarean**

POB: **Hospital**

Reason for encounter: **Open heart surgery on 9-day-old infant**

Assessment: **Transposition of great vessels**

Plan: **Will follow in hospital until d/c**

Tip: This is an inpatient procedure done by a neonatal cardiothoracic surgeon. When coding for the physician, do not report the birth status of the infant, which is reported only on the inpatient record.

1 ICD-10-CM Code _____

CPT/HCPCS Procedure Coding

Section Three: CPT/HCPCS Procedure Coding, discusses the procedure coding systems used by physicians, nonphysician providers, and outpatient facilities to bill for services. Providers establish a fee for each procedure code, which is the basis of reimbursement calculations. Diagnosis codes provide the medical justification for the reason the services are needed. Although CPT and HCPCS are completely different coding systems from ICD-10-CM, you are still able to apply the three skills of an "Ace" coder: abstract, assign, and arrange.

PROFESSIONAL PROFILE

Amy C. Riley, RHIT, CCA
Oncology Outpatient Coder II
Conifer Health Solutions

Originally, I took a short three-month course that gave me the basics of coding and enabled me to pass the certified coding associate (CCA) certification exam. I had difficulty finding employment and decided what I needed was a higher credential, so I completed a two-year online associate degree in health information management (HIM). I found that this degree gave me the thorough education I needed to obtain my registered health information technician (RHIT) credential and find employment. Employers know I have what it takes to persevere and do what is needed to succeed.

A friend of mine was a remote coder and suggested I consider coding because I have five children and she thought it would be a great opportunity to work from home. Truthfully, there is no way I could do my job with all my kids home running around needing me. I did start the schooling while the kids where littler, and now that they are older, here I am! I will admit I did start this career just as a way to stay home with my kids and not to have to work with people. But the more I learned the more passionate I became about it. I could chat with others in the profession for hours about coding and enjoy it!

In my current job, I am a coder level II. I focus on oncology outpatient facility fee coding. I read the providers' charts and code them. I also am in charge of entering the diagnoses of new patients coming to the clinic. I use information daily that I learned in school, like National Correct Coding Initiative (NCCI) edits, modifiers, and how to navigate tricky coding situations, such as transgender coding. I also cover for our radiology oncology coder when she goes on vacation.

I love discovering new codes, especially silly codes. I enjoy how each chart is a new puzzle of what to code, in what order, and what special codes need to be added.

The biggest challenge is trying to figure out the doctors' documentation. Doctors know the patient very well but do not always dictate all the details we need for coding. Sometimes I really have to dig far back into documents like pathology to find more details of a neoplasm.

I use a logic-based encoder in my job, so I enter keywords and follow the prompts for the correct codes I need to enter. A coder still has to pay attention to where the encoder is leading them because a wrong keyword will send you in the wrong code section. I also use programs like Excel, Outlook, GoToMeeting, and many other applications that help in my daily coding.

Those interested in coding should be sure to attend a recognized, accredited school. After you become certified, be sure to keep up with the required continuing education units (CEUs). Being a member of AHIMA gives me access to a members-only job board. Always strive to love what you do!

Chapter 25

Introduction to CPT Coding

Chapter Outline

- **Overview of CPT Coding**
- **Organization of the CPT Manual**
- **CPT Guidelines**
- **Abstracting Procedures for CPT Coding**
- **Assigning CPT Codes**
- **Arranging CPT Codes**
- **CPT Coding and Reimbursement**

Learning Objectives

After completing this chapter, you should have the skills to:

25.1 Spell and define the key words, medical terms, and abbreviations related to CPT coding. (Remember)

25.2 Summarize the history and purpose of CPT coding. (Understand)

25.3 Describe the organization of the CPT manual, including CPT guidelines and conventions. (Understand)

25.4 Demonstrate how to research CPT guidelines and special instructions. (Apply)

25.4 Explain how to abstract procedural information from the medical record. (Understand)

25.5 Demonstrate how to assign CPT codes. (Apply)

25.6 Utilize the guidelines for arranging (sequencing) CPT codes. (Apply)

25.7 Articulate the relationship between accurate CPT coding and reimbursement. (Apply)

Key Terms and Abbreviations

837P	common descriptor	instructional note (CPT)	semicolon (CPT)
add-on code	conversion factor	modifier (CPT)	special instructions (CPT)
bundling edit	Current Procedural	modifying term	standalone code
category (CPT)	Terminology (CPT)	parent code	subcategory (CPT)
Category I	edit	prepayment edit	subheading (CPT)
Category II	guidelines (CPT)	resequenced code	subsection (CPT)
Category III	indented code description	section (CPT)	unlisted procedure

In addition to the key terms listed here, students should know the terms defined within tables in this chapter.

INTRODUCTION

When you go shopping, each item is marked with an item number that identifies it. Similarly, procedure codes identify the procedures and services that physicians provide to patients. Procedure coding is the act of assigning a code to a patient's procedure or service. Physician procedure codes have been standardized since 1966, which has made coding more efficient and more accurate. Accuracy in procedure coding is essential because incorrect or inadequate coding may lead to denial or delay of insurance claims. Each coding system, such as ICD-10-CM and CPT, is different, so it is important to learn what information applies to all code sets and what information is unique to each. CPT uses some of the same terms as ICD-10-CM/PCS but defines them differently, so coders must understand the meanings within the context of each code set. In this chapter you learn the history, purpose, and terminology of CPT coding; the organization of the CPT manual; how to abstract, assign, and arrange (sequence) CPT codes; and the relationship between CPT codes and reimbursement.

OVERVIEW OF CPT CODING

Current Procedural Terminology (CPT) is a listing of five-character alphanumeric codes and descriptions that report outpatient medical services and procedures. CPT codes are five digits with no decimal point, such as 99215—a code that identifies a complex office visit. Certain categories of CPT codes contain a letter as the last character, such as 0500F—a special tracking code for prenatal visits. The Health Insurance Portability and Accountability Act (HIPAA) mandates the use of CPT for all covered entities that handle electronic claims related to outpatient healthcare services. As a result, CPT is the standard for communication among healthcare providers, regulators, and payers. ■ TABLE 25-1 summarizes characteristics of CPT.

Table 25-1 ■ CHARACTERISTICS OF CPT

Characteristic	CPT
Name	Current Procedural Terminology
Developed by	American Medical Association
Purpose	Outpatient procedures
Used by	Physicians, outpatient hospitals
Number of codes	10,000+
Code length	5 digits (except F, T, and U codes, which are 5 alphanumeric characters)
Modifiers	Two-digit numerical CPT modifiers, two-character alphanumeric HCPCS modifiers
Laterality	Identified with modifiers -RT, -LT, -50
Code structure	Meaning of individual characters is undefined
Code order	Most codes appear in numerical order with some resequenced codes interspersed. Evaluation and Management section appears first, out of numerical sequence.
Code descriptions	Full code descriptions include indented (dependent) descriptions and add-on codes
Decimal point	Not used

Source: © PB Resources, Inc. Used with permission.

The History of CPT Coding

Before the mid-1960s, most patients paid out of pocket for their services. When they had health insurance, they submitted their own claims to insurance companies and were reimbursed directly. There were no standard medical billing forms or procedure codes. Reimbursement was cost-based, meaning that the insurance companies paid whatever fees providers charged.

With the passage of Medicare and Medicaid in 1965, the healthcare industry recognized the need to standardize the description of services provided. The Health Care Financing Administration (HCFA), now known as the Centers for Medicare and Medicaid Services (CMS), assigned the task of developing codes to the American Medical Association (AMA). The AMA developed and published the first edition of CPT in 1966—the year that the Medicare and Medicaid programs were implemented—and has been responsible for CPT codes ever since. The first edition of CPT primarily contained surgical procedures, with limited sections on medicine, radiology, and laboratory. Codes were four digits in length.

The CPT was updated several times during the 1970s until the fourth edition—still in use today—was adopted in 1977. At that time, a process was established to update the code set on a regular basis.

In 1983, the federal government adopted CPT as part of its Healthcare Common Procedure Coding System (HCPCS) and later required that it be used to report services billed to Medicare Part B and Medicaid. CPT codes are also called Level I HCPCS codes. The passage of HIPAA in 1996 required that uniform standards for electronic transactions be established. Effective October 16, 2003, CPT was designated a mandated procedure code set for covered entities for physician services and most other types of outpatient claims, including hospital outpatient procedures.

Today, the CPT manual covers all procedures approved by the Food and Drug Administration (FDA). The CPT lists over 10,000 procedural codes. CPT is updated every year, with changes taking effect January 1. For patients seen on December 31, use the CPT manual for the old year. For patients seen on January 1 and after, use the CPT manual for the new year. The transition date for CPT differs from the transition date for the ICD-10-CM diagnosis coding manual, which is October 1.

Code changes are published by the AMA in conjunction with CMS. CPT updates are made to clarify code descriptions and incorporate new technologies and equipment. Use the edition of the CPT that was in effect on the date of service.

The Purpose of CPT Coding

Procedure codes identify billable services provided to patients. Physicians report CPT procedure codes on insurance claims—the CMS-1500 and its electronic equivalent, the 837P—to identify the services provided and the cost of those services. Refer again to Chapter 2 of this text, Figure 2-3, "Example of a completed CMS-1500 claim form." Physicians are paid for CPT codes, but diagnosis codes are required to explain the reason(s) for the encounter and/or the reason services were provided. Coders must be certain to abstract and assign at least one ICD-10-CM diagnosis code for each procedure or service billed. The same diagnosis code can be used for more than one service, but coders cannot report a service that is not supported by a diagnosis

(■ FIGURE 25-1). Any service that lacks a corresponding diagnosis code will not be paid by the insurance company.

It can be challenging to find the most appropriate and accurate code for each patient encounter. For example, patient encounters for what is commonly referred to as an "office visit" may be reported with any of 30-plus codes, depending on a number of circumstances. However, only one code is correct in any given situation, so coders must become familiar with the nuances among codes that might seem to be similar. Likewise, more than 50 codes describe sutures for a wound. The correct code is based on the location, length, and depth of the wound. Coders need to be familiar with all of the criteria for coding services offered by their office to be certain they select the accurate code.

It is improper to code for a more complex service than what was actually provided in the hope of receiving higher reimbursement. Doing so is considered fraud and carries severe penalties, including fines and possible imprisonment.

Coders must also be attentive to entering codes correctly into the computer or onto the CMS-1500 billing form. A typographic error in a code number can result in a rejected insurance claim, which must be corrected and rebilled, thus delaying the payment the office receives.

> A new patient presented in the office to establish primary care. Performed a comprehensive history, a comprehensive focused examination, and medical decision making of high complexity. Patient has a 10-year history of hypertension and 5-year history of atrial fibrillation both of which she has been taking medication for. Also complains of unknown allergies. Performed an EKG and 10 allergy patch tests. Diagnosis: hypertension, atrial fibrillation, allergic rhinitis
>
> | | |
> |---|---|
> | I10 | Essential (primary) hypertension |
> | I48.91 | Unspecified atrial fibrillation |
> | J30.9 | Allergic rhinitis, unspecified |
> | 99205 | Office or other outpatient visit for the evaluation and management of a new patient, which requires these 3 key components... |
> | 95052 | x 10 Photo patch test(s) (specify number of tests) |
> | 93000 | Electrocardiogram, routine ECG with at least 12 leads; with interpretation and report |

Figure 25-1 ■ Example of matching diagnosis codes to procedure codes. *Source: © PB Resources, Inc. Used with permission.*

Medical Terminology Used in CPT Coding

Medical terms related to procedure coding use the same word roots and combining forms as those used in diagnosis coding, but the suffixes describe procedures rather than diagnoses. Coders must be able to distinguish between medical terms that describe diagnoses and those that describe procedures. They also must understand the meaning of suffixes that describe procedures so they can accurately identify the procedure performed. ■ TABLE 25-2 lists commonly used suffixes that describe procedures. Refer to ■ TABLE 25-3 for a refresher on how to build medical terms for diagnoses and procedures related to the same anatomic site.

Table 25-2 ■ **MEDICAL TERM SUFFIXES THAT DESCRIBE PROCEDURES**

Suffix	Meaning	Example
-centesis	Surgical puncture (*withdrawal of fluid*)	Arthrocentesis (*performing surgical puncture to withdraw fluid from a joint*)
-clasis	Breaking down, fracture	Osteoclasis (*surgical fracture or refracture of a bone*)
-desis	Binding or stabilization	Arthrodesis (*stabilizing or binding together a joint*)
-desiccation	Destruction	Electrodesiccation (*destruction using electricity*)
-ectomy	Cutting out all or part of	Arthrectomy (*cutting out part of a joint*)
-graphy	Making a recording or picture/image	Radiography (*making a picture using radiation waves*)
-lysis	Loosening or destroying (*to free from adhesion*)	Arthrolysis (*surgically loosening adhesions in a joint*)
-metry	Taking a measurement, measuring	Oximetry (*measuring oxygen [in the blood]*)
-pexy	Fixating, positioning, attaching	Cystopexy (*fixation of the bladder [to the abdominal wall]*)
-plasty	Surgical repair	Arthroplasty (*repairing a joint*)
-rrhaphy	Surgically suture or repair	Cystorrhaphy (*surgical suturing of the bladder*)
-scopy	Viewing	Arthroscopy (*viewing a joint*)
-section	Cutting apart, slicing	Small-bowel resection (*cutting apart/slicing out some or all of the small intestine*)
-stasis	Stopping or controlling	Hemostasis (*stopping bleeding*)
-stomy	Creating a new opening or mouth	Colostomy (*surgical creation of an opening into the colon*)
-therapy	Treatment	Radiotherapy (*treatment using radiation waves*)
-tomy	Cutting into, opening, making an incision	Arthrotomy (*making an incision into a joint*)
-tripsy	Crushing or destroying	Lithotripsy (*crushing or destroying stones/calculi*)

Source: © PB Resources, Inc. Used with permission.

Table 25-3 ■ **EXAMPLE OF CONSTRUCTING MEDICAL TERMS FOR DIAGNOSES AND PROCEDURES**

Combining Form	Suffix	Complete Medical Term
gastr/o (*stomach*)		gastr + itis (*inflammation of the stomach*)
		gastr + ectomy (*cutting out the stomach*)
	Diagnostic:	gastro + scopy (*viewing the stomach*)
	-**itis** (*inflammation*)	
arthr/o (*joint*)	*Procedural:*	arthr + itis (*inflammation of a joint*)
	-**ectomy** (*cutting out*)	arthr + ectomy (*cutting out a joint*)
	-**scopy** (*viewing*)	arthro + scopy (*viewing a joint*)
arteri/o (*artery*)		arter + itis (*inflammation of an artery*)
		arter + ectomy (*cutting out an artery*)

ORGANIZATION OF THE CPT MANUAL

Coders need to be familiar with the organization of the CPT manual so that they can find needed information quickly. Not only do you need to understand where needed information is located, you also need to identify and interpret coding guidelines, instructional notes, and conventions. The AMA publishes several editions of the CPT, and other publishers sometimes print the CPT manual with enhanced reference information. The codes and guidelines are the same in all editions, but some organize the features differently and might include enhanced features such as diagrams, color coding, and reference information. Each CPT manual shows the year on the front cover. Always use the manual that corresponds with the calendar year of the date of service, regardless of when the billing is done. The content and labeling of specific topics can change from year to year when the manual is updated. For this reason, it is important to become familiar with the specific edition of the manual you use (■ TABLE 25-4). Open your CPT manual and locate the features and information as they are discussed in this chapter.

SUCCESS STEP

The CPT Index is located toward the back of most CPT manuals compared with the ICD-10-CM/PCS manuals, which usually place the Index in the front.

Introduction

The Introduction, or front matter, provides valuable reference material for coders. The Introduction provides a table of contents by page number, instructions for use of the codebook, and other valuable information, depending on the edition of the manual used. Possible features are a review of medical terminology and anatomic plates.

Inside the front cover or within the first few pages is a list of commonly used symbols, modifiers, and place-of-service codes. This information is provided for quick reference for users who fully understand the correct use of these items. Inside the back cover of most CPT manuals are commonly used medical abbreviations. Publishers other than the AMA may place these features in different locations or may not include them at all.

Tabular List

The Tabular List is a numerical listing of all CPT codes divided into Category I, Category II, and Category III. The Tabular List

Table 25-4 ■ **TYPICAL ORGANIZATION OF THE CPT MANUAL**

Section	Description
Introduction	Lists CPT section numbers and sequences and provides instructions for use of the CPT manual. Includes several charts and tables for commonly used information, including: • CPT symbols • Commonly used modifiers • Place-of-Service Codes for Professional Claims • Illustrated Anatomical and Procedural Review • Evaluation and Management Tables
Tabular List	Provides a numerical listing of all CPT codes, descriptions, and guidelines • Category I (Evaluation and Management, Anesthesia, Surgery, Radiology, Pathology and Laboratory, Medicine, 00100-99607) • Category II (Performance measures, 0001F-9007F) • Category III (Emerging technology, services, procedures, 0042T-0542T)
Appendices	Provides appendices that define or summarize specialized reference information
CPT Index	Provides an alphabetical listing of conditions, anatomic sites, procedures, eponyms, and acronyms with the most likely codes or code ranges in the Tabular List

provides the official descriptions of CPT codes and the guidelines for using them. When coding, first search for a code in the Index, then verify it in the Tabular List. This text uses the title *Tabular List* to refer to the numerical code listing in all coding manuals, even though CPT does not specifically use this term. Follow along in your CPT manual as features of the Tabular List are discussed.

Category I: Permanent Codes (00100-99607)

Category I codes, which comprise the bulk of the CPT, are five digits in length, numbered **00100** to **99607**. They describe widely used services and procedures approved by the FDA and are permanent codes. The CPT manual does not specifically label codes as Category I. Rather, Category I codes carry the names of the six **sections** (■ TABLE 25-5).

Although most of the sections appear in numerical order, the first section typically contains the codes **99201** through **99499**,

Table 25-5 ■ **SECTIONS OF CPT CATEGORY I CODES**

Section	Code Range(s)
Evaluation and Management (E/M)	99201–99499
Anesthesiology	00100–01999, 99100–99140
Surgery	11004–69990
Radiology	70010–79999
Pathology and Laboratory	80047–89398, 0001U and higher
Medicine	90281–99199, 99500–99607

which are Evaluation and Management (E/M) codes. E/M codes describe physician encounters such as office visits and hospital visits. They are the most frequently used codes and are used by all medical specialties, so they are placed first in the manual for convenience. Codes in other sections are used more selectively, based on the specific services provided by each office. All physicians and health professionals may report any code in the CPT manual that is within their legally mandated scope of practice and that they are qualified to perform.

Codes appear in numerical order within each section, with one general exception. Some of the codes added since 2010 are not in strict numerical order. Normally, new procedures are assigned the next unused number for the type of procedure and anatomic site. If there are no unused numbers where you would expect them, the new procedures are assigned a number that is out of sequence. These are resequenced codes and are identified with the symbol **#**. The resequenced code number appears in numerical order with an instruction that identifies the code range where the description appears. However, this cross-referenced code range can be rather broad, encompassing several code numbers. Sometimes the coder must browse multiple columns of code descriptions to locate the resequenced code.

Each section within the CPT manual is further divided into additional topics. For example, the Surgery section is divided by body system and anatomic site within each body system. The additional topics are typically organized into subsections, subheadings, categories, and subcategories based on anatomy, procedure, condition, or descriptor (■ FIGURE 25-2). The name of each division may be printed using a different size and/

Division	Title
Subsection	**Cardiovascular System (33101–37799)**
Subheading	**Heart and Pericardium (33010–33999)**
Category	**Cardiac Valves (33361–33478)**
Subcategory	**Aortic Valve (33361–33417, 33440)** **Mitral Valve (33418-33430)**
Code	**33361** Transcatheter aortic valve replacement (TAVR/TAVI) with prosthetic valve; percutaneous femoral artery approach

Figure 25-2 ■ Example of CPT Tabular List organization.

or color of text, depending on the edition and publisher of the CPT manual. In general, the print size of the headings decreases in each successive subdivision. Not all the divisions appear under every section; it depends on the amount of information in each section. All codes appear under the lowest division. Coders must be familiar with the organization of the divisions so they can locate codes and determine to which codes certain guidelines and instructions apply.

Most categories in the CPT manual also provide a code for an unlisted procedure. When physicians provide a unique service that is not adequately described by an existing CPT code, a code for an unlisted procedure can be reported. Such codes generally end with the digits **9** or **99** and appear at the end of the category or subdivision to which they apply. Unlisted procedure codes should be accompanied by a detailed report from the physician that describes the service or procedure provided so the payer can identify the service(s) provided.

> ### SUCCESS STEP
>
> Many coders find it helpful to tab their CPT manuals to make it easier to quickly locate information. Apply self-adhesive tabs to the Tabular List pages that contain codes 99201, 01000, 10000, 20000, and so on, through code 90000. Also tab Category II and III codes. Finally, tab each appendix and each letter of the alphabet in the Index.

Category II: Performance Tracking (0001F-9007F)

Category II codes are optional codes used to collect and track data for performance measurement. They consist of four numbers followed by the letter **F**, such as **1002F Anginal symptoms and level of activity assessed**. Category II codes identify certain services or test results that contribute to quality patient care and are usually included in a routine examination or other service. Examples include documentation of:

- Disease-specific assessments (heart failure, osteoarthritis)
- Certain types of care plans (prenatal flow sheet, pain management)
- Some elements of the patient history (fall history, tobacco use history)
- Components of the physical assessment (blood pressure, weight, mental status)
- Test results (mammogram, oxygen saturation)

Medical offices reduce the amount of time spent auditing charts to collect information when they use Category II codes. The codes themselves are not billable and carry no charge, but Medicare pays physicians a separate financial incentive for reporting Category II codes for data collection purposes.

Category III: Temporary (0042T-0542T)

Category III codes are temporary codes for data collection and for tracking the use of emerging technology, services, and procedures. The codes are four numbers followed by the letter **T**; for example, **0163T Total disc arthroplasty (artificial disc), anterior approach, including discectomy to prepare**

interspace (other than for decompression), each additional interspace, lumbar. If a Category III code is available, coders should report it *instead of* a Category I code. Category III technology and procedures are generally in the process of being reviewed for FDA approval. Services are items that the AMA is considering adding to Category I. For example, procedures for fenestrated endovascular aneurysm repair (FEVAR) were reported with temporary codes **0078T-0081T** from 2005 to 2013. In 2014, the procedures were assigned to Category I with a series of codes from **34841** to **34848**.

Appendices

The CPT manual has several appendices that provide reference information. Some appendices summarize codes designated with special symbols throughout the CPT manual. Other appendices provide technical information used in offices that perform specialized procedures, such as nerve conduction studies, cardiac catheterization, or genetic testing. Appendices A, B, and C are used most often by coders. Look through the other appendices in the CPT manual so you become familiar with the available information.

Appendix A: Modifiers

Appendix A presents a complete description of all modifiers applicable to the current year codes. Modifiers are two-digit alphanumeric suffixes appended to CPT codes to further describe circumstances. Most publishers print an abbreviated list of commonly used modifiers inside the front cover, but you should develop the habit of referring to Appendix A until you are familiar with the details of how a specific modifier is to be used. Use of modifiers is introduced later in the chapter.

Appendix B: Summary of Additions, Deletions, and Revisions

Appendix B lists all the changes in the current year's manual. It is useful at the beginning of the year when the new CPT codes are released. You can quickly cross-reference the CPT codes on encounter forms to Appendix B to determine how the codes commonly used in your office might be affected by the annual revision.

Appendix C: Clinical Examples

Appendix C provides examples of E/M code scenarios for many medical specialties. These should not be used for coding but for learning and understanding how various patient encounters might be coded. The most commonly used E/M codes each have at least one example.

Index

Coders should always begin to locate a code by using the CPT Index. After identifying potential codes in the Index, users should verify them in the Tabular List. Never select the final code based only on the Index, even when only one code appears. Follow along in the Index of your CPT manual as the features are discussed next.

The Index lists procedures and services in the CPT manual alphabetically by Main Term and modifying terms that aid in locating the most appropriate code or range of codes (■ FIGURE 25-3). Modifying terms, or subterms, are descriptive words in the Index that appear indented under the Main Term

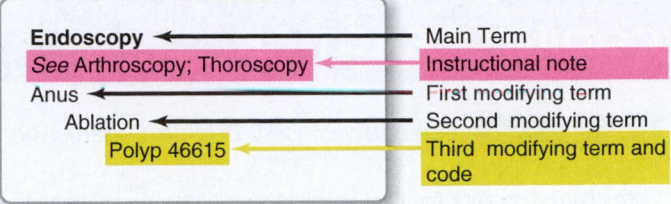

Figure 25-3 ■ Example of CPT Index organization.

to further describe the service or procedure. When modifying terms appear, it is important to review the entire list of options before selecting the most specific term.

Do not confuse the CPT expressions *modifying term* and *modifier*. Modifying terms are Index entries that add further detail to the Main Term. Modifiers are two-character suffixes that are appended to Category I codes to further explain the service provided.

The first level of modifying terms is aligned on the same margin as the Main Term but is set in smaller, nonboldfaced type. The second and third levels of modifying terms each are indented several spaces beyond the previous level. They further describe the Main Term in reference to anatomic site (e.g., **Endoscopy**, **Anus**); extent (e.g., **Excision**, **Clavicle**, **Partial**); procedure (e.g., **Electrocardiography**, **12 lead**); or similar descriptors.

When the Main Term or modifying term is too long to fit on one line, a carry-over line is used. Carry-over lines are indented the same number of spaces as the beginning of the line. It is important to read carefully to distinguish between carry-over lines and modifying terms.

Main Terms and modifying terms contain instructional notes, such as *see* or *see also*, which direct the user to synonyms for the code. For example, the entry **Pituitectomy—See Pituitary Gland, Excision** instructs the user to look under the Main Term **Pituitary Gland** and the modifying term **Excision** to locate the codes for removal of the pituitary gland. In Figure 25-3, the instructional note **See Arthroscopy; Thoroscopy** directs the user to other useful Main Terms.

Code number(s) next to a Main Term indicate the most likely applicable codes. Numbers may be single codes, a range of codes, or a nonsequential list (■ TABLE 25-6).

Table 25-6   ■   DESIGNATION OF CODES AND CODE RANGES IN THE CPT INDEX

Symbol	Purpose	Example
None	Single code	Bicarbonate 82374
Hyphen (-)	Range of codes All codes beginning with the first code number and ending with the last code number should be reviewed.	Bone Graft, Harvesting 20900-20902
Comma (,)	Nonsequential codes The specific codes listed should be reviewed, but the intervening code number(s) are not applicable or do not exist.	Biopsy, Urethra 52204, 52250, 52354, 53200

CODING PRACTICE

Exercise 25.1 Overview of CPT Coding/Organization of the CPT Manual

Instructions: Use your medical terminology skills and resources to define the following symptoms, signs, and abnormal findings, then assign the CPT code.

Follow these steps:

• Use slash marks "/" to break down each term into its root(s) and suffix.

• Define the meaning of the word, based on the meaning of each word part.

• If code(s) are listed next to the Main Term, write down the code. If no code is listed next to the Main Term, write down the first-level modifying term and the CPT code(s) listed for it.

Example: appendectomy append/ectomy   Meaning *cutting out the appendix*   First-level modifying term/code *Appendix, Excision 44950, 44955, 44960*

1. ventriculography   Meaning _____   First-level modifying term/code(s) _____

2. acetabuloplasty   Meaning _____   First-level modifying term/code(s) _____

3. ureterotomy   Meaning _____   First-level modifying term/code(s) _____

4. ileostomy   Meaning _____   First-level modifying term/code(s) _____

5. pneumonolysis   Meaning _____   First-level modifying term/code(s) _____

6. urethropexy   Meaning _____   First-level modifying term/code(s) _____

7. pericardiocentesis   Meaning _____   First-level modifying term/code(s) _____

8. lymphadenectomy   Meaning _____   First-level modifying term/code(s) _____

9. laryngoscopy   Meaning _____   First-level modifying term/code(s) _____

10. neurorrhaphy   Meaning _____   First-level modifying term/code(s) _____

CPT GUIDELINES

CPT provides guidelines at beginning of each section in the Tabular List and also provides special instructions at the beginning or many subsection and category headings. Instructional notes appear throughout the Tabular List before or after individual codes. Coders are obligated to read and understand all guidelines and instructions to ensure they abstract, assign, and arrange codes correctly.

New codes and guidelines are added or revised annually, so all coders must learn to analyze and apply updated information. This information can be challenging to understand because of the length and detail of the guidelines and special instructions. Key criteria for reading and interpreting CPT guidelines appears in ■ TABLE 25-7.

Guided Example of Researching CPT Guidelines

Use the category **Fenestrated Endovascular Repair of the Visceral and Infrarenal Aorta (34839-34848)** as an example of learning to read and understand special instructions.

The category **Fenestrated Endovascular Repair of the Visceral and Infrarenal Aorta** (34839-34848) in the CPT Cardiovascular System subsection under Surgery reports services

previously reported with Category III temporary codes. Fenestrated endovascular aneurysm repair (FEVAR) is the reinforcement of a section of the aorta weakened by a bulge, using a customized prosthesis. Holes in the prosthesis material, positioned to align with connecting arteries, allow blood flow to be maintained and allow for stents and catheters to be placed or maneuvered through the fenestration. FEVAR provides a

Table 25-7 ■ KEY CRITERIA FOR READING CPT GUIDELINES

❑ What is the purpose of the category and procedure(s)?

❑ How are anatomic sites or regions defined?

❑ How are the codes divided?

❑ What services are included in the code descriptions (not separately reportable)?

❑ What services can be reported separately?

❑ What standalone codes, indented codes, and add-on codes appear in the category?

❑ What instructional notes appear within the code descriptions in the Tabular List?

❑ What Main Term in the Index leads most directly to these codes?

Source: © PB Resources, Inc. Used with permission.

treatment alternative when the aneurysm is situated near arterial branches. Traditional endovascular aneurysm repair (EVAR), which uses a nonperforated prosthesis, is usually less successful in these situations because of its inability to provide support around the arteries.

Read through the special instructions and follow along in your CPT manual as Tanisha Riemann, CCS-P, identifies the key points.

▶ *What is the purpose of the procedure(s)?*

❑ The fenestrated (*perforated*) endoprosthesis (*prosthesis within a vessel*) is deployed (*placed*) within the visceral aorta. Fenestrations (perforations) within the fabric allow for selective catheterization of the visceral and/or renal arteries. They also allow for an endoprosthesis such as a bare metal or covered stent to be placed at a later time to maintain flow to the visceral artery.

▶ *How are anatomic sites or regions defined?*

❑ The thoracic aorta extends from the aortic valve to the aortic segment, just above the celiac artery.

❑ The visceral aorta is the upper abdominal aorta that contains the celiac, superior mesenteric, and renal arteries.

❑ The infrarenal (*below the kidney*) aorta is the lower abdominal aorta, below the renal arteries. (This definition is not stated in the special instructions but is based on anatomy.)

▶ *How are codes divided?*

❑ Codes **34839-34844** describe repairs using endoprostheses that span from the visceral aorta to the infrarenal aorta. Code descriptions specify one, two, three, or four visceral artery origins. The prostheses in these codes *do not* extend into the common iliac arteries.

❑ Codes **34845-34848** describe repairs using endoprostheses that span from the visceral aorta through the infrarenal aorta *into the common iliac arteries*. Code descriptions specify one, two, three, or four visceral artery origins.

▶ *What services are included in the code descriptions?*

❑ Proximal abdominal aortic extension prostheses and distal extension prostheses that terminate in the aorta or the common iliac arteries

❑ Placement of unilateral or bilateral docking devices used in the infrarenal aorta

❑ Introduction of guide wires and catheters in the aorta and visceral and/or renal arteries

❑ Balloon angioplasty within the target treatment zone of the endograft, either before or after endograft deployment

❑ Fluoroscopic guidance and radiological supervision and interpretation

▶ *What services can be reported separately?*

❑ Deployment of a fenestrated endograft distal to the infrarenal aorta (e.g **34845-34848**)

❑ Catheterization of the hypogastric artery(ies) and/or arterial families outside the treatment zone of the graft

❑ Exposure of the access vessels (e.g., **34812**)

❑ Extensive repair of an artery (e.g., **35226, 35286**)

❑ Other interventional procedures such as:
  ▪ Arterial embolization
  ▪ Intravascular ultrasound
  ▪ Balloon angioplasty
  ▪ Stenting of native artery(ies) outside the endoprosthesis target zone

▶ *What standalone codes, indented codes, and add-on codes appear in the category?* To answer this question, read the code descriptions in the category. Look for CPT conventions, such as indented code descriptions and the add-on code symbol (**+**). This category has two standalone codes and six indented code descriptions, as follows:

❑ Standalone code **34841** reports repair of the visceral aorta.

❑ Standalone code **34845** reports repair of both the visceral aorta and infrarenal aorta.

❑ Each standalone code reports the use of one endoprosthesis.

❑ Indented code descriptions under each standalone code report the use of two, three, or four or more endoprostheses.

▶ *What instructional notes appear within the code descriptions in the Tabular List?*

❑ Several instructional notes appear at the end of the category, after code **34848**, that identify codes that should not be reported together and provide clarification and cross-references.

▶ *What Main Term in the Index leads most directly to these codes?* The special instructions do not provide this information, so you need to investigate it yourself. To identify the best Main Term, try locating codes in the Index using the methods suggested by CPT in the introduction to the Index: anatomic site, procedure name, condition, synonym, eponym, abbreviation, or acronym.

❑ Follow the basic CPT procedure of looking first under the anatomic site, which is **Aorta**. A first-level modifying term identifies **Visceral** and additional second-level modifying terms identify **Repair, Endovascular**. The code range **34839, 34841-34848**, leads to the appropriate category in the Tabular List.

❑ As an alternative approach, look up the procedure **Endovascular Repair** as the Main Term. A first-level modifying term identifies **Visceral Aorta** with second-level modifying terms that identify the various types of endografts listed in this category.

Use a process similar to this whenever you encounter complex guidelines or special instructions. Make a list or create a summary table to help visualize the information provided.

ABSTRACTING PROCEDURES FOR CPT CODING

Coding procedures in CPT requires the three skills of an "Ace" coder—abstracting, assigning, and arranging codes. Because the CPT manual has a unique organization and unique conventions, coders must learn how using these skills differs for CPT compared with other code sets. This section of the chapter provides a guided example of coding using the CPT manual.

When abstracting for CPT, coders need to read the medical record and identify key criteria based on the services provided. Abstract only services provided during the encounter being coded. Do not code services that were previously provided or that may be planned for the future. Abstracting procedures from the patient's medical record involves three steps:

1. Identify the primary service or procedure.
2. Identify secondary services or procedures.
3. Identify the quantity of each procedure.

Identify the Primary Service or Procedure

Physicians may indicate procedure codes on the encounter form by placing a check mark next to or circling the CPT code that best describes the service provided. CPT codes may be data entered from the encounter forms directly into the practice management/billing system. However, medical offices must still audit and verify codes against the medical record on a regular basis to ensure that the documentation supports the services billed.

First, look for the chief complaint or reason for the visit, which usually provides an indication of the services that may be provided. Identify the primary procedure or the main service provided during the encounter. It is common for the E/M to be the only service provided. An E/M code includes the ongoing evaluation and management of a patient's care—specifically, taking the patient's history, conducting a physical examination, and performing the medical decision making required to create a plan of care.

When the physician orders a test to be performed at a later time, do not code for the test as part of the current encounter. Ordering the test or procedure is part of the medical decision-making component of the E/M service. Likewise, when the physician reviews test results during the encounter, do not code for the test, which was performed at a different time. The physician's review of the test results and discussion with the patient is included in the E/M code for the encounter. However, when a test is performed as part of the encounter—such as an in-office urinalysis or x-ray—code for the test in addition to the E/M service.

Identify Secondary Services or Procedures

Next, identify whether any secondary procedures were provided. Secondary procedures are any additional services documented in the medical record in addition to the primary procedure. They are abstracted and coded in the same way as the primary procedure. At the time of abstracting, coders do not necessarily know whether an additional service or procedure can be coded because it often depends on how the specific code is defined. For example, when a surgeon removes the uterus, cervix, and fallopian tubes you may be unsure how many CPT codes are required. By identifying all the structures removed when abstracting, you are prepared. When assigning codes, you learn that only one code is required to report the removal of all three structures (**58150 Total abdominal hysterectomy (corpus and cervix), with or without removal of tube(s), with or without removal of ovary(s)**).

Identify the Quantity of Each Procedure

All services must be billed with the quantity provided. Although coders may or may not be responsible for preparing the claim, they are responsible for identifying the quantity for each code because quantity is reported differently for different codes. For many procedures the quantity is one.

For services that can be repeated multiple times during one operative session, such as removal of lesions, the quantity reported with the code varies based on the code definition. You must first identify the type and number of lesions removed, as documented in the medical record, then convert the number to agree with the quantity included in the code description. For example, code **11200** for the removal of skin tags is defined as **up to and including 15 lesions**. Any quantity of lesions from 1 to 15 is reported with a quantity of **01** unit on the 837P electronic claim or Item 24G on the CMS-1500 form.

For services based on time, identify the number of minutes spent providing the service, then convert them to the unit of time required by the code description. For example, code **97035** for therapeutic ultrasound is reported in 15-minute increments. When 30 minutes of treatment are provided, report a quantity of **02** units on the 837P electronic claim or CMS-1500 form.

Refer to ■ TABLE 25-8 for general guidance on how to abstract procedures and services. These criteria apply to most services and procedures. More detailed abstracting criteria are presented for each body system throughout the CPT section of this text. Abstracting questions are a guide and not every question applies to, or can be answered for, every case. For example, complications do not occur with every patient.

Guided Example of Abstracting Procedures

Refer to the following example throughout this chapter to practice skills for abstracting, assigning, and arranging CPT codes.

OFFICE   Gender: M   Age: 32

Preprocedure diagnosis: Lesion on the back

Procedure: Prepared the area, administered local anesthesia, and excised one lesion from the back using a scalpel. Total excised area 0.7 cm. The site was closed with simple sutures.

Postprocedure diagnosis: Benign lesion on the back

Pathology report: Benign lesion 0.7 cm including margins

Table 25-8 ■ KEY CRITERIA FOR ABSTRACTING PROCEDURES (GENERAL GUIDELINES)

General Questions

❏ What service(s) were provided or procedure(s) performed at the current encounter by a physician or other qualified healthcare professional?

❏ What is the main service or procedure?

❏ What additional services or procedures were performed?

❏ What is the patient's age and gender?

Procedure-specific Questions

❏ What method, instrumentation, or approach was used?

❏ What anatomic site(s) were treated?

❏ What quantity was provided or time spent?

❏ What complications or unusual circumstances were encountered?

❏ Was more than one provider involved?

❏ What is the final diagnosis?

Source: © PB Resources, Inc. Used with permission.

Follow along as the fictitious coder, Sherry Whittle, CPC, abstracts the procedure. Check off each step after you complete it.

▶ Sherry reads through the entire record, paying special attention to the reason for the encounter and the final assessment. Sherry refers to Table 25-8, Key Criteria for Abstracting Procedures (General Guidelines).

❏ *What service(s) were provided or procedure(s) performed at the current encounter?* Removal of a lesion

❏ *What is the main service or procedure?* Removal of a lesion

❏ *What additional services or procedures were performed?* None

❏ *What is the patient's age and gender?* Male, 32

❏ *What method, instrumentation, or approach was used?* Local anesthesia, scalpel

❏ *What anatomic site(s) were treated?* Back

❏ *What quantity was provided or time spent?* One lesion, 0.7 cm

❏ *What complications or unusual circumstances were encountered?* None

❏ *Was more than one provider involved?* No

❏ *What is the final diagnosis?* Benign lesion on the back

CODING PRACTICE

Exercise 25.2 Abstracting Procedures for CPT Coding

Instructions: Read the mini-medical-record of each patient's encounter and answer the abstracting questions. Write the answer on the line provided. Do not assign any codes.

INPATIENT HOSPITAL   Gender: F   Age: 48

Preprocedure diagnosis: Metastatic breast cancer

Procedure: Left axillary lymphadenectomy, complete, using the open approach

Postprocedure diagnosis: Left breast cancer with metastasis to lymph nodes

Plan: Begin radiation therapy in 3 weeks.

1. What service(s) were provided or procedure(s) performed during the current encounter? _____

2. Describe the procedure performed in your own words. _____ _____

3. What is the patient's age and gender? _____

4. Are the patient's age and gender appropriate for the procedure? _____

5. What method, instrumentation, or approach was used? _____ _____

6. What anatomic site(s) were treated? _____
   Where is this site(s) located? _____

7. What quantity was provided? _____
   What is the extent of the service (superficial or complete)? _____

8. What service is listed in the Plan? _____
   Should it be coded? _____
   Why or why not? _____

9. What is the final diagnosis? _____

10. What is the principal diagnosis (the main reason the procedure was performed)? _____

ASSIGNING CPT CODES

Assigning CPT codes requires coders to research the procedure in the Index, then verify the code(s) in the Tabular List. Each of these processes includes several steps, which are discussed next. Never assign a code based on the Index alone, and do not turn to the Tabular List without first using the Index.

Research the Procedure in the Index

Use the Index to locate the preliminary code(s). This involves determining the Main Term, modifying terms, and codes or code ranges. Using the Index involves three steps:

1. Identify the Main Term.
2. Review the modifying terms and instructional notes.
3. Identify the preliminary code(s).

Identify the Main Term

The CPT Index is organized by Main Terms, the word(s) you look up in the Index to find the code(s). Each Main Term can stand alone or be followed by one to three modifying terms that provide added specificity. The CPT Index classifies Main Terms in four ways. Coders may use any of these methods to locate a code in the Index. If one method does not provide adequate information, then another method may be used. The four types of entries for Main Terms are:

- Procedure or service name
  - Examples: **Endoscopy, Incision, Cast**
- Organ or anatomic site
  - Examples: **Tibia, Colon, Lung**
- Condition
  - Examples: **Abscess, Clot, Fracture**
- Synonym, eponym, or abbreviation

  - Synonym examples: **Ocular Implant, Orbital Implant**
  - Eponym examples: **Nissen procedure, Fowler-Stephens procedure**
  - Abbreviation examples: **EKG, CD4**

The Main Term is always boldface, and each word begins with a capital letter. Some Main Terms are broad, with several pages of modifying terms, such as **Excision**, whereas others are quite specific, with only a single code, such as **Color Vision Examination**.

In the CPT Index, Main Terms include organs and anatomic sites, whereas in ICD-10-CM, the anatomic site is not an option in the Index. There are many choices of how to locate a Main Term, so a good guideline is to search in this order: eponym or abbreviation; procedure or service name; organ or anatomic site; disease or condition; synonym.

Review the Modifying Terms and Instructional Notes

After locating the Main Term, review the modifying terms and instructional notes. Modifying terms are entries under the Main Term that identify additional details regarding the anatomic site or procedure. Main Terms can have several levels of modifying terms. Each modifying term is a cumulative definition that includes the terms at the previous levels. For example, in Figure 25-3 the meaning of the fourth-level modifying term **Polyp** is *Endoscopy of the anus with the ablation of a polyp.*

Instructional notes list other Main Terms to look up if you cannot find what you need under the current term. They also tell you when to look up a synonym or other variation of the term. For example, when you look up an abbreviation or eponym in the CPT Index, it might redirect you to another entry, such as the fully spelled-out term or the generic name for the procedure. This feature assists coders in finding the appropriate Main Term more quickly (■ FIGURE 25-4).

Identify the Preliminary Code(s)

When the appropriate modifying terms are located, the preliminary code(s) is printed immediately to the right. It is helpful to jot down the preliminary codes before verifying in the Tabular List, being careful not to transpose any digits. Never use the Index to select the final code. Even when only one code appears, it must be verified in the Tabular List to be certain the code selection is accurate and to read any instructional notes.

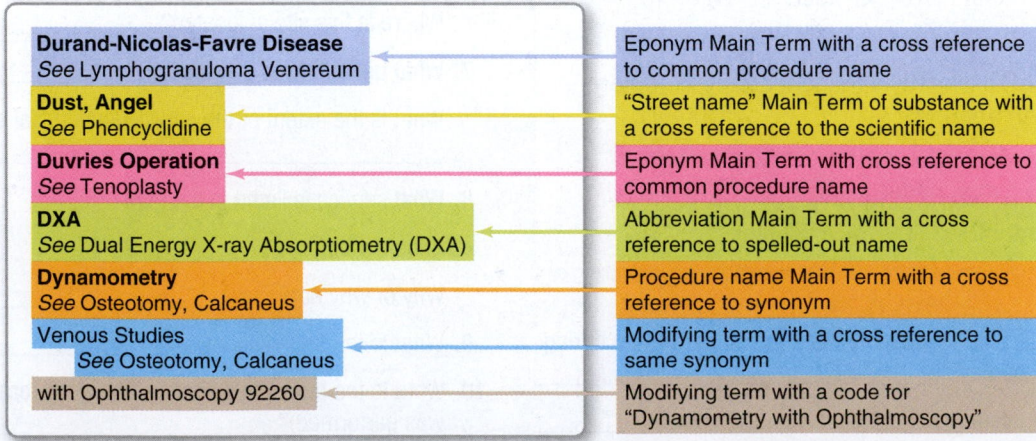

Figure 25-4 ■ Cross-reference instructional notes in CPT Index. *Source: © PB Resources, Inc. Used with permission.*

> ### CODING CAUTION
>
> Be aware of how the CPT Index differs from the ICD-10-CM Index. In the ICD-10-CM Index, each Main Term or subterm provides only one possible code. In the CPT Index, a Main Term or modifying term often provides several possible codes to consider. You must read the code descriptions and instructional notes in the Tabular List to select the final code.

Verify the Code in the Tabular List

All codes must be verified in the Tabular List to ensure that the description accurately represents the service provided. Coders also need to read the guidelines, special instructions, and instructional notes printed in the Tabular List. Verifying the code in the Tabular List involves the following steps.

1. Locate the preliminary code(s) in the Tabular List.
2. Interpret Tabular List conventions.
3. Select the code with the highest level of specificity.
4. Review the code for appropriate edits, such as bundling, add-on codes, and quantity.
5. Append modifiers, if necessary.
6. Assign the code.

Locate the Preliminary Code(s) in the Tabular List

Look for the preliminary code number in the Tabular List, where codes are arranged in numerical order. The Tabular List contains six sections, each of which is divided into subsections, subheadings, categories, and subcategories based on anatomy, procedure, condition, or descriptor. Be aware that because of the expanding nature of the code set, some codes are not in strict numerical order. These are resequenced codes and are highlighted with the symbol # for easy identification.

The CPT Index does not always list every possible code for a procedure. Sometimes it will list one or two codes from a series, and the coder must review surrounding codes in the Tabular List to locate the one needed.

Interpret Tabular List Conventions

Before coders verify and finalize the code, they first need to interpret the conventions presented with the code. The CPT code number appears on the left side of the column, with its description to the right. Tabular List conventions include formatting, punctuation, verbal instructions, and symbols. Conventions may appear on the same line with the code, above it, below it, or at the beginning of a subcategory, category, subheading, subsection, or section. Look carefully for any information that may be relevant to the preliminary code selection because this additional information can direct you to use a different code or an additional code. The Tabular List conventions of the semicolon, verbal instructions, and symbols are discussed next.

Semicolon. In the Tabular List, an important convention is the use of the semicolon (;) and indented code descriptions. To conserve space and avoid having to repeat common terminology, some of the procedure descriptors in the Tabular List are not printed in their entirety, but rather refer back to a common portion of the procedure descriptor listed in a preceding entry. The **standalone code** or **parent code** is the one whose description is left-justified and begins with a capital letter. The shared portion of the code before the semicolon is the **common descriptor**, which is shared with indented codes. The portion after the semicolon is the unique descriptor that applies to only one code number. The **indented code description** is indented three spaces and begins with a lowercase letter. This description is the unique descriptor for that code number. The unique descriptor must be combined with the shared descriptor from the standalone code to obtain a full description of the code. Within a series of indented codes, coders *must* refer back to the preceding standalone code to determine the common descriptor of the indented code(s). Indented codes describe variations of the standalone code, such as an alternative anatomic site, alternative procedure, or extent of services.

■ FIGURE 25-5 illustrates this formatting convention. The standalone code is **11400**. The words before the semicolon— **Excision, benign lesion including margins, except skin tag (unless listed elsewhere), trunk, arms or legs;**—are the common part of the description. This common descriptor should be considered part of each of the following indented codes in that series. For example, the full procedure descriptor represented by code **11401** is:

> **11401 Excision, benign lesion including margins, except skin tag (unless listed elsewhere), trunk, arms or legs; excised diameter 0.6 to 1.0 cm**

An indented code should not be billed together with the parent code unless both services were provided. These are considered

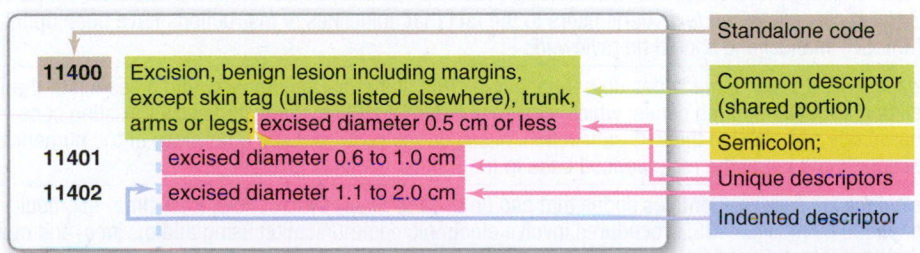

Figure 25-5 ■ Example of the semicolon convention. *Source: © PB Resources, Inc. Used with permission.*

two distinct procedures or services. The common descriptor is simply a space-saving convention in the printed book.

Narrative Instructions. The CPT manual provides several types of narrative instructions that guide coders:

• **Guidelines** are instructions that appear at the beginning of each of the six sections and apply to all codes in that section. Guidelines also list commonly used modifiers and provide subsection information.

• **Special instructions** are directions within each section describing specific rules and definitions for use of codes within a particular category or subcategory. Read and

interpret the special instructions before assigning a code, even if it means going back to the top of the page or a previous page to find them.

• **Instructional notes** appear in parentheses after a code description. They direct the user to alternative codes for closely related procedures or to codes that must or must not be used together (■ FIGURE 25-6).

Symbols. Symbols in the Tabular List alert the user to certain circumstances that can affect the use or interpretation of codes. A key appears at the bottom of each page. Coders should become familiar with these meanings (■ TABLE 25-9).

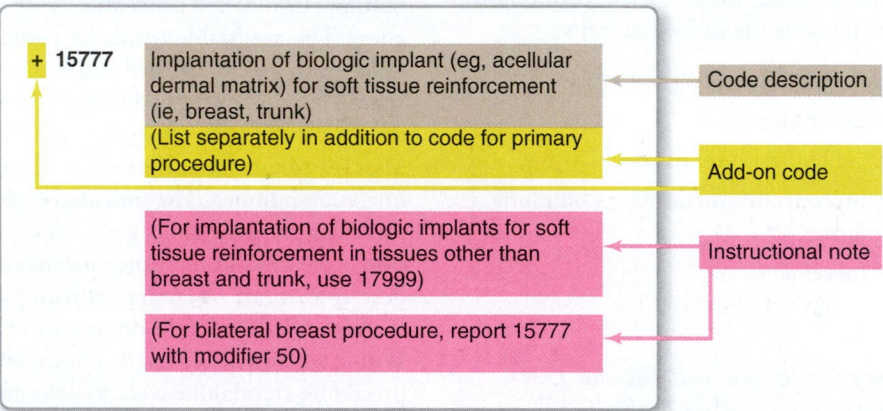

Figure 25-6 ■ Example of CPT Tabular List conventions. *Source: © PB Resources, Inc. Used with permission.*

Table 25-9 ■ **SYMBOLS USED IN THE CPT TABULAR LIST**

Symbol	Meaning
⊘	*Modifier -51 exempt.* When billing multiple procedures, a code with this symbol should not use modifier -51.
✚	*Add-on code must be used in conjunction with another CPT code.* The accepted companion codes are frequently provided in an instructional note. (When an add-on code is also an indented code, then report both the parent code and indented code.)
⟋	*FDA approval pending.* FDA approval of the vaccine described is expected to come during the current year.
( )	*Parentheses enclose synonyms, eponyms, or supplementary descriptors.* These terms do not have to appear in a physician's statement of condition to use the code.
•	*New code in this edition of the CPT manual.*
▲	*Revised code.* The code number is the same, but the descriptor has been updated for the current edition of the CPT manual. The descriptor should be reviewed to determine whether it is still appropriate.
▶◀	*Contains new or revised text.* Alerts users to the fact that guidelines or instructions have been updated in the current edition of the CPT manual and should be reviewed.
#	*Resequenced code.* Some codes do not appear in strict numerical sequence within a section of the Tabular List. Rather than deleting and renumbering codes, which was done before 2010, resequencing allows existing codes to be relocated to an appropriate place within the CPT subsection, based on the code concept, regardless of the numerical order. This symbol is appears to the left of the resequenced code in the Tabular List to help locate it.
★	*Telemedicine service.* Identifies codes that can be used to report synchronous (real-time) telemedicine services when appended by modifier -95. Procedures involve electronic communication using audio, video, and other interactive telecommunications equipment.
○	*Recycled/reinstated code.* Indicates that this code number was used in the past for a different service.

Select the Code with the Highest Level of Specificity

There is no universal rule that describes how many codes need to be reviewed to identify the one with the highest specificity. Sometimes, the best code is the first one listed; other times, there can be a dozen or more codes to review and additional ones to cross-reference. There is also no universal rule that governs how precise the description of the correct code will be. For example, many codes for the integumentary system include the size of the lesion or area treated, but the size is usually a range, such as a diameter of 1.1 to 2.0 cm or total area greater than 100 sq cm. If a lesion is *exactly* 1.5 cm, or the area is 110 sq cm, there is *not* a more specific code or modifier to describe the exact size. The medical record often contains more detail than what is coded. Only by carefully interpreting the conventions associated with each code, category, and section can one confirm the level of detail contained in a code description. As you become experienced in a particular office, you will become very familiar with the most frequently used codes.

Review the Code for Appropriate Edits

Carefully review code descriptions, instructional notes, and special instructions one more time to be certain that the code selected is accurate. Edits are specific coding and billing criteria that are checked for accuracy based on predetermined rules. Payers' computer systems reject claims that violate edit rules. Bundling, add-on codes, and quantity definitions are edits that should be reviewed.

Bundling Edits. Pay special attention to bundling edits, which are frequently triggered by the words **includes** and **not separately reportable**. These phrases indicate that multiple services are included in a single code. The words **report separately** or **use in conjunction with** indicate that additional codes should be used.

For example, the special instructions for codes **33510-33516 Venous Grafting Only for Coronary Artery Bypass** include both bundling and multiple coding situations.

- Instructions regarding bundling state: **Procurement of the saphenous vein graft is included in the description of the work for 33510-33516 and should not be reported as a separate service or co-surgery**.
- Instructions regarding multiple coding state that an additional code is needed in some situations: **To report harvesting of an upper extremity vein, use 35500 in addition to the bypass procedure**.

Add-On Codes. Add-on code are marked with a + in the CPT manual and must be reported with an additional procedure. Instructional notes appear in the Tabular List below an add-on and identify which code(s) the add-on codes should be used with. For example, when coding for discectomy of multiple disks, the code for each additional interspace is reported in addition to a specific primary procedure code. CPT add-on code **63078** should be used in conjunction with **60377**. Add-on codes may be standalone codes or indented codes, as **63078** is (■ FIGURE 25-7).

Quantity Edits. CPT codes differ regarding how the quantity of procedures is to be reported. This information is provided in the code description or special instructions. For example:

- To report removal of skin tags, a single code, **11200**, describes **up to and including 15 lesions**. Although the code is reported with a quantity of **01** in Item 24G of the CMS-1500 form, it describes any quantity from 1 to 15 lesions.
- To report shaving of epidermal or dermal lesions (**11300-11313**), each code describes a single lesion; multiple lesions of the same size and body area are reported by designating the number of lesions in Item 24G on the CMS-1500 form.
- To report end-stage renal disease services, use a single code for the entire month (**90960-90961**); the special instructions describe the scope of services included.

Codes that include a time-based element also vary in how quantity is reported. For example, codes for certain physical therapy treatments (**97032-97039**) describe 15 minutes of

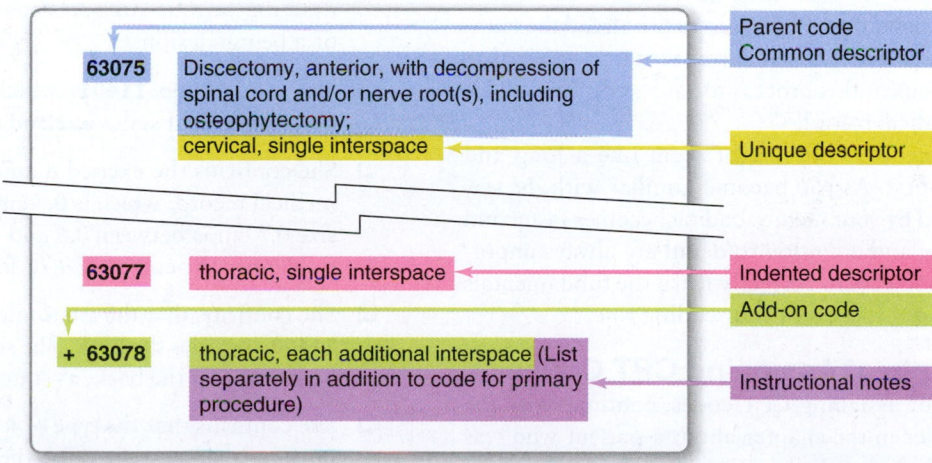

Figure 25-7 ■ Example of CPT indented and add-on codes. *Source: © PB Resources, Inc. Used with permission.*

treatment with a quantity of **01** in the appropriate electronic field for the 837P or in Item 24G on the CMS-1500 form. Thirty minutes of treatment is reported with a quantity of **02** in the appropriate electronic field for the 837P or in Item 24G on the CMS-1500 form.

Append Modifiers, If Necessary

Modifiers are two-digit suffixes used with CPT codes to report a service or procedure that has been modified by some specific circumstance without altering or modifying the basic definition or CPT code. The proper use of modifiers can speed up claims processing and increase reimbursement. Improper use of CPT modifiers may result in claim delays or denials.

Modifiers are used for a variety of reasons:

- To report only the professional component of a procedure or service
- To report a service mandated by a third-party payer
- To indicate that a procedure was performed bilaterally
- To report multiple procedures performed during the same session by the same provider
- To report a portion of a service or procedure that was reduced or eliminated at the physician's discretion
- To report a portion of the surgical package provided by someone other than the primary surgeon
- To report assistant surgeon services

Use of modifiers may be described in the instructional notes, special instructions, or guidelines. Modifiers may be necessary when the code(s) reported are affected by Medicare reimbursement rules. The experience of the coder is an important factor when determining whether the situation calls for any modifiers. A complete list of modifiers, with their full definitions, appears in Appendix A of the CPT manual.

Assign the Code

As a final check, with coding manual instructions fresh in your mind, refer back to the original documentation and verify that all conditions of the code agree with the medical record. If a discrepancy arises, work through the process again from the beginning. Write down the final code where indicated on your worksheet or documentation. Be certain to proofread the number as you wrote or keyed it to catch transcription errors that are easy to make. Repeat this process for any additional codes required by the medical record.

Selecting a procedure code might seem like a long and tedious process at first. As you become familiar with the services and codes used by your facility, coding becomes faster and easier, but accuracy and attention to detail are always important. Taking time and care to correctly learn the fundamentals helps create long-term success in your coding role.

Guided Example of Assigning CPT Codes

To practice skills for assigning CPT codes, continue with the example from earlier in the chapter about a patient who was seen for removal of a lesion. Follow along in your CPT manual as fictional coder Sherry Whittle, CPC, assigns codes. Check off each step after you complete it.

▶ First, Sherry confirms the procedure performed: excision, benign lesion 0.7 cm including margins.

▶ Sherry knows that she must search the CPT Index for the Main Term for the procedure. She has three choices for the Main Term:

- ❑ Procedure: **Excision**
- ❑ Condition: **Lesion**
- ❑ Anatomic site: **Skin**

▶ She decides to search for the condition and locates the Main Term **Lesion**.

- ❑ Immediately under the entry for **Lesion**, she reads the instructional note **See Tumor**. The patient did not have a tumor, so she does not follow the cross-reference.

- ❑ She understands that a lesion on the back is located on the skin. She locates the first-level modifying term, **Skin**.

- ❑ She locates the second-level modifying term for the procedure, **Excision**.

- ❑ Under Excision, she has a choice of **Benign** or **Malignant**, so she chooses **Benign** because it is consistent with the postprocedure diagnosis.

- ❑ She writes down the code range listed **11400-11471**. She knows she needs to reference all of these codes in the Tabular List to determine the correct code.

▶ Sherry turns to code **11400** in the Tabular List.

- ❑ First, she checks the title of the category, **Excision—Benign Lesions**, which seems to correctly match the medical record.

- ❑ She reads the code title, **11400 Excision, benign lesion including margins, except skin tag (unless listed elsewhere), trunk, arms or legs; excised diameter 0.5 cm or less**.

- ❑ She reads through the rest of the indented code descriptions through code **11471** and identifies that they describe various sizes and anatomic sites for excision of a benign lesion.

- ❑ She reads code **11401**, which is an indented code description that states **excised diameter 0.6 to 1.0 cm**.

- ❑ She confirms the excised diameter of the lesion in the medical record, which is 0.7 cm including margin. The size 0.7 cm is between 0.6 and 1.0 cm, so **11401** seems to identify the correct size of lesion.

- ❑ She confirms that the anatomic site in the parent code, **11400**, includes the back. The site of **trunk** stated in the code includes the back, as stated in the medical record.

- ❑ She confirms that the type of lesion in the parent code, **benign lesion**, agrees with the medical record.

- ❑ She combines the common portion of the parent code **11400** that comes before the semicolon with the unique description of code **11401** for a complete code description of **Excision, benign lesion including margins, except skin tag (unless listed elsewhere), trunk, arms or legs; excised diameter 0.6 to 1.0 cm**.

▶ Sherry checks for instructional notes in the Tabular List.

❏ She looks for instructional notes following the code and finds none. (Some editions of the CPT manual provide a cross-reference to the newsletter *CPT Assistant*, published by the AMA. Electronic coding programs often provide a similar reference.)

❏ She cross-references the beginning of category **Excision—Benign Lesions** and reads through the special instructions. The instructions provide the following information:

- Definition of excision as it applies to lesions
- Explanation that the lesion size includes the most narrow margins required to adequately excise the lesion.
- Clarification that the code for excision includes a simple closure (single-layer closure with sutures or staples)
- Instructions on how to code intermediate or complex closures, if required

❏ She refers back to the beginning of the subsection, **Integumentary System**, and the heading, **Skin, Subcutaneous, and Accessory Structures**, which appear before code **10030**. She finds no further instructions. She is already familiar with the **Surgery Guidelines** at the beginning of the section that include the **CPT Surgical Package Definition**. These guidelines confirm that local anesthesia is part of the surgical package and should not be coded separately.

▶ Sherry reviews the CPT code she has assigned for this case.

❏ **11401 Excision, benign lesion including margins, except skin tag (unless listed elsewhere), trunk, arms or legs; excised diameter 0.6 to 1.0 cm.**

▶ If more than one CPT code were required, she would need to determine how to sequence the codes.

▶ Sherry also assigns the ICD-10-CM diagnosis code for the lesion:

❏ **L98.9 Disorder of the skin and subcutaneous tissue, unspecified** (ICD-10-CM Index: **Lesion, skin, unspecified**).

CODING PRACTICE

Exercise 25.3 Assigning CPT Procedure Codes

Instructions: Refer to the mini-medical-record below that you abstracted in Exercise 25.2. Answer the questions to assign the CPT code. Write your answers on the lines provided.

INPATIENT HOSPITAL Gender: F Age: 48

Preprocedure diagnosis: Metastatic breast cancer

Procedure: Left axillary lymphadenectomy, complete, using the open approach

Postprocedure diagnosis: Left breast cancer with metastasis to lymph nodes

Plan: Begin radiation therapy in 3 weeks.

---

1. What is the Main Term for the procedure performed? _____

2. Look up the Main Term in the CPT Index. What first-level modifying term should you select? _____

3. What code(s) are listed next to the first-level modifying term?
_____

4. Locate the codes in the Tabular List. Which code is a standalone code? _____
_____

5. Which code is an indented code? _____
_____

6. Which code best describes the procedure performed? _____
_____

7. Write out the full description of the code. _____
_____

8. What is the name of the category in which this code appears?
_____

9. What is the name of the subheading in which this code appears? _____

ARRANGING CPT CODES

When more than one CPT code is required, secondary procedures are coded in the same way as primary procedures. CPT codes are prioritized from highest cost to lowest cost on the 837P electronic claim or CMS-1500 form. This is because many insurance companies pay the first procedure in full but often discount additional procedures performed at the same time. In general, the E/M code is identified first because the E/M code is not subject to a price reduction when multiple procedures are performed. Other services and procedures, including those subject to payment reductions, are listed after the E/M code.

CPT CODING AND REIMBURSEMENT

CPT coding has significant impact on reimbursement because fees are attached to CPT codes. Accurate coding and accurate data entry are essential to ensuring accurate reimbursement. Improper coding can result both in lower reimbursement than the provider is entitled to and in overpayment that puts the provider at risk of refunds and fines. To code accurately, coders must link procedures to diagnoses and adhere to reimbursement edits.

Diagnosis–Procedure Linking

Coders must ensure that each CPT code reported is linked, or cross-referenced, to one or more diagnosis codes that identify the medical reason each service was provided. Any CPT code not linked with an appropriate diagnosis code will not be paid by the carrier. If the coder identifies a service that does not

have documentation of a diagnosis that supports the need for the service, the provider should be queried. To query a provider involves sending the physician a message that asks for the reason the service was provided and requests the physician to amend the documentation to reflect the diagnosis.

Payers, including Medicare, maintain extensive databases of which diagnoses are considered to establish the medical necessity for each CPT code.

Coders should not manipulate codes in a manner that reports diagnoses not documented to receive reimbursement. Documentation should not be manipulated or altered to reflect diagnoses that do not actually exist. Both practices are improper and fraudulent.

On the CMS-1500 form, diagnosis codes are entered in Item 21. Date(s) of service, CPT codes, charges, and related information are entered on lines 1 through 6 of Item 24. In column 24E, enter the letter from Item 21 (A through L) that corresponds to the diagnosis that supports each service. Each service must be linked to one or more diagnosis codes. A diagnosis code can be linked to as many services as appropriate.

Reimbursement Edits

Reimbursement edits are rules regarding codes that may or may not be billed together or have special billing requirements. The purpose is to prevent overpayment associated with incorrect coding. Rules vary by payer and by region of the country. Medicare issues the largest number of reimbursement rules, summarized in ■ TABLE 25-10. Most Medicare edits are also applicable to

Table 25-10 ■ **REIMBURSEMENT EDIT CHECKS**

Name	Description	Example
National coverage determination (NCD)	Identifies the extent to which Medicare will cover specific services, procedures, or technologies on a national basis	Bariatric Surgery for Treatment of Morbid Obesity (100.1) • Specifies the types of bariatric surgery that are approved for coverage. • Specifies a list of comorbidities (*simultaneous diagnoses*), one of which must be present in addition to obesity for bariatric surgery to be approved.
National Correct Coding Initiative (NCCI)	Identifies code pairs that should not be reported together because they could not be performed during the same patient encounter because they are mutually exclusive based on anatomic, time, or gender considerations or because one code is a component of the other code	*41251 Repair of laceration 2.5 cm or less; posterior one-third of tongue* • Cannot be reported at the same time as code *12001 Simple repair of superficial wounds of scalp, neck, axillae, external genitalia, trunk, and/or extremities (including hands and feet); 2.5 cm or less.* • This would be a misuse of code 12001. 12001 can be billed with modifier -25, -57, or -59 when supported by documentation.
Medically unlikely edits (MUEs)	Identifies the maximum units of service that a provider would report under most circumstances for a single beneficiary on a single date of service	*21920 Biopsy, soft tissue of back or flank; superficial* • MUE: three units per patient per day per line. • Some MUEs can be bypassed if the code is reported on a separate line with a modifier for separate anatomic sites, global surgery package, or modifiers -27, -59, or -91 and documentation supports it.
Local coverage determination (LCD)	Identifies a decision by a Medicare administrative contractor (MAC) whether to cover a particular service or item as reasonable and necessary for providers in its region	Removal of Skin Lesion (Non-Melanoma) • Medicare allows coverage and payment for only those services that are considered to be medically reasonable and necessary. • The LCD indicates that the MAC will consider the removal of benign skin lesions as medically necessary, and not cosmetic, if a condition from a list of approved diagnoses is present and clearly documented in the medical record. It also provides a list of applicable CPT codes.

Source: © PB Resources, Inc. Used with permission.

Medicaid. Private payers can follow Medicare edits or publish their own. Medicare publishes most of its criteria for coverage and coding edits on its website, **www.cms.gov**. Medicare administrative contractors (MACs) also maintain websites for each region of the country and each contractor uses its website to publish local rules.

Reimbursement edits are automated **prepayment edits**, which means that claims are electronically scanned for compliance with the rules before the payer accepts them into the claims processing system. Depending on the specific rule and codes billed, in some cases providers can append a modifier to the code in question that will allow it to be accepted.

Medicare national coverage determination (NCD) and local coverage determination (LCD) policies that provide direction regarding specific diagnosis codes will be updated for ICD-10-CM. Most encoder software contains built-in reference information (■ FIGURE 25-8) or edit checks that screen for these rules so the error can be corrected before the provider submits

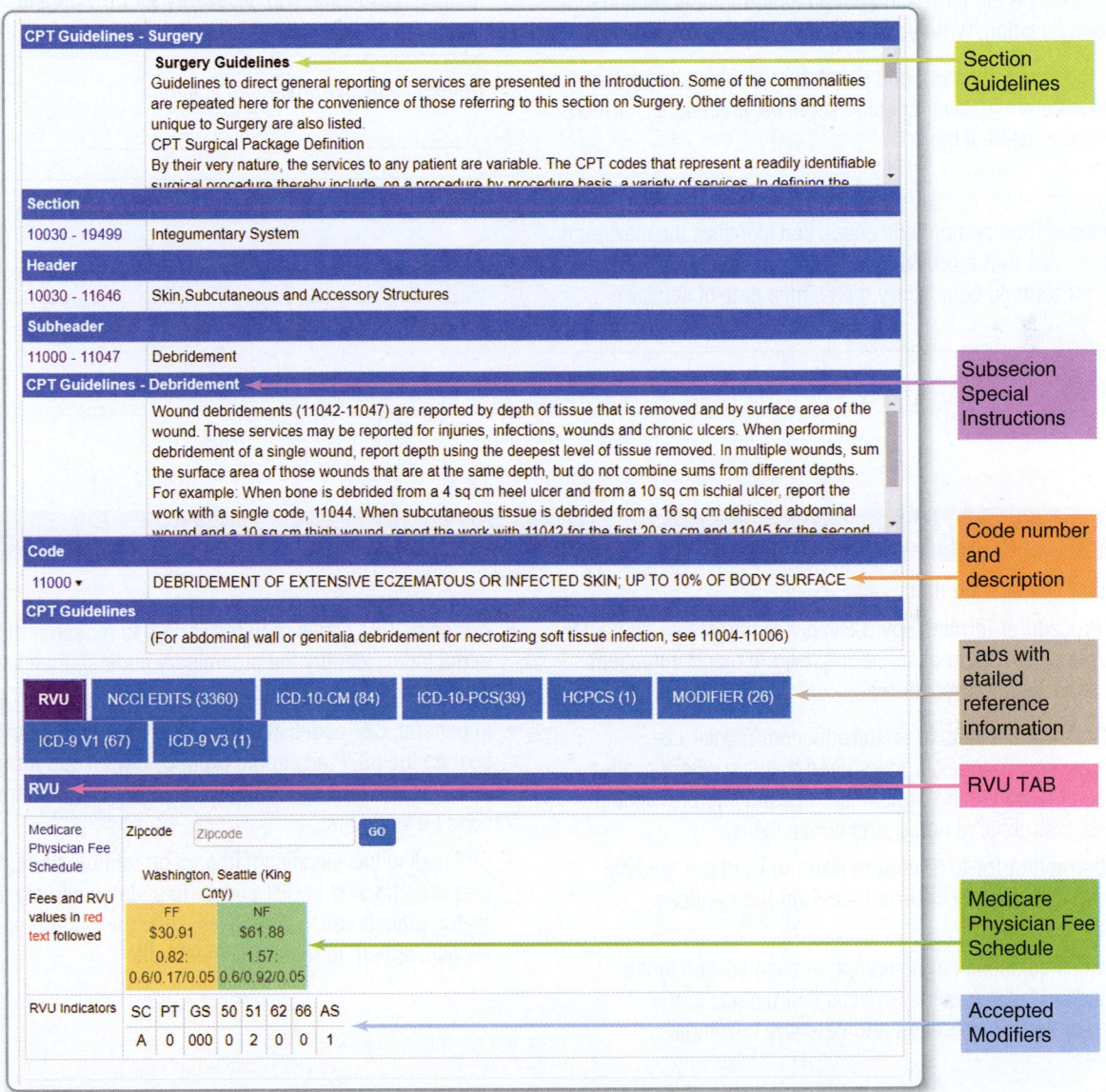

Figure 25-8 ■ Example of reimbursement edits in an encoder. *Source: SpeedeCoder, Reprinted with permission.*

the claim. Electronic claims clearinghouses, which route claims from the provider to the payers, also may scrub the claims for certain edit checks. If providers repeatedly submit claims that violate the edit checks, they may be investigated by payers for compliance.

Some medically unlikely edits (MUEs) are confidential and shared only with MACs. Providers learn by trial and error which MUEs impact them the most. Physician and outpatient hospital reimbursement is discussed in detail in Chapter 2 of this text.

CODING PRACTICE

Exercise 25.4 CPT Coding and Reimbursement

Instructions: Provide the term and abbreviation from this section that answers each question. Write your answer on the line provided.

1. What is the reimbursement edit check that identifies the extent to which Medicare will cover specific services, procedures, or technologies on a national basis?

   _____

2. What is the reimbursement edit check that identifies the maximum units of service that a provider would report under most circumstances for a single beneficiary on a single date of service?

   _____

3. What reimbursement edit check is a decision by a Medicare administrative contractor whether to cover a particular service or item as reasonable and necessary for providers in its region?

   _____

4. Define *diagnosis-procedure linking*.

   _____

   _____

5. Define *reimbursement edits*.

   _____

   _____

CHAPTER SUMMARY

In this chapter you learned that:

- Current Procedural Terminology (CPT) is a listing of five-character alphanumeric codes and descriptions used to report outpatient medical services and procedures.

- The CPT manual consists of an Introduction, Tabular List, Appendices, and an Index. Coders need to know where needed information is located and how to identify and interpret coding guidelines, instructional notes, and conventions.

- When abstracting for CPT, coders need to read the medical record and identify key criteria based on the services provided.

- CPT provides guidelines at beginning of each section in the Tabular List and also provides special instructions at the beginning or many subsection and category headings.

- Assigning CPT codes requires coders to research the procedure in the Index, identify the preliminary code(s), then verify the code(s) in the Tabular List.

- In general, CPT codes are prioritized from highest cost to lowest cost on the 837P electronic claim or CMS-1500 form, although some payers request that the Evaluation and Management (E/M) code be listed first.

- CPT coding has significant impact on reimbursement because fees are attached to CPT codes. To code accurately, coders must match procedures to diagnoses, code for the appropriate level of service, adhere to reimbursement edits.

CONCEPT QUIZ

Take a moment to look back at this introduction to CPT coding and solidify your skills. Try to answer the questions from memory first, then refer to the discussion in this chapter and the Glossary at the end of this book if you need a little extra help.

Completion

Instructions: Write the term that completes each statement based on the information you learned in this chapter. Choose from the following list. Some choices may be used more than once and some choices may not be used at all.

add-on codes	modifiers
Category I	modifying terms
Category II	parent code
Category III	prepayment edit
common descriptor	semicolon
edits	subcategory
instructional notes	

1. _____ codes comprise the bulk of CPT and describe widely used services and procedures approved by the FDA.

2. A _____ is a two-digit alphanumeric suffix appended to a CPT code to provide further description of the circumstances of an encounter.

3. _____ are Index entries that are indented under the Main Term and add further detail about the service or procedure.

4. _____ inform the coder of other Main Terms to look up, such as synonyms or other variations of the term.

5. _____ codes are optional, consist of four numbers followed by the letter *F*, and are used to collect and track data performance measurement.

6. Conventions may appear on the same line with the code, above it, below it, or at the beginning of a _____.

7. A standalone or parent code's common descriptor is shared with an indented code descriptor by the use of a _____.

8. _____ codes are temporary codes used for data collection and for tracking the use of emerging technology, services, and procedures.

9. _____ are specific coding and billing criteria that are checked for accuracy based on predetermined rules.

10. _____ codes that are marked with a + in the CPT manual and must be reported with an additional procedure code.

Multiple Choice

Instructions: Circle the letter of the best answer to each question based on the information you learned in this chapter.

1. What is the term for sending the physician a message that asks for the reason the service was provided and requests the physician to amend the documentation to reflect the diagnosis?
   A. Memo
   B. Inquiry
   C. Query
   D. Instant message

2. What is the name of the edits in which claims are electronically scanned for rules before a payer accepts them into the claims processing system?
   A. Precertification
   B. Prepayment
   C. Preview
   D. Preordered

3. In what order should CPT codes be sequenced on a claim?
   A. Ascending code number
   B. Descending code number
   C. Ascending fee
   D. Descending fee

4. What type of fee covers the cost of the physician's time?
   A. Professional fee
   B. Technical fee
   C. Facility fee
   D. Referral fee

5. What medical term means *inflammation of an artery?*
   A. Arteritis
   B. Arthritis
   C. Arterectomy
   D. Arthrectomy

6. Which edit identifies code pairs that should not be coded together?
   A. National coverage determination (NCD)
   B. National Correct Coding Initiative (NCCI)
   C. Medically unlikely edits (MUEs)
   D. Quick reference edits (QREs)

(continued)

(continued from page 461)

7. What billing format is the electronic equivalent of the CMS-1500 form?
   A. 1500E
   B. CMS-1501
   C. 837P
   D. ICD10

8. What element establishes the medical necessity of each CPT code?
   A. Modifiers
   B. Add-on codes
   C. Procedure codes
   D. Diagnosis codes

9. What is the name of the instructions that appear at the beginning of each CPT section?
   A. Guidelines
   B. Conventions
   C. Practices
   D. Edits

10. Which component of an E/M service includes ordering a test or procedure?
    A. History
    B. Medical decision making
    C. Examination
    D. Chief complaint

KEEP ON CODING

Instructions: Read the procedural statement, then use the Index and Tabular List to assign CPT procedure codes. Write the code(s) on the line provided.

1. Endoscopic placement of bronchial stent, left. CPT Code(s) _____

2. Dacryocystotomy, left. CPT Code(s) _____

3. Intermediate (layered) repair of open wound to fascia, 7.2 cm, right thigh. CPT Code(s) _____

4. Computerized tomography without contrast, head. CPT Code(s) _____

5. Swallowing function study with images. CPT Code(s) _____

6. Bone marrow biopsy from pelvic bone. CPT Code(s). _____

7. Rhinoscopy with biopsy of left sinus. CPT Code(s). _____

8. Ultrasound guidance only for biopsy of endomyocardial mass. CPT Code(s) _____

9. Transurethral prostatectomy. CPT Code(s) _____

10. Carpal tunnel release. CPT Code(s) _____

11. Diagnostic lumbar puncture. CPT Code(s) _____

12. Spirometry and evaluation. CPT Code(s) _____

13. Cardiac echography, spectral and color flow, 2D. CPT Code(s) _____

14. Endoscopic removal of foreign body from small intestine. CPT Code(s) _____

15. Excision of coccygeal pressure ulcer. CPT Code(s) _____

16. Endoscopic ablation of colon polyp. CPT Code(s) _____

17. Cast, arm below elbow for hairline fracture, right ulna. CPT Code(s) _____

18. Cystotomy with repair of ureterocele. CPT Code(s) _____

19. Screening, computer-aided mammography. CPT Code(s) _____

20. MRI, diagnostic, right hip joint. CPT Code(s)

21. Ultrasound of fetus for biophysical profile without nonstress testing. CPT Code(s) _____

22. Nasogastric feeding tube placement with fluoroscopic guidance. CPT Code(s) _____

23. Laparoscopic splenectomy. CPT Code(s) _____

24. Vascular flow study of liver (SPECT). CPT Code(s) _____

25. Aortic serialographic arteriography, abdominal. CPT Code(s) _____

CODING CHALLENGE

Instructions: Read the mini-medical-record, then answer the questions that follow to abstract, assign, and arrange ICD-10-CM diagnosis codes and CPT procedure codes.

OUTPATIENT HOSPITAL   Gender: F   Age: 54

Reason for encounter: Hematuria; patient is on insulin for type 1 diabetes

Procedure: Cystourethroscopy revealed 2.7-cm mass in bladder neck; mass resected using snare technique

Postoperative diagnosis: Pathology confirmed bladder neck mass as an adenomatoid tumor

Plan: Follow-up ultrasound in 6 weeks.

Part 1: Abstract

1. Read through the mini-medical-record. First, abstract for the diagnosis. Compare the chief complaint to the final assessment.

   a. What symptoms did the patient report in the chief complaint? _____

   b. What condition is stated in the assessment? _____

2. Review the symptom(s).

   a. What is the meaning of the medical term for the symptom?

   _____

   b. Should you code for the symptom? _____

   Why or why not? _____

3. Review the mini-medical-record for any other conditions.

   a. Is another condition documented? _____

   If so, list the condition. _____

   b. Should the condition be coded? _____

   Why or why not? _____

4. Next, abstract for the procedure.

   a. Break down the term into its two roots and suffix.

   _____/_____/_____

   b. What does this term mean? _____

   c. What instrument was used during this procedure?

   _____

   d. Through what route was the instrument inserted to reach its final objective? _____

5. Were any other procedures performed during this operative session? _____

   If so, name the additional procedure(s). _____

Part 2: Assign

6. First, assign the diagnosis codes. You can look up the conditions in any order you wish, as long as you sequence them correctly in the end based on any instructional notes and Official Guidelines for Coding and Reporting.

   a. Look up the Main Term **Tumor** in the Index of your ICD-10-CM manual, then the subterm **adenomatoid**. Are there special instructions? _____ If so, what do the special instructions tell you to do? _____

   _____

   _____

   b. Where do you locate **Neoplasm, benign, by site** in the ICD-10-CM manual? _____

   c. What first-level subterm and second-level subterm should you locate? _____

   d. What code is listed? _____

   e. Verify this code in the Tabular List. What is the final code?

   _____

7. Assign and verify the diagnosis code for diabetes. What is the correct code? _____

   _____

8. Now assign the procedure code. In the CPT manual, look up the Main Term **Excision** then the first-level modifying term **Bladder**.

   a. Is there an additional modifying term that should be referenced under Bladder? _____ If so, what is the term? _____

   b. What code or code range is listed? _____

9. Verify the code in the CPT Tabular List.

   a. Under what CPT section and subsection is this code located? Section _____ Subsection _____

   b. What is the code description? _____

   _____

   c. Does this code description accurately identify the procedure performed during this encounter? _____

   Why or why not? _____

   d. Is there an instructional note listed under this narrative? _____ If yes, what does the instructional note say?

   _____

   _____

   e. When you cross-reference code 52234, does it accurately describe the procedure? _____ Why or why not? _____

   _____

   f. Which code within the range 52234-52240 best describes the procedure performed? _____ Why? _____

   _____

   g. CPT codes can be indexed under several different Main Terms. Provide at least one additional Index path that can be used to locate this code. Main Term _____.

   Modifying terms _____

   _____

(continued)

(continued from page 463)

Part 3: Arrange

10. You identified two ICD-10-CM codes and one CPT for this case. Review your answers in the previous questions to determine the correct sequencing.

    a. Which diagnosis code is sequenced first? _____

       Why? _____

    b. Which diagnosis code is sequenced second? _____

       Why? _____

    c. What is the final procedure code? _____

    d. Is the procedure code supported by the first-listed diagnosis? _____

       Why? _____

Chapter 26

Learning Objectives

After completing this chapter, you should have the skills to:

26.1 Spell and define the key words, medical terms, and abbreviations related to HCPCS coding. (Remember)

26.2 Summarize the main characteristics of HCPCS coding. (Understand)

26.3 Describe the organization of the HCPCS manual. (Understand)

26.4 Examine and abstract procedural information from the medical record for HCPCS codes and modifiers. (Analyze)

26.5 Demonstrate how to assign codes using the HCPCS Index and Tabular List. (Apply)

Chapter Outline

- **Overview of HCPCS Codes**
- **Organization of the HCPCS Manual**
- **Abstracting for HCPCS Codes and Modifiers**
- **Assigning HCPCS Codes**

Key Terms and Abbreviations

enteral nutrition
HCPCS Index
HCPCS modifier
HCPCS Table of Drugs

HCPCS Tabular List
Healthcare Common Procedure Coding System (HCPCS)
Level I (HCPCS)

Level II (HCPCS)
millicurie
miscellaneous code
parenteral nutrition

permanent national code
temporary national code

In addition to the key terms listed here, students should know the terms defined within tables in this chapter.

INTRODUCTION

Item numbering systems differ among manufacturers, but a retailer must find ways to accommodate the various systems. Likewise, coders must adapt to multiple code sets. Procedure coding was formalized in the late 1960s and 1970s after the creation of Medicare and Medicaid. Medicare gave rise to rapid growth within the healthcare industry, and by the 1980s major updating and streamlining were needed. This led to the creation of a new coding system, the Healthcare Common Procedure Coding System (HCPCS), to classify and report services and supplies not included in the Current Procedural Terminology (CPT). This chapter introduces the HCPCS system, the organization of the HCPCS coding manual, and instructions on abstracting and assigning HCPCS codes and modifiers.

OVERVIEW OF HCPCS CODES

The Healthcare Common Procedure Coding System (HCPCS) was developed by the Center for Medicare and Medicaid Services (CMS) in conjunction with the American Medical Association (AMA) and was released in 1983. HCPCS has two divisions, or levels, of codes:

Level I—Current Procedural Terminology (CPT) codes

Level II—National Healthcare Common Procedure Coding System codes

Although CPT codes have been used since 1966, in 1983 they were updated and incorporated into the overall HCPCS system. However, they remain the property of the AMA. CPT codes are Level I codes within the HCPCS system. Most people refer to them as CPT codes, but you will sometimes encounter references to Level I codes when reading rules and regulations from Medicare or other payers.

Level II codes were a new code set in 1983 to classify services *not included in* CPT, as well as physician and nonphysician services, medical supplies, equipment, and medications. Level II codes are commonly referred to as HCPCS (pronounced "hick-picks") codes. They are owned by CMS, with the exception of codes for dental services, which are copyrighted by the American Dental Association. Examples of services, supplies, and items reported with HCPCS codes include ambulance services, medical and surgical supplies, drugs, nutrition therapy, durable medical equipment, orthotic and prosthetic procedures, and hearing and vision services.

Initially, providers were required to use HCPCS codes only for Medicare and Medicaid patients. However, many other payers found HCPCS codes to be useful and began to require that providers use them. As of 2003, HCPCS Level II became a mandated code set under the Health Insurance Portability and Accountability Act (HIPAA). CMS is responsible for maintaining Level II HCPCS codes, including yearly revisions, additions, and deletions. Updates occur quarterly throughout the year, and the full code set is published annually in January.

HCPCS codes are reported in Item 24D on the CMS-1500 form or in the comparable field on the 837P electronic claim.

Categories of HCPCS Codes

HCPCS codes have three categories:

1. Permanent national codes
2. Temporary national codes
3. Miscellaneous codes

Permanent National Codes

Permanent national codes are those that all U.S. providers and insurances can use for billing and statistical purposes. CMS created a HCPCS workgroup, which determines whether to add, revise, or delete HCPCS codes. The workgroup is responsible for maintaining the permanent codes.

Temporary National Codes

The HCPCS workgroup also creates temporary national codes for services and supplies that do not have a permanent code. The workgroup creates these codes in response to Medicare's needs, but any provider and insurance can use temporary codes. The workgroup can add temporary codes before the annual HCPCS code set update on January 1. Temporary codes remain temporary indefinitely until the workgroup decides to replace them with permanent codes. When the workgroup replaces a temporary code with a permanent one, it deletes the temporary code from the code set and provides a cross-reference to the new permanent code.

Miscellaneous Codes

Miscellaneous codes allow providers to immediately bill insurances for a service or item as soon as the FDA approves its use, even though there is no permanent or temporary code that describes it. Examples of miscellaneous or not otherwise specified codes include:

- **A9999 Miscellaneous DME supply or accessory, not otherwise specified**
- **J9999 Not otherwise classified, antineoplastic drugs**
- **V5274 Assistive listening device, not otherwise specified**

Medicare and other payers manually review claims with miscellaneous codes, so providers must submit supporting documentation to payers explaining why the patient needs the item or service. Before reporting a miscellaneous code, check with individual payers to ensure that there is not another permanent or temporary code to describe the service.

ORGANIZATION OF THE HCPCS MANUAL

There are approximately 3,000 HCPCS codes. Each is made up of a letter followed by four numbers (**A0000-V9999**). Each letter represents a group of similar services, supplies, drugs, and equipment. For example, HCPCS codes beginning with the letter **J** represent drugs, and codes beginning with the letter **D** represent dental services. The American Dental Association

(ADA) created and owns the copyright to dental codes, called *Current Dental Terminology (CDT)* codes. These codes do not appear in the HCPCS manual and must be purchased from the ADA or from a publisher who is authorized to print them as part of the full HCPCS manual. The HCPCS code set can also be located online at the CMS website (**www.cms.gov**).

Examples of specific codes and their meanings include:

- **A4206 Syringe with needle, sterile, 1 cc or less, each**
- **E0117 Crutch, underarm, articulating, spring assisted, each**
- **G0390 Trauma response team associated with hospital critical care service**
- **J0360 Injection, hydralazine HCl, up to 20 mg**

HCPCS codes are used by physicians, hospitals, pharmacies, ambulance services, and durable medical equipment suppliers.

The HCPCS manual contains six sections. The order in which the sections appear in a printed manual depends on the publisher, so it is important to become familiar with the organization of the specific HCPCS manual that you use. The sections are:

- Introduction
- Index
- Tabular List
- Table of Drugs
- Modifiers
- Appendix

CODING CAUTION

You may hear people in healthcare refer to HCPCS codes as **A** codes, **B** codes, **C** codes, and so on, based on the first letter of the code. Be careful not to confuse these codes with ICD-10-CM codes that also begin with letters. You usually can tell from the context of the conversation which code set is being referenced.

Introduction

The Introduction provides an overview of the organization of the HCPCS manual because each publisher organizes the manual a bit differently. Publisher-specific conventions, such as symbols and color coding, are identified. Brief instructions on how to use the HCPCS manual are provided.

HCPCS Index

The HCPCS Index is an alphabetical listing of services and supplies organized by Main Terms and subterms. Main Terms may consist of the name of an item (such as wheelchair), the type of service (such as hospice care), the anatomic site (such as leg), or a medication provided (such as digoxin).

The HCPCS Index uses conventions similar to other coding manuals. Main Terms are set flush left and appear in boldface type in some manuals. Subterms are indented, followed by a single code, several codes, or a range of continuous codes. Instructional notes with cross-references and other information also occur (■ FIGURE 26-1). Coders must verify all the codes listed in the Tabular List. You cannot randomly use any code listed after a subterm entry. You must research the description in the Tabular List and select the correct code that specifically describes the service or supply.

HCPCS Tabular List

The HCPCS Tabular List arranges codes in alphanumeric order, beginning with codes that start with the letter *A*, followed by four numbers (■ TABLE 26-1 page 468). Chapters are organized with subheadings that identify groups of related services. However, HCPCS does not have a formal multilevel organization scheme like other code sets. Depending on the publisher of the HCPCS manual, the Tabular List may include helpful coding notes, CMS coding and billing guidelines, and other information to help you assign the correct code, such as identifying codes with a specific color that represents additional information. These are publisher-specific conventions that are described in the Introduction to the manual. A key to symbols and color coding often appears at the bottom of each page in the Tabular List.

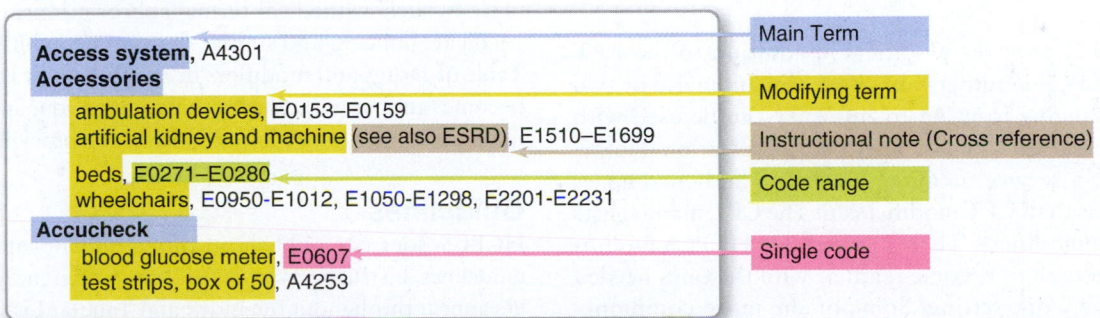

Figure 26-1 ■ Conventions in the HCPCS Index. *Source: © PB Resources, Inc. Used with permission.*

Table 26-1 ■ **ORGANIZATION OF THE HCPCS TABULAR LIST**

Code Range	Description
A0021–A9999	Transportation services such as ambulance; medical and surgical supplies, including supplies for urinary incontinence (*loss of urinary bladder control*), ostomy, respiratory, and dialysis; and radiopharmaceuticals (*radioactive substances used for diagnostic or therapeutic services*).
B4034–B9999	Supplies, equipment, and nutritional products for enteral and parenteral nutrition.
C1713–C9899	New technology procedures, drugs, biologicals, radiopharmaceuticals, magnetic resonance angiography (MRA), and devices for outpatient hospitals to report.
D Codes	Dental services. The ADA holds the copyright to D codes. They usually do not appear in the HCPCS manual.
E0100–E8002	Durable medical equipment (DME) for patients' activities of daily living, including crutches and oxygen equipment.
G0008–G9990	Procedures and services that may or may not have equivalent CPT codes, such as screening exams.
H0001–H2037	Mental health services, including treatment for alcohol and drug abuse.
J0120–J9999	Drugs that the patient does not self-administer.
K0001–K0903	DME for which there are no other HCPCS codes available, such as power wheelchairs.
L0112–L9900	Orthotics (*devices that help to regain function*) and prosthetics (*replacement body parts*), including cervical collars, lumbar support, artificial limbs, or male vacuum erection systems.
M0075–M1071	Other medical services, cardiovascular services, and quality measures.
P2028–P9615	Pathology and laboratory services and blood products.
Q0035–Q9995	Temporary codes for drugs and supplies.
R0070–R0076	Transportation of portable diagnostic radiology equipment to provider locations.
S0012–S9999	Drugs, services, and supplies for Medicaid and other non-Medicare payers.
T1000–T5999	Medicaid services and supplies.
V2020–V5364	Vision supplies, such as eyeglasses; hearing services and supplies; and speech-language pathology services.

Table of Drugs

HCPCS provides codes for generic and brand name drugs, which are organized in the **HCPCS Table of Drugs**. These codes are used to bill for drugs prescribed by a physician and administered by a healthcare provider. The Table of Drugs provides a convenient way to locate drug codes, but they usually can also be located in the Index using the name of the drug as the Main Term. Regardless of whether you identify the drug code using the Table of Drugs or the Index, all codes must be verified in the Tabular List. The Table of Drugs may be located at the end of the Index, the end of the Tabular List, or in an appendix, depending on the publisher.

Modifiers

HCPCS Level II provides modifiers in addition to the CPT modifiers. **HCPCS modifiers** are either alphanumeric or two letters long, ranging from **A1** to **ZB**. They can be used with both HCPCS and CPT codes. They provide additional information about a service, item, or procedure and encompass more situations than CPT modifiers do. The CPT manual lists some of these modifiers. There are over 300 HCPCS modifiers, so it takes time to become familiar with the ones needed in a particular work setting. Some of the more commonly used modifiers identify laterality and anatomic site and are listed in the CPT manual.

Other uses of HCPCS modifiers include:

- Reimbursement-related information, such as medical necessity requirements or patient-requested items
- Type of provider, such as nurse-midwife, clinical social worker, or principal physician of record
- Clinical indicators, such as hematocrit level or urea reduction ratio (URR)
- Ambulance services, point of origin, and destination

Appendices

Many publishers provide appendices with reference information, such as medical terms, abbreviations, excerpts from Medicare policies, and similar data. Some publishers place the Table of Drugs and modifiers in appendices. It is important to become familiar with the organization of your specific HCPCS manual so you know where to locate necessary information.

Guidelines

HCPCS does not publish an official document with coding guidelines. Instructional notes and cross-references to assist coders appear throughout the Index and Tabular List. Payment and coding policies issued by Medicare, Medicaid, and other payers provide coders with direction on how to use HCPCS codes.

CODING PRACTICE

Exercise 26.1   HCPCS Overview and Organization

Instructions: For each description of services, supplies, equipment, or drugs, write down the Main Term to look for in the HCPCS Index. Locate the appropriate subterm, then list the code(s) that appear next to the subterm.

Example: A physician provides an ankle splint to a patient. Main Term: *Splint* HCPCS Code(s): *L4392-L4398, S8451*

1. A physician orders a raised toilet seat for a patient to use at home, which the DME supplier provides. Main Term: _____ HCPCS Code(s): _____

2. A psychologist conducts a patient assessment for mental health services at an outpatient mental health facility. Main Term: _____ HCPCS Code(s): _____

3. The physician changes a lead in a patient's pacemaker, which is a transvenous VDD single pass. Main Term: _____ HCPCS Code(s) _____

4. A primary care physician (PCP) gives a patient an enteral fiber additive to assist the patient in having regular bowel movements. Main Term: _____ HCPCS Code(s): _____

5. A physician assistant administers the hepatitis B vaccine to a patient. Main Term: _____ HCPCS Code(s): _____

ABSTRACTING FOR HCPCS CODES AND MODIFIERS

The three skills of an "Ace" coder—abstracting, assigning, and arranging codes—apply to HCPCS coding. As with many areas of coding, the most challenging part of working with HCPCS codes is knowing when they are needed. It takes some experience and familiarity with HCPCS codes and Medicare regulations to learn all the situations in which a HCPCS code is required. In addition, not all payers use HCPCS codes to the same extent, so it is necessary to learn and organize the requirements for the payers and services provided in your workplace.

This section provides general guidelines for abstracting HCPCS codes and modifiers. Refer to ■ TABLE 26-2 for general abstracting criteria for HCPCS codes. An answer of *yes* to any of the abstracting questions indicates a potential need for one or more HCPCS codes. Look up the supply item or service in the HCPCS Index or look up the drug in the HCPCS Table of Drugs.

For help identifying when HCPCS modifiers are needed, refer to ■ TABLE 26-3 (page 470). When the answer to a question is *yes*, review the modifiers listed in the right-hand column. Look up the description of each modifier suggested in the HCPCS modifier list and determine which, if any, apply to the patient. Also refer to payer policies for guidance. Table 26-3 does not cover all modifiers or all situations, but it will help you get started. As with HCPCS codes, it takes a while to become familiar with all the HCPCS modifiers. In the workplace, you will learn which modifiers are used most often by your provider. Practice management system (PMS) software and encoders can be preprogrammed to alert to the potential need for modifiers.

Table 26-2 ■ **KEY CRITERIA FOR ABSTRACTING HCPCS CODES**

❑ Is the patient covered by Medicare or Medicaid?

❑ Does the patient's payer require/accept HCPCS codes?

❑ Did the patient receive durable medical equipment (DME), such as wheelchairs, crutches, hospital beds, or related accessories?

❑ Did the patient receive supplies to help treat or manage any of the following conditions:
  - Urinary incontinence
  - Ostomies
  - Respiratory problems
  - End-stage renal disease (ESRD)/dialysis
  - Need for parenteral and enteral nutrition

❑ Was radiopharmaceutical contrast administered (such as for a nuclear medicine scan)?

❑ Did the patient receive medication or drugs administered by a healthcare provider, including:
  - Injections
  - Chemotherapy drugs for cancer treatment
  - Immunosuppressive drugs for treatment of patients whose immune systems are compromised (including patients with AIDS)
  - Inhaled solutions

❑ Did the patient receive services or supplies related to orthotics or prosthetics?

❑ Did the patient receive preventive care services such as an immunization, mammogram, or colorectal cancer screening?

Source: © PB Resources, Inc. Used with permission.

Table 26-3 ■ **KEY CRITERIA FOR ABSTRACTING HCPCS MODIFIERS**

Criteria	Modifier(s)
❏ Did the patient receive a service on a paired organ or site?	LT, RT
❏ Did the patient receive a service that treated the eyelids, fingers, toes, or coronary arteries?	E1-E4, F1-FA, TA, T1-T9, LC, LD, LM, RC, RI
❏ Was chiropractic manipulation provided?	AT
❏ Were one or more wounds dressed?	A1-A9
❏ Did the patient units of service exceed those in the medically unlikely edits (MUEs)?	GD
❏ Was a waiver of liability/Advanced Beneficiary Notice (ABN) issued or required due to the possibility of a Medicare denial for lack of medical necessity?	GA, GL, GK, GU, GZ, KB
❏ Was only the technical component of a service provided by a facility?	TC
❏ Did a dialysis patient receive dialysis-related services or non-dialysis-related services?	AX, AY, CB, CD-CF, ED-EM, G1-G6, JE, V5-V7
❏ Were psychotherapy or substance abuse services provided?	H9-HZ
❏ Did a nonphysician provider deliver the service?	AE-AJ, AS, GF, QY, SB, SD
❏ Was the service provided by a substitute or locum tenens provider?	Q5-Q6
❏ Were anesthesia services provided?	AA-AD, G8-G9, P1-P6, QX-QZ
❏ Was a screening mammogram or colonoscopy converted to a diagnostic test or done on the same day as a diagnostic version of the procedure?	GG, GH, PT
❏ Was a supply item or piece or part of equipment replaced?	FB, FC, KC, KN, KM, MS, RA, RB
❏ Were services performed that are normally bundled, but should be billed separately because of a separate encounter, separate provider, separate structure or anatomic site, or other unusual circumstances?	XE, XP, XS, XU
❏ Did the physician admit the patient to a hospital or nursing facility during the encounter?	AI

Source: © PB Resources, Inc. Used with permission.

CODING PRACTICE

Exercise 26.2 Abstracting for HCPCS Codes and Modifiers

Instructions: Identify the appropriate modifier for each of the following situations. Refer to Table 26-3, Key Criteria for Abstracting HCPCS Modifiers, to locate potential modifiers. Then look up the modifiers listed in the HCPCS manual and select the correct one. Assign the modifier only. Do not assign codes.

1. A patient received an opiate substitute as part of an opioid addiction treatment program. Modifier: _____

2. A woman delivered a 6 pound, 5 ounce infant with the assistance of a nurse-midwife. Modifier: _____

3. Dressings were changed for two wounds. Modifier: _____

4. A chalazion was removed from the right upper eyelid. Modifier: ____

5. A patient's portable respiratory suction pump malfunctioned and was replaced by the supply company. Modifier: _____

ASSIGNING HCPCS CODES

Assigning HCPCS codes requires coders to use the HCPCS Index and verify codes in the HCPCS Tabular List. This section provides details and examples of assigning codes for the most common services and supplies: transportation services, medical supplies, radiopharmaceuticals, enteral and parenteral nutrition, durable medical equipment, professional services, drugs administered by clinicians, and orthotics.

Coding for Transportation Services Including Ambulance (A0021-A0999)

HCPCS codes are used for both nonemergency and emergency transportation services. Such services use specially equipped

vehicles to transport ill or injured patients. Modes of transportation include:

- Ambulance van
- Air ambulance, fixed wing (airplane), or rotary wing (helicopter)
- Wheelchair van
- Taxi
- Bus
- Automobile

Ambulance providers are either freestanding or institution-based services. Freestanding services include independently owned and operated ambulance services, volunteer fire and/or ambulance companies, and local government-run firehouse-based ambulances. Institution-based ambulance providers are owned or operated by a hospital, critical access hospital (CAH), skilled nursing facility (SNF), comprehensive outpatient rehabilitation facility (CORF), home health agency (HHA), or hospice provider.

The company or facility that owns and provides ambulance or nonemergency transportation services is the entity that codes and bills for the service. The hospital or provider that receives a patient *does not* bill for the transportation service.

Ambulances offer two levels of service to patients: basic life support (BLS) and advanced life support (ALS). BLS includes services from a certified emergency medical technician (EMT). ALS includes services from a certified EMT-Intermediate or an EMT-Paramedic. At least two people, including one EMT, must be in the ambulance.

Ambulance providers use HCPCS codes to bill payers for transportation services for transporting patients to the hospital, SNF, or other destination. They also use HCPCS modifier(s) with the transportation code. Ambulance services are paid a base rate for the level of service provided, a mileage rate, and fees for supplies or extra personnel. Refer to ■ TABLE 26-4 for guidance in abstracting information to code for transportation services.

Ambulance services appear under the Main Term **Ambulance** in the HCPCS Index. Coding for ambulance services involves the following steps (■ FIGURE 26-2):

1. Assign a HCPCS code for the type of transportation service provided, with the quantity of **1** (codes **A0225, A0426-A0434**).

2. If the ambulance is an institution-based provider, append one of the following modifiers to describe the type of arrangement.

   - **QM**—Ambulance service provided under arrangement by a provider of services

   - **QN**—Ambulance service furnished directly by a provider of services

3. Refer to the list of location codes (**D** through **X**) at the beginning of section **A** in the HCPCS manual. Using these codes, create a two-letter modifier than identifies the origin and destination.

   - The first letter of the modifier identifies the origin (where the patient was picked up).

   - The second letter of the modifier identifies the destination (where the patient was taken to).

Table 26-4 ■ KEY CRITERIA FOR ABSTRACTING AMBULANCE SERVICES

- ❏ Is the ambulance service freestanding or institution-based?
- ❏ What type of vehicle was used to transport the patient: ground (ambulance), air fixed wing (airplane), or air rotary wing (helicopter)?
- ❏ What type of services did the patient need: nonemergency, emergency, ALS, BLS, specialty care transport (SCT), or neonatal care?
- ❏ How many miles did the ambulance have to travel from its origin to its destination?
- ❏ Were extra personnel involved?
- ❏ What supplies were used?

Source: © PB Resources, Inc. Used with permission.

Branton Ambulance Service (freestanding supplier)
Patient was transported by ambulance from home to Branton Medical Center, after she collapsed on the kitchen floor.
Service provided: BLS, 12 miles.

A0429-RH Ambulance service, basic life support, emergency transport (BLS-emergency); origin-home (R); destination-hospital (H)
A0380 Basic life support mileage x 12

Figure 26-2 ■ Example of HCPCS coding for ambulance services. *Source:* © PB Resources, Inc. Used with permission.

4. Append the origin/destination modifier to the ambulance service code. Sequence this as the *second* modifier for institution-based providers.

5. Assign a code for the miles travelled (**A0380, A0390, A0425, A0435, A0436**), with a quantity that identifies the number of miles.

6. Assign a code for waiting time (**A0420**), if applicable, with a quantity based on the time increments shown before code **A0420** in the HCPCS Tabular List.

7. Assign codes for supplies used and any extra attendants, beyond two.

To code for nonemergency transport, follow these steps:

1. Assign a code for the mode of nonemergency transportation (**A0090-A0210**) with a quantity of **1**.

2. Assign a code for miles driven (**A0021-A0080**) with a quantity that identifies the number of miles driven.

SUCCESS STEP

Employment with an ambulance service can be a potential entry-level job for coders. You have the opportunity to gain experience and confidence working with a high volume of claims that have similar but very specific coding requirements.

Coding for Medical Supplies (A4206-A9300, A9900-A9999)

Healthcare providers and medical supply companies code and bill payers for supplies provided to patients. Providers can purchase supplies directly from supply companies, dispense the supply to a patient, and then bill the patient's insurance. The supply company can also provide the supply directly to the patient and then bill the patient's insurance.

Each payer, including Medicare, has unique coding, billing, and reimbursement guidelines for supplies, depending on the type of supply, the patient's diagnosis, and the circumstances involved. Some payers do not pay separately for specific supplies that they consider to be a normal part of providing a service. Instead, the payer issues one payment for the service that includes the supply costs.

To locate codes in the HCPCS Index, locate the Main Term for the supply item, such as **Catheter** or **Dressing**, or a Main Term for the condition, such as **Ostomy**.

Some payers may require providers to report the generic CPT code **99070 Supplies and materials** instead of a HCPCS code that identifies the specific supply. Coding departments should maintain a quick reference sheet of each payer's requirements. Always contact the payer directly when there are questions about how to bill supplies.

Coding for Radiopharmaceutical Drugs (A9500-A9700)

Radiopharmaceutical drugs, also called *contrasts* or *tracers*, are used in nuclear medicine procedures. They are radioactive drugs that emit radiation that can be seen on a scan to help physicians and clinicians determine an organ's structure and function (■ FIGURE 26-3). Radiopharmaceuticals are also used to treat diseases such as bone cancer. The tracer or contrast medium is billed by the radiologist, in addition to the CPT code for the procedure (■ FIGURE 26-4).

Medicare and other payers have specific guidelines regarding which radiopharmaceutical providers are permitted to code and bill in addition to the radiology service. They also have guidelines for radiopharmaceuticals that should not be separately reported because they are included with payment for the CPT code. Always check individual payer guidelines to ensure that you report the correct codes.

To locate radiopharmaceutical drugs in the HCPCS Index, use the Main Term **Radiopharmaceutical**, then locate the

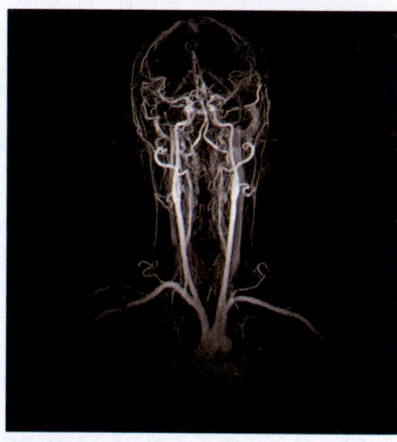

Figure 26-3 ■ Magnetic resonance angiography (MRA) of arteries in the head and neck that can be seen using a trace. *Photo credit: Bendao/Shutterstock.*

> A physician performed a positron emission tomography (PET) perfusion scan with a tracer for a patient at rest. 60 millicuries of the radiopharmaceutical Rubidium Rb-82 was used in the study.

78491	Myocardial imaging, positron emission tomography (PET), perfusion; single study at rest or stress
A9555	Rubidium Rb-82, diagnostic, per study dose, up to 60 millicuries x 1

Figure 26-4 ■ Example of coding for a radiology service and a radiopharmaceutical drug. *Source: © PB Resources, Inc. Used with permission.*

name of the substance. You can also look up the name of the substance as the Main Term or use the Table of Drugs. The unit of measurement for radiopharmaceutical drugs is the **millicurie**. Report the quantity based on the dosage measurement identified in the code description. For code **A9555**, the quantity of **1** identifies 0–60 millicuries; the quantity of **2** identifies 61–120 millicuries, and so on. All radiopharmaceutical codes should be verified in the Tabular List.

Coding for Enteral and Parenteral Therapy (B4034-B9999)

HCPCS **B** codes represent supplies, equipment, and nutritional products for parenteral and enteral nutrition. **Enteral nutrition** therapy, also called *tube feeding*, is providing nutrients to patients through a tube in one of the following sites:

- Nose using a nasogastric (NG) tube
- Stomach using a gastrostomy (G) tube
- Small intestine using a jejunostomy (J) tube

Parenteral nutrition therapy is treatment that provides nutrients intravenously because the body is unable to take in nutrients orally or by other methods. Patients who need enteral or parenteral therapy suffer from disorders or effects of surgery that prohibit them from taking food by mouth, such as swallowing disorders, neuromuscular diseases, trauma, or reconstructive procedures to treat head, neck, and bowel diseases, such as colon cancer. Patients may experience various types of infections or other complications from receiving enteral and parenteral nutrition.

Medicare and other payers may reimburse for these items when they are not part of an inpatient hospital stay, but payment depends on the place of service, the patient's diagnosis, and whether the condition is short term or long term, among other criteria.

To locate codes in the HCPCS Index, look up the Main Term for the supply item, such as **Tube**, or look up the Main Term **Parenteral nutrition** or **Enteral nutrition**, then locate the appropriate subterm. Always verify codes in the Tabular List.

Coding for Durable Medical Equipment (E0100-E8002)

HCPCS **E** codes represent DME, which includes crutches, wheelchairs, commodes, canes, walkers, hospital beds, oxygen and related respiratory equipment, pacemakers and related monitoring equipment, patient lifts and other safety equipment, fracture and traction equipment, and artificial kidney machines.

Patients must meet specific criteria of medical necessity to qualify for DME coverage by Medicare. CMS provides Certificate of Medical Necessity forms that must be completed by the DME supplier and physician to document the medical need for certain supplies and equipment (■ FIGURE 26-5). Forms can be downloaded from **www.cms.gov**. Look on the *Medicare* tab for a link to *CMS Forms*.

To locate codes in the HCPCS Index, look up the Main Term for the DME item, such as **Wheelchair** or **Oxygen**, then locate the appropriate subterm. Always verify codes in the Tabular List.

DEPARTMENT OF HEALTH AND HUMAN SERVICES
CENTERS FOR MEDICARE & MEDICAID SERVICES

Form Approved OMB
No. 0938-0679
Expires 02/2020

CERTIFICATE OF MEDICAL
NECESSITY CMS-484 OXYGEN

DME 484.03

SECTION A: Certification Type/Date: INITIAL ___/___/___ REVISED ___/___/___ RECERTIFICATION ___/___/___

PATIENT NAME, ADDRESS, TELEPHONE and MEDICARE ID	SUPPLIER NAME, ADDRESS, TELEPHONE and NSC or NPI #
(___) ____–____ Medicare ID	(___) ____–____ NSC or NPI # _____

PLACE OF SERVICE _____	Supply Item/Service Procedure Code(s):	PT DOB ___/___/___ Sex ___ (M/F) Ht. ___(in) Wt ___
NAME and ADDRESS of FACILITY if applicable (see reverse)		PHYSICIAN NAME, ADDRESS, TELEPHONE and UPIN or NPI # (___) ____–____ UPIN or NPI # _____

SECTION B: Information in this Section May Not Be Completed by the Supplier of the Items/Supplies.

EST. LENGTH OF NEED (# OF MONTHS): _____ 1–99 (99=LIFETIME) | DIAGNOSIS CODES: _____ _____ _____ _____

ANSWERS	ANSWER QUESTIONS 1–9. (Check Y for Yes, N for No, or D for Does Not Apply, unless otherwise noted.)
a) _____mm Hg b) _____% c) ___/___/___	1. Enter the result of recent test taken on or before the certification date listed in Section A. Enter (a) arterial blood gas PO2 and/or (b) oxygen saturation test; (c) date of test.
☐ 1 ☐ 2 ☐ 3	2. Was the test in Question 1 performed (1) with the patient in a chronic stable state as an outpatient, (2) within two days prior to discharge from an inpatient facility to home, or (3) under other circumstances?
☐ 1 ☐ 2 ☐ 3	3. Check the one number for the condition of the test in Question 1: (1) At Rest; (2) During Exercise; (3) During Sleep
☐ Y ☐ N ☐ D	4. If you are ordering portable oxygen, is the patient mobile within the home? If you are not ordering portable oxygen, check D.
_____LPM	5. Enter the highest oxygen flow rate ordered for this patient in liters per minute. If less than 1 LPM, enter an "X".
a) _____mm Hg b) _____% c) ___/___/___	6. If greater than 4 LPM is prescribed, enter results of recent test taken on 4 LPM. This may be an (a) arterial blood gas PO2 and/or (b) oxygen saturation test with patient in a chronic stable state. Enter date of test (c).

ANSWER QUESTIONS 7-9 ONLY IF PO2 = 56–59 OR OXYGEN SATURATION = 89 IN QUESTION 1

☐ Y ☐ N	7. Does the patient have dependent edema due to congestive heart failure?
☐ Y ☐ N	8. Does the patient have cor pulmonale or pulmonary hypertension documented by P pulmonale on an EKG or by an echocardiogram, gated blood pool scan or direct pulmonary artery pressure measurement.
☐ Y ☐ N	9. Does the patient have a hematocrit greater than 56%?

NAME OF PERSON ANSWERING SECTION B QUESTIONS, IF OTHER THAN PHYSICIAN (Please Print):

NAME_____ TITLE_____ EMPLOYER_____

SECTION C: Narrative Description of Equipment and Cost

(1) Narrative description of all items, accessories and option ordered; (2) Suppliers charge; and (3) Medicare Fee Schedule Allowance for each item, accessory, and option (see instructions on back)

SECTION D: PHYSICIAN Attestation and Signature/Date

I certify that I am the treating physician identified in Section A of this form. I have received Sections A, B and C of the Certificate of Medical Necessity (including charges for items ordered). Any statement on my letterhead attached hereto, has been reviewed and signed by me. I certify that the medical necessity information in Section B is true, accurate and complete, to the best of my knowledge, and I understand that any falsification, omission, or concealment of material fact in that section may subject me to civil or criminal liability.

PHYSICIAN'S SIGNATURE_____ DATE ___/___/___
Signature and Date Stamps Are Not Acceptable.

Form CMS–484 (02/17)

Figure 26-5 ■ Medicare Certificate of Medical Necessity for Oxygen form. (*continued*)

INSTRUCTIONS FOR COMPLETING THE CERTIFICATE OF MEDICAL NECESSITY FOR OXYGEN

SECTION A:	**(May be completed by the supplier)**
CERTIFICATION DATE:	If this is an initial certification for this patient, indicate this by placing date (MM/DD/YY) needed initially in the space TYPE/ marked "INITIAL." If this is a revised certification (to be completed when the physician changes the order, based on the patient's changing clinical needs), indicate the initial date needed in the space marked "INITIAL," and indicate the recertification date in the space marked "REVISED." If this is a recertification, indicate the initial date needed in the space marked "INITIAL," and indicate the recertification date in the space marked "RECERTIFICATION." Whether submitting a REVISED or a RECERTIFIED CMN, be sure to always furnish the INITIAL date as well as the REVISED or RECERTIFICATION date.
PATIENT INFORMATION:	Indicate the patient's name, permanent legal address, telephone number and his/her Medicare ID as it appears on his/her Medicare card and on the claim form.
SUPPLIER INFORMATION:	Indicate the name of your company (supplier name), address and telephone number along with the Medicare Supplier Number assigned to you by the National Supplier Clearinghouse (NSC) or applicable National Provider Identifier (NPI). If using the NPI Number, indicate this by using the qualifier XX followed by the 10-digit number. If using a legacy number, e.g. NSC number, use the qualifier 1C followed by the 10-digit number. (For example. 1Cxxxxxxxxxx)
PLACE OF SERVICE:	Indicate the place in which the item is being used, i.e., patient's home is 12, skilled nursing facility (SNF) is 31, End Stage Renal Disease (ESRD) facility is 65, etc. Refer to the DMERC supplier manual for a complete list.
FACILITY NAME:	If the place of service is a facility, indicate the name and complete address of the facility.
SUPPLY ITEM/SERVICE PROCEDURE CODE(S):	List all procedure codes for items ordered. Procedure codes that do not require certification should not be listed on the CMN.
PATIENT DOB, HEIGHT, WEIGHT AND SEX:	Indicate patient's date of birth (MM/DD/YY) and sex (male or female); height in inches and weight in pounds, if requested.
PHYSICIAN NAME, ADDRESS:	Indicate the PHYSICIAN'S name and complete mailing address.
PHYSICIAN INFORMATION:	Accurately indicate the treating physician's Unique Physician Identification Number (UPIN) or applicable National Provider Identifier (NPI). If using the NPI Number, indicate this by using the qualifier XX followed by the 10-digit number. If using UPIN number, use the qualifier 1G followed by the 6-digit number. (For example. 1Gxxxxxx)
PHYSICIAN'S TELEPHONE NO:	Indicate the telephone number where the physician can be contacted (preferably where records would be accessible pertaining to this patient) if more information is needed.
SECTION B:	**(May not be completed by the supplier. While this section may be completed by a non-physician clinician, or a Physician employee, it must be reviewed, and the CMN signed (in Section D) by the treating practitioner.)**
EST. LENGTH OF NEED:	Indicate the estimated length of need (the length of time the physician expects the patient to require use of the ordered item) by filling in the appropriate number of months. If the patient will require the item for the duration of his/her life, then enter "99".
DIAGNOSIS CODES:	In the first space, list the diagnosis code that represents the primary reason for ordering this item. List any additional diagnosis codes that would further describe the medical need for the item (up to 4 codes).
QUESTION SECTION:	This section is used to gather clinical information to help Medicare determine the medical necessity for the item(s) being ordered. Answer each question which applies to the items ordered, checking "Y" for yes, "N" for no, or "D" for does not apply.
NAME OF PERSON ANSWERING SECTION B QUESTIONS:	If a clinical professional other than the treating physician (e.g., home health nurse, physical therapist, dietician) or a physician employee answers the questions of Section B, he/she must print his/her name, give his/her professional title and the name of his/her employer where indicated. If the physician is answering the questions, this space may be left blank.
SECTION C:	**(To be completed by the supplier)**
NARRATIVE DESCRIPTION OF EQUIPMENT & COST:	Supplier gives (1) a narrative description of the item(s) ordered, as well as all options, accessories, supplies and drugs; (2) the supplier's charge for each item(s), options, accessories, supplies and drugs; and (3) the Medicare fee schedule allowance for each item(s), options, accessories, supplies and drugs, if applicable.
SECTION D:	**(To be completed by the physician)**
PHYSICIAN ATTESTATION:	The physician's signature certifies (1) the CMN which he/she is reviewing includes Sections A, B, C and D; (2) the answers in Section B are correct; and (3) the self-identifying information in Section A is correct.
PHYSICIAN SIGNATURE AND DATE:	After completion and/or review by the physician of Sections A, B and C, the physician's must sign and date the CMN in Section D, verifying the Attestation appearing in this Section. The physician's signature also certifies the items ordered are medically necessary for this patient.

Form CMS-484 (02/17) INSTRUCTIONS

Figure 26-5 ■ *(continued)* from previous page

Coding for Procedural/Professional Services (G0008-G9990)

HCPCS **G** codes are temporary national codes used to identify professional services and procedures that would otherwise be coded using CPT or for which no CPT code exists. Many of these codes were created for tracking by Medicare and Medicaid because they are usually more specific than CPT codes and identify services that are reimbursed in a unique way.

When a patient has Medicare or Medicaid, report the HCPCS code. CMS has specific regulations for reimbursing screening exams, including the patient's age, such as age 50 or older, and the frequency of exams, such as every 4 years (■ FIGURE 26-6).

When the patient has insurance *other than* Medicare or Medicaid, *report the CPT code* unless the payer requires the HCPCS code. Always check individual payer coding guidelines to be sure whether they require the HCPCS code or the CPT code (■ FIGURE 26-7).

A Medicare patient is seen for a screening colonoscopy using flexible sigmoidoscopy.

G0104 Colorectal cancer screening; flexible sigmoidoscopy

Figure 26-6 ■ Example of coding for a colonoscopy for a Medicare patient. *Source: © PB Resources, Inc. Used with permission.*

A patient with private insurance is seen for a screening colonoscopy using flexible sigmoidoscopy.

45330 Sigmoidoscopy, flexible, diagnostic; with or without collection of specimen(s) by brushing or washing (separate procedure)

Figure 26-7 ■ Example of coding for a colonoscopy for a private insurance patient. *Source: © PB Resources, Inc. Used with permission.*

SUCCESS STEP

Medical billing software can be programmed to identify whether each insurance company requires a HCPCS or CPT code. To activate this feature, the coding department must identify services that have both CPT and HCPCS codes, then give the computer technician a list of which payers require which code. Then, the billing staff member can enter only the CPT code, and the computer will substitute the HCPCS code for the required payers.

Coding for Drugs (J0120-J9999)

HCPCS **J** codes include drugs that the patient does not self-administer. They include injections, chemotherapy drugs for cancer treatment, immunosuppressive drugs for treatment of patients whose immune systems are compromised (including patients with AIDS), and inhaled solutions. Clinicians administer these drugs and monitor patients to ensure that there are no contraindications or side effects.

HCPCS also provides codes for drugs in sections **A**, **C**, **G**, **K**, **Q**, and **S**. In addition, there are HCPCS codes that represent

supplies used to administer drugs, such as syringes or an IV medication bag. HCPCS codes for drugs and related supplies do not include the actual service that the clinician performs to administer the drug. CPT codes identify these services.

To locate codes for drugs in the HCPCS Index, locate the Main Term for the name of the drug. You can also locate most drugs in the Table of Drugs (■ FIGURE 26-8). The Table of Drugs provides four columns. Various publishers may use different titles for the columns, but they are similar to the following:

- Column 1, Drug Name: Alphabetical list of drugs by generic and brand names. Drugs that are manufactured in more than one concentration have a separate entry for each.

- Column 2, Dose: Identifies the quantity or dose identified by the code.

- Column 3, Route: The method of administration of the substance (■ TABLE 26-5 page 476).

- Column 4, Code: The HCPCS code that must be verified in the Tabular List.

Drug	Dosage	Route	Code
Akineton, see Biperiden			
Alatrofloxacin mesylate, injection	100 mg	IV	J0200
Albuterol	0.5 mg	INH	J7620
Albuterol, concentrated form	1 mg	INH	J7610, J7611
Albuterol, unit dose form	1 mg	INH	J7609, J7613
Aldesleukin	per single use vial	IM, IV	J9015
Aldomet, see Methyldopa HCl			
Alefacept	0.5 mg	IM, IV	J0215
Alferon N, *see* Interferon alfa-n3			
Alglucerase	per 10 units	IV	J0205
Alglucosidase alfa	10 mg	IV	J0220, J0221

Figure 26-8 ■ Excerpt from the HCPCS Table of Drugs.

Table 26-5 ■ ROUTES OF DRUG ADMINISTRATION

Abbreviation	Meaning
IA	Intra-arterial administration
IV	Intravenous administration
IM	Intramuscular administration
IT	Intrathecal (into fluid around the spinal cord)
SC	Subcutaneous administration
INH	Administration by inhaled solution
VAR	Various routes of administration (joints, cavities, tissues, topical applications, other parenteral administrations)
OTH	Other routes of administration (suppositories, catheter injections)
ORAL	Administered orally

To use the Table of Drugs, locate the drug name in the left-hand column, then identify the dose in the second and the route in the third columns. The fourth column provides the suggested code. Whether you locate codes using the Index or the Table of Drugs, always verify them in the Tabular List.

Report the quantity of a drug the patient received as a multiple of the dose listed in the second column. For example, the dose for **J0205 Alglucerase** is **10 units**, as shown on the Table of Drugs and in the Tabular List. If a dose of 11-20 units is administered intravenously, report a quantity of **2** for code **J0205** on the claim (20/10 = 2).

CODING CAUTION

The HCPCS Table of Drugs is different than the ICD-10-CM Table of Drugs and Chemicals. The HCPCS Table of Drugs is used to report drugs prescribed by and administered by healthcare providers. The ICD-10-CM Table of Drugs and Chemicals is used to report injuries caused by substances and due to an adverse reaction or improper use.

Orthotics (L0112-L9900)

HCPCS **L** codes represent orthotics, devices that help a patient to regain normal functioning, and prosthetics, devices that replace a body part lost to disease or trauma. Patients with orthotics and prosthetics can include those who have been diagnosed with upper or lower musculoskeletal injuries or conditions, patients with amputated limbs, and patients with spinal deformities. Examples of these devices are collars, rib braces and belts, rib aprons with straps to immobilize and support the rib cage, orthotic devices that limit the rotation of the hip, and gelatin or silicone breast implants.

To locate codes for orthotics in the HCPCS Index, locate the Main Term for the name of the item, such as **Collar** or **Boot**, or the more general term **Orthotics**. Then locate the subterm for the specific type of device. Always verify the code in the Tabular List.

CODING PRACTICE

Exercise 26.3   Assigning HCPCS Codes

Instructions: Read the mini-medical-record of each patient's encounter and assign the correct HCPCS code(s). Write the answer on the line provided.

---

1. INPATIENT HOSPITAL   GENDER: F   AGE: 58

Reason for encounter: Anxiety disorder

Procedure: Administered Librium, 100 mg

1 HCPCS Code _____

---

2. OFFICE   Gender: F   Age: 85

Assessment: Diabetic polyneuropathy, callus formation

Procedure: Fitted patient with a pair of custom-molded shoes

Plan: Office will schedule follow-up appointment when shoes arrive.

1 HCPCS Code _____ Quantity _____

---

3. OUTPATIENT HOSPITAL   Gender: M   Age: 65

Reason for encounter: History of malignant neoplasm of the lower GI tract 4 years ago places patient at high risk of colorectal cancer

Procedure: Colorectal cancer screening

Findings: Normal

1 HCPCS Code _____

(continued)

CODING PRACTICE (continued)

4. DME SUPPLIER   Gender: M   Age: 41

Reason for encounter: Limited mobility due to morbid obesity, weight 400 pounds, BMI = 57 kg/m2

Equipment: Power wheelchair, group 2 heavy duty, sling/solid seat/back

1 HCPCS Code _____

5. OFFICE   Gender: F   Age: 21

Reason for encounter: Neck pain following automobile accident 1 week ago

Equipment: Provided patient with a cervical, flexible, nonadjustable foam collar

Plan: Return to office 1 week

1 HCPCS Code _____

CHAPTER SUMMARY

In this chapter you learned that:

- HCPCS codes are Level II codes of the Healthcare Common Procedure Coding System used to report services not included in CPT and for physician and nonphysician services, medical supplies, equipment, and medications.

- The HCPCS manual consists of an Index, Tabular List, Table of Drugs, and modifiers.

- The three skills of an "Ace" coder—abstracting, assigning, and arranging codes—apply to HCPCS coding.

- Specific methods are required to assign modifiers and codes for transportation services, medical supplies, radiopharmaceuticals, enteral and parental nutrition, durable medical equipment, professional services, drugs administered by clinicians, and orthotics. Each payer has unique guidelines.

CONCEPT QUIZ

Take a moment to look back at HCPCS coding and solidify your skills. Try to answer the questions from memory first, then refer to the discussion in this chapter and the Glossary at the end of this book if you need a little extra help.

Completion

Instructions: Write the term that completes each statement based on the information you learned in this chapter. Choose from the list below. Some choices may be used more than once and some choices may not be used at all.

AMA	facility
CMS	guidelines
contrast medium	HCPCS
CPT	Index
dental	Medicare
diagnosis	orthotics
DME	therapy
enteral nutrition therapy	

1. B codes represent supplies and products for _____.

2. D codes represent _____ supplies and products.

3. Each payer has unique coding, billing, and reimbursement _____ for supplies.

4. L codes represent _____ supplies and services.

5. _____ has specific regulations for reimbursing screening exams, including the patient's age and the frequency of exams.

6. _____ is billed by the radiologist, in addition to the CPT code for the procedure.

7. When the patient has insurance *other than* Medicare or Medicaid, report the _____ code unless the insurance requires the _____ code.

8. E codes represent supplies and products known as _____.

9. _____ codes identify the supplies used to administer drugs.

10. _____ codes identify the services to administer drugs.

Multiple Choice

Instructions: Circle the letter of the best answer to each question based on the information you learned in this chapter.

1. How would you code the following scenario? *A Medicare patient is seen for a screening colonoscopy using flexible sigmoidoscopy.*
   A. G0105
   B. G0104
   C. G0121
   D. G0122

(continued)

(continued from page 477)

2. What term does DME stand for?
   A. Diagnostic medical evaluation
   B. Durable medicine equipment
   C. Diagnostic modern equipment
   D. Durable medical equipment

3. What modifier is used to notify Medicare that the units of service exceed those in the medically unlikely edits (MUEs)?
   A. GA
   B. GD
   C. GL
   D. GZ

4. How would you code the following scenario? *A physician performed a positron emission tomography (PET) perfusion scan with a tracer for a patient at rest. 60 millicuries of the radiopharmaceutical Rubidium Rb-82 was used in the study.*
   A. 78491, A9606 x 60
   B. A9597-60
   C. 78491, A9555 x 60
   D. 78491, A9555 x 1

5. What abbreviation identifies that a drug is administered directly into the patient's vein?
   A. IV
   B. IT
   C. IA
   D. IM

6. How would you code the following scenario? *A patient was transported by ambulance from home to the hospital emergency department after she collapsed on the kitchen floor. Service provided: BLS, 12 miles.*
   A. A0429-12
   B. A0429, A0380-12
   C. A0429-RH, A0380 x 12
   D. A0429-H-ED, A0380 x 12

7. What is the format of HCPCS modifiers?
   A. Alphanumeric or two letters
   B. Two numbers
   C. Two letters ranging from AA to ZZ
   D. One number and one letter

8. Where in the HCPCS code set are drugs listed in alphabetical order?
   A. Table of Drugs
   B. List of Modifiers
   C. Index
   D. Table of Brand Drugs

9. Who administers the drugs reported by J codes?
   A. The patient
   B. A healthcare professional
   C. A friend or family member
   D. All of the above

10. What term does the acronym HCPCS stand for?
    A. Hospital Care Procedural Coding System
    B. Hospital Common Procedural Coding System
    C. Healthcare Common Procedure Coding System
    D. Healthcare Common Periodic Coding System

KEEP ON CODING

Instructions: Read the diagnostic or procedural statement, then use the appropriate Index and Tabular List to assign HCPCS codes. Write the code(s) on the line provided.

1. Injection of mitomycin, 5 mg. HCPCS Code(s) _____

2. Insulin infusion pump. HCPCS Code(s) _____

3. IV injection of paclitaxel 2 mg. HCPCS Code(s) _____

4. Foley catheter, two-way, silicone. HCPCS Code(s) _____

5. Nasogastric tube, without stylet. HCPCS Code(s) _____

6. CPAP device. HCPCS Code(s) _____

7. Alcohol wipes, one box. HCPCS Code(s) _____

8. Pair of crutches, adjustable, wood. HCPCS Code(s) _____

9. Prostate screening, rectal exam. HCPCS Code(s) _____

10. Gel mattress. HCPCS Code(s) _____

11. Helicopter transport, rotary wing, 5 miles. HCPCS Code(s) _____

12. Pediatric gait trainer, upright support. HCPCS Code(s) _____

13. Administration, influenza virus vaccine. HCPCS Code(s) _____

14. Lightweight wheelchair, high strength, detachable arms desk, swing-away detachable elevating leg. HCPCS Code(s) _____

15. Clubfoot wedge. HCPCS Code(s) _____

16. 100 units of Pitocin IV. HCPCS Code(s) _____

17. Hearing aid assessment. HCPCS Code(s) _____

18. Nasal cannula. HCPCS Code(s) _____

19. 12-volt battery and battery charger. HCPCS Code(s) _____

20. Basic life support ambulance services, nonemergency, 7 miles, from scene of accident to hospital. HCPCS Code(s) _____

21. Custom plastic artificial eye. HCPCS Code(s) _____

22. Contraceptive, cervical cap. HCPCS Code(s) _____

23. Orthotic device, Legg-Perthes, Scottish Rite type. HCPCS Code(s) _____

24. Standard metal bed pan. HCPCS Code(s) _____

25. Emergency ambulance transport with ALS-1 support from patient's home to helicopter pad, 21 miles. HCPCS Code(s) _____

CODING CHALLENGE

Instructions: Read the mini-medical-record of each patient's encounter, then abstract, assign, and arrange ICD-10-CM diagnosis codes and HCPCS procedure codes using the appropriate Index and Tabular List. Write the code(s) on the line provided.

1. EMERGENCY DEPT   Gender: F   Age: 57

Reason for encounter: Nausea and vomiting, nausea, and cramps

Assessment: Enteritis due to Escherichia coli

Service provided: Ordered ampicillin sodium and sulbactam sodium IV injections 1.5 g every 6 hours. Patient received the drug for 18 hours and then was released.

Tip: Code for the supplies only.

1 ICD-10-CM Code _____

1 HCPCS Code _____

2. EMERGENCY DEPT   Gender: F   Age: 50

Reason for encounter: Badly infected second-degree burn on her scalp that occurred in the bathroom of her home with a curling iron

Assessment: Patient has not properly cared for the wound. Treated the wound and applied an alginate dressing, 10 square inches.

Service Provided: Based on the wound's appearance and fluid oozing from it, I gave the patient two additional dressings to change once a week for two weeks and discharged home.

Tip: Code for the supplies only, not the service.

4 ICD-10-CM Codes _____

_____

1 HCPCS Code _____

3. OFFICE   Gender: M   Age: 62

Reason for encounter: Visit to adjust a colostomy bag

Procedure: Fitted a drainable, rubber colostomy with a faceplate and drain, and a protective solid skin barrier, size 4 inches square

1 ICD-10-CM Code _____

2 HCPCS Codes _____

4. OFFICE   Gender: M   Age: 55

Reason for encounter: Review of patient's diet

Assessment: Patient currently utilizes an enteral feeding supply kit due to malnutrition from neck cancer. Patient needs additional fiber in his diet.

Service: Provided patient with a fiber additive for the enteral formula

2 ICD-10-CM Codes _____

1 HCPCS Code _____

5. DME SUPPLIER   Gender: F   Age: 82

Patient diagnosis: Alzheimer dementia with behavioral disturbances. Patient is at risk of falling out of bed at night.

Equipment provided: Hospital bed with a mattress and variable-height side rails

Tip: Code for the equipment.

2 ICD-10-CM Codes _____

1 HCPCS Code _____

(continued from page 479)

6. DME SUPPLIER/HOME Gender: M Age: 68

Reason for encounter: Patient is paraplegic, needs to have his electric wheelchair motor repaired. DME repair technician makes a service call to the patient's home.

Service provided: Wheelchair motor repair, 60 minutes due to multiple nonroutine problems. Motor was running properly upon completion.

Tip: Refer to the amount of time that service was provided to calculate the units of service as stated in the code description.

1 ICD-10-CM Code _____

1 HCPCS Code _____

Quantity _____

7. OFFICE Gender: M Age: 12

Reason for encounter: Congenital scoliosis

Supplies provided: Cervical-thoracic-lumbar-sacral orthotic (CTLSO) (Milwaukee) brace

1 ICD-10-CM Code _____

1 HCPCS Code _____

8. SENIOR DAY CARE CENTER Gender: F

Age: 100

Reason for encounter: Senility

Service provided: Respite care, nursing, 1100–1600. Daughter is the regular caretaker.

Tip: Refer to the amount of time the service was provided to calculate the units of service as stated in the code description.

1 ICD-10-CM Code _____

1 HCPCS Code _____

Quantity _____

9. OFFICE Gender: M Age: 82

Reason for encounter: Difficulty hearing in right ear

Assessment: Hearing assessment shows conductive hearing loss in right ear

1 ICD-10-CM Code _____

1 HCPCS Code _____

10. TRANSPORT SERVICE GENDER: M AGE: 72

Reason for encounter: Open fracture of the neck of right femur, type I, routine healing

Service provided: Nonemergency transport in a wheelchair van from hospital to rehabilitation center

Distance traveled: 3 miles

1 ICD-10-CM Code _____

2 HCPCS Codes _____

Quantity _____

Chapter 27

CPT Modifiers

Learning Objectives

After completing this chapter, you should have the skills to:

27.1 Spell and define the key words, medical terms, and abbreviations related to CPT modifiers. (Remember)

27.2 Summarize the main characteristics of coding with CPT modifiers. (Understand)

27.3 Adhere to the coding guidelines related to CPT modifiers. (Apply)

27.4 Examine and abstract procedural information from the medical record for using CPT

27.5 Demonstrate how to assign codes using CPT modifiers. (Apply)

27.6 Utilize guidelines for arranging (sequencing) codes using CPT modifiers. (Apply)

Chapter Outline

- **Overview of CPT Modifiers**
- **Guidelines for CPT Modifiers**
- **Abstracting for CPT Modifiers**
- **Assigning Codes Using CPT Modifiers**
- **Arranging Codes with CPT Modifiers**

Key Terms and Abbreviations

Appendix A
laterality
professional component
technical component

In addition to the key terms listed here, students should know the terms defined within tables in this chapter.

INTRODUCTION

When an item in a store is part of a special offer, the storekeeper posts a special sign to bring attention to it and may even tag and ring it up with a special code. Nothing in life is exactly the same 100% of the time, and sometimes we need a way to flag an exception to the rule so that others notice it. CPT modifiers do just that. By adding modifiers to CPT codes when needed, we may eliminate the need to write a detailed letter to the insurance company to explain how a service differs from what is usually provided. This chapter introduces you to CPT modifiers and their uses. It also helps you build skills to identify when modifiers are needed and how to apply them.

OVERVIEW OF CPT MODIFIERS

CPT modifiers are two-digit suffixes entered at the end of a CPT code to identify how the service provided varies from the usual code description. Some modifiers affect payment because they identify how a service was reduced or increased from the code description. Other modifiers are informational only and do not affect payment, such as those that identify laterality, the side of the body affected.

CPT provides more than three dozen modifiers, a few of which are used only by hospital outpatient and ambulatory surgery centers. In addition to these, approximately 50 HCPCS modifiers are listed in the CPT manual for use with CPT codes. HCPCS modifiers not listed in the CPT manual can also be used with CPT codes. They can be located in the HCPCS coding manual. HCPCS modifiers are two-character alphanumeric suffixes.

You do not need to use modifiers on every CPT code. They are used most frequently with surgical codes and, sometimes, with evaluation and management (E/M) codes. Appendix A of the CPT manual provides a full definition of all modifiers. Locate and refer to Appendix A frequently as you become familiar with modifiers. A list of modifiers with shortened descriptions appears inside the front cover of most CPT manuals.

CPT modifiers consist of two numbers that are placed immediately following a CPT code number. When writing a code, it is common to place a hyphen in front of the modifier to separate it from the code number or to clarify that a modifier is being referenced (■ FIGURE 27-1). The hyphen is not used when entering the modifier into billing software or on a CMS-1500 form (■ FIGURE 27-2). The 837P electronic claim format and the CMS-1500 form allow up to four modifiers to be reported with a code.

CPT and HCPCS are the only codes that use modifiers. ICD-10-CM diagnosis codes and ICD-10-PCS inpatient procedure codes do not have modifiers. Modifiers are discussed

As established patient was evaluated for acute abdomen (*severe abdominal pain*). After a comprehensive examination and medical decision making of high complexity, the physician recommended surgery the following day.

99215-57 Office or other outpatient visit for an established patient (level 5)
Modifier 57 Decision for Surgery: An evaluation and management service that resulted in the initial decision to perform the surgery may be identified by adding modifier 57 to the appropriate level of E/M service.

Figure 27-1 ■ Example of using CPT modifiers. *Source: © PB Resources, Inc. Used with permission.*

before you learn the details of CPT coding because modifiers are used with codes throughout the CPT manual. An introduction to modifiers is presented in this chapter. Examples of applying modifiers in specific situations are provided in all CPT coding chapters of this text in the sections about assigning and arranging codes.

GUIDELINES FOR CPT MODIFIERS

The CPT manual does not provide a specific section of guidelines for modifiers. The full definitions of modifiers are listed in CPT Appendix A. Other appendices provide guidance on specific modifiers, including:

- Appendix E—Summary of CPT Codes Exempt from Modifier -51

- Appendix F—Summary of CPT Codes Exempt from Modifier -63

- Appendix P—CPT Codes that May Be Used for Synchronous Telemedicine Services (Modifier -95).

Code section guidelines and instructional notes often discuss modifier use with select codes. Read these carefully to be sure you understand how to apply modifiers in specific circumstances.

As with many areas of coding, the specific requirements regarding modifier usage vary by payer. The Medicare Physician Fee Schedule Database (MPFSDB) provides information about certain modifiers, the codes they can be used with, and the impact on reimbursement. Medicare requires certain modifiers that other payers do not, and private payers may have requirements that do not apply to Medicare. Requirements for modifier usage can vary by the region of the country, even for a specific payer, as well as the data from the MPFSDB. As you enter the workplace, you will want to learn about modifier requirements in your area and for the specific payers billed

24. A.	DATE(S) OF SERVICE					B.	C.	D. PROCEDURES, SERVICES, OR SUPPLIES		E.	F.		G.	H.	I.	J.
	From			To		PLACE OF		(Explain Unusual Circumstances)		DIAGNOSIS	$ CHARGES		DAYS OR	EPSDT Family	ID.	RENDERING
	MM	DD	YY	MM	DD	YY	SERVICE	EMG	CPT/HCPCS	MODIFIER	POINTER			UNITS	Plan	QUAL.	PROVIDER ID. #
1	01	05	YY				11		99125	57		AC	200 00	01		NPI	99 9999999

Figure 27-2 ■ How to enter modifiers on the CMS-1500 form, Item 24D.

most frequently by your facility. Medical billing software programs can often be programmed with the coding and billing requirements of individual payers. This customization provides reminder prompts to users or enters modifiers automatically, when appropriate. Specific rules for modifier use are discussed throughout this chapter of the text.

CODING PRACTICE

Exercise 27.1   Overview and Guidelines for CPT Modifiers

Instructions: Write the answers to the following questions on the lines provided.

1. What is the purpose of modifiers? _____

_____

2. Which code sets use modifiers? _____

3. What is the correct way to write code 99215 with modifier -57?

_____

4. Where in the CPT manual can you find detailed information about modifiers? _____

5. What type of CPT codes most frequently require modifiers?

_____

ABSTRACTING FOR CPT MODIFIERS

Coders need to abstract information for modifiers from the patient's medical record, in addition to abstracting for diagnoses and procedures. For help identifying when CPT modifiers are needed, refer to ■ TABLE 27-1. When the answer to a question is *yes*, review the modifiers listed in the right-hand column. When you move on to assigning modifiers and codes, you will look up the description of each modifier suggested and determine which, if any, apply to the patient. Also refer to payer policies for guidance. The fact that several modifiers are listed next to a question does not mean you can use any of them at random. Only specific modifiers are correct in any particular circumstance. For some patients, none of the modifiers might be needed. Table 27-1 is a tool to help you identify when a modifier *might* be needed and to help narrow down the modifiers that *might* apply. This table does not cover all modifiers or all situations but will help you get started. Additional criteria for abstracting modifiers relative to specific body systems are highlighted in Chapters 28-45.

Table 27-1   ■   **KEY CRITERIA FOR ABSTRACTING CPT MODIFIERS**

Criteria	Modifier(s)
Was a service provided that was more extensive than usual?	-22, -23, -47, -59
Was a service reduced or discontinued?	-52, -53
Was the service mandated (required) by a third party?	-32
Was the service bilateral (performed on both members/sides of a paired organ or site)?	-50
Was more than one surgeon involved in performing a surgical procedure?	-62, -66, -80, -81, -82
Was the service provided during the global period of a surgical procedure? Was the previous procedure performed by the physician now seeing the patient? Is the current service unrelated to the previous surgery?	-24, -25, -54, -55, -56, -79
Did the physician provide only the professional component of a service that has both technical and professional components?	-26
Was the service performed in a hospital outpatient or ambulatory surgery center?	-73, -74
Was an evaluation and management service provided on the same day or day before a surgical procedure?	-25, -57
Was the procedure repeated or a staged or unrelated procedure performed?	-58, -76, -77, -78, -79
Were surgeons other than the one who performed the surgery involved in the preoperative or postoperative care?	-54, -55, -56
Was the service habilitative or rehabilitative in nature?	-96, -97

Source: © PB Resources, Inc. Used with permission.

CODING PRACTICE

Exercise 27.2 Abstracting for CPT Modifiers

Instructions: Refer to Table 27-1, Key Criteria for Abstracting CPT Modifiers, to answer the following questions. Identify the group of modifiers that should be considered for each of the following situations based on the Key Criteria questions. Write the answer on the line provided. You do not need to select the final modifier.

Example: A colonoscopy was discontinued due to a drop in the patient's blood pressure. *-52, -53*

1. Monthly drug testing was ordered by the court as a condition of probation. _____

2. A patient had an emergency cholecystectomy while on vacation and was followed by her own physician for postoperative care. _____

3. A thoracic surgeon and a neurosurgeon performed a discectomy (*excision of an intervertebral disc*). _____

4. An E/M service was provided the day before surgery. _____

5. An appendectomy required an hour longer than usual to complete due to extensive abdominal adhesions. _____

ASSIGNING CODES USING CPT MODIFIERS

This section discusses the different purposes of modifiers for different types of services. As you learn how to code procedures for each body system, you will learn more about using modifiers for specific patient cases. An encoder or a practice management system often provides links to reference information or edit checks that identify which modifiers can be used with a particular CPT code (■ FIGURE 27-3). The MPFSDB also identifies the modifiers accepted for each CPT code. Some modifiers are used for multiple purposes, including those for anatomic sites. Others are limited to use with certain types of services, including evaluation and management (E/M), surgery, anesthesia, laboratory services, radiology, and hospital outpatient ambulatory surgery centers. Each of these types of modifiers is discussed next. A few of the most common HCPCS modifiers are also discussed.

General CPT Modifiers

Some modifiers apply to most or all classes of CPT codes (■ TABLE 27-2). Whenever a service is mandated or required by a third-party payer, court, or other authority, modifier **-32 Mandated Services** alerts the payer.

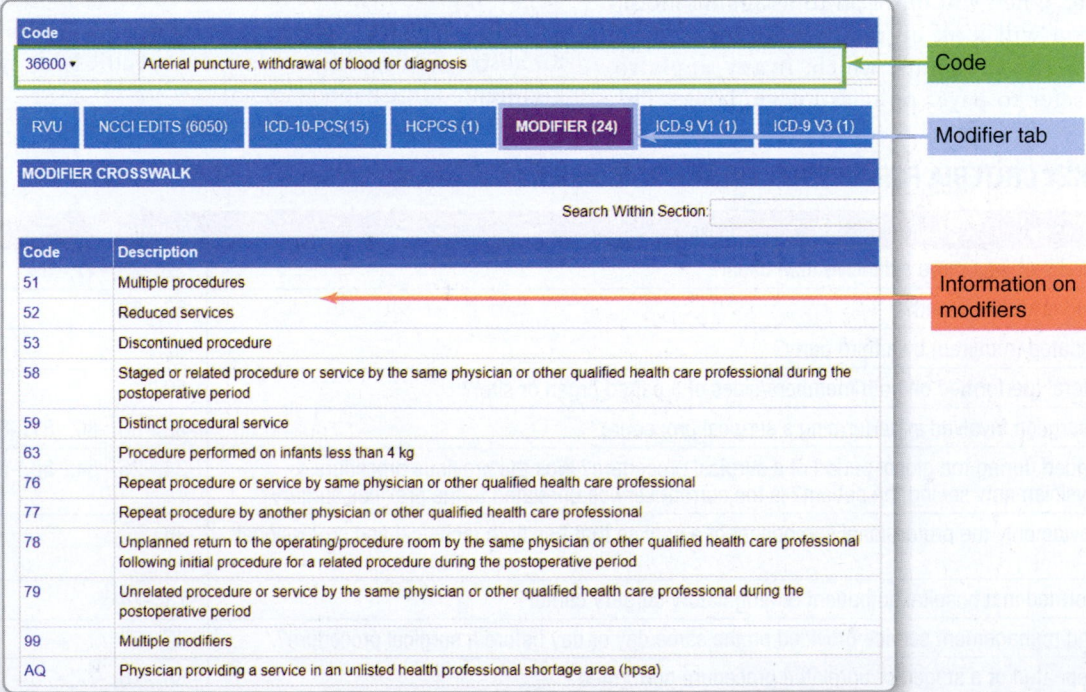

Figure 27-3 ■ Example of modifier information displayed in an encoder. *Source: SpeedeCoder, Reprinted with permission.*

Table 27-2 ■ GENERAL MODIFIERS

Modifier	Short Description
-32	Mandated services
-99	Multiple modifiers
-GA	Waiver of liability statement on file (Medicare)
-GZ	Item or service expected to be denied as not reasonable and necessary (Medicare)

When more than four modifiers are required on a single CPT code, they must be entered into a separate comments field (CMS-1500 Item 19), so modifier **-99 Multiple Modifiers** alerts the payer to look in that field for the modifiers.

Medicare requires that patients be notified in writing when a covered service might be denied because of a lack of medical necessity. Providers must have patients sign an Advance Beneficiary Notice (ABN) acknowledging the reason for the potential denial, which makes the patient financially responsible to pay for the service (■ FIGURE 27-4). Modifier **-GA** informs Medicare

A. Notifier:

B. Patient Name: **C. Identification Number:**

Advance Beneficiary Notice of Noncoverage (ABN)

__NOTE:__ If Medicare doesn't pay for D. _____ below, you may have to pay.
Medicare does not pay for everything, even some care that you or your health care provider have good reason to think you need. We expect Medicare may not pay for the **D.**_____ below.

D.	E. Reason Medicare May Not Pay:	F. Estimated Cost

WHAT YOU NEED TO DO NOW:
- Read this notice, so you can make an informed decision about your care.
- Ask us any questions that you may have after you finish reading.
- Choose an option below about whether to receive the D._____ listed above.
  Note: If you choose Option 1 or 2, we may help you to use any other insurance that you might have, but Medicare cannot require us to do this.

G. OPTIONS: Check only one box. We cannot choose a box for you.

☐ **OPTION 1.** I want the D._____ listed above. You may ask to be paid now, but I also want Medicare billed for an official decision on payment, which is sent to me on a Medicare Summary Notice (MSN). I understand that if Medicare doesn't pay, I am responsible for payment, but **I can appeal to Medicare** by following the directions on the MSN. If Medicare does pay, you will refund any payments I made to you, less co-pays or deductibles.
☐ **OPTION 2.** I want the D._____ listed above, but do not bill Medicare. You may ask to be paid now as I am responsible for payment. **I cannot appeal if Medicare is not billed**.
☐ **OPTION 3.** I don't want the D._____ listed above. I understand with this choice I am **not** responsible for payment, and **I cannot appeal to see if Medicare would pay.**

H. Additional Information:

This notice gives our opinion, not an official Medicare decision. If you have other questions on this notice or Medicare billing, call **1-800-MEDICARE** (1-800-633-4227/**TTY:** 1-877-486-2048).
Signing below means that you have received and understand this notice. You also receive a copy.

I. Signature:	J. Date:

CMS does not discriminate in its programs and activities. To request this publication in an alternative format, please call: 1-800-MEDICARE or email: AltFormatRequest@cms.hhs.gov.

According to the Paperwork Reduction Act of 1995, no persons are required to respond to a collection of information unless it displays a valid OMB control number. The valid OMB control number for this information collection is 0938-0566. The time required to complete this information collection is estimated to average 7 minutes per response, including the time to review instructions, search existing data resources, gather the data needed, and complete and review the information collection. If you have comments concerning the accuracy of the time estimate or suggestions for improving this form, please write to: CMS, 7500 Security Boulevard, Attn: PRA Reports Clearance Officer, Baltimore, Maryland 21244-1850.

Form CMSR-131 (Exp. 03/2020)   Form Approved OMB No. 0938-0566

Figure 27-4 ■ Medicare Advance Beneficiary Notice of Noncoverage form.

> A patient had a chalazion removed from the right upper eyelid.
>
> **67800-E3**
> **67800 Excision of chalazion; single**
> **Modifier E3 Upper right eyelid**

Figure 27-5 ■ Example of an anatomic modifier. *Source: © PB Resources, Inc. Used with permission.*

that the ABN has been signed and allows the provider to bill the patient if Medicare does not pay for the service. If the service is expected to be denied and the ABN was *not* signed, report modifier **-GZ**. In this case, the provider is responsible for the cost and the provider cannot bill the patient for the denied service.

Anatomic Site Modifiers

Anatomic site modifiers allow providers to specify the anatomic site more specifically than is described in a CPT code by itself. CPT codes do not specify laterality for procedures that can be performed on paired sites (■ FIGURE 27-5). Therefore, modifiers are used to distinguish laterality as follows (■ TABLE 27-3):

- All sites (right, left, or bilateral)
- Eyelids
- Fingers
- Toes
- Coronary arteries

Some CPT codes identify whether a procedure is performed on one side of the body or bilaterally. Other CPT codes do not. Laterality can be reported with modifiers **-RT Right side** or **-LT Left side**. Bilateral procedures not specified as such in the code description are reported using modifier **-50 Bilateral**. Some payers require that bilateral procedures be billed using two CPT codes: one with **-RT** and one with **-LT**. Medical billing software can often be preprogrammed with the requirements of each payer regarding how bilateral procedures should be reported. For Medicare claims, refer to the MPFS to determine whether CPT modifier **-50** is accepted with a particular procedure code.

Evaluation and Management Modifiers

Evaluation and Management (E/M) codes, which describe physician encounters such as office visits or physician hospital visits, require a modifier under certain circumstances (■ TABLE 27-4):

- A surgeon sees a patient during the postoperative period for a reason unrelated to the procedure.
- A physician provides an E/M service that should be paid separately from another service on the same day.
- The E/M service was required by a payer or legal authority (■ FIGURE 27-6).
- The E/M service resulted in a decision to perform surgery within 24 hours.
- The E/M service is the initial care provided by the admitting physician.
- Part of the E/M service is provided via real-time telemedicine service, using audio and video equipment.

Table 27-3 ■ ANATOMIC SITE MODIFIERS

Modifier	Description
All Sites	
-50	Bilateral procedure
-LT	Left side (used to identify procedures performed on the left side of the body)
-RT	Right side (used to identify procedures performed on the right side of the body)
Eyelids	
-E1	Upper left eyelid
-E2	Lower left eyelid
-E3	Upper right eyelid
-E4	Lower right eyelid
Fingers	
-FA	Left hand, thumb
-F1	Left hand, second digit
-F2	Left hand, third digit
-F3	Left hand, fourth digit
-F4	Left hand, fifth digit
-F5	Right hand, thumb
-F6	Right hand, second digit
-F7	Right hand, third digit
-F8	Right hand, fourth digit
-F9	Right hand, fifth digit
Toes	
-TA	Left foot, great toe
-T1	Left foot, second digit
-T2	Left foot, third digit
-T3	Left foot, fourth digit
-T4	Left foot, fifth digit
-T5	Right foot, great toe
-T6	Right foot, second digit
-T7	Right foot, third digit
-T8	Right foot, fourth digit
-T9	Right foot, fifth digit
Coronary Arteries	
-LC	Left circumflex coronary artery
-LD	Left anterior descending coronary artery
-LM	Left main coronary artery
-RC	Right coronary artery
-RI	Ramus intermedius coronary artery

Surgical/Procedural Modifiers

Modifiers are used on codes for medical and surgical procedures when the procedure is altered in a way that could affect its reimbursement. According to CPT guidelines, all surgical codes include specific services performed before, during, and after the procedure that are bundled into the CPT surgical

Table 27-4 ■ EVALUATION AND MANAGEMENT MODIFIERS

Modifier	Short Description
-24	Unrelated evaluation and management service by the same physician or other qualified healthcare professional during a postoperative period
-25	Significant, separately identifiable evaluation and management service by the same physician or other qualified healthcare professional on the same day of the procedure or other service
-32	Mandated services
-57	Decision for surgery
-95	Synchronous telemedicine service rendered via a real-time interactive audio and video telecommunications system. (See CPT Appendix for list of valid codes.)
-AI	Principal physician of record (Medicare)

An insurance company requires a patient to be evaluated by a consulting physician for a second surgical opinion on back surgery. The consultant performs a comprehensive history, a comprehensive examination, and medical decision making of high complexity and concurs with the opinion of the first physician.

99245-32
99245 Office consultation for a new or established patient, which requires these 3 key components: a comprehensive history; a comprehensive examination; and medical decision making of high complexity
Modifier 32 Mandated services: Services related to mandated consultation and/or related services (e.g., third party payer, governmental, legislative or regulatory requirement) may be identified by adding modifier 32 to the basic procedure.

Figure 27-6 ■ Example of the mandated services modifier.
Source: © PB Resources, Inc. Used with permission.

package or global period. When all of these services are not provided by the same physician, a modifier is required. Surgical and procedural codes require modifiers in the following situations (■ TABLE 27-5):

- The procedure is more extensive or less extensive than described by the CPT code.

- The surgeon, rather than the anesthesiologist, administers general anesthesia.

- More than one surgeon is involved in the procedure.

- Preoperative or postoperative care is provided by a different surgeon than the one who performed the procedure.

- Multiple procedures are performed during the same operative session.

- The procedure is staged, or planned to be completed over the course of several operative sessions.

- The procedure is repeated or an unplanned revision to the procedure is required (■ FIGURE 27-7 page 488).

- The surgeon who performed the procedure sees the patient for another procedure, unrelated to the first procedure, during the postoperative period.

Table 27-5 ■ SURGICAL/PROCEDURAL MODIFIERS

Modifier	Short Description
-22	Increased procedural services
-32	Mandated services
-33	Preventive service
-47	Anesthesia by surgeon
-51	Multiple procedures
-52	Reduced services
-53	Discontinued procedure
-54	Surgical care only
-55	Postoperative management only
-56	Preoperative management only
-58	Staged or related procedure or service by the same physician or other qualified healthcare professional during the postoperative period
-59	Distinct procedural service
-62	Two surgeons
-63	Procedure performed on infants less than 4 kg
-66	Surgical team
-76	Repeat procedure or service by same physician or other qualified healthcare professional
-77	Repeat procedure by another physician or other qualified healthcare professional
-78	Unplanned return to the operating/procedure room by the same physician or other qualified healthcare professional following initial procedure for a related procedure during the postoperative period
-79	Unrelated procedure or service by the same physician or other qualified healthcare professional during the postoperative period
-80	Assistant surgeon
-81	Minimum assistant surgeon
-82	Assistant surgeon (when qualified resident surgeon not available)
-99	Multiple modifiers
-BL	Special acquisition of blood and blood products
-CA	Procedure payable only in the inpatient setting when performed emergently on an outpatient who expires prior to admission
-XE	Separate encounter
-XP	Separate structure
-XS	Separate practitioner
-XU	Unusual nonoverlapping service

During the postoperative period of a malignant lesion removal, the patient returned for a re-excision of the same lesion because frozen section pathology showed the margins of excision were inadequate for complete tumor removal. The final excised diameter was 3.9 cm.

11624-58
11624 Excision, malignant lesion including margins, scalp, neck, hands, feet, genitalia; excised diameter 3.1 to 4.0 cm
Modifier 58 Staged or related procedure or service by the same physician or other qualified health care professional during the postoperative period: It may be necessary to indicate that the performance of a procedure or service during the postoperative period was: (a) planned or anticipated (staged); (b) more extensive than the original procedure; or (c) for therapy following a surgical procedure. This circumstance may be reported by adding modifier 58 to the staged or related procedure.

Figure 27-7 ■ Example of a modifier for a staged or related procedure. *Source: © PB Resources, Inc. Used with permission.*

- A distinct procedural service is provided, such as a separate encounter, separate anatomic structure, separate practitioner, or other unusual nonoverlapping service.

Anesthesia Modifiers

General anesthesia (*using drugs to render a patient completely unaware and unable to feel pain*) is normally administered by an anesthesiologist. Anesthesiologist services are coded and billed by the anesthesiologist's office, separate from those for the surgeon. Anesthesia modifiers are used in the following situations (■ Table 27-6):

- All anesthesia codes require a modifier that identifies the physical status of the patient prior to surgery (■ Figure 27-8).

- General anesthesia was used in a procedure for which it is normally not used.

- The procedure was discontinued either before or after anesthesia was administered (outpatient hospital/ambulatory surgery centers).

- HCPCS modifiers are used with Medicare patients to identify the type of anesthesia provider.

Radiology Modifiers

Modifiers are used on radiology codes when the service is reduced, discontinued, or repeated (■ Table 27-7). Radiology codes sometimes comprise two components: the **technical component**, which covers the cost of staffing and equipment, and the **professional component**, which covers the cost of a radiologist supervising the technician and interpreting the results. When the technical and professional components are provided by two different entities or individuals, modifiers are applied to identify the component of the service provided by each (■ Figures 27-9 and 27-10).

Table 27-6 ■ **ANESTHESIA MODIFIERS**

Modifier	Short Description
-P1	A normal healthy patient
-P2	A patient with mild systemic disease
-P3	A patient with severe systemic disease
-P4	A patient with severe systemic disease that is a constant threat to life
-P5	A moribund patient who is not expected to survive without the operation
-P6	A declared brain-dead patient whose organs are being removed for donor purposes
-23	Unusual anesthesia
-52	Reduced services
-53	Discontinued procedure
-59	Distinct procedural service
-73	Discontinued outpatient hospital/ambulatory surgery center (ASC) procedure prior to the administration of anesthesia
-74	Discontinued outpatient hospital/ambulatory surgery center (ASC) procedure after administration of anesthesia
-76	Repeat procedure or service by same physician or other qualified healthcare professional
-77	Repeat procedure by another physician or other qualified healthcare professional
-78	Unplanned return to the operating/procedure room by the same physician or other qualified healthcare professional following initial procedure for a related procedure during the postoperative period
-79	Unrelated procedure or service by the same physician or other qualified healthcare professional during the postoperative period
-99	Multiple modifiers
-AA	Anesthesia services performed personally by anesthesiologist
-QX	CRNA service with medical direction by a physician
-QY	Medical direction of one certified registered nurse anesthetist (CRNA) by an anesthesiologist
-QZ	CRNA service without medical direction by a physician

Anesthesia services were provided for a ventral hernia on a patient with controlled hypertension.

00752-P2
00752 Anesthesia for hernia repairs in upper abdomen; lumbar and ventral (incisional) hernias and/or wound dehiscence
Modifier P2 Patient with mild systemic disease

Figure 27-8 ■ Example of an anesthesia physical status modifier. *Source: © PB Resources, Inc. Used with permission.*

Laboratory Modifiers

Modifiers are used on laboratory codes when the service is reduced, discontinued, or repeated (■ Table 27-8). When physicians send laboratory tests to an outside laboratory for processing, the laboratory can bill the patient's insurance for the test or they can bill the physician's office and allow the

Table 27-7 ■ RADIOLOGY MODIFIERS

Modifier	Short Description
-26	Professional component
-32	Mandated services
-52	Reduced services
-53	Discontinued procedure
-59	Distinct procedural service
-76	Repeat procedure or service by same physician or other qualified healthcare professional
-77	Repeat procedure by another physician or other qualified healthcare professional
-78	Unplanned return to the operating/procedure room by the same physician or other qualified healthcare professional following initial procedure for a related procedure during the postoperative period
-79	Unrelated procedure or service by the same physician or other qualified healthcare professional during the postoperative period
-80	Assistant surgeon
-81	Minimum assistant surgeon
-82	Assistant surgeon (when qualified resident surgeon not available)
-99	Multiple modifiers
-GG	Performance and payment of a screening mammogram and diagnostic mammogram on the same patient, same day
-GH	Diagnostic mammogram converted from screening mammogram on same day
-TC	Technical component

Table 27-8 ■ LABORATORY MODIFIERS

Modifier	Short Description
-32	Mandated services
-52	Reduced services
-53	Discontinued procedure
-59	Distinct procedural service
-79	Unrelated procedure or service by the same physician or other qualified healthcare professional during the postoperative period
-90	Reference (outside) laboratory
-91	Repeat clinical diagnostic laboratory test
-92	Alternative laboratory platform testing
-99	Multiple modifiers
-QW	CLIA waived test

A physician collected the specimen for a renal function panel, which he sent to a reference laboratory for analysis. The physician billed the patient's insurance company on behalf of the lab.

36415 Collection of venous blood by venipuncture
99000 Handling and/or conveyance of specimen for transfer from the office to a laboratory
80069-90
80069 Renal function panel
Modifier 90 Reference (outside) laboratory: When laboratory procedures are performed by a party other than the treating or reporting physician or other qualified health care professional, the procedure may be identified by adding modifier 90 to the usual procedure number.

Figure 27-11 ■ Example of a modifier for use of a reference laboratory. *Source: © PB Resources, Inc. Used with permission.*

73222 Magnetic resonance (e.g., proton) imaging, any joint of upper extremity; with contrast material(s)	
Total Fee	$301.74
Professional component (-26)	$62.43
Technical component (-TC)	$239.31

Figure 27-9 ■ Example of a professional and technical component fees. *Source: © PB Resources, Inc. Used with permission.*

A radiologist supervised and interpreted a transvaginal ultrasound.

76830-26
76830 Ultrasound, transvaginal
Modifier 26 Professional component: Certain procedures are a combination of a physician or other qualified health care professional component and a technical component. When the physician or other qualified health care professional component is reported separately, the service may be identified by adding modifier 26 to the usual procedure number.

Figure 27-10 ■ Example of a professional component modifier. *Source: © PB Resources, Inc. Used with permission.*

physician to bill the patient's insurance for the amount paid to the laboratory. This practice is a convenience to the laboratory because it saves paperwork. It is usually easy for the physician's office because it will be billing the patient's insurance for other services, including specimen collection. When the physician bills on behalf of the laboratory, the physician applies modifier **-90** to the code for the laboratory test (■ FIGURE 27-11). The physician must bill the insurance company the same amount as the laboratory charged the physician. Medicare does not allow this practice and it has become less common among private payers than it once was.

Hospital Outpatient/Ambulatory Surgery Center Modifiers

A specific subset of modifiers, including three unique ones, apply to hospital outpatient and ambulatory surgery centers (■ TABLE 27-9 page 490). The unique modifiers are **-27 Multiple Outpatient Hospital E/M Encounters on the Same Date** and modifiers **-73** and **-74**, which pertain to discontinued procedures. The other modifiers approved for use by these facilities are the same ones used by other facilities.

Table 27-9 ■ **HOSPITAL OUTPATIENT/AMBULATORY SURGERY CENTER MODIFIERS**

Modifier	Short Description
-25	Significant, separately identifiable evaluation and management service by the same physician or other qualified healthcare professional on the same day of the procedure or other service
-27	Multiple outpatient hospital E/M encounters on the same date
-50	Bilateral procedure
-52	Reduced services
-58	Staged or related procedure or service by the same physician or other qualified healthcare professional during the postoperative period
-59	Distinct procedural service
-73	Discontinued outpatient hospital/ambulatory surgery center (ASC) procedure prior to the administration of anesthesia
-74	Discontinued outpatient hospital/ambulatory surgery center (ASC) procedure after administration of anesthesia
-76	Repeat procedure or service by same physician or other qualified healthcare professional
-77	Repeat procedure by another physician or other qualified healthcare professional
-78	Unplanned return to the operating/procedure room by the same physician or other qualified healthcare professional following initial procedure for a related procedure during the postoperative period
-79	Unrelated procedure or service by the same physician or other qualified healthcare professional during the postoperative period
-91	Repeat clinical diagnostic laboratory test

CODING PRACTICE

Exercise 27.3 Assigning Codes Using CPT Modifiers

Instructions: Identify the specific modifier that should be used in each of the following situations. Refer to all the tables in this chapter, as needed.

Example: An x-ray of the patient's left knee was taken. *-LT*

1. A splint was applied to the patient's right middle finger. _____

2. A patient had an emergency cholecystectomy while on vacation out of town. When she returned home, a local physician provided postoperative care. _____

3. A thoracic surgeon and a neurosurgeon performed a discectomy. _____

4. An E/M service that resulted in the decision to perform surgery was provided the day before surgery. _____

5. A surgery required an hour longer than usual to complete due to extensive abdominal adhesions. _____

6. An anesthesiologist provided anesthesia services for a patient with a mild systemic disease. _____

7. A radiologist provided the professional components of supervising and interpreting a computerized tomography (CT) scan of the head. _____

8. A clinical diagnostic laboratory test had to be repeated for the same patient on the same day. _____

9. Multiple surgical procedures were performed during the same operative session. _____

10. A bilateral procedure was performed. _____

ARRANGING CODES WITH CPT MODIFIERS

There are several considerations when arranging codes using CPT modifiers. The order in which codes are arranged sometimes determines which codes receive modifiers.

The use of modifiers and the sequence of codes can impact payment. For example, when multiple surgical procedures are performed during the same operative session, the most costly procedure is sequenced first. Depending on the description of the CPT code, the secondary procedures sometimes need modifier **-51 Multiple Procedures** and are paid at a percentage of their usual rate. The discounted payment reflects the fact that less setup time is required for the secondary procedure(s) when performed during the same session as another procedure.

When a code requires more than one modifier, the order in which modifiers are applied can affect whether the claim is processed. Modifiers that affect price or payment are generally sequenced before modifiers that are used for informational purposes. For example, a modifier such as **-26 Professional Component** affects payment because the physician does not perform all the components of code. It should be sequenced before anatomic modifiers that identify **-RT Right side** or **-LT Left side**, which are information only (■ FIGURE 27-12).

> A radiologist supervised and interpreted an MRI of the right shoulder.
>
> 73222-26-RT
> **73222 Magnetic resonance (e.g., proton) imaging, any joint of upper extremity; with contrast material(s)**
> **Modifier 26 Professional component** (affects payment)
> **Modifier RT Right side** (informational)

Figure 27-12 ■ Example of sequencing multiple modifiers.
Source: © PB Resources, Inc. Used with permission.

CHAPTER SUMMARY

In this chapter you learned that:

- CPT modifiers are two-digit suffixes entered at the end of a CPT code to identify how the service provided varies from the usual code description.

- Information on modifiers is listed in the CPT manual appendix, section guidelines, and instructional notes. Specific requirements regarding modifier usage vary by payer.

- Coders need to abstract information for modifiers from the patient's medical record, in addition to abstracting for diagnoses and procedures.

- Some modifiers are used for multiple purposes, including those for anatomic site. Others are limited to use with certain types of services, including Evaluation and Management (E/M), surgery, anesthesia, laboratory services, radiology, and hospital outpatient ambulatory surgery centers.

- The order in which codes are arranged sometimes determines which codes receive modifiers.

CONCEPT QUIZ

Take a moment to look back at CPT modifiers and solidify your skills. Try to answer the questions from memory first, then refer to the discussion in this chapter and the Glossary at the end of this book if you need a little extra help.

Completion

Instructions: Write the term that completes each statement based on the information you learned in this chapter. Choose from the list below. Some choices may be used more than once and some choices may not be used at all.

-23	anesthesia
-25	payer
-26	primary care physician
-27	professional
-32	reduced service
-50	skin lesions
-62	surgeon
-63	technical
-80	toes
-81	unusual anesthesia
-82	

1. Modifier _____ is reported by the assistant surgeon.
2. Modifier _____ is used to indicate that the procedure was performed on both sides of the body.
3. Modifier _____ reports the professional component of a radiology service.
4. _____ is reported using modifier -23.
5. Modifier _____ alerts the payer that a procedure was performed on an infant weighing less than 4 kg.
6. Modifiers are used to distinguish laterality for _____.
7. Modifier _____ is used when an E/M service is required by a payer.
8. All _____ codes require a modifier that identifies the physical status of the patient prior to surgery.
9. The _____ component modifier of a radiology code is used to cover the cost of staffing and equipment.
10. Modifier _____ applies uniquely to hospital outpatient and ambulatory surgery centers.

Multiple Choice

Instructions: Circle the letter of the best answer to each question based on the information you learned in this chapter.

1. Which of the following is a modifier?
   A. -LT
   B. -MT
   C. -NT
   D. -OT

2. When must the Medicare Advance Beneficiary Notice of Noncoverage be completed?
   A. A service is never covered by Medicare
   B. A covered service might be denied because of a lack of medical necessity
   C. After any service is denied
   D. A patient does not have a Medicare policy

3. What modifier should be used for the following scenario? *A physician manages postoperative care only for a patient who had a suboccipital craniectomy for exploration of cranial nerves.*
   A. 61458-53
   B. 61458-54
   C. 61458-55
   D. 61458-56

4. What modifier is used for interpretation of a test result?
   A. Radiology service
   B. Global service
   C. Professional component
   D. Technical component

5. What is the format of CPT modifiers?
   A. Two numbers
   B. Two letters
   C. One letter and one number
   D. One letter and one symbol

6. What modifier is used to indicate a physician performed multiple procedures at the same operative session, such as repair of a wound on the left temporal area and removal of a cyst on the right temporal area?
   A. -50
   B. -51
   C. -LT
   D. -RT

7. What services does a CPT surgical code include?
   A. All services during the global period
   B. Preoperative services and the surgical procedure only
   C. The surgical procedure only
   D. The surgical procedure and postoperative services only

8. What physical status modifier should be used for the following scenario? *A moribund patient undergoes anesthesia for direct coronary artery bypass grafting with pump oxygenator.*
   A. 00567-P3
   B. 00567-P4
   C. 00567-P5
   D. 00567-P6

9. What modifier should be used in the following scenario? *An obstetrician administers a regional anesthesia block prior to an emergency cesarean delivery.*
   A. 59514-22
   B. 59514-23
   C. 59514-47
   D. 59514-51

10. What modifier is used for a procedure with two co-surgeons?
    A. -62
    B. -58
    C. -51
    D. -66

KEEP ON CODING

Instructions: Read the modifier definition and refer to the modifier table in this chapter listed in parentheses or to the CPT manual. Look up the modifier number. Write the modifier on the line provided.

1. Decision for surgery (Evaluation and Management). CPT Modifier _____

2. Anesthesia by surgeon (Surgical). CPT Modifier _____

3. Preoperative management only (Surgical). CPT Modifier _____

4. Bilateral procedure (Anatomic Site). CPT Modifier _____

5. Mandated services (General). CPT Modifier _____

6. A patient with severe systemic disease (Anesthesia). CPT Modifier _____

7. Technical component (Radiology). CPT Modifier _____

8. Left anterior descending coronary artery (Anatomic Site). CPT Modifier _____

9. Assistant surgeon (Surgical). CPT Modifier _____

10. CLIA waived test (Laboratory). CPT Modifier _____

11. Left hand, fifth digit (Anatomic Site). CPT Modifier _____

12. Discontinued outpatient hospital/ambulatory surgery center (ASC) procedure after administration of anesthesia (Hospital Outpatient/Ambulatory Surgery Center). CPT Modifier _____

13. Discontinued procedure (Surgical). CPT Modifier _____

14. Significant, separately identifiable evaluation and management service by the same physician or other qualified healthcare professional on the same day of the procedure or other service (Evaluation and Management). CPT Modifier _____

15. Separate structure (Surgical). CPT Modifier _____

16. Waiver of liability statement on file—Medicare (General). CPT Modifier _____

17. Professional component (Radiology). CPT Modifier _____

18. Synchronous telemedicine service rendered via a real-time interactive audio and video telecommunications system (Evaluation and Management). CPT Modifier _____

19. Multiple outpatient hospital E/M encounters on the same date (Hospital Outpatient/Ambulatory Surgery Center). CPT Modifier _____

20. Right foot, great toe (Anatomic Site). CPT Modifier _____

21. Reference (outside) laboratory (Laboratory). CPT Modifier _____

22. Rehabilitative service provided (Key Criteria table). CPT Modifier _____

23. Surgical team (Surgical). CPT Modifier _____

24. CRNA service with medical direction by a physician (Anesthesia). CPT Modifier _____

25. Multiple procedures (Surgical). CPT Modifier _____

CODING CHALLENGE

Instructions: Read the mini-medical-record of each patient's encounter, then identify the modifier that should be applied. Refer to the tables provided in this chapter. Write the modifier number and name on the line provided. Do not assign any codes.

Example: *-22 Unusual anesthesia services*

---

1. INPATIENT HOSPITAL   Gender: M   Age: 57

Preoperative assessment: Abdominal hemorrhage, 1 day postoperative from open cholecystectomy

Procedure: Return to operating room for exploration of abdomen and ligation of vessels to achieve hemostasis

1 Modifier _____

---

2. OUTPATIENT HOSPITAL   Gender: M   Age: 6

Preoperative assessment: Patient had first stage of a hypospadias repair one month ago. Returns today for the second-stage repair.

Procedure: Urethroplasty with free skin graft obtained from a site other than genitalia.

1 Modifier _____

---

3. OUTPATIENT SURGERY   Gender: M   Age: 17

Preoperative diagnosis: Bulge in groin area for a few months

Procedure: Bilateral inguinal herniorrhaphy with mesh

Postoperative diagnosis: Reducible, bilateral inguinal hernias

1 Modifier _____

---

4. INPATIENT HOSPITAL   Gender: F   Age: 26

Reason for encounter: Patient pulled out central line

Procedure: Central line reinserted by the same cardiologist

1 Modifier _____

---

5. OFFICE   Gender: M   Age: 25

Reason for encounter: Follow up on test results after evaluation of proximal muscle weakness, easy bruising, weight gain

Assessment: Endogenous Cushing's syndrome due to pituitary adenoma, evaluated for surgery

Plan: Surgery scheduled to remove tumor tomorrow

1 Modifier _____

(continued)

(continued from page 493)

6. OUTPATIENT HOSPITAL   Gender: F   Age: 61

Reason for encounter: Carpal tunnel decompression

Preoperative diagnosis: Numbness, tingling, and pain in the right arm, hand, and fingers due to pinched nerve

Procedure: Carpal tunnel decompression. Regional nerve block administered by surgeon with decompression of right carpal tunnel nerve.

Postoperative diagnosis: Carpal tunnel syndrome

2 Modifiers _____

---

7. INPATIENT HOSPITAL   Gender: F   Age: 13

Preoperative diagnosis: Knee dislocated during tackle football game

Procedure: Closed reduction of dislocation of right knee

Postoperative diagnosis: Dislocation of right knee

1 Modifier _____

---

8. EMERGENCY DEPT.   Gender: M   Age: 45

Reason for encounter: Possible tibial fracture sustained when the ATV he was riding tipped over

Procedure: Supervised and interpreted x-ray of lower leg that shows a transverse fracture of shaft of the right tibia

Diagnosis: Transverse fracture, right tibia

2 Modifiers _____

---

9. OUTPATIENT SURGERY   Gender: M   Age: 48

Procedure: Cystourethroscopy with bladder biopsy. Twenty minutes into the procedure, the patient developed some arrhythmia and the surgery was stopped.

1 Modifier _____

---

10. OFFICE   Gender: F   Age: 25

Reason for encounter: Follow-up care of fracture

Assessment: Fracture of L distal femur while skiing in Colorado. The physician in Colorado performed a closed treatment of the fracture with manipulation. Patient now sees me, as a local physician, for postoperative care.

2 Modifiers _____

Evaluation and Management Services (99201-99499)

Chapter 28

Learning Objectives

After completing this chapter, you should have the skills to:

28.1 Spell and define the key words, medical terms, and abbreviations related to evaluation and management services. (Remember)

28.2 Summarize the main characteristics of coding for evaluation and management services. (Understand)

28.3 Adhere to the CPT coding guidelines in the Evaluation and Management section. (Apply)

28.4 Examine and abstract information from the medical record for coding evaluation and management services. (Analyze)

28.5 Demonstrate how to assign codes for services in the Evaluation and Management section. (Apply)

28.6 Identify guidelines for advanced coding for services in the Evaluation and Management section. (Apply)

Chapter Outline

- **Overview of Evaluation and Management Services**
- **Guidelines for Evaluation and Management Services**
- **Abstracting Evaluation and Management Services**
- **Assigning Codes for Evaluation and Management Services**
- **Advanced Coding for Evaluation and Management Services**

Key Terms and Abbreviations

chief complaint (CC) (CPT)
concurrent care (CPT)
consultation (CPT)
consulting physician (CPT)
content of service requirements (CPT)
documentation guideline (DG) (CPT)

established patient (EP) (CPT)
Evaluation and Management (E/M) (CPT)
facility fee (CPT)
history of present illness (HPI) (CPT)
initial encounter (CPT)

key component (KC) (CPT)
level of service (CPT)
new patient (NP) (CPT)
nursing facility (NF) (CPT)
past, family, and social history (PFSH) (CPT)
patient type (CPT)

place of service (POS) (CPT)
referring physician (CPT)
review of systems (ROS) (CPT)
setting (CPT)
subsequent encounter (CPT)
transfer of care (CPT)

In addition to the key terms listed here, students should know the terms defined within tables in this chapter and the definitions of all evaluation and management categories.

INTRODUCTION

You might schedule service for a household appliance—such as a washing machine, furnace, or stove—for any number of reasons. Perhaps you experience a sudden breakdown, finally get around to having a long-standing issue fixed, or schedule preventive maintenance in the hopes of avoiding a major repair.

There are also many reasons that patients seek medical care, such as to receive preventive care, check out a new symptom or health problem, manage chronic conditions, monitor hospital care, receive emergency and critical care, or request a consultative service or second opinion. Physicians also provide case management, oversight, and coordination of care services when the patient is not present. CPT provides a special section of codes—Evaluation and Management (E/M) services—to describe a wide variety of physician encounters.

OVERVIEW OF EVALUATION AND MANAGEMENT SERVICES

Patients meet with physicians for many different reasons. Encounters can take place in a wide variety of settings—clinics, hospitals, emergency departments, skilled nursing facilities, assisted living facilities, and even the patient's home. Physicians interview patients, perform physical examinations, and review medical data to determine the treatment plan. Evaluation and Management (E/M) codes describe patient encounters with a physician for the evaluation and management of a health problem. Each setting or purpose has a separate category of codes and a specific set of criteria for selecting the correct code.

E/M codes are numbered **99201** through **99499**. Although the codes begin with the numbers 99, they are located out of numerical sequence in the CPT manual. The E/M section appears first in the CPT coding manual for convenience because these are the most commonly used group of CPT codes and are used by all specialties.

During the evaluation portion of the visit, the physician does the following:

- Asks the patient questions (subjective assessment) regarding the chief complaint or reason for the encounter

- Discusses with the patient the background of the problem, symptoms or other systems affected, and past medical history, family medical history, and social (lifestyle) history

- Performs a physical examination (objective assessment) related to the patient's health and presenting problem(s)

During the management portion of the encounter, providers formulate a treatment plan—also called medical decision making—which requires them to:

- Review test results or other records that are relevant to the presenting problem.

- Order further diagnostic testing.

- Refer the patient to other providers for specialized evaluation.

- Prescribe therapeutic treatments and medication.

- Schedule follow-up appointments to monitor progress.

Together, these components are referred to as the chief complaint or presenting problem, history, examination, and medical decision making.

Physicians and nonphysician practitioners (NPPs) provide E/M services. Nonphysician practitioners can be a physician assistant (PA), nurse practitioner (NP), clinical nurse specialist (CNS), or certified nurse midwife (CNM). These providers are licensed medical professionals who have less training than a physician but can diagnose patients and bill independently. The details of nonphysician practitioners' scope of practice vary by state, training, and licensure. Some nonphysician practitioners, such as physician assistants, must practice under a physician's supervision, but nurse practitioners practice independently in most states. Nonphysician practitioners may also prescribe medication in most states. They provide a cost-effective means of delivering professional, personalized care for routine medical needs.

The provider may mark the E/M code on the encounter form or enter it into the electronic health record (EHR) (■ FIGURE 28-1). Coders need to ensure that documentation in the medical record is consistent with the codes marked by the provider. Offices should audit claims on a regular basis to verify that every detail of the E/M code is clearly documented. EHR systems can prompt the physician to document the various criteria required for E/M coding, then suggest the most appropriate code based on the physician's input.

Evaluation and management is often the only service provided, but it also can be provided at the same time as other procedures, such as a laboratory test that is performed in the office, an electrocardiogram (EKG or ECG), or x-ray.

E/M coding possesses some differences from the rest of CPT coding because E/M codes are assigned based on unique criteria. These criteria have specific definitions within the CPT guidelines that coders must adhere to. The criteria are:

- **Setting**—Where the service is provided, such as office/outpatient, hospital, emergency department, or nursing facility; also called *place of service*

RANK	Office visit	New	Est	RANK	Office procedu...
	Minimal		99211		Anoscopy
	Problem focused	99201	99212		Audiometry
	Expanded problem focused	99202	99213		Cerumen remo...
	Detailed	99203	99214		Colposcopy
	Comprehensive	99204	99215		Colposcopy w/...
	Comprehensive (new patient)	99205			ECG, w/interpre...
	Significant, separate service	-25	-25		ECG, rhythm stri...
	Well visit	**New**	**Est**		Endometrial bi...
	< 1 y		99391		Flexible sigm...
	1-4 y	99382	99392		Flexible sigmo...
	5-11 y	99383	99393		Fracture care, c...
	12-17 y	99384	99394		Site: _____
	18-39 y	99385	99395		Nebulizer
	40-64 y	99386	99396		Nebulizer dem...
	65 y +	99387	99397		Spirometry
	Medicare preventive services				Spirometry, pre...
	Pap		Q0091		Tympanometry
	Pelvic & breast		G0101		Vasectomy
	Prostate/PSA		G0103		**Skin procedu...**
	Tobacco counseling/3-10 min		99406		Burn care, init...
	Tobacco counseling/>10 min		99407		Foreign body, ...
	Welcome to Medicare exam		G0344		Foreign body, s...

Figure 28-1 ■ Encounter form showing E/M codes.
Source: Billing, Coding, and Reimbursement, 3e by Deborah Vines Copyright © 2017 by Pearson Education.

- **Patient type**–Whether the patient is new or established
- **Level of service**–The complexity or length of service provided based on the nature of the presenting problem, the history, the examination, and the medical decision making.

The E/M section is organized by the setting in which the service is provided. The divisions of the E/M section are called categories and subcategories, rather than subsections and subheadings, as is the case in most other CPT sections. A category, the first level of division in the E/M section, identifies the setting or place of service. Most categories are divided into subcategories based on patient type (new or established), age, or frequency. Each subcategory is divided into codes based on the level of service. Take a moment to review the table of contents for the E/M section that appears on page 1, before the E/M guidelines, in the CPT manual.

This chapter provides an overview of basic E/M coding by discussing the guidelines and the organization of the E/M section, followed by abstracting and assigning the most common categories of E/M codes. At the end of this chapter is information about advanced E/M coding. Advanced E/M coding is also discussed in the CPT body system chapters of this text, Chapters 29–43.

SUCCESS STEP

E/M codes used by ophthalmologists appear in the Ophthalmology subsection of the Medicine section, codes **92002** to **92014**.

GUIDELINES FOR EVALUATION AND MANAGEMENT SERVICES

Coders should understand the organization of this CPT section, section guidelines, and instructional notes in the Tabular List. This information is necessary for accurate coding. Four sources of guidelines must be considered when determining the level of E/M service provided:

- E/M Section Guidelines
- Category Special Instructions
- 1995 Documentation Guidelines for Evaluation and Management Services
- 1997 Documentation Guidelines for Evaluation and Management Services

The purpose of each set of guidelines is discussed next.

E/M Section Guidelines

Coders should understand the organization of this CPT section, section guidelines, and instructional notes in the Tabular List. This information is necessary for accurate coding. The CPT guidelines appear at the beginning of the E/M section and provide information that applies to all codes in the section. The guidelines are several pages in length and explain the overall organization of the E/M section, define commonly used terms, and provide instructions for selecting a level of E/M service. In most editions of the CPT manual, these pages are shaded for easy identification.

Category Special Instructions

Each of the categories of E/M services begins with special instructions that apply to all codes within the category. Special instructions provide the following types of information:

- Explain the purpose of the category.
- Describe the circumstances and settings for which codes in the category are to be used.
- Define terms applicable to codes in the category.
- Identify services that are and are not bundled with the codes in the category.
- Redirect the coder to other categories that may be more appropriate.

Many subcategories also provide instructions for that subset of codes. Coders must read the category and subcategory special instructions before selecting a code. Specific guidelines and instructional notes are discussed throughout this chapter of the text.

1995 Documentation Guidelines for Evaluation and Management Services

E/M codes were added to CPT in 1992 to replace "office visit" codes that were poorly defined. Rather than basing codes solely on the amount of time spent by providers during an encounter, E/M codes attempted to define the complexity of the visit. However, providers interpreted the CPT guidelines inconsistently, which resulted in confusion. To help provide clearer direction, the Centers for Medicare and Medicaid Services (CMS) and the American Medical Association (AMA) developed **documentation guidelines (DGs)** for the E/M services, titled *1995 Documentation Guidelines for Evaluation and Management Services* (1995 DG).

The document outlines general principles of medical documentation (■ FIGURE 28-2, page 498) and guidelines for documenting the history, examination, and medical decision-making components of E/M services. It also discusses how to document an encounter dominated by counseling or coordination of care. The 1995 DG lists the recognized body areas and organ systems addressed during an examination but does not clearly define the criteria for reporting the extent of the examination. 1995 DG is still used today.

1997 Documentation Guidelines for Evaluation and Management Services

After the 1995 DG was implemented, many providers desired more definition regarding how to document the physical examination. To provide clarity, CMS and the AMA developed additional guidelines, titled *1997 Documentation Guidelines for Evaluation and Management Services* (1997 DG). The 1997 DG is still in use today.

The 1997 DG further specify the requirements for a comprehensive multisystem examination, as well as single-organ system examinations frequently performed by specialists. For each type of examination, the 1997 DG provides a bulleted list of elements to be evaluated. The number of elements included in the examination determines the level of complexity of the examination: problem focused, expanded problem focused, detailed, or comprehensive.

1. The medical record should be complete and legible.
2. The documentation of each patient encounter should include:
    • reason for the encounter and relevant history, physical examination findings, and prior diagnostic test results;
    • assessment, clinical impression, or diagnosis;
    • plan for care; and
    • date and legible identity of the observer.
3. If not documented, the rationale for ordering diagnostic and other ancillary services should be easily inferred.
4. Past and present diagnoses should be accessible to the treating and/or consulting physician.
5. Appropriate health risk factors should be identified.
6. The patient's progress, response to and changes in treatment, and revision of diagnosis should be documented.
7. The CPT and [ICD-10-CM] codes reported on the health insurance claim form or billing statement should be supported by the documentation in the medical record.

Figure 28-2 ■ Principles of medical record documentation. *Source: 1995 Documentation Guidelines for Evaluation and Management Services.*

Physicians may use either the 1995 or 1997 DG as documentation criteria for any E/M encounter. They can use 1995 DG for one patient and 1997 DG for another patient. But they cannot pick and choose from both sets of guidelines for the same encounter. In general, specialists prefer the 1997 guidelines because they delineate single-organ system examinations.

Specific guidelines and instructional notes are discussed throughout this chapter. This text discusses current guidelines in the CPT manual and the 1995 and 1997 DG. CMS is expected to implement changes to physician documentation requirements and reimbursement criteria in 2019-2021. Coders should monitor updates from CMS and professional organizations, such as AHIMA and AAPC.

The 1995 DG and 1997 DG can be downloaded from the CMS website at **www.cms.gov**.

CODING PRACTICE

Exercise 28.1 Overview and Guidelines for Evaluation and Management Services

Instructions: Answer the following questions based on the information in the Overview and Guidelines sections of this chapter. Write your answer on the lines provided.

1. Where in the CPT manual are Evaluation and Management (E/M) codes located?

2. What are the three criteria that define E/M codes?

3. What guidelines describe the circumstances and settings for which codes in the category are to be used?

4. Name three examples of nonphysician practitioners.

5. What guidelines provide a bulleted list of elements to be evaluated in an examination?

ABSTRACTING EVALUATION AND MANAGEMENT SERVICES

All the information used to classify E/M services—the setting in which service was provided, the type of patient and/or frequency of the encounter, and the criteria used to determine the level of service—must be abstracted before codes can be assigned. Especially when first learning about E/M services, it is difficult to memorize and organize all the details. The guidelines and special instructions are there to help you, so do not become frustrated or impatient when reading them.

■ FIGURE 28-3 provides a flow chart/decision tree for abstracting and assigning E/M codes. Refer to columns 1, 2, and 3 as you read the following material on abstracting the E/M setting and patient type.

• Column 1: Select the general setting of service as outpatient, inpatient, without direct patient contact, or other.
• Column 2: Select the type of service (E/M category) within the setting.
• Column 3: Select the subcategory of service within the type.

Abstracting the Setting

The first piece of information to abstract for E/M codes is the setting in which service was provided. The following

E/M Flow Chart

Patient Name _____

Date of Service _____ / _____ / _____

Use this chart to help locate the correct **range** of codes. Then, refer to the CPT manual Tabular List to select and verify codes.

DO NOT code from this chart. Always read CPT code descriptions and category instructions to verify final code.

1. Identify Setting	2. Identify Category/ Type of Service	3. Identify Sub-category of Service	4. Verify Code Range	5. Identify Criteria / Key Components (KC)
Office/Outpatient	☐ Office/Outpatient *(with presenting problem)*	☐ New Patient	99201-99205	**3 KC:** H/E/MDM
		☐ Established Patient	99211-99215	**2 KC:** H/E/MDM
	☐ Preventive Medicine	☐ New Patient	99381-99387	Age
		☐ Established Patient	99391-99397	Age
		☐ Individual Counseling/Risk Factor	99401-99404	Time
		☐ Individual, Behavior Change Interventions	99406-99409	Time
		☐ Group Counseling/Risk Factor	99411-99412	Time
	☐ Consultation/ Office	☐ Office/Outpatient *(Non-Medicare)*	99241-99245	**3 KC:** H/E/MDM
	☐ Newborn Care	☐ Not in hospital or birthing center	99461	Setting
	☐ Other Office/Outpatient	☐ Life/Disability Exam	99450	NA
		☐ Work Related/Medical Disability	99455-99456	Treating or non-treating
		☐ Post-operative follow-up *(bundled)*	99024 *(located in Medicine section)*	
Hospital	☐ Emergency Dept	☐ Any Patient New/Established	99281-99285	**3 KC:** H/E/MDM
		☐ EMS direction by MD	99288	NA
	☐ Hospital Observation *(not formally admitted)*	☐ Initial (New or Estab.)	99218-99220	**3 KC:** H/E/MDM
		☐ Subsequent (New or Estab.)	99224-99226	**2 KC:** H/E/MDM
		☐ Observation Discharge	99217	NA
		☐ Same Day Admit/Discharge	99234-99236	**3 KC:** H/E/MDM
	☐ Hospital Inpatient *(admitted)*	☐ Initial Hosp Care/Admission	99221-99223	**3 KC:** H/E/MDM
		☐ Subsequent Hosp Care	99231-99233	**2 KC:** H/E/MDM
		☐ Hospital Discharge	99238-99239	Time
		☐ Same Day Admit/Discharge	99234-99236	**3 KC:** H/E/MDM
	☐ Consultation/ Inpatient	☐ Initial Inpatient *(Non-Medicare)*	99251-99255	**3 KC:** H/E/MDM
	☐ Critical Care (CC) *(life threatening condition)*	☐ 6 yr and older/ Adult	99291-99292	Time
		☐ Neonatal/Pediatric Critical Care	99466-99482	Age/Status/Service
	☐ Intensive Care	☐ Neonatal/Pediatric Intensive Care	99477-99480	Age/Status/Service
		☐ Pediatric CC Transport (<=24 mo.)	99466-99486	Time/Service
	☐ Newborn Care	☐ Normal Newborn	99460-99463	Setting
		☐ Delivery Attendance/Resuscitation	99464-99465	Type of service
Without Direct Patient Contact	☐ Non Face-to-Face Services	☐ Telephone Services	99441-99443	Time
		☐ Online Medical Evaluation	99444	NA
		☐ Interprofessional Telephone/Internet	99446-99452	Time
		☐ Remote Physiologic Monitoring	99453-99457	NA
	☐ Care Plan Oversight	☐ Domiciliary, Rest Home	99339-99340	Time
		☐ Home Health Agency Patient	99374-99375	Time
		☐ Hospice Patient	99377-99378	Time
		☐ Nursing Facility Patient	99379-99380	Time
	☐ Case Management	☐ Team Conferences	99366-99368	Face to Face/Not
	☐ Transitional Care Management	☐ Transitional Care Management	99495-99496	Complexity/Time frame
	☐ Standby - Physician	☐ Standby - Physician	99360	Time
	☐ Prolonged Service	☐ No Direct Face to Face Contact	99358-99359	Time
Other Settings	☐ Nursing Facility	☐ Initial (New or Established)	99304-99306	**3 KC:** H/E/MDM
		☐ Subsequent (New or Established)	99307-99310	**2 KC:** H/E/MDM
		☐ Discharge	99315-99316	Time
		☐ Annual Assessment	99318	**3 KC:** H/E/MDM
	☐ Domiciliary/Rest Home	☐ New Patient	99324-99328	**3 KC:** H/E/MDM
		☐ Established Patient	99334-99337	**3 KC:** H/E/MDM
	☐ Home Service	☐ New Patient	99341-99345	**3 KC:** H/E/MDM
		☐ Established Patient	99347-99350	**2 KC:** H/E/MDM
	☐ Chronic Care Management	☐ Complex Chronic Care Coordination	99487-99489	Time
	☐ Psychiatric Collaborative Care	☐ Psychiatric Collaborative Care	99492-99494	Initial/Subsequent/Time
Any Setting	☐ Prolonged Service	☐ With Direct Face to Face Contact	99354-99357	Time/Report required
	☐ Prolonged Clinical Staff Svc	☐ Clinical Staff with Physician Supervision	99415-99416	Time/Report required
	☐ Unlisted service	☐ Other/Unlisted E/M	99499	Report required

6. Evaluate Key Components
(Also refer to the Key Components Tool)

H= History   E= Exam   MDM= Medical Decision Making

For any code using H/E/MDM criteria, use the chart below to select the appropriate level of each criteria.

History	Exam	MDM
☐ Prob Focused	☐ Prob Focused	☐ Straightforward
☐ Exp Prob Focused	☐ Exp Prob Focused	☐ Low complexity
☐ Detailed	☐ Detailed	☐ Mod complexity
☐ Comprehensive	☐ Comprehensive	☐ High complexity

See CPT manual for definition of each of these levels.

2 KC= At least 2 H/E/MDM levels must meet or exceed definition
3 KC = All 3 H/E/MDM levels must meet or exceed definition

7. Evaluate Time Factor Override

Time is a factor in determining an H/E/MDM code ONLY when counseling and coordination of care occupy more than 50% of the face-to-face time.

Face to Face Time	Counseling/ Coord Care Time	Couns/Coord More than 50%?
		☐ Yes
		☐ No

See CPT code definition for typical time per level of care.

8. Determine if a Modifier is needed

☐ -24 Unrelated E/M service by same physician during post-operative period (unrelated to original procedure)
☐ -25 Significant, separately identifiable E/M service by same physician on the day (within 24 hr) of a (minor) procedure
☐ -32 Mandated services (by 3rd party)
☐ -57 Decision for surgery (major) made at time of visit
☐ -AI Admitting physician (Medicare inpatients)

See CPT manual Appendix A for full description of modifiers

9. Determine if Special Circumstances Apply

Services provided:
☐ 99050 Outside of normal office hours
☐ 99051 During regularly scheduled eve, wkend, or holiday hrs
☐ 99053 10pm - 8am at 24-hour facility
☐ 99056 Patient requests services outside of office
☐ 99058 Emergency basis, in office
☐ 99060 Emergency basis, out of office

INSTRUCTIONS

1. Identify the general setting in which service was provided.
2. Identify the type of service within the setting rows.
3. Select the subcategory of service within the category rows.
4. Reference the code range provided in the Tabular List.
5. Identify the criteria used to define the level of service and, when applicable, the # of Key Components needed.
6. Summarize the levels of the 3 KC, where applicable. Also refer to the Key Components Evaluation Tool for help.
7. Evaluate if the time factor qualifies to override the 3 KC.
8. Determine if a modifier is needed.
9. Determine if special circumstances apply.

CPT codes only © American Medical Association.
© PB Resources, Inc. All rights reserved.

Figure 28-3 ■ E/M flow chart. Source: © PB Resources, Inc. Used with permission.

information discusses the office, outpatient hospital, and inpatient hospital settings in detail, then provides an overview of other E/M settings. Office and inpatient settings include many types of E/M services. Therefore, several categories are provided for both of these settings, and coders must accurately select the correct one. The E/M section provides more than 20 categories of codes. Refer to ▪ TABLE 28-1 for a general guide in abstracting the setting or category of service.

Office-Based Evaluation and Management Services

An office or other outpatient setting is a nonresidential medical facility to which patients come for several minutes or several hours at one time. Patients are outpatients until they are formally admitted to an inpatient facility. Medical offices, clinics, urgent care clinics, outpatient hospitals, and ambulatory surgery centers qualify as office or outpatient settings. CPT provides several E/M categories for office-based and outpatient services.

In addition to encounters for the evaluation or treatment of a health problem, other E/M categories identify preventive care services, consultations, disability evaluations, and life insurance examinations provided in an office setting. The categories for office-based services do not appear next to each other within the E/M section. A description of the most commonly used outpatient E/M categories follows.

Office or Other Outpatient Services (99201-99215). Office or Other Outpatient Services (99201-99215) is the first category that appears in the E/M section, but *not all* office and outpatient services are coded here. The category **99201-99215** identifies services to diagnose or treat health problems and symptoms. The subcategory divisions are based on patient type (new or established). Within each patient type, codes are divided based on the level of service.

Office or Other Outpatient Consultations (99241-99245). A consultation is an evaluation of a patient requested by another physician to obtain a professional opinion on a specific problem. The provider who requests the consultation is the referring physician. The consulting physician, also called the *consultant*, is the one who receives the request. The consultant can recommend treatment or determine whether to accept the patient for ongoing management of one or more problems. The consulting physician reports the consultation visit using the appropriate code

from **Office or Other Outpatient Consultations (99241-99245)** to identify the level of service. The request for a consultation must be documented in the patient's medical records, kept both by the referring physician and the consulting physician. The consultant's findings or opinion must be reported back to the referring physician and also be documented in the patient's medical record(s).

Outpatient consultations include not only those provided in the office, outpatient department, or other ambulatory facility but also those provided to hospital observation patients and those at home, in the emergency department, or in a domiciliary or rest home.

A transfer of care occurs when the consulting physician assumes management of a patient's care for one or more problems or conditions. From that point forward, the physician is no longer in a consulting role and reports ongoing services with the appropriate code(s) from **Office or Other Outpatient Services (99201-99215)**. Concurrent care occurs when more than one physician treats a patient at the same time for different conditions or different aspects of the same condition. *Concurrent care* is a clinical term, rather than a coding term. It describes the general nature of the care, but there is no code or modifier to identify concurrent care.

Office or Other Outpatient Consultations (99241-99245) is a subcategory under **Consultations**. Codes are defined based on the level of care provided.

Medicare does not pay for consultation codes. When consultation services are provided for Medicare patients in the office or outpatient setting, report codes for **Office or Other Outpatient Services (99201-99215)** based on the type of patient and level of service provided. Private payers may or may not pay for consultation codes, so be sure to check which codes a specific payer requires.

Preventive Medicine Services (99381-99429). Preventive medicine services are general comprehensive checkups performed to maintain health, identify risk factors, and provide appropriate counseling, rather than to manage acute or chronic conditions. Preventive medicine subcategory divisions are based on patient type—new or established. Within each patient type, codes are divided based on the age of the patient.

Laboratory, radiology, and other screening tests can be ordered or administered during a preventive medicine visit. Vaccinations or immunizations can also be given. These services are reported with separate CPT codes, in addition to the E/M code. However, if the only service provided is a screening test or vaccination, report only that service and not an E/M code.

When a new problem is identified, or an existing problem is managed, requiring a substantial workup or evaluation, report a code from **Office or Other Outpatient Services (99201-99215)**, in addition to the preventive medicine code. Apply modifier **-25** to this code to identify that two separate E/M services were provided on the same day.

When both a preventive medicine code and a code from **Office or Other Outpatient Services (99201-99215)** are reported on the same day, be sure to assign two ICD-10-CM diagnosis codes. An ICD-10-CM code from **Z00.- Encounter for general examination without complaint, suspected or reported diagnosis** supports the preventive medicine service.

Table 28-1 ▪ KEY CRITERIA FOR ABSTRACTING THE E/M SETTING (CATEGORY)

- ❏ Where (in what setting) was the service provided: office or other outpatient, inpatient hospital, or another setting (specify)?
- ❏ Did the service require minimal or no direct patient contact?
- ❏ Is the patient a neonate or child?
- ❏ What type of service was provided: management of a health problem, preventive care, consultation only, or other?
- ❏ If outpatient, is the patient new or established?
- ❏ If inpatient, is the encounter for the admission, continuing care, or discharge?

Source: © PB Resources, Inc. Used with permission.

Also assign a code for the condition or problem to support the office or other outpatient services code (■ FIGURE 28-4).

The Preventive Medicine Services category also includes subcategories for counseling and assessments:

- Individual counseling for risk factor reduction (**99401-99404**)
- Individual behavior change treatments related to smoking and alcohol abuse (**99406-99409**)
- Group counseling for risk factor reduction (**99411-99412**)

Other Office and Outpatient Services. Other E/M services provided in the office or outpatient setting are life and disability insurance examinations, postoperative follow-up visits, and critical care.

Life and Disability Insurance Examinations (99450-99456). Physicians sometimes provide an evaluation service to establish baseline health measurements for patients before a life insurance or disability insurance policy is issued. They also perform periodic examinations of patients who are disabled and covered by either workers' compensation or a medical disability policy. The purpose of the examination is to provide information; no active treatment is provided during the encounter. Three codes are available in the category **Special Evaluation and Management Services (99450-99456)** to report these examinations.

Postoperative Follow-up (99024). Most postoperative follow-up visits are bundled, or included, with the CPT code for the procedure performed as part of the global surgery package. However, sometimes payers require that the encounters be reported. Code **99024 Postoperative follow-up visit, normally included in the surgical package** is used for this purpose. The code carries no charge. **99024** does not appear in the E/M section. It appears in the Medicine section, which is the last section in the CPT manual.

Critical Care Services (Age 6 to Adult) (99291, 99292). Critical care services can be provided in any setting that has the appropriate equipment and supplies. Critical care services are discussed in detail in the section "Inpatient Hospital Evaluation and Management Services" later in the chapter because they are most commonly provided in the inpatient setting. However, the same codes are reported for critical care services, regardless of the setting.

Prolonged Services (99354-99360, 99415-99416)

The amount of time that physicians spend with patients or coordinating their care varies widely. Most E/M codes are defined based on the level of service provided and include a general estimate of time typically spent by physicians. The actual time spent with or in relationship to a specific patient can vary widely from the estimate and, most of the time, physicians cannot charge higher fees when the estimated time is exceeded. When the amount of time actually spent exceeds more than 30 minutes above and beyond the estimate included in the code, physicians can report the extra time with a code from the category **Prolonged Services (99354-99360)**. Prolonged face-to-face time spent by clinical staff under physician supervision can be reported with codes **99415** and **99416**. Be sure to review the CPT guidelines that appear before these codes. Prolonged services less than 30 minutes beyond the usual cannot be reported separately.

For example, code **99205** includes a typical face-to-face time of 60 minutes. When the provider spends 75 minutes with the patient, there is no additional payment due for the additional time. However, when the provider spends 91 minutes or longer face to face, then it may be possible to bill for prolonged services and receive additional payment.

Prolonged service codes are add-on codes and can be used with any E/M code in any setting. This category is divided based on whether the prolonged service is direct (face to face with the patient). Codes are defined based on the amount of *excess* time. Direct patient contact codes are further defined based on whether the service was outpatient or inpatient. Refer to the category special instructions for a chart that

---

An established patient, age 58, comes in for his annual checkup. The patient complains of recent episodes of right leg numbness, tingling, and muscle weakness. The physician performed an evaluation and management service consisting of a detailed history, a comprehensive neurological examination, and medical decision making of high complexity.

Z00.01 Encounter for general adult medical examination with abnormal findings

99396 Periodic comprehensive preventive medicine reevaluation... established patient; 40–64 years

M54.17 Radiculopathy, lumbosacral region

99215-25 Office or other outpatient visit for the evaluation and management of an established patient (level 5)
-25 Significant, Separately Identifiable Evaluation and Management Service by the Same Physician or Other Qualified Health Care Professional on the Same Day of the Procedure or Other Service

Figure 28-4 ■ Example of coding preventive care and problem-oriented E/M on same day.
Source: © PB Resources, Inc. Used with permission.

provides an example of how to report various amounts of time (■ FIGURE 28-5). A report that describes the nature of the prolonged services should be submitted with the claim.

Outpatient Hospital Evaluation and Management Services

Two types of services occur in a hospital facility but are reported as outpatient services because the patient has not been admitted as an inpatient. These areas are emergency department services and hospital observation services.

Emergency Department Services (99281-99288). An emergency department (ED) is an organized, hospital-based facility that is open 24 hours per day and provides unscheduled services to patients requiring immediate medical attention, such as injury, trauma, or sudden onset of potentially life-threatening symptoms and signs. Urgent care clinics are not emergency departments, even though they may be open 24 hours per day, because they do not provide care for injuries or conditions that threaten life or limb. ED codes are divided based on the level of service provided. Patients treated in the ED are outpatients. They can be discharged, transferred, placed on outpatient observation status, or admitted as an inpatient.

When physicians treat patients in the ED then admit them, the ED services are combined with the initial inpatient services provided on the same day. Only one code, from the category **Initial Hospital Care (99221-99223)**, is reported.

Hospital Observation Services (99217-99226). Patients placed on observation status have not been formally admitted to the hospital as inpatients because they do not meet the necessary criteria for hospital admission. However, the physician wants to monitor certain symptoms or complaints that make it unsafe for a patient to be sent home. Some hospitals provide a designated observation unit and others assign observation patients to beds on inpatient units or in the emergency department. Observation status may occur for a few hours or for multiple days, until the physician decides either to admit the patient or discharge them from observation status.

Observation is an outpatient service because patients have not been formally admitted to the hospital, although they occupy hospital beds. The category **Hospital Observation Services (99217-99226)** is divided into subcategories based on patient status (initial or subsequent care) and further divided into codes based on the level of service. Separate codes are provided for **Observation Care Discharge Services (99217)** and for observation patients admitted and discharged on the same date of service (**99234-99236**).

Inpatient Hospital Evaluation and Management Services

The category **Hospital Inpatient Services (99221-99223, 99231-99239)** classifies inpatient admission, continuing follow-up visits while an inpatient, and discharges. Visits with consulting physicians and critical care services appear in other categories. The categories for inpatient services do not appear next to each other within the E/M section. A description of the most commonly used inpatient E/M categories follows.

Hospital Inpatient Services (99221-99223, 99231-99239). A hospital inpatient is a patient who has been formally admitted to a hospital. Medicare requires that the patient stay span two midnights to qualify for inpatient reimbursement. The requirements of other payers vary. Codes are divided by the type of encounter—initial or subsequent. This category does not distinguish between new and established patients. Apply HCPCS modifier **-AI Principal physician of record** to the code for **Initial hospital care (99221-99223)** when the physician admits a patient during the encounter. The modifier distinguishes the admission encounter from initial inpatient visits by consulting physicians.

Partial Hospitalization Programs. A partial hospitalization program (PHP) is a mental health program, usually provided by a hospital. It consists of an intensive ambulatory treatment service of less than 24-hour daily care, but one that most patients attend every day. Patients do not stay overnight in the hospital unless they are already an inpatient. PHPs can provide a transition from inpatient to outpatient care, shorten an inpatient stay, or eliminate the need for an inpatient admission. CPT does not provide a specific E/M category for PHPs. E/M services provided for patients in a PHP setting are always coded as **Hospital Inpatient Services (99221-99223, 99231-99239)**. PHP patients may be outpatients if they have not been formally admitted, but the service is coded as an inpatient service.

Inpatient Consultations (99251-99255). Inpatient consultations follow the same definitions as those for outpatient consultations. Codes in this category are reported for consultations provided to hospital inpatients, residents of nursing facilities,

---

A 13-year-old new patient is brought in by her mother due to recent symptoms of increased thirst, frequent urination, extreme hunger, and weight loss. The physician performs a comprehensive history, comprehensive examination, and medical decision making of high complexity. The physician diagnoses type 1 diabetes and spends 50 minutes discussing the disease and treatment options with the mother and daughter. A total of 95 minutes (1:35) is spent with the patient.

99205 New patient office visit (level 5)... Typically, 60 minutes are spent face-to-face with the patient and/or family.
(95 minutes – 60 minutes = 35 minutes of prolonged service)

99354 Prolonged service in the office or other outpatient setting requiring direct patient contact beyond the usual service; first hour

Figure 28-5 ■ Example of coding for prolonged services.

or patients in a PHP. Consulting physicians should report a consultation code only once per admission. Any follow-up or subsequent services provided during the same admission are reported with codes for **Subsequent Hospital Care (99231-99233)** or **Subsequent Nursing Facility Care (99307-99310)**.

Medicare has not paid for consultation codes since 2010. When consultation services are provided for Medicare patients in the inpatient setting, report codes for **Hospital Inpatient Services (99221-99223, 99231-99239)** based on the type of patient and level of service provided.

Critical Care Services (Age 6 to Adult) (99291-99292). Critical care is medical treatment provided for an illness or injury that impairs one or more vital organ systems and presents a high probability of imminent or life-threatening deterioration. It involves close, constant attention by a team of specially trained healthcare providers. Critical care often takes place in an intensive care unit or ED but does not have to occur in those locations to use the critical care codes. Critical care services can also be provided in an outpatient setting, such as the emergency department or clinic. Critical care codes report the time spent providing services. Special instructions for this category in the CPT manual specify the services that are included in critical care time and should not be billed in addition to the critical care codes (■ TABLE 28-2). Any service performed not included in this list should be reported separately.

All time must be one-on-one direct care by the physician but does not have to be continuous. Report the total amount of time spent during the day. When less than 30 minutes is spent delivering critical care, report the appropriate E/M code, not a critical care code. Count the time spent evaluating, managing, and providing critical care services to a critically ill or injured person. The time to be billed for critical care must be spent at the immediate bedside or elsewhere on the floor as long as the physician is available to the patient. No other patients can be cared for during the time reported for critical care of a specific patient. If the physician departs to care for another patient, the clock stops, then restarts when the physician resumes critical care for the first patient.

To report the time spent on a given date, report code **99291** once for the first 30–74 minutes of critical care time. Then, report one unit of code **99292** for *each additional 30 minutes* of care on a given date (■ FIGURE 28-6). The special instructions for codes **99291** and **99292** provide a box that shows how to report various increments of time.

These codes are used for children age six and older and adults. Critical care for children younger than six years old is reported with neonatal and pediatric intensive care codes. Study the special instructions for reporting the critical care codes carefully to ensure that all services are properly reported.

Table 28-2 ■ **SERVICES BUNDLED INTO CRITICAL CARE TIME**

- ❏ Interpretation of cardiac output measurements (93561, 93562)
- ❏ Chest x-rays (71045, 71046)
- ❏ Pulse oximetry (94760, 94761, 94762)
- ❏ Blood gases (94760-94762)
- ❏ Physiologic data stored in computers (e.g., ECGs, blood pressures, hematologic data [99090])
- ❏ Gastric intubation (43752, 43753)
- ❏ Temporary transcutaneous pacing (92953)
- ❏ Ventilatory management (94002-94004, 94660, 94662)
- ❏ Vascular access procedures (36000, 36410, 36415, 36591, 36600)

Newborns. CPT provides specially designated codes for several newborn services, including normal newborn care, intensive care, and delivery attendance or resuscitation. Neonatal critical care is reported with critical care codes.

Normal Newborn Care Services (99460-99463). Inpatient care for normal newborns is reported with codes **99460** to **99463**. Codes are divided by setting—hospital/birthing center and other—and by initial care, subsequent care, and same-day admission and discharge. Discharges occurring after the admission date are reported with the codes for inpatient discharges, **99238** and **99239**.

Delivery/Birthing Room Attendance and Resuscitation Services (99464-99465). When the physician performing a delivery requests another physician to be present during delivery and assist with stabilization of the newborn, report code **99464**. When a physician provides resuscitation or ventilation services to a newborn, report code **99465**. Read the instructional notes with these codes to identify codes that can and cannot be reported together.

Neonatal Intensive Care and Critical Care and Pediatric Critical Care (99466-99486). Neonatal and pediatric critical care codes are used for children younger than six years old. The same definition of critical care services for adults applies to neonates and children. However, codes for **Neonatal and Pediatric Critical Care Services (99466-99476)** report all services provided per day, rather than being time based, as the adult codes are. Codes are divided based on the age of the child and whether the service is initial or subsequent. The special instructions for this category identify the services that are bundled into the critical care codes. Other services should be reported separately.

A physician provided 2.5 hours of critical care time on March 15 to a patient in acute respiratory distress.

99291 Critical care, evaluation and management of the critically ill or critically injured patient; first 30–74 minutes
99292 x 3 Critical care, evaluation and management of the critically ill or critically injured patient; each additional 30 minutes

Figure 28-6 ■ Example of reporting critical care time.

Intensive care services (**99477-99480**) are provided for newborns and children who are not critically ill but require intensive observation and frequent interventions. Infants and neonates weighing less than 5,000 grams, or about four and a half pounds, often require extended cardiac and respiratory monitoring, frequent vital sign monitoring, heat maintenance, enteral and/or parenteral nutritional adjustments, laboratory and oxygen monitoring, and constant observation by the healthcare team. Review the detailed special instructions that appear in this category to ensure proper coding.

Services Without Direct Patient Contact

A number of E/M services require minimal or no direct contact between the provider and the patient. Brief descriptions of these services include:

- **Non-Face-to-Face Services (99441-99457)** report services involving the telephone, Internet, electronic health record (EHR), and digitally stored data. These services do not require in-person face-to-face contact between the patient and physician. Read the detailed special instructions provided in the CPT manual for each of these subcategories. This category includes the following types of service:

  - **Telephone Services (99441-99443)** must be initiated by and provided to an established patient, not relating to a service within the past 7 days or next 24 hours.

  - **Online Medical Evaluation (99444)** must be initiated by and provided to an established patient, not relating to a service within the past 7 days or next 24 hours

  - **Interprofessional Telephone/Internet/Electronic Health Record Consultations (99446-99452)** do not require face-to-face contact between the patient and consultant. The primary care provider must request the opinion or treatment advice of a physician with specific specialty expertise.

  - **Digitally Stored Data Services/Remote Physiologic Monitoring (99453, 99454, 99091)** codes report the set-up, patient education, collection, supply, assessment, and interpretation of data from remote monitoring of parameters such as weight, blood pressure, pulse oximetry, and respiratory flow rate during a 30-day period. CPT provides detailed instructions about when and how to report these codes. Code **99091** is resequenced from the Medicine section.

  - **Remote Physiologic Monitoring Treatment Management Services (99457)** reports using the collected data to manage a patient under a specific treatment plan.

- **Care Plan Oversight Services (99374-99380)** are reported by the primary supervising provider for patients under the care of home health, hospice, or nursing facilities. The work involves coordinating complex and multidisciplinary services and regular monitoring and updating of care plans. Services also include communication with a patient's family member or caregiver. Codes are divided by setting and time.

- **Case Management Services (99363-99368)** involve coordinating, managing access to, initiating, and supervising a range of healthcare services needed by the patient. Codes

identify medical team conferences involving at least three health professionals from three disciplines, each of whom provide direct care to the patient. One person from each discipline may report a case management code. Patients may attend some team conferences, so codes are divided based on whether the patient is present.

- **Transitional Care Management (TCM) Services (99495-99496)** are provided for assisting complex patients in making a transition from an inpatient setting to the patient's community setting, whether it is the patient's private residence or an assisted living or rest home type of facility. TCM consists of one face-to-face encounter with the patient, as well as a broad range of non-face-to-face services. Codes are divided based on complexity and when the face-to-face patient visit occurs. Read the special instructions carefully to understand how to report codes in this category.

- **Prolonged Service Without Direct Patient Contact (99358, 99359)** codes are reported for service above and beyond the normal E/M time, not involving direct patient contact. Codes are based on the total amount of time spent per day. Refer to the category special instructions for a chart that provides an example of how to report various amounts of time. A report that describes the nature of the prolonged services should be submitted with the claim.

Other Evaluation and Management Services

Other E/M services include those provided in other settings or for specialized needs. Study the guidelines and instructions that accompany these codes in the CPT manual.

- **Nursing Facility Services (99304-99318)** codes are reported for E/M services provided in a **nursing facility (NF)**, formerly known as a skilled nursing facility (SNF), intermediate care facility (ICF), or long-term care facility (LTCF). These are residential facilities that provide professional medical and nursing care. Codes are divided by type of encounter (initial or subsequent encounter) and the level of service provided by the physician during an E/M encounter. This category does not distinguish between new and established patients.

- **Domiciliary, Rest Home, Custodial (99324-99337; 99339-99340)** codes are reported for E/M services provided in custodial care settings such as a domiciliary, rest home, or assisted living facility. These facilities provide limited assistance with activities of daily living (ADLs) but do not provide professional medical or nursing care. Codes are divided by patient type (new or established) and the level of service provided by the physician during an E/M encounter.

- **Home Services (99341-99350)** codes are reported for E/M services provided in the patient's private residence, temporary lodging, or short term accommodation, such as a hotel, campground, hostel, or cruise ship. Codes are divided by patient type (new or established) and the level of service provided.

- **Complex Chronic Care Coordination Evaluation and Management Services (99487-99491)** codes are reported for patient-centered management and support services provided to an individual who resides at home or in a domiciliary, rest home, or assisted living facility. These services address the coordination of care by multiple disciplines and community service agencies. The codes are reported by the provider who oversees the management of services for all medical conditions, psychosocial needs, and activities of daily living. Codes are divided based on time spent during a calendar month. Be sure to read the detailed special instructions for this category in the CPT manual.

- **Cognitive Assessment and Care Plan Services (99483)** are provided when a patient who exhibits signs or symptoms of a cognitive impairment needs a comprehensive evaluation of their condition for further study of the diagnosis.

- **Psychiatric Collaborative Care Management Services (99492-99484)** are reported for patients who have a diagnosed psychiatric disorder that requires a behavioral health assessment, establishing or updating of a care plan, and provision of brief interventions.

- **Other Evaluation and Management Services (99499)** codes are reported only when no other E/M code adequately describes the service provided. This is a code for an unlisted procedure and should be accompanied by a detailed report that describes the services provided.

CODING CAUTION

When billing E/M services on the 837P electronic claim or CMS-1500 form, each CPT code must be associated with a two-digit **place of service (POS)** identifier, entered in Item 24B. The POS identifier must be consistent with the setting of the E/M code for the claim to be processed. For example, you cannot submit a claim for E/M code **99221** (initial hospital services) with POS 11 Office. POS codes are listed in the front of most CPT manuals.

CODING PRACTICE

Exercise 28.2   Abstracting the Setting

Instructions: Identify the E/M setting for each of the following scenarios. Write the letter of the choice on the line. Choose from:

A. Office or other outpatient

B. Inpatient

C. Services without direct patient contact

D. Other settings

1. _____ After being seen in the emergency department, a patient is admitted to the hospital.

2. _____ A mother brings her child to an urgent care clinic.

3. _____ A physician assists with a delivery in a hospital birthing room.

4. _____ A physician provides care plan oversight services for a patient in a nursing facility.

5. _____ A patient is seen in the emergency department after an automobile accident.

6. _____ A physician provides evaluation and management services to a patient in an assisted living facility.

7. _____ A patient residing at home received physician services for complex chronic care coordination.

8. _____ A patient complaining of chest pain is kept overnight in the hospital for observation.

9. _____ A patient attends a partial hospitalization program 12 hours a day and returns home at night.

10. _____ A patient preparing to move home after a three-week stay in a rehabilitation center receives transitional care management services.

Abstracting the Patient Type

Four E/M categories divide codes based on patient type or status, which means whether the patient is new or established:

- Office or Other Outpatient Services
- Preventive Medicine Services
- Domiciliary, Rest Home, or Custodial Care Services
- Home Services

CPT provides specific definitions for new and established patients. An **established patient (EP)** is one who has received professional services from the same physician, or another physician in the group of the same specialty and subspecialty, within the previous three years (■ TABLE 28-3). Any other patient is classified as a **new patients (NP)**, who has not previously received services from a particular physician or group of

---

Table 28-3 ■ **KEY CRITERIA FOR ABSTRACTING E/M ESTABLISHED PATIENT TYPE**

- ❏ Has the patient seen the same physician within the past three years?
  - *Yes*: Patient is established.
  - *No*: The next three questions must be answered *Yes* to qualify as an established patient.
- ❏ Did the patient see a physician of the exact same specialty as a previous physician in the same group?
- ❏ If previous physician was a subspecialist, did the patient see a physician of the exact same subspecialty as the previous physician in the same group?
- ❏ Does the visit with the same specialist or subspecialist occur within three years of the previous visit?

Source: © PB Resources, Inc. Used with permission.

physicians in the same specialty or subspecialty. New patient E/M services are reported with separate CPT codes than established patients. Each specialty and subspecialty has differing assessments and examinations, and new patients require a more extensive workup than established patients.

To understand the definition of an established patient, you must understand the meaning of a medical group, a medical specialty, and a subspecialty.

- A *medical group* is a business organization, such as a corporation or partnership, in which physicians share certain resources, such as space and staff. Revenue may be shared or may be allocated to individual physicians.

- A *medical specialty* is an area of study within medicine pertaining to a specific body system (cardiology), class of procedures (thoracic surgery), or patient characteristics (pediatrics). Medical specialties and subspecialties are defined by the American Board of Medical Specialties and are not listed in the CPT manual.

- A *subspecialty* is a narrower aspect of a specialty that requires additional training, such as interventional cardiology, congenital cardiac surgery, or adolescent medicine. Not all physicians have a subspecialty.

When patients are seen by the same physician within the past three years, they are established patients. If the physician has moved from one practice to another, the patient is still established with that physician if seen within three years.

When patients cannot see the same physician as before, they may accept an appointment with another physician in the same group. If the new physician is of the same specialty and subspecialty as the previous physician, then the patient is still established, as long as it has been three years or less.

However, if the specialty is different from the previous physician, the patient is **New** for CPT coding purposes. If the specialty is the same as that of the previous physician but the subspecialty is different, the patient is **New** for CPT coding purposes. The "Evaluation and Management (E/M) Services Guidelines" section in the CPT manual provides a decision tree to assist in distinguishing new and established patients.

Some E/M categories do not distinguish between new and established patient types because other criteria are more important in defining the services provided. Patient age is used to divide categories for preventive care and certain services provided to newborns and children. Frequency—such as initial care, subsequent care, or discharge—is used for certain inpatient services. Coders must be attentive to the CPT special instructions for each category of E/M service to fully understand the basis on which categories and subcategories are defined.

CODING CAUTION

The E/M categories Inpatient Hospital Services, Hospital Observation Services, and Nursing Facility Services divide codes based on whether the encounter is initial or subsequent. Initial encounter refers to the first encounter by the admitting physician during the current admission. Subsequent encounter refers to the second or later encounter by the admitting provider during the current admission and to all encounters by other than the admitting physician. CPT definitions for *initial* and *subsequent* encounters differ from those used by ICD-10-CM.

CODING PRACTICE

Exercise 28.3 Abstracting Patient Type

Instructions: Identify whether each patient is new or established. Place a checkmark in front of the correct answer.

1. A child is seen by a pediatric cardiologist, to whom he was referred by his regular pediatrician at the same clinic.
   ☐ New ☐ Established

2. A patient returns to Branton Family Practice to see her internal medicine physician, whom she last saw two years ago.
   ☐ New ☐ Established

3. A mother brings her newborn daughter to the same pediatrician who has cared for the older siblings for three years.
   ☐ New ☐ Established

4. A patient is evaluated by a thoracic surgeon prior to undergoing a coronary artery bypass graft, recommended by a cardiologist at the same clinic. ☐ New ☐ Established

5. A patient comes to Branton Family Practice for the first time to see her primary care physician, whom she last saw one year ago at another clinic. ☐ New ☐ Established

6. A patient sees a gastroenterologist for the first time at the same clinic where he goes twice a year because his previous gastroenterologist retired. ☐ New ☐ Established

7. A patient sees a general surgeon for evaluation for a hernia repair. The same surgeon repaired another hernia four years ago. ☐ New ☐ Established

8. A woman who just learned, as the result of a home pregnancy test, that she might be pregnant sees her obstetrician, who delivered her first child two years ago.
   ☐ New ☐ Established

9. A patient sees his regular dermatologist for evaluation and treatment of a new skin rash that he has never experienced before. ☐ New ☐ Established

10. A patient who has been out of the country for three years returns to the clinic to see the same physician who cared for her before she went abroad. She brings with her the medical records that cover the time she was away.
    ☐ New ☐ Established

Abstracting the Level of Service

Eight E/M categories define the level, or complexity, of service provided based on a set of three **key components (KCs)** (■ TABLE 28-4). The key components are the history, the examination, and the medical decision making, each of which can be performed at varying levels of complexity. The combinations of the three key components define three to five levels of service within each category. Criteria that include the three key components also include three contributory factors and time. Levels of service cannot be interchanged or substituted across E/M categories. For example, the criteria for the five levels of service for a new patient office visit cannot be interchanged with the criteria for the five levels of service for an established

Table 28-4   ■   E/M CATEGORIES THAT USE KEY COMPONENTS

- ❏ Consultation Services
- ❏ Domiciliary, Rest Home (e.g., Boarding Home), or Custodial Care Services
- ❏ Emergency Department Services
- ❏ Home Services
- ❏ Hospital Inpatient Services
- ❏ Hospital Observation Services
- ❏ Nursing Facility Services
- ❏ Office or Other Outpatient Services

Source: Used by permission of PB Resources, Inc.

patient office visit because the key components are combined in different ways.

Key components are also referred to as **content of service requirements** because they define the work done during the encounter, in contrast to codes based on time, patient age, or other elements.

Three Key Components

The three key components are the extent of the patient's history gathered by the physician, the extent of the physical examination, and the complexity of medical decision making. Each key component is divided into four levels, each of which describes the complexity of the service provided (■ TABLE 28-5).

Table 28-5   ■   SUMMARY OF KEY COMPONENTS AND CONTRIBUTORY FACTORS

Three Key Components	
History levels: • Problem focused • Expanded problem focused • Detailed • Comprehensive	Subjective information that the patient provides, including four elements: 1. Chief complaint (CC) 2. History of present illness (HPI) 3. Review of systems (ROS) 4. Past, family, and social history (PFSH)
Examination levels: • Problem focused • Expanded problem focused • Detailed • Comprehensive	Objective information that the physician identifies during the examination of specific body areas and/or organ systems
Medical decision making levels: • Straightforward • Low • Moderate • High	The physician renders a diagnosis and makes recommendations for treatment. Medical decision making includes reviewing and analyzing three elements: • Number of possible diagnoses and/or number of management options • Amount and/or complexity of medical records, diagnostic tests, and/or other information • Risk of significant complications, morbidity and/or mortality, and comorbidities
Three Contributory Factors	
Counseling	The physician provides counseling to a patient and/or family members regarding the patient's diagnosis, treatment, and follow-up.
Coordination of care	The physician coordinates the patient's care with other healthcare providers or agencies.
Nature of presenting problem	A symptom, complaint, condition, illness, disease, sign, finding, or injury that represents the reason for the patient's encounter.
Time	
Intraservice (face-to-face) time	Face-to-face time the physician spends with the patient for office or other outpatient services and unit/floor time for hospital and other inpatient services.

History. History refers to the discussion between the patient and physician regarding several areas that could provide information regarding the patient's medical situation. The history is subjective because it is based on what the patient tells the physician. It includes the **chief complaint (CC)**, a **history of present illness (HPI)**, a **review of systems (ROS)**, and the patient's **past, family, and social history (PFSH)**. Each of these elements (except for the CC) is also assigned a level of complexity based on the amount of information gathered.

Examination. The physical examination is objective because it is based on the physician's examination of the patient. The type of examination is determined by the patient's chief complaint and the amount of information the physician needs to collect to make a diagnosis and formulate a treatment plan. The physician can perform a general multisystem examination or an organ-specific examination. The examination can include up to seven defined body areas and 12 organ systems.

A general multisystem examination or a single organ system examination may be performed by any physician, regardless of specialty. The type (general multisystem or single organ system) and content of the examination are selected by the examining physician and are based on clinical judgment, the patient's history, and the nature of the presenting problem(s). The 1997 DG presents a bulleted list of elements in each body system that potentially can be examined for the general multisystem examination. The number of body areas and/or organ systems examined and the total number of bulleted items examined determine the level of the examination.

The 1997 DG also defines 11 single-organ examinations and provides a bulleted list of elements that can potentially be examined in each organ system. The number of bulleted items examined and documented determines the level of the examination. These criteria may vary among organ systems.

Medical Decision Making. Medical decision making refers to the complexity of establishing a diagnosis and/or selecting a management option as measured by:

- The number of possible diagnoses and/or the number of management options that must be considered

- The amount and/or complexity of medical records, diagnostic tests, or other information that must be obtained, reviewed, and analyzed

- The risk of significant complications, morbidity, or mortality, as well as comorbidities associated with the patient's presenting problem(s), the diagnostic procedure(s), and the possible management options

The number of elements required in each of these areas determines the level of complexity of the medical decision making for a specific encounter (■ FIGURE 28-7).

Contributory Factors. In addition to the key components, E/M services have three contributory factors that are important, but not all are required at every encounter. These are counseling, coordination of care, and the nature of the presenting problem.

Counseling is the time spent with the patient and family discussing management options. Coordination of care is the time spent arranging for referrals to other providers or facilities for tests and treatments. The nature of the presenting problem is the disease, condition, or other reason for the encounter. Every encounter has a presenting problem, but not every encounter requires counseling and coordination of care. All services provided during an encounter must be medically necessary based on the nature of the presenting problem.

Time. Most E/M codes based on the three key components also provide the typical amount of time spent face to face with the patient and/or family for that level of service. Normally, codes are selected based on the levels of the three key components, not the time spent. When the actual time spent exceeds the typical time stated in the E/M code, a higher-level code cannot be selected, with one exception.

When the time spent in counseling and coordination of care exceeds 50% of total face-to-face time spent during the encounter, then time is the controlling factor to qualify for a particular level of E/M service. Then, a higher level of E/M code can be assigned, even if the three key components are not met. The nature of the counseling and coordination of care,

Patient presents to the emergency department with severe abdominal pain in the right lower quadrant. A full workup including a CBC, C-reactive protein, and KUB scan, reveals acute appendicitis with rupture.

Number of possible diagnoses and/or the number of management options: New presenting problem with workup.

Amount and/or complexity of medical records, diagnostic tests, or other information that must be obtained, reviewed and analyzed: Independent visualization of image by physician performing E/M service.

Risk of significant complications, morbidity or mortality: High

Figure 28-7 ■ Example of high complexity of medical decision making.

and the time spent, must be thoroughly documented. The total face-to-face time must also be documented so the coder can determine whether the counseling and coordination of care comprised more than 50% of the total time.

Other Level of Service Criteria

E/M categories that do not use the three key components to establish the level of service define code levels in other ways, such as the amount of time spent by the physician or the patient's age. Coders must read the code descriptions and category special instructions to learn the criteria used to define code levels. Refer to ▪ TABLE 28-6 for a guide in abstracting the level of service.

When time is a criterion for selecting codes, the code descriptions provide the range of time applicable for each code, not an exact length of time. Depending on the code, time ranges can be expressed in minutes, hours, or even days. When a time range is provided, such as 31–60 minutes, no further coding or modifiers are required to define the specific number of minutes.

When age is a criterion for selecting codes, the code descriptions provide an age range applicable for each code, not one code for each age. Age may be expressed in days, months, or years.

Other criteria that are sometimes used for final code selection are the setting, whether the patient is present, the specific services provided, and other details unique to a particular group of codes. Coders must read the code descriptions and identify the differences between similar codes to determine the exact criteria needed.

This provides a general overview of the criteria for E/M coding. Additional details can be found in the E/M section guidelines in the CPT manual and professional reference resources.

Guided Example of Abstracting E/M Services

Refer to the following example throughout this chapter to practice skills for abstracting and assigning E/M codes.

Table 28-6 ▪ KEY CRITERIA FOR ABSTRACTING THE E/M LEVEL OF SERVICE

❑ What are the criteria for determining the level of service: 2/3 key components, 3/3 key components, time, or other (specify)? (*You first must identify the preliminary E/M category to answer this question.*)
- What level of history was taken by the provider?
- What level of examination was performed?
- What was the complexity of medical decision making?
- How much time was spent in counseling and coordination of care?

❑ What is the patient's age?

❑ How much time was spent providing the service?

Source: © PB Resources, Inc. Used with permission.

OFFICE   Gender: F   Age: 32   Status: Established

Chief complaint: Sinus pressure, sore throat, cough

History: Detailed. Extended HPI, extended ROS, pertinent PFSH. Patient was last seen by me 6 months ago for annual preventive exam.

Examination: Expanded problem-focused general multisystem exam

Medical decision making: Moderate complexity. New presenting problem, without workup. Sinus infection. Rx antibiotics.

Follow along as Scott Hood, CPC, abstracts the procedure. Check off each step after you complete it.

▶ Scott reads through the entire record, paying special attention to the chief complaint: Sinus pressure, sore throat, cough.

▶ Scott refers to the Key Criteria for Abstracting the E/M Setting (Category) (Table 28-1).

  ❑ *In what setting was the service provided: office or outpatient, inpatient hospital, or another setting?* Office

  ❑ *What type of service was provided: management of a health problem, preventive care, consultation only, or other?* Health problem: sinus pressure, sore throat, cough

  ❑ *If outpatient, is the patient new or established?* Established

▶ Scott refers to Key Criteria for Abstracting Established Patient Type (Table 28-3) to confirm the patient type.

  ❑ *Has the patient seen the same physician within the past three years?* Yes. Patient was last seen by me 6 months ago for annual preventive exam. The patient is established because she has been seen by the same physician within the past three years.

▶ Scott refers to Key Criteria for Abstracting the Level of Service (Table 28-6) to determine the level of service.

  ❑ *What are the criteria for determining the level of service for code selection: 3 key components, time, or other?* 3 key components

  ❑ *What level of history was taken by the provider?* Detailed

  ❑ *What level of examination was performed?* Expanded problem-focused general multisystem exam

  ❑ *What was the complexity of medical decision making?* Moderate complexity

  ❑ *How much time was spent in counseling and coordination of care?* This information was not documented

  ❑ *What is the patient's age?* 32. Age is not a factor for this type of E/M service.

  ❑ *How much time was spent providing the service?* This information was not documented.

▶ Scott has abstracted the information needed. Next, he needs to assign the E/M code.

CODING PRACTICE

Exercise 28.4 **Abstracting the Level of Service**

Instructions: Read the mini-medical-record of each patient's encounter and answer the abstracting questions. Write the answer on the line provided. Do not assign any codes.

---

1. OFFICE   Gender: F   Age: 48   Status: Established

Chief complaint: Annual preventive care visit

History: Pure hypercholesterolemia

Examination: Comprehensive preventive care exam

Medical decision making: Cholesterol seems to be well controlled. No new problems.

a. In what setting was the service provided: office or outpatient, inpatient hospital, or another setting (specify)? _____

b. What type of service was provided: management of a health problem, preventive care, consultation only, or other? _____

c. Is the patient new or established? _____

d. What code range is applicable for this type of encounter? _____

   What is the title of the subcategory? _____

e. What new problems were identified or managed? _____

f. What criteria are used to determine the level of service? _____

g. What patient information meets these criteria?

---

2. INPATIENT HOSPITAL   Gender: M   Age: 25

Chief complaint: Patient admitted by me for hematuria, severe pain in lower pelvic region

History: Detailed. Extended HPI, extended ROS, pertinent PFSH

Examination: Comprehensive GU exam

Medical decision making: Moderate complexity

a. In what setting was the service provided: office or outpatient, inpatient hospital, or another setting? _____

b. What type of service was provided: management of a health problem, preventive care, consultation only, or other? _____

c. Is the encounter initial or subsequent? _____

d. What code range is applicable for this type of encounter? _____

(continued)

---

2. (continued)

   What is the title of the subcategory? _____

e. What criteria are used to determine the level of service? _____

f. What level of history was taken by the provider? _____

g. What level of examination was performed? _____

h. What was the complexity of medical decision making? _____

i. How much time was spent in counseling and coordination of care? _____

---

3. OFFICE   Gender: M   Age: 48   Status: New

Chief complaint: Patient was referred to me (endocrinologist) by his primary care physician for diabetes management. Refer to dietician.

History: Comprehensive; diabetes is secondary to chronic pancreatitis

Examination: Comprehensive general multisystem examination

Medical decision making: High complexity. Spent 25 minutes of this 60-minute encounter counseling patient on diet management and other lifestyle changes needed to prevent serious diabetic complications.

a. In what setting was the service provided: office or outpatient, inpatient hospital, or another setting? _____

b. What type of service was provided: management of a health problem, preventive care, consultation only, or other? _____

c. Is the patient new or established? _____

d. What code range is applicable for this type of encounter? _____

   What is the title of the subcategory? _____

e. What criteria are used to determine the level of service? _____

f. What level of history was taken by the provider? _____

g. What level of examination was performed? _____

h. What was the complexity of medical decision making? _____

i. How much time was spent in counseling and coordination of care? _____

j. How much face-to-face time was spent with the patient? _____

CODING PRACTICE (continued)

4. OFFICE   Gender: F   Age: 61   Status: Established

Chief complaint: Cough and congestion

History: Expanded problem focused. Brief HPI, extended ROS, pertinent past history.

Examination: Detailed respiratory exam

Medical decision making: Moderate complexity. Chest x-ray negative for pneumonia. Rx antibiotics for acute bronchitis.

a. In what setting was the service provided: office or outpatient, inpatient hospital, or another setting?

_____

b. What type of service was provided: management of a health problem, preventive care, consultation only, or other? _____

c. Is the patient new or established? _____

d. What code range is applicable for this type of encounter? _____

   What is the title of the subcategory? _____

e. What criteria are used to determine the level of service? _____

f. What level of history was taken by the provider?

_____

g. What level of examination was performed? _____

h. What was the complexity of medical decision making?

_____

---

5. NURSING FACILITY   Gender: F   Age: 87

Chief complaint: Status post total left hip replacement

History: Problem-focused history of patient whom I saw last week

Examination: Expanded problem-focused MS exam

Medical decision making: Straightforward. Patient is improving.

a. In what setting was the service provided: office or outpatient, inpatient hospital, or another setting (specify)? _____

b. What type of service was provided: management of a health problem, preventive care, consultation only, or other? _____

c. Is the encounter initial or subsequent? _____

d. What code range is applicable for this type of encounter? _____

   What is the title of the subcategory? _____

e. What criteria are used to determine the level of service? _____

(continued)

---

5. (continued)

f. What level of history was taken by the provider?

_____

g. What level of examination was performed? _____

h. What was the complexity of medical decision making?

_____

---

6. INPATIENT HOSPITAL   Gender: M
Age: 72 (Medicare)

Chief complaint: Presented to ED with complaints of chest pain, SOB

History: Comprehensive. Extended HPI, complete ROS, complete PFSH

Examination: Comprehensive CV exam

Medical decision making: High complexity. Patient experienced a myocardial infarction while being examined and I provided 1 hour, 20 minutes of critical care in addition to the other services provided. Patient was stabilized and subsequently admitted by me.

a. In what setting was the service provided: office or outpatient, inpatient hospital, or another setting (specify)? _____

b. What type of service was provided: management of a health problem, preventive care, consultation only, or other? _____

c. Is the encounter initial or subsequent? _____

d. What code range is applicable for the basic service in type of encounter? _____

   What is the title of the subcategory? _____

e. What criteria are used to determine the basic level of service? _____

f. What level of history was taken by the provider?

_____

g. What level of examination was performed? _____

_____

h. What was the complexity of medical decision making?

_____

i. How much time was spent on additional services beyond the basic evaluation and management?

_____

j. What code range is applicable for the additional service? _____

   What is the title of the subcategory? _____

k. What criteria are used to determine the additional service? _____

ASSIGNING CODES FOR EVALUATION AND MANAGEMENT SERVICES

The majority of work in E/M coding occurs during abstracting because coders must abstract the setting, the patient type, and the level of service provided. After determining these criteria, assigning codes requires only a few decisions. Refer back to Figure 28-3, E/M Flow Chart, which outlines the steps in assigning E/M codes.

1. Identify the general setting in which the service was provided.

2. Identify the type of service within the setting rows.

3. Select the subcategory of service (usually the patient type).

4. Reference the code range provided in the Tabular List.

5. Select the level of service. Identify the criteria used to define the level of service and, when applicable, the number of key components needed.

6. Summarize the levels of the key components, where applicable. Also refer to the Key Components Evaluation Tool for help.

7. Evaluate whether contributory factors and time qualify to override the three key components.

8. Determine whether a modifier is needed.

9. Determine whether special circumstances apply.

During abstracting, you completed the first three steps: identifying the setting, the category or type of service, and the patient type. After selecting these items, refer to the code range listed in column 4 to verify your choices and select the level of service.

After you become familiar with E/M codes, these steps can also be accomplished using the CPT Index. Look for the Main Term **Evaluation and Management**, then select the first-level modifying term for the category of service, such as **Hospital Services** or **Office and Other Outpatient** (■ FIGURE 28-8). Cross-reference the code range listed. When you know the category needed but need to find the code range, use the category name as the Main Term (■ FIGURE 28-9).

Evaluate the Key Components

When you cross-reference the code range in the Tabular List, you need to identify the criteria that differentiate the codes, then select the level of service. For codes that use the three key components—history, examination, and medical decision making—follow these steps.

- Determine the extent of history: problem focused, extended problem focused, detailed, or comprehensive.

- Determine the extent of the examination: problem focused, extended problem focused, detailed, or comprehensive.

- Determine the complexity of medical decision making: straightforward, low complexity, moderate complexity, or high complexity.

- Identify the number of key components that must meet or exceed the levels listed in the code description. Usually, established patient visits must meet or exceed two of the three (2/3) components and new patient encounters must meet or exceed all three (3/3) key components.

- Match the key components to the corresponding code.

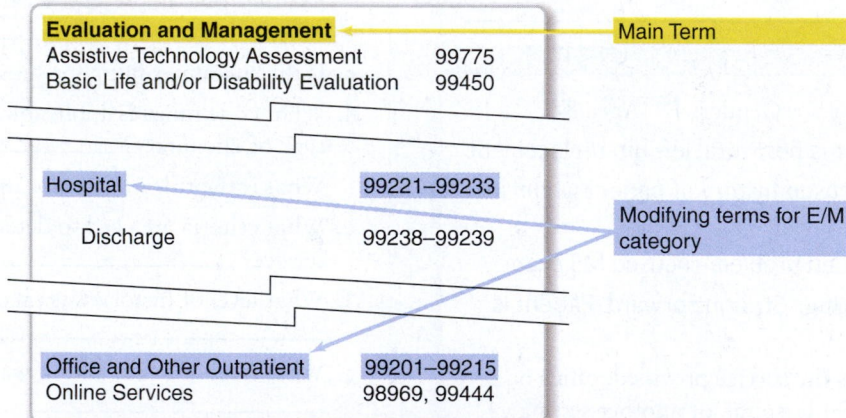

Figure 28-8 ■ CPT Index Main Term for "Evaluation and Management".
Source: © PB Resources, Inc. Used with permission. (CPT codes only © American Medical Association.)

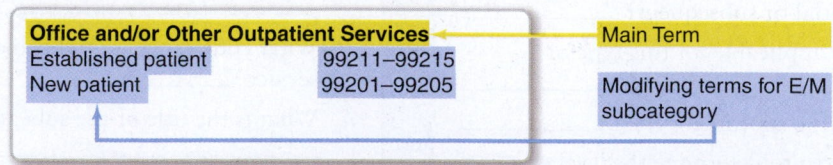

Figure 28-9 ■ CPT Index Main Term for "Office and Other Outpatient Services".
Source: © PB Resources, Inc. Used with permission. (CPT codes only © American Medical Association.)

Many times, the key component levels exactly match the levels described in a particular E/M code. In these cases, code selection is fairly clear. Code selection can be a little more confusing when the key component levels in the medical record do not exactly match those described in the code. When codes require 2/3 components, then one component can be lower than the one listed in the code, but two must meet or exceed the code. When codes require 3/3 components, then all three components must meet or exceed the levels listed in the code description.

- When a key component level in the medical record is *lower* than the one listed in the code, you must use the lower-level code.

- When a key component level in the medical record is *higher* than the one listed in the code, you cannot use the higher code unless the required number of criteria (2/3 or 3/3) match.

The Key Component Tool in ■ FIGURE 28-10 (page 514) helps you match the medical record to the CPT codes for office and inpatient hospital services. Use the tool as follows:

1. In the top left-hand box labeled Patient Summary, circle the level of each criteria in your patient case. Circle OP (outpatient) or IP (inpatient). If outpatient, circle New or Established. If inpatient, circle Initial or Subsequent.

2. Locate the corresponding grids for office services (blue) on the top half of the page or inpatient services (red) on the bottom half of the page.

3. Locate the grid for a new patient/initial service (green) or established patient/subsequent service (purple) in the appropriate quadrant.

4. Compare the boxes circled on the patient summary grid with those on the grid in the appropriate quadrant of the tool. Be mindful of whether you must match 3/3 (new patient) or 2/3 (established patient) components.

5. Select the code and verify it in the Tabular List.

Also evaluate the contributory factors—counseling, coordination of care, and the nature of the presenting problem. For outpatient services, compare the total face-to-face time with the typical time stated in the code description for which you matched the key components. For inpatient services, compare the time spent on the unit or floor with the typical time stated in the code description for which you matched the key components. When the time spent in counseling and coordination of care exceeds 50% of the face-to-face or unit/floor time, you can select the code that matches the amount of face-to-face time spent (■ FIGURE 28-11, page 515).

Determine Whether Modifiers Are Needed

Five modifiers are used on E/M codes to alert payers that an E/M service normally not payable is payable because of unique circumstances. Three of these circumstances relate to surgery. Recall that the global surgical package includes a related E/M service on the day of, or day before, a surgical procedure. It also includes related E/M services during the postoperative period of 10 or 90 days for surgical follow-up. Under normal circumstances, an E/M service reported immediately before a procedure within the postoperative period would be denied by the payer. However, there are circumstances when patients receive E/M services unrelated to the surgical procedure and the physician should be paid. Each of these situations can be explained by using the appropriate modifier.

Modifier -24

The description of modifier **-24** is **Unrelated E/M service by same physician or other qualified health care professional during post-operative period (unrelated to original procedure).** This modifier identifies that an E/M service *unrelated* to a surgical procedure was provided during a postoperative period by the *same provider* who performed the procedure. Add modifier **-24** to the E/M code and be sure to assign a diagnosis code that identifies the reason for the encounter (■ FIGURE 28-12, page 515). When the E/M service is provided by a different physician than the one who performed the surgery, a modifier is not necessary because that physician is not being paid for postoperative care.

> ### CODING CAUTION
>
> E/M modifiers are subject to the concept of the *same provider* that is used to distinguish new and established patients. *Same provider* means the provider who performed the original service, or another physician in the same group practice who has the exact same specialty and subspecialty as the physician who performed the original service. The second provider should use modifiers **-24** and **-25** in the same way as if the patient had seen the original provider.

Modifier -25

The description of modifier **-25** is **Significant, separately identifiable evaluation and management service by the same physician or other qualified health care professional on the same day of the procedure or other service.** A preoperative E/M service is part of the surgical package for all major procedures and most minor procedures. When another E/M service is provided on the same day, by the same physician, for a reason *unrelated to the procedure*, add modifier **-25** to the E/M code. This alerts the payer that the E/M service is not part of the surgical package and should be paid. Also assign a diagnosis code to identify the reason for the E/M service and link it to the E/M code on the 837P electronic claim or CMS-1500 form.

Modifier -57

The description of modifier **-57** is **Decision for surgery.** The E/M encounter in which the decision for surgery is made is payable separate from the surgical package. The global

KEY COMPONENTS TOOL

PATIENT SUMMARY:	OutPt New Estab /		InPt Initial	Subsequent
History	Problem Focused	Expanded Problem Focused	Detailed	Comprehensive
Exam	Problem Focused	Expanded Problem Focused	Detailed	Comprehensive
MDM	Straight forward	Low Complex	Moder. Complex	High Complex

Instructions: 1. Circle the patient type on the Patient Summary (Outpatient-New or Established/Inpatient-Initial or Subsequent)
2. Circle the level of each Key Component on the Pt Summary (**one** item per line).
3. Locate the corresponding Office or Inpatient chart for patient type and levels.
4. Verify that patient levels for Key Components on the Patient Summary meet or exceed those shown in the Office or Inpatient chart for the code selected.

Do NOT code from this tool. Always read CPT® code descriptions and category instructions before selecting final code.

Office or Outpatient (99201–99205)
New patient

99201 — Required Components: 3/3

History	**Problem Focused**	Expanded Problem Focused	Detailed	Comprehensive
Exam	**Problem Focused**	Expanded Problem Focused	Detailed	Comprehensive
MDM	**Straight forward**	Low Complex	Moderate Complex	High Complex

99202 — Required Components: 3/3

History	Problem Focused	**Expanded Problem Focused**	Detailed	Comprehensive
Exam	Problem Focused	**Expanded Problem Focused**	Detailed	Comprehensive
MDM	**Straightforward**	Low Complex	Moderate Complex	High Complex

99203 — Required Components: 3/3

History	Problem Focused	Expanded Problem Focused	**Detailed**	Comprehensive
Exam	Problem Focused	Expanded Problem Focused	**Detailed**	Comprehensive
MDM	Straightforward	**Low Complex**	Moderate Complex	High Complex

99204 — Required Components: 3/3

History	Problem Focused	Expanded Problem Focused	Detailed	**Comprehensive**
Exam	Problem Focused	Expanded Problem Focused	Detailed	**Comprehensive**
MDM	Straightforward	Low Complex	**Moderate Complex**	High Complex

99205 — Required Components: 3/3

History	Problem Focused	Expanded Problem Focused	Detailed	**Comprehensive**
Exam	Problem Focused	Expanded Problem Focused	Detailed	**Comprehensive**
MDM	Straightforward	Low Complex	Moderate Complex	**High Complex**

Office or Outpatient (99211–99215)
Established patient

99211 — Required Components: NA

History	
Exam	Minimal presenting problem may not require the presence of a physician. Typically, 5 minutes are spent performing or supervising these services.
MDM	

99212 — Required Components: 2/3

History	**Problem Focused**	Expanded Problem Focused	Detailed	Comprehensive
Exam	**Problem Focused**	Expanded Problem Focused	Detailed	Comprehensive
MDM	**Straightforward**	Low Complex	Moderate Complex	High Complex

99213 — Required Components: 2/3

History	Problem Focused	**Expanded Problem Focused**	Detailed	Comprehensive
Exam	Problem Focused	**Expanded Problem Focused**	Detailed	Comprehensive
MDM	Straightforward	**Low Complex**	Moderate Complex	High Complex

99214 — Required Components: 2/3

History	Problem Focused	Expanded Problem Focused	**Detailed**	Comprehensive
Exam	Problem Focused	Expanded Problem Focused	**Detailed**	Comprehensive
MDM	Straightforward	Low Complex	**Moderate Complex**	High Complex

99215 — Required Components: 2/3

History	Problem Focused	Expanded Problem Focused	Detailed	**Comprehensive**
Exam	Problem Focused	Expanded Problem Focused	Detailed	**Comprehensive**
MDM	Straightforward	Low Complex	Moderate Complex	**High Complex**

Inpatient Hospital (c–99223)
Initial hospital care

99221 — Required Components: 3/3

History	Problem Focused	Expanded Problem Focused	**Detailed**	Comprehensive
Exam	Problem Focused	Expanded Problem Focused	**Detailed**	Comprehensive
MDM	Straightforward	**Low Complex**	Moderate Complex	High Complex

99222 — Required Components: 3/3

History	Problem Focused	Expanded Problem Focused	Detailed	**Comprehensive**
Exam	Problem Focused	Expanded Problem Focused	Detailed	**Comprehensive**
MDM	Straightforward	Low Complex	**Moderate Complex**	High Complex

99223 — Required Components: 3/3

History	Problem Focused	Expanded Problem Focused	Detailed	**Comprehensive**
Exam	Problem Focused	Expanded Problem Focused	Detailed	**Comprehensive**
MDM	Straightforward	Low Complex	Moderate Complex	**High Complex**

Inpatient Hospital (99231–99233)
Subsequent hospital care

99231 — Required Components: 2/3

History	**Problem Focused**	Expanded Problem Focused	Detailed	Comprehensive
Exam	**Problem Focused**	Expanded Problem Focused	Detailed	Comprehensive
MDM	**Straightforward**	Low Complex	Moderate Complex	High Complex

99232 — Required Components: 2/3

History	Problem Focused	**Expanded Problem Focused**	Detailed	Comprehensive
Exam	Problem Focused	**Expanded Problem Focused**	Detailed	Comprehensive
MDM	Straightforward	**Low Complex**	Moderate Complex	High Complex

99233 — Required Components: 2/3

History	Problem Focused	Expanded Problem Focused	**Detailed**	Comprehensive
Exam	Problem Focused	Expanded Problem Focused	**Detailed**	Comprehensive
MDM	Straightforward	Low Complex	**Moderate Complex**	High Complex

Always read CPT code descriptions and category instructions before selecting final code.

© PB Resources, Inc. CPT©American Medical Assn.

Figure 28-10 ■ Key component tool *Source: © PB Resources, Inc. Used with permission.*

An established patient with type 2 diabetes is referred to an endocrinologist due to poor management of the condition. The endocrinologist performs a comprehensive history, comprehensive examination, and medical decision making of moderate complexity. He spends 45 minutes counseling the patient regarding diet and lifestyle management and reviews the potential risks if the diabetes is not brought under control. Total face to face time is 80 minutes.

99245 Office consultation for a new or established patient (level 5)
... Typically, 80 minutes are spent face-to-face with the patient and/or family.

The three key components qualify for code 99244 (comprehensive history; comprehensive examination; and medical decision making of moderate complexity), which has a typical face to face time of 60 minutes. Because more than half of the visit was spent in counseling and coordination of care, the code can be upgraded to 99245.

Figure 28-11 ■ Example of coding for time as the controlling factor.

Patient sees the general surgeon regarding treatment for chronic bleeding peptic ulcers. 30 days ago the same surgeon performed a laparoscopic cholecystectomy (90 day postoperative period).

K27.4 Chronic or unspecified peptic ulcer, site unspecified, with hemorrhage
99213-24 Office and other outpatient visit, established patient (level 3);
-24 Unrelated E/M service by same physician or other qualified health care professional during post-operative period (unrelated to original procedure)

Figure 28-12 ■ Example of modifier -24.

surgical package includes one preoperative encounter *after the decision for surgery is made* and on the day of or the day before the procedure. When the decision for surgery is made within a day of performing the procedure, add modifier **-57** to the E/M code to inform the payer that the encounter was not a bundled preoperative visit but, rather, the initial decision for surgery. When the decision for surgery is made several days or weeks before the procedure is performed, modifier **-57** is not required. Payers can vary in how they want modifier **-57** to be used, so it is a good idea to check the policies of individual payers.

Modifier -32

The description of modifier **-32** is **Mandated services**. When an E/M service is required by a payer, court, or other third party, use modifier **-32** to alert the payer that it should be paid, when otherwise it might not. An E/M service can be mandated when a second surgical opinion or second medical evaluation is required. You may also need to submit the letter or order form from the mandating party to document who requested the service and the reason.

Modifier -AI

The description of modifier **-AI** is **Principal physician of record**. This is a HCPCS modifier required by Medicare when a physician admits a patient to the hospital. Admitting physicians report a code from **Initial Hospital Services (99221-99223)** for the initial history and physical when they admit a patient (■ FIGURE 28-13). Consulting physicians also use these codes for an initial consultation encounter with a Medicare patient because Medicare does not pay for inpatient consultation codes. Modifier **-AI** identifies the admitting physician and differentiates her or him from a consulting physician, who does not use a modifier.

A Medicare patient was seen in the emergency department for a fractured left hip. The same physician admitted the patient. The combined services in the ED and for the admission involved a comprehensive history, a comprehensive examination, and medical decision making of high complexity.

99223-AI Initial hospital care, per day (level 3);
-AI Principal physician of record.

Figure 28-13 ■ Example of coding a hospital admission.

Determine Whether Special Circumstances Apply

CPT provides codes for special circumstances for use when services are provided at unusual times (**99050-99060**) (■ FIGURE 28-14). Although the codes begin with **99**, they do not appear in the E/M section. They appear in the Medicine section at the end of the CPT Tabular List. These can be used as additional codes with E/M services, as appropriate. Medicare does not pay an additional amount for these codes, but some payers do.

ARRANGING E/M CODES

Typically, an E/M code is listed first on a claim, then codes for other services are sequenced in descending price order. Some payers may request a different sequencing.

When two E/M codes are reported, as may occur during a preventive medicine visit when a problem is identified that requires a separate evaluation, report the preventive medicine code first because it is related to the reason for the encounter.

When an E/M code and a special circumstances code (**99050-99060**) are reported, sequence the E/M code first and the special circumstances code second.

Guided Example of Assigning E/M Codes

To practice skills for assigning codes for E/M services, continue with the example from earlier in the chapter about a patient who was seen for a sinus infection. Follow along in your CPT manual as Scott Hood, CPC, assigns codes. Check off each step after you complete it.

▶ First, Scott reviews the information he abstracted.

❑ An established patient was seen in the office for a sinus infection.

❑ The history was detailed.

❑ The examination was expanded problem focused.

❑ The medical decision making was of moderate complexity.

▶ Scott searches the Index for the Main Term **Evaluation and Management**.

❑ He locates the subterm Office and Other Outpatient.

❑ The code range is **99201-99215**.

▶ Scott turns to the Tabular List to review codes **99201** through **99215**.

❑ He reads the category title **Office or Other Outpatient** Services listed at the top of the page, before code **99201**.

❑ He reads the category special instructions and confirms that he has selected the appropriate category. He reads instructions that cross-reference him to other categories for emergency department, observation care, and inpatient care services. None of these apply because the patient was seen in the office.

❑ He reads the subcategory title **New Patient**, which appears immediately before code **99201**.

❑ He reviews the rest of the category and locates another subcategory, **Established Patient**, which begins with code **99211**. There are no additional subcategories after this one.

❑ He believes this is the correct subcategory because the patient was an outpatient seen for a health problem and is an established patient.

▶ Scott reviews the code requirements for codes in the subcategory **Established Patient 99211-99215**.

❑ Code **99211** is a minimal visit that does not require the presence of a physician.

❑ Codes **99212** through **99215** utilize the three key components: history, examination, and medical decision making.

❑ The code descriptions confirm that the codes describe office and other outpatient visits for evaluation and management of an established patient.

❑ He reads in the code descriptions that to select a code, it must meet two of the three key components at the level stated in the code or higher.

▶ Scott compares the level of each component for the patient with those listed in the coding manual.

❑ The patient's history was detailed, which qualifies for code **99214** or lower.

99050 Services provided in the office at times other than regularly scheduled office hours, or days when the office is normally closed (e.g., holidays, Saturday or Sunday), in addition to basic service

99051 Service(s) provided in the office during regularly scheduled evening, weekend, or holiday office hours, in addition to basic service

99053 Service(s) provided between 10:00 PM and 8:00 AM at 24-hour facility, in addition to basic service

99056 Service(s) typically provided in the office, provided out of the office at request of patient, in addition to basic service

99058 Service(s) provided on an emergency basis in the office, which disrupts other scheduled office services, in addition to basic service

99060 Service(s) provided on an emergency basis, out of the office, which disrupts other scheduled office services, in addition to basic service

Figure 28-14 ■ CPT codes that identify special circumstances.

❏ The patient's examination was expanded problem focused, which qualifies for code **99213** or lower.

❏ The patient's medical decision making was of moderate complexity, which qualifies for code **99214** or lower.

❏ Two of the three key components—history and medical decision making—qualify for the levels stated in code **99214**.

▶ Scott checks for any additional instructional notes under the code and finds none.

▶ Scott reconfirms the levels of the three key components to be certain they match the code, then he finalizes the E/M code.

❏ **99214 Established patient office visit, level 4.**

The full CPT code description is:

(1) **Office or other outpatient visit for the evaluation and management of an established patient, which requires at least 2 of these 3 key components: a detailed history; a detailed examination; medical decision making of low complexity.**

(2) **Counseling and/or coordination of care with other physicians, other qualified health care professionals, or agencies are provided consistent with the nature of the problem(s) and the patient's and/or family's needs. Usually, the presenting problem(s) are of low to moderate severity. Typically, 20 minutes are spent face-to-face with the patient and/or family.**

▶ Scott also assigns an ICD-10-CM diagnosis code that supports the need for the service. The confirmed diagnosis, sinus infection, is documented. He does not assign codes for the presenting symptoms because they are integral to the confirmed diagnosis. The complete coding is:

❏ **J01.90 Acute sinusitis, unspecified**

❏ **99214 Established patient office visit, level 4**

To code this case using the tools provided in this chapter, do the following.

First, refer to Figure 28-3, 'E/M Flow Chart'.

• In column 1, select *Office/Outpatient*.

• In column 2, select *Office/Outpatient (with presenting problem)*.

• In column 3, select *Established patient*.

• In column 4, select *code range 99211-99215*.

• In column 5, select *2 KC: H/E/MDM*.

• In column 6, place a checkmark next to *Detailed* in the History column. Place a checkmark next to *Exp prob focused* in the Exam column. Place a checkmark next to *Mod complexity* in the MDM column.

• In box 7, write NA because no information on time was provided.

• In box 8, draw an X across the box because none of the circumstances stated occurred for this patient.

• In box 9, draw an X across the box because none of the circumstances stated occurred for this patient.

Next, refer to Figure 28-10, Key Component Tool, to select the code.

• In the box at the top left of the page titled Patient Summary, circle *OutPt* and *Estab*.

• In the first row, History, circle *Detailed*.

• In the second row, Exam, circle *Expanded problem focused*.

• In the third row, MDM, circle *Moder. Complex*.

• Locate the section of grids labeled *Office or Outpatient (99211-99215) Established patient*. (Notice that the colors of blue for the title and purple for the subtitle match the colors of your choices on the Patient Summary grid for outpatient [blue] and established [purple].)

• Next, locate the code grid (99214) in which at least two of the highlighted key components are equal to or lower than the components circled in the Patient Summary grid.

• Verify the code in the Tabular List.

These tools provide assistance while learning about E/M coding. As you become more familiar with E/M coding, you may find that you no longer need to use both tools.

CODING PRACTICE

Exercise 28.5 Assigning Codes for Evaluation and Management Services

Instructions: Read the mini-medical-record of each patient's encounter, review the information abstracted in Exercise 28.4, and assign CPT procedure codes using the Index and Tabular List. Write the code(s) on the line provided.

---

1. OFFICE   Gender: F   Age: 48   Status: Established

Chief complaint: Annual preventive care visit

History: Pure hypercholesterolemia

Examination: Comprehensive preventive care exam

Medical decision making: Cholesterol seems to be well controlled. No new problems.

1 CPT Code _____

(continued)

CODING PRACTICE *(continued)*

2. INPATIENT HOSPITAL   Gender: M   Age: 25

Chief complaint: Patient admitted by me for hematuria, severe pain in lower pelvic region

History: Detailed. Extended HPI, extended ROS, pertinent PFSH

Examination: Comprehensive GU exam

Medical decision making: Moderate complexity

Tip: To meet 3/3 key components, all components of the encounter must be at or above the level stated in the code.

1 CPT Code _____

3. OFFICE   Gender: M   Age: 48   Status: New

Chief complaint: Patient was referred to me (endocrinologist) by his primary care physician for diabetes management

History: Comprehensive; diabetes is secondary to chronic pancreatitis

Examination: Comprehensive general multisystem examination

Medical decision making: High complexity. Spent 25 minutes of this 60-minute encounter counseling patient on diet management and other lifestyle changes needed to prevent serious diabetic complications. Refer to dietician.

Tip: When counseling and coordination of care make up more than 50% of the encounter, the level of the code can be upgraded.

1 CPT Code _____

4. OFFICE   Gender: F   Age: 61   Status: Established

Chief complaint: Cough and congestion

History: Expanded problem focused. Brief HPI, extended ROS, pertinent past history.

(continued)

4. *(continued)*

Examination: Detailed respiratory exam

Medical decision making: Moderate complexity. Chest x-ray negative for pneumonia. Rx antibiotics for acute bronchitis.

1 CPT Code _____

5. NURSING FACILITY   Gender: F   Age: 87

Chief complaint: Status post total left hip replacement

History: Problem-focused history of patient whom I saw last week in this facility

Examination: Expanded problem-focused MS exam

Medical decision making: Straightforward. Patient is improving.

1 CPT Code _____

6. INPATIENT HOSPITAL   Gender: M   Age: 72 (Medicare)

Chief complaint: Presented to ED with complaints of chest pain, SOB

History: Comprehensive. Extended HPI, complete ROS, complete PFSH

Examination: Comprehensive CV exam

Medical decision making: High complexity. Patient experienced a myocardial infarction while being examined and I provided 1 hour, 20 minutes of critical care in addition to the other services provided. Patient was stabilized and subsequently admitted by me.

Tip: A modifier is needed.

3 CPT Codes _____

_____

ADVANCED CODING FOR EVALUATION AND MANAGEMENT SERVICES

Although this chapter has covered a great deal of information, you have only scratched the surface of E/M coding. You may be asking questions such as:

• What elements make a history *problem focused* or *expanded problem focused*?

• What elements make an examination *detailed* or *comprehensive*?

• What is the difference between medical decision making of *moderate* and *high* complexity?

All E/M codes that are based on the three key components—history, examination, and medical decision making—require additional abstracting to determine the level of each component.

Physicians must document their findings for the history, examination, and medical decision making in the medical record. They cannot document a general statement such as "I conducted a problem-focused examination" or "The medical decision making was of high complexity." (Such summary information is provided in this chapter to assist in learning.) They must document the exact information for each sign, symptom, body area, organ system, and patient complaint. The coder or medical record auditor can read the documentation and count the exact number of elements recorded for each key component. This provides the basis for determining the levels of the key components.

CMS and the AMA defined specific criteria for each of the three key components in the 1995 DG and 1997 DG. The charts that follow provide an overview of how the key components are determined, but you are not expected to master these details now. You will learn more about this aspect of E/M coding as you progress through your coding studies. For further information, download and study the 1995 DG and 1997 DG.

Determining the Level of History

Analyzing the patient history is a detailed process because the history consists of three elements in addition to the chief complaint—HPI, ROS, and PFSH—and each of these elements consists of several factors. The HPI consists of eight factors, the ROS can consist of up to 14 systems, and the PFSH consists of three major factors, each with multiple components. Thus, determining the level of history requires coders to identify as many as 25 statements in the medical record. History levels and elements are summarized in ■ TABLE 28-7, then the content of each of the three elements are discussed. All information in each component must be relevant to the chief complaint. For example, a physician cannot ask a multitude of questions that are not necessary to understand the patient's chief complaint just to qualify for a higher level of history-taking.

HPI Factors

HPI consists of an interview in which the physician asks the patient questions about eight factors relating to the chief complaint. ■ TABLE 28-8 defines the factors and provides examples of each.

ROS Factors

The ROS continues the physician's interview with the patient. In this phase, the physician asks questions regarding how the chief complaint might impact other body systems. The ROS is not the physical examination. It consists of patients telling the physician what other signs and symptoms they are experiencing (■ TABLE 28-9, page 520). Refer to the 1995 DG and 1997 DG for a list of systems with examples of signs and symptoms that qualify for review.

Table 28-7 ■ **HISTORY LEVELS AND ELEMENTS**

History (3/3 required) (Chief Complaint included)	Problem Focused	Expanded Problem Focused	Detailed	Comprehensive
History of Present Illness (HPI) Location, severity, timing, modifying factors, quality, duration, context, associated signs/symptoms	Brief (1 element)	Brief (2–3 elements)	Extended (4+ elements *or* 3 chronic problems)	Extended (4+ elements *or* 3 chronic problems)
Review of Systems (ROS) Constitutional, allerg/immun, CV, ENT/M, endocrine, eyes, GI, GU, hemic/lymph, MS, neurologic, psychiatric, respiratory, skin/breast	None	Pertinent (1 system)	Extended (2–9 systems)	Complete (10+ systems)
Past, Family, and Social History (PFSH) New pt/initial hosp/consults	Pertinent (1–2 elements)	Pertinent (1–2 elements)	Pertinent (1–2 elements)	Complete (3 elements)
Established pt/subsequent hospital	Pertinent (1 element)	Pertinent (1 element)	Pertinent (1 element)	Complete (2–3 elements)

Source: Adapted with permission from Kate Gabriel-Jones, *Medical Coding Evaluation and Management*, Pearson Education, 2014.

Table 28-8 ■ **HPI FACTORS**

HPI Factors	Physician's Question	Examples
1. Location	Where is the problem/condition located?	Left leg, stomach, elbow, head
2. Quality	Can you describe how the condition feels?	Aching, burning, radiating pain, raw, itching
3. Severity	What is the level of sensation or pain on a scale of 1 to 10, with 1 being the least severe and 10 being the most severe?	10 on a pain scale of 1 to 10
4. Duration	How long have you had the condition; when did it begin?	Started three days ago; condition has lasted two weeks
5. Timing	When does the condition occur?	Constant or comes and goes
6. Context	Does the condition appear when you are engaging in a certain activity or at a certain time of the day?	Pain occurs when lifting large objects at work; pain is worse upon awakening
7. Modifying factors	What factors improve or worsen the condition?	Pain decreases when heat is applied; pain increases when standing up
8. Associated signs and symptoms	Are there any other problems that occur along with the condition?	Numbness in toes also occurs with leg pain

Table 28-9 ■ **ROS FACTORS**

ROS Level	Number of Systems*	Description	Example
Problem-pertinent	1	The physician asks about the system directly related to the problem stated in the HPI.	The patient's CC is an earache. The ROS is positive for left ear pain. The patient denies tinnitus or a feeling of fullness in the ear. In this example, the physician reviews one system, the ear.
Extended	2–9	The physician asks about the system directly related to the problem stated in the HPI and also asks about additional systems.	The patient's CC is a follow-up visit after a cardiac catheterization. The patient states, "I feel great." The patient denies chest pain, syncope, palpitations, and shortness of breath. In this example, the physician reviews two systems, cardiovascular and respiratory.
Complete	10 or more	The physician asks about the system directly related to the problem stated in the HPI and also asks about additional systems.	The patient's CC is having a "fainting spell." The ROS documents related signs and symptoms of 10 body systems.

* ROS systems: constitutional, ENT/M, respiratory, GU, skin/breast, endocrine, allergic/ immunologic, eyes, CV, GI, MS, psychiatric, neurologic, hemic/lymphatic

Table 28-10 ■ **PFSH FACTORS**

PFSH Factor	Description
Past medical history (P)	The patient's past experiences with illnesses, injuries, treatments, surgeries, hospitalizations, current medications, immunizations, and allergies
Family medical history (F)	The health history of family members (parents, siblings, children), such as diseases or conditions they have or had; cause of death of deceased family members; review of hereditary medical conditions that may place the patient at risk
Social history (S)	An age-appropriate review of the patient's past and current activities, such as marital status, employment, occupation, education, sexual history, smoking, drugs, alcohol, and tobacco

PFSH Factors

In the PFSH, the physician asks questions about the patient's past medical history, the family medical history, and the patient's lifestyle or social history, as they pertain to the chief complaint. ■ TABLE 28-10 defines each of these factors.

Determining the Level of Examination

Physicians have three options for evaluating the content of the physical examination: the 1995 DG, the general multisystem examination described in the 1997 DG, and 11 single organ system examinations, also described in the 1997 DG. ■ TABLE 28-11 summarizes the requirements of each type of examination. Refer to the 1997 DG to read the elements required in each single organ system examination for a limited, expanded problem-focused, detailed, or comprehensive examination. You will learn about the single organ system examinations as you study CPT coding for the various medical specialties.

Table 28-11 ■ **EXAMINATION LEVELS IN 1995 AND 1997 DOCUMENTATION GUIDELINES**

Examination	Problem Focused	Expanded Problem Focused	Detailed	Comprehensive
1995 DG physical examination	A limited exam of affected BA or OS (1 BA/OS)	A limited exam of affected BA or OS and other symptomatic or related OS (2–4 BA/OS)	An extended exam of affected BA or OS and other symptomatic or related OS (5–7 BA/OS)	A general multisystem exam or complete exam of a single OS and other symptomatic or related OS (8+ BA *or* OS, but they cannot be mixed)
1997 DG general multisystem examination	1–5 elements identified by a bullet	At least 6 elements identified by a bullet	At least 2 elements identified by a bullet from each of 6 areas/systems or at least 12 elements identified by a bullet in 2 or more areas/systems	Performance of all elements identified by a bullet in at least 9 BA/OS and documentation of at least 2 elements identified by a bullet in each of the examined systems
1997 DG single organ system examination	1–5 elements identified by a bullet	At least 6 elements identified by a bullet	At least 12 elements identified by a bullet Eye and psychiatric: at least 9 elements identified by a bullet	All elements identified by a bullet within each shaded border and at least 1 element identified by a bullet within each unshaded border

BA, body area(s); OS, organ system(s).

Bullet refers to a bulleted list of elements in the charts in the 1997 DG.

Shaded and *unshaded borders* refer to areas in the charts in the 1997 DG.

Source: Adapted with permission from Kate Gabriel-Jones, *Medical Coding Evaluation and Management,* Pearson Education, 2014.

All elements of the history, examination, and medical decision making must be medically necessary based on the chief complaint/presenting problem. For example, a comprehensive examination would not be medically necessary for a chief complaint of contact dermatitis. Although all the elements of a comprehensive examination may have been performed, it would be improper to code and accept payment for it, based on the diagnosis of contact dermatitis.

Determining the Level of Medical Decision Making

Medical decision making consists of three elements, each of which has multiple factors. ■ TABLE 28-12 summarizes the elements and factors required for each of the four levels of medical decision making. Also refer to the 1995 DG and 1997 DG to view the Table of Risk, which specifies additional details.

As you progress through your study of coding, you will learn more about how to read a complete medical record and analyze the elements of history, examination, and medical decision making. The tables here provide you with reference information and help you understand that very specific criteria are used to evaluate the level of service provided.

Hospital Outpatient E/M Coding

The criteria for evaluating the three key components discussed in this chapter apply to individual providers, who bill for professional services. Hospitals also use E/M codes to report emergency department visits and outpatient critical care services. The hospital fee is referred to as the facility fee. Hospitals bill for facility resources, not professional services, so the three key components do not apply. Facility resources include nursing and support staff, supplies, medication administration, social services, and the cost of space.

Hospital emergency departments assign E/M code levels based on the resources used. Types of visits that require fewer resources are assigned to lower-level E/M codes and those using more resources are assigned to higher-level E/M codes. Each facility is directed by CMS to create its own custom crosswalk based on the types of services provided, a process called E/M "leveling." For Medicare patients, the E/M codes, together with other CPT codes, are mapped to an ambulatory payment classification (APC) group based on similar clinical characteristics

and costs. APC is part of Medicare's Outpatient Prospective Payment System (OPPS), under which an all-inclusive, predetermined rate is paid to outpatient hospitals for patients with similar resource consumption. APCs for outpatient services are similar in concept to Medicare Severity Adjusted Diagnosis Related Groups (MS-DRGs) for inpatient services.

The facility service may be mapped to a higher- or lower-level E/M code than the actual professional fee. Medicare does not require or expect a correlation between the professional E/M code and the facility E/M code for the same encounter. For example, one encounter may involve two or three physicians, each of whom bills a professional fee, but the hospital bills only one facility fee. Another example of this difference is a patient who requires limited physician care but extensive facility resources (■ FIGURE 28-15). In other situations, the facility E/M level could be lower than that reported by the physician because limited facility resources are utilized but extensive physician care is required.

A patient presents to the emergency department with vomiting due to excessive alcohol intake. The physician performs a problem focused history, a problem focused exam, and medical decision making of low complexity. The physician orders a lab test to determine the BAC, then allows the patient to sleep for several hours until he is able to be discharged safely. During this time, the nurses continually monitor the condition of the patient and assist the patient to the restroom several times due to vomiting. The patient is discharged 6 hours later.

Physician coding:
99282 Emergency department visit for the evaluation and management of a patient, which requires these 3 key components: an expanded problem focused history; an expanded problem focused examination; and medical decision making of low complexity.

Facility coding:
99283 Emergency department visit for the evaluation and management of a patient (level 3)
APC 0614 Level 3 Type A Emergency Visits

Figure 28-15 ■ Example of professional and facility coding for the same encounter

Table 28-12 ■ MEDICAL DECISION-MAKING LEVELS

Medical Decision Making (2/3 required)	Straightforward	Low Complexity	Moderate Complexity	High Complexity
Number of diagnoses or management options	Established presenting problem, stable or improving	Established presenting problem, worsening	New presenting problem, without workup	New presenting problem, with workup
Amount and/or complexity of data to be reviewed	Ordering or reviewing diagnostic data	Obtaining old records or additional history from someone other than the patient	Discussion of diagnostic results with physician who performed diagnostic testing	Independent visualization of image, tracing, or scan by physician performing the E/M service
Risk of significant complications, morbidity, and/or mortality*	Minimal	Low	Moderate	High

* Refer to the Table of Risk in the 1997 DG for the criteria for minimal, low, moderate, and high risk.
Source: Adapted with permission from Kate Gabriel-Jones, *Medical Coding Evaluation and Management,* Pearson Education, 2014.

CODING PRACTICE

Exercise 28.6 Advanced Coding for Evaluation and Management Services

Instructions: Refer to the tables in this section of the chapter to identify the following information. Write your answer on the line provided.

1. Table 28-7, History Levels and Elements: What is the level of history based on 2–3 elements of HPI, 1 system in the ROS, and 1–2 elements in a new patient PFSH? _____

2. Table 28-8, HPI Factors: Which HPI factor is addressed with a description of pain that started three days ago? _____

3. Table 28-9, ROS Factors: How many systems does an extended ROS include? _____

4. Table 28-10, PFSH Factors: Which PFSH factor includes a review of the patient's tobacco and alcohol use? _____

5. Table 28-11, Examination Levels in 1995 and 1997 Documentation Guidelines: What level of examination is described by 6 bulleted items in the 1997 DG? _____

6. Table 28-11, Examination Levels in 1995 and 1997Documentation Guidelines: How many body areas or organ systems must be addressed for a detailed examination under the 1995 DG? _____

7. Table 28-12, Medical Decision-Making Levels: What type of medical decision is required when the presenting problem is established and stable or improving? _____

8. Table 28-12, Medical Decision-Making Levels: What type of medical decision is required when the treating physician discusses diagnostic results with the physician who performed diagnostic testing? _____

9. What do outpatient hospitals use as the basis for assigning E/M code levels? _____

10. What is the purpose of an APC? _____

CHAPTER SUMMARY

In this chapter you learned that:

- Physicians can provide E/M services in many settings and for a number of different purposes. Each type of encounter has a separate category of codes and a specific set of criteria for selecting the correct code.

- Four sources of guidelines must be considered when determining the level of E/M service provided: E/M Section Guidelines; Category Special Instructions; 1995 Documentation Guidelines for Evaluation and Management Services; and 1997 Documentation Guidelines for Evaluation and Management Services.

- The divisions of the E/M section are called categories and subcategories, rather than subsections and subheadings, as is the case in most other CPT sections. A category, the first level of division in the E/M section, identifies the setting of service.

- The most commonly used E/M categories for office and outpatient settings are Office or Outpatient Services, Preventive Care, Consultations, Emergency Department, and Hospital Observation.

- The most commonly used E/M categories for inpatient services are Hospital Inpatient Services, Hospital Inpatient Consultations, Critical Care Services, and Newborn, Neonatal, and Pediatric Intensive and Critical Care Services.

- An established patient is one who has received professional services from the same physician, or another physician in the group with the same specialty and subspecialty, within the previous three years. All other patients are new patients because each specialty and subspecialty has differing assessments and examinations.

- Eight E/M categories define the level, or complexity, of service provided based on a set of three key components—the history, the examination, and the medical decision making—and each key component can be performed at varying levels of complexity.

- When E/M codes require two of three key components, one component in the medical record can be lower than the one listed in the code, but two must meet or exceed the levels listed in the code description. When codes require all three components, then all three components in the medical record must meet or exceed the levels listed in the code description.

- E/M codes that are based on the three key components require additional abstracting to determine the actual level of each component. This is accomplished by following detailed instructions in the 1995 and 1997 Documentation Guidelines.

CONCEPT QUIZ

Take a moment to look back at services in the Evaluation and Management section. Try to answer the questions from memory first, then refer to the discussion in this chapter if you need a little extra help.

Completion

Instructions: Write the term that completes each statement based on the information you learned in this chapter. Choose from the list below. Some choices may be used more than once and some choices may not be used at all.

case management	observation patient
consultation	outpatient
critical care	preventive care
disability evaluation	prolonged service
emergency department	resuscitation
home services	transfer of care
inpatient	transitional care
intensive care	

1. _____ is an evaluation of a patient requested by another physician to obtain a professional opinion on a specific problem.

2. _____ services include codes for counseling and assessments.

3. _____ services are provided for assisting complex patients in making a transition from an inpatient setting to the patient's community setting.

4. _____ codes are add-on codes and can be used with any E/M code in any setting.

5. A patient treated in the ED and discharged is a(n) _____.

6. A(n) _____ is a patient who has been formally admitted to a hospital spanning at least two midnights.

7. _____ occurs when the consulting physician assumes management of a patient's care for one or more problems or conditions

8. _____ and _____ codes report the time spent providing services.

9. A patient in a partial hospitalization program is considered a(n) _____.

10. _____ codes are reported for services to newborns and children who are not critically ill but require close observation and frequent interventions.

Multiple Choice

Instructions: Circle the letter of the best answer to each question based on the information you learned in this chapter.

1. What criterion is used to divide categories for preventive care and certain services to newborns and children?
   A. Physician specialty
   B. Physician subspecialty
   C. Patient age
   D. Frequency of care

2. How would you code the following scenario? *An established patient with complaints of sinus pressure, sore throat, and cough is seen in the office. The physician performs a detailed history, expanded problem-focused examination, and moderate complexity medical decision making. A sinus infection is diagnosed and antibiotics are prescribed.*
   A. 99202
   B. 99204
   C. 99213
   D. 99214

3. What are the three key components of E/M services?
   A. Chief complaint, history, time
   B. Chief complaint, examination, medical decision making
   C. History, examination, medical decision making
   D. History, examination, time

4. An established patient is defined as one who has received professional services from the physician within how many years?
   A. One
   B. Two
   C. Three
   D. Four

5. Which key component identifies subjective information that the patient provides?
   A. History
   B. Examination
   C. Medical decision making
   D. Counseling

6. What modifier identifies the admitting physician and differentiates him from a consulting physician, who does not use a modifier?
   A. -24
   B. -25
   C. -B1
   D. -AI

7. What key component refers to the complexity of establishing a diagnosis?
   A. Chief complaint
   B. Examination
   C. History of present illness
   D. Medical decision making

(continued from page 523)

8. Which contributory factor includes the time spent arranging for referrals to another provider?
   A. Counseling
   B. Coordination of care
   C. Care management
   D. Online services

9. What step should a coder take before selecting the level of service?
   A. Identify the setting
   B. Evaluate contributory factors
   C. Determine whether time is a factor
   D. Determine whether a modifier is needed

10. How would you code the following scenario? *A patient is admitted to the hospital. The physician performs a comprehensive history, comprehensive examination, and medical decision making of moderate complexity.*
    A. 99220
    B. 99222
    C. 99223
    D. 99233

KEEP ON CODING

Instructions: Read the diagnostic or procedural statement, then use the appropriate Index and Tabular List to assign CPT procedure codes. Write the code(s) on the line provided.

1. Established patient office visit with a comprehensive history, comprehensive examination, and high-complexity medical decision making, resulting in a decision for major surgery the next day. CPT Code(s) _____

2. A 45-year-old male presents to the ER, where an open fracture of the left radius is diagnosed. Patient is admitted and ER physician requests surgery consult. Surgeon performs comprehensive history, comprehensive examination, and medical decision making of high complexity. Surgery is scheduled for the next day. (Code for the surgeon only). CPT Code(s) _____

3. A new patient was seen in the physician's office for abdominal pain. The physician performs a detailed history and comprehensive examination. Medical decision making is of moderate complexity. CPT Code(s) _____

4. A patient with rectal bleeding was seen in the office of a gastroenterologist. The patient's primary care physician requested that the gastroenterologist provide advice about this case. The specialist conducted a comprehensive history and exam, and medical decision making was high. The consultant documented his findings and communicated them via written report to the primary care physician. CPT Code(s) _____

5. An established patient is seen for his monthly B12 injection. The nurse performs the service under the physician's supervision. CPT Code(s) _____

6. A new patient is seen in the physician's office for a cough, sore throat, and fever. The physician performs a problem-focused history and exam, and medical decision making was straightforward. CPT Code(s) _____

7. Set-up and patient education regarding the use of equipment for remote monitoring of blood pressure, pulse oximetry, and respiratory flow rate. CPT Code(s) _____

8. Established patient office visit for evaluation of a hard lump on his shoulder, status post appendectomy 10 days ago. Problem-focused history, problem-focused examination, straightforward medical decision making. CPT Code(s) _____

9. Emergency department visit for a painful sunburn with blister formation on the back. Problem-focused history, problem-focused examination, straightforward medical decision making. CPT Code(s) _____

10. Referred to office by PCP for consult for avascular necrosis of the left humeral head due to trauma. Detailed history, detailed examination, and medical decision making of low complexity. CPT Code(s) _____

11. Office visit for 18-year-old new male patient with cystic acne of the face unresponsive to over-the-counter medications. Expanded problem-focused history, expanded problem-focused examination, straightforward medical decision making. CPT Code(s) _____

12. Initial hospital visit for one-day-old with cyanosis, respiratory distress, and tachypnea. CPT Code(s) _____

13. Established patient admitted for outpatient observation following medication reaction with nausea and vomiting and dizziness. Comprehensive history, comprehensive examination, moderate-complexity medical decision making. CPT Code(s) _____

14. First office visit of 20-year-old female for annual Pap test and discussion of contraception options. CPT Code(s) _____

15. Required new patient office visit for worker's compensation evaluation of acute four-extremity weakness and shortness of breath one week after exposure to toxic chemicals. Comprehensive history, comprehensive examination, medical decision making of high complexity. CPT Code(s) _____

16. Established patient seen at 6:30 P.M. by nurse after regular office hours requesting a return-to-work certificate for resolving contact dermatitis. CPT Code(s) _____

17. Initial care management for psychiatric collaborative care for a patient with bipolar I disorder, requiring a behavioral health assessment, establishment of a care plan, and brief interventions, 100 minutes during the month. CPT Code(s) _____

18. Emergency department visit for a 24-year-old who fell off a trail bike and sustained a head injury with loss of consciousness for approximately 5 minutes. Detailed history, detailed examination, medical decision making of moderate complexity. CPT Code(s) _____

19. First office visit for removal of mole. Patient also asks physician to evaluate ingrown toenail. Expanded problem-focused history, expanded problem-focused examination, straightforward medical decision making. CPT Code(s) _____

20. First hour of critical care for a patient with acute respiratory failure from acute exacerbation of chronic obstructive emphysema. CPT Code(s) _____

21. Subsequent hospital visit for maintenance of analgesia using an IV Dilaudid infusion. Expanded problem-focused history, problem-focused examination, straightforward medical decision making. CPT Code(s) _____

22. Consultation by ophthalmologist requested at a psychiatric residential treatment center for possible purulent bacterial conjunctivitis. Problem-focused history, problem-focused examination, straightforward medical decision making. CPT Code(s) _____

23. Office visit for an established patient with a history of bipolar disorder and migraine headaches complaining of auditory hallucinations. Comprehensive history, comprehensive examination, medical decision making of moderate complexity. CPT Code(s) _____

24. Established patient seen by his personal nephrologist, who was called to the emergency department at midnight because patient presented with new-onset peripheral edema and increased blood pressure three months post kidney transplant. Detailed history, comprehensive examination, medical decision making of high complexity. CPT Code(s) _____

25. Critical care services in the emergency department for a patient in respiratory failure and with congestive heart failure. Ventilator management is initiated. Physician spends 1 hour 50 minutes providing critical care for this patient. CPT Code(s) _____

CODING CHALLENGE

Instructions: Read the mini-medical-record of each patient's encounter, then abstract, assign, and arrange ICD-10-CM diagnosis codes and CPT procedure codes using the appropriate Index and Tabular List. Write the code(s) on the line provided.

1. INPATIENT HOSPITAL Gender: M Age: 67 (Medicare) Status: Initial

Chief complaint: LUQ pain and swelling, increasing over the past 3 days, indigestion. Pt is admitted.

History: Comprehensive. Pain is worse after eating; does not smoke; weekly alcohol consumption at 2–3 cases of beer 10 years.

Examination: A comprehensive GI exam; abdominal tenderness in the LUQ without masses; liver and spleen WNL

Medical decision making: Moderate complexity with stool sample collected; abdominal US; IV fluids with pain control; GI consult ordered

Assessment: Acute pancreatitis, alcohol induced

Tip: Refer to Medicare rules for billing this type of service.

1 ICD-10-CM Code _____

1 CPT Code _____

2. INPATIENT HOSPITAL Gender: F Age: 42 Status: Discharge

Reason for admission: Patient found nonresponsive. Family reports patient being on a fast.

Course of treatment: IV fluids increased to soft diet

(continued)

2. (continued)

Assessment: nondiabetic hypoglycemic coma

Plan: instructed on diet and glucometer; FU in 1 week

Time spent: 10 minutes

1 ICD-10-CM Code _____

1 CPT Code _____

3. OFFICE Gender: F Age: 42 Status: Established

Chief complaint: Blood pressure check

History: Long-time patient with hypertension, which has been difficult to control. Patient is here for her twice weekly BP check.

Examination: Blood pressure check by the nurse. BP reading is 120/72 today.

Tip: Minimal time is spent by the nurse under supervision of the physician for a routine office visit.

1 ICD-10-CM Code _____

1 CPT Code _____

4. OFFICE Gender: M Age: 52 Status: New

Chief complaint: Dizziness upon sudden standing, temporary visual dimming, numbness and tingling in arms and hands

History: History of present illness, ROS, and PFSH reviewed in detail

Examination: Detailed constitutional exam of vital signs and general appearance; detailed CV exam

(continued)

(continued from page 525)

---

4. (continued)

Medical decision making: BP to be checked daily and follow instructions related to lifestyle changes (i.e., improve diet and exercise); low complexity

Assessment: Orthostatic hypotension

Tip: Identify the setting and the type of service.

1 ICD-10-CM Code _____

1 CPT Code _____

---

5. INPATIENT HOSPITAL Gender: F

Age: 71 Status: New

Chief complaint: Patient referred by Dr. Conover for consult on peripheral autonomic neuropathy

History: Comprehensive history. The patient also has type 2 diabetes, which has been well managed with diet and lifestyle.

Examination: Comprehensive examination

Medical decision making: High complexity. Rx and tests. Return in 6 weeks. Report sent to Dr. Conover.

Assessment: Type 2 DM, peripheral neuropathy

Tip: Determine whether the neuropathy is related to the diabetes. Refer to Medicare rules for billing this type of service.

1 ICD-10-CM Code _____

1 CPT Code _____

---

6. OFFICE Gender: F Age: 4 Status: Established

Reason for encounter: Routine exam of a 4-year-old

History: Normal healthy female child; immunizations up to date; detailed history obtained

Examination: Detailed exam; no new findings

Plan: RTO in 1 year, call if any new problems

Tip: Determine the type of service for this visit.

1 ICD-10-CM Code _____

1 CPT Code _____

---

7. EMERGENCY DEPT Gender: M

Age: 24 Status: New

Chief complaint: In pain with swollen wrist, unable to bend

History: Expanded problem focused. Patient slipped walking across an icy driveway and used his right hand to break his fall.

Examination: Expanded problem focused

Medical decision making: Low. X-ray of the right arm reviewed.

(continued)

---

7. (continued)

Assessment: Fracture of the distal right radius

Tip: Injury codes should be followed by external cause codes. Sequence the external cause codes correctly.

3 ICD-10-CM Codes _____

_____

1 CPT Code _____

---

8. NURSING FACILITY Gender: F

Age: 87 Status: Established

Chief complaint: Cellulitis, left leg

History: Problem focused, cellulitis improved on IV antibiotic

Examination: Problem-focused examination limited to left leg, less swelling

Medical decision making: Discontinue IV antibiotic and start oral antibiotic; topical medication; DM and HTN stable

3 ICD-10-CM Codes _____

_____

1 CPT Code _____

---

9. INPATIENT HOSPITAL Gender: M

Age: 77 Status: Established

Chief Complaint: Acute renal failure

Treatment: Reviewed lab results and renal ultrasound; discussed possible dialysis with patient and limitations due to anteroseptal MI last week; nephrologist consulted; central line discontinued

Time spent: Critical care provided from 1700 to 1820

1 ICD-10-CM Code _____

_____

2 CPT Codes _____

---

10. OFFICE Gender: M Age: 59 Status: New

Chief complaint: Patient comes in today for a migraine, which started two days ago with aura

History: Detailed; patient is referred by his PCP for neurological evaluation of pharmacoresistant migraine

Examination: Detailed examination of multiple body areas

Medical decision making: Low complexity; Rx for zolmitriptan and Cafergot

Assessment: Migraine with aura

1 ICD-10-CM Code _____

1 CPT Code _____

Medicine Procedures (90281-99199, 99500-99607)

Learning Objectives

After completing this chapter, you should have the skills to:

29.1 Spell and define the key words, medical terms, and abbreviations related to procedures in the Medicine section. (Remember)

29.2 Summarize the fundamentals of medicine procedures. (Understand)

29.3 Adhere to the CPT coding guidelines for the Medicine section. (Apply)

29.4 Examine and abstract procedural information from the medical record for coding services in the Medicine section. (Analyze)

29.5 Demonstrate how to assign codes for procedures in the Medicine section. (Apply)

29.6 Utilize guidelines for arranging (sequencing) codes for procedures in the Medicine section. (Apply)

29.7 Determine how to code Evaluation and Management services for psychiatry. (Evaluate)

Chapter Outline

- **Medicine Procedure Basics**
- **Coding Guidelines for the Medicine Section**
- **Abstracting Medicine Procedures**
- **Assigning Codes for Medicine Procedures**
- **Arranging Codes for Medicine Procedures**
- **E/M Coding for Medicine**

Key Terms and Abbreviations

allergen immunotherapy	electrocardiogram (ECG or EKG)	interactive complexity	psychiatric diagnostic interview
allergenic extract	electroencephalogram (EEG)	manometry	psychotherapy
allergy testing	electromyogram (EMG)	minimally invasive (procedure)	push technique
antigen	hemodialysis	motility study	revascularization
catheter	immune globulin	noninvasive (procedure)	supervised modality
constant attendance modality	immunization	occlusive disease	toxoid
dialysis	immunodeficiency	otorhinolaryngological	vaccine
echocardiogram (ECC)	infusion technique	peritoneal dialysis	

In addition to the key terms listed here, students should know the terms defined within tables in this chapter.

INTRODUCTION

A department store carries a wide variety of products, such as men's, women's, and children's clothing, tools, household products, kitchen products, and perhaps even furniture. This variety is in contrast to a specialized store that carries closely related products, such as only kitchen products or only children's clothing.

Similarly, the Medicine section of the CPT manual contains codes for services provided by many medical specialties that are not suitable to the Surgery section. Any physician or qualified provider can perform procedures from the Medicine section that are within the provider's scope of practice and training.

MEDICINE PROCEDURE BASICS

Medicine procedures can be diagnostic or therapeutic, each of which can be divided into several broad types of procedures. Diagnostic procedures are performed to help analyze a patient's complaint and determine the cause of signs and symptoms. Diagnostic techniques classified in the Medicine section include an assessment or evaluation, an examination, or the use of equipment or tools to make a recording or measurement or conduct a function study.

- **Assessment/evaluation**—Asking questions to arrive at a conclusion. Examples are a psychiatric diagnostic interview and a discussion of a patient's symptoms.

- **Examination**—Performing a visual and physical inspection, with or without the assistance of instruments, to arrive at a conclusion. Examples are range-of-motion testing and any ophthalmoscopy.

- **Recording**—Creating an image of a structure or process. Examples are electrocardiography and angiography.

- **Measurement**—Using equipment or tools to quantify the body's response, reflex, or perception. Examples are a tonometer that measures intraocular pressure and an audiometer that measures the ear's response to sound.

- **Function study**—Visualizing a physiologic function in real time to observe the processes at work. Examples are a gastric motility (*movement*) study and nerve function studies.

Therapeutic procedures treat a condition to minimize its effects, eliminate it, or cure it. Therapeutic procedures classified in the Medicine section include physical, pharmacologic, immunologic, mechanical, and mental techniques.

- **Corporeal (physical)**—Applying a manual technique to the body. Examples are chiropractic manipulation or use of a hot pack.

- **Pharmacologic**—Altering the body's processes via drugs or biologicals. Examples are intravenous administration of antibiotics or intravenous administration of antineoplastic drugs.

- **Immunologic/vaccine**—Activating the body's defenses through administration of an immune globulin or vaccine. Examples are the hepatitis B immune globulin and the influenza vaccine.

- **Assistive device (mechanical)**—Using an external device to assist or perform the body's normal function. Examples are a pacemaker and a neurostimulator.

- **Psychotherapy (mental)**—Using questions, discussion, and advice to redirect mental and behavioral processes. Examples are individual, group, and family psychotherapy.

Medical Terminology

Medical terms for medical procedures combine roots for various organs or anatomic sites with prefixes and suffixes to create a term that describes a specific service or procedure. Many of the procedures in this section contain a prefix or root that identifies the organ or anatomic site that is the target of the procedure, such as heart (*cardi/o*), eye (*opt/o*), or nerve (*neur/o*). The prefix can describe the method or technique used, such as sound (*echo-*) or within a structure (*intra-*). The suffix describes the purpose of the procedure, such as measuring (*-metry*), recording an image (*-graphy*), or providing treatment (*-therapy*). Refer to ■ TABLE 29-1 for a refresher on how to build medical terms related to Medicine procedures.

Table 29-1 ■ **EXAMPLE OF CONSTRUCTING MEDICAL TERMS FOR MEDICINE PROCEDURES**

Prefix/Combining Form	Suffix	Complete Medical Term
echo- (prefix; *sound*)		**echo + cardio + graphy** (*recording of the heart using sound waves*)
		electro + cardio + graphy (*recording of the heart using electrical waves*)
psych/o (*mind*)	**-graphy** (*recording*)	**psycho + metry** (*measurement/testing of the mind*)
tympan/o (*eardrum*)	**-metry** (*measurement*)	**tympano + metry** (*measurement of the eardrum*)
electr/o (*electrical*)	**-therapy** (*treatment*)	**electro + convulsive + therapy** (*treatment using electricity to create convulsion*)
		psycho + therapy (*treatment of the mind*)

Source: © PB Resources, Inc. Used with permission.

CODING CAUTION

Be alert for medical words that are spelled similarly and have different meanings.

chemotherapy (*treatment using drugs*) and
    photochemotherapy (*treatment using drugs and light*)
plethysmography (*recording of the volume*) and
    polysomnography (*multiple recordings of sleep*)

SUCCESS STEP

You may recognize *gonioscopy* as a medical term because you know the suffix *-scopy* refers to a visual examination, but the root *goni/o* is probably unfamiliar. *Goni/o* means "angle." Gonioscopy is the visual examination of the angle between the cornea and iris (iridocorneal angle) using a specialized tool called a gonioscope.

CODING PRACTICE

Exercise 29.1   Medicine Procedure Basics

Instructions: Use your medical terminology skills and resources to define the following procedures, then identify the applicable code or code range. Follow these steps:

- Use slash marks "/" to break down the underlined term into its root(s) and suffix.
- Define the meaning of the underlined word based on the meaning of each word part.
- Use the entire phrase to identify the code or code range shown in the CPT Index.

Example: <u>audiometry</u>, comprehensive audio/metry   Meaning *measurement of hearing*   CPT Code(s) *0212T, 92557*

1. <u>electrogastrography</u>   Meaning _____   CPT Code(s) _____
2. <u>hemofiltration</u>   Meaning _____   CPT Code(s) _____
3. <u>hydrotherapy</u>, application   Meaning _____   CPT Code(s) _____
4. <u>endomyocardial</u> biopsy   Meaning _____   CPT Code(s) _____
5. allergy tests, <u>intradermal</u>, biologicals   Meaning _____   CPT Code(s) _____
6. <u>angiography</u>, bypass graft   Meaning _____   CPT Code(s) _____
7. <u>anorectal</u> biofeedback   Meaning _____   CPT Code(s) _____
8. <u>otorhinolaryngology</u>, unlisted services and procedures   Meaning _____   CPT Code(s) _____
9. infusion therapy, <u>subcutaneous</u>   Meaning _____   CPT Code(s) _____
10. <u>ophthalmoscopy</u>   Meaning _____   CPT Code(s) _____

CODING GUIDELINES FOR THE MEDICINE SECTION

Coders should understand the organization of this CPT section, section guidelines, and instructional notes in the Tabular List. This information is necessary for accurate coding. The CPT section for Medicine procedures contains 34 subsections that are divided by the type of procedure. Review the subsection and category names and code ranges listed at the beginning of the Medicine section in many CPT manuals to become familiar with the content and organization. In this list, subsections and categories followed by an asterisk (*) contain special instructions that provide guidelines for using codes in that subsection or category.

The Medicine section reports **noninvasive** (*procedures performed without puncturing the skin*) and **minimally invasive** (*procedures performed using only natural body openings, needles, or small incisions*) procedures from a wide variety of medical specialties that are not appropriate for the Surgery section. Among the procedures reported in this section are those for immunology, vaccinations, psychiatry, dialysis, gastroenterology, otorhinolaryngology, cardiovascular, pulmonology, endocrinology, neurology, dermatology, physical medicine and rehabilitation, nutrition, moderate (conscious) sedation, and home health. The Ophthalmology subsection provides evaluation and management codes, in addition to other procedures. Several subsections identify procedures from complementary medicine: acupuncture, biofeedback, osteopathic, and chiropractic. Non-face-to-face services provided by nonphysician providers appear here. Codes for qualifying circumstances for anesthesia also appear here but are discussed in Chapter 31, "Anesthesia Procedures," of this text because they are used with anesthesia codes.

Because the Medicine section lists codes from a wide range of medical specialties, diagnosis codes from nearly any chapter of the ICD-10-CM manual can be used to support these procedures. When tests are performed for diagnostic purposes, the CPT codes for outpatient procedures might require diagnosis code(s) for signs and symptoms if test results are not known and a definitive diagnosis has not yet been established. When test results, and the physician's interpretation of those results, are available when the record is coded, then assign the code for the diagnosis stated by the physician.

The principal diagnosis for inpatient procedures is the one determined, *after study*, to be chiefly responsible for the admission. *Study* includes many of the tests and procedures classified in the Medicine section. When a patient is admitted for testing to determine the cause of signs and symptoms, tests from this section may be performed. Keep in mind that the ordering physician must indicate the significance of the test result in determining the patient's diagnosis. Do not assign a diagnosis based solely on the test result.

CPT Medicine guidelines discuss add-on codes, separate procedures, unlisted services or procedures, special reports, and supplied materials.

Recall that add-on codes must be reported in addition to a primary service. Add-on codes do not require modifier -51 because they are exempt from the multiple procedure concept that reduces payment for additional procedures performed at the same time. The symbol + in front of a code designates it as an add-on code. In addition, the wording of the code description includes phrases such as **each additional** or **List separately in addition to primary procedure**.

Some procedures in this section are commonly performed as an integral part of a more extensive procedure. Codes identified with the note **(separate procedure)**, for example, **92511 Nasopharyngoscopy with endoscope (separate procedure)**, should not be reported in addition to the more extensive service. Use such a code only when it is performed as a distinct, independent procedure, such as one performed during a different patient encounter, on a separate anatomic site, or not as part of another procedure. Apply modifier -59 to alert the payer that you are reporting the code as a separate procedure.

Supplies such as procedure trays, drugs, supplies, and other materials beyond those normally included with the procedure should be reported separately. Use CPT code **99070** or a HCPCS code for the specific supply.

Because of the varied nature of procedures in the Medicine section, many subsections and categories begin with special instructions that provide additional guidelines and instructions for reporting specific procedures. Coders must read this information before assigning codes from these subsections to ensure they are using the codes properly. Frequent instructional notes in the Tabular List identify codes that may and may not be reported together, as well as cross-references to related codes. Specific guidelines and instructional notes are discussed throughout this chapter of the text.

ABSTRACTING MEDICINE PROCEDURES

Because there are so many different types of Medicine procedures, each subsection has its own abstracting rules. Some subsections require multiple sets of abstracting criteria because of

Table 29-2 ■ KEY CRITERIA FOR ABSTRACTING MEDICINE PROCEDURES

❑ What organ system or anatomic site is involved?
❑ Is the procedure diagnostic or therapeutic?
❑ What equipment and techniques are used?
❑ What is the quantity, duration, or frequency?
❑ Is the procedure part of a more extensive procedure?

Source: © PB Resources, Inc. Used with permission.

the wide variety of procedures included. In general, the information shown in ■ TABLE 29-2 provides a good starting point when approaching a case you are unfamiliar with. As you learn more about the specific services provided, refer to the specific abstracting tables in the discussion that follows. Finally, you will work through a detailed example for the Medicine section. Remember that the abstracting questions are a guide and that not every question applies to, or can be answered for, every case. For example, time is not a factor in every procedure.

Abstracting Immune Globulins and Immunizations

Providers of all specialties administer immunizations and immune globulins. Allergists and immunologists offer additional expertise. When the body's immune system fails or reduces in function, **immunodeficiency** results. Immunodeficiency can result from disease, an organ transplant, cancer treatment, or drug side effects. A person with immunodeficiency has a greater risk of becoming ill because his or her immune system cannot adequately produce antibodies to protect the body from diseases. Immunizations and immune globulins, also called *immunoglobulins*, assist the human body in achieving active and passive immunity (■ TABLE 29-3).

An **immunization** provides active immunity and consists of administering a vaccine (virus) or toxoid (bacteria). A **vaccine** contains antigens from a weakened strain of a virus so that the body will produce antibodies to fight it, but the person will not become ill. A **toxoid** contains bacteria that are nontoxic so that the immune system will produce antibodies, but the individual will not become ill. Later, if the person is exposed to the active virus or bacteria, then the immune system will recognize the pathogen and attack it.

Immune globulins provide passive immunity and consist of serum globulins or recombinant immune globulins. Serum globulins are proteins extracted from purified human blood plasma. Recombinant immune globulin products are created in a lab from human or animal proteins. Immune globulin protection wears off in a short period of time, typically a few months, and an individual could contract a specific disease after the effects of the immune globulin have worn off.

Protection against some conditions is available both as an immunization and as an immune globulin. Immunizations are administered as a preventive measure in patients who do not currently have, and have not been recently exposed to, a disease. Immune globulins are used when patients have already been exposed to a disease—called *postexposure prophylaxis*—or if their immune systems are compromised.

Table 29-3 ■ **TYPES OF IMMUNITY**

Type of Immunity	Description	Examples
Active immunity	The body's immune system produces antibodies to fight off a disease.	
Natural active immunity	A person is exposed to a disease pathogen, becomes ill, and then develops immunity toward the disease.	Chickenpox, measles, and mumps
Artificial active immunity	A person is exposed to a disease through an antigen from a vaccine or toxoid (bacteria), and then the immune system produces antibodies that attack the antigen so the person does not become ill.	Vaccines: hepatitis A, influenza virus, measles, and mumps Toxoids: diphtheria and tetanus
Passive immunity	The body's immune system receives antibodies to fight off a disease.	
Natural passive immunity	The fetus receives antibodies from the mother during gestation, which protect the baby for approximately the first six months of life.	Tetanus
Artificial passive immunity	A person receives an immune globulin that contains antibodies, which help to prevent a disease or lessen the effects of a disease to which a person has already been exposed.	Hepatitis B

■ TABLE 29-4 provides abstracting criteria for immunizations and immune globulins. Administering immunizations and immune globulins consists of two parts, both of which are documented in the medical record: (1) the work or service of administering the injection and (2) the actual immune globulin, vaccine, or toxoid product used. The service includes the route of administration and, for immunizations, whether counseling was provided to the family of a child. In addition, identify whether an additional E/M service was provided, such as a preventive care visit or evaluation of a health problem that created the need for the service.

Table 29-4 ■ **KEY CRITERIA FOR ABSTRACTING IMMUNIZATIONS AND IMMUNE GLOBULINS**

Immune Globulins
❑ Is the administration method infusion or injection?
❑ Is the route subcutaneous (SQ), intramuscular (IM), intravenous (IV), or intra-arterial (IA)?
❑ How long does the infusion last?
❑ How many substances or drugs are injected?
❑ What substance(s) or drugs(s) is given?

Immunizations
❑ What is the patient's age?
❑ Is counseling provided to the parents or family members of a child?
❑ How many vaccine components or combinations are administered?
❑ What is the route of administration of each vaccine or component?
❑ Is the vaccination provided in conjunction with a preventive medicine or other service?
❑ Is an immunization given for H1N1 influenza?

Source: © PB Resources, Inc. Used with permission.

Abstracting Psychiatry Services

Psychiatry services include diagnostic services, psychotherapy, and other services provided to an individual, family, or group. Psychiatry services are provided most often by a psychiatrist (MD), psychologist (PsyD), psychiatric mental health nurse practitioner (NP), clinical nurse specialist (CNS), or clinical social worker (CSW). Only psychiatrists and nurse practitioners can prescribe medication.

During a **psychiatric diagnostic interview**, or psychiatric exam, the provider assesses a patient's mental status by reviewing the patient's medical history, asking the patient a series of questions, and communicating with family members and other providers involved in the patient's care to determine the patient's diagnosis. The diagnostic interview is typically the first meeting with a patient to diagnose the patient and establish a plan for further treatment options. The interview may also be interactive, especially when treating children. The provider uses play equipment, such as dolls, to communicate with a patient who cannot or will not communicate verbally.

Psychotherapy involves the provider communicating face-to-face with the patient to determine the cause(s) of a specific condition and develop ways to effectively cope with it. Psychotherapy can be provided at the same time as medication management or medical evaluation and management services. The physician must document the components of an E/M service—history, exam, medical decision making—in addition to documentation of psychotherapy.

Psychotherapy can also be provided for families and in groups:

- **Family psychotherapy**—Family members meet with the clinician to discuss the patient's condition and how to help the patient. The patient may be present.

- **Group psychotherapy**—A group of patients with the same disorder meet with the clinician to share information to help one another change their behaviors. An example is

Table 29-5 ■ **KEY CRITERIA FOR ABSTRACTING PSYCHIATRY SERVICES**

- ❑ What is the duration of psychotherapy services?
- ❑ Are services provided in a group or family setting?
- ❑ Is pharmacologic management provided?
- ❑ Is the service provided for crisis?
- ❑ Is interactive complexity required?
- ❑ Is testing or other services provided?
- ❑ Are separate E/M services provided?

Source: © PB Resources, Inc. Used with permission.

group psychotherapy for patients who suffer from anxiety disorders to help them to learn techniques to deal with their anxiety.

- **Multiple-family group psychotherapy**—A group of families who share the same problems meets to discuss the issues they are having. An example is a group made up of parents with children with behavioral problems. The clinician and families discuss ways to improve the children's behavior and learn effective parenting skills.

Other treatments that can be provided include electroconvulsive therapy (ECT) and hypnotherapy.

Physicians use ECT, also called shock treatment, to treat conditions such as depression when medications and psychotherapy fail. ECT involves placing the patient under anesthesia and attaching electrodes to his or her head. The electrodes deliver shocks to the brain and cause the patient to seize for a short time. ECT remains a controversial method of treating patients, as many clinicians feel that it causes brain damage or does not improve patients' conditions.

Hypnotherapy involves hypnotizing the patient to change specific behaviors, such as to stop smoking, lose weight, or cope with anxiety.

■ TABLE 29-5 provides abstracting criteria for psychiatry services. Psychotherapy services require coders to identify the length of time spent providing the service.

Psychiatry services have a component of interactive complexity when communication is challenging because of the involvement of third parties in addition to the patient, such as a parent, language interpreter, social agency, or law enforcement. Interactive complexity also includes maladaptive communication—high anxiety, repeated questions, disagreement, unhelpful caregiver emotions or behavior, mandated reporting, and use of play equipment or other physical devices to aid in communication.

Psychotherapy for crisis is an urgent assessment for a highly complex or life-threatening problem. Service includes a history of a crisis state, a mental status examination, and a final disposition or outcome. Treatment includes mobilization of resources to stabilize the crisis situation, psychotherapy, and other interventions to minimize the potential for psychological damage.

Abstracting Dialysis and ESRD Procedures

Dialysis is filtering the blood to remove impurities and toxins when the kidneys cannot perform this function. Nephrologists perform E/M and supervisory services related to dialysis.

Hemodialysis and inpatient peritoneal dialysis treatments are provided by registered nurses (RNs) specially trained in dialysis procedures and by dialysis technicians under physician supervision. Each patient's nephrologist provides a prescription for the frequency, duration, and other parameters of dialysis treatments. Physicians monitor and evaluate patients, typically one to four times per month, and adjust the dialysis prescription as needed.

Long-term dialysis, typically administered three times per week for three to four hours at a time, is provided for patients who have end-stage renal disease (ESRD). Patients need long-term dialysis to survive and receive dialysis for the rest of their lives or until they receive a kidney transplant. The only reason for long-term dialysis is ESRD, but ESRD can be caused by numerous conditions, including diabetes, primary or secondary glomerulonephritis, vasculitis, nephritis, hypertension, neoplasms, and various congenital diseases.

Short-term dialysis, typically consisting of a few treatments to several weeks of treatment, is provided for patients with acute renal failure (ARF) or certain other situations, such as a drug overdose, in which a substance needs to be removed from the blood. Patients receive short-term dialysis to recover from an acute condition but do not need it for the rest of their lives.

Both short-term and long-term dialysis patients can receive dialysis in hospitals or outpatient dialysis clinics. When properly trained, patients can administer dialysis at home, usually using peritoneal dialysis, a process in which the peritoneal membrane is used as the filtering agent.

Hemodialysis involves connecting a patient to dialysis equipment through a dialysis access, which consists of one of the following methods:

- Inserting an intravenous (IV) catheter
- Creating an arteriovenous (AV) fistula—Anastomosis of an artery and vein to create a larger access route for blood
- Implanting an AV graft—Anastomosis of an artery and vein with a synthetic tube, called a graft, when an AV fistula does not work

Tubing is connected from the catheter, fistula, or graft to the dialysis machine. The patient's blood is circulated through an extracorporeal (*external to the body*) circuit, passed through a dialyzer fluid to filter toxins from the blood, and returned to the body, a process that takes several hours to complete.

■ TABLE 29-6 provides abstracting criteria for dialysis procedures. Coders must identify the type of service provided, the reason it was provided, the location of service, and the number of face-to-face physician encounters.

Abstracting Gastroenterology Procedures

Gastroenterologists perform gastric function studies to evaluate digestive processes. An esophageal motility study, also called manometry, evaluates muscular activity of the esophagus at rest and during swallowing to diagnose esophageal disorders involving motility or causes of heartburn.

An acid perfusion test, or Bernstein test, evaluates causes of heartburn. Physicians insert a nasogastric (NG) tube through the nose and into the esophagus. They introduce hydrochloric

Table 29-6 ■ KEY CRITERIA FOR ABSTRACTING DIALYSIS PROCEDURES

❑ What is the patient's age?

❑ Where is the service provided?

❑ Are the services ESRD related?

❑ What type of dialysis is provided: hemodialysis, peritoneal dialysis, hemofiltration, or other continuous replacement therapies?

❑ How many days of ESRD inpatient services are provided during the month?

❑ How many ESRD outpatient encounters with the physician occur during the month?

❑ Are ESRD dialysis services provided in the hospital, a clinic, or the home?

❑ Are separate evaluation and management services provided, in addition to dialysis-related evaluation and management?

❑ For inpatient dialysis, how many evaluations are required with the hemodialysis procedure?

Source: © PB Resources, Inc. Used with permission.

Table 29-7 ■ KEY CRITERIA FOR ABSTRACTING GASTROENTEROLOGY PROCEDURES

❑ What site in the gastrointestinal system is involved?

❑ What is the nature of the test?

❑ Is fluoroscopy or endoscopy used?

❑ Which components of the service are provided: professional, technical, or both?

Source: © PB Resources, Inc. Used with permission.

acid then saline solution into the esophagus to determine whether the patient experiences pain. No pain indicates a normal esophagus; pain could indicate acid reflux or another disorder, such as esophagitis.

A breath hydrogen test analyzes the patient's breath to determine normal concentrations of hydrogen and methane, followed by concentrations after introducing another substance, such as fructose (*sugar found in fruit*) or lactose (*sugar found in milk*), to determine whether the patient can adequately absorb the sugars or has an overgrowth of intestinal bacteria.

Electrogastrography uses electrodes to detect electrical activity of the stomach—gastrointestinal contractions—to diagnose stomach disorders.

■ TABLE 29-7 provides abstracting criteria for gastroenterology procedures. These are relatively straightforward to abstract because all that is needed is the nature of the test and the site involved. Identify services that involve fluoroscopy or endoscopy because these services are not coded from the Medicine section.

Abstracting Ophthalmology Services

Ophthalmology includes eye procedures such as exams, tests, and imaging. In addition to evaluation and management of eye conditions, ophthalmologists perform specialized assessments and procedures. An ophthalmologist (MD) is a physician who provides complete eye care, including medical and surgical care, and plastic surgery on the eye. An optometrist (OD) specializes in conducting eye examinations, diagnosing and treating vision disorders such as nearsightedness and farsightedness, and prescribing corrective lenses. A licensed dispensing optician (LDO) helps fit eyeglasses and contact lenses following prescriptions from ophthalmologists and optometrists. Specialized eye services include:

- **Gonioscopy**—Viewing the angle between the iris and cornea with a goniolens or gonioscope, a magnification lens with an attached mirror, to test for glaucoma.

- **Computerized corneal topography**—The clinician measures the shape and variations of the cornea when diseases or trauma cause it to be misshapen.

- **Tonometry**—Measuring intraocular pressure (IOP) in the eye with a tonometer to test for diseases such as glaucoma.

- **Ophthalmoscopy**—Viewing the inside of the eye with an ophthalmoscope, a viewing instrument with a lens and mirror.

- **Contact lens services**—Prescription, modification, and replacement of one or two contact lenses for the cornea or the cornea and sclera (corneoscleral).

- **Spectacle services**—Fitting and repairing various types of eyeglasses, depending on the type of eye disorder that the patient has.

■ TABLE 29-8 provides abstracting criteria for ophthalmology services. Although it is always necessary to abstract a diagnosis that supports the services provided, in ophthalmology, some services are diagnosis-specific, so you need to abstract the diagnosis to determine the correct CPT code. E/M services for ophthalmology appear in the Medicine section, not the Evaluation and Management section. Intermediate ophthalmological services describe evaluation of a new diagnostic or management problem that requires a new treatment program. Comprehensive ophthalmological services describe a general evaluation of the complete visual system with initiation of a new treatment program. Definitions for new and established patients are the same as for other E/M services.

Identify any specialized ophthalmological services provided. Also identify the prescription and fitting of contact lenses and eyeglasses (spectacles).

Table 29-8 ■ KEY CRITERIA FOR ABSTRACTING OPHTHALMOLOGY SERVICES

❑ Is a diagnostic and treatment program initiated? Is the patient new or established? Is the level of service intermediate or comprehensive?

❑ Is contact lens service provided?

❑ Is spectacle service provided?

❑ What ophthalmic condition(s) is treated?

❑ Is ophthalmoscopy performed?

❑ What other type(s) of ophthalmic services is provided?

❑ Is the service bilateral or unilateral?

Source: © PB Resources, Inc. Used with permission.

Abstracting Hearing Services

In addition to physicians, speech-language pathologists and audiologists also provide some **otorhinolaryngological** (*pertaining to the ear, nose, and throat*) services. A speech-language pathologist (SLP), also called a speech therapist, assesses, diagnoses, treats, and helps to prevent disorders related to speech sounds and rhythm; understanding and producing language; cognitive communication; voice pitch and tone; swallowing; and fluency. A doctor of audiology (AuD), or audiologist, diagnoses and treats a patient's hearing and balance problems using advanced technology and procedures.

Speech, language, and swallowing difficulties can result from a variety of causes, including stroke, brain injury or deterioration, developmental delays or disorders, learning disabilities, cerebral palsy, cleft palate, voice pathology, intellectual disabilities, hearing loss, or emotional problems.

Audiologists examine patients of all ages and identify those with symptoms of hearing loss and other auditory issues, difficulties with balance, and related sensory and neural problems. Using audiometers, computers, and other testing devices, audiologists measure the volume at which a person begins to hear sounds, the ability to distinguish among sounds, and the impact of hearing loss on an individual's daily life. They also use computer equipment to evaluate and diagnose balance disorders. Audiologists interpret these results and may coordinate them with medical, educational, and psychological information to make a diagnosis and determine a course of treatment. Audiologists who diagnose and treat balance disorders often work in collaboration with physicians and physical and occupational therapists.

■ TABLE 29-9 provides abstracting criteria for hearing services. Certain diagnostic and treatment procedures are included with evaluation and management services, such as otoscopy, anterior rhinoscopy, tuning fork test, and removal of impacted cerumen. Do not abstract these as separate procedures. Identify only services that are above and beyond an E/M service.

Coders must identify the specific site and function of the ear–nose–throat system that was evaluated or treated. Identifying any tools or equipment used also helps to determine the correct code.

Abstracting Cardiovascular Procedures

Cardiologists perform a variety of cardiovascular procedures to diagnose and treat heart disorders. Some of these procedures can be complex and involved.

Take time to review the anatomy of the heart and great vessels, also called the coronary arteries, because coronary anatomy provides the foundation for assigning the correct

Table 29-9 ■ **KEY CRITERIA FOR ABSTRACTING HEARING SERVICES**

- ❏ Is an evaluation and management (E/M) service provided?
- ❏ Is the service diagnostic or therapeutic?
- ❏ What anatomic site(s) is evaluated or treated?
- ❏ What specific tests are performed?
- ❏ What is the purpose of any evaluation service(s) provided?
- ❏ How much time is spent providing the evaluation?
- ❏ For speech-related services, does the service evaluate speech production and language abilities or does it evaluate the effect of residual hearing abilities on speech formation?
- ❏ What is the purpose of any therapy provided?
- ❏ What devices, tools, or equipment are used?

Source: © PB Resources, Inc. Used with permission.

procedure codes (■ FIGURE 29-1 page 536). Anatomy books may use alternative names and designations of the coronary arteries. In addition, the precise anatomy and branches of the coronary arteries varies from one person to the next. For coding purposes, CPT recognizes five major coronary arteries and up to two branches of each. The coronary arteries are listed below with the *branches* of the coronary arteries shown in italics.

- Artery: Left main (LM)
- Artery: Left anterior descending (LAD)
  - Branches: *Diagonal* (D1, D2)
- Artery: Circumflex (LCX)
  - Branches: *Marginal* (M1, M2) or *obtuse marginal* (OM1, OM2)
- Artery: Ramus intermedius (appears only in 15% of patients; is located between the LAD and LCX)
  - Branches: None
- Artery: Right coronary artery (RCA)
  - Branches: *Posterior descending* (PDA) or *posterior intraventricular* (PIV)
  - Branches: *Posteroloateral* (PLB)

Cardiovascular procedures that appear in the Medicine section are performed to diagnose a variety of cardiac conditions, which may be treated with other Medicine section procedures or may require surgical intervention (■ TABLE 29-10). Separate abstracting criteria are provided for interventional cardiology (■ TABLE 29-11, page 536), evaluation of cardiac devices (■ TABLE 29-12, page 536), electrophysiological studies (■ TABLE 29-13, page 536), and cardiac catheterization (■ TABLE 29-14, page 537).

Table 29-10   ■   **CARDIOVASCULAR PROCEDURES**

Procedure	Purpose	Description
Angiography	Diagnose blockages; visualize vessels to guide catheter placement for diagnostic or therapeutic procedures	• Use of contrast dyes and x-rays to view the inside of vessels • Performed as part of some cardiovascular procedures
Cardiac catheterization	View blood circulation and detect blockages affecting the heart, the coronary arteries, and the aorta	• Threading an IV catheter into the patient's vein (usually the femoral vein) to a site in the heart, aorta, or coronary arteries • A contrast dye is injected through the catheter, giving the physician a picture of the coronary vessel patency • The image is viewed on a monitor
Cardiopulmonary resuscitation (CPR)	Treatment to revive a patient who has stopped breathing	Use of manual chest compressions and artificial respiration
Cardiovascular stress test	Monitor the heart's activity when the patient is exercising; diagnose the causes of symptoms such as chest pain	• Placement of multiple leads on the patient's chest while patient exercises on a treadmill or bicycle • The heart's response to activity is recorded on a graph, similar to EKG tracings • Pharmacologic stress test: When a patient is unable to exercise, medication that mimics the effect of exercise on the heart is administered
Cardioversion	Treatment of arrhythmias, such as atrial fibrillation	• Use of a low electrical current to restore normal heart rhythm • With the patient under moderate sedation, patches are placed both over the heart and to the side of the heart
Echocardiography	View the anatomic structures of the heart	• Use of sound waves to create a moving picture of the heart • A transducer is placed on the external chest wall that sends sound waves through the chest • The picture is more detailed than a plain x-ray image and involves no radiation exposure
Electrocardiogram (ECG or EKG)	Monitor heart rhythm and diagnose abnormal heart rhythm	• Placement of electrode leads on the patient's chest, arms, and legs • Results are transmitted to an EKG machine that produces a graph of the electrical activity of the heart, heart rate, and any abnormal rhythm
Intracardiac electrophysiological studies (EP studies)	Diagnose and treat abnormal heart rhythms	• Any of a variety of invasive and noninvasive studies to assess the electrical activity of the heart • Can involve arrhythmia induction (causing a disturbance in the heart rhythm), mapping (visualizing the electrical activity of the heart), and ablation (selective destruction of heart tissue causing abnormalities) • Uses a combination of fluoroscopy-assisted catheterization, injection of drugs, and monitoring via EKG electrodes and other monitoring devices
Percutaneous coronary intervention (PCI)	Treatment of unstable angina, acute myocardial infarction (MI), and multivessel coronary artery disease (CAD)	• Nonsurgical restoration of circulation to the coronary vessel • The heart is accessed using a guided catheter to perform a therapeutic procedure or combination of procedures • Atherectomy: the surgeon shaves or removes plaque using tiny rotating blades or a laser on the end of a catheter • Balloon angioplasty: the physician inserts a balloon through the catheter and inflates it so that it pushes against the artery wall • Stenting: a small tube is inserted in the vessel to keep the artery open (■ FIGURE 29-2 page 536)

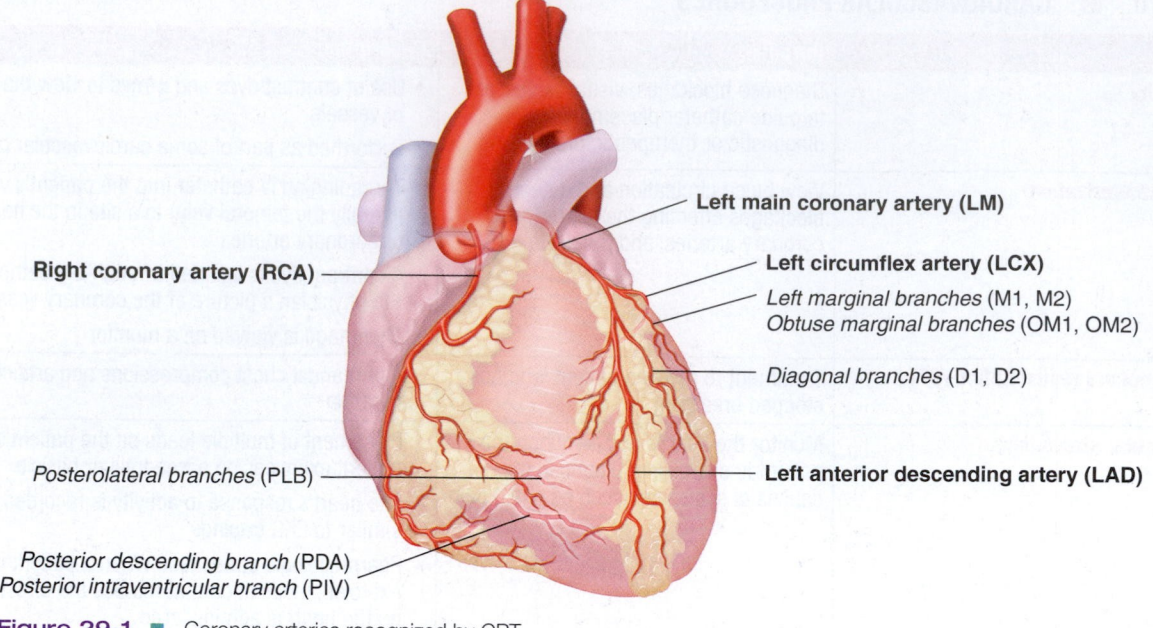

Figure 29-1 ■ Coronary arteries recognized by CPT.

Figure 29-2 ■ Balloon angioplasty procedure: (A) The balloon catheter is threaded into the affected coronary artery. (B) The balloon is positioned across the area of obstruction. (C) The balloon is inflated. (D) The balloon is removed, leaving plaque flattened against the arterial wall. (E) An x-ray angiogram of the balloon catheter. *Source: Du Cane Medical Imaging Ltd/Science Source.*

Table 29-11 ■ KEY CRITERIA FOR ABSTRACTING INTERVENTIONAL CARDIOVASCULAR PROCEDURES

❏ Is the procedure diagnostic or therapeutic (interventional)?
❏ How many and which coronary arteries are treated?
❏ Which branches of each coronary artery are treated?
❏ How many grafted vessels are treated?
❏ Is contrast dye used?
❏ Is a stent or balloon used?
❏ Is intravascular Doppler velocity or coronary flow measured?

Diagnostic Angiography

❏ Is angiography performed at the same time as a coronary interventional procedure?
❏ Has the patient previously had angiography performed?
❏ Has there been a change in the patient's clinical indicators since the previous angiography?

Source: © PB Resources, Inc. Used with permission.

Table 29-12 ■ KEY CRITERIA FOR ABSTRACTING EVALUATION OF CARDIAC DEVICES

❏ What type of device is evaluated?
❏ How many leads does the device have?
❏ What type of evaluation is performed?
❏ Are programming services performed?
❏ Which components of the service are provided: professional, technical, or both?

Source: © PB Resources, Inc. Used with permission.

Table 29-13 ■ KEY CRITERIA FOR ABSTRACTING ELECTROPHYSIOLOGICAL STUDIES

❏ Which site(s) is evaluated?
❏ Is pacing performed?
❏ Is a comprehensive electrophysiologic evaluation performed?
❏ Which specific elements are evaluated?

Source: © PB Resources, Inc. Used with permission.

Table 29-14 ■ KEY CRITERIA FOR ABSTRACTING CARDIAC CATHETERIZATION

- ❏ Is catheterization performed for congenital heart disease?
- ❏ For catheterization procedures, which site(s) is catheterized: right heart, left heart, coronary arteries, bypass grafts?
- ❏ Is contrast dye used?
- ❏ Is catheterization accompanied by any of the following?
  - Transeptal or transapical puncture
  - Pharmacological study
  - Exercise study
  - Injection procedure for selective right-ventricular or left-atrial angiography; supravalvular aortography; pulmonary angiography
- ❏ Which components of the catheterization service are provided: professional, technical, or both?
- ❏ Is another procedure such as revascularization with a stent or balloon performed?

Source: © PB Resources, Inc. Used with permission.

Tables 29-11 through 29-14 provide abstracting criteria for a variety of cardiovascular procedures.

Abstracting Noninvasive Vascular Studies

Noninvasive vascular diagnostic studies include specialized services to study veins and arteries other than the heart and great vessels. Conventional ultrasound bounces sound waves off blood vessels and a computer creates a black-and-white moving image on a screen. Doppler ultrasound uses short bursts of sound to create an image that shows the speed and direction of blood flow. The image can be color-coded to highlight blockages. Duplex scans combine conventional ultrasound with Doppler ultrasound. Duplex scans are useful to diagnose carotid artery occlusive disease, deep vein thrombosis, peripheral artery disease, aortoiliac occlusive disease, varicose veins, and abdominal aneurysms. ■ TABLE 29-15 provides abstracting criteria for noninvasive vascular studies.

Abstracting Allergy Procedures

Allergists and immunologists most commonly perform allergy procedures. An allergy is an abnormal reaction of the human immune system. It wrongly identifies certain allergens as harmful foreign bodies and produces antibodies against them. When these antibodies are produced in excess, they release histamine and other chemicals in the body, which in turn results

Table 29-15 ■ KEY CRITERIA FOR ABSTRACTING NONINVASIVE VASCULAR STUDIES

- ❏ What body region is evaluated?
- ❏ Does the study involve arteries, veins, or both?
- ❏ What technique(s) or equipment is used?
- ❏ Is the study limited or complete?
- ❏ Is the study unilateral or bilateral?

Source: © PB Resources, Inc. Used with permission.

Table 29-16 ■ KEY CRITERIA FOR ABSTRACTING ALLERGY PROCEDURES

Allergy Testing

- ❏ What method(s) of testing is used: percutaneous, intracutaneous, or inhalation?
- ❏ What type(s) of test is performed: allergenic extracts, venoms, biologicals, or food?
- ❏ How many tests of each type were performed?

Immunotherapy

- ❏ Is the service injection only, provision of antigen and injection, or provision of antigen only?

Source: © PB Resources, Inc. Used with permission.

in an allergic reaction. Allergy testing is a skin or inhalation test to expose a patient to an allergen to determine whether it causes an allergic response. Allergen immunotherapy exposes a patient to allergenic extracts or insect venoms to decrease his or her sensitivity to the allergen, a process called *desensitization*.

■ TABLE 29-16 provides abstracting criteria for allergy procedures. When immunotherapy is performed, you must identify whether the medical office or the patient provided the allergen extract.

Abstracting Neurology Procedures

Neurologists specialize in conditions that affect the nervous system. They provide a wide range of tests to diagnose and treat neurological conditions.

Sleep testing is performed while the patient sleeps to assess various body functions to diagnose sleep disorders such as sleep apnea, insomnia, narcolepsy, and somnambulism. Tests include polysomnography, which includes multiple measurements of functions and activities of the heart, muscles, brain, and eyes during sleep.

Several types of tests evaluate the function and responsiveness of nerves and muscles, including evoked potentials and reflex tests, needle electromyography (EMG), nerve conduction studies, range-of-motion studies, and other tests.

Electroencephalography (EEG) records the electrical activity of the brain and produces a graphical report. A routine EEG usually requires 20–40 minutes but can be conducted for longer amounts of time. Specialized EEG monitoring can last for several days. EEG is used to diagnose seizures, epilepsy, sleep disorders, coma, encephalopathies, and brain death.

Intraoperative neurophysiology monitoring (IONM), also called surgical neurophysiology, is used during procedures that pose a risk to the nervous system. A variety of neurological modalities, such as EEG, EMG, and evoked potentials, detect changes in nerve, spinal cord, and brain activity. This provides to the surgeon real-time information that helps avoid or minimize complications such as paralysis, hearing loss, or stroke.

Central nervous system assessments evaluate the cognitive (*intellectual*) function of the central nervous system. Several types of written tests and standardized functional assessments are used, depending on the specific type of information desired, such as reasoning ability, speech, visual response, and

Table 29-17 ■ KEY CRITERIA FOR ABSTRACTING NEUROLOGY PROCEDURES

- ❏ What site(s) is treated?
- ❏ What testing method(s) is used?
- ❏ How many studies or tests are performed?
- ❏ How long does a recording last, if performed?
- ❏ Are all services—recording, interpretation, and report—provided?

Sleep Studies

- ❏ How old is the patient?
- ❏ What parameters are measured?
- ❏ Is the testing attended, unattended, or remote?
- ❏ Which components of the service are provided: professional, technical, or both?

Source: © PB Resources, Inc. Used with permission.

so on. The tests produce quantitative data that is compiled and interpreted in a report written by a physician.

■ TABLE 29-17 provides abstracting criteria for neurology procedures.

CODING CAUTION

Be attentive to acronyms that are similar but identify different tests:

ECG/EKG—electrocardiogram—a recording of the electrical activity of the heart

ECC—echocardiogram—image of the heart made using sound waves

EEG—electroencephalogram—a recording of the electrical activity of the brain

EMG—electromyogram—a recording of the electrical activity of a muscle

---

Abstracting Infusion and Injection Procedures

Patients may need certain medications delivered under direct physician supervision, by infusion or injection, because of the nature of their condition, the type of drug needed, or other special considerations. In general, these methods deliver the medication more quickly than oral administration. The route of administration can be subcutaneous (SQ), intravenous (IV), intramuscular (IM), or intra-arterial (IA) (■ FIGURE 29-3).

Injections and infusions can be administered directly into the site or through an access port. Ports are used to avoid repeatedly penetrating the vein with a needle. An access port is a small medical appliance implanted under the skin, with a **catheter** (*small tube*) that connects to the vein. Intravenous and intra-arterial administration of drugs can be accomplished through the **infusion technique** (*a slow, steady rate of release of medication over a long period of time*) or the **push technique** (*a one-time, rapid injection of medication into the bloodstream*). When infusion is performed, a bag or bottle of solution containing the medication is hung on a stand and is connected to the site with tubing. The push technique is also called a bolus.

Physician services involve approval of the treatment plan and direct supervision of staff administering the procedure, usually an RN. Infusion services include the use of local anesthesia, starting the IV, accessing the indwelling catheter or port, flushing, and standard tubing, syringes, and supplies. A single drug or multiple drugs can be administered. Multiple drugs can be administered concurrently (*at the same time*) or sequentially (*one after the other*). The purpose of infusion can be any of the following:

- **Hydration**—Replenishing fluid lost through dehydration, such as vomiting, diarrhea, and alcohol-related illnesses
- **Therapy**—Treatment of an illness or condition, such as antibiotic administration for a serious infection
- **Prophylaxis**—Preventive purposes, such as an antibiotic before surgery
- **Diagnosis**—Diagnostic purposes, such as to measure the uptake or absorption of a substance
- **Chemotherapy**—Antineoplastic drugs, highly complex drugs, or biologic agents for treatment of cancer or other conditions, such as cyclophosphamide for autoimmune conditions. In addition to the customary subcutaneous, intramuscular, and intravenous routes, chemotherapy can be administered via additional routes, including intra-arterial, intralesional, intrathecal, subarachnoid, and into the pleural or peritoneal cavities.

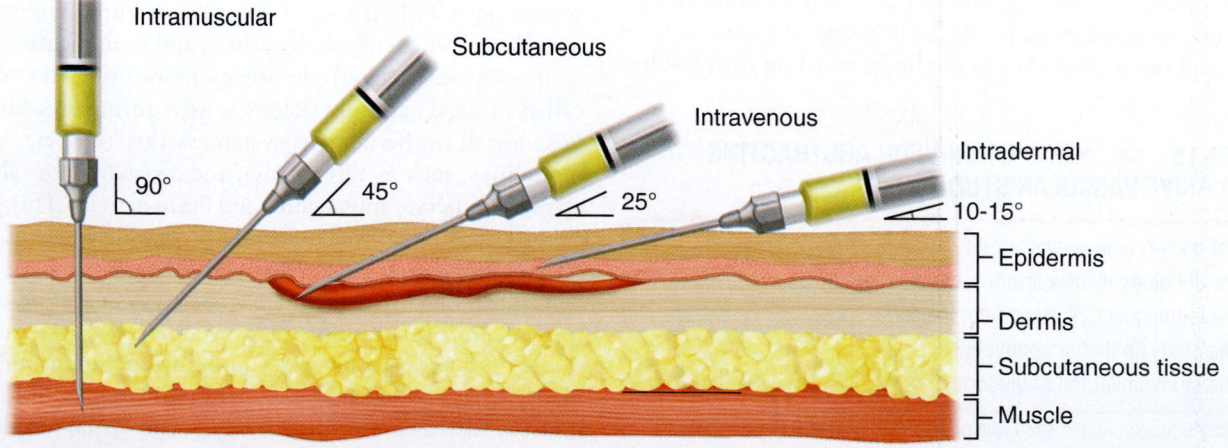

Figure 29-3 ■ Routes of injection administration.

Table 29-18 ■ KEY CRITERIA FOR ABSTRACTING INFUSION AND INJECTION PROCEDURES

- ❑ What is the purpose of the infusion?
- ❑ What is the route of administration?
- ❑ What administration technique is used?
- ❑ How long does the administration last?

Source: © PB Resources, Inc. Used with permission.

■ TABLE 29-18 provides abstracting criteria for infusion and injection procedures.

Abstracting Physical Medicine, Osteopathic, and Chiropractic

Physical medicine and rehabilitation includes physical therapy (PT), occupational therapy (OT), and athletic training and involves evaluations, exercises, tests, and wound care management, including debridement. Services are provided for patients with any number of disorders, including physical and neurological conditions. Therapists may treat patients after a stroke or motor vehicle accident to help them to regain their physical and mental strength and abilities.

An osteopathic physician (DO), or osteopath, manually performs osteopathic manipulative treatment (OMT), which involves moving joints and muscles through various methods, such as applying pressure. This treatment can help to alleviate disorders such as migraine headaches and carpal tunnel syndrome.

A doctor of chiropractic (DC), or chiropractor, is a healthcare professional who focuses on improving patients' conditions by manipulating body areas, typically the spine, to improve the structure and function of specific sites. Chiropractors manually massage, adjust, and manipulate the spinal column to treat conditions such as low-back pain. They cannot prescribe medications in most states.

■ TABLE 29-19 provides abstracting criteria for physical medicine procedures.

CODING CAUTION

A doctor of osteopathy is a DO. A doctor of optometry is an OD. An ophthalmologist is an MD.

Table 29-19 ■ KEY CRITERIA FOR ABSTRACTING PHYSICAL MEDICINE PROCEDURES

- ❑ What site(s) is treated?
- ❑ What type of evaluation or assessment is performed (if any)?
- ❑ What modality is used?
- ❑ Is the service supervised or constant attendance?
- ❑ What is the duration of treatment for each modality?
- ❑ How many spinal or body regions were treated by a chiropractor or osteopath?

Source: © PB Resources, Inc. Used with permission.

Guided Example of Abstracting Medicine Services

Refer to the following example throughout this chapter to practice skills for abstracting, assigning, and arranging Medicine codes. Cardiovascular therapy is used as an example because it is among the more challenging services to code. Coding services in each subsection of Medicine vary based on the specific type of procedure.

OUTPATIENT HOSPITAL   Gender: M   Age: 62

Preprocedure diagnosis: ASHD with angina

Procedure: Catheterization for coronary angiography and stenting. Moderate sedation was administered. Catheterization was performed with access through the right femoral artery. Dye was injected to visualize the coronary arteries, noting significant plaque in the RCA. We proceeded to open the vessel with a stent. (Professional component provided.)

Postprocedure diagnosis: 75% blockage of RCA due to lipid-rich plaque

---

Follow along as fictitious coder Ladonna Shuck, CPC, abstracts the procedure. Check off each step after you complete it.

▶ Ladonna reads through the entire record, paying special attention to the reason for the encounter and the final assessment. She refers to the Key Criteria for Abstracting Cardiac Catheterization (Table 29-14).

- ❑ She notes the preprocedure diagnosis of ASHD and the postprocedure diagnosis of 75% blockage of RCA.

- ❑ *For catheterization procedures, which site(s) is catheterized?* Coronary arteries

- ❑ *Is catheterization accompanied with any of the following?*
  - ▪ *Transeptal or transapical puncture.* No
  - ▪ *Pharmacological study.* No
  - ▪ *Exercise study.* No
  - ▪ *Injection procedure for selective right-ventricular or left-atrial angiography; supravalvular aortography; pulmonary angiography.* No

- ❑ *Is the professional component, technical component, or both components of catheterization provided?* Professional component only.

- ❑ *Is another procedure such as revascularization with a stent or balloon performed?* Yes, in the RCA

▶ At this time, Ladonna does not know which services may need to be coded, nor how many codes she will end up with. She will learn about this when she moves on to assigning codes.

CODING PRACTICE

Exercise 29.2 Abstracting for Medicine Procedures

Instructions: Read the mini-medical-record of each patient's encounter and answer the abstracting questions. Write the answer on the line provided. Do not assign any codes.

1. OFFICE   Gender: F   Age: 67

Reason for encounter: Referred by PCP due to extreme depression since death of husband 6 months ago

Procedure: Psychiatric diagnostic examination that included a history and review of diagnostic and laboratory studies

Assessment: Depressive state with tremors

a. What is the duration of psychotherapy services?

_____

b. Are services provided in a group or family setting?

_____

c. Is pharmacologic management provided?

_____

d. Is the service provided for crisis? _____

e. Is testing or other services provided?

_____

f. Are separate E/M services provided?

_____

2. INPATIENT HOSPITAL   Gender: F   Age: 31

Preprocedure diagnosis: Acute renal failure

Procedure: Hemodialysis with two evaluations due to hypotensive episode after onset of treatment

a. What is the patient's age? _____

b. Where is the service provided? _____

c. Are the services ESRD related? _____

d. What type of dialysis is provided: hemodialysis, peritoneal dialysis, hemofiltration, or other continuous replacement therapies? _____

e. Are separate evaluation and management services provided, in addition to dialysis-related evaluation and management? _____

f. For inpatient dialysis, how many evaluations are required with the hemodialysis procedure?

_____

3. HOSPITAL SLEEP LAB   Gender: F   Age: 31

Reason for encounter: "I feel tired all the time"

Assessment: Insomnia   *(continued)*

3. (continued)

Procedure: Sleep study, attended by technologist, simultaneous recording of ventilation, respiratory effort, heart rate, and oxygen saturation

Plan: Severe obstructive sleep apnea based on interpretation of sleep study. Refer to pulmonologist for further treatment

a. How old is the patient? _____

b. What parameters are measured? _____

c. Is the testing attended, unattended, or remote?

_____

4. OFFICE   Gender: F   Age: 8

Reason for encounter: Annual preventive care checkup for established patient

Procedure: Comprehensive periodic preventive medicine examination. Updated immunizations: IM injection TdaP (diphtheria, tetanus toxoid, acellular pertussis); oral poliovirus.

Plan: Counseled mother regarding potential side effects and signs to be observant for. Call office with any concerns.

a. What is the patient's age? _____

b. How many vaccine components or combinations are administered? _____

c. What is the route of administration of each vaccine or component? _____

d. Is the vaccination provided in conjunction with a preventive medicine or other service?

_____

e. Is an immunization given for H1N1 influenza?

_____

5. OFFICE (Physical therapy)   Gender: M   Age: 42

Reason for encounter: Referred by PCP for therapy for low-back strain while playing golf

Procedure: Initial physical therapy evaluation; 15 minutes of manual electrical stimulation; 15 minutes of therapeutic exercises to increase ROM and flexibility; 15 minutes of alternating hot and cold packs

Plan: Return 3x week for 2 weeks, per physician's order

a. What site(s) is treated? _____

b. What type of evaluation or assessment is performed (if any)? _____

c. What modality is used? _____

                                        (continued)

CODING PRACTICE (continued)

5. (continued)

d. Is the service supervised or constant attendance?
_____

e. What is the duration of treatment for each modality?
_____

---

6. INPATIENT HOSPITAL   Gender: M   Age: 72

Reason for admission: STEMI of LAD with thrombus

Procedure: Percutaneous transluminal revascularization during acute myocardial infarction using angiography. Stent and thrombectomy for acute total occlusion of LAD. Both diagonals show evidence

(continued)

---

6. (continued)

of chronic subtotal occlusion. Balloon angioplasty on D1 and D2 due to chronic subtotal occlusion.

a. Is the procedure diagnostic or therapeutic (interventional)? _____

b. How many and which coronary arteries are treated?
_____

c. Which branches of each coronary artery are treated?
_____

d. Is contrast dye used? _____

e. Is a stent or balloon used? _____

f. What is the extent of the occlusion in each site?
_____

ASSIGNING CODES FOR MEDICINE PROCEDURES

Because the Medicine section contains a wide range of services, coders must be certain to thoroughly read the guidelines, special instructions, and instructional notes that appear throughout the section. Follow along in your CPT manual and locate the codes and guidelines as they are discussed.

Immune Globulins and Immunizations (90281-90399, 90460-90749)

To assign CPT codes for immune globulins and immunizations, assign a code for the administration and an additional code(s) for the product(s) administered. The steps for assigning codes are discussed separately for immune globulins and immunizations. Diagnoses that support the administration of immune globulins and immunizations are often disorders from ICD-10-CM Chapter 1, "Certain Infectious and Parasitic Diseases (A00-B99);" Chapter 18, "Symptoms, Signs, Abnormal Clinical and Laboratory Findings (R00-R99);" Chapter 21, "Factors Influencing Health Status and Contact with Health Services (Z00-Z99);" or the body system chapter of the affected system.

Immune Globulins

The following information outlines the steps required to assign codes for immunization administration and the product administered.

Immune Globulin Administration. Immune globulin administration identifies the method and route of administration. Assign an administration code for each substance administered, as follows:

1. Search the Index for the Main Term **Immune Globulin Administration**.

2. Select the first-level modifying term **Intravenous Infusion** or **Injection** to identify the method. Identify the code(s) or code range.

3. In the Tabular List, review the codes to select the appropriate description of route and time or quantity.

In the Tabular List, infusion codes are subdivided by route (IV or SQ) and time. The parent codes for intravenous (**96365**) and subcutaneous (**96369**) identify the first hour of infusion. Add-on codes identify each additional hour and additional substances. Additional substances can be administered either sequentially or concurrently.

Injection codes are subdivided by route: subcutaneous or intramuscular (**96372**), intra-arterial (**96373**), and intravenous push (**96374**). Report additional injections using the same route (SQ/IM, IA) with an additional unit or quantity of the code. Add-on codes report additional IV push injections, divided by whether a new substance (**96375**) or the same substance (**96376**) is injected. Assign a separate administration code for each substance or dug administered.

Codes for administration contain a parenthetical instructional note that states (**specify substance or drug**). This note reminds coders to assign an additional code to identify the product.

SUCCESS STEP

To assign diagnosis codes for patients who receive immune globulins, determine the reason why the patient needs the immune globulin. If it is for an immunodeficiency disorder, assign a code for the type of immunodeficiency disorder the patient has. If it is because the patient was exposed to a disease but has no symptoms, search the ICD-10-CM Index for the Main Term **Exposure (to)**.

Immune Globulin Product. The immune globulin product identifies the substance administered. Assign a code for each immune globulin product, as follows:

1. Search the Index for the Main Term **Immune Globulins**.

2. Select the first-level modifying term to identify the type of substance.

Patient with primary immunodeficiency (PID) is seen at home by a home health nurse. Nurse administers human immune globulin using IV infusion, which requires 3 hours.

D84.9 Immunodeficiency, unspecified
96365 Intravenous infusion, for therapy, prophylaxis, or diagnosis (specify substance or drug); initial, up to 1 hour
96366 x 2 Intravenous infusion, for therapy, prophylaxis, or diagnosis (specify substance or drug); each additional hour
90283 Immune globulin (IgIV), human, for intravenous use

Figure 29-4 ■ Example of immune globulin coding.

3. Identify the code(s) or code range.

4. Review the code(s) in the Tabular List and select the code that identifies the proper product.

Read the product descriptions carefully because some names look similar. Some products are divided based on the intended route of administration. Products intended for intravenous administration may contain IV in the product name:

> **90281 Immune globulin (Ig), human, for intramuscular use**

> **90283 Immune globulin (IgIV), human, for intravenous use**

Refer to ■ FIGURE 29-4 to learn more about assigning codes for immune globulin administration.

CODING CAUTION

Verify that the route of administration in the administration code (SQ, IV) matches the route of administration in the immune globulin product.

Immunizations

The following information outlines the steps required to assign codes for immunization administration and the product administered. Assigning codes for immunizations for Medicare patients is also discussed.

Immunization Administration. Immunization administration identifies the method and route of administration. Assign an administration code for each substance administered, as follows:

1. Search the Index for the Main Term **Administration** or **Immunization Administration**.

2. Select the first-level modifying term **Immunization** and the second-level modifying term **One Vaccine/Toxoid**. When counseling is provided to the parents or guardians of children through age 18, select the third-level modifying term **with Counseling**. Identify the codes or code range.

3. In the Tabular List, review the codes to select the appropriate description of route and provision of counseling.

4. When more than one vaccine is provided, repeat the process, but select the second-level modifying term **Each Additional Vaccine/Toxoid**.

In the Tabular List, vaccine codes are divided by route and the provision of counseling. Assign the appropriate add-on code when more than one vaccine is administered during the encounter. Assign a separate administration code for each substance or dug administered.

- **90460** and **90461** identify the first and additional vaccinations, respectively, for patients through 18 years of age, with counseling, via any route

- **90471** and **90472** identify the first and additional vaccinations, respectively, via percutaneous, intradermal, subcutaneous, or intramuscular routes

- **90493** and **90474** identify the first and additional vaccinations, respectively, via intranasal or oral routes

A combination vaccine or toxoid contains multiple vaccine components in one injection or one intranasal or oral administration, such as diphtheria, tetanus, and pertussis. Assign one administration code and one product code for the combination.

Do not assign a code for an E/M service when a patient receives a vaccine/toxoid unless the physician performs separate E/M services, such as a comprehensive preventive care examination or evaluation and management of a health problem. If there is an E/M service along with the vaccine, then apply modifier **-25 Significant, separately identifiable E/M** to the E/M code.

Immunizations Vaccine/Toxoid Product. In addition to reporting the vaccine administration, also report the product.

1. Search the Index for the Main Term **Vaccines** for both vaccine and toxoid products.

2. Select the first-level modifying term to identify the type of substance.

3. Identify the code(s) or code range.

4. Review the code(s) in the Tabular List and select the code that identifies the proper product.

5. Do not assign modifier **-51 Multiple procedures** when assigning codes for the vaccines/toxoids in addition to the route(s) of administration.

Refer to ■ FIGURE 29-5 to learn more about assigning codes for vaccinations.

Immunizations for Medicare Patients. Medicare requires that providers report HCPCS **G** codes instead of CPT codes for administration of the following immunizations:

- **G0008 Administration of influenza virus vaccine**

- **G0009 Administration of pneumococcal vaccine**

- **G0010 Administration of hepatitis B vaccine**

> A 12 year old boy who is a new patient is seen for a preventive medicine examination. He also receives vaccinations for Tdap (intramuscular) and Meningococcal polysaccharide vaccine (subcutaneous), with counseling of side effects provided to his mother.
>
> **Z00.129 Encounter for routine child health examination without abnormal findings**
>
> **99384–25 Initial comprehensive preventive medicine evaluation and management, new patient; adolescent (age 12 through 17 years). Significant, separately identifiable evaluation and management service by the same physician or other qualified health care professional on the same day of the procedure or other service.**
>
> **90460 Immunization administration through 18 years of age via any route of administration, with counseling by physician or other qualified health care professional; first or only component of each vaccine or toxoid administered**
>
> **90461 Immunization administration through 18 years of age via any route of administration, with counseling by physician or other qualified health care professional; each additional vaccine or toxoid component administered (List separately in addition to code for primary procedure)**
>
> **90715 Tetanus, diphtheria toxoids and acellular pertussis vaccine (Tdap), when administered to individuals 7 years or older, for intramuscular use**
>
> **90733 Meningococcal polysaccharide vaccine (any group(s)), for subcutaneous use**

Figure 29-5 ■ Example of immunization coding.

Psychiatry (90785-90899)

Patients may receive only psychiatric evaluation and management services, only psychiatric diagnostic services, only psychotherapy or treatment, or any combination of these. Any combination of codes may be assigned based on the services documented in the medical record. Although most medical specialties have codes in the Surgery section as well as the Medicine section, psychiatry is a specialty that does not have a surgical component, so all services except evaluation and management are coded from this section of CPT. Psychiatric E/M services are discussed later in this chapter.

1. To assign codes for Psychiatry services, search the Index for one of the following Main Terms that best describes the service provided:

   - **Psychiatric Diagnosis**
   - **Psychiatric Treatment**
   - **Psychoanalysis**
   - **Psychotherapy**

2. Select the desired modifying term(s) under the selected Main Term for the service provided. Identify the code(s) or code range.

3. In the Tabular List, review the codes to select the appropriate service.

In the Tabular List of the Psychotherapy subsection, codes are divided based on time and whether an E/M service is also provided. Time refers to the face-to-face time between the provider and the patient and/or family member and must be documented in the medical record.

When evaluation and management services are provided in addition to psychotherapy, report both the E/M code and the appropriate psychotherapy code (**90833, 90836, 90838**). When psychotherapy is the only service provided, report the appropriate psychotherapy code (**90832, 90834, 90837**). When both an E/M service and a time-based psychiatry service are provided, the time spent providing the E/M service cannot also be counted toward the time reported in the psychiatry code. Providers must specifically document the amount of time spent providing each type of service to avoid duplicate reporting of time.

Several codes in this subsection can be provided via telemedicine and are identified with the five-pointed star symbol (★) before the code.

Diagnoses for psychiatry services are often psychiatric disorders from ICD-10-CM Chapter 5, "F01-F99 Mental, Behavioral and Neurodevelopmental Disorders;" however, some diagnoses may be found in other chapters.

Dialysis Procedures (90935-90999)

CPT provides extensive special instructions about reporting codes within each Dialysis category. Coders must read the instructions thoroughly to identify when and how various codes are to be reported. To assign codes for dialysis services, follow these steps.

1. In the Index, search for one of the following Main Terms based on the service to be coded:

   - **Dialysis**
   - **End Stage Renal Disease**
   - **Hemodialysis**
   - **Peritoneal Dialysis**

2. Identify the code(s) or code range from the Medicine section, which usually appear immediately to the right of each Main Term. Be alert for the following:

   - Modifying terms generally list dialysis-related surgical procedures, which are discussed in the corresponding CPT chapter.
   - Some Main Terms and modifying terms list Category II CPT codes that end with the letter **F**. Category II codes are reported for performance measurement and tracking and do not replace CPT codes used for billing.

3. In the Tabular List, review the codes to select the appropriate service.

Patients with ESRD may receive services as inpatients, as clinic outpatients, or self-administered in the home. Patients

ESRD patient, age 45, who receives hemodialysis service in the dialysis clinic 3 times per week, is hospitalized for 4 days. The nephrologist evaluates the patient daily while in the hospital and orders 2 hemodialysis procedures by the dialysis staff. The nephrologist also evaluates the patient 3 times as an outpatient during the month.

90935 x 2 Hemodialysis procedure with single evaluation by a physician or other qualified health care professional

90961 x 1 End-stage renal disease (ESRD) related services monthly, for patients 20 years of age and older; with 2–3 face-to-face visits by a physician or other qualified health care professional per month

Note: Also report Inpatient E/M codes (**99221–99233**) for the encounters on the two days when no hemodialysis procedure was performed.

Figure 29-6 ■ Example of coding ESRD services.

with ESRD typically receive dialysis three days per week, or 12–13 times per month. They typically are evaluated by a physician one to four times per month. Codes identify the number of face-to-face physician visits during the month, not the number of clinic encounters to receive dialysis.

Clinic and home-based services are identified using codes that identify the number of outpatient physician encounters provided during the month (**90951-90970**).

Inpatient services are reported for each face-to-face physician encounter. When a patient from a dialysis clinic is hospitalized, inpatient dialysis services are almost always provided. Report inpatient dialysis codes for a hemodialysis procedure with physician evaluation. Report partial-month outpatient dialysis services with the code that identifies the correct number of outpatient physician encounters (■ FIGURE 29-6). ■ TABLE 29-20 summarizes the division of ESRD codes by location, number of physician visits, and age.

Inpatient and outpatient services include all evaluation and management related to the dialysis procedure. E/M services not related to dialysis should be reported separately using the appropriate E/M code with modifier **-25 Significant, separately identifiable evaluation and management service**. Dialysis services eligible for telemedicine are identified with the five-pointed star (★) symbol in the Tabular List.

All patients with ESRD require a first-listed diagnosis of **N18.6 End stage renal disease** for dialysis-related services and the additional diagnosis **Z99.2 Dependence on renal dialysis**. Additional **Z** codes are available to report fitting and adjustment of a dialysis catheter (**Z49.0-**) and patient noncompliance with dialysis (**Z91.15**). In addition, physicians may identify additional diagnoses for the underlying causes of ESRD and any comorbidities.

Diagnoses for patients undergoing short-term dialysis may include acute renal failure (**N17.-**), drug overdose, and injury to the kidneys. In addition, physicians may identify additional diagnoses for the underlying causes of acute renal failure (ARF) and any comorbidities.

Gastroenterology Procedures (91010-91299)

The Gastroenterology subsection does not provide any special instructions. Frequent instructional notes appear in the Tabular List; these direct coders to codes for specific types of tests and also identify codes that can and cannot be used together. To assign codes for gastroenterology procedures, use one of the following methods to locate the Main Term in the Index.

1. Search for the Main Term **Gastric Tests**, then select the first-level modifying term, **Acid Reflux** or **Motility**, for the type of test. Identify the code(s) or code range to verify in the Tabular List.

2. Search for name or type of test as the Main Term, such as:
   - **Reflux Study**
   - **Manometric Studies**
   - **Manometry**
   - **Motility Study**

Some tests, such as manometric studies and motility studies, can be performed at a variety of anatomic sites, so be certain to select the code for the correct site. Identify the code(s) or code range to verify in the Tabular List.

Table 29-20 ■ CODES FOR HEMODIALYSIS PHYSICIAN SERVICES

Location	Number of Physician Visits	Codes by Age Group			
		<2 Years	**2–11 Years**	**12–19 Years**	**≥20 Years**
ESRD inpatient	1 evaluation per treatment	90935	90935	90935	90935
	Repeated evaluations	90937	90937	90937	90937
ESRD clinic	1 visit/month	90953	90956	90959	90962
	2–3 visits/month	90952	90955	90958	90961
	≥4 visits/month	90951	90954	90957	90960
ESRD home dialysis	Full month	90963	90964	90965	90966
ESRD clinic or home	Per day (less than a full month)	90967	90968	90969	90970
Non-ESRD	One (1) evaluation per treatment	90935-90937			

3. Search for the anatomic site as the Main Term, such as **Esophagus**. Locate an appropriate subterm for the procedure, such as **acid reflux, acid perfusion, balloon distention provocation study, imaging studies**. Some tests, such as manometric studies and motility studies, can be performed at a variety of anatomic sites, so be certain to select the code for the correct site.

In the Tabular List, review the codes in the relevant range and select the code that accurately describes the service provided. There are only a few add-on codes and indented codes in this subsection, so code selection tends to be straightforward. Read the instructional notes that identify codes that cannot be reported together.

Most of the procedures in the Gastroenterology subsection consist of technical and professional components, so the appropriate modifier **-26 Professional component** or **-TC Technical component** should be used as appropriate.

Diagnoses that support gastroenterology procedures most often come from ICD-10-CM Chapter 11, "Diseases of the Digestive System (K00-K95)," or Chapter 18, "Symptoms, Signs, Abnormal Clinical and Laboratory Findings (R00-R99)."

Ophthalmology (92002-92499) and Hearing Services (92502-92700)

Ophthalmology services include general and special ophthalmological services, as well as contact lens and spectacle services. Hearing services include a variety of evaluation and testing services.

To assign codes from these subsections, follow these steps.

1. For ophthalmological services:
   - Search the Index for the Main Term **Ophthalmology, Diagnostic.**
   - Locate the name of the specific service as the Main Term, such as **Gonioscopy** or **Contact Lens Service.**

2. For hearing services:
   - Search the Index for the Main Term **Audiologic Function Tests**, **Vestibular Function Tests**, or **Audiometry**, as appropriate.
   - To locate codes by anatomic site, locate the Main Term **Ear, Nose, and Throat**. This entry is separate from the Main Term **Ear** alone.

3. If necessary, locate the appropriate modifying term(s) that describes the specific service provided. Identify the code(s) or code range.

4. Refer to the Tabular List to select and verify the appropriate code based on the type and extent of service.

The Tabular List provides special instructions for the Ophthalmology subsection that contain detailed definitions for intermediate, comprehensive, and special ophthalmological services. Coders must be familiar with these definitions so they know the services included in each category of codes.

The subheading **General Ophthalmological Services (92002-92014)** provides codes for services that do not meet the criteria of evaluation and management (E/M) codes, such as yearly eye exams. The definitions of new and established patients are the same as for E/M codes, but the levels of service are different, as described in the special instructions. Do not assign an E/M code in addition to, or in place of, codes **92002-92014**.

Codes under the subheading **Special Ophthalmological Services (92015-92287)** describe tests that evaluate a particular part of the visual system. Assign these codes in addition to E/M codes and codes for **General Ophthalmological Services**, as appropriate.

Codes in the subheading **Contact Lens Services (92310-92326)** include the prescription, fitting, patient education, and follow-up related to contact lenses. Codes are divided by who provides the fitting and whether one eye or both eyes are treated. Report codes **92310-92313** when the fitting is provided by the same office that prescribed the lenses. Report codes **92314-92317** when the prescription is provided by one office and the fitting is performed by an independent technician. Codes **92310** and **92314** include the description **except aphakia** (*absence of a lens*) and are used when contact lenses are prescribed to supplement a person's natural lens. Append modifier **-52 Reduced Services** when a lens is prescribed for only one eye.

Codes that include the description **for aphakia** are used when the contact lens replaces a person's natural lens, as occurs with cataract removal.

The supply of the lens itself may be reported as part of the fitting service or may be reported separately using code **99070** or the appropriate HCPCS code.

Codes under the subheading **Spectacle Services (92340-92499)** include the fitting, patient education, and follow-up related to eyeglasses. Prescription of the lenses is included in code **92015 Determination of refractive state**. Codes are divided by the type of lens—monofocal, bifocal, or multifocal—and the condition: for aphakia, not for aphakia, and low-vision aids. The supply of the material is not included in the fitting service and should be reported separately using code **99070** or the appropriate HCPCS code.

Read the code descriptions to determine whether the code is unilateral or bilateral. Some services provide separate codes for one eye or both eyes, and others do not. When the code description includes the words **unilateral** or **bilateral**, select the code that describes the extent of service provided. Append the appropriate modifier, **-LT** or **-RT**, for a unilateral procedure. When the description does not specify bilateral, apply modifier **-50 Bilateral procedure**. When the procedure description states bilateral but the service was provided for only one eye, apply modifier **-52 Reduced services**.

Diagnosis codes that support the need for ophthalmological services most often come from ICD-10-CM Chapter 7, "Diseases of the Eye and Adnexa (H00-H59)," or the section **Diabetes mellitus (E08-E13)** from Chapter 4, "Endocrine, Nutritional and Metabolic Diseases (E00-E89)."

Diagnosis codes that support the need for hearing services most often come from ICD-10-CM Chapter 8, "Diseases of the Ear and the Mastoid Process (H60-H95)." Diagnosis codes for injuries to the eye and ear are in the section **Injuries to the head (S00-S09)** of ICD-10-CM Chapter 19, "Injury, Poisoning and Certain Other Consequences of External Causes."

Cardiovascular Procedures (92920-93799)

The Cardiovascular subsection contains 11 subheadings, most of which provide detailed special instructions and frequent instructional notes. Coders must thoroughly read and understand these guidelines so they can accurately assign codes. Highlights of this subsection follow.

Percutaneous Coronary Intervention (92920-92944)

Percutaneous coronary intervention (PCI) describes percutaneous procedures performed to restore blood flow to the coronary vessels that have been obstructed, usually due to occlusive disease (*a buildup of plaque or a blood clot*). This process is revascularization. To assign codes for PCI, follow these steps.

1. Search for the name of the procedure or the anatomic site where the procedure was performed, then locate the appropriate modifying term(s). There are many possible coding paths for a PCI procedure. A few examples follow.

   - For angioplasty, locate the Main Term **Angioplasty** then the first-level modifying term **Coronary Artery**. Select the appropriate second-level modifying term.

   - When a stent is placed, locate the Main Term **Stent** and the first-level modifying term **for Revascularization, Intracoronary**.

   - Locate the Main Term **Artery**, the first-level modifying term **Coronary**, and the second-level modifying term for the type of procedure, such as **Angiography** or **Atherectomy**.

2. Identify the code(s) or code range.

3. Refer to the Tabular List to select and verify the code based on the type of service(s) performed and the number of coronary arteries or branches treated.

CODING CAUTION

Codes for surgical procedures to treat occlusive disease appear in the Cardiovascular subsection of the CPT Surgery section. When coding PCI, be careful to select a code for the percutaneous procedure, which begins with **9**, and not a code for a similarly named surgical procedure, which begins with **3**.

PCI codes appear under the Tabular List category heading **Coronary Therapeutic Services and Procedures**. These codes have been updated multiple times in recent years, resulting in many resequenced codes. The category begins immediately following code **92998** in the CPT Tabular List.

In the Tabular List, PCI codes are listed in pairs consisting of a parent code, which identifies the service performed on one (or the first) vessel, and an indented code, which is also an add-on code, that identifies each additional branch treated (■ TABLE 29-21). The main coronary artery and up to two additional branches can be coded. Additional PCI in a third branch of the same coronary artery cannot be coded.

Codes include all of the elements of the procedure:

- Accessing and selectively catheterizing the vessel

- Traversing the lesion

- Radiological supervision and interpretation directly related to the intervention performed

- Closure of the arteriotomy when performed through the access sheath

- Imaging performed to document completion of the intervention

- Balloon angioplasty, when performed

Diagnostic Coronary Angiography. Diagnostic coronary angiography is included in PCI codes but may be reported separately in any of the following circumstances, which are described in the special instructions under PCI.

- A full diagnostic angiography is performed on a patient for whom a prior catheter-based angiograph is not available and a decision to intervene is based on the findings.

- The patient's condition and clinical indicators have changed since the prior angiography study.

- The prior angiography does not adequately visualize the anatomy or pathology involved.

- There is a clinical change during the procedure that requires new evaluation outside the target area of intervention.

When diagnostic coronary angiography is performed for one of these reasons, report the appropriate code from the

---

Table 29-21 ■ **CODES FOR PERCUTANEOUS CORONARY INTERVENTION**

Type of Vessel or Condition	Service(s) Included	Single Vessel	Each Additional Vessel
Native vessel	Angioplasty only	92920	92921
	Atherectomy (and angioplasty, when performed)	92924	92925
	Stent (and angioplasty, when performed)	92928	92929
	Atherectomy and stent (and angioplasty, when performed)	92933	92934
Bypass graft	Atherectomy, stent, and/or angioplasty (in any combination)	92937	92938
During myocardial infarction	Atherectomy, stent, and/or angioplasty (in any combination)	92941	92920-92938, 92943, 92944
For chronic total occlusion	Atherectomy, stent, and/or angioplasty (in any combination)	92943	92944

Source: © PB Resources, Inc. Used with permission. CPT codes © American Medical Association.

range **93454-93461**. Apply modifier **-59 Distinct procedural service** to inform the payer that the angiography was above and beyond that normally included in the PCI procedure code. PCI codes consist of a professional component only, so modifiers **-26** and **-TC** are not used.

Diagnoses that support PCI most commonly include codes from the ICD-10-CM category **Ischemic heart diseases (I20-I25)**, as well as codes for other forms of heart disease, in Chapter 10, "Diseases of the Circulatory System (I00-I99)," and codes from Chapter 18, "Symptoms, Signs, Abnormal Clinical and Laboratory Findings (R00-R99)," that could point to heart disease. CPT code **92941** should be supported with a diagnosis code for myocardial infarction (**I21-I22**). CPT codes **92937** and **92938** should be supported with a diagnosis code that identifies occlusion of a bypass graft (**I25.7-**). Patients frequently have multiple comorbidities not only in the cardiovascular system but also in other organ systems.

Cardiac Catheterization (93451-93583)

Cardiac catheterization is a diagnostic medical procedure that includes:

- Introducing and positioning a catheter within the vascular system
- Repositioning the catheter when necessary
- Recording intracardiac pressure, intravascular pressure, oxygen saturation, and cardiac output
- Final evaluation and report of procedure

To assign codes for cardiac catheterization, follow these steps.

1. In the Index, search for the Main Term **Cardiac Catheterization**.
2. Locate the first- and second-level modifying terms that identify the type of service provided. Identify the code(s) or code range.
3. Refer to the Tabular List to select and verify the code based on the site(s) treated.
4. Read the special instructions and instructional notes, which are extensive for cardiac catheterization.

5. Identify and select the code(s) for any additional services provided.
6. Refer to the CPT table titled "Cardiac Catheterization Codes" at the end of this subheading in the CPT manual, which lists the components of each catheterization code and the add-on codes that can be used. Use of this table helps ensure that you select the correct code and appropriate add-on codes.

The Tabular List provides two code families for cardiac catheterization: one for congenital heart disease and one for all other conditions. The bundling guidelines in ■ TABLE 29-22 apply to codes other than those for congenital heart disease.

Cardiac catheterization codes have a professional and a technical component, so when only one component is provided, apply the appropriate modifier: **-26 Professional component** or **-TC Technical component**.

Diagnoses that support cardiac catheterization commonly include heart valve disease, occlusive disease, arrhythmias, heart failure, myocardial infarction, endocarditis, and pericarditis. Codes **93455**, **93457**, **93459**, and **93461** should be supported by a diagnosis code that identifies the existence of or problem in a grafted vessel. Patients frequently have multiple comorbidities.

Electrophysiological Studies (93600-93662)

An intracardiac electrophysiologic study (EPS) includes invasive diagnostic tests that assess the electrical activity in the heart. The electrical activity for a normal heartbeat starts at the top of the heart and spreads down. A patient may experience cardiac arrhythmias or abnormal heart rhythms when the electrical activity in the heart starts somewhere other than at the top of the heart. To assign codes for an EPS, follow these steps:

1. In the Index, locate the Main Term **Electrophysiologic Procedure**. For ablation procedures locate the Main Term **Arrhythmogenic Focus** or the Main Term **Ablation**, the first-level modifying term **Heart**, and the second-level modifying term **Arrhythmogenic Focus**.
2. For EPS, refer to the code range listed, which includes all the codes in this subheading.

Table 29-22 ■ **CATHETERIZATION PROCEDURES AND BUNDLED SERVICES**

Procedure	Codes	Bundled Services (other than for congenital heart disease)
Cardiac catheterization	93452-93461	• Contrast injection • Imaging supervision, interpretation, and report
Left heart catheterization	93452, 93453, 93458-93461	• Intraprocedural injection(s) for left-ventricular/left-atrial angiography • Imaging supervision and interpretation
Coronary catheter placement	93454-93461	• Intraprocedural injection(s) for coronary angiography • Imaging supervision and interpretation
Catheter placement in bypass graft	93455, 93457, 93459, 93461	• Intraprocedural injection(s) for bypass graft angiography • Imaging supervision and interpretation

3. Refer to the Tabular List to select and verify the correct code based on the specific test provided.

In the Tabular List, read the special instructions at the beginning of this subheading. Three types of procedures are described in this subheading:

- **Arrhythmia induction**—Recreating the arrhythmia using electrical pacing or programmed stimulation
- **Mapping**—Recording the site of origin of the tachycardia or its electrical path through the heart
- **Ablation**—Selectively destroying cardiac tissue using radiofrequency or cryo-energy

Many times, patients with arrhythmias are evaluated and treated during the same encounter. When this occurs, report the induction and ablation with one code that bundles both procedures (**93653-93655**), but report the mapping as a separate service with an add-on code (**93609** or **93613**). Read the instructional notes in the Tabular List to verify codes that can and cannot be reported together.

The bundle of His (pronounced "hiss") recording is a test that can be performed alone or as part of an EPS. A catheter with a sensor on the end is advanced to the heart to measure the electrical activity of the bundle of His.

When more than one procedure is performed during an encounter, the second and subsequent codes from this subsection require modifier **-51 Multiple procedures**. Do not use modifier **-51** on add-on codes or codes that require modifier **-59 Distinct procedural service**.

EPS procedures are commonly supported by diagnoses for conduction disorders and cardiac arrhythmias (**I44-I49**) and signs and symptoms that may indicate the presence of these conditions. Patients might also have other cardiac conditions and a variety of comorbidities.

SUCCESS STEP

The CPT Index provides a limited number of Main Terms for specific EPS services, making them challenging to find. You may wish to write your own notes in the Index, to guide yourself. For example, write in a new entry under **B** to identify *Bundle of His 93600*. Write additional notes under **M**, **P**, and **R** to create Main Terms that seem logical, such as *Mapping*, *Pacing*, and *Recording*. For these entries, you can list the code range *93602-93662*.

Noninvasive Vascular Studies (93880-93998)

The subsection Noninvasive Vascular Diagnostic Studies includes specialized services to study veins and arteries other than the heart and great vessels.

To assign codes for noninvasive vascular diagnostic studies, follow these steps.

1. In the Index, locate the Main Term **Vascular Studies**.
2. Locate the first-level modifying term for the type of procedure or body site. Identify the code(s) or code range.

3. Refer to the Tabular List to select and verify the code for the body site and type of vessel treated.

In the Tabular List, codes are divided into subheadings by body site and whether the study involves an artery, vein, or both. The subsection provides special instructions that describe how the studies are performed and lists the components required for limited and complete studies of both the lower and upper extremities. In general, limited studies require measurements at one or two levels and complete studies require measurements at three or more levels. Examples of levels for the lower extremities are the high thigh, low thigh, calf, ankle, metatarsal, and toes. Examples of levels for the upper extremities are the arm, forearm, wrist, and digits.

Codes for extremity studies identify a bilateral study. When the study is unilateral, apply modifier **-52 Reduced services**.

Codes under the subheading Cerebrovascular Arterial Studies (**93880-93895**) are divided by methodology—either a duplex scan or transcranial Doppler (TCD) study. Parent codes identify a complete study; indented codes identify a limited or unilateral study. Codes in this subsection are comprised of professional and technical components, so apply modifiers **-26** and **-TC** as appropriate.

Diagnosis codes that support noninvasive vascular diagnostic studies are frequently found in the following sections of ICD-10-CM Chapter 10, "Diseases of the Circulatory System (I00-I99)":

- Cerebrovascular diseases (I60-I69)
- Diseases of the arteries, arterioles and capillaries (I70-I79)
- Disease of veins, lymphatic vessels and lymph nodes, not elsewhere classified (I80-89)

Allergy Procedures (95004-95199)

The subsection **Allergy and Clinical Immunology** describes services to allergy testing and allergen immunotherapy. An antigen is any natural or artificial substance that produces an immune response. An allergenic extract is a concentration of components from the allergen, such as grass or pollen. Do not confuse allergen immunotherapy with the administration of immune globulins, discussed earlier in this chapter.

To locate codes for allergy and clinical immunology, follow these steps.

1. For allergy testing, search for the Main Term **Allergy Test** in the Index.
2. Locate the first- and second-level modifying terms that identify the type of test.
3. For allergen immunotherapy, search for the Main Term **Allergen Immunotherapy**.
4. Locate the first- and second-level modifying terms that identify the type of therapy provided. Identify the code(s) or code range.
5. Refer to the Tabular List to select and verify the code based on the type of test provided.

In the Tabular List, allergy testing codes are divided by the type of test performed. When the description states **specify**

CODING CAUTION

Under the Main Term **Allergen Immunotherapy**, the first-level modifying term **Allergen** leads to codes for laboratory tests from the Pathology and Laboratory section, which begin with **8**. Codes for testing and treatment appear in the Medicine section and begin with **9**.

number of tests, report one unit of the code for each test performed. Ingestion challenge test codes are defined based on the length of time required for the test. Allergen immunotherapy is the periodic administration of antigens to increase a person's immune response to the allergen.

The antigen or allergenic extract can be provided by the physician or by the patient, purchased elsewhere. Codes **95115** and **95117** describe professional immunotherapy services when the physician *does not* provide the antigen. Codes **95120** and **95125** describe professional immunotherapy services when the physician *does* provide the antigen. The parent code (**95115** and **95120**) in each pair reports one injection. The indented code (**95117** and **95125**) in each pair reports two or more injections. It is not an add-on code and should not be reported with the respective parent code. Additional indented codes are provided for stinging insect venoms.

Codes are also provided to report professional services for the supervision of preparation and provision of antigens by the physician.

The interpretation and reporting of allergy tests is included in the code and should not be reported separately using an E/M code. E/M codes can be reported when a significant, separately identifiable E/M service is provided. Apply modifier **-25** to the E/M code.

Codes for allergy procedures are most commonly supported by a diagnosis of an inflammatory condition of the affected anatomic site, such as rhinitis, sinusitis, conjunctivitis, otitis, dermatitis, and similar conditions.

Neurology Procedures (95782-96020)

Neurology services are typically provided as E/M consultations for outpatients and inpatients. In addition, diagnostic and therapeutic procedures can be reported separately. The subsection Neurology and Neuromuscular Procedures provides codes for a wide variety of tests including sleep testing, routine and special EEG tests, nerve and muscle function tests, and intraoperative neurophysiology.

To assign codes from the Neurology subsection, follow these steps.

1. In the Index, search for the name of the test or procedure as the Main Term.

2. Review the modifying term(s) to select the appropriate code range.

3. Refer to the Tabular List to select and verify the code based on the type of test.

The Tabular List provides special instructions that describe various tests and identify codes that can and cannot be reported

together. Be attentive to how each code reports time or quantity of service.

Sleep testing (**95803-95811**) is performed while the patient sleeps to assess various body functions to diagnose sleep disorders such as sleep apnea, insomnia, narcolepsy, and somnambulism. Tests include polysomnography, which includes multiple measurements of functions and activities of the heart, muscles, brain, and eyes during sleep. Polysomnography codes are divided by the age of the patient and the number of sleep parameters evaluated.

Evoked potentials and reflex tests (**95925-95939**) are performed to diagnose neuromuscular diseases and are completed by measuring visual, auditory, and automatic nerve reflexes.

The Intraoperative Neurophysiology subheading provides two codes, **95940** and **95941**, both of which are add-on codes used in conjunction with other neurological tests performed during surgery. Code **95940** reports continuous one-on-one intraoperative monitoring in the operating room and is reported in 15-minute increments. Code **95941** reports intraoperative monitoring from a remote or nearby location outside of the operating room and is reported in one-hour increments. Read the detailed special instructions with this subheading to use the codes correctly.

Most, but not all, procedures in this subsection contain professional and technical components, so apply modifiers **-26** and **-TC** as needed. When services described as bilateral are performed unilaterally, apply modifier **-52**.

Diagnosis codes that support Neurology subsection procedures are most commonly supported by codes from ICD-10-CM Chapter 6, "Diseases of the Nervous System and Sense Organs (G00-G99)," or Chapter 18, "Symptoms, Signs, Abnormal Clinical and Laboratory Findings (R00-R99)."

Infusion and Injection Procedures (96360-96549)

Infusion and injection procedures include hydration; therapeutic, prophylactic, and diagnostic injections and infusions; and chemotherapy administration. Administration of other highly complex drugs that require close supervision and monitoring for side effects is coded with the same codes used for chemotherapy administration.

To assign codes for infusion and injection procedures, follow these steps.

1. In the Index, search for the Main Term **Infusion Therapy**.

2. Locate the first-level modifying term for the type: **Hydration**, **Intravenous**, or **Subcutaneous** (■ FIGURE 29-7 page 550).

3. For chemotherapy, locate the second-level modifying term **Chemotherapy** under **Intravenous**.

4. As an alternative, select a Main Term for the type of infusion, which leads directly to the appropriate code: **Chemotherapy**, **Hydration**, or **Intravenous Therapy**.

5. Regardless of the Main Term selected, identify the code range to verify in the Tabular List.

The Tabular List for this subsection provides detailed special instructions that identify the terms used to assign codes,

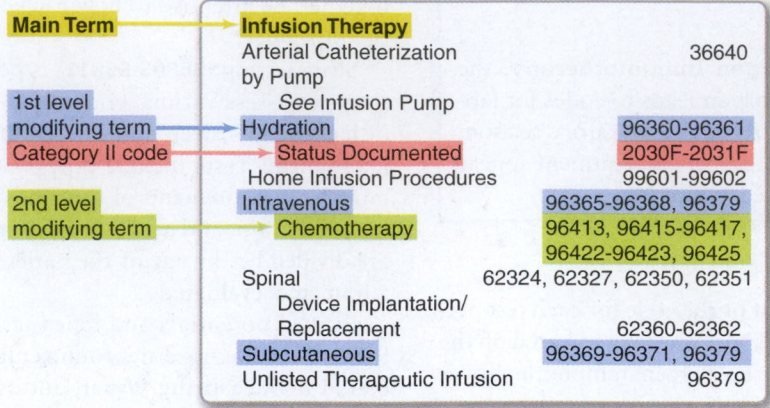

Figure 29-7 ■ CPT Index entry for "Infusion therapy." *Source: Used by permission of PB Resources, Inc.*

sequencing directions, and differences between physician coding and facility coding.

When the following services are performed to facilitate the infusion or injection, they are bundled and should not be reported separately.

- Use of local anesthesia
- Starting the IV
- Access to indwelling IV, subcutaneous catheter, or port
- Flush at conclusion of infusion
- Standard tubing, syringes, and supplies

Three categories of infusion codes identify the purpose of the service:

- Hydration **96360-96361**
- Therapeutic, prophylactic, and diagnostic services **96365-96379**
- Chemotherapy **96401-96549** (■ FIGURE 29-8)

Patient is seen for chemotherapy infusion for metastatic colon cancer. Oxaliplatin is administered through intravenous infusion for two hours followed by leucovorin for two hours. A bolus (*push*) of 5-fluorouracil (5-FU) is administered at the same access site.

Z51.11 Encounter for antineoplastic chemotherapy
C79.9 Secondary malignant neoplasm of unspecified site
C18.9 Malignant neoplasm of colon, unspecified
96413 x 1 Chemotherapy administration, intravenous; infusion technique, up to 1 hour, single or initial substance/drug
96417 x 1 Chemotherapy administration, intravenous infusion technique; each additional sequential infusion (different substance/drug), up to 1 hour
96415 x 2 Chemotherapy administration, intravenous; infusion technique, each additional hour (*Note:* One unit is the second hour of oxaliplatin infusion and one unit is the second hour of leucovorin infusion)
96411 Chemotherapy administration, intravenous; push technique

Figure 29-8 ■ Example of coding infusion services.

Except for hydration services, there are three basic types of infusion codes: initial, concurrent, and sequential.

- **Initial infusion**—Report one code per day, unless a second, separate site is required for additional infusions. Report the second code with modifier **-59**. This is a time-based code, with an add-on code for additional time.
- **Concurrent infusion**—Report a single code for infusion of a second substance or drug infused at the same time as another substance or drug. If a third substance is administered concurrently, do not report it.
- **Sequential infusion**—Report an infusion or IV push of a new substance or drug following a primary or initial service.

Physicians report infusion therapy for nonfacility or office-based services only. Physicians report the infusion that is the main reason for the encounter, regardless of the chronological order in which infusions are provided. Facilities follow a hierarchy of sequencing priorities, which is discussed later in the chapter.

A significant, separately identifiable office or other outpatient E/M service can be reported on the same day as the infusion, when performed. Apply modifier **-25** in addition to the infusion code(s) **96360-96549**.

Thousands of diagnoses can support infusion and injection procedures. Hydration services are frequently supported with codes from ICD-10-CM Chapter 4, "Endocrine, Nutritional, and Metabolic Diseases (E00-E89)," for volume depletion (**E86**) and disorders of fluid, electrolyte, and acid–base imbalance (**E87**). Chemotherapy services are often, but not always, supported by codes from ICD-10-CM Chapter 2, "Neoplasms (C00-D49)."

Physical Medicine (97010-97799), Osteopathic (98925-98929), and Chiropractic (98940-98943)

Physical medicine and rehabilitation services include physical and occupational therapy evaluations, modalities, therapeutic procedures, active wound care management, tests and measurements, and orthotic and prosthetic management.

CPT provides guidelines for coding of physical and occupational therapy evaluations, which follow different criteria than medical evaluations. Codes for physical therapy, occupational therapy, and athletic training evaluations include a history and activity profile, examination, clinical decision making, and development of a plan of care. Review the special instructions and definitions at the beginning of each category to select the correct code:

- **Physical therapy evaluations 97161-97164**
- **Occupational therapy evaluations 97165-97168**
- **Athletic training evaluations 97169-97172**

Many services can be located by searching the Index for the name of the procedure. To assign codes for physical medicine, follow these steps.

1. Search the Index for the Main Term **Physical Medicine/Therapy/Occupational Therapy**.

2. Locate the first- and second-level modifying terms for the specific service or modality, such as **Evaluation, Physical Therapy** or **Modalities, Traction**. Some services also appear directly under a Main Term for the name of the service, such as **Traction Therapy** or **Wound, Care**.

3. Identify the code(s) or code range to verify in the Tabular List.

4. In the Tabular List, select the code and determine the quantity to be reported based on the code description.

Modalities are physical therapy treatments that use thermal (*heat*), acoustic (*sound*), luminous (*light*), mechanical, or electric energy to produce beneficial changes in biologic tissue. Codes for modalities are divided into supervised and constant attendance.

Supervised modalities do not require continuous one-on-one contact with the patient by the provider. The provider sets up the treatment then can leave the room while the modality runs. Examples are the application of hot packs or mechanical traction. Supervised modality codes (**97010-97028**) are reported with one unit of service regardless of the amount of time the modality operates.

Constant attendance modalities require constant one-on-one contact with the patient by the provider. The provider personally applies the modality and is present with the patient the entire time. Examples are ultrasound and contrast baths. Constant attendance modality codes (**97032-97039**) are time-based codes in which 15 minutes equals one unit of service, 30 minutes equals two units of service, and so on.

The subheading **Therapeutic Procedures (97110-97546)** provides codes for other types of therapy, training, and activities. Code descriptions identify those that are time-based.

Read the documentation carefully to determine the exact type of service provided. Some modalities can be applied using either supervision or constant attendance. For example, electrical stimulation can be either supervised/unattended (**97014**) or constant attendance/manual (**97032**). Whirlpool (**96365**) and paraffin baths (**97018**) are supervised, and contrast baths (**97034**) and the Hubbard tank (**97036**) are constant attendance. Mechanical traction is supervised (**97012**), and manual traction is reported with a time-based code (**97140**) from the Therapeutic Procedures subheading (■ FIGURE 29-9).

Patient receives physical therapy treatment for a back sprain. The physical therapist applies unattended electrical stimulation for 15 minutes, then provides therapeutic exercises for 30 minutes. The session concludes with 15 minutes of manual therapy including traction.

S33.5XXA	Dislocation and sprain of joints and ligaments of lumbar spine and pelvis, initial encounter
97110	x 2 Therapeutic procedure, 1 or more areas, each 15 minutes; therapeutic exercises to develop strength and endurance, range of motion and flexibility
97140	x 1 Manual therapy techniques (eg, mobilization/manipulation, manual lymphatic drainage, manual traction), 1 or more regions, each 15 minutes
97014	Application of a modality to 1 or more areas; electrical stimulation (unattended)

Figure 29-9 ■ Example of coding for physical medicine.

To assign codes for chiropractic or osteopathic manipulation, locate the Main Term **Chiropractic Treatment** or **Osteopathic Manipulation**, respectively. The Tabular List provides special instructions for both of these subsections. Select codes based on the number of body regions treated, which are defined in the special instructions.

SUCCESS STEP

Medicare covers chiropractic treatment only for acute injuries supported by radiographic (x-ray) evidence. Append HCPCS modifier **-AT Acute Treatment** to the code. Contact your local Medicare Administrative Contractor (MAC) for detailed guidelines on chiropractic billing.

Diagnoses that support physical medicine services can come from many chapters of the ICD-10-CM manual because nearly every body system can be affected by conditions for which patients can be helped by physical medicine. Conditions from ICD-10-CM Chapter 19, "Injury, Poisoning and Certain Other Consequences of External Causes (S00-T88)," also frequently require physical medicine services. Chiropractic services often require codes from specific categories such as **M99 Biomechanical lesions, not elsewhere classified** or codes for **Subluxation and dislocation of** the cervical (**S13.1-**), thoracic (**S23.1-**), or lumbar (**S33.1-**) vertebra to qualify for reimbursement.

Other Medicine Procedures

The Medicine section contains many additional subsections beyond the ones discussed here. Use the three skills of an "Ace" coder—abstract, assign, and arrange—to approach new coding situations that you have not encountered before. The special instructions and instructional notes in the Tabular List provide the needed guidance for any given subsection or category.

Biofeedback (90901-90911)

Biofeedback teaches patients to regulate certain body functions through mental or physical exercises. Patients who experience increased heart rate, respirations, and blood pressure in response to stress can learn to control their mental processes to regulate their body functions. For example, patients who suffer from irritable bowel syndrome (IBS) or fecal incontinence (*inability to control the bowels*) can learn to relax or constrict their anal sphincters to manage their disorders. Many payers cover biofeedback training because biofeedback can help resolve many conditions in the long run. To locate codes for biofeedback, search the Index for the Main Term **Biofeedback Training**.

Pulmonary Procedures (94002-94799)

Pulmonologists treat conditions related to the function of the lungs. Pulmonary diagnostic testing and therapies include many different diagnostic breathing tests to identify pulmonary and respiratory disorders by assessing lung functions and therapeutic services to help patients to breathe more easily. To locate codes for pulmonary procedures, search the Index for the Main Term **Pulmonology** then the first-level modifying term **Diagnostic** or **Therapeutic**. Then locate the additional modifying term(s) for the type of procedure. Alternatively, search for the Main Term for the name of the procedure.

Endocrinology (95249-95251)

The Endocrinology subsection contains two codes for ambulatory continuous glucose monitoring of interstitial tissue fluid. Some diabetic patients need this service. A continuous monitoring device is implanted under the abdominal skin to measure glucose concentrations every five minutes for 72 hours. The device transmits the results to a monitor worn by the patient. Report codes for these services only once a month.

To locate endocrinology codes in the Index, search for the Main Term **Glucose**, the first-level modifying term **Interstitial Fluid**, and the second-level modifying term **Continuous Monitoring**. An alternative coding path is to locate the Main Term **Monitoring** then the modifying terms **Glucose** and **Interstitial Fluid**.

Non-Face-to-Face Services (98966-98969) and Special Services (99000-98969)

The Medicine section provides subsections for non-face-to-face services provided by nonphysicians, online medical evaluation, and special services, procedures, and reports. Take a few moments to review these subsections and become familiar with the codes. To locate these codes in the Index, use the subsection or category title as the Main Term.

Moderate (Conscious) Sedation (99151-99157)

Moderate, or conscious, sedation is a drug-induced depression of consciousness, during which patients are able to respond purposefully to verbal commands and breathe on their own. They do not require an anesthesia provider to maintain cardiovascular function or an open airway. Moderate sedation can be administered by the physician performing the procedure or by a second anesthesia provider. Do not assign moderate sedation codes for services listed in the Anesthesia section (**00100-01999**).

Search the Index for the Main Term Sedation, which has one first-level modifying term, Moderate. The Tabular List provides two parent codes (**99151** and **99155**), each of which has one indented code and one indented add-on code.

Codes **99151** to **99153** are reported when the physician performing the primary procedure also administers the moderate sedation. Codes **99151** and **99152** are divided by age and include up to 15 minutes of intraservice time. Code **99155** reports each additional 15 minutes of service.

Codes **99155** to **99157** are reported when a physician other than the one performing the primary procedure administers the moderate sedation. Codes **99155** and **99156** are divided by age and include up to 15 minutes of intraservice time. Code **99157** reports each additional 15 minutes of service.

Guided Example of Assigning Medicine Codes

To practice skills for assigning codes for Medicine services, continue with the example from earlier in the chapter about a patient who was seen for cardiac therapy. Follow along in your CPT manual as Ladonna Shuck, CPC, assigns codes. Check off each step after you complete it.

▶ First, Ladonna confirms cardiac catheterization of the right heart followed by balloon angioplasty of the right coronary artery.

▶ Ladonna searches the Index for the Main Term **Catheterization**.

❏ She locates the modifying term **Cardiac**, which provides a cross-reference, **See Cardiac Catheterization**. This tells her to look under a different Main Term.

❏ She locates the Main Term entry for **Cardiac Catheterization**, which provides a cross-reference, **See Catheterization, Cardiac**. This is confusing at first because that is where she just looked. Then she notices additional modifying terms that identify various anatomic sites.

❏ She reads all of the modifying terms until she locates **for Angiography**, which lists several modifying terms. She selects the second-level modifying term **Coronary** because the coronary arteries were catheterized. The codes listed for **Coronary** are 93454-93461, 93563, 93571.

▶ Ladonna locates codes **93454-93461, 93563, 93571** in the Tabular List and reads the code descriptions of each. She needs to determine the differences between the parent code and the indented codes under it (■ TABLE 29-23).

❏ **93454 Catheter placement in coronary artery(s) for coronary angiography, including intraprocedural injection(s) for coronary angiography, imaging supervision and interpretation**

❏ **93455** identifies **for bypass graft angiography**, which is not documented.

❏ **93456** identifies **with right heart catheterization**, which is not documented.

❏ **93457** identifies **for bypass graft angiography** and **right heart catheterization**, which are not documented.

❏ **93458** identifies **with left heart catheterization**, which is not documented.

❏ **93459** identifies **with left heart catheterization** and **bypass graft angiography**, which are not documented.

Table 29-23   ■   **SUMMARY OF CARDIAC CATHETERIZATION CODES (93451-93461)**

Main Site ↓	Second Site ➡			
	Right Heart	**Left Heart**	**Coronary Arteries**	**Coronary Arteries + Bypass Graft**
Right heart	93451	93453	93456	93457
Left heart	93453	93452	93458	93459
Coronary arteries	93456	93457	93454	93455
Right + left heart	93453	93453	93460	93461

Source: © PB Resources, Inc. Used with permission. CPT codes © American Medical Association.

❑ **93460** identifies **with right and left heart catheterization**, which is not documented.

❑ **93461** identifies **with right and left heart catheterization** and **bypass graft angiography**, which are not documented.

❑ **93571** is an add-on code that identifies **intravascular Doppler velocity**. She rejects this code because intravascular Doppler velocity is not documented.

▶ Ladonna concludes that code **93454** is the code that describes the procedure, but she would not have known this without reviewing all the codes listed in the Index.

▶ Ladonna checks the special instructions under the category heading **Cardiac Catheterization**.

❑ She reads the description of each target site: right heart catheterization, left heart catheterization, catheter placement in coronary arteries.

❑ She also reads that cardiac catheterization codes **include contrast injection(s), imaging supervision, interpretation, and report**, as well as **all roadmapping angiography**.

❑ She does not find any instructions that indicate the codes include balloon angioplasty or stenting.

▶ Ladonna rereads the documentation and identifies that a stent was inserted in the RCA. Because the code for catheterization does not include stenting, she knows she must find another code.

▶ Ladonna locates the Main Term **Stent** in the CPT Index.

❑ She locates the first-level modifying term **for Revascularization, Intracoronary** and identifies the codes listed: **92937-92938, 92941, 92943-92944**.

❑ Just to be sure, she also checks the Main Term **Angioplasty** and the first-level modifying term **Coronary Artery** with the second-level modifying term **with stent placement**. The same codes are listed, with the addition of **92928-92929**.

▶ Ladonna turns to the Tabular List to verify the codes.

❑ When she locates code **92928** in numerical sequence, she reads an instructional note that states: **92928 is out of numerical sequence. See 92998-93000.**

❑ She locates code **92998**, then finds **92928** in the code series that follows.

▶ Now Ladonna must identify the differences among codes **92928-92929, 92937-92938, 92941**, and **92943-92944**.

❑ **92928** and **92929** identify stenting without any qualifications or criteria. She thinks **92928** might be a possibility, but needs to read the remaining codes.

❑ **92937** and **92938** identify stenting of a **bypass graft**, which is not documented.

❑ **92941** identifies stenting during a **myocardial infarction**, which is not documented.

❑ **92943** and **92944** identify stenting to correct **chronic total occlusion**. She thinks **92943** might be a possibility, but is unsure whether 75% occlusion documented in the medical record qualifies as **chronic total occlusion**.

▶ Ladonna checks the special instructions under the category heading **Coronary Therapeutic Services and Procedures**.

❑ She reads that **Chronic total occlusion of a coronary vessel is present when there is no antegrade flow through the true lumen**. She further reads that **subtotal occlusion . . . [is] not considered chronic total occlusion**.

❑ Based on this information, she concludes that 75% occlusion is subtotal occlusion, not chronic total occlusion. Therefore, **92943** is not appropriate because it specifies **chronic total occlusion**.

❑ She selects code **92928 Percutaneous transcatheter placement of intracoronary stent(s), with coronary angioplasty when performed; single major coronary artery or branch**.

▶ Ladonna reads the rest of the special instructions before code **92920** and learns that angiography (**99354**) cannot always be reported with a code from **92920-92944**.

❑ She reads that **Diagnostic angiography performed at the time of a coronary interventional procedure may be separately reportable if: 1. No prior catheter-based coronary angiography study is available, and a full diagnostic study is performed, and a decision to intervene is based on the diagnostic angiography**.

❑ The situation she is coding meets this criterion because a full diagnostic study was performed and, based on the result, a decision was made to perform the angioplasty and stent placement. Therefore, she is confident that she can use both codes.

▶ Ladonna reviews the procedure codes she has assigned for this case.

❏ **92928 Percutaneous transcatheter placement of intracoronary stent(s), with coronary angioplasty when performed; single major coronary artery or branch**

❏ **93454 Catheter placement in coronary artery(s) for coronary angiography, including intraprocedural injection(s) for coronary angiography, imaging supervision and interpretation**

▶ Next, Ladonna must determine how to sequence the codes and whether any modifiers are needed.

CODING PRACTICE

Exercise 29.3 Assigning Codes for Medicine Procedures

Instructions: Read the mini-medical-record of each patient's encounter. Review the information abstracted in Exercise 29.2 for questions 1–3. For questions 4 and 5, do the abstracting on your own. Assign CPT procedure codes using the Index and Tabular List. Write the code(s) on the line provided.

---

1. OFFICE (Psychiatrist)   Gender: **F**   Age: **67**

Reason for encounter: **Referred by PCP due to extreme depression since death of husband 6 months ago**

Procedure: **Psychiatric diagnostic examination that included a history and review of diagnostic and laboratory studies**

Assessment: **Depressive state with tremors**

Tip: The CPT Index provides several Main Terms relating to psychiatry.

1 CPT Code _____

---

2. INPATIENT HOSPITAL   Gender: **F**   Age: **31**

Preprocedure diagnosis: **Acute renal failure**

Procedure: **Hemodialysis with two evaluations due to hypotensive episode after onset of treatment**

1 CPT Code _____

---

3. HOSPITAL SLEEP LAB   Gender: **F**   Age: **31**

Reason for encounter: **"I feel tired all the time."**

Assessment: **Insomnia**

Procedure: **Sleep study, attended by technologist, simultaneous recording of ventilation, respiratory effort, heart rate, and oxygen saturation**

Plan: **Severe obstructive sleep apnea based on interpretation of sleep study. Refer to pulmonologist for further treatment.**

(continued)

---

3. (continued)

Tip: The physician provided only the professional component of the service because the hospital provided the technical component.

1 CPT Code _____

---

4. OUTPATIENT HOSPITAL   Gender: **M**   Age: **53**

Preprocedure diagnosis: **Severe COPD**

Procedure: **Pulmonary stress test including CO_2 production, O_2 uptake, and ECG**

Plan: **Medication adjustment, RTO 6 weeks**

Tip: You did not abstract this case in Exercise 29.2, so do the abstracting before you code it. The physician provided only the professional component of the service.

1 CPT Code _____

---

5. OUTPATIENT HOSPITAL   Gender: **F**   Age: **23**

Reason for encounter: **Constant heartburn and indigestion**

Procedure: **2-hr gastroesophageal reflux test with nasal catheter intraluminal impedance electrode**

Postprocedure diagnosis: **GERD**

Tip: You did not abstract this case in Exercise 29.2, so do the abstracting before you code it. The physician provided only the professional component of the service.

1 CPT Code _____

ARRANGING CODES FOR MEDICINE PROCEDURES

Arranging codes for Medicine procedures follows general CPT sequencing rules. The first procedure code should be one of the following, based on payer requirements:

- Separate or unrelated E/M

- Procedure most related to the principal or first-listed diagnosis
- Procedure with the highest fee

Specific types of services have additional sequencing requirements, which are summarized in ■ TABLE 29-24.

Table 29-24   ■   **SEQUENCING GUIDELINES FOR MEDICINE SERVICES**

Type of Service	Sequencing Instructions
Immunizations and Immune Globulins (90281-90399, 90460-90749)	1. Unrelated E/M, when applicable
	2. Administration service
	3. Second administration service, if any
	4. First product or combination administered
	5. Second product administered, if any
Psychiatry (90785-90899)	1. E/M, when applicable
	2. Psychiatric diagnostic evaluation
	3. Psychotherapy services
Dialysis (90935-90999)	1. Inpatient ESRD services
	2. Outpatient ESRD services
Ophthalmology (92002-92499)	1. Ophthalmologic evaluation and management
	2. Special ophthalmological services
	3. Contact lens or spectacle services
Cardiovascular (92920-93799)	1. First vessel treated
	2. First "additional" branch
	3. Second "additional" branch
	4. Additional services
Allergy (95004-95199)	1. Unrelated E/M, when applicable
	2. First injection
	3. Each additional injection
Infusion and Injection (96360-96549) **Professional**	1. Initial treatment, the primary reason for the encounter
	2. Each additional hour, if applicable
	3. Initial infusion (if different than initial treatment)
	4. Concurrent infusion(s)
	5. Additional sequential infusion(s)
Infusion and Injection (96360-96549) **Facility**	1. Chemotherapy
	1.1 Infusion
	1.2 Push
	1.3 Injection
	2. Therapeutic, prophylactic, diagnostic
	2.1 Infusion
	2.2 Push
	2.3 Injection
	3. Hydration
Physical Medicine (97010-97799), Chiropractic (98925-98929), and Osteopathic (98940-98943)	*Physical therapy/rehabilitation:*
	1. Evaluation, assessment
	2. Constant attendance modalities
	3. Supervised modalities
	Chiropractic and osteopathic:
	1. Separate E/M, when applicable
	2. Number of regions treated
	3. Other physical medicine services

Source: © PB Resources, Inc. Used with permission.

Using Modifiers with Medicine Codes

Modifiers can be assigned either when assigning the code or when determining the sequencing. Sometimes the sequencing of codes dictates which ones need modifiers. Some modifiers also need to be sequenced when a code requires multiple modifiers. To streamline the presentation of material, modifiers are discussed in the section of the chapter, "Arranging Codes for Medicine Procedures." In the workplace, some modifiers can be assigned earlier in the coding process. In addition to general criteria for abstracting and assigning modifiers, services in the Medicine section should be evaluated to determine when codes require modifiers **-26, -59,** or one of the extended modifiers **-XE, -XP, -XS,** or **-XU**. Medicine section services delivered using telemedicine require modifier **-95**. Some cardiac codes require modifiers to identify the coronary arteries. Whenever an unrelated E/M service is provided on the same day as a Medicine service, apply modifier **-25 Significant, separately identifiable E/M service**. Modifier **-51 Multiple procedures** is required in some situations.

Modifier -26 Professional Component

Several, but not all, services in this section consist of both a technical and professional component. When coding for the physician, apply modifier **-26 Professional component** to report that only the professional component is provided. When coding for the facility, apply modifier **-TC Technical component** to report that only the technical component is provided. In cases where the facility also hires the medical staff, do not report either modifier, indicating that both components were provided.

Common services with both professional and technical components include:

- Cardiac catheterization
- Echocardiogram
- Electroencephalogram
- Nerve conduction studies
- Pulmonary function tests
- Reflux studies
- Sleep studies

Check the Medicare Physician Fee Schedule (MPFS) on the CMS website (**www.cms.gov**) to identify codes that have professional and technical components. Many encoders also provide this information (■ Figure 29-10). In the workplace, the billing software is usually preloaded with information about which codes have professional and technical components and which component(s) is normally provided by your company.

Modifier -59 Distinct Procedural Service

When a procedure that is normally performed as part of a larger, more extensive procedure is performed by itself, modifier **-59 Distinct procedural service** may be required to identify that the procedure performed is separate and distinct and should be paid. Payers may require one of the extended HCPCS modifiers, referred to as **-X{EPSU}** modifiers, instead of **-59** to identify why it should be considered a separate procedure:

- **-XE Separate encounter**
- **-XP Separate structure**
- **-XS Separate practitioner**
- **-XU Unusual nonoverlapping service**

Diagnostic angiography (**93454-93461**) requires modifier **-59** when performed as a separate service during the same encounter as percutaneous coronary revascularization (**92920-92944**). Special instructions before code **92920** describe when angiography can be reported with PCI. Apply modifier **-59** to the angiography code.

Modifier -95 Telemedicine Service

Telemedicine service is synchronous (real-time) use of electronic communication using interactive telecommunication equipment that includes, at a minimum, audio and video. Append modifier **-95** to the CPT code for the service when using telemedicine to perform them. A five-pointed star (★) placed in the margin to the left of the code number identifies these codes in the Tabular List. A list of eligible codes appears in a CPT appendix.

Coronary Artery Modifiers

When procedures are performed on the coronary arteries, apply a HCPCS modifier to identify the artery. The modifiers are:

-LM Left main coronary artery

-LD Left anterior descending coronary artery

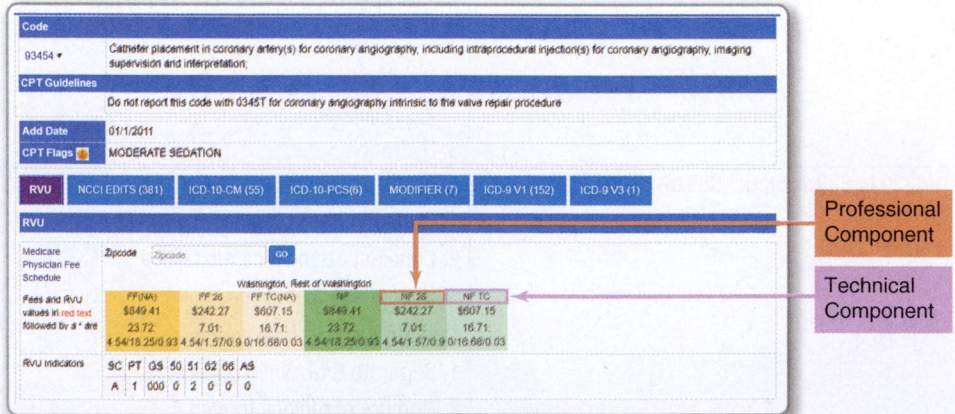

Figure 29-10 ■ Encoder screen showing professional and technical components for CPT code 93454.
Source: SpeedeCoder, Reprinted with permission.

-**LC** Left circumflex coronary artery

-**RI** Ramus intermedius coronary artery

-**RC** Right coronary artery

There are no modifiers for coronary artery branches.

Guided Example of Arranging Medicine Codes

To practice skills for arranging codes for Medical procedures, continue with the example from earlier in the chapter about the patient who was seen for cardiac therapy. Follow along in your CPT manual as Ladonna Chuck, CPC, arranges the codes. Check off each step after you complete it.

▶ Ladonna reviews the procedure codes she identified:

❏ **92928 Percutaneous transcatheter placement of intracoronary stent(s), with coronary angioplasty when performed; single major coronary artery or branch**

❏ **93454 Catheter placement in coronary artery(s) for coronary angiography, including intraprocedural injection(s) for coronary angiography, imaging supervision and interpretation**

▶ Ladonna knows that procedures should be ranked in order of descending cost on the claim.

❏ **93454** is the more extensive procedure, has the higher price, and should be sequenced first.

❏ **92928** is less extensive and should be sequenced second.

▶ Ladonna needs to determine whether modifiers are needed.

❏ She reads that modifier -**59 Distinct procedural service** is required on code **93454** to identify that the

diagnostic angiography is separate and distinct from the stent placement.

❏ Cardiac catheterization codes consist of a technical component and a professional component. Assign modifier -**26 Professional component** to indicate that the physician provided only the professional component. Sequence this as the first modifier because it affects payment.

❏ **92928** requires HCPCS modifier -**RC Right coronary artery** to identify the location of the stent.

▶ Ladonna finalizes the procedure codes and sequencing for this case:

(1) **93454-26-59 Catheter placement in coronary artery(s) for coronary angiography, including intra-procedural injection(s) for coronary angiography, imaging supervision and interpretation; -59 Distinct procedural service**

(2) **92928-RC Percutaneous transcatheter placement of intracoronary stent(s), with coronary angioplasty when performed; single major coronary artery or branch; -RC Right coronary artery**

▶ Ladonna also assigns and sequences the ICD-10-CM diagnosis codes that support the need for the service.

(1) **I25.119 Atherosclerotic heart disease of native coronary artery with unspecified angina pectoris**

(2) **I25.83 Coronary atherosclerosis due to lipid rich plaque**

CODING PRACTICE

| Exercise 29.4 | Arranging Codes for Medicine Procedures |

Instructions: Read the mini-medical-record of each patient's encounter. Review the information abstracted in Exercise 29.2 for questions 1–3. For questions 4 and 5, do the abstracting on your own. Assign CPT procedure codes using the Index and Tabular List, and arrange them correctly.

---

1. OFFICE Gender: F Age: 8

Reason for encounter: Annual preventive care checkup for established patient

Procedure: Comprehensive periodic preventive medicine examination. Updated immunizations: IM injection TdaP (diphtheria, tetanus toxoid, acellular pertussis).

(continued)

---

1. (continued)

Plan: Counseled mother regarding potential side effects and signs to be observant for. Call office with any concerns.

Tip: Code for the E/M service, vaccine administration, and vaccine products.

4 CPT Codes _____

_____

---

2. OFFICE (Physical therapy) Gender: M Age: 42

Reason for encounter: Referred by PCP for therapy for low-back strain while playing golf

Procedure: Moderate complexity physical therapy evaluation; 15 minutes of manual electrical stimulation; 15 minutes of therapeutic exercises to increase ROM and flexibility; 15 minutes of alternating hot and cold packs

(continued)

CODING PRACTICE (continued)

2. (continued)

Plan: Return 3x week for 2 weeks, per physician's order

Tip: Indicate the quantity to be reported for each modality.

4 CPT Codes _____

_____

---

3. INPATIENT HOSPITAL   Gender: M   Age: 62

Reason for admission: STEMI of LAD with thrombus

Procedure: Percutaneous transluminal revascularization during acute myocardial infarction using angiography. Stent and thrombectomy for acute total occlusion of LAD. Both diagonals show evidence of chronic subtotal occlusion. Balloon angioplasty on D1. Balloon angioplasty and atherectomy on D2.

Tip: Use a modifier to identify the coronary artery. Review the section of this chapter that discusses the coronary arteries and branches. Read the CPT special instructions about coronary artery branches and the instructional notes under the code(s) in the Tabular List.

3 CPT Codes _____

_____

---

4. OFFICE   Gender: F   Age: 32

Reason for encounter: Eye examination

Procedure: Ophthalmological examination and evaluation of established patient, intermediate; prescription and fitting of contact lens, both eyes

Assessment: Astigmatism, myopia

Tip: You did not abstract this case in Exercise 29.2, so do the abstracting before you code it. Code for the services and for supply of the product.

3 CPT Codes _____

_____

---

5. INPATIENT HOSPITAL   Gender: M   Age: 66

Preprocedure diagnosis: Single-lead pacemaker insertion for right bundle branch block

Procedure (Cardiologist): Periprocedural evaluation and programming of single-lead pacemaker before surgery. Reevaluation and parameter adjustment after surgery. Analysis, review, and report pre- and postprocedure.

Plan: FU in office 1 week

Tip: You did not abstract this case in Exercise 29.2, so do the abstracting before you code it. Read the instructional notes to determine the quantity to report. The physician provided the professional component of service.

1 CPT Code _____

_____

E/M CODING FOR MEDICINE

E/M coding for medicine services is determined by the type of examination provided. Physicians may perform a general multisystem examination or a single organ system examination, depending on the nature of the problem being addressed. This text addresses single organ system examinations within the context of each specialty.

Psychiatry is one of the few specialties in the Medicine section that does not have a counterpart in the Surgery section. The *1997 Documentation Guidelines for Evaluation and Management Services* (1997 DG), published by CMS, provides requirements for each level of a psychiatric E/M examination (■ FIGURE 29-11). To determine the appropriate E/M code, coders must review the documentation in detail and identify the specific elements documented.

- To translate the documentation into the E/M requirements for the history, refer to Chapter 28, "Evaluation and Management (E/M) Services," Tables 28-7 to 28-10, or to the 1997 DG.

- To determine the requirements for an examination, refer to Figure 29-11 or to the single organ system examination for psychiatric in the 1997 DG.

- To determine the levels for medical decision making (MDM), refer to Chapter 28, Tables 28-11 and 28-12, and to the Table of Risk in the 1997 DG.

Select the appropriate category of E/M code based on the setting in which services are provided.

- Report inpatient services E/M codes (**99221-99239**) for hospital inpatient and partial hospitalization programs.

- Report outpatient services E/M codes (**99201-99215**) for services provided in a clinic, community health center, or other outpatient facility.

- Report domiciliary/custodial care E/M codes (**99324-99337**) for services provided in a psychiatric group home or psychiatric residential treatment facility (PRTF).

- Report consultation E/M codes (**99241-99255**) for the psychiatric evaluation of a patient that includes

System/Body Area	Elements of Psychiatric Examination
Musculoskeletal	❑ Assessment of **muscle** strength and tone (e.g., flaccid, cog wheel, spastic) with notation of any atrophy and abnormal movements ❑ Examination of **gait** and station
Constitutional	❑ Measurement of any **three** of the following seven **vital** signs: • 1) sitting or standing blood pressure, • 2) supine blood pressure, • 3) pulse rate and regularity, • 4) respiration, • 5) temperature, • 6) height, • 7) weight (May be measured and recorded by ancillary staff) ❑ General **appearance** of patient (e.g., development, nutrition, body habitus, deformities, attention to grooming)
Psychiatric	❑ Description of **speech** including: rate; volume; articulation; coherence; and spontaneity with notation of abnormalities (e.g., perseveration, paucity of language) ❑ Description of **thought processes** including: rate of thoughts; content of thoughts (e.g., logical vs. illogical, tangential); abstract reasoning; and computation ❑ Description of **associations** (e.g., loose, tangential, circumstantial, intact) ❑ Description of abnormal or **psychotic thoughts** including: hallucinations; delusions; preoccupation with violence; homicidal or suicidal ideation; and obsessions ❑ Description of the patient's **judgment** (e.g., concerning everyday activities and social situations) and insight (e.g., concerning psychiatric condition) *Complete mental status examination including:* ❑ **Orientation** to time, place and person ❑ Recent and remote **memory** ❑ **Attention** span and concentration ❑ **Language** (e.g., naming objects, repeating phrases) ❑ Fund of **knowledge** (e.g., awareness of current events, past history, vocabulary) ❑ **Mood** and affect (e.g., depression, anxiety, agitation, hypomania, lability)

Total # Bullets Performed and Documented ➔	☐	# of Elements Performed and Documented	Level of Examination
		1–5	Problem focused
		6+	Expanded problem focused
		9+	Detailed
		ALL	Comprehensive (Document every element in each box with a shaded border and at least one element in each box with an unshaded border)

Figure 29-11 ■ 1997 documentation guidelines for a psychiatric examination.

examination of a patient; exchange of information with the primary physician and other parties, such as nurses or family members; and preparation of a report. Use consultation codes only for non-Medicare patients. For Medicare patients, report the appropriate outpatient or inpatient service code.

Other categories of E/M codes may also be used for psychiatric services, using the E/M definitions of each category. Prolonged services codes may not be reported with codes for psychotherapy with evaluation and management service (**90833, 90836, 90838**).

Guided Example of E/M Coding for Psychiatry

Refer to the inpatient psychiatric consultation (■ FIGURE 29-12 page 560) to practice skills for abstracting and assigning E/M codes. Follow along as fictitious coder Ladonna Shuck, CPC, abstracts the procedure. Check off each step after you complete it.

▶ First, Ladonna needs to establish the category of service so she can determine the information needed to abstract and assign the code.

❑ *What is the setting?* Inpatient hospital

❑ *What is the type of service?* The purpose of the encounter is stated as a psychiatric consultation for anxiety

❑ *What is the code range?* Ladonna refers to the CPT Index and looks up the Main Term **Consultation** and the first-level modifying term **Inpatient**. The code range listed is **99251-99255**.

❑ *How many key components are required?* Ladonna refers to the code range in the Tabular List and reads the code description of the first code, which states **Inpatient consultation for a new or established patient, which requires these 3 key components**. All codes in the category have the same requirements

INPATIENT PSYCHIATRIC CONSULTATION REPORT

HISTORY: Detailed

REASON FOR CONSULT: Anxiety.

CHIEF COMPLAINT: "I felt anxious yesterday."

Chief complaint (CC)

HPI: A 58-year-old white female with a history of metastatic breast cancer, depression, anxiety was admitted on yesterday for lightheadedness, weakness, and shortness of breath. This psychiatry consult is requested for anxiety. The patient has experienced anxiety before and had a panic attack yesterday with "syncopal episodes." She was given lorazepam 0.25 mg on a PRN basis with relief after one to two hours. The labs were reviewed and were positive for UTI. Anemia is also present. She previously responded well to trazodone for depression, poor appetite, and decreased sleep and anxiety. A low dose of clonazepam was also helpful for sedation.

MDM: Established presenting problem, worsening (Low)

HPI: Extended (4+)

ROS: Extended (2–9)

PAST MEDICAL HISTORY: Metastatic breast cancer to bone. The patient also has a history of hypertension, recurrent UTI

PFSH: Complete (3)

PAST PSYCHIATRIC HISTORY: The patient has a history of depression and anxiety. She was taking mirtazapine (*tetracyclic antidepressant*)15 mg QHS, zolpidem (*sedative*) 5 mg QHS PRN, lorazepam (*benzodiazepine antianxiety*) 0.25 mg every 6 hours PRN, and clonazepam (*benzodiazepine antianxiety*) 0.25 mg at night while she was at home.

FAMILY HISTORY: There is a family history of colorectal cancer, lung cancer, cardiac disease. Sister committed suicide 10 years ago.

SOCIAL HISTORY: The patient is married and lives at home with her husband. She has a history of smoking one pack per day for 25 years. The patient quit in 2007. The patient also drinks wine daily for the last 50 years, usually one to two drinks per day.

MEDICATIONS:
1. Clonazepam 0.25 mg PO every evening.
2. Fluconazole (*antifungal antibiotic*) 200 mg PO daily.
4. Mirtazapine 15 mg PO at bedtime.
5. Ceftriaxone (*cephalosporin antibiotic*) IV 1 g in 1/2 NS every 24 hours.

PRN MEDICATIONS:
1. Acetaminophen (*pain reliever*) 650 mg PO every 4 hours.
2. Clonazepam 0.5 mg PO every 8 hours.
3. Promethazine (*phenothiazine antipsychotic*) 12.5 mg every 4 hours.
4. Zolpidem (*sedative*) 5 mg PO at bedtime.

ALLERGIES:
Penicillin

LABORATORY DATA:
Sodium 141, potassium 4.3, glucose 95, bicarbonate 23, BUN 33, chloride 103, creatinine 1.6. RBC 3.7, WBC 35,000, hemoglobin 11.2, hematocrit 35.6, platelet count 151000. The urinalysis was positive for UTI.

MDM: Ordering or reviewing diagnostic data (Straightforward Data)

EXAMINATION: Detailed

PHYSICAL EXAMINATION:
VITALS: Sitting BP 140/90, P 80 regular, R 20. Normal muscle strength and tone. Normal gait and station

Constitutional (2)

Musculoskeletal (2)

MENTAL STATUS EXAMINATION:
ORIENTATION: Alert and oriented to person place and time. GENERAL APPEARANCE: The patient is well groomed with good hygiene. She is wearing a hospital gown and is sitting in bed during the interview. MOTOR ACTIVITY: No psychomotor retardation or agitation noted. Good eye contact. ATTITUDE: Pleasant and cooperative. ATTENTION AND CONCENTRATION: Normal. The patient does not appear to be distracted during the interview. MOOD: Okay. AFFECT: Mood congruent normal affect. THOUGHT PROCESS: Logical and goal directed. THOUGHT CONTENT: No delusions noted. PERCEPTION: Not assessed. MEMORY: Not tested. LANGUAGE: Shaky voice, stuttering. SENSORIUM: Alert. JUDGMENT: Good. INSIGHT: Good.

Psychiatric (9)

MEDICAL DECISION MAKING: Low Complexity

IMPRESSION:
1. Possibly major depression or generalized anxiety disorder.
2. Breast cancer with metastasis, anemia
3. Interpersonal stressors.
4. Difficulty in social functioning, but generally functioning pretty well and has some meaningful interpersonal relationships.

MDM: One or more chronic illnesses with mild exacerbation. Prescription drug management. (Moderate Risk)

ASSESSMENT AND PLAN:
1. Continue mirtazapine 15 mg PO at bedtime and clonazepam 0.25 mg PO at bedtime. 2. Clonazepam 0.5 mg PO on a PRN basis for panic attacks. 3. Supportive psychotherapy for anxiety.

KEY: HPI History of the present illness ROS Review of systems
PFSH Past, family, and social history MDM Medical decision making

Figure 29-12 ■ Psychiatric encounter. *Source: © PB Resources, Inc. Used with permission.*

for key components. This tells her that all three key components must meet or exceed the levels listed in the code (3/3).

▶ Next, Ladonna identifies the level of history.

❏ *What is the level of HPI?* The HPI is **extended** because four or more elements are documented

❏ *What is the level of ROS?* The ROS is **extended** because two to nine systems are documented

❏ *What is the level of PFSH?* The PFSH is **complete** because three elements are documented

❏ *Based on these factors, what is the overall level of history?* The level of history is **detailed** because the lowest of the three factors (HPI, ROS, and PFSH) determines the history level. The extended HPI and complete PFSH qualify for a comprehensive history, but the extended ROS qualifies for only a detailed history.

▶ Ladonna refers to the psychiatric examination in the 1997 DG (Figure 29-11) to abstract information needed to determine the level of examination.

❏ *What is the level of examination?* The level of examination is **detailed**. Thirteen (13) elements of the examination are documented, which exceeds the requirement of nine or more bulleted elements for a detailed examination. A comprehensive examination requires that all bulleted items be documented, which they are not.

▶ Ladonna determines the level of medical decision making. (Refer to Table 28-12, Medical Decision-Making Levels.)

❏ *What is the level of complexity of the number of diagnoses or management options, based on the presenting problem?* The level is **Low** because there is an established presenting problem that is worsening

❏ *What is the amount and/or complexity of data to be reviewed?* The level is **Straightforward** because the physician reviewed the patient's laboratory results

❏ *What is the level of risk of significant complications, morbidity, and/or mortality?* Ladonna reviews each column in the Table of Risk in the 1997 DG and determines that the level of risk is **Moderate**. The patient presents with one or more chronic illness with mild exacerbation (Moderate), clinical labs are reviewed but not ordered, and prescription drug management is required (Moderate). The single highest element in the Table of Risk determines the overall risk. The column **Management options selected** is the highest level (Moderate).

❏ *Based on these factors, what is the overall level of medical decision making?* The medical decision making is **Low complexity**. At least two of the three MDM factors are required to qualify for a specific level of MDM. Two of the three MDM factors meet or exceed **Low complexity** decision making.

▶ Now Ladonna is ready to assign the code for the inpatient psychiatric consultation. The exercise that follows guides you through additional abstracting skills and allows you to assign the correct code.

CODING PRACTICE

Exercise 29.5 **E/M Coding for Medicine**

Instructions: Refer to the *1997 Documentation Guidelines for Evaluation and Management Services* (available at **www.cms.gov**) or Chapter 28, "Evaluation and Management Services" (Tables 28-7 to 28-12), in this text. Answer the following questions about the "Psychiatric encounter" (Figure 29-12).

1. a. Which elements of the HPI are documented? Circle all that apply. Location, Quality, Severity, Duration, Timing, Context, Modifying factors, Associated signs and symptoms

   b. How many elements are documented? _____

   c. What is the level of HPI? _____

2. a. Which systems are reviewed in the ROS? Circle all that apply. Constitutional, Allergic/immunologic, CV, Endocrine, ENT/M, Eyes, GI, GU, Hemic/lymphatic, MS, Neurologic, Psychiatric, Respiratory, Skin/breast

   b. How many systems are documented? _____

   c. What is the level of ROS? _____

3. a. Which PFSH elements are documented? Circle all that apply. Past medical, Family, Social

   b. What is the level of PFSH? _____

   c. What is the overall level of history? (The lowest history factor—HPI, ROS, or PFSH—determines the level of history.)

   _____

4. Refer to Figure 29-11 (1997 DG for Psychiatric Examination).

   a. Which bulleted items are documented for the examination? (Check off the bulleted items documented.)

   b. How many bulleted items are documented? _____

   c. What is the level of the examination? _____

5. Refer to Table 28-12, Medical Decision-Making Levels, or the 1997 DG.

   a. What is the MDM level for the number of diagnoses or management options? _____

   b. What is the MDM level for the amount and/or complexity of data to be reviewed? _____

(continued)

CODING PRACTICE (continued)

c. Refer to the Table of Risk in the 1997 DG. Which elements of risk are documented for each risk factor?

1. Presenting problem: _____

2. Diagnostic procedures ordered: _____

3. Management options selected: _____

d. What is the level of risk? _____

e. What is the overall level of MDM? (2/3 MDM factors are needed to determine the overall level.) _____

6. a. What is the setting? _____

b. What is the type of service? _____

c. What is the code range? _____

d. How many key components are required? _____

e. What is the level of history? _____

f. What is the level of examination? _____

g. What is the level of medical decision making? _____

h. What is the correct code for the inpatient psychiatric consultation? _____

7. Abstract, assign, and arrange (sequence) the diagnosis code(s) that support the E/M code.

ICD-10-CM Code(s) _____

CHAPTER SUMMARY

In this chapter you learned that:

- Diagnostic techniques classified in the Medicine section include an assessment or evaluation, an examination, or the use of equipment or tools to make a recording or measurement or conduct a function study.

- Therapeutic procedures classified in the Medicine section include physical, pharmacologic, immunologic, mechanical, and mental techniques.

- Medical terms for medical procedures combine roots for various organs or anatomic sites with prefixes and suffixes to create a term that describes a specific service or procedure.

- The CPT section for Medicine procedures contains 34 subsections, divided by the type of procedure, and reports noninvasive and minimally invasive procedures from a wide variety of medical specialties that are not appropriate for the Surgery section.

- Each Medicine subsection has its own abstracting rules; some subsections require multiple sets of abstracting criteria for different types of procedures.

- Coders must be certain to thoroughly read the guidelines, special instructions, and instructional notes that appear throughout the Medicine section to guide them when assigning codes.

- Arranging codes for Medicine procedures follows general CPT sequencing rules.

- To provide E/M services for Medicine procedures, physicians may perform a general multisystem examination or a single organ system examination, depending on the nature of the problem being addressed.

CONCEPT QUIZ

Take a moment to look back at the Medicine section and solidify your skills. Try to answer the questions from memory first. Then, refer to the discussion in this chapter if you need a little extra help.

Completion

Instructions: Write the term that completes each statement based on the information you learned in this chapter. Choose from the list below. Some choices may be used more than once and some choices may not be used at all.

anesthesia

antigen

arrhythmia induction

cardioversion

chiropractor

ECT

EKG

EMG

EPS

immune globulin

immunization

mapping

medicine

nephrology

osteopathic physician

physical therapist

plethysmography

polysomnography

psychiatry

1. A(n) _____ is administered as a preventive measure in patients who do not currently have, and have not been recently exposed to, a disease.

2. A(n) _____ is any natural or artificial substance that produces an immune response.

3. _____ is used to treat arrhythmias such as atrial fibrillation.

4. _____ includes invasive diagnostic tests that assess the electrical activity in the heart.

5. A(n) _____ focuses on improving patients' conditions by manipulating body areas, typically the spine, to improve the structure and function of specific sites.

6. _____ is a recording of volume.

7. _____ is one of the few specialties in the Medicine section that does not have a counterpart in the Surgery section.

8. _____ is used to treat conditions such as depression when medications and psychotherapy fail.

9. _____ is the recording of the electrical activity of a muscle.

10. _____ is the recording of the site of origin of tachycardia or its electrical path through the heart.

Multiple Choice

Instructions: Circle the letter of the best answer to each question based on the information you learned in this chapter.

1. What physician specialist provides E/M and supervisory services for dialysis?
   A. Nephrologist
   B. Neurologist
   C. Gastroenterologist
   D. Oncologist

2. What type of immunity occurs when the body's immune system receives antibodies to fight off a disease?
   A. Artificial active
   B. Artificial passive
   C. Natural active
   D. Natural passive

3. Which modifier should a physician report to identify that only the professional component of a service was provided?
   A. -59
   B. -52
   C. -PC
   D. -26

4. What test records the electrical activity of the brain?
   A. ECC
   B. EEG
   C. EKG
   D. EMG

5. What modifier identifies the left main coronary artery?
   A. -LC
   B. -LA
   C. -LM
   D. -LT

6. For what type of service does Medicare require radiographic evidence to be eligible for coverage?
   A. Cardiac catheterization
   B. Physical therapy
   C. Dialysis
   D. Chiropractic manipulation

7. What type of procedure is performed for revascularization?
   A. PCI
   B. ECG
   C. TCD
   D. EPS

8. What type of procedure enables physicians to visualize vessels to guide catheter placement for diagnostic or therapeutic cardiac procedures?
   A. Angiography
   B. Echocardiography
   C. Intracardiac electrophysiological studies
   D. Cardiac catheterization

9. How would you code the following scenario? *A 14 year old girl receives two immunizations: an intramuscular Tdap and a subcutaneous Meningococcal polysaccharide vaccine. Counseling regarding side effects is provided to her mother.*
   A. 90460
   B. 90460, 90715, 90733
   C. 90715, 90733
   D. 90460, 90461, 90715, 90733

10. How would you code the following scenario? *The surgeon performs a percutaneous transluminal placement of an intracoronary stent with coronary angioplasty on the LAD coronary artery of an 81 year old.*
    A. 92920-LD
    B. 92924-LD
    C. 92928-LD
    D. 92943-LD

KEEP ON CODING

Instructions: Read the procedural statement, then use the Index and Tabular List to assign and sequence CPT procedure codes. Provide the correct quantity of each CPT code with more than one unit of service. Write the code(s) on the line provided.

1. IM injection for rabies human immune globulin. CPT Code(s) _____

2. Routine EKG with 12 leads. CPT Code(s) _____

3. Individual psychotherapy, 30 minutes. CPT Code(s) _____

4. Peritoneal dialysis with one evaluation by physician. CPT Code(s) _____

5. Bilateral computerized corneal topography with interpretation and report. CPT Code(s) _____

6. Color vision exam to test for color blindness. CPT Code(s) _____

7. Impedance tympanometry. CPT Code(s) _____

8. 30 minutes of acupuncture with 11 needles without electrical stimulation, with reinsertion of needles. CPT Code(s) _____

9. Scratch tests, five trees. CPT Code(s) _____

10. 45 minutes of moderate sedation by dentist for 5-year-old patient, with a trained observer to assist in monitoring. CPT Code(s) _____

11. EEG, awake and asleep, supervision, interpretation, and report. CPT Code(s) _____

12. Chemotherapy administration via IV infusion, push technique. CPT Code(s) _____

13. Professional service for gastroesophageal reflux test. CPT Code(s) _____

14. PUVA photochemotherapy. CPT Code(s) _____

15. Gait and stairs retraining, 40 minutes. CPT Code(s) _____

16. CPAP. CPT Code(s) _____

17. Psychoanalysis via telemedicine. CPT Code(s) _____

18. Chiropractic treatment, three areas of spine. CPT Code(s) _____

19. Colon motility study. CPT Code(s) _____

20. Spirometry. CPT Code(s) _____

21. Comprehensive eye exam, new patient. CPT Code(s) _____

22. IM injection of hepatitis B and 4-type HPV vaccines. CPT Code(s) _____

23. Complete bilateral study of extracranial arteries using a duplex scan. CPT Code(s) _____

24. Electronic analysis of dual lead pacemaker system. CPT Code(s) _____

25. Catheterization of right heart with measurement of oxygen saturation (professional service only). CPT Code(s) _____

CODING CHALLENGE

Instructions: Read the mini-medical-record of each patient's encounter, then abstract, assign, and arrange ICD-10-CM and CPT codes using the Index and Tabular List. Provide the correct quantity of each CPT code with more than one unit of service. Write the codes on the lines provided.

1. OUTPATIENT HOSPITAL   Gender: F   Age: 63

Reason for encounter: Intermittent chest pain

Assessment: Unspecified chest pain

(continued)

1. (continued)

Procedure: Left heart catheterization via femoral artery. I moved catheter to right and left coronary arteries during angiography. No blockage or defects noted.

1 ICD-10-CM Code _____

1 CPT Code _____

2. EMERGENCY DEPARTMENT   Gender: M   Age: 23

Reason for encounter: Patient presents with dry mouth, dry skin, minimal output during past 24 hours

Assessment: Dehydration

Procedure: IV fluids for 24 hours

Plan: No work for 24 hours, increase fluids, follow up with PCP

1 ICD-10-CM Code _____

2 CPT Codes _____

3. OUTPATIENT HOSPITAL   Gender: M   Age: 17

Reason for encounter: Family history of stroke; patient needs clearance to play basketball

Procedure: Transthoracic echocardiogram

2 ICD-10-CM Codes _____

1 CPT Code _____

4. OFFICE   Gender: F   Age: 72

Reason for encounter: Hearing aid check

Assessment: Patient has sensorineural hearing loss and wears hearing aids in both ears

Procedure: Inspection and cleaning of both hearing aids, replaced batteries

1 ICD-10-CM Code _____

1 CPT Code _____

5. OFFICE   Gender: M   Age: 85

Reason for encounter: Recheck of open-angle glaucoma

Procedure: Comprehensive ophthalmologic examination

1 ICD-10-CM Code _____

1 CPT Code _____

6. OFFICE   Gender: M   Age: 48

Reason for encounter: Pain in the right hip

Procedure: Chiropractic manipulation of the lumbar and sacroiliac spinal regions

Plan: Return to clinic in two days

1 ICD-10-CM Code _____

1 CPT Code _____

7. OUTPATIENT HOSPITAL   Gender: F   Age: 36

Reason for encounter: Chemotherapy needed for cancer of left breast that has metastasized to the spinal column

Procedure: Chemotherapy infusion administered intravenously for 90 minutes

3 ICD-10-CM Codes _____

_____

2 CPT Codes _____

8. HOME   Gender: F   Age: 58

Reason for encounter: Acute osteomyelitis of the left ankle. Patient is completing IV antibiotics at home.

Procedure: Administration of antibiotic infusion for 4 hours

Plan: I will return tomorrow to administer another dose of antibiotic.

1 ICD-10-CM Code _____

2 CPT Codes _____

9. OFFICE   Gender: M   Age: 13

Reason for encounter: Patient's mother requests allergy testing due to constant sneezing

Procedure: Percutaneous tests using 10 allergen extracts, with immediate type reaction

Plan: Tests indicate patient is allergic to animal dander. Patient should avoid close contact with animals.

1 ICD-10-CM Code _____

1 CPT Code _____

10. OUTPATIENT HOSPITAL   Gender: F   Age: 45

Reason for encounter: Patient has asthma. Lately, she has been wheezing and having difficulty catching her breath.

Procedure: Conducted vital capacity test

Plan: Rx for rescue inhaler, continue with steroids to manage asthma.

1 ICD-10-CM Code _____

1 CPT Code _____

Chapter 30

Overview of Surgery Coding (10004-10021)

Chapter Outline

- **Surgery Basics**
- **Coding Guidelines for the Surgery Section**
- **Abstracting Surgery Section Procedures**
- **Assigning Surgery Codes**
- **Arranging Surgery Codes**
- **Surgery: General Subsection (10004-10021)**

Learning Objectives

After completing this chapter, you should have the skills to:

30.1 Spell and define the key words, medical terms, and abbreviations related to procedures in the Surgery section. (Remember)

30.2 Summarize the fundamentals of surgical services. (Understand)

30.3 Adhere to CPT coding guidelines for the Surgery section. (Apply)

30.4 Examine and abstract procedural information from the medical record for coding Surgery section procedures. (Analyze)

30.5 Demonstrate how to assign codes for procedures in the Surgery section. (Apply)

30.6 Utilize guidelines for arranging (sequencing) codes for Surgery section procedures. (Apply)

Key Terms and Abbreviations

Column 1	global period	National Correct Coding Initiative (NCCI)	prepayment edit
Column 2	incision site		screening procedure
CPT surgical package	integral component	operative report	surgical approach
diagnostic procedure	Medicare global surgical package	optional surgery	surgical destruction
elective surgery	Medicare Physician Fee Schedule (MPFS)	position (patient)	surgical facility
emergency surgery		preauthorization	therapeutic procedure
fine-needle aspiration biopsy (FNAB, FNA, NAB)	Medicare Physician Fee Schedule Database (MPFSDB)		

In addition to the key terms listed here, students should know the terms defined within tables in this chapter.

INTRODUCTION

When making a purchase, you always take a few minutes to read the details of what items are included in the package and what you might need to purchase separately.

Surgical procedures are also defined as a package that includes certain services, all of which are covered in the reimbursement. Services not part of the package can be coded and billed separately. In this chapter you learn about the basics of surgery and how to abstract, assign, and arrange codes for surgical procedures. You also learn about the General subsection of Surgery. In later chapters, you learn the details of coding for surgery for each body system. You also learn how to code anesthesia services, which CPT classifies separate from surgery.

SURGERY BASICS

Surgery is the branch of medicine that treats diseases, injuries, and deformities through the use of instruments or manual techniques. A surgical procedure is a combination of a surgical method and an anatomic site. Any given method, such as incision or ablation, can be performed on many different anatomic sites.

The words *operation* and *procedure* are sometimes used interchangeably and sometimes used to indicate how invasive the procedure is. The word *operation* implies that the treatment requires the physician to create an incision. The word *procedure* can refer to an operation, but it is also used to describe treatments performed without breaking the skin, such as an endoscopy. Surgeons are physicians with advanced training in surgical methods related to a specific organ system or body region. Some surgeons specialize in a specific technique or a specific anatomic site within an organ system. For example, ophthalmologists can specialize in treating either the cornea or the retina. Heart surgeons can specialize in neonates, children, or adults and in specific sites, such as the heart valves or the front portion of the eye.

The following sections discuss the various ways that surgical procedures are classified, medical terminology for surgery, and how a surgical facility operates.

Classifications of Surgery

Surgery can be classified according to many criteria, depending on the aspect of the procedure being discussed. Four common classifications are based on method, anatomic site, urgency, and purpose.

Method

Surgery can be performed in different ways, depending on the nature of the problem being treated. The method identifies how the procedure is performed. ■ TABLE 30-1 provides the names and definitions of many common surgical methods. The same method can be performed on a variety of anatomic sites.

Anatomic Site

Anatomic site identifies the site(s) where the procedure is performed and refers not only to the organ or structure, but the specific location within the organ or structure. For example, a heart procedure is not described simply as "heart surgery" but rather "repair of the mitral valve" of the heart. Coders must also be aware of terms that relate to more than one anatomic site and identify which one the surgeon is operating on. For example, a *cervix* or *neck* occurs in several sites: the spine, the uterus, and the urinary bladder. *Bicep* refers to a muscle with two heads and could identify the *bicep brachii* in the arm or the *bicep femoris* in the leg. It is important to read operative notes carefully and identify the exact location. You also must follow the terms in the Index carefully to be sure you select the correct location. If you are unsure about an anatomic site, look it up in your reference materials.

Urgency

The classification of the urgency of surgery identifies how quickly a procedure must be performed. Surgery can be emergency, elective, or optional.

- **Emergency surgery** must be performed immediately to save a life or prevent a disability, such as loss of a limb. Examples are surgery to stop bleeding following an accident or surgery to prevent the spread of an infection, as may occur with a gangrenous appendix or necrotizing fasciitis.

- **Elective surgery** is nonemergency surgery that is medically necessary but can be delayed at least 24 hours. Some elective procedures are necessary to prolong life, such as an angioplasty or a coronary artery bypass. Others improve the quality of life, such as cataract surgery or a joint replacement.

- **Optional surgery** provides a personal benefit but provides no medical benefit, such as a cosmetic face lift or breast augmentation, and is rarely covered by insurance.

CPT does not provide modifiers or supplemental codes to identify the urgency of the procedure as emergency, elective, or optional.

Many payers require **preauthorization** or prior authorization of elective surgery. The preauthorization process determines whether the planned procedure is covered under the patient's policy and considered medically necessary by the payer. In general, the physician's office submits a preauthorization request to the payer before the procedure is performed, but the patient is ultimately responsible to ensure that the preauthorization is obtained. Payers provide a preauthorization letter or reference number to be submitted with the claim. Obtaining preauthorization does not guarantee payment. Payment is determined based on the actual claim submitted. Although emergency surgery cannot be preauthorized, most payers require that they be notified soon after it occurs, usually within 24–72 hours.

Purpose

A surgical procedure can be performed for any of three purposes: screening, diagnosis, or therapy.

- A **screening procedure** is performed to determine whether an abnormality exists in a person showing no signs or symptoms of disease. A common example is a screening colonoscopy, which is recommended to be performed every 10 years to detect early signs of malignancy.

Table 30-1 ■ **COMMON SURGICAL METHODS**

Method*	CPT Definition
Ablation	Separating, detaching, or destroying
Amputation	Cutting off all or a portion of a body part, such as a leg or arm
Anastomosis	Joining two structures that are not normally joined together
Biopsy	Removing skin, tissue, muscle, or bone to test for the presence of disease
Closure	Closing an open wound with stitches, staples, or other mechanism
Debridement	Cleaning out an area using various methods, such as scraping or irrigation, to remove contaminated or necrotic tissue
Decompression	Removing pressure
Destruction	Reducing to tiny fragments
Dilation/dilatation	Expanding or stretching an opening
Drainage	Removing fluids
Endoscopy	Viewing a body cavity using a long, narrow, hollow instrument that has a light and a camera
Excision	Cutting out all or part of an organ or tissue; sometimes used synonymously with resection
Exploration	Examining an organ or structure to determine a diagnosis
Fusion/arthrodesis	Joining together two or more bones, joints, or vertebrae
Graft	Attaching a piece of skin, fascia, muscle, or bone from one area of the body to another
Incision	Cutting with a sharp instrument
Incision and drainage (I&D)	Cutting into and releasing fluid
Injection	Forcing a fluid or other substance into a cavity, tissue, or vessel
Introduction/insertion	Putting something in place
Laparotomy	Cutting into the abdominal cavity
Ligation	Tying off using any substance, such as cotton, silk, or wire
Manipulation/reduction	Using force to move a bone
Reconstruction	Restoring or reforming a part of the body
Removal	Taking something out
Repair	Restoring damaged or diseased tissues to normal function
Resection	Removing all or part of a structure or organ; sometimes used synonymously with excision
Revision	Repairing or replacing work performed during a previous procedure
Suture	Closing a wound with stitches
Transplant	Replacing an organ or tissue with an organ or tissue from a donor

*The procedures in this table apply to CPT coding. Definitions vary from those for ICD-10-PCS Root Operations.

- A **diagnostic procedure**, or exploratory procedure, is performed to identify a suspected abnormality. An example is diagnostic colonoscopy performed to detect the cause of bleeding or to collect a specimen.

- A **therapeutic procedure** is performed to treat a condition. An example is therapeutic colonoscopy performed to remove polyps or control bleeding.

The physician performs the procedure in the same way, regardless of the purpose, except that in a therapeutic procedure additional steps may be performed to treat the problem. A diagnosis code always identifies the reason the procedure was performed. CPT does not provide modifiers or supplemental codes to identify the purpose of the procedure as screening, diagnostic, or therapeutic. For some procedures, CPT provides separate codes for screening, diagnosis, and/or treatment.

Procedures that qualify as a preventive care service under the Patient Protection and Affordable Care Act (PPACA) require modifier **-33 Preventive services** if the CPT code description does not identify the procedure as a screening or preventive in nature. A screening colonoscopy is an example.

When a procedure that is begun as screening or diagnostic becomes a therapeutic procedure during the operative session, the procedure should be coded as therapeutic if a separate code is provided. Do not assign an additional code for the diagnostic procedure performed at the same time using the same method.

Medical Terminology Used in Surgery

Medical terminology skills are essential to CPT coding. Physicians document using medical terms to identify surgical methods and anatomic sites. The CPT manual uses medical terms to classify procedures. Coders must be able to interpret unfamiliar medical terms by breaking them into the components of root, suffix, and prefix.

Medical terms for surgery combine the word roots for anatomic sites with suffixes that identify the type of procedure or methods. When analyzing an unfamiliar medical term, first identify the suffix, then identify the word root(s) for the anatomic site(s) and the prefix. Refer back to Table 25-1, "Medical Term Suffixes That Describe Procedures," to review suffixes commonly used for surgical procedures. ■ TABLE 30-2 provides a refresher on how to build medical terms using surgical suffixes. Be sure to keep immediate access to an online and hardcopy medical dictionary and medical terminology text.

CODING CAUTION

Be alert for medical suffixes that are spelled similarly and have different meanings.

-**desis** (*fusion*) and -**centesis** (*drainage*)

-**tomy** (*cutting into*) and -**stomy** (*surgical creation of an opening*)

The Surgical Facility

The **surgical facility** is the setting or location in which surgery is performed. The choice of the facility is determined by the type of procedure to be performed, patient condition and risk factors, availability, and surgeon preference. Common sites of surgery and an example of the type of procedure performed include:

- Office—Example: destruction of skin lesions
- Ambulatory surgery center (ASC)—Example: arthroscopic joint surgery
- Outpatient hospital procedure room—Example: screening or diagnostic colonoscopy
- Outpatient hospital operating room (OR)—Example: arthroscopic joint surgery
- Bedside in the inpatient hospital room—Example: wound debridement
- Inpatient operating room (OR)—Example: heart bypass, hip replacement

Physicians bill for providing the professional service of performing the surgical procedure. The facility bills for the use of the facility, supplies, and staff.

Facility Billing

The facility provides the operating room, the staff, and the instruments, drugs, and supplies used during the procedure. The facility charges an operating room fee that includes use of the room and staff. Other charges are itemized then consolidated into revenue codes (*four-digit accounting codes that summarize inpatient hospital cost center [department] charges*). For Medicare inpatients, the operating room costs are paid under the Medicare Severity-Adjusted Diagnosis Related Group (MS-DRG), a predetermined, all-inclusive amount for the inpatient admission based on the patient's diagnosis and procedure. Facility services provided to Medicare patients at an ambulatory surgery center are paid under the ambulatory payment classification (APC), a predetermined, all-inclusive amount for the outpatient procedure based on the patient's diagnosis and procedure. Private payers might use MS-DRGs and APCs but substitute their own reimbursement amounts, modify the Medicare systems, or create their own methodology, such as a per diem (*daily*) payment rate.

SUCCESS STEP

Inpatient hospitals bill procedures using ICD-10-PCS codes. All other facility locations are outpatient and bill using CPT codes.

Facility Staff

Except for minor procedures performed in the office or at the patient's bedside, surgery requires staff in addition to the surgeon. An anesthesia provider—either an anesthesiologist, certified registered nurse anesthetist (CRNA), or anesthesia assistant (AA)—administers most types of anesthesia other than local, topical, or a nerve block to the hand or foot. Types of anesthesia are discussed in detail in Chapter 31 of this text. Anesthesiologists typically belong to a medical group practice that contracts with the facility to provide anesthesia services. The group practice is responsible to code and bill for the services of

---

Table 30-2 ■ **EXAMPLES OF CONSTRUCTING MEDICAL TERMS FOR SURGERY**

Combining Form	Suffix	Complete Medical Term
nephr/o (*kidney*)		**nephr + ectomy** (*surgical removal of the kidney*)
		nephro + rraphy (*suture of the kidney*)
	-**ectomy** (*surgical removal*)	**nephro + plasty** (*surgical repair of the kidney*)
	-**rraphy** (*suture*)	**nephro + scopy** (*visual examination of the kidney with an endoscope*)
gastr/o (*stomach*)	-**plasty** (*surgical repair*)	**gastr + ectomy** (*surgical removal of the stomach*)
	-**scopy** (*visual examination*)	**gastro + rraphy** (*suture of the stomach*)
		gastro + plasty (*surgical repair of the stomach*)
		gastro + scopy (*visual examination of the stomach*)

Source: © PB Resources, Inc. Used with permission.

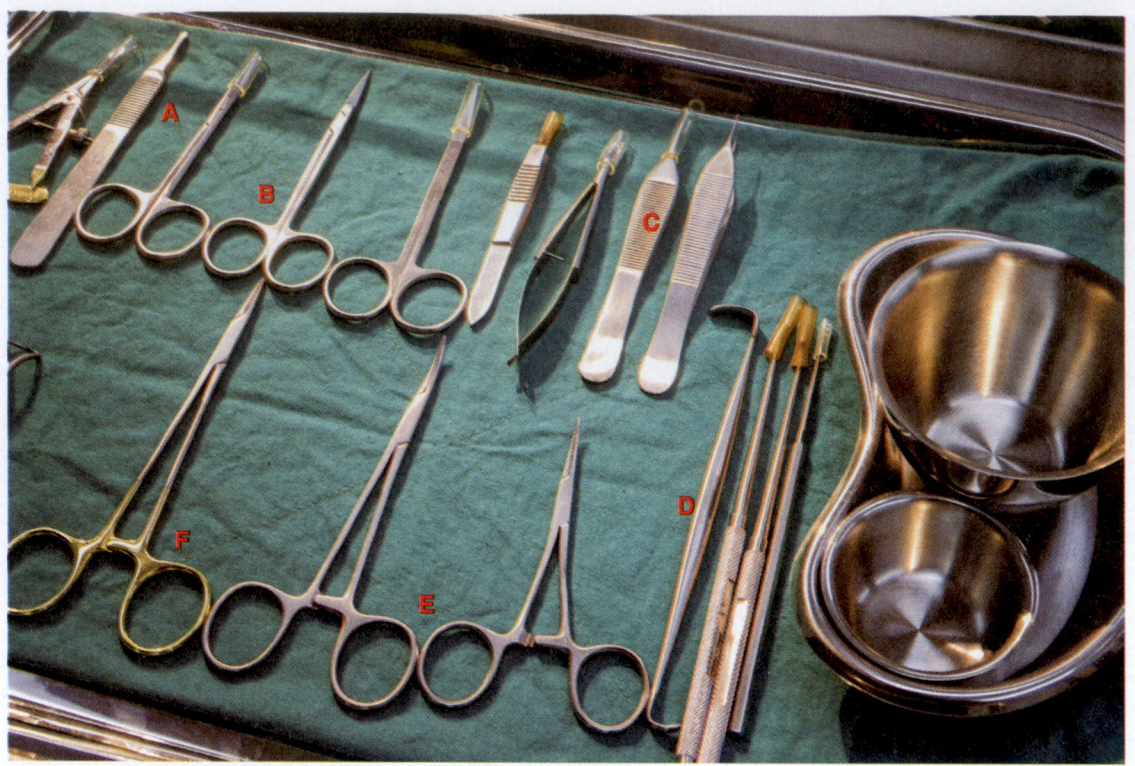

Figure 30-1 ■ Typical general surgery instruments: (A) Scalpel (B) Scissors (C) Forceps (D) Retractor. (E) Hemostats/locking forceps (F) Needle holder.

the anesthesia providers, although this task can be outsourced to a medical billing service or the hospital billing department.

The operating room staff consists of a scrub and a circulator. The scrub is a nurse or surgical technician who adopts a sterile state (*washing hands and forearms in the prescribed manner and wearing a sterile surgical gown, gloves, mask, and hair covering*), prepares the table or tray of sterile supplies and instruments (■ FIGURE 30-1), passes instruments and supplies to the surgeon, and assists the surgeon by holding retractors or anatomic sites as requested. Some surgeons provide their own scrub so they can work with the same person all the time—someone who is familiar with their operating techniques and preferences. The circulator, required to be a registered nurse (RN) in most states, is responsible for the overall nursing care, maintains safety, transfers the patient into and out of the operating room, and assists in positioning the patient and preparing the surgical site.

Variations occur for minor procedures, which do not always require a full operating room setup or a scrub and circulator, and for more extensive procedures, which can require a team of multiple surgeons, additional operating room staff, or special equipment.

CODING PRACTICE

Exercise 30.1   **Surgery Basics**

Instructions: Use your medical terminology skills and resources to define the following procedures, then identify the applicable code or code range. Follow these steps.

- Use slash marks "/" to break down the underlined term into its root(s) and suffix.
- Define the meaning of the underlined word based on the meaning of each word part.
- Use the entire phrase to identify the code or code range shown in the CPT Index.

Example: arthroplasty, ankle arthro/plasty   Meaning <u>*surgical repair of a joint*</u>   CPT Code(s) <u>27700-27703</u>

1. <u>cystourethroscopy</u> with brush biopsy   Meaning _____   CPT Code(s) _____

2. posterior <u>colporrhaphy</u>   Meaning _____   CPT Code(s) _____

(continued)

3. <u>ureterocalycostomy</u> Meaning _____ CPT Code(s) _____

4. <u>tenotomy</u>, elbow Meaning _____ CPT Code(s) _____

5. <u>hemorrhoidopexy</u> by stapling Meaning _____ CPT Code(s) _____

6. diagnostic <u>amniocentesis</u> Meaning _____ CPT Code(s) _____

7. partial <u>adrenalectomy</u> Meaning _____ CPT Code(s) _____

8. penetrating <u>keratoplasty</u> Meaning _____ CPT Code(s) _____

9. intrapleural <u>pneumonolysis</u> Meaning _____ CPT Code(s) _____

10. subtalar <u>arthrodesis</u> Meaning _____ CPT Code(s) _____

CODING GUIDELINES FOR THE SURGERY SECTION

Coders should understand the organization of this CPT section, section guidelines, and instructional notes in the Tabular List. This information is necessary for accurate coding.

The CPT **Surgery (10004-69990)** section contains 19 subsections divided by body system. Each subsection is further divided into subheadings and categories by type of procedure and anatomic site. Review the subsection names and code ranges in ■ TABLE 30-3 to become familiar with the content and organization.

Table 30-3 ■ SURGERY SUBSECTIONS

Subsection Name	Code Range
General	10004-10021
Integumentary System	10030-19499
Musculoskeletal System	20100-29999
Respiratory System	30000-32999
Cardiovascular System	33010-37799
Hemic and Lymphatic Systems	38100-38999
Mediastinum and Diaphragm	39000-39599
Digestive System	40490-49999
Urinary System	50010-53899
Male Genital System	54000-55899
Reproductive System Procedures	55920
Intersex Surgery	55970-55980
Female Genital System	56405-58999
Maternity Care and Delivery	59000-59899
Endocrine System	60000-60699
Nervous System	61000-64999
Eye and Ocular Adnexa	65091-68899
Auditory System	69000-69979
Operating Microscope	69990

Surgery section guidelines appear in the CPT manual at the beginning of the Surgery section, before the list of codes. The guidelines provide general information that applies to all codes in this section, including the definition of the **CPT surgical package**, which identifies services in addition to the operative procedure included in the procedure code. These services cannot be billed separately.

The guidelines list codes for unlisted services or procedures for the subsections and subheadings within the Surgery section. When a physician performs a unique, experimental, or new procedure not represented by a CPT Category I or Category III code, assign the corresponding code for an unlisted procedure. Submit a report with the claim that describes the service provided, including the nature of, extent of, and need for the procedure, as well as the time, effort, and equipment required.

The guidelines provide information about coding for **surgical destruction**, also called *lysis*. Destruction is the obliteration of tissue using electrosurgery, cryosurgery, laser, or chemical treatment. It is part of a surgical procedure and should not be coded separately unless the destruction technique substantially alters the standard management of a problem or condition.

The guidelines discuss CPT codes that carry the instructional note (**separate procedure**). This note identifies a procedure that sometimes is performed by itself and sometimes is part of a more extensive procedure. Assign the code for the separate procedure only when it is performed alone or is not bundled into the main procedure (■ FIGURE 30-2, page 572). When it is performed with a more extensive procedure that includes the service identified as the separate procedure, only assign a code for the more extensive procedure (■ FIGURE 30-3, page 572).

Special instructions that pertain to specific groups of codes appear at the beginning of subsections, subheadings, and categories throughout the Surgery section. Instructional notes providing further information on the use of specific codes appear in the Tabular List. Specific guidelines and instructional notes are discussed throughout this chapter of the text.

All surgical codes must be supported by the appropriate ICD-10-CM diagnosis codes that identify the reason(s) the procedure is performed.

The surgeon performs a bilateral pelvic lymphadenectomy on a patient with bladder cancer, to determine whether it has metastasized to the lymph nodes.

C67.9 Malignant neoplasm of bladder, unspecified
38770–50 Pelvic lymphadenectomy, including external iliac, hypogastric, and obturator nodes (separate procedure); –50 Bilateral procedure

Figure 30-2 ■ Example of coding a separate procedure.

The surgeon performs a complete cystectomy with a bilateral pelvic lymphadenectomy on a patient with bladder cancer with metastases to the pelvic lymph nodes.

C67.9 Malignant neoplasm of bladder, unspecified
C77.5 Secondary and unspecified malignant neoplasm of intrapelvic lymph nodes
51575 Cystectomy, complete; with bilateral pelvic lymphadenectomy, including external iliac, hypogastric, and obturator nodes

Figure 30-3 ■ Example of a separate procedure included in a more extensive procedure.

ABSTRACTING SURGERY SECTION PROCEDURES

The details of abstracting for surgery are provided for each body system in subsequent chapters of this text. Also refer to Table 25-8, Key Criteria for Abstracting Procedures (General Guidelines). The discussion that follows provides information about the nature of surgery that aids in determining which details must be abstracted.

A surgical procedure has several **integral components**, tasks that are part of the intraoperative service and are not coded or billed separately (■ TABLE 30-4). Coders must be familiar with these components and should not attempt to assign separate codes.

Three components that can be especially helpful to the coder in understanding the procedure are the patient position, surgical approach, and incision site. This information helps to identify certain details that can affect the choice of codes.

Patient Position

Patients must be arranged in a particular **position** that enables the surgeon to best access the operative site. Proper positioning of the patient helps prevent injury from loss of circulation, impaired respiration, or diminished skin integrity. The position of the patient (■ FIGURE 30-4) is not coded but can help determine whether an anterior or posterior approach is used in certain types of procedures, such as those performed on the spinal column. For example, when a patient is positioned in the prone (face-down) position, the posterior approach to the spine, through the back, is used.

Surgical Approach

The **surgical approach** identifies how the surgeon reaches the surgical site (■ TABLE 30-5). The approach must be abstracted

Table 30-4 ■ **INTEGRAL COMPONENTS OF A SURGICAL PROCEDURE**

- ❏ Assess the patient in the preoperative area to determine readiness for surgery.
- ❏ Transfer the patient to the operating room.
- ❏ Prepare the patient for surgery, including removing hair and cleaning the surgical site.
- ❏ Position the patient for surgery, including elevating specific anatomic sites, such as a knee.
- ❏ Drape the patient (cover the patient and surrounding area with a sterile surgical drape to separate sterile from nonsterile areas).
- ❏ Administer local and, sometimes, regional anesthesia (by the surgeon).
- ❏ Make a surgical incision through multiple layers to access the surgical site.
- ❏ Explore specific areas of the patient, including further investigation of an anatomic site.
- ❏ Perform lysis of lesions or adhesions necessary to access the surgical site.
- ❏ Debride or excise necrotic or contaminated tissue and remove foreign bodies.
- ❏ Perform the procedure.
- ❏ Perform lavage/irrigation (washing out).
- ❏ Achieve hemostasis (stoppage of bleeding).
- ❏ Close the incision after surgery, including closing multiple layers of tissue.
- ❏ Transfer the patient to the postoperative care area.
- ❏ Document the procedure.

because CPT provides separate codes for open procedures and those performed endoscopically. CPT code descriptions assume an open approach. An endoscopic or percutaneous approach is specified in the code description.

In operative reports, the approach is not always explicitly stated or described. For example, when a surgeon documents, *A 4-cm upper midline incision was made*, the word *open* is not used. The approach is open because an extended incision was made. Descriptions of endoscopic percutaneous procedures mention the creation of short or stab incisions, use of a trocar, and insertion of an endoscope. *Endoscopy* is a general term that often takes on the name of the anatomic site treated, such as arthroscopy, laparoscopy, colonoscopy, and so on.

Incision Site

The operative report also identifies the **incision site** (*the anatomic location at which the surgeon cuts through the skin and subcutaneous tissue*) (■ FIGURE 30-6, page 574). Although the incision site is not coded, it helps provide an understanding of the procedure and the internal structures that might be accessed.

Operative Report

At the conclusion of a procedure or operation, the physician dictates the **operative report**, which is a detailed narrative description of the procedure that includes:

- Patient name, age, and date
- Name and role of all physicians

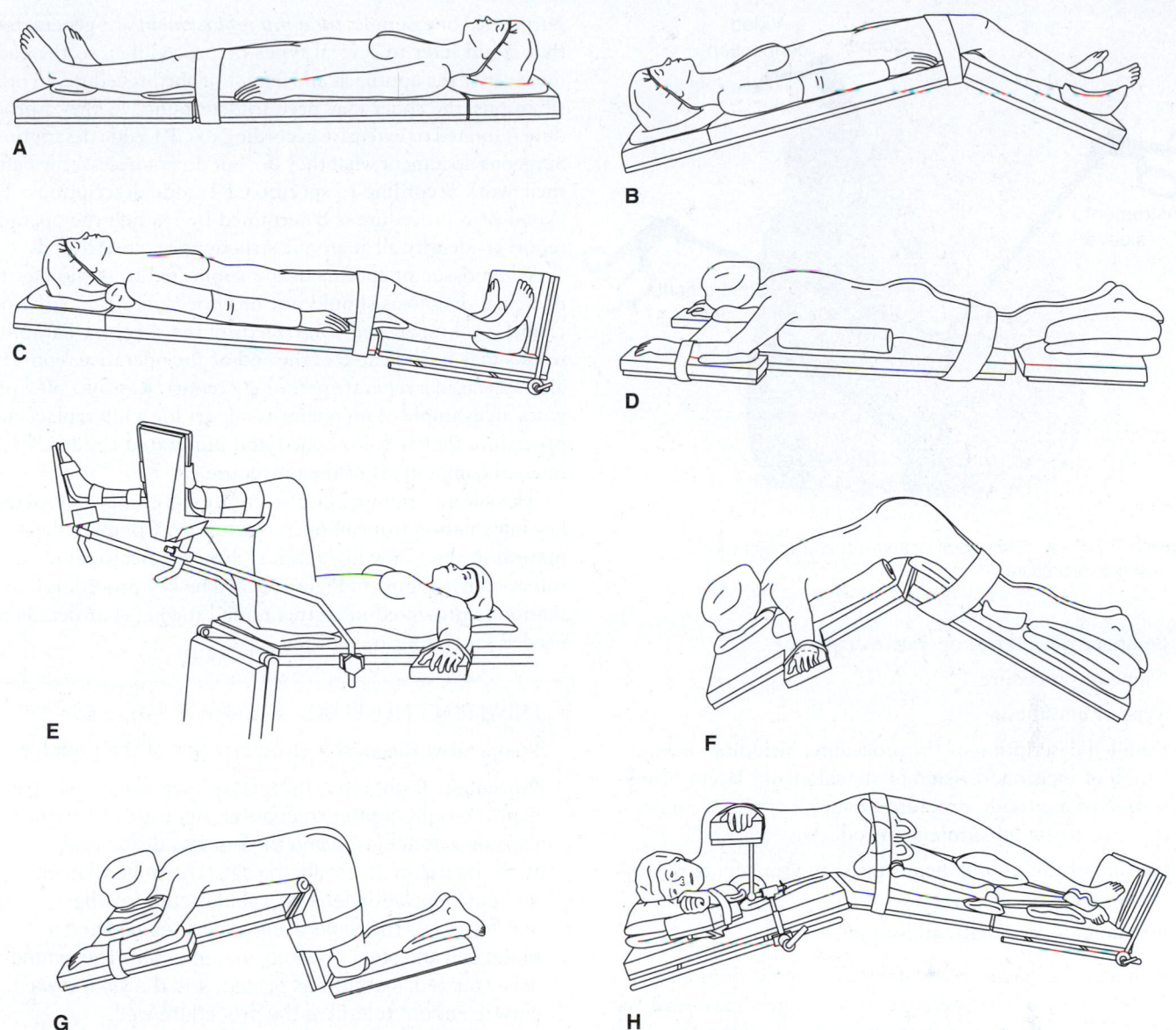

Figure 30-4 ■ Patient positions for surgery: (A) Dorsal recumbent/supine, (B) Trendelenburg, (C) Reverse Trendelenburg, (D) Prone, (E) Lithotomy, (F) Kraske/jacknife, (G) Knee–chest, (H) Lateral.

Table 30-5   ■   **TYPES OF SURGICAL APPROACH**

Name	Description	Documentation Example
Endoscopic (via natural opening)	An endoscope is inserted through an existing orifice (*body opening*), such as the nose, mouth, anus, vagina, or urethra.	A #21 French cystoscope was then used to visualize the entire urethra and bladder.
Endoscopic (percutaneous)	Several small incisions, 5–10 mm in length, are made, through which instruments and a camera, linked to an external video monitor, are inserted (■ FIGURE 30-5, page 574).	A stab incision was made within the umbilicus. The standard four trocars were inserted uneventfully.
Open	An extended incision is made through the skin, subcutaneous tissue (with division or dissection of the fascia), and muscle when necessary.	A McBurney's incision was made. A transverse right lower quadrant incision was made.
Percutaneous	A needle or other punch technique is used to penetrate the skin and subcutaneous tissue, but an incision is not made.	A long 20-gauge spinal needle was passed to the level of the foramen ovale. The needle was withdrawn.

Note: The approaches and definitions in this table vary from those defined with the ICD-10-PCS system.

Source: © PB Resources, Inc. Used with permission.

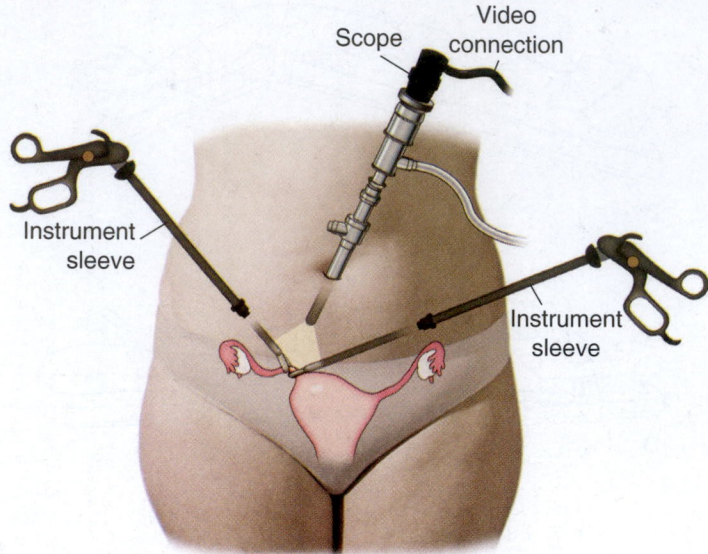

Figure 30-5 ■ Example of instruments and incisions for a laparoscopic procedure.

- Preoperative and postoperative diagnoses
- Name of procedure
- Type of anesthesia
- Detailed description of the procedure, including site and length of incision, division of subcutaneous layers, visualization of anatomic structures, removal of tissue, and new tissue or tissue substitute(s) introduced
- Closure of the wound, hemostasis, and transfer to postoperative area
- Instruments, materials, and supplies used

Although the diagnosis and name of the procedure are stated at the beginning of the operative report, coders must read and analyze the entire report to confirm the details of the procedure and diagnosis necessary for coding. The terminology used by the physician may differ from the terms in the coding manuals, so it is necessary to confirm the exact nature of the procedure and the details of the postoperative diagnosis for coding

purposes. For example, *total hip replacement* is a general term that could refer to several types of procedures, so the coder must verify the approach and extent of the procedure. In other situations, the coder may need to determine whether a procedure is limited or extensive according to CPT code descriptions. Surgeons document what they do, but do not necessarily define their work according to specific CPT code descriptions. The extent of a procedure is determined by reading the operative report to identify all anatomic structures or sites treated.

When tissue or specimens are submitted to pathology, the principal diagnosis should not be coded until the pathology results are known *and confirmed by the surgeon*. Pathology results may be indicated at the end of the operative report but also appear in a separate pathology report. ■ FIGURE 30-7 provides an example of an operative report for a hip replacement procedure that is color-coded and annotated to identify the integral components of the procedure.

The surgical mini-medical-record used in this text extracts key information from an operative report. Compare the information in the following surgical mini-medical-record to the full operative report in Figure 30-7. The key procedural information is presented in a streamlined format, but details not needed for coding are omitted.

INPATIENT HOSPITAL   Gender: F   Age: 63

Preoperative diagnosis: Osteoarthritis of the right hip

Procedure: Right hip arthroplasty. Incision was made over the right greater trochanter. Access to the joint capsule was achieved and the hip was dislocated. With the use of an oscillating saw, the femoral neck was cut. A polyethylene acetabular cup prosthesis was inserted. The femoral canal was reamed and a metal ball and stem inserted, uncemented. The wound was irrigated, a drain was placed, and the wound was closed. Patient tolerated the procedure well.

Postoperative diagnosis: Osteoarthritis of the right hip

Pathology report: Femoral head and acetabulum show evidence of osteoarthritis.

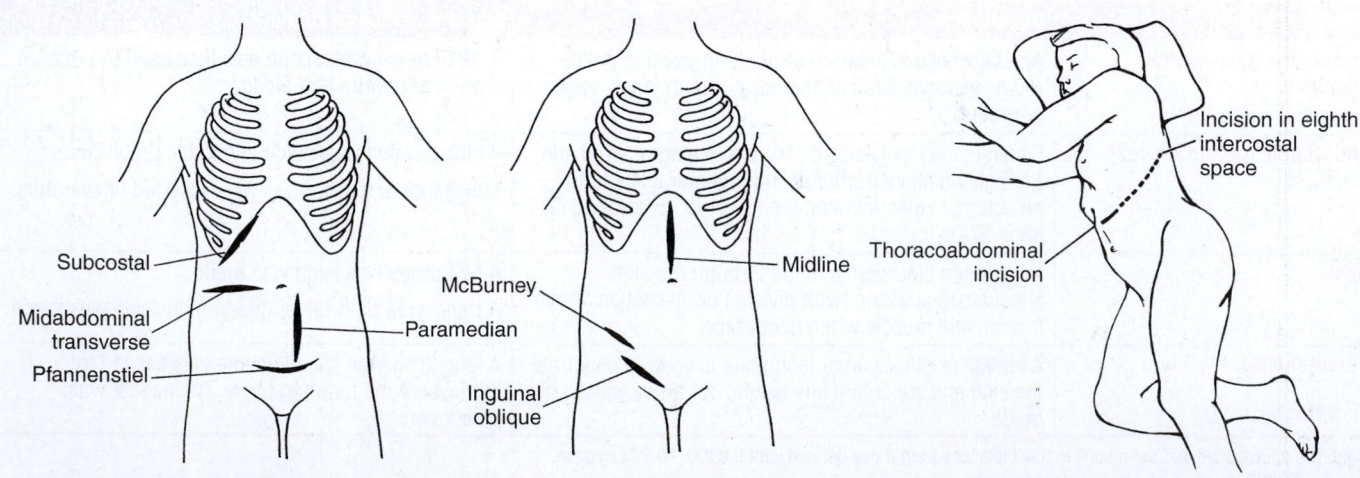

Figure 30-6 ■ Location of surgical incisions.

OPERATIVE REPORT

PREOPERATIVE DIAGNOSIS: Right hip osteoarthritis.
POSTOPERATIVE DIAGNOSIS: Right hip osteoarthritis.
PROCEDURES PERFORMED: Total hip replacement, right side using the following components:
1. Polyethylene acetabular system 10-degree elevated rim located at the 12 o'clock position.
2. Polyethylene modular acetabular system 45 mm in diameter.
3. Metal femoral head 30 mm diameter +0 mm neck length.
4. Metal offset stem, uncemented.
ANESTHESIA: Spinal.
DESCRIPTION OF PROCEDURE IN DETAIL: The patient was brought into the operating room and was placed on the operative table in a lateral decubitus position with the right side up. Kidney rests were also used because of the patient's large size. All bony prominences were well padded. Time out was performed. The right lower extremity was prepped and draped in a sterile fashion. Spinal anesthesia was administered. A 20 cm in length incision was made over the greater trochanter. This was angled posteriorly. Access to the tensor fascia lata was performed. This was incised with the use of scissors. Gluteus maximus was incised and split proximally. The bursa around the hip was identified, and the bleeders were coagulated with the use of Bovie retractor. Hemostasis was achieved. The piriformis fossa was identified, and the piriformis fossa tendon was elevated with the use of a Cobb elevator (retractor). It was detached from the piriformis fossa and tagged with 2-0 Vicryl filament. Access to the joint capsule was achieved. The capsule was excised from the posterior and superior aspects. It was released also in the front with the use of a Mayo scissors. The hip was then dislocated. With the use of an oscillating saw, the femoral neck was cut. The acetabulum was then visualized and debrided from soft tissues and osteophytes. Extensive degenerative disease was found on the femoral head as well as in the acetabulum. Reaming was initiated and completed for a 45 mm diameter cap without complications. The trial component was put in place and was found to be stable in an anatomic position. The actual component was then impacted in the acetabulum. A 10-degree polyethylene lip was also placed in the acetabular cap. Our attention was then focused to the femur. With the use of a cookie cutter, the femoral canal was accessed. The broaches were then used to prepare the femur with the appropriate amount of version. In full extension and external rotation, there was no dislocation. The actual 30 mm femoral head and stem component was inserted in place and hemostasis was achieved. The wound was irrigated with normal saline. The medium-sized Hemovac drain was placed in the wound. The wound was then closed in layers. The tensor fascia lata was closed with 0 PDS filament and the wound was closed with 2-0 Monocryl filament. Staples were used for the skin. The patient recovered from anesthesia without complications.
ESTIMATED BLOOD LOSS: 45 mL.
IV FLUIDS: 2 liters.
DRAINS: One medium-sized Hemovac.
COMPLICATIONS: None.
DISPOSITION: The patient was transferred to the PACU in stable condition.
PATHOLOGY: Femoral head and acetabulum show evidence of osteoarthritis.

COLOR KEY

Diagnosis

Procedure name

Components of the hip's replacement prosthesis

Anesthesia

Transfer of patient

Patient position

Patient prep

Draping

Anesthesia

Instruments, supplies, sutures

Incision (Open procedure)

Identification and exploration of site

Debridement (H)

Main steps of the procedure (I)

Prosthetic components

Hemostasis

Irrigation (lavage)

Wound closure

Transfer to postoperative area

Figure 30-7 ■ Example of an operative report.

CODING PRACTICE

Exercise 30.2 **Abstracting Surgery Section Procedures**

Instructions: Check-off either *Yes* or *No* to indicate whether each of the following services is an integral component of the procedure for coding purposes.

1. Obtain laboratory tests prior to the procedure.   ☐ Yes   ☐ No

2. Prepare the patient for surgery, including removing hair and cleaning the surgical site. ☐ Yes   ☐ No

3. Perform lysis of lesions or adhesions necessary to access the surgical site.   ☐ Yes   ☐ No

4. Clean and sterilize the operating room before the procedure begins.   ☐ Yes   ☐ No

5. Debride or excise necrotic or contaminated tissue and remove foreign bodies.   ☐ Yes   ☐ No

ASSIGNING SURGERY CODES

To assign Surgery codes, follow the standard process for assigning CPT codes. Refer to the preceding mini-medical-record of a right hip arthroplasty as an example of Surgery coding.

1. Locate the Main Term that describes the procedure in the Index. Search by procedure name, anatomic site, condition, synonym, eponym, or abbreviation. Examples: **Arthroplasty** (procedure name), **Replacement** (synonym), or **Hip** (anatomic site).

2. Identify the appropriate first- and second-level modifying term(s). Examples:

   - Main Term **Arthroplasty**; first-level modifying term **Hip**; second-level modifying term **Total Replacement**.
   - Main Term **Replacement**; first-level modifying term **Hip**.
   - Main Term **Hip**; first-level modifying term **Arthroplasty**.

3. Identify the code(s) or code range. Example: **27130-27132**.

4. Refer to the Tabular List to select and verify the code. Example: **27130 Arthroplasty, acetabular and proximal femoral prosthetic replacement (total hip arthroplasty), with or without autograft or allograft.** (*Note:* Code **27132** describes the conversion of a previous hip surgery to total hip arthroplasty. This example is not a conversion.)

5. Read all applicable guidelines, special instructions, and instructional notes.

6. Assign modifiers, as needed. Example: **-RT Right side**.

7. Repeat this process for each procedure performed.

Surgical Care Process

Coders must develop a good understanding of the surgical care process to help them understand the use of Surgery codes and modifiers. This understanding begins with a patient's first encounter with a physician regarding a problem and continues through the preoperative preparation, the surgical procedure, and postoperative healing and follow-up period. ■ TABLE 30-6 summarizes the major steps a patient experiences and identifies the diagnosis and procedure codes assigned by both physicians and hospitals.

This example involves a patient who is admitted as an inpatient for a total right hip replacement due to osteoarthritis. Notice the following features of the case:

- Several different physicians, each with a unique role, become involved at various stages of the process.
- The physician(s) and hospital code for different aspects of the procedure.
- The diagnosis code(s) evolves, depending on the phase of surgical care and the provider.

The codes provided are examples only. Actual codes could vary based on the actual situation and the documentation of services provided.

Table 30-6 ■ **OVERVIEW OF THE SURGICAL CARE PROCESS: TOTAL RIGHT HIP REPLACEMENT DUE TO OSTEOARTHRITIS**

Services Provided	Physician Coding	Hospital Coding
Patient with chronic osteoarthritis of the right hip presents to PCP with complaints of increased hip pain. After evaluation and discussion, patient agrees to an evaluation by an orthopedic surgeon for possible joint replacement.	PCP codes and bills for the encounter. ICD-10-CM: M16.11 Unilateral primary osteoarthritis, right hip CPT*: 99213	Not applicable.
The PCP orders an updated x-ray at the request of the orthopedic surgeon. Patient presents to the radiology department at the hospital where the x-ray will be performed.	Neither the PCP nor orthopedic surgeon codes or bills for ordering the x-ray. The service is factored into the evaluation and management (E/M) service when the patient is evaluated. The radiologist who contracts with the hospital codes for the professional component of the x-ray. ICD-10-CM: M16.11 CPT: 73502-26-RT Radiologic examination, hip, unilateral; 2-3 views; -26 Professional component; -RT Right side	Outpatient radiology codes for the technical component of the x-ray. ICD-10-CM: M16.11 CPT: 73510-TC-RT
Patient presents to the orthopedic surgeon, who evaluates the patient and determines she is a good candidate for the procedure. The patient and surgeon decide to schedule a total hip replacement procedure.	The orthopedic surgeon codes for the E/M visit for surgical evaluation. ICD-10-CM: M16.11 CPT*: 99245 Office consultation for a new or established patient, Level 5	Not applicable.
The day before the procedure, the patient presents to the orthopedic surgeon for preoperative clearance. She also reports to the hospital outpatient laboratory for preoperative tests.	The orthopedic surgeon does not charge for the preoperative visit because it is part of the global surgical package.	The outpatient laboratory codes and enters charges for the tests into the hospital's computer. The tests will be bundled into an inpatient admission.

Table 30-6   ■   (*continued*)

Services Provided	Physician Coding	Hospital Coding
The patient reports to the hospital, where she is admitted. The orthopedic surgeon performs a successful procedure, using a metal prosthesis for the proximal femoral component and a polyethylene acetabular liner.	The orthopedic surgeon codes for a total right hip replacement. ICD-10-CM: M16.11 CPT: 27130-RT Arthroplasty, acetabular and proximal femoral prosthetic replacement (total hip arthroplasty), with or without autograft or allograft; -RT Right side	The hospital codes and enters charges for the use of the operating room and supplies. The hospital enters a charge for the technical component of the pathology evaluation. ICD-10-CM: M16.11 CPT: 88304-TC; Technical component
	The anesthesiologist codes and bills for services provided during the procedure. ICD-10-CM: M16.11 CPT: 01214-P1-AA Anesthesia for open procedures involving hip joint; total hip arthroplasty; -P1 Normal healthy patient; -AA Anesthesia services performed personally by anesthesiologist	
	The pathologist codes and bills for evaluation of joint material removed from the patient during surgery. ICD-10-CM: M16.11 CPT: 88304-26 Level III - Surgical pathology, Femoral head, other than fracture; -26 Professional component	
The patient remains in the hospital for three days following surgery. The surgeon visits the patient each day and evaluates her progress.	The orthopedic surgeon does not charge for the postoperative visits because they are part of the global surgical package, which includes a 90-day postoperative period. ICD-10-CM: M16.11, Z96.641 Presence of right artificial hip joint CPT: 99024 Postoperative follow-up visit (The code is reported once for each visit with the corresponding date. There is no charge attached to reporting the postoperative follow-up visit on the claim. The code alerts the payer that the visit occurred as part of the global surgery package.)	The hospital enters charges for daily room and board, which includes nursing care.
The patient is discharged on the fourth day following surgery.	The orthopedic surgeon does not charge for the discharge because it is part of the global surgical package. ICD-10-CM: Z47.1 Aftercare following joint replacement surgery, Z96.641 CPT: 99024	The hospital generates a bill for all charges accumulated during the patient's stay. ICD-10-CM: M16.11 ICD-10-PCS*: 0SR902Z Replacement of Right Hip Joint with Metal on Polyethylene Synthetic Substitute, Open Approach
The patient follows up with the orthopedic surgeon for postoperative evaluation 2, 4, 8, and 12 weeks after surgery.	The orthopedic surgeon does not charge or bill for the postoperative visits because they are part of the global surgical package. ICD-10-CM: Z47.1, Z96.641 CPT: 99024 (The code is reported once for each postoperative visit with the corresponding date.)	Not applicable.
The orthopedic surgeon refers the patient to physical therapy at the hospital for rehabilitation.	The orthopedic surgeon does not charge or bill for writing orders because it is included in the surgical package.	The hospital's outpatient physical therapy department bills for the rehabilitative services provided during each visit, such as therapeutic exercise and gait training. ICD-10-CM: Z47.1, Z96.641 CPT*: 97110-97 Therapeutic exercises, -97 Rehabilitative Services 97116-97 Gait training

* The codes shown are examples. The actual code is determined based on documentation of the service performed.

Note: M16.11 does not require a seventh character to identify the episode of care, so report a Z code for aftercare .

Source: © PB Resources, Inc. Used with permission.

Surgical Package

The surgical package identifies a group of services that all relate to a single surgery, including preoperative, intraoperative, and postoperative services. The **global period** is the number of days during which the provider must render all services related to the surgery. Each payer establishes its own time frames for the global period for each procedure then issues one payment to cover all services performed during that time. CPT guidelines provide a definition of the CPT surgical package. Medicare defines its own global surgical package. The policies of private payers vary.

CPT Surgical Package

The Surgery guidelines, which appear at the beginning of the Surgery section in the CPT manual, provide the CPT definition of a surgical package. ■ TABLE 30-7 identifies the elements included, or bundled, in the CPT surgical package and those that can be billed separately. The required modifier, if any, for the additional services is also shown.

Medicare Global Surgical Package

Medicare providers render services that are related to the global surgical package in any setting, including hospitals, ambulatory surgery centers (ASCs), and physicians' offices.

Medicare defines services that are included in the **Medicare global surgical package**, which varies slightly from the CPT surgical package (■ TABLE 30-8).

Medicare assigns a global period of 0, 10, or 90 days to each procedure. A global period of 0 includes only the day of surgery. Minor procedures have a global period of 10 days *plus* the day of surgery. Major procedures have a global period of 90 days *plus* one day before surgery and the day of surgery itself. CMS publishes Medicare's number of global days for specific CPT codes in the **Medicare Physician Fee Schedule Database (MPFSDB)**, which can be accessed through the CMS website and many encoder software programs. The MPFSDB contains not only the relative value units (RVUs) and allowable fees for each CPT code, it also identifies other rules, such as the global period, the modifiers accepted, and reimbursement impact of modifiers. When multiple procedures are performed during one operative session, the global period is determined by the primary procedure. Add-on and secondary procedures do not add to the length of the global period.

Some private payers follow Medicare's global period, and others establish their own criteria. Check with individual payers to learn the length of the global period and the services included in the surgical package.

Table 30-7 ■ **CPT SURGICAL PACKAGE**

Services in the CPT Surgical Package	Additional Services
Before the Procedure	
Subsequent to (*after*) the decision for surgery, conducting one related E/M encounter on the date immediately prior to or on the date of procedure, including history and physical	The initial encounter, and any related tests, in which the physician evaluates the patient and the decision for surgery is made (append modifier -57 to the E/M code when the decision for surgery is made within 24 hours of the procedure)
During the Procedure	
Local anesthesia, metacarpal/metatarsal/digital block, topical anesthesia	General anesthesia is billed by the anesthesiologist using codes from the Anesthesia section. (If general anesthesia is provided by the surgeon, append modifier -47 to the surgical procedure code.)
The procedure(s) performed	
Supplies and materials usually included with the procedure	Supplies and materials over and above those usually included with the procedure (identify using CPT code 99070 or the appropriate HCPCS code)
Immediate postoperative care, including dictating operative notes and talking with the family and other physicians	Surgeries for which services performed are significantly greater than usually required (identify with modifier -22)
Evaluating the patient in the postanesthesia recovery area	Surgeries for which services performed are significantly less than usually required (identify with modifier -52)
After the Procedure	
Writing orders	Services provided by other physicians, except when the surgeon and the other physician(s) agree on the transfer of care
Typical postoperative follow-up care based on the number of days in the follow-up period as defined by the payer (identify with code 99024.)	E/M services provided by the surgeon during the postoperative period that are *unrelated* to the procedure (identify with modifier -24)
Care for typical complications from the procedure	*Unrelated* procedures performed by the same physician during the postoperative period (identify with modifier -79)
	Care of the condition for which a diagnostic procedure was performed
	Care for comorbid conditions
	Repeat procedure by the same or another physician (identify with modifier -76 or -77, respectively)
	Unplanned return to the operating room during the postoperative period (identify with modifier -78)

Source: © PB Resources, Inc. Used with permission.

The length of a month affects the end date of the postoperative period. For example, a 10-day postoperative period for a procedure performed on February 25 ends on March 7 in a non–leap year and on March 6 in a leap year. A 10-day postoperative period for a procedure performed on March 25 ends on April 4 because March has 31 days. A 90-day postoperative period for a procedure performed in June or July must take into account that both July and August contain 31 days. Remember to count the day *after* surgery as the first day of a 10- or 90-day period.

Surgery Modifiers

Modifiers provide payers with information about the services or procedures that vary from the standard protocol so that they will consider the claim for payment. (Refer to Table 27-1, Key Criteria for Abstracting CPT Modifiers.) A wide variety of surgical circumstances requires modifiers. After the decision for surgery is made, the most common use of modifiers is to report multiple procedures, multiple surgeons, or portions of the surgical package. A modifier for increased procedural services—those that require substantial additional work—is also available but should be used infrequently.

-57 Decision for Surgery

When an evaluation and management (E/M) encounter results in a decision for major surgery and the procedure is performed within 24 hours, the physician reports the E/M code and applies modifier **-57**. This indicates that the decision for

> ### SUCCESS STEP
> Place a self-adhesive tab or electronic note on this page of the text with the label *Surgery Modifiers*. Doing so will make it easy to refer back to this important information as you proceed through your coding class.

surgery occurred within the Medicare global period, which begins the day before the procedure. Commercial payers may follow different policies. Example: **99215-57**.

-22 Increased Procedural Services

When the physician work required to provide a service is substantially greater than usual, apply modifier **-22** to the usual CPT code (■ FIGURE 30-8). This modifier should be used only in the most unusual of circumstances, such as increased intensity, time, and technical difficulty of the procedure, severity of the patient's condition, and physical and mental effort required. Medicare and some private payers require that the unusual circumstance must require at least 50% more time than usual. Some payers allow it when the procedure time is increased by 25%. Increase the charge reported for the service in proportion to the increased work when the claim is billed because payers do not automatically increase the amount paid. Medicare increases payment by 18% for this modifier. Private payers may do the same or follow a different policy.

Table 30-8   ■   **MEDICARE GLOBAL PACKAGE**

Services in the Medicare Global Surgical Package	Additional Services
Before the Procedure	
For minor surgery: the initial encounter in which the physician evaluates the patient and the decision for surgery is made	For major surgery: the initial encounter in which the physician evaluates the patient and the decision for surgery is made (append modifier -57 to the E/M code when the decision for surgery is made within 24 hours of the procedure)
Preoperative visits	Diagnostic tests and procedures, including diagnostic radiology procedures
During the Procedure	
Intraoperative services (the procedure itself and any directly related services)	Splints and casting supplies
Supplies, except for those identified as exclusions by the payer	Supplies identified as exclusions by the payer
	Surgeries for which services performed are significantly greater than usually required (identify with modifier -22)
Surgical tray (for most payers) (HCPCS code A4550)	Surgeries for which services performed are significantly less than usually required (identify with modifier -52)
After the Procedure	
Complications following surgery that do not require additional trips to the operating room	Visits unrelated to the diagnosis for which the surgical procedure is performed
	Treatment for the underlying condition
Postoperative visits and services, such as dressing changes, removal of sutures, wires, drains, cases, splints, and tubes	Clearly distinct surgical procedures that are conducted during the postoperative period that are not reoperations or treatment for complications
	A more extensive procedure required when an original, less extensive procedure fails
Postsurgical pain management	Treatment for postoperative complications that requires a return trip to the operating room (identify with modifier -78)
	Immunosuppressive therapy for organ transplants
	Critical care services unrelated to the surgery where a seriously injured or burned patient is critically ill and requires the physician's constant attendance (identify with codes 99291 and 99292)

Source: © PB Resources, Inc. Used with permission.

The surgeon performs a laparoscopic cholecystectomy due to acute cholecystitis, but cannot access the gall bladder because of extensive adhesions in the abdominal cavity. He changes to an open approach and spends an additional 35 minutes lysing the adhesions. Once the gall bladder can be accessed, then he completes the procedure without further problems. The work on the adhesions increases the length of the procedure by 50% to 1 hour, 35 minutes.

K81.0 Acute cholecystitis
K66.0 Peritoneal adhesions
47600–22 Cholecystectomy; –22 Increased procedural services

Usual charge: $1,200.00
Charge for this patient: $1,800.00

Figure 30-8 ■ Example of coding with modifier -22. *Source:* © *PB Resources, Inc. Used with permission. CPT codes only* © *American Medical Association.*

Examples of unusual circumstances include morbid obesity, excessive hemorrhaging, extensive adhesions that block access to the surgical site, and medical emergencies, such as cardiac arrest. Documentation must describe in detail the nature of the unusual circumstance, the reason additional work was required, and the time spent providing the service. In addition to the diagnosis code reported for the service itself, also report diagnosis codes that describe the nature of the unique circumstance. When the reason is morbid obesity, report a diagnosis code for morbid obesity (**E66.-**).

Modifier **-22** can be used with all CPT codes except E/M services.

Multiple Procedures

When multiple procedures are performed during the same operative session or during the global period, modifiers **-50**, **-51**, and **-59** explain the circumstances. Coders also need to understand how to use the National Correct Coding Initiative (NCCI) to identify when multiple procedures can be billed and when they are bundled together. When repeat, staged, or unplanned procedures are performed during the postoperative period, CPT provides modifiers **-58**, **-76**, **-77**, **-78**, and **-79**.

-50 Bilateral Procedure. When a procedure is performed on paired anatomic sites or organs, such as both hands or both eyes, it is a bilateral procedure. To code bilateral procedures, assign the CPT code for the unilateral procedure and append modifier **-50** (■ FIGURE 30-9). Report a quantity of **1** in Item 24G on the CMS-1500 claim form or the corresponding field on the 837P electronic claim. In general, double the charge for the service, understanding that the payer may take a discount. Medicare pays the second procedure at 50% of the standard fee. Payment policies of private payers vary.

When the code description contains the word **bilateral**, do not apply modifier **-50** because the bilateral nature of the procedure is already identified. When the code description states **unilateral or bilateral**, the same code is reported whether the procedure is done on one side or both (■ FIGURE 30-10). Do not append a modifier and do not adjust the fee. The MPF-SDB identifies CPT codes for which modifier **-50** is allowed.

-51 Multiple Procedures. When more than one procedure is performed during the same operative session by the same individual, report the CPT code for the first procedure, then append modifier **-51** to the second and subsequent procedures. Modifier **-51** identifies the following situations:

- Multiple, related surgical procedures performed by the same surgeon during the same operative session

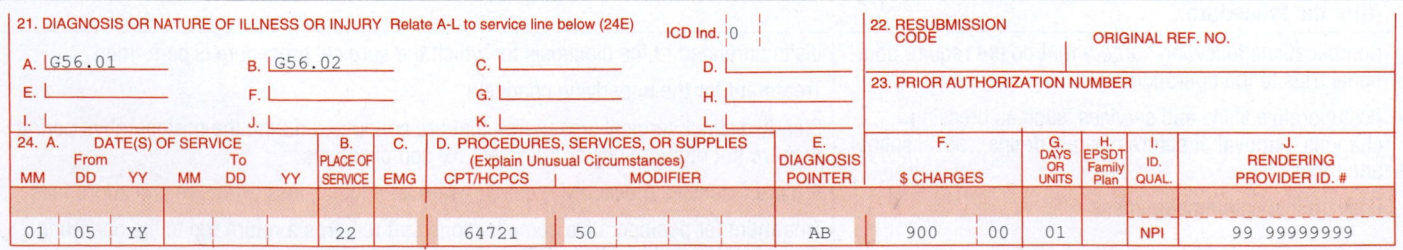

The surgeon performs carpal tunnel decompression on both hands.

G56.01 Carpal tunnel syndrome, right upper limb
G56.02 Carpal tunnel syndrome, left upper limb
64721–50 Neuroplasty and/or transposition; median nerve at carpal tunnel; –50 Bilateral procedure

A

21. DIAGNOSIS OR NATURE OF ILLNESS OR INJURY Relate A-L to service line below (24E)				ICD Ind. 0		22. RESUBMISSION CODE		ORIGINAL REF. NO.

A. G56.01   B. G56.02   C. ____   D. ____
E. ____   F. ____   G. ____   H. ____
I. ____   J. ____   K. ____   L. ____

23. PRIOR AUTHORIZATION NUMBER

24. A. DATE(S) OF SERVICE From MM DD YY To MM DD YY	B. PLACE OF SERVICE	C. EMG	D. PROCEDURES, SERVICES, OR SUPPLIES (Explain Unusual Circumstances) CPT/HCPCS | MODIFIER	E. DIAGNOSIS POINTER	F. $ CHARGES	G. DAYS OR UNITS	H. EPSDT Family Plan	I. ID. QUAL.	J. RENDERING PROVIDER ID. #
01 05 YY	22		64721 | 50	AB	900 00	01		NPI	99 99999999

Note: If usual fee for the procedure is $450.00, then bill $900.00 for a bilateral procedure, unless the payer provides other direction. For example, CMS allows 150% of the usual price of one procedure for a bilateral procedure, which would be $675.00 here.

B

Figure 30-9 ■ Example of coding a bilateral procedure with modifier -50. (A) Scenario and coding. (B) CMS-1500 form. *Source:* © *PB Resources, Inc. Used with permission. CPT codes only* © *American Medical Association.*

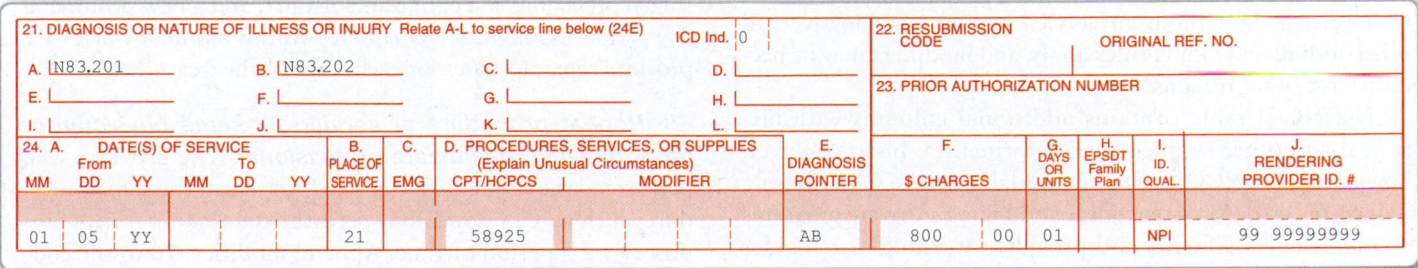

The surgeon performs a cystectomy of both ovaries.

N83.201 Unspecified ovarian cysts, right side
N83.202 Unspecified ovarian cysts, left side
58925 Ovarian cystectomy, unilateral or bilateral

A

B

Figure 30-10 ■ Example of coding a bilateral procedure that does not require modifier -50. (A) Scenario and coding. (B) CMS-1500 form.
Source: © PB Resources, Inc. Used with permission. CPT codes only © American Medical Association.

- A combination of surgical procedures that may be performed through either the same or different incisions and at either the same or a different anatomic site
- A combination of medical and surgical procedures performed during the same session

Do not report modifier **-51** on E/M codes, add-on codes (designated with the symbol + in the CPT manual), or codes exempt from modifier **-51** (designated with the symbol ø in the CPT manual). The MPFSDB identifies CPT codes for which modifier **-51** is allowed.

-59 Distinct Procedural Service. Use modifier **-59** to identify that a procedure or service is separate and distinct from other services provided during the same session. Use this modifier only when no other modifier is appropriate. It identifies services that are not normally reported together but are appropriate in the current situation because of:

- A different operative session
- A different anatomic site or organ system
- A different procedure or surgery
- A separate incision or excision
- A separate lesion
- A separate injury or separate area of injury in extensive injuries

Modifier **-59** informs the payer that although the procedure is normally bundled with another procedure, in this case it is not. Apply an extended modifier, referred to as the **-X{EPSU}** modifiers, instead of **-59** when it describes the situation:

- **-XE Separate encounter**
- **-XP Separate practitioner**
- **-XS Separate organ/structure**
- **-XU Unusual separate service**

More information about bundling and unbundling related to the National Correct Coding Initiative is discussed next.

National Correct Coding Initiative. The **National Correct Coding Initiative (NCCI)** was implemented to promote correct coding and to control improper coding leading to inappropriate payment. NCCI identifies pairs of codes that normally cannot be reported together. NCCI code pair edits are automated **prepayment edits** for Medicare and other payers, which means that the payer's computer analyzes codes before the claim is processed and flags claims that might result in improper payment. The goal is to prevent improper payment when certain codes are submitted for services covered by Medicare Part B for the same patient, on the same date, by the same provider.

The NCCI data are presented in a table that consists of several columns. **Column 1** contains a list of all payable CPT codes. **Column 2** contains the code that is not payable with a particular Column 1 code unless a modifier is permitted and submitted (■ TABLE 30-9). The column labeled Modifier Indicator identifies whether the code in Column 2 can be billed with the code in Column 1.

- 0–Not Allowed. No modifiers associated with NCCI are allowed to be used with this code pair. There are no circumstances in which both procedures of the code pair should be paid for the same beneficiary on the same day by the same provider.
- 1–Allowed. The modifiers **-25**, **-57**, or **-59** are allowed on the Column 2 code of the code pair when clinically

Table 30-9 ■ **EXAMPLES OF NCCI CODE PAIRS**

Column 1	Column 2	Modifier Indicator
39561	96375	1
39561	96376	1
39561	99155	0
39561	99156	0
39561	99157	0
39561	99211	1
39561	99212	1

Source: Centers for Medicare and Medicaid Services.

appropriate, such as when one of the circumstances listed in the preceding subheading for modifier -59 exists or when an E/M service provided during the global period is not part of the global surgical package (-25, -57).

• 9–Not Applicable. An NCCI edit does not apply to this code pair. A previous edit was deleted.

Any code *not* listed in Column 2 can be reported with the Column 1 code without any NCCI restrictions. However, all other coding and billing rules apply, and modifiers may be necessary for other reasons.

The NCCI table contains additional columns with historical and other supplemental information. Instructions on how to use the NCCI tables are available on the CMS website (**www.cms.gov**). Many encoders and billing software programs contain the NCCI edits and provide a warning or reminder when a code pair is used that is not allowed or requires a special modifier (■ FIGURE 30-11).

Staged, Repeat, and Unplanned Procedures. When staged, repeat, or unplanned procedures are performed during the postoperative period, CPT provides modifiers -58, -76, -77, -78, and -79. Multiple procedures may be performed during the postoperative period for several reasons. A modifier identifies the reason for an additional procedure and alerts the payer that it is a separate procedure that should be paid. If the appropriate modifier is not used, the payer considers the procedure to be a duplicate bill or a service included in the global surgical package and does not pay it. Coders must apply the modifiers correctly on the original claim. If a modifier is omitted that results in a denied claim, it is difficult to persuade the payer to accept the modifier retroactively.

-58 Staged or related procedure or service by the same physician or other qualified healthcare professional during the postoperative period. A series of procedures is planned to accomplish the operative objective, such as skin grafts or breast reconstruction. A procedure that is more extensive than the original is performed, such as amputation of additional gangrenous digits. A therapeutic procedure is performed following a surgical procedure, such as a mastectomy performed after a breast biopsy is positive for carcinoma. Append modifier -58 to the code for the subsequent procedure(s). The modifier alerts the payer that the staged procedure is separate and distinct, and a new postoperative period should begin. Do not report this modifier when CPT provides separate codes for each stage of the treatment.

-76 Repeat procedure or service by same physician or other qualified healthcare professional. The provider who performed the original service needs to repeat the same procedure, such as x-rays or EKGs performed for comparative purposes over a period of time. Append modifier -76 to the code for the repeat procedure reported by the same physician. The modifier alerts the payer that this is not a duplicate billing of the same procedure, but it was performed for a specific reason.

-77 Repeat procedure or service by another physician or other qualified healthcare professional. The same procedure as the original is repeated by a different provider than performed the original, such as when the original physician is not available, the patient chooses to see a different physician, or a physician of a different specialty repeats the procedure for a medically necessary reason. Append modifier -77 to the code for the repeat procedure reported by the second physician. The modifier alerts the payer that this is not a duplicate billing of the same procedure, but it was performed for a specific reason.

-78 Unplanned return to the operating/procedure room by the same physician or other qualified healthcare professional following initial procedure for a related procedure during the postoperative period. A procedure to

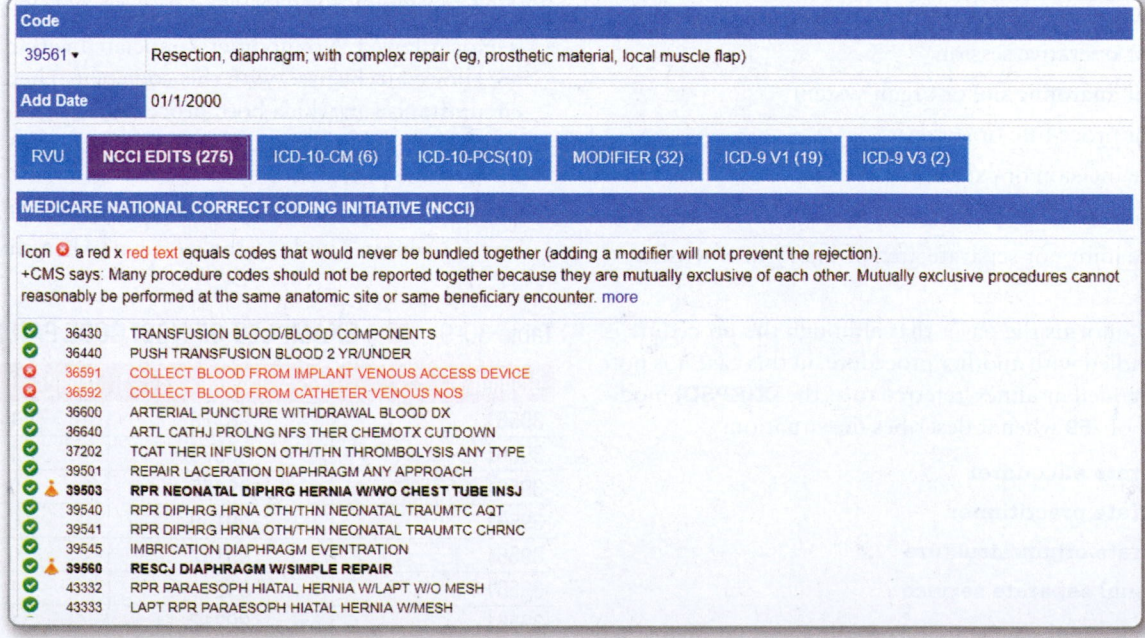

Figure 30-11 ■ Example of color-coding of NCCI edits in encoder. *Source: SpeedeCoder, Reprinted with permission.*

treat a complication arising from the original procedure is performed by the same surgeon who performed the original procedure, such as returning to the operating room to control postoperative hemorrhaging. Append modifier **-78** to the code for the unplanned procedure. The modifier alerts the payer that the procedure should be paid, even though it occurs during the global postoperative follow-up period. When the unplanned procedure is performed by a different physician, no modifier is required because the follow-up days of the global package apply only to the original physician.

-79 Unrelated procedure or service by the same physician or other qualified healthcare professional during the postoperative period. A procedure not related to the original procedure is performed by the same surgeon who performed the original procedure, such as an emergency appendectomy during the postoperative period of a cholecystectomy. Append modifier **-79** to the code for the unrelated procedure. The modifier alerts the payer that the procedure should be paid, even though it occurs during the global postoperative follow-up period, because it is unrelated to the original procedure. When the unrelated procedure is performed by a different physician, no modifier is required because the follow-up days of the global package apply only to the original physician.

Multiple Surgeons

Most surgical procedures are performed by one surgeon, but in some situations multiple surgeons are needed. Coders must understand the various roles of surgeons so that each physician's involvement in the procedure can be coded and billed correctly. The role of each physician is identified on the operative report and is reported using a modifier. Each surgeon bills the same CPT code, then appends the modifier that identifies his or her role in the procedure. The total amount of reimbursement for the procedure is prorated among all surgeons involved, based on the role of each. The MPFSDB identifies CPT codes for which each of these modifiers is allowed and how the reimbursement is prorated. Other payers can follow Medicare's criteria or develop their own.

-66 Surgical Team. A surgical team is a group of several physicians or other qualified health professionals, usually of different specialties, who work together to perform highly complex procedures, such as organ transplants or open heart surgery. Each provider performs a specific part of the procedure for which they have been specially trained. Each surgeon reports the same CPT code with modifier **-66**. Payment is split between the surgeons based on the work that each performed.

-62 Two Surgeons. Cosurgeons are two surgeons of different specialties who work together as primary surgeons to perform separate parts of a procedure. An example is spinal surgery, in which a thoracic surgeon makes the surgical incision and creates access to the spine and a neurosurgeon performs the spinal procedure. Each surgeon reports the same CPT code with modifier **-62**. Payment is split between the two surgeons based on the work that each performed.

-80 Assistant Surgeon. An assistant surgeon actively assists the primary surgeon in performing the procedure and is present for all, or a substantial portion, of the procedure. The assistant surgeon must be medically necessary. Fewer than 5% of surgical cases require an assistant surgeon. The assistant surgeon reports the same CPT code as the primary surgeon and appends modifier **-80**.

-81 Minimum Assistant Surgeon. A minimum assistant surgeon assists the surgeon for a short time during the procedure. The medical necessity of a minimum assistant surgeon must be documented, and this situation is rare.

-82 Assistant Surgeon When a Qualified Resident Is Not Available. A qualified resident surgeon is a licensed physician who is receiving advanced training after completing medical school. Hospitals with a teaching program often use a qualified resident surgeon when an assistant surgeon is needed. The cost of residents is incorporated into the overall reimbursement rates for the hospital. When a resident surgeon is not available, then another surgeon, who is not paid by the hospital or paid at a different rate, must fill the assistant surgeon role.

Assistant surgeons and minimum assistant surgeons report the same CPT code as the primary surgeon and append the appropriate modifier. The primary surgeon reports the CPT code with no modifier.

Portions of the Surgical Package

Surgeons' services include all care included in the global package. When the same surgeon does not provide all phases of the global package—preoperative, procedural, and postoperative—then each surgeon involved must use a modifier to identify the portion of the global package provided. The MPFSDB identifies the portion of the procedure fee paid to each physician who provides part of the surgical package, based on the role of each. Private payers establish their own payment criteria.

-56 Preoperative Management Only. When a surgeon provides the preoperative visit but does not perform the procedure or provide the postoperative follow-up, report the CPT code for the surgical procedure and append modifier **-56**.

-54 Surgical Care Only. When a surgeon performs the surgical procedure but does not provide preoperative and postoperative care, report the CPT code for the surgical procedure and append modifier **-54**.

-55 Postoperative Management Only. When a surgeon provides the postoperative follow-up visits, but not the preoperative visit, and does not perform the procedure, report the CPT code for the surgical procedure and append modifier **-55**.

When a surgeon provides two components of the surgical package, such as providing preoperative care and performing the procedure, report the CPT code for the surgical procedure and append the modifiers for the two components provided.

CODING PRACTICE

Exercise 30.3 Assigning Surgery Codes

Instructions: Check either *Yes* or *No* to indicate whether each of the following services is part of the CPT surgical package.

1. The initial encounter, and any related tests, in which the physician evaluates the patient and the decision for surgery is made. ☐ Yes ☐ No

2. Local anesthesia. ☐ Yes ☐ No

3. General anesthesia. ☐ Yes ☐ No

4. Care for typical complications from the procedure. ☐ Yes ☐ No

5. Care for comorbid conditions. ☐ Yes ☐ No

ARRANGING SURGERY CODES

Sequence multiple surgical procedures in descending order by the dollar charge or RVU. Ideally, both methods result in the same order because the price should reflect the RVU. The Medicare Physician Fee Schedule (MPFS) (*a listing of CPT codes and Medicare allowable fees published by the Centers for Medicare and Medicaid Services*) is based on RVUs, so price order and RVU order should be the same. Other payers may have specific instructions regarding whether price or RVU takes priority. Some payers' computer systems, including Medicare's, automatically rearrange codes to the desired order. Most payers allow the full amount of the first procedure and reduce the value of subsequent procedures that carry modifier **-51** to 50% of the allowed amount. The reduction is based on the efficiencies gained when multiple procedures are performed during the same operative session compared with being performed alone. More specific guidance on sequencing Surgery codes appears in the subsections for each body system.

SURGERY: GENERAL SUBSECTION (10004-10021)

The first and smallest subsection of the Surgery chapter is General, which includes only two codes. The codes identify fine-needle aspiration without imaging guidance and with imaging guidance.

Fine-needle aspiration biopsy (FNAB, FNA, or NAB) is a procedure in which a physician inserts a fine (*thin*), hollow needle under the skin to obtain aspirate—or suck out—a small sample of cells, tissue, or fluid. It can be performed on nearly any anatomic site to help determine the cause of a lump, mass, infection, or inflammation. The physician can use imaging, such as ultrasound, fluoroscopy, MRI, or CT, to visualize the needle and determine where to move it. The cells from the sample are placed on a glass slide and stained, and a pathologist views them under a microscope.

When abstracting for fine-needle aspiration, verify that the documentation identifies fine-needle aspiration and not another type of needle biopsy, such as a percutaneous core needle biopsy, which uses a larger needle and is classified by anatomic site (■ TABLE 30-10).

To assign codes for fine-needle aspiration, search the Index for the Main Term **Fine Needle Aspiration (FNA) Biopsy**. Locate the first-level modifying term **Lesion**, and the second-level subterm for the type of imaging guidance. If guidance is not used, select the subterm **without Guidance**.

Instructional notes in parentheses direct you to assign other codes for radiologic supervision, laboratory analysis of the sample, and percutaneous needle biopsy other than fine needle. For other types of needle biopsies, search for the Main Term **Biopsy** and the first-level modifying term for the anatomic site.

Table 30-10 ■ **KEY CRITERIA FOR ABSTRACTING FINE-NEEDLE ASPIRATION**

❏ Is the aspiration procedure specified as *fine-needle* aspiration?

❏ What type of imaging guidance, if any, is performed?

❏ Is a specimen being obtained?

Locate other codes if the answer to any of the following questions is *Yes*:

❏ Is the specimen being evaluated? (Use laboratory codes.)

❏ Does the aspirate consist of orbital contents? (Use eye codes.)

❏ Is the transendoscopic method used to obtain the aspirate from the esophagus, stomach, duodenum, or colon? (Use gastrointestinal system codes.)

❏ Is a percutaneous or core needle biopsy performed? (Use appropriate code for the anatomic site.)

Source: © PB Resources, Inc. Used with permission.

CODING PRACTICE

Exercise 30.4   Surgery: General Subsection

Instructions: Code the following services using the Index and Tabular List. Write the code(s) on the line provided.

1. Fine-needle aspiration biopsy of the pancreas, with ultrasound imaging guidance. 1 CPT Code _____

2. Percutaneous core needle biopsy of the left breast. 1 CPT Code _____

3. Transendoscopic fine-needle aspiration of the colon. 1 CPT Code _____

4. FNAB of the thyroid. 1 CPT Code _____

5. Fine-needle aspiration biopsy of the axillary lymph node with fluoroscopic guidance. 1 CPT Code _____

CHAPTER SUMMARY

In this chapter you learned that:

- Surgery is the branch of medicine that treats diseases, injuries, and deformities through the use of instruments or manual techniques. A surgical procedure is a combination of a surgical method and an anatomic site.

- Surgery section guidelines appear in the CPT manual at the beginning of the Surgery section, before the list of codes. The guidelines provide general information that applies to all codes in this section, including the definition of the CPT surgical package, which identifies services in addition to the operative procedure included in the procedure code.

- A surgical procedure has several integral components—tasks that are considered part of the procedure and are not coded or billed separately.

- Medicare defines services that are included in the Medicare global surgical package, which varies slightly from the CPT surgical package.

- To assign Surgery codes, follow the standard process for assigning CPT codes. Modifiers provide payers with more information about the services so they will consider the claim for payment.

- Sequence multiple surgical procedures in descending order by the dollar charge or relative value unit (RVU).

- The first and smallest subsection of the Surgery chapter is General, which includes codes for fine-needle aspiration biopsies.

CONCEPT QUIZ

Take a moment to look back at the Surgery section and solidify your skills. Try to answer the questions from memory first, then refer to the discussion in this chapter if you need a little extra help.

Completion

Instructions: Write the term that completes each statement based on the information you learned in this chapter. Choose from the list below. Some choices may be used more than once and some choices may not be used at all.

ablation	exploration
anastomosis	fusion
biopsy	laparotomy
decompression	ligation
dilation	reconstruction
drainage	resection
excision	suturing

1. _____ is the method used to relieve pressure.

2. _____ is cutting into the abdominal cavity.

3. _____ is joining together two or more bones, joints, or vertebrae.

4. _____ is the surgical method used to remove fluid.

5. The purpose of a(n) _____ is to remove skin, tissue, muscle, or bone to test for the presence of disease.

6. _____ may be done to examine an organ or structure to determine a diagnosis.

7. _____ is tying off using any substance, such as cotton, silk, or wire.

8. _____ describes a procedure in which all or part of a structure or organ is removed.

9. _____ is a surgical method used to separate, detach, or destroy.

10. _____ is expanding or stretching an opening.

Multiple Choice

Instructions: Circle the letter of the best answer to each question based on the information you learned in this chapter.

1. Which service is part of the CPT surgical package?
   A. The encounter in which the decision for surgery is made
   B. Care for typical complications from the procedure
   C. General anesthesia
   D. A repeat procedure by the same physician

2. How many days is the Medicare postoperative period for minor procedures?
   A. 0
   B. 5
   C. 10
   D. 15

3. What modifier is assigned when a surgeon provides the preoperative visit but does not perform the procedure or provide postoperative follow-up?
   A. -53
   B. -54
   C. -55
   D. -56

4. What modifier identifies services that are not normally billed together but are appropriate in the current situation?
   A. -59
   B. -22
   C. -80
   D. -81

5. What type of surgery is medically necessary but can be delayed at least 24 hours?
   A. Emergency
   B. Screening
   C. Optional
   D. Elective

6. Which of the following is an integral component of a surgical procedure?
   A. Anesthesia administered by a CRNA
   B. Preoperative lab work
   C. Transferring the patient to the operating room
   D. Postoperative follow-up

7. What is the surgical approach for a procedure that begins with a McBurney's incision?
   A. Percutaneous
   B. Open
   C. Endoscopic via natural opening
   D. Endoscopic percutaneous

8. Where does the coder find Medicare's number of global days for specific CPT codes?
   A. Medicare Global Period Schedule
   B. Appendix A of the CPT code book
   C. Medicare Physician Fee Schedule
   D. CPT Surgical Package Schedule

9. What is the last day of a 90-day postoperative period for a procedure performed on October 3?
   A. January 1
   B. January 2
   C. January 3
   D. January 4

10. When is it appropriate to use modifier -22?
    A. Multiple procedures are performed during the same operative session
    B. Services performed are significantly greater than usually required
    C. E/M services unrelated to an operative procedure are provided by the surgeon during the postoperative period of the procedure
    D. There is an unplanned return to the operating room during the postoperative period

KEEP ON CODING

Instructions: Read the procedure description and determine the needed modifiers. Write the modifier number on the line provided.

1. A patient presents to the radiology department for an x-ray of the left hip. Assign the modifier(s) for the radiology department. CPT Modifier(s) _____

2. A radiologist supervises an x-ray of the left hip and provides a written interpretation and report. Assign the modifier(s) for the radiologist. CPT Modifier(s) _____

3. A general surgeon evaluates a patient in the emergency department for abdominal pain and determines that immediate surgery is needed. Assign the modifier(s) for the E/M code. CPT Modifier(s) _____

4. A surgeon sees a patient who is on vacation for preoperative assessment and performs an appendectomy. The surgeon does not provide postoperative care. Assign the modifier(s) for this surgeon. CPT Modifier(s) _____

5. A surgeon sees a patient for postoperative management only because the patient had surgery elsewhere while on vacation. Assign the modifier(s) for this surgeon. CPT Modifier(s) _____

6. A cholecystectomy takes 50% longer than usual due to extensive adhesions. Assign the modifier(s) for the extra service. CPT Modifier(s) _____

7. A physician performs two tendon sheath injections at separate sites that require the same CPT code. Assign the modifier(s) to identify the second injection is performed at a separate site. CPT Modifier(s) _____

8. A surgical team performs a coronary artery bypass graft procedure on the left circumflex coronary artery. Assign the modifier(s) to be reported by all members of the surgical team. CPT Modifier(s) _____

9. A surgeon removes benign lesions on the trunk and hands, which arc reported with separate CPT codes. Assign the modifiers(s) to identify that multiple procedures were performed at one operative session. CPT Modifier(s) _____

10. A surgeon takes a patient back to the operating room to treat postoperative hemorrhaging after a bowel resection by the same surgeon the previous day. Assign the modifier(s) for this unplanned return to the operating room. CPT Modifier(s) _____

Chapter 31

Anesthesia Procedures (00100-01999)

Chapter Outline

- **Anesthesia Basics**
- **Coding Guidelines for the Anesthesia Section**
- **Abstracting Anesthesia Procedures**
- **Assigning Anesthesia Codes**
- **Arranging Anesthesia Codes**

Learning Objectives

After completing this chapter, you should have the skills to:

31.1 Spell and define the key words, medical terms, and abbreviations related to anesthesia. (Remember)

31.2 Explain the types of anesthesia services. (Understand)

31.3 Adhere to CPT coding guidelines in the Anesthesia section. (Apply)

31.4 Examine and abstract procedural information from the medical record for coding Anesthesia section procedures. (Analyze)

31.5 Demonstrate how to assign codes for procedures in the Anesthesia section. (Apply)

31.6 Utilize guidelines for arranging (sequencing) codes for Anesthesia section procedures. (Apply)

Key Terms and Abbreviations

anesthesia
anesthesia code package
anesthesia conversion factor (CF)
anesthesia time

anesthesiologist
base unit (B)
certified registered nurse anesthetist (CRNA)
controlled hypotension

Mallampati score
modifying unit (M)
monitored anesthesia care (MAC)
patient-controlled analgesia (PCA)

physical status score
postoperative anesthesia care unit (PACU)
time unit (T)
total-body hypothermia

In addition to the key terms listed here, students should know the terms defined within tables in this chapter.

INTRODUCTION

When you take a car to the repair shop, mechanics can begin work immediately, without advance preparation to protect the vehicle. However, when people need surgery, they must be protected from pain and discomfort through the use of anesthesia. In this chapter you learn about the specialized area of anesthesia services and how to code for them, including the unique anesthesia payment formula. Although the Anesthesia section appears before the Surgery section in the CPT manual, this text presents the introduction to the Surgery section first so that you understand the basics of surgery before tackling anesthesia services.

ANESTHESIA BASICS

Anesthesia is a medical specialty that works in conjunction with surgical specialties to manage a patient's status during a surgical procedure. The surgeon is solely responsible for performing the operative procedure; the anesthesia provider keeps the patient immobile and unaware of pain while the procedure is performed. Coders must be familiar with the types of anesthesia providers, the anesthesia patient care cycle, and the various types of anesthesia.

Anesthesia Providers

Anesthesia providers include anesthesiologists, certified registered nurse anesthetists, and anesthesiologist assistants. **Anesthesiologists** are physicians who specialize in providing perioperative care, developing anesthesia plans, and administrating anesthetics. Some anesthesiologists specialize in anesthesia for cases in pediatrics, obstetrics, cardiothoracic, neurosurgical, orthopedics, critical care, trauma, organ transplant, ambulatory, and pain management. Most procedures require only one anesthesia provider. Anesthesiologists also supervise other anesthesia providers, such as certified registered nurse anesthetists and anesthesiologist assistants.

A **certified registered nurse anesthetist (CRNA)** is a registered nurse with advanced education and training in the field of anesthesia. CRNAs can work alone on cases, with other CRNAs, or under the supervision of an anesthesiologist. An anesthesiologist has more education and training than a CRNA and is licensed to practice medicine. CRNAs can work in hospitals and ambulatory surgery centers, as well as surgery suites, physician offices, and pain management clinics.

An anesthesiologist assistant (AA) is a specialty physician assistant who assists the anesthesiologist and can also work alongside a CRNA. An anesthesia technician, certified anesthesia technician, and certified anesthesia technologist assist the anesthesiologist, AA, and CRNA. AAs also operate, maintain, and monitor equipment and oversee supplies.

The Centers for Medicare and Medicaid Services (CMS) requires that anesthesia services be provided by one of the following providers to qualify for reimbursement:

- Anesthesiologist
- Physician other than an anesthesiologist, including licensed residents and fellows
- Dentist, oral surgeon, or podiatrist who is qualified to administer anesthesia under state law

- CRNA under the supervision of the operating surgeon or an anesthesiologist who is immediately available if needed, meaning that they are physically located in the same area
- AA under the supervision of an anesthesiologist who is immediately available if needed

Anesthesia providers work in a facility, such as an inpatient hospital, outpatient hospital, ambulatory surgery center (ASC), or pain clinic. In most cases, anesthesia providers are not employed by the facility. Individual providers belong to a group practice that contracts with one or more facilities to provide anesthesia services. They bill using CPT codes. Billing is done by the group practice staff or is contracted out to a billing service or a hospital's billing department. Payment is issued to the anesthesia practice.

Anesthesia Care Cycle

The patient care cycle for anesthesia services includes preoperative, intraoperative, and postoperative services.

Preoperative care includes evaluation of the patient's current health and readiness for anesthesia. The **physical status score** identifies the patient's health status at the time anesthesia begins, on a scale of 1 through 5. The **Mallampati score** rates the potential difficulty of endotracheal intubation on a scale of I through IV. Preoperative care also includes placing monitoring devices on the patient and facilitating anesthesia administration with other equipment, such as an endotracheal tube. Anesthesia administration begins when the anesthesia provider induces the patient; it includes monitoring the patient's vital signs to ensure that the patient receives the correct amount of anesthesia and has no adverse reactions.

Intraoperative anesthesia care involves monitoring and managing the patient's physiological status during a procedure and ensuring the patient's safety. If a patient experiences complications from anesthesia, then the anesthesia provider must render appropriate care to the patient, including life-saving interventions, such as cardiopulmonary resuscitation, restoration of fluids and blood, and respiratory therapy. Routine monitoring includes electrocardiography (ECG, EKG), oximetry (*measurement of the concentration of oxygen in the blood*), capnography (*measurement of the concentration of carbon dioxide in the blood*), and mass spectrometry (*measurement of the amount of gases and anesthetics the patient inhales and exhales*), as well as monitoring of temperature and blood pressure. In unusual situations, monitoring may be performed using an intra-arterial catheter (*one inserted into an artery*), a Swan-Ganz (*a catheter inserted into the pulmonary artery*), and a central venous catheter (CVC) (*one inserted into one of the large veins near the heart*).

Physicians use the lowest level of anesthesia necessary to keep the patient comfortable and pain free because of the risks inherent in anesthesia administration. For example, regional—rather than general—anesthesia is used whenever possible because it poses less risk to the patient. For many patients even major joint procedures, such as total hip replacement, can be performed using regional anesthesia. The nature and extent of some procedures leave no option other than general anesthesia.

After surgery is complete, the patient is taken to a **postoperative anesthesia care unit (PACU)** or other area to recover from the surgical procedure and effects of anesthesia. Anesthesia administration ends when the anesthesia provider turns over the care and supervision of the patient to PACU nursing staff. After the anesthesia provider and PACU staff ensure that the patient has no negative effects or complications, the patient is moved out of the PACU. Outpatients are discharged to home. Inpatients are transferred to an inpatient room, where they are monitored for one or more days until discharged by the attending physician.

Types of Anesthesia

Anesthesia is a temporary state, induced by drugs, of unconsciousness, loss of memory, lack of pain, and/or muscle relaxation. The three components of anesthesia are analgesia (*pain relief*), amnesia (*loss of memory*), and immobilization (■ TABLE 31-1). Some drugs may achieve all three components, but often a combination of drugs is used, each with a unique effect (■ TABLE 31-2). General anesthetics cause a reversible loss of consciousness, and local anesthetics cause a reversible loss of sensation in a limited region of the body while maintaining consciousness. Additional drugs, called reversal agents,

are administered to reverse the effects of anesthesia when the procedure is complete.

Anesthesia providers give patients anesthesia through various methods, including intravenous injection or infusion, a face mask, an endotracheal tube, intranasal spray, or an injection directly into the anatomic site where surgery will occur. Patients receive specific types of anesthesia depending on the procedure performed, their physical condition and health history, and the potential for possible complications (■ TABLE 31-3).

Although advances in anesthesia enable providers to eliminate patients' pain during many types of surgeries, anesthesia is not without risks. Patients with comorbidities are at a greater risk for developing complications from anesthesia than are normal, healthy patients. Risks also depend on the complexity of a procedure and the type of anesthesia administered.

Monitored Anesthesia Care

Monitored anesthesia care (MAC) is a planned procedure during which the patient undergoes local anesthesia together with sedation and analgesia. MAC is the first choice in 10–30% of surgical procedures because it is less physically demanding and allows for faster recovery than general anesthesia. The fundamental principles of MAC are safe sedation, anxiety control, and pain control.

Table 31-1   ■   EXAMPLE OF CONSTRUCTING MEDICAL TERMS FOR ANESTHESIA

Combining Form	Prefix/Suffix	Complete Medical Term
algesi/o (*sense of pain*) **esthesi/o** (*nervous sensation*) **mnesi/o** (*memory*)	**a-/an-** (prefix; *lack of*) **-ia** (suffix; *condition*)	**an + alges + ia** (*condition of lack of pain*) **an + esthes + ia** (*condition of lack of nervous sensation*) **a + mnes + ia** (*condition of lack of memory*)

Source: © PB Resources, Inc. Used with permission.

Table 31-2   ■   COMMONLY USED ANESTHETIC DRUGS

Generic Name (Brand Name)	Drug Class
Articaine/epinephrine (Septocaine, Orabloc, Articadent, Zorcaine)	Local anesthetic
Bupivacaine (Marcaine, Sensorcaine)	Local anesthetic
Cisatracurium (Nimbex)	Neuromuscular blocking agent
Dexamethasone (Baycadron, DexPak, Zema Pak, etc.)	Corticosteroid
Fentanyl (Sublimaze)	Narcotic analgesic
Flumazenil (Romazicon)	Reversal agent
Hyoscyamine (Anaspaz, Cystospaz, etc.)	Anticholinergic/antispasmodic
Ketamine (Ketalar)	General anesthetic
Lidocaine (Anestacaine, Xylocaine, etc.)	Topical anesthetic
Meperidine (Demerol)	Narcotic analgesic
Mepivacaine (Carbocaine, Polocaine, Scandonest)	Local or regional anesthetic
Methohexital (Brevital Sodium)	Barbiturate
Midazolam (Versed)	Benzodiazepine sedative
Naloxone (Narcan)	Reversal agent
Prilocaine (AgonEaze, Emla, Oraqix, etc.)	Topical anesthetic
Propofol (Diprivan)	General anesthetic
Succinylcholine (Anectine, Quelicin)	Neuromuscular blocking agent

Table 31-3 ■ **TYPES OF ANESTHESIA**

Type	Description	Examples/Uses
Topical	Numbs the surface area of a body part.	Removal of a foreign object from the eye.
Local	Numbs a small area of a body part. Patient is awake and alert.	Cyst removal from the skin Tooth extraction.
Moderate (conscious) sedation	Uses a mild sedative to relax the patient and pain medicine to relieve pain. Patient stays awake but may not remember the procedure afterward.	Colonoscopy or endoscopy, dental reconstructive surgery or dental prosthetics.
Regional	Epidural, spinal, and peripheral nerve blocks. Blocks pain in an area of the body, such as an arm or leg. Patient feels nothing in that area of the body.	Cesarean delivery, many orthopedic procedures.
General	Affects the whole body, including the brain. Patient feels nothing and has no memory of the procedure afterward.	Open-heart surgery, abdominal surgery.

MAC may include varying levels of sedation as necessary. The provider of monitored anesthesia care must be prepared and qualified to convert to general anesthesia when necessary. If the patient loses consciousness and the ability to respond purposefully, the anesthesia care is a general anesthetic, irrespective of whether airway instrumentation is required.

Third-party payers reimburse for MAC services only when they are medically necessary based on the patient's condition and medical history and patient information documented in the anesthesia record.

Special Anesthesia Techniques

Anesthesia providers occasionally use controlled hypotension and total-body hypothermia to help reduce patients' risk pertaining to certain conditions.

Controlled hypotension, also called *induced hypotension* or *hypotensive anesthesia*, is a technique that lowers the mean arterial blood pressure (MAP) by 30% during surgery, with the goal of reducing intraoperative blood loss and minimizing the risk of fluid overload. This reduces the need for blood transfusions and may also decrease the risk of fluid-related complications, such as edema and deep vein thrombosis (DVT) (*the formation of blood clots in the legs*). Hypotension is accomplished by administering vasodilators (*drugs that widen the diameter of blood vessels*). It is most often used with patients at high risk of these conditions who are undergoing orthopedic, spinal, or maxillofacial surgery.

Total-body hypothermia, also called *induced hypothermia* or *hypothermic anesthesia*, is a technique that lowers the core body temperature below 35°C (95°F) during surgery, with the goal of protecting neurons from injury or degeneration. Hypothermia is accomplished by administering antipyretics (*drugs that lower fever*) and using various physical mechanisms such as ice packs, fans, and cooling blankets and caps. It is most often used with comatose cardiac arrest survivors, head injury victims, and patients with neonatal encephalopathy.

Patient-Controlled Analgesia

Patient-controlled analgesia (PCA) is a method of pain control that patients can administer in response to the level of pain experienced. A PCA pump is an electronically controlled analgesia pump that delivers pain medication intravenously. The patient pushes a button on a hand-held device to direct the pump to deliver the medication. The provider sets a limit on the maximum amount of medication that the pump can deliver to the patient during a specific time interval. PCA pumps help postoperative and terminally ill patients with pain control.

CODING PRACTICE

Exercise 31.1 Anesthesia Basics

Instructions: Use your medical terminology skills and resources to define the following procedures, then identify the applicable code or code range. Follow these steps:

- Use slash marks "/" to break down the underlined term into its root(s) and suffix.
- Define the meaning of the underlined word based on the meaning of each word part.
- Locate the Main Term *Anesthesia* in the CPT Index, then identify the code(s) shown for the procedure in the CPT Index.

Example: anesthesia, <u>angiography</u> angio/graphy   Meaning <u>*recording of vessels*</u>   CPT Code <u>01920</u>

1. Anesthesia, <u>cystolithotomy</u>   Meaning _____   CPT Code _____

2. Anesthesia, <u>vitreoretinal</u> surgery   Meaning _____   CPT Code _____

3. Anesthesia, <u>tenodesis</u>   Meaning _____   CPT Code _____

4. Anesthesia, <u>abdominoperineal</u> resection   Meaning _____   CPT Code _____

(continued)

CODING PRACTICE (continued)

5. Anesthesia, <u>urethrocystoscopy</u>   Meaning _____   CPT Code _____

6. Anesthesia, <u>retropharyngeal</u> tumor excision   Meaning _____   CPT Code _____

7. Anesthesia, <u>vulvectomy</u>   Meaning _____   CPT Code _____

8. Anesthesia, <u>lymphadenectomy</u>   Meaning _____   CPT Code _____

9. Anesthesia, <u>colporrhaphy</u>   Meaning _____   CPT Code _____

10. <u>Omphalocele</u>   Meaning _____   CPT Code _____

CODING GUIDELINES FOR THE ANESTHESIA SECTION

Coders should understand the organization of this CPT section, section guidelines, and instructional notes in the Tabular List. This information is necessary for accurate coding. The CPT **Anesthesia (00100-01999)** section contains 19 subsections, most of which are divided by anatomic site. The last four subsections are divided by the type of procedure: radiological, burn excisions or debridement, obstetric, and other. Review the subsection names and code ranges listed at the beginning of the Anesthesia section in the CPT manual to become familiar with the content and organization.

This chapter includes codes reported by anesthesia providers for the administration of anesthesia services. Do not report codes from this section when the surgeon administers anesthesia. Instead, append modifier **-47 Anesthesia by surgeon** to the CPT code for the procedure. Codes for moderate sedation appear in the **Moderate (Conscious) Sedation (99151-99157)** category of the Medicine section. Moderate sedation codes are discussed in Chapter 29, "Medicine Procedures," in this text.

Codes in the Anesthesia section are supported by the same diagnosis code(s) reported by the surgeon.

CPT Anesthesia section guidelines provide information regarding time reporting, supplied materials, multiple procedures, anesthesia modifiers, and qualifying circumstances. These guidelines are discussed throughout this chapter.

None of the categories in the Anesthesia section provide special instructions.

Instructional notes in the Tabular List redirect coders to other codes for specific procedures, as appropriate, and provide instructions regarding codes that may and may not be reported together. Specific guidelines and instructional notes are discussed throughout this chapter of the text.

ABSTRACTING ANESTHESIA PROCEDURES

Abstracting for anesthesia services is more extensive than abstracting only the surgical procedure. First, identify the surgical procedure performed, then abstract the additional details

needed to assign anesthesia codes and modifiers. Necessary documentation includes:

- Preanesthesia evaluation form (■ FIGURE 31-1), completed by the anesthesia provider
- Anesthesia record (■ FIGURE 31-2, page 594), completed by the anesthesia provider
- Postanesthesia record, completed by the anesthesia provider and the PACU team
- Operative report, completed by the surgeon

In this text, key information from these reports is summarized in the mini-medical-record.

The medical record of anesthesia includes details about the patient's anesthesia administration and monitoring from the beginning of a procedure to the time the patient is recovering postoperatively. The anesthesia provider documents intraoperative anesthesia services including administration and monitoring of anesthesia, drugs administered, techniques used, fluids or blood products given, vital signs, complications, and adverse reactions. The anesthesia provider also documents postanesthesia information in the patient's medical record.

Refer to ■ TABLE 31-4 (page 595) for guidance on how to abstract Anesthesia procedures. Remember that the abstracting questions are a guide and that not every question applies to, or can be answered for, every case. For example, anesthesiologists do not *always* supervise other anesthesia providers. The following information discusses how to abstract anesthesia time and the patient's physical status.

To abstract the surgical procedure, identify the anatomic site, type of procedure, and approach, such as open or closed. If more than one surgical procedure is performed, abstract only the primary or principal procedure. Calculate the anesthesia time for the total duration of all procedures. Anesthesia time begins when the anesthesia provider begins to prepare the patient for the induction of anesthesia and ends when the anesthesia provider is no longer in personal attendance and the patient can be safely placed under postoperative supervision. Anesthesia time is always greater than the time it takes the surgeon to perform the procedure. The start and stop times for anesthesia are documented on the anesthesia record.

PRE-ANESTHESIA EVALUATION

AGE	SEX	HEIGHT	WEIGHT	PRE-PROCEDURE VITAL SIGNS
	☐ M ☐ F	in./cm.	lb./kg.	B/P P R T

PROPOSED PROCEDURE

PREVIOUS ANESTHESIA/OPERATIONS *(If none, check here ☐)*

CURRENT MEDICATIONS *(If none, check here ☐)*

FAMILY HISTORY OF ANESTHESIA COMPLICATIONS *(If none, check here ☐)*

ALLERGIES *(If NKDA, check here ☐)*

AIRWAY/TEETH/HEAD AND NECK

HISTORY FROM
☐ PARENT/GUARDIAN   ☐ POOR HISTORIAN   ☐ CHART
☐ SIGNIFICANT OTHER   ☐ PATIENT

SYSTEM	WNL	COMMENTS	PERTINENT STUDY RESULTS
RESPIRATORY Asthma Pneumonia Bronchitis Productive cough COPD Recent cold Dyspnea SOB Orthopnea Tuberculosis	☐	Tobacco Use: ☐ No ☐ Yes ____ Pack/Day for ____ Years	Chest X-ray Pulmonary Studies
CARDIOVASCULAR Angina MI Arrhythmia Murmur CHF MVP Exercise Tolerance Pacemaker Hypertension Rheumatic fever	☐		EKG
HEPATO/GASTROINTESTINAL Bowel obstruction Jaundice Cirrhosis N&V Hepatitis Reflux/heartburn Histal hernia Ulcers	☐	Ethanol Use: ☐ No ☐ Yes Frequency_____	
NEURO/MUSCULOSKELETAL Arthritis Paresthesia Back problems Syncope CVA/stroke Seizures DJD TIAs Headaches Weakness Loss of consciousness Neuromuscular disease Paralysis	☐		
RENAL/ENDOCRINE Diabetes Renal failure/Dialysis Thyroid disease Urinary retention Urinary tract infection Weight loss/gain	☐		
OTHER Anemia Bleeding tendencies Hemophilia Pregnancy Sickle cell trait Transfusion history			

PROBLEM LIST/DIAGNOSES	ASA PS	LAB STUDIES Hgb/HcT/CBC Electrolytes Urinalysis
	1	
	2	
PLANNED ANESTHESIA/SPECIAL MONITORS	3	Other
	4	
	5	
	E	**POST-ANESTHESIA NOTE**

PRE-ANESTHESIA MEDICATIONS ORDERED

SIGNATURE OF EVALUATOR(S)

Signed   Date   Time

OPTIONAL FORM 517 BACK

Figure 31-1 ■ Example of a preanesthesia evaluation form. *Source: US General Services Administration (OF517).*

AUTHORIZED FOR LOCAL REPRODUCTION

MEDICAL RECORD–ANESTHESIA

PROCEDURE

ITEM	START	STOP
Anesthesia		
Procedure		

DATE	OR NO.	PAGE OF	SURGEON(S)

PRE–PROCEDURE
- ☐ Identified ☐ ID Band ☐ Questioning
- ☐ Chart Review ☐ Permit Signed
- ☐ NPO Since
- Pre-anesthetic State: ☐ Calm
- ☐ Awake ☐ Asleep
- ☐ Apprehensive ☐ Confused
- ☐ Uncooperative ☐ Unresponsive

PATIENT SAFETY
- ☐ Anes. Machine # _____ Checked
- ☐ Safety Belt On ☐ Axillary Roll
- ☐ Arm Restraints ☐ Arms Tucked
- ☐ Pressure points checked and padded
- ☐ Eye Care: ☐ Ointment ☐ Saline
- ☐ Taped ☐ Pads ☐ Goggles

TIME:

MONITORS AND EQUIPMENT
- ☐ Steth ☐ Esoph ☐ Precord ☐ Other
- ☐ Non-Invasive B/P ☐ Nerve Stimulator
- ☐ Continuous EKG ☐ V Lead EKG
- ☐ Pulse Oximeter ☐ Oxygen Analyzer
- ☐ End Tidal CO_2 ☐ Resp Gas Anlyzr
- ☐ Temp _____ ☐ EEG
- ☐ Warming Blanket ☐ Fluid Warmer
- ☐ Airway Humidifier ☐ _____
- ☐ NG/OG Tube ☐ Foley Catheter
- ☐ Art Line _____
- ☐ CVP _____
- ☐ PA Line _____
- ☐ IV(s) _____
- ☐ _____

ANESTHETIC TECHNIQUES
- Method: ☐ General ☐ Spinal
- ☐ Epidural ☐ Caudal ☐ Brachial
- ☐ Bier Block ☐ Ankle Blk ☐ M.A.C.
- General: ☐ Pre-O_2 ☐ L.T.A.
- ☐ Rapid Sequence ☐ Cricoid Pressure
- ☐ Intravenous ☐ Inhalation
- ☐ Intramuscular ☐ Rectal
- Regional: ☐ Position _____
- ☐ Prep _____ ☐ Local _____
- ☐ Needle _____
- ☐ Drug(s) _____
- ☐ Dose _____ ☐ Attempts x ___
- ☐ Site _____ ☐ Level _____
- ☐ Catheter _____ ☐ See Remarks

AIRWAY MANAGEMENT
- ☐ Intubation ☐ Oral ☐ Nasal
- ☐ Direct Vision ☐ Magill's ☐ Blind
- ☐ Diff. see Rmks ☐ Fiber Op ☐ Stylet
- ☐ Attempts x ___ ☐ Blade ___
- ☐ Tube size ___ ☐ Endobronchial
- ☐ Regular ☐ RAE ☐ Armored ☐ Laser
- ☐ Cuffed ☐ Min. occ. pres. ☐ Air ☐NS
- ☐ Uncuffed, leaks at ___ cm H_2O
- ☐ Secured at ___ ☐ ET CO_2 Present
- ☐ Breath Sounds _____
- ☐ Circuit: ☐ Circle ☐ Non-rebreathing
- ☐ Airway: ☐ Oral ☐ Nasal ☐ Natural
- ☐ Mask Case ☐ Via Tracheostomy
- ☐ Nasal Cannula ☐ Simple O_2 Mask

RECOVERY ROOM
Time	B/P	O_2 Sat.
☐ PACU	P	R	T
☐ ICU ☐ L&D		

- ☐ Awake ☐ Spont Resp ☐ Oral Airway
- ☐ Asleep ☐ Ventilator ☐ Nasal Airway
- ☐ Stable ☐ Extubated ☐ Face Shield O_2
- ☐ Unstable ☐ Intubated ☐ T-Piece O_2

CONTROLLED DRUGS
Drug	Used	Destroyed	Returned

Provider	Witness

AGENTS
- ☐ Hal ☐ Enf ☐ Iso (%)
- ☐ N_2O ☐ Air (L/min)
- Oxygen (L/min)
- ( )
- ( )
- ( )
- ( )
- ( )

TOTALS

FLUIDS

MONITORS
- Urine (ml)
- EBL (ml)
- EKG
- % O_2 Inspired (FIO_2)
- O_2 Saturation (SaO_2)
- End Tidal CO_2
- Temp: ☐ °C ☐ °F

SYMBOLS
- × ANESTHESIA
- ⊙ OPERATION
- ∨ ∧ B/PCUFF PRESSURE
- ⊥ ⊤ ARTERIAL LINE PRESSURE
- Δ MEAN ARTERIAL PRESSURE
- ● PULSE
- O SPONTANEOUS RESP
- ∅ ASSISTED RESP
- ⊗ CONTROLLED RESP
- ⊤ TOURNIQUET

VITAL SIGNS

Baseline Values: 200, 180, 160, 140, 120, 100, 80, 60, 40, 20

B/P
P
R

VENT
- Tidal Vol. (ml)
- Resp. Rate
- Peak Pres. (cm H_2O)
- PEEP (cm H_2O)

Symbols for Remarks

Position

ANESTHESIA PROVIDER(S)

REMARKS

PATIENT'S IDENTIFICATION (For typed or written entries give: Name–last, first, middle: ID No. (SSN or other); hospital or medical facility.)

ANESTHESIA
Medical Record
OPTIONAL FORM 517 (7–95)
Prescribed by GSA/ICMR,
FPMR (41 CFR) 101–11.203(b)(10)

Figure 31-2 ■ Example of an anesthesia record. *Source: U.S. General Services Administration (OF517).*

Table 31-4 ■ KEY CRITERIA FOR ABSTRACTING ANESTHESIA PROCEDURES

- ❏ What is anatomic site, type of procedure, and approach for the main procedure performed?
- ❏ What is the diagnosis(es)?
- ❏ How old is the patient?
- ❏ What type of anesthesia is provided (local, regional, general)?
- ❏ How long was anesthesia care provided?
- ❏ What is the health status of the patient?
- ❏ What type of anesthesia provider is in attendance?
- ❏ Are anesthesia services provided personally by the anesthesiologist?
- ❏ How many anesthesia providers did the physician supervise, if any?
- ❏ Did the surgeon provide anesthesia services?
- ❏ Is total-body hypothermia provided?
- ❏ Is controlled hypotension used?
- ❏ Is anesthesia complicated by emergency conditions?
- ❏ Are any unusual forms of monitoring used (intra-arterial, central venous, Swan-Ganz)?
- ❏ Is moderate sedation provided?
- ❏ Is monitored anesthesia care (MAC) provided?

Source: © PB Resources, Inc. Used with permission.

The physical status of the patient, also documented on the anesthesia record, is expressed in categories defined by the American Society of Anesthesiologists (ASA) as follows:

- **-P1 A normal healthy patient**
- **-P2 A patient with mild systemic disease**
- **-P3 A patient with severe systemic disease**
- **-P4 A patient with severe systemic disease that is a constant threat to life**
- **-P5 A moribund patient who is not expected to survive without the operation**
- **-P6 or E (expired) A declared brain-dead patient whose organs are being removed for donor purposes**

Verify that documentation includes diagnoses to support any systemic diseases and comorbidities identified by the physical status category

Guided Example of Abstracting Anesthesia Codes

Refer to the following example throughout this chapter to practice skills for abstracting, assigning, and arranging Anesthesia section codes.

Follow along as Jacob Bates, CCS, abstracts the procedure. Check off each step after you complete it.

INPATIENT HOSPITAL   Gender: F   Age: 76
Status: P3
Anesthesia Provider: MD   Start time: 1200   Stop time: 1510
Anesthesia Type: Epidural
Monitoring: Percutaneous catheter in the left radial artery for monitoring
Diagnosis: Osteoarthritis, generalized. CHF.
Procedure: Total joint replacement, right hip

▶ Jacob reads through the entire record, paying special attention to the name of the procedure and the type of anesthesia. He refers to the Key Criteria for Abstracting Anesthesia Procedures (TABLE 31-4).

- ❏ *What is anatomic site, type of procedure, and approach for the main procedure performed?* Total joint replacement, right hip, open
- ❏ *What is the diagnosis(es)?* Osteoarthritis, generalized; CHF
- ❏ *How old is the patient?* 76
- ❏ *What type of anesthesia is provided?* Epidural, which is a type of regional anesthesia
- ❏ *How long was anesthesia care provided?* 3 hours, 10 minutes
- ❏ *What is the health status of the patient?* P3
- ❏ *What type of anesthesia provider is in attendance?* MD
- ❏ *Are anesthesia services provided personally by the anesthesiologist?* Yes
- ❏ *How many other anesthesia providers did the physician supervise, if any?* None
- ❏ *Is total-body hypothermia provided?* No
- ❏ *Did the surgeon provide anesthesia services?* No
- ❏ *Is controlled hypotension used?* No
- ❏ *Is anesthesia complicated by emergency conditions?* No
- ❏ *Are any unusual forms of monitoring used (intra-arterial, central venous, Swan-Ganz)?* Intra-arterial monitoring with access through the left radial artery
- ❏ *Is moderate sedation provided?* No
- ❏ *Is monitored anesthesia care provided?* No

▶ Next, Jacob must assign the codes and modifiers.

CODING PRACTICE

Exercise 31.2 **Abstracting Anesthesia Procedures**

Instructions: Read the mini-medical-record of each patient's encounter and answer the abstracting questions. Write the answer on the line provided. Do not assign any codes.

---

1. OUTPATIENT HOSPITAL Gender: **M** Age: **67**
Status: **P1**

Start time: **0900** Stop time: **1115**

Anesthesia provider: **CRNA without medical direction**

Anesthesia type: **Patient requested general anesthesia rather than conscious sedation because he was anxious about remaining awake for the procedure**

Diagnosis: **Corneal edema that is a sequela of an automobile accident five years ago**

Procedure: **Corneal transplant, right eye**

a. What is the anatomic site and type of procedure for the main procedure performed? _____

b. What is the diagnosis(es)? _____

c. How old is the patient? _____

d. What type of anesthesia is provided (local, regional, general)? _____

e. How long was anesthesia care provided? _____

f. What is the health status of the patient? _____

g. What type of anesthesia provider is in attendance?

_____

---

2. INPATIENT HOSPITAL Gender: **M** Age: **28**
Status: **P4**

Start time: **0600** Stop time: **0930**

Anesthesia provider: **MD in personal attendance**

Anesthesia type: **General**

Diagnosis: **ESRD**

Procedure: **Kidney transplant, open**

a. What is the anatomic site, type of procedure, and approach for the main procedure performed? _____

_____

b. What is the diagnosis(es)? _____

c. How old is the patient? _____

d. What type of anesthesia is provided (local, regional, general)? _____

e. How long was anesthesia care provided? _____

(continued)

---

2. (continued)

f. What is the health status of the patient? _____

g. What type of anesthesia provider is in attendance?

_____

h. Are anesthesia services provided personally by the anesthesiologist? _____

i. How many anesthesia providers did the physician supervise, if any? _____

---

3. OUTPATIENT HOSPITAL Gender: **M** Age: **66**
Status: **P1**

Start time: **1115** Stop time: **1330**

Anesthesia provider: **CRNA under medical direction of an anesthesiologist**

Anesthesia type: **Spinal**

Diagnosis: **Benign prostatic hyperplasia (BPH)**

Procedure: **Transurethral resection of the prostate (TURP)**

a. What is the anatomic site, type of procedure, and approach for the main procedure performed? _____

_____

b. What is the diagnosis(es)? _____

c. How old is the patient? _____

d. What type of anesthesia is provided (local, regional, general)? _____

e. How long was anesthesia care provided? _____

f. What is the health status of the patient? _____

g. What type of anesthesia provider is in attendance?

_____

h. Are anesthesia services provided personally by the anesthesiologist? _____

---

4. OUTPATIENT HOSPITAL Gender: **M** Age: **78**
Status: **P3**

Start time: **1315** Stop time: **1500**

Anesthesia provider: **CRNA without medical direction**

Anesthesia type: **General**

Diagnosis: **Cardiac arrhythmia**

Procedure: **Pacemaker insertion**

(continued)

CODING PRACTICE (continued)

4. (continued)

a. What is the anatomic site, type of procedure, and approach for the main procedure performed?

_____

b. What is the diagnosis(es)? _____

c. How old is the patient? _____

d. What type of anesthesia is provided (local, regional, general)? _____

e. How long was anesthesia care provided? _____

f. What is the health status of the patient? _____

g. What type of anesthesia provider is in attendance?

_____

---

5. INPATIENT HOSPITAL   Gender: M   Age: 54
Status: P4

Start time: 1415   Stop time: 1945

Anesthesia provider: CRNA under medical direction of an MD who is supervising 3 cases

Anesthesia type: General

Diagnosis: Third-degree burns are the result of a house fire that occurred last week

Procedure: Burn excision and debridement of the trunk involving 20% of total body surface area. Supplemental monitoring provided using a CVC (nontunneled).

a. What is the anatomic site, type of procedure, and approach for the main procedure performed? _____

_____

b. What is the diagnosis(es)? _____

c. How old is the patient? _____

d. What type of anesthesia is provided (local, regional, general)? _____

e. How long was anesthesia care provided? _____

f. What is the health status of the patient? _____

g. What type of anesthesia provider is in attendance?

_____

(continued)

---

5. (continued)

h. Are anesthesia services provided personally by the anesthesiologist? _____

i. How many anesthesia providers did the physician supervise, if any? _____

j. Are any unusual forms of monitoring used (intra-arterial, central venous, Swan-Ganz)? _____

---

6. INPATIENT HOSPITAL   Gender: F   Age: 79
Status: P4

Start time: 1015   Stop time: 1245

Anesthesia provider: MD in personal attendance

Anesthesia type: General, with Swan-Ganz monitoring and controlled hypotension

Diagnosis: Fracture of the neck of the left scapula, hypertension, DVT

Procedure: Open scapula repair with controlled hypotension

a. What is the anatomic site, type of procedure, and approach for the main procedure performed? _____

_____

b. What is the diagnosis(es)? _____

c. How old is the patient? _____

d. What type of anesthesia is provided (local, regional, general)? _____

e. How long was anesthesia care provided? _____

f. What is the health status of the patient? _____

g. What type of anesthesia provider is in attendance?

_____

h. Are anesthesia services provided personally by the anesthesiologist? _____

i. How many anesthesia providers did the physician supervise, if any? _____

j. Is controlled hypotension used? _____

k. Are any unusual forms of monitoring used (intra-arterial, central venous, Swan-Ganz)?

_____

ASSIGNING ANESTHESIA CODES

The **anesthesia code package** includes preoperative visits, administration of anesthesia, intraoperative monitoring (■ TABLE 31-5), and postoperative services. Drugs, tray supplies, and materials above and beyond those usually included with the service are reported in addition to the basic service. These are usually reported by the facility, not the anesthesia provider. Assigning codes for anesthesia services requires the following steps, which are discussed in the next sections.

1. Identify the surgical procedure.
2. Assign the Anesthesia code.
3. Assign the physical status modifier.
4. Assign any qualifying circumstances code(s).
5. Assign any moderate sedation code(s).
6. Assign CPT and HCPCS modifiers.
7. Assign codes for any unusual monitoring services.
8. Calculate the anesthesia payment formula.

Identify the Surgical Procedure

The actual surgical procedure was identified during abstracting, but do not assign a code for it. You do need to know the anatomic site, the type of procedure, and the approach to accurately assign the code for anesthesia services. Anesthesia codes are less specific than Surgery codes. CPT provides fewer than 300 Anesthesia codes but thousands of Surgery codes. Thus, a single Anesthesia code is intended to be used with a large number of Surgery codes.

SUCCESS STEP

The ASA publication "American Society of Anesthesiologists. (2018). *CROSSWALK: A Guide for Surgery/Anesthesia CPT Codes.* Schaumburg, IL" links CPT Surgery codes to the appropriate Anesthesia code(s) and provides tips for code selection.

Assign the Anesthesia Code

Anesthesia providers report only one Anesthesia code per operative session, with the exception of Anesthesia add-on codes for burn excisions or debridement and obstetric services. Report an Anesthesia code for the most extensive or most complex procedure performed.

Table 31-5 ■ **INTRAOPERATIVE SERVICES INCLUDED IN THE ANESTHESIA CODE PACKAGE**

- ❑ Blood administration
- ❑ Fluid administration
- ❑ Electrocardiogram (ECG, EKG)
- ❑ Temperature
- ❑ Blood pressure
- ❑ Oximetry
- ❑ Capnography
- ❑ Mass spectrometry

Coders also must identify the circumstances for which they should *not* assign codes from the Anesthesia section.

- Topical or local anesthesia and metacarpal/metatarsal/digital blocks are included in the CPT surgical package.
- Anesthesia administered by the surgeon, rather than an anesthesia provider, is reported with modifier **-47** appended to the Surgery section code.
- Moderate sedation is reported with Medicine section codes **99151-99157**.

Locating Anesthesia Codes

To assign codes for anesthesia services, search for the Main Term **Anesthesia** in the Index (■ FIGURE 31-3). Most procedures are indexed in multiple ways under the **Anesthesia** entry: by anatomic site, type of procedure, and, often, synonym. First-level modifying terms that identify the anatomic site provide a second-level modifying term for the procedure (e.g., **Anesthesia, Hip, Arthroplasty**). First-level modifying terms that identify the procedure provide a second-level modifying term for the anatomic site (e.g., **Anesthesia, Arthroplasty, Hip**). Some procedures are indexed both by the medical term and the synonym (e.g., **Anesthesia, Replacement, Hip**).

Do not use the actual procedure name as the Main Term because the Main Term for a procedure, such as **Angiography**, leads to the code for the procedure, not the related anesthesia services.

The Tabular List of the Anesthesia section provides a separate category for each anatomic region. Codes within an anatomic region are divided by the specific site and/or the general type of procedure.

Add-on Codes for Burn and Cesarean Delivery Procedures

The Anesthesia section provides three add-on codes: one for burn excisions or debridement and two for cesarean deliveries. Anesthesia for burn excision or debridement is reported based on the percentage of total body surface area (TBSA) treated. Two codes identify treatment of less than 4% of TBSA (**01951**) and 4–9% of TBSA (**01952**). The add-on code **01953** reports each additional 9% of TBSA, or portion thereof, beyond the first 9%.

The Obstetric category provides two add-on codes to be used with code **01967 Neuraxial labor analgesia/anesthesia for planned vaginal delivery**.

- Code **01968** identifies **Anesthesia for cesarean delivery following neuraxial labor analgesia/anesthesia**.
- Code **01969** identifies **Anesthesia for cesarean hysterectomy following neuraxial labor analgesia/anesthesia**.

Assign the Physical Status Modifier (P1-P6)

A physical status modifier must be assigned for each anesthesia patient. It is appended to the Anesthesia code for the primary or most extensive procedure performed. The CPT modifiers correspond with the ASA physical status indicators discussed earlier in this chapter. The ASA category is

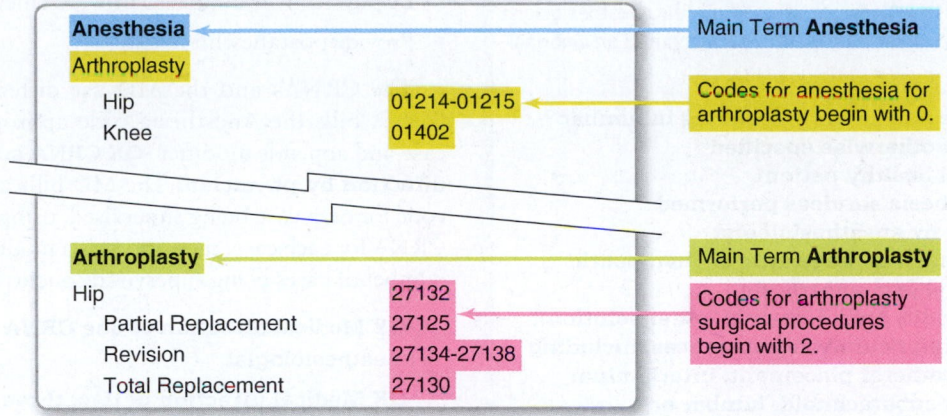

Figure 31-3 ■ CPT Index entries for "*Anesthesia–arthroplasty*" and "*Arthroplasty*". *Source: Annotations © PB Resources, Inc. Used with permission. CPT codes only © American Medical Association.*

documented on the anesthesia record; coders do not determine the physical status based on patients' diagnoses. The modifiers also appear in the CPT guidelines at the beginning of the Anesthesia section.

Assign Any Moderate Sedation Codes (99151-99157)

When an anesthesia provider provides moderate sedation, assign the appropriate code(s) from the Medicine section except for services listed in the Anesthesia section **00100-01999**. Moderate sedation is discussed in detail in Chapter 29, "Medicine Procedures," in this text.

Assign Any Qualifying Circumstances Codes (99100-99140)

Qualifying circumstances codes are add-on codes that identify four situations that increase the difficulty of anesthesia administration. They include codes for age younger than 1 year or older than 70 (**99100**) (■ FIGURE 31-4); use of total-body hypothermia (**99116**); use of controlled hypotension (**99135**); and emergency circumstances (**99140**). Do not use the code for age younger than one year when the Anesthesia code already includes the age. Qualifying circumstance codes appear in the CPT guidelines at the beginning of the Anesthesia section and can also be located under the Main Term **Anesthesia** and the first-level modifying term **Special Circumstances**. In the Tabular List, they appear in numerical order in the Medicine section.

Do not append modifiers to codes for qualifying circumstances.

Assign CPT and HCPCS Modifiers

In addition to physical status modifiers, Anesthesia codes accept both CPT and HCPCS modifiers. Do not use modifiers for laterality (-50, -RT, -LT) on Anesthesia codes, even if a paired anatomic site, such as one arm or leg, receives a regional block.

Unusual Procedural Circumstances

CPT modifiers describe unusual procedural circumstances, such as those for unusual anesthesia (**-23**), discontinued procedures (**-53**), reduced services (**-52**), distinct procedural service (**-59, -XE, -XP, -XS, -XU**) (■ FIGURE 31-5, page 600), repeat procedures (**-76, -77**), and unplanned returns to the operating room (**-78, -79**). Report modifier **-23** when a procedure that normally requires no anesthesia or local anesthesia instead requires general anesthesia. Two modifiers used specifically by outpatient hospitals and ASCs report discontinued procedures:

-73 Discontinued outpatient hospital/ambulatory surgery center (ASC) procedure prior to the administration of anesthesia

-74 Discontinued outpatient hospital/ambulatory surgery center (ASC) procedure after administration of anesthesia

Refer to Appendix A of the CPT manual for full descriptions of these modifiers.

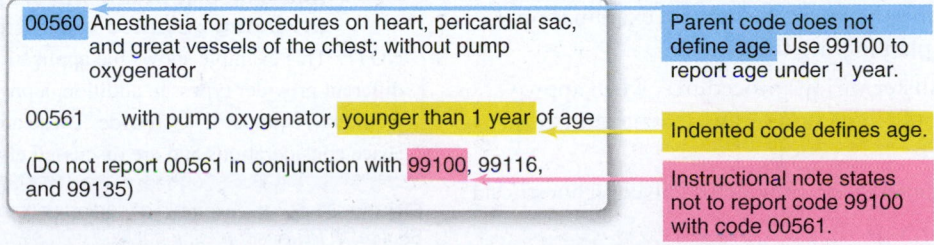

Figure 31-4 ■ Example of Anesthesia codes that do and do not specify age.

Following a lumbar disk replacement procedure, the anesthesiologist administered an epidural for postoperative pain control on a normal healthy patient (P1).

00630-P1-AA Anesthesia for procedures in lumbar
        region; not otherwise specified
        -P1 Normal healthy patient
        -AA Anesthesia services performed
        personally by anesthesiologist
62322-59 Injection(s), of diagnostic or therapeutic
        substance(s) (e.g. anesthetic,
        antispasmodic, opioid, steroid, other solution),
        not including neurolytic substances, including
        needle or catheter placement, interlaminar
        epidural or subarachnoid, lumbar or
        sacral (caudal), without imaging.
        -59 Separate procedure

Figure 31-5 ■ Example of using modifier -59 with anesthesia services.

Monitored Anesthesia Care

When MAC is provided, report one of the following HCPCS modifiers:

-QS MAC (monitored anesthesia care, informational)

-G8 Monitored anesthesia care (MAC) for deep complex, complicated, or markedly invasive surgical procedures.

-G9 Monitored anesthesia care for patient who has history of severe cardiopulmonary condition

Anesthesia Providers and Medical Direction

Anesthesiologists may personally provide services to some patients and provide only medical direction for other patients whose direct anesthesia provider is a CRNA or anesthesiologist assistant.

When the anesthesiologist personally provides anesthesia services, assign the appropriate Anesthesia code for the procedure and append modifier -AA Anesthesia services performed personally by anesthesiologist.

In some states, and for some payers, CRNAs can provide anesthesia services independently, without medical direction. In this situation, assign the appropriate Anesthesia code for the procedure and append modifier -QZ CRNA service: without medical direction by a physician.

Medicare and some other payers, and some states, require CRNAs to work under the medical direction of an anesthesiologist. To qualify for medical direction, physicians must meet the following criteria:

- Perform the preanesthesia evaluation and examination and develop the plan for anesthesia

- Personally administer various procedures, when appropriate, including the induction of and emergence from anesthesia

- Oversee another anesthesia provider involved in anesthesia care

- Frequently monitor anesthesia care of the patient

- Be physically available to provide emergency care if needed

- Provide postanesthesia care

The CRNAs and the MD use different modifiers. Each CRNA bills the Anesthesia code appropriate for his or her case and appends modifier -QX CRNA service: with medical direction by physician. The MD bills a separate Anesthesia code for each case being supervised, using the same code as the CRNA for each case, then appends a modifier that identifies the number of cases being supervised concurrently (■ Figure 31-6):

-QY Medical direction of one CRNA by an anesthesiologist

-QK Medical direction of two, three, or four concurrent anesthesia procedures involving qualified individuals

-AD Medical supervision by a physician: more than four concurrent anesthesia procedures

The payment for anesthesia services is prorated between the MD and the CRNA for each case.

An anesthesiologist provides medical direction of three CRNAs, each providing anesthesia services for a different patient.

Patient #1: Pancreatectomy
00794 Anesthesia for intraperitoneal procedures in
        upper abdomen including laparoscopy;
        pancreatectomy, partial or total (e.g., Whipple
        procedure)
CRNA: 00794-QX CRNA service: with medical direction
        by physician
MD: 00794-QK Medical direction of two, three, or four
        concurrent anesthesia procedures involving
        qualified individuals

Patient #2: Ventral hernia repair
00832 Anesthesia for hernia repairs in lower abdomen;
        ventral and incisional hernias
CRNA: 00832-QX CRNA service: with medical direction
        by physician
MD: 00832-QK Medical direction of two, three, or four
        concurrent anesthesia procedures involving
        qualified individuals

Patient #3: Vaginal hysterectomy
00944 Anesthesia for vaginal procedures (including
        biopsy of labia, vagina, cervix or endometrium);
        vaginal hysterectomy
CRNA: 00944-QX CRNA service: with medical direction
        by physician
MD: 00944-QK Medical direction of two, three, or
        four concurrent anesthesia procedures
        involving qualified individuals

NOTE: This example shows the application of modifiers for different provider types. In addition, a physical status modifier would be required on each code. These are not shown here for space considerations and are discussed elsewhere in this chapter.

Figure 31-6 ■ Example of coding anesthesia medical direction.
Source: © PB Resources, Inc. Used with permission. CPT codes only © American Medical Association.

Assign Code(s) for Any Unusual Monitoring Services

Assign codes for unusual monitoring services not included in the Anesthesia package when the catheter insertion is separate and distinct from the operative procedure (■ TABLE 31-6). Do not assign a separate code when the catheter is inserted as part of the operative procedure. Assign a code for insertion of a Swan-Ganz catheter when it is inserted through an existing CVC. Do not assign a code for the existing CVC because it was not inserted during the current treatment.

Calculate the Anesthesia Payment Formula

Anesthesia services are reimbursed using a unique payment formula, which varies slightly between Medicare and commercial payers (■ FIGURE 31-7, page 602). Payment for Anesthesia codes uses **base units (B)**, rather than relative value units (RVUs), as with other CPT codes. The ASA assigns base unit values to Anesthesia section codes, qualifying circumstances codes, and physical status modifiers, and publishes updates in the *Relative Value Guide* (RVG). The components of the anesthesia payment formula are three unit values and an anesthesia conversion factor expressed as $(B + T + M) \times CF$.

- Base units (B)—A number that represents the complexity of the anesthesia, the risk to the patient, and the skills needed by the anesthesia provider to render services for each CPT Anesthesia code. Use the base units for the most complex or extensive Anesthesia service provided. (Assign a minimum of five units for procedures of the head, neck, or shoulder girdle that require field avoidance and procedures performed in a position other than supine or lithotomy.)

- Time units (T)—The total minutes of anesthesia service provided for all procedures divided by 15.

- Modifying units (M)—Numbers assigned to each physical status modifier and each qualifying circumstance code to represent the added difficulty of the procedure (■ TABLE 31-7, page 602). Some payers, including Medicare, do not pay extra for modifying units.

- Anesthesia conversion factor (CF)—A dollar value, adjusted for geographic differences in cost, that Medicare (and other payers) assigns to one base unit of anesthesia. The anesthesia conversion factor is different than the overall conversion factor established by Medicare (and other payers) for other CPT codes. This amount is updated annually.

To compute the payment or allowable amount, follow these steps (■ FIGURE 31-8, page 602).

1. Look up the numbers for the base units, time units, and modifying units (physical status and qualifying circumstances).

2. Add the number of units together to arrive at a total.

3. Multiply the total number of units by the anesthesia conversion factor.

4. The resulting number is the payment or allowable amount for the procedure.

When reporting Anesthesia services on a claim, report only time units in Item 24G on the CMS-1500 form or the corresponding field on the 837P electronic claim. Payers' claims processing systems automatically calculate the base units and modifying units using preloaded data. Some payers might require that actual minutes be reported instead of time units. In some areas of the country, time longer than four hours is calculated in 10-minute intervals.

> ### SUCCESS STEP
>
> Base units and conversion factors can be downloaded from the Anesthesiologists Center on the CMS website (www.cms.gov). Most medical billing systems automatically calculate the anesthesia payment formula based on preloaded data, even though it is not entered on the CMS-1500 form or 837P electronic claim.

Guided Example of Assigning Anesthesia Codes

To practice skills for assigning codes from the Anesthesia section, continue with the example from earlier in the chapter about a patient who was seen for a total hip replacement with regional anesthesia. Follow along in your CPT manual as Jacob Bates, CCS, assigns codes. Check off each step after you complete it.

► First, Jacob confirms the procedure of a total hip replacement performed under regional anesthesia.

► Second, Jacob assigns the code for anesthesia services.

   ❑ He searches the Index for the Main Term **Anesthesia**.

   ❑ He locates the first-level modifying term **Arthroplasty** and the second-level modifying term **Hip**.

Table 31-6 ■ ASSIGNING CODES FOR CATHETER MONITORING DURING ANESTHESIA

Catheter Type	Main Term	Modifying Terms	Code(s)
Central venous (CVC) (centrally inserted)	Central Venous Catheter Placement	Insertion, Central, Non-Tunneled	36555 Patient <5 years old 36556 Patient ≥5 years
Peripherally inserted central venous (PICC)	Central Venous Catheter Placement	Insertion, Peripheral, without Port or Pump	36568 Patient <5 years old 36569 Patient ≥5 years
Intra-arterial (A-line)	Catheterization	Arterial System	36625 Cutdown 36620 Percutaneous
Swan-Ganz	Swan-Ganz Catheter	Insertion	93503

Source: © PB Resources, Inc. Used with permission. CPT codes only © American Medical Association.

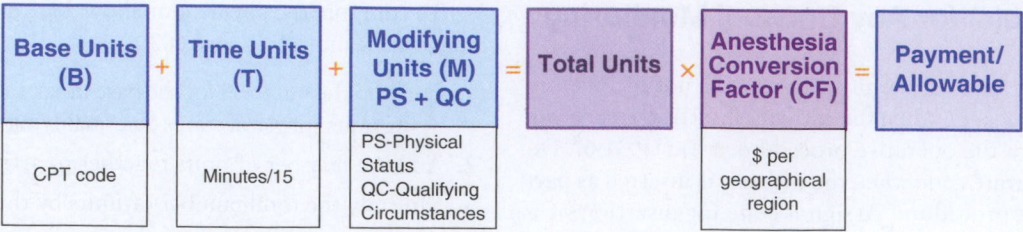

Figure 31-7 ■ Anesthesia payment formula. *Source: © PB Resources, Inc. Used with permission.*

Table 31-7 ■ SUMMARY OF ANESTHESIA UNITS FOR MODIFYING FACTORS

Modifier	Modifying Units
-P1, -P2, -P6	0
-P3	1
-P4	2
-P5	3

Code	Modifying Units
99100	1
99116	5
99135	5
99140	2

An anesthesiologist provides anesthesia services for a pancreatectomy. The physical status is P1, a normal healthy patient. Total anesthesia time is 3 hours (180 minutes).

00794-P1-AA Anesthesia for intraperitoneal procedures in upper abdomen including laparoscopy; pancreatectomy, partial or total (eg, Whipple procedure). -P1 Normal healthy patient. -AA Anesthesia services performed personally by anesthesiologist

1. *Look up the numbers for the base units, time units, and modifying units.*
   B-Base units: 8
   T-Time units: 180/15 = 12
   M-Modifying units: 0
2. *Add the number of units together to arrive at a total.*
   Total units: 8 + 12 = 20
   CF-Anesthesia conversion factor: $22.04
3. *Multiply the total number of units times the anesthesia conversion factor.*
   Payment or allowable: 20 × $22.04 = $480.80
4. *The resulting number is the payment or allowable amount for the procedure.*
   $440.80

Figure 31-8 ■ Example of calculating anesthesia payment. *Source: © PB Resources, Inc. Used with permission. CPT codes only © American Medical Association.*

❑ He writes down the code range listed: **01214-01215**.

❑ As a double-check, he also looks under the Main Term **Anesthesia** and the first-level modifying term **Hip**. The same codes are listed: **01214-01215**.

▶ Jacob consults the Tabular List to verify codes **01214-01215** and select the appropriate code.

❑ He notices that both codes are indented codes under the parent code **01210 Anesthesia for open procedures involving hip joint**.

❑ He reads the description for **01214 Total hip arthroplasty** and compares it with code **01215 Revision of total hip arthroplasty**.

❑ Because code **01215** describes a revision of a previous hip arthroplasty, it does not apply to this case.

▶ Jacob checks for instructional notes in the Tabular List and finds none.

❑ As a double-check, he scans the rest of the codes under the category **Upper Leg (Except Knee)**. The other codes for open procedures are not for a total hip arthroplasty. The remaining codes describe closed procedures, which do not describe this case.

❑ The full description of code **01214 is Anesthesia for open procedures involving hip joint; total hip arthroplasty**.

▶ Third, Jacob assigns the physical status modifier that is appended to the anesthesia code.

❑ He verifies the physical status modifier in the medical record, **P3 A patient with severe systemic disease**.

❑ He verifies that the description is consistent with congestive heart failure.

▶ Fourth, Jacob assigns a qualifying circumstances code because of the patient's age.

❑ **99100 Anesthesia for patient of extreme age, younger than 1 year and older than 70**

▶ Fifth, Jacob must assign a code for the intra-arterial monitoring.

❑ He locates the Main Term **Catheterization** and the first-level modifying term **Arterial system**.

❑ He reviews the second-level modifying terms and selects **Percutaneous 36620**.

❑ He verifies code **36620 Arterial catheterization or cannulation for sampling, monitoring or transfusion (separate procedure); percutaneous**.

❏ He makes note of the symbol ø which identifies that this code is exempt from modifier **-51 Multiple procedures**.

▶ Sixth, Jacob assigns CPT and HCPCS modifiers.

❏ Code **01214** requires the modifier **-P3** to identify the physical status of the patient at the beginning of the procedure.

❏ Code **01214** also requires modifier **-AA Anesthesia services performed personally by anesthesiologist**.

❏ Code **99100** does not require any modifiers. Modifiers **-P3** and **-AA** are assigned to the Anesthesia service code only.

❏ Code **36620** does not require any modifiers because it is exempt from modifier **-51**. National Correct Coding Initiative (NCCI) edits do not place any restrictions on these codes being reported together.

▶ Seventh, Jacob calculates the anesthesia payment formula.

❏ The base units for this procedure are 8.

❏ The time units for 3 hours, 10 minutes are 190 minutes/15 = 13 (12.66 rounded up).

❏ The modifying unit for the physical status **P3** is 1.

❏ The modifying unit for qualifying circumstances code **99100** is 1.

❏ The total units are 8 + 13 + 1 + 1 = 23.

❏ The conversion factor for the local geographic region is $22.03.

❏ The total payment or allowable is 23 units × $22.03 = $506.69.

❏ Code **36620** will be paid in addition to the anesthesia payment.

▶ Next, Jacob must determine how to sequence the codes.

CODING PRACTICE

Exercise 31.3 Assigning Anesthesia Codes

Instructions: Each question has three parts.

Part a: Read the mini-medical-record of each patient's encounter. Review the information abstracted in Exercise 31.2 for questions 1–3. For questions 4–6, abstract the case on your own. Assign CPT codes using the Index and Tabular List, and arrange the codes in the proper sequence. Assign modifiers for physical status, type of provider, and any other applicable circumstances. Write the code(s) and modifier(s) on the line provided.

Part b: Determine the time units.

Part c: Calculate the modifying units. PS is the number of physical status units. QC is the number of qualifying circumstances units.

---

1. OUTPATIENT HOSPITAL   Gender: M   Age: 67
Status: P1

Start time: 0900   Stop time: 1115

Anesthesia provider: CRNA without medical direction

Anesthesia type: Patient requested general anesthesia rather than conscious sedation because he was anxious about remaining awake for the procedure

Diagnosis: Corneal edema that is a sequela of an automobile accident five years ago

Procedure: Corneal transplant, right eye

(continued)

---

1. (continued)

Tip: Assign a modifier for unusual anesthesia.

a. 1 CPT Code _____

b. Anesthesia time (minutes) _____/15 =
Time units

c. PS _____ + QC _____ =
_____ Modifying units

---

2. INPATIENT HOSPITAL   Gender: M   Age: 28
Status: P4

Start time: 0600   Stop time: 0930

Anesthesia provider: MD in personal attendance

Anesthesia type: General

Diagnosis: ESRD

Procedure: Kidney transplant, open

a. 1 CPT Code _____

b. Anesthesia time (minutes) _____/15 =
Time units

c. PS _____ + QC _____ =
_____ Modifying units

CODING PRACTICE (continued)

3. OUTPATIENT HOSPITAL Gender: M Age: 66
Status: P1

Start time: 1115 Stop time: 1330

Anesthesia provider: CRNA under medical direction of an anesthesiologist

Anesthesia type: Spinal

Diagnosis: Benign prostatic hyperplasia (BPH)

Procedure: Transurethral resection of the prostate (TURP)

Tip: Code only for the CRNA.

a. 1 CPT Code _____

b. Anesthesia time (minutes) _____/15 =
   Time units

c. PS _____ + QC _____ =
   _____ Modifying units

---

4. INPATIENT HOSPITAL Gender: F Age: 3 months Status: P4

Start time: 0700 Stop time: 1245

Anesthesia provider: MD in personal attendance

Anesthesia type: General

Diagnosis: Atrial septal defect

Procedure: Open-heart surgery with pump oxygenator

Tip: Abstract this scenario on your own before coding.

a. 1 CPT Code _____

b. Anesthesia time (minutes) _____ /15 = Time units

c. PS _____ + QC _____ =
   _____ Modifying units

---

5. INPATIENT HOSPITAL Gender: M Age: 61
Status: P5

Start time: 0345 Stop time: 0845

Anesthesia provider: MD in personal attendance

Anesthesia type: General

Diagnosis: Dissecting abdominal aortic aneurysm

Procedure: Emergency repair of AAA

Tip: Abstract this scenario on your own before coding. The abdominal aorta is a major abdominal blood vessel. Assign one code for the anesthesia and one code for the qualifying circumstances.

a. 2 CPT Codes _____

b. Anesthesia time (minutes) _____/15 =
   Time units

c. PS _____ + QC _____ =
   _____ Modifying units

---

6. INPATIENT HOSPITAL Gender: F Age: 34
Status: P3

Start time: 1345 Stop time: 1700

Anesthesia provider: Anesthesiologist in personal attendance

Anesthesia type: General with MAC due to morbid obesity, which significantly increased the complexity of the procedure

Diagnosis: Morbid obesity, obstructive sleep apnea, hypertension

Procedure: Gastric banding

Tip: Abstract this scenario on your own before coding.

a. 1 CPT Code _____

b. Anesthesia time (minutes) _____/15 =
   Time units

c. PS _____ + QC _____ =
   _____ Modifying units

ARRANGING ANESTHESIA CODES

Many times anesthesia cases require only one code. Even when multiple surgical procedures are performed, only one anesthesia code—the one for the most complex procedure—is assigned. Multiple codes are required when there is a qualifying circumstance or an additional anesthesia service not included in the anesthesia package. When this occurs, sequence the codes as follows:

1. Anesthesia service (**00100-01999**) with **P** modifier
2. Additional services
3. Qualifying circumstances (**99100-99140**)

When a code requires multiple modifiers, remember to sequence the modifiers that affect payment before those that are informational only.

Guided Example of Arranging Anesthesia Codes

To practice skills for arranging codes for the Anesthesia section, continue with the example from earlier in the chapter about the patient who was seen for a total right hip arthroplasty. Follow along in your CPT manual as Jacob Bates, CCS, arranges (sequences) the codes. Check off each step after you complete it.

▶ Jacob reviews the sequencing guidelines for Anesthesia.

❑ The Anesthesia code **01214** is the primary service provided and has the highest price, so should be sequenced first. The code requires two modifiers, **-P3** and **-AA**. Modifier **-P3** is required on Anesthesia codes and affects payment because it adds modifying units to the payment formula. **-AA** is informational only and does not affect payment, so **-P3** is sequenced first, followed by **-AA**.

❑ The modifying circumstances code **99100** has no RVU or monetary value, so it is sequenced last.

❑ Code **36620** for the arterial line monitoring is sequenced second. The MFPS assigns 1.47 RVUs to this code.

▶ Jacob finalizes the procedure codes, modifiers, and sequencing for this case:

(1) **01214-P3-AA Anesthesia for open procedures involving hip joint; total hip arthroplasty. -P3 A patient with severe systemic disease. -AA Anesthesia services performed personally by anesthesiologist**

(2) **36620 Arterial catheterization or cannulation for sampling, monitoring or transfusion (separate procedure); percutaneous**

(3) **99100 Anesthesia for patient of extreme age, younger than 1 year and older than 70**

▶ Jacob assigns and sequences the ICD-10-CM diagnosis codes that support the need for the service.

(1) **M16.11 Unilateral primary osteoarthritis, right hip**

(2) **I50.9 Heart failure, unspecified**

CODING PRACTICE

Exercise 31.4 Arranging Anesthesia Codes

Instructions: **Part a.** Read the mini-medical-record of each patient's encounter. Review the information abstracted in Exercise 31.2 for questions 1–3. For questions 4–6, abstract the case on your own. Assign CPT codes using the Index and Tabular List, and arrange the codes in the proper sequence. Assign modifiers for physical status, type of provider, and any other applicable circumstances. Write the code(s) and modifier(s), if any, on the line provided.

Part b: Calculate the time and modifying units. Using the base units provided in the *Tip* and a conversion factor of $22.04, calculate the anesthesia payment formula. Base units (B) + Time units (T) + Modifying units (M) = Total units (TU) × $22.04 = Anesthesia payment/allowable.

---

1. OUTPATIENT HOSPITAL   Gender: M   Age: 78
Status: P3

Start time: 1315   Stop time: 1500

Anesthesia provider: CRNA without medical direction

Anesthesia type: General

Diagnosis: Cardiac arrhythmia

Procedure: Pacemaker insertion

Tip: Base units = 4.

a. 2 CPT Codes _____

b. B _____ + T _____ +
M _____ = _____ TU ×
$22.04 = $ _____

---

2. INPATIENT HOSPITAL   Gender: M   Age: 54
Status: P4

Start time: 1415   Stop time: 1945

Anesthesia provider: CRNA under medical direction of an MD who is supervising 3 cases

Anesthesia Type: General

Diagnosis: Third-degree burns are the result of a house fire that occurred last week

Procedure: Burn excision and debridement of the trunk involving 20% of total body surface area. Supplemental monitoring provided using a CVC (nontunneled).

Tip: Base units = 7. Provide the quantity for the anesthesia codes. Code for the CRNA only.

a. 3 CPT Codes (CRNA) _____ × _____,
_____ × _____, _____

b. B _____ + T _____ + M
_____ = _____ TU × $22.04 = $ _____

---

3. INPATIENT HOSPITAL   Gender: F   Age: 79
Status: P4

Start time: 1015   Stop time: 1245

Anesthesia provider: MD in personal attendance

Anesthesia Type: General, with Swan-Ganz monitoring and controlled hypotension

(continued)

CODING PRACTICE (continued)

3. (continued)

Diagnosis: Fracture of the neck of the left scapula, hypertension, DVT

Procedure: Open scapula repair with controlled hypotension

Tip: Base units = 3. Sequence the code for the Swan-Ganz catheter second.

a. 4 CPT Codes _____

b. B _____ + T _____ + M _____
   = _____ TU × \$22.04 = \$ _____

---

4. INPATIENT HOSPITAL   Gender: F   Age: 26   Status: P1

Start time: 1215   Stop time: 1345

Anesthesia provider: MD in personal attendance

Anesthesia Type: Anesthesia for cesarean delivery following neuraxial labor analgesia for planned vaginal delivery

Diagnosis: Cephalopelvic disproportion and obstructed labor

Procedure: Cesarean delivery after planned vaginal delivery, 1 healthy baby boy delivered

Tip: Abstract this scenario on your own before coding. Base units = 7.

a. 2 CPT Codes _____

b. B _____ + T _____ + M _____
   = _____ TU × \$22.04 = \$ _____

---

5. OUTPATIENT HOSPITAL   Gender: M   Age: 9 months   Status: P1

Start time: 1030   Stop time: 1300

Anesthesia provider: CRNA under medical direction of an anesthesiologist. MD provides medical direction to 5 cases.

Anesthesia Type: General

Diagnosis: Undescended left testicle

Procedure: Open orchiopexy

Tip: Abstract this scenario on your own before coding. Assign codes for both the CRNA and anesthesiologist (MD).

a. 2 CPT Codes (CRNA) _____
   2 CPT Codes (MD) _____

b. Anesthesia time (minutes) _____/15 = _____ Time units

c. PS _____ + QC = _____ Modifying units

---

6. DENTAL OFFICE   Gender: M   Age: 25   Status: P1

Start time: 0945   Stop time: 1100

Anesthesia provider: CRNA without medical direction provided general anesthesia, monitoring, and observation while dentist performed the procedure

Anesthesia Type: General

Diagnosis: Impacted wisdom teeth

Procedure: Tooth extraction #1, 16, 17, 32

Tip: Abstract this scenario on your own before coding. Base units = 5.

a. 1 CPT Code _____

b. B _____ + T _____ + M _____
   = TU × \$22.04 = \$ _____

CHAPTER SUMMARY

In this chapter you learned that:

- Anesthesia is a medical specialty that works in conjunction with surgical specialties to manage the patient's status during a surgical procedure by keeping the patient immobile and unaware of pain while the procedure is performed.

- CPT Anesthesia section guidelines provide information regarding time reporting, supplied materials, multiple procedures, anesthesia modifiers, and qualifying circumstances. Codes are used by anesthesia providers for the administration of anesthesia services.

- Abstracting for anesthesia services differs from abstracting for the actual surgical procedure because first you need to identify the actual surgical procedure performed, then you need to abstract the additional details needed to assign anesthesia codes and modifiers.

- The anesthesia code package includes preoperative visits, administration of anesthesia, intraoperative monitoring, and postoperative services; several steps are required to assign all required codes and modifiers.

- Multiple Anesthesia section codes are required when there is a qualifying circumstance or an additional anesthesia service not included in the anesthesia package.

CONCEPT QUIZ

Take a moment to look back at Anesthesia section coding and solidify your skills. Try to answer the questions from memory first, then refer to the discussion in this chapter if you need a little extra help.

Completion

Instructions: Write the term that completes each statement based on the information you learned in this chapter. Choose from the following list. Some choices may be used more than once and some choices may not be used at all.

amnesia	moderate (conscious) sedation
analgesia	monitored anesthesia care (MAC)
anesthesia	
capnography	oximetry
central venous	patient care cycle
controlled hypotension	patient-controlled analgesia
immobilization	provider
intra-arterial	regional
Mallampati	Swan-Ganz
medical specialty	total-body hypothermia

1. The _____ score rates the potential difficulty of endotracheal intubation on a scale of I through IV.

2. The _____ for anesthesia services includes pre-, intra-, and postoperative services.

3. The three components of anesthesia care are _____, _____, and _____.

4. _____ is a planned procedure during which the patient undergoes local anesthesia together with sedation and analgesia.

5. _____ is the technique that lowers mean arterial blood pressure to reduce intraoperative blood loss and minimize the risk of fluid overload.

6. _____, _____ and _____ monitoring are considered unusual forms of anesthesia monitoring.

7. _____ is the measurement of the concentration of carbon dioxide in the blood.

8. A method of pain control that patients can administer in response to the level of pain they are experiencing is _____.

9. Epidural, spinal, and peripheral nerve blocks are examples of _____ anesthesia.

10. _____ is a technique that lowers the core body temperature during surgery to protect neurons from injury or degeneration.

Multiple Choice

Instructions: Circle the letter of the best answer to each question based on the information you learned in this chapter.

1. What class of drug is ketamine?
   A. Neuromuscular blocking agent
   B. Reversal agent
   C. General anesthetic
   D. Narcotic analgesic

2. How would you code the following procedure? *An anesthesiologist provides general anesthesia for 70-year old patient with a severe systemic disease undergoing total hip arthroplasty.*
   A. 01214-AA-P3, 99100
   B. 01214-P3-AA, 99100
   C. 99100-P3-AA, 01214-AA-P3
   D. 01214-AA, 99100-P3

3. How would you code the following procedure? *A CRNA provides anesthesia services with medical direction by physician to a normal healthy 35-year-old patient undergoing repair of ventral and incisional hernias.*
   A. 00832-P1-QX
   B. 00832-P1-QY
   C. 00832-P1-QZ
   D. 00832, 99100

4. What is the designation for a registered nurse with advanced education and training in the field of anesthesia?
   A. RNFA
   B. AA
   C. ARN
   D. CRNA

5. What score identifies a patient's health status on a scale of 1 through 5 at the time anesthesia is begun?
   A. Anesthesia score
   B. Physical status score
   C. Apgar score
   D. Mallampati score

6. What is the first step in assigning codes for anesthesia services?
   A. Identify the surgical procedure.
   B. Select the qualifying circumstances code(s).
   C. Calculate the anesthesia payment formula.
   D. Determine the physical status modifier.

7. What is the anesthesia payment formula?
   A. $B + T + M + CF$
   B. $B + PS + QC$
   C. $(B + T + QC) \times CF$
   D. $(B + T + M) \times CF$

(continued)

(continued from page 607)

8. What is the name of the dollar value that Medicare assigns to one base unit of anesthesia?
   A. Anesthesia geographic factor
   B. Anesthesia allowable amount
   C. Anesthesia conversion factor
   D. Anesthesia payment formula

9. How would you code the following procedure? *An anesthesiologist provides general anesthesia for a patient with a mild systemic disease undergoing a total cystectomy (removal of the urinary bladder).*
   A. 00870-P2-AA
   B. 00864-P2-AA
   C. 51570-P2-AA
   D. 51530-P2-AA

10. When is more than one anesthesia code reported?
    A. An anesthesia add-on code is required
    B. More than one anesthesiologist participates in the procedure
    C. More than one surgical procedure is performed during the same operative session
    D. Complications arise due to the anesthesia

KEEP ON CODING

Instructions: Read the procedural statement, then use the Index and Tabular List to assign and sequence CPT procedure codes. Assign modifiers and qualifying circumstances codes as appropriate. Do not calculate the time. Write the code(s) on the line provided.

1. Anesthesia for an otherwise healthy patient for removal of bladder calculus by incision with bladder spoon and anesthesia provided by CRNA with medical direction from physician; status P1. CPT Code(s) _____

2. Anesthesia for an otherwise healthy patient for left carpal tunnel release; anesthesia provided by CRNA without medical direction; status P1. CPT Code(s) _____

3. Anesthesia for a warfarin patient for arthroscopic partial medial meniscectomy; anesthesia supervised by physician with five concurrent anesthesia procedures; status P2. CPT Code(s) _____

4. Anesthesia for a patient with mild hypertension has right hemilaminectomy of L1 and L2 and discectomy of L1; anesthesia personally provided by anesthesiologist; status P2. CPT Code(s) _____

5. Anesthesia for a controlled diabetic patient for right ankle arthrodesis, open; anesthesia provided by CRNA without physician supervision; status P2. CPT Code(s) _____

6. Anesthesia for an oncology patient for radical hysterectomy, bilateral salpingo-oophorectomy, extended pelvic lymphadenectomy; anesthesia personally provided by anesthesiologist; status P4. CPT Code(s) _____

7. Anesthesia for a mild congestive heart failure patient for arthroscopic removal of an osteochondritis dissecans of right glenohumeral joint; anesthesia provided by CRNA without physician supervision; status P2. CPT Code(s) _____

8. Anesthesia for a patient with severe carotid stenosis for left carotid endarterectomy with bovine patch angioplasty; anesthesia provided by a physician providing medical direction of three concurrent anesthesia procedures involving qualified individuals; status P4. CPT Code(s) _____

9. Anesthesia for a 78-year-old patient for craniotomy to evacuate frontal hematoma; anesthesia personally provided by anesthesiologist; status P4. CPT Code(s) _____

10. Anesthesia for an emergency patient for debridement of second-degree burn of 6% total body surface area; anesthesia provided by CRNA without direction by a physician; status P1. CPT Code(s) _____

11. Anesthesia for an oncology patient for the Whipple procedure; anesthesia provided by physician providing medical direction of three concurrent anesthesia procedures involving qualified individuals; status P3. CPT Code(s) _____

12. Anesthesia for a healthy pregnant female for vaginal delivery; supervision of two concurrent services under the anesthesiologist's direction; status P1. CPT Code(s) _____

13. Anesthesia provided by the surgeon for open reduction and internal fixation of proximal femoral shaft fracture for a patient with systemic lupus erythematous. CPT Code(s) _____

14. Anesthesia for a patient with severe hypertension for arthroscopic removal of bone fragment in the left elbow joint; anesthesia provided by CRNA without physician direction; status P4. CPT Code(s) _____

15. Anesthesia for a patient with 90% occlusion in the left carotid artery for balloon angioplasty and stent placement; anesthesia personally performed by the anesthesiologist; status P4. CPT Code(s) _____

16. Anesthesia for a brain-dead patient on life support for harvesting organs for donor purposes; medical direction of one concurrent anesthesia procedure by qualified individuals; status P6. CPT Code(s) _____

17. Anesthesia for a patient with 100% coronary artery blockage for CABG without pump oxygenator; anesthesia provided by CRNA without direction by a physician; status P4. CPT Code(s) _____

18. Anesthesia for an obese patient for therapeutic right L5 and L6 nerve blocks in lateral decubitus position; anesthesia provided by a physician with medical direction of one CRNA; status P3. CPT Code(s) _____

19. Anesthesia for a 21-year-old female patient with intellectual disabilities for vaginal examination and Pap test; anesthesia provided by CRNA with medical direction by physician; status P1. CPT Code(s) _____

20. Anesthesia for an emergency patient for pulmonary thromboendarterectomy with pump oxygenator, controlled hypotension and hypothermia, and cardiac arrest; anesthesia personally performed by the anesthesiologist; status P5. CPT Code(s) _____

21. Anesthesia for an oncology patient for breast reconstruction with implants (complicated procedure) and monitored anesthesia care; status P3. CPT Code(s) _____

22. Anesthesia for an otherwise healthy orthopedic patient for fusion across the sacroiliac joint; anesthesiologist performs anesthesia services; status P1. CPT Code(s) _____

23. Anesthesia for a healthy 71-year-old patient for smaller saphenous varicose vein procedure; anesthesia performed under medical direction of one CRNA by anesthesiologist; status P1. CPT Code(s) _____

24. Anesthesia for an otherwise healthy 15-year-old girl for tonsillectomy; anesthesia performed by anesthesiologist; status P1. CPT Code(s) _____

25. Anesthesia for a patient with Cushing's disease due to left adrenal gland adenoma for unilateral adrenalectomy; anesthesia performed by anesthesiologist; status P2. CPT Code(s) _____

CODING CHALLENGE

Instructions: Read the mini-medical-record of each patient's encounter, then abstract, assign, and arrange ICD-10-CM and CPT codes using the Index and Tabular List.

1. Append physical status modifiers and any applicable CPT modifiers.
2. Assign applicable qualifying circumstances codes.
3. Assign HCPCS modifiers identifying the anesthesia provider and/or MAC.
4. Report the total elapsed time in hours and minutes and the number of time units for the procedure (15 minutes = 1 time unit).

---

1. INPATIENT HOSPITAL   Gender: F   Age: 32
Status: P1

Start time: 0800   Stop time: 1300

Anesthesia provider: CRNA without medical direction

Anesthesia type: General

Diagnosis: Lumbar spondylolisthesis

Procedure: Posterior lumbar interbody fusion (PLIF), L3-L4

1 ICD-10-CM Code _____

1 CPT Code _____

Time _____ hours _____ minutes.
Time units _____

---

2. INPATIENT HOSPITAL   Gender: M   Age: 74
Status: P4

Start time: 1245   Stop time: 1900

(continued)

---

2. (continued)
Anesthesia provider: MD in personal attendance

Anesthesia type: General, with induced hypothermia

Diagnosis: Coronary atherosclerosis

Procedure: CABG with pump oxygenator

1 ICD-10-CM Code _____

3 CPT Code(s) _____

Time _____ hours _____ minutes.
Time units _____

---

3. INPATIENT HOSPITAL   Gender: F   Age: 42
Status: P4

Start time: 0603   Stop time: 0718

Anesthesia provider: CRNA

Anesthesia type: Spinal, general

Diagnosis: Preterm premature rupture of membranes (PPROM), 33 weeks 2 days, primigravida, hypertensive chronic renal disease stage 1

Procedure: Low transverse cesarean delivery following attempted vaginal delivery

Tip: Assign codes for PPROM, supervision of pregnancy, weeks of gestation, outcome of delivery, hypertensive kidney disease in pregnancy, and the stage of CKD.

7 ICD-10-CM Codes _____

2 CPT Codes _____

Time _____ hours _____ minutes.
Time units _____

(continued)

(continued from page 609)

4. OUTPATIENT SURGERY   Gender: M   Age: 63
Status: P2

Start time: 0915   Stop time: 1145

Anesthesia provider: Anesthesiologist assistant under direction of the anesthesiologist who is supervising one other concurrent procedure

Anesthesia type: Conscious sedation

Diagnosis: Sinoatrial node dysfunction, mild congestive heart failure

Procedure: Radiofrequency sinus node ablation

2 ICD-10-CM Codes _____

1 CPT Code _____

Time _____ hours _____ minutes.

Time units _____

5. OFFICE   Gender: M   Age: 19   Status: P3

Start time: 0930   Stop time: 1245

Anesthesia provider: Oral surgeon personally administers the local anesthetic

Anesthesia type: Local

Diagnosis: Gingival hyperplasia, mandibular; type 1 diabetes

Procedure: Excision of lesion of gum with one suture

2 ICD-10-CM Codes _____

1 CPT Code _____

Time _____ hours _____ minutes.

Time units _____

6. OUTPATIENT SURGERY   Gender: M   Age: 71
Status: P4

Start time: 1330   Stop time: 1415

Anesthesia provider: Anesthesiologist in personal attendance

Anesthesia type: Monitored anesthesia care (MAC)

Diagnosis: Morbid obesity (BMI = 47 kg/m^2); obstructive sleep apnea; hypertension

(continued)

6. (continued)

Procedure: Laparoscopic placement of gastric band

4 ICD-10-CM Codes _____

2 CPT Codes _____

Time _____ hours _____ minutes.

Time units _____

7. INPATIENT HOSPITAL   Gender: F   Age: 66
Status: P3

Start time: 0745   Stop time: 1145

Anesthesia provider: CRNA under medical direction of an anesthesiologist

Anesthesia type: General

Diagnosis: Left breast cancer, primary

Procedure: Radical mastectomy—removal of the breast, pectoral muscles, axillary lymph nodes, and associated skin and subcutaneous tissue

1 ICD-10-CM Code _____

1 CPT Code _____

Time _____ hours _____ minutes.

Time units _____

8. INPATIENT HOSPITAL   Gender: M   Age: 21 days   Status: P4

Start time: 1415   Stop time: 1845

Anesthesia provider: Anesthesiologist in personal attendance

Anesthesia type: General

Diagnosis: Atrial septal defect

Procedure: Open repair interarterial septal defect with pump oxygenator

1 ICD-10-CM Code _____

1 CPT Code _____

Time _____ hours _____ minutes.

Time units _____

9. OUTPATIENT SURGERY   Gender: F   Age: 14
Status: P1

Start time: 1015   Stop time: 1115

Anesthesia provider: Anesthesiologist in personal attendance

Anesthesia type: Monitored anesthesia care (MAC)

Diagnosis: Calcaneal bone spur, right

Procedure: Excision of calcaneal bone spur, right

1 ICD-10-CM Code _____

1 CPT Code _____

Time _____ hours _____ minutes.

Time units _____

10. OUTPATIENT HOSPITAL   Gender: M   Age: 47
Status: P2

Start time: 0750   Stop time: 0935

Anesthesia provider: MD supervising 3 other concurrent procedures

Anesthesia type: Regional, peripheral block

Diagnosis: Ganglion cyst of left wrist, hypercholesterolemia

Procedure: Arthroscopic excision of lesion, left wrist

2 ICD-10-CM Codes _____

1 CPT Code _____

Time _____ hours _____ minutes.

Time units _____

Chapter 32

Digestive System Procedures (40490-49999)

Chapter Outline

- **Digestive System Procedure Basics**
- **Coding Guidelines for Digestive System Procedures**
- **Abstracting Digestive System Procedures**
- **Assigning Codes for Digestive System Procedures**
- **Arranging Codes for Digestive System Procedures**
- **E/M Coding for Gastroenterology**

Learning Objectives

After completing this chapter, you should have the skills to:

32.1 Spell and define the key words, medical terms, and abbreviations related to digestive system procedures. (Remember)

32.2 Summarize the fundamentals of digestive system procedures. (Understand)

32.3 Adhere to CPT coding guidelines in the Digestive System subsection. (Apply)

32.4 Examine and abstract procedural information from the medical record for coding procedures in the Digestive System subsection. (Analyze)

32.5 Demonstrate how to assign codes for Digestive System subsection procedures. (Apply)

32.6 Utilize guidelines for arranging (sequencing) codes for Digestive System subsection procedures. (Apply)

32.7 Determine how to code Evaluation and Management services for gastroenterology. (Evaluate)

Key Terms and Abbreviations

allotransplantation	capsule endoscopy	proximal	transnasal
anastomosis	incidental appendectomy	pull-through	transoral
by report	multiple endoscopy rule	reducible	

In addition to the key terms listed here, students should know the terms defined within tables in this chapter.

INTRODUCTION

It is exciting when a favorite store offers a BOGO sale—buy one, get one at half-price. Insurance companies require a similar discount when physicians bill for multiple procedures done at the same time. Coders indicate this circumstance with a modifier. Modifiers and multiple endoscopy payment rules are among the skills to be mastered when using codes from the CPT subsection Digestive System.

DIGESTIVE SYSTEM PROCEDURE BASICS

Gastroenterology is a subspecialty of internal medicine that specializes in the digestive system. Gastroenterologists perform medical procedures such as endoscopies and gastric function studies, but they do not perform surgery. General surgeons perform surgery on digestive system organs and structures. Plastic surgeons perform reconstructive repairs involving the lips and mouth, such as cleft palate repair. Oral and maxillofacial surgeons (OMSs) perform surgery on the face, mouth, and jaw.

For procedural purposes, the digestive system is divided into four parts:

- Upper gastrointestinal (GI) tract—Lips through ileum
- Lower gastrointestinal (GI) tract—Cecum through anus
- Accessory organs—Salivary glands, liver, gallbladder, and pancreas
- Surrounding structures—Abdomen, peritoneum, and omentum

Physicians use a variety of dividing points between the upper and lower GI tract, depending on the context:

- Diagnosis of bleeding—Bleeding above the duodenal junction is classified as upper GI bleeding, and bleeding below the duodenal junction is classified as lower GI bleeding.
- Endoscopic access—An upper GI endoscopy includes the mouth through the duodenum, and a lower GI endoscopy includes the cecum through the anus. The jejunum and ileum are not accessible to endoscopy procedures.
- Embryonic development—Developmentally, the GI tract is divided into three parts—the upper, from the mouth to the major duodenal papilla (*opening of the pancreatic duct into the duodenum*); middle, from the duodenal papilla

to the midtransverse colon; and lower, from the midtransverse colon to the anus—based on the derivation from the foregut, midgut, and hindgut, respectively.

Because the digestive, or alimentary, tract consists of and connects several anatomic sites, medical terms frequently contain word roots of multiple sites, which are combined with a procedural suffix. To understand terminology, identify the suffix, then break down each word into the combining forms for each site. Refer to ■ TABLE 32-1 for a refresher on how to build medical terms related to digestive system procedures.

Procedures commonly performed on each section of the digestive system are discussed next. Refer to detailed anatomic diagrams of specific parts of the digestive system when you need to refresh your memory of the relationship of organs and sites to each other. Chapter 8 of this text provides information on digestive system anatomy and conditions.

CODING CAUTION

Be alert for medical terms that are spelled similarly and have different meanings.

cholecystectomy (*excision of the gall bladder*) and **choledochocystectomy** (*excision of the common bile duct*)

laparotomy (*cutting into the abdomen*) and **laparoscopy** (*visual examination of the abdomen*)

an/o (combining form for *anus*) and **an-** (prefix meaning "none")

Procedures of the Upper GI Tract

Procedures commonly performed on the upper GI tract are summarized in ■ TABLE 32-2 (page 614). In particular, coders need to understand upper GI endoscopy, anastomosis, and foreign body removal.

Upper GI Endoscopy

Endoscopy is a procedure that is performed for screening, diagnostic, and therapeutic purposes. In the upper GI tract, the endoscope access can be **transoral** (*through the oral cavity*) or **transnasal** (*through the nose*) and can access the esophagus, stomach, and duodenum. Transnasal procedures are performed with a rigid endoscope. Transoral procedures can be performed

---

Table 32-1 ■ **EXAMPLE OF CONSTRUCTING MEDICAL TERMS FOR DIGESTIVE SYSTEM PROCEDURES**

Combining Form	Suffix	Complete Medical Term
esophag/o (*esophagus*)	-**scopy** (*visual examination*) -**ectomy** (*excision*)	**esophago + scopy** (*visual examination of the esophagus*)
		gastro + scopy (*visual examination of the stomach*)
		duodeno + scopy (*visual examination of the duodenum*)
gastr/o (*stomach*)		**esophago + gastro + duodeno + scopy** (*visual examination of the esophagus, stomach, and duodenum*)
		esophag + ectomy (*excision of the esophagus*)
duoden/o (*duodenum*)		**gastr + ectomy** (*excision of the stomach*)
		duoden + ectomy (*excision of the duodenum*)

Source: © PB Resources, Inc. Used with permission.

Table 32-2 ■ **COMMON PROCEDURES OF THE UPPER GASTROINTESTINAL TRACT**

Procedure Name	Definition	Reason Performed
Antrectomy • Distal gastrectomy	The distal (*lowest*) portion of the stomach is excised. (Open approach)	Gastric ulcers, neoplasms
Billroth I • Gastroduodenostomy	The pylorus is removed and the **proximal** (*toward the center of the body*) stomach is anastomosed (*connected*) directly to the duodenum in an end-to-end manner. (Open approach)	Reestablish gastrointestinal continuity after excision of portions of one or more organs
Billroth II • Gastrojejunostomy	The greater curvature of the stomach is connected to the first part of the jejunum in a side-to-side manner. (Open approach)	Reestablish gastrointestinal continuity after excision of portions of one or more organs
Cleft lip/cleft palate repair	Abnormally oriented and attached muscles are repositioned to repair the functionality of soft palate musculature. (Open approach)	Cleft lip or cleft palate (*incomplete formation of the lip or roof of the mouth*)
Endoscopic balloon dilation (EBD)	Through-the-scope (TTS) balloon dilators or plastic dilators are moved over a guide wire to stretch the esophagus, pyloric valve, or duodenum. (Endoscopic approach)	Stricture (*narrowing*) of the esophagus, pylorus, or duodenum due to a variety of conditions (e.g., gastric outlet obstruction [GOO], peptic ulcers, Crohn's disease)
Endoscopic sclerotherapy	A solution that causes inflammation and scarring is injected into a vein to close it off. (Endoscopic approach)	Esophageal varices
Esophagectomy • Transhiatal esophagectomy (THE) • Transthoracic esophagectomy (TTE)	All or part of the esophagus is surgically removed. (Open approach)	Barrett's esophagus, localized esophageal cancer
Esophagogastroduodenoscopy (EGD) • Upper gastrointestinal endoscopy	The endoscope is inserted through the mouth and moved down the throat into the esophagus, stomach, and duodenum. (Endoscopic approach)	Esophagitis, gastritis, gastroesophageal reflux disease (GERD), esophageal stricture (*narrowing*), varices, Barrett's esophagus, hiatal hernia, ulcers, cancer
Foreign body removal (FBR)	An object is retrieved from within the body. (Endoscopic or open approach)	Removal of an object from outside the body that has made its way into the body, usually into a hollow organ, such as the nose, ear, or throat
Gastric bypass	The stomach is divided to create a small pouch and causes food to bypass part of the small intestine. (Laparoscopic or open approach)	Reduce calorie absorption
Heller myotomy • Esophagomyotomy	The esophageal sphincter muscle is cut. (Laparoscopic approach)	Achalasia (*a disorder of the esophagus that makes it difficult for foods and liquids to pass into the stomach*)
Laparoscopically adjustable gastric banding (LABG) • Lap-band • A-band • Gastric restriction	An inflatable silicon device is placed around the top portion of the stomach to divide it into a smaller pouch and a larger pouch. (Laparoscopic or open approach)	Slow and reduce food consumption
Nissen fundoplication	The upper part of the stomach is wrapped around the lower esophageal sphincter (LES). (Laparoscopic or open approach)	Strengthen the sphincter, prevent acid reflux, repair a hiatal hernia
Paraesophageal hernia repair • Hiatal hernia repair • Hiatus hernia repair • Fundoplication	The diaphragm is repaired using sutures or mesh; part of the stomach may be wrapped around the esophagus (fundoplication). (Laparoscopic or open approach)	Paraesophageal hernia (part of the stomach bulges through the hiatus [*opening in the diaphragm*])
Percutaneous endoscopic gastrostomy (PEG)	A tube is passed into a patient's stomach through the abdominal wall. (Percutaneous approach)	Feed patients who cannot swallow due to conditions such as stroke and neurological diseases
Roux-en-Y (RNY) • Gastrojejunostomy	The stomach and small bowel are joined using an end-to-side anastomosis. (Laparoscopic or open approach)	Reestablish gastrointestinal continuity after excision of portions of one or more organs
Sialolithotomy	Calculus is removed from the salivary gland(s). (Open approach)	Sialolithiasis (*calculi in the salivary gland*)
Tonsillectomy/adenoidectomy (T&A)	The tonsils and adenoids are surgically removed. (Open approach)	Acute tonsillitis, obstructive sleep apnea, nasal airway obstruction, peritonsillar abscess
Vagotomy • Truncal vagotomy (TV) • Selective vagotomy (SV) • Highly selective vagotomy (HSV)	A portion of the vagus nerve in the stomach is excised. (Laparoscopic or open approach)	Peptic ulcer disease

Source: © PB Resources, Inc. Used with permission.

with either a rigid or flexible endoscope. Rigid endoscopes provide excellent lighting and visualization and have tips of varying angles and sizes. They enable tissue collection, surgery, and procedures such as cauterization. Flexible endoscopes are smaller in diameter and can be manipulated in tight areas but require two hands to operate. Among procedures most commonly performed with an endoscope are:

- Collection of specimens by brushing or washing
- Injections
- Biopsies
- Removal of foreign bodies
- Dilation of strictures
- Removal of tumors or polyps
- Electrocauterization
- Hemostasis
- Ultrasound examination
- Cyst drainage
- Resection

Endoscopes cannot access the jejunum or ileum, so physicians may opt to use capsule endoscopy to examine the small intestine. **Capsule endoscopy** is a technology in which patients swallow a video capsule the size of a large pill that contains a video microchip, light bulb, battery, and radio transmitter. As the capsule moves through the alimentary tract, it takes about 14 photographs per second and transmits them to a receiver worn by the patient. When the capsule passes through the anus, it is flushed down the toilet. The physician downloads thousands of photographs from the receiver and analyzes them to formulate a diagnosis or plan for further testing.

Anastomosis

Sometimes all or part of a digestive organ must be removed because of disease. The excision interrupts the continuous flow of the GI tract, so continuity is reestablished through anastomosis. **Anastomosis** is a surgical connection between two, usually tubular, structures such as the organs in the digestive tract or blood vessels. Several techniques can be used to join the structures:

- End-to-end—The ends of both tubes are connected
- End-to-side—The end of one tube is connected to an opening in the side of another
- Side-to-side—The sides of two tubes are connected with an opening between them

The choice of technique depends on the condition, the exact sites removed, and the surgeon's preference (■ FIGURE 32-1).

In an operative note, anastomosis can be described as a pull-through, which means that the surgeon removes the diseased portion of organ and connects the healthy segment to the adjacent organ. The **pull-through** procedure was originally developed to treat Hirschsprung disease (*nerve cells normally present in the wall of the intestine do not form properly during fetal development*). Part of the colon is excised, then joined to the anus in a posterior sagittal anorectoplasty (PSARP) procedure. The pull-through became preferred over a colostomy, and the technique was eventually adapted for use in other portions of the digestive tract.

SUCCESS STEP

An anastomosis is described with the suffix -*stomy* for the creation of a new opening and word roots that identify the two body parts joined. For example, *gastro/duodeno/stomy* describes the joining of the stomach and the duodenum.

Foreign Body Removal

Foreign bodies can enter the digestive tract through the mouth. They can pass through the system without incident or become lodged. Some objects, such as a coin, normally pass through without a problem and are excreted. An object that becomes lodged can create an obstruction or perforation and pose a medical risk. Objects that are potentially poisonous must be removed immediately. For example, ingested batteries have potential for corrosive injury. X-rays are used to identify the type and location of foreign objects. Many can be retrieved endoscopically, but others require an open procedure to access the site.

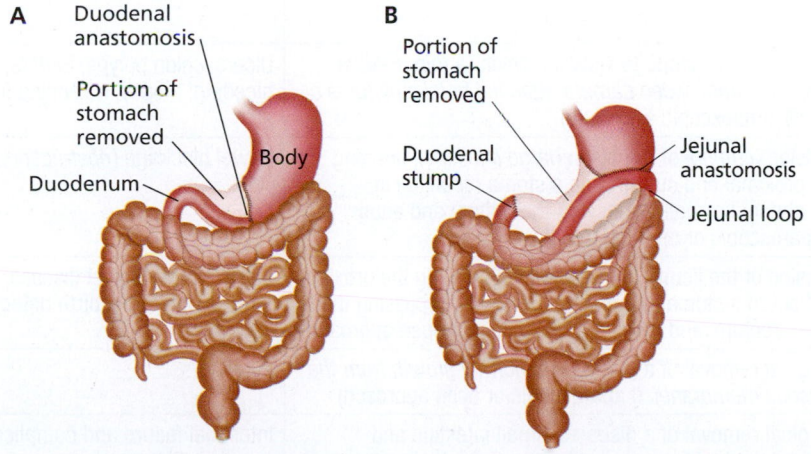

Figure 32-1 ■ Types of anastomoses: (A) End-to-end gastroduodenostomy. (B) End-to-side gastrojejunostomy.

Procedures of the Lower GI Tract

Procedures commonly performed on the lower GI tract are summarized in ■ TABLE 32-3. Endoscopy and ostomy procedures of the lower GI tract require special attention from coders.

Lower GI Endoscopy

Endoscopy of the lower GI tract is named after the sites examined: anoscopy (*endoscopy of the anus*), proctosigmoidoscopy (*endoscopy of the anus, rectum, and part of the descending colon*), sigmoidoscopy (*endoscopy of the anus, rectum, and part of the sigmoid colon*), and colonoscopy (*endoscopy of the entire colon from the rectum to the cecum and possibly the terminal ileum*). A colonoscopy is the preferred method of screening for colorectal cancer, which is recommended by the Centers for Disease Control and Prevention (CDC) every 10 years from ages 50 to 75. When abnormalities are found by a screening colonoscopy, such as polyps that are removed, it becomes a therapeutic, or surgical, procedure.

Ostomy

An *ostomy* is a temporary or permanent surgically created opening that connects an internal organ to the surface of the body. In the lower GI tract, ostomies are performed most commonly to reroute the contents of the ileum or colon because of rectal cancer or inflammatory bowel disease. A temporary ostomy may be performed when the intestinal tract cannot be properly prepared for surgery, as occurs when it is blocked by disease (e.g., tumors) or scar tissue, or when inflammation or an operative wound needs to heal without contamination by stool. Temporary ostomies can usually be reversed with minimal or no loss of intestinal function. A permanent ostomy may be required when disease, or its treatment, impairs normal intestinal function or when the pelvic and anal sphincter muscles that control elimination do not work properly. After the procedure, an ostomy appliance (*a bag or pouch that is adhered to the body with an adhesive*) collects bowel contents. The appliance is quite secure and is emptied or changed as needed. Whenever a portion of the small or large intestines is removed, the excision procedure must be followed by an anastomosis or ostomy.

Table 32-3   ■   **COMMON PROCEDURES OF THE LOWER GASTROINTESTINAL TRACT**

Procedure Name	Definition	Reason Performed
Appendectomy	Surgical removal of the appendix. (Laparoscopic or open approach)	Appendicitis
Colectomy • Bowel resection • Total colectomy • Partial (subtotal) • Hemicolectomy • Proctocolectomy	Surgical removal of all or part of the large intestine. (Laparoscopic or open approach)	Bleeding, bowel obstruction, Crohn's disease, colon cancer, ulcerative colitis, diverticulitis
Colonoscopy	Use of an endoscope to view the colon (*a thin, flexible tube with small video camera attached to take pictures or video*). (Endoscopic approach)	Ulcers, colon polyps, tumors, and areas of inflammation or bleeding; biopsy, screening for malignant neoplasm
Colostomy	Division (*cutting*) of the colon (*large intestine*), bringing the proximal end out through a stoma (*opening*) in the abdominal wall, bypassing the rectum and anus. (Laparoscopic or open approach)	Bowel blockage (*obstruction*), bowel resection, injuries
Ileostomy • Enterostomy	Division of the ileum (*small intestine*) bringing the proximal end out to a stoma in the abdominal wall, bypassing the colon, rectum, and anus. (Laparoscopic or open approach)	Inflammatory bowel disease, colon or rectal cancer, familial polyposis, birth defects involving the intestines, injuries
Polypectomy	Surgical removal of a polyp(s) (*abnormal growth from the mucous membrane*). (Laparoscopic or open approach)	Polyps
Small bowel transplant	Surgical removal of a diseased small intestine and replacement with some or all of a small intestine from a healthy person. (Open approach)	Intestinal failure and complications related to parenteral nutrition (PN)

Source: © PB Resources, Inc. Used with permission.

Procedures of the Accessory Digestive Organs

Commonly performed procedures on the accessory digestive organs are summarized in ■ TABLE 32-4. In particular, coders need to be familiar with procedures on the biliary tract and transplant procedures.

Biliary Tract

The biliary tract, or biliary tree, consists of the gall bladder, cystic duct, common bile duct, extrahepatic ducts, and pancreatic duct (■ FIGURE 32-2). The sphincter of Oddi is a muscular valve that joins the biliary tree to the duodenum. Any of these structures can become inflamed or obstructed, requiring surgery that may involve multiple components. A cholecystectomy can be either a laparoscopic or open procedure. It can be performed alone, aided by cholangiography, with exploration and/or excision of the common bile duct, with anastomosis of the intestinal tract, and with a sphincteroplasty or sphincterotomy. Calculi can occur in the gall bladder, common bile duct, or both. When gallstones become symptomatic, they must be excised or destroyed using a method such as lithotripsy.

Transplantation

The six organs that can be transplanted between individuals are, in descending order of frequency, kidney, liver, heart, lung, pancreas, and intestine. Organ transplantation involves three

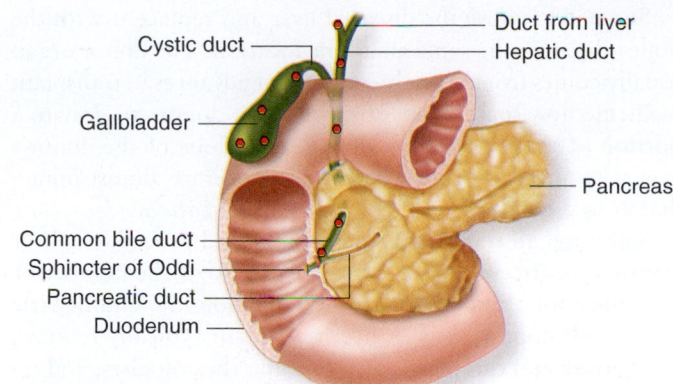

Figure 32-2 ■ Biliary tract (red dots identify common sites of calculi).

distinct components: harvesting the donor organ, backbench work to prepare the organ, and recipient **allotransplantation** (*receiving an organ from another person*).

Liver transplantation is the replacement of a diseased liver with some or all of a healthy liver from another person. It is a viable treatment option for acute liver failure and end-stage liver disease, which can be caused by cirrhosis (*scarring of the liver*), chronic hepatitis B or C, bile duct diseases, genetic diseases, autoimmune liver diseases, primary liver cancer, alcoholic liver disease, and fatty liver disease.

Table 32-4 ■ COMMON PROCEDURES OF ACCESSORY DIGESTIVE ORGANS

Procedure Name	Definition	Reason Performed
Autologous islet cell transplantation	The pancreas is surgically removed and the islet cells are isolated then injected into the portal vein. (Open approach)	Prevent or minimize the risk of diabetes after a pancreatectomy
Cholecystectomy	Surgical removal of the gallbladder. (Laparoscopic or open approach)	Gallstones, infected or inflamed gallbladder
Common bile duct (CBD) exploration	Injection of a dye into the duct, visualization on an x-ray, removal of calculi, and introduction of a drainage bag when necessary (Laparoscopic approach)	Obstructive jaundice, stones in bile ducts
Endoscopic retrograde cholangiopancreatography (ERCP)	Injection of contrast medium into the bile ducts via a tube through the ampulla of Vater to visualize the entire biliary tree (*pancreatic, common bile, cystic, and hepatic ducts*). (Percutaneous approach)	Obstructive jaundice, stones in bile ducts, pancreatitis, biliary strictures due to cancer
Hepatectomy • Liver resection	Surgical removal of all or part of the liver. (Open approach)	Donor for, or recipient of, liver transplantation, usually due to neoplasms of the liver or cirrhosis
Lithotripsy of gallstones	Use of high-frequency sound waves to break up gallstones. (External approach)	Cholelithiasis, choledocholithiasis
Liver biopsy	Surgical removal of a small piece of the liver. (Percutaneous, transvenous, or laparoscopic approach)	Determine the presence of liver disease
Liver transplant	Surgical removal of a diseased liver and replacement with some or all of a healthy liver from another person. (Open approach)	Acute and end-stage liver failure, usually due to neoplasms of the liver or cirrhosis
Pancreatectomy	Surgical removal of all or part of the pancreas. (Open approach)	Chronic pancreatitis, malignant neoplasm
Pancreaticoduodenectomy • Whipple procedure	Surgical removal of parts of the pancreas, duodenum, common bile duct, and, if required, portions of the stomach. (Open approach)	Pancreatic cancer, neuroendocrine (islet cell) tumors, chronic pancreatitis, cancer of the ampulla of Vater (ampullary cancer), duodenal cancer, cancer of the distal bile duct

Source: © PB Resources, Inc. Used with permission.

Surgeons remove the diseased liver and replace it with the donor organ in the same anatomic location. The donor organ usually comes from a cadaver, but recent advances in transplant medicine now make it possible for living donors to donate a portion of their liver. Typically, the right lobe of the donor's liver is removed. The liver begins to regenerate almost immediately and continues to do so for about a year.

Although all transplants are complicated procedures, liver transplants are even more intricate because of the number of disconnections and reconnections of abdominal and hepatic tissue and blood vessels. A liver transplant typically requires 4–12 hours and three surgeons, two anesthesiologists, and up to four nurses.

Pancreas transplants are provided for diabetic patients, often in conjunction with a kidney transplant. The diseased pancreas is not removed during the operation. The donor pancreas is usually placed in the right lower part of the patient's abdomen. Blood vessels from the new pancreas are anastomosed to the patient's blood vessels. Pancreas transplant surgery takes about 3 hours; a combination kidney/pancreas transplant requires about six hours.

Pancreatic islets, also called islets of Langerhans, are tiny clusters of cells scattered throughout the pancreas. Autologous (*from the same person*) islet cell transplantation is an option for patients who require a pancreatectomy because of chronic pancreatitis that cannot be managed by other treatments. The surgeon removes the pancreas from the patient, extracts and purifies islets, and infuses them into the patient's liver using a catheter. The goal is to give the body enough healthy islets to make insulin. Type 1 diabetics cannot receive autologous islet cell transplants because their beta cells (*islet cells that produce insulin*) do not function. Allotransplantation from a cadaver is an experimental procedure approved for limited use by the Food and Drug Administration (FDA) and is being tested as an option for type 1 diabetics.

Procedures on the Abdominal Structures

Procedures commonly performed on the abdominal structures that surround the digestive organs are summarized in ■ TABLE 32-5. When extensive adhesions impede access to an operative site, surgeons must perform adhesiolysis as part of the procedure.

Hernias can occur in several locations and are named by site (■ FIGURE 32-3). Some hernias are **reducible**, which means they can be corrected by the physician pushing the tissue back into place. Other hernias require surgical repair, suturing, or insertion of a mesh prosthesis to reinforce the abdominal wall.

This section provides a general reference to help understand the most common digestive system procedures. Remember to keep standard reference books handy in case you get stuck.

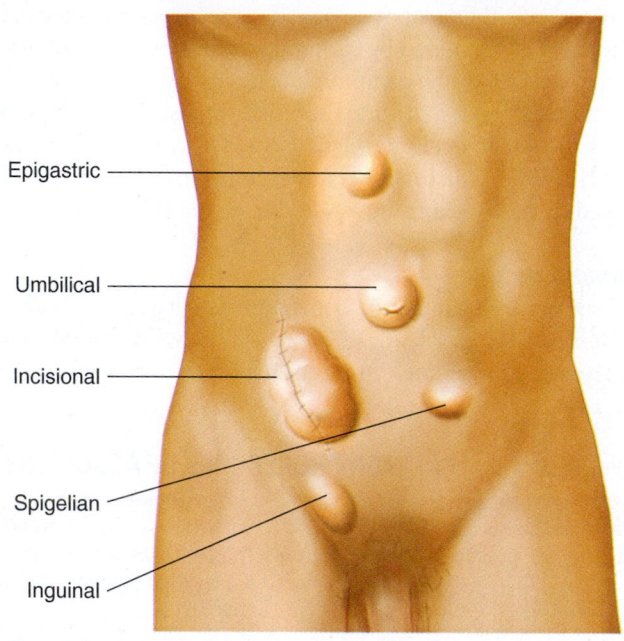

Epigastric

Umbilical

Incisional

Spigelian

Inguinal

Figure 32-3 ■ Common types of hernias.

Table 32-5 ■ COMMON PROCEDURES WITHIN THE ABDOMINAL CAVITY

Procedure Name	Definition	Reason Performed
Adhesiolysis	Use of scalpel or electric current to destroy or cut free adhesions (*scar tissue between organs or structures*). (Laparoscopic or open approach)	Abdominal adhesions
Hernia repair • Hernioplasty • Herniorrhaphy • Herniotomy	Surgical correction of a hernia through the use of manual manipulation, sutures, or mesh. (External, laparoscopic, or open approach)	Bulging of internal organs or tissues through a defect in the wall of a body cavity
Omental flap	Removal of part of the omentum with blood vessel supply intact. (Open approach)	Reconstruction of other anatomic sites, such as the chest wall or abdomen
Paracentesis	A surgical puncture of a body cavity to remove ascites (*excess fluid*). (Percutaneous approach)	Remove excess fluid caused by conditions such as infection, inflammation, cirrhosis, cancer, or injuries.

Source: © PB Resources, Inc. Used with permission.

CODING PRACTICE

Exercise 32.1   Digestive System Procedure Basics

Instructions: Use your medical terminology skills and resources to define the following procedures, then identify the applicable code or code range. Follow these steps:

- Use slash marks "/" to break down the underlined term into its root(s) and suffix.
- Define the meaning of the underlined word based on the meaning of each word part.
- Use the entire phrase to identify the code(s) or code range shown in the CPT Index.

Example: appendectomy, laparoscopic   Meaning *cutting out of the appendix*   CPT Code *44970*
append/ectomy

1. operculectomy   Meaning _____   CPT Code_____

2. pancreatorrhaphy   Meaning _____   CPT Code_____

3. sialodochoplasty   Meaning _____   CPT Code_____

4. anus, sphincter, sphincterectomy   Meaning _____   CPT Code_____

5. proctosigmoidoscopy, biopsy   Meaning _____   CPT Code_____

6. cholangiopancreatography, endoscopic   Meaning _____   CPT Code_____
   retrograde, with papillotomy

7. vermilionectomy   Meaning _____   CPT Code_____

8. pyloromyotomy   Meaning _____   CPT Code_____

9. enterolysis   Meaning _____   CPT Code_____

10. cheiloplasty   Meaning _____   CPT Code_____

CODING GUIDELINES FOR DIGESTIVE SYSTEM PROCEDURES

Coders should understand the organization, guidelines, and instructional notes in the Tabular List of this CPT subsection. This information is necessary for accurate coding. The CPT Surgery subsection **Digestive System (40490-49999)** contains 18 subheadings divided by anatomic site. Anatomic sites are arranged by the order in which they occur in the alimentary (*digestive*) tract, beginning with the lips and ending with the anus (■ TABLE 32-6). The last four subheadings identify sites that aid in digestion but are not part of the alimentary tract: the liver, biliary tract, pancreas, and abdomen/peritoneum/omentum. Each subheading contains categories divided by the type of procedure, such as incision, excision, introduction, endoscopy, destruction, repair, and other procedures. The specific category titles vary by subheading based on what is applicable to a particular anatomic site. Review the subheadings, categories, and code ranges listed at the beginning of the Digestive System subsection in many CPT manuals, to become familiar with the content and organization.

This chapter includes invasive, minimally invasive, and non-invasive surgical procedures on the digestive system. Codes for diagnostic tests on the digestive system appear in the Medicine section. The medical necessity of any procedure codes must always be supported by diagnosis codes. CPT codes in the Digestive System subsection are frequently supported by diagnosis codes from ICD-10-CM Chapter 11, "Diseases of the Digestive System (K00-K95)", as well as neoplasms, symptoms

Table 32-6   ■   **DIGESTIVE SYSTEM SUBHEADINGS**

Subheading	Code Range
Lips	40490-40799
Vestibule of Mouth	40800-40899
Tongue and Floor of Mouth	41000-41599
Dentoalveolar Structures	41800-41899
Palate and Uvula	42000-42299
Salivary Gland and Ducts	42300-42699
Pharynx, Adenoids, and Tonsils	42700-42999
Esophagus	43020-43499
Stomach	43500-43999
Intestines (Except Rectum)	44005-44799
Meckel's Diverticulum and the Mesentery	44800-44899
Appendix	44900-44979
Colon and Rectum	45000-45999
Anus	46020-46999
Liver	47000-47399
Biliary Tract	47400-47999
Pancreas	48000-48999
Abdomen, Peritoneum, and Omentum	49000-49999

Table 32-7 ■ **LOCATING ICD-10-CM AND ADDITIONAL CPT CODES FOR THE DIGESTIVE SYSTEM**

Type of Code	Codes
ICD-10-CM Digestive System–Related Codes	
Digestive system conditions	K00-K95
Neoplasms	C00-C26
Symptoms and signs	R10-R19
Injuries	S09.93, S19.9, S36.-, T28.-
CPT Digestive System–Related Codes	
Medicine procedures	91010-91299
Radiologic procedures	
• Diagnostic radiology	74210-74363
• Diagnostic ultrasound	76700-76776, 76975
• Radiologic guidance	77001-77022
• Nuclear medicine, diagnostic	78201-78299
Laboratory organ/disease panels	80074-80076

Source: © PB Resources, Inc. Used with permission.

and signs, and injuries (■ TABLE 32-7). ICD-10-CM classifies injuries of the lips, mouth, and tongue with injuries of the face. Injuries of the throat are classified with injuries of the neck. These are the most commonly used codes to support procedures on the digestive system; however, diagnosis codes from any ICD-10-CM chapter are permissible.

CPT guidelines at the beginning of the Surgery section apply to Digestive System procedures. There are no special instructions at the beginning of this subsection, but there are some for subheadings and categories that provide definitions and coding information. A special instruction that appears in each endoscopy or laparoscopy category is that a surgical endoscopy or laparoscopy always includes a diagnostic endoscopy or laparoscopy. To report a diagnostic laparoscopy as a separate procedure, use code **49320**. Endoscopic procedures on the digestive system are often performed with moderate sedation. When this occurs, assign the appropriate moderate sedation code(s) (**99151-99157**).

Instructional notes appear throughout the Tabular List to alert coders to the need for modifiers, provide cross-references to codes for similar procedures on other sites, identify when additional codes might be needed for radiological services, and highlight resequenced and recently deleted codes. Specific guidelines and instructional notes are discussed throughout this chapter of the text.

ABSTRACTING DIGESTIVE SYSTEM PROCEDURES

Abstracting digestive system procedures requires paying special attention to the detailed anatomy of the digestive system and the order of the digestive organ within the GI tract, starting from either end. Knowledge of the order of the alimentary tract is necessary to determine the path of an endoscope and the farther site reached. Refer to Chapter 8, "Diseases of the Digestive System," in this text for a refresher on digestive system anatomy.

In addition to familiarity with each structure, coders must be able to locate specific anatomic landmarks within the

mouth, salivary glands, stomach (■ FIGURE 32-4), or colon. Coders need to read operative or procedure reports and determine the exact organ(s) and site(s) accessed, treated, excised, and/or reconnected to another site.

Refer to ■ TABLE 32-8 for guidance on how to abstract procedures on the Digestive System, then work through the detailed example that follows. Remember that the abstracting questions are a guide and that not every question applies to, or can be answered for, every case. For example, anastomosis is not performed in every procedure. Age is a factor for tonsillectomies and some hernia repairs.

Guided Example of Abstracting Digestive System Procedures

Refer to the following example throughout this chapter to practice skills for abstracting, assigning, and arranging Digestive System procedure codes.

OUTPATIENT HOSPITAL   Gender: M   Age: 57

Preoperative diagnosis: Hematochezia

Procedure: Colonoscopy, polypectomy, hemorrhoidectomy. Moderate sedation provided by surgeon with a trained observer present for monitoring. Intraservice time of 60 minutes. Inspection of anus immediately revealed internal hemorrhoids. Colonoscopic examination identified 2 polyps in the sigmoid colon at 20 cm that were removed with hot forceps and one polyp in the transverse colon at 100 cm that was removed with a snare. Remainder of colon to cecum was unremarkable. Hemorrhoids were ligated with rubber bands. Patient tolerated procedure well and was transferred to the recovery area. Polyps were submitted to pathology.

Postoperative diagnosis: Internal first-degree hemorrhoids, colonic polyps

Pathology report: Benign adenomatous polyps

Follow along as fictitious coder Jill Hynes, CPC, abstracts the procedure. Check off each step after you complete it.

▶ Jill reads through the entire record, paying special attention to the reason for the encounter, the procedure performed, and the postoperative diagnosis. She refers to the Key Criteria for Abstracting Digestive System Procedures (Table 32-8).

❏ She notes the preoperative diagnosis, hematochezia (*bloody stool*).

❏ *What is the patient's age?* 57

❏ *What site is treated?* Colon

❏ *What primary procedure is performed?* Colonoscopy

❏ *What other procedure(s), if any, are performed?* Polypectomy, hemorrhoidectomy

❏ *Is the treatment screening, diagnostic, or therapeutic?* Diagnostic because of hematochezia

❏ *What is the approach?* Through the anal opening

Figure 32-4 ■ Anatomic landmarks of the stomach.

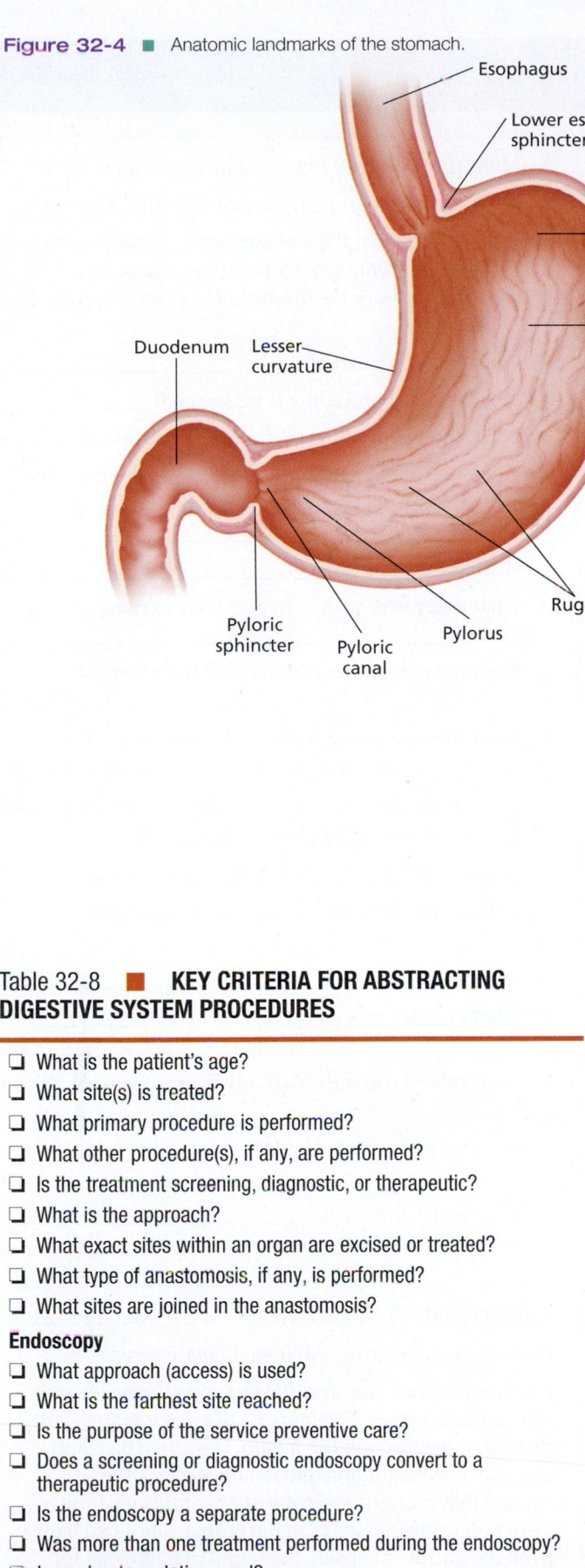

Table 32-8 ■ KEY CRITERIA FOR ABSTRACTING DIGESTIVE SYSTEM PROCEDURES

- ❏ What is the patient's age?
- ❏ What site(s) is treated?
- ❏ What primary procedure is performed?
- ❏ What other procedure(s), if any, are performed?
- ❏ Is the treatment screening, diagnostic, or therapeutic?
- ❏ What is the approach?
- ❏ What exact sites within an organ are excised or treated?
- ❏ What type of anastomosis, if any, is performed?
- ❏ What sites are joined in the anastomosis?

Endoscopy
- ❏ What approach (access) is used?
- ❏ What is the farthest site reached?
- ❏ Is the purpose of the service preventive care?
- ❏ Does a screening or diagnostic endoscopy convert to a therapeutic procedure?
- ❏ Is the endoscopy a separate procedure?
- ❏ Was more than one treatment performed during the endoscopy?
- ❏ Is moderate sedation used?
- ❏ Is the patient covered by Medicare?

Source: © PB Resources, Inc. Used with permission.

- ❏ *What exact sites within an organ are excised or treated?* Anus, sigmoid colon, transverse colon

- ❏ *What is the farthest site reached?* Cecum

- ❏ *Is the purpose of the service preventive care?* No

- ❏ *Does a screening or diagnostic endoscopy convert to a therapeutic procedure?* Yes, polyps were removed

- ❏ *Is the endoscopy a separate procedure?* Yes, because no other procedures were performed

- ❏ *Was more than one treatment performed during the endoscopy?* Yes, two methods of polyp removal: hot forceps and snare

- ❏ *Is moderate sedation used?* Yes, with trained observer. Intraservice time is 60 minutes.

▶ At this time, Jill does not know which of these procedures may need to be coded, nor how many codes she will end up with. She will learn about this when she moves on to assigning codes.

CODING PRACTICE

Exercise 32.2 **Abstracting Digestive System Procedures**

Instructions: Read the mini-medical-record of each patient's encounter and answer the abstracting questions. Write the answer on the line provided. Do not assign any codes.

---

1. OUTPATIENT HOSPITAL Gender: M Age: 57

Preprocedure diagnosis: Screening colonoscopy

Procedure: Flexible colonoscopy, two polyps in descending segment, one polyp in transverse segment, remainder of colon to cecum was clear. Polyps were removed with bipolar cautery and submitted to pathology

Postprocedure diagnosis: Adenomatous polyps per pathology report

a. What site(s) is treated? _____

b. What primary procedure is performed? _____

c. What approach (access) is used? _____

d. What is the farthest site reached? _____

e. Is the purpose of the service preventive care? _____

f. Does a screening or diagnostic endoscopy convert to a therapeutic procedure? _____

g. Is the endoscopy a separate procedure? _____

h. Was more than one treatment performed during the endoscopy? _____

---

2. INPATIENT HOSPITAL Gender: F Age: 33

Diagnosis: Morbid obesity, BMI = 43 kg/m²

Procedure: Laparoscopic gastric bypass and Roux-en-Y gastroenterostomy (100 cm)

a. What site(s) is treated? _____

b. What primary procedure is performed? _____

c. What other procedure(s), if any, are performed? _____

d. Is the treatment screening, diagnostic, or therapeutic? _____

e. What is the approach? _____

f. What exact sites within an organ are excised or treated? _____

g. What type of anastomosis, if any, is performed? _____

h. What sites are joined in the anastomosis? _____

---

3. INPATIENT HOSPITAL Gender: F Age: 48

Diagnosis: Squamous cell carcinoma of the esophagus

Procedure: Near-total esophagectomy, thoracotomy, end-to-side pharyngogastrostomy (*restructuring of the pathway from the throat to the stomach after esophagectomy*)

a. What site(s) is treated? _____

b. What primary procedure is performed? _____

c. What other procedure(s), if any, are performed? _____

d. Is the treatment screening, diagnostic, or therapeutic? _____

e. What is the approach? _____

f. What exact sites within an organ are excised or treated? _____

g. What type of anastomosis, if any, is performed? _____

h. What sites are joined in the anastomosis? _____

---

4. OUTPATIENT HOSPITAL Gender: M Age: 64

Diagnosis: Initial incarcerated incisional hernia

Procedure: Incarcerated incisional hernia repair with mesh

a. What site(s) is treated? _____

b. What primary procedure is performed? _____ _____

c. What other procedure(s), if any, are performed? _____

d. Is the treatment screening, diagnostic, or therapeutic? _____

e. What is the approach? _____

---

5. OUTPATIENT HOSPITAL Gender: M Age: 61

Preoperative diagnosis: Melena, hematemesis

Procedure: Moderate sedation by second provider with intraservice time of 75 minutes. EGD was initiated with flexible scope through the mouth. Identified bleeding ulcers in esophagus and duodenum, which were successfully cauterized. Features of chronic gastritis were noted. No masses or hiatal hernia. Obtained biopsy from the antrum. Biopsies submitted to pathology for

(continued)

CODING PRACTICE (continued)

5. (continued)

H&E (*hematoxylin and eosin stain test to detect cancer*) and CLO (test for Campylobacter H. pylori).

Postoperative diagnosis: Bleeding esophageal ulcer and bleeding peptic ulcer

Pathology report: Biopsies negative for H. pylori and carcinoma

a. What site(s) is treated? _____

b. What primary procedure is performed? _____

c. What is the approach? _____

d. What is the farthest site reached? _____

e. Does a screening or diagnostic endoscopy convert to a therapeutic procedure? _____

f. Was more than one treatment performed during the endoscopy? If so, name the additional procedures. _____

g. Is moderate sedation provided? _____
Who provides the moderate sedation? _____
What is the intraservice time? _____

6. INPATIENT HOSPITAL   Gender: M
Age: 3 months

Diagnosis: Bilateral cleft lip and nasal deformity

Procedure: Primary repair of a bilateral cleft lip and nasal deformity; repair of soft tissue of cleft palate and closure of alveolar ridge

a. What site(s) is treated? _____

b. What primary procedure is performed? _____

c. What other procedure(s), if any, are performed? ____ _____

d. Is the treatment screening, diagnostic, or therapeutic? _____

e. What is the approach? _____

f. What exact sites within an organ are excised or treated? _____

ASSIGNING CODES FOR DIGESTIVE SYSTEM PROCEDURES

This section reviews coding rules for several commonly performed Digestive System procedures: tonsillectomy, appendectomy, anastomosis, endoscopy, transplants, and repairs. Learning about these procedures will reinforce basic coding skills that you can use throughout the CPT manual.

Tonsillectomy

Tonsillectomy and adenoidectomy (**42820-42870**) provide several coding options based on patient age and the combination of procedures performed. Codes *do not* distinguish among the surgical method used: tonsillotome (*scalpel*), cryosurgery, laser, or electrocautery.

To assign codes, search the Index for the Main Term **Tonsillectomy**; **Tonsils** with the first-level modifying term **Excision**; or **Adenoids** with the first-level modifying term **Excision**. Review and verify the codes in the Tabular List based on the following criteria.

When a tonsillectomy and adenoidectomy are performed together, select the code based on patient age: **42820** for **younger than 12** and **42821** for **age 12 or over**.

When only a tonsillectomy is performed, select the code based on patient age: **42825** for **younger than 12** and **42826** for **age 12 or over**.

When only an adenoidectomy is performed, determine whether the procedure is primary (*the patient's first*

adenoidectomy) or secondary (*the patient's second adenoidectomy performed to remove regrowth after a previous surgery*). Then select the code based on the patient's age. Codes **42830** and **42831** identify a primary adenoidectomy; codes **42835** and **42836** identify a secondary adenoidectomy.

Codes for other tonsil procedures, such as radical resection, excision of tonsil tags, and excision of the lingual tonsil, are also provided.

CODING CAUTION

Although the tonsils are made of lymphoid tissue, CPT classifies procedures on the tonsils under the digestive system. ICD-10-CM classifies diagnoses for the tonsils under the respiratory system (**J02.-** and **J35.-**). ICD-10-PCS classifies inpatient procedures on the tonsils as part of the PCS body system **Mouth and Throat (C)**.

Appendectomy

Although there are only six codes in the Appendix subheading, they are used frequently, and coders must understand the differences. To locate codes in the Index, search for the Main Term **Appendix** or **Appendectomy**. In the Tabular List, CPT provides one code for **Incision and drainage of appendiceal abscess, open** (**44900**), three codes for open appendectomies, and one code for a laparoscopic appendectomy (plus a code for an unlisted laparoscopic procedure).

An incidental appendectomy is the removal of the appendix as a preventive measure during another procedure, such as a cholecystectomy. Incidental appendectomies are usually not coded.

When an appendectomy is performed for an indicated (specific) reason, assign the code as follows. Refer to the CPT manual to observe the formatting of codes and read the full code descriptions.

- When an open appendectomy is performed and the appendix has not ruptured, assign **44950**.

- When an open appendectomy is performed for a ruptured appendix with abscess or generalized peritonitis, assign **44960**.

- When an open appendectomy is done for an indicated reason at the same time as another procedure, assign the add-on code **44955**.

- For a laparoscopic appendectomy, assign **44970**.

Anastomosis

Anastomosis is not a standalone procedure; it is performed in conjunction with a total or partial excision of an organ. When an excision is performed on the alimentary tube or a duct, either an anastomosis or an ostomy is almost always necessary.

To locate codes in the Index, search for the Main Term **Anastomosis**, a first-level modifying term for the site treated, and a second-level modifying term for the site connected to.

Refer to the Tabular List to select the correct code based on the details of the procedure. Read the code options to determine how anastomosis is to be coded:

- Bundled into the code for the main procedure

- An indented code under the main code

- An add-on code

- A separate standalone code

Identify the two sites that are connected and the type of connection created, such as Roux-en-Y, end-to-end, end-to-side, and side-to-end. The specific type of connection is sometimes, but not always, coded.

Endoscopy

CPT differentiates between endoscopy and laparoscopy in the Digestive System subsection. Endoscopy codes describe access through the mouth, nose, or rectum. Laparoscopy codes describe percutaneous access through the abdomen. The subheadings **Esophagus** and **Intestines** provide codes for both endoscopy and laparoscopy. The subheading **Anus** provides endoscopy codes only. The subheadings **Stomach**; **Appendix**; **Liver**; and **Abdomen, Peritoneum, and Omentum** provide laparoscopy codes only because these sites, except for the stomach, cannot be reached endoscopically. Endoscopy of the stomach and duodenum is classified with the esophagus because the stomach and duodenum are examined in conjunction with the esophagus.

Each category for endoscopy or laparoscopy presents special instructions that define the extent of the examinations for the respective anatomic sites. The special instructions also direct that a surgical scope procedure always includes a diagnostic scope procedure. This means that when an endoscopic or laparoscopic procedure begins as a screening or diagnostic procedure and is converted to a surgical procedure, only the surgical procedure should be coded.

For example, during a screening colonoscopy, the physician may remove a polyp. The polypectomy coverts the procedure from screening to surgical. Only one code—the one for the polypectomy—should be reported.

Assign endoscopy codes based on the farthest site accessed. In the upper GI system, when the esophagus, stomach, and duodenum are examined, assign a code for esophagogastroduodenoscopy only; do not also assign a code for esophagoscopy. In the lower GI system, when the entire colon is examined, assign a code for colonoscopy only; do not also assign codes for anoscopy, proctosigmoidoscopy, and sigmoidoscopy, even if procedures were done in those areas (■ FIGURE 32-5).

Multiple Endoscopy Rule

The multiple endoscopy rule explains how to assign endoscopy codes when more than one procedure is performed during the same session. Endoscopy codes are divided into families, each with a base code. The base code is a screening/diagnostic endoscopy for a particular region. The other codes in the family are therapeutic/surgical procedures, such as biopsy, dilation, or tumor excision. You may assign as many surgical codes from one family as necessary, but do not assign the *base* diagnostic endoscopy code together with a *surgical* endoscopy code. The Medicare Physician Fee Schedule Database (MPFSDB) identifies the codes subject to this rule and the corresponding base codes (■ TABLE 32-9). The descriptions of the base codes include the designation (**separate procedure**), which means that the base code should be reported only when it is done as a distinct procedure and not as part of a more extensive surgical procedure. Each code in the family includes the work RVU and price of the base code service, plus the additional work and price for the surgical procedure. Although more than one surgical endoscopy code from the same family can be billed, a special endoscopy payment formula excludes the price of the base service from all but the first code reported (■ FIGURE 32-6, page 626).

Upper GI Endoscopy

CPT provides endoscopy codes for esophagoscopy and esophagogastroduodenoscopy. Special instructions at the beginning of the Endoscopy category define an esophagoscopy as extending from the upper esophageal sphincter to the gastroesophageal junction. When only the esophagus is examined, assign a code for esophagoscopy (43191-43232). Esophagoscopy codes are divided based on whether the endoscope is rigid (parent code **43191**) or flexible. Flexible endoscopy codes are divided based on whether the access is transnasal (parent code **43197**) or transoral (parent code **43200**). Each of these code families is subdivided based on the additional procedures performed during the examination, such as a biopsy, foreign body removal, or polyp removal.

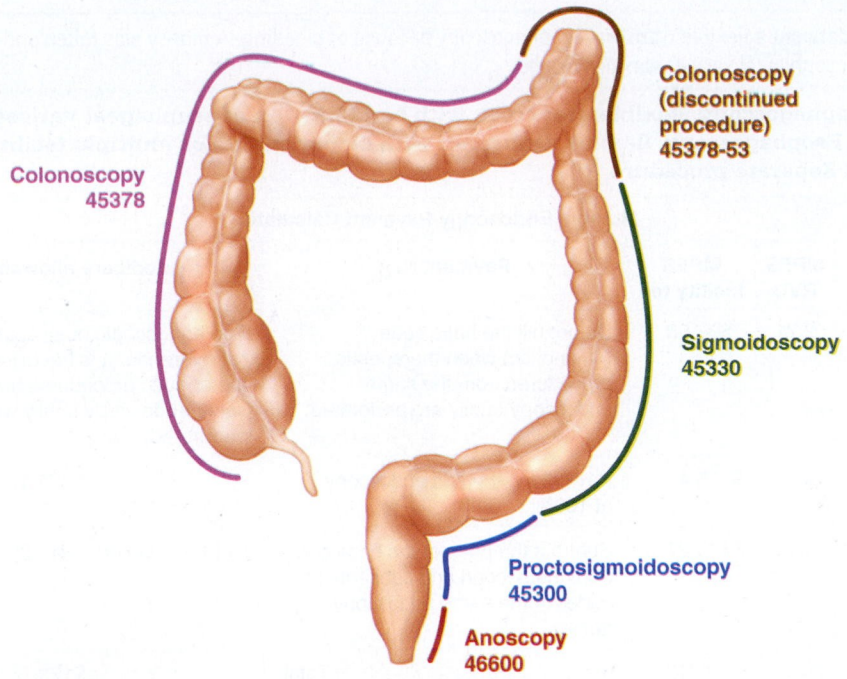

Figure 32-5 ■ Lower GI endoscopy codes.

Table 32-9 ■ **ENDOSCOPIC CODE FAMILIES FOR THE DIGESTIVE SYSTEM**

Base Code	Short Description	Code Family
43191	Esophagoscopy, rigid, transoral; diagnostic	43192-43196
43197	Esophagoscopy, flexible, transnasal; diagnostic	43198
43200	Esophagoscopy, flexible, transoral; diagnostic	43201-43232
43235	Esophagogastroduodenoscopy, flexible, transoral; diagnostic	43236-43259, 43233, 43266, 43270, 43210
43260	Endoscopic retrograde cholangiopancreatography (ERCP); diagnostic	43261-43265, 43274-43278
44360	Small intestinal endoscopy, enteroscopy beyond second portion of duodenum, not including ileum; diagnostic	44361-44373
44376	Small intestinal endoscopy, enteroscopy beyond second portion of duodenum, including ileum; diagnostic	44377-44379
44380	Ileoscopy through stoma; diagnostic	44381-44386
44388	Colonoscopy through stoma; diagnostic	44389-44408
45300	Proctosigmoidoscopy, rigid; diagnostic	45303-45327
45330	Sigmoidoscopy, flexible; diagnostic	45331-45350
45378	Colonoscopy, flexible; diagnostic	45379-45398
46600	Anoscopy; diagnostic	46601-46615
47552	Biliary endoscopy, percutaneous via T-tube or other tract; diagnostic	47553-47556
49320	Laparoscopy, abdomen, peritoneum, and omentum; diagnostic	49321-49327

Source: © PB Resources, Inc. Used with permission. CPT codes only © American Medical Association.

When the stomach and duodenum are examined, assign a code for esophagogastroduodenoscopy (**43235-43259**). Do not also assign a code for esophagoscopy because the service is included in the code for the esophagogastroduodenoscopy. Code **43235** is the parent code for this code family. Codes are divided based on the additional procedures performed during the examination. CPT provides an important instructional note at the beginning of the esophagogastroduodenoscopy code family. When the examination includes the stomach but not the duodenum, assign a code for esophagogastroduodenoscopy

Patient underwent a flexible transoral esophagoscopy because of bleeding. A biopsy was taken and band ligation of esophageal varices was performed.

43205 Esophagoscopy, flexible, transoral; with band ligation of esophageal varices facility

43202-59 Esophagoscopy, flexible, transoral; with biopsy, single or multiple facility;
   -59 Separate procedure

Multiple Endoscopy Payment Calculation

Code	MPFS RVU	MPFS facility fee	Payment rule	Medicare allowable
Endoscopic base code 43200	2.71	$97.08	Do not bill the base code (diagnostic) when therapeutic procedures from the same endoscopy family are performed.	The endoscopic base code is used for reference. It is not billed because therapeutic procedures from the same endoscopy family were performed.
43205	4.34	$155.47	Pay (allow) the first endoscopy at 100%	$155.47
43202	3.19	$114.27	Subtract the price of the base code from the second and subsequent codes in the same endoscopy family.	$114.27 - 97.08 = $17.29
			Total	$172.76

Figure 32-6 ■ Example of the multiple endoscopy payment rule. *Source: © PB Resources, Inc. Used with permission. CPT codes only © American Medical Association.*

with modifier **-52** or **-53**. The choice of modifier depends on whether the physician intends to repeat the examination to include the duodenum.

- When the duodenum is not examined because it is not considered clinically relevant to the reason for the procedure, assign modifier **-52 Reduced services** (■ FIGURE 32-7).

- When the duodenum is not examined because an issue, such as retained gastric contents, prevents safe access to the duodenum, and the physician plans to repeat the procedure under better conditions, assign modifier **-53 Discontinued procedure** (■ FIGURE 32-8).

- When a repeat examination is not planned, assign modifier **-52 Reduced services**.

CODING CAUTION

Many codes in the Digestive System subsection have been resequenced. The cross-referencing instruction provided in the Tabular List does not always lead to the exact location of the resequenced code. It is worthwhile to take a few minutes to locate the new code, then write a note next to where the code number appears in numerical order. For example, the cross-reference next to code **46945** states **See 46200-46288**. Because this is a large range to search, next to **46945** write *see after code 46221* so you can immediately locate the resequenced code.

Medicare Colonoscopy Coding

Medicare has special rules for coding screening colonoscopies. The code for a screening colonoscopy for non-Medicare patients is **45378**. Medicare requires that a HCPCS Level II code be used. **G0105** identifies a screening for an individual

Patient underwent an endoscopic examination of the esophagus and stomach because of suspected reflux disease. The physician does not examine the duodenum because it is not clinically pertinent.

43235-52 Esophagogastroduodenoscopy, flexible, transoral; diagnostic, including collection of specimen(s) by brushing or washing, when performed (separate procedure); -52 Reduced services

Figure 32-7 ■ Example of coding an EGD with modifier -52.

Patient underwent an esophagogastroduodenoscopy for peptic ulcers. The physician cannot move the endoscope past the gastroduodenal junction because the patient did not prepare properly and there is still food in the duodenum. The patient is instructed about the necessity of proper preparation. The procedure is rescheduled for next week.

43235-53 Esophagogastroduodenoscopy, flexible, transoral; diagnostic, including collection of specimen(s) by brushing or washing, when performed (separate procedure); -53 Discontinued procedure

Figure 32-8 ■ Example of coding an EGD with modifier -53.

at high risk of developing colon cancer, which Medicare has established specific criteria for. **G0121** is used for a screening colonoscopy for a person who does not meet Medicare's high-risk criteria. Medicare also provides HCPCS Level II codes for other types of colorectal cancer screening: fecal occult blood testing, flexible sigmoidoscopy, colonoscopy, and screening barium enema (■ TABLE 32-10). Medicare provides detailed instructions regarding how these codes should be used and the diagnoses needed to support them.

Table 32-10 ■ HCPCS LEVEL II CODES FOR COLON CANCER SCREENING

HCPCS Code	HCPCS Code Descriptor
G0104	Colon cancer screening; flexible sigmoidoscopy
G0105	Colon cancer screening; colonoscopy on individual at high risk
G0106	Colon cancer screening; alternative to G0104, screening sigmoidoscopy, barium enema
G0120	Colon cancer screening; alternative to G0105, screening colonoscopy, barium enema
G0121	Colon cancer screening; colonoscopy for individuals not meeting criteria for high risk
G0122	Colon cancer screening; barium enema (noncovered)
G0328	Colon cancer screening; fecal occult blood test, immunoassay, 1–3 simultaneous determinations

Source: Centers for Medicare and Medicaid Services.

When a screening colonoscopy is converted to a diagnostic or surgical endoscopy—for example, when polyps are removed—assign the HCPCS Level II modifier -**PT Colorectal cancer screening test, converted to diagnostic test or other procedure** (■ FIGURE 32-9).

Transplants

Each type or organ transplant has three groups of codes for the three main parts of the transplant process: donor organ harvesting, backbench work, and recipient transplantation. Special instructions at the beginning of each transplant category (liver, pancreas, and small intestine) describe the division and use of codes.

Physician performs a screening colonoscopy on a patient not at high risk. During the procedure, two polyps were found and removed using hot forceps.

G0121-PT Colon cancer screening; colonoscopy for individuals not meeting criteria for high risk; -PT Colorectal cancer screening test, converted to diagnostic test or other procedure

Figure 32-9 ■ Example of coding for a Medicare screening colonoscopy.

For liver transplants, different codes are used for a cadaver hepatectomy (**47133**) than for a living donor. Codes for a living donor hepatectomy are divided based on which segments of the liver are removed (**47140-47142**). Codes for backbench preparation and reconstruction are divided based on the extent of work performed (**47143-47147**). Recipient codes are divided based on whether the transplant is orthotopic (*the transplanted organ is placed in the same position as the original organ*) or heterotopic (*the transplanted organ is placed in a position other than that of the original organ*) (**47135-47136**).

The donor and recipient require different diagnosis codes. A living donor is assigned a **Z** code indicating the donor status. Diagnosis codes for the organ recipient identify the condition(s) that describes why the transplant is necessary, as well as any comorbid conditions.

Multiple physicians are usually involved in various parts of the transplantation process. Each physician reports the appropriate code(s) for the services personally provided (■ FIGURE 32-10).

A living donor match is found for a pediatric patient with congenital biliary atresia who has been on the liver transplant list. The transplant team consists of two surgeons. Surgeon A performs a hepatectomy of the left lateral segment on the living donor. Surgeon B performs the backbench reconstruction with two venous anastomoses and two arterial anastomoses. Both surgeons transplant the liver segment into the patient recipient. The transplant is orthotopic .

Surgeon A
Living donor:
Z52.6 Liver donor
47140 Donor hepatectomy (including cold preservation), from living donor; left lateral segment only (segments II and III)

Surgeon B
Backbench reconstruction:
Q44.2 Atresia of bile ducts
47147 × 2 Backbench reconstruction of cadaver or living donor liver graft prior to allotransplantation; arterial anastomosis, each
47146-51 × 2 Backbench reconstruction of cadaver or living donor liver graft prior to allotransplantation; venous anastomosis, each; -51 Multiple procedures

Surgeon A and Surgeon B
Transplant recipient:
Q44.2 Atresia of bile ducts
47135-66 Liver allotransplantation; orthotopic, partial or whole, from cadaver or living donor, any age; -66 Surgical team

Figure 32-10 ■ Example of coding a liver transplant. *Source:* © PB Resources, Inc. Used with permission. CPT codes only © American Medical Association.

Modifier rules vary among the six types of organ transplants. Carefully review the MPFSDB to determine which transplant codes accept modifier **-66 Surgical team** and which codes require modifier **-51 Multiple procedures**.

Repairs

Repair involves closing an opening—such as a laceration, fistula, or ostomy—or restructuring/reconstructing an anatomic site. This is in contrast to an incision made for drainage or to create an opening and in contrast to an excision, which removes tissue. Most Digestive System subheadings provide a category for repair. To locate Repair codes in the Index, search for the one of the following:

- The Main Term **Repair** and a first-level modifying term for the anatomic site
- The name of the procedure, which usually ends with the suffix -*plasty*, -*rraphy*, or -*pexy*
- The name of the anatomic site and a first-level modifying term for **Repair**

In the Tabular List, review the details of the codes to select the one that describes the details of the procedure. Repair codes may appear as a parent code with several indented codes that describe variations of the procedure (■ FIGURE 32-11).

Adhesions

When performing procedures in the abdominal cavity, surgeons frequently encounter adhesions resulting from scarring from previous surgeries or inflammation. They must loosen, excise, or destroy the adhesions to reach the surgical site. CPT guidelines state that surgical destruction is part of a surgical procedure and, usually, should not be reported separately. This includes adhesions. When adhesions are so extensive that the surgeon spends a significant amount of time destroying or removing them to enable access to the surgical site, it might be possible to append modifier **-22 Increased procedural services** to the CPT code for the procedure. Documentation must identify the amount of excess time required, describe in detail what the surgeon did, and explain why the added time was necessary. In general, modifier **-22** should be used only when the added work has increased the operative time by 50% or more.

Separate codes for adhesiolysis are reported in the unusual circumstance when lysis is performed as a separate procedure. To locate adhesiolysis codes in the Index, search for the Main Term **Adhesions** and the first-level modifying term for the anatomic site.

Surgeon performs an esophagoplasty and closes a tracheoesophageal fistula using the thoracic approach.

43312 Esophagoplasty (plastic repair or reconstruction), thoracic approach; with repair of tracheoesophageal fistula

---

Figure 32-11 ■ Example of coding a repair on the esophagus.

Guided Example of Assigning Digestive System Procedure Codes

To practice skills for assigning codes from the Digestive System subsection, continue with the guided example from earlier in the chapter about a patient who was seen for a colonoscopy. Follow along in your CPT manual as Jill Hynes, CPC, assigns codes. Check off each step after you complete it.

▶ First, Jill confirms the procedures: colonoscopy, polypectomy, hemorrhoidectomy.

▶ Jill searches the Index for the Main Term **Colonoscopy**.

❑ She locates the first-level modifying term **Flexible**.

❑ She locates the second-level modifying term **Removal**, then **Polyp**.

❑ She identifies the codes to verify: **45384, 45385**.

▶ Jill turns to the Tabular List to review and verify codes **45384-45385**.

❑ She notices that **45384-45385** are indented codes, so she traces back through the Tabular List to locate the parent code, **45378**.

❑ She reads the common part of code **45378** that appears before the semicolon: **Colonoscopy, flexible**. This code describes the basic colonoscopy provided, which extended from the anus to the cecum. She reads the second part of the code description—**diagnostic, including collection of specimen(s) by brushing or washing, when performed (separate procedure)**—and confirms that it does not describe this procedure because a therapeutic procedure was also performed.

❑ She reads the indented description for code **45384, with removal of tumor(s), polyp(s), or other lesion(s) by hot biopsy forceps** and confirms that this accurately describes the two polyps found in the sigmoid colon.

❑ She reads the indented description for code **45385, with removal of tumor(s), polyp(s), or other lesion(s) by snare technique** and confirms that this accurately describes the polyp found in the transverse colon.

▶ Jill checks for instructional notes in the Tabular List.

❑ She looks for instructional notes after the parent code, **45378**, and the indented codes she plans to use, **45384** and **45385**, and finds none.

❑ She refers to the beginning of the category **Endoscopy**, which appears before code **45300**, and reviews the special instructions that include definitions of endoscopic procedures on the colon.

❑ She understands that even though a polypectomy occurred in the sigmoid segment of the colon, she should not report a sigmoidoscopy; she should assign codes based on the farthest extent of the procedure, which was the entire length of the colon from the rectum to the cecum.

- ❏ She also reads the statement **Surgical endoscopy always includes diagnostic endoscopy.** This tells her that she should not use a separate code for the diagnostic portion of the procedure in addition to the codes for the polypectomies.

- ❏ She checks for special instructions at the beginning of the Digestive System subsection, before code **40490**, and finds none.

- ❏ She reviews the Surgery section guidelines that appear before code **10004** but does not find any information specific to endoscopies.

▶ Jill returns to the codes for the polypectomies: **45384** and **45385**.

- ❏ Because these codes share the same parent code (**45378**), she needs to determine whether they can both be reported.

- ❏ She confirms that there were no instructional notes directing her not to use the codes together.

- ❏ She recalls the multiple endoscopy rule that permits multiple codes from the same code family to be reported together. Both of these codes belong to the code family with the base code **43578**, so she knows that she can report both codes.

▶ Jill turns her attention to the hemorrhoidectomy.

▶ Jill searches the Index for the Main Term **Hemorrhoidectomy**.

- ❏ She locates the first-level modifying term **Ligation**.

- ❏ She identifies the code range to verify: **46221, 46945-46946**.

▶ Jill turns to the Tabular List to review and verify the codes.

- ❏ First, she locates code **46221** and notices that codes **46945-46946** appear next because they are resequenced codes. She likes being able to review and compare all three codes together.

- ❏ She reads the description for code **46221, Hemorrhoidectomy, internal, by rubber band ligation(s)**. This sounds like the right description but she checks the other codes to be certain.

- ❏ She notices that code **46945** is a parent code for **46946**, and the common descriptor is **Hemorrhoidectomy, internal, by ligation other than rubber band;**

- ❏ She double-checks the documentation and confirms the ligation method: Hemorrhoids were ligated with rubber bands. The documentation confirms that **46221** is the correct code because the code specifies **by rubber band ligation**.

▶ Jill reviews the Tabular List for instructional notes and finds two.

- ❏ The first instructional note appears after code **46221: (Do not report 46221 in conjunction with 45350,**

45398). This note does not apply because she already determined that she is not reporting code **45350** or **45398**.

- ❏ The second instructional note appears after code **46946: (Do not report 46221, 46945, and 46946, in conjunction with 0249T.)** This note does not apply because she is not using code **0249T**.

- ❏ Jill also reviews the special instructions at the beginning of the subheading **Anus**, before code **46020**. The special instructions define the codes to use for various types of hemorrhoids and confirm that she selected the correct code for ligation of internal hemorrhoids.

▶ Jill assigns the codes for moderate sedation by the provider performing the service with an independent observer.

- ❏ She searches the Index for **Moderate Sedation**, which refers her to the entry for **Sedation**. The Main Term **Sedation** lists a first-level modifying term for **Moderate** and lists the code range **99151-99153, 99155-99157**.

- ❏ She selects the code range **99151-99153** because it identifies that the sedation was provided by the same physician performing the procedure.

- ❏ She assigns **99152 Moderate sedation services provided by the same physician or other qualified health care professional performing the diagnostic or therapeutic service that the sedation supports, requiring the presence of an independent trained observer to assist in the monitoring of the patient's level of consciousness and physiological status; initial 15 minutes of intraservice time, patient age 5 years or older** for the initial 15 minutes.

- ❏ She assigns **99153 Moderate sedation services provided by the same physician or other qualified health care professional performing the diagnostic or therapeutic service that the sedation supports, requiring the presence of an independent trained observer to assist in the monitoring of the patient's level of consciousness and physiological status; each additional 15 minutes intraservice time (List separately in addition to code for primary service)** with a quantity of **3** for the remaining 45 minutes.

▶ Jill reviews the procedure codes she has assigned for this case.

- ❏ **46221 Hemorrhoidectomy, internal, by rubber band ligation(s)**

- ❏ **45384 Colonoscopy, flexible; with removal of tumor(s), polyp(s), or other lesion(s) by hot biopsy forceps**

- ❏ **45385 Colonoscopy, flexible; with removal of tumor(s), polyp(s), or other lesion(s) by snare technique**

❏ **99152 Moderate sedation services provided by the same physician or other qualified health care professional performing the diagnostic or therapeutic service that the sedation supports...; initial 15 minutes of intraservice time, patient age 5 years or older**

❏ **99153 × 3 Moderate sedation services provided by the same physician or other qualified health care...; each additional 15 minutes intraservice time**

▶ Next, Jill must determine what modifiers are needed and how to sequence the codes.

CODING PRACTICE

Exercise 32.3 Assigning Codes for Digestive System Procedures

Instructions: Read the mini-medical-record of each patient's encounter. Review the information abstracted in Exercise 32.2 for questions 1–3. For questions 4–6, do the abstracting on your own. Assign CPT procedure codes using the Index and Tabular List. Write the code(s) on the line provided.

---

1. OUTPATIENT HOSPITAL Gender: M Age: 57

Preprocedure diagnosis: Screening colonoscopy

Procedure: Flexible colonoscopy, 2 polyps in descending segment, 1 polyp in transverse segment, remainder of colon to cecum was clear. Polyps were removed with bipolar cautery and submitted to pathology.

Postprocedure diagnosis: Adenomatous polyps per pathology report

Tip: Apply a modifier to identify this as a preventive service.

1 CPT Code _____

---

2. INPATIENT HOSPITAL Gender: F Age: 33

Diagnosis: Morbid obesity, BMI = 43 kg/m^2

Procedure: Laparoscopic gastric bypass and Roux-en-Y gastroenterostomy (100 cm)

Tip: Identify the meaning of *gastroenterostomy* to determine the Roux-en-Y sites.

1 CPT Code _____

---

3. INPATIENT HOSPITAL Gender: F Age: 48

Diagnosis: Squamous cell carcinoma of the esophagus

Procedure: Near-total esophagectomy, thoracotomy, end-to-side pharyngogastrostomy (*restructure of the pathway from the throat to the stomach after esophagectomy*)

1 CPT Code _____

---

4. EMERGENCY DEPT Gender: M Age: 2

Reason for encounter: Mother brings in her son, who swallowed a toy piece

Procedure: Rigid esophagoscopy through the mouth, retrieved plastic toy piece, no damage or laceration apparent

Diagnosis: Esophagoscopy with foreign body removal

Tip: Abstract this procedure on your own before attempting to assign codes.

1 CPT Code _____

---

5. EMERGENCY DEPT Gender: F Age: 26

Diagnosis: Abscess under the tongue

Procedure: Superficial sublingual incision and drainage

Tip: Abstract this procedure on your own. Do not confuse the sublingual site within the mouth with the sublingual salivary gland.

1 CPT Code _____

---

6. LOCATION Gender: M Age: 36

Preprocedure diagnosis: Rectal mass

Procedure: Transsacral proctotomy to excise rectal tumor

Postprocedure diagnosis: Stage I carcinoma of the rectum

Tip: Abstract this procedure on your own before attempting to assign codes.

1 CPT Code _____

ARRANGING CODES FOR DIGESTIVE SYSTEM PROCEDURES

When more than one procedure is performed during an operative session, coders must be attentive to modifiers and how to arrange (sequence) codes. The order of codes sometimes determines the modifiers needed. Some modifiers can be assigned at the same time the code is assigned, and some modifiers cannot be assigned until the codes are sequenced. Certain modifiers are required even when only one procedure is performed.

In general, multiple surgical procedures are sequenced in descending order of RVU, which corresponds to the complexity and price of the procedure. RVUs are provided in the MPFSDB and in most encoders and billing software programs.

Modifiers

Modifiers that have a special application for specific Digestive System codes have been discussed throughout this chapter and examples have been provided. This section summarizes those modifiers and introduces some new ones. These are not the only modifiers that can be used with Digestive System subsection codes. Refer to Appendix A of the CPT manual and to Chapters 27 and 30 of this text for more information about modifiers.

-33 Preventive Service

Modifier **-33** identifies certain procedures, such as a screening colonoscopy, as preventive care services under the Patient Protection and Affordable Care Act (PPACA). The United States Preventive Services Task Force (USPSTF) assigns one of five letter grades (A, B, C, D, or I) to recommend the likelihood of the net benefit of providing a preventive service. The PPACA requires that services rated as A or B be covered in full by private health plans. Copayments, coinsurances, and deductibles are not owed for these services under PPACA.

When a service on the approved list does not have a CPT code specifically described as preventive, assign modifier **-33** to indicate that the service was provided for preventive care. For example, CPT provides codes for preventive medicine E/M visits, so those codes do not need modifier **-33**. However, CPT does not provide a dedicated code for screening colonoscopies, so the code for a diagnostic colonoscopy (**45378**) must be reported. Append modifier **-33** to identify the colonoscopy as preventive in

nature. The insurance company will waive the patient's copayment, coinsurance, and deductible and pay 100% of the allowed fee to the provider (■ FIGURE 32-12). A copayment may still apply if preventive care is not the *primary* purpose of the office visit or other services that require copayment are provided.

-51 Multiple Procedures

When multiple procedures are performed at the same operative session by the same provider, modifier **-51** indicates that payment should be reduced on the second and subsequent procedures because of the efficiencies gained. Procedures should be ordered in descending order by RVU, so that the most extensive procedure is paid in full and payment is reduced for the less extensive procedures. The standard Medicare rule for payment of multiple surgeries is to allow the full amount of the first procedure and allow the second through fifth procedures at 50% of the Medicare Physician Fee Schedule (MPFS) rate. Multiple procedures beyond six are priced **by report** (*based on a report submitted by the physician*). Private payers establish their own guidelines for payment of multiple procedures.

Do not append modifier **-51** to add-on codes or to codes with the symbol (**modifier-51 exempt**). The MPFSDB and most encoders identify the codes for which this modifier is applicable.

-52 Reduced Services

The subcategory **Esophagogastroduodenoscopy** provides special instructions regarding modifier **-52** that appear before code **43235**. When the duodenum is not examined because it is

---

Physician performs a routine screening colonoscopy on a patient, age 50.

45378-33 Colonoscopy, flexible, proximal to splenic flexure; diagnostic, with or without collection of specimen(s) by brushing or washing, with or without colon decompression (separate procedure); -33 Preventive services

Modifier -33 Payment Calculation					
Code	Modifier	Allowed fee	Patient co-insurance	Patient pays	Insurance pays
45378	33	$400.00	Waived	$0.00	$400.00
45378	None	$400.00	20%	$80.00	$320.00

Figure 32-12 ■ Example of using modifier -33. *Source: © PB Resources, Inc. Used with permission. CPT codes only © American Medical Association.*

not judged clinically relevant, append modifier **-52**. Likewise, if the duodenum cannot be examined for some other reason, such as retention of gastric contents, and a repeat examination is not planned, append modifier **-52**. Reduce the fee to be billed based on the extent of the service actually provided. Use of this modifier is required.

Special instructions at the beginning of the **Endoscopy** category for **Colon and Rectum** provide further direction on modifier **-52**. There are times when a therapeutic colonoscopy cannot proceed all the way to the cecum or small intestine, usually due to retained fecal matter. In this situation, append modifier **-52** to the therapeutic colonoscopy code. Submit appropriate documentation with the claim to explain the reason the procedure was reduced.

-53 Discontinued Procedure

The special instructions for the subcategory **Esophagogastroduodenoscopy** also include directions about modifier **-53**. In the situation that the duodenum cannot be examined and a repeat examination *is planned*, append modifier **-53**.

CPT special instructions at the beginning of the **Endoscopy** category for **Colon and Rectum** provide additional guidance regarding this modifier. When a screening colonoscopy cannot proceed all the way to the cecum or small intestine, report the code for the full colonoscopy and append modifier **-53** to indicate that the procedure could not be completed. Use of this modifier is required. Reduce the fee to be billed based on the extent of the service actually provided. Submit appropriate documentation with the claim to explain the reason the procedure was discontinued.

-59 Distinct Procedural Service

Modifier **-59** is used to clarify that two procedures that might be considered to be bundled were performed on distinct sites or lesions or through distinct procedures. When the NCCI assigns the indicator 1 to a pair of surgical codes, modifier **-59** identifies that two separate services were provided. A common example of this with procedures from the Digestive System subsection is when multiple therapeutic procedures from the same endoscopic code family are performed, as described under the multiple endoscopy rule discussed earlier in this chapter. Both indented codes are reported and modifier **-59** is appended to the second code of the pair.

In 2015, the Centers for Medicare and Medicaid (CMS) introduced four HCPCS modifiers to selectively identify subsets of procedures that would otherwise be reported with modifier **-59**. They are referred to as **-X{EPSU}** modifiers and describe specific reasons that services should be considered as separate and distinct. When appropriate, use one of the following modifiers instead of modifier **-59** for Medicare patients. Check with other payers to learn how they want these modifiers applied:

- **-XE Separate Encounter**—A service that is distinct because it occurred during a separate encounter

- **-XP Separate Practitioner**—A service that is distinct because it was performed by a different practitioner

- **-XS Separate Structure**—A service that is distinct because it was performed on a separate organ/structure

- **-XU Unusual Non-Overlapping Service**—The use of a service that is distinct because it does not overlap usual components of the main service

-66 Surgical Team

Surgical teams are used for liver and pancreas transplants. Each surgeon reports modifier **-66** on the code for the recipient transplantation. Payment is prorated among the surgeons based on the role of each documented in the operative report. Surgical teams are not paid for all components of a transplant. For example, harvesting a cadaver organ or backbench preparation may not qualify for a surgical team. Intestinal transplants do not qualify for a surgical team. In some cases, a cosurgeon (modifier **-62**) or assistant surgeon (modifier **-80**) is allowed. The MPFSDB identifies the modifiers accepted for each code. Many encoders and billing software programs also provide modifier information.

-PT Colorectal Cancer Screening Test, Converted to Diagnostic Test or Other Procedure

Assign this HCPCS Level II modifier for Medicare patients when a screening colonoscopy or other colorectal cancer screening test is converted to a diagnostic or therapeutic procedure. This includes any time that a treatment is performed during the screening, including removing a polyp, cauterization, dilation, and so on.

Guided Example of Arranging Digestive System Procedure Codes

To practice skills for assigning modifiers and arranging codes for procedures from the Digestive System subsection, continue with the example from earlier in the chapter about the patient who was seen for a colonoscopy. Follow along in your CPT manual as Jill Hynes, CPC, arranges the codes. Check off each step after you complete it.

▶ First, Jill confirms the CPT codes.

❑ **46221 Hemorrhoidectomy, internal, by rubber band ligation(s)**

❑ **45384 Colonoscopy, flexible; with removal of tumor(s), polyp(s), or other lesion(s) by hot biopsy forceps**

❑ **45385 Colonoscopy, flexible; with removal of tumor(s), polyp(s), or other lesion(s) by snare technique**

❑ **99152 Moderate sedation services provided by the same physician or other qualified health care professional performing the diagnostic or therapeutic service that the sedation supports...; initial 15 minutes of intraservice time, patient age 5 years or older**

❑ **99153 × 3 Moderate sedation services provided by the same physician or other qualified health care...; each additional 15 minutes intraservice time**

▶ Jill reviews the RVUs for each code. She selects the facility RVUs because the physician is performing the procedure at an outpatient hospital facility rather than at a location he personally owns and operates. The RVU schedule defines *facility RVU* as a facility owned by a third party (other than the physician). Facility RVUs are used when the physician performing the service does not own the facility where the procedure is performed. Nonfacility RVUs are used when the physician performing the service owns the location where the procedure is performed. The facility RVUs and pricing do not reimburse the physician for facility-related costs, so they are lower than nonfacility RVUs and pricing, which reimburse the physician for facility-related costs, such as those for the building, equipment, and staff. (*Note:* Although this is not a Medicare patient, the MPFSDB is used because many private payers use Medicare RVUs and assign their own prices. In the workplace, follow the rules of each payer.)

❏ Moderated sedation codes (**99152** and **99153**) are not subject to multiple procedure fee reductions, so they are sequenced first.

❏ Code **45385** for the polypectomy using the snare technique is the most extensive service, with a facility RVU of 8.78. She sequences this code third.

❏ Code **45384** for the polypectomy using hot forceps is the second most extensive service, with a facility RVU of 7.74. She sequences this code fourth. Although two polyps were removed, the code description identifies the entire procedure. It does not provide direction to assign multiple occurrences of the code for each polyp removed, so she reports this code only once.

❏ Code **46221** for the hemorrhoid ligation is the least extensive service, with a facility RVU of 5.46. She sequences this code fifth.

▶ Jill reviews the codes to determine the need for modifiers. (Refer to Table 27-1, Key Criteria for Abstracting CPT Modifiers, in this text or Appendix A in the CPT manual.)

❏ Code **45385** does not require any modifiers because it is the primary procedure performed. She will link a diagnosis code for a polyp of the transverse colon to support this procedure.

❏ Code **45384** requires modifier **-XS Separate structure** to clearly identify that the hot forceps polypectomy was a different lesion than the snare polypectomy. This will be clarified further when she links the diagnosis code for a polyp of the sigmoid colon. This procedure will be paid under the multiple endoscopy rule, not the multiple procedures rule, so modifier **-51 Multiple procedures** is not needed. (Some private payers might require modifier **-51** in addition to modifier **-XS**.)

❏ Code **46221** requires modifier **-51 Multiple procedures** because the hemorrhoidectomy was performed during the same session as the colonoscopy. The payment will be reduced to 50% of the usual fee.

❏ Code **99152** is marked with the symbol ⊘, indicating **Exempt from modifier -51** in the CPT manual. The symbol means the code is not subject to multiple procedure fee reductions. Code **99153** is an add-on code, so it does not require modifier **-51**. The moderate sedation codes are sequenced first because they are not subject to a multiple fee reduction.

▶ Jill finalizes the procedure codes, modifiers, and sequencing for this case (■ FIGURE 32-13):

(1) **99152 Moderate sedation services provided by the same physician or other qualified health care professional performing the diagnostic or therapeutic service that the sedation supports, requiring the presence of an independent trained observer to assist in the monitoring of the patient's level of consciousness and physiological status; initial 15 minutes of intraservice time, patient age 5 years or older**

21. DIAGNOSIS OR NATURE OF ILLNESS OR INJURY Relate A-L to service line below (24E)			ICD Ind. 0	22. RESUBMISSION CODE	ORIGINAL REF. NO.
A. D12.3	B. D12.5	C. K64.0	D.	23. PRIOR AUTHORIZATION NUMBER	
E.	F.	G.	H.		
I.	J.	K.	L.		

24. A. DATE(S) OF SERVICE From MM DD YY To MM DD YY	B. PLACE OF SERVICE	C. EMG	D. PROCEDURES, SERVICES, OR SUPPLIES (Explain Unusual Circumstances) CPT/HCPCS / MODIFIER	E. DIAGNOSIS POINTER	F. $ CHARGES	G. DAYS OR UNITS	H. EPSDT Family Plan	I. ID. QUAL.	J. RENDERING PROVIDER ID. #
1 01 05 YY	22		99152	ABC	52 37	01		NPI	99 99999999
2 01 05 YY	22		99153	ABC	11 15	03		NPI	99 99999999
3 01 05 YY	22		45385	A	314 52	01		NPI	99 99999999
4 01 05 YY	22		45384 XS	B	277 27	01		NPI	99 99999999
5 01 05 YY	22		46221 51	C	195 59	01		NPI	99 99999999

Figure 32-13 ■ CMS-1500 form billing for the "Guided Example". *Source: © PB Resources, Inc. Used with permission. CPT codes only © American Medical Association.*

(2) **99153 × 3 Moderate sedation services provided by the same physician or other qualified health care professional performing the diagnostic or therapeutic service that the sedation supports, requiring the presence of an independent trained observer to assist in the monitoring of the patient's level of consciousness and physiological status; each additional 15 minutes intraservice time**

(3) **45385-XS Colonoscopy, flexible; with removal of tumor(s), polyp(s), or other lesion(s) by snare technique**

(4) **45384 Colonoscopy, flexible; with removal of tumor(s), polyp(s), or other lesion(s) by hot biopsy forceps; -XS Separate structure**

(5) **46221-51 Hemorrhoidectomy, internal, by rubber band ligation(s); -51 Multiple procedures**

▶ Jill also assigns and sequences the ICD-10-CM diagnosis codes that support the need for the service.

(1) **D12.3 Benign neoplasm of transverse colon**

(2) **D12.5 Benign neoplasm of sigmoid colon**

(3) **K64.0 First degree hemorrhoids**

CODING PRACTICE

Exercise 32.4 Arranging Codes for Digestive System Procedures

Instructions: Read the mini-medical-record of each patient's encounter, and review the information abstracted in Exercise 32.2 for questions 1–3. For questions 4–6, do the abstracting on your own. Assign CPT codes and modifiers using the Index and Tabular List, and arrange the codes in proper sequence. Write the code(s) on the line provided.

---

1. OUTPATIENT HOSPITAL   Gender: M   Age: 64

Diagnosis: Initial incarcerated incisional hernia

Procedure: Incarcerated incisional hernia repair with mesh

2 CPT Codes _____

---

2. OUTPATIENT HOSPITAL   Gender: M   Age: 61

Preoperative diagnosis: Melena, hematemesis

Procedure: Moderate sedation by second provider with intraservice time of 75 minutes. EGD was initiated with flexible scope through the mouth. Identified bleeding ulcers in esophagus and duodenum, which were successfully cauterized. Features of chronic gastritis were noted. No masses or hiatal hernia. Obtained biopsy from the antrum. Biopsies submitted to pathology for H&E (*hematoxylin and eosin stain test to detect cancer*) and CLO (test for Campylobacter H. pylori).

Postoperative diagnosis: Bleeding esophageal ulcer and bleeding peptic ulcer

Pathology report: Biopsies negative for H. pylori and carcinoma

(continued)

---

2. (continued)

Tip: Code for both the provider of moderate sedation and the performing provider. EGD with control of bleeding has a higher RVU than EGD with biopsy.

a. 2 CPT codes (Performing physician) _____

b. 2 CPT Codes (Sedation provider) _____,
_____ x _____

---

3. INPATIENT HOSPITAL   Gender: M   Age: 3 months

Diagnosis: Bilateral cleft lip with nasal deformity and cleft palate

Procedure: Primary repair of a bilateral cleft lip and nasal deformity; repair of soft tissue of cleft palate and closure of alveolar ridge

Tip: Primary repair identifies a one-stage procedure.

2 CPT Codes _____

---

4. HOSPITAL   Gender: F   Age: 58

Preprocedure diagnosis: Breast cancer with metastasis to the ileum and abdominal cavity

Procedure: Made a midline incision in the abdominal cavity. Excised tumors of 5 cm, 7 cm, 9 cm, and 12 cm in diameter from the peritoneum. Turned our attention to the ileum, from which a 75-cm segment was resected, and the healthy bowel was anastomosed in an end-to-end manner.

Tip: Abstract this procedure on your own. To locate the Main Term, use the medical term for cutting out part of the small intestine.

2 CPT Codes _____

CODING PRACTICE (continued)

5. INPATIENT HOSPITAL   Gender: M   Age: 57

Diagnosis: Malignant ascites

Procedure: Under general anesthesia, created trocar ports in the abdomen and chest. Using the laparoscope, we inserted a tunneled intraperitoneal catheter, then inserted a subcutaneous extension from the catheter to exit from the chest.

Tip: Abstract this procedure on your own. A trocar is a sharp tool used to create openings and hold instruments used for laparoscopic surgery.

2 CPT Codes _____

6. INPATIENT HOSPITAL   Gender: M   Age: 74

Diagnosis: Dysphagia following stroke

Procedure: Administered moderate sedation. Injected contrast medium. Under fluoroscopic guidance created gastrostomy, inserted feeding tube, and then converted to gastrojejunostomy tube.

Tip: Abstract this procedure on your own. The surgeon provided the image documentation and report.

2 CPT Codes _____

E/M CODING FOR GASTROENTEROLOGY

The *1997 Documentation Guidelines for Evaluation and Management Services* (1997 DG), published by CMS, do not provide guidelines for a single-system gastroenterology examination. Gastroenterologists use the multisystem examination criteria (■ FIGURE 32-14, page 636). To determine the appropriate E/M code, coders must review the documentation in detail and identify the specific elements documented.

- To translate the documentation into the E/M requirements for the history, refer back to Chapter 28, "Evaluation and Management Services (99201-99499)," Tables 28-7 to 28-10, or the 1997 DG.

- To determine the requirements for an examination, refer to or to the general multisystem examination in the 1997 DG.

- To determine the levels for medical decision making (MDM), refer to Chapter 28, Table 28-12, and to the Table of Risk in the 1997 DG.

Guided Example of E/M Coding for Gastroenterology

Refer to ■ FIGURE 32-15, (page 638) Gastroenterology Encounter, to practice skills for abstracting and assigning E/M codes. Follow along as fictitious coder Jill Hynes, CPC, abstracts the procedure. Check off each step after you complete it.

▶ First, Jill needs to establish the category of service so she can determine the information needed to abstract and assign the code.

- ❑ *What is the setting?* Office

- ❑ *What is the type of service?* The encounter qualifies as a consultation because the gastroenterologist's advice is requested by the referring physician and the gastroenterologist sends a report back to the referring physician at the conclusion of the encounter.

- ❑ *What is the code range?* Jill refers to the CPT Index and looks up the Main Term **Evaluation and Management**

and the subterm **Consultation**. The code range listed is **99241-99255**.

- ❑ *How many key components are required?* Jill refers to the code range in the Tabular List and notices that the Consultation subheading is divided into two categories: **Office or other outpatient** and **Inpatient**. She selects the **Office or other outpatient** category and reads the code description of the first code, which states **Office consultation for a new or established patient, which requires these 3 key components**. All codes in the category have the same requirements for key components. This tells her that all three key components must meet or exceed the levels listed in the code (3/3).

▶ Next, Jill identifies the level of history.

- ❑ *What is the level of HPI?* The HPI is **extended** because seven elements are documented

- ❑ *What is the level of ROS?* The ROS is **extended** because four systems are documented

- ❑ *What is the level of PFSH?* The PFSH is **complete** because three elements are documented

- ❑ *Based on these factors, what is the overall level of history?* The level of history is **detailed** because the lowest of the three factors (HPI, ROS, and PFSH) determines the history level. The HPI and PFSH qualify for a comprehensive history, but the ROS qualifies for only a detailed history.

▶ Jill refers to the multisystem examination in the 1997 DG (FIGURE 32-14) to abstract information needed to determine the level of the examination.

- ❑ *What is the level of examination?* The level of examination is **detailed**. Nineteen (19) elements in four organ systems are documented, which exceeds the requirement of 12 or more elements in two organ systems for a detailed examination. A comprehensive examination

System/Body Area	Elements of Multi-System Examination
Constitutional	❑ Measurement of any <u>three</u> of the following seven **vital** signs: • 1) sitting or standing blood pressure, • 2) supine blood pressure, • 3) pulse rate and regularity, • 4) respiration, • 5) temperature, • 6) height, • 7) weight (May be measured and recorded by ancillary staff) ❑ General **appearance** of patient (eg, development, nutrition, body habitus, deformities, attention to grooming)
Eyes	❑ Inspection of **conjunctivae** and **lids** ❑ Examination of **pupils** and **irises** (eg, reaction to light and accommodation, size and symmetry) ❑ Ophthalmoscopic examination of **optic discs** (eg, size, C/D ratio, appearance) and posterior segments (eg, vessel changes, exudates, hemorrhages
Ears, Nose, Mouth and Throat	❑ External **inspection** of ears and nose (eg, overall appearance, scars, lesions, masses) ❑ Otoscopic examination of external **auditory canals** and **tympanic membranes** ❑ Assessment of **hearing** (eg, whispered voice, finger rub, tuning fork) ❑ Inspection of **nasal mucosa, septum** and **turbinates** ❑ Inspection of **lips, teeth** and **gums** ❑ Examination of **oropharynx:** oral mucosa, salivary glands, hard and soft palates, tongue, tonsils and posterior pharynx
Neck	❑ Examination of **neck** (eg, masses, overall appearance, symmetry, tracheal position, crepitus) ❑ Examination of **thyroid** (eg, enlargement, tenderness, mass)
Respiratory	❑ Assessment of **respiratory effort** (eg, intercostal retractions, use of accessory muscles, diaphragmatic movement) ❑ **Percussion** of chest (eg, dullness, flatness, hyperresonance) ❑ **Palpation** of chest (eg, tactile fremitus) ❑ **Auscultation** of lungs (eg, breath sounds, adventitious sounds, rubs)
Cardiovascular	❑ **Palpation of heart** (eg, location, size, thrills) ❑ **Auscultation** of heart with notation of abnormal sounds and murmurs Examination of: ❑ **carotid arteries** (eg, pulse amplitude, bruits) ❑ **abdominal aorta** (eg, size, bruits) ❑ **femoral arteries** (eg, pulse amplitude, bruits) ❑ **pedal pulses** (eg, pulse amplitude) ❑ **extremities** for edema and/or varicosities
Chest (Breasts)	❑ **Inspection** of breasts (eg, symmetry, nipple discharge) ❑ **Palpation** of breasts and axillae (eg, masses or lumps, tenderness)
Gastrointestinal (Abdomen)	❑ Examination of **abdomen** with notation of presence of masses or tenderness ❑ Examination of **liver** and **spleen** ❑ Examination for presence or absence of **hernia** ❑ Examination (when indicated) of **anus, perineum** and **rectum,** including sphincter tone, presence of hemorrhoids, rectal masses ❑ Obtain **stool sample** for occult blood test when indicated
Genitourinary	**MALE:** ❑ Examination of the **scrotal contents** (eg, hydrocele, spermatocele, tenderness of cord, testicular mass) ❑ Examination of the **penis** ❑ Digital rectal examination of **prostate** gland (eg, size, symmetry, nodularity, tenderness) **FEMALE:** Pelvic examination (with or without specimen collection for smears and cultures), including ❑ Examination of **external genitalia** (eg, general appearance, hair distribution, lesions) and **vagina** (eg, general appearance, estrogen effect, discharge, lesions, pelvic support, cystocele, rectocele) ❑ Examination of **urethra** (eg, masses, tenderness, scarring) ❑ Examination of **bladder** (eg, fullness, masses, tenderness) Cervix (eg, general appearance, lesions, discharge) ❑ **Uterus** (eg, size, contour, position, mobility, tenderness, consistency, descent or support) ❑ **Adnexa**/parametria (eg, masses, tenderness, organomegaly, nodularity)

Figure 32-14 ■ 1997 documentation guidelines for multisystem examination. *Source: Centers for Medicare and Medicaid Services, 1997 Documentation Guidelines for Evaluation and Management Services (with formatting adjustments).*

Lymphatic	Palpation of lymph nodes in **two or more** areas: ❏ Neck ❏ Axillae ❏ Groin ❏ Other
Musculoskeletal	❏ Examination of **gait and station** ❏ Inspection and/or palpation of **digits** and **nails** (eg, clubbing, cyanosis, inflammatory conditions, petechiae, ischemia, infections, nodes) Examination of joints, bones and muscles of <u>one or more</u> of the following six areas: ❏ 1) head and neck; ❏ 2) spine, ribs and pelvis; ❏ 3) right upper extremity; ❏ 4) left upper extremity; ❏ 5) right lower extremity; and ❏ 6) left lower extremity. The examination of a given area includes: • Inspection and/or palpation with notation of presence of any **misalignment,** asymmetry, crepitation, defects, tenderness, masses, effusions • Assessment of **range of motion** with notation of any pain, crepitation or contracture • Assessment of **stability** with notation of any dislocation (luxation), subluxation or laxity • Assessment of muscle **strength** and **tone** (eg, flaccid, cog wheel, spastic) with notation of any atrophy or abnormal movements
Skin	❏ **Inspection** of skin and subcutaneous tissue (eg, rashes, lesions, ulcers) ❏ **Palpation** of skin and subcutaneous tissue (eg, induration, subcutaneous nodules, tightening)
Neurologic	❏ Test **cranial nerves** with notation of any deficits ❏ Examination of **deep tendon reflexes** with notation of pathological reflexes (eg, Babinski) ❏ Examination of **sensation** (eg, by touch, pin, vibration, proprioception)
Psychiatric	❏ Description of the patient's **judgment** and **insight** *Brief assessment of mental status including:* ❏ **Orientation** to time, place and person ❏ Recent and remote **memory** ❏ **Mood** and affect (eg, depression, anxiety, agitation, hypomania, lability)

Total # Bullets Performed and Documented →	☐	# of Elements Performed and Documented	Level of Examination
		1–5	Problem focused
		6+	Expanded problem focused
		6 organ systems/body areas @ 2 bullet points each OR: 12 elements in at least 2 organ systems/body areas	Detailed
		ALL	Comprehensive (Perform all elements identified by a bullet in **at least nine** organ systems or body areas and document **at least two elements** identified by a bullet from **each of nine** areas/systems)

Figure 32-14 ■ *(continued)*

requires documentation of at least two elements identified by a bullet from each of nine systems, which they are not.

▶ Jill determines the level of medical decision making. (Refer to Table 28-12, Medical Decision-Making Levels, in Chapter 28 of this text.)

❏ *What is the level of complexity of the number of diagnoses or management options based on the presenting problem?* The level is **moderate** because there is a new presenting problem without a workup by this provider. The workup was done by the referring provider.

❏ *What is the amount and/or complexity of data to be reviewed?* The level is **Straightforward** because diagnostic data were reviewed.

❏ *What is the level of risk of significant complications, morbidity, and/or mortality?* She reviews each column in the Table of Risk in the 1997 DG and determines that the level of risk is **Moderate** because the patient has an acute illness with systemic symptoms and elective major surgery is agreed to. The patient has no identified risk factors. The single highest element in the Table of Risk determines the overall risk. Both of these risk elements are classified as **Moderate.**

GASTROENTEROLOGY ENCOUNTER

HISTORY: Detailed

Chief complaint (CC)

CHIEF COMPLAINT: Nausea and abdominal pain after eating.

HPI: The patient is a 33 year old white female, came to the office. She is referred to me by her internal medicine physician for evaluation for a cholecystectomy. Patient complains of pain after eating fatty food, dark colored urine, subjective chills, subjective low-grade fever, nausea and sharp stabbing pain. Symptoms started about 2 months ago. Symptoms are relieved when lying on right side and with antacids. Prior workup by internist includes abdominal ultrasound positive for cholelithiasis without CBD obstruction. Laboratory studies include elevated total bilirubin and elevated WBC.

HPI: Extended (4+)

Consultation referral

MDM Management: New presenting problem, without workup (Moderate Management Options)

MDM Data: Ordering or reviewing diagnostic data (Straightforward Data)

PAST MEDICAL HISTORY: No significant past medical problems.
PAST SURGICAL HISTORY: Diagnostic laparoscopic exam for pelvic pain/adhesions.
ALLERGIES: No known drug allergies.
CURRENT MEDICATIONS: No current medications.
SOCIAL HISTORY: Marital status: married. Patient states smoking history of 1 pack per day. Patient quit smoking 1 year ago. Admits to no history of using alcohol. States use of no illicit drugs.
FAMILY MEDICAL HISTORY: There is no significant, contributory family medical history.
OB GYN HISTORY: LMP: 4/03/YY. Gravida: 2. Para: 2. Date of last pap smear: 8/25/YY.

PFSH: Complete (3)

REVIEW OF SYSTEMS:
Cardiovascular: Denies angina, MI history, dysrhythmias, palpitations, murmur, pedal edema, orthopnea, TIAs, stroke.
Pulmonary: Denies cough, hemoptysis, wheezing, dyspnea, bronchitis, emphysema, TB exposure or treatment.
Neurological: Denies seizures and ataxia.
Skin: Denies scaling, rashes, blisters, photosensitivity.

ROS: Extended (2–9)

PHYSICAL EXAMINATION:
Appearance: Healthy appearing. Moderately overweight.
HEENT: Normocephalic. EOMs (*extraocular movements*) intact. PERRLA. Oral pharynx without lesions.
Neck: Neck mobile. Trachea is midline.
Lymphatic: No apparent cervical, supraclavicular, axillary or inguinal adenopathy.
Breast: Normal appearing breasts bilaterally, nipples everted. No nipple discharge, skin changes.
Chest: Normal breath sounds heard bilaterally without rales or rhonchi. No pleural rubs. No scars.
Cardiovascular: Regular heart rate and rhythm without murmur or gallop. No signs of edema.
Abdominal: Bowel sounds are high pitched.
Extremities: Lower extremities are normal in color, touch and temperature. No ischemic changes are noted. Range of motion is normal.
Skin: Normal color, temperature, turgor and elasticity; no significant skin lesions.

EXAMINATION: Detailed
(12 elements in at least 2 organ systems/body areas)

IMPRESSION: Abdominal pain due to acute cholecystitis.

DISCUSSION: Reviewed laparoscopic cholecystectomy procedure sheet and answered questions. The patient gave verbal and written consent for the procedure.

MEDICAL DECISION MAKING: Moderate Complexity

MDM Risk: Acute illness with systemic symptoms, Elective major surgery (open, percutaneous or endoscopic) with no identified risk factors (Moderate Risk)

PLAN: We will proceed with laparoscopic cholecystectomy with intraoperative cholangiogram. Report sent to the referring physician with my assessment and recommendation.

MEDICATIONS PRESCRIBED: None.

Consultation report

PROCEDURES SCHEDULED: Laparoscopic cholecystectomy scheduled in 2 weeks on 5/11/YY at outpatient surgery center.

KEY: HPI History of the present illness   ROS Review of systems
PFSH Past, family, and social history   MDM Medical decision making

Figure 32-15 ■ Gastroenterology encounter. *Source:* © PB Resources, Inc. Used with permission.

❏ *Based on these factors, what is the overall level of medical decision making?* The medical decision making is **Moderate complexity**. At least two of the three MDM factors are required to qualify for a specific level of MDM. Two of the three MDM factors meet or exceed moderate decision making.

Now Jill is ready to assign the code for the GI encounter. The exercise that follows guides you through additional abstracting skills and allows you to assign the correct code.

CODING CAUTION

Verify that the physician signature is present in the medical record and is legible. If it is not, the physician must sign an attestation statement, which identifies the author. If the documentation for an encounter is not signed or attested to, Medicare considers the claim to be *insufficiently documented* and can deny or recoup payment.

CODING PRACTICE

Exercise 32.5   E/M Coding for Gastroenterology

Instructions: Refer to the *1997 Documentation Guidelines for Evaluation and Management Services* (available at **www.cms.gov**) or Chapter 28, "Evaluation and Management Services (99201-99499)," Tables 28-7 to 28-12, in this text. Answer the following questions about the figure "Gastroenterology encounter" (Figure 32-15).

1. a. Which elements of the HPI are documented? Circle all that apply. Location, Quality, Severity, Duration, Timing, Context, Modifying factors, Associated signs and symptoms

    b. How many elements are documented? _____

    c. What is the level of HPI? _____

2. a. Which systems are reviewed in the ROS? Circle all that apply. Constitutional, Allergic/immunologic, CV, Endocrine, ENT/M, Eyes, GI, GU, Hemic/lymphatic, MS, Neurologic, Psychiatric, Respiratory, Skin/breast

    b. How many systems are documented? _____

    c. What is the level of ROS? _____

3. a. Which PFSH elements are documented? Circle all that apply. Past medical, Family, Social

    b. What is the level of PFSH? _____

    c. What is the overall level of history? (The lowest history factor—HPI, ROS, or PFSH—determines the level of history.) _____

4. a. Refer to ("1997 documentation guidelines for multisystem examination."). Which bulleted items are documented for the examination? (Check off the items documented.)

    b. How many bulleted items are documented? _____

    c. What is the level of the examination? _____

5. Refer to Table 28-12, Medical Decision-Making Levels, in Chapter 28 of this text or the 1997 DG.

    a. What is the MDM level for the number of diagnoses or management options? _____

    b. What is the MDM level for the amount and/or complexity of data to be reviewed? _____

    c. Refer to the Table of Risk in the 1997 DG. Which elements of risk are documented for each risk factor?

        1. Presenting problem: _____

        2. Diagnostic procedures ordered: _____

        3. Management options selected: _____

    d. What is the level of risk? _____

    e. What is the overall level of MDM? (2 of the 3 MDM factors are needed to determine the overall level.) _____

6. a. What is the setting? _____

    b. What type of service? _____

    c. What is the code range? _____

    d. How many key components are required? _____

    e. What is the level of history? _____

    f. What is the level of examination? _____

    g. What is the level of medical decision making? _____

    h. What is the correct code? _____

    i. Is modifier -57 required? _____ Why or why not? _____

7. Abstract, assign, and arrange (sequence) the diagnosis codes that support the E/M code.

    1 ICD-10-CM Code _____

CHAPTER SUMMARY

In this chapter you learned that:

- Because the digestive, or alimentary, tract consists of and connects several anatomic sites, medical terms frequently contain word roots of multiple sites, which are combined with a procedural suffix.

- The CPT Surgery subsection Digestive System (40490-49999) contains 18 subheadings divided by anatomic site. Anatomic sites are arranged by the order in which they occur in the

alimentary (digestive) tract, beginning with the lips and ending with the anus.

- The Digestive System does not have any subsection guidelines or special instructions, but some subheadings and categories provide definitions and coding information. A special instruction that appears in each endoscopy or laparoscopy category directs that a surgical endoscopy or laparoscopy always includes a diagnostic one.

(*continued*)

(continued from page 639)

- Abstracting Digestive System procedures requires special attention to the detailed anatomy of the digestive system and the order of the digestive organs within the GI tract, starting from either end.

- Coding for tonsillectomy, appendectomy, anastomosis, endoscopy, transplants, and repairs reinforces basic coding skills that you can use throughout the CPT manual.

- The order of codes sometimes determines the modifiers needed. Some modifiers can be assigned at the same time the code is assigned, and some cannot be assigned until the codes are sequenced. Certain modifiers are required even when only one procedure is performed.

- Gastroenterologists use the multisystem examination criteria because the *1997 Documentation Guidelines for Evaluation and Management Services* do not provide guidelines for a single-system gastroenterology examination.

CONCEPT QUIZ

Take a moment to look back at the Digestive System subsection and solidify your skills. Try to answer the questions from memory first, then refer to the discussion in this chapter if you need a little extra help.

Completion

Instructions: Write the term that completes each statement based on the information you learned in this chapter. Choose from the list below. Some choices may be used more than once and some choices may not be used at all.

anastomosis	lap band
antrectomy	lithotripsy
colostomy	Nissen fundoplication
endoscopic sclerotherapy	paracentesis
ERCP	Roux-en-Y
gastric bypass	transthoracic esophagectomy
herniorrhaphy	vagotomy
ileostomy	

1. During a(n) _____, the upper part of the stomach is wrapped around the lower esophageal sphincter (LES).

2. A(n) _____ may be created to relieve a bowel blockage or obstruction in the large intestine.

3. _____ is a surgical puncture of a body cavity to remove excess fluid.

4. A(n) _____ is also called a gastrojejunostomy.

5. A(n) _____ may be performed to repair bulging of internal organs or tissues through a defect in the wall of a body cavity.

6. A(n) _____ may be used to treat Barrett's esophagus.

7. _____ consists of high-frequency sound waves used to break up gallstones.

8. A(n) _____ is the removal of the distal portion of the stomach due to gastric ulcers.

9. A(n) _____ may be performed to reestablish gastrointestinal continuity after excision of portions of one or more organs.

10. An open or laparoscopic _____ may be performed to relieve acid secretion when treating peptic ulcer disease.

Multiple Choice

Instructions: Circle the letter of the best answer to each question based on the information you learned in this chapter.

1. How would you code the following procedure? *A physician performs a screening colonoscopy on a Medicare patient at high risk for colorectal cancer.*
   A. G0104
   B. G0105
   C. 45378
   D. 45330

2. What procedure is an examination of the rectum, sigmoid colon, and part of the descending colon?
   A. Proctosigmoidoscopy
   B. Anoscopy
   C. Sigmoidoscopy
   D. Colonoscopy

3. What is the collective name for the salivary glands, liver, gall bladder, and pancreas?
   A. Accessory organs
   B. Omentum
   C. Hepatic system
   D. Digestive tract

4. What is the special instruction that appears in each endoscopy category?
   A. Surgical endoscopy always includes diagnostic endoscopy.
   B. Refer to CPT coding guidelines, Endoscopy.
   C. Surgical endoscopy codes should not be used with surgical laparoscopy codes.
   D. Surgical endoscopy includes radiologic guidance.

5. How would you code the following procedure? *A physician performs a diagnostic endoscopic retrograde cholangiopancreatography with biopsy.*
   A. 43260
   B. 43261
   C. 43274
   D. 43277

6. What abstracting question should be answered for an endoscopic procedure on the digestive system?
   A. Does the surgeon administer general anesthesia?
   B. How long does the procedure take?
   C. Is the procedure open or closed?
   D. What is the farthest site reached?

7. How are multiple surgical procedures sequenced?
   A. In numerical order
   B. In descending order of complexity and price
   C. In the order listed by the surgeon in the operative report
   D. According to the modifier(s) used

8. What modifier should be used when the duodenum is not examined during an EGD because it is not judged clinically relevant?
   A. -51
   B. -52
   C. -53
   D. -58

9. What action does *pull-through* refer to?
   A. A surgical approach for an open procedure
   B. A type of laparoscopic procedure
   C. An anastomosis technique
   D. An ostomy technique

10. How would you code the following procedure? *A physician performs ligation of internal hemorrhoids and a colonoscopy at the same operative session.*
    A. 45378, 46221-51
    B. 45378-51, 46221
    C. 45378-51, 46221-58
    D. 45378-22, 46221-59

KEEP ON CODING

Instructions: Read the procedural statement, then use the appropriate Index and Tabular List to assign CPT procedure codes. Write the code(s) on the line provided.

1. Percutaneous endoscopic colostomy. CPT Code(s) _____

2. Transnasal biopsy of esophagus. CPT Code(s) _____

3. Transoral esophagogastroduodenoscopy with cold forceps biopsy. CPT Code(s) _____

4. Hemiglossectomy. CPT Code(s) _____

5. Laparoscopic appendectomy converted to open due to extensive intestinal adhesions, which were lysed to provide access to the appendix. Enterolysis increased the time for the procedure by 50%. CPT Code(s) _____

6. Endoscopic retrograde cholangiopancreatography with stent placement. CPT Code(s) _____

7. Orthotopic liver transplantation by a surgical team. CPT Code(s) _____

8. Open drainage of subphrenic abscess. CPT Code(s) _____

9. Left colon resection with colorectal anastomosis; complete mobilization of the splenic flexure. CPT Code(s) _____

10. Laparoscopic cholecystectomy with needle biopsy of liver. CPT Code(s) _____

11. Repair of nasolabial fistula. CPT Code(s) _____

12. Small-bowel resection for congenital atresia, approximately 1.5 feet; jejunostomy; placement of durable abdominal negative pressure wound dressing, wound surface area 20 sq cm. CPT Code(s) _____

13. Parotid gland needle biopsy. CPT Code(s) _____

14. Incarcerated ventral hernia repair. CPT Code(s) _____

15. Excision of full-thickness lip lesion with local flap reconstruction. CPT Code(s) _____

16. Flexible sigmoidoscopy with removal of foreign body. CPT Code(s) _____

17. Esophagogastroduodenoscopy with esophageal variceal band ligation, with 45 minutes of intraservice time for moderate sedation provided by the surgeon, with an independent observer, patient over 5 years of age. CPT Code(s) _____

18. Pelvic exenteration for colorectal malignancy with proctectomy and colostomy. CPT Code(s) _____

19. Revision of ileostomy. CPT Code(s) _____

20. Endoscopic ultrasound of sigmoid colon. CPT Code(s) _____

21. Gastric lavage. CPT Code(s) _____

22. EGD with dilation of gastric outlet for obstruction and biopsy of esophagus. CPT Code(s) _____

23. Closure of gastrostomy. CPT Code(s) _____

24. Gastrotomy with suture of bleeding gastric ulcer. CPT Code(s) _____

25. Closure of anal fistula with rectal advancement flap. CPT Code(s) _____

CODING CHALLENGE

Instructions: Read the mini-medical-record of each patient's encounter, then abstract, assign, and arrange ICD-10-CM diagnosis codes and CPT procedure codes using the appropriate Index and Tabular List. Write the code(s) on the line provided.

1. OUTPATIENT HOSPITAL   Gender: F   Age: 61

Diagnosis: Recurrent inguinal hernia on the right side

Procedure: Right inguinal herniorrhaphy

1 ICD-10-CM Code _____

1 CPT Code _____

2. OFFICE   Gender: M   Age: 52

Reason for encounter: Lump and tenderness in jaw

Assessment: Abscess, submandibular salivary gland; heavy current tobacco use

Procedure: Incision and drainage of abscess

Tip: Read the instructional note under the code for the salivary gland abscess to identify the second code.

2 ICD-10-CM Codes _____

1 CPT Code _____

3. INPATIENT HOSPITAL   Gender: M   Age: 38

Diagnosis: Fecal incontinence due to nontraumatic anal sphincter tear, which has not improved

Procedure: Sphincteroplasty

Tip: Read the instructional notes under the code for nontraumatic anal sphincter tear to identify the second code.

2 ICD-10-CM Codes _____

1 CPT Code _____

4. INPATIENT HOSPITAL   Gender: F   Age: 52

Reason for encounter: RUQ pain, T 102 degrees, vomiting

Diagnosis: Ultrasound revealed acute cholecystitis with CBD calculus causing obstruction

Procedure: Laparoscopic cholecystectomy

1 ICD-10-CM Code _____

1 CPT Code _____

5. OUTPATIENT HOSPITAL   Gender: M   Age: 47

Reason for encounter: Foreign body–like sensation in his proximal esophagus after a meal

Assessment: Evaluated with lateral C-spine films and soft-tissue films without any evidence of perforation. The patient then was taken to the endoscopy suite.

Procedure: EGD with removal of a foreign body from gastroesophageal junction (piece of fish bone)

1 ICD-10-CM Code _____

1 CPT Code _____

6. OUTPATIENT HOSPITAL   Gender: F   Age: 57

Assessment: Multiple severe external hemorrhoids

Procedure: Removal of external hemorrhoids

1 ICD-10-CM Code _____

1 CPT Code _____

7. OUTPATIENT HOSPITAL   Gender: M   Age: 67

Reason for encounter: Screening colonoscopy

Procedure: Colonoscopy with snare removal of two adenomatous polyps, biopsy of suspicious lesion in transverse colon to rule out malignancy. 60 minutes of moderate sedation intraservice time provided by a CRNA.

Pathology report: Benign polyps, benign lesion

Tip: Refer to the OGCR for sequencing guidelines for the diagnoses codes. In addition to the physician's procedure codes, assign codes for the moderate sedation service provided by the CRNA.

3 ICD-10-CM Codes _____

_____

2 CPT Codes (physician) _____

2 CPT codes (CRNA) _____ × 1,

_____ × 3

8. OUTPATIENT HOSPITAL   Gender: M   Age: 9

Diagnosis: Chronic hypertrophic tonsillitis and adenoiditis, chronic otitis media refractory to antibiotics, left ear

Procedure: Tonsillectomy and adenoidectomy, insertion of myringotomy tube under general anesthesia

2 ICD-10-CM Codes _____

2 CPT Codes _____

9. INPATIENT HOSPITAL   Gender: F   Age: 49

Diagnosis: Ulcerative colitis involving primarily the rectosigmoid, unresponsive to steroids

Procedure: Laparoscopic total abdominal colectomy with end ileostomy; splenorrhaphy to repair accidental puncture of spleen

2 ICD-10-CM Codes _____

2 CPT Codes _____

10. INPATIENT HOSPITAL   Gender: M   Age: 53

Assessment: Admitted to the intensive care unit with complaints of abdominal pain and unstable vital signs

Procedure: Repair of perforated duodenal ulcer, gastrojejunostomy and feeding jejunostomy placement

Postoperative diagnosis: Perforated duodenal ulcer

1 ICD-10-CM Code _____

3 CPT Codes _____

_____

Chapter 33

Endocrine System Procedures (60000-60699)

Chapter Outline

- **Endocrine System Procedure Basics**
- **Coding Guidelines for Endocrine System Procedures**
- **Abstracting Endocrine System Procedures**
- **Assigning Codes for Endocrine System Procedures**
- **Arranging Codes for Endocrine System Procedures**
- **E/M Coding for Endocrinology**

Learning Objectives

After completing this chapter, you should have the skills to:

33.1 Spell and define the key words, medical terms, and abbreviations related to endocrine system procedures. (Remember)

33.2 Summarize the fundamentals of endocrine system procedures. (Apply)

33.3 Adhere to CPT coding guidelines in the Endocrine System subsection. (Apply)

33.4 Examine and abstract procedural information from the medical record for coding Endocrine System subsection procedures. (Analyze)

33.5 Demonstrate how to assign codes for procedures in the Endocrine System subsection. (Apply)

33.6 Utilize guidelines for arranging (sequencing) codes for Endocrine System subsection procedures. (Apply)

33.7 Determine how to code Evaluation and Management services for endocrinology. (Evaluate)

Key Terms and Abbreviations

cervical approach	dorsal approach	secondary thyroidectomy	total thyroidectomy
complete thyroidectomy	neck dissection	subtotal thyroid lobectomy	transabdominal approach
contralateral lobectomy	partial thyroid lobectomy	total thyroid lobectomy	transthoracic approach

In addition to the key terms listed here, students should know the terms defined within tables in this chapter.

INTRODUCTION

Although everyone loves the drama of opening a large package, small packages often contain the most impressive or most powerful items. Such is the case with the endocrine system. Endocrine glands are among the smallest in the body, but they provide the power and balance to keep the body functioning properly because of the hormones they secrete.

ENDOCRINE SYSTEM PROCEDURE BASICS

Endocrinology is a subspecialty of internal medicine that specializes in the endocrine system. Endocrinologists diagnose and manage endocrine conditions. They perform medical procedures such as glucose monitoring studies and order laboratory tests to analyze endocrine system function, but they do not perform surgery. Otolaryngologists perform surgery on some endocrine glands, such as the thyroid. General surgeons also perform surgery on the endocrine system.

Medical terms for endocrine system procedures consist of the name of the gland and the suffix that identifies the procedure, which is usually an excision. Word parts describing direction, together with the word part for an anatomic site, identify the approach used to access the operative site. Refer to ■ TABLE 33-1 for a refresher on how to build medical terms related to the Endocrine System. Chapter 9 of this text provides information on endocrine system anatomy and conditions.

CODING CAUTION

Be alert for medical terms that are used with more than one body system.

- A **lobectomy** (*surgical removal of a lobe*) can be performed on the thyroid gland, the liver, the brain, or the lungs.
- An **isthmus** (*a narrow connection between two larger organs or sites*) exists in the thyroid, the eustachian tube, the uterus, the pharynx, the brain, and the aorta.

Procedures on the Endocrine System

■ TABLE 33-2 summarizes procedures of the endocrine system. In particular, coders must be familiar with the terminology related to a thyroidectomy, the most commonly performed procedure on the endocrine system.

Excision procedures on the parathyroid glands are sensitive to perform. These glands are small, surgeons must work in a restricted space, and the thyroid gland is adjacent to the trachea (■ FIGURE 33-1) and the superior and recurrent laryngeal nerves. Surgeons must take great care not to damage any of these sites.

A thyroidectomy is excision of all or part of the thyroid gland, usually performed due to carcinoma, hyperthyroidism (*overactive thyroid*), Graves' disease (*most common type of hyperthyroidism*), nodules, or goiter (*enlarged thyroid*). The amount of the thyroid gland excised depends upon the extent of the patient's disease or condition. After surgery, many patients must take synthetic hormones to replace the hormones that the thyroid produces.

Table 33-2 ■ **COMMON PROCEDURES OF THE ENDOCRINE SYSTEM**

Procedure Name	Definition	Reason Performed
Adrenalectomy	Surgical removal of all or most of an adrenal gland(s). (Open or laparoscopic approach)	Cushing's syndrome, tumor, malignancy
Lobectomy	Surgical removal of all or part of one lobe of the thyroid gland. (Open approach)	Thyroid nodules
Parathyroid autotransplantation	Surgical removal of the four parathyroid glands and their transplantation into a muscle in the neck or forearm. (Open approach)	Secondary parathyroidism, parathyroid hyperplasia, parathyroid reoperation
Parathyroidectomy	Surgical removal of all or part of the parathyroid glands. (Open approach)	Hyperparathyroidism (*parathyroid glands produce too much parathyroid hormone [PTH]*)
Thymectomy	Surgical removal of all/most of the thymus gland. (Open approach)	Myasthenia gravis
Thyroidectomy	Surgical removal of all/most of the thyroid gland. (Open approach)	Hyperthyroidism, malignancy, tumor, goiter
Thyroidectomy, substernal	Surgical removal of an enlarged thyroid that has grown behind the sternum. (Open approach)	Hyperthyroidism, goiter
Thyrotomy	Cutting into the thyroglossal duct. (Open approach)	Abscess, cyst

Source: © PB Resources, Inc. Used with permission.

Table 33-1 ■ **EXAMPLE OF CONSTRUCTING MEDICAL TERMS FOR ENDOCRINE SYSTEM PROCEDURES**

Combining Form	Prefix/Suffix	Complete Medical Term
thyr/o (*thyroid*)	**trans-** (prefix; *across*)	**thyroid + ectomy** (*excision of the thyroid*)
gloss/o (*tongue*)		**thyro + gloss + al** (*pertaining to the thyroid and the tongue*)
cervic/o (*neck*)	**-ectomy** (suffix; *excision*)	**trans + abdomin + al** (*pertaining to across the abdomen*)
abdomin/o (*abdomen*)	**-al** (suffix; *pertaining to*)	**trans + cervic + al** (*pertaining to across the neck*)

Source: © PB Resources, Inc. Used with permission.

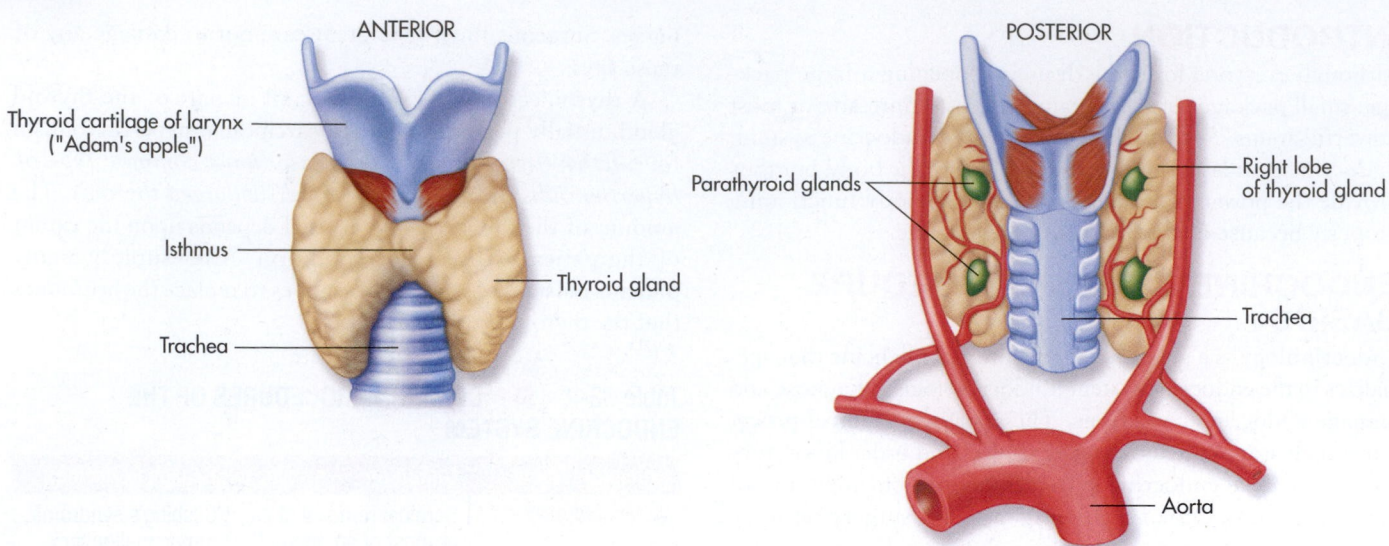

Figure 33-1 ■ Thyroid and parathyroid glands.

Excision of the thyroid is described based on the extent of the thyroid removed. Types of thyroid removal include:

- A **partial thyroid lobectomy** is excision of less than two-thirds of one lobe of the thyroid gland.

- A **subtotal thyroid lobectomy** is excision of more than two-thirds of one lobe but less than the entire lobe.

- A **total thyroid lobectomy** is the excision of one entire lobe of the thyroid gland.

- A **contralateral lobectomy** is excision of part of the opposite or second lobe in addition to a partial, subtotal, or total lobectomy of the first lobe.

- A **total** or **complete thyroidectomy** is excision of both lobes of the thyroid gland in their entirety.

- A **secondary thyroidectomy** is a second operation to excise remaining thyroid tissue following a previous thyroidectomy; it is also called a completion thyroidectomy.

A thyroidectomy can be performed with limited, modified, or radical **neck dissection**, which involves excising lymph nodes and surrounding tissue from the neck. The physician also examines the larynx and additional tissue during a neck dissection. Types of neck dissections are based on the extent of lymph node removal:

- Radical neck dissection (RND)—Excision of lymphatic tissue in the first five regions of lymph nodes of the neck, including the internal jugular vein (IJV), spinal accessory nerve (SAN), and sternocleidomastoid muscle (SCM)

- Modified radical neck dissection (MRND)—Excision of tissue in the first five regions of lymph nodes of the neck with preservation of the IJV, SAN, and SCM

- Selective neck dissection—Excision of three regions of cervical lymph nodes

- Limited neck dissection—Excision of one or two regions of cervical lymph nodes

CODING PRACTICE

Exercise 33.1   **Endocrine System Overview**

Instructions: Use your medical terminology skills and resources to define the following procedures, then identify the applicable code or code range. Follow these steps:

- Use slash marks "/" to break down the underlined term into its root(s) and suffix.
- Define the meaning of the underlined word based on the meaning of each word part.
- Use the entire phrase to identify the code or code range shown in the CPT Index.

Example: <u>thyroidectomy</u>, secondary thyroid/ectomy   Meaning <u>*excision of the thyroid gland*</u>   CPT Code <u>60260</u>

1. <u>parathyroidectomy</u>   Meaning _____   CPT Code _____

2. <u>thymectomy</u>, partial   Meaning _____   CPT Code _____

3. <u>adrenalectomy</u>, complete   Meaning _____   CPT Code _____

4. parathyroid gland <u>autotransplantation</u>   Meaning _____   CPT Code _____

5. <u>thyroglossal</u> duct cyst excision   Meaning _____   CPT Code _____

CODING GUIDELINES FOR ENDOCRINE SYSTEM PROCEDURES

Coders should understand the organization, guidelines, and instructional notes in the Tabular List of this CPT subsection. This information is necessary for accurate coding. The CPT subsection **Endocrine System (60000-60699)** contains two subheadings that are divided by anatomic site (■ TABLE 33-3). Review the subheadings, categories, and code ranges listed at the beginning of the Endocrine System subsection in the CPT manual to become familiar with the content and organization. This subsection has approximately 30 codes.

The Endocrine System subsection includes invasive and minimally invasive surgical procedures on four of the nine endocrine glands: the thyroid, parathyroid, thymus, and adrenal glands. Procedures for removal of a tumor from the carotid body (*a small cluster of chemoreceptor cells near the bifurcation [splitting in two] of the carotid artery in the neck*) also appear in this subsection. The carotid body is considered an endocrine gland because it secretes erythropoiesis hormones. Although the pancreas appears in the second subheading title, no procedures on the pancreas appear in the Tabular List. Several endocrine glands also function as part of other organ systems. Procedures on five endocrine glands appear in other Surgery subsections, as follows:

- Ovaries—Female Genital System (58600-58960)
- Pancreas—Digestive System (48000-48999)
- Pineal gland—Nervous System (61105-61576)
- Pituitary gland—Nervous System (61546-61548)
- Testes—Male Genital System (54500-56499)

Codes for diagnostic tests on the endocrine system appear in the Medicine section. Many endocrine conditions are managed medically, so patients may have codes only for Evaluation and Management (E/M) encounters. CPT codes in the Endocrine System subsection are frequently supported by diagnosis codes from ICD-10-CM Chapter 4, "Endocrine, Nutritional, and Metabolic Diseases (E00-E89)," as well as neoplasms, symptoms and signs, and injuries (■ TABLE 33-4). These codes are most commonly assigned to support procedures on the endocrine system; however, diagnosis codes from any ICD-10-CM chapter are permissible.

CPT guidelines for the Surgery section apply to the Endocrine System subsection. This subsection has no additional guidelines or special instructions. Instructional notes in the Tabular List redirect coders when different or additional codes are required. One add-on code, for parathyroid autotransplantation, appears in this section. An instructional note identifies the standalone codes it can be reported with. Specific guidelines and instructional notes are discussed throughout this chapter of the text.

Table 33-3 ■ ENDOCRINE SYSTEM SUBHEADINGS

Subheading	Code Range
Thyroid Gland	60000-60300
Parathyroid, Thymus, Adrenal Glands, Pancreas, and Carotid Body	60500-60699

Table 33-4 ■ LOCATING ICD-10-CM AND CPT CODES FOR THE ENDOCRINE SYSTEM

Type of Code	Codes
ICD-10-CM Endocrine System–Related Codes	
Endocrine system conditions	E00-E89
Neoplasms	C73-75, C78.89, D09.3, D35, D44
Symptoms and signs	R62, R94.7
Screening	Z13.2
CPT Endocrine System–Related Codes	
Medicine procedures	95249-95251
Radiologic procedures	
• Diagnostic ultrasound	76536
• Nuclear medicine	78012-78099
Laboratory tests	
• Organ/disease panels	80047-80050
• Chemistry	80400-80439, 81506, 84431-84445

Source: © PB Resources, Inc. Used with permission.

ABSTRACTING ENDOCRINE SYSTEM PROCEDURES

Surgical approach always identifies the technique used, such as open, endoscopic, or external. The anatomic approach identifies the site of the incision and the direction from which the surgical site is accessed. Certain thyroidectomy and thymectomy procedures can be performed through an incision in the neck, which is a **cervical approach**, or through an incision in the chest, which is a **transthoracic approach**. An adrenalectomy can be performed through an incision in the abdomen, which is a **transabdominal approach**; the lower back, which is a lumbar approach; or the midback, which is a **dorsal approach**.

Refer to ■ TABLE 33-5 for guidance on how to abstract procedures on the Endocrine System, then work through the detailed example that follows. Remember that the abstracting questions are a guide and that not every question applies to, or can be answered for, every case. For example, some, but not all, codes are divided based on whether the purpose of an excision is to remove a malignancy.

Table 33-5 ■ KEY CRITERIA FOR ABSTRACTING ENDOCRINE SYSTEM PROCEDURES

- ❏ What endocrine gland is treated?
- ❏ What is the surgical approach (e.g., open, endoscopic)?
- ❏ What is the anatomic approach (e.g., cervical, thoracic)?
- ❏ Is the procedure partial, subtotal, or total/complete?
- ❏ Is the procedure done to remove a malignancy?
- ❏ Were any adjacent tumors removed?
- ❏ What is the extent of lymph node excision, if any?

Source: © PB Resources, Inc. Used with permission.

Guided Example of Abstracting Endocrine System Procedures

Refer to the following example throughout this chapter to practice skills for abstracting, assigning, and arranging Endocrine System codes.

> INPATIENT HOSPITAL   Gender: F   Age: 35
>
> Preoperative diagnosis: Suspected carcinoma per result of fine-needle aspiration (FNA) done last week
>
> Procedure: Thyroidectomy with radical neck dissection. With the patient in the supine position, a horizontal 10-cm incision was made just below the larynx. The skin flaps were separated and the muscle and fascia were divided, exposing the thyroid gland. Being diligent to protect the recurrent laryngeal nerve from trauma, all of both thyroid lobes and the first five regions of bilateral cervical lymph nodes and the internal jugular vein (IJV), spinal accessory nerve (SAN), and sternocleidomastoid muscle (SCM). Hemostasis was achieved, the operative wound was closed, and the patient was transferred to postoperative care in stable condition. Tissue was submitted to pathology.
>
> Postoperative diagnosis: Differentiated thyroid cancer (DTC) with lymph node metastases
>
> Pathology report: Papillary thyroid cancer, metastatic cancer in lymph nodes (confirmed as clinically significant by surgeon)

Follow along as fictitious coder, Tamara Brownlee, CCS-P, abstracts the procedure. Check off each step after you complete it.

▶ Tamara reads through the entire record, paying special attention to the reason for the encounter, the procedure performed, and the postoperative diagnosis. She refers to the Key Criteria for Abstracting Endocrine System Procedures (Table 33-5).

❏ She notes the preoperative diagnosis. She does not code the FNA because it was performed last week and coded at that time.

❏ *Which gland is treated?* Thyroid

❏ *What is the surgical approach?* Open, as indicated by the excision

❏ *What is the anatomic approach?* Cervical

❏ *Is the procedure partial, subtotal, or total/complete?* Total because all of both thyroid lobes was removed

❏ *Is the procedure done to remove a malignancy?* Yes, suspected carcinoma, confirmed by pathology

❏ *Were any adjacent tumors removed?* No

❏ *What was the extent of lymph node excision, if any?* Radical; first five regions of cervical lymph nodes

▶ Tamara also reviews the general criteria for abstracting procedures(Table 25-6).

❏ *Is the name of the procedure consistent with the documented details?* Yes, a total thyroidectomy involves excision of all, or nearly all, of the thyroid. An RND involves excision of cervical lymph nodes I–V and the internal jugular vein (IJV), spinal accessory nerve (SAN), and sternocleidomastoid muscle (SCM).

❏ *What is the final diagnosis?* differentiated thyroid cancer (DTC) with lymph node metastases

▶ At this time, Tamara does not know how many codes she will end up with. She will learn about this when she moves on to assigning codes.

CODING PRACTICE

Exercise 33.2   Abstracting Endocrine System Procedures

Instructions: Read the mini-medical-record of each patient's encounter and answer the abstracting questions. Write the answer on the line provided. Do not assign any codes.

> 1. OUTPATIENT HOSPITAL   Gender: F   Age: 4
>
> Preprocedure diagnosis: Abscess, thyroglossal duct
>
> Procedure: I&D, cyst in the thyroglossal duct. Punctured the cyst with a needle, drained exudate, and applied a sterile dressing.
>
> Postprocedure diagnosis: Infected thyroglossal duct cyst
>
> *(continued)*

1. (continued)

a. What endocrine gland is treated? _____

b. What is the surgical approach? _____

c. What is the anatomic approach? _____

d. What procedure is performed? _____

e. Is the procedure done to remove a malignancy?

_____

f. Were any adjacent tumors removed?

_____

g. What was the extent of lymph node excision, if any?

_____

CODING PRACTICE (continued)

2. INPATIENT HOSPITAL   Gender: F   Age: 45

Preoperative diagnosis: Myasthenia gravis, thymoma

Procedure: Transthoracic thymectomy. Made a length-wise incision in the chest slightly left of the midline. Explored the chest and excised the entire thymus gland. No adjacent structures were disturbed. Inspected the surgical field to ensure no residual thymic tissue. Closed surgical wound and transferred patient to the postoperative area in stable condition.

Postoperative diagnosis: Thymoma, benign

a. What endocrine gland is treated? _____

b. What is the surgical approach? _____

c. What is the anatomic approach? _____

d. What procedure is performed? _____

e. Is the procedure done to remove a malignancy?

_____

f. Were any adjacent tumors removed? _____

g. What was the extent of lymph node excision, if any?

_____

3. OUTPATIENT HOSPITAL   Gender: M   Age: 35

Preoperative diagnosis: Adrenal adenoma, Cushing syndrome

Procedure: Laparoscopic adrenalectomy, right adrenal gland

Postoperative diagnosis: Benign adrenal tumor

a. What endocrine gland is treated? _____

b. What is the surgical approach? _____

c. What procedure is performed? _____

d. On which side of the body is the procedure performed? _____

e. Is the procedure done to remove a malignancy?

_____

f. Were any adjacent tumors removed? _____

_____

g. What was the extent of lymph node excision, if any?

_____

4. INPATIENT HOSPITAL   Gender: F   Age: 38

Preoperative diagnosis: Hyperthyroidism

Procedure: Excision of both lobes of the thyroid gland through an incision in the neck

(continued)

4. (continued)

Postoperative diagnosis: Thyroid tissue negative for malignancy

a. What endocrine gland is treated? _____

b. What is the surgical approach? _____

c. What is the anatomic approach? _____

d. What procedure is performed? _____

e. Is the procedure done to remove a malignancy?

_____

f. Were any adjacent tumors removed? _____

g. What was the extent of lymph node excision, if any?

_____

5. INPATIENT HOSPITAL   Gender: F   Age: 47

Diagnosis: Four-gland hyperparathyroidism

Procedure: Transthoracic parathyroidectomy with mediastinal exploration and parathyroid autotransplantation, left forearm

a. What endocrine gland is treated? _____

b. What is the surgical approach? _____

c. What is the anatomic approach? _____

d. What is the primary procedure? _____

e. What is the secondary procedure? _____

f. Is the procedure done to remove a malignancy?

_____

g. Were any adjacent tumors removed? _____

h. What was the extent of lymph node excision, if any?

_____

i. What is the site of autotransplantation? _____

6. OUTPATIENT HOSPITAL   Gender: F   Age: 42

Diagnosis: Recurrent nodular goiter

Procedure: Secondary thyroidectomy, cervical, bilateral

a. What endocrine gland is treated? _____

b. What is the surgical approach? _____

c. What is the anatomic approach? _____

d. What procedure is performed? _____

e. What is the laterality? _____

f. Is the procedure done to remove a malignancy?

_____

g. Were any adjacent tumors removed? _____

h. What was the extent of lymph node excision, if any?

_____

ASSIGNING CODES FOR ENDOCRINE SYSTEM PROCEDURES

To locate codes for Endocrine System procedures in the Index, search for the Main Term that identifies the gland, such as **Thyroid Gland, Adrenal Gland, Parathyroid Gland,** or **Thymus Gland,** then locate the appropriate first-level modifying term and second-level modifying term that describe the procedure. Alternatively, search for the Main Term that identifies the procedure, such as **Thyroidectomy, Lobectomy, Adrenalectomy,** or **Thymectomy,** and the appropriate modifying terms.

When verifying codes in the Tabular List, be alert for indented codes and the parent codes they are paired with. Although there are only 30 codes in this subsection, you must still navigate the Tabular List carefully to identify variations described by indented codes. Codes for thyroid lobectomy procedures are divided based on whether tissue is removed from one or both lobes and whether the excision of one lobe is partial, subtotal, or complete (■ FIGURE 33-2). When all tissue is removed from both lobes, assign a code for a total thyroidectomy (**60240-60274**).

Adrenalectomy codes are divided based on whether the procedure is open (**60540, 60545**) or laparoscopic (**60550**). A surgical laparoscopy includes a diagnostic laparoscopy, when performed. One code encompasses several variations of an adrenalectomy procedure:

- Partial or complete
- Exploratory with or without biopsy
- Transabdominal, lumbar, or dorsal approach

Open adrenalectomy has an indented code for use when a retroperitoneal tumor is excised at the same time as the adjacent adrenal gland (**60545**).

Guided Example of Assigning Endocrine System Procedure Codes

To practice skills for assigning codes for the Endocrine System, continue with the example from earlier in the chapter about a patient who was seen for a thyroidectomy. Follow along in your CPT manual as Tamara Brownlee, CCS-P, assigns codes. Check off each step after you complete it.

▶ First, Tamara confirms the procedure, thyroidectomy with radical neck dissection.

▶ Tamara searches the Index for the Main Term **Thyroidectomy**.

❑ She locates the first-level modifying term **Total**.

❑ She locates the second-level modifying term **for Malignancy** and the indented term **Radical Neck Dissection**.

❑ She identifies the code **60254**.

▶ Tamara verifies code **60254** in the Tabular List.

❑ She reads the code title for **60254 with radical neck dissection** and recognizes this as an indented code because the description is indented two spaces and begins with a lowercase letter.

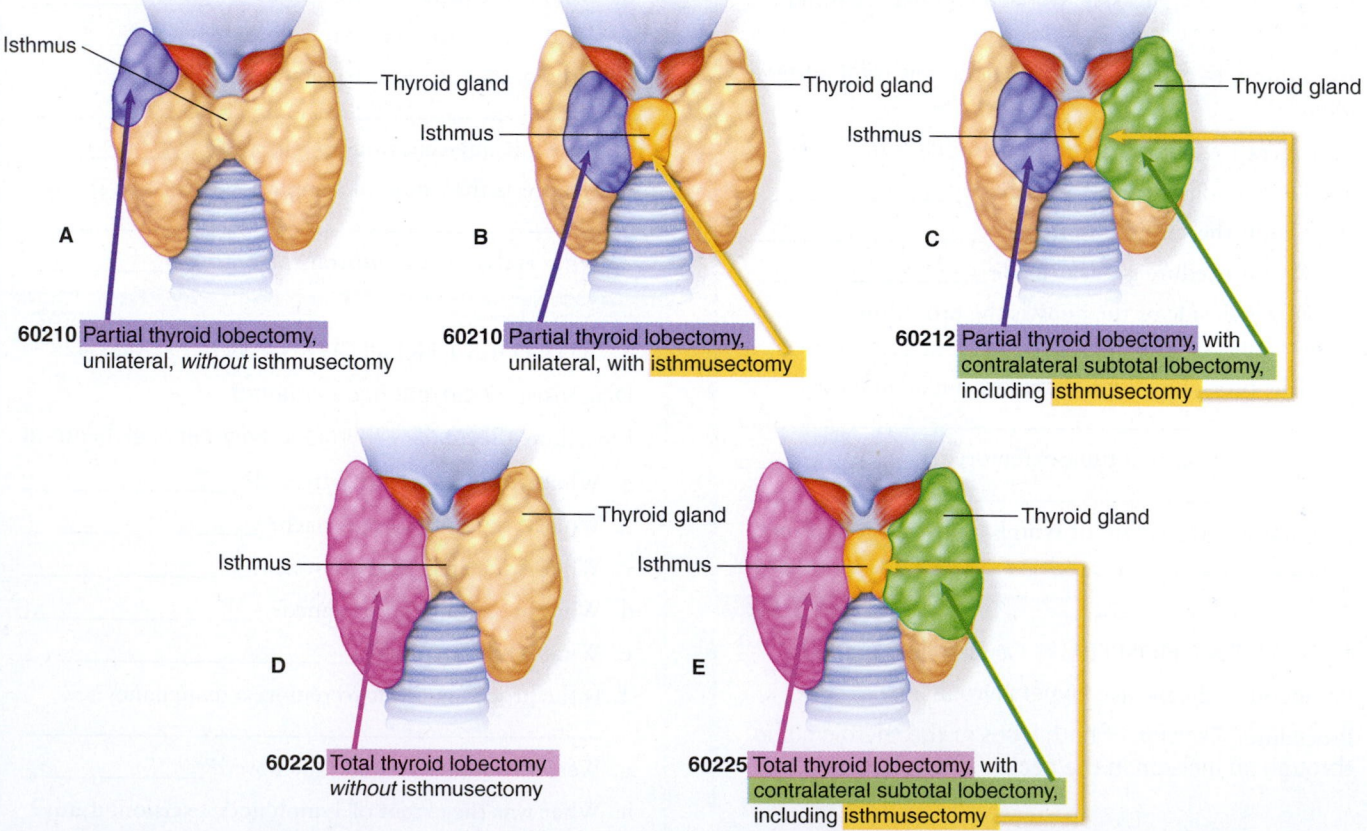

Figure 33-2 ■ Coding thyroid lobectomy procedures. *Source: Annotations © PB Resources, Inc. CPT codes only © American Medical Association.*

❏ She identifies that the preceding code, **60252**, is a parent code because the description is left justified, begins with a capital letter, and contains a semicolon. The parent code description reads **Thyroidectomy, total or subtotal for malignancy; with limited neck dissection**. The portion of the description before the semicolon is the common descriptor that applies to the indented code. The only difference between the parent code and the indented code is that the parent code describes a *limited* neck dissection and the indented code describes a *radical* neck dissection.

❏ She confirms that the medical record describes a radical neck dissection and concludes that **60254** accurately describes the procedure.

❏ She combines the common descriptor from the parent code with the descriptor from the indented code to arrive at the full description for code **60254 Thyroidectomy, total or subtotal for malignancy; with radical neck dissection**.

▶ Tamara checks for instructions in the Tabular List.

❏ She looks for instructional notes immediately before and after the code family **60252-60254** and finds none.

❏ She cross-references the beginning of the subcategory **Excision** and the category **Excision** and verifies that there are no special instructions.

❏ She cross-references the beginning of the subheading **Endocrine** and verifies that there are no special instructions.

❏ She cross-references the beginning of the **Surgery** section and reviews the guidelines. She determines that there are no further instructions or guidelines to direct the coding of this case.

▶ Tamara double-checks the medical record to determine whether there are any other procedures that she should code. Because the lymphadenectomy is included in the code for the thyroidectomy, she does not need to assign a separate code.

▶ Next, Tamara must determine whether she needs a modifier.

CODING PRACTICE

Exercise 33.3 Assigning Codes for Endocrine System Procedures

Instructions: Read the mini-medical-record of each patient's encounter. Review the information abstracted in Exercise 33.2. Assign CPT codes and modifiers using the Index and Tabular List. Write the code(s) on the line provided.

---

1. OUTPATIENT HOSPITAL   Gender: F   Age: 4

Preprocedure diagnosis: Abscess, thyroglossal duct

Procedure: I&D, cyst in the thyroglossal duct. Punctured the cyst with a needle, drained exudate, and applied a sterile dressing.

Postprocedure diagnosis: Infected thyroglossal duct cyst

Tip: You need to distinguish between I&D and excision of a cyst.

1 CPT Code _____

---

2. INPATIENT HOSPITAL   Gender: F   Age: 45

Preoperative diagnosis: Myasthenia gravis, thymoma

Procedure: Transthoracic thymectomy. Made a length-wise incision in the chest slightly left of the midline. Explored the chest and excised the entire thymus gland. No adjacent structures were disturbed. Inspected the surgical field to ensure no residual thymic tissue. Closed surgical wound and transferred patient to the postoperative area in stable condition.

Postoperative diagnosis: Thymoma, benign

1 CPT Code _____

---

3. OUTPATIENT HOSPITAL   Gender: M   Age: 35

Preoperative diagnosis: Adrenal adenoma, Cushing's syndrome

Procedure: Laparoscopic adrenalectomy, right adrenal gland

Postoperative diagnosis: Benign adrenal tumor

Tip: Assign a modifier for laterality.

1 CPT Code _____

ARRANGING CODES FOR ENDOCRINE SYSTEM PROCEDURES

The endocrine section has several specific situations in which coders must use multiple codes and/or modifiers. These include bilateral procedures, separate procedures, modified radical neck dissection, and imaging guidance.

Bilateral Procedures

Although the thyroid gland contains two lobes, it is a single organ and is not coded as bilateral. Code excision of the lobes as follows:

- When a single lobe is excised, assign a code for a lobectomy.
- When both lobes are excised at the same time, assign a code for thyroidectomy.
- When one lobe is removed and the next day the other lobe is removed, assign a code for a lobectomy for the first procedure and a code for secondary thyroidectomy for the second procedure. Assign modifier **-50 Bilateral procedure** to the secondary thyroidectomy when tissue is removed from both sides.

Lymph nodes are bilateral because they occur in paired chains on either side of the body. Cervical lymph nodes occur on both sides of the neck. When a thyroidectomy includes bilateral neck dissection with excision of lymph nodes, assign modifier **-50 Bilateral procedure**. Per the National Correct Coding Initiative (NCCI), Medicare does not pay additional for a bilateral lymphadenectomy performed with a thyroidectomy. However, the *CPT Assistant* newsletter, published by the American Medical Association, directs coders to apply the bilateral modifier (November 2000, volume 10, issue 11). Therefore, for private payers, use modifier **-50** for thyroidectomy with bilateral neck dissection and lymph node removal. Payment policies vary by payer.

The adrenal glands are bilateral organs because one adrenal gland exists suprarenally (*at the top of the kidneys*) on each side of the body. An instructional note in the Tabular List following code **60545** directs **For bilateral procedure, report 60540 with modifier 50**.

-59 Distinct Procedural Service

The Endocrine System subheading contains four codes with the designation **(separate procedure)** as part of the code description: **60520, 60521, 60522** (thymectomy) and **60540** (adrenalectomy). An adrenalectomy is often performed as part of a nephrectomy and is bundled into the nephrectomy code. When the adrenal gland(s) is removed as an independent procedure, assign code **60540**.

A thymectomy is a separate procedure when performed with most thyroidectomy procedures because the two procedures require separate incisions. Append modifier **-59 Distinct procedural service** when a thymectomy is performed with a thyroidectomy (■ FIGURE 33-3) to indicate that it is separate from the thyroidectomy. The exception is when a transthoracic thyroidectomy (**60270**) is performed; then, the thymectomy (**60520-60522**) can be performed through the same incision. Because the thymus gland is located in the upper portion of the thorax, it can be accessed through

Surgeon performs a total thyroidectomy and a transcervical thymectomy through a separate incision in the lower neck.

60240 Thyroidectomy, total
60520-59 Thymectomy, partial or total; transcervical approach (separate procedure); -59 separate procedure

Figure 33-3 ■ Example of coding a thyroidectomy with a thymectomy. *Source:* © PB Resources, Inc. Used with permission. CPT codes only © American Medical Association.

same incision as a transthoracic thyroidectomy, so the procedures are bundled.

Append one of the extended modifiers **-X{EPSU}** instead of **-59** when applicable. These modifiers are discussed in greater detail in Chapter 27, "CPT Modifiers," Chapter 29, "Medicine Procedures," and Chapter 32, "Digestive System Procedures," of this text.

Modified Radical Neck Dissection

CPT provides combination codes for a thyroidectomy with a limited or radical neck dissection. When a modified neck dissection is performed, report two codes: one for the thyroidectomy and one for a modified radical neck dissection (■ FIGURE 33-4). The modified radical neck dissection is worth 41.83 RVUs, compared with 26.48 RVUs for the thyroidectomy, so the lymph node dissection is sequenced first. Append modifier **-50** to the bilateral lymphadenectomy. Append modifier **-51** to the thyroidectomy. Although the thyroidectomy is the main reason surgery is performed, it is not sequenced by physicians as the primary procedure because the code with the highest RVU is sequenced first.

Both modifiers **-50** and **-51** can impact payment. Payers might allow up to a 50% increase in payment for bilateral procedures. At the same time, they might reduce payment for a secondary procedure by as much as 50% (■ TABLE 33-6).

Surgeon performs a total thyroidectomy with a bilateral modified radical neck dissection.

38724-50 Cervical lymphadenectomy (modified radical neck dissection); -50 bilateral procedure
60240-51 Thyroidectomy, total; -51 multiple procedures

Figure 33-4 ■ Example of coding a thyroidectomy with modified radical neck dissection. *Source:* © PB Resources, Inc. Used with permission. CPT codes only © American Medical Association.

Table 33-6 ■ **IMPACT OF CODE SEQUENCING AND MODIFIERS ON REIMBURSEMENT**

CPT Code	Fee Schedule	Modifier Adjustment	Allowed Amount
38724-50	$1,501.22	150%	$2,251.83
60240-51	$950.33	50%	$475.16
Total	**$2,451.55**		**$2,727.00**

Source: © PB Resources, Inc. Used with permission. CPT codes only © American Medical Association.

Imaging Guidance

When imaging guidance is performed to assist with a percutaneous core needle biopsy, assign an additional code from the Radiology section. An instructional note following code **60100** identifies the appropriate Radiology codes (**76942, 77002, 77012, 77021**) based on the type of imaging required (■ FIGURE 33-5).

Guided Example of Arranging Endocrine System Procedure Codes

Continue with the example from earlier in the chapter about the patient who was seen for a thyroidectomy. Although no sequencing is required because only one code is needed, modifiers must be reviewed. Follow along in your CPT manual as Tamara Brownlee, CCS-P, finalizes the coding. Check off each step after you complete it.

Surgeon performs a percutaneous core needle biopsy of the thyroid with fluoroscopic guidance.

60100 Biopsy thyroid, percutaneous core needle
77002 Fluoroscopic guidance for needle placement (eg, biopsy, aspiration, injection, localization device)

Figure 33-5 ■ Example of coding thyroid biopsy with fluoroscopic guidance. *Source:* © PB Resources, Inc. Used with permission. CPT codes only © American Medical Association.

▶ First, Tamara confirms the procedure **60254 Thyroidectomy, total or subtotal for malignancy; with radical neck dissection**.

- ❏ She confirms that no additional procedure codes are needed.
- ❏ She reviews the procedure to determine the need for modifiers.
- ❏ She identifies that the thyroidectomy procedure does not require a bilateral modifier.
- ❏ She confirms that the radical neck dissection was performed on both sides and assigns modifier -50 **Bilateral procedure**.

▶ Tamara finalizes the procedure code and modifier for this case:

(1) **60254-50 Thyroidectomy, total or subtotal for malignancy; with radical neck dissection; -50 Bilateral procedure**

▶ Tamara also assigns and sequences the ICD-10-CM diagnosis codes that support the need for the procedure.

(1) **C73 Malignant neoplasm of thyroid gland**
(2) **C77.0 Secondary and unspecified malignant neoplasm of lymph nodes of head, face and neck**

CODING PRACTICE

Exercise 33.4 Arranging Codes for Endocrine System Procedures

Instructions: Read the mini-medical-record of each patient's encounter. Review the information abstracted in Exercise 33.2. Assign CPT codes and modifiers using the Index and Tabular List, and arrange the codes in the proper sequence. Write the code(s) on the line provided.

---

1. INPATIENT HOSPITAL Gender: F Age: 38

Preoperative diagnosis: Hyperthyroidism

Procedure: Excision of both lobes of the thyroid gland through an incision in the neck

Postoperative diagnosis: Thyroid tissue negative for malignancy

1 CPT Code _____

---

2. INPATIENT HOSPITAL Gender: F Age: 47

Diagnosis: Four-gland hyperparathyroidism

Procedure: Transthoracic parathyroidectomy with mediastinal exploration and parathyroid autotransplantation, left forearm

2 CPT Codes _____

---

3. OUTPATIENT HOSPITAL Gender: F Age: 42

Diagnosis: Recurrent nodular goiter

Procedure: Secondary thyroidectomy, cervical, bilateral

Tip: Read the instructional note following this code in the Tabular List.

1 CPT Code _____

E/M CODING FOR ENDOCRINOLOGY

Neither the *1995* nor *1997 Documentation Guidelines for Evaluation and Management Services* (DG) provide a single organ system examination for the endocrine system. Endocrinologists use a multisystem E/M physical examination (■ FIGURE 33-6, page 654). Documentation guidelines for the history and medical decision making are the same for the 1995 DG and the 1997 DG. The requirements of the physical examination vary. Physicians and their coders can use either the 1995 DG or 1997 DG for any encounter. They can assign an E/M code based on whichever set of criteria is most beneficial, but they cannot be combined or intermixed for the same encounter. They do not need to use

Body Areas (BA)	Organ Systems (OS)
❑ Head, including the face ❑ Neck ❑ Chest, including breasts and axillae ❑ Abdomen ❑ Genitalia, groin, buttocks ❑ Back, including spine Each extremity: ❑ Right arm ❑ Left arm ❑ Right leg ❑ Left leg	❑ Constitutional (e.g., vital signs, general appearance) ❑ Eyes ❑ Ears, nose, mouth, and throat ❑ Cardiovascular ❑ Respiratory ❑ Gastrointestinal ❑ Genitourinary ❑ Musculoskeletal ❑ Skin ❑ Neurologic ❑ Psychiatric ❑ Hematologic/lymphatic/immunologic
(A) Total number of body areas:	(B) Total number of organ systems:

(A) + (B)	(C)	# of ❑ Elements Performed and Documented	Level of Examination
Total # body areas + organ systems →	▢	1 body area or organ system (C)	Problem focused
		2–4 body areas and/or organ systems (C)	Expanded problem focused
		5–7 body areas and/or organ systems (C)	Detailed
		8+ body areas (A) _or_ 8+ organ systems (B), but they cannot be combined	Comprehensive

Figure 33-6 ■ 1995 documentation guidelines for multisystem examination. *Source: © PB Resources, Inc. Used with permission. Based on Centers for Medicare and Medicaid Services, 1995 Documentation Guidelines for Evaluation and Management Services.*

the same DG for all patients. To determine the appropriate E/M code using the 1995 DG, coders must review the documentation in detail and identify the specific elements documented.

- To translate the documentation into the E/M requirements for the history, refer back to Chapter 28, "Evaluation and Management Services (99201-99499)," Tables 28-7 to 28-10, or to the 1995 DG.

- To determine the requirements for an examination, refer to Figure 33-6. The 1995 DG provide general examination criteria but do not quantify the number of elements required. This chapter reviews the 1995 DG multisystem examination and follows the generally accepted quantitative guidelines for each examination level shown in the figure.

- To determine the levels for medical decision making (MDM), refer to Chapter 28, Table 28-12, and to the Table of Risk in the 1995 DG.

Guided Example of E/M Coding for Endocrinology

Refer to the endocrinology encounter (■ FIGURE 33-7) to practice skills for abstracting and assigning E/M codes. This example demonstrates use of the 1995 DG. Follow along as fictitious coder Tamara Brownlee, CCS-P, abstracts the service. Check off each step after you complete it.

▶ First, Tamara needs to establish the category of service so she can determine the information needed to abstract and assign the code.

❑ *What is the setting?* Endocrine clinic (office)

❑ *What is the type of service?* Established patient

❑ *What is the code range?* Tamara refers to the CPT Index and looks up the Main Term **Evaluation and Management**. She must determine whether the encounter should be coded as a consultation or an office visit. She reviews the definition of a consultation, which requires that one physician request the opinion of another physician with a report back on the findings. This patient is established with the endocrinology clinic and is returning for a six-month checkup. Management of the patient's diabetes is under the ongoing care of the endocrinologist, so this is not a consultation.

❑ Tamara returns to the CPT Index and locates the subterm **Office and other outpatient**. The code range listed is **99201-99215**. Tamara refers to the code range in the Tabular List and notices that the code range is divided into two categories: **New Patient** and **Established Patient**. She selects the code range for **Established patient 99211-99215**.

❑ *How many key components are required?* Tamara refers to the code range in the Tabular List. The first code, **99211**, is described as a minimal visit that does not require the presence of a physician; it probably does not apply to this encounter because the patient met with the physician and the service was more than

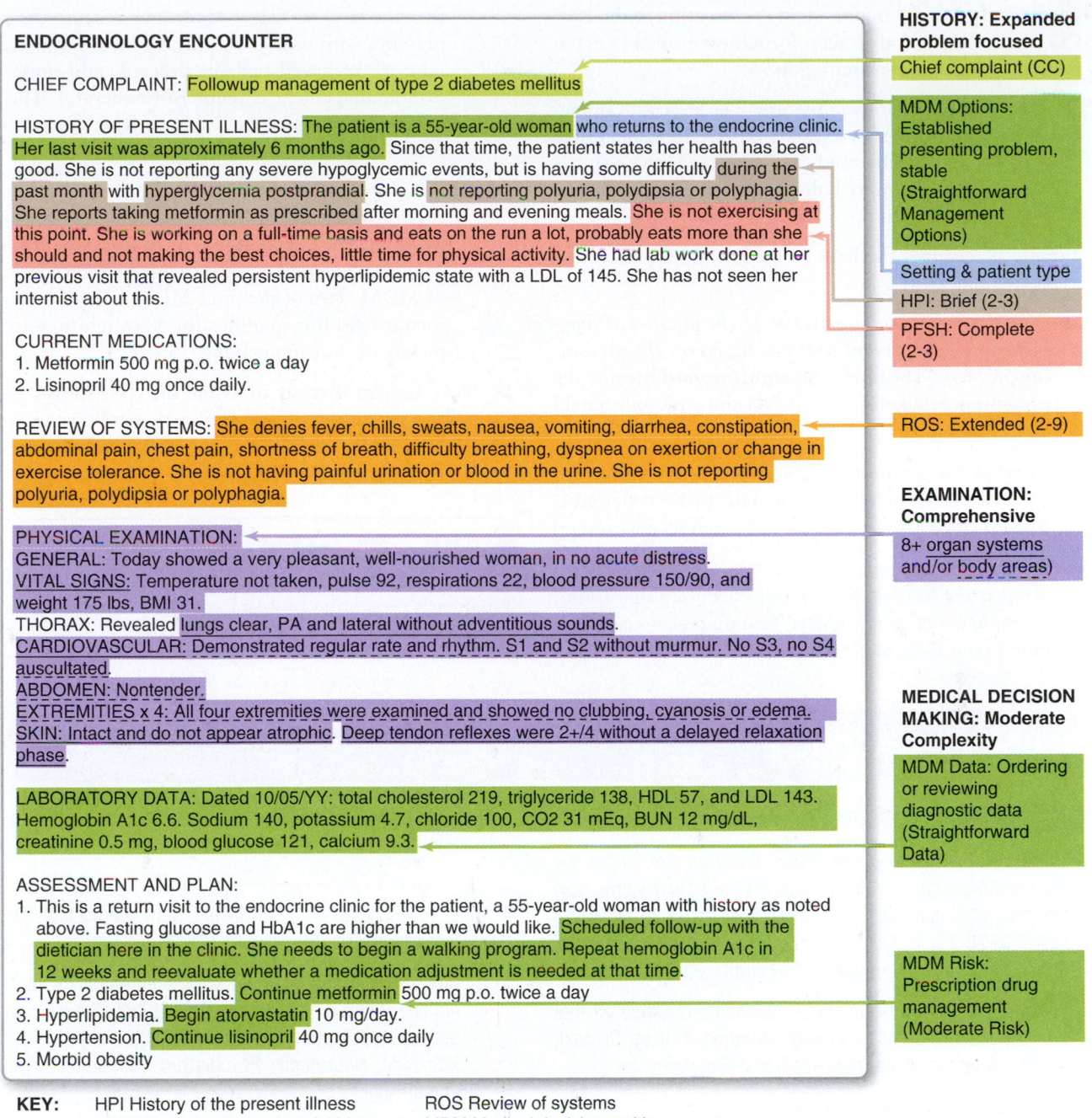

ENDOCRINOLOGY ENCOUNTER

CHIEF COMPLAINT: Followup management of type 2 diabetes mellitus

HISTORY OF PRESENT ILLNESS: The patient is a 55-year-old woman who returns to the endocrine clinic. Her last visit was approximately 6 months ago. Since that time, the patient states her health has been good. She is not reporting any severe hypoglycemic events, but is having some difficulty during the past month with hyperglycemia postprandial. She is not reporting polyuria, polydipsia or polyphagia. She reports taking metformin as prescribed after morning and evening meals. She is not exercising at this point. She is working on a full-time basis and eats on the run a lot, probably eats more than she should and not making the best choices, little time for physical activity. She had lab work done at her previous visit that revealed persistent hyperlipidemic state with a LDL of 145. She has not seen her internist about this.

CURRENT MEDICATIONS:
1. Metformin 500 mg p.o. twice a day
2. Lisinopril 40 mg once daily.

REVIEW OF SYSTEMS: She denies fever, chills, sweats, nausea, vomiting, diarrhea, constipation, abdominal pain, chest pain, shortness of breath, difficulty breathing, dyspnea on exertion or change in exercise tolerance. She is not having painful urination or blood in the urine. She is not reporting polyuria, polydipsia or polyphagia.

PHYSICAL EXAMINATION:
GENERAL: Today showed a very pleasant, well-nourished woman, in no acute distress.
VITAL SIGNS: Temperature not taken, pulse 92, respirations 22, blood pressure 150/90, and weight 175 lbs, BMI 31.
THORAX: Revealed lungs clear, PA and lateral without adventitious sounds.
CARDIOVASCULAR: Demonstrated regular rate and rhythm. S1 and S2 without murmur. No S3, no S4 auscultated.
ABDOMEN: Nontender.
EXTREMITIES x 4: All four extremities were examined and showed no clubbing, cyanosis or edema.
SKIN: Intact and do not appear atrophic. Deep tendon reflexes were 2+/4 without a delayed relaxation phase.

LABORATORY DATA: Dated 10/05/YY: total cholesterol 219, triglyceride 138, HDL 57, and LDL 143. Hemoglobin A1c 6.6. Sodium 140, potassium 4.7, chloride 100, CO2 31 mEq, BUN 12 mg/dL, creatinine 0.5 mg, blood glucose 121, calcium 9.3.

ASSESSMENT AND PLAN:
1. This is a return visit to the endocrine clinic for the patient, a 55-year-old woman with history as noted above. Fasting glucose and HbA1c are higher than we would like. Scheduled follow-up with the dietician here in the clinic. She needs to begin a walking program. Repeat hemoglobin A1c in 12 weeks and reevaluate whether a medication adjustment is needed at that time.
2. Type 2 diabetes mellitus. Continue metformin 500 mg p.o. twice a day
3. Hyperlipidemia. Begin atorvastatin 10 mg/day.
4. Hypertension. Continue lisinopril 40 mg once daily
5. Morbid obesity

HISTORY: Expanded problem focused

Chief complaint (CC)

MDM Options: Established presenting problem, stable (Straightforward Management Options)

Setting & patient type

HPI: Brief (2-3)

PFSH: Complete (2-3)

ROS: Extended (2-9)

EXAMINATION: Comprehensive

8+ organ systems and/or body areas)

MEDICAL DECISION MAKING: Moderate Complexity

MDM Data: Ordering or reviewing diagnostic data (Straightforward Data)

MDM Risk: Prescription drug management (Moderate Risk)

KEY: HPI History of the present illness   ROS Review of systems
PFSH Past, family, and social history   MDM Medical decision making

Figure 33-7 ■ Endocrinology encounter.

minimal. She reads the code description of the second code, **99212**, which states **Office or other outpatient visit for the evaluation and management of an established patient, which requires at least 2 of these 3 key components.** Codes **99212-99215** have the same requirements for key components. This tells her that two out of three (2/3) key components must meet or exceed the levels listed in the code.

▶ Next, Tamara identifies the level of history.

❏ *What is the level of HPI?* The HPI is **Extended** because four elements are documented.

❏ *What is the level of ROS?* The ROS is **Extended** because two to nine systems are documented.

❏ *What is the level of PFSH?* The PFSH is **Complete** because two to three elements are documented, which qualifies as a complete PFSH for an established patient.

❏ *Based on these factors, what is the overall level of history?* The level of history is **Expanded problem-focused** because the lowest of the three factors (HPI, ROS, and PFSH) determines the history level. The ROS and PFSH qualify for a higher level of history, but the HPI qualifies for only an **Expanded problem-focused** history.

▶ Tamara refers to the multisystem examination in the 1995 DG (Figure 33-6) to abstract information needed to determine the level of the examination.

❑ *What is the level of examination?* The level of examination is **Comprehensive**. Ten (10) body areas and organ systems are documented, which exceeds the requirement of eight or more bulleted elements for a comprehensive examination.

▶ Tamara determines the level of medical decision making (refer to Table 28-12).

❑ *What is the level of complexity of the number of diagnoses or management options, based on the presenting problem?* The level is **Straightforward** because the presenting problem is established and with only a mild exacerbation.

❑ *What is the amount and/or complexity of data to be reviewed?* The amount of data to be reviewed is **Straightforward** because the physician reviews several laboratory tests.

❑ *What is the level of risk of significant complications, morbidity, and/or mortality?* Tamara reviews each column in the Table of Risk in the 1995 DG. She identifies that the level of risk is **Moderate** because the patient presents with one stable chronic illness (low), clinical labs are reviewed but not ordered, and prescription drug management is required (moderate). The single highest element in the Table of Risk determines the overall risk.

❑ *Based on these factors, what is the overall level of medical decision making?* The medical decision making is **Straightforward complexity**. At least two of the three MDM factors are required to qualify for a specific level of MDM. Two of the three MDM factors are straightforward, so this qualifies for a straightforward complexity of decision making.

▶ Now Tamara is ready to assign the code for the endocrinology encounter. The exercise that follows guides you through additional abstracting skills and allows you to assign the correct code.

SUCCESS STEP

Physicians use their clinical judgment and the nature of the patient's presenting problem(s) to determine the depth of history needed to complete the service.

CODING PRACTICE

Exercise 33.5 E/M Coding for Endocrinology

Instructions: Refer to the *1995 Documentation Guidelines for Evaluation and Management Services* (available at **www.cms.gov**) or Chapter 28, "Evaluation and Management Services (99201-99499)," Tables 28-7 to 28-12, in this text. Answer the following questions about the "Endocrinology encounter" (■ Figure 33-7).

1. a. Which elements of the HPI are documented? Circle all that apply. Location, Quality, Severity, Duration, Timing, Context, Modifying factors, Associated signs and symptoms

   b. How many elements are documented? _____

   c. What is the level of HPI? _____

2. a. Which systems are reviewed in the ROS? Circle all that apply. Constitutional, Allergic/ immunologic, CV, Endocrine, ENT/M, Eyes, GI, GU, Hemic/lymphatic, MS, Neurologic, Psychiatric, Respiratory, Skin/breast

   b. How many systems are documented? _____

   c. What is the level of ROS? _____

3. a. Which PFSH elements are documented? Circle all that apply. Past medical, Family, Social

   b. What is the level of PFSH? _____

   c. What is the overall level of history? (The lowest history factor—HPI, ROS, or PFSH—determines the level of history.)

   _____

4. Refer to Figure 33-6 "1995 documentation guidelines for multisystem examination."

   a. How many organ systems are documented for the examination? Circle all that apply. Constitutional (e.g., vital signs, general appearance); Eyes; ENT/M; CV; Respiratory; GI; GU; MS; Skin; Neurologic; Psychiatric; Hematologic/lymphatic/ immunologic

   b. How many body areas are documented for the examination? Circle all that apply. Head, including the face; Neck; Chest, including breasts and axillae; Abdomen; Genitalia, groin, buttocks; Back, including spine; Each extremity (×4)

   c. What is the total number of body areas and organ systems documented? _____

   d. What is the level of the examination? _____

5. Refer to Table 28-12, Medical Decision-Making Levels, or the 1995 DG.

   a. What is the MDM level for the number of diagnoses or management options? _____

   b. What is the MDM level for the amount and/or complexity of data to be reviewed? _____

CODING PRACTICE *(continued)*

c. Refer to the Table of Risk in the 1995 DG. Which elements of risk are documented for each risk factor?

   1. Presenting problem: _____

   2. Diagnostic procedures ordered: _____

   3. Management options selected: _____

d. What is the level of risk? (The highest of the three risk factors determines the overall level of risk.) _____

e. What is the overall level of MDM? (2/3 MDM factors are needed to determine the overall level.) _____

6. a. What is the setting? _____

   b. What is the patient (or service) type? _____

   c. What is the code range? _____

d. How many key components are required? _____

e. What is the level of history? _____

f. What is the level of examination? _____

g. What is the level of medical decision making? _____

h. What is the correct code? _____

7. Abstract, assign, and arrange (sequence) the diagnosis codes that support the E/M code.

   Tip: Hyperlipidemia is also known as hyperlipemia.

   5 ICD-10-CM Code(s) _____

   _____

CHAPTER SUMMARY

In this chapter you learned that:

- Endocrinologists perform medical procedures such as glucose monitoring studies and order laboratory tests to analyze endocrine system function; general surgeons perform surgery on the endocrine system.

- The Endocrine System subsection includes invasive and minimally invasive surgical procedures on four of the nine endocrine glands: the thyroid, parathyroid, thymus, and adrenal glands.

- The Endocrine System subsection has no additional guidelines or special instructions beyond the Surgery section guidelines. Instructional notes in the Tabular List redirect coders when different or additional codes are required.

- The anatomic approach identifies the site of the incision and the direction from which the surgical site is accessed, such as cervical, transthoracic, or transabdominal.

- To locate codes for Endocrine System procedures in the Index, search for the Main Term that names the gland, such as *Thyroid Gland*, *Adrenal Gland*, *Parathyroid Gland*, or *Thymus Gland*, then locate the appropriate first-level modifying term and second-level modifying term that describe the procedure.

- Coders must know when to code a bilateral procedure for a thyroidectomy and when to report a separate procedure when coding an adrenalectomy or thymectomy.

- Endocrinologists use a multisystem E/M physical examination because neither the *1995* nor *1997 Documentation Guidelines for Evaluation and Management Services* (DG) provide a single organ system examination for the endocrine system.

CONCEPT QUIZ

Take a moment to look back at the Endocrine System subsection and solidify your skills.

Completion

Instructions: Write the term that completes each statement. Choose from the following list. Some choices may be used more than once and some may not be used at all.

adrenalectomy	subtotal thyroid lobectomy
contralateral lobectomy	thymectomy
limited neck dissection	thyrotomy
lobectomy	total thyroid lobectomy
partial thyroid lobectomy	total thyroidectomy
selective neck dissection	

1. A(n) _____ is excision of one entire lobe of the thyroid gland.

2. A _____ is excision of part of the opposite or second lobe in addition to a partial, subtotal, or total lobectomy of the first lobe.

3. Excision of one or two regions of cervical lymph nodes is classified as a(n) _____.

4. Surgical removal of all or most of the thymus gland is described as _____.

5. A _____ procedure can be performed on the thyroid gland, the liver, the brain, or the lungs

6. A(n) _____ is excision of less than two-thirds of one lobe of the thyroid gland.

(continued)

(continued from page 657)

7. _____ is excision of three regions of cervical lymph nodes.

8. A _____ is cutting into the thyroglossal duct.

9. A _____ is performed on patients with a goiter.

10. A _____ is excision of more than two-thirds of one lobe but less than the entire lobe.

Multiple Choice

Instructions: Circle the letter of the best answer to each question based on the information you learned in this chapter.

1. What type of dissection is excision of tissue in the first five regions of lymph nodes, including the IJV, SAN, and SCM?
   A. Radical neck dissection
   B. Modified radical neck dissection
   C. Selective neck dissection
   D. Limited neck dissection

2. What procedure is surgical removal of an enlarged thyroid that has grown behind the sternum?
   A. Thyroidectomy
   B. Thyrotomy
   C. Thyroidectomy, substernal
   D. Lobectomy

3. How would you code the following procedure? *A surgeon performs a percutaneous core needle biopsy of the thyroid with fluoroscopic guidance.*
   A. 60100, 77002-51
   B. 60100, 77002-59
   C. 60100, 77002
   D. 60100-51

4. What is the name of an operation to remove remaining thyroid tissue after a thyroidectomy?
   A. Total thyroidectomy
   B. Secondary thyroidectomy
   C. Complete thyroidectomy
   D. Thyroidectomy

5. What approach to a thyroidectomy is performed through the midback?
   A. Cervical
   B. Transthoracic
   C. Dorsal
   D. Substernal

6. How would you code the following procedure? *A surgeon performs a total thyroidectomy and a transcervical thymectomy through a separate incision in the lower neck.*
   A. 60240, 60520-51
   B. 60240-51, 60520-59
   C. 60240-59, 60520-59
   D. 60240, 60520-59

7. What is the medical term for surgical removal of all or most of the thymus gland?
   A. Thyrotomy
   B. Lobectomy
   C. Isthmusectomy
   D. Thymectomy

8. How would you code the following procedure? *A surgeon performs a total thyroidectomy with a bilateral modified radical neck dissection.*
   A. 38724-51, 60240-50
   B. 38724-50, 60240-51
   C. 60240-50, 38724-51
   D. 60240-51, 38724-50

9. What procedure involves surgical removal of the four parathyroid glands and their transplantation into a muscle in the neck or forearm?
   A. Parathyroid autotransplatnation
   B. Hyperparathyroidism
   C. Radical lobectomy
   D. Radical lymphadenctomoy

10. What named body part is found in the thyroid, eustachian tube, uterus, pharynx, brain, and aorta?
    A. Cervix
    B. Lobe
    C. Isthmus
    D. Chamber

KEEP ON CODING

Instructions: Read the procedural statement, then use the appropriate Index and Tabular List to assign CPT procedure codes. Write the code(s) on the line provided.

1. Subtotal thyroidectomy for carcinoma with limited neck dissection. CPT Code(s) _____

2. Unilateral total thyroid lobectomy with contralateral subtotal lobectomy and isthmusectomy and parathyroid autotransplantation. CPT Code(s) _____

3. Excision of carotid body tumor. CPT Code(s) _____

4. Reexploration of parathyroid glands. CPT Code(s) _____

5. Laparoscopic adrenalectomy with biopsy, left side, lumbar approach. CPT Code(s) _____

6. Parathyroidectomy. CPT Code(s) _____

7. Excision of cyst in thyroglossal duct. CPT Code(s) _____

8. Aspiration of a thyroid cyst. CPT Code(s) _____

9. Bilateral thyroidectomy including substernal thyroid, cervical approach. CPT Code(s) _____

10. Partial thymectomy, sternal approach, with radical mediastinal dissection (separate procedure). CPT Code(s) _____

CODING CHALLENGE

Instructions: Read the mini-medical-record of each patient's encounter, then abstract, assign, and arrange ICD-10-CM diagnosis codes and CPT procedure codes using the appropriate Index and Tabular List. Write the code(s) on the line provided.

---

1. OFFICE   Gender: F   Age: 45

Diagnosis: Chronic thyroiditis due to cyst

Procedure: Aspiration of thyroid cyst. Made 1-cm skin incision, inserted catheter, and drained cyst.

1 ICD-10-CM Code _____

1 CPT Code _____

---

2. INPATIENT HOSPITAL   Gender: M   Age: 62

Diagnosis: Anaplastic thyroid cancer; metastatic to cervical lymph nodes

Procedure: Thyroidectomy and lymphadenectomy due to malignancy. Removed all of both lobes, including isthmus. Performed with modified radical dissection of cervical lymph nodes on both sides.

1 ICD-10-CM Code _____

1 CPT Code _____

---

3. OUTPATIENT HOSPITAL   Gender: M   Age: 33

Diagnosis: Thyroid nodule

Procedure: Percutaneous core needle biopsy. Using ultrasound guidance, positioned the core needle (*an automatic spring–powered device with a hollow inner needle*) over the nodule and extracted tissue sample. Tissue submitted to pathology for analysis.

Pathology report: Negative

1 ICD-10-CM Code _____

2 CPT Codes _____

---

4. OUTPATIENT HOSPITAL   Gender: M   Age: 24

Preoperative diagnosis: Difficulty swallowing due to large thyroid nodule

Procedure: Removal of colloid cyst in thyroid

Postoperative diagnosis: Malignant neoplasm of thyroid

Pathology report: Positive for malignant neoplasm of thyroid

1 ICD-10-CM Code _____

1 CPT Code _____

(continued)

INTRODUCTION

When you buy beverages such as soda, you can choose among various sizes and packaging: single cans, liter bottles, six-packs, twelve-packs, mini cans, and so on. Each package has one price, regardless of the number of bottles or cans it contains. CPT codes often work the same way. When coding for removal of lesions in the integumentary system, the number of lesions described by a single CPT varies from 1 to 15, depending on the type of lesion and method of removal.

INTEGUMENTARY SYSTEM PROCEDURE BASICS

Dermatologists diagnose and treat disorders of the skin and also perform surgical procedures. Plastic surgeons perform both **reconstructive** (*relating to restoring normal function or appearance*) procedures and **cosmetic** (*relating to aesthetics or appearance*) procedures. Podiatrists diagnose and treat conditions of the foot, including the skin of the foot and the toenails.

Review the anatomic structure of the skin and the associated medical terms for the layers in Chapter 10 of this text. This knowledge helps in determining the extent and complexity of many procedures. Refer to ■ TABLE 34-1 for a refresher on how to build medical terms for integumentary system procedures.

Procedures of the Integumentary System

Procedures commonly performed on the integumentary system are summarized in ■ TABLE 34-2. Coders must understand the basic principles of measurements when working with excision procedures and wound repair. Reviewing the wound healing process is also helpful. Additional procedures to be familiar with are Mohs

CODING CAUTION

Be alert for combining forms that are spelled similarly and have different meanings.

ungu/o (*nail*) and **lingu/o** (*tongue*)

xen/o (*stranger, foreign material*) and **xanth/o** (*yellow*) and **xer/o** (*dryness*)

hydr/o (*water*) and **hidr/o** (*sweat*)

micrographic surgery, burns, tissue transfer and skin replacement, and breast removal and reconstruction. These are discussed next.

Measurements

Working with the integumentary system requires knowledge of measurements because many procedures are classified by size. Lesions and wound repairs are described by linear measurements, tissue repairs are classified by area, and burn treatments are classified by the percentage of total body surface area (TBSA). Linear and area measurements are reported using the metric system, which consists of meters (m), centimeters (cm), and millimeters (mm). A **linear measurement** identifies the distance between two points and is used to classify the length of wound repairs and the diameter (*distance from one side to the other*) of excised lesions. An **area measurement** describes the space inside a boundary and is used to classify the amount of skin treated in a tissue repair or skin graft. Area is calculated as the length multiplied by the width of the affected tissue (L × W) and is expressed in square centimeters (sq cm) (■ FIGURE 34-1). The details of how to use measurements to assign codes are discussed later in this chapter.

Table 34-1 ■ **EXAMPLE OF CONSTRUCTING MEDICAL TERMS FOR INTEGUMENTARY SYSTEM PROCEDURES**

Combining Form	Suffix	Complete Medical Term
derm/o (*skin*)	**-plasty** (*surgical repair, formation*) **-lysis** (*surgical destruction, loosening*)	**dermo + plasty** (*surgical repair of the skin*)
		lipo + plasty (*surgical formation of fat*)
lip/o (*fat*) **electr/o** (*electrical*)		**dermo + lysis** (*surgical loosening of the skin*)
		lipo + lysis (*surgical destruction of fat*)
		electro + lysis (*surgical destruction using electricity*)

Source: © PB Resources, Inc. Used with permission.

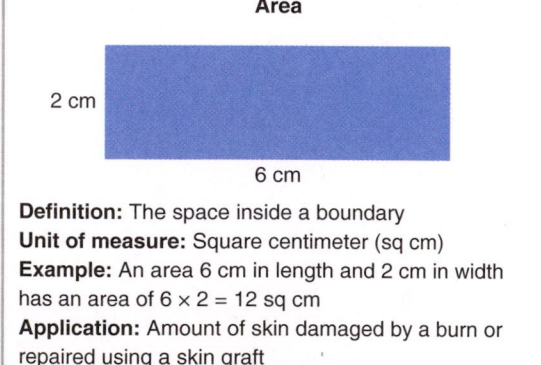

Length

6 cm

Definition: The distance between two points
Unit of measure: Linear centimeter (cm)
1 cm = 0.39 inches. 1 inch = 2.54 cm.
Examples: 2 cm or 5.5 cm
Application: Length of a wound, diameter of a lesion

Area

2 cm

6 cm

Definition: The space inside a boundary
Unit of measure: Square centimeter (sq cm)
Example: An area 6 cm in length and 2 cm in width has an area of 6 × 2 = 12 sq cm
Application: Amount of skin damaged by a burn or repaired using a skin graft

Figure 34-1 ■ Length and area.

Table 34-2 ■ **COMMON PROCEDURES OF THE INTEGUMENTARY SYSTEM**

Procedure Name	Definition	Reason Performed
Adjacent tissue transfer/ rearrangement (ATT/R)	Transfer of a section of skin or flap from that immediately next to the damaged skin and that can be moved without completely detaching it	Repair or replace damaged skin
Autograft	Use of a patient's own tissue from one site to replace damaged tissue at another site	Repair or replace damaged skin
Avulsion	Forceful tearing of the nail plate	Treat onychocryptosis (*ingrown toenail*), perform a biopsy, or treat an infection
Chemosurgery	Use of a chemical agent (e.g., trichloroacetic acid, hydroxy acid, silver nitrate) to destroy tissue	Remove lesions
Cryotherapy	Use of liquid nitrogen to destroy tissue	Remove lesions
Destruction	Rendering tissue into tiny fragments	Remove lesions
Electrocauterization	Use of a hot instrument to destroy tissue	Remove lesions
Electrosurgical destruction	Use of high-frequency electric current to destroy tissue	Remove lesions
Excision	Use of scissors, scalpel, or other sharp instrument to cut out tissue	Full-thickness removal of diseased or damaged tissue
Flap transfer	Moving a section of skin and subcutaneous tissue (sometimes including muscle, fascia, and bone), with blood vessels intact, from one site to another; with anastomosis to vessels at the recipient site	Repair or replace damaged skin and vasculature
Intralesional injection	Injection of a drug, such as a corticosteroid, into a skin lesion	Treat keloids, psoriasis, hypertrophic scars, cystic acne, and eczema
Ligature	Tying off a skin tag at its base with thread, eliminating blood flow to the skin tag; it eventually dies and falls off	Remove skin tags
Mohs micrographic surgery	A multistage procedure in which a malignant lesion is excised in microscopic layers. The physician performing the procedure also performs pathological evaluation of each tissue layer. When no further malignancy is found, the site is closed.	Basal cell carcinoma, squamous cell carcinoma
Paring/cutting/curettement	Use of a scalpel, blade, or curette (*surgical instrument with a scoop or ring at the end*) to scrape away the tissue	Remove dead or infected tissue
Shaving	Use of a sharp instrument	Remove an epidermal or dermal lesion without a full-thickness excision
Skin replacement	Use of skin from the patient's own body or a donor to replace damaged skin that cannot be repaired with sutures alone	Repair or replacement of damaged skin
Skin substitute	Use of synthetic (*artificial*) material to replace damaged skin	Temporary repair or replacement of damaged skin while the body generates new skin tissue
Tattooing	Injection of a colored pigment into the skin	Hide a discoloration caused by disease, a congenital deformity, injury, or trauma; create color for an areola and nipple after breast reconstruction; create color for eyebrows and eyelashes for patients with hair loss from cancer or alopecia
Tissue expander	A temporary inflatable or saline implant placed under the skin to stretch it and allow growth of new skin cells	Create new skin needed to perform surgery and/or to replace skin on areas of the body where skin was lost from burns, trauma, or injury
Wound repair–intermediate	Layered closure of one or more of the deeper layers of subcutaneous tissue and superficial (*nonmuscle*) fascia, in addition to the skin (*epidermal and dermal*) closure; also includes extensive cleaning/ decontamination of wounds otherwise requiring single-layer closure	Clean and close deep wounds
Wound repair–simple	One-layer closure of epidermis, dermis, or subcutaneous tissue without significant involvement of deeper structures; includes local anesthesia and electrocauterization, when used	Close lacerations and wounds
Wound repair–complex	A layered closure that also requires scar revision, debridement, extensive undermining (*freeing the skin from the underlying tissue along lateral edge of the wound*), stents, or retention sutures (*reinforcing sutures placed around the primary suture line*)	Restructure or reinforce deep wounds

Source: © PB Resources, Inc. Used with permission.

Physicians are trained to use metric units in documentation, but understanding the relationship between the metric system and the English system is helpful for coders so they can spot potential errors, such as a misplaced decimal. A comparison of metric measures and English measures follows:

- 1 meter = 3.28 feet (*3 feet, 3 inches*)
- 1 centimeter (*1/100th [written as 0.01] of a meter*) = 0.39 inches (*just less than ½ inch*)
- 1 millimeter (*1/1000th of a meter [written as 0.001] or 1/10th [written as 0.10] of a centimeter*) = 0.039 inches (*1/25th of an inch*)

> ## CODING CAUTION
> Metric numbers less than 1 should be written with a 0 in front of the decimal, such as 0.25, to avoid potential confusion with a similar whole number, such as 25.

Wound Healing

Wound healing is an intricate process in which the body regenerates skin cells; it can be summarized in four basic phases (■ TABLE 34-3). External assistance helps to speed the healing process and prevent infection. Physicians use three types of wound healing protocols based on the severity of the wound.

- **Primary intention healing** is wound closure performed with sutures, staples, or adhesive tape or glue. It is used for uncomplicated lacerations and healing after most surgeries.

Table 34-3 ■ **SUMMARY OF THE PHASES OF WOUND HEALING**

Phase	Name	Description	Time Frame (After Injury)
1	Hemostasis	Platelets stop bleeding	1–60 minutes
2	Inflammation	Neutrophils, mast cells, and macrophages phagocytize (*clean up or digest cells*) wound debris to prevent infection	6 hours to 4 days
3	Proliferation/granulation	Fibroblasts rebuild the base of the wound and pericytes regenerate the outer layers of capillaries (angiogenesis), endothelial cells rebuild the lining (granulation), keratinocytes create new epithelial tissue (epithelialization), and the wound begins to close (contracture)	5–21 days
4	Maturation/remodeling	Fibroblasts rebuild, reinforce, and strengthen dermal tissues	3 weeks to 2 years

- **Secondary intention healing** is an extended process in which the wound is not closed with sutures but left open to granulate (*generate new connective tissue and vasculature*). The surgeon may pack the wound with gauze or use a drainage system. Wound care is performed daily to remove wound debris and allow for granulation. It is used for tooth extraction sockets burns, severe lacerations, and pressure ulcers.

- **Tertiary intention healing** is delayed primary closure. The wound is initially cleaned, debrided, and left open for observation for several days before closure. It is used for healing after a tissue graft.

Negative-pressure wound therapy (NPWT) is a treatment in which a sealed wound dressing is connected to a vacuum pump that removes fluids, debris, and infectious materials from the wound. The process helps promote granulation and is used with secondary or tertiary intention healing protocols. The type of healing undertaken provides information on the type of procedure performed. For example, when a physician documents, "The wound was left to close by secondary intention," you know that no suturing was performed.

Mohs Micrographic Surgery

Mohs micrographic surgery is an advanced technique used to excise skin cancer lesions and is considered highly successful. It is used to remove large, complex, rapidly growing, recurring, or ill-defined skin cancer and requires that 100% of the surgical margin be examined. The roots of a skin cancer may extend beyond the visible portion of the tumor. If these roots are not removed, the cancer will recur. Examination of the surgical margin helps determine whether the entire malignancy has been removed.

The Mohs technique is unique because one physician functions as both surgeon and pathologist. After the affected area has been numbed, the surgeon removes the visible tumor and a margin. This margin tissue is subdivided, put on slides, and examined under a microscope by the surgeon. If there is evidence of cancer, another layer of tissue is taken from the area where the cancer was detected. This ensures that only cancerous tissue is removed during the procedure, minimizing the loss of healthy tissue. These steps are repeated until all samples are free of cancer. Most tumors require one to three stages for complete removal.

Burns

Burns are classified based on the percentage of TBSA affected. Physicians estimate the extent, depth, and percentage of burns using the **Lund-Browder classification,** a system that identifies the percentage of the total body comprised by various body areas (■ FIGURE 34-2). It is similar in concept to the Rule of Nines used in diagnosis coding but is considered more accurate because it divides the body into smaller

Area	Age (years)					% 1°	% 2°	% 3°	% Total
	0–1	1–4	5–9	10–15	Adult				
Head	19	17	13	10	7				
Neck	2	2	2	2	2				
Ant. trunk	13	13	13	13	13				
Post. trunk	13	13	13	13	13				
R. buttock	2½	2½	2½	2½	2½				
L. buttock	2½	2½	2½	2½	2½				
Genitalia	1	1	1	1	1				
R.U. arm	4	4	4	4	4				
L.U. arm	4	4	4	4	4				
R.L. arm	3	3	3	3	3				
L.L. arm	3	3	3	3	3				
R. hand	2½	2½	2½	2½	2½				
L. hand	2½	2½	2½	2½	2½				
R. thigh	5½	6½	8½	8½	9½				
L. thigh	5½	6½	8½	8½	9½				
R. leg	5	5	5½	6	7				
L. leg	5	5	5½	6	7				
R. foot	3½	3½	3½	3½	3½				
L. foot	3½	3½	3½	3½	3½				
									Total

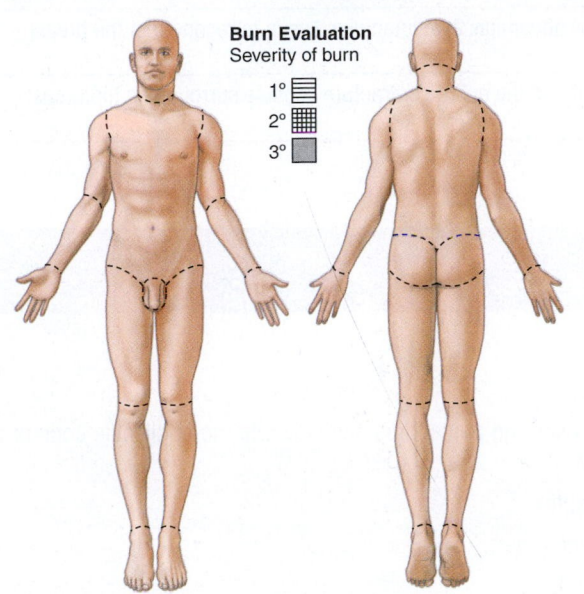

Burn Evaluation
Severity of burn

1°
2°
3°

Figure 34-2 ■ Lund-Browder classification chart for burns.

areas and accommodates the varying proportions of the body as children grow. Using a preprinted or electronic chart, the physician shades a diagram to show the areas of the body affected by first-, second-, and third-degree burns then determines the percentage of TBSA affected using the data in the accompanying table.

Tissue Transfer and Skin Replacement

When an area of skin is damaged to the extent that it will not heal on its own, a tissue transfer, skin graft, or skin substitute might be used. In an **adjacent tissue transfer/rearrangement (ATT/R)**, part of the skin transferred remains connected to its original site to maintain the blood supply when it is attached to the new site.

Skin replacement and skin substitutes include skin grafts and other materials to repair defects and replace skin. In an **autograft**, skin is removed from one area of the body—the donor site—and transferred to the recipient site, where the wound or defect exists. Autografts consist of grafts, flaps, and skin substitutes. In a **split-thickness skin graft (STSG)** (*a skin graft consisting of the epidermis and a portion of the dermis or a mucosal graft consisting of only a partial thickness of mucosa*) or **full-thickness skin graft (FTSG)** (*a skin graft consisting of the epidermis and the full depth of the dermis*), skin from the donor site is completely removed from its connecting blood supply before the physician transfers it to the recipient site. In a **flap**, the blood supply remains intact or the physician removes the skin and blood vessels and connects them to the recipient site. Flaps can also involve subcutaneous tissue, muscle, fascia, and bone.

Skin substitutes can be an **allograft** (*skin from another person*), **xenograft** (*skin from another species, such as a pig*), or a synthetic substitute. These materials are used for temporary coverage while the patient grows new skin because they are foreign materials and the body will not accept them long term, and they must be replaced with an autograft.

Skin replacement procedures are generally named based on the visual configuration of the tissue, such as Z-plasty, W-plasty, rotation flap, or tubed flap. Refer to a pathophysiology text or reliable Internet resource to learn more about the specific types of grafts and flaps.

Breast Removal and Reconstruction Procedures

Although physiologically the breast is classified as part of the reproductive system, breast procedures are classified with the Integumentary System subsection in CPT because they involve the skin and subcutaneous tissue. Procedures are identified based on the extent of skin, breast tissue, lymph nodes, and/or chest muscles removed. Breast reconstruction is performed using other muscles and tissue to replace the tissue removed. Procedures are named based on the technique and specific muscles used. ■ TABLE 34-4 (page 666) identifies breast treatment and reconstruction procedures in progressive order, from least to most complex.

This section provides a general reference to help understand the most common integumentary system procedures. Remember to keep standard reference books handy in case you get stuck.

Table 34-4   ■   **BREAST PROCEDURES**

Procedure	Description
Treatment Procedures	
Mastotomy	Incision and drainage of a breast abscess
Partial mastectomy (lumpectomy, tylectomy)	Removal of only enough breast tissue to ensure that the margins of the specimen are free of malignant cells
Subcutaneous mastectomy	Excision of breast tissue but not the overlying skin, nipple, and areola, making it possible for the breast form to be reconstructed
Simple complete mastectomy	Removal of only the breast tissue, nipple, and a small portion of the overlying skin, also called *simple mastectomy* and *total mastectomy*
Modified radical mastectomy	A simple mastectomy plus removal of axillary lymph nodes but not the pectoralis major muscle
Radical mastectomy	Removal of the breast, pectoralis major and minor muscles, axillary lymph nodes, and associated skin and subcutaneous tissue
Repair and Reconstruction Procedures	
Mastopexy	A skin reduction with removal or reduction of underlying breast muscles to reorient the breasts into a higher position
Mammaplasty	Repair or reconstruction of the breast
Latissimus dorsi (LD) flap	Use of a latissimus dorsi muscle flap, often commonly combined with a tissue expander or implant, to reconstruct the breast
Deep inferior epigastric perforator (DIEP) flap	Use of blood vessels called *deep inferior epigastric perforators (DIEPs)* and the skin and connected fat, or skin only (but no muscle), from the wall of the lower belly to rebuild the breast
Transverse rectus abdominis myocutaneous (TRAM) flap	Use of the transverse rectus abdominis myocutaneous tissue to reconstruct the breast
Periprosthetic capsulectomy	Removal of a breast implant and the entire contracture capsule surrounding the breast implant

Source: © PB Resources, Inc. Used with permission.

CODING PRACTICE

Exercise 34.1   Integumentary System Procedure Basics

Instructions: Use your medical terminology skills and resources to define the following procedures, then identify the applicable code or code range. Follow these steps:

- Use slash marks "/" to break down the underlined term into its root(s) and suffix.
- Define the meaning of the underlined word, based on the meaning of each word part.
- Use the entire phrase to identify the code or code range shown in the CPT Index.

Example: <u>mastectomy</u>, partial mast/ectomy   Meaning <u>*surgical removal of the breast*</u>   CPT Code(s) <u>19301-19302</u>

1. <u>cryotherapy</u>, acne   Meaning _____   CPT Code(s) _____

2. <u>mammaplasty</u>, reduction   Meaning _____   CPT Code(s) _____

3. <u>ischiectomy</u>, with pressure ulcer excision   Meaning _____   CPT Code(s) _____

4. <u>rhytidectomy</u>, forehead   Meaning _____   CPT Code(s) _____

5. <u>mastopexy</u>   Meaning _____   CPT Code(s) _____

6. <u>blepharoplasty</u>   Meaning _____   CPT Code(s) _____

7. <u>hidradenitis</u>, excision   Meaning _____   CPT Code(s) _____

8. evacuation of hematoma, <u>subungual</u>   Meaning _____   CPT Code(s) _____

9. <u>escharotomy</u>, graft site   Meaning _____   CPT Code(s) _____

10. skin graft and flap, <u>fasciocutaneous</u>   Meaning _____   CPT Code(s) _____

CODING GUIDELINES FOR INTEGUMENTARY SYSTEM PROCEDURES

Coders should understand the organization, guidelines, and Tabular List instructional notes in this CPT subsection. This information is necessary for accurate coding. The CPT subsection **Integumentary System (10030-19499)** contains seven subsections that are divided by anatomic site and type of procedure (Table 34-5). Review the subheading and category names and code ranges listed in the Integumentary System table of contents, which appears at the beginning of the Integumentary System in the CPT manual, immediately after the Surgery section guidelines. Become familiar with the content and organization of this subsection. In this list, subheadings and categories followed by an asterisk (*) contain special instructions that provide guidelines for using codes in that subheading or category.

This chapter includes invasive, minimally invasive, and noninvasive surgical procedures on the skin, subcutaneous tissue, nails, and breast. Codes for diagnostic tests on the skin appear in the Medicine section. CPT codes in the Integumentary System subsection are frequently supported by diagnosis codes from ICD-10-CM Chapter 12, "Diseases of the Skin and Subcutaneous Tissue (L00-L99)," and Chapter 14, "Diseases of the Genitourinary System, Disorders of the Breast (N60-N65)." Diagnosis codes for neoplasms, symptoms and signs, and superficial injuries (■ TABLE 34-6) also support integumentary system procedures. ICD-10-CM codes for superficial injuries appear throughout the injury chapter (**S00-T88**) because injury codes are organized by anatomic site from head to foot, and the skin covers all sites. These are the codes most commonly used to support procedures on the integumentary system; however, diagnosis codes from any ICD-10-CM chapter are permissible.

CPT guidelines for the Surgery section apply to the Integumentary System subsection. In addition, be alert for special instructions that provide definitions and coding guidelines at the beginning of many categories. Coding rules vary quite a bit for specific types of procedures within the Integumentary System, so the special instructions explain the relevant rules for each code category. In particular, study the special instructions for excision of benign and malignant lesions, wound repairs, and various types of flaps and grafts.

Instructional notes appear throughout the Tabular List to alert coders to the need for modifiers, provide cross-references to codes for similar procedures on other sites, identify when additional codes might be needed, and highlight resequenced

Table 34-5 ■ INTEGUMENTARY SYSTEM SUBHEADINGS

Subheading	Code Range
Skin, Subcutaneous, and Accessory Structures	10030-11646
Nails	11719-11765
Pilonidal Cyst	11770-11772
Introduction	11900-11983
Repair (Closure)	12001-16036
Destruction	17000-17999
Breast	19000-19499

Table 34-6 ■ LOCATING ICD-10-CM AND ADDITIONAL CPT CODES FOR THE INTEGUMENTARY SYSTEM

Type of Code	Codes
ICD-10-CM Integumentary System-Related Codes	
Integumentary system conditions	L00-L99, N60-N65
Neoplasms	C43-C44
Symptoms and signs	R20-R23
Injuries (superficial)	S00-T88
CPT Integumentary System-Related Codes	
Medicine procedures	96900-96999, 97597-97610
Radiologic procedures	
• Diagnostic radiology	77046-77067

Source: © PB Resources, Inc. Used with permission.

and recently deleted codes. Specific guidelines and instructional notes are discussed throughout this chapter of the text.

The Integumentary System Tabular List contains many parent/indented code families and add-on codes. Indented code descriptions identify alternative anatomic sites where the parent code procedure can be performed, as well as alternative quantities, lengths, or sizes (square centimeters) of the affected area. Add-on codes identify additional quantities or sizes to be reported in addition to those of the standalone code.

ABSTRACTING INTEGUMENTARY SYSTEM PROCEDURES

Although the Integumentary System subsection includes a variety of procedures, a few basic concepts apply to most procedures: site, complexity, size, method, and quantity. The details of these criteria vary for different classes of procedures, such as excisions, repairs, and grafts. As discussed earlier, the size for lesion excisions is reported as diameter, wound repairs as length, and grafts as area, but size is still the basic criteria. The complexity of burns is expressed as first, second, or third degree, whereas the complexity of wound repairs is expressed as wound depth and type of closure.

Refer to ■ TABLE 34-7 for guidance on how to abstract procedures on the integumentary system, then work through the detailed example that follows. Remember that the abstracting questions are a guide and that not every question applies to, or can be answered for, every case. For example, not every procedure requires a length or area measurement.

Table 34-7 ■ KEY CRITERIA FOR ABSTRACTING INTEGUMENTARY SYSTEM PROCEDURES

- ❏ What is the procedure?
- ❏ What is the anatomic site?
- ❏ What is the depth or complexity of the repair or treatment?
- ❏ What is the size (length or area) of the site treated?
- ❏ What method is used?
- ❏ What is the quantity?
- ❏ Is a malignancy involved?

Source: © PB Resources, Inc. Used with permission.

INPATIENT HOSPITAL Gender: F Age: 84

Preoperative diagnosis: Stage 4 pressure ulcer, right hip

Procedure: Excision of pressure ulcer with ischiectomy and flap closure, 30 sq cm. After administration of anesthesia, an incision was made around the ulcerated region of the ischium. The skin was cut in an elliptical fashion around the wound and the ulcerated tissue was excised down to the ischium bone; 1 cm of the ischium was excised. Purulent drainage was copiously irrigated. Defect area was 5 cm by 6 cm, needing a 30-sq cm repair. The patient's skin integrity adjacent to the ulcer was compromised, and I felt that an adjacent transfer rotational flap was contraindicated. The abdominal tissue was intact, so a myocutaneous flap was created from the abdomen and relocated to cover the wound on the ischium. The surgical site was closed with staples and a 1/0 Jackson-Pratt drain was placed. The donor site, measuring 30 sq cm, was closed with an adjacent transfer rotational flap of 32 sq cm. Patient tolerated the procedure well and was transferred to postoperative care in stable condition. The excised tissue and bone fragments were sent to pathology.

Pathology report: Tissue consistent with decubitus ulcer. Bone fragments show evidence of osteomyelitis.

Postoperative diagnosis: Stage 4 pressure ulcer, right hip. Acute osteomyelitis of the ischium.

Guided Example of Abstracting Integumentary System Procedures

Refer to the following example throughout this chapter to practice skills for abstracting, assigning, and arranging Integumentary System codes.

Follow along as fictitious coder Joshua Grider, CPC, abstracts the procedure. Check off each step after you complete it.

▶ Joshua reads through the entire record, paying special attention to the reason for the encounter, the procedure performed, and the postoperative diagnosis. He refers to the Key Criteria for Abstracting Integumentary System Procedures (Table 34-7).

❏ He notes the diagnosis of Stage 3 pressure ulcer, right hip.

❏ *What is the anatomic site?* Skin, right hip; Joshua understands that although the pressure ulcer is on the right hip, the organ system treated is the skin

❏ *What is the primary procedure performed?* Excision of pressure ulcer

❏ *What is the depth or complexity of the repair or treatment?* Stage 4 pressure ulcer

❏ *What method is used?* Excision

❏ *What is the quantity?* One

❏ *Is a malignancy involved?* No

❏ *What additional procedure is performed?* Ischiectomy

❏ *What additional procedure is performed?* Full-thickness myocutaneous flap closure

❏ *What is the size (area) of the site treated?* 30 sq cm

CODING PRACTICE

Exercise 34.2 Abstracting Integumentary System Procedures

Instructions: Read the mini-medical-record of each patient's encounter and answer the abstracting questions. Write the answer on the line provided. Do not assign any codes.

1. OFFICE Gender: F Age: 39

Preprocedure diagnosis: Rough scaly lesions on arms, face, and neck

Procedure: Surgical curettement of 20 lesions ranging in size from 2 to 6 mm

Pathology report: Premalignant actinic keratoses

Postprocedure diagnosis: Premalignant actinic keratoses

a. What is the procedure? _____

b. What is the anatomic site? _____

(continued)

1. (continued)

c. What is the size of the lesions? _____

d. What method is used? _____

e. What is the quantity? _____

f. Is a malignancy involved? _____

2. INPATIENT HOSPITAL Gender: M Age: 26

Preprocedure diagnosis: Multiple second-degree burns nearly covering both lower legs and feet

Procedure: Removed blisters, debrided necrotic tissue, and applied dressings

Postprocedure diagnosis: Leg burns, 21% TBSA second-degree

a. What is the procedure? _____

b. What is the anatomic site? _____

(continued)

CODING PRACTICE (continued)

2. (continued)

c. What is the depth or complexity of the repair or treatment? _____

d. What is the size (length or area) of the site treated? _____

e. What method is used? _____

3. INPATIENT HOSPITAL   Gender: F   Age: 35

Diagnosis: Facial nerve paralysis from Bell's palsy

Procedure: Harvested a fascia lata (*deep thigh*) free graft from right leg and applied to face to restore facial nerve function. Defect area 20 sq cm

a. What is the procedure? _____

b. Where is the recipient site? _____

c. Where is the donor site? _____

d. What type of donor tissue is used? _____

e. What is the size (length or area) of the site treated? _____

f. What method is used? _____

4. OUTPATIENT SURGERY   Gender: M   Age: 46

Preprocedure diagnosis: Chronic infection and necrosis of the abdominal wall from internal dehiscence (*splitting open*) following a hernia repair 3 weeks ago

Procedure: Removed the mesh prosthesis from the hernia repair, then, using a curette, debrided 30 sq cm of subcutaneous tissue, fascia, and muscle in the abdominal wall. Applied antibiotics and packed with saline-soaked gauze for healing by secondary intention.

Postprocedure diagnosis: Infection due to mesh prosthesis and internal wound dehiscence following ventral hernia repair

a. What is the primary procedure? _____

b. What is the anatomic site? _____

c. What is the depth or complexity of the repair or treatment? _____

d. What is the area of the site treated? _____

e. What method is used? _____

f. What additional procedure is performed? _____

g. What is the site of the secondary procedure? _____

5. OFFICE   Gender: F   Age: 37

Preprocedure diagnosis: Suspicious lesions on back, arm, and hand

Procedure: Excised two lesions from the back, 1.5 and 2.1 cm including margins. One lesion from the arm, 0.5 cm including margins. One lesion from the hand, 0.4 cm including margins. All sites sutured in one layer. Tissue was submitted to pathology.

Pathology: Four specimens received, all consistent with malignant melanoma

Postprocedure diagnosis: Malignant melanoma on back, arm, and hand

a. What is the procedure? _____

b. What is the anatomic site(s)? _____

c. What is the depth or complexity of the repair or treatment? _____

d. What is the size (length or area) of the site treated? _____

e. What method is used? _____

f. What is the quantity? _____

g. Is a malignancy involved? _____

6. EMERGENCY DEPT   Gender: F   Age: 16

Preprocedure diagnosis: Multiple lacerations from crash that occurred when she was driving an off-road vehicle in the woods

Procedure: Closed a 7.0-cm wound on the neck with a one-layer closure, a 2.5-cm wound on the face with heavy contamination requiring extensive debris removal and a simple closure, and a 10.2-cm wound on the right forearm with complex closure with debridement

Postprocedure diagnosis: Lacerations

a. What is the procedure? _____

b. What is the anatomic site? _____

c. What is the complexity of each repair? _____

d. What is the length of each wound? _____

e. What is the quantity? _____

▶ At this time, Joshua does not know which of these procedures may need to be coded, nor how many codes he will end up with. He will learn about this when he moves on to assigning codes.

ASSIGNING CODES FOR INTEGUMENTARY SYSTEM PROCEDURES

In addition to locating Main Terms and modifying terms for Integumentary System subsection procedures in the Index, coders must understand how code families are organized in this subsection and how to determine the quantity applicable to the code. After reviewing the basics of using the Index and interpreting code families, this chapter discusses coding for lesions, wound repair, mastectomy procedures, and skin grafts and flaps.

Using the Index

To locate codes in the Integumentary System subsection, search first for the Main Term **Skin**, then a first-level modifying term for the procedure, and finally a second-level modifying term for the details of the procedure. Use the Main Term **Skin** rather than the anatomic site, such as back or arm. Main Terms for anatomic sites generally lead to codes about procedures on the structure itself, not on the skin covering the structure. If a Main Term for the procedure, such as **Excision**, or condition, such as **Lesion**, is selected, be sure to locate a first-level modifying term for **Skin**. This is the most direct path to the code because the code ranges listed in the Index are more detailed under **Skin** than under other potential Main Terms (■ FIGURE 34-3).

In addition to the Main Term **Skin**, the CPT Index provides separate Main Term entries for **Skin Graft and Flap** and **Skin Substitute Graft**, so be sure to look for these entries when coding these procedures. Procedures not performed directly on the skin are indexed under Main Terms that identify the site, such as **Nails** and **Pilonidal Cyst**.

Code Families

The Tabular List organizes many codes into code families divided by anatomic site and size, area, and/or complexity. Code families are clusters of parent codes and indented codes. The common descriptor (*the portion before the semicolon*) in the parent code applies to the indented codes and is part of the description of the indented code, even though it is not reprinted for each code number. Code families follow a specific structure within many code categories of the Integumentary System subsection (■ FIGURE 34-4).

- The first portion of the parent code's common descriptor describes the *type of procedure* for category and is *similar* for all parent codes in the category.

- The second portion of the parent code common descriptor describes the *anatomic sites* included in the code family and applies to all codes in one family. However, this portion is *different* for each parent code in the category.

- The unique descriptor in the parent code and each indented code identifies the characteristics of the specific code, such as *size* or *quantity*. The unique descriptors tend to be *similar for all code families* within a category.

Determining Quantity

Coders must evaluate how the number of lesions or area of skin relates to the number of units identified in the code description to determine the correct code in the integumentary system. Methods of determining quantity include single quantity, single quantity by size and/or type, multiple quantities, and add-together quantities. To understand the method used in a specific code family, read the code description and identify the unit of measure. Also read the surrounding codes for indented and add-on codes that report additional quantities and identify the type of quantities described.

Single Quantity

Single quantity refers to codes for which one unit is reported for each service performed. This is the default method for reporting CPT codes. Categories of skin procedures that use a single quantity include:

- Incision and drainage (I&D)
  - For example: **10140 Incision and drainage of hematoma, seroma or fluid collection**
- Some nail procedures
  - For example: **11760 Repair of nail bed**

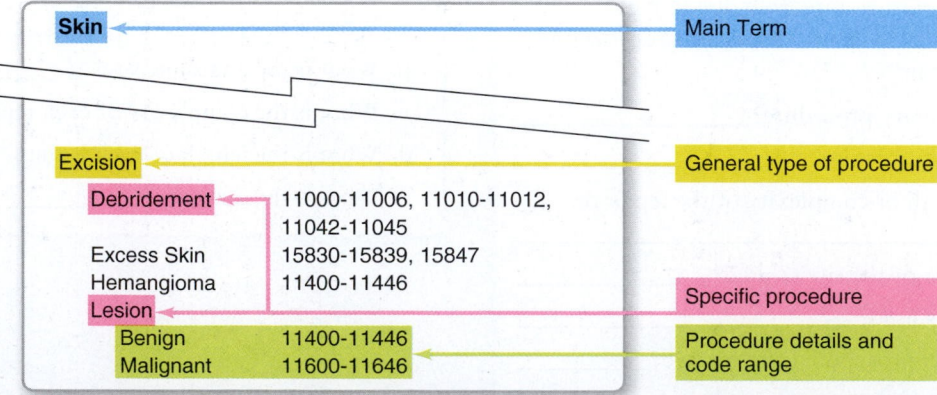

Figure 34-3 ■ CPT Index entry for the Main Term "Skin." *Source: © PB Resources, Inc. Used with permission. CPT codes only © American Medical Association.*

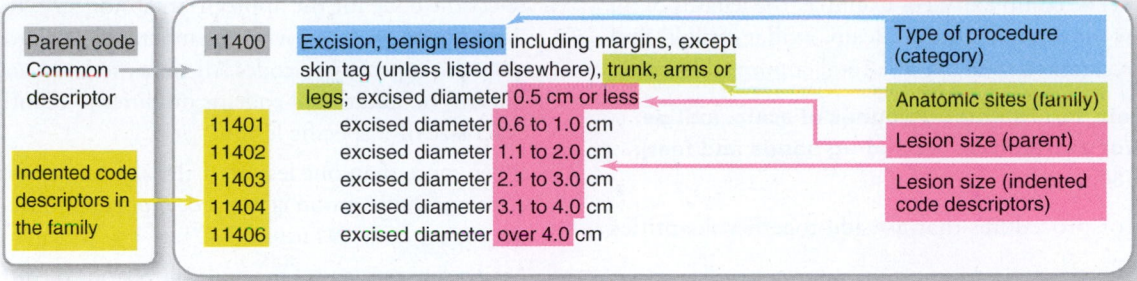

Figure 34-4 ■ Example of a code family in the Integumentary System subsection. *Source: Formatting © PB Resources, Inc. Used with permission. CPT codes only © American Medical Association.*

For example:

- **11760 Repair of nail bed**
- **10140 Incision and drainage of hematoma, seroma or fluid collection**

Single Quantity By Size and/or Site

Single quantity codes can be divided by size and/or site. Each code identifies a quantity of one, and separate codes identify different anatomic sites and/or sizes.

For example:

- **11601 Excision, malignant lesion including margins, trunk, arms, or legs; excised diameter 0.6 to 1.0 cm**
- **11621 Excision, malignant lesion including margins, scalp, neck, hands, feet, genitalia; excised diameter 0.6 to 1.0 cm**

Anatomic sites are grouped together based on the difficulty of treating the area. For example, the trunk, arms, and legs are often grouped together. Sizes or areas are reported in ranges. For example, lesions ranging in size from 0.6 to 1.0 cm are grouped together by site. Lesions of the same anatomic group and size range can be coded with multiple units. Categories of skin procedures that use a single quantity by size and site include:

- Shaving of epidermal or dermal lesions
- Excision of benign and malignant lesions
- Destruction of malignant lesions
- Some nail procedures

Details on assigning codes for lesions using this type of quantity are discussed later in this chapter.

Multiple Quantity Ranges

A code family can be organized to report quantities of more than one for a particular procedure. Each code in the family reports a different quantity or range. Coders must read all the code descriptions in the code family to determine the correct range to use. For example:

- **11720 Debridement of nail(s) by any method(s); 1 to 5**
- **11721 Debridement of nail(s) by any method(s); 6 or more**

Select the code that identifies the quantity of the service performed. Categories of procedures that use a multiple quantity with add-ons include:

- Debridement of nails
- Paring or cutting
- Incision and drainage

Multiple Quantity, Base Quantity with Add-on Quantities

Some code families provide a standalone code that identifies a base quantity followed by one or more add-on codes that identify additional quantities. Report one unit of the base code and as many units of the add-on code as necessary to report the rest of the service. Categories of procedures that use a multiple quantity with add-ons include:

- Destruction of benign or premalignant lesions
- Removal of skin tags
- Tissue transfer and replacement

In the example in ■ Figure 34-5, codes for skin tag removal include all methods, so the 33 lesions can be combined for coding purposes. Report **11200** for the first 15 lesions, leaving 18 lesions. Each unit of **11201** reports up to 10 lesions, so the first unit reports the 16th to 25th lesions; the second unit reports the 26th to 33rd lesions. Do not append modifier **–51** to code **11201** because it is an add-on code.

Add-Together Quantities

Procedures that involve measurement of length and area require that multiple measurements be added together. Sum the measurement of areas in the same anatomic grouping and

---

Physician removes 10 skin tags using electrosurgical destruction and 23 skin tags using chemical destruction, for a total of 33.

11200 Removal of skin tags, multiple fibrocutaneous tags, any area; up to and including 15 lesions

11201 × 2 Removal of skin tags, multiple fibrocutaneous tags, any area; each additional 10 lesions, or part thereof (List separately in addition to code for primary procedure)

Figure 34-5 ■ Example of coding multiple quantities.

of the same level of complexity. For example, the lengths of all intermediate wound repairs on the scalp, axillae, trunk, and extremities are summed to arrive at a total combined length:

- **12036 Repair, intermediate, wounds of scalp, axillae, trunk and/or extremities (excluding hands and feet); 20.1 cm to 30.0 cm**

Categories of procedures that use add-together quantities include:

- Wound repair
- Skin replacement surgery
- Adjacent tissue transfer or rearrangement
- Skin flaps
- Burns, local treatment

Details about how to assign codes for these types of procedures are discussed later in this chapter.

> ### SUCCESS STEP
>
> Annotate your CPT coding manual to help yourself navigate the extensive list of parent and indented code families. In each parent code description, highlight the anatomic sites included. In each indented description, highlight the size. Highlight *selected* words within each description, rather than the entire description, so it is easier to identify the differences. This helps you code faster and more accurately.

Lesion Removal

To assign codes for lesion removal, you need to determine the following criteria:

- Method of removal
- Whether the lesion is benign, premalignant, or malignant
- Anatomic site
- Size

To locate codes in the Index, search for the Main Term **Skin**; the first-level modifying term for the method used, such as **Destruction**, **Excision**, **Shaving**, **Paring**, or **Removal**; and additional modifying terms, if necessary, for the type of lesion. The modifying term **Removal** is used for skin tags. Identify the code range and turn to the Tabular List to select and verify the code(s).

The Tabular List provides detailed special instructions at the beginning of categories for lesion removal. Take time to read and understand these definitions and instructions. To select a code in the Tabular List, follow these steps.

1. Confirm that you have the correct category based on the method of removal, type of lesion, and benign or malignant status.
2. Review the parent codes in the code families to identify the correct anatomic group. Lesion sites are grouped into three code families: (1) trunk, arms, and legs; (2) sites on the face; (3) scalp, neck, hands, feet, and genitalia (■ FIGURE 34-6).

3. Select the code for the appropriate lesion size. Read the size options provided with the indented codes to determine the appropriate code. All sizes are given as a range. There is no additional code or modifier to identify the exact size of a specific lesion.
4. When more than one lesion of the same size range in the same anatomic group is excised, report a multiple quantity for the code (■ FIGURE 34-7).
5. Assign separate codes for multiple lesions of different sizes or different anatomic groups.

A physician measures the size of the lesion before removing it. In excisions, size is determined by the diameter of the lesion itself plus the most narrow margin (*healthy tissue around the lesion*) required to adequately excise it, based on the physician's judgment (■ FIGURE 34-8). Adequate margins are necessary to prevent regrowth of the lesion and are especially important with malignant lesions. Lesion measurements are reported in centimeters.

The global surgical package concept applies to codes for lesion removal. Codes for shaving of epidermal and dermal lesions have a postoperative global period of zero days. Codes for removal of skin tags and excision of lesions and most codes for destruction of a lesion have a 10-day postoperative global period. Destruction of cutaneous vascular proliferative lesions (**17103-17108**) has a 90-day global period. Local anesthesia and simple, non-layered closure of the operative wound is included in the code. Do not assign additional codes for these bundled services. When a wound resulting from an excision requires an intermediate or complex closure, assign an additional code for the repair. Repair codes are discussed later in this section of the chapter.

When the physician uses electrocautery to remove the entire lesion, do not assign a code for shaving. Instead, assign a code for destruction of a lesion (**17000–17250**). Shaving does not require suture closure of the wound.

> ### SUCCESS STEP
>
> All parent codes for anatomic groupings have indented codes for similar sizes, so do not look only for the size. Identify the correct anatomic code family *first*, then select the code for lesion size.

Mohs Micrographic Surgery

To assign codes for Mohs, search the Index for the Main Term **Mohs Micrographic Surgery**, then refer to the code range in the Tabular List. To select codes in the Tabular List, determine the number of blocks (*each division of the tissue*) and stages (*each phase of excision*) involved in the procedure.

The code category includes special instructions that define the process and five codes. The two parent codes (**17311** and **17313**) are divided based on anatomic site and include up to five tissue blocks. The *first* stage of excision is described by the parent code. Each *additional* stage is reported with add-on codes (**17312** and **17314**). When more than five tissue blocks are examined, report add-on code **17315** for each additional block.

The procedure is no longer Mohs when either function of surgeon or pathologist is delegated to a physician who reports codes separately. Do not assign codes for Mohs surgery in this case.

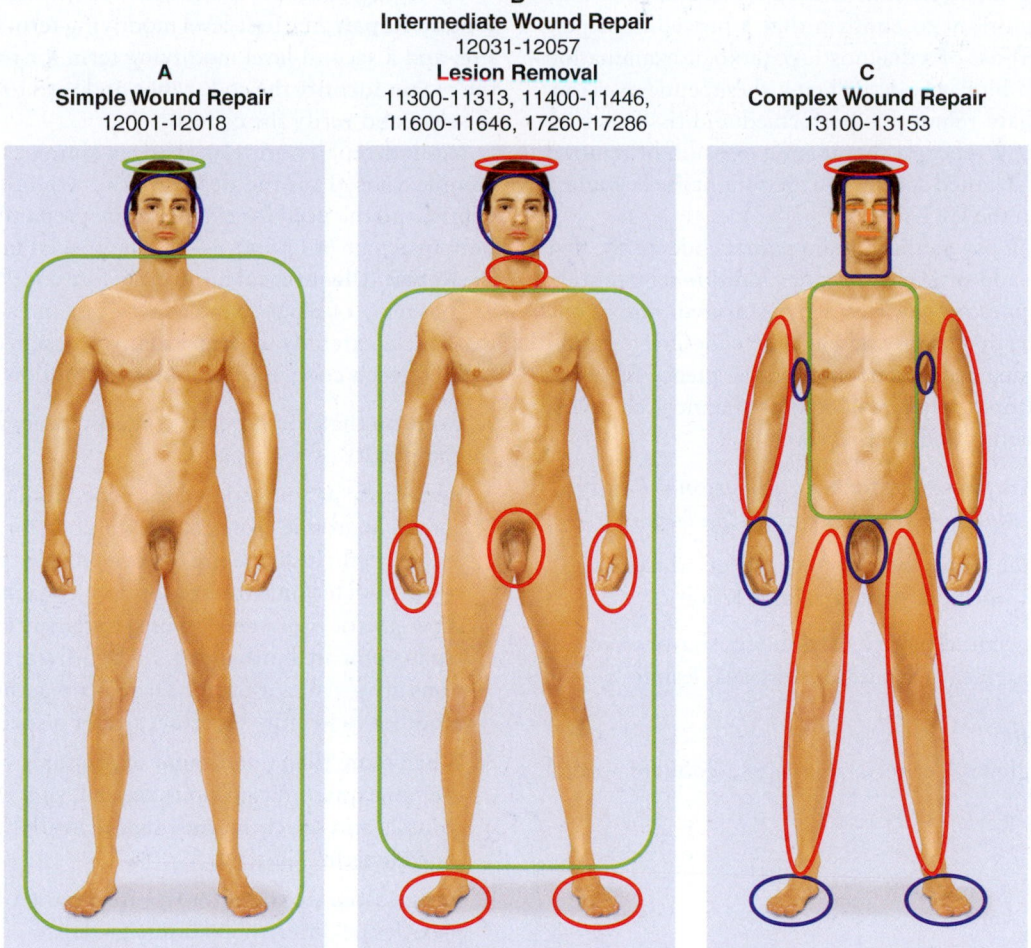

A
Simple Wound Repair
12001-12018

B
Intermediate Wound Repair
12031-12057
Lesion Removal
11300-11313, 11400-11446,
11600-11646, 17260-17286

C
Complex Wound Repair
13100-13153

Figure 34-6 ■ Code families for lesion removal and wound repair.

Biopsy

A biopsy is a procedure performed to obtain tissue solely for diagnostic purposes and sent to a laboratory for histopathologic examination. To assign codes **11102-11107**, the procedure must be distinct and separate from other services. Biopsies performed on distinct lesions or different sites on the same date of service can be reported separately.

CPT provides codes for three types of biopsies:

- **Tangential biopsy**—Performed with a sharp blade, oblique scalpel, or curette to remove a sample of the epidermis with or without the underlying dermis. It is a superficial sample and does not remove any underlying lesion in deeper tissues. A tangential biopsy can be described as *shave, scoop, saucerize,* or *curettage*. When shave removal is performed with a therapeutic intent to remove the lesion, use codes **11300-11313**.

- **Punch biopsy**—Requires a punch tool to remove a full-thickness cylindrical tissue sample. The codes include simple closure.

- **Incisional biopsy**—Requires the use of a sharp blade, other than a punch tool, to remove a full-thickness sample of tissue. The surgeon makes a vertical incision or wedge and penetrates deep into the subcutaneous tissue. The codes include simple closure.

Physician excises the two benign lesions, one of 0.75 cm from the right arm and one of 1.0 cm from the right leg.

11401-51 × 2 Excision, benign lesion including margins, except skin tag (unless listed elsewhere), trunk, arms or legs; excised diameter 0.6 to 1.0 cm

Figure 34-7 ■ Example of coding excision of a lesion.

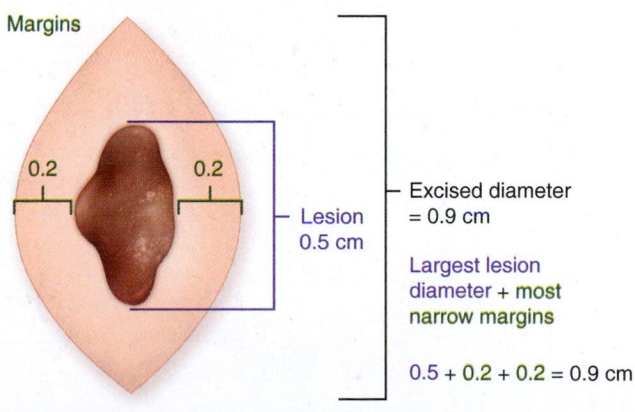

Margins

0.2   0.2

Lesion 0.5 cm

Excised diameter = 0.9 cm

Largest lesion diameter + most narrow margins

0.5 + 0.2 + 0.2 = 0.9 cm

Figure 34-8 ■ How to calculate lesion size.

Similar cutting methods can be used for therapeutic purposes, so it is important to confirm that a procedure is performed for the purpose of a diagnostic pathologic examination before assigning a biopsy code. When a therapeutic excision, destruction, or shave removal is performed and tissue is submitted to pathology, report a therapeutic excision or removal code. Refer to the detailed special instructions at the beginning of this category in the CPT manual.

Each of these biopsy methods has a parent code for the first procedure and an add-on code to report additional quantities. When different types of biopsies are performed, report one parent code for the first biopsy and add-on codes for the additional biopsies using a different method. Sequence the most complex method first, with incisional as the most complex, followed by tangential, and, lastly, punch.

> EXAMPLE: *A surgeon performs an incisional biopsy and two tangential biopsies of separate skin lesions.*
>
> 11106 Incisional biopsy of skin (eg, wedge) (including simple closure, when performed); single lesion
>
> 11103 × 2 Tangential biopsy of skin (eg, shave, scoop, saucerize, curette); each separate/additional lesion

Wound Repair

Determine the following criteria to assign a code for wound repair:

- Anatomic site
- Complexity of the repair
- Length

To locate codes in the Index, search for the Main Term **Wound Repair**, the first-level modifying term for the anatomic site, and a second-level modifying term for the complexity of the repair. Identify the code range and turn to the Tabular List to select and verify the code(s).

Wound repairs are classified as simple, intermediate, or complex based on the depth of the wound, the amount of debris, and the need for extensive site preparation, reconstruction, or repair (■ FIGURE 34-9). The special instructions under the **Repair (Closure)** subheading, before code **12001**, define the various types of repair, bundled services, and additional coding. Read these carefully to ensure that you assign codes accurately.

To select a code in the Tabular List, follow these steps.

1. Confirm that you have the correct category based on the complexity of the repair.

2. Review the parent codes in the code families to identify the correct anatomic group. Select the code for the appropriate lesion length. Read the size options provided with the indented codes to determine the appropriate code. ■ FIGURE 34-10 shows metric measurements used to classify lengths of wound repair compared to an adult's arm. All sizes in code descriptions are given as a range. There is no additional code or modifier to identify the exact size of a specific wound.

3. When more than one wound of the same complexity in the same anatomic group is excised, sum the lengths of all wounds and select the code that identifies the total combined length.

4. Assign separate codes for wound repairs of different complexities or different anatomic groups.

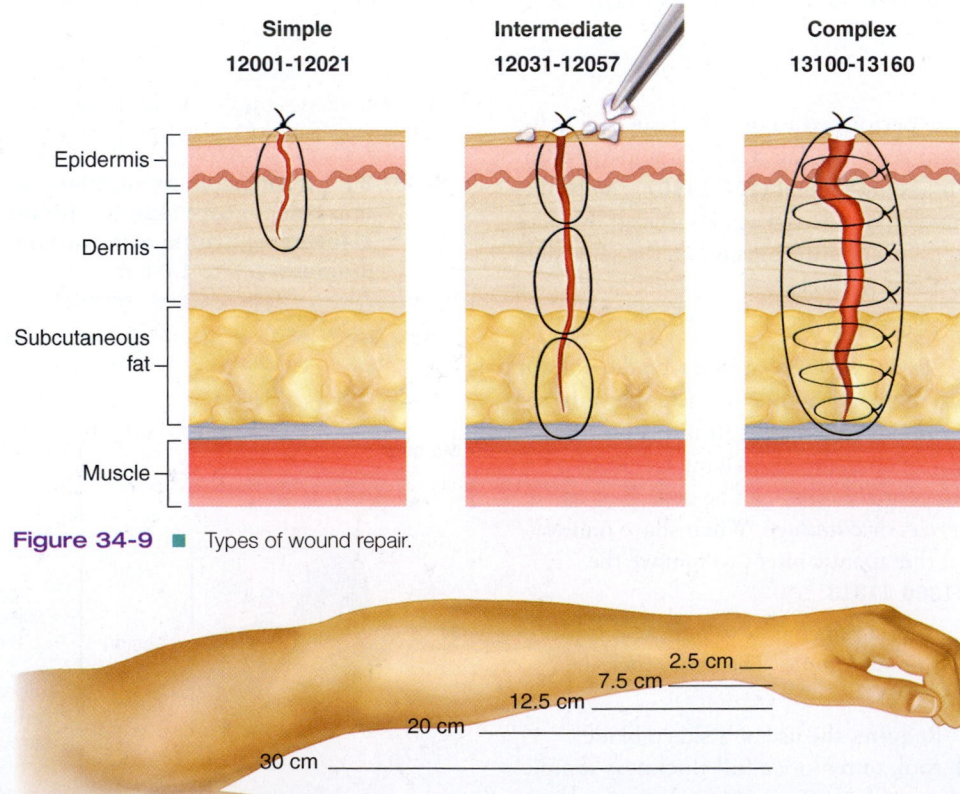

Figure 34-9 ■ Types of wound repair.

Figure 34-10 ■ Approximate lengths relative to an adult arm.

The anatomic sites for wound repair codes are different for each type of repair. Read the parent code of each code family within the category to determine how the sites are grouped:

- Simple repair—Two code families: (1) all sites except the face and (2) sites on the face (see Figure 34-6A)

- Intermediate repair—Three code families: (1) trunk, arms, and legs; (2) sites on the face; and (3) scalp, neck, hands, feet, and genitalia (see Figure 34-6B)

- Complex repair—Four code families: (1) trunk; (2) scalp, arms, and legs; (3) forehead, cheeks, chin, mouth, neck, axillae, genitalia, hands, and feet; and (4) eyes, nose, mouth, and ears (see Figure 34-6C)

In the example in ■ FIGURE 34-11, the two intermediate repairs occur within the same anatomic group (scalp, axillae, trunk, and/or extremities), so the lengths of the wounds are added together (7.5 + 8.0 = 15.5) to arrive at the correct code, **12035**.

If either wound were coded alone as the only repair, the codes would be as follows:

- For the 7.5-cm wound on the right arm: **12032 Repair, intermediate, wounds of scalp, axillae, trunk and/or extremities (excluding hands and feet); 2.6 cm to 7.5 cm**

- For the 8.0-cm wound on the right leg: **12034 Repair, intermediate, wounds of scalp, axillae, trunk and/or extremities (excluding hands and feet); 7.6 cm to 12.5 cm**

Do not report the two codes separately when the procedures are performed at the same time because CPT special instructions state: **When multiple wounds are repaired, add together the lengths of those in the same classification (see above) and from all anatomic sites that are grouped together into the same code descriptor.**

Do not combine repairs of different complexity, such as a simple repair and an intermediate repair, and do not combine repairs of different anatomic groupings, such as an intermediate repair of the trunk and an intermediate repair of the face.

The global surgical package concept applies to codes for wound repair, which have a 10-day postoperative global period. Local anesthesia is included in the code.

Simple closure of operative wounds for excision of lesions is included in the lesion removal. When a wound resulting from an excision requires an intermediate or complex closure, assign a code for the repair in addition to the code for the lesion removal.

Breast Procedures

Breast procedures include biopsy, cyst and lesion excision, mastectomy, repair, and reconstruction. To assign codes, locate the Main Term **Breast** in the Index, then locate the first-level modifying term for the type of procedure. Second-level modifying

terms identify details of the procedure and provide the code(s) or code range.

The Breast subheading in the Tabular List provides special instructions for the **Excision** and **Introduction** categories. The **Excision** instructions also provide guidelines for **Mastectomy**, even though it is a separate category.

Biopsy procedures can be percutaneous or open (incisional) and with or without imaging guidance. Imaging guidance modalities include stereotactic mammography (*specialized mammography imaging from two angles at the same time*), ultrasound (US), and magnetic resonance imaging (MRI). In addition, a localization device such as a clip, wire, or metallic pellet can be placed in conjunction with a biopsy or as a separate procedure. Imaging is also used for placement of a localization device. The localization device guides the surgeon to the site of the tumor during surgery performed at a later time.

Biopsy and introduction codes are divided based on the type of imaging guidance used. When more than one site is biopsied or more than one device placed, the parent code identifies the first lesion, and an add-on code is assigned for each additional lesion.

Mastectomy codes are divided based on the extent of tissue removed, so coders must read the details of the operative note and identify the specific structures affected. The types of mastectomy are:

- Lumpectomy or partial mastectomy (**19301**)—Part of the breast

- Partial mastectomy and lymphadenectomy (**19302**)—Part of the breast and axillary lymph nodes (■ FIGURE 34-12A, page 676)

- Simple mastectomy, complete (**19303**)—The entire breast, including skin (Figure 34-12B, page 676)

- Subcutaneous mastectomy (**19304**)—The breast tissue under the skin but not the skin itself (Figure 34-12C, page 676)

- Modified radical mastectomy (**19307**)—The breast, pectoralis minor (but not pectoralis major) muscle, and axillary lymph nodes (Figure 34-12D, page 676)

- Radical mastectomy (**19305**)—The breast, pectoralis major and minor muscles, and axillary lymph nodes

- Radical mastectomy (Urban-type operation) (**19306**)—The breast, pectoralis major and minor muscles, axillary lymph nodes, and internal mammary lymph nodes (Figure 34-12D, page 676)

Repair and reconstruction codes are divided based on the type of reconstructive technique and type of flap. Refer to the documentation to identify the technique used, then select the corresponding code.

Mastectomy codes are unilateral, so when the same type of procedure is performed on both breasts, assign modifier **-50 Bilateral procedure**. When a different type of mastectomy is performed on each breast, assign the appropriate code for each side with the modifier **-RT** or **-LT** to identify the laterality.

Skin Replacements

CPT provides separate coding paths for various types of skin replacement procedures. To assign codes for adjacent tissue transfers, search the Index for the Main Term **Skin** and the

---

> Physician performs intermediate repair of two wounds: 7.5 cm on the right arm and 8 cm on the right leg.
>
> **12035 Repair, intermediate, wounds of scalp, axillae, trunk and/or extremities (excluding hands and feet); 12.6 cm to 20.0 cm**

Figure 34-11 ■ Example of adding together repair lengths.

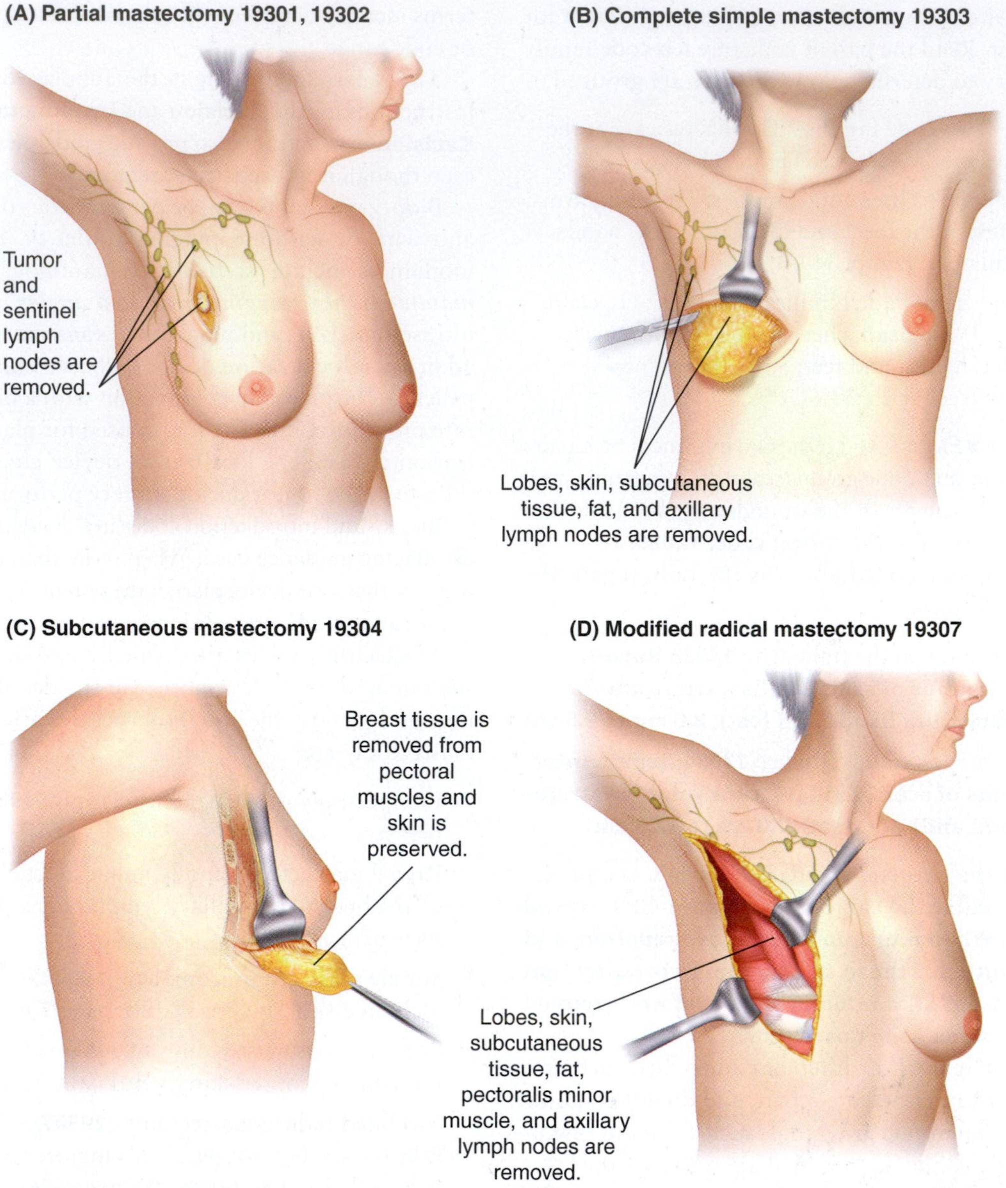

(A) Partial mastectomy 19301, 19302

Tumor and sentinel lymph nodes are removed.

(B) Complete simple mastectomy 19303

Lobes, skin, subcutaneous tissue, fat, and axillary lymph nodes are removed.

(C) Subcutaneous mastectomy 19304

Breast tissue is removed from pectoral muscles and skin is preserved.

(D) Modified radical mastectomy 19307

Lobes, skin, subcutaneous tissue, fat, pectoralis minor muscle, and axillary lymph nodes are removed.

Figure 34-12 ■ Types of mastectomy procedures.

first-level modifying term **Adjacent tissue transfer**. One code range is provided, so turn to the Tabular List to select and verify the code. Codes are divided into code families by anatomic site, then are arranged by size within the site. The size identifies the area of the defect. Adjacent tissue transfers include lesion excisions, so do not report them separately. Adjacent tissue transfers include simple repair; however, when the physician performs intermediate or complex repair, report the repair separately, in addition to the tissue transfer.

To assign codes for skin grafts and flaps, search the Index for the Main Term **Skin Graft and Flap**, which is a separate Main Term entry after **Skin**. Locate the first-level modifying term for the type of graft or flap. The Tabular List provides extensive special instructions for this category, which includes codes **15002** through **15278**. The special instructions define the terminology necessary for code selection and identify procedures that are bundled and those that are coded separately. Codes are divided by the type of graft, such as epidermal, dermal, split thickness, full thickness, and tissue culture, then by

anatomic site and size. Many of the code families for anatomic site provide a parent code for a specific area, such as 25 or 100 sq cm, and an add-on code for each additional unit of the same size. The parent code has a higher RVU than the add-on codes.

To assign codes for skin substitute grafts, search the Index for the Main Term **Skin Substitute Graft**, which is a separate Main Term entry after the entries for **Skin** and **Skin Graft and Flap**. Locate the first-level modifying term for the anatomic site. The Tabular List special instructions at the beginning of the category **Skin Replacement Surgery** apply to the subcategory for **Skin Substitute Grafts**. Codes are divided by anatomic site and size. Many of the code families for anatomic site provide a parent code for a specific area, such as 100 sq cm, and an add-on code for each additional unit of the same size. Coding instructions state that the areas listed in code descriptors identify the recipient site, not the donor site.

Codes are provided for surgical preparation or creation of a recipient site—which involves cleaning the site and ensuring that the surface is appropriate for repair of the defect—for a graft, flap, skin replacement, or skin substitute (**15002–15005**). Do not report codes **15002–15005** for surgical preparation and debridement of a wound left to heal by secondary intention because it is a wound without surgical closure that heals on its own. Instead, report wound management or debridement codes.

When the physician must repair a donor site with a skin graft or local flap, assign one code for the recipient site procedure and an additional code for the donor site repair.

Guided Example of Assigning Integumentary System Procedure Codes

To practice skills for assigning codes for the Integumentary System subsection, continue with the example from earlier in the chapter about a patient who was seen for a pressure ulcer. Follow along in your CPT manual as Joshua Grider, CPC, assigns codes. Check off each step after you complete it.

▶ First, Joshua confirms the procedures, Excision of pressure ulcer with ischiectomy and myocutaneous graft closure, 30 sq cm.

❏ He is not sure if he needs three codes—one for the pressure ulcer excision, one for the ischiectomy, and one for the skin graft closure—or if one or more procedures might be reported with a combination code.

❏ He needs to look up each procedure in the Index to learn how the codes are structured.

▶ Joshua searches the Index for the Main Term **Pressure**.

❏ He locates the first-level modifying term **Ulcer (Decubitus)**.

❏ He locates the third-level modifying term for the procedure, **Excision**.

❏ He locates the third-level modifying term for the site, **Ischial**.

❏ He identifies the code ranges **15940-15941, 15944-15946**.

▶ Joshua locates codes **15940-15941, 15944-15946** in the Tabular List.

❏ He reads the category title **Pressure Ulcers (Decubitus Ulcers)** to confirm that he is in the location he would expect.

❏ He reviews the range of five contiguous codes. All codes begin with the words **Excision, ischial pressure ulcer**, which describes the procedure performed, excision of pressure ulcer, so he needs to determine the differences among them.

❏ He observes that codes **15940** and **15944** are parent codes, each with an indented code, **15941** and **15945**, respectively, that states **with ostectomy (ischiectomy)**. Code **15946** is a standalone code that also includes **with ostectomy**.

❏ The procedure he is coding includes with ischiectomy and 1 cm of the ischium was excised. He must read the remaining portion of the code descriptions to select the most appropriate code.

❏ To determine the difference between codes **15941** and **15945**, he knows that he must refer to the common

descriptor in each parent code because it also applies to the indented code. He identifies that the difference between the parent codes is the nature of the wound closure. Code **15940** describes **with primary suture** and code **15944** describes **with skin flap closure**. He thinks this might be the right code, but knows he should also check code **15946**.

❏ The description for code **15946** states **in preparation for muscle or myocutaneous flap or skin graft closure**.

❏ He refers to the documentation to verify the nature of the closure. The documentation states a myocutaneous flap was created.

❏ He rereads the code title for **15946 Excision, ischial pressure ulcer, with ostectomy, in preparation for muscle or myocutaneous flap or skin graft closure** and confirms that this accurately describes the procedure.

▶ Joshua checks for instructions in the Tabular List.

❏ Under code **15946** he reads the special instructions that state: (**For repair of defect using muscle or myocutaneous flap, use code(s) 15734 and/or 15738 in addition to 15946.**) This information provides an answer to Joshua's question about how many codes are needed by telling him to assign an additional code for the myocutaneous flap.

❏ He locates codes **15734** and **15738** in the Tabular List and notices they are indented codes. He reads the unique descriptor in the parent code **15733 Muscle, myocutaneous, or fasciocutaneous flap;** and determines that it accurately describes the base procedure.

❏ He identifies that the indented codes identify alternate sites but is unsure whether the sites refer to the donor site or the recipient site. He reads the special instructions at the beginning of the category **Flaps (Skin and/or Deep Tissues)**. The instructions provide guidance for a variety of situations, and he locates the statement that applies to the code family he needs to use: **Codes 15733-15738 are described by donor site of the muscle, myocutaneous, or fasciocutaneous flap.**

❏ The special instructions confirm that he should select the indented code that identifies the donor site, which, according to the documentation, is the abdomen. He reviews the indented codes again and selects code **15734 Muscle, myocutaneous, or fasciocutaneous flap; trunk**. The abdomen is located on the trunk and there is not a code specifically for the abdomen.

❏ He rereads the special instructions and notices a comment about repair of the donor site: **A repair of a donor site requiring a skin graft or local flaps is considered an additional separate procedure.** He checks the documentation and identifies: The donor site … was closed with an adjacent transfer rotational flap.

❏ Because the donor site was closed with a local flap, he needs to assign an additional code. Instructional notes below the special instructions provide a cross-reference: **(For adjacent tissue transfer flaps, see 14000-14302)**.

▶ Joshua needs to assign a code for the adjacent transfer rotational flap at the donor site.

❑ He locates codes **14000-14302** and reviews how they are organized. He identifies several pairs of parent codes and indented codes. He determines that the parent codes are divided by anatomic site and the indented codes are divided by defect size.

❑ He identifies that the common descriptor in parent code **14000** includes the trunk: **Adjacent tissue transfer or rearrangement, trunk;**. The area defined by **14000** is a **defect 10 sq cm or less** and the area defined by the indented code **14001** is a **defect 10.1 sq cm to 30.0 sq cm**.

❑ He refers to the documentation to verify the size of the defect, which is 5 cm by 6 cm, needing a 30-sq cm repair. This information points to code **14001** because it includes the appropriate area.

❑ Joshua reads the special instructions for the category **Adjacent Tissue Transfer or Rearrangement**. He reads the last paragraph that begins with the statement **Skin graft necessary to close secondary defect is considered an additional procedure**. As he reads the rest of the paragraph, he learns that he might have incorrectly determined the size of the defect area. He had previously identified the size of the defect at the recipient site, but the special instructions state that he should determine the area of the secondary, or donor, site and that the measurement includes the size of the defect *plus* the size of the transfer necessary to repair it.

❑ He refers to the documentation again and locates the measurements of the secondary (donor) site: The donor site, measuring 30 sq cm, was closed with an adjacent transfer rotational flap of 32 sq cm. The secondary defect is 30 sq cm and the transfer necessary to repair it is 32 sq cm, for a total of 62 sq cm. Now he must determine how to code the new size of the repair.

❑ When he rereads code **14001**, he determines that this code is no longer appropriate because it describes a **defect 10.1 sq cm to 30.0 sq cm**. Because it does not say *each additional 30.0 sq cm*, he knows that he cannot report multiple units of this code, such as ×2 or ×3.

❑ He reviews all the codes in the category **14000-14350** to look for possible add-on codes.

❑ He locates code **14301 Adjacent tissue transfer or rearrangement, any area; defect 30.1 sq cm to 60.0 sq cm**. He recognizes that this code is used to report an ATT larger than the 30 sq cm allowed by code **14001**. However, the total secondary defect is 62 sq cm, so he still needs an additional code.

❑ He identifies the add-on code **14302 Adjacent tissue transfer or rearrangement, any area; each additional 30.0 sq cm, or part thereof** and the instructional note that follows: **(Use 14302 in conjunction with 14301)**. This instructional note directs him to report code **14302** for the **additional 30 sq cm** with code **14301**, *not* code **14002**.

❑ He reviews all the code descriptions, special instructions, and instructional notes again and is confident he has selected the appropriate codes.

▶ Joshua reviews the procedure codes he has assigned for this case.

❑ **14301 Adjacent tissue transfer or rearrangement, any area; defect 30.1 sq cm to 60.0 sq cm**

❑ **14302 Adjacent tissue transfer or rearrangement, any area; each additional 30.0 sq cm, or part thereof (List separately in addition to code for primary procedure)**

❑ **15946 Excision, ischial pressure ulcer, with ostectomy, in preparation for muscle or myocutaneous flap or skin graft closure**

❑ **15734 Muscle, myocutaneous, or fasciocutaneous flap; trunk**

▶ Next, Joshua must determine how to sequence the codes.

CODING PRACTICE

Exercise 34.3 Assigning Codes for Integumentary System Procedures

Instructions: Read the mini-medical-record of each patient's encounter. Review the information abstracted in Exercise 34.2 for questions 1–3. For questions 4–6, abstract the case on your own. Assign CPT codes, quantities, and modifiers using the Index and Tabular List. Write the code(s) on the line provided.

1. OFFICE   Gender: F   Age: 39

Preprocedure diagnosis: Rough scaly lesions on arms, face, and neck

Procedure: Surgical curettement of 20 lesions ranging in size from 2–6 mm

Pathology report: Premalignant actinic keratoses

Postprocedure diagnosis: Premalignant actinic keratoses

1 CPT Code _____

CODING PRACTICE *(continued)*

2. INPATIENT HOSPITAL Gender: M Age: 26

Preprocedure diagnosis: Multiple second-degree burns nearly covering both lower legs and feet

Procedure: Removed blisters, debrided necrotic tissue, and applied dressings

Postprocedure diagnosis: Leg burns, 21% TBSA second-degree

1 CPT Code _____

---

3. INPATIENT HOSPITAL Gender: F Age: 35

Diagnosis: Facial nerve paralysis from Bell's palsy

Procedure: Harvested a fascia lata (*deep thigh*) free graft from right leg and applied to face to restore facial nerve function. Defect area 20 sq cm

1 CPT Code _____

---

4. OUTPATIENT SURGERY Gender: M Age: 4

Preprocedure diagnosis: Wound, right thigh

Procedure: Applied acellular dermal replacement on the right thigh as a temporary repair. Defect was measured and consists of 1% of the patient's body area

(continued)

---

4. *(continued)*

Postprocedure diagnosis: Wound, to heal by secondary intention, RTO 1 week

1 CPT Code _____

---

5. OFFICE Gender: M Age: 16

Diagnosis: Acne

Procedure: Chemical exfoliation (*peeling off layers of skin*). Applied salicylic acid over the acne with a cotton-tipped swab, let rest for a few seconds to desquamate (*peel off*) the acne. Treatment was successful.

1 CPT Code _____

---

6. OFFICE Gender: F Age: 55

Preprocedure diagnosis: Breast reconstruction following a left breast mastectomy

Procedure: Tattooed nipples on both breasts, total area of 15 sq cm

1 CPT Code _____

ARRANGING CODES FOR INTEGUMENTARY SYSTEM PROCEDURES

Multiple coding is common for Integumentary System procedures because more than one lesion removal or wound repair often is performed at the same time. Multiple procedures can be identified by reporting multiple quantities of one code, using add-on codes, using additional standalone codes, and/or appending modifier(s). Read code descriptions carefully to determine which method should be used with any specific code. Although codes are usually arranged (sequenced) based on complexity, or RVU value, the process is not as intuitive as it might be with other types of procedures.

Sequencing Excision of Lesion Codes

The complexity of Integumentary System subsection procedures is affected both by the size of the lesion or defect and by the anatomic site. For lesions of differing sizes but the same anatomic code family, excision of the larger lesion always has a higher RVU. For lesions of the same size but different anatomic code families, excision of lesions of the trunk, arm, or legs has the lowest RVU; excision of lesions of the scalp, neck, hands, and feet has the next highest RVU; and excision of lesions of the face, ears, eyelids, mouth, lips, and mucous membrane has the highest RVU. Excision of a malignant lesion has a higher RVU than excision of a benign lesion of the same size and same anatomic site. However, when lesions are different sizes and of different anatomic code families, no general rule applies.

Identify the quantity as **× 2** when two procedures are performed and both are described by the same code.

EXAMPLE: *Excision of benign lesions, 0.6 cm on the arm and 0.75 cm on the leg:* **11401 × 2**

Append modifier **-51 Multiple procedures** to the second and subsequent codes (■ FIGURE 34-13, page 680). The lesions of the right arm and right leg are identified by the same code, so two units of code **11401** are reported. Sequence codes in descending RVU order. Append modifier **-51** to the second and third codes.

CODING CAUTION

Add together the lengths of similar repairs or the areas of similar grafts, but *do not* add together the diameters of multiple excised lesions. Report each lesion separately.

Physician excises the following benign lesions: 0.3 from the trunk; 0.75 from the right arm; 1.0 from the right leg; and 0.5 from the neck.

11420 Excision, benign lesion including margins, except skin tag (unless listed elsewhere), scalp, **neck**, hands, feet, genitalia; excised diameter **0.5 cm or less** (Facility RVU 3.14)

11401-51 × 2 Excision, benign lesion including margins, except skin tag (unless listed elsewhere), trunk, **arms or legs**; excised diameter **0.6 to 1.0 cm** (Facility RVU 2.93)

11400-51 Excision, benign lesion including margins, except skin tag (unless listed elsewhere), **trunk**, arms or legs; excised diameter **0.5 cm or less** (Facility RVU 2.25)

Figure 34-13 ■ Example of sequencing codes for excision of lesions. *Source:* © *PB Resources, Inc. Used with permission. CPT codes only* © *American Medical Association.*

Physician repairs the following wounds: 3 cm, simple, on the trunk; 7.5 cm, intermediate, on the right arm; 8 cm, intermediate, on the right leg; and 1.5 cm, complex, on the neck.

12035 Repair, **intermediate**, wounds of scalp, axillae, trunk and/or **extremities** (excluding hands and feet); 12.6 cm to 20.0 cm (Facility RVU 6.91)

13100-51 Repair, **complex, neck**; 1.1 cm to 2.5 cm (Facility RVU 5.9)

12002-51 **Simple** repair of superficial wounds of scalp, neck, axillae, external genitalia, **trunk** and/or extremities (including hands and feet); 2.6 cm to 7.5 cm (Facility RVU 1.67)

Figure 34-14 ■ Example of sequencing wound repair codes. *Source:* © *PB Resources, Inc. Used with permission. CPT codes only* © *American Medical Association.*

Sequencing Wound Repair Codes

The RVUs for repair codes are affected by the complexity of the repair, the length, and the anatomic code family. A small complex repair can have a lower RVU value than a longer simple or intermediate repair. No general rule applies, so the Medicare Physician Fee Schedule Database (MPFSDB)—or other payer's source—must be consulted to obtain RVU information.

Compare the facility RVU for the intermediate repair code **12053** for a 5.1- to 7.5-cm wound to complex repair codes for 1.1- to 2.5-cm wounds. Code **12053** for an intermediate repair of 5.1 to 7.5 cm has a *higher* RVU than code **13100** but a *lower* RVU than code **13120**:

- **12053 Repair, intermediate, wounds of face, ears, eyelids, nose, lips and/or mucous membranes; 5.1 cm to 7.5 cm** (6.26 RVU)

- **13100 Repair, complex, trunk; 1.1 cm to 2.5 cm** (5.9 RVU)

- **13120 Repair, complex, scalp, arms, and/or legs; 1.1 cm to 2.5 cm** (6.78 RVU)

After adding together wound repairs of the same anatomic code family and same complexity, sequence codes in descending RVU order. Append modifier **-51 Multiple procedures** to the second and third codes (■ FIGURE 34-14).

Using Modifiers with Integumentary System Codes

Several modifiers are commonly used when coding procedures from the Integumentary System subsection. These include modifier **-25**, which might be used on an E/M code in conjunction with an integumentary system procedure; several laterality and anatomic modifiers; modifier **-51** for multiple procedures; modifier **-58** for staged procedures; and modifier **-59** to identify a separate procedure in certain circumstances. These modifiers are discussed next.

-25 Significant, Separately Identifiable E/M

Removal of lesions is often a relatively simple procedure and may be done when a patient is being seen for another reason, such as an annual physical. When a separately identifiable E/M service is

provided at the same time as lesion removal (or any procedure), assign an E/M code in addition to the procedure. Append modifier **-25 Significant, separately identifiable evaluation and management service by the same physician or other qualified health care professional on the same day of the procedure or other service** to the E/M code only. Do not apply the modifier to the procedure code. The modifier informs the payer that the E/M is a separate service that should be paid. To use this modifier, the E/M service should be a separate and significant workup, in addition to the evaluation of the lesion (■ FIGURE 34-15).

Laterality Modifiers

Because the skin is not a bilateral organ, do not use modifiers **-50 Bilateral procedure**, **-RT Right**, and **-LT**, except on the breast.

> EXAMPLE: *Mastotomy of the left breast with drainage of an abscess, deep:* **19020-LT**

> EXAMPLE: *Simple repair of a 2.5-cm laceration on the left cheek:* **12011**

Use HCPCS Level II modifiers **FA-F9** for the fingernails, but not for the skin on the fingers; use modifiers **TA-T9** for the toenails, but not for the skin on the toes.

> EXAMPLE: *Evacuation of a subungual hematoma on the right great toe:* **11740-T5**

> EXAMPLE: *Shaving of an epidermal lesion on the right great toe:* **11300**

-51 Multiple Procedures

Use modifier **-51 Multiple procedures** when two different procedures are performed on the same date by the same provider. Append **-51** to the second procedure only.

> EXAMPLE: *Excision of benign lesions, 0.6 cm on arm and 1.5 cm on leg:* **11402, 11401-51**

-58 Staged Procedure

A staged procedure is one that is usually planned in advance to be performed during the postoperative period of another related procedure. The staged procedure may be planned or anticipated, be more extensive than the original procedure, or represent a therapy following the original surgical procedure. Modifier **-58 Staged or related procedure or service by the**

A 37 year old male patient is seen for an annual physical. During the examination, the patient asks about a dark spot on the neck that "comes and goes." The physician identifies the lesion as benign seborrheic keratosis, removes it using cryotherapy, and instructs the patient that if it returns, they should shave it.

99395-25 Periodic comprehensive preventive medicine reevaluation and management of an individual including an age and gender appropriate history, examination, counseling/anticipatory guidance/risk factor reduction interventions, and the ordering of laboratory/diagnostic procedures, established patient; 18-39 years; -25 Significant, separately identifiable evaluation and management service

17110 Destruction (eg, laser surgery, electrosurgery, cryosurgery, chemosurgery, surgical curettement), of benign lesions other than skin tags or cutaneous vascular proliferative lesions; up to 14 lesions

Figure 34-15 ■ Example of using modifier -25 with the Integumentary System subsection.

same physician or other qualified health care professional during the postoperative period alerts the payer that the second procedure was performed as part of the overall treatment for the condition and is not part of the global surgical package.

Examples of staged procedures that may be performed on the integumentary system include the insertion of a prosthesis after a skin graft, removal of a malignancy following a biopsy, or breast reconstruction following a mastectomy (■ FIGURE 34-16).

Do not use modifier **-58** in the following circumstances. Instead, code as indicated.

- A problem related to the first procedure that requires a return to the operating room during the global period. Use modifier **-78 Unplanned Return to the Operating/Procedure Room by the Same Physician**.

- Procedures during the global period that are *unrelated* to the original procedure. Use modifier **-79 Unrelated Procedure or Service by the Same Physician**.

- Related procedures with a global period of zero days performed during the global period of another procedure. Report these as part of the surgical package.

- Procedures described as staged in the code descriptor, such as Mohs micrographic surgery. Report the code(s) for the procedures performed, following CPT special instructions.

- Procedures following a related procedure that has a global period of zero days, such as some biopsies. Report the second procedure without a modifier.

-59 Distinct Procedural Service

Use modifier **-59 Distinct procedural service** to report two procedures performed at the same time but not normally

6/6/yy: Surgeon performs a quadrantectomy on the right breast of a 47 year old woman, after an incisional biopsy done on 6/1/yy was positive for carcinoma. (The incisional breast biopsy procedure (19101) has a global period of 10 days.)

19301-58-RT Mastectomy, partial (eg, lumpectomy, tylectomy, quadrantectomy, segmentectomy); -58 Staged procedure; -RT Right side

Figure 34-16 ■ Example of using modifier -58 with the Integumentary System subsection.

performed together, such as a different site, different lesion, different incision/excision, or codes that can be reported only when performed as a separate and distinct procedure; the phrase (**separate procedure**) often appears in the code description.

EXAMPLE: *Radical resection of a 3-cm sarcoma from the forearm and excision of a separate, benign lesion 0.6 cm from the forearm during the same session:* **25077, 11404-59**

Some payers may require that one of the extended HCPCS modifiers **-X{EPSU}** be reported instead of modifier **-59**. For example, **-XS Separate structure** identifies that a second site was treated. The extended modifiers are discussed in greater detail in Chapter 27, "CPT Modifiers," Chapter 29, "Medicine Procedures," and Chapter 32, "Digestive System Procedures," of this text.

Guided Example of Arranging Integumentary System Procedure Codes

To practice skills for arranging codes for procedures in the Integumentary System subsection, continue with the example from earlier in the chapter about the patient who was seen for a pressure ulcer excision. Follow along in your CPT manual as Joshua Grider, CPC, arranges the codes. Check off each step after you complete it.

▶ First, Joshua confirms the procedure, area, and anatomic sites.

❏ Excision of pressure ulcer with ischiectomy, myocutaneous flap closure, 30 sq cm

❏ Myocutaneous flap created from the abdomen, donor site 30 sq cm, closed with an adjacent transfer rotational flap of 32 sq cm

▶ Joshua reviews the procedure codes.

❏ **14301 Adjacent tissue transfer or rearrangement, any area; defect 30.1 sq cm to 60.0 sq cm**

❏ **14302 Adjacent tissue transfer or rearrangement, any area; each additional 30.0 sq cm, or part thereof (List separately in addition to code for primary procedure)**

❏ **15946 Excision, ischial pressure ulcer, with ostec-tomy, in preparation for muscle or myocutaneous flap or skin graft closure**

❏ **15734 Muscle, myocutaneous, or fasciocutaneous flap; trunk**

▶ Joshua arranges the codes in descending RVU order according to the Medicare Physician Fee Schedule Data-base (MPFSDB). He uses the facility RVU because the procedure was performed at the hospital, not at the phy-sician's office. The RVU order is consistent with what Joshua intuitively expected; however, this is not always the case.

❏ **15946** Facility RVU = 47.09

❏ **15734** Facility RVU = 37.90

❏ **14301** Facility RVU = 25.25

❏ **14302** Facility RVU = 6.37

▶ Joshua reviews the codes to determine the need for modifi-ers. (Refer to Table 27-1, Key Criteria for Abstracting CPT Modifiers, or Appendix A in the CPT manual.)

❏ Code **15946** does not require a modifier because it is the primary procedure and there are no extenuating circumstances. A modifier for laterality is not required because the skin is not a bilateral organ.

❏ Code **15734** requires modifier **-51 Multiple procedures** because it was performed during the same operative

session as another procedure. The payment will be reduced to 50% of the usual fee.

❏ Code **14301** requires modifier **-51 Multiple procedures** because it was performed during the same operative session as another procedure. The payment will be reduced to 50% of the usual fee.

❏ Code **14302** does not require a modifier because it is an add-on code.

▶ Joshua finalizes the procedure codes and sequencing for this case:

(1) **15946 Excision, ischial pressure ulcer, with ostec-tomy, in preparation for muscle or myocutaneous flap or skin graft closure**

(2) **15734-51 Muscle, myocutaneous, or fasciocutaneous flap; trunk; -51 Multiple procedures**

(3) **14301-51 Adjacent tissue transfer or rearrange-ment, any area; defect 30.1 sq cm to 60.0 sq cm; -51 Multiple procedures**

(4) **14302-51 Adjacent tissue transfer or rearrange-ment, any area; each additional 30.0 sq cm, or part thereof (List separately in addition to code for pri-mary procedure)**

▶ Joshua also assigns and sequences the ICD-10-CM diagno-sis codes that support the need for the service.

(1) **L89.214 Pressure ulcer of right hip, stage 4**

(2) **M86.059 Other acute osteomyelitis, unspecified femur**

CODING PRACTICE

Exercise 34.4   **Arranging Codes for Integumentary System Procedures**

Instructions: Read the mini-medical-record of each patient's encoun-ter. Review the information abstracted in Exercise 34.2 for questions 1–3. For questions 4–6, abstract the case on your own. Assign CPT codes, quantities, and modifiers using the Index and Tabular List, and arrange the codes in proper sequence. Write the code(s) on the line provided.

---

1. OUTPATIENT SURGERY   Gender: M   Age: 46

Preprocedure diagnosis: Chronic infection and necrosis of the abdominal wall from internal dehiscence (*splitting open*) following a hernia repair 3 weeks ago

Procedure: Removed the mesh prosthesis from the hernia repair, then, using a curette, debrided 30 sq cm of subcutaneous tissue, fascia, and muscle in the abdominal wall. Applied antibiotics and packed with saline-soaked gauze for healing by secondary intention.

(continued)

---

1. (continued)

Postprocedure diagnosis: Infection due to mesh prosthesis and internal wound dehiscence following ventral hernia repair

Tip: A modifier is needed because this procedure was performed during the 90-day global period for the hernia repair.

2 CPT Codes _____

---

2. OFFICE   Gender: F   Age: 37

Preprocedure diagnosis: Suspicious lesions on back, arm, and hand

Procedure: Excised two lesions from the back, 1.5 and 2.1 cm, including margins. One lesion from the arm, 0.5 cm including margins. One lesion from the hand, 0.4 cm including margins. All sites sutured in one layer. Tissue was submitted to pathology.

Pathology: Four specimens received, all confirmed as malignant melanoma

(continued)

CODING PRACTICE (continued)

2. (continued)

Postprocedure diagnosis: Malignant melanoma on back, arm, and hand

Tip: In this exercise, codes for the larger lesions earn higher RVUs. RVUs for codes of the *same size range* but different families are ranked as follows: The code family for the scalp, neck, hands, feet, and genitalia has the highest RVUs. The code family for trunk, arms, or legs has the lowest RVUs.

4 CPT Codes _____

_____

---

3. EMERGENCY DEPT   Gender: F   Age: 16

Preprocedure diagnosis: Multiple lacerations from crash that occurred when she was driving an off-road vehicle in the woods

Procedure: Closed a 7.0-cm wound on the neck with a one-layer closure, a 2.5-cm wound on the face with heavy contamination requiring extensive debris removal and a simple closure, and a 10.2-cm wound on the right forearm with complex closure with debridement

Postprocedure diagnosis: Lacerations

Tip: Add together the length of wounds in the same code family of related anatomic sites.

4 CPT Codes _____

_____

---

4. OFFICE   Gender: F   Age: 14

Preprocedure diagnosis: Multiple lesions

Procedure: 1.0 cm with 0.5-cm margins from the cheek, 2.1 cm with 1.0-cm margins from the neck, and 3.0 cm with 0.5-cm margins from the forehead

Pathology report: Benign lesions

Postprocedure diagnosis: Benign lesions

2 CPT Codes _____

---

5. OFFICE   Gender: F Age: 23

Preprocedure diagnosis: Epidermal lesions

Procedure: Injected local anesthesia and, using a #15 scalpel, performed shave removal of a 0.5-cm lesion from the right eyelid, a 0.6-cm lesion from the left eyelid, and a 1.0-cm lesion from the left cheek

Pathology report: 3 specimens submitted, all benign lesions

Postprocedure diagnosis: Benign epidermal lesions

Tip: Identify the code family(ies), determine the number of lesions in each code family, then identify the number of lesions in the size range listed in each code.

2 CPT Codes _____

---

6. OFFICE   Gender: F   Age: 23

Preprocedure diagnosis: Malignant lesions

Procedure: Mohs micrographic surgery. Removed lesion from right arm, prepared six tissue blocks, which under microscopic examination showed clear margins. Removed lesion from hand, prepared three tissue blocks. Margins were not clear under microscopic examination, so removed additional tissue, which was divided into two tissue blocks. Both blocks were clear under microscopic examination. All sites closed with sutures.

Postprocedure diagnosis: Squamous cell carcinoma

Tip: Two procedures were performed: one that required one stage and one that required two stages. Assign a code for each procedure's first stage. Assign a code for each additional stage. Determine the number of tissue blocks examined for each code and assign a code for any excess blocks. Sequence codes by descending RVU: 17311 (18.82 RVU), 17312 (11.07 RVU), 17313 (17.6 RVU), 17314 (10.30 RVU), 17315 (2.28 RVU).

4 CPT Codes _____

_____

E/M CODING FOR DERMATOLOGY

The *1997 Documentation Guidelines for Evaluation and Management Services* (1997 DG), published by CMS, provides requirements for each level of an examination of the skin (■ FIGURE 34-17, page 684). Dermatologists are not limited to using the guidelines for a skin examination only. They can also use guidelines for a general multiorgan system examination, or any other single organ system examination, based on what is most advantageous for a specific encounter. However, physicians cannot combine elements from more than one type of examination for a given encounter. The skin examination guidelines typically provide the best results when a detailed skin examination is performed.

To determine the appropriate E/M code, coders must review the documentation in detail and identify the specific elements documented.

System/Body Area	Elements of Skin Examination
Constitutional	❑ Measurement of any **three** of the following seven **vital** signs: • 1) sitting or standing blood pressure, • 2) supine blood pressure, • 3) pulse rate and regularity, • 4) respiration, • 5) temperature, • 6) height, • 7) weight (May be measured and recorded by ancillary staff) ❑ General **appearance** of patient (eg, development, nutrition, body habitus, deformities, attention to grooming)
Eyes	❑ Inspection of **conjunctivae** and **lids**
Ears, Nose, Mouth and Throat	❑ Inspection of **teeth** and **gums** ❑ Examination of **oropharynx:** oral mucosa, salivary glands, hard and soft palates, tongue, tonsils and posterior pharynx
Neck	❑ Examination of **thyroid** (eg, enlargement, tenderness, mass)
Cardiovascular	❑ Examination of **peripheral vascular system** • **observation** (eg, swelling, varicosities) and • **palpation** (eg, pulses, temperature, edema, tenderness)
Gastrointestinal (Abdomen)	❑ Examination of **liver** and **spleen** ❑ Examination of **anus** for condyloma and other lesions
Lymphatic	❑ Palpation of lymph nodes • Neck • Axillae • Groin • Other
Extremities	❑ Inspection and palpation of **digits and nails** (eg, clubbing, cyanosis, inflammation, petechiae, ischemia, infections, nodes)
Skin	❑ Palpation of scalp and inspection of hair of scalp, eyebrows, face, chest, pubic area (when indicated) and extremities ❑ Inspection and/or palpation of skin and subcutaneous tissue (eg, rashes, lesions, ulcers, susceptibility to and presence of photo damage) in **eight** of the following ten areas: • Head, including the face • Neck • Chest, including breasts and axillae • Abdomen • Genitalia, groin, buttocks • Back • Right upper extremity • Left upper extremity • Right lower extremity • Left upper extremity • NOTE: For the **comprehensive** level, the examination of at least eight anatomic areas must be performed and documented. ■ For the **three lower levels** of examination, each body area is counted separately. For example, inspection and/or palpation of the skin and subcutaneous tissue of the right upper extremity and the left upper extremity constitutes two elements. ❑ Inspection of eccrine and apocrine glands of skin and subcutaneous tissue with identification and location of any hyperhidrosis, chromhidroses or bromhidrosis
Neurological/ Psychiatric	Brief assessment of mental status including: ❑ **Orientation** to time, place and person ❑ **Mood** and affect (eg, depression, anxiety, agitation, hypomania, lability)

Total # Bullets Performed and Documented →	☐	# of ❑ Elements Performed and Documented	Level of Examination
		1–5	Problem focused
		6–11	Expanded problem focused
		12	Detailed
		ALL	Comprehensive (Document **every** element in each box with a shaded border **AND** at least **one** element in each box with an unshaded border)

Figure 34-17 ■ 1997 documentation guidelines for skin examination. *Source:* Centers for Medicare and Medicaid Services, *1997 Documentation Guidelines for Evaluation and Management Services (with formatting adjustments).*

- To translate the documentation into the E/M requirements for the history, refer back to Chapter 28, "Evaluation and Management (E/M) Services (99201-99499)," Tables 28-7 to 28-10, or to the 1997 DG.

- To determine the requirements for an examination, refer to Figure 34-17 or to the single organ system examination for the skin in the 1997 DG.

- To determine the levels for medical decision making (MDM), refer to Chapter 28, Tables 28-11 and 28-12, and also to the Table of Risk in the 1997 DG.

Guided Example of E/M Coding for Integumentary System

Refer to the dermatology encounter (■ Figure 34-18) to practice skills for abstracting and assigning E/M codes. Follow along as fictitious coder Joshua Grider, CPC, abstracts the procedure. Check off each step after you complete it.

▶ First, Joshua needs to establish the category of service so he can determine the information needed to abstract and assign the code.

❏ *What is the setting?* Urgent care clinic, which is office or other outpatient

❏ *What is the type of service?* Established

❏ *What is the code range?* Joshua refers to the CPT Index and looks up the Main Term **Office or Other Outpatient Services** and the first-level modifying term **Office visit**, then the second-level modifying term **Established patient**. The code range listed is **99211-99215**.

❏ *How many key components are required?* Joshua refers to the code range in the Tabular List and reads the code description of the first full code (**99211** is a nurse-only visit), which states **Office or other outpatient visit for the evaluation and management of an established patient, which requires at least 2 of these 3 key components**. Codes **99212-99215** in the category have the same requirements for key components. This tells him that two of three key components must meet or exceed the levels listed in the code (2/3).

▶ Next, Joshua identifies the level of history.

❏ *What is the level of HPI?* The HPI is **Extended** because four or more elements are documented.

❏ *What is the level of ROS?* There is no ROS because no systems are documented

❏ *What is the level of PFSH?* The PFSH is **Pertinent** because one element is documented

❏ *Based on these factors, what is the overall level of history?* The level of history is **Problem focused** because the lowest of the three factors (HPI, ROS, and PFSH) determines the history level. The ROS qualifies for a problem-focused history. Although the HPI and PFSH qualify for higher levels of history, Joshua is restricted to selecting the overall history level based on the ROS, which is the lowest.

▶ Joshua refers to the Skin examination in the 1997 DG (Figure 34-17) to abstract information needed to determine the level of the examination.

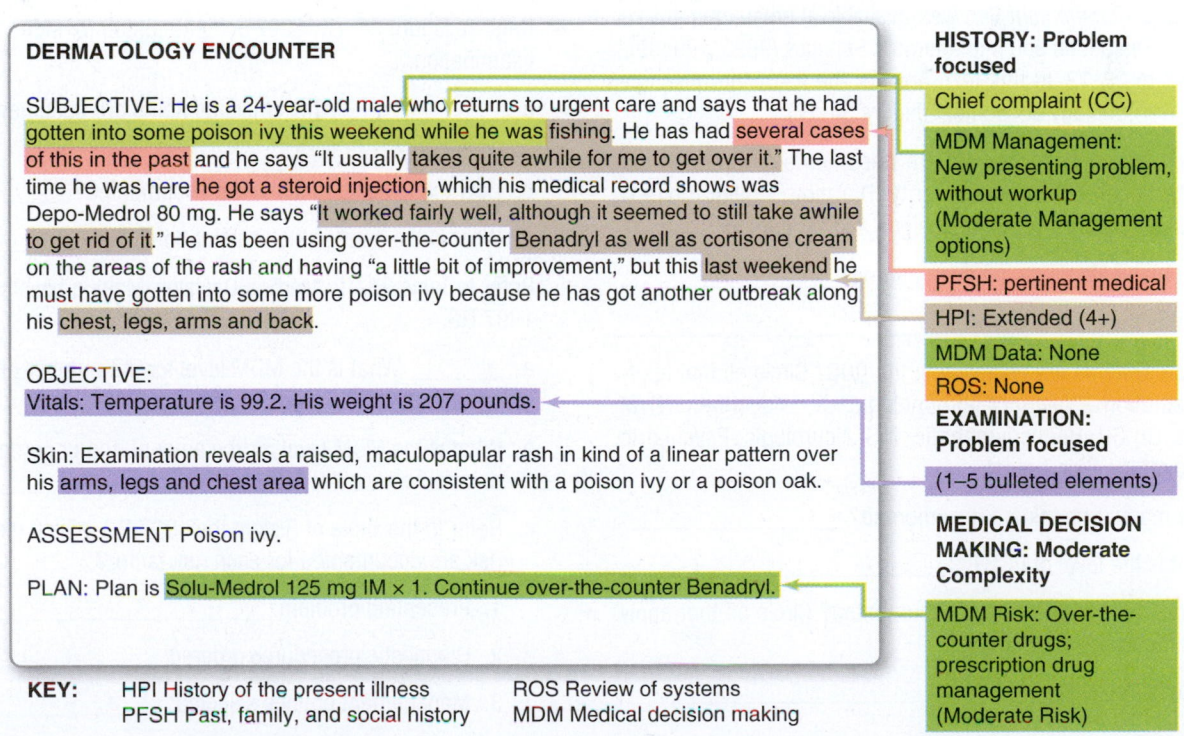

DERMATOLOGY ENCOUNTER

SUBJECTIVE: He is a 24-year-old male who returns to urgent care and says that he had gotten into some poison ivy this weekend while he was fishing. He has had several cases of this in the past and he says "It usually takes quite awhile for me to get over it." The last time he was here he got a steroid injection, which his medical record shows was Depo-Medrol 80 mg. He says "It worked fairly well, although it seemed to still take awhile to get rid of it." He has been using over-the-counter Benadryl as well as cortisone cream on the areas of the rash and having "a little bit of improvement," but this last weekend he must have gotten into some more poison ivy because he has got another outbreak along his chest, legs, arms and back.

OBJECTIVE:
Vitals: Temperature is 99.2. His weight is 207 pounds.

Skin: Examination reveals a raised, maculopapular rash in kind of a linear pattern over his arms, legs and chest area which are consistent with a poison ivy or a poison oak.

ASSESSMENT Poison ivy.

PLAN: Plan is Solu-Medrol 125 mg IM × 1. Continue over-the-counter Benadryl.

HISTORY: Problem focused

Chief complaint (CC)

MDM Management: New presenting problem, without workup (Moderate Management options)

PFSH: pertinent medical

HPI: Extended (4+)

MDM Data: None

ROS: None

EXAMINATION: Problem focused

(1–5 bulleted elements)

MEDICAL DECISION MAKING: Moderate Complexity

MDM Risk: Over-the-counter drugs; prescription drug management (Moderate Risk)

KEY:	HPI History of the present illness	ROS Review of systems
	PFSH Past, family, and social history	MDM Medical decision making

Figure 34-18 ■ Dermatology encounter. *Source: © PB Resources, Inc. Used with permission.*

❏ *What is the level of examination?* The level of examination is **Problem focused**. One bulleted element of the examination is documented, which meets the requirement of one to five bulleted elements for a problem-focused examination.

▶ Joshua determines the level of medical decision making. (Refer to Table 28-12, Medical Decision-Making Levels.)

❏ *What is the level of complexity of the number of diagnoses or management options, based on the presenting problem?* The level is **Moderate** because there is a new presenting problem, without workup

❏ *What is the amount and/or complexity of data to be reviewed?* No data are reviewed

❏ *What is the level of risk of significant complications, morbidity, and/or mortality?* He reviews each column in the Table of Risk in the 1995 DG and determines that the level of risk is **Moderate**. The patient presents with one stable chronic illness (Low), clinical labs are reviewed but not ordered, and prescription drug management is required (Moderate). The single highest element in the Table of Risk determines the overall risk. The column **Management options selected** is the highest level (Moderate).

❏ *Based on these factors, what is the overall level of medical decision making?* The medical decision making is **Moderate complexity**. At least two of the three MDM factors are required to qualify for a specific level of MDM. Two of the three MDM factors—the nature of the presenting problem and the level of risk—meet moderate-level decision making. Although the data factor is at a lower level (none), it can be disregarded because two of the three factors meet the criteria for **Moderate complexity**.

Now Joshua is ready to assign the code for the dermatology encounter. The exercise that follows guides you through additional abstracting skills and allows you to assign the correct code.

> ### CODING CAUTION
>
> A study conducted by the Office of the Inspector General (OIG) revealed that 26% of Medicare physician claims for E/M services were upcoded, meaning that a code was assigned for a higher level of service than supported by the documentation. Upcoding results in overpayments that can potentially lead to fines and charges or fraud or abuse.

CODING PRACTICE

Exercise 34.5   E/M Coding for Dermatology

Instructions: Refer to the *1997 Documentation Guidelines for Evaluation and Management Services* (available at **www.cms.gov**) or Chapter 28, "Evaluation and Management Services (99201-99499)," Tables 28-7 to 28-12, in this text. Answer the following questions about the "Dermatology encounter" (Figure 34-18).

1. a. Which elements of the HPI are documented? Circle all that apply. Location, Quality, Severity, Duration, Timing, Context, Modifying factors, Associated signs and symptoms

   b. How many elements are documented? _____

   c. What is the level of HPI? _____

2. a. Which systems are reviewed in the ROS? Circle all that apply. Constitutional, Allergic/ immunologic, CV, Endocrine, ENT/M, Eyes, GI, GU, Hemic/lymphatic, MS, Neurologic, Psychiatric, Respiratory, Skin/breast

   b. How many systems are documented? _____

   c. What is the level of ROS? _____

3. a. Which PFSH elements are documented? Circle all that apply. Past medical, Family, Social

   b. What is the level of PFSH? _____

c. What is the overall level of history? (The lowest history factor—HPI, ROS, or PFSH—determines the level of history.)

   _____

4. Refer to Figure 34-17 "1997 documentation for skin examination."

   a. _____ Which bulleted items are documented for the examination? (Check off the items documented.)

   b. How many bulleted items are documented? _____

   c. What is the level of the examination? _____

5. Refer to Table 28-12, Medical Decision-Making Levels, or the 1997 DG.

   a. _____ What is the MDM level for the number of diagnoses or management options?

   b. What is the MDM level for the amount and/or complexity of data to be reviewed? _____

   c. Refer to the Table of Risk in the 1997 DG. Which elements of risk are documented for each risk factor?

   1. Presenting problem: _____

   2. Diagnostic procedures ordered: _____

   3. Management options selected: _____

CODING PRACTICE *(continued)*

d. What is the level of risk? (The highest of the three areas determines the overall level of risk.) _____

e. What is the overall level of MDM? (2/3 MDM factors are needed to determine the overall level.) _____

6. a. What is the setting? _____

b. What is the patient (or service) type? _____

c. What is the code range? _____

d. How many key components are required? _____

e. What is the level of history? _____

f. What is the level of examination? _____

g. What is the level of medical decision making? _____

h. What is the correct code? _____

7. Abstract, assign, and arrange (sequence) the diagnosis code that supports the E/M code.

1 ICD-10-CM Code(s) _____

CHAPTER SUMMARY

In this chapter you learned that:

- Coders must understand the basic principles of measurements and wound healing when working with excision procedures and wound repair. Additional procedures to be familiar with are Mohs micrographic surgery, burns, tissue transfer and skin replacement, and breast removal and reconstruction.

- CPT provides special instructions and instructional notes throughout the Integumentary System subsection that define terminology and bundling rules. Although the Integumentary System subsection includes a variety of procedures, a few basic concepts apply to most procedures: site, complexity, size, method, and quantity.

- To locate codes in the Integumentary System subsection, search for the Main Term *Skin*, a first-level modifying term for the

procedure and a second-level modifying term for the details of the procedure. The Tabular List organizes many codes into code families divided by anatomic site and size, area, and/or complexity.

- Multiple coding is common for Integumentary System subsection procedures because more than one lesion removal or wound repair is often performed at the same time. Read code descriptions carefully to determine whether multiple procedures require reporting of multiple quantities of one code, use of add-on codes, use of additional standalone codes, and/or modifier(s).

- The *1997 Documentation Guidelines for Evaluation and Management Services* (1997 DG), published by CMS, provides requirements for each level of an examination of the skin.

CONCEPT QUIZ

Take a moment to look back at the Integumentary System subsection and solidify your skills. Try to answer the questions from memory, first, then refer to the discussion in this chapter if you need a little extra help.

Completion

Instructions: Write the term that completes each statement based on the information you learned in this chapter. Choose from the following list. Some choices may be used more than once and some choices may not be used at all.

abrasion	incisional
adjacent tissue transfer/ rearrangement	intermediate
	ligature
allograft	Mohs micrographic surgery
autograft	shaving
cryotherapy	simple
destruction	skin replacement
excision	skin substitute
flap graft	tangential
flap transfer	

1. A(an) _____ biopsy uses a sharp blade, oblique scalpel, or curette to remove a sample of the epidermis.

2. _____ is moving a section of skin and subcutaneous tissue from one site to another, with blood vessels intact, and anastomosis to vessels at the recipient site.

3. _____ uses a sharp instrument to remove an epidermal or dermal lesion without a full-thickness excision.

4. _____ is a procedure that removes skin tags by tying off the skin tag at its base with thread.

5. _____ is using liquid nitrogen to remove lesions by destroying the tissue.

6. _____ involves relocating a section of skin or flap from a donor site that is immediately next to the damaged skin and can be moved without completely detaching it.

7. A(n) _____ uses a patient's own tissue from one site to replace damaged tissue at another site.

8. A(n) _____ wound repair is a one-layered closure of epidermis, dermis, or subcutaneous tissue without significant involvement of deeper structures.

(continued)

(continued from page 687)

9. _____ is a multistage procedure in which a malignant lesion is excised in microscopic layers and the physician performing the procedure also performs the pathological evaluation of each tissue layer.

10. A(n) _____ is the use of synthetic (artificial) material to temporarily repair or replace damaged skin.

Multiple Choice

Instructions: Circle the letter of the best answer to each question based on the information you learned in this chapter.

1. What type of measurement identifies the distance between two points and is used to classify length of wound repairs and diameter of excised lesions?
   A. Metric unit
   B. Total body surface area
   C. Area measurement
   D. Linear measurement

2. How would you code the following procedure? *A physician excises two benign lesions from the left arm with excised diameters of 0.5 cm and 1.0 cm respectively.*
   A. 11402
   B. 11401, 11400
   C. 11602
   D. 11601, 11600

3. What tool helps physicians estimate the extent, depth, and percentage of body area affected by burns?
   A. Complexity of burns chart
   B. Total body surface area formula
   C. Lund-Browder classification
   D. Burn rate chart

4. How would you code the following procedure? *A surgeon performs a subcutaneous mastectomy on the right breast.*
   A. 19304
   B. 19307
   C. 19303
   D. 19301

5. Which type of procedure restores normal function or appearance as it relates to the Integumentary System?
   A. Restorative
   B. Repair
   C. Cosmetic
   D. Reconstructive

6. What type of graft involves skin from another species, such as a pig, and is used for temporary coverage while the patient grows new skin?
   A. Free flap graft
   B. Autograft
   C. Xenograft
   D. Flap transfer graft

7. What type of measurement defines a space inside a boundary and is used to classify the amount of skin treated in a tissue repair or skin graft?
   A. Area conversion
   B. Area measurement
   C. Add-on code
   D. Intermediate unit

8. What type of procedure obtains tissue for pathologic examination and is performed independently or is unrelated or distinct from other procedures/services provided at that time?
   A. Biopsy
   B. Excision
   C. Paring/cutting
   D. Shaving

9. What type of skin graft consists of the epidermis and a portion of the dermis?
   A. Punch graft
   B. Split-thickness skin graft
   C. Pedicle flap skin graft
   D. Rotational flap skin graft

10. How would you code the following procedure? *A physician performs intermediate repair of two wounds: 7.5 cm on the right arm and 8 cm on the right leg.*
    A. 12034, 12032
    B. 12031 × 2
    C. 12035
    D. 12016

KEEP ON CODING

Instructions: Read the procedural statement, then use the appropriate Index and Tabular List to assign CPT procedure codes. Write the code(s) on the line provided.

1. Lumpectomy of breast. CPT Code(s) _____

2. Removal of lesion using Mohs procedure, left thorax; first stage, eight blocks; second stage, four blocks. CPT Code(s) _____

3. Excision of pressure ulcer of hip, partial ostectomy of the trochanter, and a skin flap closure. CPT Code(s) _____

4. One-layer repair, 1.6-cm laceration of forehead. CPT Code(s) _____

5. Excision of pilonidal cyst, coccygeal region, extensive. CPT Code(s) _____

6. Removal of subungual hematoma by evacuation. CPT Code(s) _____

7. Cryotherapy to remove malignant melanomas of skin; 0.9-cm lesion on back; 1.3-cm lesion on thigh; 0.4-cm lesion on upper eyelid. CPT Code(s) _____

8. Debridement and application of dressing for second-degree burn, calf; 3% TBSA. CPT Code(s) _____

9. Application of skin substitute graft to anterior trunk (65 sq cm) and arm (33 sq cm). CPT Code(s) _____

10. Breast reduction, bilateral. CPT Code(s) _____

11. Superficial fascial repair of 2.7-cm open wound of thigh. CPT Code(s) _____

12. Intralesional injection of skin of scalp, four lesions. CPT Code(s) _____

13. Excision of umbilical hidradenitis with intermediate repair. CPT Code(s) _____

14. Needle biopsy of breast. CPT Code(s) _____

15. Destruction of 2-sq cm cutaneous vascular lesion of neck using laser. CPT Code(s) _____

16. Application of split-thickness tissue-cultured skin autograft to adult trunk (85 sq cm) and legs (52 sq cm). CPT Code(s) _____

17. Layered closure of 1.2 cm of abdomen, 0.3 cm of foot, and 1.2 cm of shoulder. CPT Code(s) _____

18. Excision of malignant skin lesions including margins; 0.5 cm on scalp, 0.8 cm on neck, 1.4 cm on shoulder. CPT Code(s) _____

19. Removal of 3 epidermal lesions by shaving. 0.2 cm on one hand, 0.7 on the cheek, 1.15 cm on the other hand. CPT Code(s) _____

20. One tangential biopsy and two incisional biopsies of separate skin lesions. CPT Code(s) _____

21. Stereotactic guidance to place radioactive seeds into breast lesion; first lesion (Localization device placement). CPT Code(s) _____

22. Removal of 19 skin tags on upper back and 8 on the neck. CPT Code(s) _____

23. Paring of three corns on toes. CPT Code(s) _____

24. Incision and drainage of breast abscess. CPT Code(s) _____

25. Wound debridement and layered closure of 1.3-cm cheek wound. CPT Code(s) _____

CODING CHALLENGE

Instructions: Read the mini-medical-record of each patient's encounter, then abstract, assign, and arrange ICD-10-CM diagnosis codes and CPT procedure codes using the appropriate Index and Tabular List. Assign quantities and modifiers where needed. Write the code(s) on the line provided.

---

1. OUTPATIENT SURGERY   Gender: M   Age: 39

Preprocedure diagnosis: Male pattern baldness

Procedure: Hair transplant, 21 punch grafts

1 ICD-10-CM Code _____

1 CPT Code _____

---

2. OUTPATIENT SURGERY   Gender: M   Age: 22

Preprocedure diagnosis: Ingrown toenail, right great toe

Procedure: Wedge excision of the skin of the nail fold, right great toe

Postprocedure diagnosis: Ingrowing nail, right great toe

1 ICD-10-CM Code _____

1 CPT Code _____

---

3. OFFICE   Gender: M   Age: 43

Preprocedure diagnosis: Skin lesion, left forearm; two skin lesions, left shoulder region

Procedure: Punch biopsy of three lesions

Postprocedure diagnosis: Blue nevus, left forearm; blue nevus, left shoulder region ×2

Pathology report: 3 lesions consistent with blue nevi

Tip: Obtaining tissue specifically for pathologic examination is distinct and unrelated to any other procedure/services provided during this encounter.

1 ICD-10-CM Code _____

3 CPT Codes _____

_____

---

4. EMERGENCY DEPARTMENT   Gender: F   Age: 26

Preprocedure diagnosis: Multiple lacerations from a motor vehicle accident where she was a passenger in a car

Procedure: Layered closure of a 20.3-cm laceration of the face; one-layer closure of a 4.0-cm laceration of the neck; one-layer closure of a 5.5-cm laceration of the face; layered closure (superficial fascia) of a 15.2-cm laceration of the face

(continued)

(continued from page 689)

4. (continued)

Postprocedure diagnosis: Wound repair of multiple lacerations of the face and neck

Tip: ICD-10-CM: Remember to code the External Cause and Intent of the reported injury(ies).

CPT: When multiple wounds are repaired, add together the lengths of those in the same classification and from all anatomic sites that are grouped together.

3 ICD-10-CM Codes _____

_____

3 CPT Codes _____

_____

---

5. OUTPATIENT SURGERY   Gender: F   Age: 57

Preprocedure diagnosis: Suspected carcinoma of the skin; two lesions on each arm and one lesion on the forehead

Procedure: Performed Mohs procedure on two lesions on each arm, first stage, 3 blocks on each lesion. Pathology confirmed. Performed Mohs procedure on one lesion on forehead; first stage, 2 blocks.

Postprocedure diagnosis: Basal cell carcinoma of the skin of both arms and the skin of the forehead

Pathology report: Confirms basal cell carcinoma of the skin on each arm and the skin of the forehead

Tip: The surgeons treated a total of 12 blocks in first stage for both arms (2 lesions on each arm = 4 lesions × 3 blocks each = 12)

3 ICD-10-CM Codes _____

_____

3 CPT Codes _____

_____

---

6. INPATIENT HOSPITAL   Gender: F   Age: 46

Preprocedure diagnosis: Left breast cancer with metastasis to the regional axillary lymph nodes

Procedure: Removed the entire left breast, pectoral muscles, and left axillary lymph nodes

Postprocedure diagnosis: Invasive ductal carcinoma, left breast with metastasis to the regional axillary lymph nodes

2 ICD-10-CM Codes _____

1 CPT Code _____

---

7. OFFICE   Gender: F   Age: 41

Preprocedure diagnosis: Annual checkup, established patient

Procedure: During the examination, the patient asked to have skin tags removed. Removed 9 skin tags from the right side of the neck; removed 7 skin tags from the left side of the neck; removed 12 skin tags from the chest. Separate E/M services were not performed for the skin tags. Patient is otherwise healthy.

Tip: Remember to add the appropriate modifier to the E/M code for the additional service provided at the time of the annual checkup.

2 ICD-10-CM Code _____

3 CPT Codes _____

_____

---

8. INPATIENT HOSPITAL   Gender: M   Age: 82

Preprocedure diagnosis: Stage 4 pressure ulcer of the sacral region

Procedure: 22-sq cm excision of the pressure ulcer with partial excision of sacrum. A 24-sq cm myocutaneous flap graft was placed on the defect. An adjacent tissue transfer of 26 sq cm was performed and this defect was closed using a single-layered closure. Bone from sacrum was sent to pathology.

Postprocedure diagnosis: Stage 4 pressure ulcer; sacral region; osteomyelitis of the sacrum

Pathology report: Osteomyelitis of the sacrum

Tip: Remember to sum the size of the graft and the size of the adjacent tissue transfer for the total defect size.

2 ICD-10-CM Codes _____

3 CPT Codes _____

_____

---

9. INPATIENT HOSPITAL   Gender: M   Age: 31

Preprocedure diagnosis: Second-degree burns to both upper arms, subsequent encounter

Procedure: Debridement of blisters and skin on both upper arms measuring 180 sq cm. A skin substitute was applied.

Tip: Remember that a second-degree burn is also called a partial-thickness burn.

2 ICD-10-CM Codes _____

4 CPT Codes _____

_____

10. OUTPATIENT HOSPITAL   Gender: F   Age: 64

Preprocedure diagnosis: Squamous cell carcinoma, skin of right hand and left cheek

Procedure: Used laser to destroy 2 lesions of cheek: first lesion 0.2-cm excised diameter, second lesion 0.5-cm excised diameter, and 1 lesion of hand, 1.1-cm excised diameter

Postprocedure diagnosis: Squamous cell carcinoma, skin of hand; two premalignant lesions on skin of cheek

Pathology report: Confirms squamous cell carcinoma on the skin of hand; finds two lesions on skin of face are actinic keratosis (premalignant)

2 ICD-10-CM Codes _____

3 CPT Codes _____

_____

Chapter 35

Musculoskeletal System Procedures (20100-29999)

Chapter Outline

- **Musculoskeletal System Procedure Basics**
- **Coding Guidelines for Musculoskeletal System Procedures**
- **Abstracting Procedures for the Musculoskeletal System**
- **Assigning Codes for Musculoskeletal System Procedures**
- **Arranging Codes for Musculoskeletal System Procedures**
- **E/M Coding for Orthopedics**

Learning Objectives

After completing this chapter, you should have the skills to:

35.1 Spell and define the key words, medical terms, and abbreviations related to musculoskeletal procedures. (Remember)

35.2 Summarize the fundamentals of musculoskeletal procedures. (Understand)

35.3 Adhere to CPT coding guidelines into the Musculoskeletal System subsection. (Apply)

35.4 Examine and abstract procedural information from the medical record for coding Musculoskeletal System subsection procedures. (Analyze)

35.5 Demonstrate how to assign codes for procedures in the Musculoskeletal System subsection. (Apply)

35.6 Utilize guidelines for arranging (sequencing) codes for Musculoskeletal System subsection procedures. (Apply)

35.7 Determine how to code Evaluation and Management services for orthopedics. (Evaluate)

Key Terms and Abbreviations

chondroplasty	level (spinal)	reduction	transfer
external fixation	manipulation	release	uniplane fixator
hemiarthroplasty	multiplane fixator	repair	vertebral segment
internal fixation	multiple endoscopy rule	stabilization	
interspace	reconstruction	synovectomy	

In addition to the key terms listed here, students should know the terms defined within tables in this chapter.

INTRODUCTION

Someone shopping in a hardware store might be bewildered by the vast array of tools and fasteners, yet each is designed for a specific purpose. The table of surgical instruments in an orthopedic operating room might look like a hardware store to some people because orthopedic surgeons use saws, drills, screwdrivers, and fasteners to perform repairs on the musculoskeletal system.

MUSCULOSKELETAL SYSTEM PROCEDURE BASICS

Several medical specialties focus on the musculoskeletal (MS) system. Orthopedic (also spelled *orthopaedic*) surgeons evaluate, treat, and perform surgery related to trauma, sports injuries, degenerative diseases, infections, tumors, and congenital disorders of the musculoskeletal system. Orthopedic surgeons can specialize in one or more specific anatomic sites, such as the knee, shoulder, back, or hip. When patients seek orthopedic surgery, it is important that they work with a surgeon who specializes in the specific site and problem. Any given orthopedic procedure can be performed using a variety of techniques, which can involve specific types of sutures and bone anchors aimed at promoting maximum stability and preventing reinjury. Patients need to discuss the surgeon's technique and choose the one they are most comfortable with.

Because the nerves are closely related to the function of the musculoskeletal system, neurologists may be part of the surgical team. For example, spinal surgery may be necessary when a bone deformity impacts neurological function. In general, orthopedic surgeons perform procedures related to deformities or injuries to the bone and muscle. Neurosurgeons perform procedures involving the nerves, brain, and spinal cord. Podiatrists perform procedures on the foot. Oral maxillofacial surgeons (OMSs) perform procedures on the face and mouth bones, such as for facial injuries, dental implants, oral cancer, and tumors and cysts of the jaws.

Orthopedic surgeons receive referrals from other medical specialties, such as primary care physicians, physiatrists (*physical medicine and rehabilitation physicians*), rheumatologists, pain medicine physicians, and athletic trainers. They may refer postsurgical patients to any of these specialists, as well as to physical therapists, psychologists, and psychiatrists.

Medical terminology related to Musculoskeletal System procedures can be challenging because of the number of bones, muscles, and connecting structures involved. Chapter 11 of this text provides additional information on musculoskeletal system anatomy and conditions. Joints are named for the two bones they connect, such as the radioulnar joint, which consists of the ends of the radius and ulna. Muscles, tendons, and ligaments are often named for the sites they connect or their shape (■ Figure 35-1, page 694). For example, the sternocleidomastoid muscle connects the sternum, clavicle (*cleido-*), and mastoid process. The iliofemoral tendon joins the ilium and femur. The deltoid muscle is triangular in shape, named after the Latin word *delta*, meaning "triangle." The anterior and posterior cruciate ligaments form a crosslike shape and are named after the Latin terms *cruc-* or *crux*, meaning "cross." Although you may not be able to specifically name every bone, muscle, tendon, and ligament, you can use your knowledge of combining forms to understand the location of unfamiliar structures.

Refer to ■ Table 35-1 for a refresher on how to build medical terms related to the musculoskeletal system.

CODING CAUTION

Be alert for anatomic terms that are spelled similarly and have different meanings.

metacarp/o (*long bone of the hand that connects the carpus [wrist bones] to the phalanges [fingers]*) and **metatars/o** (*long bone of the foot that connects the tarsus [ankle bones] to the phalanges [toes]*)

ilium (*uppermost and largest bone of the pelvis*) and **ischium** (*lower and back part of the hip bone*)

patella (*kneecap*) and **palate** (*roof of the mouth*)

Table 35-1 ■ **EXAMPLE OF CONSTRUCTING MEDICAL TERMS FOR MUSCULOSKELETAL SYSTEM PROCEDURES**

Combining Form	Suffix	Complete Medical Term
capsul/o (*joint capsule, a thin membrane around the joint that contains synovial fluid*)	**-desis** (*surgical fusion*) **-ectomy** (*excision*) **-tomy** (*cutting into*)	**capsulo + desis** (*surgical fusion of the joint capsule*) **arthro + desis** (*surgical fusion of the joint*)
		capsul + ectomy (*surgical excision of the joint capsule*) **arthr + ectomy** (*surgical excision of the joint*)
arthr/o (*joint, the location where bones meet*)		**capsulo + tomy** (*cutting into the joint capsule*) **arthro + tomy** (*cutting into the joint*)

Source: © PB Resources, Inc. Used with permission.

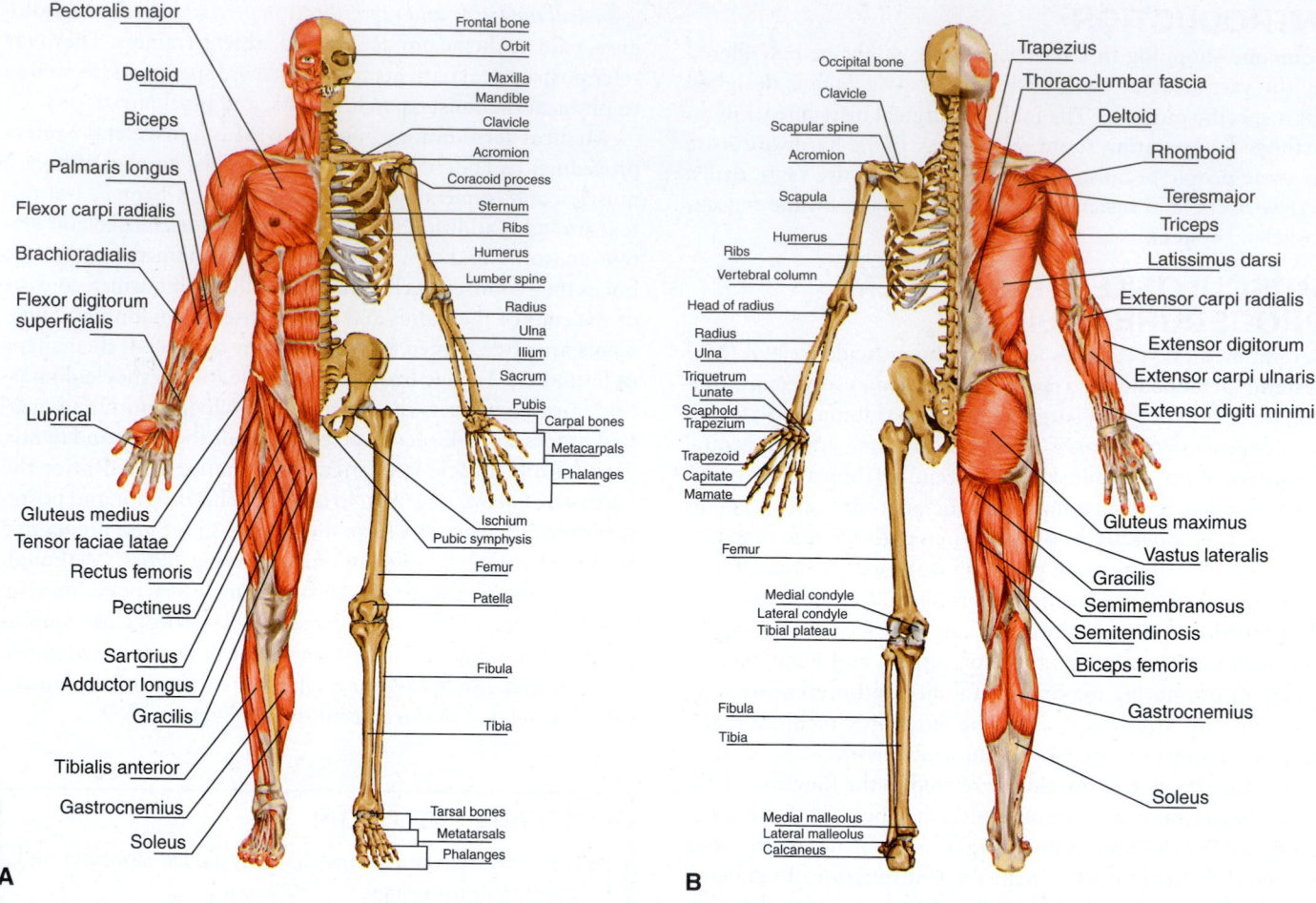

Figure 35-1 ■ The musculoskeletal system. (A) Anterior view. (B) Posterior view.

Procedures of the Musculoskeletal System

Procedures commonly performed on the Musculoskeletal System are summarized in ■ TABLE 35-2. In particular, coders need to understand arthroscopy, joint replacement, fracture treatment, and soft-tissue repair and reconstruction.

Arthroscopy

Knee arthroscopy is the most commonly performed procedure on the musculoskeletal system. Arthroscopy is also performed on other major joints, such as the shoulder, elbow, wrist, hip, and ankle. Although arthroscopy can be done as an independent procedure for diagnostic purposes, therapeutic procedures are often performed at the same time. These may include aspiration of fluid, **chondroplasty** (*reshaping of cartilage*), **synovectomy** (*surgical removal of the synovial membrane*), debridement, and a variety of repairs. Repairs can be performed using either an open or arthroscopic approach.

Joint Replacement

The most commonly replaced joints are the knee, hip, and shoulder. The most common reason for joint replacement is osteoarthritis. Pathologic hip fractures due to osteoporosis can

also result in joint replacement. In a total joint replacement, also called arthroplasty, the patient's anatomy is replaced with artificial ball-and-socket components that perform the same function. The ends of the long bone(s) forming the joint are cut off and replaced with a ball on a stem that inserts into the remaining bone. In the knee the distal end of the femur and the proximal end of the tibia are replaced; in the hip the head of the femur is replaced; in the shoulder the head of the humerus is replaced. The cup or socket is also reamed out and replaced with a prosthetic component. In the knee the patella is replaced; in the hip the acetabulum is replaced; in the shoulder the glenoid is replaced.

The surgeon selects the type of prosthetic material—metal alloy, ceramic, or polyethylene—based on a number of factors, such as the patient's activity level, age, weight, and health. The same material can be used for all components or a different material used for the ball than the socket. The implant may be cemented (*attached to the bone with surgical cement*) or cementless (*attached to the bone with a fine mesh into which the bone grows*), or a different method can be used on each component.

Joint replacement procedures have many variations. Some patients require that only one component of the joint be

Table 35-2 ■ **COMMON PROCEDURES OF THE MUSCULOSKELETAL SYSTEM**

Procedure Name	Definition	Reason Performed
Anterior cruciate ligament (ACL) reconstruction	Replacement of the ACL with a graft	Torn ACL
Arthrocentesis	Aspiration of a small joint or bursa (*a fluid-filled sac that helps movement of bones, tendons, and muscles*) or collection of synovial fluid from a joint with a needle	Diagnose disorders such as infections; alleviate pain
Biopsy	Removal of a sample of bone, muscle, fascia, or other tissue	Determine the presence of disease
Chondroplasty	Reshaping and cleaning the cartilage in a joint to remove uneven surfaces and fragments	Knee or shoulder injury
Decompression	Cutting into a muscle, joint, or fascia to relieve tension or pressure	Compartment syndrome, shoulder impingement syndrome
External fixation	Installation of a rigid device, external to the body, attached to the bone with pins and screws to stabilize it	Open fractures, closed fractures with severe soft-tissue injuries, infected nonunion of fracture, limb lengthening, stabilization
Fasciotomy	Cutting into the fascia to relieve pressure or tension	Compartment syndrome (Compartment: an anatomic segment that involves muscles, nerves, and vessels confined by a fascia membrane)
Fracture reduction (manipulation)	The use of force to move parts of a bone into normal alignment	Fracture
Injection	Administration of a medication using a needle	Treat inflammation and pain with steroids or anesthetics
Joint replacement	Removal of a natural joint and insertion of an artificial ball and cup made of metal, ceramic, polyethylene, or other artificial material	Hip fracture, osteoarthritis of the hip or knee
Meniscectomy	Shaving, debriding, or excising all or part of the meniscus	Torn or damaged meniscus
Replantation	Reattachment of an amputated body member	Accidental amputation of an arm, forearm, hand, digit, thumb, or foot
Skeletal traction	Placing pins and/or wires through broken bones and connecting them to stirrups, ropes, pulleys, and weights outside the body to secure bones in place until they heal	Fracture
Skull traction	Applying cranial tongs or calipers to the head and attaching them to ropes and weights on the outside, which secure the spine into place	Cervical spine factures and dislocations; immobilize head for stereotactic radiosurgery or radiation therapy
Spinal fusion	Joining together two vertebrae to stabilize them and help alleviate persistent pain	Herniated disk, stenosis, or spinal injury
Tendon repair	Sewing together the damaged or torn ends of a tendon	Torn or damaged tendon
Wound exploration	Enlargement, dissection, and examination of a wound to determine the wound depth or perform a procedure	Foreign body removal; debridement; repair of tissue, fascia, muscle, or blood vessel

Source: © PB Resources, Inc. Used with permission.

replaced, which is called a partial joint replacement or **hemiarthroplasty**. Prosthetic material wears down through use, just as the natural components do, and may require replacement or modification in the future. Technology related to joint replacements is constantly advancing, so new techniques and materials continue to be developed.

Patients participate in physical therapy after a joint replacement procedure to help rebuild strength and develop stability.

Most patients experience significant pain relief and increased mobility after joint replacement.

Fracture Treatment

Fractures comprise approximately 16% of all musculoskeletal injuries in the United States each year, accounting for 3.5 million visits to the emergency department, according to the United States Bone and Joint Initiative. The most common fracture site for people younger than age 75 is the wrist, whereas the most common fracture site for people older than age 75 is the hip. Although the treatment of fractures varies based on the site, type of fracture, and patient health, it generally consists of stabilization and/or restorative treatment.

Stabilization. Stabilization involves immobilizing the fracture site to prevent further injury and allow for healing. Fractures can be stabilized using straps, splints, or a variety of casts. Sometimes stabilization is the only treatment needed. In other situations, stabilization is an initial or temporary measure taken until restorative treatment can be performed. The physician who stabilizes the fracture may provide that service only or may also provide all the follow-up care.

Restorative Treatment. Restorative treatment is surgical repair or manipulation of displaced bones. Not all fractures result in displaced bones, but when they do, the bones must be realigned. Manipulation or reduction is the realignment of bone fragments or segments. Closed reduction is performed through the direct application of force. Open reduction requires a surgical incision to expose the bone, then realign it.

After reduction, the bones are stabilized with a cast, fixation device, or traction so they heal in the proper position. External fixation is the use of a rigid frame, external to the body, which is attached to the bone(s) using screws and pins. It may be used temporarily until the patient is able to withstand surgery or may be the primary mode of treatment and left in place until the fracture heals. A uniplane fixator has a single external rod that runs parallel to a long bone and is used almost exclusively on fractures of the shaft. A multiplane fixator has a ring-shaped frame that surrounds the treatment site. Wires apply tension to the frame to hold it in position. Internal fixation is the use of special implants, such as plates, screws, nails, rods, and/or wires, applied directly to the bone(s). The implants may be removed when the fracture has healed or may be left in permanently.

Open and closed reductions are identified based on the surgical approach used to realign displaced bones. The terms have no bearing on whether the fracture itself is open (*piercing the skin*) or closed (*not piercing the skin*). For example, a closed displaced fracture may be treated with either open or closed reduction and either external or internal fixation.

Fracture Follow-up. Surgeons monitor patients during the postoperative follow-up period, which is usually 90 days for Medicare. They may take x-rays to ensure the bones maintain correct alignment during healing. In the event of nonunion, malunion, or infection, additional treatment may be required.

Soft-Tissue Repair and Reconstruction

Muscles, tendons, and ligaments may need to be repaired because of injury, disease, or deformity. In a release, the tissue is freed from surrounding adhesions so that it can move freely within the tendon sheath; for example, tenolysis of the ankle. In a repair, a torn or damaged tissue, such as a muscle, is sewn together; for example, suturing of a ruptured hamstring muscle. In a transfer, one end of a muscle or tendon is moved to a new site to replace a damaged or nonfunctional muscle or tendon; for example, transfer of the iliopsoas muscle from the lesser trochanter of the femur to the greater trochanter to compensate for weak hip abductor muscles. In reconstruction, the original tissue is replaced with grafted tissue to create a new structure; for example, replacement of the anterior cruciate ligament (ACL) with a graft from the patellar tendon.

This section provides a general reference to help understand the most common musculoskeletal system procedures. Remember to keep standard reference books handy in case you get stuck.

CODING PRACTICE

Exercise 35.1 Musculoskeletal System Procedure Basics

Instructions: Use your medical terminology skills and resources to define the following procedures related to the Musculoskeletal System, then identify the code(s) or code range listed in the CPT Index. Follow these steps:

- Use slash marks "/" to break down each term into its root(s) and suffix.
- Define the meaning of the word based on the meaning of each word part.
- Identify the CPT code(s) or code range listed in the CPT Index.
- Use the entire phrase to identify the code or code range shown in the CPT Index.

Example: <u>arthrodesis</u>, knee arthro/desis   Meaning *fusion of a joint*   CPT Code <u>27580</u>

  1. <u>tenomyotomy</u>   Meaning _____   CPT Code _____

  2. <u>sesamoidectomy</u>, finger   Meaning _____   CPT Code _____

CODING PRACTICE (continued)

3. patellectomy, complete   Meaning _____   CPT Code _____

4. osteoplasty, ulna   Meaning _____   CPT Code _____

5. tenolysis, foot   Meaning _____   CPT Code _____

6. orbitocraniofacial reconstruction, secondary   Meaning _____   CPT Code _____

7. fasciotomy, palm   Meaning _____   CPT Code _____

8. capsulorrhaphy, posterior   Meaning _____   CPT Code _____

9. talus, diaphysectomy   Meaning _____   CPT Code _____

10. synovectomy, glenohumeral joint   Meaning _____   CPT Code _____

CODING GUIDELINES FOR MUSCULOSKELETAL SYSTEM PROCEDURES

Coders should understand the organization, guidelines, and instructional notes in the Tabular List of this CPT subsection. This information is necessary for accurate coding. The CPT section/subsection **Musculoskeletal System (20100-29999)** contains 15 subheadings that are divided by anatomic site (■ TABLE 35-3). Within each anatomic site, codes are divided by the type of procedure, such as incision, excision, introduction, and so on. Review the subheading and category names and code ranges listed in the Musculoskeletal System subsection to become familiar with the content and organization. Some editions of the CPT manual provide a summary list of the subheadings and categories at the beginning of the Musculoskeletal System subsection, which also displays an asterisk (*) next to categories that contain special instructions.

This chapter includes invasive, minimally invasive, and noninvasive surgical procedures on the Musculoskeletal System. Codes for diagnostic tests on the Musculoskeletal System appear in the Medicine section. CPT codes in the Musculoskeletal System subsection are frequently supported by diagnosis codes from ICD-10-CM Chapter 13, "Diseases of the Musculoskeletal System and Connective Tissue (M00-M99)," as well as neoplasms, symptoms, and signs, and injuries (■ TABLE 35-4).

Table 35-3 ■ MUSCULOSKELETAL SYSTEM SUBHEADINGS

Subheading	Code Range
General	20100-20999
Head	21010-21499
Neck (Soft Tissues) and Thorax	21501-21899
Back and Flank	21920-21936
Spine (Vertebral Column)	22010-22899
Abdomen	22900-22999
Shoulder	23000-23929
Humerus (Upper Arm) and Elbow	23930-24999
Forearm and Wrist	25000-25999
Hand and Fingers	26010-26989
Pelvis and Hip Joint	26990-27299
Femur (Thigh Region) and Knee Joint	27301-27599
Leg (Tibia and Fibula) and Ankle Joint	27600-27899
Foot and Toes	28001-28899
Application of Casts and Strapping	29000-29799
Endoscopy/Arthroscopy Procedures	29800-29999

Table 35-4 ■ LOCATING ICD-10-CM AND ADDITIONAL CPT CODES FOR THE MUSCULOSKELETAL SYSTEM

Type of Code	Codes
ICD-10-CM Musculoskeletal System-Related Codes	
Musculoskeletal system conditions	M00-M99
Neoplasms	C40-C41, D16, D21
Symptoms and signs	R25-R29
Injuries	S00-T89
CPT Musculoskeletal System-Related Codes	
Medicine procedures	96000-96004, 97161-97799, 97810-97814, 98925-98929, 98940-98943
Radiologic procedures	
• Diagnostic radiology	70010-73725
• Radiologic guidance	77001-77022
• Diagnostic ultrasound	76506-76642, 76801-76857, 76881-76886
• Bone/joint studies	77071-77086
• Nuclear medicine, diagnostic	78300-78399
Laboratory organ/disease panels	None are applicable specifically to the musculoskeletal system.

Source: © PB Resources, Inc. Used with permission.

These are the codes most commonly used to support procedures on the Musculoskeletal System; however, diagnosis codes from any ICD-10-CM chapter are permissible. CPT codes must always be linked with diagnosis codes that support the medical necessity of the procedure.

CPT guidelines for the Surgery section apply to the Musculoskeletal System subsection.

Special instructions at the beginning of the Musculoskeletal System subsection provide definitions and coding guidelines for treatment of fractures and excision of tumors. This information applies to all codes within the Musculoskeletal System subsection and should be studied before attempting to assign codes for these procedures. Additional special instructions appear at the beginning of many categories throughout the subsection. The **Spine (Vertebral Column)** subheading in particular provides numerous instructions regarding the use of modifiers and multiple coding.

Instructional notes appear throughout the Tabular List to alert coders to the need for modifiers, provide cross-references to codes for similar procedures on other sites, identify when additional codes for radiological services might be needed, and highlight resequenced and recently deleted codes. Specific guidelines and instructional notes are discussed throughout this chapter of the text.

ABSTRACTING PROCEDURES FOR THE MUSCULOSKELETAL SYSTEM

Because the Musculoskeletal System is a combination of two systems, separate abstracting guidelines are provided. Abstracting for skeletal system procedures (■ TABLE 35-5) requires special attention not only to the general anatomic site, such as the tibia, but also sometimes the specific location, such as the shaft, neck, or head. Abstract information about any implants, prostheses, hardware, or cement used and left in place. Spinal procedures require identification of the procedural approach, such as open, percutaneous, or endoscopic, as well as the anatomic approach, such as anterior, posterior, or posterolateral. Abstracting for fractures and dislocations (■ TABLE 35-6) also requires that coders take note of the types of reduction, stabilization, fixation, and traction provided.

For muscular system procedures, identify the specific type of procedure, for example, an excision, repair, transfer, release, or reconstruction; the type of soft tissue treated; and the deepest layer reached (■ TABLE 35-7). Remember that the abstracting questions are a guide and that not every question applies to, or can be answered for, every case. For example, materials and prostheses are not used in all cases.

Table 35-5 ■ KEY CRITERIA FOR ABSTRACTING SKELETAL SYSTEM PROCEDURES

- ❏ What is the general anatomic site?
- ❏ What is the specific location and/or compartment within the anatomic site?
- ❏ What is the laterality?
- ❏ What is the procedural approach (open or endoscopic)?
- ❏ What is the anatomic approach for spine procedures (posterior, anterior, anterolateral, or a combination)?
- ❏ What is the purpose of the procedure (diagnostic or therapeutic)?
- ❏ Is a foreign body removed?
- ❏ What type(s) of materials are used and/or prostheses/devices implanted?
- ❏ Which components of a joint are replaced (total or partial)?

Source: © PB Resources, Inc. Used with permission.

Table 35-6 ■ KEY CRITERIA FOR ABSTRACTING TREATMENT OF FRACTURES AND DISLOCATIONS

- ❏ What bone is fractured or dislocated?
- ❏ What site on the bone is fractured?
- ❏ What is the laterality?
- ❏ What type of reduction is provided (open or closed)?
- ❏ What general type of stabilization is provided (fixation or immobilization)?
- ❏ What type of fixation is provided (internal or external/percutaneous)?
- ❏ What type of traction is provided (skeletal or skin)?
- ❏ Is re-reduction of the injury required?

Application of Casts and Strapping

- ❏ What anatomic site is treated?
- ❏ Is the service an initial treatment?
- ❏ Is restorative treatment provided?
- ❏ Is restorative treatment provided by the same individual who applied the cast/strapping?
- ❏ Is the cast removed or repaired by the same individual who applied it?

Source: © PB Resources, Inc. Used with permission.

Table 35-7 ■ KEY CRITERIA FOR ABSTRACTING MUSCULAR SYSTEM PROCEDURES

- ❏ Is the procedure an excision, release, repair, transfer, or reconstruction or other type of procedure?
- ❏ Is the tissue a muscle, tendon, ligament, fascia, or other?
- ❏ What is the anatomic site?
- ❏ What is the laterality?
- ❏ What is the deepest layer of tissue treated?
- ❏ Is a foreign body removed?
- ❏ Is a malignancy involved?

Source: © PB Resources, Inc. Used with permission.

Guided Example of Abstracting Musculoskeletal System Procedures

Refer to the following example throughout this chapter to practice skills for abstracting, assigning, and arranging Musculoskeletal System subsection codes. ■ FIGURE 35-2 provides a review of the anatomy of the knee.

OUTPATIENT SURGERY   Gender: M   Age: 37

Preoperative diagnosis: Current tear of medial meniscus, chondromalacia of the patella, right knee

Procedure: Right knee arthroscopy with partial medial meniscectomy and lateral meniscorrhaphy. A #11-blade stab incision was made, followed by the insertion of a trocar. An arthroscopy probe was inserted and a systematic tour of the knee compartments was performed. All menisci were probed. All articular cartilage surfaces of the tibia, femur, and patella were probed. A posterior horn tear of the medial meniscus was complex in nature. Due to the tear being irreparable, it was debrided back to a stable margin using an arthroscopy meniscal biter and a #4.0 shaver. A separate peripheral tear in the lateral meniscus also was visualized in the red-red zone. This was not identified on the previous MRI and appeared amenable to repair. The edges were reduced with electrocautery and approximated, then closed with 6-0 Vicryl sutures. The chondromalacia changes were all stable and did not require any chondroplasty. Patient tolerated the procedure well and was transferred to PACU in stable condition.

Postoperative diagnosis: 1) Complex posterior horn tear around medial meniscus in the white-white to white-red zone. 2) peripheral tear in the lateral meniscus in the red-red zone. 3) Chondromalacia changes of grade 2 of the patellofemoral compartment.

Postoperative plan: Oral analgesics, oral anti-inflammatory medications. Ice and elevation of the limb. Weight bearing as tolerated. RTO 6-10 days for postoperative wound examination, suture removal, and referral to physical therapy.

Follow along as fictitious coder, Jacob Bates, CCS, abstracts the procedure. Check off each step after you complete it.

► Jacob reads through the entire record, paying special attention to the reason for the encounter, the procedure performed, and the postoperative diagnosis. He refers to the

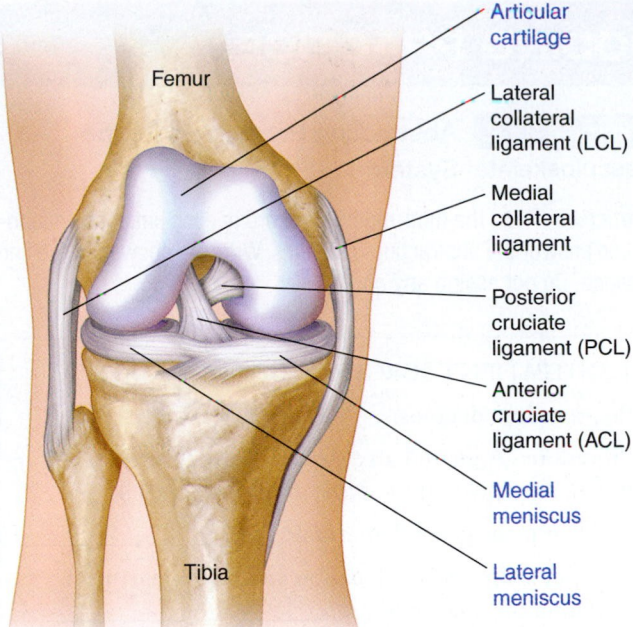

Figure 35-2 ■ Anatomy of the knee.

Key Criteria for Abstracting Muscular System Procedures (Table 35-7).

❏ He notes the preoperative diagnosis: Tear of medial meniscus, chondromalacia of the patella

❏ *Is the site a joint or a bone?* Joint

❏ *What procedure is performed?* Partial medial meniscectomy

❏ *What is the anatomic site?* Knee/medial meniscus

❏ *What is the laterality?* Right

❏ *What is the procedural approach (open or endoscopic)?* Endoscopic (arthroscopy)

❏ *What additional procedure was performed?* Lateral meniscorrhaphy

❏ *What is the anatomic site?* Knee/lateral meniscus

❏ *What is the laterality?* Right

❏ *What is the procedural approach (open or endoscopic)?* Endoscopic (arthroscopy)

❏ *What is the purpose of the procedure (diagnostic or therapeutic)?* Both diagnostic (exploratory/examination) and therapeutic (debridement, suturing) services are provided, so the procedure is classified as therapeutic.

► At this time, Jacob does not know which of these procedures may need to be coded, nor how many codes he will end up with. He will learn about this when he moves on to assigning codes.

CODING PRACTICE

Exercise 35.2 Abstracting Procedures for the Musculoskeletal System

Instructions: Read the mini-medical-record of each patient's encounter and answer the abstracting questions. Write the answer on the line provided. Do not assign any codes.

---

1. OUTPATIENT SURGERY Gender: M Age: 33

Preprocedure diagnosis: Fracture of left tibia shaft

Procedure: Adjusted an external fixation system, including replacing the pins, under anesthesia

a. What is the general anatomic site? _____

b. What is the specific location and/or compartment within the anatomic site? _____

c. What is the laterality? _____

d. What is the procedural approach? _____

e. What type(s) of materials are used and/or prostheses/devices implanted? _____

---

2. OFFICE Gender: M Age: 12

Preprocedure diagnosis: Fracture, left radius. Cast applied by another physician while the boy was attending summer camp.

Procedure: Removal of long arm cast

a. What anatomic site is treated? _____

b. Is the service an initial treatment? _____

c. Is restorative treatment provided? _____

d. Is the cast removed or repaired by the same individual who applied it? _____

---

3. INPATIENT HOSPITAL Gender: F Age: 46

Preprocedure diagnosis: Mass, abdominal wall

Procedure: Excised a tumor from the intramuscular tissue of the right anterior abdominal wall. The tumor measures 4.0 cm in diameter.

Pathology report: Benign desmoid tumor

a. Is the procedure an excision, release, repair, transfer, or reconstruction or other type of procedure? _____
_____

b. Is the tissue a muscle, tendon, ligament, fascia, or other? _____

(continued)

---

3. (continued)

c. What is the anatomic site? _____

d. What is the laterality? _____

e. What is the deepest layer of tissue treated? _____
_____

f. Is a foreign body removed? _____

g. Is a malignancy involved? _____

---

4. INPATIENT HOSPITAL Gender: M Age: 65

Preprocedure diagnosis: Pain in the thoracic spine due to degenerated and protruding discs

Procedure: Arthrodesis on T9–T10 and T10–T11 interspace using an anterolateral approach

Postprocedure diagnosis: Degeneration and protrusion, T9–T10 and T10–T11

a. What is the general anatomic site? _____

b. What is the specific location and/or compartment within the anatomic site? _____

c. What is the laterality? _____

d. What is the procedural approach (open or endoscopic)? _____

e. What is the anatomic approach (posterior, anterior, anterolateral, or a combination)? _____

f. What is the purpose of the procedure (diagnostic or therapeutic)? _____

---

5. EMERGENCY DEPARTMENT Gender: M Age: 25

Preprocedure diagnosis: Index finger and middle finger on right hand were completely amputated during automobile accident.

Procedure: Reattach both fingers, including distal tip to sublimis tendon insertion

a. What is the general anatomic site? _____

b. What is the specific location within the anatomic site? _____

c. What is the laterality? _____

d. What is the procedural approach? _____

e. What type(s) of materials are used and/or prostheses/devices implanted? _____

CODING PRACTICE *(continued)*

6. INPATIENT HOSPITAL   Gender: F   Age: 42

Preprocedure diagnosis: Chronic lower back pain due to degenerative disc disease

Procedure: Arthroplasty L4-L5 and L5-L6. Using an anterior approach excised the entire disc L4-L5 and inserted an implant. We then moved to L5-L6 where we also excised the entire disc L4-L5 and inserted an implant. Patient tolerated procedure well and was moved to PACU in stable condition.

Postprocedure diagnosis: Intervertebral disc degeneration L4-L5, L5-L6

(continued)

6. (continued)

a. What is the general anatomic site? _____

b. What is the specific location and/or compartment within the anatomic site? _____

c. What is the laterality? _____

d. What is the procedural approach (open or endoscopic)? _____

e. What is the anatomic approach (posterior, anterior, anterolateral, or a combination)? _____

f. What is the purpose of the procedure (diagnostic or therapeutic)? _____

ASSIGNING CODES FOR MUSCULOSKELETAL SYSTEM PROCEDURES

Whenever possible, search the Index for the name of the specific muscle or bone treated because these Main Terms usually provide the most detail and lead most directly to the desired code. In addition to searching for a specific site, such as **Ulna**, you can also search for a more general anatomic term, such as **Arm**; however, the results may not be as specific. Other alternatives are to search for the name of the procedure or condition. When you have difficulty locating the appropriate code, remember to search for it using an alternative Main Term. Two areas requiring special attention are using the Index to locate the appropriate anatomic site and coding for fracture care.

Indexing of Joints and Bones

The Index sometimes provides multiple Main Term entries for a joint, each with a different nuance. Therefore, coders must read beyond the first applicable Main Term entry they locate. For example, Index entries for the knee include **Knee**, **Knee Joint**, **Knee Prosthesis**, and **Kneecap**. The Main Term **Knee** classifies procedures on the tissues of the knee, such as the muscles and ligaments, whereas the entries for the Main Term **Knee Joint** classify procedures on the bony structure of the knee, including joint replacement. Arthroscopy appears only under **Knee** because arthroscopy is performed in the knee compartments, not on the bone itself. The Main Term **Knee** also provides an instructional note **See Femur; Fibula; Patella; Tibia**, so refer to these additional Main Terms if you cannot find an appropriate code. The Main Term **Knee Prosthesis** provides a cross reference to the Main Term **Prosthesis** and the first-level modifying term **Knee**. These codes classify prosthesis introduction and removal procedures. The Main Term **Kneecap** classifies procedures on the patella itself.

The Index also provides multiple Main Terms for **Hip** and **Hip Joint**, as well as **Shoulder** and **Shoulder Joint**. When locating Main Terms for the back, distinguish between the **Back** (soft tissue), **Spine** (bone), **Spinal Cord** (bundle of nerves), **Vertebra** (each bony segment of the spine), and **Intervertebral Disc** (pad of fibrocartilage between the vertebrae). Procedures on the back, spine, and vertebrae are classified under the Musculoskeletal System, whereas procedures on the spinal cord and intervertebral discs are classified under the Nervous System. Most of these Main Term entries also provide cross-references to more specific sites, so take the time to review the entries in detail and follow all cross-references, especially when you are having difficulty locating the appropriate code.

In the Tabular List, codes for the spinal column are often divided by the section of the spine—cervical, thoracic, and lumbar—with add-on code(s) for each additional vertebra, also called a level or vertebral segment. When coding for procedures on the spine, distinguish between vertebrae and intervertebral discs. In documentation, each vertebra is identified by a letter–number combination, such as C4 for the fourth cervical vertebra, L2 for the second lumbar vertebra, and so on. An intervertebral disc, or interspace, is the space between two vertebrae and is identified by the vertebrae above and below. For example, the L2-L3 interspace is the disc situated between the second and third lumbar vertebrae. On a vertebral procedure, L2-L3 refers to *two* vertebrae (■ FIGURE 35-3, page 702), whereas on disc procedures, L2-L3 refers to *one* interspace (■ FIGURE 35-4, page 702). This distinction is important when assigning quantity and codes to spinal procedures.

Assigning Codes for Fracture Care

Assigning codes for fracture care depends on careful abstracting of who performs the service, as well as the extent of services provided. According to the National Correct Coding Initiative (NCCI), the initial encounter for fracture care with a 90-day global period usually involves an Evaluation and Management (E/M) code, a treatment code, and HCPCS codes for the materials used or the generic CPT code **99070 Supplies**.

> Surgeon performed an osteotomy on L2, L3, and L4 using the posterolateral approach.
>
> **22214 Osteotomy of spine, posterior or posterolateral approach, 1 vertebral segment; lumbar**
> **22216 × 2 Osteotomy of spine, posterior or posterolateral approach, 1 vertebral segment; each additional vertebral segment**

Figure 35-3 ■ Example of coding procedures on multiple vertebrae.

> Surgeon replaced artificial discs at L2-L3 and L3-L4 using the anterior approach.
>
> **22862 Revision including replacement of total disc arthroplasty (artificial disc), anterior approach, single interspace; lumbar**
> **0165T Revision including replacement of total disc arthroplasty (artificial disc), anterior approach, each additional interspace, lumbar**

Figure 35-4 ■ Example of coding procedures on multiple discs.

CPT provides separate codes for restorative treatment and casting. For procedures with a global period of 0 or 10 days, the initial evaluation is considered to be included in the treatment code. The exception is the application of casts and strapping, in which case an E/M code can be reported, subject to documentation and the nature of the service provided. Medicare administrative contractors (MACs) and private insurance companies may have additional claim edits that apply.

To locate codes for restorative fracture care, search the Index for the Main Term that identifies the bone(s) involved, such as **Tibia** or **Clavicle**, then locate the first-level modifying term **Fracture**. Additional modifying terms identify the type of treatment provided. Codes for restorative treatment include services such as open or closed treatment, with or without manipulation, and application of internal or external fixation. The subheadings for each anatomic site within the Musculoskeletal System subsection contain a category titled **Fracture and/or Dislocation**.

To locate codes for the application of casts and strapping, search the Index for the Main Term **Cast**, then locate the first-level modifying term for the type of cast. Codes are divided based on the region of the body, such as **Below knee to toes** or **Finger**, but not for specific bones. If you cannot find the description needed as a first-level modifying term, look under the first-level modifying term **Type**, then locate the specific cast in the list of second-level modifying terms.

In the Tabular List, all codes for casting and strapping appear under the subheading **Application of Casts and Strapping 29000-29799**. Codes are divided by the upper and lower extremities, with subdivisions for casts, splints, and straps. Special instructions appear before code **29000** and provide guidance regarding when cast application and strapping should be coded separately from the E/M code and/or restorative treatment.

- When the *same* provider applies the initial cast or strapping and also provides restorative treatment for the fracture and all follow-up care, assign a code for the restorative treatment that identifies the type of service provided. The initial cast application is included in the code for restorative care. Coding is as follows:
  - An E/M code for the type of service provided
  - A code from the category for the anatomic site that describes the type of restorative treatment provided
  - A HCPCS code or code **99070 Supplies** for the materials used

- When *different providers* perform the preoperative care, restorative treatment, and/or postoperative care, assign the code for the restorative treatment with the corresponding modifier(s) to identify the phase of care: **-54 Surgical care only, -55 Postoperative management only, -56 Preoperative management only**. Temporary cast application is not classified as preoperative care by CPT. Only the provider who performs the preoperative management codes an E/M code, which identifies the preoperative encounter at which the initial evaluation is performed and the decision for surgery is made (■ FIGURE 35-5).

- When cast application or strapping is the *only* service provided, and no other treatment is performed or anticipated, assign codes as follows (■ FIGURE 35-6):
  - An E/M code for the type of service provided
  - A code from **29000-29799** that describes the type of cast or strapping applied
  - A HCPCS code or CPT code **99070 Supplies** for the materials used

- When cast application or strapping is a *replacement* procedure during or after follow-up care, assign a code from **29000-29584** for the type of cast or strapping applied.

- When the cast is *removed* or repaired by a different individual than the one who applied it, assign a code from the category **Removal or Repair 29700-29750**.

SUCCESS STEP

When the E/M service is provided on the same day as the restorative treatment and results in a decision for surgery, apply modifier **-57 Decision for surgery** to the E/M code.

Guided Example of Assigning Musculoskeletal System Procedure Codes

To practice skills for assigning codes for the Musculoskeletal System subsection, continue with the example from earlier in the chapter about a patient who was seen for a right knee arthroscopy. Follow along in your CPT manual as Jacob Bates, CCS, assigns codes. Check off each step after you complete it.

▶ First, Jacob confirms right knee arthroscopy with partial medial meniscectomy and lateral meniscorrhaphy.

Physician A evaluates the patient's fractured tibia, left leg, in the emergency department. He performs an expanded problem focused history, an expanded problem focused examination, and medical decision making of moderate complexity. X-rays reveal a fracture of the distal tibia. Physician A performs closed treatment with manipulation, and applies a short leg cast. The patient was on vacation at the time. When she returns home, Physician B provides the postoperative followup care, including x-rays to monitor proper healing and cast removal.

Physician A

99283-57 Emergency department visit for the evaluation and management of a patient, which requires these 3 key components: An expanded problem focused history; An expanded problem focused examination; and Medical decision making of moderate complexity. -57 Decision for surgery

27825-54-56-LT Closed treatment of fracture of weight bearing articular portion of distal tibia (eg, pilon or tibial plafond), with or without anesthesia; with skeletal traction and/or requiring manipulation; -54 Surgical care only; -56 Preoperative management only; -LT Left

Physician B

27825-55-LT Closed treatment of fracture of weight bearing articular portion of distal tibia (eg, pilon or tibial plafond), with or without anesthesia; with skeletal traction and/or requiring manipulation; -55 Postoperative management only; -LT Left

Figure 35-5 ■ Example of coding for fracture care by multiple providers. *Source: © PB Resources, Inc. Used with permission. CPT codes only © American Medical Association.*

A patient presents to urgent care with right wrist pain. The patient reports that he fell yesterday and braced himself with his hand. The physician performs an expanded problem focused history, and examination, and medical decision making of moderate complexity. X-rays reveal no fracture. The physician diagnoses a sprain and applies a static short arm splint to stabilize the joint. No further treatment is planned.

99282-57 Emergency department visit for the evaluation and management of a patient, which requires these 3 key components: An expanded problem focused history; An expanded problem focused examination; and Medical decision making of moderate complexity. -57 Decision for surgery

29125-RT Application of short arm splint (forearm to hand); static; -RT Right

Figure 35-6 ■ Example of coding for application of casts and strapping. *Source: © PB Resources, Inc. Used with permission. CPT codes only © American Medical Association.*

▶ Jacob searches the Index for the Main Term **Knee**. Because both procedures are arthroscopic procedures on the right knee, he thinks that he will find the codes close together, so he begins with a general search on the knee and will refine it later, as needed.

❏ He locates the first-level modifying term **Arthroplasty**. Then he locates another first-level modifying term, **Arthroscopy**. He notices that different codes are listed after each entry, so he must decide which entry is preferred. He recalls that the default approach for surgical procedures is open and then recognizes that **Arthroplasty** identifies an open procedure, whereas **Arthroscopy** identifies an endoscopic procedure. An arthroscopy was performed, so **Arthroscopy** is the Main Term he needs.

❏ He reads the second-level modifying terms **Diagnostic** and **Surgical**. The procedure performed has both diagnostic and surgical features. He recognizes that surgical procedures always include diagnostic procedures at the same site, so he selects the modifying term **Surgical**.

❏ He identifies the relevant codes **29866-29868, 29871, 29873-29877, 29879-29889**. He recognizes that numerous codes and code ranges are provided, so he will need to research the Tabular List carefully to be certain he doesn't miss anything. He also notices that, in the Index, there are no modifying terms to help distinguish between the meniscectomy and meniscorrhaphy.

▶ Jacob turns to the Tabular List to review and select the codes. He decides to begin with **29866**, the first code listed.

❏ He notices that the first three codes (**29866-29868**) are a code family that describes **osteochondral autografts, allografts,** and **meniscal transplantation.** Although the meniscus was treated, a transplantation was not involved. Therefore, none of these codes are correct for this case.

❏ He identifies that the next code, **29871,** is a parent code for all entries through code **29887.** The common descriptor states **Arthroscopy, knee, surgical.** He reads all the indented code descriptions to identify one that describes the procedure performed.

■ Code **29877** describes **debridement/shaving of articular cartilage (chondroplasty).** Debridement was performed, so he identifies this code as a possibility.

■ Codes **29880** and **29881** describe **meniscectomy.** A medial meniscectomy was performed, so he identifies these codes as a possibility.

■ Codes **29882** and **29883** describe **meniscus repair.** The lateral meniscus was sutured, so he identifies this code as a possibility.

❏ The final two codes listed in the Index, **29899** and **29899,** describe the **anterior** and **posterior cruciate ligaments,** respectively. These ligaments were not treated, so these codes are not correct.

▶ Jacob reviews the five codes he identified as possibilities.

❏ Although code **29877** describes debridement and shaving, the site is articular cartilage, not the medial meniscus. He refers to the documentation and confirms that the articular cartilage was probed and evaluated and did not require any chondroplasty. Therefore, he determines that this code is not correct.

❏ Code **29880** describes **meniscectomy** and **meniscal shaving** but identifies the **medial AND lateral** ligaments. Although both the medial and lateral menisci were treated, only the medial meniscus was debrided. Jacob determines that this code is probably not correct.

❏ Code **29881** describes **meniscectomy** and **meniscal shaving** and identifies the **medial OR lateral** ligaments. Because only the medial meniscus was debrided, he thinks this code could be the one he needs. However, he knows he must review all the codes to determine if there is another code that accurately describes both procedures. He reads in the code description that the code includes **debridement/shaving of articular cartilage (chondroplasty) . . . when performed.** He recognizes that the words **when performed** do not require that a chondroplasty be performed to use this code.

❏ Codes **29882** and **29883** describe **meniscus repair.** Jacob refers to the documentation and determines that no repair was performed on the medial meniscus because the damage was irreparable. That is the reason the debridement was performed. The lateral meniscus was repaired with sutures, so he thinks one of these codes could be correct.

❏ He compares the descriptions of codes. Code **29882** describes **meniscus repair** and identifies **medial OR lateral.** Because only the lateral meniscus was debrided, he determines that this code is probably correct.

❏ Code **29883** describes **meniscus repair** and identifies **medial AND lateral.** He determines this code is not correct because, although both the medial and lateral menisci were treated, only the lateral meniscus was repaired.

❏ After reviewing all codes listed in the code range and verifying the details of anatomic site and procedure with the documentation, Jacob determines that code **29881** is the correct code for partial medial meniscectomy and code **29882** is the correct code for the lateral meniscorrhaphy.

❏ He must combine the *common descriptor* portion of parent code **29871** with the *unique descriptors* of codes **29881** and **29882** to arrive at the complete code descriptions.

▶ Jacob checks for instructions in the Tabular List.

❏ He looks for instructional notes immediately before or after codes **29881** and **29882** to identify any information about whether the two codes can be used together. After careful checking, he does not find any warnings or instructions that prohibit reporting both codes.

❏ He cross-references the special instructions at the beginning of **Endoscopy/Arthroscopy** that state **Surgical endoscopy/arthroscopy always includes a diagnostic endoscopy/arthroscopy.** This confirms that the diagnostic inspection of the rest of the knee compartment and the articular cartilage surfaces is bundled with the code for the surgical procedures and should not be coded separately.

❏ He cross-references the special instructions at the beginning of the subcategory **Musculoskeletal System** and verifies that there are no additional instructions that apply to this procedure.

▶ Jacob reviews the procedure code he has assigned for this case.

❏ **29881** Arthroscopy, knee, surgical; with meniscectomy (medial OR lateral, including any meniscal shaving) including debridement/shaving of articular cartilage (chondroplasty), same or separate compartment(s), when performed

❏ **29882** Arthroscopy, knee, surgical; with meniscus repair (medial OR lateral)

▶ Next, Jacob must determine how to sequence the codes.

CODING PRACTICE

Exercise 35.3   Assigning Codes for Musculoskeletal System Procedures

Instructions: Read the mini-medical-record of each patient's encounter. Review the information abstracted in Exercise 35.2 for questions 1–3. For questions 4–6, abstract the case on your own. Assign CPT codes, quantities, and modifiers using the Index and Tabular List. Write the code(s) on the line provided.

---

1. OUTPATIENT SURGERY   Gender: M   Age: 33

Preprocedure diagnosis: Fracture of left tibia shaft

Procedure: Adjusted an external fixation system, including replacing the pins, under anesthesia

Tip: Adjustment of an external fixation requires the same code, regardless of anatomic site, so use *External Fixation* as the Main Term.

1 CPT Code _____

---

2. OFFICE   Gender: M   Age: 12

Preprocedure diagnosis: Fracture, left radius. Cast applied by another physician while the boy was attending summer camp.

Procedure: Removed long arm cast

1 CPT Code _____

---

3. INPATIENT HOSPITAL   Gender: F   Age: 46

Preprocedure diagnosis: Mass, abdominal wall

Procedure: Excised a tumor from the intramuscular tissue of the right anterior abdominal wall. The tumor measures 4.0 cm in diameter.

Pathology report: Benign desmoid tumor

1 CPT Code _____

---

4. EMERGENCY DEPT   Gender: F   Age: 12

Preprocedure diagnosis: Dislocated fracture of carpometacarpal right thumb, jammed in car door

Procedure: Manipulated thumb under anesthesia and restored the thumb to normal function

Tip: Code only for the treatment, not the E/M or supplies.

1 CPT Code _____

---

5. EMERGENCY DEPT   Gender: M   Age: 32

Preprocedure diagnosis: Dislocated right shoulder

Procedure: Closed treatment with manipulation, applied sling

1 CPT Code _____

---

6. EMERGENCY DEPT   Gender: M   Age: 21

Preprocedure diagnosis: Closed Colles' fracture (radius), right, that the patient sustained when he fell off a horse he was riding.

Procedure: Performed closed reduction and applied a gauntlet cast (*a cast from the lower forearm to the hand*)

Postprocedure diagnosis: Referred to orthopedic surgeon for follow-up care and cast removal

Tip: Append modifiers to identify the portion of the surgical package provided by the ED. Code only for the treatment, not the E/M or supplies.

1 CPT Code _____

ARRANGING CODES FOR MUSCULOSKELETAL SYSTEM PROCEDURES

Special instructions that appear at the beginning of and throughout the Musculoskeletal System subsection provide detailed guidance regarding multiple coding and the use of modifiers, particularly in the **Spine (Vertebral Column)** subheading. Coders must take the time to study all of the special instructions and instructional notes relevant to the codes they are researching to ensure accurate coding. Specific instructions include:

- Report bone grafting procedures (**20900-20939**) separately, in addition to arthrodesis.

- Report spinal instrumentation codes (**22840-22852**) in addition to the primary procedure.

- Report exploration of spinal fusion (**22830**) in addition to the code for the definitive procedure, including arthrodesis.

Modifiers

The Musculoskeletal System subsection provides specific direction regarding the use of modifiers **-51**, **-52**, and **-62**. This information appears in special instructions and instructional notes throughout the subsection.

-51 Multiple Procedures

When exploration of spinal fusion (**22830**) is reported with other definitive procedures, including arthrodesis, append modifier **-51** to **22830**.

When arthroscopy is performed with arthrotomy, append modifier **-51** to the endoscopy code.

Do not report modifier **-51** with add-on codes.

-52 Reduced Services

Modifier **-52** identifies a service or procedure that is partially reduced or eliminated at the discretion of the physician. When replantation is performed on an incomplete amputation, see the specific codes for the repairs performed, such as repair of bones, ligaments, tendons, nerves, or blood vessels, and report modifier **-52** to identify that less than the usual service was performed. This provides a means of reporting reduced services without disturbing the identification of the basic service.

-62 Two Surgeons

Two surgeons may work together as primary surgeons on orthopedic procedures, each performing a separate and equal component of the procedure. For example, because some spinal procedures use an anterior approach, a general surgeon may create the surgical access and an orthopedic surgeon performs the spinal procedure. Both surgeons report the same procedure code and each appends modifier **-62** to identify that he or she performed a portion of the procedure. Append modifier **-62** not only to the primary procedure but also to any additional procedures, including add-on codes, unless directed otherwise and as long as the two surgeons continue to work together as primary surgeons. Special instructions in the Tabular List identify procedures that accept modifier **-62** and, in some cases, those that do not.

• When bone grafts are performed with arthrodesis, only the surgeon performing the bone graft reports the bone graft code and does not append modifier **-62** (■ FIGURE 35-7).

• Spinal instrumentation codes (**22840-22852**) do not accept modifier **-62**.

Such instructions appear in the **Grafts (or Implants)** category (**20900-20938**) as well as in multiple places under the **Spine (Vertebral Column)** subheading.

Guided Example of Arranging Musculoskeletal System Procedure Codes

To practice skills for arranging codes for procedures of the Musculoskeletal System subsection, continue with the example from earlier in the chapter about the patient who was seen for a knee arthroscopy. Follow along in your CPT manual as Jacob Bates, CCS, arranges the codes. Check off each step after you complete it.

▶ First, Jacob confirms the procedure, anatomic sites, approach, and laterality.

❏ Arthroscopy

❏ Right knee

❏ Medial meniscectomy

❏ Lateral meniscus repair

▶ Jacob reviews the codes he assigned and confirms the details with the medical record.

❏ **29881 Arthroscopy, knee, surgical; with meniscectomy (medial OR lateral, including any meniscal shaving) including debridement/shaving of articular cartilage (chondroplasty), same or separate compartment(s), when performed**

❏ **29882 Arthroscopy, knee, surgical; with meniscus repair (medial OR lateral)**

▶ Jacob arranges the codes in descending RVU order according to the Medicare Physician Fee Schedule Database

---

> Two surgeons performed an anterior interbody arthrodesis on L4-L5. The general surgeon made a midline abdominal incision and prepared the approach to the lumbar spine. The orthopedic surgeon performed the discectomy and osteophytectomy (*removed a bone spur*). He then performed a local autograft using the spinous process and inserted the interbody fusion device. The general surgeon closed the fascia, abdominal muscles, subcutaneous tissues, and skin in layers with sutures.
>
> General surgeon:
> **22558-62 Arthrodesis, anterior interbody technique, including minimal discectomy to prepare interspace (other than for decompression); lumbar. -62 Two surgeons**
>
> Orthopedic surgeon:
> **22558-62 Arthrodesis, anterior interbody technique, including minimal discectomy to prepare interspace (other than for decompression); lumbar. -62 Two surgeons**
> **20936 Autograft for spine surgery only (includes harvesting the graft); local (eg, ribs, spinous process, or laminar fragments) obtained from same incision**

Figure 35-7 ■ Example of using modifier -62 with an anterior approach. *Source: © PB Resources, Inc. Used with permission. CPT codes only © American Medical Association.*

(MPFSDB). He uses the facility RVU because the procedure was performed at the outpatient surgery center, not at the physician's office.

- ❏ **29882** Facility RVU = 20.19
- ❏ **29881** Facility RVU = 15.56

▶ Jacob examines the need for modifiers. (Refer to Table 27-1, Key Criteria for Abstracting CPT Modifiers, or Appendix A in the CPT manual.)

- ❏ Code **29882** requires two modifiers. Modifier **-RT** identifies the right knee. The NCCI identifies **29882** as a Column 2 code when reported with code **29881**. This designation means that the lateral meniscus repair should be specifically identified as distinct from meniscectomy on the medial meniscus because it was performed to correct a separate injury at a separate site and in a different compartment of the knee. Modifier **-XS Separate site** reports this information. This is an extended **-X{EPSU}** modifier that replaces modifier **-59 Distinct procedural service**. There are no additional modifiers that identify each different knee compartment or meniscus. The Column 2 indicator identifies that code **29882** is bundled into code **29881** when both are done on the same site. It is unusual that code **29882**, the

code with the higher RVU, is bundled into code **29881**, which has a lower RVU. Jacob sequences modifier **-XS** first because it provides information used for determining payment. Modifier **-RT** is informational only.

- ❏ Code **29881** requires modifiers **-RT Right** to identify the right knee. This code is unusual because it has a lower RVU value even though it is actually the more extensive procedure. Jacob appends modifier **-51 Multiple procedures** because it was performed during the same operative session as another procedure. Jacob is reminded by the encoder he uses that because arthroscopy was performed, the codes are subject to the **multiple endoscopy rule** for modifier **-51** (■ FIGURE 35-8). The multiple endoscopy rule states that when two codes from the same code family are reported, 100% is allowed on the first procedure and the allowed amount for the second procedure is the *difference* in price between the second code and the endoscopic base code, which in this case is **29870** (facility RVU = 11.82). The MPFSDB identifies the endoscopic base code for each code family. (Refer to Figure 33-6, "Example of Multiple Endoscopy Payment Rule".) Jacob sequences modifier **-51** first because it provides information used to calculate payment. Modifier **-RT** is informational only.

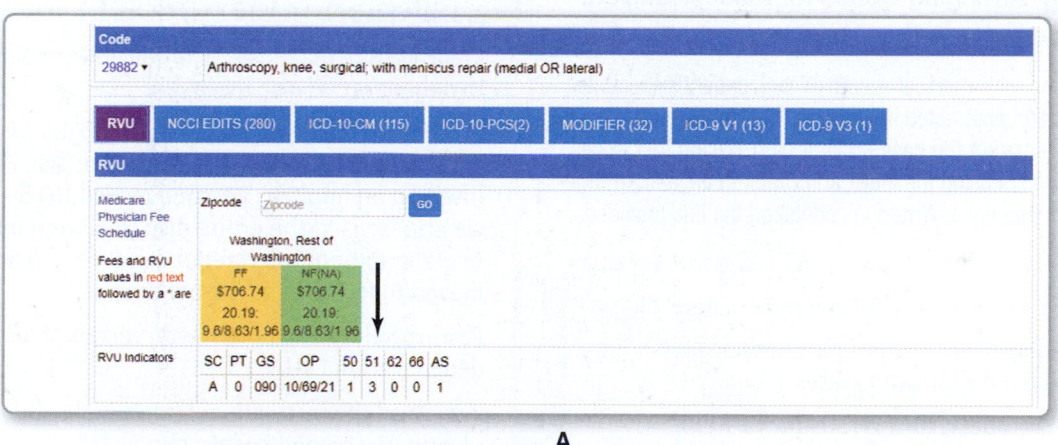

A

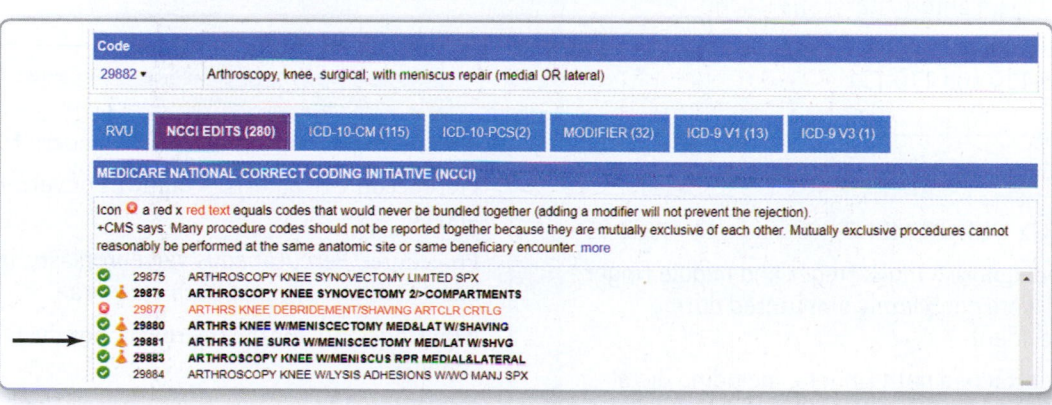

B

Figure 35-8 ■ Example of encoder screens for code 29882. (A) The indicator number 3 that appears below modifier -51 identifies that the code is subject to the multiple endoscopy rule. (B) The orange icon is a user-friendly method of displaying the significance of NCCI indicator 1, meaning that if the two codes are reported together, a modifier must be applied to indicate the reason. *Source: SpeedeCoder, Reprinted with permission.*

❏ He sequences code **29882** first because it has the higher RVU value, even though it requires modifier **-XS**.

❏ He sequences code **29881** second because it has a lower RVU value and thus a lower payment.

▶ Jacob finalizes the procedure codes and sequencing for this case:

(1) **29882-XS-RT Arthroscopy, knee, surgical; with meniscus repair (medial OR lateral); -XS Separate site; -RT Right**

(2) **29881-51-RT Arthroscopy, knee, surgical; with meniscectomy (medial OR lateral, including any meniscal shaving) including debridement/shaving of articular cartilage (chondroplasty), same or separate compartment(s), when performed; -51 Multiple procedures; -RT Right**

▶ Jacob also assigns and sequences the ICD-10-CM diagnosis codes that support the need for the service. He sequences the diagnosis code for the tear of the lateral meniscus first because the repair of the lateral meniscus is the first-listed procedure. He understands that it is acceptable to report diagnoses in a different order than they appear in the post-operative diagnosis in the operative report, based on coding and billing guidelines. A diagnosis for chondromalacia is reported, even though the condition was not directly treated, because it is part of the diagnostic evaluation and the physician documents it as significant in the operative report.

(1) **S83.261A Peripheral tear of lateral meniscus, current injury, right knee, initial encounter**

(2) **S83.231A Complex tear of medial meniscus, current injury, right knee, initial encounter**

(3) **M94.261 Chondromalacia, right knee**

SUCCESS STEP

If you do not have an encoder available, you can search the MPFSDB to identify the modifier indicator and the NCCI database to identify the NCCI bundling rules. Both databases are available at **www.cms.gov**.

CODING PRACTICE

Exercise 35.4 Arranging Codes for Musculoskeletal System Procedures

Instructions: Read the mini-medical-record of each patient's encounter. Review the information abstracted in Exercise 35.2 for questions 1–3. For questions 4–6, abstract the case on your own. Assign CPT codes, quantities, and modifiers using the Index and Tabular List, and arrange the codes in proper sequence. Write the code(s) on the line provided.

1. INPATIENT HOSPITAL Gender: M Age: 65

Preprocedure diagnosis: Pain in the thoracic spine due to degenerated and protruding discs

Procedure: Arthrodesis on T9-T10 and T10-T11 interspace using an anterolateral approach

Postprocedure diagnosis: Degeneration and protrusion, T9-T10 and T10-T11

2 CPT Codes _____

2. EMERGENCY DEPARTMENT Gender: M Age: 25

Preprocedure diagnosis: Index finger and middle finger on right hand were completely amputated during automobile accident.

Procedure: Reattached both fingers, including distal tip to sublimis tendon insertion

Tip: Identify the quantity to be reported with the code. Assign modifiers to identify the digits treated.

1 CPT Code _____

3. INPATIENT HOSPITAL Gender: F Age: 42

Preprocedure diagnosis: Chronic lower back pain due to degenerative disc disease

Procedure: Arthroplasty L4-5 and L5-L6. Using an anterior approach excised the entire disc L4-L5 and inserted an implant. We then moved to L5-L6 where we also excised the entire disc L4-L5 and inserted an implant. Patient tolerated procedure well and was moved to PACU in stable condition.

Postprocedure diagnosis: Intervertebral disc degeneration L4-L5, L5-L6

Tip: Read the instructional notes in the Tabular List to identity the second code.

2 CPT Codes _____

4. OUTPATIENT HOSPITAL Gender: F Age: 33

Preprocedure diagnosis: Fractures of vertebrae L3 and L4

Procedure: Percutaneous vertebroplasty, injected bone cement bilaterally into both vertebrae

Tip: Code only for the treatment, not the E/M or supplies.

2 CPT Codes _____

CODING PRACTICE *(continued)*

5. EMERGENCY DEPARTMENT   Gender: M   Age: 22

Preprocedure diagnosis: ATV accident, open fracture of the distal clavicle and deeply embedded debris in left shoulder

Procedure: Reduced fracture and applied internal fixation device consisting of wire and screws to stabilize bone. Excised debris from subcutaneous and subfascial tissue in left shoulder.

Tip: The treatment is open because internal fixation was applied.

2 CPT Codes _____

6. OUTPATIENT HOSPITAL   Gender: F   Age: 26

Preprocedure diagnosis: Right PCL avulsion

Procedure: Arthroscopically aided open repair of the right posterior cruciate ligament. Used an assistant surgeon (from the same medical group).

Tip: Code for both the surgeon and the assistant surgeon, using the appropriate modifier.

2 CPT Codes _____

E/M CODING FOR ORTHOPEDICS

The *1997 Documentation Guidelines for Evaluation and Management Services* (1997 DG), published by the Centers for Medicare and Medicaid Services (CMS), provides requirements for each level of a musculoskeletal E/M examination (■ Figure 35-9, page 710). Orthopedists are not limited to using the guidelines for a musculoskeletal examination only. They can also use guidelines for a general multiorgan system examination, or any other single organ system examination, based on what is most advantageous for a specific encounter. However, physicians cannot combine elements from more than one type of examination for a given encounter. The musculoskeletal examination guidelines typically provide the best results when a detailed musculoskeletal examination is performed.

To determine the appropriate E/M code, coders must review the documentation in detail and identify the specific elements documented.

- To identify the category and type of service, identify whether the encounter is a consultation—a service requested by another physician with a report back—or an office or inpatient visit in which the orthopedist is managing the care of the problem.
- To translate the documentation into the E/M requirements for the history, refer back to Chapter 28, "Evaluation and Management Services (99201-99499)," Tables 28-7 to 28-10, or to the 1997 DG.
- To determine the requirements for an examination, refer to Figure 35-9 or to the single organ system examination for the musculoskeletal system in the 1997 DG.
- To determine the levels for medical decision making (MDM), refer to Chapter 28, Table 28-12, and also the Table of Risk in the 1997 DG.

Guided Example of E/M Coding for the Musculoskeletal System

Refer to the orthopedic encounter (■ Figure 35-10, page 711) to practice skills for abstracting and assigning E/M codes. Follow along as fictitious coder Jacob Bates, CCS, abstracts the procedure. Check off each step after you complete it.

▶ First, Jacob needs to establish the category of service so he can determine the information needed to abstract and assign the code.

❑ *What is the setting?* Office.

❑ *What is the type of service?* Established patient

❑ *What is the code range?* Jacob refers to the CPT Index and looks up the Main Term **Evaluation and Management** and the subterm **Office and other outpatient**. The code range listed is **99201-99215**.

❑ *How many key components are required?* Jacob refers to the code range in the Tabular List and identifies that **99211-99215** identify established patient visits. All codes in the category except **99211** have the same requirements for key components. He reads the code description of the second code, which states **two out of three**. This tells him that two of three key components must meet or exceed the levels listed in the code (2/3).

▶ Next, Jacob identifies the level of history.

❑ *What is the level of HPI?* The HPI is **Extended** because four elements are documented.

❑ *What is the level of ROS?* The ROS is **Pertinent** because one system is documented.

❑ *What is the level of PFSH?* The PFSH is **Pertinent** because one element is documented.

System/Body Area	Elements of Musculoskeletal System Examination
Constitutional	❑ Measurement of any **three** of the following seven **vital** signs: • 1) sitting or standing blood pressure, • 2) supine blood pressure, • 3) pulse rate and regularity, • 4) respiration, • 5) temperature, • 6) height, • 7) weight (May be measured and recorded by ancillary staff) ❑ General **appearance** of patient (eg, development, nutrition, body habitus, deformities, attention to grooming)
Cardiovascular	❑ **Examination of peripheral vascular system by** • **observation** (eg, swelling, varicosities) • **palpation** (eg, pulses, temperature, edema, tenderness)
Lymphatic	Palpation of lymph nodes in **two or more** areas: ❑ Neck ❑ Axillae ❑ Groin ❑ Other
Musculoskeletal	❑ Examination of **gait** and **station** Examination of joints, bones and muscles of **four** of the following six areas: ❑ 1) head and neck; ❑ 2) spine, ribs and pelvis; ❑ 3) right upper extremity; ❑ 4) left upper extremity; ❑ 5) right lower extremity; and ❑ 6) left lower extremity. The examination of a given area includes: • Inspection and/or palpation with notation of presence of any **misalignment**, asymmetry, crepitation, defects, tenderness, masses, effusions • Assessment of **range of motion** with notation of any pain, crepitation or contracture • Assessment of **stability** with notation of any dislocation (luxation), subluxation or laxity • Assessment of muscle **strength** and **tone** (eg, flaccid, cog wheel, spastic) with notation of any atrophy or abnormal movements NOTE: For the **comprehensive** level of examination: all four of the **elements** identified by a bullet must be performed and documented for **each of four anatomic** areas. For the **problem focused, expanded problem focused, and detailed levels** of examination: Count each element **separately** for each body area. For example, assessing range of motion in two extremities constitutes two elements.
Skin	**Inspection and/or palpation** of skin and subcutaneous tissue (eg, scars, rashes, lesions, cafe-au-lait spots, ulcers) in **four** of the following six areas: ❑ 1) head and neck; ❑ 2) spine, ribs and pelvis; ❑ 3) right upper extremity; ❑ 4) left upper extremity; ❑ 5) right lower extremity; and ❑ 6) left lower extremity. NOTE: For the **comprehensive** level of examination: the examination of all **four anatomic** areas must be performed and documented. For the **problem focused, expanded problem focused, and detailed levels** of examination: Count each body area **separately**. For example, inspection and/or palpation of the skin and subcutaneous tissue of two extremities constitutes two elements.
Neurological/ Psychiatric	❑ Test **coordination** (eg, finger/nose, heel/ knee/shin, rapid alternating movements in the upper and lower extremities, evaluation of fine motor coordination in young children) ❑ Examination of **deep tendon reflexes** and/or nerve stretch test with notation of pathological reflexes (eg, Babinski) ❑ Examination of **sensation** (eg, by touch, pin, vibration, proprioception) Brief assessment of **mental status** including ❑ **Orientation** to time, place and person ❑ **Mood** and **affect** (eg, depression, anxiety, agitation)

Total # Bullets Performed and Documented →	⬜	# of ❑ **Elements Performed and Documented**	**Level of Examination**
		1–5	Problem focused
		6–11	Expanded problem focused
		12	Detailed
		ALL	Comprehensive (Document **every** element in each box with a shaded border and at least **one** element in each box with an unshaded border)

Figure 35-9 ■ 1997 documentation guidelines for musculoskeletal system examination.
Source: Centers for Medicare and Medicaid Services, 1997 Documentation Guidelines for Evaluation and Management Services (with formatting adjustments).

ORTHOPEDIC ENCOUNTER

CHIEF COMPLAINT: Left wrist pain.

HISTORY OF PRESENT PROBLEM: The patient has a previous history of a left traumatic wrist injury, which has left him with a chronic scapholunate problem and possibly other problems in his wrist, which I have seen him for multiple times over the past five years, most recently about 18 months ago. He was doing relatively fine and tolerating the wrist soreness that he had, which varies day to day, but it has not gotten much worse until this most recent injury. He lifted a box out of the back of his car three weeks ago and it started to hurt with a sharp stabbing pain. Since then he was significantly more affected than he was before, and now he reports a dull aching pain on the ulnar side of his wrist. He presents to my office for evaluation.

CLINICAL/PHYSICAL EXAMINATION:
Musculoskeletal: An examination of the left wrist shows that the patient has point tenderness to palpation along the ulnar styloid extensor carpi ulnaris (ECU) ridge with some minor tenderness at the triangular fibrocartilage complex (TFC) region, as well as the lunotriquetral joint. There is some minor soreness, but not nearly as sore at the scapholunate (SL) ligament with dorsiflexion 30°, palmar flexion 30°, radial deviation 5° and ulnar deviation 0°. Supination/pronation grossly intact without significant signs of instability. Negative piano key sign compared to the contralateral side.
Skin: No skin breakdown or hyperhidrosis.
Neurologic: Negative signs of compressive median nerve neuropathy.
Vascular: Intact.

RADIOLOGICAL/LABORATORY EXAM: X-rays, three views of the wrist of good penetrance and quality, reveal scapholunate widening of a slack wrist with a possible ulnar styloid nonunion, with a possible occult distal radius fracture fibrous union. MRI report reviewed.

EVALUATION/TREATMENT PLAN: The MRI is consistent with edema and swelling in the ulnar styloid region, which is consistent with the injury pattern that he is claiming and where he is most sore. He has a chronic problem that needs to potentially be addressed. Sometimes with these acute on chronic problems, what was tolerated initially may no longer be tolerated by the patient, which we talked about. Our focus still should be on the initial injury which brought him in at this time. It is a three-week-old injury. Given the MRI, we probably have seen on radiographs a fibrous union between that ulnar styloid and the remaining portion of the ulna, which may have been torn or injured, especially consistent with the MRI. Therefore, I would cast him initially to get that to heal, and then reassess. All questions were answered, and we will make the treatment plans accordingly. He will followup in two weeks. We casted him.

HISTORY: Problem focused
Chief complaint (CC)
PFSH: Pertinent (1)
ROS: None (0)
MDM Management: Established presenting problem, worsening (Low Complexity Management Options)
HPI: Extended (4+)
Setting & patient type

EXAMINATION: Problem focused
(1-5 elements)

MDM Data: Independent visualization of image, tracing, or scan by physician performing the E/M service (High Complexity Data)

MEDICAL DECISION MAKING: Moderate Complexity
MDM Risk: Acute illness with systemic symptoms, Elective major surgery (open, percutaneous or endoscopic) with no identified risk factors (Moderate Risk)

KEY: HPI History of the present illness   ROS Review of systems
      PFSH Past, family, and social history   MDM Medical decision making

Figure 35-10 ■ Orthopedic encounter. *Source: © PB Resources, Inc. Used with permission.*

❏ *Based on these factors, what is the overall level of history?* The level of history is **Expanded problem focused** because the lowest of the three factors (HPI, ROS, and PFSH) determines the history level. The HPI qualifies for a detailed history but the ROS and PFSH qualify for an expanded problem-focused history.

▶ Jacob refers to the musculoskeletal system examination in the 1997 DG (Figure 35-9) to abstract information needed to determine the level of examination.

❏ *What is the level of examination?* The level of examination is **Problem focused**. Three (3) elements of the examination are documented, which exceeds the requirement of one to five bulleted elements for a problem-focused examination.

▶ Jacob determines the level of medical decision making. (Refer to Table 28-12, Medical Decision-Making Levels.)

❏ *What is the level of complexity of the number of diagnoses or management options, based on the presenting problem?* The level is **Low complexity** because there is an established presenting problem that is worsening as a result of a recent exacerbation.

❏ *What is the amount and/or complexity of data to be reviewed?* The level is **High complexity** because the physician providing the E/M service performed an independent visualization of the x-rays and MRI.

❏ *What is the level of risk of significant complications, morbidity, and/or mortality?* Jacob reviews each column in the Table of Risk in the 1997 DG and determines that the level of risk is **Moderate**. The patient presents with a chronic condition with mild exacerbation (Moderate), x-rays and an MRI were ordered (Minimal), and casting was performed (Minimal). The single highest element in the Table of Risk determines the overall risk. The column **Presenting problem** is the highest level (Moderate).

❏ *Based on these factors, what is the overall level of medical decision making?* The medical decision making is

Moderate complexity. At least two of the three MDM factors are required to qualify for a specific level of MDM. Because the complexity of data to be reviewed is high and the risk of complications is moderate, two of the three MDM factors meet or exceed moderate decision making.

Now Jacob is ready to assign the code for the orthopedic encounter. The exercise that follows guides you through additional abstracting skills and allows you to assign the correct code.

CODING PRACTICE

Exercise 35.5 E/M Coding for Orthopedics

Instructions: Refer to the *1997 Documentation Guidelines for Evaluation and Management Services* (available at **www.cms.gov**) or Chapter 28, "Evaluation and Management Services," Tables 28-7 to 28-12, in this text. Answer the following questions about the "Orthopedic encounter" (Figure 35-10).

1. a. Which elements of the HPI are documented? Circle all that apply. Location, Quality, Severity, Duration, Timing, Context, Modifying factors, Associated signs and symptoms

   b. How many elements are documented? _____

   c. What is the level of HPI? _____

2. a. Which systems are reviewed in the ROS? Circle all that apply. Constitutional, Allergic/ immunologic, CV, Endocrine, ENT/M, Eyes, GI, GU, Hemic/lymphatic, MS, Neurologic, Psychiatric, Respiratory, Skin/breast

   b. How many systems are documented? _____

   c. What is the level of ROS? _____

3. a. Which PFSH elements are documented? Circle all that apply. Past medical, Family, Social

   b. What is the level of PFSH? _____

   c. What is the overall level of history? (The lowest history factor—HPI, ROS, or PFSH—determines the level of history.)

   _____

4. Refer to Figure 35-9, "1997 documentation guidelines for musculoskeletal system examination."

   a. Which bulleted items are documented for the examination? (Check off the items documented.)

   b. How many bulleted items are documented? _____

   c. What is the level of the examination? _____

5. Refer to Table 28-12, Medical Decision-Making Levels, or the 1997 DG.

   a. What is the MDM level for the number of diagnoses or management options? _____

   b. What is the MDM level for the amount and/or complexity of data to be reviewed? _____

   c. Refer to the Table of Risk in the 1997 DG. Which elements of risk are documented for each risk factor?

   1. Presenting problem: _____

   2. Diagnostic procedures ordered: _____

   3. Management options selected: _____

   d. What is the level of risk? (The highest of the three risk factors determines the overall level of risk.) _____

   e. What is the overall level of MDM? (2/3 MDM factors are needed to determine the overall level.) _____

6. a. What is the setting? _____

   b. What is the patient (or service) type? _____

   c. What is the code range? _____

   d. How many key components are required? _____

   e. What is the level of history? _____

   f. What is the level of examination? _____

   g. What is the level of medical decision making? _____

   h. What is the correct code? _____

   i. What modifier(s) is required? _____

7. Abstract and assign the diagnosis code that supports the E/M code. There are no appropriate external cause codes.

   1 ICD-10-CM Code _____

CHAPTER SUMMARY

In this chapter you learned that:

- Any given orthopedic procedure can be performed using a variety of techniques, which can involve specific types of sutures and bone anchors aimed at promoting maximum stability and preventing reinjury.

- CPT provides guidelines about fracture treatment and excision of muscular system tumors at the beginning of the Musculoskeletal System subsection. Detailed special instructions and instructional notes throughout the subsection provide guidance regarding coding spinal procedures, modifiers, and multiple coding.

- Because the Musculoskeletal System is a combination of two systems, separate abstracting guidelines are provided for skeletal system, fractures and dislocations, and muscular system procedures.

- Two areas requiring special attention when assigning codes are using the Index to locate the appropriate anatomic site and coding for fracture care.

- Special instructions that appear at the beginning of and throughout the Musculoskeletal System subsection provide detailed guidance regarding multiple coding and the use of modifiers, particularly in the *Spine (Vertebral Column)* subheading.

- The *1997 Documentation Guidelines for Evaluation and Management Services* (1997 DG), published by CMS, provides requirements for each level of a musculoskeletal E/M examination, but orthopedists are not limited to using the guidelines for a musculoskeletal examination only.

CONCEPT QUIZ

Take a moment to look back at the Musculoskeletal System subsection and solidify your skills. Try to answer the questions from memory first, then refer to the discussion in this chapter if you need a little extra help.

Completion

Instructions: Write the term that completes each statement based on the information you learned in this chapter. Choose from the list below. Some choices may be used more than once and some choices may not be used at all.

arthroplasty	internal fixation
biopsy	interspace
chondroplasty	manipulation
decompression	reconstruction
discectomy	replantation
external fixation	spinal fusion
fasciotomy	tenolysis
hemiarthroplasty	vertebral segment

1. _____ is another term for fracture stabilization with a rigid frame and one or more screws.

2. _____ is the use of force to move parts of a bone into normal alignment.

3. To relieve shoulder impingement a(n) _____ may be performed.

4. _____ is removing a sample of muscle to determine the presence of disease such as muscular dystrophy.

5. In a(n) _____, two vertebrae are joined together to provide stabilization.

6. A(n) _____ may be performed when a knee injury requires reshaping and cleaning of the cartilage.

7. _____ is a partial replacement of a joint.

8. _____ is the release of a tendon.

9. _____ is a reattachment of a complete amputation of a thumb.

10. On disc procedures, L2-L3 refers to one _____.

Multiple Choice

Instructions: Circle the letter of the best answer to each question based on the information you learned in this chapter.

1. What is the medical term for surgical excision of a joint?
   A. Arthrotomy
   B. Arthroplasty
   C. Arthrectomy
   D. Arthrodesis

2. Which type of treatment involves manipulation of displaced bones?
   A. Restorative
   B. Palliative
   C. Stabilization
   D. External fixation

3. What is the Main Term that classifies procedures on the patella?
   A. Knee
   B. Knee joint
   C. Knee bone
   D. Kneecap

4. How would you code the following procedure? *A neurosurgeon and an orthopedic surgeon each perform a portion of an anterior cervical discectomy and fusion at C5-C6.*
   A. 22558-80
   B. 22558-51
   C. 22558-62
   D. 22558 × 2

(continued)

(continued from page 713)

5. What resource helps the coder to determine sequencing of CPT codes?
   A. Multiple Endoscopy Rule
   B. Medicare Physician Fee Schedule
   C. Appendix A of the CPT code book
   D. Appendix G of the CPT code book

6. How would you code the following procedure? *During a procedure for open reduction with internal fixation (ORIF) of the left femur, the patient developed tachycardia and the procedure was terminated.*
   A. No code
   B. 27269-52-LT
   C. 27269-53-LT
   D. 27269-54-LT

7. What type of codes never use modifier -51?
   A. Arthroscopy codes
   B. Add-on codes
   C. Fracture codes
   D. Spine codes

8. When should a code for cast application be reported?
   A. When the cast is removed or repaired by a different individual than the one who applied it
   B. When different providers perform the preoperative care, restorative treatment, and/or postoperative care
   C. When the provider who applies the initial cast or strapping also provides restorative treatment for the fracture and all follow-up care
   D. When cast application or strapping is the only service provided and no other treatment is anticipated

9. How would you code the following procedure? *A surgeon performs arthrocentesis of the right hip and right ankle during the same surgical episode.*
   A. 20610-RT × 2
   B. 20605-RT × 2
   C. 20610-RT, 20605-51-RT
   D. 20610-51-RT, 20605-51-RT

10. What resource identifies bundling rules?
    A. MPFS
    B. RVU
    C. OPPS
    D. NCCI

KEEP ON CODING

Instructions: Read the procedural statement, then use the appropriate Index and Tabular List to assign CPT procedure codes, quantities, and modifiers. Write the code(s) on the line provided.

1. Cemented right total hip replacement. CPT Code(s) _____

2. Kyphoplasty, T3, T4. CPT Code(s) _____

3. Endoscopic repair of left rotator cuff tendon. CPT Code(s) _____

4. Arthroscopic repair of left and right medial menisci. CPT Code(s) _____

5. Arthroscopic repair of the anterior cruciate ligament, left knee. CPT Code(s) _____

6. Arthroscopic capsulorrhaphy, right shoulder. CPT Code(s) _____

7. Arthroscopic medial meniscectomy, right knee. CPT Code(s) _____

8. Removal of Stableloc external fixator from left wrist. CPT Code(s) _____

9. Left total knee replacement. CPT Code(s) _____

10. Hemiarthroplasty, right side femoral neck fracture. CPT Code(s) _____

11. Sternal debridement for bone infection. CPT Code(s) _____

12. Aspiration of three ganglion cysts of the wrist. CPT Code(s) _____

13. Complete amputation of second toe of left foot at the metatarsophalangeal joint. CPT Code(s) _____

14. ORIF right proximal humeral head. CPT Code(s) _____

15. Percutaneous drainage of right knee fluid. CPT Code(s) _____

16. Posterior interbody arthrodesis of lumbar vertebrae L1-L2. CPT Code(s) _____

17. Repair of fracture of the left femoral shaft with intramedullary rod. CPT Code(s) _____

18. Replacement of a short leg walking cast on the right leg during aftercare. CPT Code(s) _____

19. ORIF bimalleolar fracture, right. CPT Code(s) _____

20. Osteotomy of T2 with discetomy of the T2-T3 disc using the anterior approach. CPT Code(s) _____

21. Open reduction internal fixation of left ulnar shaft fracture with placement of long arm cast. CPT Code(s) _____

22. Radical resection of a 2.5-cm sarcoma of the scalp. CPT Code(s) _____

23. Incision and drainage with extensive debridement, left shoulder, with removal of prosthesis. CPT Code(s) _____

24. Removal of ulnar nail implant. CPT Code(s) _____

25. Open intramedullary nail fixation with locking screws of a left tibial shaft fracture. CPT Code(s) _____

CODING CHALLENGE

Instructions: Read the mini-medical-record of each patient's encounter, then abstract, assign, and arrange ICD-10-CM diagnosis codes and CPT procedure codes using the appropriate Index and Tabular List. Assign quantities and modifiers where needed. Write the code(s) on the line provided.

1. OUTPATIENT SURGERY   Gender: M   Age: 12

Preprocedure diagnosis: Malunion, proximal humerus fracture, right arm

Procedure: Repair of malunion of the right proximal humerus with internal fixation using a 2-hole, 16-mm pin plate

1 ICD-10-CM Code _____

1 CPT Code _____

2. OUTPATIENT SURGERY   Gender: F   Age: 56

Preprocedure diagnosis: Chronic diabetic ulcer of left midfoot with muscle necrosis

Procedure: Below-the-knee amputation, left leg

Postprocedure diagnosis: Diabetic ulcer of plantar surface of the left midfoot with muscle necrosis

2 ICD-10-CM Codes _____

1 CPT Code _____

3. OUTPATIENT SURGERY   Gender: F   Age: 27

Preprocedure diagnosis: Contractures due to excessive scarring of the tendon bed of the 4th and 5th fingers of the left hand from previous knife injury

Procedure: Excision of flexor tendon of 4th and 5th fingers and implantation of synthetic rods, left hand

Postprocedure diagnosis: Excessive scarring of the tendon bed of the 4th and 5th fingers of the left hand

Tip: Identify the digits using modifiers.

1 ICD-10-CM Code _____

2 CPT Codes _____

4. OUTPATIENT SURGERY   Gender: F   Age: 49

Preprocedure diagnosis: Hammer toe deformity of left foot, third and fourth digits

Procedure: Arthroplasty of the third and fourth digits proximal interphalangeal joint laterally of left foot

Postprocedure diagnosis: Hammer toe deformity of left foot, third and fourth digits

1 ICD-10-CM Code _____

2 CPT Codes _____

5. EMERGENCY DEPT   Gender: M   Age: 26

Reason for encounter: Worsening pain ×3 days in right lower leg extending to the foot, expanded problem-focused history, expanded problem-focused examination, low-complexity medical decision making

Procedure: Short leg splint applied for stabilization

Assessment: Acute right ankle sprain, possible small avulsion fracture

Plan: Immobilize the ankle and make an appointment with the orthopedic surgeon in the next three days

Tip: Code only for the treatment, not the E/M or supplies.

1 ICD-10-CM Code _____

1 CPT Code _____

6. PHYSICIAN OFFICE   Gender: F   Age: 66

Reason for encounter: Pathologic fracture of right radius, return to office for short arm cast change

Procedure: Replaced short arm cast with a fiberglass gauntlet cast

Assessment: Right radial fracture healing as expected

Plan: Return to office in two weeks

Tip: Code for the service and the supply.

1 ICD-10-CM Code _____

1 CPT Code _____

1 HCPCS Code _____

(continued)

(continued from page 715)

---

7. INPATIENT HOSPITAL   Gender: F   Age: 50

Reason for encounter: Chronic plantar fasciitis, right foot; morbidly obese at 327 lb; insulin-dependent diabetic

Procedure: Open plantar fasciotomy, right foot

Assessment: Failed conservative care; patient desires corrective surgery

Plan: Walker boot post-op with full weight bearing, return to office in 4 days

4 ICD-10-CM Codes _____

_____

1 CPT Code _____

---

8. INPATIENT HOSPITAL   Gender: F   Age: 58

Preprocedure diagnosis: Probable osteomyelitis

Procedure: Open biopsy of left upper femur

Postprocedure diagnosis: Acute and chronic osteomyelitis of the femur

Pathology report: Acute and chronic osteomyelitis

Tip: Review the guidelines for anatomic modifiers.

2 ICD-10-CM Codes _____

1 CPT Code _____

---

9. PHYSICIAN OFFICE   Gender: M   Age: 52

Preprocedure diagnosis: Subpatellar bursitis, left knee

Procedure: Aspiration of fluid from bursa; excision of suspicious 0.4 cm mole on left thigh

Postprocedure diagnosis: Subpatellar bursitis, left knee; septic knee ruled out; malignant melanoma of thigh

2 ICD-10-CM Codes _____

2 CPT Codes _____

---

10. EMERGENCY DEPT   Gender: F   Age: 62

Reason for encounter: Fall at home after stepping on a dog toy, now with pain and swelling of the left lower arm

Procedure: Closed reduction of left ulnar olecranon process

Assessment: X-ray reveals a nondisplaced fracture of the left ulnar olecranon process

Plan: Referred to orthopedic surgeon for follow-up

Tip: Code for the diagnosis and the external cause. Apply seventh characters as required. Code only for the treatment, not the E/M or supplies.

3 ICD-10-CM Codes _____

_____

1 CPT Code _____

Cardiovascular System Procedures (33010-37799)

Learning Objectives

After completing this chapter, you should have the skills to:

36.1 Spell and define the key words, medical terms, and abbreviations related to cardiovascular procedures. (Remember)

36.2 Summarize the fundamentals of cardiovascular procedures. (Understand)

36.3 Adhere to the CPT coding guidelines into the Cardiovascular System subsection. (Apply)

36.4 Examine and abstract procedural information from the medical record for coding Cardiovascular System subsection procedures. (Analyze)

36.5 Demonstrate how to assign codes for procedures in the Cardiovascular System subsection. (Apply)

36.6 Utilize guidelines for arranging (sequencing) codes for Cardiovascular System subsection procedures. (Apply)

36.7 Determine how to code Evaluation and Management services for cardiology. (Evaluate)

Chapter Outline

- **Cardiovascular System Procedure Basics**
- **Coding Guidelines for Cardiovascular System Procedures**
- **Abstracting Cardiovascular System Procedures**
- **Assigning Codes for Cardiovascular System Procedures**
- **Arranging Codes for Cardiovascular System Procedures**
- **E/M Coding for Cardiology**

Key Terms and Abbreviations

bypass graft	contralateral	nonselective catheter placement	selective catheter placement
cardiopulmonary bypass (CPB)	ipsilateral	open heart surgery	vascular family

In addition to the key terms listed here, students should know the terms defined within tables in this chapter.

INTRODUCTION

Traveling to a shopping destination may take you through a network of roads and streets. A primary destination, such as a mall, may be located next to a main highway, but to reach a small neighborhood shop you probably need to make turns onto a series of side streets. In a similar way, the cardiovascular system is a hierarchy of vessels, each leading to a more remote site than the previous one.

CARDIOVASCULAR SYSTEM PROCEDURE BASICS

Cardiology is a subspecialty of internal medicine that specializes in the cardiovascular system. Cardiologists perform medical procedures such as cardiac function tests and cardiac catheterization but do not perform surgery. Cardiothoracic surgeons perform surgery on the heart and surrounding structures, including the lung when necessary. Vascular surgeons perform surgery on the vessels. Some surgeons specialize further in areas such as heart valve surgery, neonatal cardiac surgery, and pediatric cardiac surgery. Chapter 13 of this text provides more information on cardiovascular system anatomy and conditions. Refer to ■ TABLE 36-1 for a refresher on how to build medical terms related to the cardiovascular system.

CODING CAUTION

Be alert for medical terms that are spelled similarly and have different meanings.

en**darter**ectomy (*excision of the lining of a vessel*) and **enter**ectomy (*excision of the intestine*)

arteriotomy (*incision into an artery*) and **ar**t**hro**tomy (*incision into a joint*)

val**vulo**plasty (*surgical repair of a valve*) and **vulvulo**plasty (*surgical repair of the vulva*)

Procedures of the Cardiovascular System

Procedures commonly performed on the cardiovascular system are summarized in ■ TABLE 36-2. After discussing approaches to heart surgery, this section discusses procedures for pacemakers, catheterization, and congenital heart defects.

Approaches to Heart Surgery

Heart surgery is performed to correct structural and functional problems with the heart anatomy and to improve the flow of blood to and through the heart. Surgeons can operate on the heart using open-heart surgery, off-pump heart surgery, and minimally invasive heart surgery.

Open Heart Surgery. Open heart surgery involves exposing the heart through a 15- to 20-cm (6- to 8-inch) incision in the chest wall that requires cutting through the sternum. For some types of surgery, the surgeon also may open the heart, but the term *open* refers to the chest, not the heart. After the heart is exposed, the patient is connected to a **cardiopulmonary** (*heart–lung*) **bypass (CPB)** machine that takes over the pumping action of the heart. A specialist oversees the CPB machine. It moves blood away from the heart, allowing the surgeon to operate on a heart that is not beating and does not have blood flowing through it. A breathing tube is placed through the throat into the lungs and is connected to a ventilator. After the procedure is completed, blood flow is restored to the heart and the patient is disconnected from the equipment. The sternum is closed with wires that remain in the body permanently. Open heart surgery is used to perform CABGs, repair or replace heart valves, treat atrial fibrillation, do heart transplants, and implant VADs and TAHs.

Off-Pump Heart Surgery. Off-pump coronary artery bypass (OPCAB) surgery is also an open procedure, but a CPB machine is not used. The surgeon steadies the heart with a mechanical device and operates while blood is pumping through it. Although OPCAB is believed to reduce certain risks and complications associated with open heart surgery, it requires special training for the surgeon, and not all patients are candidates.

Minimally Invasive Heart Surgery. For minimally invasive heart surgery, a surgeon makes small incisions (10–12 cm [4–5 inches] in length) in the side of the chest between the ribs. The surgeon connects a graft to diseased coronary arteries on a beating heart without any artificial support to the circulation. Because of the nature of the operation, suturing must be done under direct vision and the coronary artery to be bypassed must lie directly beneath the incision. Consequently, this procedure is only designed to bypass one or two coronary arteries. This procedure provides the most minimally invasive heart surgery alternative to limited CABG and angioplasty currently practiced.

Minimally invasive heart surgery is used to do some bypass and maze surgeries. Surgeons also used this approach to repair or replace heart valves, insert pacemakers or implantable cardioverter-defibrillators (ICDs), or harvest a vein or artery to use as a **bypass graft** (*inserting a new vessel to permanently redirect blood flow to avoid a blockage in an artery*) for CABG.

Table 36-1 ■ **EXAMPLE OF CONSTRUCTING MEDICAL TERMS FOR CARDIOVASCULAR PROCEDURES**

Root/Combining Form	Suffix	Complete Medical Term
angi/o (*vessel*)		**phlebo + tomy** (*cutting into a vein*)
		veni + puncture (*piercing a vein*)
arteri/o (*artery*)	**-tomy** (*cutting into*)	**arterio + tomy** (*cutting into an artery*)
	-puncture (*piercing*)	**arterial + puncture** (*piercing an artery*)
ven/o (*vein*)	**-graphy** (*recording*)	**angio + graphy** (*recording of a vessel*)
		veno + graphy (*recording of a vein*)
phleb/o (*vein*)		**arterio + graphy** (*recording of an artery*)

Source: © PB Resources, Inc. Used with permission.

Table 36-2 ■ **COMMON PROCEDURES OF THE CARDIOVASCULAR SYSTEM**

Procedure Name	Definition	Reason Performed
Arteriovenous (AV) fistula creation	Creation of a connection between an artery and vein	Hemodialysis access
Arteriovenous (AV) fistula repair	Closure of an abnormal connection between two vessels	Congenital or acquired AV fistula
Atherectomy	Threading through the veins a catheter that has a rotating shaver on its tip to cut away plaque from the artery	Atherosclerosis
Catheter ablation/radiofrequency ablation	Use of a fluoroscopy-guided catheter to the exact site of arrhythmia in the heart to emit radiofrequency energy that destroys heart muscle cells in a very small area (about 1/5 of an inch)	Arrhythmia, supraventricular tachyarrhythmia
Coronary artery bypass grafting (CABG)	Grafting (*connecting*) a healthy artery or vein from elsewhere in the body to a blocked coronary artery	Coronary artery disease (CAD), arterial stenosis, lesions, atherosclerosis, or peripheral vascular occlusive disease
Endovascular aneurysm repair (EVAR)	Replacement of a weak section of an artery or heart wall with a patch, stent, or graft	Aneurysm
Excisional embolectomy/ thrombectomy	Incision into a vein or artery and removal of a clot	Embolus (*a moving blood clot or obstruction*) or thrombus (*a stationery blood clot*)
Fenestrated endovascular aneurysm repair (FEVAR)	Reinforcement of a weak section of the aorta with a stent that has holes customized to accommodate arterial branches	Aneurysm located at a site where a traditional stent would block one or more arteries
Heart transplant	Replacement of a diseased heart with a healthy heart from a deceased donor	End-stage heart failure
Maze surgery	Creation of new paths for the heart's electrical signals to travel through	Atrial fibrillation
Mechanical thrombectomy	A transcatheter procedure that uses a thrombolytic agent, radiological guidance, and a small blade or water jet to fragment, then suction out, a clot from an artery or vein	Thrombus
Pacemaker insertion	Placement under the skin of the chest or abdomen of a small device with wires connected to the heart chambers that transmit low-energy electrical pulses to control heart rhythm	Arrhythmia
Total artificial heart (TAH) implantation	Insertion of a device that replaces the ventricles	End-stage heart failure
Transmyocardial revascularization (TMR)	Use of lasers to make small channels through the heart muscle and into the left ventricle	Angina
Valve repair or replacement	Opening or tightening flaps on a heart valve	Valvular stenosis, regurgitation, or prolapse
Ventricular assist device (VAD) implantation	Insertion of a mechanical pump used to support heart function and blood flow	End-stage heart failure

Source: © PB Resources, Inc. Used with permission.

This type of procedure is also known as limited-access coronary artery surgery and includes port-access coronary artery bypass (PACAB or PortCAB), which uses a heart–lung machine, and minimally invasive direct coronary artery bypass graft (MIDCAB), which does not.

CODING CAUTION

Remember to distinguish between the terms *bypass graft* and *cardiopulmonary bypass*. A bypass graft refers to the *procedure* of inserting a new vessel to permanently redirect blood flow to avoid a blockage in an artery. Cardiopulmonary bypass refers to use of a *machine* to temporarily replace the function of the heart during surgery by directing the flow of blood away from the heart, through the bypass pump, and back into the body.

Pacemaker Procedures

Pacemakers and ICDs are small devices with a battery-operated pulse generator connected to leads (*wires*). Electrodes are attached to the leads, which then are attached to the heart. Physicians implant pacemakers in a skin pocket in the chest or abdomen to help control abnormal heart rhythms. They place leads directly on the epicardium (*outer layer of the heart*) through a thoracoscopy (*thoracotomy with endoscopy*) or transvenously (*through a vein*) and then into the right atrium or right ventricle (■ FIGURE 36-1, page 720). ICD electrodes are usually placed transvenously, but some can also be placed in a subcutaneous pocket with the pulse generator.

A pacemaker or ICD monitors heart rhythm and sends electrical pulses or shocks during an emergent situation to prompt the heart to beat at a normal rate. These devices are for patients with arrhythmias, disorders of heart rhythm including tachycardia and bradycardia. A pacemaker also records the

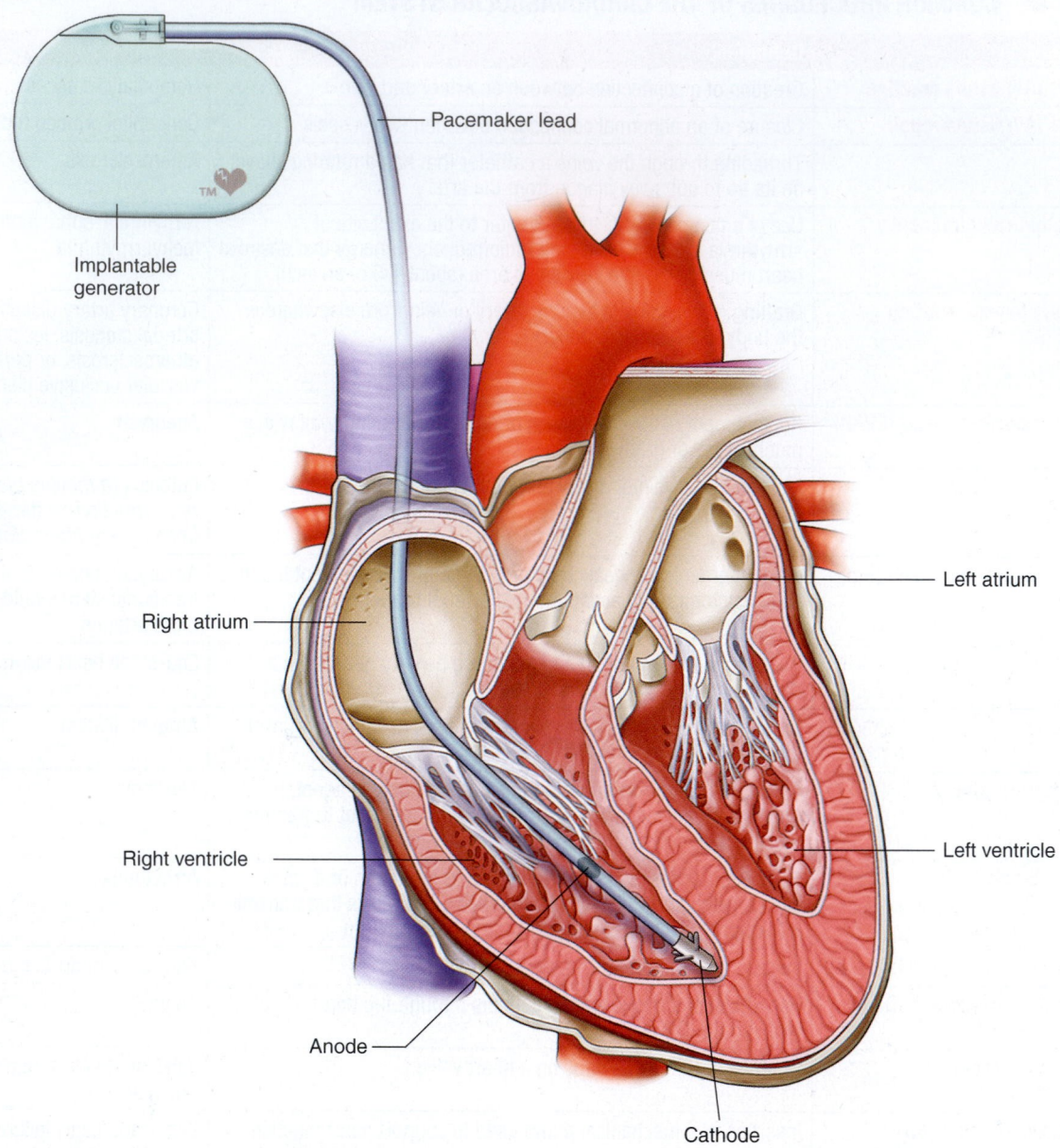

Figure 36-1 ■ Pacemaker components.

heart's electrical activity and rhythm. The physician analyzes the recordings to adjust a patient's pacemaker so that it functions well.

Pacemakers have one to three wires that are placed in different chambers of the heart.

- The wires in a single-chamber pacemaker usually carry pulses between the right ventricle and the pulse generator.

- The wires in a dual-chamber pacemaker carry pulses between the right atrium and the right ventricle and the pulse generator. The pulses help coordinate the timing of these two chambers' contractions using two leads.

- The wires in a biventricular pacemaker, also called a cardiac resynchronization therapy (CRT) device, carry pulses between an atrium and both ventricles and the generator. The pulses help coordinate electrical signaling between the two ventricles using three leads.

Pacemakers can be temporary or permanent. Temporary pacemakers are used to treat temporary heartbeat problems, such as a slow heartbeat caused by a heart attack, heart surgery, or an overdose of medicine. Temporary pacemakers are also used during emergencies until a permanent pacemaker can be implanted or until the temporary condition subsides. Permanent pacemakers are used to control long-term heart rhythm problems.

Pacemaker batteries last between 5 and 15 years, with an average of 7 years, depending on how active the pacemaker is. Physicians replace both the pulse generator and the battery before the battery starts to run down. Replacing the generator and battery is less involved than the original surgery to implant the pacemaker. Eventually, the pacemaker's wires may also need to be replaced.

An ICD sends electrical pulses and shocks to the ventricles of the heart, called defibrillation. An ICD helps treat more serious heart disorders, such as cardiac arrest. An ICD can

Table 36-3 ■ **CONGENITAL HEART DEFECT REPAIR PROCEDURES**

Name	Condition	Procedure(s)
Atrial septal defect (ASD) repair	A hole in the wall between the left and right upper chambers of the heart	• Open heart surgery to close the hole with sutures or a patch • Transcatheter placement of metal clamp or plug to close the hole
Coarctation of the aorta repair	Presence of a coarctation (*an abnormally narrow section*) in the aorta	• Synthetic (Gore-Text) or autologous (subclavian artery) graft to widen the vessel • Removal of the coarctation followed by anastomosis • Creation of a bypass around the coarctation using a tube • Stent placement to widen the lumen
Hypoplastic left heart syndrome (HLHS) repair	Underdeveloped aorta and left ventricle in which the aortic and mitral valves are either too small to allow sufficient blood flow or are completely atretic (*closed*)	3-stage repair: • Creation of one blood vessel from the pulmonary artery and the aorta to carry blood to the lungs and the rest of the body (Norwood procedure) • Connect the superior vena cava directly to pulmonary arteries (Glenn shunt or hemi-Fontan procedure) • Connect the inferior vena cava directly to the pulmonary arteries (Fontan procedure)
Patent ductus arteriosus (PDA) ligation	Failure of the ductus arteriosus (*a blood vessel in the fetus that connects the aorta and the pulmonary artery*) to close after birth	• Medication • Insertion of a metal coil to block the opening • Surgery to divide and ligate the vessel
Tetralogy of Fallot repair	Presence of four defects: • Ventricular septal defect (VSD) • Pulmonary stenosis (*obstructed outflow of blood from the right ventricle to the lungs*) • Dextroposition/overriding aorta (*blood flow from the aorta into both ventricles*) • Right-ventricular hypertrophy (*thickened wall of the right ventricle*)	• Widening the pulmonary stenosis • Patching the right ventricle and pulmonary artery • Closing the VSD • Replacing the pulmonary valve • Shunting to move blood flow
Total anomalous pulmonary venous return (TAPVR) correction	The pulmonary veins bring oxygen-rich blood from the lungs back to the right side of the heart instead of the left	Route pulmonary veins back to the left side of the heart; close any abnormal connections; ligate PDA, if present
Transposition of the great vessels repair	The placement of the aorta and pulmonary artery are switched, preventing pulmonary circulation	Arterial switch: divide the aorta and pulmonary artery; connect pulmonary artery to right ventricle; connect aorta and coronary arteries to left ventricle
Tricuspid atresia repair	Narrowed, deformed, or absent tricuspid valve	• Medication (temporary) • Repair or replace tricuspid valve • One or a series of shunts to direct blood to the lungs
Truncus arteriosus repair	The aorta, coronary arteries, and pulmonary artery all come out of one common trunk	Separate pulmonary arteries from the aortic trunk; patch defects; close VSD, if present
Ventricular septal defect (VSD) repair	A hole in the wall between the left and right lower chambers of the heart	Place a patch through open heart surgery or using a guidewire

Source: © PB Resources, Inc. Used with permission.

deliver higher-energy electrical pulses than a pacemaker and, as a result, is used for more serious heart disorders, whereas a pacemaker can deliver only low-energy electrical pulses.

Catheterization Procedures

The Medicine section of CPT classifies catheterization procedures performed on the heart. The Cardiovascular System subsection classifies catheterization procedures performed on the vessels. Vascular injection procedures involve injecting contrast dye for radiological imaging or injecting medication into blood vessels. Catheter placement may be nonselective or selective and may be performed for injection procedures, angioplasty, atherectomy, or stent placement in the vascular system. The most frequently used access sites are the common femoral artery (CFA) and brachial arteries. **Nonselective catheter placement** is the insertion of a catheter that remains in the accessed vessel or the aorta. **Selective catheter placement** is the insertion of a catheter into a vessel, moving it to the aorta, then moving it through one or more arteries that branch off the aorta to reach the specific vessel needing treatment.

Vessels connect to one another through branches, or vascular families, and are categorized in groups, called first-, second-, or third-order vessels. A **vascular family** is a network of vessels branching off the same primary vessel. A first-order branch is the first division off of the primary vessel, such as the aorta. The first artery that divides off the aorta is a first-order branch; an artery that divides off the first-order artery is a second-order branch; an artery that divides off a second-order artery is a third-order branch; any additional branches are referred to as beyond third-order.

In normal human anatomy, the aortic arch has three branches or vascular families: brachiocephalic (also called innominate), left subclavian, and left common carotid. Some people have a bovine arch, an anatomic variation with two branches off the aorta called the brachiocephalic and left subclavian branches. In this anatomy, the left common carotid artery branches off of the brachiocephalic artery rather than the aorta. Other variations also occur.

Angiography and other injection procedures on the head and extremities are defined as occurring on the ipsilateral or contralateral side. These terms refer to the side on which the circulation is examined in relation to the site of catheterization.

The prefix *ipsi-* means "same," and *lateral* means "pertaining to the side," so an *ipsilateral* examination refers to the examination of circulation on the same side on which the catheterization was performed. *Contralateral* means "the opposite side."

Congenital Heart Defect Procedures

Surgery to correct congenital heart defects corrects misplaced and/or misconfigured vessels and other structural anomalies in an attempt to restore normal cardiac anatomy and function to the greatest extent possible. Procedures may require that surgeons reposition vessels, close holes with sutures or a patch, create openings, divide fistulas, and create new divisions or structures, depending on the specific anomaly or combination of anomalies (■ TABLE 36-3, page 721).

This section provides a general reference to help understand the most common cardiovascular procedures. Remember to keep standard reference books handy in case you get stuck.

CODING PRACTICE

| Exercise 36.1 | Cardiovascular System Procedure Basics

Instructions: Use your medical terminology skills and resources to define the following procedures related to the cardiovascular system, then identify the code(s) or code range listed in the CPT Index. Follow these steps:

- Use slash marks "/" to break down each underlined term into its root(s) and suffix.
- Define the meaning of the underlined word based on the meaning of each word part.
- Identify the CPT code(s) or code range listed in the CPT Index.

Example: <u>aortoplasty</u> aorto/plasty   Meaning *surgical repair of the aorta*   CPT Code *33417*

1. <u>pericardiocentesis</u>   Meaning _____   CPT Code _____

2. <u>thrombolysis</u>, cranial vessels   Meaning _____   CPT Code _____

3. ablation, heart <u>arrhythmogenic</u> focus   Meaning _____   CPT Code _____

4. <u>valvotomy</u>, mitral valve   Meaning _____   CPT Code _____

5. <u>septoplasty</u>   Meaning _____   CPT Code _____

6. aneurysm repair, <u>thoracoabdominal</u> aorta   Meaning _____   CPT Code _____

7. <u>thromboendarterectomy</u>, brachial artery   Meaning _____   CPT Code _____

8. <u>angioscopy</u>, noncoronary vessels   Meaning _____   CPT Code _____

9. <u>endovascular</u> repair, vena cava, repositioning   Meaning _____   CPT Code _____

10. <u>arteriovenous</u> fistula, revision, without thrombectomy   Meaning _____   CPT Code _____

CODING GUIDELINES FOR CARDIOVASCULAR SYSTEM PROCEDURES

Coders should understand the organization guidelines, and instructional notes in the Tabular List of this CPT section. This information is necessary for accurate coding. The CPT subsection **Cardiovascular System (33010-37799)** contains two subheadings (■ TABLE 36-4). The subsection **Heart and Pericardium (33010-33999)** includes procedures on the conduction system. Each subheading contains numerous categories divided by the anatomic site, condition, and type of procedure. Review the subheading and category names and code ranges listed in the Cardiovascular System subsection to become familiar with the content and organization. Some editions of the CPT manual provide a summary list of the subheading and categories at the beginning of the Cardiovascular System subsection and also display an asterisk (*) next to categories that contain special coding instructions.

This chapter includes invasive, minimally invasive, and noninvasive surgical procedures on the cardiovascular system. Codes for diagnostic tests on the cardiovascular system appear in the Medicine section. Procedures represented by CPT codes must be linked on a claim with diagnosis codes to support their medical necessity. CPT codes in the Cardiovascular System subsection are frequently supported by diagnosis codes from ICD-10-CM Chapter 9, "Diseases of the Circulatory System (I00-I99)," as well as symptoms and signs and congenital malformations (■ TABLE 36-5); however, diagnosis codes from any ICD-10-CM chapter are permissible.

CPT guidelines for the Surgery section apply to the Cardiovascular System subsection.

Special instructions at the beginning of the subsection direct how to code for catheterization within a vascular family. The CPT appendix **Vascular Families** shows the designation of first-, second-, and third-order branches within vascular families for catheterization beginning at the aorta.

Detailed special instructions and coding tables appear in the CPT manual for several categories, including **Pacemaker or Implantable Defibrillator (33202-33273)** procedures, **Extracorporeal Membrane Oxygenation or Extracorporeal Life Support (ECMO/ ECLS) Services (33946-33989)**, **Vascular Injection Procedures (36000-36598)**, and **Dialysis Circuit (36901-37183)**.

Minimally invasive procedures on the cardiovascular system, such as pacemaker insertion and selective catheter placement, may be performed with moderate sedation. When this occurs, assign the appropriate moderate sedation code(s) **(99151-99157)**.

Instructional notes appear throughout the Tabular List to alert coders to the need for modifiers, provide cross-references to codes for similar procedures on other sites, identify when additional codes for radiological services might be needed, and highlight resequenced and recently deleted codes. Specific guidelines and instructional notes are discussed throughout this chapter of the text.

ABSTRACTING CARDIOVASCULAR SYSTEM PROCEDURES

Various types of cardiovascular procedures require unique abstracting criteria. Criteria for procedures on the heart (■ TABLE 36-6) include specialized criteria for CABG and central venous access procedures. Pacemaker procedures and ICD procedures can be abstracted using similar criteria (■ TABLE 36-7, page 724). Vascular procedures include specialized criteria for catheterization and vascular injection procedures (■ TABLE 36-8, page 724).

Guided Example of Abstracting Cardiovascular System Procedures

Refer to the following example throughout this chapter to practice skills for abstracting, assigning, and arranging Cardiovascular System subsection codes.

Table 36-4   ■   **CARDIOVASCULAR SUBHEADINGS**

Subheading	Code Range
Heart and Pericardium	33010-33999
Arteries and Veins	34001-37799

Table 36-5   ■   **LOCATING ICD-10-CM AND ADDITIONAL CPT CODES FOR THE CARDIOVASCULAR SYSTEM**

Type of Code	Codes
ICD-10-CM Cardiovascular System-Related Codes	
Cardiovascular system conditions	I00-I99
Congenital malformations	Q20-Q28
Symptoms and signs	R00, R01, R50-R69
CPT Cardiovascular System-Related Codes	
Medicine procedures	92920-93999
Radiologic procedures	
• Diagnostic radiology	75557-75989
• Diagnostic ultrasound	76604-76642, 76881-76886
• Radiologic guidance	77001-77022
• Nuclear medicine, diagnostic	78414-78499
Laboratory organ/disease panels	80050, 80053, 80061

Source: © PB Resources, Inc. Used with permission. CPT codes only © American Medical Association.

Table 36-6   ■   **KEY CRITERIA FOR ABSTRACTING CARDIAC PROCEDURES**

❑ What type of procedure is performed?
❑ What is the anatomic site?
❑ Is a device implanted or removed?
❑ Is imaging supervision and interpretation provided by the surgeon?
❑ Is moderate sedation used?

Coronary Artery Bypass Graft

❑ How many grafted vessels are used?
❑ How many and which arteries are used for grafting?
❑ How many and which veins are used for grafting?
❑ Is a venous graft obtained endoscopically?
❑ How many distal anastomoses are performed?
❑ Is cardiopulmonary bypass used?

Central Venous Access Procedures

❑ What type of procedure is performed (insertion, repair, partial or complete replacement, removal)?
❑ Is the catheter inserted centrally or peripherally?
❑ Is the centrally inserted catheter tunneled or nontunneled?
❑ Is a pump or port included?
❑ What is the age of the patient?

Source: © PB Resources, Inc. Used with permission.

TABLE 36-7 ■ KEY CRITERIA FOR ABSTRACTING PACEMAKER AND ICD PROCEDURES

❏ What is the type of device (pacemaker, implantable [transvenous] cardioverter-defibrillator, or subcutaneous cardioverter-defibrillator)?

❏ What type of procedure is performed (initial placement, removal, replacement, upgrade, or repair)?

❏ Which components are involved (pulse generator and/or lead)?

❏ How many and which chambers are involved?

❏ What type of leads does the pulse generator have (atrial, ventricular, dual, multiple)?

❏ How many leads are removed and/or inserted transvenously? How many leads are reused?

❏ What approach is used L (open [thoracotomy], endoscopic, or transvenous)?

❏ Is the device temporary or permanent?

❏ What other related services are provided (device evaluation, skin pocket relocation, defibrillator threshold testing)?

❏ Is moderate sedation used?

Source: © PB Resources, Inc. Used with permission.

TABLE 36-8 ■ KEY CRITERIA FOR ABSTRACTING VASCULAR PROCEDURES

❏ What site is treated?

❏ Is a catheter used?

❏ What type of procedure is performed?

❏ What is the surgical approach?

❏ Is a stent, filter, or other prosthesis used?

❏ Is moderate sedation used?

Vascular Injection Procedures

❏ Is the catheterization nonselective, selective, or both?

❏ How many access sites are used?

❏ What is the point(s) of access (e.g., femoral, radial, jugular, brachial)?

❏ Does the procedure begin at the aorta?

❏ Which vascular family(ies) is accessed?

❏ What is the first-order branch?

❏ Is more than one first-order branch (family) accessed?

❏ What is the second-order branch?

❏ What is the site of the examination/injection (e.g., ipsilateral or contralateral)?

❏ What is the most distal anatomic site to where the catheter is manipulated?

❏ What imaging studies are performed?

Source: © PB Resources, Inc. Used with permission.

Follow along as fictitious coder, Tanisha Riemann, CCS-P, abstracts the procedure. Check off each step after you complete it.

▶ Tanisha reads through the entire record, paying special attention to the reason for the procedure, the procedure

---

INPATIENT HOSPITAL   Gender: M   Age: *67*

Preoperative diagnosis: Chronic unstable angina, acute STEMI right inferoposterior wall

Procedure: Coronary artery bypass grafting (CABG) times three utilizing the left internal mammary artery (LIMA) to the left anterior descending (LAD) artery and two segments of the reversed autologous great saphenous vein graft (SVG) to the posterior descending (PDA) branch of the right coronary artery (RCA) and the obtuse marginal (OM) branch of the left main (LM) coronary artery, total cardiopulmonary bypass (CPB), cold blood potassium cardioplegia (*introduction of a solution to stop the heart*) for myocardial protection. The sternotomy was performed, the heart was physically stabilized, and the pericardium was entered. The PDA branch of the right coronary artery was identified, opened, and anastomosed in an end-to-side fashion to the reversed autologous SV. The OM was identified and opened and end-to-side anastomosis was performed to a second segment of the reversed autologous SV. The LIMA was clipped distally, divided, and spatulated (*spread open*) for anastomosis. The LAD was identified and opened. End-to-side anastomosis was performed through the LIMA. The mammary pedicle was sutured to the heart. Aortotomies were made and the veins were cut to fit these and sutured in place. Ventricular and atrial pacing wires were placed. The patient was fully warmed and weaned from CPB. Good hemostasis was noted. A single mediastinal and left pleural chest tube was placed. The sternum was closed with interrupted wire, and the linea alba, sternal fascia, and subcutaneous tissue were closed. The patient tolerated the procedure well and was transferred to PACU in stable condition.

Postoperative diagnosis: Acute STEMI right inferoposterior wall; atherosclerotic heart disease of RCA with 95% blockage in PDA; 85% blockage in OM; and 90% blockage in LAD, with unstable angina due to 50 years of cigarette nicotine dependence

---

performed, and the postoperative diagnosis. She refers to the Key Criteria for Abstracting Cardiac Procedures (Table 36-6).

❏ She notes preoperative diagnosis: chronic unstable angina, acute STEMI right inferoposterior wall

❏ *What is the patient's age?* 67

❏ *What site is treated?* Heart

❏ *What is the primary procedure performed?* Coronary artery bypass grafting

❑ *What is (are) the harvested vessels?* Left internal mammary artery (LIMA) and two segments of the reversed autologous great saphenous vein

❑ *How many grafted vessels are used?* Coronary artery bypass grafting times three

❑ *How many distal anastomoses are performed?* Three, identified as follows: (1) The PDA branch of the right coronary artery was identified, opened, and anastomosed in an end-to-side fashion to the reversed autologous SV. (2) The OM was identified and opened and end-to-side anastomosis was performed to a second

segment of the reversed autologous SVG. (3) The LAD was identified and opened. End-to-side anastomosis was performed through the LIMA.

❑ *Is a venous graft obtained endoscopically?* No

❑ *Is cardiopulmonary bypass used?* Yes, total cardiopulmonary bypass (CPB)

▶ At this time, Tanisha does not know which of these procedures may need to be coded, nor how many codes she will end up with. She will learn about this when she moves on to assigning codes.

CODING PRACTICE

Exercise 36.2   **Abstracting Cardiovascular System Procedures**

Instructions: Read the mini-medical-record of each patient's encounter and answer the abstracting questions. Write the answer on the line provided. Do not assign any codes.

---

1. OUTPATIENT HOSPITAL   Gender: F   Age: 64

Preprocedure diagnosis: Arrhythmia

Procedure: Administered moderate sedation (60 minutes by same provider with observer) and implanted a subcutaneous cardiac rhythm monitor

a. What type of procedure is performed? _____
_____

b. What is the anatomic site? _____

c. Is a device implanted or removed? _____

d. Is moderate sedation used? _____

---

2. OUTPATIENT HOSPITAL   Gender: M   Age: 79

Preprocedure diagnosis: Pulmonary edema with acute pericardial effusion

Procedure: Using ultrasound guidance provided by the radiologist, advanced the needle into the pericardial space. Aspirated fluid from the pericardial sac into a syringe. Patient tolerated procedure well.

a. What type of procedure is performed? _____
_____

b. What is the anatomic site? _____

c. Is a device implanted or removed? _____

d. Was imaging supervision and interpretation provided by the surgeon? _____

e. What is the medical term for this procedure? _____
_____

---

3. INPATIENT HOSPITAL   Gender: M   Age: 57

Preprocedure diagnosis: Acute anterior wall MI

Procedure: CABG ×1 using radial artery bypass, aorta to LAD. Patient placed on CPB.

a. What type of procedure is performed? _____
_____

b. What is the anatomic site? _____

c. Is a device implanted or removed? _____

d. How many grafted vessels are used? _____

e. How many and which arteries are used for grafting?
_____

f. How many and which veins are used for grafting? ___
_____

g. Is a venous graft obtained endoscopically? _____

h. How many distal anastomoses are performed? _____

i. Is cardiopulmonary bypass used? _____

---

4. INPATIENT HOSPITAL   Gender: M   Age: 63

Preprocedure diagnosis: Coronary artery disease

Procedure: CABG ×4; left radial artery from the aorta to the PDA branch of the RC; LIMA from the aorta to the ramus intermedius coronary artery (RI) and then sequentially to the diagonal branch of the LAD; left saphenous vein graft to the obtuse marginal branch of the left circumflex (LCX). The assistant surgeon performed an endoscopic video-assisted harvesting of the saphenous vein.

a. What type of procedure is performed? _____

b. What is the anatomic site? _____

c. Is a device implanted or removed? _____

d. How many grafted vessels are used? _____

(continued)

CODING PRACTICE (continued)

4. (continued)

e. How many and which arteries are used for grafting?

_____

f. How many and which veins are used for grafting? ___

_____

g. Is a venous graft obtained endoscopically? _____

h. How many distal anastomoses are performed? _____

_____

i. Is cardiopulmonary bypass used? _____

5. (continued)

l. Is more than one first-order branch (family) accessed?

_____

m. What is the second-order branch? _____

n. What is the site of the examination/injection (e.g., ipsilateral or contralateral)? _____

o. What is the most distal anatomic site to where the catheter is manipulated? _____

p. What imaging studies are performed? _____

---

5. OUTPATIENT HOSPITAL   Gender: M   Age: 47

Preprocedure diagnosis: Occlusion and stenosis of carotid artery vascular family with cerebral infarction

Procedure: Selective catheter placement with angiography and stent. Inserted catheter percutaneously in the left femoral artery and maneuvered it to the aorta, where angiography was performed on the cervicocerebral arch. Moved catheter into the left common carotid artery, proceeded to the internal carotid artery then into the left middle cerebral branch. Performed angiography of the ipsilateral common carotid circulation. Radiological supervision and interpretation done by surgeon

Postprocedure diagnosis: Occlusion and stenosis of left middle cerebral artery with cerebral infarction

a. What site is treated? _____

b. Is a catheter used? _____

c. What type of procedure is performed? _____

d. What is the surgical approach? _____

e. Is a stent, filter, or other prosthesis used? _____

f. Is the catheterization nonselective, selective, or both?

_____

g. How many access sites are used? _____

h. What is the point(s) of access (e.g., femoral, radial, jugular, brachial)? _____

i. Does the procedure begin at the aorta? _____

j. Which vascular family(ies) is accessed? _____

k. What is the first-order branch? _____

(continued)

---

6. INPATIENT HOSPITAL   Gender: F   Age: 68

Preprocedure diagnosis: ICD that was implanted two years ago for ventricular tachycardia

Procedure: Upgrade ICD in right ventricle to dual chamber. Removed pulse generator in the subcutaneous pocket in the chest. Tested existing lead, which was found to be in good condition, so it was reused. Under fluoroscopic guidance, threaded a new lead into the right ventricle and right atrium. Inserted new pulse generator.

a. What is the type of device (pacemaker or implantable cardioverter-defibrillator)? _____

b. What type of procedure is performed (initial placement, removal, replacement, upgrade, or repair)?

_____

c. Which components are involved (pulse generator and/or lead)? _____

d. How many and which chambers are treated? _____

_____

e. How many leads are removed and/or inserted transvenously? How many leads are reused? _____

f. What approach is used (open [thoracotomy], endoscopic, or transvenous)? _____

g. Is the device temporary or permanent? _____

_____

h. What other related services were provided (device evaluation, skin pocket relocation, defibrillator threshold testing)? _____

ASSIGNING CODES FOR CARDIOVASCULAR SYSTEM PROCEDURES

The Cardiovascular System subsection provides extensive special instructions throughout the Tabular List that clarify definitions, code assignment, and bundling rules. This section discusses coding highlights for blood draws, pacemaker procedures, catheterization, congenital heart defect procedures, and CABG. The guided example introduced earlier in the chapter, about a patient who was seen for CABG, is continued.

Blood Collection

The collection of a blood specimen submitted for laboratory tests is coded from the Cardiovascular System subsection. Blood specimens can be collected from a capillary, vein, or artery, an implantable venous access device, or an established catheter (■ TABLE 36-9). To locate codes for blood collection in the Index, search for the Main Term **Collection and Processing**, then the subterm **Specimen**. Alternatively, search for the Main Term **Specimen Collection**, then the subterm **Specimen**. Then locate the source of the specimen. To locate blood collection using an arterial puncture, search for the Main Term **Puncture**, then the subterm **Artery**.

SUCCESS STEP

The CPT Index does not provide a Main Term for "Blood Draw" or "Blood Collection." However, you can create your own reminder by writing the words *Blood Draw* under *B* in your CPT Index, then writing a cross-reference such as *See "Collection and Processing, Specimen"* or *See "Specimen Collection."* This will direct you to the correct Main Terms.

Pacemaker Procedures

To locate codes in the Index for pacemaker or ICD procedures, search for the Main Term **Pacemaker** or **Implantable Defibrillator**. Subterms identify the type of procedure performed. Subcutaneous devices are coded with temporary Category III codes.

The number of codes required varies based on the procedure. Some procedures are reported with a single code, whereas others require separate codes for each component, that is, the pulse generator and the lead(s). Refer to the chart of pacemaker and ICD procedures that appears before or near code **33202** when verifying codes in the Tabular List. To use this chart, follow these steps:

1. In the first column, identify the type of transvenous procedure performed.

2. Select code(s) from the second (Pacemaker) or third (ICD) column that corresponds to the type of device in use.

3. Verify the code descriptions in the Tabular List.

4. Read the instructional notes following the code for variations of the procedure and bundling rules.

5. Review the special instructions for this category and ensure that all guidelines are followed.

Nonselective and Selective Catheterization

Vascular catheterization consists of inserting a catheter at a specific point and moving it through the arteries or veins to arrive at the site the physician wishes to examine or treat. Arterial catheterization most often begins at the femoral or radial artery then proceeds to the aorta, from where the desired vessel(s) are accessed. Central venous access is made through the inferior vena cava or the jugular, subclavian, or femoral veins. Peripheral venous access is made through other sites, such as the basilic or cephalic vein.

When coding for selective catheter placement, code for the most distal anatomic site reached (■ FIGURE 36-2). The procedure report should identify the access point and the path the catheter takes, naming each successive branch accessed (■ FIGURE 36-3, page 728). The CPT appendix **Vascular Families** lists vascular families and the first-, second-, and third-order branches. It is a useful reference to help identify the names of the vessels and the order they represent. ■ FIGURE 36-4 (page 728) illustrates how to follow the hierarchical progression within vascular families. Begin identifying vascular families at the point where the examination begins. Do not code the movement of the catheter from the access point to the beginning point of the examination. For example, when the catheter is inserted in the femoral artery and moved to the aorta, where the examination is begun, begin coding the vascular family branches at the aorta.

Table 36-9 ■ **CODES FOR OBTAINING BLOOD SAMPLES**

Source of Blood Sample	Code(s)
Artery (puncture)	36600
Capillary	36416
Implantable venous access device	36591
Vein (venipuncture)	36415 (routine)
	36420 (cutdown <1 year)
	36400-36410 (nonroutine)
Venous catheter (established)	36592

Catheter was threaded from the aorta into the brachiocephalic artery (*first-order*), through the subclavian artery (*second-order*), and into the right vertebral artery (*third-order*).

36217 Selective catheter placement, arterial system; initial third order or more selective thoracic or brachiocephalic branch, within a vascular family

Figure 36-2 ■ Example of coding selective catheterization to a third-order branch.

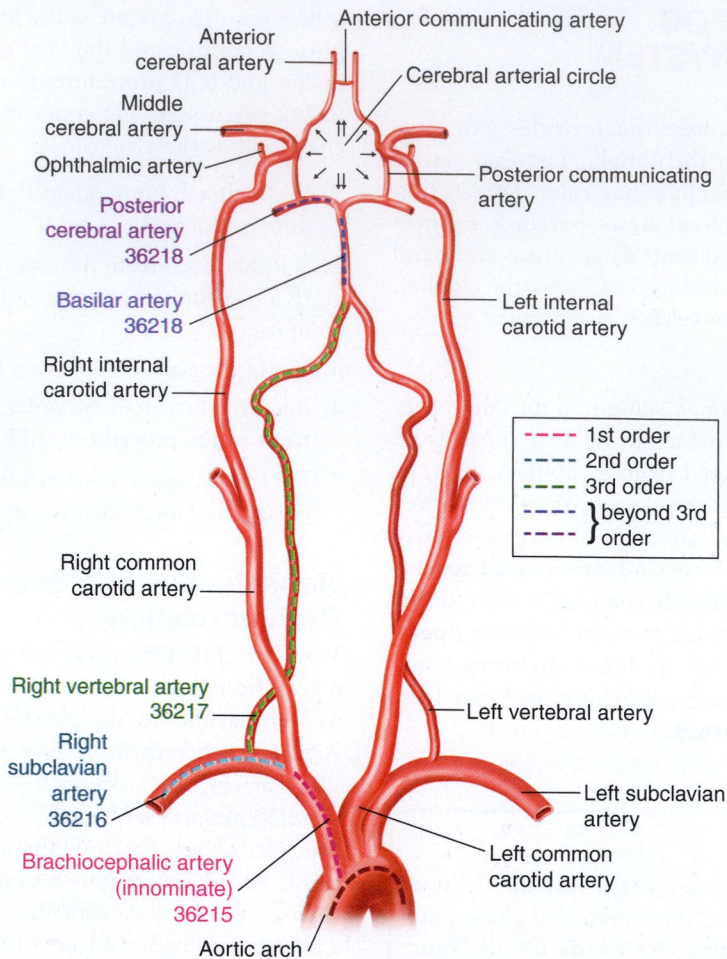

Figure 36-3 ■ Anatomy of selective catheterization coding.

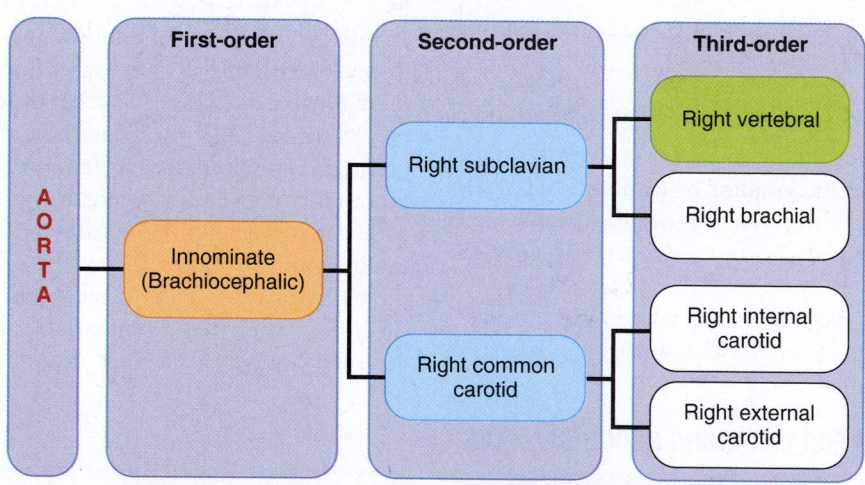

Figure 36-4 ■ Branches of a vascular family (partial).

When the catheter is partially retracted then redirected through an additional branch of the same vascular family, assign an additional code for the most distal anatomic site reached in the additional branch (■ FIGURE 36-5).

To locate codes for vascular procedures, search the Index for the Main Term **Artery** or **Vein** and the first-level modifying term for the specific vessel. Identify the second-level modifying term for the type of procedure performed. In some cases, the first-level modifying term identifies the procedure, rather than the vessel.

The CPT Tabular List divides codes based on whether catheterization is performed in arteries or veins and whether

Catheter was threaded from the aorta into the brachiocephalic artery (*first-order*), through the subclavian artery (*second-order*), and into the right vertebral artery (*third-order*). It was then retracted back to the brachiocephalic artery and threaded into the right common carotid artery (*additional second-order*).

36217 Selective catheter placement, arterial system; initial third order or more selective thoracic or brachiocephalic branch, within a vascular family

36218 Selective catheter placement, arterial system; additional second order, third order, and beyond, thoracic or brachiocephalic branch, within a vascular family (List in addition to code for initial second or third order vessel as appropriate)

Figure 36-5 ■ Example of coding multiple selective catheterizations.

the upper or lower body, as divided at the diaphragm, is accessed. Review code descriptions to identify separate codes for specific arteries accessed and the extent of the catheterization: first-, second-, third-order and beyond branches. Many vessels are referred to by more than one name. For example, the *innominate* artery listed in CPT appendix **Vascular Families** is the same as the *brachiocephalic* artery named in the Tabular List.

Codes for angiography include catheter placement, angiography, and all associated radiological supervision and interpretation, so these services should not be reported separately. However, assign codes for additional imaging studies performed. ■ TABLE 36-10 summarizes the rules for catheterization coding.

SUCCESS STEP

Vascular families are similar to a highway system. If you think of the aorta as analogous to an interstate highway, the first-order branch would be the first main road turned onto from an exit ramp. When you turn off of the main road onto a secondary road, it is similar to a second-order branch. Turning onto a side street is similar to a third-order branch, and so on.

Table 36-10 ■ **SUMMARY OF RULES FOR CATHETERIZATION CODING**

- ❑ Code each access site separately.
- ❑ Code each vascular family separately.
- ❑ Code additional second- or third-order catheterizations within a family.
- ❑ Code additional imaging studies within a family above the basic examination included in the code.
- ❑ Do not code both selective and nonselective catheter placement from the same access and in the same vascular family. Code only the selective catheterization.

Congenital Heart Defect Procedures

To locate codes for repair of a congenital heart anomaly, search the Index for the name of the condition as the Main Term. Read the modifying terms, if any, to identify the appropriate code range. The Tabular List often provides several codes that describe variations of a procedure, so coders must read the details of the operative report to determine the code that best describes the operation.

Coronary Artery Bypass Graft

To locate codes for a coronary artery bypass, search the Index for the Main Term **Artery**, then the first-level modifying term **Coronary** and the second-level modifying term **Bypass**. The Index provides the code range **33510-33536**. In the Tabular List, select the category that identifies the type of graft used:

- Use of venous grafts only (**33510-33516**)
- Use of both arterial and venous grafts (**33517-33523**)
- Use of arterial grafts only (**33533-33536**)

Within each category, codes are divided based on the number of grafts performed. The number of grafts reported is identified by the number of distal anastomoses. The proximal anastomosis connects the graft to the aorta. The distal anastomosis connects the graft to a coronary artery beyond the blockage or to another graft. To report combined arterial-venous grafting, report a standalone code(s) for the arterial graft(s) and an add-on code(s) for the venous graft(s). Refer to ■ FIGURE 36-6 (page 730) to better understand arterial and venous grafting.

Review the summary below to determine when harvesting of the vessel to be used for grafting is reported separately:

- Upper extremity artery—Report harvesting with code **35600** in addition to the bypass procedure
- Upper extremity vein—Report harvesting with code **35500** in addition to the bypass procedure
- Femoropopliteal vein segment—Report harvesting with code **35572** in addition to the bypass procedure
- Saphenous vein—Harvesting is included in the description of the work for **33517-33523** and should not be reported separately
- Artery (other than upper extremity)—Harvesting is included in the description of the work for **33533-33536** and should not be reported separately
- Video-assisted harvesting—Report code **33508** in addition to the bypass procedure, including when the procurement is otherwise bundled (e.g., saphenous vein)

When a surgical assistant performs arterial and/or venous graft procurement, add modifier **-80** to codes **33517-33523** and **33533-33536**. Refer to the special instructions for each CABG category for more information.

When the left internal mammary artery (LIMA) is used for the graft, report **4110F** in addition to the category I code. Code **4110F** is a category II code for supplemental tracking. Studies over the past 20 years have shown better long-term patency (*remaining unobstructed*) rates and survival in patients undergoing CABG with LIMA to the LAD, making it the preferred method for CABG worldwide.

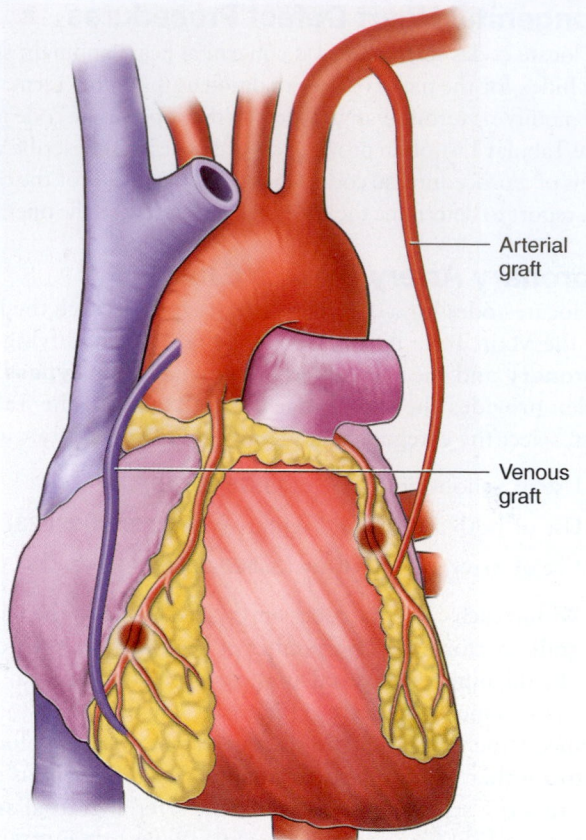

A Venous and arterial grafts

B Graft bypassing the diseased vessel

Figure 36-6 ■ Coronary artery bypass grafting.

SUCCESS STEP

To locate codes for a *peripheral* artery or venous bypass, search the Index for the Main Term **Artery** or **Vein**, then the first-level modifying term for the name of the vessel and the second-level modifying term **Bypass Graft**.

Guided Example of Assigning Cardiovascular System Procedure Codes

To practice skills for assigning codes for the Cardiovascular System subsection, continue with the example from earlier in the chapter about a patient who was seen for CABG. Follow along in your CPT manual as Tanisha Riemann, CCS-P, assigns codes. Check off each step after you complete it.

▶ First, Tanisha confirms the procedure CABG ×3.

▶ Tanisha searches the Index for the Main Term **Coronary Artery Bypass Graft (CABG)**.

❑ She locates the first-level modifying term **Arterial-Venous Graft** because both an artery (LIMA) and a vein (SV) were used. If only an artery had been used, she would select the subterm **Arterial Bypass**. If only a vein had been used, she would select the subterm **Venous Bypass**.

❑ She identifies the code range **33517-33519, 33521-33523**.

▶ Tanisha turns to the Tabular List to select and verify the code(s).

❑ She notices that all the codes in the category **Combined Arterial-Venous Grafting for Coronary Bypass** are add-on codes. She is a little confused because she knows that add-on codes cannot be used alone but must be used in conjunction with a standalone code.

❑ She notices special instructions at the beginning of the category, so decides to read them to see whether she can learn more about how to code the CABG. The special instructions state that:

  ▪ The codes in this category **may NOT be used alone**.

  ▪ **Two codes must be reported**: one from this category for the combined arterial-venous graft and one from code **33533-33536** for the arterial graft.

  ▪ **Procurement of the saphenous vein graft is included in codes 31517-33523 and should not be reported as a separate service.**

  ▪ **Procurement of the artery for grafting is included in codes 33533-33536 and should not be reported as a separate service.**

❑ Before beginning to select codes, she refers to the category **Arterial Grafting for Coronary Artery Bypass**, which contains the standalone codes **33533-33536**, to review the special instructions. The special instructions state that:

- The codes in this category are used **to report coronary artery bypass procedures using either arterial grafts only or a combination of arterial-venous grafts**.
- The codes **include the use of the internal mammary artery**, as well as several other arteries.
- **It is necessary to report two codes**, as stated in the previous instructions.
- **Procurement of the artery for grafting** is included in codes from this category.

❑ This category provides the standalone code needed, so Tanisha reads the code descriptions for the arterial graft to select this code first.

- Codes **33533-33536** are divided by the number of arterial grafts used.
- She refers to the documentation and confirms that the only arterial graft was the LIMA and it was used for one anastomosis. (The LAD was identified and opened. End-to-side anastomosis was performed through the LIMA.)
- She reads the code title for **33533, Coronary artery bypass, using arterial graft(s); single arterial graft**, and confirms that this accurately describes the principal procedure.

▶ Next, Tanisha needs to select the code for the venous grafting from the code ranges **33517-33519, 33521-33523**.

❑ Codes in this category are divided by the number of venous grafts used.

❑ The common portion of the descriptor appears in code **33517 Coronary artery bypass, using venous graft(s) and arterial graft(s).**

❑ She refers to the documentation and confirms that the great saphenous vein was procured. It was used for two anastomoses (two segments of the reversed autologous great saphenous vein graft [SVG] to the posterior descending [PDA] branch of the right coronary artery [RCA] and the obtuse marginal [OM] coronary artery).

❑ She selects code **33518, 2 venous grafts (List separately in addition to code for primary procedure).**

❑ She reads the instructional note under this code, which states (**Use 33518 in conjunction with 33533-33536**), and confirms that she has followed this rule.

▶ Tanisha rechecks the special instructions in the Tabular List.

❑ She cross-references the special instructions that she read previously to be certain that she did not miss any details.

❑ She cross-references the beginning of the subheading **Heart and Pericardium** and verifies that there are no special instructions.

❑ She cross-references the beginning of the subsection **Cardiovascular System** and reviews the special instructions. She determines that these instructions apply to selective catheterization and not to CABG.

▶ Tanisha has learned through her experience coding for cardiac surgery that a Category II code can be reported as an optional code when the LIMA is used for a CABG.

❑ To locate the code, she searches the Index for the Main Term **Artery**, the first-level modifying term **Coronary**, and the second-level modifying term **Bypass**. Under **Bypass**, she locates **Internal Mammary Artery** and the Category II code **4110F**.

❑ She verifies the code description in the Category II Tabular List, which appears after code **99607**.

▶ Tanisha reviews the procedure codes she has assigned for this case.

❑ **33518 Coronary artery bypass, using venous graft(s) and arterial graft(s); 2 venous grafts**

❑ **33533 Coronary artery bypass, using arterial graft(s); single arterial graft**

❑ **4110F Internal mammary artery graft performed for primary, isolated coronary artery bypass graft procedure**

▶ Next, Tanisha must determine how to sequence the codes.

CODING PRACTICE

Exercise 36.3   Assigning Codes for Cardiovascular System Procedures

Instructions: Read the mini-medical-record of each patient's encounter. Review the information abstracted in Exercise 36.2 for questions 1–3. For questions 4–6, abstract the case on your own. Assign CPT codes, quantities, and modifiers using the Index and Tabular List. Write the code(s) on the line provided.

1. OUTPATIENT HOSPITAL   Gender: F   Age: 64

Preprocedure diagnosis: Arrhythmia

Procedure: Administered moderate sedation (60 minutes by same provider with observer) and implanted a subcutaneous cardiac rhythm monitor

Tip: Assign one CPT code for the procedure and two codes for moderate sedation with appropriate quantity. Refer to the main term *Cardiac Assist Devices* in the CPT Index.

3 CPT Codes _____

_____

(continued)

CODING PRACTICE *(continued)*

---

2. OUTPATIENT HOSPITAL   Gender: M   Age: 79

Preprocedure diagnosis: Pulmonary edema with acute pericardial effusion

Procedure: Using ultrasound guidance provided by the radiologist, advanced the needle into the pericardial space. Aspirated fluid from the pericardial sac into syringe. Patient tolerated procedure well.

1 CPT Code _____

---

3. INPATIENT HOSPITAL   Gender: M   Age: 57

Preprocedure diagnosis: Acute anterior wall MI

Procedure: CABG ×1 using radial artery bypass, aorta to LAD. Patient placed on CPB.

Tip: Report harvesting of the radial artery in addition to the CABG.

2 CPT Codes _____

---

4. INPATIENT HOSPITAL   Gender: F   Age: 46

Preprocedure diagnosis: Blood clot in right leg

Procedure: Thrombectomy of the femoral artery using a leg incision. The vascular return is reestablished.

1 CPT Code _____

---

5. INPATIENT HOSPITAL   Gender: M   Age: 66

Preprocedure diagnosis: Visceral and infrarenal AAA

Procedure: FEVAR repair involving endoprostheses in the visceral aorta for the celiac and renal arteries and infrarenal repair extending to the right and left iliac arteries

1 CPT Code _____

---

6. OUTPATIENT SURGERY   Gender: M   Age: 43

Preprocedure diagnosis: ESRD

Procedure: Created AV fistula for dialysis in left upper arm between the brachial artery and cephalic vein using an autogenous graft.

Tip: AV fistulas can be created directly by anastomosing an artery to a vein or indirectly by using an autogenous or synthetic graft.

1 CPT Code _____

ARRANGING CODES FOR CARDIOVASCULAR SYSTEM PROCEDURES

Multiple cardiac procedures are often performed together, and there is no set pattern for what is normally done because each patient's circumstances are unique. Follow the standard CPT guidelines for sequencing codes in descending RVU order. In addition, there are special considerations in coding for associated radiological services and multiple surgeons.

Radiology Services

Many services in the Cardiovascular System subsection involve radiological imaging, supervision, and interpretation. Read the code descriptions, special instructions, and instructional notes to identify when radiological services are bundled in the code and when they should be reported separately.

When radiological services are to be reported separately, code them only if the physician for whom you are coding provided the radiological service. If you are coding for the cardiac surgeon and the radiological services are provided by a radiologist from another practice, do not assign radiology codes because they will be coded by the radiologist's coder.

Multiple Surgeons

Cardiac surgery may involve multiple physicians, so remember to append the appropriate modifiers to identify the role of the physician for whom you are coding. When two surgeons work together as primary surgeons, each physician reports the same CPT code and appends modifier **-62 Two surgeons**. Each surgeon receives 50% of the payment. When a surgical team, usually consisting of distinct specialists, works together to perform a procedure, such as a CABG, each surgeon reports the same CPT code and appends modifier **-66 Surgical team**. Payment is split between the surgeons based on the work that each performed. When an assistant surgeon participates in a procedure with a primary surgeon, the assistant surgeon reports the same CPT code as the primary surgeon and appends modifier **-80 Assistant surgeon**. When the assistant surgeon independently performs a distinct and separately billable procedure, such as video-assisted harvesting of a vessel, then the assistant surgeon reports only the CPT code for the service performed and appends modifier **-80**.

Not all CPT codes are eligible for payment for multiple physicians. The Medicare Physician Fee Schedule Database (MPFSDB) identifies the modifiers accepted for each procedure.

Laterality

Most veins and arteries occur in pairs on opposite sides of the body. Use modifiers **-RT Right side** and **-LT Left side** to identify the laterality of vascular procedures. Do not assign laterality modifiers to procedures on the heart, heart chambers, or valves.

Coronary Arteries

HCPCS modifiers identify each of the coronary arteries:

- **-LC Left circumflex coronary artery**
- **-LD Left anterior descending coronary artery**
- **-LM Left main coronary artery**
- **-RC Right coronary artery**
- **-RI Ramus intermedius coronary artery**

Assign these modifiers when procedures are performed on the coronary arteries, including CABG.

Guided Example of Arranging Cardiovascular System Procedure Codes

To practice skills for arranging codes for procedures of the Cardiovascular System subsection, continue with the example from earlier in the chapter about the patient who was seen for CABG. Follow along in your CPT manual as Tanisha Riemann, CCS-P, arranges the codes. Check off each step after you complete it.

▶ Tanisha reviews the procedure codes she has assigned for this case.

❑ **33518 Coronary artery bypass, using venous graft(s) and arterial graft(s); 2 venous grafts**

❑ **33533 Coronary artery bypass, using arterial graft(s); single arterial graft**

❑ **4110F Internal mammary artery graft performed for primary, isolated coronary artery bypass graft procedure**

▶ Tanisha recalls that the Tabular List and special instructions provide sequencing guidance for these codes.

❑ **33518** is an add-on code, so it cannot be sequenced first.

❑ The code description for **33518** states (**List separately in addition to code for primary procedure**). Code **33533** for the arterial graft is the primary procedure.

❑ The instructional note after code **33518** states (**Use 33518 in conjunction with 33533-33536**).

❑ Because the informational code **4110F** does not affect payment, she sequences it last.

▶ Tanisha examines the need for modifiers. (Refer to Table 27-1, Key Criteria for Abstracting CPT Modifiers, or Appendix A in the CPT manual.)

❑ Neither of these codes requires a modifier because add-on codes do not require a modifier for a multiple or separate procedure. No other extenuating circumstances exist.

▶ Tanisha finalizes the procedure codes and sequencing for this case:

(1) **33533-LD-LC Coronary artery bypass, using arterial graft(s); single arterial graft;**

(2) **33518-RC Coronary artery bypass, using venous graft(s) and arterial graft(s); 2 venous grafts;**

(3) **4110F Internal mammary artery graft performed for primary, isolated coronary artery bypass graft procedure**

▶ Tanisha also assigns and sequences the ICD-10-CM diagnosis codes that support the need for the service.

(1) **I21.11 ST elevation (STEMI) myocardial infarction involving right coronary artery**

(2) **I25.110 Atherosclerotic heart disease of native coronary artery with unstable angina pectoris**

(3) **F17.218 Nicotine dependence, cigarettes, with other nicotine-induced disorders**

CODING PRACTICE

Exercise 36.4 Arranging Codes for Cardiovascular System Procedures

Instructions: Read the mini-medical-record of each patient's encounter. Review the information abstracted in Exercise 36.2 for questions 1–3. For questions 4–6, abstract the case on your own. Assign CPT codes, quantities, and modifiers using the Index and Tabular List, and arrange the codes in the proper sequence. Write the code(s) on the lines provided.

---

1. INPATIENT HOSPITAL   Gender: M   Age: 63

Preprocedure diagnosis: Coronary artery disease

Procedure: CABG ×4; left radial artery from the aorta to the PDA branch of the RC; LIMA from the aorta to the ramus intermedius coronary artery (RI) and then sequentially to the diagonal branch of the LAD; left saphenous vein graft to the obtuse marginal branch of the left circumflex (LCX). The assistant surgeon performed an endoscopic video-assisted harvesting of the saphenous vein.

Tip: Code for the primary surgeon who performed the CABG and the assistant surgeon's graft procurement.

5 CPT Codes _____
_____

(continued)

CODING PRACTICE (continued)

2. OUTPATIENT HOSPITAL Gender: M Age: 47

Preprocedure diagnosis: Occlusion and stenosis of carotid artery vascular family with cerebral infarction

Procedure: Selective catheter placement with angiography and stent. Inserted catheter percutaneously in the left femoral artery and maneuvered it to the aorta, where angiography was performed on the cervicocerebral arch. Moved catheter into the left common carotid artery, proceeded to the internal carotid artery then into the left middle cerebral branch. Performed angiography of the ipsilateral common carotid circulation. Radiological supervision and interpretation done by surgeon.

Postprocedure diagnosis: Occlusion and stenosis of left middle cerebral artery with cerebral infarction

Tip: The left middle cerebral vertebral artery is an intra-cranial branch of the left internal carotid artery.

2 CPT Codes _____

3. INPATIENT HOSPITAL Gender: F Age: 68

Preprocedure diagnosis: ICD that was implanted two years ago for ventricular tachycardia

Procedure: Upgrade ICD in right ventricle to dual chamber. Removed pulse generator in the subcutaneous pocket in the chest. Tested existing lead, which was found to be in good condition, so it was reused. Under fluoroscopic guidance, threaded a new lead into the right ventricle and right atrium. Inserted new pulse generator.

Tip: Refer to the pacemaker/ICD coding chart in the CPT manual.

2 CPT Codes _____

4. INPATIENT HOSPITAL Gender: M Age: 64

Preprocedure diagnosis: Arteriosclerosis

Procedure: Percutaneous revascularization of the right common iliac artery with transluminal angioplasty; revascularization of the ipsilateral external iliac artery with angioplasty and transluminal stent placement

3 CPT Codes _____

_____

5. INPATIENT HOSPITAL Gender: F Age: 35

Preprocedure diagnosis: Pain and swelling in both legs

Procedure: Femoral vein valvuloplasty in both legs

1 CPT Code _____

6. OUTPATIENT SURGERY Gender: M Age: 71

Preprocedure diagnosis: Heart failure

Procedure: Conversion of existing pacemaker system to biventricular. Removed the current pulse generator and replaced with a new pulse generator with a multiple-lead system with biventricular pacing capabilities. Inserted left ventricular pacing electrode at the same time.

Tip: Code for the replacement of the pulse generator and insertion of the LV lead.

2 CPT Codes _____

E/M CODING FOR CARDIOLOGY

The *1997 Documentation Guidelines for Evaluation and Management Services* (1997 DG), published by Centers for Medicare and Medicaid Services (CMS), provides requirements for each level of a cardiovascular E/M examination (■ FIGURE 36-7). Specialists are not limited to using only the guidelines for a cardiovascular examination. They can also use guidelines for a general multiorgan system examination or any other single organ system examination based on what is most advantageous for a specific encounter. However, physicians cannot combine elements from more than one type of examination for a given encounter. Typically, the cardiovascular examination guidelines provide the best results when a detailed examination is performed.

To determine the appropriate E/M code, coders must review the documentation in detail and identify the specific elements documented.

- To translate the documentation into the E/M requirements for the history, refer back to Chapter 28, "Evaluation and Management Services (99201-99499)," Tables 28-7 to 28-10, or to the 1997 DG.

- To determine the requirements for an examination, refer to Figure 36-7 or to the single organ system examination for the cardiovascular system in the 1997 DG.

- To determine the levels for medical decision making (MDM), refer to Chapter 28, Table 28-12, and also to the Table of Risk in the 1997 DG.

System/Body Area	Elements of Cardiovascular Examination
Constitutional	❑ Measurement of any <u>**three**</u> of the following seven **vital** signs: • 1) sitting or standing blood pressure, • 2) supine blood pressure, • 3) pulse rate and regularity, • 4) respiration, • 5) temperature, • 6) height, • 7) weight (May be measured and recorded by ancillary staff) ❑ General **appearance** of patient (eg, development, nutrition, body habitus, deformities, attention to grooming)
Eyes	❑ Inspection of **conjunctivae** and **lids** (eg, xanthelasma)
Ears, Nose, Mouth and Throat	❑ Inspection of **lips, teeth, gums** and **palate** ❑ Inspection of **oral mucosa** with notation of presence of **pallor** or **cyanosis**
Neck	❑ Examination of **jugular veins** (eg, distension; a, v or cannon a waves) ❑ Examination of **thyroid** (eg, enlargement, tenderness, mass)
Respiratory	❑ Assessment of **respiratory effort** (eg, intercostal retractions, use of accessory muscles, diaphragmatic movement) ❑ **Auscultation** of lungs (eg, breath sounds, adventitious sounds, rubs)
Cardiovascular	❑ **Palpation of heart** (eg, location, size, and forcefulness of the point of maximal impact; thrills; lifts; palpable S3 or S4) ❑ **Auscultation** of heart with notation of abnormal sounds and murmurs ❑ Measurement of **blood pressure in two or more extremities** when indicated (eg, aortic dissection, coarctation) Examination of: ❑ **carotid arteries** (eg, pulse amplitude, bruits) ❑ **abdominal aorta** (eg, size, bruits) ❑ **femoral arteries** (eg, pulse amplitude, bruits) ❑ **pedal pulses** (eg, pulse amplitude) ❑ **extremities** for edema and/or varicosities
Gastrointestinal (Abdomen)	❑ Examination of **abdomen** with notation of presence of masses or tenderness ❑ Examination of **liver** and **spleen** ❑ Obtain **stool sample** for occult blood from patients who are being considered for thrombolytic or anticoagulant therapy
Musculoskeletal	❑ Examination of the **back** with notation of **kyphosis** or **scoliosis** ❑ Examination of **gait** with notation of ability to undergo **exercise** testing and/or participation in exercise programs ❑ Assessment of **muscle strength** and **tone** (eg, flaccid, cog wheel, spastic) with notation of any atrophy and abnormal movements
Extremities	❑ Inspection and palpation of **digits** and **nails** (eg, clubbing, cyanosis, inflammation, petechiae, ischemia, infections, Osler's nodes)
Skin	❑ Inspection and/or palpation of **skin and subcutaneous tissue** (eg, stasis dermatitis, ulcers, scars, xanthomas)
Neurological/ Psychiatric	Brief assessment of mental status including: ❑ **Orientation** to time, place and person ❑ **Mood** and affect (eg, depression, anxiety, agitation)

Total # Bullets Performed and Documented →	☐	# of ❑ Elements Performed and Documented	Level of Examination
		1–5	Problem focused
		6–11	Expanded problem focused
		12	Detailed
		ALL	Comprehensive (Document **every** element in each box with a shaded border and at least **one** element in each box with an unshaded border)

Figure 36-7 ■ 1997 documentation guidelines for cardiovascular examination. *Source: Centers for Medicare and Medicaid Services, 1997 Documentation Guidelines for Evaluation and Management Services (with formatting adjustments).*

Guided Example of E/M Coding for Cardiology

Refer to the "Cardiology encounter" (■ FIGURE 36-8) to practice skills for abstracting and assigning E/M codes. This guided example illustrates the 1997 DG for cardiovascular examination. In the workplace, coders must evaluate each encounter against the 1995 DG, the 1997 general multisystem DG, and the single organ system DG to identify the criteria that provide the optimal level of coding. Follow along as fictitious coder Tanisha Riemann, CCS-P, abstracts the procedure. Check off each step after you complete it.

▶ First, Tanisha needs to establish the category of service so she can determine the information needed to abstract and assign the code.

❏ *What is the setting?* Admitted to hospital last evening

❏ *What is the type of service?* Hospital inpatient services

❏ *What is the code range?* Tanisha refers to the CPT Index and looks up the Main Term **Evaluation and Management** and the subterm **Hospital**. The code range **99221-99233** is listed.

CARDIOLOGY ENCOUNTER

HISTORY OF PRESENT ILLNESS: The patient is a charming and delightful 46-year-old woman admitted to this hospital last evening with palpitations and presyncope. This is my first encounter with the patient.

The patient is active and a previously healthy young woman, who has had seven years of occasional heart palpitations. Symptoms occur three to four times per year and follow no identifiable pattern. She has put thought and effort in trying to identify precipitating factors or circumstances but has been unable to do so. Symptoms can last for an hour or more and she feels as if her heart is going very rapidly. She said that has not measured her heart rate. The last two episodes, the most recent of which was yesterday, she also "felt lightheaded and dizzy." On neither occasion did she lose consciousness.

Yesterday, she had a modestly active morning taking a walk with her dogs and performing her normal routines. While working on a computer, she had a spell. Palpitations persisted for a short time thereafter as outlined in the hospital's admission note prompting her to seek evaluation at the hospital. She was in sinus rhythm on arrival and has been asymptomatic since.

No history of exogenous substance abuse, alcohol abuse, or caffeine abuse. She does have a couple of sodas and a few cups of coffee daily. She is a nonsmoker. She is a mother of one. There is no family history of congenital heart disease. She has had no history of thoracic trauma. No symptoms to suggest thyroid disease.

No known history of diabetes, hypertension, or dyslipidemia. Family history is negative for ischemic heart disease. She underwent an ACL repair 15 years ago, complicated by contact urticaria from a neoprene cast.
No regular medications prior to admission.
The only allergy is the neoprene reaction outlined above.

PHYSICAL EXAMINATION: Vital signs as charted. Pupils are reactive. Sclerae nonicteric. Mucous membranes are moist. Neck veins not distended. No bruits. Lungs are clear. Cardiac exam is regular without murmurs, gallops, or rubs. Abdomen is soft without guarding, rebound masses, or bruits. Extremities well perfused. No edema. Strong and symmetrical distal pulses.

A 12-lead EKG shows sinus rhythm with normal axis and intervals. No evidence of preexcitation.

LABORATORY STUDIES: Unremarkable. No evidence of myocardial injury. Thyroid function is pending.

Two-dimensional echocardiogram shows no evidence of clinically significant structural or functional heart disease.

IMPRESSION/PLAN: Episodic palpitations over a seven-year period. Outpatient workup would be appropriate after discharge. Event recorder should be obtained and the patient can be seen again in the office upon completion of that study. Suppressive medication (beta-blocker or Cardizem) was discussed with the patient for symptomatic improvement, though this would be unlikely to be a curative therapy. The patient expresses a preference to avoid medical therapy if possible. Caffeine avoidance was discussed.

Thank you for this consultation. We will be happy to follow her both during this hospitalization and following discharge.

Annotations (right margin):

HISTORY: Detailed

Chief complaint (CC)

Setting & patient type

HPI: Extended (4+)

ROS: Extended (2-9)

PFSH: Complete (3)

EXAMINATION: Expanded Problem Focused

(6-11 bulleted elements)

MEDICAL DECISION MAKING: Moderate Complexity

MDM Risk: Undiagnosed new problem with uncertain prognosis (Moderate Risk)

MDM Data: Independent visualization of image (High Data)

MDM Management: New presenting problem, with workup (Moderate Management Options)

KEY: HPI History of the present illness   ROS Review of systems
PFSH Past, family, and social history   MDM Medical decision making

Figure 36-8 ■ Cardiology encounter.

- Tanisha refers to the code range in the Tabular List and notices that the **Hospital Inpatient Services** subsection is divided by **Initial Hospital Care** and **Subsequent Hospital Care**. She reads the special instructions for the category **Initial Hospital Care** that state, in part, **The following codes are used to report the first hospital inpatient encounter with the patient by the admitting physician. For initial inpatient encounters by physicians other than the admitting physician, see initial inpatient consultation codes (99251-99255) or subsequent hospital care codes (99231-99233) as appropriate.**

- The special instructions tell Tanisha that because this is not the admission encounter and the physician is not documented as the admitting physician, she should not use the **Initial Hospital Care** category, despite the fact that this is the physician's first encounter with the patient.

- Although the documentation uses the term *consultation* at the end of the report, this encounter does not meet the criteria for a consultation code because there is no documentation of a request for the cardiologist's evaluation or a report back to the requesting physician. Therefore, Tanisha understands that she must code this as **Subsequent Hospital Care (99231-99233)**.

❑ *How many key components are required?* Tanisha reads the code description of the first code, which states **2 of these 3 key components**. All codes in the category have the same requirements for key components. This tells her that two of the three key components must meet or exceed the levels listed in the code (2/3).

▶ Next, Tanisha identifies the level of history.

❑ *What is the level of HPI?* The HPI is **Extended** because five elements are documented.

❑ *What is the level of ROS?* The ROS is **Extended** because five systems are documented.

❑ *What is the level of PFSH?* The PFSH is **Complete** because three elements are documented.

❑ *Based on these factors, what is the overall level of history?* The level of history is **Detailed** because the lowest of the three factors (HPI, ROS, and PFSH)

determines the history level. The HPI and ROS qualify for a detailed history, and the PFSH qualifies for a detailed or comprehensive history.

▶ Tanisha refers to the cardiovascular examination in the 1997 DG (Figure 36-7) to abstract information needed to determine the level of the examination.

❑ *What is the level of examination?* The level of examination is **Expanded Problem Focused**. Eight elements of the examination are documented, which exceeds the requirement of six or more bulleted elements for an expanded problem-focused examination. A detailed examination requires that 12 bulleted items be documented, which they are not.

▶ Tanisha determines the level of medical decision making. (Refer to Table 28-12, Medical Decision-Making Levels.)

❑ *What is the level of complexity of the number of diagnoses or management options, based on the presenting problem?* The level is **Moderate** because there is a new presenting problem, without workup.

❑ *What is the amount and/or complexity of data to be reviewed?* The level is **High** because the physician provided independent visualization of the CT scan.

❑ *What is the level of risk of significant complications, morbidity, and/or mortality?* Tanisha reviews each column in the Table of Risk in the 1997 DG and determines that the level of risk is **Moderate**. The patient presents with an undiagnosed new problem with uncertain prognosis illness (Moderate), clinical labs are reviewed and an event recorder is ordered (Minimal), and prescription drugs are discussed but not implemented (Moderate). The single highest element in the Table of Risk determines the overall risk. The column **Presenting problem** is the highest level (Moderate).

❑ *Based on these factors, what is the overall level of medical decision making?* The medical decision making is **Moderate complexity**. At least two of the three MDM factors are required to qualify for a specific level of MDM. Two of the three MDM factors meet or exceed Moderate decision making.

Now Tanisha is ready to assign the code for the cardiovascular encounter. The exercise that follows guides you through additional abstracting skills and allows you to assign the correct code.

CODING PRACTICE

Exercise 36.5 E/M Coding for Cardiology

Instructions: Refer to the *1997 Documentation Guidelines for Evaluation and Management Services* (available at **www.cms.gov**) or Chapter 28, "Evaluation and Management (E/M) Services (99201-99499)," Tables 28-7 to 28-12, in this text. Answer the following questions about the "Cardiology encounter" (Figure 36-8).

1. a. Which elements of the HPI are documented? Circle all that apply. Location, Quality, Severity, Duration, Timing, Context, Modifying factors, Associated signs and symptoms

    b. How many elements are documented? _____

    c. What is the level of HPI? _____

2. a. Which systems are reviewed in the ROS? Circle all that apply. Constitutional, Allergic/ immunologic, CV, Endocrine, ENT/M, Eyes, GI, GU, Hemic/lymphatic, MS, Neurologic, Psychiatric, Respiratory, Skin/breast

    b. How many systems are documented? _____

    c. What is the level of ROS? _____

3. a. Which PFSH elements are documented? Circle all that apply. Past medical, Family, Social

    b. What is the level of PFSH? _____

    c. What is the overall level of history? (The lowest history factor—HPI, ROS, or PFSH—determines the level of history.) ___ _____

4. Refer to Figure 36-7, "1997 documentation guidelines for cardiovascular examination."

    a. Which bulleted items are documented for the examination? (Check off the items documented.) _____

    b. How many bulleted items are documented? _____

    c. What is the level of the examination? _____

5. Refer to Table 28-12, Medical Decision-Making Levels, or the 1997 DG.

    a. What is the MDM level for the number of diagnoses or management options? _____

    b. What is the MDM level for the amount and/or complexity of data to be reviewed? _____

    c. Refer to the Table of Risk in the 1997 DG. Which elements of risk are documented for each risk factor?

       1. Presenting problem: _____

       2. Diagnostic procedures ordered: _____

       3. Management options selected: _____

    d. What is the level of risk? (The highest of the three risk factors determines the overall level of risk.) _____

    e. What is the overall level of MDM? (2/3 MDM factors are needed to determine the overall level.) _____

6. a. What is the setting? _____

    b. What is the patient (or service) type? _____

    c. What is the code range? _____

    d. How many key components are required? _____

    e. What is the level of history? _____

    f. What is the level of examination? _____

    g. What is the level of medical decision making? _____

    h. What is the correct code? _____

7. Abstract and assign the diagnosis code that supports the E/M code.

    ICD-10-CM Code _____

CHAPTER SUMMARY

In this chapter you learned that:

- Cardiology is a subspecialty of internal medicine that specializes in the cardiovascular system. Cardiothoracic surgeons perform surgery on the heart and surrounding structures, including the lung when necessary. Vascular surgeons perform surgery on the vessels.

- Surgeons can operate on the heart using open heart surgery, off-pump heart surgery, and minimally invasive heart surgery.

- The CPT subsection *Cardiovascular System (33010-37799)* contains two subheadings: *Heart and Pericardium (33010-33999)*, which includes procedures on the conduction system, and *Arteries and Veins (34001-36556)*. Each subheading contains numerous categories divided by the type of anatomic site, condition, and type of procedure.

- Various types of cardiovascular procedures require unique abstracting criteria, including coronary artery bypass grafts, central venous access procedures, pacemakers and implantable cardiodefibrillators, and vascular procedures.

- The Cardiovascular System subsection provides extensive special instructions throughout the Tabular List that clarify definitions, code assignments, and bundling rules. Detailed special instructions and coding tables appear in the CPT manual for several categories, including Pacemaker or Implantable Defibrillator (33202-33273) procedures, Extracorporeal Membrane Oxygenation or Extracorporeal Life Support Services (33946-33989), Vascular Injection Procedures (36000-36598) and Dialysis Circuit (36901-37183).

- Multiple cardiac procedures are often performed together, and there is no set pattern for what is normally done because each patient's circumstances are unique. Follow the standard CPT guidelines for sequencing codes in descending RVU order. In addition, there are special considerations when coding associated radiological services and multiple surgeons.

- The *1997 Documentation Guidelines for Evaluation and Management Services* (1997 DG), published by CMS, provides requirements for each level of a cardiovascular E/M examination.

- Special instructions at the beginning of the subsection direct how to code for catheterization within a vascular family. The CPT appendix "Vascular Families", shows the designation of first-, second-, and third-order branches within vascular families for catheterization beginning at the aorta.

CONCEPT QUIZ

Take a moment to look back at the Cardiovascular System subsection and solidify your skills. Try to answer the questions from memory first, then refer to the discussion in this chapter if you need a little extra help.

Completion

Instructions: Write the term that completes each statement based on the information you learned in this chapter. Choose from the list below. Some choices may be used more than once and some choices may not be used at all.

abdominal aortic aneurysm	patent ductus arteriosus ligation
arterial	synthetic
autologous	tetralogy of Fallot
endovascular aneurysm repair	total artificial heart implantation
fenestrated stent	transmyocardial revascularization
heart transplant	
hemodialysis	ventricular assist device implantation
maze surgery	ventricular septal defect

1. When the ductus arteriosus fails to close after birth, a(n) _____ is performed.

2. If a traditional stent would block one or more arteries in the repair of an aneurysm, a(n) _____ can be used.

3. One treatment for atrial fibrillation that creates new paths for the heart's electrical signal is _____.

4. A(n) _____ employs the use of lasers in the treatment of angina.

5. A(n) _____ is repaired through placement of a patch through open heart surgery or using a guidewire.

6. One of the four defects found in _____ is pulmonary stenosis.

7. A patch, stent, or graft may be used to replace a weak section of an artery during a(n) _____.

8. A(n) _____ or autologous graft may be used to widen the vessel in coarctation of the aorta.

9. A(n) _____ uses a device to replace the ventricles in end-stage heart failure.

10. _____ access can be created using an AV fistula.

Multiple Choice

Instructions: Circle the letter of the best answer to each question based on the information you learned in this chapter.

1. What reference table appears in the Cardiovascular System subsection?
   A. The Central Venous Access Procedures Table
   B. The Coronary Artery Bypass Graft Table
   C. The Vascular Family Branches Table
   D. The EVAR/FEVAR Table

2. What term is used to describe interventional procedures?
   A. Therapeutic
   B. Operative
   C. Invasive
   D. Selective

3. What branch order is the subclavian artery when a catheter is threaded from the aorta into the brachiocephalic artery, through the subclavian artery, and into the right vertebral artery?
   A. First
   B. Second
   C. Third
   D. Additional third order

4. What is the starting point for vascular families when determining the branch order?
   A. Femoral artery
   B. Inferior vena cava
   C. Radial artery
   D. Aorta

5. How would you code the following procedure? *A surgeon is a member of a surgical team that performs a CABG of the LAD using the LIMA.*
   A. 33533-51-LT
   B. 33533-58-LM
   C. 33533-66-LD, 4110F
   D. 33533-62-LD

6. How would you code the following procedure? *A catheter was threaded from the aorta into the brachiocephalic artery (first-order), through the subclavian artery (second-order), and into the right vertebral artery (third-order).*
   A. 36215
   B. 36216
   C. 36217
   D. 36215, 36218

(continued)

(continued from page 739)

7. How would you code the following procedure? *An assistant surgeon procures a graft from the great saphenous vein for use in a CABG.*
   A. 33517-51
   B. 33517-80
   C. 33517-81
   D. 33517-82

8. Where does arterial catheterization most often begin?
   A. Aorta
   B. Femoral or radial artery
   C. Inferior vena cava
   D. Basilic or cephalic vein

9. Which graft procurement can be coded separately in addition to a bypass procedure?
   A. Greater saphenous vein
   B. Tibial vein
   C. Radial artery
   D. Femoropopliteal artery

10. What information should the coder identify to determine the total number of grafts that a surgeon performs?
    A. Number of grafts harvested
    B. Percentage of blockage of the artery(ies)
    C. Distal anastomoses performed
    D. Amount of time on CPB

KEEP ON CODING

Instructions: Read the procedural statement, then use the appropriate Index and Tabular List to assign CPT procedure codes, quantities, and modifiers. Write the code(s) on the line provided.

1. Aortobifemoral bypass using a bifurcated Hemashield graft. CPT Code(s) _____

2. Open repair of infrarenal aortic aneurysm, plus repair of associated arterial trauma, following unsuccessful endovascular repair wtih a tube prosthesis. CPT Code(s)_____

3. Right carotid endarterectomy with patch angioplasty. CPT Code(s) _____

4. Thrombectomy, left forearm arteriovenous Gore-Tex bridge fistula. CPT Code(s) _____

5. Initiation of veno-arterial ECMO. CPT Code(s) _____

6. Resection of right internal carotid artery aneurysm with transposition of external to internal carotid artery and patch angioplasty. CPT Code(s) _____

7. Transvenous dual-chamber ICD implantation. CPT Code(s) _____

8. Popliteal embolectomy and a fem-pop bypass with harvested saphenous vein. CPT Code(s) _____

9. Three saphenous vein grafts in a coronary artery bypass procedure for arteriosclerosis of native arteries. CPT Code(s) _____

10. Heelstick by physician assistant. CPT Code(s) _____

11. Popliteal artery thromboendarterectomy. CPT Code(s) _____

12. Endoscopic ligation of perforator veins, subfascial. CPT Code(s) _____

13. Percutaneous internal carotid angiography and angioplasty. CPT Code(s) _____

14. Endovascular insertion of IVC filter. CPT Code(s) _____

15. Distal revascularization and internal ligation (DRIL) of the upper extremity. CPT Code(s) _____

16. Ligation and stripping of left greater saphenous vein to the level of the knee. CPT Code(s) _____

17. Embolization of the uterine arteries for management of hemorrhage. CPT Code(s) _____

18. Coronary artery bypass graft ×3, including left internal mammary artery to the left anterior descending artery, saphenous vein graft to the first diagonal artery, and saphenous vein graft to the circumflex artery. CPT Code(s) _____

19. Return to the operating room for control of postoperative hemorrhage following carotid endarterectomy. CPT Code(s) _____

20. Insertion of dual-chamber rate-modulated (DDDR) permanent pacemaker with pulse generator and transvenous electrode placement. CPT Code(s) _____

21. Intravenous tPA (*tissue plasminogen activator*) for cerebral thrombolysis. CPT Code(s) _____

22. Repair of ruptured aneurysm in the common femoral artery. CPT Code(s) _____

23. Replacement of a peripherally inserted central catheter (PICC) through the same access. CPT Code(s) _____

24. Percutaneous removal of intra-aortic balloon pump (IABP). CPT Code(s) _____

25. Repair of congenital atrial septal defect, secundum, with bypass and patch. CPT Code(s) _____

CODING CHALLENGE

Instructions: Read the mini-medical-record of each patient's encounter, then abstract, assign, and arrange ICD-10-CM diagnosis codes and CPT procedure codes using the appropriate Index and Tabular List. Assign quantities and modifiers where needed. Write the code(s) on the line provided.

1. INPATIENT HOSPITAL   Gender: F   Age: 47

Preprocedure diagnosis: Metastatic breast cancer needing vascular access for chemotherapy

Procedure: Percutaneous placement of a single-lumen Hickman central venous access catheter through the left subclavian vein with fluoroscopic guidance

Postprocedure diagnosis: Metastatic breast cancer

Tip: Know the age of the patient and whether the catheter is tunneled or nontunneled to select the right code.

2 ICD-10-CM Codes _____

2 CPT Codes _____

2. OUTPATIENT HOSPITAL   Gender: M   Age: 54

Preprocedure diagnosis: Left superficial femoral artery subtotal stenosis; arterial insufficiency, left lower extremity

Procedure: Left lower extremity angiogram; left superficial femoral artery laser atherectomy; left superficial femoral artery percutaneous transluminal balloon angioplasty

Postprocedure diagnosis: Total stenosis, left superficial femoral artery; arterial insufficiency, left lower extremity

Tip: Be sure to read the instructional guidelines for endovascular revascularization (open or percutaneous, transcatheter).

2 ICD-10-CM Codes _____

1 CPT Code _____

3. OUTPATIENT HOSPITAL   Gender: F   Age: 68

Reason for encounter: Insertion of pacemaker due to tachybrady syndrome with chronic atrial fibrillation

Procedure: Implantation of a single-chamber pacemaker, right ventricular lead placement under fluoroscopic guidance by a radiologist. Moderate sedation provided by CRNA, 60 minutes intraservice time.

Assessment: Successful implantation of pacemaker, pacing and sensing appropriately

(continued)

3. (continued)

Plan: Admit overnight for observation; chest x-ray to verify lead position and rule out pneumothorax

Tip: Assign codes for the physician, the radiologist performing the fluoroscopic guidance, and the CRNA providing moderate sedation.

2 ICD-10-CM Code _____

1 CPT Code (physician) _____

1 CPT code (radiologist) _____

CPT codes (CRNA) _____ ×1, _____ ×3

4. OUTPATIENT SURGERY   Gender: F   Age: 45

Reason for encounter: End-stage hypertensive renal failure; on chronic hemodialysis with thrombosed dialysis access

Procedure: Thrombectomy and open revision of left forearm AV fistula

Assessment: Thrombosed AV fistula, awaiting kidney transplant

Plan: Continue dialysis three times a week

Tip: Follow the instructions in the ICD-10-CM Tabular List to *Use additional code*.

5 ICD-10-CM Codes _____

_____

1 CPT Code _____

5. INPATIENT HOSPITAL   Gender: M   Age: 78

Reason for encounter: Pacemaker battery at end of life

Procedure: Pulse generator replacement, removal of a Medtronic unit and insertion of Biotronik Stratos LV with biventricular port

Assessment: Previous aortic valve replacement with subsequent insertion of a dual-chamber pacemaker for underlying chronic atrial fibrillation, and now the pacemaker has shown signs of battery at the end of life

Plan: Potential need for biventricular pacemaker

3 ICD-10-CM Codes _____

_____

1 CPT Code _____

(continued)

(continued from page 741)

6. OUTPATIENT HOSPITAL   Gender: F   Age: 17

Reason for encounter: Congenital renal arteriovenous malformation; uncontrolled secondary hypertension

Procedure: Angiographically guided embolization of the malformation with absolute alcohol

Assessment: Renal angiogram of the right kidney revealed a large lower-pole congenital AVM amenable to embolization

Plan: Embolization followed by regulation of hypertension

2 ICD-10-CM Codes _____

1 CPT Code _____

---

7. HOSPITAL OUTPATIENT   Gender: M   Age: 72

Preprocedure diagnosis: Bilateral carotid artery occlusive disease; peripheral vascular disease

Procedure: Bilateral carotid cerebral angiogram and right femoral-popliteal angiogram

Tip: A modifier is used for both procedures.

2 ICD-10-CM Codes _____

2 CPT Codes _____

---

8. INPATIENT HOSPITAL   Gender: M Age: 62

Preprocedure diagnosis: Postoperative femoral-tibial bypass thrombus formation in saphenous vein graft

Procedure: Return to surgery for thrombectomy

Tip: Assign a modifier to report the return to surgery.

1 ICD-10-CM Code _____

1 CPT Code _____

---

9. HOSPITAL INPATIENT   Gender: M   Age: 84

Reason for encounter: Second-degree protein–calorie malnutrition due to end-stage kidney disease

Procedure: Insertion of a tunneled femoral triple lumen catheter for TPN

Assessment: Protein–calorie malnutrition, moderate

Plan: Central venous access for total parenteral nutrition

2 ICD-10-CM Codes _____

1 CPT Code _____

---

10. HOSPITAL INPATIENT   Gender: F   Age: 68

Reason for encounter: Mitral valve regurgitation

Procedure: Mitral valve replacement with a 27-mm CarboMedics mechanical valve with cardiopulmonary bypass; intraoperative transesophageal echocardiogram to assess new valve for continued regurgitation

Assessment: Mitral valve regurgitation, cardiomyopathy with left-ventricular failure

Plan: Monitor in cardiovascular intensive care unit

3 ICD-10-CM Codes _____

_____

2 CPT Codes _____

Hemic and Lymphatic Systems (38100-38999) and Mediastinum and Diaphragm Procedures (39000-39599)

Chapter
37

Learning Objectives

After completing this chapter, you should have the skills to:

37.1 Spell and define the key words, medical terms, and abbreviations related to hemic and lymphatic systems, mediastinum, and diaphragm procedures. (Remember)

37.2 Summarize the fundamentals of hemic and lymphatic systems, mediastinum, and diaphragm procedures. (Understand)

37.3 Adhere to the CPT coding guidelines in the Hemic and Lymphatic Systems subsection and the Mediastinum and Diaphragm subsection. (Apply)

37.4 Examine and abstract procedural information from the medical record for coding hemic and lymphatic systems, mediastinum, and diaphragm procedures. (Analyze)

37.5 Demonstrate how to assign codes for procedures in the Hemic and Lymphatic Systems subsection and the Mediastinum and Diaphragm subsection. (Apply)

37.6 Utilize guidelines for arranging (sequencing) codes for procedures in the Hemic and Lymphatic Systems subsection and the Mediastinum and Diaphragm subsection. (Apply)

37.7 Determine how to code Evaluation and Management services for the hemic and lymphatic systems, mediastinum, and diaphragm. (Evaluate)

Chapter Outline

- **Hemic and Lymphatic Systems Procedure Basics**
- **Coding Guidelines for Hemic and Lymphatic Systems Procedures**
- **Abstracting Hemic and Lymphatic Systems Procedures**
- **Assigning Codes for Hemic and Lymphatic Systems Procedures**
- **Arranging Codes for Hemic and Lymphatic Systems Procedures**
- **E/M Coding for the Hemic and Lymphatic Systems**

Key Terms and Abbreviations

allogeneic	diaphragm	lymph chain	sentinel lymph node
autologous	hemic	lymph node	T-lymphocytes
bone marrow	lymph	mediastinum	

In addition to the key terms listed here, students should know the terms defined within tables in this chapter.

INTRODUCTION

The shelves of drugstores and health food stores are lined with products to boost your immune system and ward off illness. Such products may support the lymphatic and hemic systems, which are central to fighting many illnesses and diseases. For the sake of brevity, this chapter refers to the hemic and lymphatic systems, mediastinum, and diaphragm collectively as the hemic and lymphatic systems.

HEMIC AND LYMPHATIC SYSTEMS PROCEDURE BASICS

The **hemic** (*blood*) and lymphatic systems are studied together because blood and lymph are two of the body's main fluids, which are circulated through two separate but interconnected vessel systems. The hemic system consists of the blood, whereas the cardiovascular/circulatory system consists of the heart, great vessels, and blood vessels. Blood is circulated through arteries, veins, and capillaries by the pumping action of the heart. Chapter 14 of this text provides additional information on the anatomy and conditions of the hemic system.

The lymphatic system is part of the body's immune system, or defense against invading organisms. It transports **lymph** (*a clear fluid containing proteins, salts, organic substances, and water*) from body tissues to the blood. The lymphatic system consists of vessels or channels, nodes, ducts, and the accessory organs of the tonsils, adenoids, thymus, and spleen (■ FIGURE 37-1).

Lymph nodes are small masses of tissue that range from the size of a pinhead to about one inch in diameter and are located along the lymph vessels. Lymph nodes assist the bone marrow to produce lymphocytes, which in turn produce antibodies to defend the body against disease, bacteria, and viruses. **Lymph chains** are sequential groupings of lymph nodes along lymph vessels, occurring in sites where the body is most vulnerable to infection. Lymph nodes and lymph chains are identified by the general anatomic area where they occur, such as cervical or pelvic, but each anatomic area is generally subdivided into several levels of nodes based on the flow of lymphatic fluid. A **sentinel lymph node** is the first node or group of nodes in a chain.

The lymphatic system is one of the avenues by which cancer metastasizes (*spreads*) to areas of the body distant from its origin. Surgeons often sample lymph nodes to help stage cancer (*evaluate how far cancer has spread*) and usually remove affected nodes to help diminish further spread of the malignancy.

Lymph fluid drains from lymphatic capillaries in body tissue, through lymph vessels, and into the large veins of the circulatory system located in the upper chest. Lymph fluid is not pumped and does not circulate in the same way blood does. Muscles contract around the lymph vessels to move the fluid forward. Valves within the lymphatic system provide for a one-way flow created by muscular action.

The thymus contributes to the production of **T-lymphocytes**, which are white blood cells that protect against viruses and bacteria. The thymus decreases in size after a person reaches puberty. The thymus also performs endocrine functions.

Bone marrow is soft, spongy tissue inside bones. The body produces red blood cells (RBCs), white blood cells (WBCs),

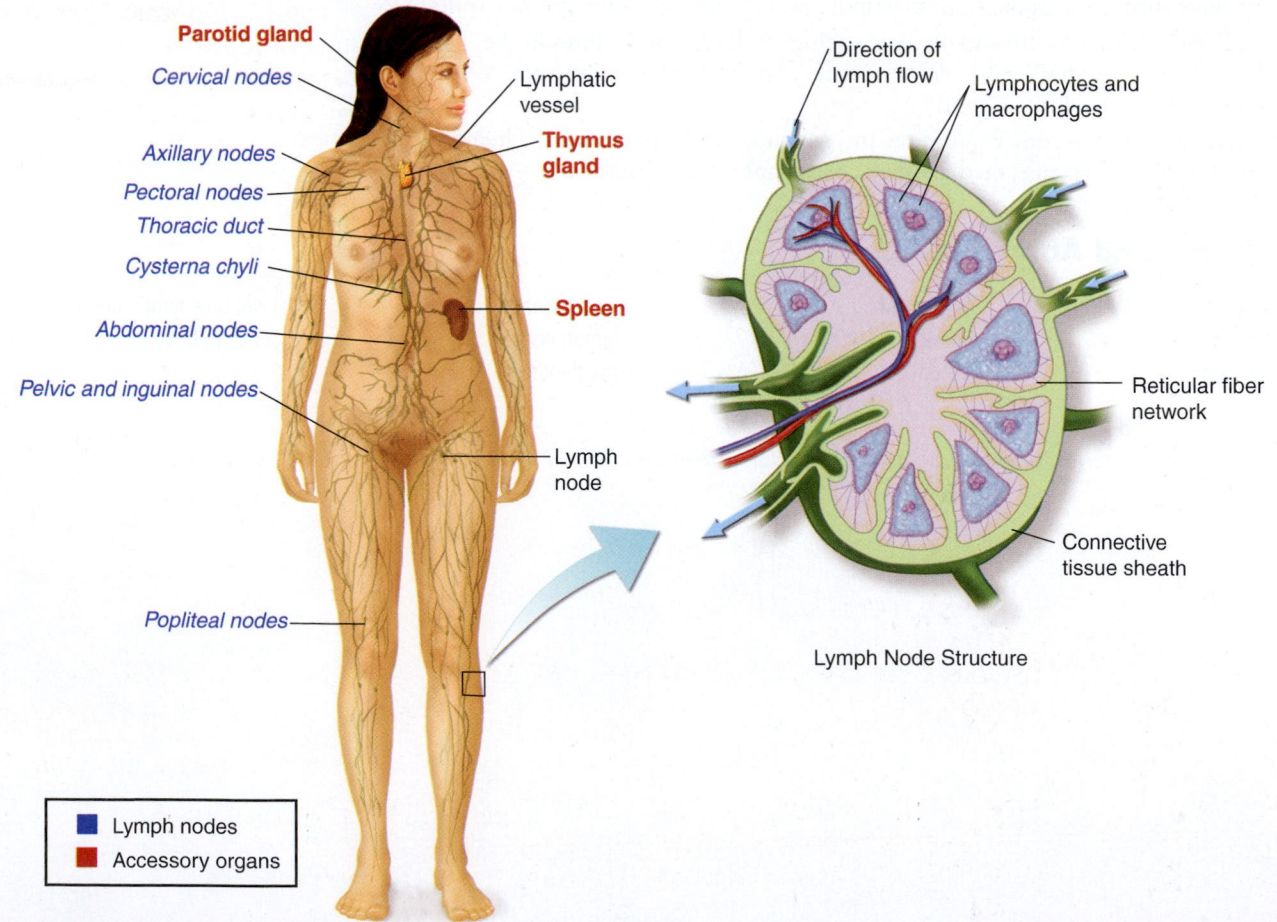

Parotid gland
Cervical nodes
Lymphatic vessel
Thymus gland
Axillary nodes
Pectoral nodes
Thoracic duct
Cysterna chyli
Spleen
Abdominal nodes
Pelvic and inguinal nodes
Lymph node
Popliteal nodes

■ Lymph nodes
■ Accessory organs

Direction of lymph flow
Lymphocytes and macrophages
Reticular fiber network
Connective tissue sheath

Lymph Node Structure

Figure 37-1 ■ The lymphatic system.

platelets, and stem cells in bone marrow. Stem cells help the body to repair damaged tissue and can grow to become other types of cells through a process called differentiation. Red bone marrow produces blood cells and platelets, and yellow marrow is made up of fat cells.

Anatomy of the Mediastinum and Diaphragm

The mediastinum and diaphragm are anatomically separate from the hemic and lymphatic systems. There are a small number of codes and CPT lists them in a contiguous section, so they are covered in this textbook chapter.

Refer to ■ FIGURE 37-2 to visualize the location of the mediastinum and diaphragm in relationship to other structures in the thoracic cavity. The mediastinum is located in the thorax and is surrounded by connective tissue. It separates the lungs and contains the esophagus, heart, and superior and inferior vena cava and aorta. Procedures performed on the mediastinum include removal of tumors and treatment of infections such as mediastinitis.

The diaphragm is a muscle shaped like half of a dome and is located between the thoracic and abdominal cavities.

It contracts and flattens during inhalation and relaxes during exhalation. Procedures on the diaphragm include repairs of diaphragmatic hernias, a paralyzed phrenic nerve (*a sensory and motor nerve that conveys signals to the pleura, pericardium, and diaphragm*), and eventration (*a congenital anomaly of poor diaphragmatic muscle development*). Refer to ■ TABLE 37-1 for a refresher on how to build medical terms related to the hemic and lymphatic systems.

Procedures commonly performed on the hemic and lymphatic systems are discussed next.

CODING CAUTION

Be alert for medical word roots that are spelled similarly and have different meanings.

globin (*a by-product of hemoglobin*) and **globulin** (*a protein molecule that comprises immunoglobulins*)

erythrocyte (*red blood cell*) and **erythema** (*redness*) and **erythremia** (*polycythemia vera—a circulatory disorder*)

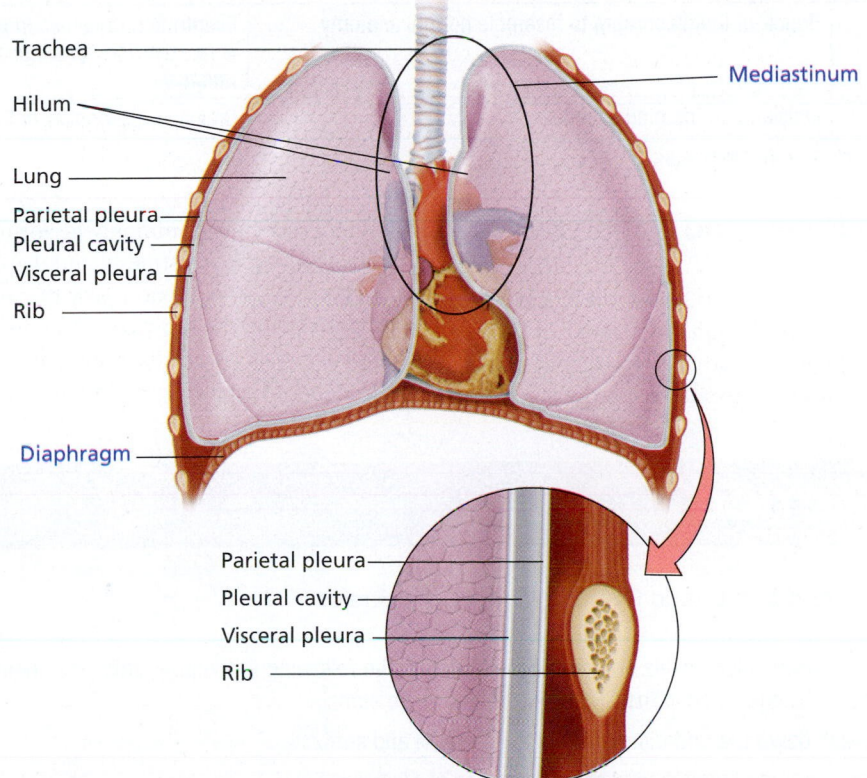

Figure 37-2 ■ The mediastinum and diaphragm.

Labels: Trachea, Hilum, Lung, Parietal pleura, Pleural cavity, Visceral pleura, Rib, Diaphragm, Mediastinum

Inset labels: Parietal pleura, Pleural cavity, Visceral pleura, Rib

---

Table 37-1 ■ **EXAMPLE OF CONSTRUCTING MEDICAL TERMS FOR HEMIC AND LYMPHATIC SYSTEMS PROCEDURES**

Combining Form	Suffix	Complete Medical Term
lymph/o (*lymph fluid*)	**-ectomy** (*excision*)	**lymph + aden + ectomy** (*surgical excision of a lymph gland*)
angi/o (*vessel*)	**-graphy** (*recording*)	**lymph + angio + graphy** (*recording a lymph vessel*)
aden/o (*gland*)	**-pheresis** (*removal*)	
hemat/o (*blood*)	**-poiesis** (*formation*)	**hema + pheresis** (*removal of blood*)
hem/e (*blood*)		**hemato + poiesis** (*formation of blood*)

Source: © PB Resources, Inc. Used with permission.

Table 37-2 ■ **COMMON PROCEDURES OF THE HEMIC AND LYMPHATIC SYSTEMS, MEDIASTINUM, AND DIAPHRAGM**

Procedure Name	Definition	Reason Performed
Hemic and Lymphatic Systems		
Cannulation of thoracic duct	Insertion of a tube (cannulation) into the thoracic duct to collect lymph	Diagnosis of disorders of lymph flow
Limited lymphadenectomy	Removal of lymph nodes	Staging or treatment of cancer
Lymphangiography	Radiology procedure where contrast medium is injected into the patient to visualize lymph nodes and lymph circulation	Diagnosis of diseases, such as cancer
Lymphangiotomy	Incision into a vessel of the lymphatic system	Drainage of an abscess
Radical lymphadenectomy	Removal of lymph nodes and nearby structures	Staging or treatment of cancer
Splenectomy	Total or partial excision of the spleen	Injury, cancer, blood disorders such as idiopathic thrombocytopenic purpura (ITP; *an autoimmune condition in which antibodies target blood platelets*)
Splenorrhaphy	Repair of ruptured spleen, with or without partial splenectomy	Injured or ruptured spleen
Transplantation	Replacement of bone marrow or hematopoietic progenitor cells (HPCs; *stem cells in the umbilical cord and bone marrow*), including harvesting, cryopreservation, thawing, and specific cell depletion, allogeneic (*from a different person*) or autologous (*from the same person*)	Treatment of various conditions, such as cancer
Mediastinum and Diaphragm		
Imbrication of the diaphragm	Repair of the diaphragm to resemble normal anatomy	Eventration (*a condition in which the diaphragm is relaxed and not shaped like a dome, leading to paralysis*)
Mediastinotomy	Incision into the mediastinum	Drainage, exploration, or foreign body removal

Source: © PB Resources, Inc. Used with permission.

Procedures of the Hemic and Lymphatic Systems

Depending on the patient's condition and severity of illness, diagnosing and treating disorders of the lymphatic system may involve an immunologist, an oncologist, or other types of physicians. General surgeons perform surgical procedures on the lymphatic system. Procedures commonly performed on the hemic and lymphatic systems, mediastinum, and diaphragm are summarized in ■ TABLE 37-2. This section provides a general reference to help you understand the most common procedures of the hemic and lymphatic systems, mediastinum, and diaphragm. Remember to keep standard reference books handy in case you get stuck.

CODING PRACTICE

Exercise 37.1 Hemic and Lymphatic Systems Procedure Basics

Instructions: Use your medical terminology skills and resources to define the following procedures related to hemic and lymphatic systems, then identify the code(s) or code range listed in the CPT Index. Follow these steps:

• Use slash marks "/" to break down the underlined term into its root(s) and suffix.

• Define the meaning of the underlined word based on the meaning of each word part.

• Use the entire phrase to identify the code or code range shown in the CPT Index.

Example: <u>splenoplasty</u> spleno/plasty   Meaning *repair of the spleen*   CPT Code *38115*

1. <u>splenectomy</u>, total   Meaning _____   CPT Code _____

2. <u>splenorrhaphy</u>   Meaning _____   CPT Code _____

3. <u>lymphadenectomy</u>, cervical   Meaning _____   CPT Code _____

4. <u>splenoportography</u>, injection procedure   Meaning _____   CPT Code _____

5. <u>retroperitoneal</u> transabdominal lymphadenectomy   Meaning _____   CPT Code _____

6. injection for <u>lymphangiography</u>   Meaning _____   CPT Code _____

CODING PRACTICE (continued)

7. <u>mediastinotomy</u>, cervical approach   Meaning _____   CPT Code _____

8. <u>lymphangiotomy</u>   Meaning _____   CPT Code _____

9. excision of cystic <u>hygroma</u>   Meaning _____   CPT Code _____

10. bone marrow harvesting, <u>allogeneic</u>   Meaning _____   CPT Code _____

CODING GUIDELINES FOR HEMIC AND LYMPHATIC SYSTEMS PROCEDURES

Coders should understand the organization, guidelines, and instructional notes in the Tabular List of these CPT subsections. This information is necessary for accurate coding. The CPT subsection **Hemic and Lymphatic Systems (38100-38999)** contains codes that represent procedures related to the spleen, bone marrow, blood, lymph nodes, and lymphatic channels (vessels). It has several subheadings divided by anatomic site (■ TABLE 37-3). Each subheading contains several categories based on the type of procedure. The CPT subsection **Mediastinum and Diaphragm (39000-39599)** contains two subheadings—**Mediastinum** and **Diaphragm**—each with categories for the type of procedure.

Review the subheading and category names and code ranges listed in both of these subsections to become familiar with the content and organization. Some editions of the CPT manual provide a summary list of the subheadings and categories at the beginning of each subsection, which also displays an asterisk (*) next to categories that contain special coding instructions.

Codes for diagnostic tests on the hemic and lymphatic systems appear in the Medicine, Laboratory, and Radiology sections. The medical necessity of procedures represented by CPT codes must be justified by diagnosis codes. CPT codes in the Hemic and Lymphatic Systems subsection are frequently supported by diagnosis codes from ICD-10-CM Chapter 1, "Certain Infectious and Parasitic Diseases (A00-B99)," as well as selected sections of the circulatory and integumentary systems chapters, neoplasms, symptoms and signs, and injuries (■ TABLE 37-4). These are the codes used most commonly to support procedures on the hemic and lymphatic systems; however, diagnosis codes from any ICD-10-CM chapter are permissible.

Table 37-3 ■ HEMIC AND LYMPHATIC SYSTEMS, MEDIASTINUM, AND DIAPHRAGM SUBHEADINGS

Subheading	Code Range
Hemic and Lymphatic Systems	
Spleen	38100-38200
General	38204-38232
Transplantation and Post-Transplantation Cellular Infusions	38240-38243
Lymph Nodes and Lymphatic Channels	38300-38999
Mediastinum and Diaphragm	
Mediastinum	39000-39499
Diaphragm	39501-39599

Table 37-4 ■ LOCATING ICD-10-CM AND ADDITIONAL CPT CODES ON THE HEMIC AND LYMPHATIC SYSTEMS

Type of Code	Codes
ICD-10-CM Hemic and Lymphatic System-Related Codes	
Hematological conditions	D50-D89
Lymphatic/immune conditions	A00-B99, I88-I89, L03-L04
Neoplasms	C81-C96, D18, D46-D47
Symptoms and signs	R50-R69, R70-R79
Injuries	S35, S36
CPT Hemic and Lymphatic System-Related Codes	
Medicine procedures	90281-90756, 93880-93998
Radiologic procedures	
• Diagnostic radiology	75600-75989
• Radiologic guidance	77001-77022
• Diagnostic ultrasound	76506-76642, 76801-76857, 76881-76886
• Nuclear medicine, diagnostic	78102-78199
Laboratory organ/disease panels, tests	80047, 80050, 80074, 80075, 85002-85999, 86000-86849

Source: © PB Resources, Inc. Used with permission.

CPT guidelines for the Surgery section apply to the Hemic and Lymphatic Systems subsections as well as the Mediastinum and Diaphragm subsection. There are no additional guidelines at the beginning of these subsections.

Special instructions that describe how the codes should be reported appear at the beginning of the categories **Bone Marrow or Stem Cell Services/Procedures** and **Transplantation and Post-Transplantation Cellular Infusions**.

Instructional notes appear throughout the Tabular List to alert coders to the need for modifiers, provide cross-references to codes for similar procedures on other sites, identify bundled services, determine when additional codes might be needed for radiological services, and highlight resequenced and recently deleted codes. Specific guidelines and instructional notes are discussed throughout this chapter of the text.

ABSTRACTING HEMIC AND LYMPHATIC SYSTEMS PROCEDURES

Familiarity with the anatomy of the lymphatic system is fundamental to abstracting because coding is based on the site and extent of treatment. Lymph nodes are identified by the anatomic region where they occur. Procedures on the lymph nodes

Table 37-5   ■   **KEY CRITERIA FOR ABSTRACTING HEMIC AND LYMPHATIC SYSTEMS PROCEDURES**

- ❑ What is the procedure?
- ❑ What is the anatomic site?
- ❑ What is the surgical approach?
- ❑ Is the procedure performed during the same operative session as another major procedure?
- ❑ Is the harvest allogeneic or autologous?
- ❑ How many donors are used?
- ❑ What components are depleted or removed?
- ❑ Is the service a biopsy, limited removal for staging, or radical resection?
- ❑ Which specific nodes and/or chains are removed?
- ❑ Is the procedure bilateral (where applicable)?

Source: © PB Resources, Inc. Used with permission.

can be performed to determine the stage of cancer metastasis; they can also be described as radical, complete, partial, or superficial depending on the specific structures treated. Codes depend on these descriptions of extent and/or on the specific sites of nodes excised. Refer to ■ TABLE 37-5 for guidance on how to abstract procedures on the hemic and lymphatic systems, then work through the detailed example that follows. Remember that the abstracting questions are a guide and that not every question applies to, or can be answered for, every case.

OUTPATIENT HOSPITAL   Gender: M   Age: 32

Preoperative diagnosis: Stage 4 Hodgkin's lymphoma involving multiple lymph nodes above and below the diaphragm

Procedure: Prepared hematopoietic progenitor cells (HPCs) for transplant, including thawing and washing previously frozen harvests from two allogeneic donors, and performed specific T-cell (lymphocyte) depletion within both harvests. Proceeded with the transplantation of both harvests using sequential injections into an intravenous (IV) drip.

Guided Example of Abstracting Hemic and Lymphatic Systems Procedures

Refer to the following example throughout this chapter to practice skills for abstracting, assigning, and arranging Hemic and Lymphatic Systems codes. Follow along as fictitious coder Scott Hood, CPC, abstracts the procedure. Check off each step after you complete it.

▶ Scott reads through the entire record, paying special attention to the preoperative diagnosis and the procedure performed. He refers to the Key Criteria for Abstracting Hemic and Lymphatic Systems Procedures (Table 37-5) and takes note of the added criteria for bone marrow and stem cell services.

- ❑ He notes preoperative diagnosis: Hodgkin's lymphoma involving multiple lymph nodes
- ❑ *What is the patient's age?* 32
- ❑ *What is the procedure?* Prepare hematopoietic progenitor cells (HPCs) for transplant and allogeneic transplantation.
- ❑ *What is the anatomic site?* Hematopoietic progenitor cells
- ❑ *What is the surgical approach?* The approach does not apply to the preparation. The transplantation is performed using injections into an intravenous (IV) drip.
- ❑ *Is the procedure performed during the same operative session as another major procedure?* Two HPC procedures are performed: thawing and washing and specific T-cell (lymphocyte) depletion within harvests. In addition, the transplant is performed. No other procedures are performed.
- ❑ *What components are depleted or removed?* T-cell (lymphocyte) depletion
- ❑ *Is the harvest allogeneic or autologous?* Allogeneic
- ❑ *How many donors are used?* Two

▶ At this time, Scott does not know which of these procedures may need to be coded, nor how many codes he will end up with. He will learn about this when he moves on to assigning codes.

CODING PRACTICE

Exercise 37.2   Abstracting Hemic and Lymphatic Systems Procedures

Instructions: Read the mini-medical-record of each patient's encounter and answer the abstracting questions. Write the answer on the line provided. Do not assign any codes.

---

1. INPATIENT HOSPITAL   Gender: M   Age: 32

Preprocedure diagnosis: Lacerated spleen sustained as a result of automobile accident

Procedure: Laparoscopic splenectomy

a. What is the procedure? _____

b. What is the anatomic site? _____

c. What is the surgical approach? _____

d. Is the procedure performed during the same operative session as another major procedure? _____

CODING PRACTICE (continued)

2. OUTPATIENT HOSPITAL Gender: F Age: 45

Preprocedure diagnosis: Leukemia

Procedure: Bone marrow aspiration from the sternum, diagnostic

a. What is the procedure? _____

b. What is the anatomic site? _____

c. What is the surgical approach? _____

d. Is the procedure performed during the same operative session as another major procedure? _____

3. INPATIENT HOSPITAL Gender: F Age: 37

Preprocedure diagnosis: Mediastinal tumor

Procedure: Substernal mediastinectomy, open

Postprocedure diagnosis: Benign tumor

a. What is the procedure? _____

b. What is the anatomic site? _____

c. What is the surgical approach? _____

d. Is the procedure performed during the same operative session as another major procedure? _____

4. INPATIENT HOSPITAL Gender: F Age: 56

Preprocedure diagnosis: Metastasis of lung cancer (middle lobe)

Procedure: Complete axillary lymphadenectomy, bilateral

Postprocedure diagnosis: Metastasis of lung cancer (middle lobe)

a. What is the procedure? _____

b. What is the anatomic site? _____

c. What is the surgical approach? _____

d. Is the procedure performed during the same operative session as another major procedure? _____

e. Is the service a biopsy, limited removal for staging, or radical resection? _____

f. Which specific nodes and/or chains are removed?

_____

g. Is the procedure bilateral (where applicable)? _____

5. INPATIENT HOSPITAL Gender: M Age: 46

Preprocedure diagnosis: CT scan shows evidence of ruptured spleen following automobile accident

Procedure: Splenectomy; incised the abdomen below the left ribs and exposed the spleen. Rupture and parenchymal fragmentation was evident. Ligated and divided splenic arteries and veins. Freed the spleen from surrounding structures and ligaments. Removed the spleen in its entirety. Irrigated the surgical site, placed a drain, and performed a layered closure. Patient tolerated procedure well.

Postprocedure diagnosis: Splenic rupture with parenchymal fragmentation

a. What is the procedure? _____

b. What is the anatomic site? _____

c. What is the surgical approach? _____

d. Is the procedure partial or total? _____

6. OUTPATIENT SURGERY Gender: M Age: 28

Preprocedure diagnosis: Acute myeloid leukemia

Procedure: Thawed previously frozen HPCs harvested from a single donor, without washing, and performed RBC depletion for HPC boost, which was administered by IV

Postprocedure diagnosis: Acute myeloid leukemia

a. What is the procedure? _____

b. What is the surgical approach? _____

c. Is the procedure performed during the same operative session as another major procedure? _____

d. Is the harvest allogeneic or autologous? _____

e. How many donors are used? _____

f. What components are depleted or removed?

_____

ASSIGNING CODES FOR HEMIC AND LYMPHATIC SYSTEM PROCEDURES

To assign codes for procedures from the Hemic and Lymphatic Systems subsection, and the Mediastinum and Diaphragm subsection, search the Index for the Main Term of the anatomic site, such as **Spleen**, **Mediastinum**, or **Diaphragm**. Locate the first-level modifying term for the type of procedure and the second-level modifying term for any additional details, as required. Verify codes in the Tabular List, paying special attention to the code descriptions and instructional notes. Additional considerations for coding bone marrow/stem cell services, transplant-related cellular infusions, and lymphadenectomies are discussed next.

Bone Marrow/Stem Cell/Transplantation Procedures

To locate codes for bone marrow or stem cell services, procedures, and cellular infusions, search the Index for the Main Term **Bone Marrow** or **Stem Cell**. Locate the first-level modifying term for the type of service or procedure provided and identify the code(s) or code range to be verified in the Tabular List. In the Tabular List, codes for these services appear under the subheading **General** in the subsection **Hemic and Lymphatic Systems**. Codes are divided into two categories.

The category **Bone Marrow or Stem Cell Services/Procedures** contains codes that describe the steps used to harvest, preserve, prepare, and purify bone marrow or stem cells, also called HPCs, for a transplant or reinfusion procedure. Special instructions at the beginning of the category state that codes in this category are reported only once per patient per day, regardless of the quantity of cells treated. The exception is codes whose descriptions contain the phrase **per donor**. When cells from more than one donor are thawed, report one code for each donor (■ FIGURE 37-3). After cells are harvested from a donor, they are frozen and stored for later use. When needed for a procedure, they are thawed and usually washed to remove the preserving solution and other impurities. Components of the harvest might be removed or reduced to create a product suitable for the transplant recipient. Separate codes report each of these services.

Physician thawed and washed previously frozen HPC harvests from two separate donors, then performed plasma volume depletion on each.

38214 × 1 Transplant preparation of hematopoietic progenitor cells; plasma (volume) depletion
38209 × 2 Transplant preparation of hematopoietic progenitor cells; thawing of previously frozen harvest, with washing, <mark>per donor</mark>

Figure 37-3 ■ Example of reporting separate transplant codes for each donor. *Source: © PB Resources, Inc. Used with permission. CPT codes only © American Medical Association.*

The category **Transplantation and Post-Transplantation Cellular Infusions** contains four codes for the actual transplantation or infusion procedure. The special instructions at the beginning of the category outline the services and activities included in the code descriptions and those that can be reported separately. Separately reportable services include management of post-transplant adverse reactions and administration of medications and/or hydration *unrelated* to the transplant. Codes in this category are divided based on whether the procedure is a transplant, post-transplant boost, or lymphocyte infusion. Transplant codes are divided based on whether the harvest is autologous or allogeneic. Allogeneic transplants are reported per donor harvest when harvests are administered sequentially.

CODING CAUTION

Medicare publishes a medically unlikely edit (MUE) of 1 for allogeneic transplantation (**38240 Hematopoietic progenitor cell (HPC); allogeneic transplantation per donor**), meaning that the code can be reported only once per day, despite the code descriptor stating **per donor**. Some private carriers follow Medicare MUEs, whereas others do not, so checking with individual carriers regarding how to report this service is helpful.

Lymphadenectomy

To locate codes for procedures on the lymphatic system, search the Index for the Main Term **Lymph Duct**, **Lymph Nodes**, **Lymph Vessels**, or **Lymphadenectomy**. The Main Term **Lymph Nodes** provides the most detailed code listing. Identify the first-level modifying term for the anatomic site and/or type of procedure. In the Tabular List, codes for procedures on the lymph nodes and lymphatic channels are divided by the type and extent of the procedure. Within each procedure category, unique codes are provided for distinct anatomic regions and sites. A lymphadenectomy can be performed as a biopsy, a cancer staging procedure, or a complete excision. When staging is performed, the surgeon first injects a radioactive dye to identify the sentinel lymph node. Code the injection procedure in addition to the staging procedure.

A lymphatic biopsy and/or lymphadenectomy is often performed in conjunction with the partial or total excision of another organ—such as the breast, ovary(ies), prostate, or colon—because of the presence of cancer. The procedures most commonly performed with a lymphadenectomy often include code options for bundled lymphadenectomy in the CPT subsection for the primary organ. However, when a lymphadenectomy is performed in conjunction with procedures on the esophagus, trachea, thyroid, and parathyroid, the lymphadenectomy is usually reported separately. Coders must refer to the documentation, code descriptions, and instructional notes to determine when the lymphadenectomy is reported as a standalone procedure (■ FIGURE 37-4), when it is bundled with another procedure (■ FIGURE 37-5), and when it is reported separately (■ FIGURE 37-6).

Surgeon injects a radioactive tracer to identify the sentinel node then performs a limited pelvic lymphadenectomy for staging of prostate cancer.

38562 Limited lymphadenectomy for staging (separate procedure); pelvic and para-aortic

38792-51 Injection procedure; radioactive tracer for identification of sentinel node; -51 Multiple procedures

Figure 37-4 ■ Example of coding a standalone lymphadenectomy. *Source: © PB Resources, Inc. Used with permission. CPT codes only © American Medical Association.*

Surgeon performs a radical perineal prostatectomy, including a limited excision of pelvic lymph nodes, to treat prostate cancer.

55812 Prostatectomy, perineal radical; with lymph node biopsy(s) (limited pelvic lymphadenectomy)

Figure 37-5 ■ Example of coding a bundled lymphadenectomy. *Source: © PB Resources, Inc. Used with permission. CPT codes only © American Medical Association.*

Surgeon performs a transthoracic thyroidectomy, including substernal thyroid, and a thoracic lymphadenectomy via thoracotomy of the low cervical and upper paratracheal nodes.

60270 Thyroidectomy, including substernal thyroid; sternal split or transthoracic approach

38746 Thoracic lymphadenectomy by thoracotomy, mediastinal and regional lymphadenectomy (List separately in addition to code for primary procedure)

Figure 37-6 ■ Example of coding a separate lymphadenectomy. *Source: © PB Resources, Inc. Used with permission. CPT codes only © American Medical Association.*

Guided Example of Assigning Hemic and Lymphatic Systems Procedure Codes

To practice skills for assigning procedure codes for the hemic and lymphatic systems, continue with the example from earlier in the chapter about a patient who was seen for an HPC transplant. Follow along in your CPT manual as Scott Hood, CPC, assigns codes. Check off each step after you complete it.

▶ First, Scott confirms the procedures:

❏ Thawing and washing of previously frozen harvests

❏ Specific T-cell (lymphocyte) depletion

❏ Transplantation of both harvests

▶ Scott searches the Index for the Main Term **Transplantation**.

❏ He locates the first-level modifying term **Stem Cells** and identifies the code range **38240-38242**.

❏ He reviews the second-level modifying terms and locates entries for **T-cell depletion 38210** and **Thawing 38208-38209**.

❏ He believes that these entries will address everything that was done during the procedure, but just to be certain he also looks up **Stem Cells** as a Main Term. He locates the first-level modifying terms for **T-cell depletion 38210**, **Thawing 38208-38209, 88241**, and **Transplantation 38240-38242**. He also notices a first-level modifying term for **Hematopoietic Progenitor Cells** that cross-references him to a Main Term entry for the same. This Main Term entry provides similar first- and second-level modifying terms with the same code ranges.

▶ Scott verifies the codes in the Tabular List. Because they are located close together, he can check all the codes in one search.

▶ He begins with thawing because that is the first procedure completed. According to the Index, he has two choices for thawing: codes **38208** and **38209**.

❏ In the Tabular List, he notices that both these codes are indented codes under the parent code **38207**. The common portion of the descriptor for code **38207** is **Transplant preparation of hematopoietic progenitor cells;**

❏ He compares the descriptions of codes and identifies that code **38208** is **thawing of previously frozen harvest, without washing, per donor** and code **38209** is the same description except **with washing**.

❏ Scott refers to the medical record and confirms that this thawing was performed with washing, so he selects code **38209**.

❏ He also identifies that the code description identifies the quantity as **per donor**. He refers to the medical record again to verify that two donors were used, which means that he will need to report the quantity as 2.

❏ He reads the full code title for code **38209** by combining the common descriptor portion of the parent code with the descriptor of the standalone code and confirms that this accurately describes the procedure: **Transplant preparation of hematopoietic progenitor cells; thawing of previously frozen harvest, with washing, per donor.**

❏ He reads the instructional note in the Tabular List after code **38208** that states **(For diagnostic thawing and expansion of frozen cells, use 88241)**. Code **88241** is reported by laboratories for processing the specimen and appears in the Index entry for the Main Term **Stem Cells** and subterm **Thawing**.

▶ Next, Scott assigns the code for specific T-cell (lymphocyte) depletion within both harvests. The Index directs him to code **38210**, which is also indented under the parent code **38207**.

❏ The unique descriptor for code **38210** is **specific cell depletion within harvest, T-cell depletion.**

❏ He refers to the medical record and confirms that the description correctly reflects the documentation.

▶ Finally, Scott must assign a code for the actual transplantation procedure. The Index directs him to the code range **38240-38242**.

❏ In the Tabular List, he notices that code **38240** is the parent code for **38241**. The common portion of the descriptor for code **38240** is **Hematopoietic progenitor cells;**

❏ He compares the unique descriptors for both and identifies that code **38240** is **allogeneic transplantation per donor** and code **38241** is **autologous transplantation.**

❏ He refers to the medical record and confirms that the transplant is from two allogeneic donors, so he believes that code **38240** is correct. However, the Index also listed **38242** as an option, so he reads that code before making a final decision.

❏ The description for code **38242** is **Allogeneic lymphocyte infusions.** This is not what was done, so he confirms the selection of **38240.**

❏ He also identifies that the code description for **38240** identifies the quantity as **per donor.** He refers to the medical record again to verify that two donors were used, which means that he will need to enter the quantity as "2" on the claim.

▶ Scott checks for special instructions and instructional notes in the Tabular List.

❏ He already read the instructional note following codes **38207** and **38208**, which did not apply, and does not find any notes after code **38209.**

❏ He reads several instructional notes following code **38242.** They all direct the coder to alternative codes for procedures not performed during this encounter, so they do not apply.

❏ Next, he cross-references the beginning of the category **Transplantation and Post-Transplantation Cellular Infusions** and finds extensive special instructions. He uses a highlighter to mark information that applies to this case:

  ▪ **Hematopoietic cell transplantation (HCT) refers to the infusion of hematopoietic progenitor cells**

(HPC) obtained from bone marrow, peripheral blood apheresis, and/or umbilical cord blood.

  ▪ **HCT may be autologous (when the HPC donor and recipient are the same person) or allogeneic (when the HPC donor and recipient are not the same person). Code 38241 is used to report any autologous transplant while 38240 is used to report an allogeneic transplant.**

  ▪ **In some cases allogeneic transplants involve more than one donor and cells from each donor are infused sequentially whereby one unit of 38240 is reported for each donor infused.**

❏ Other information in these guidelines applies to other codes or to the bundling and reporting of services not documented for this case.

❏ He cross-references the beginning of the category **Bone Marrow or Stem Cell Services/Procedures** and finds more special instructions, which apply to all codes in this category, **38204-38232. Each code may be reported only once per day regardless of the quantity of bone marrow/stem cells manipulated.**

❏ When Scott reviews the codes he selected from this category, he identifies that code **38209** specifically states to assign the code once **per donor.** However, code **38210** does not include the designation *per donor*, so he confirms that code **38210** should be reported **once per day.** He cross-references the beginning of the section **Hemic and Lymphatic Systems** and verifies that there are no special instructions.

▶ Scott reviews the procedure codes and quantities he has assigned for this case.

❏ **38209 × 2 Transplant preparation of hematopoietic progenitor cells; thawing of previously frozen harvest, with washing, per donor**

❏ **38210 × 1 Transplant preparation of hematopoietic progenitor cells; specific cell depletion within harvest, T-cell depletion**

❏ **38240 × 2 Hematopoietic progenitor cell (HPC); allogeneic transplantation per donor**

▶ Next, Scott must determine how to sequence the codes.

CODING PRACTICE

Exercise 37.3 Assigning Codes for Hemic and Lymphatic Systems Procedures

Instructions: Read the mini-medical-record of each patient's encounter. Review the information abstracted in Exercise 37.2 for questions 1–3. For questions 4–6, abstract the case on your own. Assign CPT codes, quantities, and modifiers using the Index and Tabular List. Write the code(s) on the line provided.

1. INPATIENT HOSPITAL   Gender: M   Age: 32

Preprocedure diagnosis: Lacerated spleen sustained as a result of automobile accident

Procedure: Laparoscopic splenectomy

1 CPT Code _____

2. OUTPATIENT HOSPITAL   Gender: F   Age: 45

Preprocedure diagnosis: Leukemia

Procedure: Bone marrow aspiration from the sternum, diagnostic

1 CPT Code _____

3. INPATIENT HOSPITAL   Gender: F   Age: 37

Preprocedure diagnosis: Mediastinal tumor

Procedure: Substernal mediastinectomy, open

Postprocedure diagnosis: Benign tumor

1 CPT Code _____

4. OUTPATIENT HOSPITAL   Gender: F   Age: 41

Preprocedure diagnosis: Leukocytosis

Procedure: Bone marrow biopsy. Inserted the trocar through the skin over the iliac crest and pushed the needle into the bone marrow. Confirmed needle position was accurate, then proceeded to excise the bone marrow, which was transferred to a specimen container and sent to pathology.

1 CPT Code _____

5. OUTPATIENT SURGERY   Gender: M   Age: 22

Preprocedure diagnosis: Tenderness and swelling in neck

Procedure: I & D of a cervical lymph node abscess, extensive

Postprocedure diagnosis: Abscess, cervical lymph node

1 CPT Code _____

6. INPATIENT HOSPITAL   Gender: M   Age: 61

Preprocedure diagnosis: Prostate cancer

Procedure: Limited pelvic lymphadenectomy for staging

Pathology report: Sentinel nodes are negative for metastasis

Postprocedure diagnosis: Carcinoma of the prostate with no metastasis to lymph nodes

1 CPT Code _____

ARRANGING CODES FOR HEMIC AND LYMPHATIC SYSTEMS PROCEDURES

Many codes in the Hemic and Lymphatic Systems subsection can be performed at the same time as another major procedure. The instructional note **(separate procedure)** at the end of a code description reminds coders to assign the code only when the procedure is not bundled with another one or is performed at a separate site or through a separate incision. When the code description for the primary procedure includes lymph node excision, do not assign an additional code from the Hemic and Lymphatic Systems subsection.

Modifiers

In addition to modifier **-51 Multiple procedures**, modifiers for laterality and distinct procedural services are important to proper coding for the lymphatic and hemic systems.

Laterality

Most lymph nodes occur in pairs on opposite sides of the body, similar to many blood vessels. Append modifiers for laterality (**-50 Bilateral procedure, -RT Right side**, or **-LT Left side**) for procedures on lymph nodes that occur bilaterally, such as suprahyoid (**38700**), cervical (**38720, 38724**), axillary (**38740, 38745**), inguinofemoral (**38760, 38765**), and pelvic (**38770**). Laterality does not apply to thoracic and abdominal lymphadenectomies.

Coders should assign laterality whenever a site or structure occurs bilaterally. Although CPT does not usually provide instructional notes to assign laterality, it does so occasionally when laterality might be overlooked. CPT instructional notes that direct coders to report modifier -50 for bilateral procedures appear below the codes for inguinofemoral and pelvic lymphadenectomies. The lack of such a laterality note below

Surgeon performs a complete cervical lymphadenectomy on the right side and biopsy of the cervical nodes on the left side.

38720-RT Cervical lymphadenectomy (complete)
38500-59-LT Biopsy or excision of lymph node(s); open, superficial

Figure 37-7 ■ Example of using modifier -59 with the lymphatic system. *Source: © PB Resources, Inc. Used with permission. CPT codes only © American Medical Association.*

suprahyoid, cervical, and axillary lymphadenectomies does not mean that laterality modifiers are unnecessary for these codes.

-59 Distinct Procedural Service

When the surgeon performs a complete lymphadenectomy on one side but a lesser procedure—such as a biopsy—on the contralateral side or using a separate incision, assign separate codes to each service that describes the work done. Append modifier -59 to the less extensive service. Laterality modifiers help clarify that the procedures are classified as separate because they were performed on contralateral sites (■ FIGURE 37-7). Medicare and some other payers may request that modifier -XS Separate structure may be reported instead of modifier -59.

Guided Example of Arranging Hemic and Lymphatic Systems Procedure Codes

To practice skills for arranging codes for procedures on the hemic and lymphatic systems, continue with the example from earlier in the chapter about a patient who was seen for an HPC transplant. Follow along in your CPT manual as Scott Hood, CPC, arranges the codes. Check off each step after you complete it.

▶ First, Scott confirms the procedure codes he assigned.

❑ **38209 × 2 Transplant preparation of hematopoietic progenitor cells; thawing of previously frozen harvest, with washing, per donor**

❑ **38210 × 1 Transplant preparation of hematopoietic progenitor cells; specific cell depletion within harvest, T-cell depletion**

❑ **38240 × 2 Hematopoietic progenitor cell (HPC); allogeneic transplantation per donor**

▶ Scott arranges the codes in descending RVU order according to the Medicare Physician Fee Schedule Database (MPFSDB) and the patient's insurance carrier. He uses the facility RVU because the procedure was performed at the hospital rather than the physician's office.

❑ **38240** Facility RVU = 6.46

❑ **38210** Facility RVU = 2.27

❑ **38209** Facility RVU = 0.34

▶ Scott examines the need for modifiers. (Refer to Table 27-1, Key Criteria for Abstracting CPT Modifiers, or Appendix A in the CPT manual.)

❑ Code **38240** does not require modifiers because it is the first-listed code and no unusual circumstances apply.

❑ Code **38210** requires modifier **-51 Multiple procedures** because it is an additional procedure and is not an add-on code.

❑ Code **38209** requires modifier **-51 Multiple procedures** because it is an additional procedure and is not an add-on code.

▶ Scott finalizes the procedure codes and sequencing for this case:

(1) **38240 × 2 Hematopoietic progenitor cell (HPC); allogeneic transplantation per donor**

(2) **38210-51 × 1 Transplant preparation of hematopoietic progenitor cells; specific cell depletion within harvest, T-cell depletion**

(3) **38209-51 × 2 Transplant preparation of hematopoietic progenitor cells; thawing of previously frozen harvest, with washing, per donor**

▶ Scott also assigns the ICD-10-CM diagnosis code that supports the need for the service.

(1) **C81.98 Hodgkin lymphoma, unspecified, lymph nodes of multiple sites**

CODING PRACTICE

Exercise 37.4 Arranging Codes for Hemic and Lymphatic System Procedures

Instructions: Read the mini-medical-record of each patient's encounter. Review the information abstracted in Exercise 37.2 for questions 1–3. For questions 4–6, abstract the case on your own. Assign CPT codes, quantities, and modifiers using the Index and Tabular List, and arrange the codes in proper sequence. Write the code(s) on the line provided.

1. INPATIENT HOSPITAL Gender: F Age: 56

Preprocedure diagnosis: Metastasis of lung cancer (middle lobe)

Procedure: Complete axillary lymphadenectomy, bilateral

Postprocedure diagnosis: Metastasis of lung cancer (middle lobe)

1 CPT Code _____

CODING PRACTICE (continued)

2. INPATIENT HOSPITAL   Gender: M   Age: 46

Preprocedure diagnosis: CT scan shows evidence of ruptured spleen following automobile accident

Procedure: Splenectomy; incised the abdomen below the left ribs and exposed the spleen. Rupture and parenchymal fragmentation was evident. Ligated and divided splenic arteries and veins. Freed the spleen from surrounding structures and ligaments. Removed the spleen in its entirety. Irrigated the surgical site, placed a drain, and performed a layered closure. Patient tolerated procedure well.

Postprocedure diagnosis: Splenic rupture with parenchymal fragmentation

1 CPT Code _____

3. OUTPATIENT SURGERY   Gender: M   Age: 28

Preprocedure diagnosis: Acute myeloid leukemia

Procedure: Thawing previously frozen HPC harvest from a single donor, without washing, and performed RBC depletion for HPC boost, which was administered by IV

Postprocedure diagnosis: Acute myeloid leukemia

Tip: An HPC boost is an additional infusion of stem cells from the original donor after the initial transplant.

3 CPT Codes _____

_____

4. INPATIENT HOSPITAL   Gender: F   Age: 55

Preprocedure diagnosis: Edema of her left side, splenic mass

Procedure: Partial splenectomy, abdominal lymph node biopsy

Pathology report: Benign neoplasm of the spleen

Postprocedure diagnosis: Benign splenic neoplasm as indicated by pathology report, sentinel node negative for malignancy

2 CPT Codes _____

5. EMERGENCY DEPT   Gender: M   Age: 25

Preprocedure diagnosis: A piece of metal is embedded in the mediastinum, creating an open wound

Procedure: Laceration repair of the diaphragm, transthoracic mediastinotomy

Postprocedure diagnosis: Embedded foreign object

2 CPT Codes _____

6. INPATIENT HOSPITAL   Gender: F   Age: 42

Preprocedure diagnosis: Suspected metastases

Procedure: Pelvic diagnostic laparoscopy followed by bilateral total pelvic lymphadenectomy also performed with laparoscope

Postprocedure diagnosis: Metastasis of carcinoma of the bladder per pathology

1 CPT Code _____

E/M CODING FOR THE HEMIC AND LYMPHATIC SYSTEMS

The *1997 Documentation Guidelines for Evaluation and Management Services* (1997 DG), published by the Centers for Medicare and Medicaid Services (CMS), provides requirements for each level of a hematologic/lymphatic/immunologic E/M examination (■ FIGURE 37-8, page 756). Hematologists are not limited to using the guidelines for the hematologic/lymphatic/immunologic examination only. They can also use guidelines for a general multiorgan system examination, or any other single organ system examination, based on what is most advantageous for a specific encounter. However, physicians cannot combine elements from more than one type of examination for a given encounter. The hematologic/lymphatic/immunologic examination guidelines typically provide the best results when a detailed examination is performed.

To determine the appropriate E/M code, coders must review the documentation in detail and identify the specific elements documented.

- To translate the documentation into the E/M requirements for the history, refer back to Chapter 28, "Evaluation and Management Services (99201-99499)," Tables 28-7 to 28-10, or to the 1997 DG.

- To determine the requirements for an examination, refer to Figure 37-8 or to the single organ system examination for hematologic/lymphatic/immunologic in the 1997 DG.

- To determine the levels for medical decision making (MDM), refer to Chapter 28, Table 28-12, and the Table of Risk in the 1997 DG.

System/Body Area	Elements of Hematologic/Lymphatic/Immunologic Examination

Constitutional	❏ Measurement of any **three** of the following seven **vital** signs:
	  • 1) sitting or standing blood pressure,
	  • 2) supine blood pressure,
	  • 3) pulse rate and regularity,
	  • 4) respiration,
	  • 5) temperature,
	  • 6) height,
	  • 7) weight (May be measured and recorded by ancillary staff)
	❏ General **appearance** of patient (eg, development, nutrition, body habitus, deformities, attention to grooming)

Head and Face	❏ Palpation and/or percussion of **face** with notation of presence or absence of **sinus tenderness**
Eyes	❏ Inspection of **conjunctivae** and **lids**
Ears, Nose, Mouth and Throat	❏ Otoscopic examination of external **auditory canals** and **tympanic membranes** ❏ Inspection of **nasal mucosa, septum** and **turbinates** ❏ Inspection of **teeth** and **gums** ❏ Examination of **oropharynx:** oral mucosa, salivary glands, hard and soft palates, tongue, tonsils and posterior pharynx
Neck	❏ Examination of **neck** (eg, masses, overall appearance, symmetry, tracheal position, crepitus) ❏ Examination of **thyroid** (eg, enlargement, tenderness, mass)
Respiratory	❏ Assessment of **respiratory effort** (eg, intercostal retractions, use of accessory muscles, diaphragmatic movement) ❏ **Auscultation** of lungs (eg, breath sounds, adventitious sounds, rubs)
Cardiovascular	❏ **Auscultation** of heart with notation of abnormal sounds and murmurs ❏ Examination of **peripheral vascular system** by observation (eg, swelling, varicosities) and palpation (pulses, temperature, edema, tenderness)
Gastrointestinal (Abdomen)	❏ Examination of **abdomen** with notation of presence of masses or tenderness ❏ Examination of **liver** and **spleen**
Lymphatic	❏ Palpation of **lymph nodes** in neck, axillae, groin, and/or other location
Extremities	❏ Inspection and palpation of **digits** and **nails** (eg, clubbing, cyanosis, inflammation, petechiae, ischemia, infections, nodes)
Skin	❏ Inspection and/or palpation of **skin** and **subcutaneous tissue** (eg, rashes, lesions, ulcers, ecchymoses, bruises)
Neurological/ Psychiatric	Brief assessment of mental status including: ❏ **Orientation** to time, place and person ❏ **Mood** and affect (eg, depression, anxiety, agitation)

Total # Bullets Performed and Documented →	☐	# of ❏ Elements Performed and Documented	Level of Examination
		1–5	Problem focused
		6–11	Expanded problem focused
		12	Detailed
		ALL	Comprehensive (Document **every** element in each box with a shaded border and at least **one** element in each box with an unshaded border)

Figure 37-8 ■ 1997 documentation guidelines for hematologic/lymphatic/immunologic examination.
Source: Centers for Medicare and Medicaid Services, 1997 Documentation Guidelines for Evaluation and Management Services (with formatting adjustments).

Guided Example of E/M Coding for the Hemic and Lymphatic Systems

Refer to the hematology encounter (■ FIGURE 37-9) to practice skills for abstracting and assigning E/M codes. Follow along as fictitious coder Scott Hood, CPC, abstracts the procedure. Check off each step after you complete it.

▶ First, Scott needs to establish the category of service so he can determine the information needed to abstract and assign the code.

❏ *What is the setting?* Hospital inpatient

❏ *What is the type of service?* Subsequent care

HEMATOLOGY ENCOUNTER

CHIEF COMPLAINT: Newly diagnosed high-risk acute lymphoblastic leukemia; extensive deep vein thrombosis, right iliac vein and inferior vena cava (IVC), status post balloon angioplasty, and mechanical and pharmacologic thrombolysis following placement of a vena caval filter.

HISTORY OF PRESENT ILLNESS: The patient was transferred to this hospital the evening of 3/13/20YY from another hospital with a new diagnosis of high-risk acute lymphoblastic leukemia based on confirmation by flow cytometry of peripheral blood lymphoblasts that afternoon. History related to this illness probably dates back to last October when he had onset of swelling and discomfort in the left testicle with what he described as a residual "lump" posteriorly. The left testicle has continued to be painful off and on since. In early November, he developed pain in the posterior part of his upper right leg, which he initially thought was related to skateboarding and muscle strain. Physical therapy was prescribed and the discomfort temporarily improved. In December, he noted onset of increasing fatigue. He used to work out regularly, lifting weights, doing abdominal exercises, and playing basketball and found he did not have energy to pursue these activities. He has lost 10 pounds since December and feels his appetite has decreased. Night sweats and cough began in December, for which he was treated with a course of Augmentin. However, both of these problems have continued. He also began taking Accutane for persistent acne in December (this agent was stopped on 3/9/YY). Despite increasing fatigue and lethargy, he continues his studies at University of Denver, has a biology major (he aspires to be an ophthalmologist).

on 2/9/20YY, he in the morning awakened with severe right inguinal and right lower quadrant pain. He was seen in Emergency Room where it was noted that he had an elevated WBC of 18,000. CT scan of the abdomen was obtained to rule out possible appendicitis and on that CT, a large clot in the inferior vena cava extending to the right iliac and femoral veins was found. He promptly underwent appropriate treatment in interventional radiology with the above-noted angioplasty and placement of a vena caval filter followed by mechanical and pharmacologic thrombolysis. Repeat ultrasound there on 3/10/20YY showed no evidence of deep venous thrombosis (DVT). Continuous intravenous unfractionated heparin infusion was continued. Because there was no obvious cause of this extensive thrombosis, occult malignancy was suspected. Appropriate blood studies were obtained and he underwent a PET/CT scan as part of his diagnostic evaluation. This study showed moderately increased diffuse bone marrow metabolic activity. Because the WBC continued to rise and showed a preponderance of lymphocytes, the smear was reviewed by pathologist and flow cytometry was performed on the peripheral blood. These studies became available the afternoon of 3/13/20YY, and confirmed the diagnosis of precursor-B acute lymphoblastic leukemia. The patient was transferred here that evening after stopping of the continuous infusion heparin and receiving a dose of Lovenox 60 mg subcutaneously for further diagnostic evaluation and management of the acute lymphoblastic leukemia (ALL).

ALLERGIES: NO KNOWN DRUG ALLERGIES. HE DOES SEEM TO REACT TO CERTAIN ADHESIVES.

CURRENT MEDICATIONS:
1. Lovenox 60 mg subcutaneously q.12h. initiated.
2. Coumadin 5 mg p.o., was administered on 3/9/20YY and 3/12/20YY.
3. Protonix 40 mg intravenous (IV) daily.
4. Vicodin p.r.n.
5. Levaquin 750 mg IV on 3/13/20YY.

IMMUNIZATIONS: Up-to-date.

PAST SURGICAL HISTORY: The treatment of the thrombosis as noted above on 3/9/20YY and 3/10/20YY.

FAMILY HISTORY: Two half-brothers, ages 26 and 28, both in good health. Parents are in good health. A maternal great-grandmother had a deep venous thrombosis (DVT) of leg in her 40s. A maternal great-uncle developed leukemia around age 50. A maternal great-grandfather had bone cancer around age 80. His paternal grandfather died of colon cancer at age 73, which he had had since age 68. Adult-onset diabetes is present in distant relatives on both sides.

SOCIAL HISTORY: The patient is a student at the University majoring in biology. He lives in a dorm there. His parents live in Breckenridge. He admits to having smoked marijuana off and on with friends and drinking beer off and on as well.

REVIEW OF SYSTEMS: He has had emesis off and on related to Vicodin and constipation since 3/9/20YY, also related to pain medication. He has had acne for about two years, which he describes as mild to moderate. He denied shortness of breath, chest pain, hemoptysis, dyspnea, headaches, joint pains, rashes, except where he has had dressings applied, and extremity pain except for the right leg pain noted above.

Sidebar annotations:

HISTORY: Detailed

Chief complaint (CC)

Setting & patient type

MDM Management: New presenting problem, intensive workup (High Management Options)

HPI: Extended (4-9)

ROS

MDM Data: Ordering or reviewing diagnostic data (Straightforward Data)

MEDICAL DECISION MAKING: High Complexity

MDM Risk: management options include drug therapy of therapeutic heparin maintenance that requires intensive monitoring for toxicity (High Risk)

PFSH: Complete (3)

ROS: Extended (2-9)

Figure 37-9 ■ Hematology encounter. *Source: © PB Resources, Inc. Used with permission.*

(continued on page 758)

PHYSICAL EXAMINATION: GENERAL: Alert, cooperative, moderately ill-appearing young man.
VITAL SIGNS: At the time of admission, pulse was 89, respirations 21, blood pressure 125/65, temperature 98.6, height 5'10", weight 170 pounds, and pulse oximetry on room air 95%.
HAIR AND SKIN: Mild facial acne.
HEENT: Extraocular muscles (EOMs) intact. Pupils equal, round, and reactive to light and accommodation (PERRLA), fundi normal.
CARDIOVASCULAR: A 2/6 systolic ejection murmur (SEM), regular sinus rhythm (RSR).
LUNGS: Clear to auscultation with an occasional productive cough.
ABDOMEN: Soft with mild lower quadrant tenderness, right more so than left; liver and spleen each decreased 4 cm below their respective costal margins.
MUSCULOSKELETAL: Mild swelling of the dorsal aspect of the right foot and distal right leg. Mild tenderness over the prior catheter entrance site in the right popliteal fossa and mild tenderness over the right medial upper thigh.
GENITOURINARY: Testicle exam disclosed no firm swelling with mild nondiscrete fullness in the posterior left testicle.
NEUROLOGIC: Exam showed him to be oriented ×4. Normal fundi, intact cranial nerves II through XII with downgoing toes, symmetric muscle strength, and decreased patellar deep tendon reflexes (DTRs).

EXAMINATION:
Expanded problem focused

(6-11 elements)

LABORATORY DATA: White count 24,800 (26 neutrophils, 1 band, 7 lymphocytes, 1 monocyte, 1 myelocyte, 64 blasts), hemoglobin 14.3, hematocrit 39.8, and 323,000 platelets. Electrolytes, BUN, creatinine, phosphorus, uric acid, AST, ALT, alkaline phosphatase, and magnesium were all normal. LDH was elevated to 1925 units/L (upper normal 670), and total protein and albumin were both low at 6.1 and 3.2 g/dL respectively. Calcium was also slightly low at 8.7 mg/dL. Low molecular weight heparin test was low at 0.25 units/mL. PT was 11.9, INR 1.2, and fibrinogen 369. Urinalysis was normal.

ASSESSMENT: 1. Newly diagnosed high-risk acute lymphoblastic leukemia.
2. Deep vein thrombosis of the distal iliac and common femoral/right femoral and iliac veins, status post vena caval filter placement and mechanical and thrombolytic therapy, on continued anticoagulation.
3. Probable chronic left epididymitis.

MDM Risk

PLAN: 1. Proceed with diagnostic bone marrow aspirate/biopsy and lumbar puncture as soon as these procedures can be safely done with regard to the anticoagulation status.
2. Prompt reassessment of the status of the deep venous thrombosis with Doppler studies.
3. Ultrasound/Doppler of the testicles.
4. Maintain therapeutic anticoagulation as soon as the diagnostic procedures for ALL can be completed.

KEY: HPI History of the present illness ROS Review of systems
PFSH Past, family, and social history MDM Medical decision making

Figure 37-9 ■ (continued)

▶ Scott refers to the CPT Index and looks up the Main Term **Evaluation and Management** and the subterm **Hospital**. The code range listed is **99221-99233**.

❏ *How many key components are required?* Scott refers to the code range in the Tabular List and identifies two categories: **Initial Hospital Care** and **Subsequent Hospital Care**. This encounter is not documented as the initial encounter because the patient was admitted the previous evening, so he selects the category **Subsequent Hospital Care** and reads the description of the first code, which states **requires at least 2 of these 3 key components**. All codes in the category have the same requirements for key components. This tells him that two key components must meet or exceed the levels listed in the code (2/3).

▶ Next, Scott identifies the level of history.

❏ *What is the level of HPI?* The HPI is **Extended** because four or more elements are documented.

❏ *What is the level of ROS?* The ROS is **Extended** because two to nine systems are documented.

❏ *What is the level of PFSH?* The PFSH is **Complete** because two to three elements are documented.

❏ *Based on these factors, what is the overall level of history?* The level of history is **Detailed** because all three factors (HPI, ROS, and PFSH) qualify for this level.

▶ Scott refers to the hematologic/lymphatic/immunologic examination in the 1997 DG (Figure 37-8) to abstract information needed to determine the level of the examination.

❏ *What is the level of examination?* The level of examination is **Expanded problem focused**. Eight elements of the examination are documented, which exceeds the requirement of 6–11 bulleted elements for an expanded problem-focused examination. A comprehensive examination requires that 12 bulleted items be documented, which they are not.

▶ Scott determines the level of medical decision making. (Refer to Table 28-12, Medical Decision-Making Levels.)

❏ *What is the level of complexity of the number of diagnoses or management options based on the presenting problem?* The level is **High** because there is a new presenting problem, with workup.

❏ *What is the amount and/or complexity of data to be reviewed?* The level is **Straightforward** because the physician reviewed a previous summary of CT/PET and ultrasound tests and reviewed laboratory results, but there was no documented indication of an independent review of images.

❑ *What is the level of risk of significant complications, morbidity, and/or mortality?* Scott reviews each column in the Table of Risk in the 1997 DG and determines that the level of risk is **High**. The patient presents with one or more chronic illnesses with mild exacerbation, progression, or side effects of treatment illness (Moderate), diagnostic procedures ordered include obtaining bone marrow aspirate from lumbar puncture (Moderate), and management options include drug therapy of therapeutic heparin maintenance, which requires intensive monitoring for toxicity (High). The single highest element in the Table of Risk determines the overall risk. The column **Management Options Selected** is the highest level (High).

❑ *Based on these factors, what is the overall level of medical decision making?* The medical decision making is **High complexity**. At least two of the three MDM factors are required to qualify for a specific level of MDM. Two of the three MDM factors —the number of diagnosis/management options and the risk of complications, morbidity, mortality—meet high-complexity decision making.

Now Scott is ready to assign the code for the hematology encounter. The exercise that follows guides you through additional abstracting skills and allows you to assign the correct code.

CODING CAUTION

CMS requires that the medical record be authenticated with either a handwritten or electronic signature. If the signature in the medical record is illegible or missing, the physician must attest to (*verify*) the signature. If the physician does not provide an attestation statement, CMS then considers the claim to be insufficiently documented and can deny payment.

CODING PRACTICE

Exercise 37.5   E/M Coding for the Hemic and Lymphatic Systems

Instructions: Refer to the *1997 Documentation Guidelines for Evaluation and Management Services* (available at **www.cms.gov**) or Chapter 28, "Evaluation and Management Services (99201-99499)", Tables 28-7 to 28-12, in this text. Answer the following questions about the "Hematology encounter" (Figure 37-9).

1. a. Which elements of the HPI are documented? Circle all that apply. Location, Quality, Severity, Duration, Timing, Context, Modifying factors, Associated signs and symptoms

   b. How many elements are documented? _____

   c. What is the level of HPI? _____

2. a. Which systems are reviewed in the ROS? Circle all that apply. Constitutional, Allergic/immunologic, CV, Endocrine, ENT/M, Eyes, GI, GU, Hemic/lymphatic, MS, Neurologic, Psychiatric, Respiratory, Skin/breast

   b. How many systems are documented? _____

   c. What is the level of ROS? _____

3. a. Which PFSH elements are documented? Circle all that apply. Past medical, Family, Social

   b. What is the level of PFSH? _____

   c. What is the overall level of history? (The lowest history factor—HPI, ROS, or PFSH—determines the level of history.)
   _____

4. Refer to Figure 37-8, 1997 DG for Hematologic/Lymphatic/Immunologic Examination.

   a. Which bulleted items are documented for the examination? (Check off the items documented.)

   b. How many bulleted items are documented? _____

   c. What is the level of the examination? _____

5. Refer to Table 28-12, Medical Decision-Making Levels, or the 1997 DG.

   a. What is the MDM level for the number of diagnoses or management options? _____

   b. What is the MDM level for the amount and/or complexity of data to be reviewed? _____

   c. Refer to the Table of Risk in the 1997 DG. Which elements of risk are documented for each risk factor?

      1. Presenting problem: _____

      2. Diagnostic procedures ordered: _____

      3. Management options selected: _____

   d. What is the level of risk? (The highest of the three risk factors determines the overall level of risk). _____

   e. What is the overall level of MDM? (2/3 MDM factors are needed to determine the overall level.) _____

(continued)

CODING PRACTICE *(continued)*

6. a. What is the setting? _____

   b. What is the patient (or service) type? _____

   c. What is the code range? _____

   d. How many key components are required? _____

   e. What is the level of history? _____

   f. What is the level of examination? _____

   g. What is the level of medical decision making? _____

   h. What is the correct code? _____

7. Abstract, assign, and arrange (sequence) the diagnosis code(s) that supports the E/M code.

   5 ICD-10-CM Code(s) _____

   _____

CHAPTER SUMMARY

In this chapter you learned that:

- The hemic and lymphatic systems are studied together because blood and lymph are two of the body's main fluids, which are circulated through two separate but interconnected vessel systems.

- The CPT subsection Hemic and Lymphatic Systems (38100-38999) contains codes that represent procedures related to the bone marrow, blood, lymph nodes, and lymphatic channels (vessels) and contains three subheadings for the spleen, general, and lymph nodes and lymphatic channels. The CPT subsection Mediastinum and Diaphragm (39000-39599) contains two subheadings—one for the mediastinum and one for the diaphragm—each with categories for the type of procedure.

- CPT provides guidelines and instructional notes to alert coders to the need for modifiers, provide cross-references to codes for similar procedures on other sites, identify bundled services, determine when additional codes might be needed for radiological services, and highlight resequenced and recently deleted codes.

- Familiarity with the anatomy of the lymphatic system is fundamental to abstracting because coding is based on the site and extent of treatment.

- To assign codes for procedures on the hemic and lymphatic systems, mediastinum, and diaphragm, search the Index for the Main Term of the anatomic site, then locate the first-level modifying term for the type of procedure.

- The instructional note at the end of a code description reminds coders to assign the code only when the procedure is not bundled with another one or is performed at a separate site or through a separate incision.

- The *1997 Documentation Guidelines for Evaluation and Management Services (*1997 DG), published by CMS, provides requirements for each level of a hematologic/lymphatic/immunologic E/M examination.

CONCEPT QUIZ

Take a moment to look back at the hemic and lymphatic systems, mediastinum, and diaphragm and solidify your skills. Try to answer the questions from memory first, then refer to the discussion in this chapter if you need a little extra help.

Completion

Instructions: Write the term that completes each statement based on the information you learned in this chapter. Choose from the following list. Some choices may be used more than once and some choices may not be used at all.

cannula

cannulation

differentiation

eventration

limited lymphadenectomy

lymph nodes

lymphangiography

lymphangiotomy

mediastinotomy

radical lymphadenectomy

respiratory

splenectomy

splenorrhaphy

stem cells

transplantation

1. A(n) _____ is used to treat idiopathic thrombocytopenic purpura.

2. A physician may perform a/an _____ to diagnose cancer.

3. A(n) _____ is a repair of the diaphragm to resemble normal anatomy.

4. Stem cells repair damaged tissues through _____.

5. _____ is performed to replace bone marrow or HPCs.

6. A physician may insert a/an _____ to diagnose disorders of lymph flow.

7. A physician may perform a/an _____ to stage cancer.

8. The function of the _____ is to produce antibodies to defend the body.

9. A(n) _____ is performed to repair a ruptured spleen.

10. A physician may perform a/an _____ to drain an abscess.

Multiple Choice

Instructions: Circle the letter of the best answer to each question based on the information you learned in this chapter.

1. How often can a code for allogeneic transplantation be reported, according to the MUE?
   A. Up to three times a day
   B. Once per donor
   C. Once per day
   D. Only one time

2. How would you code the following procedure? *A surgeon injects a radioactive tracer to identify the sentinel node then performs a limited pelvic lymphadenectomy for staging of prostate cancer.*
   A. 38562, 38792-51
   B. 38792, 38562-51
   C. 38792
   D. 38562

3. What is the name of the first node or group of nodes in a chain?
   A. Primary lymph node
   B. Sentinel node
   C. Lymph chain
   D. T-lymphocyte

4. How would you code the following procedure? *A surgeon performs a complete cervical lymphadenectomy on the right side and biopsy of the cervical nodes on the left side.*
   A. 38720-22
   B. 38500-LT, 38720-51-RT
   C. 38720-50
   D. 38720-RT, 38500-59-LT

5. What structure separates the lungs and contains the esophagus and heart?
   A. Abdominal cavity
   B. Diaphragm
   C. Thoracic cavity
   D. Mediastinum

6. What type of transplant uses tissue or cells from a person other than the patient?
   A. Autogeneic
   B. Autologous
   C. Allogeneic
   D. Allologous

7. How many bulleted elements must be performed and documented for a physical examination to meet the criteria of a detailed hematologic/lymphatic/immunologic system E/M examination?
   A. 10
   B. 11
   C. 12
   D. 13

8. What is the name for a group of lymph nodes in a limited area along lymph vessels where the body is most prone to infection?
   A. Lymph node
   B. Lymph chain
   C. Lymphocyte
   D. Sentinel lymph node

9. How would you code the following procedure? *A physician thawed and washed previously frozen HPC harvests from two separate donors, then performed plasma volume depletion on each.*
   A. 38209 × 2
   B. 38214, 38209-51
   C. 38214 × 1, 38209 × 2
   D. 38214 × 2, 38209 × 2

10. What type of structure are hematopoietic progenitor cells?
    A. Stem cells
    B. Lymphocytes
    C. White bone marrow
    D. T-cells

KEEP ON CODING

Instructions: Read the procedural statement, then use the appropriate Index and Tabular List to assign CPT procedure codes, quantities, and modifiers. Write the code(s) on the line provided.

1. Aortic lymphadenectomy. CPT Code(s)_____

2. Diagnostic bone marrow aspiration and biopsy. CPT Code(s)_____

3. Partial splenectomy. CPT Code(s)_____

4. Total splenectomy, en bloc, for extensive disease. CPT Code(s)_____

5. Management of recipient hematopoietic progenitor cell donor search and cell acquisition. CPT Code(s)_____

6. Mediastinoscopy. CPT Code(s)_____

7. Drainage of right axilla lymph node abscess. CPT Code(s)_____

8. Ligation of the thoracic lymph duct using abdominal approach. CPT Code(s)_____

9. Repair hernia of diaphragm in neonate. CPT Code(s)_____

10. Superficial needle biopsy of left inguinal lymph node. CPT Code(s)_____

11. Bone marrow harvest for autologous transplant. CPT Code(s)_____

(continued)

(continued from page 761)

12. Right inguinofemoral lymphadenectomy, superficial, including Cloquet's node. CPT Code(s)_____

13. Laparoscopic bilateral total pelvic lymphadenectomy and peri-aortic lymph node sampling. CPT Code(s)_____

14. Suprahyoid lymphadenectomy, bilateral. CPT Code(s)_____

15. Transplant of patient's own bone marrow. CPT Code(s)_____

16. Open biopsy of the left deep axillary nodes. CPT Code(s)_____

17. Transplantation of allogeneic stem cells. CPT Code(s)_____

18. Open excision of right inguinofemoral lymph nodes. CPT Code(s)_____

19. Mediastinoscopy with mediastinal lymph node biopsy for lung cancer staging. CPT Code(s)_____

20. Surgical laparoscopy with retroperitoneal lymph node sampling, single. CPT Code(s)_____

21. Stem cell thawing, with washing. CPT Code(s)_____

22. Injection procedure for splenoportography. CPT Code(s)_____

23. Repair of chronic diaphragmatic hernia. CPT Code(s)_____

24. Transplantation of platelet depletion stem cells. CPT Code(s)_____

25. Exploration of mediastinum with mediastinotomy for drainage via cervical area. CPT Code(s)_____

CODING CHALLENGE

Instructions: Read the mini-medical-record of each patient's encounter, then abstract, assign, and arrange ICD-10-CM diagnosis codes and CPT procedure codes using the appropriate Index and Tabular List. Assign quantities and modifiers where needed. Write the code(s) on the line provided.

1. INPATIENT HOSPITAL Gender: M Age: 18

Preprocedure diagnosis: Benign neoplasm of mediastinum

Procedure: Resection of mediastinal tumor

1 ICD-10-CM Code _____

1 CPT Code _____

2. OUTPATIENT SURGERY Gender: F Age: 47

Preprocedure diagnosis: Malignant neoplasm, upper-inner quadrant left breast

Procedure: Injection for identification of left sentinel node

1 ICD-10-CM Code _____

1 CPT Code _____

3. OUTPATIENT SURGERY Gender: M Age: 12

Preprocedure diagnosis: Iron-deficiency anemia

Procedure: Bone marrow aspiration

1 ICD-10-CM Code _____

1 CPT Code _____

4. OUTPATIENT SURGERY Gender: F Age: 33

Preprocedure diagnosis: Volunteer for bone marrow donation

Procedure: Bone marrow harvesting

1 ICD-10-CM Code _____

1 CPT Code _____

5. OUTPATIENT SURGERY Gender: F Age: 72

Preprocedure diagnosis: Postoperative bleeding following partial splenectomy

Procedure: Additional repair of the spleen

Tip: A modifier is needed.

1 ICD-10-CM Code _____

1 CPT Code _____

6. EMERGENCY DEPARTMENT
Gender: M Age: 63

Preprocedure diagnosis: Lacerated diaphragm, initial encounter

Procedure: Repair of diaphragm with sutures

1 ICD-10-CM Code _____

1 CPT Code _____

7. OUTPATIENT SURGERY   Gender: F   Age: 22

Preprocedure diagnosis: Sarcoidosis of lymph nodes

Procedure: Endoscopy of mediastinum with lymph node biopsy

1 ICD-10-CM Code _____

1 CPT Code _____

---

8. OUTPATIENT SURGERY   Gender: F   Age: 27

Preprocedure diagnosis: Subsequent encounter for foreign body in median sternum

Procedure: Median sternotomy to remove foreign body

1 ICD-10-CM Code _____

1 CPT Code _____

---

9. INPATIENT HOSPITAL   Gender: F   Age: 46

Preprocedure diagnosis: Acute diaphragmatic hernia

Procedure: Repair of acute traumatic diaphragmatic hernia

1 ICD-10-CM Code _____

1 CPT Code _____

---

10. INPATIENT HOSPITAL   Gender: F   Age: 26

Preprocedure diagnosis: Spontaneous ruptured spleen

Procedure: Repair of ruptured spleen with partial splenectomy

1 ICD-10-CM Code _____

1 CPT Code _____

Chapter 38

Respiratory System Procedures (30000-32999)

Chapter Outline

- **Respiratory System Procedure Basics**
- **Coding Guidelines for Respiratory System Procedures**
- **Abstracting Respiratory System Procedures**
- **Assigning Codes for Respiratory System Procedures**
- **Arranging Codes for Respiratory System Procedures**
- **E/M Coding for Pulmonology**

Learning Objectives

After completing this chapter, you should have the skills to:

38.1 Spell and define the key words, medical terms, and abbreviations related to respiratory system procedures. (Remember)

38.2 Summarize the fundamentals of respiratory system procedures. (Understand)

38.3 Adhere to CPT coding guidelines in the Respiratory System subsection. (Apply)

38.4 Examine and abstract procedural information from the medical record for coding Respiratory System subsection procedures. (Analyze)

38.5 Demonstrate how to assign codes for procedures in the Respiratory System subsection. (Apply)

38.6 Utilize guidelines for arranging (sequencing) codes for Respiratory System subsection procedures. (Apply)

38.7 Determine how to code Evaluation and Management services for pulmonology. (Evaluate)

Key Terms and Abbreviations

accessory sinus	frontal sinus	paranasal sinus	transnasal
bilobectomy	internal approach	pneumonectomy	transoral
ethmoid sinus	lobectomy	rigid endoscope	transorbital
external approach	maxillary sinus	segmentectomy	wedge excision
flexible endoscope	operating endoscope	sphenoid sinus	

In addition to the key terms listed here, students should know the terms defined within tables in this chapter.

INTRODUCTION

Many prescription and nonprescription products that treat respiratory conditions are advertised on television and in stores. These include sinus, throat, and lung conditions. When a respiratory condition cannot be treated medically, a procedure might provide relief or correction. This chapter provides an introduction to coding procedures on the respiratory system.

RESPIRATORY SYSTEM PROCEDURE BASICS

Pulmonology is a subspecialty of internal medicine that specializes in the respiratory system. Pulmonologists perform medical procedures such as endoscopies and pulmonary function studies but do not perform surgery. Thoracic surgeons perform surgery on respiratory system organs and structures. Otolaryngologists perform procedures on the nose and throat. Because the respiratory and cardiovascular systems function interdependently, procedures that involve both the lungs and the heart are often performed.

When working with respiratory system procedures, you will find that some medical word roots can have more than one meaning; for example, *thorac/o* can mean thorax, chest, or the pleural space. Medical word roots can also have multiple forms; for example, both *pneum/o* and *pneumon/o* refer to the lung. Multiple word roots can be used interchangeably; for example, both *thorac/o* and *pleur/o* can refer to the pleural cavity. Such variations exist because medical terms are derived from both Greek and Latin, as well as other languages, and word usage tends to evolve from the original literal meaning over time. Chapter 15 of this text provides additional information on the anatomy and conditions of the respiratory system.

CODING CAUTION

Be alert for medical terms that are spelled similarly and have different meanings.

<u>rhin</u>/o (*nose*) and <u>ronch</u>/o (*snore*)

or/o (*mouth*) and o<u>x</u>/o (*oxygen*)

-<u>phyma</u> (*nodule, swelling*) and -<u>pnea</u> (*breathing*)

Refer to ■ TABLE 38-1 for a refresher on how to build medical terms related to the respiratory system.

Understanding the anatomy of the paranasal sinuses, also called accessory sinuses, is important because codes are divided based on the location of the sinus. (Other structures of the respiratory system are discussed in Chapter 15, "Diseases of the Respiratory System," of this text.) The sinus cavity contains air-filled chambers, or spaces, called paranasal sinuses, inside the skull and face bones. The sinus membrane lines the sinuses and produces mucus, which prevents bacteria, dirt, and dust in the air from entering the body. It also moistens the air and warms it. Cilia are small hairs that line the sinus membrane and move mucus from the sinus cavity to the nasal cavity.

The four paranasal sinuses, which occur in pairs on the right and left sides of the head, are (■ FIGURE 38-1):

* Frontal sinuses—Located above the eyes
* Maxillary sinuses—Located below the eyes
* Ethmoid sinuses—Located between the eyes and nose
* Sphenoid sinuses—Located at the center of the base of the skull, at the back of the nose

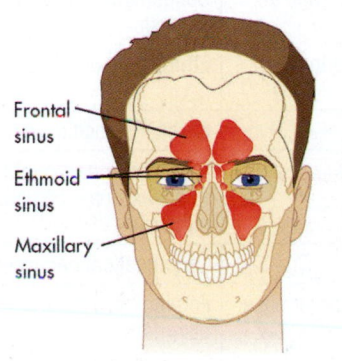
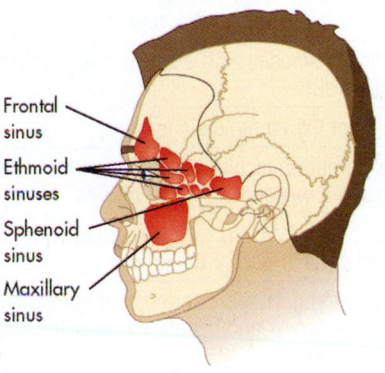

Frontal sinus
Ethmoid sinus
Maxillary sinus

Frontal sinus
Ethmoid sinuses
Sphenoid sinus
Maxillary sinus

Figure 38-1 ■ Paranasal sinuses.

Table 38-1   ■   **EXAMPLE OF CONSTRUCTING MEDICAL TERMS FOR RESPIRATORY SYSTEM PROCEDURES**

Combining Form	Suffix	Complete Medical Term
thor/a, thorac/o (*thorax, chest, pleural space*)		**thora + centesis** (*withdrawal of fluid from the thoracic cavity*)
		pleura + centesis (*withdrawal of fluid from the pleural cavity/thoracic cavity*)
		pneumo + centesis (*withdrawal of fluid from the lung*)
pleur/o/a (*membrane that lines the thoracic cavity and lungs*)	**-centesis** (*withdrawal of fluid*) **-tomy** (*incision*)	**thoraco + tomy** (*incision into the thoracic cavity*)
		pleuro + tomy (*incision into the pleural cavity/thoracic cavity*)
		pneumo + tomy (*incision into the lung*)
pneum/o, pneumon/o (*air, lung, respiration*)		**pneumo + thorax** (*air in the pleural space*)

Source: © PB Resources, Inc. Used with permission.

Procedures commonly performed on each section of the respiratory system are discussed next. Refer to detailed anatomic diagrams of specific parts of the respiratory system when you need to refresh your memory of the relationship of organs and sites to each other.

Procedures of the Respiratory System

Procedures commonly performed on the Respiratory System are summarized in ■ TABLE 38-2. In particular, coders need to understand the types of lung procedures and the types of endoscopies.

Recall that there are two lungs with a total of five lobes: the right lung has three lobes, whereas the left lung has two lobes. Procedures on the lung are defined based on the extent of tissue removed:

- Pneumonectomy—Surgical excision of an entire lung
- Lobectomy—Surgical excision of one lobe
- Bilobectomy—Surgical excision of two lobes
- Segmentectomy or wedge excision—Surgical excision of tissue from part of one lobe

Endoscopy is the preferred approach for respiratory system procedures whenever possible because it is minimally invasive and can be used to perform a wide variety of procedures. A rigid endoscope consists of a hard tube with a series of prisms and lenses that reflect the image. A flexible endoscope is a soft tube with fiber-optic bundles that transmit the image. An operating endoscope is equipped with irrigation and suction channels, as well as channels for inserting special instruments, such as biopsy forceps, to obtain tissue samples. Specialized endoscopes are sized and configured for various sites within the respiratory system and are named after the site they are designed to access, such as a laryngoscope—used to access the larynx; a bronchoscope—used to access the bronchi and lungs; and a thoracoscope—used to access the lung and chest cavity through the chest wall. An endoscopy can be diagnostic or therapeutic. It may be done to perform an examination, obtain a specimen or biopsy, place a stent or catheter, or perform surgical excision or repair. Fluoroscopic guidance, in which a live x-ray image of the region being accessed is viewed on a monitor, is used in some endoscopic procedures to assist the surgeon to visualize the correct placement and maneuvering of the endoscope.

This section provides a general reference to help you understand the most common respiratory system procedures. Remember to keep standard reference books handy in case you get stuck.

Table 38-2 ■ COMMON PROCEDURES OF THE RESPIRATORY SYSTEM

Procedure Name	Definition	Reason Performed
Caldwell-Luc procedure	Incision of the gum and bone to create an opening to the maxillary sinus	Chronic sinusitis; removal of antrochoanal (*in the maxillary sinus*) polyps, cysts, or lesions
Cricoid split	Incision of the cricoid cartilage (*ring-shaped cartilage at the larynx base*) to open the airway	Congenital or acquired subglottic (*below the glottis*) stenosis
Displacement therapy (Proetz type)	Irrigation of sinuses with a saline solution that is then suctioned out	Ethmoiditis or allergies
Ethmoidectomy	Opening of the ethmoid sinus cavity	Chronic sinusitis; removal of an obstruction
Laryngeal reinnervation by neuromuscular pedicle	Use of a neuromuscular pedicle (*a graft consisting of a nerve and a muscle*) to restore nerves	Dystonia (*a neuromuscular disorder that causes the patient to speak in a whispered or strained voice*); vocal fold paralysis
Laryngectomy	Excision of all or part of the larynx	Laryngeal cancer, trauma
Laryngoscopy (direct)	Use of a laryngoscope inserted through the mouth or nose to view the larynx and hypolarynx/subglottis (*area below the vocal cords*)	Foreign body removal; swallowing, breathing, and bleeding disorders
Laryngoscopy (indirect)	Use of a mirror to view the base of the tongue, larynx, and hypolarynx	Foreign body removal; swallowing, breathing, and bleeding disorders
Lateral rhinotomy	Creation of an incision along the nose from the inner eyebrow to the nasolabial fold (*the crease that runs from the bottom of each nostril to the corner of the mouth*)	Foreign body removal
Lavage	Irrigation of the maxillary or sphenoid sinus by puncturing the antrum or creating an ostium (*opening*)	Removal of infected mucus from chronic sinusitis, a tooth infection that spread to the sinus, or trauma that does not improve with antibiotics
Maxillectomy	Removal of all or part of the upper jaw bone	Malignant neoplasm
Pleurodesis	Use of an irritant to create inflammation within the pleural space to cause the two pleura to adhere together	Prevention of pleural effusion (*excess fluid in the pleural cavity*)
Pneumonolysis	Separation of the parietal pleura from the fascia of the chest wall	Permit the collapse of a lung; formerly used to treat tuberculosis

Table 38-2 ■ *(continued)*

Procedure Name	Definition	Reason Performed
Rhinoplasty (primary)	Surgical repair of the nose	Congenital deformity, such as a cleft lip or cleft palate; carcinoma; aesthetics (*elective or due to trauma*)
Rhinoplasty (secondary)	A second rhinoplasty that may be more complex than the primary one, including grafts of cartilage, bone, or tissue to reconstruct the nose or repair the nasal septum	Unsuccessful primary rhinoplasty; trauma to the nose following the initial procedure; patient dissatisfaction with the outcome of the initial procedure
Septoplasty	Surgical repair of the nasal septum, with or without cartilage scoring (*incising*), contouring, or replacement with graft	Deviated, or displaced, nasal septum
Thoracentesis/pleural tap	Withdrawal of air or fluid from the pleural space using a needle or tube	Cancer, pneumonia, pneumothorax (*air or gas in the pleural space*), hemothorax (*blood in the pleural space*), or congestive heart failure
Thoracoscopy	Insertion of an endoscope through a small incision in the chest wall	Examination of the lungs, pleura, or mediastinum; biopsy; removal of fluid, cysts, or lung tissue
Thoracostomy	Creation of an opening through the chest to place a chest tube or intercostal catheter into the pleural space	Empyema (*pus in the pleural space*) or pneumothorax (*air or gas in the pleural space*)
Thoracotomy	Incision into the pleural space	Procedures on the heart and lungs, including removing neoplasms and foreign bodies and performing a biopsy
Tracheobronchoscopy	Insertion of an endoscope through an established tracheostomy incision to view the trachea and bronchi	Diagnosis of causes of tracheal stenosis
Tracheostomy	Creation of an opening in the trachea through which a breathing tube is inserted	Obstructed airway, respiratory failure
Tracheotomy	Incision through the neck into the trachea	Preoperative airway clearance; emergency treatment for the inability to breathe
Video-assisted thoracoscopic surgery (VATS)	Use of an endoscope and video camera to perform procedures traditionally performed using a thoracotomy (*incision in the chest wall*)	Management of pulmonary, mediastinal, and pleural conditions

Source: © PB Resources, Inc. Used with permission.

CODING PRACTICE

Exercise 38.1 **Respiratory System Procedure Basics**

Instructions: Use your medical terminology skills and resources to define the following procedures related to the Respiratory System, then identify the code(s) or code range listed in the CPT Index. Follow these steps:

- Use slash marks "/" to break down the underlined term into its root(s) and suffix.
- Define the meaning of the underlined word based on the meaning of each word part.
- Use the entire phrase to identify the code or code range shown in the CPT Index.

Example: <u>thoracoscopy</u>, diagnostic, without   Meaning *visual examination of the chest cavity*   CPT Code *32601*
biopsy thorac/o/scopy

1. <u>septoplasty</u>   Meaning _____   CPT Code _____

2. lateral <u>rhinotomy</u>   Meaning _____   CPT Code _____

3. planned <u>tracheostomy</u>   Meaning _____   CPT Code _____

4. maxillary <u>sinusotomy</u>   Meaning _____   CPT Code _____

5. <u>arytenoidopexy</u>   Meaning _____   CPT Code _____

6. <u>sphenoidotomy</u>   Meaning _____   CPT Code _____

7. thorascopic <u>pleurodesis</u>   Meaning _____   CPT Code _____

8. <u>pharyngolaryngectomy</u>   Meaning _____   CPT Code _____

9. <u>tracheobronchoscopy</u>   Meaning _____   CPT Code _____

10. <u>pneumonolysis</u>   Meaning _____   CPT Code _____

Table 38-3 ■ **RESPIRATORY SYSTEM SUBHEADINGS**

Subheading	Code Range
Nose	30000-30999
Accessory Sinuses	31000-31299
Larynx	31300-31599
Trachea and Bronchi	31600-31899
Lungs and Pleura	32035-32999

CODING GUIDELINES FOR RESPIRATORY SYSTEM PROCEDURES

Coders should understand the organization, guidelines, and instructional notes in Tabular List of this CPT subsection. This information is necessary for accurate coding. The CPT section/subsection **Respiratory System (30000-32999)** contains five subheadings that are divided by anatomic site (■ TABLE 38-3). Within each anatomic site, codes are divided by the type of procedure, such as incision, excision, introduction, and so on. Review the subheading and category names and code ranges listed in the Respiratory System subsection to become familiar with the content and organization. Some editions of the CPT manual provide a summary list of the subheadings and categories at the beginning of the Respiratory System subsection; these also display an asterisk (*) next to categories that contain special coding instructions.

This chapter includes invasive, minimally invasive, and noninvasive surgical procedures on the respiratory system. Codes for diagnostic tests on the respiratory system appear in the Medicine section. CPT codes in the Respiratory System subsection are frequently supported by diagnosis codes from ICD-10-CM Chapter 10, "Diseases of the Respiratory System (J00-J99)," as well as neoplasms, symptoms and signs, and injuries (■ TABLE 38-4).

Table 38-4 ■ **LOCATING ICD-10-CM AND ADDITIONAL CPT CODES FOR THE RESPIRATORY SYSTEM**

Type of Code	Codes
ICD-10-CM Respiratory System–Related Codes	
Respiratory system conditions	J00-J99
Neoplasms	C30-C39
Symptoms and signs	R00-R09, R47-R49
Injuries	S20-S29
CPT Respiratory System–Related Codes	
Medicine procedures	94002-94799
Radiologic procedures	
• Diagnostic radiology	70045-70559, 71010-71555
• Radiologic guidance	77001-77022
• Diagnostic ultrasound	76506-76642
• Nuclear medicine, diagnostic	78579-78599
Laboratory organ/disease panels	None are applicable specifically to the respiratory system.

Source: © PB Resources, Inc. Used with permission. CPT codes only © American Medical Association.

CPT guidelines for the Surgery section apply to the Respiratory System subsection. Special instructions provide definitions and coding guidelines at the beginning of many categories. The subheading **Lungs and Pleura** provides detailed special instructions about lung resections and biopsies. The categories **Stereotactic Radiation Therapy** and **Lung Transplantation** provide detailed definitions and coding instructions.

Bronchoscopy procedures may be performed with moderate sedation. When this occurs, assign the appropriate moderate sedation code(s) (**99151-99157**).

Instructional notes appear throughout the Tabular List to alert coders to the need for modifiers, provide cross-references to codes for similar procedures on other sites, identify when additional codes might be needed for radiological services, and highlight resequenced and recently deleted codes.

ABSTRACTING RESPIRATORY SYSTEM PROCEDURES

Abstracting for the respiratory system requires attention to the anatomic approach and procedure type or variation. Abstracting criteria include a section on endoscopy procedures, in addition to questions that apply to all respiratory procedures.

Anatomic Approach

In addition to classifying procedures based on the surgical approach—open, endoscopic, or percutaneous—CPT also classifies Respiratory System procedures based on the anatomic approach. Some procedures on the nose can be performed using an **external approach** (*through the skin on the outside of the nasal structure*) or **internal approach** (*from within the nasal passage or through the mucous membrane inside the nasal passage*). For example, some excision and destruction procedures can be performed externally, by making an incision along the fold of the nose, or internally, by making an incision into the mucous membrane of the nasal passage.

Most sites within the respiratory system can be accessed through multiple routes, so the procedure description often identifies the route used. The route is described using word roots that identify the structures accessed and/or prefixes that identify the action. For example, endoscopy can be performed using a **transnasal** (*through the nose*) or **transoral** (*through the mouth*) approach or through an established tracheostomy. The frontal sinus can be accessed using a transnasal or a **transorbital** (*through an incision in the orbit of the eye*) route. When you encounter an unfamiliar term, remember to break it down into word parts; then you can usually envision the action and site being described. Also refer to a medical terminology text or a medical dictionary for clarification.

Procedure Type, Extent, or Variation

Procedures are sometimes described by their type, extent, or other variation.

• Many procedures are classified by difficulty, such as simple or complex; the definition is dependent on the specific procedure performed. For example, a simple revision of a tracheostoma does not include a flap rotation, whereas a complex revision does.

Table 38-5 ■ KEY CRITERIA FOR ABSTRACTING RESPIRATORY SYSTEM PROCEDURES

- ❏ What is the anatomic site?
- ❏ What is the procedure?
- ❏ What is the surgical approach (open, endoscopic, external)?
- ❏ What is the anatomic approach (transnasal, transthoracic, latero-vertical, etc.)?
- ❏ What is the purpose or variation of the procedure?
- ❏ What is the extent of the procedure (partial, total, etc.)?
- ❏ What is the laterality?
- ❏ What additional procedures were performed during the same session?

Endoscopy Procedures

- ❏ What type of endoscope is used?
- ❏ Is the procedure diagnostic, surgical, or both?
- ❏ Is moderate sedation used?
- ❏ What procedure(s) are performed during the endoscopy?
- ❏ Is the endoscopy a preoperative survey or scout?
- ❏ Is an endoscopic procedure converted to an open procedure?
- ❏ Is a decision made to perform an additional procedure during the same encounter based on the results of the endoscopy?
- ❏ What is the farthest anatomic site reached with the endoscope?

Source: © PB Resources, Inc. Used with permission.

- Procedures can be described by extent, such as limited or complete or partial and total, and definitions are dependent on the specific procedure. For example, a simple sinus excision involves a portion of a sinus cavity, whereas a complete excision involves the entire cavity.

- The technique or type of equipment can affect code classification. For example, a laryngoscopy can be direct—using an endoscope—or indirect, using a mirror and a light.

- Multiple procedures can be performed at the same time. For example, a bronchoscopy can have many variations depending on its purpose and other procedures performed, such as the type of biopsy or specimen collection, placement of a stent or catheter, removal of a foreign body, and so on.

Coders must be attentive to the details of each procedure and each code description. When you are reading and abstracting a medical record for a procedure that is unfamiliar, you may not always be certain of what information you will need to assign the code. Remember that you may need to cross-reference between the medical record and the coding manual several times before identifying all the information needed to assign the correct code. This is a normal part of the coding process.

Refer to ■ TABLE 38-5 for guidance on how to abstract procedures on the respiratory system, then work through the detailed example that follows. Remember that the abstracting questions are a guide and that not every question applies to, or can be answered for, every case. For example, not all procedures are described by extent, such as total or partial.

Guided Example of Abstracting Respiratory System Procedures

Refer to the following example throughout this chapter to practice skills for abstracting, assigning, and arranging Respiratory System codes.

OUTPATIENT HOSPITAL   Gender: M   Age: 58

Preoperative diagnosis: Lung mass on CT scan

Procedure: Diagnostic bronchoscopy with biopsy a. CRNA administered moderate sedation for 75 minutes of intraservice time. When patient was comfortable, advanced flexible bronchoscope into the left lower lobe of the lung, where a mass was visualized on CT. Acquired a biopsy of the nodule in that lobe. Specimen was submitted to pathology.

Postoperative diagnosis: Carcinoma of the lower left lobe

Pathology report: Carcinoma

Follow along as fictitious coder Leanne Riehl, CCS, abstracts the procedure. Check off each step after you complete it.

▶ Leanne reads through the entire record, paying special attention to the reason for the encounter, the procedure performed, and the postoperative diagnosis. She refers to the Key Criteria for Abstracting Respiratory System Procedures (Table 38-5).

- ❏ She notes the preoperative diagnosis as lung mass on CT scan

- ❏ *What is the patient's age?* 58

- ❏ *What site is treated?* Lung

- ❏ *What primary procedure is performed?* Diagnostic bronchoscopy with biopsy

- ❏ *What type of endoscope is used?* Flexible bronchoscope

- ❏ *Is the procedure diagnostic, surgical, or both?* Diagnostic

- ❏ *Is moderate sedation provided?* Yes, by CRNA for 75 minutes of intraservice time.

- ❏ *What procedure(s) are performed during the endoscopy?* Biopsy

- ❏ *Is the endoscopy a preoperative survey or scout?* No

- ❏ *Is an endoscopic procedure converted to an open procedure?* No

- ❏ *Is a decision made to perform an additional procedure during the same encounter based on the results of the endoscopy?* No

- ❏ *What is the farthest anatomic site reached with the endoscope?* Left lower lobe of the lung

▶ At this time, Leanne does not know which of these procedures may need to be coded, nor how many codes she will end up with. She will learn about this when she moves on to assigning codes.

CODING PRACTICE

Exercise 38.2 Abstracting Respiratory System Procedures

Instructions: Read the mini-medical-record of each patient's encounter and answer the abstracting questions. Write the answer on the line provided. Do not assign any codes.

1. EMERGENCY DEPT Gender: F Age: 48

Preprocedure diagnosis: Patient presents with complaints of nasal pain, edema, and purulent (pus) discharge. CT scan and lab tests reveal a nasal septum abscess

Procedure: Incision and drainage (I & D) nasal septum abscess; made small incision within the nasal septum over the abscess. Suctioned purulent fluid and flushed with sterile saline. Packed the nasal cavity with gauze.

Postprocedure diagnosis: Nasal septum abscess due to Staphylococcus aureus

a. What is the anatomic site? _____

b. What is the procedure? _____

c. What is the surgical approach (open, endoscopic, external)? _____

d. What is the purpose or variation of the procedure?

_____

2. EMERGENCY DEPT Gender: F Age: 4

Preprocedure diagnosis: Child is brought in by her mother who noticed her pressing her nose and picking at it. When questioned, child said a marble fell up her nose.

Procedure: Examined the nose and identified an object lodged in such a way that general anesthesia was required to remove.

Postprocedure diagnosis: Foreign body in nose

a. What is the anatomic site? _____

b. What is the procedure? _____

c. What is the surgical approach (open, endoscopic, external)? _____

d. Was anesthesia required? _____

3. OFFICE Gender: M Age: 54

Preprocedure diagnosis: Patient states: "I can't stop coughing and always feel that there is a lump in my throat." Hoarseness is evident.

Procedure: Transoral direct laryngoscopy under general anesthesia; inserted laryngoscope into the throat and visualized tumor. Excised tumor with a scalpel. Used forceps to strip the epithelium of the vocal cords. Patient tolerated procedure well. Submitted specimens to pathology.

Postprocedure diagnosis: Carcinoma of the larynx per pathology report

a. What is the anatomic site? _____

b. What is the procedure? _____

c. What is the surgical approach (open, endoscopic, external)? _____

d. What is the anatomic approach (transnasal, transthoracic, laterovertical, etc.)? _____

e. What is the purpose or variation (direct/indirect) of the procedure? _____

f. What additional procedures were performed during the same session? _____

4. EMERGENCY DEPT Gender: M Age: 28

Preprocedure diagnosis: Uncontrolled bilateral epistaxis

Procedure: Limited cautery and packing of nasal hemorrhage. Used nasal speculum to locate site of bleeding in the right anterior nasal passage, cleaned, and applied silver nitrate stick to cauterize. Repeated on the left anterior passage. Hemostasis was achieved.

Postprocedure diagnosis: Epistaxis

a. What is the anatomic site? _____

b. What is the procedure? _____

c. What is the surgical approach (open, endoscopic, external)? _____

d. What is the anatomic approach (transnasal, transthoracic, laterovertical, etc.)? _____

e. What is the purpose or variation of the procedure?

_____

f. What is the laterality? _____

CODING PRACTICE (continued)

5. OUTPATIENT SURGERY   Gender: M   Age: 36

Preprocedure diagnosis: Mucocele frontal sinus

Procedure: Left transorbital frontal sinusotomy; made an incision along the inner wall of the orbit of eye to reach the ethmoid sinus. Made an opening into the ethmoid sinus to reach the frontal sinus. Removed mucocele from the frontal sinus using curette. Performed layered closure.

a. What is the anatomic site? _____

b. What is the procedure? _____

c. What is the surgical approach (open, endoscopic, external)? _____

d. What is the anatomic approach (transnasal, transthoracic, laterovertical, etc.)? _____

e. What is the purpose or variation of the procedure?
_____

f. What is the laterality? _____

g. What additional procedures were performed during the same session? _____

6. LOCATION   Gender: M   Age: 68

Preprocedure diagnosis: Hemoptysis

Procedure: Conscious sedation was administered, and when the patient was comfortable we inserted flexible fiber optic bronchoscope through nose and examined nasal passages, with no findings. Advanced into the larynx, where no abnormalities were noted. Advanced to the trachea, where no abnormalities were noted, then to the right bronchus, which was also negative.

(continued)

6. (continued)

Retracted bronchoscope, then advanced to left bronchus. Dried blood was visualized in the alveoli. We placed a fiducial marker near the apparent source and performed bronchial alveolar lavage to cleanse area and obtain specimens. Bronchoscope was withdrawn and specimens were submitted to pathology. Patient tolerated procedure well.

Postprocedure diagnosis: Bronchial hemorrhage, pathology pending

a. What is the anatomic site? _____

b. What is the procedure? _____

c. What is the surgical approach (open, endoscopic, external)? _____

d. What is the anatomic approach (transnasal, transthoracic, laterovertical, etc.)? _____

e. What type of endoscope is used? _____

f. Is the procedure diagnostic, surgical, or both? _____

g. What procedure(s) are performed during the endoscopy? _____

h. What is the laterality? _____

i. Is the endoscopy a preoperative survey or scout? _____
_____

j. Is an endoscopic procedure converted to an open procedure? _____

k. Is a decision made to perform an additional procedure at the same encounter based on the results of the endoscopy? _____

l. What is the farthest anatomic site reached with the endoscope? _____

ASSIGNING CODES FOR RESPIRATORY SYSTEM PROCEDURES

To assign codes from 1the Respiratory System subsection, search the Index for the Main Term for the anatomic site, the first-level modifying term for the type of procedure, and a second-level modifying term for variations of the procedure. In the Tabular List, select the appropriate code for the anatomic approach and the variation of the procedure performed. Review instructional notes in the Tabular List carefully because they provide valuable guidance on bundling and redirect you to alternative codes for similar procedures.

The National Correct Coding Initiative (NCCI) provides extensive guidelines regarding the bundling of procedures on the respiratory system. The following sections discuss how to assign codes for procedures on adjacent sites or systems, biopsies, and endoscopies. Other topics addressed by NCCI are control of bleeding, intubation, and chest tube procedures.

Adjacent Sites or Systems

Some procedures on the nose and mouth may be performed near the mucocutaneous (*pertaining to the skin and mucous membranes*) margins and could potentially be coded as a procedure on the respiratory system, digestive system, or integumentary system. The exact site of the procedure—such as a lesion removal or biopsy—determines the system under which the procedure is classified. Internal procedures on the mucous membrane of the nose are classified as respiratory system procedures, whereas external procedures on the skin of the nose are generally classified as integumentary system procedures. Procedures on the larynx are classified as respiratory system procedures, whereas procedures on the pharynx and mucous membranes of the oral cavity are classified as digestive system procedures.

Sometimes procedures from multiple systems are bundled into a single code. For example, CPT provides a Respiratory System code for septoplasty that includes the graft in the code descriptor. Assign only the code from the Respiratory System: **30520 Septoplasty or submucous resection, with or without cartilage scoring, contouring or replacement with graft**. Do not also assign a code from the Integumentary System subsection for the tissue transfer because the service is included in the Respiratory System code.

When a procedure is performed near the border of two distinct sites, you may need to review codes and guidelines from both sites to determine the best code to assign. Never assign separate codes from each site for the same procedure.

Biopsy

Do not code a nasal or sinus biopsy in addition to the more extensive procedure it is performed in conjunction with. Code only the more extensive procedure (■ FIGURE 38-2). The exception is to code both procedures when the biopsy results are the reason the more extensive procedure is performed (■ FIGURE 38-3).

Endoscopy

Many procedures on the nose, sinuses, larynx, bronchi, and lungs are performed endoscopically. A surgical endoscopy

---

Patient presents with an obstruction in the ethmoid sinus that was identified on a CT scan. The surgeon performs an endoscopic anterior right ethmoidectomy and sends a tissue specimen to pathology upon completion of the procedure.

31254-RT Nasal/sinus endoscopy, surgical; with ethmoidectomy, partial (anterior); -RT Right side

Figure 38-2 ■ Example of coding for a more extensive procedure only. *Source: © PB Resources, Inc. Used with permission. CPT codes only © American Medical Association.*

Patient presents with several intranasal lesions that are not interfering with her breathing. The surgeon performs a biopsy of one lesion and sends it to pathology where a frozen section is performed. Pathology determines that the lesion is malignant, so the surgeon proceeds with complete removal of the initial lesion, as well as three additional similar lesions.

30117 × 4 Excision or destruction (eg, laser), intranasal lesion; internal approach
30100-51 Biopsy, intranasal; -51 Multiple procedures

Figure 38-3 ■ Example of coding for a biopsy and a more extensive procedure. *Source: © PB Resources, Inc. Used with permission. CPT codes only © American Medical Association.*

---

includes a diagnostic endoscopy, so when both are performed, report only the code for the surgical endoscopy. This is stated in special instructions at the beginning of the **Endoscopy** category for each anatomic site. In addition, special instructions under the **Endoscopy** category for **Sinus** state that a **surgical sinus endoscopy (when appropriate) includes a sinusotomy and diagnostic sinus endoscopy**. In most cases, only the surgical sinus endoscopy should be reported, not the sinusotomy or diagnostic endoscopy.

The findings of a diagnostic endoscopy may lead to the decision to perform a nonendoscopic surgical procedure during the same patient encounter. Assign two codes: one for the endoscopy and one for the surgical procedure.

An endoscopy should not be reported separately when the endoscope is used to survey or scout the surgical field before an open procedure. This preoperative check is considered part of the surgical procedure and is not coded as a diagnostic endoscopy.

Endoscopy of one site includes examination of all the sites accessed as the endoscope passes through to reach the final site. Report an endoscopy code only for the farthest site reached. For example, a transnasal endoscopy of the sinuses includes examination of the nose. A transoral endoscopy of the lungs includes examination of the larynx, trachea, and bronchi. The exception is when it is medically appropriate to perform distinct procedures using different types of endoscopes on separate sites. Append modifier -**59 Distinct procedural service** to identify that these were separate procedures (■ FIGURE 38-4).

When an endoscopic procedure cannot be completed and is converted to an open procedure, code only the open procedure. Do not code the endoscopy.

To locate codes for endoscopy, search the Index for the Main Term for the anatomic site and the first-level modifying term **Endoscopy**. Alternatively, search the Index for the Main Term **Endoscopy** and the first-level modifying term for the anatomic site. Review the second-level modifying terms and code descriptions in the Tabular List carefully because endoscopy codes are divided based on the purpose of the procedure, such as tumor excision, biopsy, lavage, foreign body removal, and so on.

Guided Example of Assigning Respiratory System Procedure Codes

To practice skills for assigning codes for the Respiratory System subsection, continue with the example from earlier in the

---

Physician uses a fiberoptic laryngoscope to perform a diagnostic laryngoscopy for a laryngeal mass. She then uses a fiberoptic bronchoscope to examine a lung mass.

31622 Bronchoscopy, rigid or flexible, including fluoroscopic guidance, when performed; diagnostic, with cell washing, when performed
31575-XS Laryngoscopy, flexible; diagnostic; -XS Separate structure

Figure 38-4 ■ Example of coding two endoscopie. *Source: © PB Resources, Inc. Used with permission. CPT codes only © American Medical Association.*

chapter about a patient who was seen for a bronchoscopy. Follow along in your CPT manual as Leanne Riehl, CCS, assigns codes. Check off each step after you complete it.

▶ Leanne searches the Index for the Main Term **Bronchoscopy**.

❑ She locates the first-level modifying term for the first procedure, **Biopsy**.

❑ She identifies the code ranges **31625-31629, 31632-31633**.

▶ Leanne turns to the Tabular List to review, select, and verify the code.

❑ She identifies that all the codes listed for the first-level modifying term **Biopsy** are indented codes under code **31622**.

▪ She knows she must refer to the common portion of code **31622** to understand the full description of the other codes: **Bronchoscopy, rigid or flexible, including fluoroscopic guidance, when performed;**. This accurately describes the basic procedure performed, flexible bronchoscopy.

▪ The indented codes describe additional procedures done during the bronchoscopy.

❑ She reads through the unique descriptors for the codes listed in the Index—**31625-31629, 31632-31633**—to identify possible codes for acquiring a biopsy of the nodule in the left lobe of the lung. She identifies three potential codes: **31625, 31628, 31632**. She compares the code descriptions to determine the differences between them.

▪ Code **31625** describes a bronchoscopy **with bronchial or endobronchial biopsy(s), single or multiple sites**.

▪ Code **31628** describes a bronchoscopy **with transbronchial lung biopsy(s), single lobe**.

▪ Code **31632** describes a bronchoscopy **with transbronchial lung biopsy(s), each additional lobe (List separately in addition to code for primary procedure)**.

▪ She identifies the differences: code **31625** identifies a bronchial or *endo*bronchial biopsy, which is a biopsy of or *within* a bronchus; code **31638** identifies a *trans*bronchial biopsy of the lung, in which the lung is accessed *through* the bronchus; and code **31632** identifies transbronchial lung biopsies in *more* than one lobe.

❑ She refers to the medical record to confirm that a biopsy was taken from a single lobe, then verifies the full code title for **31628, Bronchoscopy, rigid or flexible, including fluoroscopic guidance, when performed; with transbronchial lung biopsy(s), single lobe** and confirms that this accurately describes the procedure.

❑ She reads the instructional note that appears below the code description in the Tabular List that states (**31628 should be reported only once regardless of how many transbronchial lung biopsies are performed in a lobe**). Only one biopsy in this lobe was documented, so the note does not apply. If more than one biopsy had been performed in the lower left lobe, this note tells her that they would not be reported separately. However, if an additional biopsy had been performed in another lobe, she would report it using add-on code **31632** that she reviewed earlier.

▶ Leanne checks for additional instructions in the Tabular List. She has already reviewed the instructional notes that follow the codes selected.

❑ She cross-references the beginning of the category **Endoscopy** and reads the special instructions. The instructions provide direction regarding how to code multiple anatomic sites, surgical and diagnostic bronchoscopies performed by the same physician during the same encounter, and the use of fluoroscopic guidance. None of these criteria apply to this patient case because only one site was examined and neither surgery nor fluoroscopy was performed.

❑ She cross-references the beginning of the subheading **Trachea and Bronchi** and verifies that there are no instructional notes.

❑ She cross-references the beginning of the subsection **Respiratory** and verifies that there are no instructional notes.

▶ Leanne reviews the procedure code she has assigned for this case.

❑ **31628 Bronchoscopy, rigid or flexible, including fluoroscopic guidance, when performed; with transbronchial lung biopsy(s), single lobe**

▶ Next, Leanne must determine whether a modifier is needed and select the moderate sedation codes for the CRNA.

CODING PRACTICE

Exercise 38.3 Assigning Codes for Respiratory System Procedures

Instructions: Read the mini-medical-record of each patient's encounter. Review the information abstracted in Exercise 38.2 for questions 1–3. For questions 4–6, abstract the case on your own. Assign CPT codes, quantities, and modifiers using the Index and Tabular List. Write the code(s) on the line provided.

---

1. EMERGENCY DEPT   Gender: F   Age: 48

Preprocedure diagnosis: Patient presents with complaints of nasal pain, edema, and purulent (pus) discharge. CT scan and lab tests reveal a nasal septum abscess.

Procedure: Incision and drainage (I & D) nasal septum abscess; made small incision within the nasal septum over the abscess. Suctioned purulent fluid and flushed with sterile saline. Packed the nasal cavity with gauze.

Postprocedure diagnosis: Nasal septum abscess due to Staphylococcus aureus

1 CPT Code _____

---

2. EMERGENCY DEPT   Gender: F   Age: 4

Preprocedure diagnosis: Child is brought in by her mother, who noticed her pressing her nose and picking at it. When questioned, child said a marble fell up her nose.

Procedure: Examined the nose and identified an object lodged in such a way that general anesthesia was required to remove.

Postprocedure diagnosis: Foreign body in nose

1 CPT Code _____

---

3. OFFICE   Gender: M   Age: 54

Preprocedure diagnosis: Patient states: "I can't stop coughing and always feel that there is a lump in my throat." Hoarseness is evident.

Procedure: Transoral direct laryngoscopy under general anesthesia; inserted laryngoscope into the throat and visualized tumor. Excised tumor with a scalpel. Used forceps to strip the epithelium of the vocal cords. Patient tolerated procedure well. Submitted specimens to pathology.

Postprocedure diagnosis: Carcinoma of the larynx per pathology report

1 CPT Code _____

---

4. OUTPATIENT HOSPITAL   Gender: F   Age: 38

Preprocedure diagnosis: Chronic cough and chest pain

Procedure: Bronchoscopy with endobronchial biopsies of the right upper and lower lobes.

Postprocedure diagnosis: Acute bronchitis per pathology report

1 CPT Code _____

---

5. OUTPATIENT SURGERY   Gender: F   Age: 2

Preprocedure diagnosis: Congenital obstruction of the nasolacrimal duct

Procedure: Fractured the turbinates bilaterally and then repositioned them

1 CPT Code _____

---

6. OUTPATIENT SURGERY   Gender: M   Age: 68

Preprocedure diagnosis: Extensive scarring on tracheostoma

Procedure: Reconstructed tracheostoma; removed scar tissue and repaired with a rotation flap

1 CPT Code _____

ARRANGING CODES FOR RESPIRATORY SYSTEM PROCEDURES

Information about bundling, multiple coding, code sequencing, and modifiers in the Respiratory System subsection appears in special instructions, instructional notes, and code descriptions. Special instructions at the beginning of several categories, especially those for endoscopy, provide direction about when multiple codes are needed and when multiple services are bundled into a single code. Extensive instructional notes throughout the subsection identify specific codes that cannot be reported together, those that should be reported together, and when additional codes might be needed.

Code descriptions identify whether the quantity for procedures on the lungs is reported as one per procedure, per lung, per lobe, or per segment or using another unit of measure. Be attentive to the occurrence of a parent code that has multiple indented codes, each with a different unit for reporting quantity.

Although the variations in how quantity is reported may seem confusing at first, they are dependent on the type of procedure, so no general rule exists. Coders must give special consideration to this portion of the descriptor to be certain they are accurately reporting the quantity.

Modifiers

Because multiple procedures on the respiratory system can be performed during the same encounter, coders should review the use of modifiers **-59** and **-51** and laterality modifiers. These modifiers and examples are discussed next.

-59 Distinct Procedural Service

Append modifier **-59 Distinct procedural service** to codes for services that are usually bundled but are performed as a separate procedure at a distinct site, through a separate incision, or during a different operative session. Medicare and some private payers may require the use of a HCPCS **-X{EPSU}** extended

modifier instead of modifier **-59** to provide more specific information, such as:

- **-XE Separate encounter**
- **-XS Separate structure**
- **-XP Separate practitioner**
- **-XU Unusual non-overlapping service**

-51 Multiple Procedures

When more than one procedure is performed during the same operative session, remember to append modifier **-51 Multiple procedures** to the second and subsequent codes. Do not append modifier **-51** to add-on codes or codes designated with the symbol for **Modifier-51 exempt**.

Laterality

The use of modifiers to identify laterality varies for Respiratory System procedures. Because the paranasal sinuses are paired sites, assign the modifier **-LT Left side**, **-RT Right side**, or **-50 Bilateral procedure**. Most bilateral sinus procedures qualify for reimbursement at 150% of the rate for a unilateral procedure by most payers. This is indicated by an instructional note that states **(To report bilateral procedure, use . . . with modifier 50)** following several procedures (■ FIGURE 38-5).

Procedures involving the bronchi, including transbronchial procedures performed on the lung, do not accept laterality or bilateral modifiers. Transbronchial lung procedures are reported with add-on codes for each additional lobe treated, but laterality modifiers **-LT**, **-RT**, and **-50** are not reported. Because the left lung has two lobes and the right lung has three lobes, some procedures are reported separately for each lobe, but the lobe itself is not identified (■ FIGURE 38-6). When one left lobe and one right lobe are treated, do not append modifier **-50** for a bilateral procedure.

Procedures on the lungs using an approach other than transbronchial are often reported with modifiers **-RT** and **-LT** to

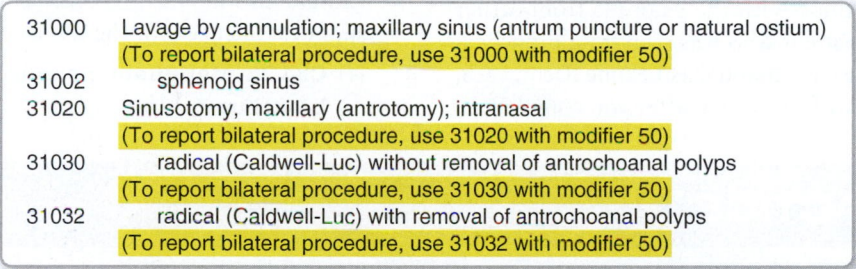

Figure 38-5 ■ Example of Tabular List instructional note to report modifier -50.
Source: © PB Resources, Inc. Used with permission. CPT codes only © American Medical Association.

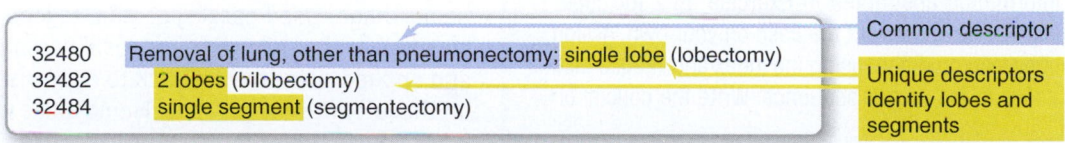

Figure 38-6 ■ Example of Tabular List entry to report lung lobes and segments. *Source: © PB Resources, Inc. Used with permission. CPT codes only © American Medical Association.*

Surgeon performed a thoracotomy and acquired two wedge biopsies of nodules in the left lung and one wedge biopsy of a nodule in the right lung.

32097-RT Thoracotomy, with diagnostic biopsy(ies) of lung nodule(s) or mass(es) (eg, wedge, incisional), unilateral; -RT Right side
32097-LT Thoracotomy, with diagnostic biopsy(ies) of lung nodule(s) or mass(es) (eg, wedge, incisional), unilateral; -LT Left side

Figure 38-7 ■ Example of coding separately for each lung. *Source: © PB Resources, Inc. Used with permission. CPT codes only © American Medical Association.*

identify laterality, but not modifier **-50** for bilateral procedures. Such procedures are followed by an instructional note to not report the procedure more than once per lung, which means that a separate code/modifier combination should be reported for each procedure performed (■ FIGURE 38-7).

When procedures are followed by instructional notes that specify to use modifier **-50** to report a bilateral procedure, the code can be reported once with modifier **-50** to indicate the procedure was performed on both sides.

When a procedure that is inherently bilateral is performed on only one side, append modifier **-52 Reduced services**.

SUCCESS STEP

This text provides general guidelines for reporting laterality. Various payers establish their own guidelines for how to report laterality. In the workplace you can refer to payer guidelines and the Medicare Physician Fee Schedule Database (MPFSDB) for more detailed information.

Guided Example of Arranging Respiratory System Procedure Codes

To practice skills for arranging codes for procedures of the Respiratory System, continue with the example from earlier in the chapter about the patient who was seen for a bronchoscopy. Follow along in your CPT manual as Leanne Riehl, CCS, arranges the codes. Check off each step after you complete it.

▶ First, Leanne confirms the procedure code **31628**, which describes the bronchoscopy and biopsy.

▶ Leanne examines the need for modifiers. (Refer to Table 27-1, Key Criteria for Abstracting CPT Modifiers, or Appendix A in the CPT manual.)

 ❏ Code **31628** does not require a modifier because laterality modifiers are not used for transbronchial lung procedures.

▶ Leanne assigns the moderate sedation codes for the CRNA:

 ❏ She looks up the Main Term **Sedation** in the CPT Index, then locates the subterm **Moderate**. The Index entry lists codes **99151-99153**.

 ❏ She refers to the code range in the Tabular List and reads the choices. She confirms that someone other than the physician performing the procedure provided the moderate sedation service. She notes in the medical record that 75 minutes of intraservice time was provided, which equates to five 15-minute segments. She assigns code **99156** for the first 15 minutes of intraservice time, and 4 units of code **99157** for the final 60 minutes of intraservice time.

▶ Leanne finalizes the procedure codes and sequencing for this case:

 (1) Physician code: **31628 Bronchoscopy, rigid or flexible, including fluoroscopic guidance, when performed; with transbronchial lung biopsy(s), single lobe**

 (2) CRNA codes: **99156 × 1 Moderate sedation services provided by a physician or other qualified health care professional other than the physician or other qualified health care professional performing the diagnostic or therapeutic service that the sedation supports; initial 15 minutes of intraservice time, patient age 5 years or older**

 99157 × 4 each additional 15 minutes intraservice time

▶ Leanne also assigns the ICD-10-CM diagnosis code that supports the need for the service.

 (1) **C34.32 Malignant neoplasm of lower lobe, left bronchus or lung**

CODING PRACTICE

Exercise 38.4 Arranging Codes for Respiratory System Procedures

Instructions: Read the mini-medical-record of each patient's encounter. Review the information abstracted in Exercise 38.2 for questions 1–3. For questions 4–6, abstract the case on your own. Assign CPT codes, quantities, and modifiers using the Index and Tabular List, and arrange the codes in the proper sequence. Write the code(s) on the line provided.

---

1. EMERGENCY DEPT   Gender: M   Age: 28

Preprocedure diagnosis: Uncontrolled bilateral epistaxis

Procedure: Limited cautery and packing of nasal hemorrhage. Used nasal speculum to locate site of bleeding in the right anterior nasal passage, cleaned, and applied silver nitrate stick to cauterize. Repeated on the left anterior passage. Hemostasis was achieved.

Postprocedure diagnosis: Epistaxis

1 CPT Code _____

CODING PRACTICE (continued)

2. OUTPATIENT SURGERY   Gender: M   Age: 36

Preprocedure diagnosis: Mucocele frontal sinus

Procedure: Left transorbital frontal sinusotomy; made an incision along the inner wall of the orbit of eye to reach the ethmoid sinus. Made an opening into the ethmoid sinus to reach the frontal sinus. Removed mucocele from the frontal sinus using curette. Performed layered closure.

1 CPT Code _____

3. OUTPATIENT SURGERY   Gender: M   Age: 68

Preprocedure diagnosis: Hemoptysis

Procedure: Conscious sedation was administered, and when the patient was comfortable we inserted a flexible fiber optic bronchoscope through the nose and examined nasal passages with no findings. Advanced into the larynx, where no abnormalities were noted. Advanced to the trachea, where no abnormalities were noted, then to the right bronchus, which was also negative. Retracted bronchoscope, then advanced to left bronchus. Dried blood was visualized in the alveoli. We placed a fiducial marker near the site and performed bronchial alveolar lavage to cleanse area and obtain specimens. Bronchoscope was withdrawn and specimens were submitted to pathology. Patient tolerated procedure well.

Postprocedure diagnosis: Bronchial hemorrhage, pathology pending

Tip: Laterality modifiers are not required.

2 CPT Codes _____

4. OFFICE   Gender: M   Age: 33

Preprocedure diagnosis: Nasal congestion and facial pain

Procedure: Performed a bilateral nasal endoscopy and excised two polyps on the right and three polyps on the left

Postprocedure diagnosis: Nasal polyps

1 CPT Code _____

5. OFFICE   Gender: F   Age: 63

Preprocedure diagnosis: Lifelong cigarette smoker, personal history of breast cancer with R breast mastectomy six years ago. Recent hemoptysis, loss of appetite, and shortness of breath

Procedure: Thoracotomy with biopsy of nodules in both right and left lungs

Postprocedure diagnosis: Metastatic CA to lung

Tip: Assign separate codes and modifiers for each lung.

2 CPT Codes _____

6. LOCATION   Gender: F   Age: 22

Preprocedure diagnosis: Cystic fibrosis, double-lung transplant candidate

Procedure: Double-lung transplant including cadaver pneumonectomy, backbench preparation, and transplantation of both lungs into recipient with use of a heart–lung machine.

Tip: Assign codes for the pneumonectomy, the backbench preparation, and the transplant.

3 CPT Codes _____

_____

E/M CODING FOR PULMONOLOGY

The *1997 Documentation Guidelines for Evaluation and Management Services* (1997 DG), published by the Centers for Medicare and Medicaid Services (CMS), provides requirements for each level of a respiratory E/M examination (■ FIGURE 38-8, page 778). Pulmonologists are not limited to using the guidelines for a skin examination only. They can also use guidelines for a general multiorgan system examination, or any other single organ system examination, based on what is most advantageous for a specific encounter. However, physicians cannot combine elements from more than one type of examination for a given encounter. The respiratory examination guidelines typically provide the best results when a detailed respiratory examination is performed.

To determine the appropriate E/M code, coders must review the documentation in detail and identify the specific elements documented.

- To translate the documentation into the E/M requirements for the history, refer back to Chapter 28, "Evaluation and Management Services (99201-99499)," Tables 28-7 to 28-10, or to the 1997 DG.

- To determine the requirements for an examination, refer to Figure 38-8 or to the single organ system examination for respiratory in the 1997 DG.

- To determine the levels for medical decision making (MDM), refer to Chapter 28, Table 28-12, and to the Table of Risk in the 1997 DG.

Guided Example of E/M Coding for Pulmonology

Refer to the pulmonology encounter (■ FIGURE 38-9, page 779) to practice skills for abstracting and assigning E/M codes. Follow along as fictitious coder Leanne Riehl, CCS, abstracts the procedure. Check off each step after you complete it.

System/Body Area	Elements of Respiratory System Examination
Constitutional	❑ Measurement of any **three** of the following seven **vital** signs: • 1) sitting or standing blood pressure, • 2) supine blood pressure, • 3) pulse rate and regularity, • 4) respiration, • 5) temperature, • 6) height, • 7) weight (May be measured and recorded by ancillary staff) ❑ General **appearance** of patient (eg, development, nutrition, body habitus, deformities, attention to grooming)
Ears, Nose, Mouth and Throat	❑ Inspection of **nasal mucosa, septum** and **turbinates** ❑ Inspection of **teeth** and **gums** ❑ Examination of **oropharynx:** oral mucosa, salivary glands, hard and soft palates, tongue, tonsils and posterior pharynx
Neck	❑ Examination of **neck** (eg, masses, overall appearance, symmetry, tracheal position, crepitus) ❑ Examination of **thyroid** (eg, enlargement, tenderness, mass) ❑ Examination of **jugular veins** (eg, distention, a, v or cannon a waves)
Respiratory	❑ **Inspection** of chest with notation of symmetry and expansion ❑ Assessment of **respiratory effort** (eg, intercostal retractions, use of accessory muscles, diaphragmatic movement) ❑ **Percussion** of chest (eg, dullness, flatness, hyperresonance) ❑ **Palpation** of chest (eg, tactile fremitus) ❑ **Auscultation** of lungs (eg, breath sounds, adventitious sounds, rubs)
Cardiovascular	❑ **Auscultation** of heart with notation of abnormal sounds and murmurs ❑ Examination of peripheral vascular system by observation (eg, swelling, varicosities) and palpation (pulses, temperature, edema, tenderness)
Gastrointestinal (Abdomen)	❑ Examination of **abdomen** with notation of presence of masses or tenderness ❑ Examination of **liver** and **spleen**
Lymphatic	Palpation of lymph nodes in **two or more** areas: ❑ Neck ❑ Axillae ❑ Groin ❑ Other
Musculoskeletal	❑ Assessment of muscle **strength** and **tone** (eg, flaccid, cog wheel, spastic) with notation of any atrophy or abnormal movements ❑ Examination of **gait** and **station**
Extremities	❑ Inspection and/or palpation of **digits** and **nails** (eg, clubbing, cyanosis, inflammatory conditions, petechiae, ischemia, infections, nodes)
Skin	❑ **Inspection** of skin and subcutaneous tissue (eg, rashes, lesions, ulcers)
Neurologic/ Psychiatric	*Brief assessment of mental status including:* ❑ **Orientation** to time, place and person ❑ **Mood** and affect (eg, depression, anxiety, agitation, hypomania, lability)

Total # Bullets Performed and Documented →		# of ❑ **Elements Performed and Documented**	**Level of Examination**
		1–5	Problem focused
		6–11	Expanded problem focused
		12	Detailed
		ALL	Comprehensive (Document **every** element in each box with a shaded border and at least **one** element in each box with an unshaded border)

Figure 38-8 ■ 1997 documentation guidelines for respiratory system examination. *Source: Centers for Medicare and Medicaid Services, 1997 Documentation Guidelines for Evaluation and Management Services (with formatting adjustments).*

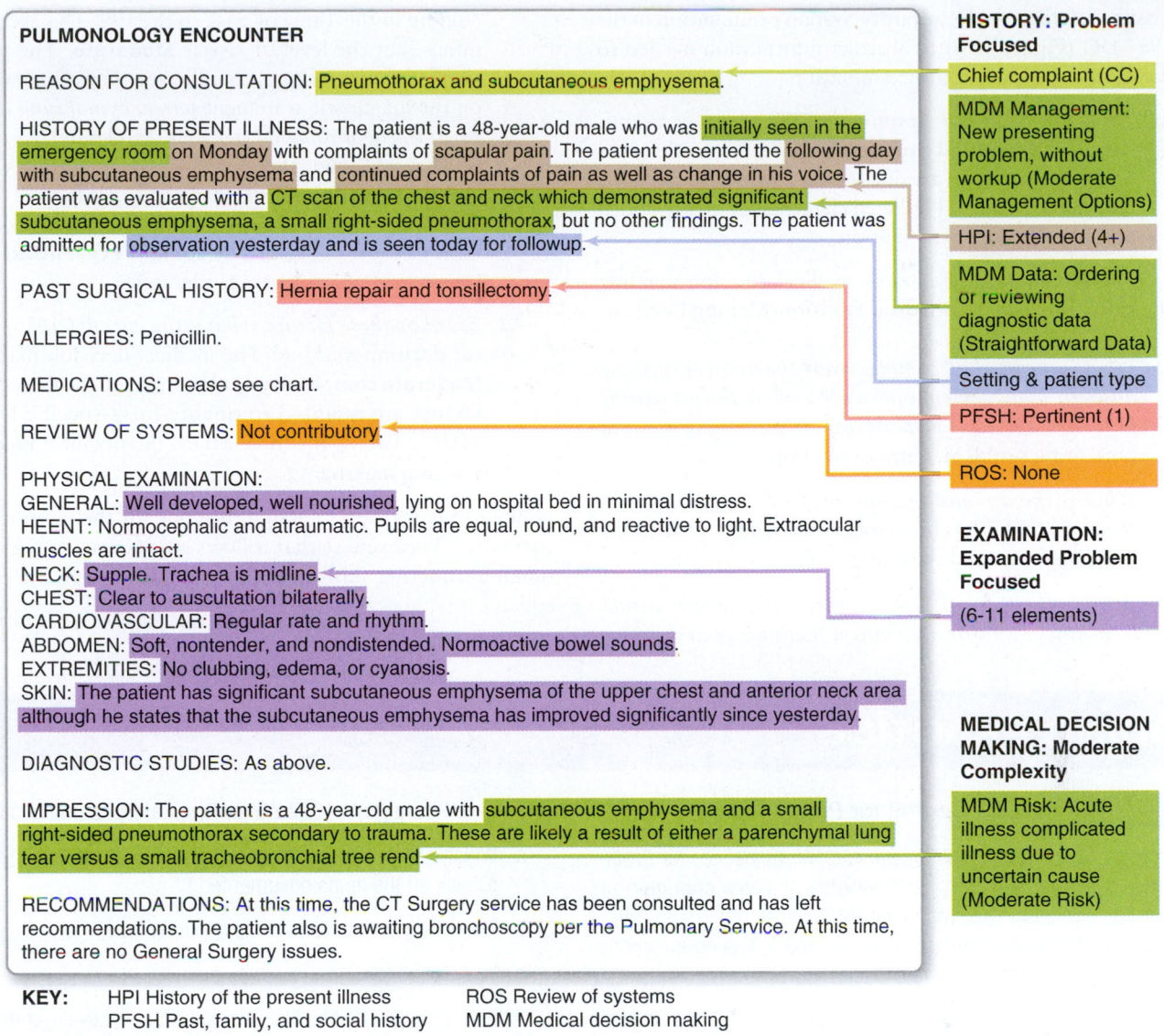

PULMONOLOGY ENCOUNTER

REASON FOR CONSULTATION: Pneumothorax and subcutaneous emphysema.

HISTORY OF PRESENT ILLNESS: The patient is a 48-year-old male who was initially seen in the emergency room on Monday with complaints of scapular pain. The patient presented the following day with subcutaneous emphysema and continued complaints of pain as well as change in his voice. The patient was evaluated with a CT scan of the chest and neck which demonstrated significant subcutaneous emphysema, a small right-sided pneumothorax, but no other findings. The patient was admitted for observation yesterday and is seen today for followup.

PAST SURGICAL HISTORY: Hernia repair and tonsillectomy.

ALLERGIES: Penicillin.

MEDICATIONS: Please see chart.

REVIEW OF SYSTEMS: Not contributory.

PHYSICAL EXAMINATION:
GENERAL: Well developed, well nourished, lying on hospital bed in minimal distress.
HEENT: Normocephalic and atraumatic. Pupils are equal, round, and reactive to light. Extraocular muscles are intact.
NECK: Supple. Trachea is midline.
CHEST: Clear to auscultation bilaterally.
CARDIOVASCULAR: Regular rate and rhythm.
ABDOMEN: Soft, nontender, and nondistended. Normoactive bowel sounds.
EXTREMITIES: No clubbing, edema, or cyanosis.
SKIN: The patient has significant subcutaneous emphysema of the upper chest and anterior neck area although he states that the subcutaneous emphysema has improved significantly since yesterday.

DIAGNOSTIC STUDIES: As above.

IMPRESSION: The patient is a 48-year-old male with subcutaneous emphysema and a small right-sided pneumothorax secondary to trauma. These are likely a result of either a parenchymal lung tear versus a small tracheobronchial tree rend.

RECOMMENDATIONS: At this time, the CT Surgery service has been consulted and has left recommendations. The patient also is awaiting bronchoscopy per the Pulmonary Service. At this time, there are no General Surgery issues.

HISTORY: Problem Focused

Chief complaint (CC)

MDM Management: New presenting problem, without workup (Moderate Management Options)

HPI: Extended (4+)

MDM Data: Ordering or reviewing diagnostic data (Straightforward Data)

Setting & patient type

PFSH: Pertinent (1)

ROS: None

EXAMINATION: Expanded Problem Focused

(6-11 elements)

MEDICAL DECISION MAKING: Moderate Complexity

MDM Risk: Acute illness complicated illness due to uncertain cause (Moderate Risk)

KEY: HPI History of the present illness   ROS Review of systems
       PFSH Past, family, and social history   MDM Medical decision making

Figure 38-9 ■ Pulmonology encounter. *Source: © PB Resources, Inc. Used with permission.*

▶ First, Leanne needs to establish the category of service so she can determine the information needed to abstract and assign the code.

❏ *What is the setting?* Hospital observation

❏ *What is the type of service?* Subsequent, because patient was admitted yesterday

❏ *What is the code range?* Leanne refers to the CPT Index and looks up the Main Term **Evaluation and Management** and the subterm **Hospital Services Observation Care**. The codes listed are **99217-99220, 99224-99226, 99234-99236.**

❏ *How many key components are required?* Leanne refers to the code ranges in the Tabular List and identifies **99224-99226** as the correct category because this is subsequent observation care. She reads the code description of the first code, which states **at least 2 of these 3 key components.** All codes in the category have the

same requirements for key components. This tells her that two key components must meet or exceed the levels listed in the code (2/3).

▶ Next, Leanne identifies the level of history.

❏ *What is the level of HPI?* The HPI is **Extended** because four elements are documented.

❏ *What is the level of ROS?* No systems are documented for the ROS. The physician's statement, *not contributory*, does not describe what the physician did.

❏ *What is the level of PFSH?* The PFSH is **Pertinent** because one element is documented.

❏ *Based on these factors, what is the overall level of history?* The level of history is **Problem focused** because the lowest of the three factors (HPI, ROS, and PFSH) determines the history level. The HPI and PFSH qualify for a detailed history, but the ROS qualifies for only a problem-focused history.

▶ Leanne refers to the Respiratory System examination in the 1997 DG (Figure 38-8) to abstract information needed to determine the level of the examination.

❏ *What is the level of examination?* The level of examination is **Expanded problem focused**. Seven elements of the examination are documented, which exceeds the requirement of 6–11 bulleted elements for an expanded problem-focused examination.

▶ Leanne determines the level of medical decision making. (Refer to Table 28-12, Medical Decision-Making Levels.)

❏ *What is the level of complexity of the number of diagnoses or management options, based on the presenting problem?* The level is **Moderate** because there is a new presenting problem, without workup.

❏ *What is the amount and/or complexity of data to be reviewed?* The level is **Straightforward** because the physician reviewed the patient's CT report.

❏ *What is the level of risk of significant complications, morbidity, and/or mortality?* Leanne reviews each

column in the Table of Risk in the 1997 DG and determines that the level of risk is **Moderate**. The patient presents with an acute, complicated illness/injury based on the diagnostic statement *parenchymal lung tear vs. small tracheobronchial tree rent* (Moderate), a CT scan is reviewed (Low), and the management option is minor elective surgery with no identified risk factors (Low). The single highest element in the Table of Risk determines the overall risk. The column **Presenting Problem** is the highest level (Moderate).

❏ *Based on these factors, what is the overall level of medical decision making?* The medical decision making is **Moderate complexity**. At least two of the three MDM factors are required to qualify for a specific level of MDM. Two of the three MDM factors meet moderate decision making.

Now Leanne is ready to assign the code for the pulmonology encounter. The exercise that follows guides you through additional abstracting skills and allows you to assign the correct code.

CODING PRACTICE

Exercise 38.5 **E/M Coding for Pulmonology**

Instructions: Refer to the *1997 Documentation Guidelines for Evaluation and Management Services* (available at **www.cms.gov**) or Chapter 28, "Evaluation and Management Services (99201-99499)," Tables 28-7 to 28-12, in this text. Answer the following questions about the "Pulmonology encounter" (Figure 38-9).

1. a. Which elements of the HPI are documented? Circle all that apply. Location, Quality, Severity, Duration, Timing, Context, Modifying factors, Associated signs and symptoms

   b. How many elements are documented? _____

   c. What is the level of HPI?_____

2. a. Which systems are reviewed in the ROS? Circle all that apply. Constitutional, Allergic/ immunologic, CV, Endocrine, ENT/M, Eyes, GI, GU, Hemic/lymphatic, MS, Neurologic, Psychiatric, Respiratory, Skin/breast

   b. How many systems are documented?_____

   c. What is the level of ROS? _____

3. a. Which PFSH elements are documented? Circle all that apply. Past medical, Family, Social

   b. What is the level of PFSH? _____

   c. What is the overall level of history? (The lowest history factor—HPI, ROS, or PFSH—determines the level of history.)

   _____

4. Refer to Figure 38-8, 1997 DG for Respiratory Examination.

   a. Which bulleted items are documented for the examination? (Check off the items documented.)

   b. How many bulleted items are documented?_____

   c. What is the level of the examination? _____

5. Refer to Table 28-12, Medical Decision-Making Levels, or the 1997 DG.

   a. What is the MDM level for the number of diagnoses or management options? _____

   b. What is the MDM level for the amount and/or complexity of data to be reviewed? _____

   c. Refer to the Table of Risk in the 1997 DG. Which elements of risk are documented for each risk factor?

      1. Presenting problem: _____

      2. Diagnostic procedures ordered: _____

      3. Management options selected: _____

   d. What is the level of risk? (The highest of the three risk factors determines the overall level of risk.) _____

   e. What is the overall level of MDM? (2/3 MDM factors are needed to determine the overall level.) _____

6. a. What is the setting? _____

   b. What is the patient (or service) type? _____

c. What is the code range? _____

d. How many key components are required? _____

e. What is the level of history? _____

f.   What is the level of examination? _____

g. What is the level of medical decision making? _____

h. What is the correct code? _____

i.   What modifier(s) is required? _____

7. Abstract, assign, and arrange (sequence) the diagnosis code(s) that support the E/M code.

ICD-10-CM Code(s) _____

CHAPTER SUMMARY

In this chapter you learned that:

- It is important to understand the anatomy of the paranasal sinuses, also called accessory sinuses, because codes are divided based on the location of the sinus.

- CPT provides guidelines and instructional notes throughout the Tabular List to alert coders to the need for modifiers, provide cross-references to codes for similar procedures on other sites, identify when additional codes might be needed for radiological services, and highlight resequenced and recently deleted codes.

- Abstracting for the respiratory system requires attention to the anatomic approach and procedure type or variation. Abstracting criteria include a special section on endoscopy procedures, in addition to questions that apply to all respiratory procedures.

- To assign codes for the Respiratory System subsection, search the Index for the Main Term for the anatomic site, the first-level modifying term for the type of procedure, and a second-level modifying term for variations of the procedure. In the Tabular List, select the appropriate code for the anatomic approach and the variation of the procedure performed.

- Information about bundling, multiple coding, code sequencing, and modifiers in the Respiratory System subsection appears in special instructions, instructional notes, and code descriptions.

- The *1997 Documentation Guidelines for Evaluation and Management Services* (1997 DG), published by CMS, provides requirements for each level of a respiratory E/M examination.

CONCEPT QUIZ

Take a moment to look back at the Respiratory System subsection and solidify your skills. Try to answer the questions from memory first, then refer to the discussion in this chapter if you need a little extra help.

Completion

Instructions: Write the term that completes each statement based on the information you learned in this chapter. Choose from the list below. Some choices may be used more than once and some choices may not be used at all.

Caldwell-Luc procedure	pneumothorax
congenital subglottic stenosis	rhinoplasty
dystonia	septoplasty
ethmoidectomy	thoracentesis
laryngoscopy	thoracotomy
maxillectomy	tracheostomy
pleurodesis	tracheotomy
pneumonolysis	VATS

1. A malignant neoplasm of the upper jaw may require a partial _____.

2. _____ is surgical repair of the nose.

3. Laryngeal reinnervation by neuromuscular pedicle may be performed to treat _____.

4. A(n) _____ creates an opening to the maxillary sinus by incising the gum and bone.

5. A(n) _____ is a minimally invasive procedure to access the pleural cavity.

6. _____ can be performed to remove fluid from the pleural space using a needle.

7. _____ is the creation of an opening through the chest to place an intercostal catheter.

8. _____ introduces an irritant in the pleural cavity to prevent pleural effusion.

9. A(n) _____ is an incision through the neck into the windpipe.

10. An indirect _____ uses a mirror to view the base of the tongue, larynx, and the hypolarynx.

Multiple Choice

Instructions: Circle the letter of the best answer to each question based on the information you learned in this chapter.

1. What approach identifies access from within the nasal passage or through the mucous membrane inside the nasal passage?
    A. Chemical
    B. External
    C. Internal
    D. Lateral

(continued)

(continued from page 781)

2. How would you code the following procedure? *A physician uses a fiberoptic laryngoscope to perform a diagnostic laryngoscopy for a laryngeal mass. She then uses a fiberoptic bronchoscope to examine a lung mass.*
   A. 31622, 31575-59
   B. 31622
   C. 31575

3. Where are the ethmoid sinuses located?
   A. Over the eyes
   B. Under the eyes
   C. Between the eyes
   D. At the back of the nose

4. How would you code the following procedure? *A surgeon performed a thoracotomy and acquired two wedge biopsies of nodules in the left lung and one wedge biopsy of a nodule in the right lung.*
   A. 32097-51
   B. 32097-50
   C. 32097-RT × 2, 32097-LT
   D. 32097-RT, 32097-LT

5. How would you code the following procedure? *A patient presents with several intranasal lesions that are not interfering with her breathing. The surgeon performs a biopsy of one lesion and sends it to pathology where a frozen section is performed. Pathology determines that the lesion is malignant, so the surgeon proceeds with complete removal of the initial lesion, as well as three additional similar lesions.*
   A. 30117 × 3
   B. 30117 × 4, 30100-51
   C. 30100 × 3
   D. 30117, 30100

6. What site is examined using a laryngoscope?
   A. Hypopharynx
   B. Trachea
   C. Oral cavity
   D. Nasal passage

7. What term describes surgical excision of tissue from part of one lobe?
   A. Pneumonectomy
   B. Lobectomy
   C. Bilobectomy
   D. Segmentectomy

8. What does the abbreviation VATS stand for?
   A. Video access thoracoscopic surgery
   B. Video-assisted thoracoscopic surgery
   C. Video-assisted therapeutic surgery
   D. Video access thoracic surgery

9. What abstracting criterion does laterovertical describe?
   A. Surgical approach
   B. Anatomic approach
   C. Extent of procedure
   D. Laterality

10. What is the typical reimbursement rate for bilateral procedures?
    A. 50% of a unilateral procedure
    B. 100% of a unilateral procedure
    C. 150% of a unilateral procedure
    D. 200% of a unilateral procedure

KEEP ON CODING

Instructions: Read the procedural statement, then use the appropriate Index and Tabular List to assign CPT procedure codes, quantities, and modifiers. Write the code(s) on the line provided.

1. Bilateral nasal endoscopy with total ethmoidectomy. CPT Code(s) _____

2. Direct laryngoscopy with stripping of vocal cords. CPT Code(s) _____

3. Bronchoalveolar lavage. CPT Code(s) _____

4. Flexible fiber-optic laryngoscopy performed for removal of a dime lodged in the patient's larynx. CPT Code(s) _____

5. Flexible bronchoscopy with cell washings, brushings, and biopsy. CPT Code(s) _____

6. Cadaver donor pneumonectomy. CPT Code(s) _____

7. Tracheostomy with division of thyroid isthmus. CPT Code(s) _____

8. Ultrasound-guided thoracentesis, left lower lobe. CPT Code(s) _____

9. Percutaneous needle biopsy of the right upper lobe of the lung. CPT Code(s) _____

10. Rhinoplasty. CPT Code(s) _____

11. Cauterization of epistaxis, left nasal septum; fiber-optic nasal laryngoscopy. CPT Code(s) _____

12. Fluoroscopy-guided bronchoalveolar lavage. CPT Code(s) _____

13. Diagnostic bronchoscopy and limited left thoracotomy with partial pulmonary decortication and insertion of 2 chest tubes. CPT Code(s) _____

14. Bronchoscopy with laser destruction of a lesion of the bronchus. CPT Code(s) _____

15. Ultrasound-guided right pleurocentesis, right lower lobe. CPT Code(s) _____

16. Tracheostomy tube change. CPT Code(s) _____

17. Flexible laryngoscopy with biopsy. CPT Code(s) _____

18. Flexible bronchoscopy with thermoplasty, right middle lobe and left upper lobe, with moderate sedation provided by same physician performing the procedure with an independent observer to monitor the patient, 45 minutes of intraservice time. CPT Code(s) _____

19. Backbench preparation of one cadaver donor lung. CPT Code(s) _____

20. Partial excision of the inferior turbinates, right side. CPT Code(s) _____

21. Emergency endotracheal intubation. CPT Code(s) _____

22. VATS wedge resection of left lung, upper and lower lobes. CPT Code(s) _____

23. Revision of tracheostomy scar. CPT Code(s) _____

24. Bilateral endoscopic nasal polypectomy. CPT Code(s) _____

25. Laryngoscopy with excision of a vocal cord polyp using an operating microscope. CPT Code(s) _____

CODING CHALLENGE

Instructions: Read the mini-medical-record of each patient's encounter, then abstract, assign, and arrange ICD-10-CM diagnosis codes and CPT procedure codes using the appropriate Index and Tabular List. Assign quantities and modifiers where needed. Write the code(s) on the line provided.

1. OFFICE   Gender: F   Age: 2

Reason for encounter: Father noticed child place an object into her nose

Procedure: Under mild sedation, a pebble was removed from her nasal passage

Assessment: Toddler noted to have an object in her nostril

Plan: Parents given signs and symptoms of complications to watch for and instructions to give the child acetaminophen for pain.

1 ICD-10-CM Code _____

1 CPT Code _____

2. OUTPATIENT SURGERY   Gender: F   Age: 60

Preprocedure Diagnosis: bilateral pulmonary infiltrates

Procedure: Fiber optic bronchoscopy with transbronchial biopsies ×3 from various subsegments of both the right lower lobe and right middle lobe under fluoroscopic guidance

Postprocedure diagnosis: Diffuse tracheobronchitis; bilateral pneumonia

Tip: Pay attention to the instructional note under Endoscopy in the tabular list.

2 ICD-10-CM Codes _____

2 CPT Codes _____

3. INPATIENT HOSPITAL   Gender: M   Age: 56

Preprocedure diagnosis: Squamous cell carcinoma of the supraglottis; two pack per day cigarette smoker

Procedure: Total laryngectomy; bilateral modified radical neck dissection, type 1

Postprocedure diagnosis: Squamous cell carcinoma of the supraglottis

Tip: Follow the instruction at the diagnosis category in the Tabular List to identify the second diagnosis code.

2 ICD-10-CM Codes _____

1 CPT Code _____

4. OUTPATIENT SURGERY   Gender: M   Age: 38

Preprocedure diagnosis: Nasal septal deviation with bilateral inferior turbinate hypertrophy

Procedure: Nasal septoplasty; bilateral submucous resection of the inferior turbinates

Postprocedure diagnosis: Nasal septal deviation with bilateral inferior turbinate hypertrophy

2 ICD-10-CM Codes _____

2 CPT Codes _____

(continued)

(continued from page 783)

---

5. INPATIENT HOSPITAL   Gender: F   Age: 74

Preprocedure diagnosis: Left malignant pleural effusion secondary to a left lung adenocarcinoma

Procedure: Left video thoracoscopy, drainage of pleural effusion and talc poudrage

Postprocedure diagnosis: Left malignant pleural effusion secondary to a left lung adenocarcinoma

Tip: Be sure to follow the instruction in the Tabular List to sequence the diagnosis codes correctly.

2 ICD-10-CM Codes _____

1 CPT Code _____

---

6. OUTPATIENT SURGERY   Gender: M   Age: 17

Preprocedure diagnosis: Hyperhidrosis involving the soles of the feet, hands, and underarms

Procedure: Bilateral endoscopic thoracic sympathectomy

Postprocedure diagnosis: Hyperhidrosis involving the soles of the feet, hands, and underarms

3 ICD-10-CM Codes _____

1 CPT Code _____

---

7. INPATIENT HOSPITAL   Gender: F   Age: 38

Preprocedure diagnosis: Pancoast tumor of the right pulmonary apex. Patient is a former smoker for 20 years and stopped 1 year ago. Chemotherapy and radiotherapy have successfully reduced the size. No metastasis has been found.

Procedure: Resected tumor and the upper right lung. Also resected a portion of the chest wall. Performed neurovascular dissection where needed. Reconstructed affected section of chest wall. Tissue was sent to pathology.

Postprocedure diagnosis: Pancoast tumor, right upper lobe

Tip: A Pancoast tumor is a rare malignant neoplasm of the upper tip of the lung.

2 ICD-10-CM Codes _____

1 CPT Codes _____

---

8. INPATIENT HOSPITAL   Gender: F   Age: 64

Preprocedure diagnosis: Left lung mass; rule out primary lung cancer

Procedure: Fiber optic bronchoscopy with bronchioalveolar lavage; exploratory left thoracotomy; left lower lobe wedge resection for frozen section; left pneumonectomy.

Postprocedure diagnosis: Squamous cell carcinoma, left lower lobe

Tip: Read the instructional notes for Lungs and Pleura in the CPT Tabular List to help decide which codes to use.

1 ICD-10-CM Code _____

3 CPT Codes _____

_____

---

9. OUTPATIENT SURGERY   Gender: M   Age: 33

Reason for encounter: Patient is a cocaine addict, now with a large perforated septum

Procedure: A nasal button was inserted in the opening and fastened in place with sutures to repair the septum

Assessment: Perforated nasal septum

Plan: Patient is in a rehab facility and in remission of his cocaine dependence; see in office in one week

2 ICD-10-CM Codes _____

1 CPT Code _____

---

10. INPATIENT HOSPITAL   Gender: M   Age: 46

Preprocedure diagnosis: Sinus pain, facial numbness

Procedure: Maxillary endoscopy with antrostomy and removal of squamous cell carcinoma (SCCA) of the right maxillary sinus.

Postprocedure diagnosis: Squamous cell carcinoma of maxillary sinus

Plan: To be followed with radiotherapy and chemotherapy.

1 ICD-10-CM Code _____

1 CPT Code _____

Chapter 39

Nervous System Procedures (61000-64999)

Learning Objectives

After completing this chapter, you should have the skills to:

39.1 Spell and define the key words, medical terms, and abbreviations related to nervous system procedures. (Remember)

39.2 Summarize the types of nervous system procedures. (Understand)

39.3 Adhere to CPT coding guidelines in the Nervous System subsection. (Apply)

39.4 Examine and abstract procedural information from the medical record for coding Nervous System subsection procedures. (Analyze)

39.5 Demonstrate how to assign codes for procedures in the Nervous System subsection. (Apply)

39.6 Utilize guidelines for arranging (sequencing) codes for Nervous System subsection procedures. (Apply)

39.7 Determine how to code Evaluation and Management services for neurology. (Evaluate)

Chapter Outline

- **Nervous System Procedure Basics**
- **Coding Guidelines for Nervous System Procedures**
- **Abstracting Nervous System Procedures**
- **Assigning Codes for Nervous System Procedures**
- **Arranging Codes for Nervous System Procedures**
- **E/M Coding for Neurology**

Key Terms and Abbreviations

annulus fibrosus	endovascular therapy	intervertebral disc	nucleus pulposus
approach procedure (skull base)	facet	lamina	process
craniotomy	foramen	laminectomy	vertebral body
definitive procedure (skull base)	hemilaminectomy	laminotomy	

In addition to the key terms listed here, students should know the terms defined within tables in this chapter.

INTRODUCTION

When going into a store for the first time, it might take a while to learn how it is configured and how to locate what you are looking for. You might rely on your experience of common store layouts to help navigate the new setting. When coding for the nervous system, you might encounter unfamiliar medical terms and anatomic designations. By using your knowledge of medical terminology and the three skills of an "Ace" coder—abstracting, assigning, and arranging codes—you can apply what you already know to help navigate the new and sometimes complex material in this chapter.

NERVOUS SYSTEM PROCEDURE BASICS

Neurological surgery, or neurosurgery, is a medical discipline and surgical specialty that provides care for patients in the treatment of pain or disease processes that affect the nervous

system. Coders should be familiar with the organization of the nervous system, including the central nervous system (CNS) and peripheral nervous system (PNS) (■ FIGURE 39-1). The supporting structures include the meninges (*a three-layer membrane around the brain and spinal cord consisting of the dura mater, arachnoid mater, and pia mater*) (■ FIGURE 39-2), skull, skull base, and vertebral column; the vascular supply includes intracranial, extracranial, and spinal blood vessels.

Operative procedures include endovascular surgery, functional and restorative surgery, stereotactic radiosurgery, and spinal fusion and instrumentation. Neurosurgeons might concentrate their practice on procedures in a particular anatomic region, such as the brain or spinal cord. Because the nervous system and musculoskeletal system are closely related, orthopedic surgeons perform some procedures involving the nervous

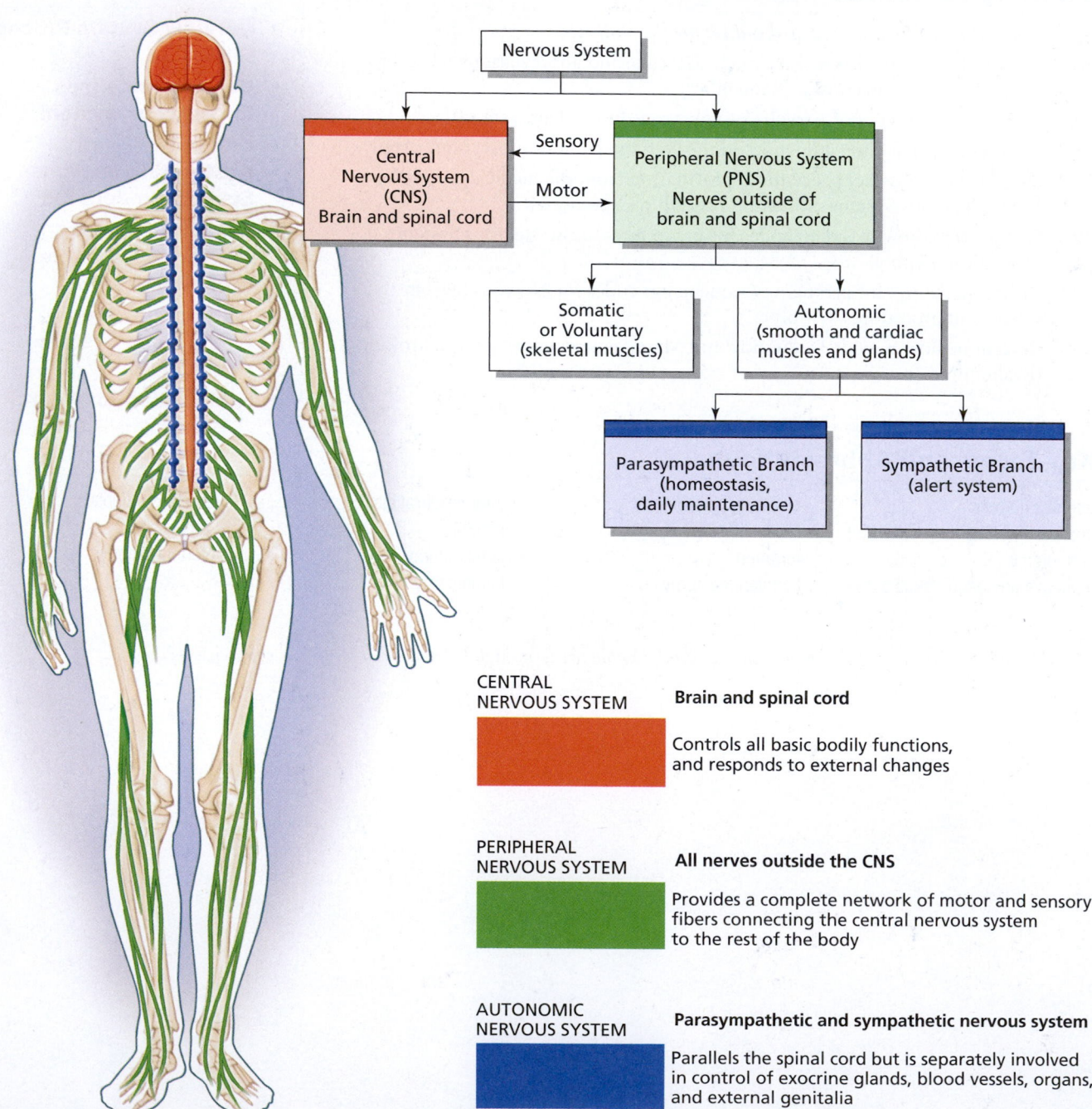

Figure 39-1 ■ The meninges of the brain and spinal cord.

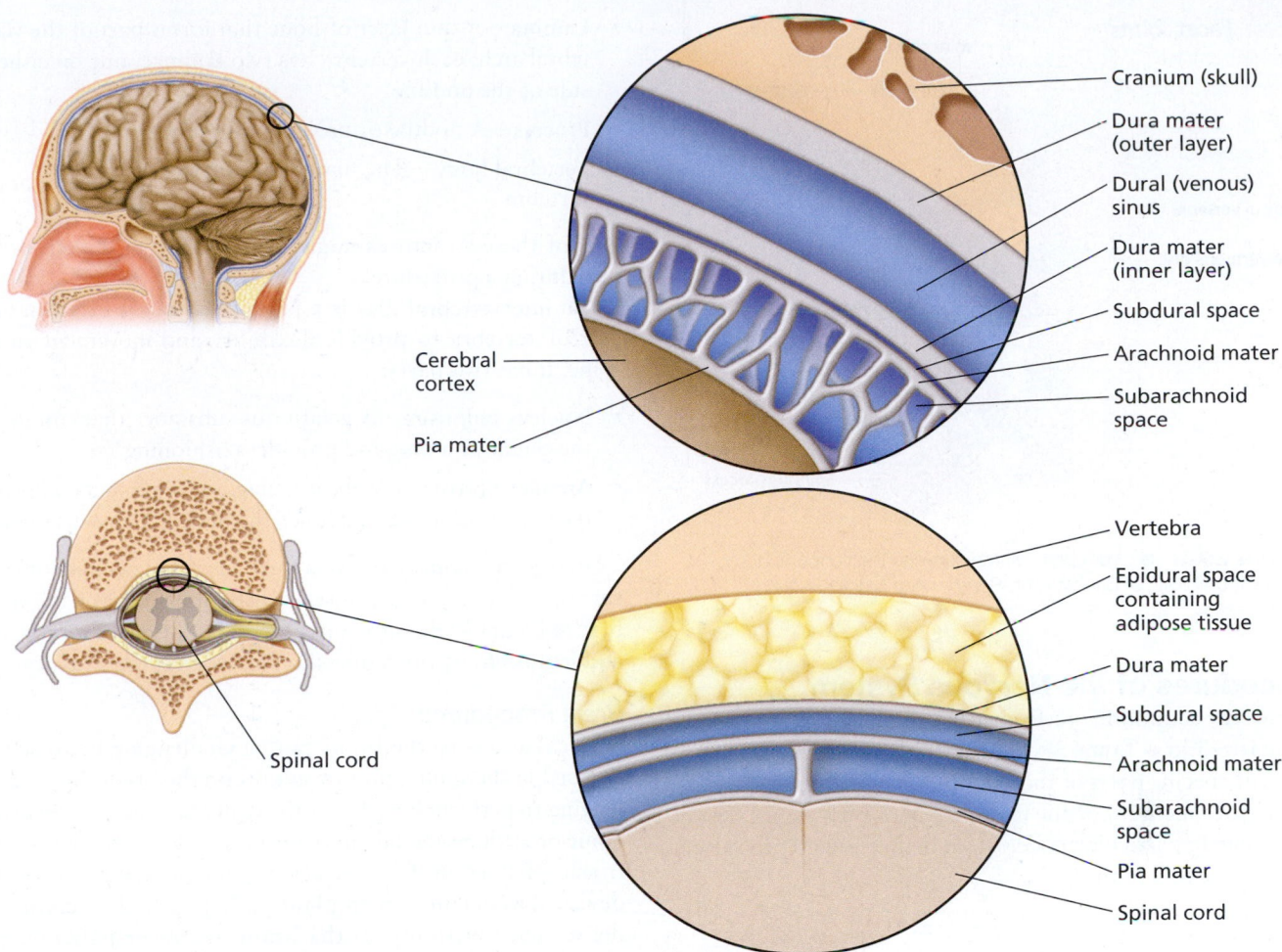

Cranium (skull)

Dura mater
(outer layer)

Dural (venous)
sinus

Dura mater
(inner layer)

Subdural space

Arachnoid mater

Subarachnoid
space

Cerebral
cortex

Pia mater

Vertebra

Epidural space
containing
adipose tissue

Dura mater

Subdural space

Arachnoid mater

Subarachnoid
space

Pia mater

Spinal cord

Spinal cord

Figure 39-2 ■ Organization of the nervous system.

system, such as spinal fusion. Neurosurgeons must consider possible problems that could arise during or after surgery and must work with an interdisciplinary team of otolaryngologists, ophthalmologists, plastic surgeons, and physical and occupational therapists to effectively manage patients' care.

Chapter 16 of this text provides more information on the anatomy and conditions of the nervous system. Refer to ■ TABLE 39-1 for a refresher on how to build medical terms related to the nervous system.

> ### CODING CAUTION
> Be alert for medical terms that are spelled similarly and have different meanings.
> **aphagia** (*lack of ability to swallow*) and **aphasia** (*lack of ability to speak*)
> **ataxia** (*lack of coordination*) and **apraxia** (*inability to perform motor tasks*)

Table 39-1   ■   EXAMPLE OF CONSTRUCTING MEDICAL TERMS FOR NERVOUS SYSTEM PROCEDURES

Combining Form	Suffix	Complete Medical Term
neur/o (*nerve*)		**neur + ectomy** (*excision of a nerve*)
		crani + ectomy (*excision of part of the skull*)
		lamin + ectomy (*excision of the lamina*)
crani/o (*skull*)	**-ectomy** (*excision*)	**neuro + tomy** (*incision into a nerve*)
	-tomy (*incision into*)	**cranio + tomy** (*incision into the skull*)
	-plasty (*repair*)	**lamino + tomy** (*incision into the lamina*)
lamin/o (*lamina*)		**neuro + plasty** (*repair of a nerve*)
		cranio + plasty (*repair of part of the skull*)
		lamino + plasty (*repair of the lamina*)

Source: © PB Resources, Inc. Used with permission.

Facet Joints

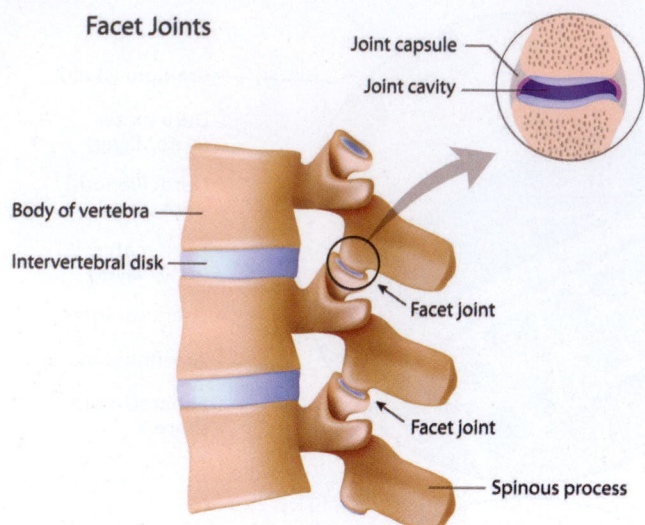

Figure 39-3 ■ Vertebral column showing the vertebral body, intervertebral disc, and facet joint. *Source: Alila Medical Media/ Shutterstock*

Procedures of the Nervous System

Procedures commonly performed on the Nervous System are summarized in ■ TABLE 39-2. Refer to detailed anatomic diagrams of specific parts of the nervous system when you need to refresh your memory of the relationship of organs and sites to each other. In particular, coders need to understand procedures on the spine and brain.

Spine Procedures

Spine procedures can be performed on the vertebrae (*the 26 bones of the spine*), the intervertebral discs (*the soft tissue between the vertebrae*), or the spinal cord (*the band of nerve tissue that extends from the brain to the lower back through the foramina [openings in the vertebrae]*). The prominent features of a vertebra used to describe procedures include:

- **Facet**—A flat surface on the edge of the spinous process that forms the connection between vertebrae (■ FIGURE 39-3)

- **Foramen**—An opening in the vertebra that surrounds the spinal cord (■ FIGURE 39-4)

- **Lamina**—A thin layer of bone that forms part of the vertebral arch; each vertebra has two laminae, one on either side of the midline

- **Process**—A nodule or projection of a bone

- **Vertebral body**—The main anterior bony part of a vertebra

Any of these structures might be removed, modified, or cut into during a procedure.

An **intervertebral disc** is a plate that occurs between each pair of vertebra to provide flexibility and movement to the spine. It has two parts:

- **Nucleus pulposus**—A gelatinous substance that comprises the center of a disc and provides cushioning

- **Annulus fibrosus**—A fibrocartilaginous ring that comprises the outside of a disc and holds the nucleus pulposus in place

Injury and damage to discs can cause pain because of pressure on the spinal cord or loss of cushioning between the vertebrae (■ Figure 39-4). Surgeons perform a variety of discectomy and laminectomy procedures to help correct the situation.

Brain Procedures

Surgical access to the brain can be challenging because it is encased in the skull, and procedures on the brain can be challenging to perform because of the delicate structures involved. Some procedures include implanting a catheter, reservoir, electroencephalogram (EEG) electrodes, and a pressure-recording device. Physicians can implant catheters and reservoirs to deliver chemotherapy to the brain in cancer patients, and catheters can also be used to drain cerebrospinal fluid (CSF). Implanted EEG electrodes monitor brain functions in patients with seizures and brain damage, and pressure-recording devices help physicians to detect intracranial pressure.

Aspiration procedures include removing CSF to test it for specific disorders, such as meningitis, or removing excess fluid caused by hydrocephalus or head trauma. The physician orders a CT scan or MRI first to determine the extent of CSF present and then withdraws fluid or directs it elsewhere in the body.

In a **craniotomy**, a physician drills or cuts into the skull to drain a hematoma or abscess or to remove part of the bone of

THE VERTEBRAL COLUMN

THORACIC VERTEBRA (SIDE VIEW)

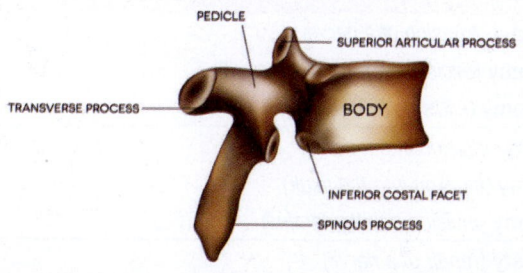

THORACIC VERTEBRA (OVERHEAD VIEW)

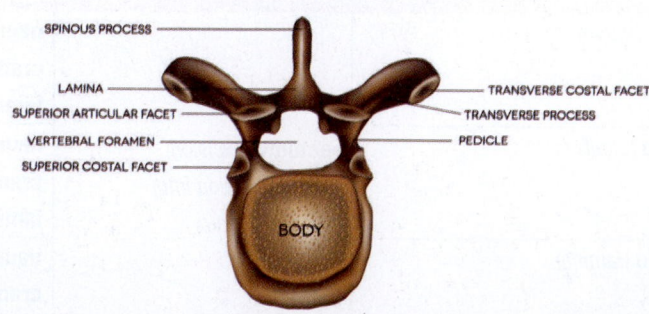

Figure 39-4 ■ A vertebra with the vertebral body, foramen, and lamina. *Source: Tefi/Shutterstock.*

Table 39-2 ■ **COMMON PROCEDURES OF THE NERVOUS SYSTEM**

Procedure Name	Definition	Reason Performed
Carpal tunnel release	Cutting of the transverse carpal ligament to release pressure on the median nerve	Carpal tunnel syndrome
Catheter procedures	Implantation, revision, or repositioning of a tunneled intrathecal or epidural catheter	Long-term medication administration; removal of an intrathecal or epidural catheter
Cerebrospinal fluid (CSF) shunt	Creation, removal, or reprogramming of a shunt and replacement or irrigation of a catheter that transports fluid from one area of the body to another (■ Figure 39-5)	Drainage of CSF from one area of the body into another (such as from the ventricles to the peritoneum)
Chemodenervation	Injection of a substance into a muscle group or glands to stop overactivity	Overactivity, such as muscle spasms or hyperhidrosis
Cisternal puncture	Withdrawal of CSF from the cisterna magna (*space between the pia mater and arachnoid membrane [thin layer of tissue covering the brain and spinal cord]*)	Diagnostic testing
Decompression	Excision of part of the skull or other body site	Drainage, excess pressure, such as from excess CSF
Deep brain stimulation (DBS)	Implantation of electrodes into a patient's brain to provide electrical stimulation to specific locations in the brain and reduce or eliminate involuntary movements	Parkinson's disease, essential tremor (*hand tremors*), dystonia (*repeated muscle contractions*), torticollis (*rotation and tilting of neck muscles*)
Discectomy	Removal of all or part of an intervertebral disc	Herniated disc
Electrocorticography	Implantation of electrodes on the brain to record electrical impulses and identify areas to surgically remove	Epilepsy
Facetectomy	Excision of the vertebral facet	Nerve decompression, pain
Hemispherectomy	Excision of one of the two cerebral hemispheres	Epilepsy
Laminectomy	Excision of the lamina	Removal of neoplasms or abnormal intervertebral discs
Lobectomy	Excision of a lobe of the brain	Epilepsy
Nerve block	Introduction or injection of an anesthetic agent	Diagnosis of source of pain or treatment of pain
Neuroendoscopy	Use of an endoscope to visualize the CNS	Dissect adhesions, remove foreign bodies, excise tumors
Neuroplasty	Any of a variety of surgical procedures to repair or alter a nerve	Nerve decompression, adhesiolysis
Neurostimulator procedures	Implantation of electrodes under the skin; removal or revision of spinal electrodes, plates, or paddles; insertion, replacement, revision, or removal of a spinal pulse generator or receiver	Intractable pain
Reservoir/pump implantation	Implantation, replacement, or removal of subcutaneous reservoir or pump; electronic analysis of programmable implanted pump	Intrathecal or epidural drug infusion
Spinal tap or puncture	Insertion of a needle into the lumbar back to collect a sample of CSF	Diagnostic testing
Stereotactic radiosurgery	Use of narrow beams of radiation with three-dimensional guidance to target lesions in difficult-to-treat areas	Brain tumors or lesions
Subdural tap	Withdrawal of CSF through a fontanelle (*a soft spot, or gap, in an infant's skull where bones have not yet formed*)	Diagnostic testing
Tractotomy	Incision of a nerve tract (*group of nerve fibers*) in the brainstem or spinal cord	Chronic pain
Ventricular puncture	Withdrawal of CSF from the ventricles of the brain by drilling a hole in the skull	Diagnostic testing

Source: © PB Resources, Inc. Used with permission.

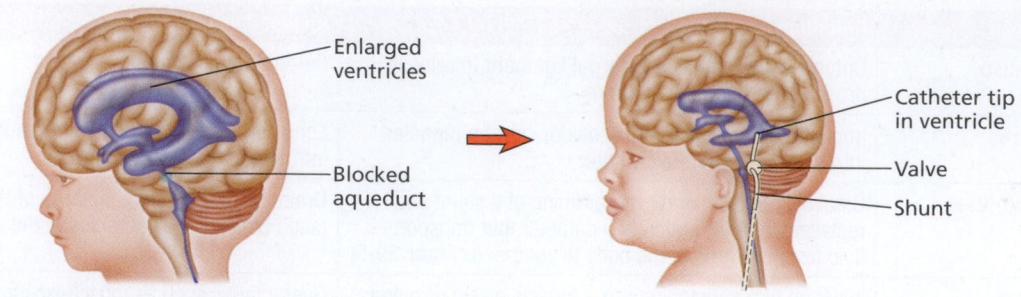

Figure 39-5 ■ Cerebrospinal fluid shunt.

the skull to gain access to perform further surgery. The procedures are named for the equipment that a physician uses to perform them—a burr and a trephine are types of saws, and a twist drill has a drill bit that is twisted.

Endovascular therapy involves inserting microcatheters (*small catheters*) into blood vessels to treat aneurysms, lesions, and neoplasms, including intracranial tumors. Treatment includes inserting balloons and stents into blood vessels or performing embolizations. In endovascular therapy neurosurgeons work with interventional radiologists to coordinate a patient's treatment and care.

This section provides a general reference to help understand the most common nervous system procedures. Remember to keep standard reference books handy in case you get stuck.

CODING CAUTION

A *ventricle* is a cavity in a body part or organ. Both the heart and the brain have ventricles, so when the term is used, remember to identify what type of ventricle is being referenced.

CODING PRACTICE

Exercise 39.1 Nervous System Procedure Basics

Instructions: Use your medical terminology skills and resources to define the following procedures related to the nervous system, then identify the code(s) or code range listed in the CPT Index. Follow these steps:

- Use slash marks "/" to break down the underlined term into its root(s) and suffix.
- Define the meaning of the underlined word based on the meaning of each word part.
- Use the entire phrase to identify the code or code range shown in the CPT Index.

Example: <u>neuroplasty</u>, cranial nerve
    neuro/plasty   Meaning <u>*surgical repair of a nerve*</u>   CPT Code <u>64716</u>

1. <u>discectomy</u>, cervical   Meaning _____ CPT Code _____

2. <u>corpectomy</u>   Meaning _____ CPT Code _____

3. <u>neurorrhaphy</u>, peripheral nerve, conduit   Meaning _____ CPT Code _____

4. <u>cranioplasty</u>, autograft   Meaning _____ CPT Code _____

5. <u>myelomeningocele</u>, repair   Meaning _____ CPT Code _____

6. <u>sympathectomy</u>, cervical   Meaning _____ CPT Code _____

7. <u>neurolysis</u>, internal   Meaning _____ CPT Code _____

8. <u>myelography</u>, spine, thoracic   Meaning _____ CPT Code _____

9. <u>cordotomy</u>, thoracic   Meaning _____ CPT Code _____

10. <u>hemilaminectomy</u>   Meaning _____ CPT Code _____

CODING GUIDELINES FOR NERVOUS SYSTEM PROCEDURES

Coders should understand the organization, guidelines, and instructional notes in the Tabular List of this CPT subsection. This information is necessary for accurate coding. The CPT subsection **Nervous System (61000-64999)** contains three subheadings that are divided by anatomic site (■ TABLE 39-3). Within each anatomic site subheading, categories are divided by the type of procedure, such as injection, repair, or excision; some categories are further divided into subcategories to provide more specific information. Review the subheading and category names and code ranges listed in the Nervous System subsection to become familiar with the content and organization. Some editions of the CPT manual provide a summary list of the subheadings and categories at the beginning of the Nervous System subsection, which also displays an asterisk (*) next to categories that contain special coding instructions.

The Nervous System subsection includes invasive, minimally invasive, and noninvasive surgical procedures on the nervous system. Codes for diagnostic tests on the nervous system appear in the Medicine section. CPT codes in the Nervous System subsection are frequently supported by diagnosis codes from ICD-10-CM Chapter 6, "Nervous System (G00-G99)," as well as neoplasms, symptoms and signs, and injuries (■ TABLE 39-4). These are the codes most commonly used to support

procedures on the nervous system; however, diagnosis codes from any ICD-10-CM chapter are permissible.

CPT guidelines for the Surgery section apply to the Nervous System.

Special instructions provide definitions and coding guidelines at the beginning of many categories, including:

- **Surgery of Skull Base**
- **Injection, Drainage, or Aspiration** category located under the **Spine and Spinal Cord** subheading
- **Endoscopic Decompression of Neural Elements and/or Excision of Herniated Intervertebral Discs** category
- **Posterior Extradural Laminotomy or Laminectomy for Exploration/Decompression of Neural Elements or Excision of Herniated Intervertebral Discs** category
- **Stereotactic Radiosurgery** and **Neurostimulators** categories, both of which occur under multiple subheadings

Remember to study these guidelines thoroughly to understand how to code accurately for these procedures. Instructional notes appear throughout the Tabular List to alert coders to the need for modifiers, provide cross-references to codes for similar procedures on other sites, identify when additional codes for radiological services might be needed, and highlight new, resequenced, and recently deleted codes. Specific guidelines and instructional notes are discussed throughout this chapter of the text.

Table 39-3 ■ NERVOUS SYSTEM SUBHEADINGS

Subheading	Code Range
Skull, Meninges, and Brain	61000-62258
Spine and Spinal Cord	62263-63746
Extracranial Nerves, Peripheral Nerves, and Autonomic Nervous System	64400-64999

Table 39-4 ■ LOCATING ICD-10-CM AND ADDITIONAL CPT CODES FOR THE NERVOUS SYSTEM

Type of Code	Codes
ICD-10-CM Nervous System–Related Codes	
Nervous system conditions	G00-G99
Neoplasms	C7A, C7B, C47, C71-C72, C79.3, C79.4
Symptoms and signs	R25-R29, R40-R49
Injuries	S00-T88
CPT Nervous System–Related Codes	
Medicine procedures	95782-96020
Radiologic procedures	
• Diagnostic radiology	70010-73725
• Radiologic guidance	77001-77022
• Diagnostic ultrasound	76506-76536, 76800
• Nuclear medicine, diagnostic	78600-78699
Laboratory/drug assays	80305-80377

Source: © PB Resources, Inc. Used with permission. CPT codes only © American Medical Association.

ABSTRACTING NERVOUS SYSTEM PROCEDURES

When abstracting for nervous system procedures, coders must pay special attention to the anatomic approach used to access the surgical site because distinct codes often identify each approach. The anatomic approach identifies the direction from which the surgical site is accessed and is often described in relation to nearby anatomic structures (■ TABLE 39-5, page 792). Approach descriptions vary based on the anatomic site being accessed because the nearby anatomic structures are different. Some spine and brain procedures are accessed from two directions, such as anterior and posterior.

SUCCESS STEP

When you encounter an approach description you are unfamiliar with, look for a prefix that identifies the direction and the root that identifies the structure. A quick Internet search for the medical term can help locate images to visualize the approach.

Refer to ■ TABLE 39-6 (page 792) for guidance on how to abstract procedures on the nervous system, then work through the detailed example that follows. Supplemental questions are provided to help identify the many variations of spine procedures. Remember that the abstracting questions are a guide and that not every question applies to, or can be answered for, every case. For example, laterality is reported for a laminectomy or laminotomy because two laminae are present—one on each side of the midline of a vertebra—but not for a discectomy because there is only one disc between each pair of vertebrae.

Table 39-5 ■ **ANATOMIC APPROACHES FOR NERVOUS SYSTEM PROCEDURES**

Approach	Definition
Anterior	From the front
Bicoronal	Through both coronal sutures (*junction of the frontal bone with the two parietal bones*) in the skull
Costovertebral	Pertaining to a rib and its adjoining vertebra
Dural	Relating to the dura mater
Epidural	From outside the dura mater
Extracranial	From outside the skull
Extradural	From outside the dura mater but within the skull
Infratentorial	Beneath the tentorium cerebelli (*fissure that divides the cerebrum and cerebellum*)
Intracranial	From within the cranium
Intradural	Within or between the membranes of the dura mater
Orbitocranial zygomatic	From the eye socket and cheek bone
Posterior	From the back
Posterolateral	From the side, toward the back
Subarachnoid	Under the arachnoid membrane
Subdural	Under the dura mater or between the dura mater and the arachnoid
Subtentorial	Same as *infratentorial*
Supratentorial	Above the tentorium cerebelli
Transcochlear	Through the cochlea
Transcondylar	Through the far lateral side of the jaw
Transcranial	Through the skull
Transorbital	Through the eye socket
Transpedicular	Through the pedicle (*base*) of a vertebra
Transpetrosal	Through a large arch extending from the temporal bone, to above and around the ear, to behind the base of the ear
Transtemporal	Through the mastoid bone

Source: © PB Resources, Inc. Used with permission.

Guided Example of Abstracting Nervous System Procedures

Refer to the following example throughout this chapter to practice skills for abstracting, assigning, and arranging Nervous System codes.

Follow along as fictitious coder Angelia Harkey, CPC, abstracts the procedure. Check off each step after you complete it.

Table 39-6 ■ **KEY CRITERIA FOR ABSTRACTING NERVOUS SYSTEM PROCEDURES**

❏ What procedure is performed?
❏ What is the anatomic site(s)?
❏ What is the surgical approach (open, closed, percutaneous, endoscopic)?
❏ What is the anatomic approach (anterior, posterior, epidural, subdural, etc.)?
❏ Is this an initial procedure or a revision/replacement?
❏ What other procedures are performed during the same encounter?

Vertebral Procedures (Laminectomy, Discectomy, Corpectomy)

❏ Which part(s) of the vertebra is treated (vertebral body, lamina, foramen, facet, disc, etc.)?
❏ How many and which segments or interspaces are treated?
❏ What is the purpose of the procedure?
❏ Is a facetectomy performed at the same time as another vertebral procedure?
❏ What is the laterality?

Source: © PB Resources, Inc. Used with permission.

INPATIENT HOSPITAL   Gender: M   Age: 45

Preoperative diagnosis: Spinal stenosis L3-L4 and L4-L5 visualized on imaging studies

Procedure: Bilateral laminotomy with decompression of nerve root and partial facetectomy at L3-L4, posterior approach, open with endoscopic assistance; right laminotomy with decompression of nerve root, partial facetectomy, and foraminotomy at L4-L5, posterior approach, open with endoscopic assistance; followed by arthrodesis of L3-L4-L5, posterior approach.

► Angelia reads through the entire record, paying special attention to the reason for the encounter, the procedure performed, and the postoperative diagnosis. She refers to the Key Criteria for Abstracting Nervous System Procedures (Table 39-6).

❏ She notes the preoperative diagnosis spinal stenosis

❏ *What is the patient's age?* 45

❏ *What site is treated?* Spine

❏ *How many and which segments or interspaces are treated?* Two interspaces: L3-L4 and L4-L5

❏ *What is the primary procedure performed?* Laminotomy

❏ *What other procedures are performed during the same encounter?* Decompression of nerve root and partial facetectomy; decompression of nerve root, partial facetectomy, and foraminotomy; arthrodesis

❏ *What is the anatomic site of the* **first** *laminotomy?* L3-L4

❏ *What is the purpose of the procedure?* Decompression of nerve root

❏ *What is the surgical approach (open, closed, percutaneous)?* Open with endoscopic assistance

❏ *What is the anatomic approach (anterior, posterior, epidural, subdural, etc.)?* Posterior

❏ *Is this an initial procedure or a revision/replacement?* Initial

❏ *Which part(s) of the vertebra is treated (vertebral body, lamina, foramen, facet, disc, etc.)?* Lamina, nerve root, and facet

❏ *Is a facetectomy performed at the same time as another vertebral procedure?* Yes

❏ *What is the laterality?* Bilateral

❏ *What is the anatomic site of the* **second** *laminotomy?* L4-L5

❏ *What is the purpose of the procedure?* Decompression of nerve root

❏ *What is the surgical approach (open, closed, percutaneous)?* Open with endoscopic assistance

❏ *What is the anatomic approach (anterior, posterior, epidural, subdural, etc.)?* Posterior

❏ *Is this an initial procedure or a revision/replacement?* Initial

❏ *Which part(s) of the vertebra is treated (vertebral body, lamina, foramen, facet, disc, etc.)?* Lamina, nerve root, facet, and foramen

❏ *Is a facetectomy performed at the same time as another vertebral procedure?* Yes

❏ *What is the laterality?* Right

❏ *What additional procedures are performed?* Arthrodesis

❏ *What is the site?* L3-L4 and L4-L5

❏ *What is the anatomic approach?* Posterior

❏ *Is a cage or device used?* No

▶ At this time, Angelia does not know which of these procedures may need to be coded, nor how many codes she will end up with. She will learn about this when she moves on to assigning codes.

CODING PRACTICE

Exercise 39.2   **Abstracting Nervous System Procedures**

Instructions: Read the mini-medical-record of each patient's encounter and answer the abstracting questions. Write the answer on the line provided. Do not assign any codes.

---

1. INPATIENT HOSPITAL   Gender: F   Age: 23

Preprocedure diagnosis: Skull fracture with hemorrhage

Procedure: Exploratory craniotomy with catheter placement. Created multiple burr holes supratentorially to explore for the source of bleeding; inserted a catheter to close off the hemorrhaging blood vessel.

a. What procedure is performed? _____

b. What is the anatomic site(s)? _____

c. What is the surgical approach (open, closed, percutaneous, endoscopic)? _____

d. What is the anatomic approach (anterior, posterior, epidural, subdural, etc.)? _____

e. Is this an initial procedure or a revision/replacement? _____

f. What other procedures are performed during the same encounter?_____

---

2. INPATIENT HOSPITAL   Gender: M   Age: 18

Preprocedure diagnosis: Congenital hydrocephalus with a ventricular shunt in place to divert CSF; recently developed headaches and visual disturbances

Procedure: Punctured the shunt tube to aspirate the excess CSF

a. What procedure is performed? _____

b. What is the anatomic site(s)? _____

c. What is the surgical approach (open, closed, percutaneous, endoscopic)? _____

d. What is the anatomic approach (anterior, posterior, epidural, subdural, etc.)?_____

e. What other procedures are performed during the same encounter?_____

(continued)

CODING PRACTICE (continued)

---

3. INPATIENT HOSPITAL Gender: F Age: 87

Preprocedure diagnosis: Cerebral meninges adhesions

Procedure: Intracranial neuroendoscopy. Created burr hole and introduced neuroendoscope through the trocar. Dissected adhesions. We removed the trocar and connected the ventricular catheter to an external collection bag. Closed and dressed the wound. Patient tolerated procedure well.

a. What procedure is performed? _____

b. What is the anatomic site(s)? _____

c. What is the surgical approach (open, closed, percutaneous, endoscopic)? _____

d. What is the anatomic approach (anterior, posterior, epidural, subdural, etc.)? _____

e. What other procedures are performed during the same encounter? _____

---

4. INPATIENT HOSPITAL Gender: F Age: 30

Preprocedure diagnosis: Nerve root compression of the cervical spine

Procedure: Cervical neck discectomy, anterior approach C3-C4, C4-C5

a. What procedure is performed? _____

b. What is the anatomic site(s)? _____

c. What is the surgical approach (open, closed, percutaneous, endoscopic)? _____

d. What is the anatomic approach (anterior, posterior, epidural, subdural, etc.)? _____

e. Is this an initial procedure or a revision/replacement?

f. What other procedures are performed during the same encounter? _____

g. Which part(s) of the vertebra is treated (vertebral body, lamina, foramen, facet, disc, etc.)? _____

h. How many and which segments or interspaces are treated? _____

i. What is the purpose of the procedure? _____

j. Is a facetectomy performed at the same time as another vertebral procedure? _____

k. What is the laterality? _____

---

5. OUTPATIENT SURGERY Gender: M Age: 35

Preprocedure diagnosis: Lacerations to the right thumb and index finger

Procedure: Neurorrhaphy to the right thumb and index finger

a. What procedure is performed? _____

b. What is the anatomic site(s)? _____

c. What is the surgical approach (open, closed, percutaneous, endoscopic)? _____

d. What is the anatomic approach (anterior, posterior, epidural, subdural, etc.)? _____

e. Is this an initial procedure or a revision/replacement?

f. What is the laterality? _____

---

6. INPATIENT HOSPITAL Gender: F Age: 48

Preprocedure diagnosis: Stenosis C4-C5, foraminal stenosis L5-S1

Procedure: Right hemilaminectomy at C4-C5, posterior approach; left hemilaminectomy with foraminotomy at L5-S1, posterior approach

a. What procedure is performed? _____

b. What is the anatomic site(s)? _____

c. What is the surgical approach (open, closed, percutaneous, endoscopic)? _____

d. What is the anatomic approach (anterior, posterior, epidural, subdural, etc.)? _____

e. Is this an initial procedure or a revision/replacement?

f. What other procedures are performed during the same encounter? _____

g. Which part(s) of the vertebra is treated (vertebral body, lamina, foramen, facet, disc, etc.)? _____

h. How many and which segments or interspaces are treated? _____

i. What is the purpose of the procedure? _____

j. Is a facetectomy performed at the same time as another vertebral procedure? _____

k. What is the laterality? _____

ASSIGNING CODES FOR NERVOUS SYSTEM PROCEDURES

To assign codes for Nervous System subsection procedures, search the Index for the Main Term for the anatomic site, such as **Skull** or **Nerve**, then locate the first-level modifying term and any second-level modifying terms for the type of procedure. If you cannot find the necessary procedure under the anatomic site, then search for the Main Term for the name of the procedure, such as **Laminectomy**.

The Tabular List does not list separate procedures for each individual nerve. Major nerve branches may be covered by the same code or commonly treated nerves might be specifically identified in separate codes, depending on the procedure. Coders need to read the codes in the Tabular List carefully and be able to identify the general location of major nerve branches.

> EXAMPLE: *The surgeon performed neuroplasty on the ulnar nerve at the elbow.*
> 64718 Neuroplasty and/or transposition; ulnar nerve at elbow

> EXAMPLE: *The surgeon excised a neuroma from the ulnar nerve.*
> 64784 Excision of neuroma; major peripheral nerve, except sciatic

Coders should pay special attention to assigning codes for basilar (*pertaining to the base*) skull procedures and laminectomies. These procedures are discussed next.

Assigning Codes for Basilar Skull Procedures

Procedures in the category of **Surgery of Skull Base** include removal of many different types of lesions of the skull base (■ TABLE 39-7). The surgery is difficult, involved, and time-consuming because the skull base is not easily accessible. The procedure often requires a team of specialized surgeons to perform various components of the surgery. Skull base surgery often requires more than one CPT code.

CPT provides detailed guidelines about coding skull base procedures. Codes are divided by the three parts of a skull base procedure, listed as the subcategories **Approach Procedures**, **Definitive Procedure**, and **Repair or Reconstruction Procedure**.

Approach Procedure

The **approach procedure** is performed to access or expose the lesion. It is described based on the anatomic site—the location where the physician gains access to a lesion in the skull base. Approach procedure codes (**61580-61598**) are divided as follows:

- Anterior cranial fossa—Procedures on the anterior lobe of the brain
- Middle cranial fossa—Procedures on the temporal lobes of the brain
- Posterior cranial fossa—Procedures on the occipital lobes of the brain

Table 39-7 ■ **TYPES OF SKULL BASE LESIONS**

Type of Lesion	Description
Aneurysm	Excessive blood vessel dilation, which could lead to a ruptured blood vessel or vein
Arteriovenous malformation (AVM)	Abnormal connection between arteries and veins, usually congenital
Basilar skull fracture	A linear fracture in the anterior or middle skull base or the posterior fossa
CSF fistula	An abnormal connection between the subarachnoid space around the brain and either the sinuses or the ear that allows the passage of CSF
Giant-cell bone tumor	A rare, aggressive, benign tumor, generally occurring in adults between the ages of 20 and 40 years
Neurofibroma	A benign tumor of nerve fibers and connective tissue
Orbital tumor	A benign or malignant tumor in the eye socket or tissues that surround the eyeball; sometimes originating from the surrounding paranasal sinuses, brain, or nasal cavity
Pituitary tumor	An abnormal growth in the pituitary gland that is usually benign

Source: © PB Resources, Inc. Used with permission.

Codes are further divided by the anatomic approach to access the specific part of the cranial fossa, such as craniofacial or infratemporal. Approach procedures can also include other procedures that the physician must perform at the same time, such as a rhinotomy (*incision into the nose*).

Definitive Procedure

The **definitive procedure** is performing the repair, biopsy, resection, or excision of a lesion. It includes primary closure of the dura, mucous membranes, and skin. CPT arranges definitive procedures (**61600-61616**) by anatomic site: the base of the anterior, middle, or posterior cranial fossa. Codes are further divided based on the approach, such as extradural or intradural.

Repair or Reconstruction Procedure

Repair and reconstruction procedures are reported if extensive dural grafts, cranioplasty, local myocutaneous pedicle flaps (*skin flap with muscle attached*), or extensive skin grafts are required. There are only two codes for a repair/reconstruction procedure: repair by free tissue graft (**61618**) and repair by pedicle or myocutaneous flap (**61619**).

Assigning Codes for Multiple Procedures or Multiple Surgeons

To assign codes for the approach or definitive skull base procedure, search the Index for the Main Term **Skull Base Surgery**, then locate the first-level modifying term of the location, including anterior cranial fossa, middle cranial fossa, or posterior cranial fossa. Locations are further divided by second-level modifying terms that identify the type of approach, such as bicoronal or craniofacial. To assign codes for a skull base repair/reconstruction procedure, search the Index for the Main Term **Skull Base Surgery**, then locate the first-level modifying term **Dura** and the second-level modifying term **Repair of cerebrospinal fluid leak**.

To assign codes for multiple skull base procedures and/or multiple surgeons, follow these guidelines:

- When separate physicians each perform distinct parts of a skull base procedure, identified by separate CPT codes, each physician should report a code for the procedure that he or she completes (■ FIGURE 39-6).

- When multiple surgeons work together to perform a single procedure, both report the same CPT code and append the appropriate modifier to indicate their respective roles. Modifiers are discussed later in this chapter.

- When one physician performs more than one part of a skull base procedure and each part is identified by separate CPT codes, report a code for each procedure, sequencing the most complex procedure first and appending modifier **-51 Multiple procedures** to the lesser procedure(s).

Assigning Codes for Laminectomy Procedures

Laminotomy and laminectomy are spinal decompression surgeries involving the lamina, a thin bony layer that covers and protects the spinal canal and spinal cord. Laminotomy, also called a hemilaminectomy, is the partial removal of the lamina, whereas laminectomy is the complete removal of the lamina. CPT indexes *laminotomy* under the Main Term **Hemilaminectomy** and *laminectomy* under the Main Term **Laminectomy**. Each of these Main Terms leads to separate codes in the Tabular List. The terms are often used interchangeably in noncoding matters, so it is important to understand the work performed and to review the code descriptions thoroughly.

A laminectomy is often done in conjunction with another procedure to resolve a problem, such as disc compression or a herniated disk (■ FIGURE 39-7). Procedures such as foraminotomy, facetectomy, discectomy, and/or bone grafts are often bundled into a single code. Therefore, in both the Index and Tabular List coders must be alert for code variations. Also be alert for procedures that should be coded separately, such as arthrodesis (■ FIGURE 39-8).

To locate codes for spinal procedures, search the Index for either the anatomic site or the procedure name. When searching by anatomic site, if the desired procedure or site does not appear under the Main Term **Spine**, refer to a Main Term for the appropriate part of the spine, such as **Spinal Cord**, **Intervertebral Disc**, or **Vertebra**. Using procedure names such as **Laminectomy**, **Hemilaminectomy**, or **Discectomy** as the Main Term often more directly leads to the desired code.

Many Index entries list codes for both nervous system and musculoskeletal system procedures. Nervous system procedures begin with 6, whereas musculoskeletal procedures begin with 2. Review code descriptions carefully to be sure you select the correct code based on the documentation.

In the Tabular List one or more parent codes may appear with slightly different variations of a laminectomy, followed by indented codes for alternative regions of the spine. Codes for vertebral corpectomy provide separate parent codes for each spinal region, with an add-on for additional segments in the same region. To select and verify codes, follow these steps:

1. Compare the unique descriptors of the parent codes to locate the correct code family.

2. Identify the correct indented code to identify the appropriate spinal region.

3. Locate add-on codes for additional vertebra or interspaces, when applicable.

4. Read instructional notes to identify any procedures, such as arthrodesis, that might need to be coded separately.

Dr. A and Dr. B work together to treat a patient with a carotid aneurysm. Dr. A performs the access to the cavernous sinus using an infratemporal post-auricular approach to middle cranial fossa. Dr. B dissects and ligates the carotid aneurysm, reapproximates the scalp, and sutures the wound closed.

Dr. A—Approach procedure:
61591 Infratemporal post-auricular approach to middle cranial fossa (internal auditory meatus, petrous apex, tentorium, cavernous sinus, parasellar area, infratemporal fossa) including mastoidectomy, resection of sigmoid sinus, with or without decompression and/or mobilization of contents of auditory canal or petrous carotid artery

Dr. B—Definitive procedure:
61613 Obliteration of carotid aneurysm, arteriovenous malformation, or carotid-cavernous fistula by dissection within cavernous sinus

Figure 39-6 ■ Example of coding skull base procedures. *Source: © PB Resources, Inc. Used with permission. CPT codes only © American Medical Association.*

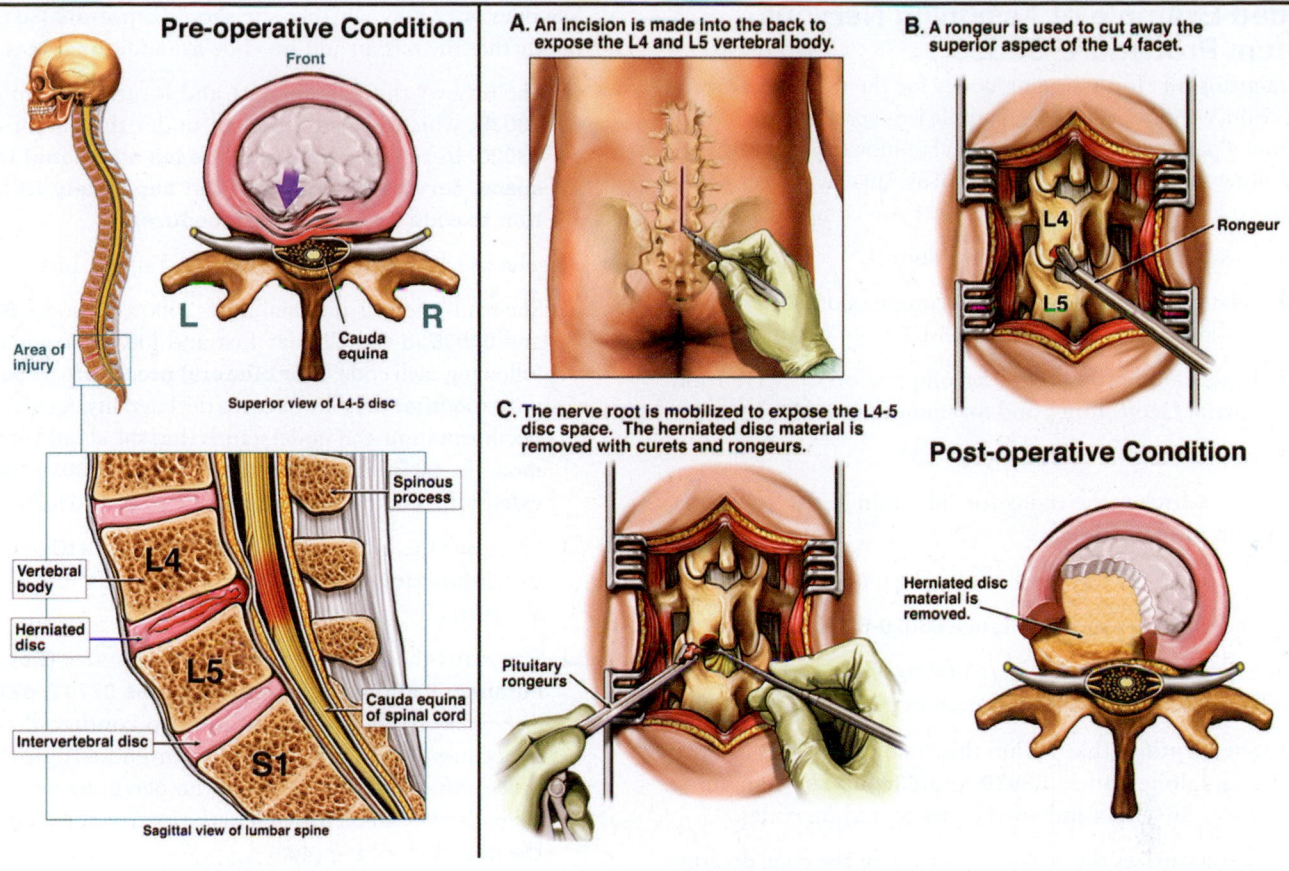

Pre-operative Condition

Front

L   R

Cauda
equina

Superior view of L4-5 disc

Area of
injury

Spinous
process

Vertebral
body   L4

Herniated
disc

L5

Cauda equina
of spinal cord

Intervertebral disc   S1

Sagittal view of lumbar spine

A. An incision is made into the back to expose the L4 and L5 vertebral body.

B. A rongeur is used to cut away the superior aspect of the L4 facet.

L4

Rongeur

L5

C. The nerve root is mobilized to expose the L4-5 disc space. The herniated disc material is removed with curets and rongeurs.

Post-operative Condition

Herniated disc
material is
removed.

Pituitary
rongeurs

Figure 39-7 ■ Discectomy procedure. *Source: Nucleus Medical Media Inc/Alamy Stock Photo.*

Pre-operative Condition

L3

Vertebral body

Intervertebral
disc   L4

Cauda equina
of spinal cord

L5

S1

L5-S1 spondylolisthesis

Sagittal view of lumbosacral spine

A. Bone graft is harvested from the posterior left iliac crest.

Bone
graft

B. A midline incision is made in the back allowing access to the L5-S1 area.

C. A laminectomy is performed at L5-S1. Pedicle and sacral screws are placed.

Fixation
screws

L4

Cauda equina
of spinal cord   L5

S1

D. Fixation rods are secured into the pedicle screws and iliac bone graft is applied for final fusion.

Fixation
hardware

Post-operative Condition

L3

L4

L5

S1

Lateral view

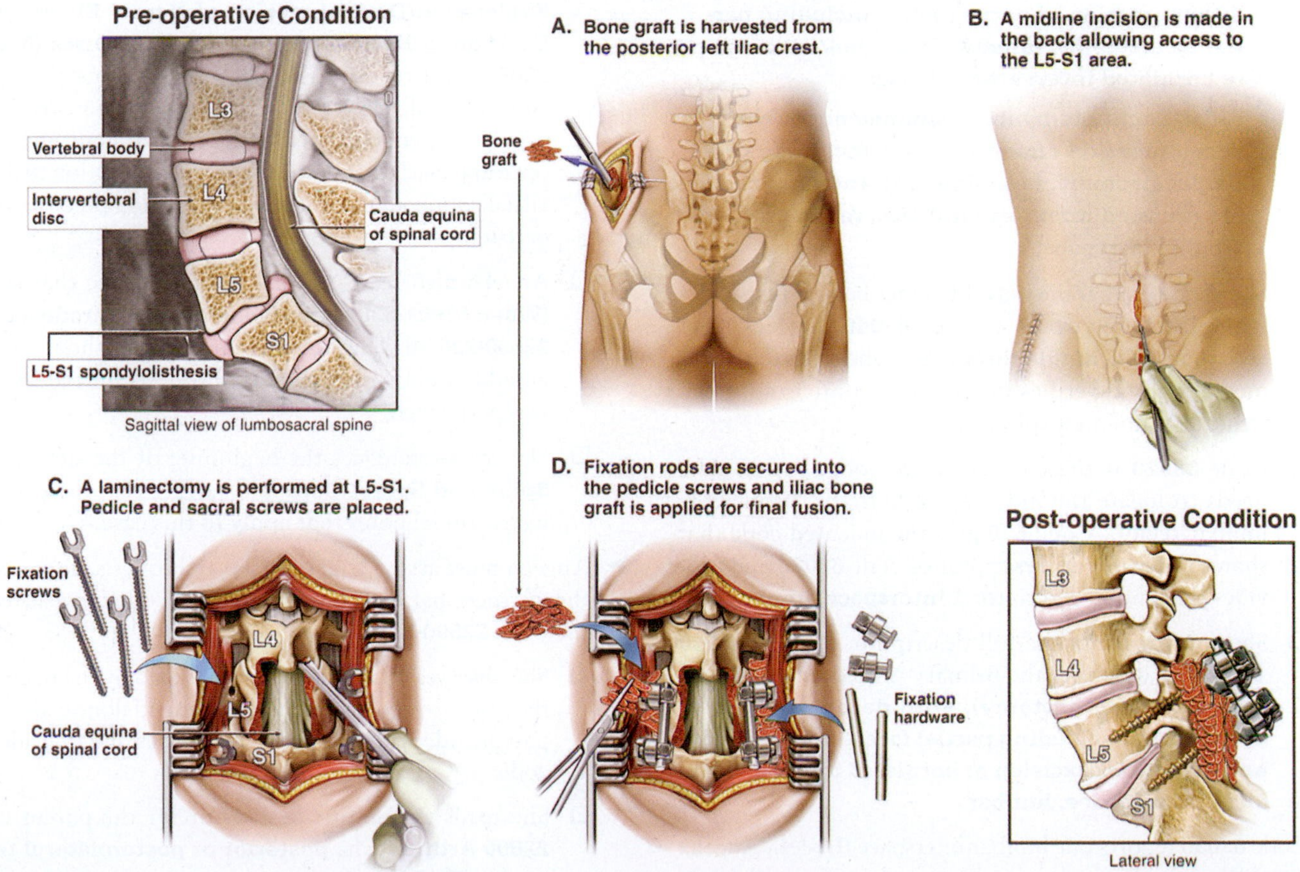

Figure 39-8 ■ Laminectomy procedure with bone graft and fixation. *Source: © Nucleus Medical Media Inc/Alamy Stock Photo.*

Guided Example of Assigning Nervous System Procedure Codes

To practice skills for assigning codes for the Nervous System subsection, continue with the example from earlier in the chapter about a patient who was seen for a laminotomy and arthrodesis. Follow along in your CPT manual as Angelia Harkey, CPC, assigns codes. Check off each step after you complete it.

▶ First, Angelia confirms the procedures:

❏ Bilateral laminotomy with decompression of nerve root and partial facetectomy at L3-L4

❏ Right laminotomy with decompression of nerve root, partial facetectomy, and foraminotomy at L4-L5

❏ Arthrodesis of L3-L4 and L4-L5

▶ Angelia searches the Index for the Main Term **Hemilaminectomy**.

❏ There are no first-level modifying terms.

❏ She identifies the code range **63020-63044**.

▶ Angelia turns to the Tabular List to select and verify the codes needed for both laminotomies.

❏ She identifies that within this code range there are two standalone codes: **63020** and **63040**. The remaining codes are either indented codes or add-on codes.

❏ She compares the common portion of the code descriptions word for word:

▪ **63020 Laminotomy (hemilaminectomy), with decompression of nerve root(s), including partial facetectomy, foraminotomy and/or excision of herniated intervertebral disc;**

▪ **63040 Laminotomy (hemilaminectomy), with decompression of nerve root(s), including partial facetectomy, foraminotomy and/or excision of herniated intervertebral disc, reexploration, single interspace;**

❏ She identifies that the only difference between the codes is the last three words of code **63040** that describes **reexploration, single interspace**. She reads the documentation and verifies that the procedure is an initial treatment, not a reexploration.

❏ Code **63020** is the correct parent code, but Angelia needs to locate the indented code that identifies the lumbar region. Code **63030** is the indented code that shares the common descriptor of code **63020** and provides the unique descriptor **1 interspace, lumbar**.

❏ She confirms that the full description of code **63030** accurately describes the primary procedure: **Laminotomy (hemilaminectomy), with decompression of nerve root(s), including partial facetectomy, foraminotomy and/or excision of herniated intervertebral disc; 1 interspace, lumbar**.

▶ Code **63030** reports one lumbar interspace (L3-L4). Angelia must determine how to report the second interspace (L4-L5).

She does not know whether she should report **63030** twice or whether there is an add-on code for additional sites.

❏ She reviews the Tabular List and locates add-on code **63035**, which is also indented under the parent code **63020**. Its unique descriptor is **each additional interspace, cervical or lumbar (List separately in addition to code for primary procedure)**.

▶ Angelia checks for instructions in the Tabular List.

❏ She reads the instructional notes following codes **63030** and **63035** in the Tabular List and locates a statement following each code: **(For bilateral procedure, report … with modifier 50)**. She refers to the laterality details in the documentation and understands that she should append modifier **-50 Bilateral procedure** to code **63030** and, by extension, modifier **-RT Right side** to code **63035**.

❏ She reads the instructional note that states **(Use 63035 in conjunction with 63020-63030)**. This verifies that she correctly applied the add-on code.

❏ She reads the instructional note that states **(For percutaneous endoscopic approach, see 0274T, 0275T)**. She refers to the documentation to confirm that the procedure approach is open with endoscopic assistance, which is different than the percutaneous endoscopic approach mentioned in the instructional note, so the note does not apply.

❏ She cross-references the beginning of category **Posterior Extradural Laminotomy or Laminectomy for Exploration/Decompression of Neural Elements or Excision of Herniated Intervertebral Discs (63001-63051)** and reads the special instructions regarding endoscopically assisted laminotomy. The instructions clarify that endoscopically assisted laminotomy is an open approach that uses endoscopy in addition to direct visualization and confirms that she should not report a percutaneous endoscopy procedure.

❏ Angelia also reads the instructional note that states **(When 63001-63048 are followed by arthrodesis, see 22590-22614)**. This note tells her that she should report an additional code for the arthrodesis procedure that was performed.

❏ She cross-references the beginning of the subheading **Spine and Spinal Cord** and verifies that there are no instructional notes that apply to this case.

▶ Angelia must assign codes for the arthrodesis, as stated in the instructional note. She refers to the code range listed in the note, **22590-22614**.

❏ She observes that the codes are divided by the region of the spine treated and include two standalone codes: one parent code with three indented codes and one add-on code.

❏ She reads the unique descriptor for the parent code **22600 Arthrodesis, posterior or posterolateral technique, single level;**

❏ She locates the indented code description for the lumbar spine, **22612 Arthrodesis, posterior or posterolateral technique, single level; lumbar (with lateral transverse technique, when performed)**. This code accurately describes the first arthrodesis procedure performed. However, because two interspaces were fixated, she needs a second code.

❏ She locates an add-on code that reports the second interspace treated: **22614 Arthrodesis, posterior or posterolateral technique, single level; each additional vertebral segment (List separately in addition to code for primary procedure)**.

❏ She reads the instructional notes that appear after the codes. She also reads the special instructions for the subcategory **Posterior, Posterolateral or Lateral Transverse Process Technique**. These instructions provide definitions of vertebral segment and an interspace.

▶ Angelia reviews the procedure codes she has assigned for this case.

❏ **22612 Arthrodesis, posterior or posterolateral technique, single level; lumbar (with lateral transverse technique, when performed)**

❏ **22614 Arthrodesis, posterior or posterolateral technique, single level; each additional vertebral segment**

❏ **63030 Laminotomy (hemilaminectomy), with decompression of nerve root(s), including partial facetectomy, foraminotomy and/or excision of herniated intervertebral disc; 1 interspace, lumbar**

❏ **63035 Laminotomy (hemilaminectomy), with decompression of nerve root(s), including partial facetectomy, foraminotomy and/or excision of herniated intervertebral disc; each additional interspace, cervical or lumbar**

▶ Next, Angelia must assign modifiers and determine how to sequence the codes.

CODING PRACTICE

Exercise 39.3   Assigning Codes for Nervous System Procedures

Instructions: Read the mini-medical-record of each patient's encounter. Review the information abstracted in Exercise 39.2 for questions 1–3. For questions 4–6, abstract the case on your own. Assign CPT codes, quantities, and modifiers using the Index and Tabular List. Write the code(s) on the line provided.

1. INPATIENT HOSPITAL   Gender: F   Age: 23

Preprocedure diagnosis: Skull fracture with hemorrhage

Procedure: Exploratory craniotomy with catheter placement. Created multiple burr holes supratentorially to explore for the source of bleeding; inserted a catheter to close off the hemorrhaging blood vessel.

1 CPT Code _____

2. INPATIENT HOSPITAL   Gender: M   Age: 18

Preprocedure diagnosis: Congenital hydrocephalus with a ventricular shunt in place to divert CSF; recently developed headaches and visual disturbances

Procedure: Punctured the shunt tube to aspirate the excess CSF

Tip: The Main Term is the anatomic site where the shunt is placed.

1 CPT Code _____

3. INPATIENT HOSPITAL   Gender: F   Age: 87

Preprocedure diagnosis: Cerebral meninges adhesions

Procedure: Intracranial neuroendoscopy. Created burr hole and introduced neuroendoscope through the trocar. Dissected adhesions. We removed the trocar and connected the ventricular catheter to an external collection bag. Closed and dressed the wound. Patient tolerated procedure well.

1 CPT Code _____

4. EMERGENCY DEPT   Gender: M   Age: 16

Preprocedure diagnosis: Injury to hand from broken glass

Procedure: Sutured the right ulnar motor nerve

1 CPT Code _____

5. INPATIENT HOSPITAL   Gender: F   Age: 27

Preprocedure diagnosis: Depressed skull fracture

Procedure: Repair of dura to elevate skull

1 CPT Code _____

6. INPATIENT HOSPITAL   Gender: M   Age: 63

Preprocedure diagnosis: 14-mm arteriosclerotic brain aneurysm in the frontal portion of skull

Procedure: Removed the aneurysm by intracranial and cervical occlusion of the carotid artery

1 CPT Code _____

ARRANGING CODES FOR NERVOUS SYSTEM PROCEDURES

Many spinal procedures are grouped into code families with separate parent codes describing the procedure at a single vertebral level in the cervical, thoracic, or lumbar region of the spine. Within some code families an add-on code reports the same procedure at each additional level, but the spinal region is not specified. Surgeons may operate on various combinations of spinal regions and vertebral levels. The National Correct Coding Initiative (NCCI) provides the following instructions for reporting procedures on multiple vertebral segments or multiple interspaces:

* When vertebral levels from different spinal regions are treated, report a parent code for each spinal region treated.

  EXAMPLE: When both C4 and T3 are treated, report a parent code for the cervical region and a parent code for the thoracic region.

* When multiple procedures from one code family are performed at contiguous vertebral levels, report the parent code for one level and add-on codes for any additional levels within the same family.

  EXAMPLE: When C3, C4, and C5 are treated, report the parent code for the cervical region and the add-on code times two.

* When the contiguous levels are in two different spinal regions, report the parent code from the first spinal region for the first level and an add-on code for the second level.

  EXAMPLE: When T12 and L1 are treated, report the parent code for the thoracic region and one add-on code because these segments are contiguous.

Remember that vertebrae are identified singly, such as the C4 or L2 vertebral segment. Interspaces and discs are identified by the vertebrae above and below the space, such as the C4-C5 interspace. Assign only one code for each interspace, even though it is identified using the two adjacent vertebrae.

Modifiers

Among the more commonly used modifiers for Nervous System procedures are those for multiple procedures, laterality, and multiple surgeons.

-51 Multiple Procedures

Append modifier **-51** when more than one procedure is performed during the same operative session by the same surgeon, except for add-on codes. Only one code (**61107**) in the Nervous System subsection is exempt from modifier **-51**, indicated by the symbol ⊘. Do not append modifier **-51** when two procedures are performed, each by a different surgeon.

Laterality

Report laterality for paired nerves or paired anatomic sites, including laminae. Be alert for instructional notes in the Tabular List that direct when to use modifier **-50 Bilateral**

procedure. Do not report laterality for procedures on vertebrae or discs.

Multiple Surgeons

Nervous system procedures may involve multiple surgeons, including a surgical team, cosurgeons, or a primary and assistant surgeon. The operative report should identify the name and role of each surgeon. In the workplace you will be coding for a specific surgeon or for all surgeons from a specific practice, but you will not code for surgeons from other practices. When two or more surgeons perform distinct parts of one procedure with one CPT code, assign a modifier to identify the role of the specific surgeon for whom you are coding. The most commonly used modifiers in this situation are:

* **-62 Two surgeons**
* **-66 Surgical team**
* **-80 Assistant surgeon**

When two surgeons each perform a different procedure, each with a different CPT code, as may occur with skull base procedures, a modifier is not necessary.

Guided Example of Arranging Nervous System Procedure Codes

To practice skills for arranging codes for procedures of the Nervous System subsection, continue with the example from earlier in the chapter about the patient who was seen for a laminotomy and arthrodesis. Follow along in your CPT manual as Angelia Harkey, CPC, arranges the codes. Check off each step after you complete it.

▶ First, Angelia reviews the procedure codes she has assigned for this case.

   ❏ **22612 Arthrodesis, posterior or posterolateral technique, single level; lumbar (with lateral transverse technique, when performed)**

   ❏ **22614 Arthrodesis, posterior or posterolateral technique, single level; each additional vertebral segment**

   ❏ **63030 Laminotomy (hemilaminectomy), with decompression of nerve root(s), including partial facetectomy, foraminotomy and/or excision of herniated intervertebral disc; 1 interspace, lumbar**

   ❏ **63035 Laminotomy (hemilaminectomy), with decompression of nerve root(s), including partial facetectomy, foraminotomy and/or excision of herniated intervertebral disc; each additional interspace, cervical or lumbar**

▶ The laminotomy is the primary procedure, so code **63030** is sequenced first, followed by the related add-on code for the second laminotomy, **63035**.

▶ The arthrodesis procedures are secondary, so code **22612** is sequenced next, followed by the related add-on code for the second interspace **22614**.

► Angelia examines the need for modifiers. (Refer to Table 27-1, Key Criteria for Abstracting CPT Modifiers, or Appendix A in the CPT manual.)

❑ Both of these codes require laterality modifiers. She verifies the procedures in the medical record and confirms that **63030** is a bilateral procedure, so she appends modifier **-50**.

❑ Code **63035** identifies a procedure performed on the right side, so she appends modifier **-RT**. Although the code description specifies cervical or lumbar interspace, there is no CPT modifier used to identify the spinal region is treated.

❑ Arthrodesis procedures are performed on the full interspace, so laterality modifiers are not required.

❑ Code **22612** is a standalone code and is an additional procedure performed during the same operative session, so modifier **-51 Multiple procedures** is required. Use of this modifier is discussed in the special instructions in the subheading **Arthrodesis** that appears before code **22532** in the Tabular List.

❑ Code **22614** is an add-on code, so modifier **-51** is not used.

► Angelia finalizes the procedure codes and sequencing for this case:

(1) **63030-50 Laminotomy (hemilaminectomy), with decompression of nerve root(s), including partial facetectomy, foraminotomy and/or excision of herniated intervertebral disc; 1 interspace, lumbar; -50 Bilateral procedure**

(2) **63035-RT Laminotomy (hemilaminectomy), with decompression of nerve root(s), including partial facetectomy, foraminotomy and/or excision of herniated intervertebral disc; each additional interspace, cervical or lumbar; -RT Right side**

(3) **22612-51 Arthrodesis, posterior or posterolateral technique, single level; lumbar (with lateral transverse technique, when performed); -51 Multiple procedures**

(4) **22532 Arthrodesis, posterior or posterolateral technique, single level; each additional vertebral segment**

► Angelia also assigns and sequences the ICD-10-CM diagnosis codes that support the need for the service.

(1) **M48.061 Spinal stenosis, lumbar region without neurogenic claudication**

CODING PRACTICE

Exercise 39.4   Arranging Codes for Nervous System Procedures

Instructions: Read the mini-medical-record of each patient's encounter. Review the information abstracted in Exercise 39.2 for questions 1–3. For questions 4–6, abstract the case on your own. Assign CPT codes, quantities, and modifiers using the Index and Tabular List, and arrange the codes in proper sequence. Write the code(s) on the line provided.

1. INPATIENT HOSPITAL   Gender: F   Age: 30

Preprocedure diagnosis: Nerve root compression of the cervical spine

Procedure: Cervical neck discectomy, anterior approach C3-C4, C4-C5

2 CPT Codes _____

2. OUTPATIENT SURGERY   Gender: M   Age: 35

Preprocedure diagnosis: Lacerations to the right thumb and index finger

Procedure: Neurorrhaphy to the right thumb and index finger

Tip: A digital nerve is one in the finger.

2 CPT Codes _____

3. INPATIENT HOSPITAL   Gender: F   Age: 48

Preprocedure diagnosis: Stenosis C4-C5, foraminal stenosis L5-S1

Procedure: Right hemilaminectomy at C4-C5, posterior approach; left hemilaminectomy with foraminotomy at L5-S1, posterior approach

Tip: The two procedures are performed on different spinal regions, so assign separate parent codes.

2 CPT Codes _____

4. INPATIENT HOSPITAL   Gender: M   Age: 84

Preprocedure diagnosis: Return to the operating room because of a subdural hematoma following surgery I performed yesterday

Procedure: Craniotomy to evacuate the hematoma; used a skull trephine craniotome to access the hematoma, then, under direct visualization, suctioned out the hematoma

Tip: Use the Main Term *Craniotomy*. Append a modifier for the return to the operating room.

1 CPT Code _____

(continued)

CODING PRACTICE *(continued)*

5. INPATIENT HOSPITAL Gender: M Age: 68

Preprocedure diagnosis: Primary malignant neoplasm of the cranial fossa

Procedure: Surgeon A: Resection of the posterior cranial fossa, extradural; removed entire tumor

Surgeon B: Performed the transtemporal approach

Tip: Code for both surgeons.

Surgeon A: 1 CPT Code _____

Surgeon B: 1 CPT Code _____

6. OUTPATIENT SURGERY Gender: M Age: 28

Preprocedure diagnosis: Lumbar back pain

Procedure: Fluoroscopic-guided destruction of paravertebral facet joint nerves bilaterally at L2 and L3 with use of a neurolytic agent

Tip: Read the instructional notes in the Tabular List regarding the use of a modifier.

2 CPT Codes _____

E/M CODING FOR NEUROLOGY

The *1997 Documentation Guidelines for Evaluation and Management Services* (1997 DG), published by the Centers for Medicare and Medicaid Services (CMS), provides requirements for each level of a neurological E/M examination (■ FIGURE 39-9). Neurologists are not limited to using the guidelines for a neurology examination only. They can also use guidelines for a general multiorgan system examination, or any other single organ system examination, based on what is most advantageous for a specific encounter. However, physicians cannot combine elements from more than one type of examination for a given encounter. The neurological examination guidelines typically provide the best results when a detailed neurological examination is performed.

To determine the appropriate E/M code, coders must review the documentation in detail and identify the specific elements documented.

- To translate the documentation into the E/M requirements for the history, refer back to Chapter 28, "Evaluation and Management Services (99201-99499)," Tables 28-7 to 28-10, or to the 1997 DG.

- To determine the requirements for an examination, refer to ■ Figure 39-9 or to the single organ system examination for neurology in the 1997 DG.

- To determine the levels for medical decision making (MDM), refer to Chapter 28, Table 12, and the Table of Risk in the 1997 DG.

Guided Example of E/M Coding for Neurology

Refer to the neurology encounter (■ FIGURE 39-10, page 804) to practice skills for abstracting and assigning E/M codes. Follow along as fictitious coder Angelia Harkey, CPC, abstracts the procedure. Check off each step after you complete it.

▶ First, Angelia needs to establish the category of service so she can determine the information needed to abstract and assign the code.

❑ *What is the setting?* Physician office

❑ *What is the type of service?* This is a consultation because the patient was referred by her primary care physician (PCP) and a report of the visit is sent to the PCP.

❑ *What is the code range?* Angelia refers to the CPT Index and looks up the Main Term **Evaluation and Management** and the subterm **Consultation**. The code range listed is **99241-99255**.

❑ *How many key components are required?* Angelia refers to the code range in the Tabular List and locates the category **Office or Other Outpatient Consultations, New or Established Patient**. She reads the description of the first code, which states **requires these 3 key components**. All codes in the category have the same requirements for key components. This tells her that all three key components must meet or exceed the levels listed in the code (3/3).

▶ Next, Angelia identifies the level of history.

❑ *What is the level of HPI?* The HPI is **Extended** because four elements are documented.

❑ *What is the level of ROS?* The ROS is **Complete** because 10 systems were examined. Although the specific systems have not been documented, the documentation provides adequate information to support an extended ROS. However, it would be best for the physician to specify the exact systems reviewed.

❑ *What is the level of PFSH?* The PFSH is **Complete** because three elements are documented.

❑ *Based on these factors, what is the overall level of history?* The level of history is **Comprehensive** because all three factors (HPI, ROS, and PFSH) meet the criteria for a comprehensive history.

System/Body Area	Elements of Neurological Examination
Constitutional	❑ Measurement of any <u>**three**</u> of the following seven **vital** signs: • 1) sitting or standing blood pressure, • 2) supine blood pressure, • 3) pulse rate and regularity, • 4) respiration, • 5) temperature, • 6) height, • 7) weight (May be measured and recorded by ancillary staff) ❑ General **appearance** of patient (eg, development, nutrition, body habitus, deformities, attention to grooming)
Eyes	❑ Ophthalmoscopic examination of **optic discs** (eg, size, C/D ratio, appearance) and posterior segments (eg, vessel changes, exudates, hemorrhages
Cardiovascular	❑ Examination of **carotid arteries** (eg, pulse amplitude, bruits) ❑ **Auscultation** of heart with notation of abnormal sounds and murmurs ❑ Examination of **peripheral vascular system** by observation (eg, swelling, varicosities) and palpation (eg, pulses, temperature, edema, tenderness)
Musculoskeletal	❑ Examination of **gait** and **station** ❑ Inspection and/or palpation of **digits** and **nails** (eg, clubbing, cyanosis, inflammatory conditions, petechiae, ischemia, infections, nodes) Assessment of motor function including: ❑ Muscle strength in upper and lower extremities ❑ Muscle tone in upper and lower extremities (eg, flaccid, cog wheel, spastic) with notation of any atrophy or abnormal movements (eg, fasciculation, tardive dyskinesia)
Extremities	[See musculoskeletal]
Neurological	Evaluation of higher integrative functions including: ❑ **Orientation** to time, place and person ❑ Recent and remote **memory** ❑ **Attention span** and concentration ❑ **Language** (eg, naming objects, repeating phrases, spontaneous speech) ❑ **Fund of knowledge** (eg, awareness of current events, past history, vocabulary) Test the following cranial nerves: ❑ **2nd** cranial nerve (eg, visual acuity, visual fields, fundi) ❑ **3rd, 4th** and **6th** cranial nerves (eg, pupils, eye movements) ❑ **5th** cranial nerve (eg, facial sensation, corneal reflexes) ❑ **7th** cranial nerve (eg, facial symmetry, strength) ❑ **8th** cranial nerve (eg, hearing with tuning fork, whispered voice and/or finger rub) ❑ **9th** cranial nerve (eg, spontaneous or reflex palate movement) ❑ **11th** cranial nerve (eg, shoulder shrug strength) ❑ **12th** cranial nerve (eg, tongue protrusion) ❑ Examination of **sensation** (eg, by touch, pin, vibration, proprioception) ❑ Examination of **deep tendon reflexes** in upper and lower extremities with notation of pathological reflexes (eg, Babinski) ❑ Test **coordination** (eg, finger/nose, heel/knee/shin, rapid alternating movements in the upper and lower extremities, evaluation of fine motor coordination in young children)

Total # Bullets Performed and Documented →	☐	# of ❑ Elements Performed and Documented	Level of Examination
		1–5	Problem focused
		6–11	Expanded problem focused
		12+	Detailed
		ALL	Comprehensive (Perform **all** elements identified by a bullet; document **every** element in each box with a shaded border and at least **one** element in each box with an unshaded border.)

Figure 39-9 ■ 1997 documentation guidelines for neurological examination. *Source: Centers for Medicare and Medicaid Services, 1997 Documentation Guidelines for Evaluation and Management Services (with formatting adjustments).*

NEUROLOGY ENCOUNTER

REASON FOR CONSULTATION: New-onset seizure.

HISTORY OF PRESENT ILLNESS: The patient is a 3 year old female seen in my office on referral by her primary care physician because of new-onset seizure. She has a history of known febrile seizures and was placed on Keppra oral solution at 150 mg b.i.d. to help prevent febrile seizures. Although this has been a very successful treatment in terms of her febrile seizure control, she is now having occasional brief periods of pauses and staring, where she becomes unresponsive, but does not lose her postural tone. The typical spell according to father lasts anywhere from 10 to 15 seconds, mother says 3 to 4 minutes, which likely means probably somewhere in the 30- to 40-second period of time. Mom did note that an episode had happened outside of a store recently, was associated with some perioral cyanosis, but there has never been a convulsive activity noted. There have been no recent changes in her Keppra dosing and she is currently only at 20 mg/kg per day, which is overall a low dose for her.

PAST MEDICAL HISTORY: Born at 36 weeks' gestation by C-section delivery at 8 pounds 3 ounces. She does have a history of febrile seizures and what parents reported as an abdominal migraine, but on further questioning, it appears to be more of a food intolerance issue.

PAST SURGICAL HISTORY: She has undergone no surgical procedures.

FAMILY MEDICAL HISTORY: There is a strong history of epilepsy on the maternal side of family including mom with some nonconvulsive seizure during childhood and additional seizures in maternal great grandmother and a maternal great aunt. There is no other significant neurological history on the paternal side of the family.

SOCIAL HISTORY: Currently lives with both parents and two siblings. She is at home full time and does not attend day care.

REVIEW OF SYSTEMS: Clear review of 10 systems are taken and revealed no additional findings other than those mentioned in the history of present illness.

PHYSICAL EXAMINATION:

Vital Signs: Weight was 15.6 kg. She was afebrile. Other vital signs were stable and within normal ranges for her age as per the medical record.

General: She was awake, alert, and oriented. She was in no acute distress, only slightly flustered when trying to place the EEG leads.

HEENT: Showed normocephalic and atraumatic head. Her conjunctivae were nonicteric and sclerae were clear. Her eye movements were conjugate in nature. Her tongue and mucous membranes were moist.

Neck: Trachea appeared to be in the midline.

Chest: Clear to auscultation bilaterally without crackles, wheezes or rhonchi.

Cardiovascular: Showed a normal sinus rhythm without murmur.

Abdomen: Showed soft, nontender, and nondistended, with good bowel sounds. There was no hepatomegaly or splenomegaly, or other masses noted on examination.

Extremities: Showed IV placement in the right upper extremity with appropriate restraints from the IV. There was no evidence of clubbing, cyanosis or edema throughout. She had no functional deformities in any of her peripheral limbs.

Neurological: From neurological standpoint, her cranial nerves were grossly intact throughout. Her strength was good in the bilateral upper and lower extremities without any distal to proximal variation. Her overall resting tone was normal. Sensory examination was grossly intact to light touch throughout the upper and lower extremities. Reflexes were 1+ in bilateral patella. Toes were downgoing bilaterally. Coordination showed accurate striking ability and good rapid alternating movements. Gait examination was deferred at this time due to EEG lead placement.

ASSESSMENT: A 3 year old female with history of febrile seizures, now with concern for spells of unclear etiology, but somewhat concerning for partial complex seizures and to a slightly lesser extent nonconvulsive generalized seizures.

RECOMMENDATIONS

1. For now, we will go ahead and try to capture EEG as long as she tolerates it; however, if she would require sedation, I would defer the EEG until further adjustments to seizure medications are made and we will see her response to these medications.

2. As per the above, I will increase her Keppra to 300 mg p.o. b.i.d. bringing her to a total daily dose of just under 40 mg/kg per day. If further spells are noted, we may increase upwards again to around 4.5 to 5 mL each day.

3. I do not feel like any specific imaging needs to be done at this time until we see her response to the medication and review her EEG findings. EEG, hopefully, will be able to be reviewed first thing tomorrow morning; however, I would not delay discharging the patient to wait on the EEG results. The patient has been discharged and we will contact the family as an outpatient.

4. The patient will need followup arrangement with me in 5 to 6 weeks' time, so we may recheck and see how she is doing and arrange for further followup then.

5. Report on the above has been sent to her primary care provider.

HISTORY:
Comprehensive

Chief complaint (CC)

Setting & patient type

HPI: Extended (4+)

ROS: Complete (10+)

PFSH: Complete (3)

EXAMINATION:
Detailed

(12 elements in at least 2 organ systems/body areas)

MEDICAL DECISION MAKING: Moderate Complexity

MDM Risk: Uncertain diagnosis, unclear prognosis (Moderate Risk)

MDM Data: Ordering or reviewing diagnostic data (Straightforward Data)

MDM Management: New presenting problem, with workup (High Management Options)

KEY: HPI History of the present illness   ROS Review of systems
        PFSH Past, family, and social history   MDM Medical decision making

Figure 39-10 ■ Neurology encounter. *Source: © PB Resources, Inc. Used with permission.*

▶ Angelia refers to the neurological examination in the 1997 DG (Figure 39-9) to abstract information needed to determine the level of the examination.

❏ *What is the level of examination?* The level of examination is **Detailed**. Eighteen elements of the examination are documented. A comprehensive examination requires that all bulleted items within the shaded borders be documented, but they are not. Therefore, the examination meets the requirement of 12 or more bulleted items for the detailed level.

▶ Angelia determines the level of medical decision making. (Refer to Table 28-12, Medical Decision-Making Levels.)

❏ *What is the level of complexity of the number of diagnoses or management options based on the presenting problem?* The level is **Moderate** because there is a new presenting problem, with workup.

❏ *What is the amount and/or complexity of data to be reviewed?* The level is **Straightforward** because the physician reviewed the patient's medical record and ordered tests.

❏ *What is the level of risk of significant complications, morbidity, and/or mortality?* Angelia reviews each column in the Table of Risk in the 1997 DG and determines that the level of risk is **Moderate**. The patient presents with an undiagnosed new problem with uncertain prognosis illness (Moderate), an EEG is ordered (Minimal), and prescription drug management is provided (Moderate). The single highest element in the Table of Risk determines the overall risk. The columns **Presenting Problem** and **Management Options Selected** both are the same level (Moderate).

❏ *Based on these factors, what is the overall level of medical decision making?* The medical decision making is **Moderate complexity**. At least two of the three MDM factors are required to qualify for a specific level of MDM. Two of the three MDM factors meet moderate decision making.

Now Angelia is ready to assign the code for the neurology encounter. The exercise that follows guides you through additional abstracting skills and allows you to assign the correct code.

CODING PRACTICE

Exercise 39.5   **Evaluation and Management Coding for Neurology**

Instructions: Refer to the *1997 Documentation Guidelines for Evaluation and Management Services* (available at **www.cms.gov**) or Chapter 28, "Evaluation and Management Services (99201-99499)," Tables 28-7 to 28-12, in this text. Answer the following questions about the "Neurology encounter" (Figure 39-10).

1. a. Which elements of the HPI are documented? Circle all that apply. Location, Quality, Severity, Duration, Timing, Context, Modifying factors, Associated signs and symptoms

   b. How many elements are documented? _____

   c. What is the level of HPI? _____

2. a. Which systems are reviewed in the ROS? Circle all that apply. Constitutional, Allergic/immunologic, CV, Endocrine, ENT/M, Eyes, GI, GU, Hemic/lymphatic, MS, Neurologic, Psychiatric, Respiratory, Skin/breast

   b. How many systems are documented? _____

   c. What is the level of ROS? _____

3. a. Which PFSH elements are documented? Circle all that apply. Past medical, Family, Social

   b. What is the level of PFSH? _____

   c. What is the overall level of history? (The lowest history factor—HPI, ROS, or PFSH—determines the level of history.)

   _____

4. Refer to Figure 39-9, 1997 DG for Neurological Examination.

   a. Which bulleted items are documented for the examination? (Check off the items documented.) _____

   b. How many bulleted items are documented? _____

   c. What is the level of the examination? _____

5. Refer to Table 28-12, Medical Decision-Making Levels, or the 1997 DG.

   a. What is the MDM level for the number of diagnoses or management options? _____

   b. What is the MDM level for the amount and/or complexity of data to be reviewed? _____

   c. Refer to the Table of Risk in the 1997 DG. Which elements of risk are documented for each risk factor? _____

      1. Presenting problem: _____

      2. Diagnostic procedures ordered: _____

      3. Management options selected: _____

   d. What is the level of risk? (The highest of the three risk factors determines the overall level of risk.) _____

   e. What is the overall level of MDM? (2/3 MDM factors are needed to determine the overall level.) _____

6. a. What is the setting? _____

   b. What is the patient (or service) type? _____

(continued)

CODING PRACTICE *(continued)*

c. What is the code range? _____

d. How many key components are required? _____

e. What is the level of history? _____

f. What is the level of examination? _____

g. What is the level of medical decision making? _____
_____

h. What is the correct code? _____

i. Why can a code for a higher-level visit not be assigned?
_____

7. Abstract, assign, and arrange (sequence) the diagnosis code(s)
that support the E/M code.

3 ICD-10-CM Code(s) _____
_____

CHAPTER SUMMARY

In this chapter you learned that:

- Neurological surgery, or neurosurgery, is a medical discipline and surgical specialty that provides care for patients in the treatment of pain or disease processes that affect the nervous system.

- Special instructions at the beginning of many categories provide definitions and coding guidelines. Instructional notes appear throughout the Tabular List to alert coders to important coding rules and cross-references.

- When abstracting for nervous system procedures, coders must pay special attention to the anatomic approach used to access the surgical site because distinct codes often identify each approach.

- Coders should pay special attention to assigning codes for basilar skull procedures and laminectomies.

- Many spinal procedures are grouped into code families with separate parent codes describing the procedure at a single vertebral level in the cervical, thoracic, or lumbar region of the spine.

- The *1997 Documentation Guidelines for Evaluation and Management Services* (1997 DG), published by CMS, provides requirements for each level of a neurologic E/M examination.

CONCEPT QUIZ

Take a moment to look back at the Nervous System subsection and solidify your skills. Try to answer the questions from memory first, then refer to the discussion in this chapter if you need a little extra help.

Completion

Instructions: Write the term that completes each statement based on the information you learned in this chapter. Choose from the list below. Some choices may be used more than once and some choices may not be used at all.

anterior	laminae
aphagia	nerve block
aphasia	neurostimulator
ataxia	posterior
chemodenervation	posterolateral
craniotomy	stereotactic
facets	subdural
hemispherectomy	

1. _____ is the medical term for lack of coordination.

2. Intractable pain can be alleviated by _____ procedures such as implantation of electrodes under the skin.

3. _____ refers to in-between membranes of the dura mater.

4. The _____ approach is performed from the front.

5. _____ radiosurgery is used to target lesions in difficult-to-treat areas, such as brain tumors.

6. _____ is injection of a substance into a muscle group or glands to stop overactivity.

7. _____ is the loss of the ability to swallow.

8. Each vertebra has two _____, one on either side of the midline.

9. In a(n) _____, a physician drills or cuts into the skull.

10. A(n) _____ approach is from the side, toward the back.

Multiple Choice

Instructions: Circle the letter of the best answer to each question based on the information you learned in this chapter.

1. How does CPT arrange definitive procedures in the range of 61600-61616?
   A. Alphabetically
   B. Numerically
   C. Anatomically
   D. By complexity

2. What is the gelatinous substance that comprises the center of a disc and provides cushioning?
   A. Nucleus pulposus
   B. Annulus fibrosus
   C. Lamina
   D. Spinal cord

3. How would you code the following procedure? *A surgeon performs a bilateral laminotomy with decompression of nerve root and partial facetectomy at L3-L4, posterior approach, open with endoscopic assistance.*
   A. 62380-50
   B. 63020, 63030
   C. 63090
   D. 63030-50

4. What is the operative approach through the far lateral side of the jaw called?
   A. Transcochlear
   B. Transcondylar
   C. Transcranial
   D. Transpedicular

5. Which of the following is a surgical approach?
   A. Endoscopic
   B. Anterior
   C. Posterior
   D. Extradural

6. How would you code the following procedure? *A physician injects an anesthetic agent into the cervical plexus.*
   A. 64400
   B. 64413
   C. 64490
   D. 64553

7. In what type of procedure do neurosurgeons work with interventional radiologists to coordinate a patient's treatment and care?
   A. Musculoskeletal surgery
   B. Spinal fusion instrumentation
   C. Restorative surgery
   D. Endovascular surgery

8. Which of the following is an anatomic approach?
   A. Open
   B. Subdural
   C. Percutaneous
   D. Endoscopic

9. How would you code the following procedure? *A physician excises a neuroma from the left ulnar nerve.*
   A. 64718-LT
   B. 64774-LT
   C. 64784-LT
   D. 64790-LT

10. What code(s) should be reported when vertebral levels from different spinal regions are treated, according to the NCCI?
    A. Report a parent code for each spinal region treated.
    B. Report the parent code for one level and add-on codes for any additional levels within the same family.
    C. Report the parent code from the first spinal region for the first level and an add-on code for the second level.
    D. Report the parent code with modifier -51, multiple procedures, appended.

KEEP ON CODING

Instructions: Read the procedural statement, then use the appropriate Index and Tabular List to assign CPT procedure codes, quantities, and modifiers. Write the code(s) on the line provided.

1. Injection of lidocaine, right brachial plexus. CPT Code(s) _____

2. Decompression craniectomy for treatment of intracranial hypertension. CPT Code(s) _____

3. Neuroplasty of the right ring finger. CPT Code(s) _____

4. Excision of neuroma of peripheral nerve of left foot. CPT Code(s) _____

5. Repair of 6-cm myelomeningocele. CPT Code(s) _____

6. Laminectomy and excision of intradural lumbar lesion. CPT Code(s) _____

7. Suture repair of left posterior tibial nerve. CPT Code(s) _____

8. Sciatic neuroplasty, left leg. CPT Code(s) _____

9. Ventriculoperitoneal shunt procedure. CPT Code(s) _____

10. Suture of digital nerves to the right thumb and second finger. CPT Code(s) _____

11. Therapeutic lumbar spinal tap for drainage of fluid. CPT Code(s) _____

(continued)

(continued from page 807)

12. Burr holes for drainage of subdural hematoma. CPT Code(s) _____

13. Stellate ganglion block, right. CPT Code(s) _____

14. Removal of intrathecal infusion pump. CPT Code(s) _____

15. Lumbar laminectomy for decompression with foraminotomies L3-L4, L4-L5, L5-S1 microtechniques; all sites bilateral; repair of CSF fistula, microtechniques L5-S1, application of DuraSeal. CPT Code(s) _____

16. Endoscopy-assisted transsphenoidal exploration and radical excision of pituitary adenoma. CPT Code(s) _____

17. Frontal craniotomy for placement of deep-brain stimulator electrode. CPT Code(s) _____

18. Subcutaneous left ulnar nerve transposition, at elbow. CPT Code(s) _____

19. Neuroendoscopic placement of left ventriculostomy catheter via twist drill. CPT Code(s) _____

20. Percutaneous balloon angioplasty, basilar artery. CPT Code(s) _____

21. Anastomosis of the facial-phrenic nerves. CPT Code(s) _____

22. Craniotomy for evacuation of cerebral hematoma. CPT Code(s) _____

23. Stereotactic stimulation of spinal cord at T3. CPT Code(s) _____

24. Bifrontal cranioplasty, 11-cm defect. CPT Code(s) _____

25. C4-C5, C5-C6 anterior cervical discectomy. CPT Code(s) _____

CODING CHALLENGE

Instructions: Read the mini-medical-record of each patient's encounter, then abstract, assign, and arrange ICD-10-CM diagnosis codes and CPT procedure codes using the appropriate Index and Tabular List. Assign quantities and modifiers where needed. Write the code(s) on the line provided.

1. OUTPATIENT SURGERY   Gender: F   Age: 32

Preoperative diagnosis: Left carpal tunnel syndrome

Procedure: Release of left carpal tunnel under general anesthesia. The median nerve was freed up along the bands from the ligament. Subcutaneous tissue and skin were closed and a dressing applied.

1 ICD-10-CM Code _____

1 CPT Code _____

2. OUTPATIENT SURGERY   Gender: M   Age: 45

Preoperative diagnosis: C6 radiculopathy confirmed by EMG

Procedure: Posterior right cervical laminoforaminotomy. Decompressive hemilaminectomy performed, with the neural elements freely mobile. The wound was irrigated and closed with sutures.

1 ICD-10-CM Code _____

1 CPT Code _____

3. HOSPITAL INPATIENT   Gender: F   Age: 29

Preoperative diagnosis: Chronic lumbar pain due to displaced disc at L3-4, which resulted from a back injury two years ago

Procedure: Percutaneous neurostimulator implant. The spinal cord stimulator electrode was placed though the spinal cord stimulator needle into the epidural space and advanced under fluoroscopic guidance. Multiple electrode settings were applied with excellent stimulation.

Tip: Review OGCR I.C.6.b.1)(a) and (b)(ii) for diagnosis sequencing instructions.

2 ICD-10-CM Codes _____

1 CPT Code _____

4. OUTPATIENT HOSPITAL   Gender: F   Age: 34

Preoperative diagnosis: Right occipital arteriovenous malformation

Procedure: CT-guided frameless stereotactic radiosurgery for the right occipital arteriovenous malformation using dynamic tracking. The patient underwent stereotactic radiosurgery to deliver 20 Gy to the AVM margin.

Plan: MRI scan in 6 months

1 ICD-10-CM Code _____

1 CPT Code _____

5. INPATIENT HOSPITAL   Gender: F   Age: 81

Preoperative diagnosis: Acute subdural hematoma 100%, right, with herniation syndrome. This procedure is being done as a life-saving emergency procedure.

Procedure: Right frontotemporoparietal craniotomy, evacuation of acute subdural hematoma. A single burr hole was made at the frontoparietal junction. The subdural hematoma was evacuated and while we were closing the dura the patient went into cardiac arrest and could not be resuscitated.

Postoperative diagnosis: Pronounced dead in the operating room

2 ICD-10-CM Codes _____

1 CPT Code _____

6. OFFICE   Gender: F   Age: 47

Preoperative diagnosis: Traumatic complete amputation of the right arm at the elbow six months ago. The stump has healed well. Seen today for relief of pain. Here for a lumbar sympathetic block to manage phantom limb pain.

Procedure: Lumbar sympathetic block injection at L3. After locating the L3 spinous process, anesthetic was slowly injected. Patient tolerated procedure well and was sent home in good condition.

2 ICD-10-CM Codes _____

1 CPT Code _____

7. INPATIENT HOSPITAL   Gender: M   Age: 9

Preoperative diagnosis: Malfunction of ventriculoatrial shunt with recurring headaches, problems with balance, poor coordination, gait disturbances

Procedure: Endoscopic ventriculoatrial shunt irrigation. Proximal shunt was partially obstructed with debris at the lumen. Debris was removed and shunt flushed normally, with no need to replace. Wound closed and sterile dressing applied. Patient was transferred to ICU in stable condition.

1 ICD-10-CM Code _____

2 CPT Codes _____

8. OUTPATIENT SURGERY   Gender: F   Age: 18

Preoperative diagnosis: Possible symptomatic hydrocephalus; patient has been followed in the office for 6 months complaining of headaches, now with ataxic gait.

Procedure: Placement of lumbar drain for CSF drainage under regional anesthesia. Tuohy needle inserted at the L4-L5 interspace. Catheter was inserted through the needle, and 12 mL of CSF was drained. Catheter was connected to a drainage system, which we will leave in place for the next 2–3 days to continue drainage.

1 ICD-10-CM Code _____

1 CPT Code _____

9. INPATIENT HOSPITAL   Gender: M   Age: 59

Preoperative diagnosis: Admitted from the ED due to laceration of superficial branch of the lateral plantar nerve and flexor digiti minimi brevis tendon, left foot. Loss of sensation across the side of the foot, with obvious open injury. Taken immediately to the OR for repair. Of note, the patient takes warfarin for prophylaxis due to atrial fib.

Procedure: A 2-cm piece of sural nerve was harvested to serve as graft to the proximal and distal ends of the lateral plantar nerve. Following this the tendon was repaired and the wound closed. Patient was admitted for overnight observation.

3 ICD-10-CM Codes _____

2 CPT Codes _____

10. OUTPATIENT SURGERY   Gender: M   Age: 56

Preoperative diagnosis: Recurrent intractable low back and left lower extremity pain following L4-L5 discectomy three months ago. No radiculopathy noted. MRI showed epidural fibrosis with lower spinal nerve root compression as the cause of patient's pain.

Procedure: Under IV sedation using an operating microscope, I performed a left L4-L5 transforaminal neuroplasty with nerve root decompression and lysis of adhesions. Procedure was well tolerated.

Plan: Discharge home and see in the office in two weeks

Tip: Use of the operating microscope should not be coded separately, per NCCI guidelines.

2 ICD-10-CM Codes _____

2 CPT Codes _____

Chapter 40

Eye and Ocular Adnexa Procedures (65091-68899)

Chapter Outline

- **Eye Procedure Basics**
- **Coding Guidelines for Eye Procedures**
- **Abstracting Eye Procedures**
- **Assigning Codes for Eye Procedures**
- **Arranging Codes for Eye Procedures**
- **E/M Coding for Ophthalmology**

Learning Objectives

After completing this chapter, you should have the skills to:

40.1 Spell and define the key words, medical terms, and abbreviations related to eye and ocular adnexa procedures. (Remember).

40.2 Summarize the types of eye and ocular adnexa procedures. (Understand)

40.3 Adhere to CPT coding guidelines in the Eye and Ocular Adnexa subsection. (Apply)

40.4 Examine and abstract procedural information from the medical record for coding Eye and Ocular Adnexa subsection procedures. (Analyze)

40.5 Assign codes for procedures in the Eye and Ocular Adnexa procedures subsection. (Apply)

40.6 Utilize guidelines for arranging (sequencing) codes for Eye and Ocular Adnexa subsection procedures. (Apply)

40.7 Determine how to code Evaluation and Management services for ophthalmology. (Evaluate)

Key Terms and Abbreviations

intraocular lens (IOL)	OD	OS
intraocular pressure (IOP)	operating microscope	OU

In addition to the key terms listed here, students should know the terms defined within tables in this chapter.

INTRODUCTION

Big gifts sometimes come in small packages. The eye is a small package but contains complex working mechanisms plus muscles, nerves, and blood vessels. Coding eye procedures requires knowledge of anatomic sites and terminology not encountered in other organ systems. In this chapter you learn about the unique aspects of coding for procedures on the eye and ocular adnexa.

EYE PROCEDURE BASICS

Ophthalmology is the branch of medicine that studies and treats diseases of the eye. Ophthalmologists are licensed medical doctors (MD) who provide medical evaluation of eye conditions and perform surgery to correct eye problems. Subspecialties of ophthalmology are cornea and external disease, glaucoma, neuro-ophthalmology, ophthalmic pathology, ophthalmic plastic surgery, pediatric ophthalmology, and vitreoretinal diseases. Cornea ophthalmologists might be referred to as specializing in the front of the eye and vitreoretinal ophthalmologists might be referred to as specializing in the back of the eye. Neurologists treat diseases of the ocular nerves and orthopedic surgeons might treat disorders of the surrounding bones, such as fracture of the ocular orbit. Optometrists conduct vision testing; opticians fit patients for corrective lenses; and ocularists fit patients with eye prostheses, also known as ocular implants.

CODING CAUTION

Be alert for medical terms that are spelled similarly and have different meanings.

trichiasis (*turning inward of the eyelashes*) and **trichinosis** (*a disease caused by trichinae parasites*)

pupil (*the opening in the iris that dilates and constricts*) and **papilla** (*a small vascular protrusion of connective tissue or skin*)

retinal (*pertaining to the retina*) and **renal** (*pertaining to the kidney*)

Chapter 18 of this text provides additional information on the anatomy, diseases, and conditions of the eye. Figure 18-1 depicts the internal structures of the eye. Refer to ■ TABLE 40-1 for a refresher on how to build medical terms related to the eye.

Procedures of the Eye and Ocular Adnexa

Procedures commonly performed on the eye and ocular adnexa are summarized in ■ TABLE 40-2 (page 812). In particular, coders need to understand the various types of keratoplasty (*corneal repair or transplant*) (■ TABLE 40-3, page 813). Physicians transplant corneas for patients whose corneas are damaged by trauma or disease that results in corneal scarring or corneal edema that causes partial or complete blindness. The corneal endothelium pumps fluid from the cornea, resulting in clear vision. Patients with corneal edema have corneas that are unable to pump fluid, and the fluid accumulates on the cornea, causing hazy, white, cloudy, or smoky vision.

A corneal transplant, also called a cornea graft, is removal of the damaged or diseased cornea and replacement with a cadaveric cornea. Penetrating keratoplasty (PKP) is removal of the entire cornea and transplantation of a full-thickness cornea. Lamellar keratoplasty is a partial-thickness transplant involving a graft of only specific corneal layers. PKP, which involves suturing the entire cornea in place, has been the standard corneal transplant for many years. Recovery from PKP is a long process, and it can take several months to two years for a patient to fully recover visually and completely heal from the procedure.

A newer corneal transplant procedure, called Descemet's stripping endothelial keratoplasty (DSEK), is replacing PKP. It involves stripping Descemet's membrane and removing only the corneal endothelium layer, replacing it with a cadaveric endothelium. In DSEK surgery, the physician uses an air bubble, instead of sutures, to hold the new corneal cells in place. Patients experience a much shorter recovery time with improved vision relatively quickly.

This section provides a general reference to help understand the most common eye procedures. Remember to keep standard reference books handy in case you get stuck.

Table 40-1   ■   EXAMPLE OF CONSTRUCTING MEDICAL TERMS FOR EYE PROCEDURES

Combining Form	Suffix	Complete Medical Term
kerat/o (*cornea*)		**kerato + plasty** (*repair of the cornea*)
		irido + plasty (*repair of the iris*)
	-plasty (*repair*)	**conjunctivo + plasty** (*repair of the conjunctiva*)
irid/o (*iris*)	**-ectomy** (*excision*)	**kerat + ectomy** (*excision of the cornea*)
conjunctiv/o (*conjunctiva*)		**irid + ectomy** (*excision of the iris*)
		conjunctiv + ectomy (*excision of the conjunctiva*)

Source: © PB Resources, Inc. Used with permission.

Table 40-2 ■ **COMMON PROCEDURES OF THE EYE AND OCULAR ADNEXA**

Procedure Name	Definition	Reason Performed
Chemocauterization	Destruction of tissue by using chemicals	Lesion
Cyclectomy	Partial excision of the ciliary body	Glaucoma, lesions
Enucleation	Removal of the eyeball without removing the ocular contents of the orbit or muscles	Tumor, trauma, endophthalmitis unresponsive to antibiotics, improvement of appearance of a blind eye, painful blind eye
Evisceration	Removal of the ocular contents and removal of the cornea; the sclera and extraocular muscles are not removed	Endophthalmitis unresponsive to antibiotics, improvement of appearance of a blind eye, painful blind eye
Exenteration	Removal of the eyeball, including the ocular contents; may include removal of bone and muscle or myocutaneous flap	Large orbital tumors or orbital extension of intraocular tumors
Extracapsular cataract extraction	Removal of the lens of the eye while leaving the elastic capsule that covers the lens partially intact to allow implantation of an intraocular lens (IOL) (*an artificial lens inserted into the lens capsule*) (■ FIGURE 40-1)	Cataract
Fistulization	Creation of a passageway, or opening, in the sclera by incising the iris and allowing the aqueous humor to drain	Glaucoma, infection, or trauma
Goniotomy	Placement of a goniolens (gonioscope) on the patient's cornea to view the iris and cornea; allows the physician to see and open the trabecular meshwork to drain aqueous humor and reduce intraocular pressure (IOP) (*pressure of fluid within the eye*)	Congenital glaucoma
Intravitreal injection	Injection of medication into the vitreous body	Diabetic retinopathy, macular edema, macular degeneration
Iridectomy	Excision of the iris	Lesion, glaucoma
Iridencleisis	Implantation of part of the iris in the cornea	Glaucoma
Iridotasis	Stretching of the iris	Glaucoma
Iridotomy	Incision of the iris to drain aqueous humor; can include transfixion (*piercing to move a part into a new position*) for iris bombé (*protrusion of the iris from excess aqueous humor in the posterior chamber*)	Glaucoma, enlargement of the pupil
Ocular implant	Insertion of a small sphere into the orbit where the natural eye used to be	Tumor, trauma
Orbital implant	Insertion of glass, plastic, or acrylic placed under an ocular implant	Tumor, trauma
Phacoemulsification	Destruction, usually with ultrasound, of a natural lens, which is then suctioned out of the eye	Cataract
Photocoagulation	Use of a laser to seal tears	Diabetic retinopathy, age-related macular degeneration, retinal ischemia, neovascularization of the choroid or retina, glaucoma
Recession	Cutting a muscle from the surface of the eye and reattaching it farther back from the front of the eye to weaken or lengthen the muscle	Strabismus
Thermocauterization	Destruction of tissue by applying heat	Lesion
Trabeculectomy	Surgical excision of a small portion of the trabecular tissue lying between the anterior chamber of the eye and the canal of Schlemm	Glaucoma
Trabeculotomy, trabeculoplasty	Incision and repair of the trabecular meshwork to improve aqueous humor outflow and reduce IOP	Glaucoma

Source: © PB Resources, Inc. Used with permission.

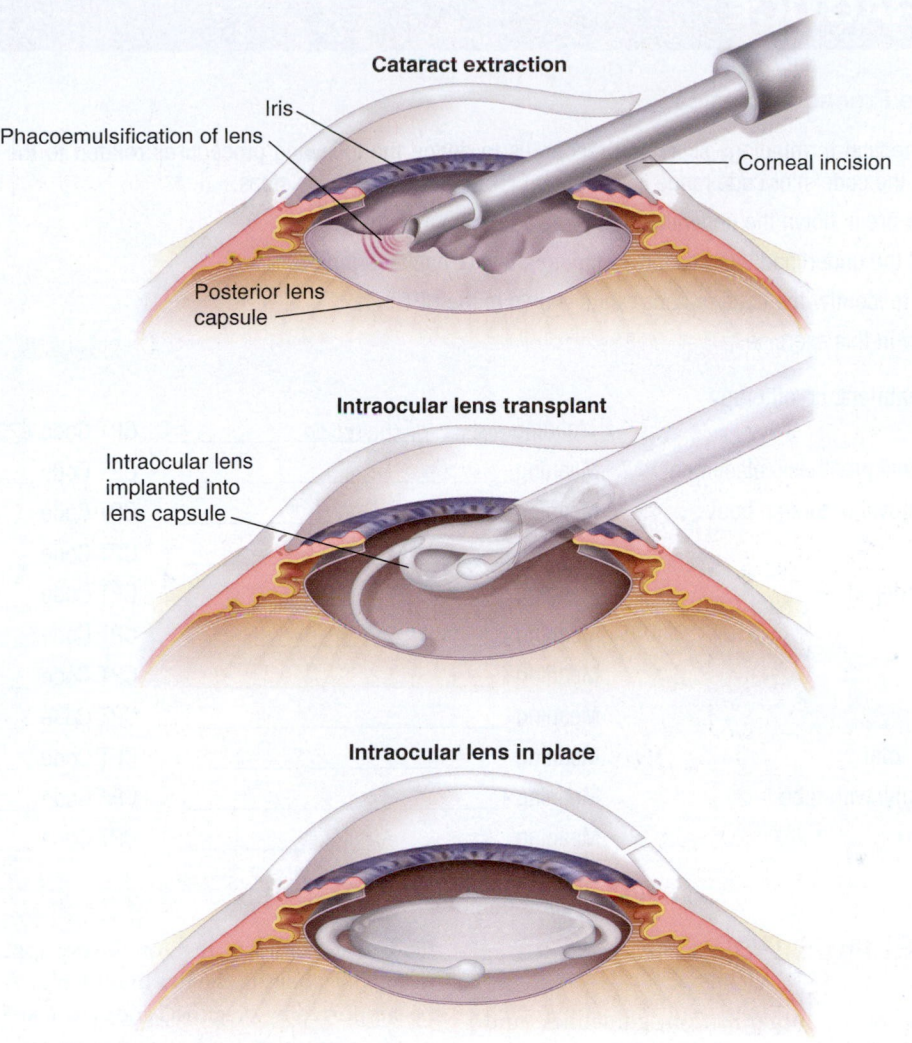

Cataract extraction

Iris

Phacoemulsification of lens

Corneal incision

Posterior lens capsule

Intraocular lens transplant

Intraocular lens implanted into lens capsule

Intraocular lens in place

Figure 40-1 ■ Cataract phacoemulsification.

Table 40-3   ■   **TYPES OF KERATOPLASTY**

Procedure Name	Definition	Reason Performed
Descemet's stripping endo-thelial keratoplasty (DSEK)	Removal of only the corneal endothelium layer and replacement with a donor (cadaver) endothelial graft	Corneal trauma or disease
Epikeratoplasty	Transplantation of donor corneal epithelium onto a patient's cornea	Refractive defect such as myopia (*nearsightedness*), presbyopia (*farsightedness*), or astigmatism
Keratomileusis	A form of keratoplasty in which a slice of the cornea is removed, reshaped (often with a laser), and placed back onto the cornea	Refractive defect
Keratophakia	Reshaping and transplantation of donor corneal tissue onto a patient's cornea	Refractive defect
Lamellar keratoplasty	Partial-thickness transplant involving a graft of only specific corneal layers	Corneal trauma or disease
Penetrating keratoplasty (PKP)	Removal of the entire cornea and transplantation of a full-thickness cornea	Corneal trauma or disease
Radial keratotomy	Flattening of the cornea by making a series of incisions in a radial pattern resembling the spokes of a wheel	Myopia

Source: © PB Resources, Inc. Used with permission.

CODING PRACTICE

Exercise 40.1 Eye Procedure Basics

Instructions: Use your medical terminology skills and resources to define the following procedures related to the Eye and Ocular Adnexa subsection, then identify the code(s) or code range listed in the CPT Index. Follow these steps:

- Use slash marks "/" to break down the underlined term into its root(s) and suffix.
- Define the meaning of the underlined word based on the meaning of each word part.
- Use the entire phrase to identify the code or code range shown in the CPT Index.
- Do not assign laterality in this exercise.

Example: <u>retinopathy</u>, treatment, cryotherapy

retino/pathy   Meaning <u>*disease of the retina*</u>   CPT Code <u>*67229*</u>

1. <u>vitrectomy</u>, with retinal prosthesis placement   Meaning _____   CPT Code _____
2. <u>orbitotomy</u>, with removal of foreign body   Meaning _____   CPT Code _____
3. <u>tarsorrhaphy</u>   Meaning _____   CPT Code _____
4. <u>trabeculotomy</u>, ab externo   Meaning _____   CPT Code _____
5. <u>keratoprosthesis</u>   Meaning _____   CPT Code _____
6. <u>canthoplasty</u>   Meaning _____   CPT Code _____
7. <u>pupillometry</u>   Meaning _____   CPT Code _____
8. <u>dacryoadenectomy</u>, total   Meaning _____   CPT Code _____
9. <u>conjunctivorhinostomy</u>, with tube   Meaning _____   CPT Code _____
10. <u>blepharoptosis</u>, repair   Meaning _____   CPT Code _____

CODING GUIDELINES FOR EYE PROCEDURES

Coders should understand the organization, guidelines, and instructional notes in the Tabular List of this CPT subsection. This information is necessary for accurate coding. The CPT subsection **Eye and Ocular Adnexa (65091-68899)** contains five subheadings that are divided by anatomic site (■ TABLE 40-4). Within each subheading, codes are further divided by more specific anatomic sites and the type of procedure, such as incision, excision, repair, destruction, and so on. Review the subheading and category names and code ranges listed in the Eye and Ocular Adnexa subsection to become familiar with the content and organization. Some editions of the CPT manual provide a summary list of the subheading and categories at the beginning of the Eye and Ocular Adnexa subsection, which also displays an asterisk (*) next to categories that contain special coding instructions.

This CPT subsection includes invasive, minimally invasive, and noninvasive surgical procedures on the eye and ocular adnexa.

Table 40-4 ■ **EYE AND OCULAR ADNEXA SUBHEADINGS**

Subheading	Code Range
Eyeball	65091-65290
Anterior Segment	65400-66999
Posterior Segment	67005-67299
Ocular Adnexa	67311-67999
Conjunctiva	68020-68899

Codes for diagnostic tests on the eye appear in the Medicine section. CPT codes in the Eye and Ocular Adnexa subsection must be supported by diagnosis codes to justify the medical necessity of the procedure. Codes for eye procedures are frequently supported by diagnosis codes from ICD-10-CM Chapter 7, "Diseases of the Eye and Adnexa (H00-H59)," as well as neoplasms, symptoms and signs, and injuries (■ TABLE 40-5). These are the codes used most commonly to support procedures on the eye; however, diagnosis codes from any ICD-10-CM chapter are permissible.

CPT guidelines for the Surgery section apply to the Eye and Ocular Adnexa subsection.

Special instructions identify services that are bundled with certain codes and also identify codes that should and should not be reported together. Subcategories with special instructions include:

- **Anterior Segment, Cornea, Keratoplasty (65710-65757)**
- **Anterior Segment, Cornea, Other Procedures (65760-65782)**
- **Anterior Segment, Lens, Removal (66830-66940)**
- **Posterior Segment, Retina or Choroid, Prophylaxis (67141-67145)**
- **Posterior Segment, Retina or Choroid, Destruction (67208-67229)**
- **Ocular Adnexa, Eyelids, Excision, Destruction (67800-67850)**
- **Ocular Adnexa, Eyelids, Excision, Reconstruction (67930-67975)**

Table 40-5 ■ LOCATING ICD-10-CM AND ADDITIONAL CPT CODES FOR THE EYE

Type of Code	Codes
ICD-10-CM Eye-Related Codes	
Eye and ocular adnexa conditions	H00-H59
Neoplasms	C69, D09, D31
Symptoms and signs	Most eye signs and symptoms are classified in H00-H59
Injuries	S00-S09, T26
CPT Eye-Related Codes	
Medicine procedures	92002-92499
Radiologic procedures	
• Diagnostic radiology	70010-70559
• Radiologic guidance	77001-77022
• Diagnostic ultrasound	76506-76536
Laboratory organ/disease panels	None

Source: © PB Resources, Inc. Used with permission.

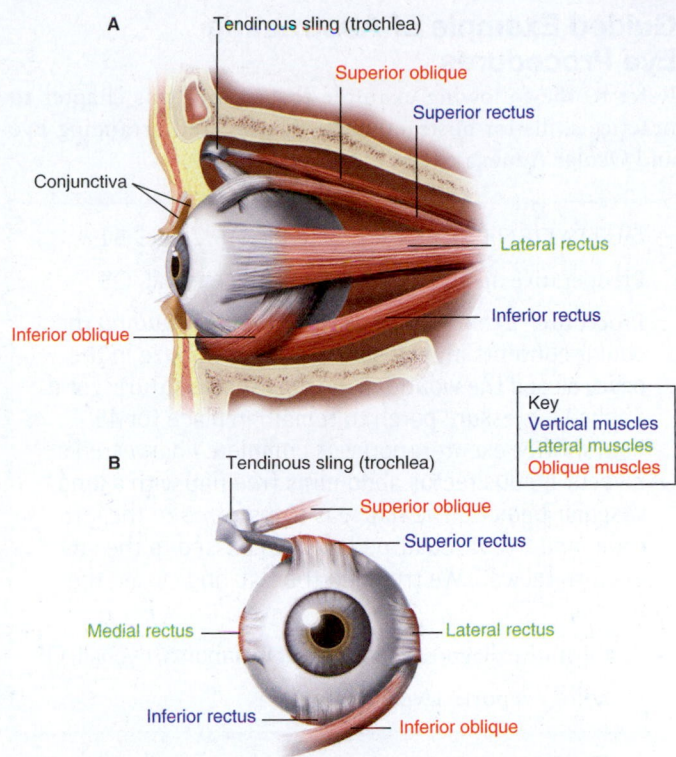

Figure 40-2 ■ Extraocular muscles, left eye. (A) Lateral view. (B) Anterior view.

Instructional notes appear throughout the Tabular List to alert coders to the need for modifiers, provide cross-references to codes for similar procedures on other sites, identify when additional codes for radiological services might be needed, and highlight resequenced and recently deleted codes. Specific guidelines and instructional notes are discussed throughout this chapter of the text.

ABSTRACTING EYE PROCEDURES

Some operative techniques used in eye procedures are rarely used to treat other body systems, such as phacoemulsification and recession. Although the eye is a small structure compared with other organs, it has numerous specific sites that affect the choice of codes, such as the pars plana, trabecular network, and extraocular muscles. The direction of extraocular muscles—vertical, lateral, or oblique—must be identified (■ FIGURE 40-2). Be aware of these unique procedures and detailed anatomy when abstracting and coding procedures on the eye. Refer to your medical resources to understand terms you may be unfamiliar with.

Laterality is always relevant for eye procedures. For procedures on the eyelid, also abstract whether the upper or lower lid is treated. In addition, identify procedures in which a graft or prosthesis—such as an IOL or implant—is used.

Some clinicians might use Latin-based abbreviations to designate the laterality of the eyes: OD (*oculus dexter*) for the right eye; OS (*oculus sinister*) for the left eye; OU (*oculus uterque*) for each eye or both eyes. These abbreviations are not on The Joint Commission's (TJC) required *Do Not Use List.* However, they are on TJC's supplemental list of abbreviations that they suggest institutions may wish to prohibit through internal policy. They also appear on the list *Error-Prone Abbreviations, Symbols, and Dose Designations* published by the Institute for Safe Medication Practices (ISMP).

Refer to ■ TABLE 40-6 for guidance on how to abstract procedures on the Eye and Ocular Adnexa, then work through

the detailed example that follows. Take note of the specialized questions for procedures on the eyelids and keratoplasty. Remember that the abstracting questions are a guide and that not every question applies to, or can be answered for, every case. For example, when a prosthesis is used, you must identify its type, but not every procedure requires a prosthesis.

Table 40-6 ■ KEY CRITERIA FOR ABSTRACTING EYE PROCEDURES

❏ What is the procedure?
❏ What part(s) of the eye is affected?
❏ What is the laterality?
❏ What is the surgical approach?
❏ What is the anatomic approach?
❏ What type of prosthesis is used?

Eyelid Procedures

❏ Is the upper or lower lid involved?
❏ Is only the skin involved, or are parts of the eye and adnexa also involved?

Keratoplasty Procedures

❏ How much of the cornea is removed (endothelium, epithelium, slice, partial thickness, full thickness)?
❏ Is the cornea reshaped?
❏ Is the patient's cornea reinserted or is a donor graft used?
❏ Is a graft secured with sutures or an air bubble?

Source: © PB Resources, Inc. Used with permission.

Guided Example of Abstracting Eye Procedures

Refer to the following example throughout this chapter to practice skills for abstracting, assigning, and arranging Eye and Ocular Adnexa codes.

> OUTPATIENT SURGERY   Gender: F   Age: 51
>
> Preoperative diagnosis: Cancer of the eyeball, OS
>
> Procedure: Exenteration of the left eye, including the ocular contents and muscle; placed dry gauze in the orbit, closed the wound using absorbable sutures, and applied a pressure patch to remain in place for 48 hours. After exenteration was complete I harvested a myocutaneous rectus abdominis free flap with a long vascular pedicle. The flap was transferred to the left orbit, and the vascular pedicle was passed to the lateral orbital wall. We trimmed the flap and closed the incision.
>
> Postoperative diagnosis: Malignant melanoma, eyeball, OS
>
> Pathology report: Uveal melanoma

Follow along as fictitious coder Megan Scheidler, CCS-P, abstracts the procedure. Check off each step after you complete it.

▶ Megan reads through the entire record, paying special attention to the reason for the encounter, the procedure performed, and the postoperative diagnosis. She refers to the Key Criteria for Abstracting Eye Procedures (Table 40-6).

❏ She notes preoperative diagnosis cancer of the eyeball, OS.

❏ *What is the patient's age?* 51

❏ *What site is treated?* Left eye

❏ *What is the primary procedure performed?* Exenteration

❏ *What is the laterality?* Left eye

❏ *What part(s) of the eye is affected?* Ocular contents and muscle

❏ *What is the surgical approach?* Open

❏ *What is the anatomic approach?* Not applicable

❏ *What type of prosthesis is used?* A prosthesis is not inserted at this time

❏ *What other procedures are performed?* Myocutaneous rectus abdominis free flap

▶ At this time, Megan does not know which of these procedures may need to be coded, nor how many codes she will end up with. She will learn about this when she moves on to assigning codes.

CODING PRACTICE

Exercise 40.2   Abstracting Eye Procedures

Instructions: Read the mini-medical-record of each patient's encounter and answer the abstracting questions. Write the answer on the line provided. Do not assign any codes.

> **1. OFFICE**   Gender: F   Age: 27
>
> Preprocedure diagnosis: Perforating laceration to the left cornea. Cannot see out of her left eye and has severe eye pain. She was hit in the eye with a softball bat during a softball game.
>
> Procedure: Repaired the corneal laceration, OS. The uveal tissue and the vascular layer beneath the sclera were intact.
>
> Plan: Steroid eye drops and antibiotics
>
> a. What is the procedure? _____
>
> b. What part(s) of the eye is affected? _____
>
> c. What is the laterality? _____
>
> d. What is the surgical approach? _____
>
> e. What is the anatomic approach? _____
>
> f. What type of prosthesis is used? _____

> **2. EMERGENCY DEPT**   Gender: F   Age: 53
>
> Preprocedure diagnosis: Partial retinal detachment with multiple defects in the OD
>
> Procedure: Retinal repair, right eye. Applied scleral buckle using encircling procedure, with drainage of subretinal fluid
>
> a. What is the procedure? _____
>
> b. What part(s) of the eye is affected? _____
>
> c. What is the laterality? _____
>
> d. What is the surgical approach? _____
>
> e. What is the anatomic approach? _____
>
> f. What type of prosthesis is used? _____

(continued)

CODING PRACTICE (continued)

3. EMERGENCY DEPT   Gender: F   Age: 67

Preprocedure diagnosis: Spontaneous hemorrhage obscuring vision, OD

Procedure: Mechanical vitrectomy; removed vitreous fluid from the eye through incisions in the pars plana

a. What is the procedure? _____

b. What part(s) of the eye is affected? _____

c. What is the laterality? _____

d. What is the surgical approach? _____

e. What is the anatomic approach? _____

f. What type of prosthesis is used? _____

4. OUTPATIENT SURGERY   Gender: M   Age: 72

Preprocedure diagnosis: Cataract, right eye

Procedure: Extracapsular cataract removal with lens implantation, right eye. Performed phacoemulsification using hydrodissection to separate the lens nucleus by injecting fluid into the capsule, then suctioned out the lens and fluid. Inserted an intraocular lens in the posterior chamber and checked for leakage.

a. What is the procedure? _____

b. What part(s) of the eye is affected? _____

c. What is the laterality? _____

d. What is the surgical approach? _____

e. What is the anatomic approach? _____

f. What type of prosthesis is used? _____

5. OFFICE   Gender: M   Age: 83

Preprocedure diagnosis: Diabetic macular edema, right eye

Procedure: Injects triamcinolone acetonide 10 mg into the Tenon's capsule (*a membrane covering the eyeball behind the conjunctiva*)

a. What is the procedure? _____

b. What part(s) of the eye is affected? _____

c. What is the laterality? _____

d. What is the surgical approach? _____

e. What is the anatomic approach? _____

f. What type of prosthesis is used? _____

6. OFFICE   Gender: M   Age: 5

Preprocedure diagnosis: Exotropia (*eye turns outward*), left eye

Procedure: Strabismus surgery, recession (*lengthening*) of left lateral rectus muscle. Placed adjustable sutures to adjust alignment postoperatively when muscles are not affected by anesthesia.

a. What is the procedure? _____

b. What part(s) of the eye is affected? _____

c. What is the laterality? _____

d. What is the surgical approach? _____

e. What is the anatomic approach? _____

f. What type of prosthesis is used? _____

ASSIGNING CODES FOR EYE PROCEDURES

To locate codes for eye procedures, search the Index for the Main Term of the anatomic site, such as **Cornea** or **Retina**, and identify the first-level modifying term for the type of procedure or condition, such as **Astigmatism** or **Removal**. This approach usually leads to the largest selection of codes. However, you may search the Index for the Main Term of the procedure, such as **Keratoplasty** or **Vitrectomy**, and identify the first-level modifying term for the variation of the procedure, which might specify the anatomic approach, such as **Anterior** or **Pars plana**.

Remember that CPT uses a variety of Main Terms to index procedures, including anatomic site, procedure name, condition, synonym, eponym, and abbreviation. If you cannot find what you are looking for using one approach, try a different one, because not all possible codes are indexed the same under all possible Main Terms. Always read the code description in the Tabular List, including any parent codes and even surrounding codes not listed in the Index. Also read the instructional notes that appear after the code and special instructions that appear at the beginning of the category to help identify the correct code.

Many eye procedures involve the use of an operating microscope, which is a specially designed microscope used to assist in the performance of delicate microsurgical procedures, such as operations on the eye, middle ear, or nerves. Code **69990** is an add-on code to report use of the operating microscope: **Microsurgical techniques, requiring use of operating microscope.** An instructional note at the beginning of the Eye and Ocular Adnexa subsection states (**Do not report code 69990 in addition to codes 65091-68850**). This instruction tells you that the operating microscope is bundled into codes and should not be reported separately, even when documented.

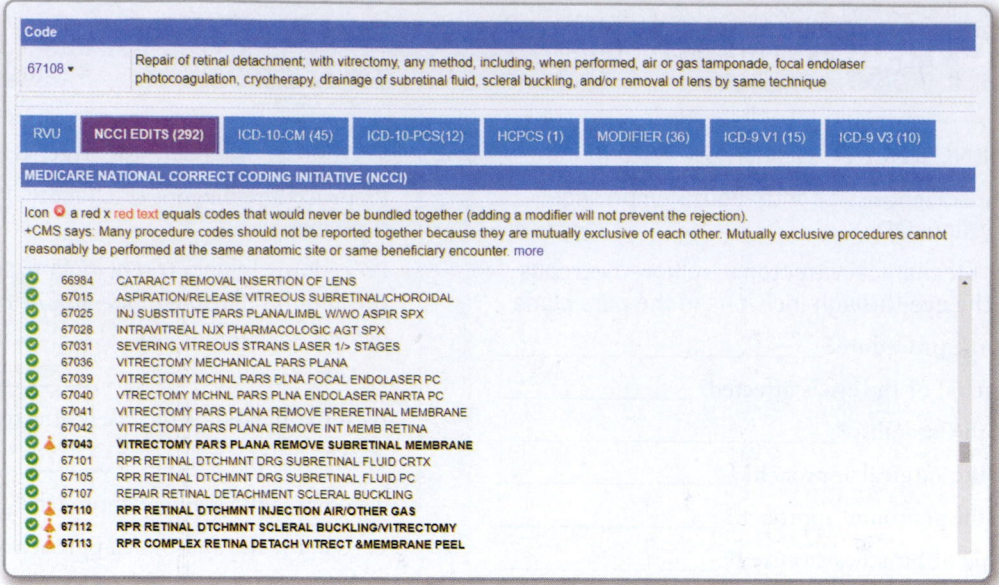

Figure 40-3 ■ Example of encoder screen with NCCI edits for code 67108. *Source: SpeedeCoder, Reprinted with permission.*

Pay special attention to the details of blepharoplasty, cataract removal, and iridectomy.

- Identify whether a blepharoplasty procedure involves the eyelid margin, tarsus, or conjunctiva or only the skin of the eyelids. Procedures that involve the lid margin, tarsus, or conjunctiva are classified under the Eye and Ocular Adnexa (**67930-67975**) and are usually performed by ophthalmologists. Blepharoplasty that involves only the skin of the eyelids is classified under the Integumentary System (**15820-15823**) and is usually performed by plastic surgeons.

- CPT codes describing cataract removal (**66982-66986**) are mutually exclusive of each other, so report only one code for cataract removal for the same eye on the same date of service.

- CPT codes describing repair of retinal detachment (**67101-67113**) are mutually exclusive of each other, so report only one code for retinal detachment repair for the same eye on the same date of service. Some retinal detachment repair procedures include procedures on the vitreous body, which are not separately reportable, unless justified by the clinical circumstances. For example, the procedure described by CPT code **67108** includes the procedures described by CPT codes **67015, 67025, 67028, 67031, 67036, 67039,** and **67040.** If the clinical circumstances warrant both procedures, append a modifier that identifies the reason for two separate procedures. The exclusions are not identified in the CPT manual but do appear in the National Correct Coding Initiative (NCCI) and, as such, are flagged by many encoders (■ FIGURE 40-3). Be sure to read the notes and explanation of formatting and icons provided by the encoder.

Guided Example of Assigning Eye Procedure Codes

To practice skills for assigning codes for the Eye and Ocular Adnexa subsection, continue with the example from earlier in the chapter about a patient who was seen for orbital exenteration.

Follow along in your CPT manual as Megan Scheidler, CCS-P, assigns codes. Check off each step after you complete it.

▶ First, Megan confirms the procedure: exenteration of the left eye.

▶ Megan searches the Index for the Main Term **Eye**.

   ❏ She locates the first-level modifying term **Exenteration**.

   ❏ She identifies the potential codes **65110, 65112, 65114.**

▶ Megan turns to the Tabular List to review the codes.

   ❏ She identifies that code **65110** is a parent code with the unique descriptor **Exenteration of orbit (does not include skin graft), removal of orbital contents**.

   ❏ She identifies that codes **65112** and **65114** are indented codes in the same code family. She reviews the unique descriptors to determine the differences between the codes.

      ▪ Code **65110** describes **removal of the orbital contents only**.

      ▪ Code **65112** describes **therapeutic removal of bone**.

      ▪ Code **65114** describes **with muscle or myocutaneous flap**.

   ❏ She refers to the documentation and confirms a myocutaneous flap was part of the procedure, so code **65114** correctly describes the procedure. The descriptor also tells her that she does not need an additional code to report the myocutaneous flap.

▶ Megan checks for instructions in the Tabular List.

   ❏ She reads the instructional notes that follow code **65114** in the Tabular List:

- (For skin graft to orbit (split skin), see 15120, 15121; free, full thickness, see 15260, 15261)

  - (For eyelid repair involving more than skin, see 67930 et seq)

❏ Although a myocutaneous graft was performed and is bundled with the procedure, a skin graft or other eyelid repair was not performed, so these notes do not apply to this case.

❏ She cross-references the beginning of the category **Removal of the Eye** and verifies that there are no special instructions.

❏ She cross-references the beginning of the subheading **Eyeball** and verifies that there are no instructional notes.

❏ She cross-references the beginning of the subsection **Eye and Ocular Adnexa** and reviews the instructional notes. She determines that they do not apply because the operating microscope was not used.

▶ Megan appends modifier **-LT Left side** to identify the laterality.

▶ Megan reviews the procedure code she has assigned for this case.

  (1) **65114-LT Exenteration of orbit (does not include skin graft), removal of orbital contents; with muscle or myocutaneous flap; -LT Left side**

▶ Megan also assigns and sequences the ICD-10-CM diagnosis code that supports the need for the service.

  (1) **C69.92 Malignant neoplasm of unspecified site of left eye**

▶ Next, Megan codes a follow-up procedure.

CODING PRACTICE

Exercise 40.3   Assigning Codes for Eye Procedures

Instructions: Read the mini-medical-record of each patient's encounter. Review the information abstracted in Exercise 40.2 for questions 1–3. For questions 4–6, abstract the case on your own. Assign CPT codes, quantities, and modifiers using the Index and Tabular List. Write the code(s) on the line provided.

1. OFFICE   Gender: F   Age: 27

Preprocedure diagnosis: Perforating laceration to the left cornea. Cannot see out of her left eye and has severe eye pain. She was hit in the eye with a softball bat during a softball game.

Procedure: Repaired the corneal laceration, OS. The uveal tissue and the vascular layer beneath the sclera were intact.

Plan: Steroid eye drops and antibiotics

1 CPT Code _____

2. EMERGENCY DEPT   Gender: F   Age: 53

Preprocedure diagnosis: Partial retinal detachment with multiple defects, OD

Procedure: Retinal repair, OD. Applied scleral buckle using encircling procedure, with drainage of subretinal fluid.

Tip: A scleral buckle is a silicone strap applied around the eyeball.

1 CPT Code _____

3. EMERGENCY DEPT   Gender: F   Age: 67

Preprocedure diagnosis: Spontaneous hemorrhage obscuring vision, OD

Procedure: Mechanical vitrectomy, OD, removed vitreous fluid from the eye through incisions in the pars plana

Tip: The pars plana is a narrow area between the iris and the choroid.

1 CPT Code _____

4. OUTPATIENT SURGERY   Gender: F   Age: 17

Preprocedure diagnosis: Tearing, eyelash encrustation with probable tear duct obstruction, OS

Procedure: Nasolacrimal duct, OS, explored under general anesthesia. Some mild resistance was found distally and we were able to navigate through this using the probe. Patency was confirmed through the naris.

Postprocedure diagnosis: Distal nasolacrimal duct stenosis with obstruction, OS

1 CPT Code _____

(continued)

CODING PRACTICE (continued)

---

5. OFFICE   Gender: M   Age: 27

Preprocedure diagnosis: Eye infections for the past year that have been resistant to multiple antibiotic therapies

Procedure: Expressed conjunctival follicles in both eyes in an attempt to determine the cause

Postprocedure diagnosis: Follicular conjunctivitis OU

1 CPT Code _____

---

6. OUTPATIENT SURGERY   Gender: M   Age: 74

Preprocedure diagnosis: Open angle glaucoma, OD, uncontrolled by maximum tolerated medical therapy

Procedure: Fistulization of sclera with trabeculectomy ab externo, OD. At the end of the procedure the anterior chamber was filled with balanced salt solution; it was noted that there was a very small amount of fluid trickling out of the scleral flap, and the pressure in the anterior chamber was considered adequate. Eye patch and eye shield were placed over the eye.

Postprocedure diagnosis: Open angle glaucoma, OD

1 CPT Code _____

ARRANGING CODES FOR EYE PROCEDURES

The NCCI provides direction for when separate procedures should be reported with cataract removal. When an iridectomy is performed to complete a cataract extraction, it is an integral part of the cataract procedure and is not separately reportable. Similarly, the minimal vitreous loss occurring during routine cataract extraction does not represent a vitrectomy and is not separately reportable.

When an iridectomy or vitrectomy that is separate and distinct from the cataract extraction is performed for an unrelated reason during the same patient encounter, the iridectomy and/or vitrectomy may be reported separately with an NCCI-associated modifier, such as modifier **-59 Distinct procedural service**. Some payers may require use of an extended **-X{EPSU}** modifier instead of modifier **-59** to identify the reason a separate procedure is reported. The medical record must document the distinct medical necessity of each procedure.

The descriptors for CPT code **67108** (**Repair of retinal detachment...**) and **67113** (**Repair of complex retinal detachment...**) include removal of lens, if performed. CPT codes for removal of lens or cataract extraction (**66830-66984**) should not be reported separately.

A trabeculectomy is separately reportable with a cataract extraction when performed for a purpose unrelated to the cataract extraction, such as glaucoma (■ FIGURE 40-4). However, when a trabeculectomy is performed as a preventative service for an expected temporary increase in intraocular pressure after cataract removal, without documentation of glaucoma, it is *not* separately reportable (■ FIGURE 40-5).

Surgeon performs an extracapsular cataract phacoemulsification and implants a posterior IOL in the right eye. During the same operative session, he performs a bilateral trabeculectomy to treat the patient's longstanding glaucoma.

66170-50 Fistulization of sclera for glaucoma; trabeculectomy ab externo in absence of previous surgery; -50 Bilateral procedure

66984-59-RT Extracapsular cataract removal with insertion of intraocular lens prosthesis (1 stage procedure), manual or mechanical technique (eg, irrigation and aspiration or phacoemulsification);-59 Distinct procedural service; -RT Right eye

V2632-RT Posterior chamber intraocular lens

Figure 40-4 ■ Example of multiple coding for cataract removal and trabeculectomy.
Source: © PB Resources, Inc. Used with permission. CPT codes only © American Medical Association.

Surgeon performs an extracapsular cataract phacoemulsification and implants a posterior IOL in the right eye. During the same operative session, he performs a right trabeculectomy as a precaution, to prevent any potential rise in IOP postoperatively.

66984-RT Extracapsular cataract removal with insertion of intraocular lens prosthesis (1 stage procedure), manual or mechanical technique (eg, irrigation and aspiration or phacoemulsification)

V2632-RT Posterior chamber intraocular lens

Figure 40-5 ■ Example of coding for trabeculectomy bundled with cataract removal. *Source: © PB Resources, Inc. Used with permission. CPT codes only © American Medical Association.*

Guided Example of Arranging Eye Procedure Codes

To practice skills for arranging codes for procedures on the Eye and Ocular Adnexa, continue with the example from earlier in the chapter about the patient who was seen for exenteration of the eye. Follow along in your CPT manual as Megan Scheidler, CCS-P, codes for a follow-up procedure six weeks after the exenteration service. Check off each step after you complete it.

OUTPATIENT SURGERY   Gender: F   Age: 51

Preoperative diagnosis: Exenteration of the left eye, including the ocular contents and muscle

Procedure: Orbital implant, OS. Attached the prosthetic eyeball outside of the muscle cone (*the gathering point of the extraocular muscles that move the eye*) of the left eye.

Plan: Refer to ocularist for ocular implant.

▶ First, Megan performs the abstracting for the follow-up procedure and determines that this procedure involves insertion of an orbital implant, a prosthetic eyeball.

▶ Megan searches the Index for the Main Term **Orbital Implant**.

❑ She notices the cross-reference instruction under the Main Term that says **See Ocular Implant**. She knows she can disregard this instruction because an ocular implant is the glass, plastic, or acrylic cover that will be inserted by the ocularist over the orbital implant and under the eyelid.

❑ She locates the subterm **Insertion** and notes the only code, **67550**.

▶ Megan turns to the Tabular List to verify code **67550**.

❑ The code description is **Orbital implant (implant outside muscle cone); insertion** and correctly describes the procedure performed.

❑ The other code in this code family, **67560**, describes **removal or revision** of the orbital implant, which was not performed.

▶ Megan appends modifier **-LT Left side** to identify the laterality.

▶ Megan refers to the global surgery schedule provided by the patient's insurance company. The exenteration procedure has a global period of 90 days. The global period means that any additional services performed during this time period are assumed to be bundled with the original procedure.

❑ Megan knows she needs a modifier to alert the payer that the orbital implant is a planned and legitimate procedure, separate from the exenteration. (Refer to Table 27-1, Key Criteria for Abstracting CPT Modifiers, or Appendix A in the CPT manual.)

❑ She appends modifier **-58 Staged or related procedure or service by the same physician or other qualified health care professional during the postoperative period.**

▶ Megan finalizes the procedure codes and sequencing for this case:

(1) **67550-58-LT Orbital implant (implant outside muscle cone); insertion; -58 Staged or related procedure or service by the same physician or other qualified health care professional during the postoperative period; -LT Left side**

▶ Megan also assigns and sequences the ICD-10-CM diagnosis codes that support the need for the service. She needs a code to identify the postoperative status of the patient and a code to identify the history of the malignant neoplasm. She assigns a history code, rather than one for a current neoplasm, because the neoplasm was removed in its entirety.

(1) **Z98.890 Other specified postprocedural states**

(2) **Z85.840 Personal history of malignant neoplasm of eye**

CODING PRACTICE

Exercise 40.4 Arranging Codes for Eye Procedures

Instructions: Read the mini-medical-record of each patient's encounter. Review the information abstracted in Exercise 40.2 for questions 1–3. For questions 4–6, abstract the case on your own. Assign CPT codes, quantities, and modifiers using the Index and Tabular List, and arrange the codes in proper sequence. Write the code(s) on the line provided.

---

1. OUTPATIENT SURGERY Gender: M Age: 72

Preprocedure diagnosis: Cataract, right eye

Procedure: Extracapsular cataract removal with lens implantation, right eye. Performed phacoemulsification using hydrodissection to separate the lens nucleus by injecting fluid into the capsule, then suctioned out the lens and fluid. Inserted intraocular lens in the posterior chamber and checked for leakage.

Tip: Assign a CPT code for the procedure and a HCPCS code for the lens.

2 CPT/HCPCS Codes _____

---

2. OFFICE Gender: M Age: 83

Preprocedure diagnosis: Diabetic macular edema, right eye

Procedure: Injected triamcinolone acetonide 10 mg into the Tenon's capsule (*a membrane covering the eyeball behind the conjunctiva*)

Tip: Assign a CPT code for the procedure and a HCPCS code for the drug.

2 CPT/HCPCS Codes _____

---

3. OFFICE Gender: M Age: 5

Preprocedure diagnosis: Exotropia (*eye turns outward*), left eye

Procedure: Strabismus surgery, recession (*lengthening*) of left lateral rectus muscle. Placed adjustable sutures to adjust alignment postoperatively when muscles are not affected by anesthesia.

Tip: The left lateral rectus muscle is a horizontal muscle.

2 CPT Codes _____

---

4. OFFICE Gender: M Age: 59

Preprocedure diagnosis: Significant pterygium, right eye

Procedure: Pterygium excision with graft, right eye, with 0.2 mg mitomycin. The pterygium was excised over the conjunctiva with Westcott scissors and undermined to sclera. Hemostasis was maintained with cautery. A sponge with approximately 0.2 mg mitomycin was placed over the previous pterygium site over the sclera. This was held in place for approximately one minute. Upon conclusion of the procedure the eye was patched.

Tip: Assign a CPT code for the procedure and a HCPCS code for the drug.

2 CPT/HCPCS Codes _____

---

5. INPATIENT HOSPITAL Gender: F Age: 48

Preprocedure diagnosis: Blind, painful right eye with conjunctival scarring

Procedure: Evisceration with implant, right eye; conjunctivoplasty, right eye; frost suture for temporary tarsorrhaphy. The conjunctivoplasty began by carefully unrolling and dissecting the conjunctiva back around the muscle insertion to carefully release scar bands and to maximize the length of the conjunctiva. The technical difficulty of this procedure required substantially more time to complete. Frost suture consisting of #6-0 silk was placed, going to the tarsal plates of the upper and lower eyelids to achieve temporary eyelid closure.

Postprocedure diagnosis: Blind painful eye, right eye, with conjunctival scarring; microcornea, right eye

3 CPT Codes _____

_____

---

6. OFFICE Gender: M Age: 8

Preprocedure diagnosis: Left orbital pseudotumor

Procedure: Anterior orbitotomy with excision of lacrimal sac, left orbit. Sharp dissection through the orbicularis muscle was continued to the level of the orbital septum, where the pseudotumor was excised. The orbital portion of the lacrimal gland prolapsed through the wound. Partial excision of the lacrimal gland was performed. Pseudotumor and lacrimal tissue sent to pathology.

Pathology report: Left orbital pseudotumor, normal lacrimal tissue

2 CPT Codes _____

System/Body Area	Elements of Eye Examination
Eyes	❑ Test **visual acuity** (Does not include determination of refractive error) ❑ **Gross visual field** testing by confrontation ❑ Test **ocular motility** including primary gaze alignment ❑ Inspection of bulbar and palpebral **conjunctivae** ❑ Examination of **ocular adnexae** including lids (eg, ptosis or lagophthalmos), lacrimal glands, lacrimal drainage, orbits and preauricular lymph nodes ❑ Examination of **pupils and irises** including shape, direct and consensual reaction (afferent pupil), size (eg, anisocoria) and morphology ❑ Slit lamp examination of the **corneas** including epithelium, stroma, endothelium, and tear film ❑ Slit lamp examination of the **anterior chambers** including depth, cells, and flare ❑ Slit lamp examination of the **lenses** including clarity, anterior and posterior capsule, cortex, and nucleus ❑ Measurement of **intraocular pressures** (except in children and patients with trauma or infectious disease) Ophthalmoscopic examination of: ❑ **Optic discs** including size, C/D ratio, appearance (eg, atrophy, cupping, tumor elevation) and nerve fiber layer ❑ **Posterior segments** including retina and vessels (eg, exudates and hemorrhages)
Neurological/ Psychiatric	Brief assessment of mental status including: ❑ **Orientation** to time, place and person ❑ **Mood** and affect (eg, depression, anxiety, agitation, hypomania, lability)

Total # Bullets Performed and Documented →	☐	# of ❑ Elements Performed and Documented	Level of Examination
		1–5	Problem focused
		6–8	Expanded problem focused
		9+	Detailed
		ALL	Comprehensive (Document **every** element in each box with a shaded border and at least **one** element in each box with an unshaded border)

Figure 40-6 ■ 1997 documentation guidelines for eye examination. *Source: Centers for Medicare and Medicaid Services, 1997 Documentation Guidelines for Evaluation and Management Services (with formatting adjustments).*

E/M CODING FOR OPHTHALMOLOGY

The *1997 Documentation Guidelines for Evaluation and Management Services* (1997 DG), published by the Centers for Medicare and Medicaid Services (CMS), provides requirements for each level of an ophthalmologic E/M examination (■ FIGURE 40-6). Ophthalmologists are not limited to using the guidelines for an eye examination only. They can also use guidelines for a general multiorgan system examination, or any other single organ system examination, based on what is most advantageous for a specific encounter. However, physicians cannot combine elements from more than one type of examination for a given encounter. The eye examination guidelines typically provide the best results when a detailed eye examination is performed.

To determine the appropriate E/M code, coders must review the documentation in detail and identify the specific elements documented.

- To translate the documentation into the E/M requirements for the history, refer back to Chapter 28, "Evaluation and Management Services (99201-99499)," Tables 28-7 to 28-10, or to the 1997 DG.
- To determine the requirements for an examination, refer to Figure 40-6, 1997 DG for Eye Examination, or to the single organ system examination for the eye in the 1997 DG.

- To determine the levels for medical decision making (MDM), refer to Chapter 28, Table 28-12, and the Table of Risk in the 1997 DG.

Guided Example of E/M Coding for Ophthalmology

Refer to the ophthalmology encounter (■ FIGURE 40-7, page 824) to practice skills for abstracting and assigning E/M codes. Follow along as fictitious coder Megan Scheidler, CCS-P, abstracts the procedure. Check off each step after you complete it.

▶ First, Megan needs to establish the category of service so she can determine the information needed to abstract and assign the code.

❑ *What is the setting?* Office

❑ *What is the type of service?* New patient

❑ *What is the code range?* Megan refers to the CPT Index and looks up the Main Term **Evaluation and Management** and the subterm **Office and other outpatient.** The code range listed is **99201-99215.**

❑ *How many key components are required?* Megan refers to the code range in the Tabular List and locates the

OPHTHALMOLOGY ENCOUNTER

Patient is an 85-year-old white female who presents to the eye clinic today for the first time because of decreased vision in the left eye over the past week.

She has a past ocular history including cataract extraction with lens implants in both eyes 10 years ago. She also has a history of glaucoma diagnosed 25 years ago and macular degeneration. She has been followed at home and is here visiting family and was brought in on an urgent basis today.

Her past medical history includes hypertension and hypercholesterolemia and hypothyroidism.

Her medications include betaxolol hydrochloride 0.5% eye drops to both eyes twice a day and pilocarpine 2% OU three times a day. She took both the drops this morning. She takes levothyroxine for hypothyroidism and felodipine for blood pressure.

She is allergic to penicillin.

She has a family history of blindness in her brother as well as glaucoma and hypertension.

Her visual acuity today at distance without correction is 20/25 in the right and count fingers at 3 feet in the left eye. Manifest refraction showed no improvement in either eye. The intraocular pressures by applanation were 8 in the right eye and 17 in the left eye. Gonioscopy showed grade 4 open angles in both eyes. Humphrey visual field testing done elsewhere showed diffuse reduction in sensitivity in both eyes. The lids were normal bilaterally. She has mild dry eye bilaterally. The corneas are clear bilaterally. The anterior chamber is deep and quiet bilaterally. Irides appear normal. The lenses show well centered posterior chamber intraocular lenses bilaterally.

Dilated fundus exam shows clear vitreous bilaterally. The optic nerves are normal in size. They both appear to have mild pallor. The optic cups in both eyes are shallow. The cup-to-disc ratio in the right eye is not overtly large, would estimate to be 0.5 to 0.6; however, she does have very thin rim tissue inferotemporally in the right eye. In the left eye, the glaucoma appears to be more advanced to the larger cup-to-disc ratio and a thinner rim tissue.

The macula on the right shows drusen (yellow deposits under the retina) with focal areas of retinal pigment epithelial (RPE) atrophy. I do not see any evidence of neovascularization such as subretinal fluid, lipid or hemorrhage. She does have a punctate area of RPE atrophy which is just adjacent to the fovea of the right eye. In the left eye, she has also several high-risk drusen, but no evidence of neovascularization. The RPE in the left eye does appear to be more diffusely abnormal although these changes do appear somewhat mild. I do not see any dense or focal areas of frank RPE atrophy or hypertrophy.

The peripheral retinas are attached in both eyes.

She has pseudophakia bilaterally which is stable and she is doing well in this regard. She has advanced stage open-angle glaucoma, which likely is worse in the left eye and also likely explains her poor vision in the left eye. The intraocular pressure in the mid-to-high teens in the left eye is probably high for her. She has allergic reaction to penicillin. I will recommend starting latanoprost ophthalmic OS nightly. I think the intraocular pressure in the right eye is acceptable and is probably a stable pressure for her OD. She will need followup at home in the next 1 or 2 months after starting the new medication which is latanoprost.

Regarding the drusen macular degeneration, she has had high-risk changes in both eyes. The vision in the right eye is good, but she does have a very concerning area of RPE atrophy just adjacent to the fovea of the right eye. I strongly recommend that she see a retina specialist as soon as possible to fully discuss prophylactic measures to prevent worsening of her macular degeneration in the right eye.

KEY: HPI History of the present illness   ROS Review of systems
         PFSH Past, family, and social history   MDM Medical decision making

HISTORY: Problem focused
Setting & patient type
HPI: Brief (2-3)
Chief complaint (CC)

PFSH: Pertinent (1-2)
ROS: Problem focused (None)

EXAMINATION: Detailed
(9+ elements performed and documented)

MEDICAL DECISION MAKING: Moderate Complexity
MDM Data: Ordering or reviewing diagnostic data (Straightforward Data)

MDM Risk: Acute illness with significant risk, Prescription drug management (Moderate Risk)

MDM Management: New presenting problem with strong recommendation for workup (Moderate Management Options

Figure 40-7 ■ Ophthalmology encounter. *Source: © PB Resources, Inc. Used with permission.*

category **New Patient**. She reads the code description of the first code, which states **requires these 3 key components**. All codes in the category have the same requirements for key components. This tells her that all three key components must meet or exceed the levels listed in the code (3/3).

▶ Next, Megan identifies the level of history.

❏ *What is the level of HPI?* The HPI is **Brief** because two elements are documented.

❏ *What is the level of ROS?* The ROS is **Problem focused** because no systems are documented.

❏ *What is the level of PFSH?* The PFSH is **Pertinent** because two elements are documented.

❏ *Based on these factors, what is the overall level of history?* The level of history is **Problem focused** because the lowest of the three factors (HPI, ROS, and PFSH) determines the history level. The HPI and PFSH qualify for an expanded problem-focused history, but the ROS qualifies for only a problem-focused history.

▶ Megan refers to the eye examination in the 1997 DG (Figure 40-6) to abstract information needed to determine the level of the examination.

❏ *What is the level of examination?* The level of examination is **Detailed**. Twelve elements of the examination are documented, which exceeds the requirement of one or more bulleted elements for a detailed examination. A comprehensive examination requires that all bulleted items with a shaded border be documented—which they are—plus one bulleted element from a box with an unshaded border, which is not. The DG for the Eye Examination contains only two bulleted elements from a box with an unshaded border. If the physician had examined and documented at least one of these, the criteria for a comprehensive examination would have been met and the encounter would qualify for higher reimbursement.

▶ Megan determines the level of medical decision making. (Refer to Table 28-12, Medical Decision-Making Levels.)

❏ *What is the level of complexity of the number of diagnoses or management options based on the presenting problem?* The level is **High** because there is a new presenting problem, with strong recommendation for workup.

❏ *What is the amount and/or complexity of data to be reviewed?* The level is **Straightforward** because the physician reviewed the patient's intraocular pressure.

❏ *What is the level of risk of significant complications, morbidity, and/or mortality?* Megan reviews each column in the Table of Risk in the 1997 DG and determines that the level of risk is **Moderate**. The patient presents with a new problem that poses a significant risk to the patient (Moderate), no clinical labs are ordered, and prescription drug management is provided (Moderate). The single highest element in the Table of Risk determines the overall risk. The column **Management Options Selected** is the highest level (Moderate).

❏ *Based on these factors, what is the overall level of medical decision making?* The medical decision making is **moderate complexity**. At least two of the three MDM factors are required to qualify for a specific level of MDM. Two of the three MDM factors meet moderate-complexity decision making.

Now Megan is ready to assign the code for the ophthalmology encounter. The exercise that follows guides you through additional abstracting skills and allows you to assign the correct code.

CODING PRACTICE

Exercise 40.5 **Evaluation and Management Coding for the Eye**

Instructions: Refer to the *1997 Documentation Guidelines for Evaluation and Management Services* (available at **www.cms.gov**) or Chapter 28, "Evaluation and Management Services (99201-99499)," Table 28-7 to 28-12, in this text. Answer the following questions about the "Ophthalmology encounter" (Figure 40-7).

1. a. Which elements of the HPI are documented? Circle all that apply. Location, Quality, Severity, Duration, Timing, Context, Modifying factors, Associated signs and symptoms

   b. How many elements are documented? _____

   c. What is the level of HPI? _____

2. a. Which systems are reviewed in the ROS? Circle all that apply. Constitutional, Allergic/immunologic, CV, Endocrine, ENT/M, Eyes, GI, GU, Hemic/lymphatic, MS, Neurologic, Psychiatric, Respiratory, Skin/breast

   b. How many systems are documented? _____

   c. What is the level of ROS? _____

3. a. Which PFSH elements are documented? Circle all that apply. Past medical, Family, Social

   b. What is the level of PFSH? _____

   c. What is the overall level of history? (The lowest history factor—HPI, ROS, or PFSH—determines the level of history.) _____

4. Refer to Figure 40-6, 1997 DG for Eye Examination.

   a. Which bulleted items are documented for the examination? (Check off the items documented.)

   b. How many bulleted items in the shaded box are documented? _____

   c. How many bulleted items in the unshaded box are documented? _____

   d. What is the level of the examination? _____

(continued)

CODING PRACTICE (continued)

5. Refer to Table 28-12, Medical Decision-Making Levels, or the 1997 DG.

   a. What is the MDM level for the number of diagnoses or management options? _____

   b. What is the MDM level for the amount and/or complexity of data to be reviewed? _____

   c. Refer to the Table of Risk in the 1997 DG. Which elements of risk are documented for each risk factor?

      1. Presenting problem: _____

      2. Diagnostic procedures ordered: _____

      3. Management options selected: _____

   d. What is the level of risk? (The highest of the three risk factors determines the overall level of risk.) _____

   e. What is the overall level of MDM? (2/3 MDM factors are needed to determine the overall level.) _____

6. a. What is the setting? _____

   b. What is the patient (or service) type? _____

   c. What is the code range? _____

   d. How many key components are required? _____

   e. What is the level of history? _____

   f. What is the level of examination? _____

   g. What is the level of medical decision making? _____

   h. What is the correct code? _____

   i. Which key component has the greatest impact on code selection for this case, based on the documentation? _____

7. Abstract, assign, and arrange (sequence) the diagnosis code(s) that support the E/M code.

   4 ICD-10-CM Code(s) _____

CHAPTER SUMMARY

In this chapter you learned that:

- Ophthalmologists are MDs who provide medical evaluation of eye conditions and perform surgery to correct eye problems; subspecialties of ophthalmology are cornea and external disease, glaucoma, neuro-ophthalmology, ophthalmic pathology, ophthalmic plastic surgery, pediatric ophthalmology, and vitreoretinal diseases.

- Special instructions in the Eye and Ocular Adnexa subsection identify services that are bundled with certain codes and also identify codes that should and should not be reported together.

- Although the eye is a small structure compared with other organs, it has numerous specific sites that affect the choice of codes, such as the pars plana, trabecular network, and extraocular muscles.

- To locate codes for eye procedures, search the Index for the Main Term of the anatomic site, then identify the first-level modifying term for the type of procedure or condition. Alternatively, use the procedure name as the Main Term when necessary.

- The NCCI provides direction for when separate procedures should be reported with cataract removal.

- The *1997 Documentation Guidelines for Evaluation and Management Services* (1997 DG), published by CMS, provides requirements for each level of an ophthalmologic E/M examination.

CONCEPT QUIZ

Take a moment to look back at the eye and ocular adnexa and solidify your skills. Try to answer the questions from memory first, then refer to the discussion in this chapter if you need a little extra help.

Completion

Instructions: Write the term that completes each statement based on the information you learned in this chapter. Choose from the list that follows. Some choices may be used more than once and some choices may not be used at all.

DSEK	iridotomy
enucleation	ocular implant
evisceration	phacoemulsification
exenteration	photocoagulation
fistulization	PKP
goniotomy	radial keratotomy
intravitreal	recession
IOL	trabeculectomy
IOP	trabeculotomy

1. A(n) _____ procedure removes the eyeball, including the ocular contents, and may include removal of bone and muscle or a myocutaneous flap.

2. One reason for a(n) _____ injection is to treat diabetic retinopathy.

3. A(n) _____ procedure is flattening the cornea by making a series of incisions in a radial pattern resembling the spokes of a wheel.

4. The _____ procedure, used to treat strabismus, is the cutting of a muscle from the surface of the eye and reattaching it farther back from the front of the eye to weaken or lengthen the muscle.

5. A(n) _____ procedure is removal of the eyeball without removing the ocular contents of the orbit or muscles.

6. A(n) _____ is implanted in the eye during cataract surgery after the cataract has been removed.

7. A(n) _____ is the incision and repair of the trabecular meshwork to improve aqueous humor outflow and reduce intraocular pressure.

8. _____ is the destruction of a natural lens, which is then suctioned out of the eye.

9. _____ is the fluid pressure inside the eye.

10. _____ describes removal of only the corneal endothelium layer and replacement with a cadaver endothelium graft.

Multiple Choice

Instructions: Circle the letter of the best answer to each question based on the information you learned in this chapter.

1. Which eye muscle is a lateral muscle?
   A. Superior rectus
   B. Superior oblique
   C. Iridoplasty
   D. Inferior rectus

2. What is the name for corneal repair or transplant?
   A. Keratoplasty
   B. Corneoplasty
   C. Iridoplasty
   D. Conjunctivoplasty

3. Where does CPT classify codes for blepharoplasty that involves only the skin of the eyelids?
   A. Eye and Ocular Adnexa
   B. Nervous System
   C. General Surgery
   D. Integumentary System

4. How would you code the following procedure? *A surgeon performs an exenteration of the right eye including the ocular contents with muscle or myocutaneous flap.*
   A. 65091-RT
   B. 65101-RT
   C. 65114-RT
   D. 65110-RT

5. What part of the eye is removed in a phacoemulsification?
   A. Cornea
   B. Lens
   C. Iris
   D. Ciliary body

6. How would you code the following procedure? *A surgeon performs a bilateral trabeculectomy to treat a patient's longstanding glaucoma.*
   A. 66150-50
   B. 65855-50
   C. 65850-50
   D. 66170-50

7. What procedure is typically performed by an ocularist?
   A. Ocular implant
   B. Orbital implant
   C. IOL implant
   D. Phacoemulsification

8. What type of eye procedures does CPT classify in codes 92002-92499?
   A. Diagnostic radiology
   B. Laboratory panels
   C. Medical
   D. Injuries

9. How would you code the following procedure? *A surgeon repairs a retinal detachment of the left eye with vitrectomy and scleral buckling.*
   A. 67107-LT
   B. 67108-LT
   C. 67107-LT, 67108-LT
   D. 67101-LT

10. In what list do the abbreviations OU, OS, and OD appear?
    A. *Do Not Use List*
    B. HCPCS modifiers list
    C. *Latin Abbreviations Accepted for Medical Use* list
    D. *Error-Prone Abbreviations, Symbols, and Dose Designations* list

KEEP ON CODING

Instructions: Read the procedural statement, then use the appropriate Index and Tabular List to assign CPT procedure codes, quantities, and modifiers. Write the code(s) on the line provided.

1. Repair of retina using cryotherapy without drainage of subretinal fluid, left eye. CPT Code(s) _____

2. Mechanical vitrectomy, pars plana approach, to remove a spontaneous hemorrhage, right eye. CPT Code(s). _____

3. Severing of vitreous face adhesions using a laser, bilateral. CPT Code(s) _____

4. Strabismus correction with surgery on the superior oblique muscle and the inferior rectus muscle, left eye. CPT Code(s) _____

5. Excisional tarsal wedge repair for entropion, right upper eyelid. CPT Code(s) _____

6. Bilateral canthoplasty. CPT Code(s) _____

7. Removal of embedded foreign body of left upper eyelid. CPT Code(s) _____

8. Incision and drainage of abscess of right lacrimal gland. CPT Code(s) _____

9. Conjunctival follicles expressed, bilateral. CPT Code(s) _____

10. Plastic laceration repair of the lacrimal canaliculi, left eye. CPT Code(s) _____

11. Fistulization of sclera to release IOP due to glaucoma, right eye. CPT Code(s) _____

12. Correction of presbyopia by epikeratoplasty, left eye. CPT Code(s) _____

13. Photocoagulative treatment of diabetic retinopathy, two sessions, right eye. CPT Code(s) _____

14. Peripheral excision of iris due to glaucoma, left eye. CPT Code(s) _____

15. Excision of multiple chalazion on both the upper and lower lids of the right eye while under anesthesia. CPT Code(s) _____

16. Suture of laceration of left upper eyelid. CPT Code(s) _____

17. Exenteration of right orbit with myocutaneous graft. CPT Code(s) _____

18. Removal of foreign body from anterior chamber of left eye. CPT Code(s) _____

19. Reconstruction of ocular surface using amniotic membrane transplantation with multiple layers, right cornea. CPT Code(s) _____

20. Paracentesis of anterior chamber of left eye with removal of blood, with irrigation. CPT Code(s) _____

21. Prophylactic photocoagulation of retinal detachment using a laser, bilateral. CPT Code(s) _____

22. Decompression of optic nerve by incision, right. CPT Code(s) _____

23. Tarsorrhaphy with Frost sutures, left eyelids. CPT Code(s) _____

24. Probing and irrigation of nasolacrimal duct, bilateral. CPT Code(s) _____

25. Insertion of ocular implant after right enucleation with muscles attached to implant, secondary procedure. CPT Code(s) _____

CODING CHALLENGE

Instructions: Read the mini-medical-record of each patient's encounter, then abstract, assign, and arrange ICD-10-CM diagnosis codes and CPT procedure codes using the appropriate Index and Tabular List. Assign quantities and modifiers where needed. Write the code(s) on the line provided.

1. OFFICE   Gender: M   Age: 42

Preprocedure diagnosis: Metal foreign body of conjunctiva, right eye, initial encounter

Procedure: Removal of metal foreign body embedded in the conjunctiva, right eye. Washed out the eye with sterile saline and identified the location of a small metal fragment. Wiped away FB with a cotton-tipped applicator.

1 ICD-10-CM Code _____

1 CPT Code _____

2. EMERGENCY DEPT   Gender: M   Age: 19

Preprocedure diagnosis: Traumatic perforation of left cornea while playing softball, initial encounter

Procedure: Repair of corneal perforation, left eye

Tip: Assign a diagnosis code to identify the patient's activity at the time of the injury.

2 ICD-10-CM Codes _____

1 CPT Code _____

3. OUTPATIENT SURGERY   Gender: F   Age: 31

Preprocedure diagnosis: Corneal scarring due to corneal herpes simplex, left eye

Procedure: PKP, left eye. Used a trephine to remove the corneal tissue. Removed the entire thickness of the cornea and replaced it with a new disc from the donor eye. Applied running sutures around the corneal disc to secure.

2 ICD-10-CM Codes _____

1 CPT Code _____

---

4. OUTPATIENT SURGERY   Gender: F   Age: 41

Preprocedure diagnosis: Staphyloma, left eye

Procedure: Repair of sclera of left eye with graft. Made incision in the left conjunctiva and sclera where the uveal tissue was protruding. Identified the staphyloma and excised it. Sutured a scleral graft, administered a topical antibiotic to the eye, and applied an eye pressure patch. Patient tolerated procedure well.

1 ICD-10-CM Code _____

1 CPT Code _____

---

5. OUTPATIENT SURGERY   Gender: M   Age: 57

Preprocedure diagnosis: Anterior synechiae, right eye; borderline glaucoma with increased IOP, bilateral

Procedure: Trabeculotomy ab externo to decrease IOP; used the same incision to access and sever anterior synechiae of the right eye

2 ICD-10-CM Codes _____

2 CPT Codes _____

---

6. OFFICE   Gender: F   Age: 67

Preprocedure diagnosis: Neoplasm of uncertain behavior on cornea, left

Procedure: Excision of lesion, left cornea

Postprocedure diagnosis: Malignant melanoma, left cornea

Pathology report: Corneal tissue submitted is positive for malignant melanoma

1 ICD-10-CM Code _____

1 CPT Code _____

---

7. OFFICE   Gender: M   Age: 79

Preprocedure diagnosis: Hypermature extracapsular cataracts, bilateral

Procedure: Phacoemulsification of extracapsular cataracts with insertion of anterior IOL, bilateral

Tip: Report a HCPCS code for the IOL.

1 ICD-10-CM Code _____

2 CPT Codes _____

---

8. OUTPATIENT SURGERY   Gender: F   Age: 57

Preprocedure diagnosis: Retinal detachment, right eye

Procedure: Photocoagulation repair of retinal detachment with drainage of subretinal fluid, right eye

1 ICD-10-CM Code _____

1 CPT Code _____

---

9. OFFICE   Gender: M   Age: 37

Preprocedure diagnosis: Cyst of the ciliary body, left eye

Procedure: Destruction of ciliary body cyst, left eye

Postprocedure diagnosis: Ciliary body cyst of the pars plana, left eye

1 ICD-10-CM Code _____

1 CPT Code _____

---

10. OFFICE   Gender: F   Age: 64

Preprocedure diagnosis: Macular degeneration, bilateral

Procedure: Injection of vitreous substitute, right eye

1 ICD-10-CM Code _____

1 CPT Code _____

Chapter Outline

- **Auditory System Procedure Basics**
- **Coding Guidelines for Auditory System Procedures**
- **Coding for the Operating Microscope**
- **Abstracting Auditory System Procedures**
- **Assigning Codes for Auditory System Procedures**
- **Arranging Codes for Auditory System Procedures**
- **E/M Coding for Otolaryngology**

Learning Objectives

After completing this chapter, you should have the skills to:

41.1 Spell and define the key words, medical terms, and abbreviations related to auditory system procedures. (Remember)

41.2 Summarize the types of auditory system procedures. (Understand)

41.3 Adhere to CPT coding guidelines in the Auditory System subsection. (Apply)

41.4 Adhere to CPT coding guidelines in the Operating Microscope subsection. (Apply)

41.5 Examine and abstract procedural information from the medical record for coding Auditory System subsection procedures. (Analyze)

41.6 Demonstrate how to assign codes for procedures in the Auditory System subsection. (Apply)

41.7 Utilize guidelines for arranging (sequencing) codes for Auditory System subsection procedures. (Apply)

41.8 Determine how to code Evaluation and Management services for otolaryngology. (Evaluate)

Key Terms and Abbreviations

AD	middle fossa approach	postauricular	translabyrinthine
AS	operating microscope	transcanal	transmastoid
AU	osseointegrated implant	transcranial	

In addition to the key terms listed here, students should know the terms defined within tables in this chapter.

INTRODUCTION

Advertisements and news constantly overload our sense of hearing to the point that mute buttons are available on television remotes, computers, and phones. The main function of the external ear is to collect and funnel sound waves to the middle and inner ear, where they are transmitted to the brain to create meaningful communication. The ear contains elements of the integumentary, cardiovascular, nervous, lymph, and musculoskeletal systems. In addition to the Auditory System subsection, this chapter also discusses the Operating Microscope subsection, which consists of one code and immediately follows the Auditory System subsection in the CPT manual.

AUDITORY SYSTEM PROCEDURE BASICS

Otolaryngology is a subspecialty of internal medicine that specializes in the ears and throat. Otolaryngologists, otologists, and neuro-otologists are physicians that perform medical procedures and surgery on the ear. Plastic surgeons perform reconstructive repairs involving the external ear. Audiologists are nonphysician healthcare professionals who specialize in hearing, balance, and related disorders. Speech-language pathologists (SLPs), also known as speech therapists, specialize in the evaluation and treatment of communication disorders and swallowing disorders. They can assist people with hearing disorders with their speech production.

When working with medical terms, first identify the literal meaning of the term based on the meaning of roots, suffixes, and prefixes. Then, interpret the procedure being described within the context of the body system and procedures actually performed. The practical meaning sometimes varies from the literal meaning. Some medical terms with different suffixes are used as synonyms, such as *myringotomy* and *myringostomy*, both of which describe making an incision into the eardrum to drain fluid. *Myringotomy* is the more commonly used term because the incision is temporary. The word roots *myring/o* and *tympan/o* both mean eardrum or tympanic membrane, with the only difference being that *myring/o* is derived from Latin and *tympan/o* is derived from Greek. The terms *myringoplasty* and *tympanoplasty* are used synonymously, but *myringotomy* and *tympanostomy* are different procedures because of the different suffixes. Myringotomy involves an incision into the ear drum only, whereas tympanostomy includes both an incision into the eardrum and the creation of a longer-term opening with the use of tubes in the tympanic membrane.

Coders must refer to the CPT manual and other medical references to understand how the terms are used in any particular situation. Refer to ■ TABLE 41-1 for a refresher on how to build medical terms related to the auditory system.

CODING CAUTION

Be alert for medical terms that are pronounced similarly and have different meanings.

<u>aural</u> (*pertaining to the ear*) and <u>oral</u> (*pertaining to the mouth*)

<u>cerumen</u> (*earwax*) and <u>semen</u> (*fluid containing sperm*)

<u>cochlea</u> (*a coiled canal in the inner ear*) and <u>cholera</u> (*an acute gastrointestinal disease*)

electro<u>cochle</u>ography (*recording of electrical activity of the cochlea*) and **electro<u>encephalo</u>graphy** (*recording of electrical activity of the brain*)

mast<u>oid</u>ectomy (*cutting out of the mastoid bone/process*) and **mastectomy** (*cutting out of breast tissue*)

Procedures commonly performed on each section of the auditory system are discussed next. Refer to detailed anatomic diagrams of specific parts of the ear when you need to refresh your memory on the location of specific structures or sites. Chapter 16 of this text provides additional information about the anatomy and conditions of the ear.

Procedures of the Auditory System

Procedures commonly performed on the auditory system are summarized in ■ TABLE 41-2 (page 832). In particular, coders need to understand the variations of mastoidectomy. *Mastoidectomy* is an example of a single term that can refer to a variety of techniques and requires a verbal modifier, such as simple or complete, to fully describe the procedure (■ TABLE 41-3, page 832). A mastoidectomy, which literally means "surgical excision of the mastoid bone," can be described as partial, complete, modified radical, or radical, based on the extent of the bone and surrounding structures removed. Therefore, coders must read the details of the operative report to identify the structures removed and assign the corresponding CPT code.

This section provides a general reference to help understand the most common auditory system procedures. Remember to keep standard reference books handy in case you get stuck.

Table 41-1 ■ **EXAMPLE OF CONSTRUCTING MEDICAL TERMS FOR AUDITORY SYSTEM PROCEDURESS**

Combining Form	Suffix	Complete Medical Term
myring/o (*eardrum, tympanic membrane*)		**myring + plasty** (*surgical repair of the eardrum*)
		tympano + plasty (*surgical repair of the eardrum*)
	-plasty (*surgical repair*)	**myring + ectomy** (*excision of the eardrum*)
tympan/o (*eardrum, tympanic membrane*)	**-ectomy** (*excision*)	**tympan + ectomy** (*excision of the eardrum*)
	-tomy (*incision*)	**myringo + tomy** (*incision into the eardrum*)
		tympano + tomy (*incision into the eardrum*)

Source: © PB Resources, Inc. Used with permission.

Table 41-2 ■ **COMMON PROCEDURES OF THE AUDITORY SYSTEM**

Procedure Name	Definition	Reason Performed
Cochlear device implantation	Implantation of a receiver into bone, which sends signals to electrodes implanted in the cochlea	Severe hearing loss, deafness
Fenestration semicircular canal	Creation of an opening in the semicircular canal	Otosclerosis
Labyrinthotomy	Surgical incision into the labyrinth of the ear, sometimes with administration/injection of drugs	Ménière's disease
Myringoplasty/tympanoplasty	Repair of the tympanic membrane, involving the drumhead and donor area, usually with a graft of living tissue such as fat or fascia	Otitis media
Myringotomy	Drainage of fluid or pus from the eardrum	Serous otitis media
Petrous apicectomy	Excision of the petrous apex (*part of the temporal bone*), including radical resection of the entire mastoid part of the posterior temporal bone	Acute petrositis, impaired mobility of the malleus, cholesteatoma/cholesteatosis of the middle ear and mastoid
Repair of oval window or round window	Closure of an opening with soft tissue such as fat or fascia	Fistula between the middle and inner ear
Stapedectomy	Excision of the stapes bone	Otosclerosis
Stapedotomy	Incision into the footplate of the stapes; may also involve inserting a prosthesis for hearing loss	Otosclerosis
Tympanolysis	Destruction of tympanic membrane adhesions, granulation tissue, or scar tissue	Adhesions, granulation tissue, or scar tissue
Tympanostomy	Creation of an opening in the eardrum to insert a plastic or metal ventilating tube to drain fluid from the middle ear	Serous otitis media

Source: © PB Resources, Inc. Used with permission.

Table 41-3 ■ **TYPES OF MASTOIDECTOMY PROCEDURES**

Procedure Name	Definition	Reason Performed
Simple mastoidectomy/ transmastoid antrotomy	Incision of the mastoid antrum (*the space between the mastoid cells and the upper part of the middle ear*) with dissection of the mastoid process (*the protruding bone behind the ear at the skull base*)	Infection such as mastoiditis or chronic otitis
Complete mastoidectomy	A simple mastoidectomy with more extensive removal of the mastoid process	Acute/chronic mastoiditis, diffuse cholesteatosis, cholesteatoma of the middle ear and mastoid
Modified radical mastoidectomy	A mastoidectomy that includes reconstruction of the eardrum and leaves a few middle ear bones intact	Suppurative otitis media
Radical mastoidectomy	Removal of the entire mastoid, tympanum, middle ear, and possibly the mastoid part of the posterior temporal bone	Cholesteatoma, neoplasms of the ear canal
Revision mastoidectomy	Total mastoidectomy following a previous mastoidectomy that failed to resolve the patient's condition	Cholesteatoma or infection

Source: © PB Resources, Inc. Used with permission.

CODING PRACTICE

Exercise 41.1   Auditory System Procedure Basics

Instructions: Use your medical terminology skills and resources to define the following procedures related to the auditory system, then identify the code(s) or code range listed in the CPT Index. Follow these steps:

- Use slash marks "/" to break down the underlined term into its root(s) and suffix.
- Define the meaning of the underlined word based on the meaning of each word part.
- Use the entire phrase to identify the code or code range shown in the CPT Index.

Example: <u>oto/plasty</u>, comprehensive oto/plasty   Meaning *surgical repair of the ear*   CPT Code *69300*

1. <u>mastoidectomy</u> with tympanoplasty, simple   Meaning _____   CPT Code _____

2. <u>tympanostomy</u>, general anesthesia   Meaning _____   CPT Code _____

3. <u>stapedotomy</u>, revision   Meaning _____   CPT Code _____

4. <u>tympanolysis</u>   Meaning _____   CPT Code _____

5. antrotomy, <u>transmastoid</u>   Meaning _____   CPT Code _____

6. <u>labyrinthectomy</u>   Meaning _____   CPT Code _____

7. <u>apicectomy</u>, with mastoidectomy   Meaning _____   CPT Code _____

8. ear, <u>exostosis</u> excision   Meaning _____   CPT Code _____

9. <u>meatoplasty</u>, external auditory canal   Meaning _____   CPT Code _____

10. <u>myringotomy</u>   Meaning _____   CPT Code _____

CODING OVERVIEW OF AUDITORY SYSTEM PROCEDURES

Coders should understand the organization, guidelines, and instructional notes in the Tabular List of this CPT subsection. This information is necessary for accurate coding. The CPT subsection **Auditory System (69000-69970)** contains four subheadings that are divided by anatomic site (■ TABLE 41-4). Within each anatomic site, codes are divided by the type of procedure, such as incision, excision, repair, and so on. Review the subheading and category names and code ranges listed in the Auditory System subsection to become familiar with the content and organization. Some editions of the CPT manual provide a summary list of the subheadings and categories at the beginning of the Auditory System subsection.

The Auditory System subsection includes codes for invasive, minimally invasive, and noninvasive surgical procedures on the auditory system. Codes for diagnostic tests on the auditory system appear in the Medicine section. Remember that when billing a claim, CPT codes must be linked with one or more diagnosis codes to justify the medical necessity of a procedure. CPT codes in this subsection are frequently supported by diagnosis codes

from ICD-10-CM Chapter 8, "Diseases of the Ear and Mastoid Process (H60-H95)," as well as neoplasms, symptoms and signs, and injuries (■ TABLE 41-5). These are the codes most commonly used to support procedures on the auditory system; however, diagnosis codes from any ICD-10-CM chapter are permissible.

CPT guidelines for the Surgery section apply to the Auditory System subsection. Instructional notes appear throughout the Tabular List to alert coders to the need for modifiers,

Table 41-4   ■   AUDITORY SYSTEM SUBHEADINGS

Subheading	Code Range
External Ear	69000-69399
Middle Ear	69420-69799
Inner Ear	69801-69949
Temporal Bone, Middle Fossa Approach	69950-69979

Table 41-5   ■   LOCATING ICD-10-CM AND ADDITIONAL CPT CODES FOR THE AUDITORY SYSTEM

Type of Code	Codes
ICD-10-CM Auditory System-Related Codes	
Auditory system conditions	H60-H95
Neoplasms	C30, C44.2, C72.4, D02.3, D03.2, D04.2, D16, D22.2, D23.2
Symptoms and signs	R47-R49
Injuries	S00-S09, T20, T28.41, T28.91, T33.01, T34.01
CPT Auditory System-Related Codes	
Medicine procedures	92502-92700
Radiologic procedures	
• Diagnostic radiology	70010-70559
• Radiologic guidance	77001-77022
• Diagnostic ultrasound	76506-76536
Laboratory organ/disease panels	Not applicable

Source: © PB Resources, Inc. Used with permission. CPT codes only © American Medical Association.

provide cross-references to codes for similar procedures on other sites, identify when additional codes for radiological services might be needed, and highlight resequenced and recently deleted codes. Specific guidelines and instructional notes are discussed throughout this chapter of the text.

CODING FOR THE OPERATING MICROSCOPE

The CPT subsection **Operating Microscope (69990)** is the subsection in the **Surgery** section layout and contains only one code. It is an add-on code used with codes from multiple organ systems.

An operating microscope is a microscope that a physician uses to see small structures, such as in eye or ear surgery. Surgeons also use microdissection for blood vessels and nerve repair, including free tissue transfer (■ FIGURE 41-1).

When a surgery requires an operating microscope and the physician cannot perform the surgery without it, the microscope is an integral component of the procedure and should not be coded separately. When it is not an integral component of a procedure, assign code **69990**, which is an add-on code, to report use of the operating microscope. Refer to ■ TABLE 41-6 for guidance in abstracting operating microscope procedures.

To locate the code for use of the operating microscope, search the Index for the Main Term **Operating Microscope**. One code is provided. Always verify the code in the Tabular List so that you can check the special instructions. Coders who frequently report the operating microscope quickly memorize the code number.

The CPT Tabular List provides instructional notes and special instructions regarding the use of code **69990** throughout the Surgery section, but notes do not appear consistently with all codes for which the operating microscope might be used. A summary of operating microscope guidelines follows.

Table 41-6 ■ KEY CRITERIA FOR ABSTRACTING OPERATING MICROSCOPE PROCEDURES

❏ What is the primary procedure performed?
❏ Is use of the operating microscope documented?
❏ Do CPT guidelines or instructional notes indicate that the use of the operating microscope is included in the primary procedure?
❏ Does the NCCI prohibit coding for the operating microscope in conjunction with the primary procedure?

Source: © PB Resources, Inc. Used with permission.

- A special instruction before code **69990** in the Tabular List identifies codes for which the operating microscope is an inclusive component. Do not assign code **69990** with any of these codes.

- Instructional notes throughout the Surgery section in the Tabular List sometimes, but not always, appear after the primary procedure code, reminding you not to code the operating microscope separately.

- An instructional note at the beginning of the subsection **Eye and Ocular Adnexa** states (**Do not report code 69990 in addition to codes 65091-68850**). This instruction applies globally to all procedures in this code range.

- For procedures that do not have instructional notes prohibiting reporting of the operating microscope, report code **69990** when documented.

- CPT provides an instructional note following some procedure codes that states (**For operating microscope, use 69990**). Assign code **69990** when the operating microscope is used with these procedures because it is not bundled.

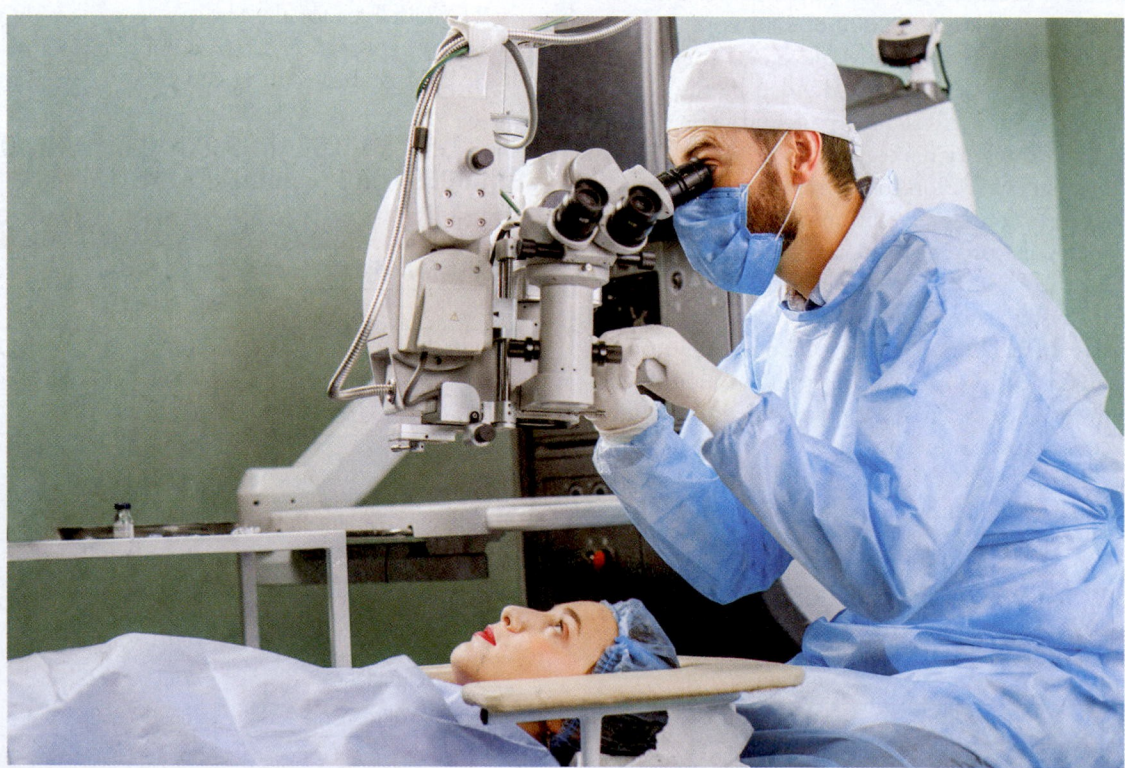

Figure 41-1 ■ A surgeon uses an operating microscope to view a patient's eye.

Code **69990** reports the work required to set up, calibrate, position, and adjust the operating microscope when it is brought into the surgical field. Therefore, it is reported once per operative session, even if it is used for multiple procedures on the same patient.

Because code **69990** is an add-on code, do not append modifier **-51 Multiple procedures**. It should be sequenced as a secondary code.

CODING CAUTION

The National Correct Coding Initiative (NCCI) prohibits the use of code **69990** for many procedures for Medicare patients, even though it is not excluded by CPT. Be aware of private payers' rules regarding reporting of the operating microscope because they might have more flexible guidelines.

CODING PRACTICE

Exercise 41.2   Coding for the Operating Microscope

Instructions: Read the mini-medical-record of each patient's encounter and use the Key Criteria for Abstracting Operating Microscope Procedures (Table 41-6) to abstract the case. Assign CPT codes, quantities, and modifiers using the Index and Tabular List and arrange the codes as required. Write the code(s) on the line provided.

1. INPATIENT HOSPITAL   Gender: F   Age: 27

Preprocedure diagnosis: Herniated disk, L2-L3

Procedure: Left hemilaminectomy L2-L3, foraminotomy, with use of operating microscope for microdissection

a. What is the primary procedure performed?

b. Is use of the operating microscope documented?

c. Do CPT guidelines or instructional notes indicate that the use of the operating microscope is included in the primary procedure?

2 CPT Codes _____

2. OUTPATIENT SURGERY   Gender: F   Age: 54

Preprocedure diagnosis: Congenital bilateral esotropia

Procedure: Bilateral medial rectus recession with microscopic control, 8 mm, both eyes

a. What is the primary procedure performed?

b. Is use of the operating microscope documented?

c. Do CPT guidelines or instructional notes indicate that the use of the operating microscope is included in the primary procedure?

2 CPT Codes _____

3. OUTPATIENT SURGERY   Gender: F   Age: 54

Preprocedure: Airway compromise; rule out squamous cell carcinoma of the larynx

Procedure: Direct laryngoscopy with biopsy using a Zeiss operating microscope

Postprocedure diagnosis: Squamous cell carcinoma of the larynx

a. What is the primary procedure performed?

b. Is use of the operating microscope documented?

c. Do CPT guidelines or instructional notes indicate that the use of the operating microscope is included in the primary procedure?

1 CPT Code _____

ABSTRACTING AUDITORY SYSTEM PROCEDURES

Laterality is always relevant for ear procedures. Some clinicians might use Latin-based abbreviations to designate the laterality of the ear: **AD** (*auris dexter*) for the right ear, **AS** (*auris sinister*) for the left ear, **AU** (*auris uterque*) for each ear or both ears. These abbreviations are not on The Joint Commission's (TJC) required *Do Not Use List*; however, they are on TJC's supplemental list of abbreviations that it suggests, but does not require, that institutions prohibit through internal policy. The abbreviations also appear on the list *Error-Prone Abbreviations, Symbols, and Dose Designations* published by the Institute for Safe Medication Practices (ISMP). Therefore, it is best not to use these abbreviations, but coders should know what they mean if they encounter them.

The anatomic approach to ear procedures describes the path the surgeon uses to access the middle ear and inner ear. Some of the commonly used approaches include:

• **Middle fossa approach**—Through-incision and partial removal of the bone above the ear

- **Postauricular**—Behind the ear
- **Transcanal**—Through the ear canal
- **Transcranial**—Through the skull
- **Translabyrinthine**—Through the labyrinth
- **Transmastoid**—Through the mastoid bone

Refer to ■ TABLE 41-7 for guidance on how to abstract procedures on the Auditory System, then work through the detailed example that follows. Remember that the abstracting questions are a guide and that not every question applies to, or can be answered for, every case. For example, the type of anesthesia affects the coding of some, but not all, Auditory System procedures.

Guided Example of Abstracting Auditory System Procedures

Refer to the following example throughout this chapter to practice skills for abstracting, assigning, and arranging Auditory System codes.

OUTPATIENT SURGERY   Gender: F   Age: 7

Preoperative diagnosis: Recurrent acute suppurative otitis media, bilateral middle ear effusions. Chronic rhinitis. Recurrent adenoiditis with adenoid hypertrophy. Both parents are cigarette smokers.

Procedure: Bilateral myringotomies. Placement of ventilating tubes. Nasal endoscopy. Adenoidectomy. General anesthesia was administered by the CRNA. Inspected ears bilaterally with an operating microscope, which was also used for the procedure. Proceeded with anterior inferior quadrant myringotomy incisions, then evacuated a modest amount of serous and mucoid material. Inserted PE tubes. Instilled antibiotic drops. Examined nasal passageways with endoscope. Acute purulent adenoiditis was evident. Shaved back the adenoids and flushed the area. Some material remained, which we resected, guided by the nasal endoscope. Submitted adenoid tissue to pathology. Patient tolerated procedure well.

Table 41-7 ■ KEY CRITERIA FOR ABSTRACTING AUDITORY SYSTEM PROCEDURES

- ❑ What is the procedure?
- ❑ What part(s) of the ear is affected?
- ❑ What is the laterality?
- ❑ What is the surgical approach?
- ❑ What is the anatomic approach?
- ❑ What type of anesthesia is used?
- ❑ What additional procedures are performed during the same operative session?

Source: © PB Resources, Inc. Used with permission.

Follow along as fictitious coder Gabriella Javiera, CPC, abstracts the procedure. Check off each step after you complete it.

▶ Gabriella reads through the entire record, paying special attention to the reason for the encounter, the procedure performed, and the postoperative diagnosis. She refers to the Key Criteria for Abstracting Auditory System Procedures (Table 41-7).

- ❑ She notes several preoperative diagnoses: recurrent acute otitis media, bilateral middle ear effusions, chronic rhinitis, and recurrent adenoiditis with adenoid hypertrophy.

- ❑ *What is the procedure?* Myringotomies, placement of ventilating tubes

- ❑ *What part(s) of the ear is affected?* Middle ear

- ❑ *What is the laterality?* Bilateral

- ❑ *What is the surgical approach?* Open

- ❑ *What is the anatomic approach?* Anterior

- ❑ *What type of anesthesia is used?* General anesthesia

- ❑ *What additional procedures are performed during the same operative session?* Nasal endoscopy, adenoidectomy

▶ At this time, Gabriella does not know which of these procedures may need to be coded, nor how many codes she will end up with. She will learn about this when she moves on to assigning codes.

CODING PRACTICE

Exercise 41.3   Abstracting Auditory System Procedures

Instructions: Read the mini-medical-record of each patient's encounter and answer the abstracting questions. Write the answer on the line provided. Do not assign any codes.

---

1. OFFICE   Gender: F   Age: 2

Preprocedure diagnosis: Pea lodged in left ear

Procedure: Foreign body removal with forceps, auditory canal, left ear. Local anesthesia was used.

a. What is the procedure? _____

b. What part(s) of the ear is affected? _____

c. What is the laterality? _____

d. What is the surgical approach? _____

e. What is the anatomic approach? _____

f. What type of anesthesia is used? _____

g. What additional procedures are performed during the same operative session? _____

---

2. OUTPATIENT SURGERY   Gender: M   Age: 13

Preprocedure diagnosis: Macrotia

Procedure: Under general anesthesia, performed otoplasty to reduce the size of the ears, bilateral

a. What is the procedure? _____

b. What part(s) of the ear is affected? _____

c. What is the laterality? _____

d. What is the surgical approach? _____

e. What is the anatomic approach? _____

f. What type of anesthesia is used? _____

g. What additional procedures are performed during the same operative session? _____

---

3. OUTPATIENT HOSPITAL   Gender: M   Age: 43

Preprocedure diagnosis: Hearing loss due to otosclerosis of the otic capsule in the right ear

(continued)

---

3. (continued)

Procedure: Right stapedectomy with footplate (*part of the stapes*) drill out. Administered general anesthesia. Made an incision in the posterior ear canal via the ear canal opening and, using microscopic visualization, moved the skin flap and posterior eardrum forward. Created an opening in the thickened footplate and inserted a prosthetic replacement, which was stabilized with a piece of fascia on the incus.

a. What is the procedure? _____

b. What part(s) of the ear is affected? _____

c. What is the laterality? _____

d. What is the surgical approach? _____

e. What is the anatomic approach? _____

f. What type of anesthesia is used? _____

g. What additional procedures are performed during the same operative session? _____

---

4. OFFICE   Gender: M   Age: 52

Preprocedure diagnosis: Vertigo due to Ménière's disease

Procedure: Endolymphatic sac exploration with shunt, bilateral. General anesthesia was administered. Made an incision exposing the right mastoid bone. Opened the mastoid and removed the bony cover of the sigmoid sinus. Worked our way down to the inner ear, taking great care to preserve all landmarks. When the endolymphatic sac was exposed, made an incision to drain it. Placed a tube between the endolymphatic sac and the mastoid cavity of the middle ear. Repeated procedure on the left ear with no problems. Patient tolerated procedure well.

a. What is the procedure? _____

b. What part(s) of the ear is affected? _____

c. What is the laterality? _____

d. What is the surgical approach? _____

e. What is the anatomic approach? _____

f. What type of anesthesia is used? _____

g. What additional procedures are performed during the same operative session? _____

ASSIGNING CODES FOR AUDITORY SYSTEM PROCEDURES

To assign codes for Auditory System subsection procedures, search the Index for the Main Term **Ear**; the first-level modifying term for the site within the ear—**External Ear, Inner Ear, Middle Ear**, or **Temporal Bone**; then the second-level modifying term for the type of procedure. Cross-reference notes after the first-level modifying term **Drum** and the entry **External Ear, Tympanic Membrane** redirect you to the Main Term **Tympanic Membrane**. Alternatively, use the name of the procedure as the Main Term.

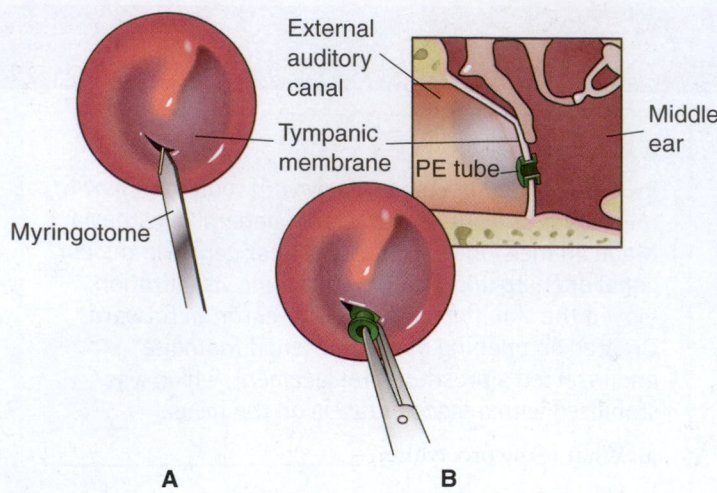

Figure 41-2 ■ (A) Myringotomy and (B) Tympanostomy procedures.

Assigning Codes for Myringotomy and Tympanostomy

Myringotomy and tympanostomy are among the most commonly performed procedures on children and are used to treat ear infections. In a myringotomy, the physician uses a myringotome to make an incision in the tympanic membrane to drain fluid from the middle ear. In a tympanostomy, a ventilating tube, also called a pressure-equalization (PE) tube, is inserted through the incision to form a permanent opening in the middle ear (■ FIGURE 41-2). The tube usually falls out on its own but in some cases might be surgically removed by the physician.

To assign codes for myringotomy or tympanostomy, search the Index for the Main Term that describes the procedure: **Myringotomy** when only drainage is performed and **Tympanostomy** when tubes are also inserted. In the Tabular List, codes for both procedures are divided by whether general anesthesia is provided (■ FIGURE 41-3). Administration of general anesthesia is not included in codes **69421** or **69436**. The anesthesiologist bills for administration of anesthesia separate from the surgeon's bill for the procedure. When the surgeon administers the anesthesia, append modifier **-47 Anesthesia by surgeon** to the primary procedure code.

Assigning Codes for Removal of Foreign Bodies and Impacted Cerumen

The ear is a common entrance site for foreign bodies, especially among young children. CPT provides codes for removal of a foreign body from the external auditory canal with and without the use of general anesthesia (**69200, 69205**). To locate codes for removal of a foreign body from the ear, search the Index for the Main Term **Ear**, the first-level modifying term **External Ear**, and the second-level modifying term **Removal**, then **Foreign Body**. Refer to the Tabular List to select the appropriate code based on whether general anesthesia is used.

Impacted cerumen is reported with a separate code, rather than the code for foreign body removal, because it is a natural by-product rather than a foreign object. Report code **69210 Removal impacted cerumen requiring instrumentation, unilateral** only when instrumentation is required. When cerumen is not impacted or can be removed by irrigation, report only the appropriate code from the Evaluation and Management (E/M) section, not a code from the Auditory System subsection. This guideline is discussed in the instructional note that follows code **69210** in the Tabular List.

Assigning Codes for the Middle and Inner Ear

The category **Other Procedures** under the subheading **Middle Ear** provides codes for hearing devices, such as the implantation, removal, or replacement of an electromagnetic bone-conduction hearing device or an osseointegrated (*integrated with bone*) **implant**. These codes represent the professional service. HCPCS codes identify the specific devices implanted (■ FIGURE 41-4) and may be billed by the facility where the procedure is performed, not by the physician. To locate these codes in the HCPCS manual, search the HCPCS Index for the Main Term **Auditory osseointegrated device**, then refer to the Tabular List to select the appropriate code.

69420	Myringotomy including aspiration and/or eustachian tube inflation	Anesthesia not specified, defaults to local or topical
69421	Myringotomy including aspiration and/or eustachian tube inflation requiring general anesthesia	General anesthesia specified
69424	Ventilating tube removal requiring general anesthesia	
69433	Tympanostomy (requiring insertion of ventilating tube), local or topical anesthesia	Local or topical anesthesia specified
69436	Tympanostomy (requiring insertion of ventilating tube), general anesthesia	General anesthesia specified

Figure 41-3 ■ CPT Tabular List entries for myringotomy and tympanostomy. *Source: © PB Resources, Inc. Used with permission. CPT codes only © American Medical Association.*

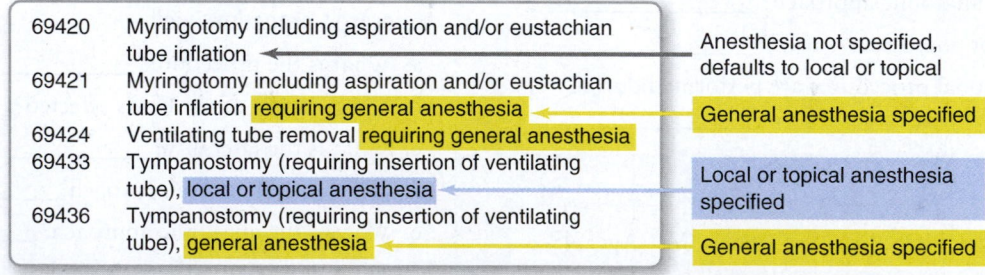

L8690 Auditory osseointegrated device, includes all internal and external components
L8691 Auditory osseointegrated device, external sound processor, excludes transducer/actuator, replacement only, each
L8692 Auditory osseointegrated device, external sound processor, used without osseointegration, body worn, includes headband or other means of external attachment
L8693 Auditory osseointegrated device abutment, any length, replacement only

Figure 41-4 ■ HCPCS Tabular List codes for osseointegrated hearing implants.

> Surgeon implants a cochlear device into the patient's right ear. The surgeon also provides the device.
>
> **69930-RT Cochlear device implantation, with or without mastoidectomy; -RT Right side**
> **L8614 Cochlear device, includes all internal and external components**

Figure 41-5 ■ Example of coding for a cochlear implant.
Source: © PB Resources, Inc. Used with permission. CPT codes only © American Medical Association.

The subheading **Inner Ear** includes procedures on the labyrinth, cochlea, vestibular chamber, and semicircular canals. In a cochlear implant procedure the physician implants a receiver into bone, which sends signals to electrodes implanted in the cochlea. The procedure destroys all residual natural hearing in the ear, so it is usually performed in only one ear. The implant device is usually provided by the facility where the procedure is performed, but if the surgeon supplies it, assign the appropriate HCPCS codes. Also remember to identify laterality (■ FIGURE 41-5).

Guided Example of Assigning Auditory System Procedure Codes

To practice skills for assigning codes for the Auditory System subsection, continue with the example from earlier in the chapter about a patient who was seen for myringotomies. Follow along in your CPT manual as Gabriella Javiera, CPC, assigns codes. Check off each step after you complete it.

▶ First, Gabriella confirms the procedures performed: bilateral myringotomies, placement of ventilating tubes, nasal endoscopy, and adenoidectomy.

▶ Gabriella begins by coding the myringotomies. She identifies that because ventilating tubes also were placed, the procedure is coded as a tympanostomy. She searches the Index for the Main Term **Tympanostomy**.

  ❏ She locates the first-level modifying term General Anesthesia.

  ❏ She identifies code **69436**.

▶ Gabriella turns to the Tabular List to review, select, and verify the code.

  ❏ She reads the title for code **69436 Tympanostomy (requiring insertion of ventilating tube), general anesthesia** and confirms that this accurately describes the primary procedure.

  ❏ She reads the instructional note following the procedure description that states (**For bilateral procedure, report 69436 with modifier 50**).

▶ Gabriella checks for instructions in the Tabular List.

  ❏ She cross-references the beginning of the subcategory **Incision** and verifies that there are no special instructions.

  ❏ She cross-references the beginning of the subheading **Middle Ear** and verifies that there are no instructional notes.

  ❏ She cross-references the beginning of the subsection **Auditory System**. The only instructional note is a cross-reference to codes for diagnostic services that does not apply to this patient.

▶ Gabriella notices that use of an operating microscope is documented.

  ❏ She turns to the Index and locates the Main Term Operating Microscope, which directs her to code **69990 Microsurgical techniques, requiring use of operating microscope**.

  ❏ In the Tabular List, she reads the special instructions under the subsection title **Operating Microscope** and confirms that code **69436** is not listed as a bundled code. She also checks with the patient's payer to confirm that the code is allowed, even though it is excluded from Medicare by NCCI.

▶ Next, Gabriella needs to code for the adenoidectomy. This procedure was performed endoscopically, and a diagnostic nasal endoscopy was also performed. She recognizes that surgical endoscopy includes diagnostic endoscopy, so because both endoscopies used the nasal passage for access, she does not code for the diagnostic nasal endoscopy.

  ❏ She searches the Index for the Main Term **Adenoids** and the first-level modifying term **Excision**. She identifies the code range **42830-42836**.

  ❏ She turns to the Tabular List to review and verify the code selection.

  ❏ She identifies that codes **42830** and **42831** are for a primary adenoidectomy. Codes **42835** and **42836** are for a secondary adenoidectomy. She recalls that a secondary adenoidectomy refers to a follow-up adenoidectomy on the same patient to remove additional tissue that was missed during the original procedure. This is not the situation with this patient, so Gabriella needs a code for primary adenoidectomy.

  ❏ She reviews the codes for primary adenoidectomy and notices that they are divided by patient age: **younger than 12** and **age 12 or over**. She confirms in the medical record that the current patient is 7 years old, so she selects code **42830 Adenoidectomy, primary; younger than age 12**.

  ❏ She checks for instructional notes below the code and for special instructions at the beginning of the category, subheading, and subsection and finds none.

▶ Gabriella reviews the procedure codes she has assigned for this case.

  ❏ **42830 Adenoidectomy, primary; younger than age 12**

  ❏ **69436-50 Tympanostomy (requiring insertion of ventilating tube), general anesthesia; bilateral procedure**

  ❏ **69990 Microsurgical techniques, requiring use of operating microscope**

▶ Next, Gabriella must determine how to sequence the codes.

CODING PRACTICE

Exercise 41.4   Assigning Codes for Auditory System Procedures

Instructions: Read the mini-medical-record of each patient's encounter. Review the information abstracted in Exercise 41.3 for questions 1 and 2. For questions 3 and 4, abstract the case on your own. Assign CPT codes, quantities, and modifiers using the Index and Tabular List. Write the code(s) on the line provided.

1. OFFICE   Gender: F   Age: 2

Preprocedure diagnosis: Pea lodged in left ear

Procedure: Foreign body removal with forceps, auditory canal, left ear. Local anesthesia was used.

1 CPT Code _____

2. OUTPATIENT SURGERY   Gender: M   Age: 13

Preprocedure diagnosis: Macrotia

Procedure: Under general anesthesia, performed otoplasty to reduce the size of the ears, bilateral

1 CPT Code _____

3. OUTPATIENT SURGERY   Gender: F   Age: 51

Preprocedure diagnosis: Profound mixed sensorineural conductive hearing loss, right side

Procedure: Right middle ear exploration with a Goldenberg TORP reconstruction

1 CPT Code _____

4. OUTPATIENT SURGERY   Gender: M   Age: 68

Preprocedure diagnosis: Squamous cell carcinoma of right temporal bone/middle ear space

Procedure: Right temporal bone resection

1 CPT Code _____

ARRANGING CODES FOR AUDITORY SYSTEM PROCEDURES

The Auditory System subsection does not provide any unique guidelines for sequencing codes. Coders must be careful not to unbundle procedures that are integral to a code.

Unbundling

Do not assign multiple codes for procedures included in the primary procedure. For example, in a labyrinthotomy procedure the surgeon makes an incision into the labyrinth of the ear, and sometimes injects drugs, to treat Ménière's disease. CPT instructional notes state **(Do not report 69801 more than once per day)** and also provide a list of codes that should not be reported together with a labyrinthotomy on the same ear. Vestibular function testing is performed for monitoring during the procedure and should not be reported separately. Diagnostic vestibular function testing is performed on a different date of service before the need for the procedure is determined. Diagnostic testing should not be reported with a labyrinthotomy procedure code on the same date of service.

Procedures that include a mastoidectomy should not be reported with a separate code for mastoidectomy, for example, codes **69910 Labyrinthectomy; with mastoidectomy** or **69530 Petrous apicectomy including radical mastoidectomy**.

-47 Anesthesia by Surgeon

For some procedures, CPT provides separate codes based on whether general anesthesia is provided. When general anesthesia is provided, and is provided by the operating surgeon, append modifier **-47 Anesthesia by surgeon**.

Guided Example of Arranging Auditory System Procedure Codes

To practice skills for arranging codes for procedures from the Auditory System subsection, continue with the example from earlier in the chapter about the patient who was seen for myringotomies. Follow along in your CPT manual as Gabriella Javiera, CPC, arranges the codes. Check off each step after you complete it.

▶ First, Gabriella reviews the procedure codes she has assigned for this case.

❏ **42830 Adenoidectomy, primary; younger than age 12**

❏ **69436-50 Tympanostomy (requiring insertion of ventilating tube), general anesthesia, bilateral procedure**

❏ **69990 Microsurgical techniques, requiring use of operating microscope**

▶ Gabriella arranges the codes in descending RVU order according to the Medicare Physician Fee Schedule Database (MPFSDB). Although the patient is not covered by Medicare, the payer follows the Medicare RVUs. She uses the facility RVU because the procedure was performed at an outpatient surgery facility, not at the physician's office.

- ❏ **42830** Facility RVU = 5.97

- ❏ **69990** Facility RVU = 6.43

- ❏ **69436** Facility RVU = 4.58

▶ Gabriella examines the need for modifiers. (Refer to Table 27-1, Key Criteria for Abstracting CPT Modifiers, or Appendix A in the CPT manual.)

- ❏ Code **42830** does not require modifiers because no special circumstances exist.

- ❏ Code **69990** does not require modifiers because, as an add-on code, it does not accept modifier **-51 Multiple procedures**

- ❏ **Code 69436** requires modifier **-51** because it is not an add-on code. It also requires modifier **-50 Bilateral procedure**

▶ Gabriella finalizes the procedure codes and sequencing for this case:

(1) **42830 Adenoidectomy, primary; younger than age 12**

(2) **69990 Microsurgical techniques, requiring use of operating microscope**

(3) **69436-51-50 Tympanostomy (requiring insertion of ventilating tube), general anesthesia; -51 Multiple procedures; -50 Bilateral procedure**

▶ Gabriella also assigns and sequences the ICD-10-CM diagnosis codes that support the need for the service.

(1) **H66.003 Acute suppurative otitis media without spontaneous rupture of ear drum, bilateral**

(2) **J35.02 Chronic adenoiditis**

(3) **J31.0 Chronic rhinitis**

(4) **Z77.22 Contact with and (suspected) exposure to environmental tobacco smoke (acute) (chronic)**

CODING PRACTICE

Exercise 41.5   Arranging Codes for Auditory System Procedures

Instructions: Read the mini-medical-record of each patient's encounter. Review the information abstracted in Exercise 41.3 for questions 1 and 2. For questions 3 and 4, abstract the case on your own. Assign CPT codes, quantities, and modifiers using the Index and Tabular List, and arrange the codes in proper sequence. Write the code(s) on the line provided.

1. OUTPATIENT HOSPITAL   Gender: M   Age: 43

Preprocedure diagnosis: Hearing loss due to otosclerosis of the otic capsule in the right ear

Procedure: Right stapedectomy with footplate (*part of the stapes*) drill out. Administered general anesthesia. Made an incision in the posterior ear canal via the ear canal opening and, using microscopic visualization, moved the skin flap and posterior eardrum forward. Created an opening in the thickened footplate and inserted a prosthetic replacement, which was stabilized with a piece of fascia on the incus.

1 CPT Code _____

2. OFFICE   Gender: M   Age: 52

Preprocedure diagnosis: Vertigo due to Ménière's disease

Procedure: Endolymphatic sac exploration with shunt, bilateral. General anesthesia was administered. Made an incision exposing the right mastoid bone. Opened the mastoid and removed the bony cover of the sigmoid sinus. Worked our way down to the inner ear, taking great care to preserve all landmarks. When the endolymphatic sac was exposed, made an incision to drain it. Placed a tube between the endolymphatic sac and the mastoid cavity of the middle ear. Repeated procedure on the left ear with no problems. Patient tolerated procedure well.

1 CPT Code _____

3. OUTPATIENT SURGERY   Gender: M   Age: 6

Preprocedure diagnosis: Bilateral chronic otitis media and possible cholesteatoma, left middle ear

Procedure: Bilateral myringotomy with insertion of tubes; middle ear exploration via myringotomy, left ear. Under general anesthesia, a right anterior inferior myringotomy was performed and a tube placed in the myringotomy site. Two myringotomies were performed

(continued)

3. (continued)

on the left: one anterior and one inferior. Anterior view revealed a small mass, which was aspirated in part and sent to pathology. Patient tolerated the procedure well.

Postprocedure diagnosis: Bilateral chronic otitis media, cholesteatoma, left middle ear

Tip: Assign the laterality separately for each procedure.

2 CPT Codes _____

4. OUTPATIENT SURGERY   Gender: F   Age: 54

Preprocedure diagnosis: Chronic eustachian tube dysfunction; dizziness

Procedure: Tympanostomy under local anesthesia. The old tube on her right side was removed and the cerumen cleaned out. On the left we saw a retracted tympanic membrane and made an inferior anterior incision to place a ventilating tube. The procedure was completed without complication.

2 CPT Codes _____

E/M CODING FOR OTOLARYNGOLOGY

The *1997 Documentation Guidelines for Evaluation and Management Services* (1997 DG), published by the Centers for Medicare and Medicaid Services (CMS), provides requirements for each level of an ear, nose, and throat E/M examination (■ FIGURE 41-6). Otolaryngologists are not limited to using the guidelines for an ear, nose, and throat examination only. They can also use guidelines for a general multiorgan system examination, or any other single organ system examination, based on what is most advantageous for a specific encounter. However, physicians cannot combine elements from more than one type of examination for a given encounter. The ear examination guidelines typically provide the best results when a detailed ear examination is performed.

To determine the appropriate E/M code, coders must review the documentation in detail and identify the specific elements documented.

- To translate the documentation into the E/M requirements for the history, refer back to Chapter 28, "Evaluation and Management Services (99201-99499)," Tables 28-7 to 28-10, or to the 1997 DG.

- To determine the requirements for an examination, refer to Figure 41-6 or to the single organ system examination for an ear, nose, and throat examination in the 1997 DG.

- To determine the levels for medical decision making (MDM), refer to Chapter 28, Table 28-12, and the Table of Risk in the 1997 DG.

Guided Example of E/M Coding for Otolaryngology

Refer to the otolaryngology encounter (■ FIGURE 41-7, page 844) to practice skills for abstracting and assigning

E/M codes. Follow along as fictitious coder Gabriella Javiera, CPC, abstracts the procedure. Check off each step after you complete it.

▶ First, Gabriella needs to establish the category of service so she can determine the information needed to abstract and assign the code.

❑ *What is the setting?* Office

❑ *What is the type of service?* New patient

❑ *What is the code range?* Gabriella refers to the CPT Index and looks up the Main Term **Evaluation and Management** and the subterm **Office and Other Outpatient**. The code range listed is **99201-99215**.

❑ *How many key components are required?* Gabriella refers to the code range in the Tabular List and identifies that the category New Patient comprises codes **99201-99215**. She reads the code description of the first code, which states **requires these 3 key components**. All codes in the category have the same requirements for key components. This tells her that all three key components must meet or exceed the levels listed in the code (3/3).

▶ Next, Gabriella identifies the level of history.

❑ *What is the level of HPI?* The HPI is **Extended** because four or more elements are documented.

❑ *What is the level of ROS?* The ROS is **Extended** because two to nine systems are documented.

❑ *What is the level of PFSH?* The PFSH is **Complete** because three elements are documented.

❑ *Based on these factors, what is the overall level of history?* The level of history is **Detailed** because the lowest of the three factors (HPI, ROS, and PFSH) determines

System/Body Area	Elements of Ear, Nose, and Throat Examination
Constitutional	☐ Measurement of any **three** of the following seven **vital** signs: • 1) sitting or standing blood pressure, • 2) supine blood pressure, • 3) pulse rate and regularity, • 4) respiration, • 5) temperature, • 6) height, • 7) weight (May be measured and recorded by ancillary staff) ☐ General **appearance** of patient (eg, development, nutrition, body habitus, deformities, attention to grooming) ☐ Assessment of ability to communicate (eg, use of sign language or other communication aids) and quality of voice
Head and Face	☐ Inspection of **head** and **face** (eg, overall appearance, scars, lesions and masses) ☐ Palpation and/or percussion of face with notation of presence or absence of **sinus** tenderness ☐ Examination of **salivary glands** ☐ Assessment of **facial strength**
Eyes	☐ Test ocular motility including primary gaze alignment
Ears, Nose, Mouth and Throat	☐ Otoscopic examination of external **auditory canals** and **tympanic membranes** ☐ Assessment of **hearing** with tuning forks and clinical speech reception thresholds (eg, whispered voice, finger rub) ☐ External **inspection** of ears and nose (eg, overall appearance, scars, lesions, masses) ☐ Inspection of **nasal mucosa, septum** and **turbinates** ☐ Inspection of **lips, teeth** and **gums** ☐ Examination of **oropharynx:** oral mucosa, salivary glands, hard and soft palates, tongue, tonsils and posterior pharynx (eg, asymmetry, lesions, hydration of mucosal surfaces) ☐ Inspection of **pharyngeal walls** and **pyriform sinuses** (eg, pooling of saliva, asymmetry, lesions) ☐ Examination by mirror of **larynx** including the condition of the epiglottis, false vocal cords, true vocal cords and mobility of larynx (Use of mirror not required in children) ☐ Examination by mirror of **nasopharynx** including appearance of the mucosa, adenoids, posterior choanae and eustachian tubes (Use of mirror not required in children)
Neck	☐ Examination of **neck** (eg, masses, overall appearance, symmetry, tracheal position, crepitus) ☐ Examination of **thyroid** (eg, enlargement, tenderness, mass)
Respiratory	☐ Inspection of **chest** including symmetry, expansion and/or assessment of respiratory effort (eg, intercostal retractions, use of accessory muscles, diaphragmatic movement) ☐ Auscultation of **lungs** (eg, breath sounds, adventitious sounds, rubs)
Cardiovascular	☐ **Auscultation** of heart with notation of abnormal sounds and murmurs ☐ Examination of **peripheral vascular system** by observation (eg, swelling, varicosities) and palpation (eg, pulses, temperature, edema, tenderness)
Lymphatic	☐ Palpation of **lymph nodes** in neck, axillae, groin and/or other location
Neurological/ Psychiatric	☐ Test **cranial nerves** with notation of any deficits *Brief assessment of mental status including:* ☐ **Orientation** to time, place and person ☐ **Mood** and affect (eg, depression, anxiety, agitation)

Total # Bullets Performed and Documented →	☐	# of ☐ **Elements Performed and Documented**	**Level of Examination**
		1–5	Problem focused
		6–11	Expanded problem focused
		12	Detailed
		ALL	Comprehensive (Document **every** element in each box with a shaded border and at least **one** element in each box with an unshaded border)

Figure 41-6 ■ 1997 documentation guidelines for ear, nose, and throat examination. *Source: Centers for Medicare and Medicaid Services, 1997 Documentation Guidelines for Evaluation and Management Services (with formatting adjustments).*

OTOLARYNGOLOGY ENCOUNTER

HISTORY: Detailed

Setting & patient type

PRESENTATION: New patient, 13 years old, comes to the office with his mother complaining about severe ear pain bilaterally. He awoke during the night with severe ear pain, and mom states that this is the third time this year he has had earaches.

Chief complaint (CC)

HPI: Extended (4+)

HISTORY OF PRESENT ILLNESS: Patient reports that he felt good after taking antibiotics with each earache episode and has recently started on the wrestling team. Mom reports that patient has been afebrile with each of the earache episodes, and he has not had upper respiratory symptoms. Patient denies any head trauma associated with wrestling practice.

BIRTH AND DEVELOPMENTAL HISTORY: Patient's mother reports a normal pregnancy with no complications, having received prenatal care from 12 weeks. Vaginal delivery was uneventful with a normal perinatal course. Patient sat alone at 6 months, crawled at 9 months, and walked at 13 months. His verbal and motor developmental milestones were as expected.

FAMILY/SOCIAL HISTORY: Patient lives with both parents and two siblings (brother – age 11 years, sister – age 15 years). He reports enjoying school, remains active in scouts, and is very excited about being on the wresting team. Mom reports that he has several friends, but she is concerned about the time required for the wrestling team. Patient is in 8th grade this year and an A/B student. Both siblings are healthy. His Dad has hypertension. Mom is healthy and has asthma.

PFSH: Complete (3)

PAST MEDICAL HISTORY: Patient has been seen in the clinic yearly for well child exams. He has had no major illnesses or hospitalizations. He had one emergency room visit 2 years ago for a knee laceration. Patient has been healthy except for the past year when he had two episodes of otitis media not associated with respiratory infections. He received antibiotic therapy (amoxicillin) for the otitis media and both episodes resolved without problems.

ROS: Extended (2-9)

PHYSICAL EXAM:
Height/weight: Patient weighs 109 pounds (60th percentile) and is 69 inches tall (93rd percentile). He is following the growth pattern he established in infancy.
Vital signs: BP 110/60, T 99.2, HR 70, R 16.
General: Alert, cooperative but a bit shy.
Neuro: DTRs symmetric, 2+, negative Romberg, able to perform simple calculations without difficulty, short-term memory intact. He responds appropriately to verbal and visual cues, and movements are smooth and coordinated.
HEENT: Normocephalic, PEERLA, red reflex present, optic disk and ocular vessels normal. TMs deep red, dull, landmarks obscured, full bilaterally. Post auricular and submandibular nodes on left are palpable and slightly tender.
Lungs: CTA, breath sounds equal bilaterally, excursion and chest configuration normal.
Cardiac: S1, S2 split, no murmurs, pulses equal bilaterally.
Abdomen: Soft, rounded, reports no epigastric tenderness. Bowel sounds active in all quadrants. No hepatosplenomegaly or tenderness. No CVA tenderness.
Musculoskeletal: Full range of motion, all extremities. Spine straight, able to perform jumping jacks and duck walk without difficulty.

EXAMINATION: Expanded Problem Focused

(6-11 bulleted elements)

LABS: Normal CBC and urinalysis.

MEDICAL DECISION MAKING: Moderate Complexity

MDM Data: Ordering or reviewing diagnostic data (Straightforward Data)

ASSESSMENT: Chronic otitis media due to a penicillin resistant organism would be the obvious diagnosis in this case. It is rare for an adolescent to have otitis media with no precipitating factor such as being on a swim team or otherwise exposed to unusual organisms or in an unusual environment. It is certainly unusual for him to have three episodes in 1 year.

MDM Management: Established problem that is worsening (Low Management Options)

PLAN: He was given a prescription for 10 days of Augmentin and a follow-up appointment for 2 weeks if not improved.

MDM Risk: Prescription management (Moderate Risk)

KEY: HPI History of the present illness
PFSH Past, family, and social history
ROS Review of systems
MDM Medical decision making

Figure 41-7 ■ Otolaryngology encounter.

the history level. The PFSH qualifies for a comprehensive history, but the HPI and ROS qualify for only a detailed history.

▶ Gabriella refers to the Ear, Nose, and Throat examination in the 1997 DG (Figure 41-6) to abstract information needed to determine the level of the examination.

❏ *What is the level of examination?* The level of examination is **Expanded problem focused**. Nine elements of the examination are documented, which exceeds the requirement of 6–11 or more bulleted elements for an expanded problem-focused examination. A comprehensive examination requires that every element in each box with a shaded border and at least one element in each box with an unshaded border be documented, which they are not.

▶ Gabriella determines the level of medical decision making. (Refer to Table 28-12, Medical Decision-Making Levels.)

❏ *What is the level of complexity of the number of diagnoses or management options, based on the presenting problem?* The level is **Low** because there is an established problem that is worsening.

❏ *What is the amount and/or complexity of data to be reviewed?* The level is **Straightforward** because clinical labs were ordered.

❏ *What is the level of risk of significant complications, morbidity, and/or mortality?* Gabriella reviews each column in the Table of Risk in the 1997 DG and determines that the level of risk is **Moderate**. The patient presents with a chronic illness with mild exacerbation (Moderate), clinical labs ordered are CBC and urinalysis (Straightforward), and prescription drug management is provided (Moderate). The single highest element in the Table of Risk determines the overall risk. The columns **Presenting Problem** and **Management Options Selected** are both Moderate.

❏ *Based on these factors, what is the overall level of medical decision making?* The medical decision making is **Low complexity**. At least two of the three MDM factors are required to qualify for a specific level of MDM. Two of the three MDM factors meet or exceed low-level decision making.

Now Gabriella is ready to assign the code for the audiology encounter. The exercise that follows guides you through additional abstracting skills and allows you to assign the correct code.

CODING PRACTICE

Exercise 41.6   E/M Coding for Otolaryngology

Instructions: Refer to the *1997 Documentation Guidelines for Evaluation and Management Services* (available at **www.cms.gov**) or Chapter 28, "Evaluation and Management Services (99201-99499)," Tables 28-7 to 28-12, in this text. Answer the following questions about the "Otolaryngology encounter" (Figure 41-7).

1. a. Which elements of the HPI are documented? Circle all that apply. Location, Quality, Severity, Duration, Timing, Context, Modifying factors, Associated signs and symptoms

   b. How many elements are documented? _____

   c. What is the level of HPI? _____

2. a. Which systems are reviewed in the ROS? Circle all that apply. Constitutional, Allergic/immunologic, CV, Endocrine, ENT/M, Eyes, GI, GU, Hemic/lymphatic, MS, Neurologic, Psychiatric, Respiratory, Skin/breast

   b. How many systems are documented? _____

   c. What is the level of ROS? _____

3. a. Which PFSH elements are documented? Circle all that apply. Past medical, Family, Social

   b. What is the level of PFSH? _____

   c. What is the overall level of history? (The lowest history factor—HPI, ROS, or PFSH—determines the level of history.)
   _____

4. Refer to Figure 41-6, 1997 DG for Ear, Nose, and Throat Examination.

   a. Which bulleted items are documented for the examination? (Check off the items documented.)

   b. How many bulleted items are documented? _____

   c. What is the level of the examination? _____

5. Refer to Table 28-12, Medical Decision-Making Levels, or the 1997 DG.

   a. What is the MDM level for the number of diagnoses or management options? _____

   b. What is the MDM level for the amount and/or complexity of data to be reviewed? _____

   c. Refer to the Table of Risk in the 1997 DG. Which elements of risk are documented for each risk factor?

      1. Presenting problem: _____

      2. Diagnostic procedures ordered: _____

      3. Management options selected: _____

   d. What is the level of risk? (The highest of the three risk factors determines the overall level of risk.) _____

   e. What is the overall level of MDM? (2/3 MDM factors are needed to determine the overall level.) _____

6. a. What is the setting? _____

   b. What is the patient (or service) type? _____

   c. What is the code range? _____

   d. How many key components are required? _____

   e. What is the level of history? _____

   f. What is the level of examination? _____

   g. What is the level of medical decision making? _____

   h. What is the correct code? _____

7. Abstract, assign, and arrange (sequence) the diagnosis code(s) that support the E/M code.

   2 ICD-10-CM Code(s) _____

CHAPTER SUMMARY

In this chapter you learned that:

- When working with medical terms, first identify the literal meaning, then interpret the procedure being described within the context of the body system and procedures performed.

- When a surgery requires an operating microscope and the physician cannot perform the surgery without it, the microscope is an integral component of the procedure and should not be coded separately; when it is not an integral component of a procedure, assign code *69990*.

- CPT provides guidelines and instructional notes on the operating microscope. Instructional notes appear throughout the Auditory System Tabular List to alert coders to the need for modifiers, provide cross-references to codes for similar procedures on other sites, identify when additional codes for radiological services might be needed, and highlight resequenced and recently deleted codes.

- Laterality is always relevant for ear procedures, but coders should be aware of the abbreviations AD, AS, and AU that providers are discouraged from using.

- To assign codes for Auditory System procedures, search the Index for the Main Term *Ear*, the first-level modifying term for the site within the ear—*External Ear*, *Inner Ear*, *Middle Ear*, or *Temporal Bone*—then the second-level modifying term for the type of procedure.

- Coders must be careful not to unbundle Auditory System procedures that are integral to a code.

- The *1997 Documentation Guidelines for Evaluation and Management Services* (1997 DG), published by CMS, provides requirements for each level of an ear, nose, and throat E/M examination.

CONCEPT QUIZ

Take a moment to look back at the Auditory System subsection and solidify your skills. Try to answer the questions from memory first, then refer to the discussion in this chapter if you need a little extra help.

Completion

Instructions: Write the term that completes each statement based on the information you learned in this chapter. Choose from the list below. Some choices may be used more than once and some choices may not be used at all.

AD	operating microscope
AS	osseointegrated implant
AU	otologists
audiologists	postauricular
BI	RT
cochlear device implantation	transcranial
LT	translabyrinthine
middle fossa approach	transmastoid

1. _____ is a surgical approach conducted through the skull.

2. The use of a(n) _____ is coded separately when it is not an integral component of the procedure.

3. _____ is a procedure where a receiver is implanted into bone, which sends signals to electrodes implanted in the cochlea.

4. _____ is the abbreviation for right ear.

5. _____ is a through-incision and partial removal of the bone above the ear.

6. _____ is the approach conducted through the labyrinth.

7. _____ is the approach conducted through the mastoid bone.

8. _____ is the abbreviation for left ear.

9. _____ are nonphysician healthcare professionals who specialize in hearing, balance, and related disorders.

10. _____ is the abbreviation for both ears.

Multiple Choice

Instructions: Circle the letter of the best answer to each question based on the information you learned in this chapter.

1. What procedure is performed to repair the tympanic membrane, involving the drumhead and donor area, usually with a graft of living tissue such as fat or fascia?
   A. Tympanostomy
   B. Stapedectomy
   C. Myringotomy
   D. Myringoplasty

2. What procedure is performed due to Ménière's disease, involving an incision into the labyrinth of the ear, and may involve administration/injection of drugs?
   A. Radical mastoidectomy
   B. Labyrinthectomy
   C. Labyrinthotomy
   D. Simple transmastoid antrotomy

3. How would you code the following procedure? *A surgeon implants a cochlear device into the patient's right ear and also provides the device.*
   A. 69930-RT
   B. L8614-RT
   C. L8614-RT, 69930-RT
   D. 69930-RT, L8614

4. What procedure is used to treat adhesions or scar tissue where tympanic membrane adhesions are destroyed?
   A. Tympanolysis
   B. Tympanogram
   C. Tympanostomy
   D. Tympanoplasty

5. What procedure is a mastoidectomy with more extensive removal of the mastoid process?
   A. Complete mastoidectomy
   B. Simple mastoidectomy
   C. Total mastoidectomy
   D. Radical mastoidectomy

6. How would you code the following procedure? *A surgeon performs a labyrinthectomy on the right ear with complete mastoidectomy.*
   A. 69905-RT, 69502-51-RT
   B. 69910-RT
   C. 69502-RT
   D. 69801-RT, 69502-51-RT

7. What procedure includes total mastoidectomy following a prior mastoidectomy that did not resolve the patient's condition?
   A. Revision mastoidectomy
   B. Radical mastoidectomy
   C. Complete mastoidectomy
   D. Simple mastoidectomy

8. What procedure is used to treat impaired mobility of the malleus and includes excision of part of the temporal bone and radical resection of the entire mastoid part of the posterior temporal bone?
   A. Tympanolysis
   B. Tympanostomy
   C. Petrous apicectomy
   D. Radical mastoidectomy

9. What procedure is commonly performed when neoplasms are present in the ear canal?
   A. Petrous apicectomy
   B. Radical mastoidectomy
   C. Tympanolysis
   D. Fenestration semicircular canal

10. How would you code the following procedure? *A surgeon performs bilateral myringotomies with placement of ventilating tubes using the operating microscope to inspect the ears for a 10-year-old patient.*
    A. 69436-51
    B. 69436, 69990
    C. 69990-51-50, 69436-51-50
    D. 69990, 69436-51-50

KEEP ON CODING

Instructions: Read the procedural statement, then use the appropriate Index and Tabular List to assign CPT procedure codes, quantities, and modifiers. Write the code(s) on the line provided.

1. Single stage reconstruction of left external auditory canal for congenital atresia. CPT Code(s) _____

2. Repair oval window fistula. CPT Code(s) _____

3. Revision of stapedotomy. CPT Code(s) _____

4. Ear piercing. CPT Code(s) _____

5. Decompression of internal auditory canal. CPT Code(s) _____

6. Simple mastoidectomy, right ear. CPT Code(s) _____

7. Biopsy of earlobe. CPT Code(s) _____

8. Facial nerve repair, medial/geniculate, left. CPT Code(s) _____

9. Simple incision and drainage of abscess, left external auditory canal. CPT Code(s) _____

10. Complete bilateral mastoidectomy. CPT Code(s) _____

11. Routine cleaning of right mastoid cavity. CPT Code(s) _____

12. Removal of tumor from temporal bone, right side. CPT Code(s) _____

13. Myringoplasty, left. CPT Code(s) _____

14. Bilateral removal of impacted cerumen using forceps. CPT Code(s) _____

15. Repair of oval window fistula, left ear. CPT Code(s) _____

16. Amputation, left external ear. CPT Code(s) _____

17. Excision, left extratemporal glomus tumor. CPT Code(s) _____

18. Use of operating microscope. CPT Code(s) _____

19. Resection, left temporal bone. CPT Code(s) _____

(continued)

(continued from page 847)

20. Excision, aural polyp. CPT Code(s) _____

21. Complex debridement of mastoid cavity under general anesthesia. CPT Code(s) _____

22. Excision, external left ear, simple repair. CPT Code(s) _____

23. Mastoidectomy with tympanoplasty, reconstruct left ossicular chain. CPT Code(s) _____

24. Myringotomy with aspiration under general anesthesia. CPT Code(s) _____

25. Myringotomy with eustachian tube inflation. CPT Code(s) _____

CODING CHALLENGE

Instructions: Read the mini-medical-record of each patient's encounter, then abstract, assign, and arrange ICD-10-CM diagnosis codes and CPT procedure codes using the appropriate Index and Tabular List. Assign quantities and modifiers where needed. Write the code(s) on the line provided.

1. OUTPATIENT SURGERY   Gender: F   Age: 22

Assessment: Chronic suppurative otitis media right ear

Procedure: Tympanoplasty with mastoidectomy, with ossicular chain reconstruction

1 ICD-10-CM Code _____

1 CPT Code _____

2. EMERGENCY DEPARTMENT   Gender: M   Age: 2

Reason for encounter: Bead in external right ear canal

Procedure: Removal of foreign body using conscious sedation

1 ICD-10-CM Code _____

1 CPT Code _____

3. OUTPATIENT SURGERY   Gender: F   Age: 45

Reason for encounter: Labyrinthitis becoming worse, right ear

Procedure: Labyrinthectomy with mastoidectomy, postauricular incision, right ear

1 ICD-10-CM Code _____

1 CPT Code _____

4. OUTPATIENT SURGERY   Gender: F   Age: 21

Reason for encounter: Foreign body in right auditory canal

Procedure: Removal of foreign body under general anesthesia, initial encounter

1 ICD-10-CM Code _____

1 CPT Code _____

5. OUTPATIENT SURGERY   Gender: M   Age: 53

Assessment: Ruptured left ear drum

Procedure: Repair of left tympanic membrane perforation using synthetic patch

1 ICD-10-CM Code _____

1 CPT Code _____

6. OUTPATIENT SURGERY   Gender: M   Age: 39

Assessment: Cyst, right external ear

Procedure: Excision of right external ear cyst

1 ICD-10-CM Code _____

1 CPT Code _____

7. OUTPATIENT SURGERY   Gender: M   Age: 71

Assessment: Tinnitus, left ear

Procedure: Exploration of middle ear via postauricular incision, left ear

1 ICD-10-CM Code _____

1 CPT Code _____

8. OUTPATIENT SURGERY   Gender: F   Age: 8

Assessment: 80% conductive hearing loss, right ear

Procedure: Cochlear implantation

1 ICD-10-CM Code _____

1 CPT Code _____

9. OUTPATIENT SURGERY   Gender: M   Age: 11

Reason for encounter: Ears are severely protruding

Procedure: Bilateral otoplasty

1 ICD-10-CM Code _____

1 CPT Code _____

10. OUTPATIENT SURGERY   Gender: F
Age: 18 months

Assessment: Chronic otitis media in left ear

Procedure: Myringotomy with tube insertion

1 ICD-10-CM Code _____

1 CPT Code _____

Chapter 42

Urinary (50010-53899), Male Genital System Procedures (54000-55899), Reproductive System (55920), and Intersex Surgery (55970-55980) Procedures

Chapter Outline

- **Urinary and Male Genital System Procedure Basics**
- **Coding Guidelines for Urinary System Procedures**
- **Coding Guidelines for Male Genital System and Other Reproductive Procedures**
- **Abstracting Procedures for the Urinary and Male Genital Systems**
- **Assigning Codes for Urinary and Male Genital System Procedures**
- **Arranging Codes for Urinary and Male Genital System Procedures**
- **E/M Coding for Urology**

Learning Objectives

After completing this chapter, you should have the skills to:

42.1 Spell and define the key words, medical terms, and abbreviations related to urinary and male genital system procedures. (Remember)

42.2 Summarize the types of procedures on the urinary and male genital systems. (Understand)

42.3 Adhere to CPT coding guidelines in the Urinary and Male Genital System subsections. (Apply)

42.4 Examine and abstract procedural information from the medical record for coding procedures in the Urinary and Male Genital System subsections. (Analyze)

42.5 Demonstrate how to assign codes for procedures in the Urinary and Male Genital Systems subsections. (Apply)

42.6 Utilize guidelines for arranging (sequencing) codes for procedures in the Urinary and Male Genital Systems subsections. (Apply)

42.7 Determine how to code Evaluation and Management services for urology. (Evaluate)

Key Terms and Abbreviations

antegrade	obstructive uropathy	retrograde	transpubic
gender data mismatch	ostomy	retroperitoneal	transurethral
ileal conduit	penile	retropubic	transvaginal
indwelling (catheter)	perineum	transcatheter	
nonindwelling (catheter)	perirenal	transperineal	

In addition to the key terms listed here, students should know the terms defined within tables in this chapter.

INTRODUCTION

Advertisements for products and pharmaceuticals related to urinary system problems appear frequently on television and in magazines. These health conditions present tangible limitations on many people's daily functioning.

This chapter discusses several related CPT subsections. The **Urinary System** subsection is discussed under chapter subtitles with the same name. Subtitles for the Male Genital System discuss three CPT subsections: **Male Genital System**, **Reproductive System Procedures**, and **Intersex Surgery**. The CPT subsections **Female Genital System** and **Maternity Care and Delivery** are discussed in Chapter 43 of this text.

URINARY AND MALE GENITAL SYSTEM PROCEDURE BASICS

Urology is a surgical specialty that deals with diseases of the male and female urinary tract and the male reproductive organs. Although urology is classified as a surgical specialty, a knowledge of internal medicine, pediatrics, gynecology, and other specialties is required because of the wide variety of clinical problems encountered. The American Urological Association identifies seven areas of clinical focus:

- Pediatric urology
- Urologic oncology
- Renal transplantation
- Male infertility
- Calculi
- Female urology—Urinary incontinence and pelvic outlet relaxation disorders
- Neurourology—Voiding disorders, urodynamic evaluation of patients, and erectile dysfunction or impotence

Refer to ■ TABLE 42-1 for a refresher on how to build medical terms related to the urinary system. Refer to ■ TABLE 42-2 for a refresher on how to build medical terms related to the male genital system.

> ### CODING CAUTION
>
> Be alert for medical words that are spelled similarly and have different meanings.
>
> **glomerul/o** (*globular tuft* [*formed by capillaries in the kidney*]) and **globulin** (*a type of protein used by the body*)
>
> **pyle/o** (*renal pelvis*) and **pylor/o** (*most distal part of the stomach*)
>
> **diuresis** (*excessive urination*) and **dialysis** (*separation of waste material* [*from the blood*])
>
> **epididymis** (*spermatic duct*) and **epidermis** (*outer layer of the skin*)
>
> **perirenal** (*surrounding the kidney*) and **perineal** (*surrounding the perineum* [*the area between the anus and external genitalia*])

Commonly performed procedures on the urinary and male genital systems are discussed next. Refer to detailed anatomic diagrams when you need to refresh your memory of the relationship of organs and sites to each other. Chapters 21 and 22 of this text provide additional information on the anatomy and conditions of the urinary system and male and female reproductive systems. Procedures commonly performed on the urinary system are summarized in ■ TABLE 42-3 (page 852–853). Procedures commonly performed on the male genital system are summarized in ■ TABLE 42-4 (page 853). In particular, coders need to understand treatment of obstructive uropathy (*the inability of urine to flow*), calculi (*stones*), congenital anomalies, and bladder reconstruction.

Table 42-1 ■ EXAMPLE OF CONSTRUCTING MEDICAL TERMS FOR URINARY SYSTEM PROCEDURES

Combining Form	Suffix	Complete Medical Term
nephr/o (*kidney*)		**nephro + scopy** (*visual examination of the kidney*)
		cysto + scopy (*visual examination of the urinary bladder*)
		uretero + scopy (*visual examination of the ureters*)
cyst/o (*urinary bladder*)	**-scopy** (*visual examination*) **-ectomy** (*excision*)	**nephr + ectomy** (*excision of the kidney*)
		cyst + ectomy (*excision of the bladder*)
		ureter + ectomy (*excision of the ureters*)
ureter/o (*ureter*)		

Source: © PB Resources, Inc. Used with permission.

Table 42-2 ■ EXAMPLE OF CONSTRUCTING MEDICAL TERMS FOR MALE GENITAL SYSTEM PROCEDURES

Combining Form	Suffix	Complete Medical Term
prostat/o (*prostate*)		**prostato + tomy** (*incision into the prostate*)
	-tomy (*incision into*) **-ectomy** (*excision*)	**vaso + tomy** (*incision into the vas deferens*)
vas/o (*vas deferens*)		**prostat + ectomy** (*excision of the prostate*)
		vas + ectomy (*excision of the vas deferens*)

Source: © PB Resources, Inc. Used with permission.

Table 42-3 ■ **COMMON PROCEDURES OF THE URINARY SYSTEM**

Procedure Name	Definition	Reason Performed
Aspiration of bladder	Removal of urine using a needle, a trocar, or a catheter	Urinary retention
Cutaneous vesicostomy	Temporary surgical procedure to create an opening in the umbilicus (*lower abdomen*), which allows urine to continuously drain from the bladder	Bladder neck obstruction, hypertonicity of the bladder, congenital atresia and stenosis of the urethra and bladder neck
Cystectomy	Partial or complete excision of the bladder; may also involve other procedures, including removing surrounding lymph nodes	Bladder cancer
Cystolithotomy	Incision of the bladder to remove calculi	Bladder calculi
Cystometrogram	Use of a manometer (*pressure-measuring device*) to evaluate bladder function; the bladder is emptied using a catheter, then filled using a smaller catheter	Voiding dysfunction
Cystostomy	Creation of an opening in the bladder, with possible removal of the bladder neck	Neoplasm
Cystotomy	Incision into the bladder	Cryosurgical lesion destruction, catheter or stent insertion, diverticulum, tumor, or ureterocele
Extracorporeal shock wave lithotripsy (ESWL)	Use of lithotriptor to aim pulsating sound waves at a kidney stone to break it into pieces	Calculi
Nephrectomy	Partial or complete removal of a kidney	Neoplasm, end-stage hydronephrosis
Nephrolithotomy	Incision of the kidney to remove a kidney calculus	Kidney calculi
Nephrorrhaphy	Suture of kidney wound or injury	Laceration
Nephrostomy	Creation of an opening in the kidney with percutaneous catheter insertion, with imaging guidance	Ureter occlusion, such as kidney calculi, neoplasm; tear in the ureter that allows urine to leak
Nephrotomy	Incision into the kidney	Obstruction, hemorrhage, neoplasm
Pelvic exenteration	Excision of the bladder, urethra, ureters, lymph nodes, prostate/vagina, uterus, colon, and rectum; may also include a hysterectomy and resecting the rectum and colon	Neoplasm
Pyeloplasty	Repair of the renal pelvis (complicated if it involves a congenital kidney abnormality, a secondary pyeloplasty, solitary kidney, or calycoplasty [*repair of the calyx*])	A ureteropelvic junction obstruction
Pyelotomy	Incision into the renal pelvis	Diagnose disorders; drain urine from the renal pelvis; calculi
Renal endoscopy	Endoscopy through an established nephrostomy, pyelostomy, nephrotomy, or pyelotomy	Biopsy, ureteral catheterization, removal of a foreign body or calculus, or tumor fulguration
Renal transplant	Implantation of a cadaver or living donor kidney to take over the function of the patient's natural kidney. Consists of a donor nephrectomy; backbench work to dissect and remove fat and prepare attached ureters, veins, and arteries for transplantation; and transplantation into the recipient	End-stage renal disease (ESRD)
Transurethral resection of prostate (TURP)	Insertion of a resectoscope via the urethra and removal of a portion of the prostate; may include cystoscopy, meatotomy, and urethral dilation	Benign prostatic hypertrophy (BPH)
Ureterectomy	Excision of the ureter	Neoplasm
Ureterolithotomy	Incision into a ureter	Calculi
Ureteroplasty	Repair of the ureter; may include excision of a portion of the ureter, then anastomosis of the ends that were not removed or grafting of tissue from the bladder	Ureteral stricture
Ureterotomy	Incision into the ureter; may include stent placement	Occlusion, stenosis

Table 42-3   ■   *(continued)*

Procedure Name	Definition	Reason Performed
Urethroneocystostomy	Repair of a defect in the bladder and urethra, with reimplantation of one or both of the ureters into the bladder	Incontinence, stricture
Urodynamic tests	A variety of tests that measure the contraction of the bladder muscle as it fills and empties, ranging from simple visual observation to precise measurements using sophisticated instruments	Lower urinary tract symptoms (LUTSs)
Vesicourethropexy, Marshall-Marchetti-Krantz (MMK) procedure, Burch procedure	Suturing of the vaginal wall to the urethra or bladder neck, with anchoring to the pubic bone or Cooper ligament	Stress urinary incontinence (SUI), cystocele, urethrocele

Source: © PB Resources, Inc. Used with permission.

Obstructive Uropathy

Obstructive uropathy can affect anyone from infants with congenital anomalies to older adults. Surgeons perform a variety of procedures depending on the cause of the problem, such as obstructed posterior urethral valves or obstructed ureteropelvic junction, bladder outlet obstruction, or benign prostatic hyperplasia.

Calculi

Treatment of kidney stones and bladder stones has benefitted from advances in technology that have eliminated the need for most surgeries to treat these problems. The use of rigid and flexible ureteroscopy enables urologists to extract calculi with forceps or a basket. Management of stones in the kidney has progressed with the introduction of percutaneous methods to disintegrate and extract kidney stones. Extracorporeal shock wave lithotripsy (ESWL) uses shock waves to break a kidney stone into small pieces that can more easily travel through the urinary tract and pass from the body. In addition, urologists can help reduce the risk of stone formation because of advances in the diagnosis and metabolic management of recurrent nephrolithiasis.

Congenital Anomalies

The urinary tract is affected by congenital anomalies more than any other organ system. Conditions range from the relatively common problem of cryptorchidism (*failure of testes to descend*) to the complex area of intersexuality. Most urologists surgically repair many congenital anomalies in children, but the more complex problems are often referred to subspecialists in pediatric urology.

Bladder Reconstruction

According to the National Institutes of Health, urinary bladder cancer is the sixth most common cancer in the United States. Surgical removal of tumors or, in some cases, the entire bladder is often the first step of treatment. Surgeons may reconstruct the bladder using a portion of the intestine and creating an **ileal conduit** (*a channel that joins the ureters to the ileum*). In some cases a cutaneous ostomy (*opening on the skin of the abdomen*) and a collection appliance might be used.

This section provides a general reference to help understand the most common urinary system procedures. Remember to keep standard reference books handy in case you get stuck.

Table 42-4   ■   **COMMON PROCEDURES OF THE MALE GENITAL SYSTEM**

Procedure Name	Definition	Reason Performed
Electroejaculation	Insertion of an electrostimulator probe into the patient's rectum next to the prostate to transmit an electrical current and stimulate ejaculation	In vitro fertilization, paralysis, retrograde ejaculation
Epididymovasostomy	Removal of a portion of the vas deferens and attachment of the vas deferens to the epididymis	Obstruction of spermatic flow
Ligation	Excision or tying-off of dilated vein(s) using a laparoscopic approach	Varicocele (*dilated vein in the scrotum*)
Prostatectomy	Removal of the prostate gland, including possible biopsy or removal of the lymph nodes	Prostate cancer or BPH
Vasectomy	Cutting out a piece of the vas deferens and cauterizing or suturing the ends closed	Sterilization
Vesiculectomy	Removal of one of the seminal vesicles	Chronic infection, prostate cancer

Source: © PB Resources, Inc. Used with permission.

CODING PRACTICE

Exercise 42.1   Urinary and Male Genital System Procedure Basics

Instructions: Use your medical terminology skills and resources to define the following procedures related to the urinary and male genital system, then identify the code(s) or code range listed in the CPT Index. Follow these steps:

- Use slash marks "/" to break down the underlined term into its root(s) and suffix.
- Define the meaning of the underlined word based on the meaning of each word part.
- Identify the CPT code(s) or code range listed in the CPT Index.

Example: nephrotomy nephro/tomy   Meaning *making an incision into the kidney*   CPT Code *50040-50045*

Urinary System

1. cystourethroscopy, biopsy, brush   Meaning _____   CPT Code _____
2. calycoplasty   Meaning _____   CPT Code _____
3. ureteroureterostomy   Meaning _____   CPT Code _____
4. pyelolithotomy   Meaning _____   CPT Code _____
5. urethrorrhaphy   Meaning _____   CPT Code _____
6. cystometrogram   Meaning _____   CPT Code _____
7. vesicourethropexy   Meaning _____   CPT Code _____

Male Genital System

8. epididymectomy, bilateral   Meaning _____   CPT Code _____
9. penis, plethysmography   Meaning _____   CPT Code _____
10. vesiculectomy   Meaning _____   CPT Code _____

CODING GUIDELINES FOR URINARY SYSTEM PROCEDURES

Coders should understand the organization, guidelines, and instructional notes in the Tabular List of these CPT subsections. This information is necessary for accurate coding. The CPT subsection **Urinary System (50010-53899)** contains four subheadings that are divided by anatomic site (■ TABLE 42-5). Within each anatomic site, codes are divided by the type of procedure, such as incision, excision, introduction, and so on. Review the subheading and category names and code ranges listed in the Urinary System subsection to become familiar with the content and organization. Some editions of the CPT manual provide a summary list of the subheadings and categories at the beginning of the Urinary System subsection, which also displays an asterisk (*) next to categories that contain special coding instructions.

This subsection includes invasive, minimally invasive, and noninvasive surgical procedures on the Urinary System.

Codes for diagnostic tests on the urinary system appear in the Medicine section. CPT codes in the Urinary System subsection are frequently supported by diagnosis codes from ICD-10-CM Chapter 14, "Diseases of the Genitourinary System (N00-N99)," as well as neoplasms, symptoms and signs, and injuries (■ TABLE 42-6). These are the codes most commonly used to support procedures on the Urinary System; however, diagnosis codes from any ICD-10-CM chapter are permissible. CPT codes must always be linked on claims with one or more diagnosis codes to justify the medical necessity of the service.

CPT guidelines for the Surgery section apply to the Urinary System subsection. Special instructions provide definitions and coding guidelines at the beginning of many categories. Special instructions are provided for **Laparoscopy** and **Endoscopy** categories in several places throughout the Urinary System, as well as for **Renal Transplantation (50300-50380)**, **Bladder-Urodynamics (51725-51798)**, and **Ureter and Pelvis (52320-52356)**.

Instructional notes appear throughout the Tabular List to alert coders to the need for modifiers, provide cross-references to codes for similar procedures on other sites, identify when additional codes for radiological services might be needed, and highlight resequenced and recently deleted codes.

Most codes in the Urinary System subsection apply to both males and females, although some are gender-specific, such as those for procedures on the prostate. Due to anatomic

Table 42-5   ■   URINARY SYSTEM SUBHEADINGS

Subheading	Code Range
Kidney	50010-50593
Ureter	50600-50980
Bladder	51020-52700
Urethra	53000-53899

Table 42-6 ■ LOCATING ICD-10-CM AND ADDITIONAL CPT CODES FOR THE URINARY AND MALE GENITAL SYSTEM

Type of Code	Codes
ICD-10-CM Urinary and Male Genital System-Related Codes	
Urinary system conditions	N00-N39
Male genital system conditions	N40-N65, Z31
Neoplasms	C50, C60-C63, C64-C68
Symptoms and signs	R30-R39
Injuries	S37-S39
CPT Urinary and Male Genital System-Related Codes	
Medicine procedures	90935-90999, 96040
Radiologic procedures	
• Diagnostic radiology	74400-74485
• Radiologic guidance	77001-77022
• Diagnostic ultrasound	76700-76776
• Nuclear medicine, diagnostic	78700-78799
Laboratory organ/disease panels	80047, 80048, 80050, 80053, 80069

Source: © PB Resources, Inc. Used with permission. CPT codes only © American Medical Association.

Table 42-7 ■ MALE GENITAL SYSTEM SUBHEADINGS

Subheading	Code Range
Penis	54000-54450
Testis	54500-54699
Epididymis	54700-54901
Tunica Vaginalis	55000-55060
Scrotum	55100-55180
Vas Deferens	55200-55400
Spermatic Cord	55500-55559
Seminal Vesicles	55600-55680
Prostate	55700-55899

differences in the urethra between males and females, some codes for procedures on the urethra are also gender-specific. Such codes are discussed later in this chapter.

CODING GUIDELINES FOR MALE GENITAL SYSTEM AND OTHER REPRODUCTIVE PROCEDURES

This chapter discusses three CPT subsections that describe the Male Genital System and other reproductive procedures. The first subsection, **Male Genital System (54000-55899)**, contains nine subheadings that are divided by anatomic site (■ TABLE 42-7). Within each anatomic site, codes are divided by the type of procedure, such as incision, excision, introduction, and so on. Review the subheading and category names and code ranges listed in the Male Genital System subsection to become familiar with the content and organization. Special instructions are provided for **Laparoscopy** and **Endoscopy** categories in several places throughout the Male Genital System subsection.

The second subsection, **Reproductive System Procedures (55920)**, contains one code that identifies **Placement of needles or catheters into pelvic organs and/or genitalia (except prostate) for subsequent interstitial radioelement application**.

The third subsection, **Intersex Surgery (55970-55980)**, contains two codes: one for male-to-female intersex surgery and one for female-to-male intersex surgery.

These three CPT subsections are discussed in the remainder of this chapter under the subtitles for the Male Genital System.

This subsection includes invasive, minimally invasive, and noninvasive surgical procedures on the male genital system and other reproductive system procedures. Codes for diagnostic tests on the male genital system appear in the Medicine section. CPT codes in the Male Genital System subsection are frequently supported by diagnosis codes from ICD-10-CM Chapter 14, "Diseases of the Genitourinary System (N00-N99)," as well as neoplasms, symptoms and signs, and injuries. These are the codes most commonly used to support procedures in the Male Genital System subsection; however, diagnosis codes from any ICD-10-CM chapter are permissible.

CPT guidelines for the Surgery section apply to the Male Genital System subsection.

Special instructions provide definitions and coding guidelines at the beginning of many categories.

Instructional notes appear throughout the Tabular List to alert coders to the need for modifiers, provide cross-references to codes for similar procedures on other sites, identify when additional codes for radiological services might be needed, and highlight resequenced and recently deleted codes. Specific guidelines and instructional notes are discussed throughout this chapter of the text.

Codes for the male genital system are gender-specific and apply only to males.

ABSTRACTING PROCEDURES FOR THE URINARY AND MALE GENITAL SYSTEMS

Abstracting for urinary and male genital system procedures uses similar processes. For both systems, coders must identify the anatomic approach and the patient's gender. Refer to ■ TABLE 42-8 (page 856) for guidance on how to abstract procedures on the urinary system. Refer to ■ TABLE 42-9 (page 856) for guidance on how to abstract procedures on the male genital system. A detailed guided example on abstracting skills follows. Remember that the abstracting questions are a guide and that not every question applies to, or can be answered for, every case. For example, anastomosis is not always performed, but when it is, you must identify the structures that are joined.

Abstracting the Anatomic Approach

As is the case with procedures in many body systems, procedures on the urinary and male genital systems often use a specific anatomic approach to access the surgical site. Coders

Table 42-8 ■ **KEY CRITERIA FOR ABSTRACTING URINARY SYSTEM PROCEDURES**

- ❏ What is the procedure?
- ❏ What is the patient's gender?
- ❏ What is the anatomic site?
- ❏ What structures outside the urinary system are involved, if any?
- ❏ What is the surgical approach?
- ❏ What is the anatomic approach?
- ❏ What is the laterality?
- ❏ What type of obstruction is treated, if any?
- ❏ What structures are joined in an anastomosis, if performed?
- ❏ Is a stoma created?

Source: © PB Resources, Inc. Used with permission.

must understand and be able to identify the correct anatomic approach based on the documentation. Commonly used anatomic approaches include:

- **Penile**—In or through the penis (male only)
- **Perirenal**—In tissues surrounding the kidney
- **Retroperitoneal**—Behind the peritoneal membrane that covers the abdominal and pelvic organs
- **Retropubic**—Behind the pubic bone
- **Ostomy**—Through an existing stoma
- **Transcatheter**—Through an existing catheter
- **Transperineal**—Through the **perineum** (*the area between the anus and external genitalia*)
- **Transpubic**— Through the pubic bone
- **Transurethral**—Through the urethra
- **Transvaginal**—Through the vagina (female only)

Table 42-9 ■ **KEY CRITERIA FOR ABSTRACTING MALE GENITAL SYSTEM PROCEDURES**

- ❏ What is the procedure?
- ❏ What is the patient's gender?
- ❏ What is the anatomic site?
- ❏ What structures outside the male genital system are involved, if any?
- ❏ What is the surgical approach?
- ❏ What is the anatomic approach?
- ❏ What is the laterality?
- ❏ What type of obstruction is treated, if any?
- ❏ What structures are joined in an anastomosis, if performed?

Source: © PB Resources, Inc. Used with permission.

Abstracting Gender

Coders must always be attentive to the patient's gender, especially when abstracting for the urinary and reproductive systems. A **gender data mismatch** occurs when the patient's documented gender is inconsistent with the procedure coded. This is most likely to occur with procedures that are gender-specific, such as a prostatectomy, and those that use a gender-specific anatomic approach—such as penile or transvaginal. A gender data mismatch can be caused by data entry errors or confusion of names, so coders must verify the patient's gender against any gender-specific edits for a code. When the gender does not match the procedure described, refer back to any source documents, such as patient registration forms, to confirm the correct information. In most cases, claims that contain a gender data mismatch cannot be transmitted for payment because they are flagged by the electronic claims processing system as containing invalid data. If they are transmitted, they may not be processed by the payer. Either way, the error causes delays and added processing time for the medical office. Sometimes, rejected or unprocessable claims are not corrected immediately but are added to the medical facility's backlog of claims that need to be resubmitted and might be neglected for weeks or months. A quick double-check by the coder to verify the patient's gender while abstracting can save significant time and money later in the claims process.

A patient's gender on the medical record and/or insurance card might differ from his or her anatomic structure due to a gender identity preference or postprocedural gender reassignment status. When this happens, refer to facility and payer policies regarding how to prepare the claim for processing.

Guided Example of Abstracting Urinary System Procedures

Refer to the following example throughout this chapter to practice skills for abstracting, assigning, and arranging urinary system codes.

> OUTPATIENT HOSPITAL   Gender: M   Age: 40
>
> Preprocedure diagnosis: Red, swollen penis
>
> Procedure: Ureterography; inserted bilateral ureteral catheters percutaneously through each renal pelvis using imaging guidance, injected contrast medium through catheter using imaging guidance, and viewed both ureters. Provided radiological supervision, reviewed findings, and dictated report for radiological procedure.
>
> Postprocedure diagnosis: Ureteral stricture

Follow along as fictitious coder Chrystal Crago, CCA, abstracts the procedure. Check off each step after you complete it.

► Chrystal reads through the entire record, paying special attention to the reason for the encounter, the procedure performed, and the postprocedure diagnosis. She refers to the Key Criteria for Abstracting Urinary System Procedures (Table 42-8).

  ❏ She notes preoperative diagnosis of a red, swollen penis and the postprocedure diagnosis of ureteral stricture.

❑ *What is the procedure?* Ureterography

❑ *What is the patient's gender?* Male

❑ *What is the anatomic site?* Ureter

❑ *What structures outside the urinary system are involved, if any?* None

❑ *What is the surgical approach?* Percutaneous

❑ *What is the anatomic approach?* Transcatheter

❑ *What is the laterality?* Bilateral because physician "viewed both ureters"

❑ *What type of obstruction is treated, if any?* A ureteral stricture was identified as the diagnosis, but it was not treated

❑ *What additional procedure is performed?* Radiological supervision

▶ At this time, Chrystal does not know which of these procedures may need to be coded, nor how many codes she will end up with. She will learn about this when she moves on to assigning codes.

CODING PRACTICE

Exercise 42.2   Abstracting Procedures for the Urinary and Male Genital Systems

Instructions: Read the mini-medical-record of each patient's encounter and answer the abstracting questions. Write the answer on the line provided. Do not assign any codes.

---

1. INPATIENT HOSPITAL   Gender: M   Age: 69

Preprocedure diagnosis: Urinary incontinence

Procedure: Sling operation. Made an incision in the perineum to advance a synthetic sling under the bladder and attached it to the muscles surrounding the urethra.

a. What is the procedure? _____

b. What is the patient's gender? _____

c. What is the anatomic site? _____

d. What structures outside the urinary system are involved, if any? _____

e. What is the surgical approach? _____

f. What is the anatomic approach? _____

g. What is the laterality? _____

h. What type of obstruction is treated, if any? _____

i. What structures are joined in an anastomosis, if performed? _____

j. Is a stoma created? _____

---

2. OUTPATIENT SURGERY   Gender: M   Age: 29

Preprocedure diagnosis: Infected seminal vesicles due to E. coli

Procedure: Vesiculotomy; incised both seminal vesicles to drain infection. Complex dissection was required due to scar tissue in the area.

a. What is the procedure? _____

b. What is the patient's gender? _____

c. What is the anatomic site? _____

d. What structures outside the male genital system are involved, if any? _____

e. What is the surgical approach? _____

f. What is the anatomic approach? _____

g. What is the laterality? _____

h. What type of obstruction is treated, if any? _____

i. What structures are joined in an anastomosis, if performed? _____

---

3. OUTPATIENT SURGERY   Gender: M   Age: 58

Preprocedure diagnosis: Residual tissue 60 days post-TURP that was performed by the same surgeon due to BPH

Procedure: TURP to remove residual tissue; advanced flexible cystourethroscope through the external opening of the urethra to the prostate and located the residual prostate tissue that continues to partially obstruct the urethra. Excised tissue using blunt and sharp dissection. A catheter was placed. Patient tolerated procedure well.

a. What is the procedure? _____

(continued)

CODING PRACTICE (continued)

3. (continued)

b. What is the patient's gender? _____

c. What is the anatomic site? _____

d. What structures outside the urinary system are involved, if any? _____

e. What is the surgical approach? _____

f. What is the anatomic approach? _____

g. What is the laterality? _____

h. What type of obstruction is treated, if any? _____

i. Was the procedure provided within the global period of another procedure by the same physician? _____

4. INPATIENT HOSPITAL   Gender: M   Age: 46

Preprocedure diagnosis: Bladder cancer; previously removed the bladder and created an ileal conduit (*use of a segment of the ileum to connect the ureters to a stoma on the abdominal wall*)

Procedure: Ureteropyelography; injected contrast medium through the existing stoma to view the ureters and ileal conduit. Supervised the radiology procedure and dictated the interpretation report.

Preprocedure diagnosis: Ileal conduit was visualized to be functioning properly

a. What is the procedure? _____

b. What is the patient's gender? _____

c. What is the anatomic site? _____

d. What structures outside the urinary system are involved, if any? _____

e. What is the surgical approach? _____

f. What is the anatomic approach? _____

g. What structures are joined in an anastomosis, if performed? _____

h. Is a stoma created? _____

i. Was radiological supervision and interpretation provided by the same physician? _____

5. INPATIENT HOSPITAL   Gender: M   Age: 67

Preprocedure diagnosis: Bladder cancer of contiguous sites of the bladder with metastasis to the colon and rectum

Procedure: Functioned as a member of a surgical team; completely excised the urinary bladder; created

(continued)

5. (continued)

a ureteroileal conduit and intestinal anastomosis; performed bilateral pelvic lymphadenectomy including external iliac, hypogastric, and obturator nodes; performed an open total colectomy with a complete proctectomy

Tip: Code for one surgeon who is working as part of the surgical team.

a. What is the anatomic site? _____

b. What is the first procedure? _____

c. What is the second procedure? _____

d. What is the third procedure? _____

e. What is the fourth procedure? _____

f. What structures outside the urinary system are involved, if any? _____

g. What is the surgical approach? _____

h. What structures are joined in an anastomosis, if performed? _____

i. Is a stoma created? _____

6. OFFICE/OUTPATIENT HOSPITAL   Gender: M   Age: 72

Reason for encounters: New patient with complaints of urinary incontinence

Procedure (Tuesday): Conducted a comprehensive history and exam with moderate-complexity medical decision making. Recommended further testing and discussed treatment options with patient.

Procedure (Friday): Performed postvoid residual (PVR) ultrasound test to measure the amount of urine left in the bladder after the patient urinates

Plan: Incontinence sling surgery

a. What service is provided on Tuesday? _____

b. What is the setting? _____

c. What is the patient type? _____

d. What is the level of history? _____

e. What is the level of examination? _____

f. What is the level of medical decision making? _____

g. What procedure is performed on Friday? _____

h. What is the anatomic site? _____

i. What testing modality is used? _____

j. What is the laterality? _____

k. What is the plan? _____

ASSIGNING CODES FOR URINARY AND MALE GENITAL SYSTEM PROCEDURES

Coders must be aware of gender-specific codes when assigning codes from the Urinary and Male Genital System subsections. They must also be familiar with coding for urinary catheterization and radiological guidance and radiological supervision and interpretation (RS&I). These skills are discussed next, followed by the continuation of the guided example.

Assigning Gender-Specific Codes

Because of the anatomic differences between the male and female urethra, some procedures are gender-specific. Differences include the longer length of the female urethra and the types of anatomic approach, such as transvaginal, prostatic, or penile. Gender edits are not identified in the official CPT manual, although some third-party publishers provide enhanced manuals with annotations or symbols. Some encoders and medical billing software programs also provide an alert for gender edits. If you do not have access to these resources, rely on the code description to identify gender-specific codes (■ TABLE 42-10).

Assigning Codes for Urinary Catheterization

Urinary catheters are hollow, flexible tubes used to drain urine from the bladder into an external collection bag. Codes for urinary catheterization are divided based on the type of catheter, the anatomic site of catheter insertion, and, in some cases, the reason for the bladder catheter. The codes differentiate between indwelling and nonindwelling catheters, which are defined as follows:

- Indwelling—A flexible, hollow tube inserted into the urinary bladder left in short or long term to provide continuous urine flow; may be inserted through the urethra or ureters

- Nonindwelling—Includes two types of catheters that are not left in the bladder: a condom catheter placed outside the body to catch urine or a straight catheter inserted into the bladder only to drain the urine then removed; also called an external catheter

Refer to ■ TABLE 42-11 to learn about the various types of urinary catheters.

Insertion of a urinary bladder catheter is a component of the global surgical package and is not separately reportable when performed at the time of or just prior to the procedure. However, when the catheter is inserted due to unforeseen circumstances after the patient has left the operating room, report the CPT code that identifies the type of catheter inserted. Electronic edit checks for claims processing often automatically deny a catheterization on the same date as a procedure. Insurance companies might request the use of modifier **-59 Distinct procedural service**, an extended modifier **-X{EPSU}**, a separate diagnosis code, or a special report that clearly identifies the problem necessitating the catheterization.

To assign codes for urinary catheterization, search the Index for the Main Term **Catheterization**, then locate the first-level modifying term **Bladder**. Refer to the Tabular List to select and

Table 42-11   ■   TYPES OF URINARY CATHETERS

Type of Catheter	Description
Balloon catheter	An urethral catheter with an inflatable balloon near the tip to hold the catheter in place and/or dilate the urethra
Condom catheter	A nonindwelling catheter consisting of a sac that fits over the penis to collect urine and drain it through a tube that leads to a collection bag; is left in place
Coudé catheter	A type of elbowed catheter with a slightly curved tip
Elbowed catheter, prostatic catheter	A urethral catheter with a sharp bend near the intake; used to navigate past obstructions in the urinary tract
Female catheter	A short urethral catheter for passage through the female urethra
Foley catheter	The most commonly used design of indwelling balloon catheter
Nephrostomy catheter	A catheter inserted through an existing nephrostomy
Olive-tip catheter	A ureteral catheter with an olive-shaped end, used to dilate a constricted ureter
Straight catheter	A nonindwelling catheter consisting of a short, rigid tube that is inserted via the urethra to allow for drainage of urine, then removed
Suprapubic catheter	An indwelling catheter inserted into the bladder through a laparotomy incision a few inches below the navel; less likely to harbor infection than indwelling urethral catheters
Ureteral catheter	An indwelling catheter inserted into the ureter, either through the urethra and bladder or posteriorly through the kidney
Urethral catheter	An indwelling catheter inserted through the urethra into the urinary bladder, percutaneously or through an existing ostomy
Winged catheter	A urethral catheter that is retained in the bladder by winglike projections on the end

Source: © PB Resources, Inc. Used with permission.

Table 42-10   ■   EXAMPLES OF GENDER EDITS FOR THE URINARY SYSTEM

Gender	CPT Code
Male	53410 Urethroplasty, 1-stage reconstruction of male anterior urethra
Male	53415 Urethroplasty, transpubic or perineal, 1-stage, for reconstruction or repair of prostatic or membranous urethra
Female	53430 Urethroplasty, reconstruction of female urethra
Female	53500 Urethrolysis, transvaginal, secondary, open, including cystourethroscopy (eg, postsurgical obstruction, scarring)
Both	53200 Biopsy of urethra
Both	53431 Urethroplasty with tubularization of posterior urethra and/or lower bladder for incontinence (eg, Tenago, Leadbetter procedure)

Source: © PB Resources, Inc. Used with permission. CPT codes only © American Medical Association.

verify the correct code. Codes are divided based on the use of a cystotomy (**51045**), suprapubic catheter (**51102**), nonindwelling catheter (**51701**), or indwelling catheter (**51702, 51703**). Indwelling catheter codes are divided based on the extent of the procedure as simple or complicated. A complicated catheterization should be documented as such by the physician and may include working with abnormal anatomy, retrieving a fractured (*broken*) catheter or balloon, or treating another complicating circumstance that requires an extensive amount of time to complete.

To locate codes for ureteral catheterization, search the Index for the Main Term **Ureter** and the first-level modifying term **Catheterization**.

When a ureteral catheter is inserted endoscopically, search the Index for the Main Term **Catheterization**, the first-level modifying term **Ureter**, and the second-level modifying term **Endoscopic**.

Although these two coding paths seem similar, they lead to different codes in the CPT Index.

Another option is to search the Index for the Main Term **Insertion**, the first-level modifying term **Catheter**, and the second-level modifying terms **Bladder**, **Kidney**, **Ureter**, or **Urethra**. Remember that when you cannot easily locate a code that accurately describes the procedure using your preferred coding path, try searching for a different Main Term.

SUCCESS STEP

A *catheter* is a thin, flexible, hollow tube used in many types of medical procedures. In addition to being used for urinary system procedures, catheters are used in procedures on the heart, vascular system, lung, and brain. When you see a catheter mentioned in documentation, always identify the type and purpose of the catheter being used.

Assigning Codes Requiring Radiologic Guidance

Some urinary system procedures are performed with radiologic guidance, such as fluoroscopy, to project a real-time x-ray image of anatomic structures onto a screen while the surgeon is manipulating instruments. Radiologic guidance can be provided by the same surgeon performing the procedure or by a radiologist, and it is almost always reported as a separate procedure with a code from the Radiology section of CPT. In the Tabular List, codes for procedures that are frequently performed with imaging guidance may be accompanied by an instructional note that directs coders to the corresponding Radiology section code. The wording of the instructional note varies. Keep in mind the following information when assigning codes for imaging procedures (■ Table 42-12):

- Instructional notes may appear at the beginning of a code range or category or immediately after a code in the Tabular List.

- The instructional note might list one code or multiple codes.

- Always verify the codes in the Radiology section of the Tabular List.

- Multiple Radiology section codes are listed when more than one type of imaging procedure is potentially applicable. Review *all* codes listed and select the *one* that describes the specific procedure performed. Do not randomly assign a code without confirming that it accurately describes the procedure.

- When the code description of the primary procedure states that imaging guidance is included, do not assign a separate Radiology section code.

- Most Radiology section codes include a professional component (*physician supervision, interpretation, and*

Table 42-12   ■   **EXAMPLES OF CODE DESCRIPTIONS AND INSTRUCTIONAL NOTES FOR RADIOLOGICAL SERVICES**

Description	Code Example
Bundled fluoroscopy	50389 Removal of nephrostomy tube, requiring fluoroscopic guidance (eg, with concurrent indwelling ureteral stent) (Removal of nephrostomy tube not requiring fluoroscopic guidance is considered inherent to E/M services. Report the appropriate level of E/M service provided.)
Fluoroscopy coded separately	50081 Percutaneous nephrostolithotomy or pyelostolithotomy, with or without dilation, endoscopy, lithotripsy, stenting, or basket extraction; over 2 cm (For fluoroscopic guidance, see 76000, 76001.)
Multiple code options for RS&I	50390 Aspiration and/or injection of renal cyst or pelvis by needle, percutaneous (For radiological supervision and interpretation, see 74425, 74470, 76942, 77002, 77012, 77021.)
Radiologic service not bundled	52010 Cystourethroscopy, with ejaculatory duct catheterization, with or without irrigation, instillation, or duct radiography, exclusive of radiologic service (For radiological supervision and interpretation, use 74440.)
Single code option for RS&I	50684 Injection procedure for ureterography or ureteropyelography through ureterostomy or indwelling ureteral catheter (For radiological supervision and interpretation, use 74425.)
Multiple code options for imaging guidance	55876 Placement of interstitial device(s) for radiation therapy guidance (eg, fiducial markers, dosimeter), prostate (via needle, any approach), single or multiple (For imaging guidance, see 76942, 77002, 77012, 77021.)

Source: © PB Resources, Inc. Used with permission.

written report) and a technical component (*facility, staffing, and equipment*). The Radiology section code may require a modifier based on the service being provided. (Review Chapters 27 and 44 in this text for more information and examples.)

- When coding for a physician who provides both components, assign the code with no modifiers.

- When coding for a physician who provides only the professional component, append modifier **-26 Professional component** to the Radiology section code.

- When coding for a facility that provides only the technical component, append modifier **-TC Technical component** to the Radiology section code.

Guided Example of Assigning Urinary System Procedure Codes

To practice skills for assigning codes for the Urinary System subsection, continue with the example from earlier in the chapter about a patient who was seen for ureterography. Follow along in your CPT manual as Chrystal Crago, CCA, assigns codes. Check off each step after you complete it.

▶ First, Chrystal confirms the procedure: transcatheter ureterography with imaging guidance.

▶ Chrystal searches the Index for the Main Term **Ureterography**.

❏ She locates the first-level modifying term **Injection Procedure**.

❏ She identifies the codes listed: **50430, 50431, 50684**.

▶ Chrystal reviews the code descriptions in the Tabular List to determine which one identifies the scenario: inserted bilateral ureteral catheters percutaneously through each renal pelvis using imaging guidance, injected contrast medium through catheter using imaging guidance, and viewed both ureters

❏ She verifies code **50430** in the Tabular List. When she locates the code in numerical sequence after code **50405**, she reads the note **50430 Code is out of numerical sequence. See 50390-50435.** This tells her the code has been resequenced and she needs to scan the Tabular List code range to locate the description for code **50430**. She finds that code **50430** appears after code **50396** and notices the symbol #, which CPT uses to highlight a resequenced code.

❏ She reads the description for code **50430 Injection procedure for antegrade nephrostogram and/or ureterogram, complete diagnostic procedure including imaging guidance (eg, ultrasound and fluoroscopy) and all associated radiological supervision and interpretation; new access**

❏ This seems to fit the case because all components of the procedure are described, including the creation of a new access for the catheter placement.

❏ She confirms that the procedure is performed in an **antegrade** (*the normal or forward direction of flow*) manner because the renal pelvis is located above the ureters. This is in contrast to a **retrograde** procedure, which would be performed "upstream" or against the normal direction of flow.

❏ She compares code **50431** and notes that it identifies the same procedure using an existing access, so rejects it.

❏ She looks up the code title for **50684 Injection procedure for ureterography or ureteropyelography through ureterostomy or indwelling ureteral catheter**. It identifies access through an ureterostomy or indwelling catheter, so she rejects the code.

▶ Chrystal checks for instructions in the Tabular List for code **50430**.

❏ She reads the instructional note that appears after code **50431**. The note applies to both **50430** and **50431** because this is a pair of a parent code and indented child code. The instructional note states **(Do not report 50430, 50431 in conjunction with 50432, 50433, 50434, 50435, 50693, 50694, 50695, 74425 for the same renal collecting system and/or associated ureter)**. This tells her the codes that cannot be used with this one. At this time, she is not planning on using any of the prohibited codes.

▶ Next, she reads the detailed special instructions at the beginning of the subcategory **Other Introduction (Injection/Change/Removal) Procedures**. The instructions clarify the components of the procedure included in this code:

❏ **injection(s) of contrast material**

❏ **all associated radiological supervision and interpretation**

❏ **procedural imaging guidance**

❏ that **the renal pelvis and its associated ureter are considered a single entity for reporting purposes**

❏ that the code is **reported once for each renal collecting system/ureter accessed**.

▶ This review of the instructions confirms that one code is needed for creating the percutaneous catheter access, performing the procedure, and radiological supervision and interpretation.

❏ A radiology code for physician supervision and interpretation is not necessary because code **50431** includes **all associated radiological supervision and interpretation** provided by the physician.

❏ She also notes that because this is a bilateral procedure, the code can be reported twice.

▶ Chrystal reviews the procedure codes she has assigned for this case.

▶ Next, Chrystal must determine whether modifiers are needed.

CODING PRACTICE

Exercise 42.3 Assigning Codes for Urinary and Male Genital System Procedures

Instructions: Read the mini-medical-record of each patient's encounv1–3. For questions 4–6, abstract the case on your own. Assign CPT codes, quantities, and modifiers using the Index and Tabular List. Write the code(s) on the line provided.

---

1. INPATIENT HOSPITAL   Gender: M   Age: 69

Preprocedure diagnosis: Urinary incontinence

Procedure: Sling operation. Made an incision in the perineum to advance a synthetic sling under the bladder and attached it to the muscles surrounding the urethra.

1 CPT Code _____

---

2. OUTPATIENT SURGERY   Gender: M   Age: 29

Preprocedure diagnosis: Infected seminal vesicles due to E. coli

Procedure: Vesiculotomy; incised both seminal vesicles to drain infection. Complex dissection was required due to scar tissue in the area.

Tip: The documentation of complex dissection qualifies this as a *complicated* procedure.

1 CPT Code _____

---

3. OUTPATIENT SURGERY   Gender: M   Age: 58

Preprocedure diagnosis: Residual tissue 60 days post-TURP that was performed by same surgeon due to BPH

Procedure: TURP to remove residual tissue; advanced flexible cystourethroscope through the external opening of the urethra to the prostate and located the residual prostate tissue that continues to partially obstruct the urethra. Excised tissue using blunt and sharp dissection. A catheter was placed. Patient tolerated procedure well.

Tip: TURP has a 90-day global period.

1 CPT Code _____

---

4. OUTPATIENT SURGERY   Gender: M   Age: 54

Preprocedure diagnosis: Carcinoma of the prostate

Procedure: Cryoablation of the prostate. Ultrasound used to assist with cryoprobe placement. A double freeze–thaw cycle was performed, with excellent evidence of freezing obtained. Monitoring probes were withdrawn.

1 CPT Code _____

---

5. OUTPATIENT SURGERY   Gender: M   Age: 24

Preprocedure diagnosis: Phimosis

Procedure: Circumcision. Under general anesthesia, heavy scissors used to cut the foreskin and retract over the glans. A cut was made around the glans and penile shaft to excise the foreskin. Hemostasis obtained with cautery. Shaft skin reapproximated. Patient sent to recovery room.

1 CPT Code _____

---

6. OUTPATIENT SURGERY   Gender: M   Age: 61

Preprocedure diagnosis: Bladder mass

Procedure: Cystoscopy with transurethral resection of 0.6-cm bladder tumor

Postprocedure diagnosis: Cystoscope used to identify the presence of the bladder tumor. Resectoscope inserted into the bladder to resect the tumor off the posterior wall. Hemostasis achieved with cautery. Scope removed and patient taken to recovery.

1 CPT Code _____

ARRANGING CODES FOR URINARY AND MALE GENITAL SYSTEM PROCEDURES

Coders must be familiar with rules for bundling and multiple coding related to endoscopy procedures. Also, be informed about how to apply modifiers for laterality and ESWL. These guidelines are discussed next, followed by the conclusion of the guided example.

Endoscopy Coding

Endoscopy is performed to visualize and treat components of the urinary system. The only natural opening of the urinary system is the urethra, which is used for endoscopic access to the urinary bladder. Laparoscopic access through an abdominal or pelvic incision into the desired site, such as the bladder, ureters, or kidney, is used for some procedures because the urethra is quite narrow and structures above the urinary bladder are difficult to reach endoscopically. Physicians also use an established ostomy access when one is available.

Coders must be familiar with the National Correct Coding Initiative (NCCI) rules and private payer rules regarding endoscopy coding. Always check with the patient's payer regarding endoscopy billing rules. The information presented in this chapter reflects the NCCI. Individual payer policies may vary.

Review the following NCCI guidelines regarding multiple coding of endoscopies applied to the genitourinary system:

- Surgical endoscopy/laparoscopy always includes a diagnostic endoscopy/laparoscopy performed at the same time using the same access. Report a code only for the surgical endoscopy/laparoscopy.

- When an endoscopic procedure is converted to an open procedure, report only the open procedure.

- When endoscopic visualization of the urinary system involves several regions, such as the kidney, renal pelvis, calyx, and ureter, assign the CPT code based on the anatomic approach, such as nephrostomy, pyelostomy, or ureterostomy. The approach is identified in the CPT code description, as in the following examples:

  - **50551 Renal endoscopy through established nephrostomy or pyelostomy, with or without irrigation, instillation, or ureteropyelography, exclusive of radiologic service**

  - **50951 Ureteral endoscopy through established ureterostomy, with or without irrigation, instillation, or ureteropyelography, exclusive of radiologic service**

- When multiple endoscopic approaches are utilized to attempt the same procedure, report the code for the completed approach.

- When multiple endoscopic approaches are *medically reasonable and necessary* to perform *different* procedures at the same patient encounter, report each separately and

append modifier -51 to the less extensive procedure code. The separate endoscopies may be linked to the same or different diagnosis codes (■ FIGURE 42-1).

Cystoscopy Procedures

Cystoscopy is a common component of many more complex procedures. CPT code definitions or NCCI edits often bundle cystoscopy into the codes for more complex procedures. Under some circumstances, you can break the bundles and separately report the cystoscopy performed with another procedure(s). In most cases, a modifier is required. Review the following examples for a patient who had a TURP performed and returns to the physician because of hematuria during the 90-day global period. In each example the physician performs a cystoscopy, but it is billed differently based on the reason it was performed and the diagnosis (■ FIGURES 42-2 and 42-3).

Laterality Modifiers

Some urinary system and male genital system codes involve paired anatomic sites, such as the kidneys, ureters, testes, and epididymides. Coders must read code descriptions carefully to determine how a code reports laterality and whether a modifier

Physician performs separate endoscopies due to left kidney cancer. He performs a renal endoscopy of the left kidney through a nephrostomy. He also performs a cystourethroscopy and inserts a suction and irrigation probe to evacuate multiple obstructing clots.

C64.2 Malignant neoplasm of left kidney, except renal pelvis

52001 Cystourethroscopy with irrigation and evacuation of multiple obstructing clots

50551-51-LT Renal endoscopy through established nephrostomy or pyelostomy, with or without irrigation, instillation, or ureteropyelography, exclusive of radiologic service; -51 Multiple procedures; -LT Left side

Figure 42-1 ■ Example of coding multiple endoscopies.
Source: © PB Resources, Inc. Used with permission. CPT codes only © American Medical Association.

A surgeon performs a cystoscopic examination to evaluate prolonged postoperative bleeding during the 90-day global period of a TURP for BPH.

The cystoscopy is an evaluation of a postoperative complication and not billable for Medicare and many other payers.
R31.9 Hematuria
99024 Postoperative follow-up visit, normally included in the surgical package, to indicate that an evaluation and management service was performed during a postoperative period for a reason(s) related to the original procedure

Figure 42-2 ■ Example of coding a bundled cystoscopy.
Source: © PB Resources, Inc. Used with permission. CPT codes only © American Medical Association.

Patient presents with complaints of hematuria during the postoperative period of a TURP. The physician performs a problem focused history; a detailed examination; and medical decision making of moderate complexity. She performs a cystoscopic examination and discovers benign bladder tumors.

Report the cystoscopy because this is a separately identifiable problem from the TURP.

R31.9 Hematuria

D30.3 Benign neoplasm of bladder

99214-24-25 Office or other outpatient visit for the evaluation and management of an established patient, which requires at least 2 of these 3 key components: A detailed history; A detailed examination; Medical decision making of moderate complexity; -24 Unrelated E/M service by the same physician or other qualified health care professional during a postoperative period); -25 Significant, separately identifiable E/M service by the same physician or other qualified health care professional on the same day of the procedure or other service

52000-79 Cystourethoscopy (separate procedure); -79 Unrelated procedure or service by the same physician or other qualified health care professional during the postoperative period

A

21. DIAGNOSIS OR NATURE OF ILLNESS OR INJURY Relate A-L to service line below (24E)		ICD Ind. 0			

A. R31.9   B. D30.3   C.   D.
E.   F.   G.   H.
I.   J.   K.   L.

22. RESUBMISSION CODE   ORIGINAL REF. NO.

23. PRIOR AUTHORIZATION NUMBER

24. A. DATE(S) OF SERVICE						B. PLACE OF SERVICE	C. EMG	D. PROCEDURES, SERVICES, OR SUPPLIES (Explain Unusual Circumstances)		E. DIAGNOSIS POINTER	F. $ CHARGES	G. DAYS OR UNITS	H. EPSDT Family Plan	I. ID. QUAL.	J. RENDERING PROVIDER ID. #
From MM	DD	YY	To MM	DD	YY			CPT/HCPCS	MODIFIER						
1 05	05	YY				11		99214	24 25	A	175 00	01		NPI	99 99999999
2 05	05	YY				11		52000	79	B	277 00	01		NPI	99 99999999

B

Figure 42-3 ■ Example of coding a separate cystoscopy: (A) Case study. (B) CMS-1500 billing format. *Source: © PB Resources, Inc. Used with permission. CPT codes only © American Medical Association.*

is needed. Review the following variations for reporting laterality based on the code description.

- One CPT code is used regardless of whether the procedure is unilateral or bilateral. Do not append any laterality modifiers.

  - **55250 Vasectomy, unilateral or bilateral (separate procedure), including postoperative semen examination(s)**

- Separate CPT codes are provided for unilateral and bilateral procedures. Report modifier **-RT Right side** or **-LT Left side** for unilateral procedures for informational purposes. Do not report modifier **-50 Bilateral procedure** for bilateral procedures because it is part of the code description and the payment is based on the higher RVUs for the bilateral procedure.

  - **54860 Epididymectomy; unilateral**

  - **54861 Epididymectomy; bilateral**

- The code description identifies a unilateral procedure. Report modifier **-RT** or **-LT** for informational purposes. For bilateral procedures, report the same code and append modifier **-50** as directed in the instructional note that follows the code.

  - **50593 Ablation, renal tumor(s), unilateral, percutaneous, cryotherapy**

    (50593 is a unilateral procedure. For bilateral procedure, report 50593 with modifier 50)

Modifiers for ESWL

ESWL is one of the most frequently performed procedures in urology practices. It is an effective, noninvasive treatment for kidney stones, which may be located in the renal pelvis, the calyx, the ureteropelvic junction, and/or the ureter. These sites are bilateral so report the code **50590 Lithotripsy, extracorporeal shock wave** once per side, regardless of how many sites contain stones. When stones are present in multiple locations on one side, assign only one occurrence of code **50590**.

When stones occur bilaterally, each side is often treated separately. One side is treated first, then a second appointment to treat the contralateral side is scheduled for several weeks later. The second appointment is usually preplanned to occur within the 90-day global period of the first procedure, meeting the definition of a staged procedure. The physician must clearly document this prospective planning for a staged procedure in the preoperative note, the medical record, or the operative note for the first procedure. Append the appropriate laterality modifier, **-RT Right side** or **-LT Left side**, to each occurrence of the procedure code **50590**. Append modifier **-58 Staged or related procedure or service by the same physician or other qualified health care professional during the postoperative period** to the second procedure (■ FIGURE 42-4).

In the event that stones are treated on both sides at the same time, append modifier **-50 Bilateral procedure** to code **50590**.

Patient presents with calculi in both kidneys and the left ureter. Physician plans to treat each kidney separately. On March 1, he performs ESWL on the left kidney and ureter. On April 15, he performs ESWL on the right kidney

March 1
N20.2 Calculus of kidney with calculus of ureter
50590-LT Lithotripsy, extracorporeal shock wave;
    -LT Left side
April 15
N20.0 Calculus of kidney
50590-58-RT Lithotripsy, extracorporeal shock wave;
    -58 Staged or related procedure or service by the
    same physician or other qualified health care
    professional during the postoperative period;
    -RT Right side

Figure 42-4 ■ Example of coding for ESWL *Source: © PB Resources, Inc. Used with permission. CPT codes only © American Medical Association.*

CODING CAUTION

Remember that ICD-10-CM diagnosis codes justify the medical necessity of a procedure. The most frequently used ICD-10-CM codes for renal calculus are **N20.0 Calculus of kidney**, **N20.1 Calculus of ureter**, and **N20.2 Calculus of kidney with calculus of ureter**. Diagnosis codes for calculi do not identify laterality.

Guided Example of Arranging Urinary System Procedure Codes

To practice skills for arranging codes for procedures of the Urinary System, continue with the example from earlier in the chapter about a patient who was seen for urography. Follow along in your CPT manual as Chrystal Crago, CCA, arranges the codes. Check off each step after you complete it.

▶ First, Chrystal confirms the codes she assigned.

❏ **50430 Injection procedure for antegrade nephrostogram and/or ureterogram, complete diagnostic procedure including imaging guidance (eg, ultrasound**

Table 42-13 ■ **EXAMPLE OF REIMBURSEMENT CALCULATION FOR MODIFIER -50**

Criterion	Value
Allowed rate (example)—CPT code 50340	$980
Adjustment for modifier -50	150%
Example calculation	$980 × 1.50 = $1,470.00
Final payment	**$1,470.00**

Source: © PB Resources, Inc. Used with permission.

and fluoroscopy) and all associated radiological supervision and interpretation; new access

▶ Chrystal examines the need for modifiers. (Refer to Table 27-1, Key Criteria for Abstracting CPT Modifiers, or Appendix A in the CPT manual.)

❏ This code requires modifier **-50 Bilateral procedure** because both ureters were catheterized. The payer will reimburse 150% of its usual rate for a bilateral procedure (■ TABLE 42-13).

▶ Modifier **-26 Professional component** does not apply to **50430** because this code does not have separate professional and technical components. (Some radiology codes have both components.)

▶ Chrystal finalizes the procedure code and modifier for this case:

(1) **50430-50 Injection procedure for antegrade nephrostogram and/or ureterogram, complete diagnostic procedure including imaging guidance (eg, ultrasound and fluoroscopy) and all associated radiological supervision and interpretation; new access; -50 Bilateral procedure**

▶ Chrystal also assigns the ICD-10-CM diagnosis code that supports the need for the service.

(1) **N13.5 Crossing vessel and stricture of ureter without hydronephrosis**

CODING PRACTICE

Exercise 42.4   Arranging Codes for Urinary and Male Genital System Procedures

Instructions: Read the mini-medical-record of each patient's encounter. Review the information abstracted in Exercise 42.2 for questions 1–3. For questions 4–6, abstract the case on your own. Assign CPT codes, quantities, and modifiers using the Index and Tabular List, and arrange the codes in proper sequence. Write the code(s) on the line provided.

1. INPATIENT HOSPITAL   Gender: M   Age: 46

Preprocedure diagnosis: Bladder cancer; previously removed the bladder and created an ileal conduit (*use of a segment of the ileum to connect the ureters to a stoma on the abdominal wall*)

Procedure: Ureteropyelography; injected contrast medium through the existing stoma to view the ureters and ileal conduit. Supervised the radiology procedure and dictated the interpretation report.

(continued)

CODING PRACTICE (continued)

1. (continued)

Preprocedure diagnosis: Ileal conduit was visualized to be functioning properly

Tip: Read the instructional note following the code for the ureteropyelography to help determine the second code.

2 CPT Codes _____

2. INPATIENT HOSPITAL Gender: M Age: 67

Preprocedure diagnosis: Bladder cancer of contiguous sites of the bladder with metastasis to the colon and rectum

Procedure: Functioned as a member of a surgical team; completely excised the urinary bladder; created a ureteroileal conduit and intestinal anastomosis; performed bilateral pelvic lymphadenectomy including external iliac, hypogastric, and obturator nodes; performed an open total colectomy with a complete proctectomy

Tip: Code for one surgeon who is working as part of the surgical team and apply the appropriate modifier. Apply other modifiers as needed.

2 CPT Codes _____

3. OFFICE/OUTPATIENT HOSPITAL Gender: M Age: 72

Reason for encounters: New patient with complaints of urinary incontinence

Procedure (Tuesday): Conducted a comprehensive history and exam with moderate-complexity medical decision making. Recommended further testing and discussed treatment options with patient.

Procedure (Friday): Performed postvoid residual (PVR) ultrasound test to measure the amount of urine left in the bladder after the patient urinates

Plan: Incontinence sling surgery

Tip: Assign one code for Tuesday and one code for Friday.

2 CPT Codes (Tuesday) _____
(Friday) _____

4. OUTPATIENT SURGERY Gender: M Age: 54

Preprocedure diagnosis: Bladder calculi; urethral calculus

Procedure: Cystolitholapaxy; left ureteral stent placement. Cystoscope used to examine the bladder. Telescope inserted through urethra into the bladder. Stones broken using crushing forceps. Next, the ureteral orifice was entered and a left ureteral stent placed. Urine was clear pink at termination of procedure.

2 CPT Codes _____

5. OFFICE Gender: M Age: 55

Preprocedure diagnosis: Penoscrotal abscess

Procedure: Incision and drainage of abscess sites. The deep open sore on the right side of the penis was opened to allow pus to drain. A second incision and drainage was performed at the proximal scrotum. A tight scrotal Kling bandage was applied.

2 CPT Codes _____

6. OFFICE Gender: M Age: 47

Preprocedure diagnosis: Recurrent dysuria, most consistent with interstitial cystitis

Procedure: Cystourethroscopy, bladder biopsies, bilateral retrograde pyelography. Cystoscope inserted and advanced into the bladder under direct visualization. Submucosal glomerulations on the lateral wall of the bladder were biopsied and sent to pathology. Bilateral retrograde pyelograms were obtained using an 8-French cone-tip catheter. The right collecting system was normal based on retrograde pyelography.

Postprocedure diagnosis: Bladder lesions, interstitial cystitis

Tip: Include the correct modifier for the professional component of the pyelography.

2 CPT Codes _____

E/M CODING FOR UROLOGY

The *1997 Documentation Guidelines for Evaluation and Management Services* (1997 DG), published by the Centers for Medicare and Medicaid Services (CMS), provide requirements for each level of a genitourinary E/M examination (■ FIGURE 42-5, page 868). Urologists are not limited to using the guidelines for a genitourinary examination only. They can also use guidelines for a general multiorgan system examination, or any other single organ system examination, based on what is most advantageous for a specific encounter. However, physicians cannot combine elements from more than one type of examination for a given encounter. Typically, the genitourinary examination guidelines provide the best results when a detailed genitourinary examination is performed.

To determine the appropriate E/M code, coders must review the documentation in detail and identify the specific elements documented.

- To translate the documentation into the E/M requirements for the history, refer back to Chapter 28, "Evaluation and Management Services (99201-99499)," Tables 28-7 to 28-10, or to the 1997 DG.

- To determine the requirements for an examination, refer to Figure 42-5 (page 868) or to the single organ system examination for genitourinary in the 1997 DG.

- To determine the levels for medical decision making (MDM), refer to Chapter 28, Table 28-12, and also to the Table of Risk in the 1997 DG.

Guided Example of E/M Coding for Urology

Refer to the urology encounter (■ FIGURE 42-6, page 869) to practice skills for abstracting and assigning E/M codes. Follow along as fictitious coder Chrystal Crago, CCA, abstracts the procedure. Check off each step after you complete it.

▶ First, Chrystal needs to establish the category of service so she can determine the information needed to abstract and assign the code.

❏ *What is the setting?* Emergency department

❏ *What is the type of service?* New or established patient

❏ *What is the code range?* Chrystal refers to the CPT Index and looks up the Main Term **Evaluation and Management** and the subterm **Emergency Department**. The code range listed is **99281-99288**.

❏ *How many key components are required?* Chrystal refers to the code range in the Tabular List and reads the code description of the first code, which states **requires these 3 key components**. All codes in the category have the same requirements for key components. This tells her that all three key components must meet or exceed the levels listed in the code (3/3).

▶ Next, Chrystal identifies the level of history.

❏ *What is the level of HPI?* The HPI is **Extended** because four elements are documented.

❏ *What is the level of ROS?* The ROS is **Complete** because 10 or more systems are documented.

❏ *What is the level of PFSH?* The PFSH is **Pertinent** because two elements are documented.

❏ *Based on these factors, what is the overall level of history?* The level of history is **Detailed** because the lowest of the three factors (HPI, ROS, and PFSH) determines the history level. The HPI and ROS qualify for a comprehensive history, but the PFSH qualifies for only a detailed history.

▶ Chrystal refers to the genitourinary examination in the 1997 DG (Figure 42-5) to abstract information needed to determine the level of the examination.

❏ *What is the level of examination?* The level of examination is **Detailed**. Fourteen (14) elements of the examination are documented, which exceeds the requirement of 12 or more bulleted elements for a genitourinary examination. A comprehensive examination requires that every element in each box with a shaded border and at least one element in each box with an unshaded border be documented, which they are not.

▶ Chrystal determines the level of medical decision making. (Refer to Table 28-12, Medical Decision-Making Levels.)

❏ *What is the level of complexity of the number of diagnoses or management options based on the presenting problem?* The level is **High** because there is a new presenting problem, with workup.

❏ *What is the amount and/or complexity of data to be reviewed?* The level is **Straightforward** because clinical labs were reviewed.

❏ *What is the level of risk of significant complications, morbidity, and/or mortality?* She reviews each column in the Table of Risk in the 1997 DG and determines that the level of risk is **High**. The patient presents with an acute or chronic illness that poses a risk to a bodily function (High), several clinical labs are ordered and reviewed (Minimal), and the decision to de-escalate care because of a poor prognosis was reconfirmed (High). The single highest element in the Table of Risk determines the overall risk. Two columns, **Presenting Problem** and **Management Options Selected**, are at the highest level (High).

❏ *Based on these factors, what is the overall level of medical decision making?* The medical decision making is **High complexity**. At least two of the three MDM factors are required to qualify for a specific level of MDM. Two of the three MDM factors meet or exceed high-complexity decision making.

Now Chrystal is ready to assign the code for the urology encounter. The exercise that follows guides you through additional abstracting skills and allows you to assign the correct code.

System/Body Area	Elements of Genitourinary Examination
Constitutional	❏ Measurement of any **three** of the following seven **vital** signs: • 1) sitting or standing blood pressure, • 2) supine blood pressure, • 3) pulse rate and regularity, • 4) respiration, • 5) temperature, • 6) height, • 7) weight (May be measured and recorded by ancillary staff) ❏ General **appearance** of patient (eg, development, nutrition, body habitus, deformities, attention to grooming)
Neck	❏ Examination of **neck** (eg, masses, overall appearance, symmetry, tracheal position, crepitus) ❏ Examination of **thyroid** (eg, enlargement, tenderness, mass)
Respiratory	❏ Assessment of **respiratory effort** (eg, intercostal retractions, use of accessory muscles, diaphragmatic movement) **Auscultation** of lungs (eg, breath sounds, adventitious sounds, rubs)
Cardiovascular	❏ **Auscultation** of heart with notation of abnormal sounds and murmurs ❏ Examination of **peripheral vascular system** by observation (eg, swelling, varicosities) and palpation (e.g. pulses, temperature, edema, tenderness)
Chest (Breasts)	See genitourinary (female)
Gastrointestinal (Abdomen)	❏ Examination of **abdomen** with notation of presence of masses or tenderness ❏ Examination for presence or absence of **hernia** ❏ Examination of **liver** and **spleen** ❏ Obtain **stool sample** for occult blood test when indicated
Genitourinary	**MALE:** ❏ Inspection of **anus** and **perineum** Examination (with or without specimen collection for smears and cultures) of genitalia including: ❏ **Scrotum** (eg, lesions, cysts, rashes) ❏ **Epididymides** (eg, size, symmetry, masses) ❏ **Testes** (eg, size, symmetry, masses) ❏ **Urethral meatus** (eg, size, location, lesions, discharge) ❏ **Penis** (eg, lesions, presence or absence of foreskin, foreskin retractability, plaque, masses, scarring, deformities) **Digital rectal** examination including: ❏ Prostate gland (eg, size, symmetry, nodularity, tenderness) ❏ Seminal vesicles (eg, symmetry, tenderness, masses, enlargement) ❏ Sphincter tone, presence of hemorrhoids, rectal masses **FEMALE:** Includes at least **seven of the following eleven elements** identified by bullets: ❏ Inspection and palpation of **breasts** (eg, masses or lumps, tenderness, symmetry, nipple discharge) ❏ **Digital rectal** examination including sphincter tone, presence of hemorrhoids, rectal masses Pelvic examination (with or without specimen collection for smears and cultures), including: ❏ **External genitalia** (eg, general appearance, hair distribution, lesions) ❏ **Urethral meatus** (eg, size, location, lesions, prolapse) ❏ **Urethra** (eg, masses, tenderness, scarring) ❏ **Bladder** (eg, fullness, masses, tenderness) ❏ **Vagina** (eg, general appearance, estrogen effect, discharge, lesions, pelvic support, cystocele, rectocele) ❏ **Cervix** (eg, general appearance, lesions, discharge) ❏ **Uterus** (eg, size, contour, position, mobility, tenderness, consistency, descent or support) ❏ **Adnexa**/parametria (eg, masses, tenderness, organomegaly, nodularity) ❏ **Anus** and **perineum**
Lymphatic	Palpation of **lymph nodes** in neck, axillae, groin and/or other location
Skin	❏ **Inspection** and/or **palpation** of skin and subcutaneous tissue (eg, rashes, lesions, ulcers)
Neurological/ Psychiatric	*Brief assessment of mental status including:* ❏ **Orientation** to time, place and person ❏ **Mood** and affect (eg, depression, anxiety, agitation, hypomania, lability)

Total # Bullets Performed and Documented →	☐	# of ❏ Elements Performed and Documented	Level of Examination
		1–5	Problem focused
		6–11	Expanded problem focused
		12	Detailed
		ALL	Comprehensive (Perform **all** elements identified by a bullet. Document **every** element in each box with a shaded border and at least **one** element in each box with an unshaded border)

Figure 42-5 ■ 1997 documentation guidelines for genitourinary examination. *Source: Centers for Medicare and Medicaid Services, 1997 Documentation Guidelines for Evaluation and Management Services (with formatting adjustments).*

UROLOGY ENCOUNTER

HISTORY: Detailed

CHIEF COMPLAINT: Blood in urine.

Chief complaint (CC)

HISTORY OF PRESENT ILLNESS: This is a 78-year-old male who presents to the Emergency Department with blood in his urine since yesterday. He has prostate cancer with metastatic disease to his bladder and several locations throughout the skeletal system including the spine and shoulder. The patient has had problems with hematuria in the past, but states that this episode began yesterday, and today he has been passing principally blood with very little urine. The patient has already completed chemotherapy and is beyond treatment for his cancer at this time. He is receiving radiation therapy targeted to the bones for symptomatic relief of skeletal pain. It is not intended to treat and cure the cancer. The patient is not enlisted in hospice, but the principle around the patient's current treatment management is focusing on comfort care measures.

Setting & patient type

ROS

HPI: Extended (4+)

MDM Risk

MDM Management

REVIEW OF SYSTEMS: CONSTITUTIONAL: No fever or chills. The patient does report generalized fatigue and weakness over the past several days. HEENT: No headache, no neck pain, no rhinorrhea, no sore throat. CARDIOVASCULAR: No chest pain. RESPIRATIONS: No shortness of breath or cough, although the patient does get easily winded with exertion over these past few days. GASTROINTESTINAL: Denies any abdominal pain. No nausea or vomiting. No changes in the bowel movement. No melena or hematochezia. GENITOURINARY: A gross hematuria since yesterday as previously described. Able to pass urine without difficulty. Denies any groin pain. The patient denies any other changes to the genital region. MUSCULOSKELETAL: The chronic lower back pain which has not changed over these past few days. The patient does have multiple other joints that cause him discomfort, but there have been no recent changes. SKIN: No rashes or lesions. No easy bruising. NEUROLOGIC: No focal weakness or numbness. No incontinence of urine or stool. No saddle paresthesia. No dizziness, syncope or near-syncope. ENDOCRINE: No polyuria or polydipsia. No heat or cold intolerance. HEMATOLOGIC/LYMPHATIC: The patient does not have a history of easy bruising or bleeding, but has had previous episodes of hematuria.

ROS: Complete (10+)

PAST MEDICAL HISTORY: Prostate cancer with metastatic disease as previously described.

PAST SURGICAL HISTORY: TURP.

PFSH: Pertinent (2)

CURRENT MEDICATIONS: Morphine, Darvocet, Flomax, Avodart and ibuprofen.

ALLERGIES: VICODIN.

SOCIAL HISTORY: The patient is a nonsmoker. Denies any alcohol or illicit drug use. The patient does live with his family.

EXAMINATION: Detailed

PHYSICAL EXAMINATION: VITAL SIGNS: Temperature is 98.8 oral, blood pressure is 108/65, pulse is 109, respirations 16, oxygen saturation is 97% on room air and interpreted as normal. CONSTITUTIONAL: The patient is well nourished, well developed. The patient appears to be pale, but otherwise looks well. The patient is calm, comfortable. The patient is pleasant and cooperative. HEENT: Eyes normal with clear conjunctivae and corneas. Nose is normal without rhinorrhea or audible congestion. Mouth and oropharynx normal without any sign of infection. Mucous membranes are moist. NECK: Supple. Full range of motion. No JVD. CARDIOVASCULAR: Heart is mildly tachycardic with regular rhythm without murmur, rub or gallop. Peripheral pulses are +2. RESPIRATIONS: Clear to auscultation bilaterally. No shortness of breath. No wheezes, rales or rhonchi. Good air movement bilaterally. GASTROINTESTINAL: Abdomen is soft, nontender, nondistended. No rebound or guarding. No hepatosplenomegaly. Normal bowel sounds. No bruit. No masses or pulsatile masses. GENITOURINARY: The patient has normal male genitalia, uncircumcised. There is no active bleeding from the penis at this time. There is no swelling of the testicles. There are no masses palpated to the testicles, scrotum or the penis. There are no lesions or rashes noted. There is no inguinal lymphadenopathy. Normal male exam. MUSCULOSKELETAL: Back is normal and nontender. There are no abnormalities noted to the arms or legs. The patient has normal use of the extremities. SKIN: The patient appears to be pale, but otherwise the skin is normal. There are no rashes or lesions. NEUROLOGIC: Motor and sensory are intact to the extremities. The patient has normal speech. PSYCHIATRIC: The patient is alert and oriented x4. Normal mood and affect. HEMATOLOGIC/LYMPHATIC: There is no evidence of bruising noted to the body. No lymphadenitis is palpated.

(12+ bulleted elements)

EMERGENCY DEPARTMENT TESTING: CBC was done, which had a hemoglobin of 7.7 and hematocrit of 22.6. Neutrophils were 81%. The RDW was 18.5, and the rest of the values were all within normal limits and unremarkable. Chemistry had a sodium of 134, a glucose of 132, calcium is 8.2, and rest of the values are unremarkable. Alkaline phosphatase was 770 and albumin was 2.4. Rest of the values all are within normal limits of the LFTs. Urinalysis was grossly bloody with a large amount of blood and greater than 50 RBCs. The patient also had greater than 300 of the protein reading, moderate leukocytes, 30-50 white blood cells, but no bacteria were seen. Coagulation profile study had a PT of 15.9, PTT of 43 and INR of 1.3.

MEDICAL DECISION MAKING: High Complexity

MDM Data: Ordering or reviewing diagnostic data (Straightforward Data)

Figure 42-6 ■ Urology encounter. *Source: © PB Resources, Inc. Used with permission.*

(continued on page 870)

EMERGENCY DEPARTMENT COURSE: The patient was given normal saline 2 liters over 1 hour without any adverse effect and multiple doses of morphine to maintain his comfort while here in the emergency room without any adverse effect. The morphine did relieve his pain and make him pain free. I spoke with the patient's urologist about most appropriate step for the patient. He said he would be happy to care for the patient in the hospital and do urologic scopes if necessary and surgery if necessary and blood transfusion. It was all a matter of what the patient wished to do given the advanced stage of his cancer. I spoke with the patient and his son about what he would like to do and what the options were from doing nothing from keeping him comfortable with pain medicines to admitting him to the hospital with the possibility of scopes and even surgery being done as well as the blood transfusion. The patient and his son chose a middle ground in which he would be transfused with 2 units of blood here in the emergency room and go home tonight. The patient was transfused 2 units of packed red blood cells after appropriately typed and match. The patient did not have any adverse reaction at any point with his transfusion. There was no fever, no shortness of breath, and at the time of disposition, the patient stated he felt a little better and felt like he had a little more strength. Over the course of the patient's several-hour stay in the emergency room, the patient did end up developing enough problems with clotted blood in his bladder that he had a urinary obstruction. Foley catheter was placed, which produced bloody urine and relieved the developing discomfort of a full bladder. The patient was given a leg bag and the Foley catheter was left in place.

MDM Management: New problem with workup (High Management Options)

MDM Risk: Acute/chronic illness that poses risk to patient (High Risk)

DIAGNOSES
1. HEMATURIA.
2. PROSTATE CANCER WITH BONE AND BLADDER METASTATIC DISEASE.
3. SIGNIFICANT ANEMIA.
4. URINARY OBSTRUCTION.

CONDITION ON DISPOSITION: Fair, but improved.

DISPOSITION: To home with his son.

PLAN: Patient is to follow up with his urologist in 2 days for reevaluation. He was encouraged to drink extra water. I gave discharge instructions on hematuria and asked him to return to the emergency room should he have any worsening of his condition or develop any other problems or symptoms of concern.

KEY: HPI History of the present illness   ROS Review of systems
      PFSH Past, family, and social history MDM Medical decision making

Figure 42-6 ■ (continued)

CODING PRACTICE

Exercise 42.5 **Evaluation and Management Coding for Urology**

Instructions: Refer to the *1997 Documentation Guidelines for Evaluation and Management Services* (available at **www.cms.gov**) or Chapter 28, "Evaluation and Management Services (99201-99499)," Tables 28-7 to 28-12, in this text. Answer the following questions about the "Urology encounter" (Figure 42-6).

1. a. Which elements of the HPI are documented? Circle all that apply. Location, Quality, Severity, Duration, Timing, Context, Modifying factors, Associated signs and symptoms

   b. How many elements are documented? _____

   c. What is the level of HPI? _____

2. a. Which systems are reviewed in the ROS? Circle all that apply. Constitutional, Allergic/immunologic, CV, Endocrine, ENT/M, Eyes, GI, GU, Hemic/lymphatic, MS, Neurologic, Psychiatric, Respiratory, Skin/breast

   b. How many systems are documented? _____

   c. What is the level of ROS? _____

3. a. Which PFSH elements are documented? Circle all that apply. Past medical, Family, Social

   b. What is the level of PFSH? _____

   c. What is the overall level of history? (The lowest history factor—HPI, ROS, or PFSH—determines the level of history.) _____

4. Refer to Figure 42-6, Urology Encounter.

   a. Which bulleted items are documented for the examination? (Check off the items documented.)

   b. How many bulleted items are documented? _____

   c. What is the level of the examination? _____

5. Refer to Table 28-12, Medical Decision-Making Levels, or the 1997 DG.

   a. What is the MDM level for the number of diagnoses or management options? _____

   b. What is the MDM level for the amount and/or complexity of data to be reviewed? _____

CODING PRACTICE *(continued)*

c. Refer to the Table of Risk in the 1997 DG. Which elements of risk are documented for each risk factor?

1. Presenting problem: _____

2. Diagnostic procedures ordered: _____

3. Management options selected _____

d. What is the level of risk? (The highest of the three risk factors determines the overall level of risk.) _____

e. What is the overall level of MDM? (2/3 MDM factors are needed to determine the overall level.) _____

6. a. What is the setting? _____

b. What is the patient (or service) type? _____

c. What is the code range? _____

d. How many key components are required? _____

e. What is the level of history? _____

f. What is the level of examination? _____

g. What is the level of medical decision making? _____

h. What is the correct code? _____

7. Abstract, assign, and arrange (sequence) the diagnosis code(s) that support the E/M code.

6 ICD-10-CM Code(s) _____

CHAPTER SUMMARY

In this chapter you learned that:

- Although urology is classified as a surgical specialty, a knowledge of internal medicine, pediatrics, gynecology, and other specialties is required because of the wide variety of clinical problems encountered.

- Coders need to understand treatment of obstructive uropathy, calculi, congenital anomalies, and bladder reconstruction.

- The CPT subsection *Urinary System (50010-53899)* contains three subheadings that are divided by anatomic site. CPT special instructions provide definitions and coding guidelines at the beginning of many categories.

- The CPT subsection *Male Genital System (54000-55899)* contains nine subheadings that are divided by anatomic site. CPT special instructions provide definitions and coding guidelines at the beginning of many categories.

- Abstracting for urinary and male genital system procedures uses similar processes. For both systems, coders must identify the anatomic approach and the patient's gender.

- Coders must be aware of gender-specific codes when coding for the Urinary and Male Genital Systems. They must also be familiar with coding for urinary catheterization and radiological guidance and supervision/interpretation.

- Coders must be familiar with rules for bundling and multiple coding related to endoscopy procedures, as well as how to apply modifiers for laterality and ESWL.

- The *1997 Documentation Guidelines for Evaluation and Management Services* (1997 DG), published by CMS, provides requirements for each level of a genitourinary E/M examination.

(continued)

CONCEPT QUIZ

Take a moment to look back at Urinary and Male Genital System subsection procedures and solidify your skills. Try to answer the questions from memory first, then refer to the discussion in this chapter if you need a little extra help.

Completion

Instructions: Write the term that completes each statement based on the information you learned in this chapter. Choose from the list below. Some choices may be used more than once and some choices may not be used at all.

catheter	nephrorrhaphy
cystometrogram	resectoscope
electroejaculation	trocar
epididymovasostomy	ureterolithotomy
lithotripter	ureterotomy
manometer	vasectomy
nephrolithotomy	vesicourethropexy
nephrorrhaphy	vesiculectomy

1. A(n) _____ is a pressure-measuring device used to evaluate bladder function.
2. A(n) _____ is used to treat stress urinary incontinence.
3. _____ is removal of one of the seminal vesicles.
4. A(n) _____ is used via the urethra to remove a portion of the prostate.
5. Aspiration of the bladder can be done using a needle, a trocar, or a(n) _____.
6. _____ is a procedure that can be done through an incision to remove a kidney stone.
7. An obstruction of spermatic flow can be treated with a(n) _____.
8. A(n) _____ is removal of a ureteral stone through an incision into the ureter.
9. _____ is the medical term for suturing a laceration of the kidney.
10. A(n) _____ aims pulsating sound waves at a kidney stone to break it into pieces.

Multiple Choice

Instructions: Circle the letter of the best answer to each question based on the information you learned in this chapter.

1. How would you code the following procedure? *A surgeon uses percutaneous cryotherapy for ablation of tumors on both kidneys.*
   A. 50593
   B. 50593-50
   C. 50593-RT-LT
   D. 50593 × 2

2. Which of the following categories in the Urinary System subsection has special instructions unique to that section?
   A. Excision
   B. Repair
   C. Laparoscopy
   D. Introduction

3. What type of catheter is placed in the urethra temporarily to allow the drainage of urine?
   A. Ureteral catheter
   B. Suprapubic catheter
   C. Foley catheter
   D. Straight catheter

4. How would you code the following procedure? *A surgeon begins an endoscopic radical right nephrectomy which must be converted to an open approach to complete the procedure.*
   A. 50545-RT
   B. 50230-RT
   C. 50545-RT, 50230-RT
   D. 50230-RT, 50545-RT

5. What modifier(s) is used when coding for a physician who provides both the professional and technical components of a radiology procedure?
   A. -26
   B. -26, -TC
   C. -59
   D. No modifier is used.

6. Which of the following would be considered an invasive urological procedure?
   A. Pelvic exenteration
   B. Percutaneous nephrolithotomy
   C. Vasectomy
   D. Vesiculectomy

7. How would you code the following procedure? *ESWL treatment was planned to be performed in two stages. Today, a surgeon performs ESWL on the right kidney two months after the same procedure was done on the left kidney.*
   A. 50590-50
   B. 50590-58
   C. 50590-58-RT
   D. 50590-RT-LT

8. Which codes are reported when multiple endoscopic approaches are utilized to attempt the same procedure?
   A. A code for the completed approach
   B. A code for the approach that reached the farthest point
   C. A code for each approach attempted
   D. A code for the open procedure only

9. What anatomic approach can be used for urinary and male genital system procedures?
   A. Endoscopic
   B. Laparoscopic
   C. Percutaneous
   D. Retropubic

10. Which of the following modifiers increases the usual reimbursement when appended to a surgical code?
    A. -25
    B. -27
    C. -50
    D. -51

KEEP ON CODING

Instructions: Read the procedural statement, then use the appropriate Index and Tabular List to assign CPT procedure codes, quantities, and modifiers. Write the code(s) on the line provided.

Urinary System

1. Percutaneous dilation of renal tract before an endourologic procedure including fluoroscopy imaging guidance, radiological supervision and interpretation, and new access into the renal collecting system. CPT Code(s) _____

2. Closure of ureterocutaneous fistula. CPT Code(s) _____

3. Ablation of renal tumor using radiofrequency. CPT Code(s) _____

4. Cryosurgical ablation of the prostate. CPT Code(s) _____

5. Cystometrogram. CPT Code(s) _____

6. Transurethral resection of a 2-cm bladder tumor. CPT Code(s) _____

7. Complete laser coagulation of prostate including vasectomy. CPT Code(s) _____

8. Pyeloscopy and biopsy of right renal pelvis. CPT Code(s) _____

9. Takedown of ureteroileal conduit. CPT Code(s) _____

10. Laparoscopic donor nephrectomy. CPT Code(s) _____

11. EMG of urethral sphincter. CPT Code(s) _____

12. Retropubic radical prostatectomy with pelvic lymph node biopsies. CPT Code(s) _____

13. Aspiration of the bladder with insertion of a suprapubic catheter. CPT Code(s) _____

14. Insertion of prosthetic urethral sphincter. CPT Code(s) _____

15. Cystoscopy with dilation of constricted bladder neck under local anesthesia. CPT Code(s) _____

16. Cystotomy with excision of bladder diverticulum. CPT Code(s) _____

17. Bilateral epididymectomy. CPT Code(s) _____

18. Insertion of straight catheter. CPT Code(s) _____

19. Cystourethroscopy, left ureteroscopy with laser lithotripsy. CPT Code(s) _____

20. Extracorporeal shock wave lithotripsy, bladder stone. CPT Code(s) _____

Male Genital System

21. Insertion of a multicomponent, inflatable penile prosthesis. CPT Code(s) _____

22. Removal of previously implanted semirigid penile implant and replacement with new semirigid implant. CPT Code(s) _____

23. Simple bilateral orchiectomy with insertion of prosthesis using scrotal approach. CPT Code(s) _____

24. Revision of circumcision to repair adhesions with urethral meatoplasty. CPT Code(s) _____

25. Excision of right spermatocele. CPT Code(s) _____

CODING CHALLENGE

Instructions: Read the mini-medical-record of each patient's encounter, then abstract, assign, and arrange ICD-10-CM diagnosis codes and CPT procedure codes using the appropriate Index and Tabular List. Assign quantities and modifiers where needed. Write the code(s) on the line provided.

Urinary System

1. OUTPATIENT SURGERY   Gender: M   Age: 56

Preprocedure diagnosis: Right-side renal calculi

Procedure: Cystoscope was inserted into the urethra, which was normal. The bladder was free of neoplasm, infection, or calculus. A guidewire was introduced into the right ureteral orifice and advanced to the right renal-collecting system without difficulty. A balloon was used to dilate the ureter and a scope was introduced. The gravel from the stone being fragmented was washed out. The stent was inserted. Patient was transferred to the recovery room in stable condition.

1 ICD-10-CM Code_____

2 CPT Codes _____

2. OFFICE   Gender: M   Age: 32

Preprocedure diagnosis: Recurrent bladder tumors of the posterior wall

Procedure: Cystoscopy with biopsy and fulguration of the bladder tumors and transurethral incision of vesical neck. The cystourethroscope was used to identify the location of the bladder tumors. A resectoscope was inserted after dilating the urethra and the bladder neck was incised; 0.4-cm and 1.5-cm tumors were biopsied and then fulgurated. A Foley catheter was placed and the patient sent to the recovery room.

1 ICD-10-CM Code _____

2 CPT Codes _____

3. OFFICE   Gender: F   Age: 41

Preprocedure diagnosis: Recurrent UTIs possibly related to left ureteral stent placed about 7 weeks ago

Procedure: Patient placed in dorsal lithotomy position, given IV pain med. Cystoscopy was performed using graspers. The stent was removed without difficulty and a new stent was inserted. Patient to continue on antibiotics and new stent to remain in place for 3 months.

Tip: Refer to the OGCR for Outpatient Services for help selecting the right code.

1 ICD-10-CM Code _____

1 CPT Code _____

4. OUTPATIENT SURGERY   Gender: M   Age: 65

Preprocedure diagnosis: Bladder calculus obstructing prostate

Procedure: Holmium laser cystolithotripsy; planned transurethral resection of his prostate was not performed as planned. A 27-French Olympus rectoscope was passed via the urethra into the bladder. He had a large 3.5-cm bladder calculus. Holmium laser with the largest fiber through the continuous flow resectoscope and sheath was used to break up the stone. Most of the chips were able to be irrigated out of the bladder. The TURP was not performed due to the substantial amount of time needed to break up the stone.

1 ICD-10-CM Code _____

1 CPT Code _____

5. INPATIENT HOSPITAL   Gender: M   Age: 56

Preprocedure diagnosis: Multi-invasive bladder cancer

Procedure: Laparoscopic radical cystectomy with bilateral pelvic lymph node dissections and orthotopic neobladder. After port placement, the bladder was meticulously dissected free and removed. Right and left obturator and pelvic lymph nodes were dissected next. The continent urinary diversion was performed by Dr. Alfred and is reported separately.

Tip: Use a modifier to report that two surgeons performed distinct parts of the procedure.

1 ICD-10-CM Code _____

1 CPT Code _____

6. OUTPATIENT SURGERY   Gender: F   Age: 39

Preprocedure diagnosis: Right distal ureteral stone. A stent had been placed two months ago due to a 5-mm ureteral stone. KUB showed stent in place and the stone in the same location as two months ago.

Procedure: Right semirigid ureteroscopy with basket stone extraction. The stent was removed and a semirigid scope was placed in the right ureter. Basket was used to retrieve the stone without incident.

Tip: Removal of the stent is bundled with the surgery at the time the stent is inserted.

1 ICD-10-CM Code _____

1 CPT Code _____

7. OFFICE   Gender: M   Age: 51

Preprocedure diagnosis: Adenocarcinoma of the prostate

Procedure: Implant of I-125 seeds into the prostate. Under fluoroscopic and ultrasound guidance, 19 needles were inserted into the prostate based on a premeasured template. Approximately 70 I-125 seeds were placed into the prostate. The patient tolerated the procedure well.

1 ICD-10-CM Code _____

1 CPT Code _____

Male Genital System

8. OUTPATIENT SURGERY   Gender: M   Age: 48

Preprocedure diagnosis: Normal-volume azoospermia

Procedure: Bilateral testis biopsies; bilateral scrotal explorations; bilateral vasograms; right-to-left crossover vasoepididymostomy using the operating microscope. The left vas deferens was transected through a scrotal incision. Vasogram revealed the vas was not patent. Testis biopsy on the left was positive for motile sperm. The same procedure was performed on the right testis; however, the biopsy was negative for motile sperm. At this point the left vas deferens was ligated and, using the operating microscope, a right-to-left crossover vasoepididymostomy performed. The testis and epididymis were placed back in the scrotal sac and then closed. The patient tolerated the procedure well.

1 ICD-10-CM Code _____

5 CPT Codes _____

_____

9. OUTPATIENT SURGERY   Gender: M   Age: 5

Preprocedure diagnosis: Sudden severe testicular pain, possible testicular detorsion on the left

Procedure: Left scrotal exploration with detorsion and orchidopexy. With a transverse incision, a dartos pouch was created before opening the tunica vaginalis of the testis. After detorsion of the testis, it was found to be viable, and bilateral orchidopexy was done to prevent future torsion and to preserve fertility.

1 ICD-10-CM Code _____

1 CPT Code _____

10. OUTPATIENT SURGERY   Gender: M   Age: 37

Preprocedure diagnosis: Fractured penis

Procedure: Repair of fractured penis; placement of Foley catheter. Patient taken to the OR emergently to repair the tear. An incision was made circumferentially on the ventral aspect of the penis secondary to this being the area of the hematoma. Dissecting along the urethra, we placed a Foley catheter. There was a large amount of bright blood coming from the penis, indicating the point of tear. The tear of the corpus cavernosum was repaired and a leak test showed no extravasation. The Buck fascia was repaired and skin reapproximated, dressing applied.

1 ICD-10-CM Code _____

1 CPT Code _____

Chapter Outline

- **OB/GYN Procedure Basics**
- **Coding Guidelines for OB/GYN Procedures**
- **Abstracting OB/GYN Procedures**
- **Assigning Codes for OB/GYN Procedures**
- **Arranging Codes for OB/GYN Procedures**
- **E/M Coding for OB/GYN**

Learning Objectives

After completing this chapter, you should have the skills to:

43.1 Spell and define the key words, medical terms, and abbreviations related to female genital system and obstetric procedures. (Remember)

43.2 Summarize the types of female genital system and obstetric procedures. (Understand)

43.3 Adhere to CPT coding guidelines in the Female Genital System and Maternity Care and Delivery Procedures subsections. (Apply)

43.4 Examine and abstract procedural information from the medical record for coding for coding procedures in the Female Genital System and Maternity Care and Delivery Procedures subsections. (Analyze)

43.5 Demonstrate how to assign codes for procedures in the Female Genital System and Maternity Care and Delivery Procedures subsections. (Apply)

43.6 Utilize guidelines for arranging (sequencing) codes for procedures in the Female Genital System and Maternity Care and Delivery Procedures subsections. (Apply)

43.7 Determine how to code Evaluation and Management services for gynecology. (Evaluate)

Key Terms and Abbreviations

global obstetric package	intraperitoneal	supracervical	transperineal
intrapartum fetal hypoxia	paravaginal	transcervical	transvaginal

In addition to the key terms listed here, students should know the terms defined within tables in this chapter.

INTRODUCTION

You may wish to purchase a vacation as an all-inclusive package or you may wish to purchase the airline tickets and hotel separately. Similarly, physicians can bill a global obstetric package for all routine antepartum, delivery, and postpartum services, or they can bill certain components separately if not all services are provided by the same practice. In this chapter, you learn about coding for obstetrics and gynecology.

Procedures to evaluate and treat a woman before conception, such as fertility procedures, are classified as gynecology or Female Genital System subsection procedures, whereas procedures to evaluate and treat a woman after conception are classified as obstetrics or Maternity Care and Delivery subsection procedures. For the sake of brevity, the abbreviation OB/GYN is sometimes used in this chapter to refer to both CPT subsections collectively.

OB/GYN PROCEDURE BASICS

Obstetrics and gynecology (OB/GYN) is a discipline that specializes in diseases and routine physical care of the reproductive system of women. Obstetricians and gynecologists (OB/GYNs) may choose a scope of practice ranging from primary ambulatory health care to a concentration in a focused area of specialization. Recognized subspecialties are gynecologic oncology, female pelvic medicine and reconstructive surgery, reproductive endocrinology and infertility, and maternal–fetal medicine. OB/GYNs may work closely with oncologists to treat cancer and with general surgeons to perform complicated procedures in the abdominopelvic cavity. An obstetrician is a physician whose practice is focused on caring for women during pregnancy, delivery, and the postpartum period. Obstetricians may work closely with cardiologists, endocrinologists, and other medical specialists for the management of chronic health conditions—such as hypertension and diabetes—during pregnancy. Newborn infants are typically cared for by a pediatrician. Health plans are required to recognize OB/GYN physicians as primary care providers (PCPs), so that women can seek care from them without a referral or preauthorization.

The United States faces an increasing shortage of obstetricians, largely because of the rising cost of malpractice insurance premiums, which are the second most costly of any specialty, behind neurosurgeons. This shortage is most acute in rural and economically underserved areas.

When working with medical and procedural terms, remember that word roots often describe a shape, so structures of that shape can occur at multiple sites in the body. For example, *salping/o* means "tube" and can refer to a fallopian tube or a eustachian tube. *Cervic/o* means "neck" and can refer to the neck of the uterus or the neck of the spine. Read the context in which the word is used or look for adjectives to identify the exact site being discussed. Refer to ■ TABLE 43-1 for a refresher on how to build medical terms related to the female genital system and obstetrics.

CODING CAUTION

Be alert for medical terms that are spelled similarly and have different meanings.

colporrhaphy (*suturing of the vagina*) and **colorrhaphy** (*suturing of the colon*)

vaginotomy (*making an incision into the vagina*) and **vagotomy** (*making an incision into the vagus nerve*)

uter/o (*uterus*) and **ureter/o** (*ureter*)

trachel/o (*necklike structure*) and **trache/o** (*trachea, windpipe*)

Procedures commonly performed on each section of the female genital system and obstetrics are discussed next. Refer to detailed anatomic diagrams of specific parts of the female genital system when you need to refresh your memory of the relationship of organs and sites to each other.

Procedures of the Female Genital System

Procedures commonly performed on the female genital system are summarized in ■ TABLE 43-2 (page 878). Most of these procedures are performed on women without regard to their pregnant state (*whether or not they are pregnant*). Some procedures, such as cerclage or dilation and curettage (D&C), can be performed for obstetrical (*relating to pregnancy*) or nonobstetrical purposes, with different codes assigned based on the purpose.

Refer to Chapter 21 of this text for additional information and anatomic diagrams related to the genitourinary system.

Table 43-1   ■   EXAMPLE OF CONSTRUCTING MEDICAL TERMS FOR FEMALE GENITAL SYSTEM AND OBSTETRIC PROCEDURES

Combining Form	Suffix	Complete Medical Term
hyster/o (*uterus*)		**hystero + scopy** (*visual examination of the uterus*)
		oophoro + scopy (*visual examination of the ovary*)
		salpingo + scopy (*visual examination of the fallopian tube*)
oophor/o (*ovary*)	**-scopy** (*visual examination*) **-ectomy** (*excision*)	**hyster + ectomy** (*excision of the uterus*)
		oophor + ectomy (*excision of the ovary*)
		salping + ectomy (*excision of the fallopian tube*)
		hystero + oophoro + salping + ectomy (*excision of the uterus, ovary, and fallopian tube*)
salping/o (*[fallopian] tube*)		

Source: © PB Resources, Inc. Used with permission.

Table 43-2 ■ **COMMON PROCEDURES OF THE FEMALE GENITAL SYSTEM**

Procedure Name	Definition	Reason Performed
Cerclage (nonobstetrical)	Extensive suturing around the cervix to make the opening smaller	Cervical incompetence (dilated, weakened cervix)
Clitoroplasty	Reduction of the size of an enlarged clitoris	Congenital anomaly
Colpocentesis	Puncture of the posterior vaginal wall with a needle to withdraw fluid from the peritoneal cul-de-sac (*area between the uterus and rectum*)	Abscess
Colpopexy/vaginofixation	Suture of the vagina to another structure, such as the abdominal wall	Vaginal prolapse
Colporrhaphy	Suture of the vagina	Cystocele, rectocele
Colpotomy	Incision into the wall of the vagina; may also include draining an abscess	Lesion, abscess
Conization of cervix	Removal of a cone-shaped piece of tissue from the uterine cervix	Diagnostic testing, precancerous cell removal, cancer
Dilation and curettage (D&C) (nonobstetrical)	Widening of the cervix and scraping of the uterine wall	Biopsy; remove retained products of conception
Endocervical curettage	Scraping tissue from the endocervical canal (which joins the cervix and uterus)	Diagnostic testing
Fallopian tube catheter introduction	Insertion of a catheter through the cervix and uterus into the fallopian tube(s)	Diagnosis and treatment of infertility, repeated miscarriages, dysmenorrhea, tumors, polyps, or fibroids; eliminate a tube occlusion or stricture
Fimbrioplasty	Opening an obstructed fallopian tube to save the function of the fimbriae (*border of the fallopian tube entrance*) for transporting an oocyte	Infertility
Hymenotomy	Incision of the hymen (*the fold of mucous membrane that partially covers the external opening of the vagina*)	Allow for the release of menstrual fluid and sexual intercourse
Hysterectomy	Removal of the uterus and/or related structures, such as the ovaries and fallopian tubes	Cancer, uterine fibroids, endometriosis, abnormal vaginal bleeding, uterine prolapse
Hysteroplasty	Repair of a malformed uterus	Congenital anomaly
Hysterorrhaphy (nonobstetrical)	Suturing the uterus	Perforated or ruptured uterus
Hysterosalpingography	X-ray of the uterus and fallopian tubes after injecting contrast dye	Diagnose blockage or abnormality
Hysteroscopy	Visualization of the cervix and uterus using a hysteroscope, passing it through the vagina into the cervix and uterine cavity	Diagnostic testing, biopsy, polyp removal
In vitro fertilization	Removal of an egg from the female patient, which is manually fertilized with sperm and then returned to the fallopian tube or implanted in the uterus	Infertility; assisted reproductive technology (ART)
Lysis of labial adhesions	Destruction or freeing of adhesions between the labia minor and major	Adhesions, which often occur as a result of fibrous bands of scar tissue; a common pediatric procedure
Marsupialization	To incise a cyst or abscess by cutting a slit into it to drain it and then suturing the edges to surrounding tissue; the surgical formation of a pouch-like sac (marsupialization) on the Bartholin's gland	Creation of a pouch-like sac for continued drainage and healing; prevention of recurrent cysts or infections
Mesh/prosthesis insertion	Repair of tissues that are too weak to be repaired without inserting a mesh or other prosthesis to strengthen them	Pelvic floor defect
Myomectomy	Removal of uterine fibroid tumors without removing healthy uterine tissue	Uterine fibroids
Pereyra procedure	Elevation of the bladder by attaching it to abdominal fascia	Stress urinary incontinence
Perineoplasty	Repair of the tissues of the perineum	Tissue damage during childbirth

Table 43-2   ■   (*continued*)

Procedure Name	Definition	Reason Performed
Pessary insertion/fitting	Evaluation and placement of a rubber, silicone, or plastic device into the vagina to support surrounding structures	Prolapsed uterus or rectum
Plastic repair introitus	Restoration of the vaginal opening to its original size	Vaginal introitus hypertrophy, often due to childbirth
Salpingostomy	Surgical creation of an opening in a fallopian tube to restore its patency	Treatment of infection or inflammation
Sonohysterography	Ultrasound of uterus after a saline solution is infused into the uterus	Fibroids, polyps, lesions
Sperm washing	Separation of the sperm from seminal fluid and removing chemicals that can be harmful to the uterus	Artificial insemination
Trachelectomy/cervicectomy	Removal of the uterine cervix	Cancer
Trachelorrhaphy	Suture of a laceration of the uterine cervix	Laceration
Uterine suspension	Shortening of the ligament that suspends the uterus by plicating (*folding*) and tacking it back in place; may also include presacral sympathectomy (*surgical excision or chemical destruction of the presacral nerve in the sympathetic nervous system; the nerve is anterior to the sacrum at the base of the spine*)	Uterine or uterovaginal prolapse; malposition of the uterus; dysmenorrhea
Vulvectomy	Surgical removal of part of the vulva	Cancer

Source: © PB Resources, Inc. Used with permission.

Maternity Care and Delivery Procedures

Common maternity care and delivery procedures are summarized in ■ TABLE 43-3. These procedures are performed on pregnant women specifically. Procedures on an unborn fetus are coded as procedures performed on the mother. After birth, the newborn constitutes a separate patient, so procedures on the newborn are coded separately from the mother using codes from the Surgery subsection for the appropriate body system.

This section provides a general reference to help understand the most common OB/GYN procedures. Remember to keep standard reference books handy in case you get stuck. Refer to Chapter 21 of this text for additional information and anatomic diagrams related to pregnancy and delivery.

Table 43-3   ■   **COMMON MATERNITY CARE AND DELIVERY PROCEDURES**

Procedure Name	Definition	Reason Performed
Abdominal hysterotomy	Surgical incision into the lower portion of the uterus	Abortion; removal of hydatidiform mole (*a grape-like cluster that represents a nonviable fetus*)
Amniocentesis	Surgical puncture into the amniotic sac to remove amniotic fluid	Remove excess amniotic fluid; diagnose fetal disorders
Assisted vaginal delivery (AVD)	The birth of an infant through the vagina, with the use of drugs or techniques to induce labor and/or with forceps or vacuum extraction to aid in moving the infant through the birth canal	Preferred outcome for pregnancy when delivery cannot be accomplished without assistance
Cephalic version	Turning the fetus so the head is oriented toward the cervix	Malposition of fetus (breech)
Cerclage (obstetrical)	Suturing the cervix closed during pregnancy	Incompetent (weak) cervix; to reduce the risk of miscarriage
Cervical dilator insertion	Transcatheter administration of a substance into the cervix to widen it. Substances used include prostaglandins, a sticky gel, and laminaria, a sterile rod made of kelp, which both expand when placed inside the cervix and help the uterus to contract	Abortion; predelivery cervical ripening (*thinning, softening, and widening*)
Cesarean delivery	Incision into the abdomen and uterus to deliver an infant	Delivery risks such as obstructed labor, fetal or maternal distress, postterm pregnancy

(*continued*)

Table 43-3 ■ *(continued)*

Procedure Name	Definition	Reason Performed
Chorionic villus sampling (CVS)	Aspiration of fetal tissue under ultrasonic guidance, by catheter through the cervix or by needle through the mother's abdominal and uterine walls into the uterine cavity	Diagnose chromosomal abnormalities and biochemical disorders
Cordocentesis/percutaneous umbilical blood sampling (PUBS)	Use of ultrasound to detect the umbilical cord and removal of a sample of fetal blood from the cord	Diagnose abnormalities
Curettage (obstetrical)	Scraping away the uterine lining	Retained placenta, abortion
Episiotomy (obstetrical)	Surgical incision into the perineum and vagina	Prevention of traumatic tear during delivery
Evacuation	Suctioning the fetus and placenta out of the uterus with a suctioning instrument placed through the vagina, into the cervix, and into the uterus	Abortion
Fetal nonstress test (NST)	Monitoring of the fetal heartbeat and oxygenation	Postterm or high-risk pregnancy
Fetal scalp blood sampling	Obtaining a blood specimen from the scalp of the fetus through the dilated cervix	Diagnose intrapartum fetal hypoxia *(insufficient amount of oxygen to the fetus during labor and delivery)*
Normal spontaneous vaginal delivery (NSVD)	The birth of an infant through the vagina, without the use of drugs or techniques to induce labor, without forceps, vacuum extraction, or cesarean delivery	Preferred outcome for pregnancy
Repeat cesarean	Performing a cesarean delivery for a mother who had a cesarean delivery with a previous pregnancy	Risk of rupturing scar of previous cesarean
Vaginal delivery after cesarean (VBAC)	Performing a vaginal delivery for a mother who had a cesarean delivery with a previous pregnancy	Preferred outcome for pregnancy when there is no risk of rupturing scar of previous cesarean
Vesicocentesis	Prenatal aspiration of fetal urine	Diagnose birth defects; remove excess urine

Source: © PB Resources, Inc. Used with permission.

CODING PRACTICE

Exercise 43.1 OB/GYN Procedure Basics

Instructions: Use your medical terminology skills and resources to define the following OB/GYN procedures, then identify the code(s) or code range listed in the CPT Index. Follow these steps:

- Use slash marks "/" to break down the underlined term into its root(s) and suffix.
- Define the meaning of the underlined word based on the meaning of each word part.
- Use the entire phrase to identify the code or code range shown in the CPT Index.

Example: hysterectomy, abdominal,
supracervical hyster/ectomy   Meaning *excision of the uterus*   CPT Code *58180*

1. vaginoscopy, biopsy   Meaning _____   CPT Code _____

2. colpoperineorrhaphy   Meaning _____   CPT Code _____

3. fistula, urethrovaginal   Meaning _____   CPT Code _____

4. oophorectomy   Meaning _____   CPT Code _____

5. vulvectomy, simple, complete   Meaning _____   CPT Code _____

6. clitoroplasty, intersex state   Meaning _____   CPT Code _____

CODING PRACTICE (continued)

7. ovariolysis	Meaning _____	CPT Code _____
8. hysterosalpingography, catheterization	Meaning _____	CPT Code _____
9. colpopexy, laparoscopic	Meaning _____	CPT Code _____
10. salpingostomy	Meaning _____	CPT Code _____

CODING GUIDELINES FOR OB/GYN PROCEDURES

Coders should understand the organization of this CPT section, section guidelines, and instructional notes in the Tabular List. This information is necessary for accurate coding. The CPT subsection **Female Genital System (56405-58999)** contains seven subheadings that are divided by anatomic site (■ TABLE 43-4). Within each anatomic site, codes are divided by the type of procedure, such as incision, excision, introduction, and so on.

The CPT subsection **Maternity Care and Delivery (59000-59899)** contains nine subheadings that are divided by anatomic site (■ TABLE 43-5). Within each anatomic site, codes are divided by the type of procedure, such as excision, vaginal delivery, cesarean delivery, and so on.

Table 43-4 ■ **FEMALE GENITAL SYSTEM SUBHEADINGS**

Subheading	Code Range
Vulva, Perineum and Introitus	56405-56821
Vagina	57000-57426
Cervix Uteri	57452-57800
Corpus Uteri	58100-58579
Oviduct/Ovary	58600-58770
Ovary	58800-58960
In Vitro Fertilization	58970-58999

Table 43-5 ■ **MATERNITY CARE AND DELIVERY SUBHEADINGS**

Subheading	Code Range
Antepartum and Fetal Invasive Services	59000-59076
Excision	59100-59160
Introduction	59200
Repair	59300-59350
Vaginal Delivery, Antepartum and Postpartum Care	59400-59430
Cesarean Delivery	59510-59525
Delivery Procedures After Previous Cesarean Delivery	59610-59622
Abortion	59812-59857
Other Procedures	59866-59899

Review the subheading and category names and code ranges listed in each subsection to become familiar with the content and organization. Some editions of the CPT manual provide a summary list of the subheadings and categories at the beginning of each subsection, which also displays an asterisk (*) next to categories that contain special coding instructions. Special instructions are provided for the subheading **Vulva, Perineum, and Introitus** under the Female Genital System subsection, as well as for the **Laparoscopy** and **Endoscopy** categories in several places throughout this subsection. Guidelines are provided at the beginning of the Maternity Care and Delivery subsection and for the category **Delivery After Previous Cesarean Delivery**.

These subsections include invasive, minimally invasive, and noninvasive surgical procedures on the female genital system and obstetrics. Codes for diagnostic tests on these systems appear in the Medicine section. When billing, the medical necessity of procedures must be justified by diagnosis codes. CPT codes in the Female Genital System subsection are frequently supported by diagnosis codes from ICD-10-CM Chapter 14, "Diseases of the Genitourinary System (N00-N99)," as well as neoplasms, symptoms and signs, and injuries (■ TABLE 43-6 (page 882)). These are the codes used most commonly to support procedures reported in the Female Genital System subsection; however, diagnosis codes from any ICD-10-CM chapter are permissible.

CPT codes in the Maternity Care and Delivery subsection are frequently supported by diagnosis codes from ICD-10-CM Chapter 15, "Pregnancy, Childbirth and the Puerperium (O00-O9A)" (Table 43-6). These are the codes used most commonly to support procedures procedures in the Maternity Care and Delivery subsection; however, diagnosis codes from other ICD-10-CM chapters are used to document the presence of non-obstetric-related conditions.

CPT guidelines for the Surgery section apply to the Female Genital System and Maternity Care and Delivery subsections.

The Maternity Care and Delivery subsection provides detailed special instructions regarding the bundling of antepartum, delivery, and postpartum procedures.

Instructional notes appear throughout the Tabular List to alert coders to the need for modifiers, provide cross-references to codes for similar procedures on other sites, identify when additional codes for radiological services might be needed, and highlight resequenced and recently deleted codes. Specific guidelines and instructional notes are discussed throughout this chapter of the text.

Table 43-6 ■ LOCATING ICD-10-CM AND ADDITIONAL CPT CODES FOR OB/GYN

Type of Code	Codes
ICD-10-CM OB/GYN-Related Codes	
Female genital system conditions	N70-N99
Neoplasms	C50, C51-58
Symptoms and signs	R30-R39
Injuries	S37-S39
Maternity Care and Delivery	O00-O9A, Z30-Z39
CPT OB/GYN-Related Codes	
Medicine procedures	None applicable
Radiologic procedures:	
• Diagnostic radiology	74710-74775
• Radiologic guidance	77001-77022
• Diagnostic ultrasound	76700-76776, 76801-76857
• Breast mammography	77046-77067
• Nuclear medicine, diagnostic	78700-78799
Laboratory organ/disease panels	80055, 80081

Source: © PB Resources, Inc. Used with permission.

Table 43-7 ■ KEY CRITERIA FOR ABSTRACTING FEMALE GENITAL SYSTEM PROCEDURES

- ❏ What is the patient's gender?
- ❏ What procedure is performed?
- ❏ What is the anatomic site?
- ❏ What additional sites are treated?
- ❏ What is the surgical approach?
- ❏ What is the anatomic approach?
- ❏ Is the procedure obstetrical or nonobstetrical?
- ❏ What is the extent of the procedure?
- ❏ What is the laterality?
- ❏ What additional procedure(s) are performed?

Source: © PB Resources, Inc. Used with permission.

ABSTRACTING OB/GYN PROCEDURES

Coders must abstract anatomic approaches used with OB/GYN procedures. They also must identify the extent of the procedure with regard to the structures affected. Separate abstracting criteria are provided for gynecology procedures and obstetric procedures.

Anatomic Approach

The anatomic approach identifies the physical route used to access the surgical site. Most approaches can be used with either open or laparoscopic procedures. When you encounter an approach description that is unfamiliar, identify the word root to identify the anatomic site, then identify the prefix to identify the direction. Commonly used anatomic approaches for gynecological procedures include:

- Abdominal—Through the abdomen
- Intraperitoneal—Within the peritoneum
- Paravaginal—Adjacent to the vagina or part of the vagina
- Supracervical—Above the cervix uteri
- Transcervical—Through the cervix uteri
- Transperineal—Through the perineum
- Vaginal/transvaginal—Through the vagina

Extent of Procedure

Some procedures are described based on the extent, such as partial or complete, simple or extensive, and so on. When abstracting, always identify the anatomic sites, or portions of sites, treated. Then, read the code descriptions when assigning codes to learn how a particular code defines the extent. You

should refer back to the medical record to interpret the procedure description in light of the coding manual definitions.

The descriptions and definition of extent vary and are not uniform for all procedures. The definition of extent often appears within the code description or may appear in special instructions at the beginning of the category. When abstracting a procedure for the first time, you may not be aware of the CPT options and definitions for the extent because you have not yet identified the code options.

For example, when abstracting a vulvectomy you may read in the operative note that the physician *excised 70% of the vulvar area*. When you assign the code for vulvectomy in the Tabular List, you will read special instructions before code **56405** that state **A partial procedure is the removal of less than 80% of the vulvar area**. This definition, along with other elements in the code description, guides you in assigning the correct code.

Refer to ■ TABLE 43-7 for guidance on how to abstract procedures in the Female Genital System and Maternity Care and Delivery subsections. ■ TABLE 43-8 identifies additional abstracting questions for only Maternity Care and Delivery subsection procedures. Remember that the abstracting questions are a guide and that not every question applies to, or can be answered for, every case. For example, not every gynecological procedure is divided by extent and not every obstetrical procedure includes identification of the trimester.

SUCCESS STEP

The weeks of gestation, and sometimes the trimester, must be abstracted to assign ICD-10-CM diagnosis codes for obstetric patients but are not necessarily required on CPT codes.

Guided Example of Abstracting OB/GYN Procedures

Refer to the following example throughout this chapter to practice skills for abstracting, assigning, and arranging OB/GYN codes.

Table 43-8 ■ KEY CRITERIA FOR ABSTRACTING MATERNITY CARE AND DELIVERY PROCEDURES

These criteria are specific to Maternity Care and Delivery subsection procedures. Also review the criteria for Female Genital System subsection procedures.

Delivery Procedures

❏ What is the trimester?

❏ How many weeks of gestation have been completed?

❏ How many infants were delivered?

❏ What is the method of delivery for each infant?

❏ Is a vaginal delivery attempted before cesarean delivery is performed?

❏ Has the patient had a previous cesarean delivery?

❏ What services are provided at the time of delivery in addition to the delivery itself?

❏ Is more than one physician involved in the antepartum care, delivery, and postpartum care?

If Yes:

• Which part of the process is provided by the current physician?

• How many antepartum visits were provided by the same physician?

Abortions

❏ What is the trimester?

❏ How many weeks of gestation have been completed?

❏ Is the abortion induced?

❏ What method is used (evacuation, D&C, or drug administration)?

❏ Is the abortion complete or incomplete?

Source: © PB Resources, Inc. Used with permission.

INPATIENT HOSPITAL   Gender: F   Age: 28

Gravida: 2   Para: 3   EGA: 39

Reason for admission: Full-term labor

Assessment: Cord entanglement and compression of fetus 2

Delivery: Fetus 1 (boy) TBLC NSVD with third-degree tear that required repair, fetus 2 (girl) TBLC vaginal delivery converted to cesarean d/t cord entanglement

Note: The patient's first delivery was vaginal. The physician provided all antepartum and postpartum care for this patient.

Follow along as fictitious coder Daphne Wittman, CCS-P, abstracts the procedure. Check off each step after you complete it.

▶ Daphne reads through the entire record, paying special attention to the reason for the encounter, the procedure performed, and the postoperative diagnosis. She refers to the Key Criteria for Abstracting Maternity Care and Delivery Procedures (Table 43-8).

❏ She notes the reason for admission, full-term labor, and identifies that a delivery of twins occurred.

❏ *What is the patient's gender?* She confirms that the medical record shows the correct gender, female.

❏ *What is the trimester?* The EGA of 39 is the third trimester.

❏ *How many weeks of gestation have been completed?* 39

❏ *How many infants were delivered?* Two

❏ *What is the method of delivery for each infant?* Fetus 1 (boy) TBLC NSVD, fetus 2 (girl) TBLC vaginal delivery converted to cesarean

❏ *Is a vaginal delivery attempted before cesarean delivery is performed?* Yes, fetus 2 (girl) TBLC vaginal delivery converted to cesarean

❏ *Has the patient had a previous cesarean delivery?* No, the patient's first delivery was vaginal

❏ *What services are provided at the time of delivery in addition to the delivery itself?* Third-degree tear that required repair

❏ *Is more than one physician involved in the antepartum care, delivery, and postpartum care?* No

▶ At this time, Daphne does not know which of these procedures may need to be coded, nor how many codes she will end up with. She will learn about this when she moves on to assigning codes.

CODING PRACTICE

Exercise 43.2   Abstracting OB/GYN Procedures

Instructions: Read the mini-medical-record of each patient's encounter and answer the abstracting questions. Write the answer on the line provided. Do not assign any codes.

1. INPATIENT HOSPITAL   Gender: F   Age: 84

Preoperative diagnosis: Vaginal prolapse and stress incontinence

(continued)

1. (continued)

Procedure: LeForte-type procedure (colpocleisis); after preparing the patient, we used forceps to grasp the cervix and prolapse the vagina. After removing segments of the pubocervical and posterior rectovaginal fascia, we stitched together underlying supporting layers of the fascia with circular stitches. The prolapse was reduced back into the patient's vagina and pelvis. Patient tolerated the procedure well.

(continued)

CODING PRACTICE (continued)

1. (continued)

a. What is the patient's gender? _____

b. What procedure is performed? _____

c. What is the anatomic site? _____

d. What additional sites are treated? _____

e. What is the surgical approach? _____

f. What is the anatomic approach? _____

g. Is the procedure obstetrical or nonobstetrical? _____
_____

h. What is the laterality? _____

i. What additional procedure(s) are performed?
_____

2. INPATIENT HOSPITAL   Gender: F   Age: 32

Gravida: 2   Para: 2   EGA: 39

Preprocedure diagnosis: Full-term labor

Procedure: Attended the delivery and performed routine antepartum and postpartum care

Delivery: NSVD, TBLC, 1 boy, 7 lb., 2 oz.

a. What is the patient's gender? _____

b. Is the procedure obstetrical or nonobstetrical? _____
_____

c. What is the trimester? _____

d. Is delivery performed? _____

e. What is the method of delivery? _____

f. Is a vaginal delivery attempted before cesarean delivery is performed? _____

g. Has the patient had a previous cesarean delivery?
_____

h. What services are provided at the time of delivery in addition to the delivery itself? _____

i. Is more than one physician involved in the antepartum care, delivery, and postpartum care? _____

j. Which part of the process is provided by the current physician? _____

3. OFFICE   Gender: F   Age: 28

Gravida: 2   Para: 1   EGA: 28

Reason for encounter: Prenatal checkup

Assessment: No pregnancy complications

Plan: Patient is moving out of town, where she will continue care with a different physician. This office provided five antepartum visits.

a. What is the patient's gender? _____

b. What service is provided? _____

c. Is the service obstetrical or nonobstetrical? _____
_____

d. What additional procedure(s) are performed? _____
_____

e. What is the trimester? _____

f. Is delivery performed? _____

g. Is more than one physician involved in the antepartum care, delivery, and postpartum care? _____

h. Which part of the process is provided by the current physician? _____

i. How many antepartum visits were provided by the same physician? _____

4. OUTPATIENT SURGERY   Gender: F   Age: 38

Preoperative diagnosis: Hydatidiform mole; patient also states that she desires no future pregnancies and requests that sterilization be performed at the same time

Procedure: Hysterotomy for excision of hydatidiform mole. Made a horizontal incision in the lower abdominal wall and entered the uterus through the lower uterine segment. Identified and removed hydatidiform mole, along with remaining membranes and placenta from the uterine cavity. After hemostasis was achieved, we sutured the uterine incisions. We then turned our attention to the fallopian tubes, using the stapler to divide each tube and then, using a needle, relocated both tube ends in the uterus. Closed the abdominal incision. Patient tolerated procedure well.

Postoperative diagnosis: Hydatidiform mole

a. What is the patient's gender? _____

b. What procedure is performed? _____

(continued)

CODING PRACTICE (continued)

4. (continued)

c. What is the anatomic site? _____

d. What additional sites are treated? _____

e. What is the surgical approach? _____

f. What is the anatomic approach? _____

g. Is the procedure obstetrical or nonobstetrical? _____
_____

h. What additional procedure(s) are performed? _____
_____

---

5. OFFICE   Gender: F   Age: 37

Preprocedure diagnosis: Vulvar lesions

Procedure: Biopsies of three vulvar lesions; used scalpel to excise three lesions with margins from the base of the vulva. Total excised diameters were 0.5 cm, 0.75 cm, and 1.0 cm. Sent to pathology for analysis.

Pathology report: Vulvar intraepithelial neoplasia—moderate (VIN II) precancerous abnormal cell growth

Postprocedure diagnosis: VIN II

a. What is the patient's gender? _____

b. What procedure is performed? _____

c. What is the anatomic site? _____

d. What additional sites are treated? _____

e. What is the surgical approach? _____

f. What is the anatomic approach? _____

g. Is the procedure obstetrical or nonobstetrical? _____
_____

(continued)

---

5. (continued)

h. What is the extent of the procedure? _____

i. What is the laterality? _____

j. What additional procedure(s) are performed? _____
_____

---

6. INPATIENT HOSPITAL   Gender: F   Age: 78

Preoperative diagnosis: Rectocele

Procedure: Posterior colporrhaphy with mesh reinforcement. Inserted speculum into the vagina to hold it open during the procedure. Evaluated the extent of the rectocele. Made an incision in the posterior vaginal wall from the top of the vagina to the levator muscles. Plicated the fascia and approximated the edges together and sutured them, making sure to include the levator muscle in the repair. Unable to repair the perineal muscles due to lack of viable tissue, so we elected to insert a prosthetic graft over the anterior vaginal wall.

a. What is the patient's gender? _____

b. What procedure is performed? _____

c. What is the anatomic site? _____

d. What additional sites are treated? _____

e. What is the surgical approach? _____

f. What is the anatomic approach? _____

g. Is the procedure obstetrical or nonobstetrical? _____
_____

h. What additional procedure(s) are performed? _____
_____

ASSIGNING CODES FOR OB/GYN PROCEDURES

To assign codes for Female Genital System subsection procedures, search the Index for the anatomic site, such as **Vulva**, and the first-level modifying term for the condition or type of procedure, such as **Lesion** or **Excision**. Alternatively, look up the Main Term for the name of the procedure, such as **Vulvectomy**, then read through the first-level modifying terms to locate the one that best describes the procedure performed. Refer to the Tabular List to read any guidelines and instructional notes, and select and verify the code.

Coders should also be familiar with how to assign codes for hysterectomy procedures, the global obstetric package, and multiple births. These skills are discussed next.

Assigning Codes for Hysterectomy

Hysterectomy, the second most common surgical procedure performed in the United States, is the removal of the uterus

and, sometimes, related structures such as the ovaries and fallopian tubes. Physicians perform hysterectomies to treat cancer, uterine fibroid tumors, endometriosis, abnormal vaginal bleeding, and uterine prolapse. CPT provides multiple codes for hysterectomy that are divided based on the following criteria:

- Surgical approach—Laparoscopic or open
- Anatomic approach—Abdominal, vaginal
- Associated structures removed—Ovaries, fallopian tubes, lymph nodes
- Extent—Total, subtotal, radical, or partial
- Weight of uterus—For vaginal hysterectomies

To assign codes for a hysterectomy, search the Index for the Main Term **Uterus**, the first-level modifying term **Excision**, and the second-level modifying term for the type of procedure based on approach or extent, such as **Laparoscopic, Total,**

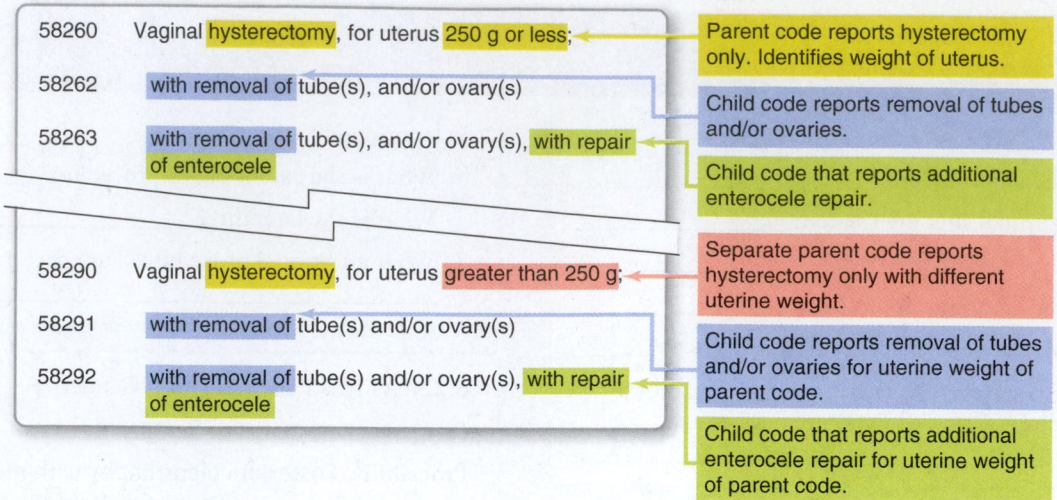

Figure 43-1 ■ CPT Tabular List entries for vaginal hysterectomy. *Source:* © *PB Resources, Inc. Used with permission. CPT codes only* © *American Medical Association.*

Vaginal, and so on. In the Tabular List, read code descriptors carefully to identify the specific criteria for each code. Identify any additional procedures listed in code descriptors to ensure that you do not separately code for services already included with the hysterectomy.

For example, code **58150** describes **Total abdominal hysterectomy (corpus and cervix), with or without removal of tube(s), with or without removal of ovary(s)**. The words **with or without** mean the same code is reported regardless of whether the physician removes the fallopian tubes and ovaries.

Codes for vaginal hysterectomy (**58260-58270, 58275-58285, 58290-58294**) and laparoscopic hysterectomy (**58541-58554**) are divided by whether or not the fallopian tubes and/or ovaries are removed in addition to the uterus. If only the uterus is removed, one code is reported; if either the tubes or ovaries or both are removed, a different code is reported, but the same code reports either structure. Codes for vaginal and laparoscopic hysterectomies are divided based on the weight of the uterus (■ FIGURES 43-1 and 43-2).

Assigning Codes for the Global Obstetric Package

Coders must understand the scope of the global obstetric package, which includes routine antepartum, delivery, and postpartum care. Report the global obstetric package code when one physician or medical group provides all services within the

package. Report additional codes for additional or nonroutine services not part of the global obstetric package are provided. ■ TABLE 43-9 identifies the elements included—or bundled—in the global obstetric package and those that can be billed separately. The required modifier, if any, for the additional services is also shown. Report global obstetric package codes at the time of delivery, not during antepartum visits.

To assign codes for the global obstetric package, search the Index for the Main Term **Obstetrical Care** and the first-level modifying term for the type of delivery, such as **Vaginal delivery** or **Cesarean delivery**, and the second-level modifying term **Routine**. Refer to the Tabular List to verify the code or review the code range to select the applicable code. More information is provided in the following paragraphs.

To assign codes for nonroutine obstetric procedures not included in the global package, search the Index for the Main Term that identifies the procedure, such as **Amniocentesis** or **Ultrasound**. Select the first-level modifying term **Obstetrical** when available, or select another appropriate modifying term. For example, the first-level modifying term under **Ultrasound** is **Pregnant uterus**. Verify the code in the Tabular List and review all available codes to select the most specific. Apply the appropriate modifier, if any, as illustrated in Table 43-9.

Follow the usual procedure to assign codes for E/M services not included in the global package. Search the Index for the Main Term **Evaluation and Management** and locate the first-level modifying term for the location of service. Refer to the Tabular List to select the appropriate code based on the three key components of an E/M service or other criteria as specified by the code description. Apply the appropriate modifier, if any, as illustrated in Table 43-9.

CPT provides four codes for the global obstetric package based on the type and circumstances of delivery (**59400, 59510, 59610**, and **59618**). Vaginal and cesarean methods of delivery require different amounts of physician work and skill, so separate codes, with different RVU values, are provided. Delivery

---

Physician performs a vaginal hysterectomy with removal of both fallopian tubes and the left ovary. The uterus weighs 280 grams.

58291 Vaginal hysterectomy, for uterus greater than 250 g; with removal of tube(s) and/or ovary(s)

Figure 43-2 ■ Example of coding vaginal hysterectomy. *Source:* © *PB Resources, Inc. Used with permission. CPT codes only* © *American Medical Association.*

Table 43-9 ■ **ELEMENTS OF THE GLOBAL OBSTETRIC PACKAGE**

Global Obstetric Package/Routine Services	Additional/Nonroutine Services
Antepartum Care	
Initial and subsequent history	Venipuncture and lab tests performed, other than routine chemical urinalysis
Physical exams	Procedures for problems related to the pregnancy
Recording weight, blood pressures, fetal heart tones	*Examples:*
	• Amniocentesis
Routine chemical urinalysis	• Chronic villous sampling
Monthly visits up to 28 weeks' gestation	• Cordocentesis
Biweekly visits from 29–36 weeks' gestation	• Fetal stress testing
Weekly visits from 37 weeks until delivery	• Fetal nonstress testing
	• OB ultrasounds (limited or complete)
	• Fetal biophysical profile
	• Fetal electrocardiography
	• Rh immune globulin administration
	E/M for complications of pregnancy
	Examples:
	• Preterm labor (PTL)
	• Decreased fetal movement (FM)
	• Preeclampsia
	• Diabetes
	• Gestational diabetes
	• Hyperemesis
	E/M and/or procedures for conditions unrelated to pregnancy
	Examples:
	• Urinary tract infection
	• Upper respiratory infection
	• Influenza
	• Vaginitis
	• Fractures, sprains
	• Any other medical condition
	Append modifier *-24 Unrelated evaluation and management service by the same physician during the global period* to alert the payer that the E/M service(s) is unrelated to the global OB package
Delivery Care	
Hospital admission	E/M services that occur more than 24 hours before the delivery may be separately reported.
Admission history and physical exam	Report multiple-gestation vaginal births, or a combination of vaginal and cesarean births, using additional codes for each infant delivered. (Append modifier *-51 Multiple procedures* to a vaginal delivery code when done with a cesarean. Append modifier *-59 Distinct procedural service* to multiple vaginal deliveries.)
Management of uncomplicated labor	
One delivery, vaginal or cesarean	
Any E/M services provided within 24 hours of delivery	Report one cesarean delivery regardless of the number of infants born because only one incision is made, and append modifier *-22 Increased procedural services* to identify the increased difficulty of the procedure when more than one fetus is delivered by cesarean delivery.
Induction labor using pitocin or oxytocin	
Artificial rupturing of membranes	Treatment of surgical complications of pregnancy, labor, and delivery such as appendectomy, hernia, or ovarian cyst
Insertion of a cervical dilator for vaginal deliveries (on the same date as the delivery)	Additional OB/GYN procedures performed at time of delivery such as hysterectomy or tubal ligation
Delivery of the placenta	Insertion of a cervical dilator for vaginal deliveries (on a separate date from the delivery)
Repair of any minor lacerations (first or second degree)	Delivery of placenta separate from delivery of baby, such as for a delivery that occurs outside of the hospital
Episiotomy, forceps, or vacuum assistance in delivery	

(continued)

Table 43-9 ■ *(continued)*

Global Obstetric Package/Routine Services	Additional/Nonroutine Services
	Repair of extensive lacerations (third or fourth degree). Append modifier *-22 Increased procedural services.*
	Laceration repaired by a provider who is not the attending
	Append modifier *-78* for unplanned return to the operating room.
	Scalp blood sampling on the newborn
	External cephalic version
	Administration of anesthesia such as an epidural
Postpartum Care	
Inpatient, office, or other outpatient visits after vaginal or cesarean delivery	Complications of postpartum care *Examples:* • Delayed postpartum hemorrhage • Infection (e.g., UTI, URI, endometritis) • Mastitis
	Procedures performed by the same physician during the postpartum period that are unrelated to the delivery (identify with modifier *-79*)
	E/M services provided by the same physician during the postoperative period that are unrelated to the delivery (identify with modifier *-24*)

Source: © PB Resources, Inc. Used with permission.

methods are further divided based on whether the mother has had a cesarean delivery with a previous pregnancy and whether a vaginal delivery was attempted before performing a cesarean for the current delivery (■ TABLE 43-10).

Portions of the Global Package

CPT provides codes for specific parts of the global obstetric package, such as the provision of *only* antepartum care, delivery, or postpartum care. When only some of the services in the package are provided, report the code(s) provided for those services (■ TABLE 43-11). Codes for the delivery and postpartum portions of the global obstetric package are indented codes under a parent code for the global package based on the type of delivery.

Table 43-10 ■ CODES FOR THE GLOBAL OBSTETRIC PACKAGE

Previous Delivery	Codes Reported for Current Delivery	
	Vaginal Delivery	Cesarean Delivery
No previous delivery	59400	59510
Previous vaginal delivery	59400	59510
Previous cesarean delivery	59610	59510
Failed vaginal delivery with previous cesarean delivery	Not applicable	59618

Source: © PB Resources, Inc. Used with permission.

The allocation of work across various aspects of the global package varies based on the type of delivery. For example, for code **59400**, which describes a normal vaginal delivery, the breakdown is:

- Antepartum care 41%
- Intrapartum (labor) care 36%
- Vaginal delivery 15%
- Postpartum care 8%

To locate codes for the global obstetric package, or portions of it, search the Index for the Main Term **Cesarean Delivery** or **Vaginal Delivery**. Locate the first-level modifying term that identifies the portion of the global package provided, such as **Antepartum care** or **Delivery only**. For the full global package, locate the first- or second-level modifying term **Routine Care**. Refer to the Tabular List to select and verify the final code using the guidelines just discussed (■ FIGURE 43-3).

CODING CAUTION

Read the third digit of the code number for the global obstetric package carefully because it is often the only way to distinguish between similar codes. For example, 59410, 59510, and 59610 all are codes related to various types of delivery, and it is easy to misread the third digit that distinguishes between them.

Table 43-11 ■ SUMMARY OF CODES FOR PROVIDING A PORTION OF THE GLOBAL OBSTETRIC PACKAGE

Services Provided	CPT Code(s)
Antepartum Care Only	
Antepartum care only; 7 or more visits	59426
Antepartum care only; 4–6 visits	59425
Antepartum care only; 1–3 visits	E/M codes
Delivery Care Only	
Vaginal delivery	59409
Cesarean delivery	59514
VBAC	59612
Repeat cesarean delivery	59620
Antepartum Care Plus Delivery	
Assign the appropriate codes for antepartum care only, based on the number of visits provided.	Antepartum: 59425-59426
Also assign the appropriate delivery code, based on the type of delivery.	Delivery: 59409, 59514, 59612, 59620
Delivery Plus Postpartum Care	
Vaginal delivery and postpartum care	59410
Cesarean delivery and postpartum care	59515
VBAC and postpartum care	59614
Repeat cesarean delivery after failed vaginal delivery and postpartum care	59622
Postpartum Care	
Postpartum care only	59430

Source: © PB Resources, Inc. Used with permission.

Table 43-12 ■ SUMMARY OF CODE ASSIGNMENT FOR TWIN BIRTHS

Type of Delivery	Code for Baby A	Code for Baby B
Vaginal delivery	59400 (Vaginal delivery, global package)	59409-59 (Vaginal delivery only, distinct procedural service)
Vaginal delivery after previous cesarean (VBAC)	59610 (Vaginal delivery after cesarean, global package)	59612-59 (Vaginal delivery after cesarean, delivery only, distinct procedural service)
Vaginal delivery for baby A, cesarean delivery for baby B	59409-51 (Vaginal delivery only, multiple procedures)	59510 (Cesarean delivery, global package)
Cesarean delivery	59510-22 (Cesarean delivery, global package, increased procedural services because of twin birth; one code reports both births)	
Cesarean delivery with failed vaginal delivery after previous cesarean delivery	59618-22 (Cesarean delivery with failed vaginal delivery after cesarean delivery, global package, increased procedural services because of twin birth; one code reports both births)	

Source: © PB Resources, Inc. Used with permission. CPT codes only © American Medical Association.

and additional codes for the delivery only, again based on the method of delivery.

When all births are vaginal, report modifier **-59 Distinct procedural service** with the second and subsequent delivery codes to clarify that the same birth is not being reported twice (■ FIGURE 43-4).

When all births are cesarean, report only one delivery code because only one incision is made. Append modifier **-22 Increased procedural services** to identify the additional work required for the additional delivery(s) and attach a report that explains the circumstances.

When multiple births are mixed—at least one vaginal and one cesarean—follow specific rules to the report all components of the procedure:

1. Assign the global obstetric package code for the cesarean delivery because it has a higher RVU.

Multiple Births

When multiple births occur due to a multiple-gestation pregnancy, report all deliveries but only one global package (■ TABLE 43-12). This usually requires reporting one code for the global obstetric package, based on the method of delivery,

---

Physician A provides 38 weeks of antepartum care for a woman who previously had a cesarean delivery and delivers this infant vaginally (VBAC). She then moves to another town and sees Physician B for the delivery, and postpartum care.

Physician A:
59426 Antepartum care only; 7 or more visits
Physician B:
59614 Vaginal delivery only, after previous cesarean delivery (with or without episiotomy and/or forceps); including postpartum care

Figure 43-3 ■ Example of coding portions of the global obstetric package. Source: © PB Resources, Inc. Used with permission. CPT codes only © American Medical Association.

Patient delivered twins vaginally. The physician provided all services in the global obstetric package.

59400 Routine obstetric care including antepartum care, vaginal delivery (with or without episiotomy, and/or forceps) and postpartum care
59409-59 Vaginal delivery only (with or without episiotomy and/or forceps); -59 Distinct procedural service

Figure 43-4 ■ Example of coding multiple births. Source: © PB Resources, Inc. Used with permission. CPT codes only © American Medical Association.

2. Report vaginal deliveries using code **59409** or **59610** for vaginal delivery only.

3. Sequence the code for the cesarean global package first, even though the cesarean delivery occurs after the vaginal delivery(s) chronologically.

4. Append modifier **-51 Multiple procedures** to the first vaginal delivery.

5. If there is more than one vaginal delivery, append modifier **-59** to the second and subsequent vaginal deliveries.

SUCCESS STEP

General CPT guidelines are discussed here. Individual payers have differing requirements about how to report codes when only a portion of the global obstetric package is provided. Checking with payers before submitting a claim saves time and money.

Guided Example of Assigning Obstetrical Procedure Codes

To practice skills for assigning codes for the Maternity Care and Delivery subsection, continue with the example from earlier in the chapter about a patient who was seen for the birth of twins. Follow along in your CPT manual as Daphne Wittman, CCS-P, assigns codes. Check off each step after you complete it.

▶ First, Daphne confirms that a twin birth occurred, one NSVD and one vaginal delivery converted to cesarean.

▶ Daphne searches the Index for the Main Term **Cesarean delivery**.

❏ She locates the first-level modifying term **Routine Care**. Because a cesarean delivery is more extensive and has a higher RVU than a vaginal delivery, she associates the routine care for the global obstetric package with the cesarean delivery.

❏ She identifies the code **59510**.

❏ She notices a second-level modifying term, **Unsuccessful attempted vaginal delivery**, and wonders if she should select this code. She notices that it appears under the first-level modifying term **Previous cesarean delivery**. Because this patient's first pregnancy resulted in a vaginal delivery, she does not think this code applies, but makes a note of the code **59618** for routine care so she can check it in the Tabular List.

▶ Daphne verifies code **59510** in the Tabular List.

❏ She reads the code title for **59510 Routine obstetric care including antepartum care, cesarean delivery, and postpartum care** and confirms that this accurately describes the principal procedure and that the physician provided all services in the global obstetric package.

❏ She also compares code **59618 Routine obstetric care including antepartum care, cesarean delivery, and postpartum care, following attempted**

vaginal delivery after previous cesarean delivery. The code clearly describes a cesarean delivery **following attempted vaginal delivery after previous cesarean delivery**. Although there was an attempted vaginal delivery, it did not occur after a previous cesarean delivery, so **59618** is not an accurate code for this patient.

❏ She reads through the descriptions for codes in the **Cesarean Delivery** category, but does not find any others that describe a cesarean following an attempted vaginal delivery. Therefore, she stays with her original choice of code **59510**.

▶ Daphne checks for instructions in the Tabular List.

❏ She cross-references the beginning of category **Cesarean Delivery** and verifies that there are no special instructions. There are two instructional notes that provide cross-references to other codes, but they do not apply to this case.

❏ She cross-references the beginning of the subsection **Maternity Care and Delivery** and reviews the instructions about bundled services in the global obstetric package.

▶ Next, Daphne codes for the vaginal delivery. She searches the Index for the Main Term **Vaginal Delivery**.

❏ She locates the first-level modifying term **Delivery Only** because the routine care for the global obstetric package, which consists of antepartum and postpartum care, was included in the code for the cesarean delivery.

❏ She identifies the code **59409**.

▶ Daphne verifies code **59409** in the Tabular List.

❏ She reads the code title for **59409, Vaginal delivery only (with or without episiotomy and/or forceps)** and confirms that this accurately describes the delivery.

▶ Daphne checks for instructions in the Tabular List.

❏ She cross-references the beginning of category **Vaginal Delivery** and verifies that there are no special instructions.

▶ Daphne reviews the medical record and identifies that the patient also sustained a third-degree tear that required repair. This service does not require a separate code, but does qualify for a modifier. She makes a note to review this further when she arranges the codes and assigns modifiers.

▶ Daphne reviews the procedure codes she has assigned for this case.

❏ **59409 Vaginal delivery only (with or without episiotomy and/or forceps)**

❏ **59510 Routine obstetric care including antepartum care, cesarean delivery, and postpartum care**

▶ Next, Daphne must determine how to sequence the codes.

CODING PRACTICE

Exercise 43.3   **Assigning Codes for OB/GYN Procedures**

Instructions: Read the mini-medical-record of each patient's encounter. Review the information abstracted in Exercise 43.2 for questions 1–3. For questions 4–6, abstract the case on your own. Assign CPT codes, quantities, and modifiers using the Index and Tabular List. Write the code(s) on the line provided.

---

1. INPATIENT HOSPITAL   Gender: F   Age: 84

Preoperative diagnosis: Vaginal prolapse and stress incontinence

Procedure: LeForte-type procedure (colpocleisis); after preparing the patient, we used forceps to grasp the cervix and prolapse the vagina. After removing segments of the pubocervical and posterior rectovaginal fascia, we stitched together underlying supporting layers of the fascia with circular stitches. The prolapse was reduced back into the patient's vagina and pelvis. Patient tolerated the procedure well.

Tip: The suffix *-cleisis* means "closure."

1 CPT Code _____

---

2. INPATIENT HOSPITAL   Gender: F   Age: 32

Gravida: 2   Para: 2   EGA: 39

Preprocedure diagnosis: Full-term labor

Procedure: Attended the delivery and performed routine antepartum and postpartum care

Delivery: NSVD, TBLC, 1 boy, 7 lb., 2 oz.

1 CPT Code _____

---

3. OFFICE   Gender: F   Age: 28

Gravida: 2   Para: 1   EGA: 28

Reason for encounter: Prenatal checkup

Assessment: No pregnancy complications

Plan: Patient is moving out of town, where she will continue care with a different physician. This office provided five antepartum visits.

1 CPT Code _____

---

4. OUTPATIENT HOSPITAL   Gender: F   Age: 33

Gravida: 2   Para: 1   EGA: 37-2/7 weeks

Reason for encounter: Oxytocin stress test after abnormal nonstress test last week

Assessment: IV oxytocin administered in increasing doses until patient had three contractions within 10 minutes lasting longer than 45 seconds. Oxytocin augmented with intermittent nipple stimulation. Monitor applied and fetal heart rate and uterine contractions recorded. No late decelerations.

Plan: Expect fetus to be able to handle stress of labor and vaginal delivery planned

1 CPT Code _____

---

5. HOSPITAL INPATIENT   Gender: F   Age: 33

Preprocedure diagnosis: Desires sterilization

Procedure: Laparoscopic tubal fulguration. Veress needle inserted through the infraumbilical incision. Abdomen insufflated and laparoscope inserted. Bipolar cautery used to fulgurate the right and left fallopian tubes distal to the uterine crown. A second fulguration completed bilaterally at a point distal to lateral point. Instruments removed, incisions repaired.

1 CPT Code _____

---

6. OUTPATIENT SURGERY   Gender: F   Age: 42

Gravida: 4   Para: 0   EGA: 12 weeks

Reason for encounter: Elderly primipara with incomplete miscarriage

Procedure: Dilation and evacuation of fetal tissue. Visible products of conception removed with forceps. Anterior lip of cervix grasped and suction curettage x2 was completed.

Plan: Return to the office in two weeks

1 CPT Code _____

ARRANGING CODES FOR OB/GYN PROCEDURES

Arranging codes for the Female Genital System and Maternity Care and Delivery subsections follows the general CPT rules. Sequence codes in descending RVU order, particularly those that are reported as multiple procedures using modifier **-51**. This helps ensure that the most costly procedure is paid in full and the multiple procedure reduction is applied to less costly procedures.

Sequence codes for multiple births in descending RVU order, rather than by birth order. For example, a cesarean delivery has a higher RVU value than a vaginal delivery. If infant one is born vaginally and its twin is delivered by cesarean, sequence the cesarean delivery first. If the global obstetric package was provided by the delivering physician, associate the global package with the cesarean delivery and sequence it first.

Modifiers Commonly Used with OB/GYN Codes

CPT does not provide any unique modifiers for use with procedures in the Female Genital System and Maternity Care and Delivery subsections. Use standard CPT modifiers when needed to further describe the circumstances of a procedure or service. In some cases, the literal description of a modifier is interpreted with reference to obstetrics. For example, modifiers pertaining to the postoperative period are understood to refer to the period of the global obstetric package.

Always check with the payer to identify the services covered under a particular modifier, and submit a special report with the claim that describes the circumstances in detail.

In addition to the usual guidelines for using modifiers that apply to all OB/GYN encounters, obstetric encounters use modifiers for the following purposes.

-22 Increased Procedural Services

Use modifier **-22** when billing for cesarean delivery of multiple fetuses. Report only one CPT code for the delivery or global obstetric package because only one surgical incision is made. The modifier identifies the additional work involved in delivering multiple infants via cesarean. Do not use modifier **-22** for multiple vaginal deliveries because each vaginal delivery is assigned a separate CPT code for the delivery or global obstetric package; the second and subsequent vaginal deliveries are reported with modifier **-51** appended.

Modifier **-22** is also used to report excessive antepartum visits beyond those typically included in the global obstetric package and for other complications of pregnancy or delivery.

When the physician repairs a third- or fourth-degree perineal laceration, append modifier **-22** to the delivery code. Do not report a separate repair code. Do not report modifier **-22** for first- or second-degree repairs.

-24 Unrelated E/M During Global Obstetric Period

When the physician supervising the pregnancy and performing the delivery also sees the patient for reasons unrelated to the pregnancy, append modifier **-24** to identify that the visit is not part of the global obstetric package. Examples include abdominal pain, genital tract infection, yeast infection, and pelvic inflammatory disease.

99203-24 Office or other outpatient visit for the evaluation and management of a new patient, which requires these 3 key components: A detailed history; A detailed examination; Medical decision making of low complexity. -24 Unrelated E/M

99213-24 Office or other outpatient visit for the evaluation and management of an established patient, which requires at least 2 of these 3 key components: An expanded problem focused history; An expanded problem focused examination; Medical decision making of low complexity. -24 Unrelated E/M

Figure 43-5 ■ Example of coding antepartum visits with modifier -24. *Source: © PB Resources, Inc. Used with permission. CPT codes only © American Medical Association.*

When a physician provides three or fewer antepartum visits, report them with E/M code(s). CPT does not provide separate E/M codes for antepartum visits. Append modifier **-24** to identify that they are not part of a global obstetric package that will be billed at the time of delivery (■ FIGURE 43-5). A special report may also be needed so the payer does not assume that the encounters are part of a global obstetric package.

-51 Multiple Procedures

When multiple births occur with one or more cesarean deliveries and one or more vaginal deliveries with one or more cesarean deliveries at the same time, report the first vaginal birth with modifier **-51** because different CPT codes are used. Report the second and subsequent vaginal births with modifier **-59**.

-52 Reduced Services

Report the code for the global package with modifier **-52** when a physician provides all services in the global obstetric package, but fewer than seven antepartum visits. This is more efficient than reporting three separate codes for the antepartum, delivery, and postpartum services.

-59 Distinct Procedural Service

Report multiple vaginal deliveries with modifier **-59** on the second and subsequent deliveries to clarify that the same procedure is not being reported twice. Some payers may require HCPCS modifier **-XS Separate Structure**, instead of **-59**, to identify that the delivery was performed on a separate infant.

When there are multiple vaginal deliveries in addition to one or more cesarean deliveries, apply modifiers as follows:

- One cesarean delivery: no modifier
- Multiple cesarean deliveries: append modifier **-22** to the code for the cesarean delivery

- One vaginal delivery followed by cesarean delivery(ies):
  - Append modifier **-51** to the vaginal delivery
  - Append modifier **-22** to the cesarean delivery if there are multiple cesarean births
- Multiple vaginal deliveries followed by cesarean delivery(ies):
  - Append modifier **-51** to the first vaginal delivery
  - Append modifier **-59** to the second and subsequent vaginal deliveries
  - Append modifier **-22** to the cesarean delivery if there are multiple cesarean births

-80 Assistant Surgeon

When cesarean deliveries use a primary surgeon and an assistant surgeon, the assistant surgeon bills the code for the delivery only with modifier **-80**. In typical surgical procedures, an assistant surgeon bills the same procedure code as the primary surgeon and appends modifier **-80**. However, in obstetrics, the assistant surgeon should report a code for the delivery only rather than the code for the global obstetric package reported by the primary surgeon, because the assistant surgeon does not provide the global package.

Guided Example of Arranging OB/GYN Procedure Codes

To practice skills for assigning codes for the Maternity Care and Delivery subsection, continue with the example from earlier in the chapter about a patient who was seen for the birth of twins. Follow along in your CPT manual as Daphne Wittman, CCS-P, arranges the codes. Check off each step after you complete it.

▶ First, Daphne confirms the procedure codes she assigned:

❏ **59409 Vaginal delivery only (with or without episiotomy and/or forceps)**

❏ **59510 Routine obstetric care including antepartum care, cesarean delivery, and postpartum care**

▶ She sequences code **59510** first because it is the more extensive code, based on the global obstetric package and the cesarean delivery. She understands that codes for deliveries are not sequenced in chronological order but in descending order according to RVU or price.

▶ Daphne examines the need for modifiers. (Refer to Table 27-1, Key Criteria for Abstracting CPT Modifiers, or Appendix A in the CPT manual.)

❏ Code **59510** does not require modifiers because there are no alterations to the service or special circumstances.

❏ Code **59409** requires modifier **-51 Multiple procedures** and will be subject to a 50% reduction in payment because it is the second procedure/delivery reported at the same encounter.

❏ Code **59409** also requires modifier **-22 Increased procedural services** to report the additional work involved in repairing the third-degree perineal laceration. She knows that she needs to assign a diagnosis code to support the need for the modifier and that she will also need to prepare a special report describing the need for the service.

▶ Daphne finalizes the procedure codes and sequencing for this case:

(1) **59510 Routine obstetric care including antepartum care, cesarean delivery, and postpartum care**

(2) **59409-51-22 Vaginal delivery only (with or without episiotomy and/or forceps); -51 Multiple procedures; -22 Increased procedural services**

▶ Daphne also assigns and sequences the ICD-10-CM diagnosis codes that support the need for the service.

(1) **O69.2XX2 Labor and delivery complicated by other cord entanglement, with compression** (Index: Delivery, complicated by, cord, entanglement, with compression, fetus 2)

(2) **O30.043 Twin pregnancy, dichorionic/diamniotic, third trimester** (Index: Pregnancy, twin, dichorionic/diamniotic, third trimester)

(3) **O70.20 Third degree perineal laceration during delivery** (Index: Laceration, perineum, female, during delivery, third degree)

(4) **Z37.2 Twins, both liveborn** (Index: Outcome of delivery, twins, both liveborn)

(5) **Z3A.39 39 weeks gestation of pregnancy** (Index: Pregnancy, weeks of gestation, 39 weeks)

CODING PRACTICE

Exercise 43.4 Arranging Codes for OB/GYN Procedures

Instructions: Read the mini-medical-record of each patient's encounter. Review the information abstracted in Exercise 43.2 for questions 1–3. For questions 4–6, abstract the case on your own. Assign CPT codes, quantities, and modifiers using the Index and Tabular List, and arrange the codes in proper sequence. Write the code(s) on the line provided.

1. OUTPATIENT SURGERY Gender: F Age: 38

Preoperative diagnosis: Hydatidiform mole; patient also states that she desires no future pregnancies and requests that sterilization be performed at the same time

(continued)

CODING PRACTICE (continued)

1. (continued)

Procedure: Hysterotomy for excision of hydatidiform mole. Made a horizontal incision in the lower abdominal wall and entered the uterus through the lower uterine segment. Identified and removed hydatidiform mole, along with remaining membranes and placenta from the uterine cavity. After hemostasis was achieved, we sutured the uterine incisions. We then turned our attention to the fallopian tubes, using the stapler to divide each tube and then, using a needle, relocated both tube ends in the uterus. Closed the abdominal incision. Patient tolerated procedure well.

Postoperative diagnosis: Hydatidiform mole

Tip: Tubal ligation is, by definition, a bilateral procedure, so a modifier is not required.

2 CPT Codes _____

---

2. OFFICE   Gender: F   Age: 37

Preprocedure diagnosis: Vulvar lesions

Procedure: Biopsies of three vulvar lesions; used scalpel to excise three lesions with margins from the base of the vulva. Total excised diameters were 0.5 cm, 0.75 cm, and 1.0 cm. Sent to pathology for analysis.

Pathology report: Vulvar intraepithelial neoplasia—moderate (VIN II) precancerous abnormal cell growth

Postprocedure diagnosis: VIN II

Tip: Identify the quantity for each code.

2 CPT Codes _____

---

3. INPATIENT HOSPITAL   Gender: F   Age: 78

Preoperative diagnosis: Rectocele

Procedure: Posterior colporrhaphy with mesh reinforcement. Inserted speculum into the vagina to hold it open during the procedure. Evaluated the extent of the rectocele. Made an incision in the posterior vaginal wall from the top of the vagina to the levator muscles. Plicated the fascia and approximated the edges together and sutured them, making sure to include the levator muscle in the repair. Unable to repair the perineal muscles due to lack of viable tissue, so we elected to insert a prosthetic graft over the anterior vaginal wall

2 CPT Codes _____

---

4. OUTPATIENT SURGERY   Gender: F   Age: 24

Preprocedure diagnosis: Chronic pelvic pain

Procedure: Laparoscopic right ovarian, paratubal cystectomy; omentectomy resection of abdominal hematoma. Inspection of the pelvic region revealed a right paratubal ovarian cyst with torsion and a 4- to 5-cm hematoma within the omentum. Omentectomy carried out and the paratubal ovarian cyst excised. Good hemostasis noted before removing instruments.

2 CPT Codes _____

---

5. INPATIENT HOSPITAL   Gender: F   Age: 59

Preprocedure diagnosis: Symptomatic leiomyomatous uterus; pelvic endometriosis

Procedure: Laparoscopic-assisted vaginal hysterectomy of 240-g uterus with right salpingo-oophorectomy; ablation of pelvic endometriosis. Pelvic exam revealed uterine size of 7- to 9-week gestation consistent with fibroid uterus. Under laparoscopic guidance implants of endometriosis were coagulated with the Harmonic scalpel. Our attention turned to the uterus, which was dissected free with care to preserve the ovaries. The specimen was delivered through the vagina. The laparoscopic instruments were removed and incisions closed. There were no complications.

2 CPT Codes _____

---

6. INPATIENT HOSPITAL   Gender: F   Age: 38

Gravida: 4   Para: 3   EGA: 36 + 5

Preprocedure diagnosis: Previous ultrasound confirmation of fetus in a frank breech position in this multiparous young woman

Procedure: Nonstress test completed to document fetal status prior to the version. Tocolytic injection given to relax the uterus and prevent contractions. External cephalic version performed by rolling the fetus to a head-down position. The fetal heart rate was monitored throughout and remained in normal range, with no distress noted.

Postprocedure diagnosis: Fetus in cephalic position

2 CPT Codes _____

E/M CODING FOR OB/GYN

The *1997 Documentation Guidelines for Evaluation and Management Services* (1997 DG), published by the Centers for Medicare and Medicaid Services (CMS), provides requirements for each level of a genitourinary E/M examination, with separate criteria for males and females (■ FIGURE 43-6, page 896). A separate obstetric examination does not exist. Gynecologists are not limited to using the guidelines for a genitourinary examination only. They can also use guidelines for a general multiorgan system examination, or any other single organ system examination, based on what is most advantageous for a specific encounter. However, physicians cannot combine elements from more than one type of examination for a given encounter. Typically the genitourinary examination guidelines provide the best results when a detailed genitourinary examination is performed.

To determine the appropriate E/M code, coders must review the documentation in detail and identify the specific elements documented.

- To translate the documentation into the E/M requirements for the history, refer back to Chapter 28, "Evaluation and Management Services (99201-99499)," Tables 28-7 to 28-10, or to the 1997 DG.

- To determine the requirements for an examination, refer to Figure 43-6 or to the single organ system examination for genitourinary in the 1997 DG.

- To determine the levels for medical decision making (MDM), refer to Chapter 28, Table 28-12, and also to the Table of Risk in the 1997 DG.

Guided Example of E/M Coding for Gynecology

Refer to the gynecology encounter (■ FIGURE 43-7, page 897) to practice skills for abstracting and assigning E/M codes. Follow along as fictitious coder Daphne Wittman, CCS-P, abstracts the procedure. Check off each step after you complete it.

▶ First, Daphne needs to establish the category of service so she can determine the information needed to abstract and assign the code.

❑ *What is the setting?* Office

❑ *What is the type of service?* This is a consultation because the patient was referred by the primary care physician for an opinion and a report was sent back by the consulting physician.

❑ *What is the code range?* Daphne refers to the CPT Index and looks up the Main Term **Evaluation and Management** and the subterm **Consultation**. The code range listed is **99241-99255**.

❑ *How many key components are required?* Daphne refers to the code range in the Tabular List. The subheading **Consultations** is divided into two categories: **Office or other outpatient consultations** and **Inpatient consultations**. She locates the code rage

99241-99245 for office consultations and reads the code description of the first code, which requires **these 3 key components**. All codes in the category have the same requirements for key components. This tells her that all three key components must meet or exceed the levels listed in the code (3/3).

▶ Next, Daphne identifies the level of history.

❑ *What is the level of HPI?* The HPI is **Extended** because four or more elements are documented.

❑ *What is the level of ROS?* The ROS is **Extended** because two to nine systems are documented.

❑ *What is the level of PFSH?* The PFSH is **Complete** because two elements are documented.

❑ *Based on these factors, what is the overall level of history?* The level of history is **Detailed** because the lowest of the three factors (HPI, ROS, and PFSH) determines the history level. The PFSH qualifies for a comprehensive history, but the HPI and ROS qualify for only a detailed history.

▶ Daphne refers to the genitourinary examination in the 1997 DG (Figure 43-6) to abstract information needed to determine the level of the examination.

❑ *What is the level of examination?* The level of examination is **Detailed**. Fourteen elements of the examination are documented, which exceeds the requirement of 12 or more bulleted elements for a Detailed examination. A comprehensive examination requires that every element in each box with a shaded border and at least one element in each box with an unshaded border be documented, which they are not.

▶ Daphne determines the level of medical decision making. (Refer to Table 28-12, Medical Decision-Making Levels.)

❑ *What is the level of complexity of the number of diagnoses or management options, based on the presenting problem?* The level is **High** because there is a new presenting problem, without workup.

❑ *What is the amount and/or complexity of data to be reviewed?* The level is **Low** because the physician reviewed the patient's past medical record.

❑ *What is the level of risk of significant complications, morbidity, and/or mortality?* She reviews each column in the Table of Risk in the 1997 DG and determines that the level of risk is **Moderate**. The patient presents with an undiagnosed new problem with uncertain prognosis (Moderate), clinical labs are reviewed (Minimal), and a diagnostic endoscopy is performed (Moderate). The single highest element in the Table of Risk determines the overall risk. The columns **Presenting problem** and **Diagnostic procedure(s) ordered** are the highest level (Moderate).

System/Body Area	Elements of Genitourinary Examination

Constitutional	❑ Measurement of any <u>**three**</u> of the following seven **vital** signs:
	  • 1) sitting or standing blood pressure,
	  • 2) supine blood pressure,
	  • 3) pulse rate and regularity,
	  • 4) respiration,
	  • 5) temperature,
	  • 6) height,
	  • 7) weight (May be measured and recorded by ancillary staff)
	❑ General **appearance** of patient (eg, development, nutrition, body habitus, deformities, attention to grooming)

Neck	❑ Examination of **neck** (eg, masses, overall appearance, symmetry, tracheal position, crepitus) ❑ Examination of **thyroid** (eg, enlargement, tenderness, mass)
Respiratory	❑ Assessment of **respiratory effort** (eg, intercostal retractions, use of accessory muscles, diaphragmatic movement) **Auscultation** of lungs (eg, breath sounds, adventitious sounds, rubs)
Cardiovascular	❑ **Auscultation** of heart with notation of abnormal sounds and murmurs ❑ Examination of **peripheral vascular system** by observation (eg, swelling, varicosities) and palpation (e.g. pulses, temperature, edema, tenderness)
Chest (Breasts)	See genitourinary (female)
Gastrointestinal (Abdomen)	❑ Examination of **abdomen** with notation of presence of masses or tenderness ❑ Examination for presence or absence of **hernia** ❑ Examination of **liver** and **spleen** ❑ Obtain **stool sample** for occult blood test when indicated
Genitourinary	**MALE:** ❑ Inspection of **anus** and **perineum** Examination (with or without specimen collection for smears and cultures) of genitalia including: ❑ **Scrotum** (eg, lesions, cysts, rashes) ❑ **Epididymides** (eg, size, symmetry, masses) ❑ **Testes** (eg, size, symmetry, masses) ❑ **Urethral meatus** (eg, size, location, lesions, discharge) ❑ **Penis** (eg, lesions, presence or absence of foreskin, foreskin retractability, plaque, masses, scarring, deformities) **Digital rectal** examination including: ❑ Prostate gland (eg, size, symmetry, nodularity, tenderness) ❑ Seminal vesicles (eg, symmetry, tenderness, masses, enlargement) ❑ Sphincter tone, presence of hemorrhoids, rectal masses ❑ <mark>**FEMALE:**</mark> Includes at least **seven of the following eleven elements** identified by bullets: ❑ Inspection and palpation of **breasts** (eg, masses or lumps, tenderness, symmetry, nipple discharge) ❑ **Digital rectal** examination including sphincter tone, presence of hemorrhoids, rectal masses Pelvic examination (with or without specimen collection for smears and cultures), including ❑ **External genitalia** (eg, general appearance, hair distribution, lesions) ❑ **Urethral meatus** (eg, size, location, lesions, prolapse) ❑ **Urethra** (eg, masses, tenderness, scarring) ❑ **Bladder** (eg, fullness, masses, tenderness) ❑ **Vagina** (eg, general appearance, estrogen effect, discharge, lesions, pelvic support, cystocele, rectocele) ❑ **Cervix** (eg, general appearance, lesions, discharge) ❑ **Uterus** (eg, size, contour, position, mobility, tenderness, consistency, descent or support) ❑ **Adnexa**/parametria (eg, masses, tenderness, organomegaly, nodularity) ❑ **Anus** and **perineum**
Lymphatic	Palpation of **lymph nodes** in neck, axillae, groin and/or other location
Skin	❑ **Inspection** and/or **palpation** of skin and subcutaneous tissue (eg, rashes, lesions, ulcers)
Neurological/Psychiatric	*Brief assessment of mental status including:* ❑ **Orientation** to time, place and person ❑ **Mood** and affect (eg, depression, anxiety, agitation, hypomania, lability)

Total # Bullets Performed and Documented →	☐	# of ❑ **Elements Performed and** <u>**Documented**</u>	**Level of Examination**
		1–5	Problem focused
		6–11	Expanded problem focused
		12	Detailed
		ALL	Comprehensive (Perform **all** elements identified by a bullet. Document **every** element in each box with a shaded border and at least **one** element in each box with an unshaded border)

Figure 43-6 ■ 1997 documentation guidelines for genitourinary examination. *Source: Centers for Medicare and Medicaid Services,* 1997 Documentation Guidelines for Evaluation and Management Services *(with formatting adjustments).*

❑ *Based on these factors, what is the overall level of medical decision making?* The medical decision making is **Moderate complexity.** At least two of the three MDM factors are required to qualify for a specific level of MDM. Two of the three MDM factors meet or exceed moderate decision making.

Now Daphne is ready to assign the codes for the gynecology encounter. The exercise that follows guides you through additional abstracting skills and allows you to assign the correct codes.

GYNECOLOGY ENCOUNTER

The patient is a 42-year-old G2, P2, LMP 3 weeks ago. She comes in to the office today in consultation from her primary care physician for an ASCUS (atypical squamous cells of undetermined significance) Pap smear.

Pap smear in last month showed atypical squamous cells of undetermined significance. She has a history of an abnormal Pap smear. At that time, she was diagnosed with CIN 3 as well as vulvar intraepithelial neoplasia. She underwent a cone biopsy that per her report was negative for any pathology. She had no vulvar treatment at that time. Since that time, she has had normal Pap smears. She denies abnormal vaginal bleeding, discharge, or pain. She uses Yaz for birth control. She reports one sexual partner since for 20 years and she is a nonsmoker.

She states that she has a tendency to have yeast infections and bacterial vaginosis. She is also being evaluated for a possible interstitial cystitis because she gets frequent urinary tract infections. She had a normal mammogram done in 6 months ago and a history of perirectal condyloma that have been treated by another physician. She also has a history of chlamydia when she was in college.

PAST MEDICAL HX: Depression.
PAST SURGICAL HX: None.
MEDICATIONS: Lexapro 10 mg a day and Yaz.
ALLERGIES: NO KNOWN DRUG ALLERGIES.
OB HX: Normal spontaneous vaginal delivery at term 10 years ago and 12 years ago, first child weighed 7 pounds 8 ounces and second child weighed 9 pounds 8 ounces.
FAMILY HX: Paternal grandfather had a MI which she reports is secondary to tobacco and alcohol use. He currently has metastatic melanoma, mother with hypertension and depression, father with alcoholism.
SOCIAL HX: She is a marketing consultant. She is a nonsmoker, drinks infrequent alcohol and does not use drugs.

PE: VITALS: Height: 5 feet 7 inches. Weight: 145 lb. BMI: 22.7. Blood Pressure: 106/62.
GENERAL: She is well-developed and well-nourished with normal habitus and no deformities. She is alert and oriented to time, place, and person and her mood and affect is normal. NECK: Without thyromegaly or lymphadenopathy. LUNGS: Clear to auscultation bilaterally. HEART: Regular rate and rhythm without murmurs. BREASTS: Deferred. ABDOMEN: Soft, nontender, and nondistended. There is no organomegaly or lymphadenopathy. PELVIC: Normal external female genitalia. Vulva, vagina, and urethra, within normal limits. Cervix is status post cone biopsy; however, the transformation zone grossly appears normal and cervical discharge is clear and normal in appearance. GC and chlamydia cultures as well as a repeat Pap smear were done.

Colposcopy is then performed without and with acetic acid. This shows an entirely normal transformation zone, so no biopsies are taken. An endocervical curettage is then performed with Cytobrush and curette and sent to pathology. Colposcopy of the vulva is then performed again with acetic acid. There is a thin strip of acetowhite epithelium located transversely on the clitoral hood that is less than a centimeter in diameter. There are absolutely no abnormal vessels within this area. The vulvar colposcopy is completely within normal limits.

A/P: ASCUS Pap smear with history of a cone biopsy 21 years ago and normal followup.

We will check the results of the Pap smear, in addition we have ordered DNA testing for high-risk HPV. We will check the results of the ECC. She will return in two weeks for test results. If these are normal, she will need two normal Pap smears six months apart, and I think followup colposcopy for the vulvar changes.

Consultation report was sent to her PCP.

Side annotations:
HISTORY: Detailed
Setting & patient type
Chief complaint (CC)
MDM Data: Ordering or reviewing diagnostic data (Straightforward Data)
HPI: Extended (4+)
ROS: Extended (2-9)
PFSH: Complete (3)
EXAMINATION: Detailed
(12+ bulleted elements)
MEDICAL DECISION MAKING: Moderate Complexity
MDM Management: New problem with work-up (High Management Options)
MDM Risk: Undiagnosed new problem with uncertain prognosis (Moderate Risk)

KEY: HPI History of the present illness   ROS Review of systems
PFSH Past, family, and social history   MDM Medical decision making

Figure 43-7 ■ Gynecology encounter. *Source: © PB Resources, Inc. Used with permission.*

CODING PRACTICE

Exercise 43.5 E/M Coding for OB/GYN

Instructions: Refer to the *1997 Documentation Guidelines for Evaluation and Management Services* (available at **www.cms.gov**) or Chapter 28, "Evaluation and Management Services (99201-99499)," Tables 28-7 to 28-12, in this text. Answer the following questions about the "Gynecology encounter" (Figure 43-7).

1. a. Which elements of the HPI are documented? Circle all that apply. Location, Quality, Severity, Duration, Timing, Context, Modifying factors, Associated signs and symptoms

   b. How many elements are documented? _____

   c. What is the level of HPI? _____

2. a. Which systems are reviewed in the ROS? Circle all that apply. Constitutional, Allergic/immunologic, CV, Endocrine, ENT/M, Eyes, GI, GU, Hemic/lymphatic, MS, Neurologic, Psychiatric, Respiratory, Skin/breast

   b. How many systems are documented? _____

   c. What is the level of ROS? _____

3. a. Which PFSH elements are documented? Circle all that apply. Past medical, Family, Social

   b. What is the level of PFSH? _____

   c. What is the overall level of history? (The lowest history factor—HPI, ROS, or PFSH—determines the level of history.)
   _____

4. Refer to Figure 43-6, 1997 Documentation Guidelines for Genito-urinary Examination.

   a. Which bulleted items are documented for the examination? (Check off the items documented.)

   b. How many bulleted items are documented? _____

   c. What is the level of the examination? _____

5. Refer to Table 28-12, Medical Decision-Making Levels, or the 1997 DG.

   a. What is the MDM level for the number of diagnoses or management options? _____

   b. What is the MDM level for the amount and/or complexity of data to be reviewed? _____

   c. Refer to the Table of Risk in the 1997 DG. Which elements of risk are documented for each risk factor?

      1. Presenting problem: _____

      2. Diagnostic procedures ordered: _____

      3. Management options selected: _____

   d. What is the level of risk? (The highest of the three risk factors determines the overall level of risk.) _____

   e. What is the overall level of MDM? (2/3 MDM factors are needed to determine the overall level.) _____

6. a. What is the setting? _____

   b. What is the patient (or service) type? _____

   c. What is the code range? _____

   d. How many key components are required? _____

   e. What is the level of history? _____

   f. What is the level of examination? _____

   g. What is the level of medical decision making?
   _____

   h. What is the correct code? _____

   i. What modifier is required? _____

7. a. What procedure was performed in addition to the E/M?
   _____

   b. 1 CPT code _____

8. Abstract, assign, and arrange (sequence) the diagnosis code(s) that support the E/M code.

   2 ICD-10-CM Code(s) _____

CHAPTER SUMMARY

In this chapter you learned that:

- Most procedures in the Female Genital System subsection are performed on women without regard to their pregnant state, although some procedures, such as cerclage or dilation and curettage, can be performed for obstetrical or nonobstetrical purposes, with different codes assigned based on the purpose.

- Maternity Care and Delivery subsection procedures are performed on pregnant women; procedures on the unborn fetus are coded as procedures performed on the mother.

- The CPT subsection *Female Genital System (56405-58999)* contains seven subheadings that are divided by anatomic site.

The CPT subsection *Maternity Care and Delivery (59000-59899)* contains nine subheadings that are divided by anatomic site. The *Maternity Care and Delivery* subsection provides detailed special instructions regarding the bundling of antepartum, delivery, and postpartum procedures.

- Coders must abstract anatomic approaches and the extent of the procedure for OB/GYN procedures.

- Coders should be familiar with how to assign codes for hysterectomy procedures and the global obstetric package.

- Use standard CPT modifiers when needed to further describe the circumstances of a procedure or service, but be aware that the literal description of a modifier may be interpreted slightly differently than usual with reference to obstetrics.

- The *1997 Documentation Guidelines for Evaluation and Management Services* (1997 DG), published by CMS, provides requirements for each level of a genitourinary E/M examination, with separate criteria for males and females; a separate obstetric examination does not exist.

CONCEPT QUIZ

Take a moment to look back at the Female Genital System and Maternity Care and Delivery subsections and solidify your skills. Try to answer the questions from memory first, then refer to the discussion in this chapter if you need a little extra help.

Completion

Instructions: Write the term that completes each statement based on the information you learned in this chapter. Choose from the list below. Some choices may be used more than once and some choices may not be used at all.

amniocentesis	hysteroscopy
cerclage	hysterotomy
colpocentesis	in vitro fertilization
colpocleisis	mesh
colpotomy	myomectomy
conization	sperm washing
cordocentesis	stress test
episiotomy	version

1. The removal of uterine fibroid tumors without removing healthy uterine tissue is called a(n) _____.

2. A uterine polyp can be removed vaginally via _____.

3. _____ is a type of assisted reproductive technology.

4. _____ may be inserted to strengthen an area if surrounding tissues are too weak to be repaired.

5. A(n) _____ may be done early in the pregnancy to diagnose fetal disorders.

6. _____ is removal of fetal blood from the umbilical cord.

7. _____ may be done to prevent injury to the perineum during delivery.

8. _____ may be performed to remove precancerous cervical tissue.

9. A cephalic _____ might need to be performed if the fetus is in an abnormal position.

10. An obstetrical _____ involves closing the cervix with sutures during the pregnancy.

Multiple Choice

Instructions: Circle the letter of the best answer to each question based on the information you learned in this chapter.

1. What procedure is performed to diagnose a blockage or abnormality of the fallopian tubes?
   - A. Hysterosalpingography
   - B. Salpingostomy
   - C. Sonohysterography
   - D. Fimbrioplasty

2. How is the oxygen level of the fetus monitored during labor and delivery?
   - A. Vesicocentesis
   - B. Cordocentesis
   - C. Chorionic villus sampling
   - D. Fetal scalp blood sampling

3. What procedure can be done to treat a prolapsed uterus or rectum?
   - A. Pereyra procedure
   - B. Pessary insertion
   - C. Perineoplasty
   - D. Hysteroscopy

4. How would you code the following procedure? *A physician performs a vaginal hysterectomy with removal of both fallopian tubes and the left ovary. The uterus weighs 280 grams.*
   - A. 58150
   - B. 58260
   - C. 58290
   - D. 58291

5. How would you code the following procedure? *A patient delivered twins vaginally. The physician provided all services in the global obstetric package.*
   - A. 59400
   - B. 59400 x 2
   - C. 59400-22
   - D. 59400, 59409-59

6. What instrument is used for direct visualization of the peritoneal cavity, ovaries, and the outer surfaces of the fallopian tubes and uterus?
   - A. Laparoscope
   - B. Hysteroscope
   - C. Colposalpingoscope
   - D. Peritoneoscope

(continued)

(continued from page 899)

7. What procedure treats urinary stress incontinence by elevating the bladder and attaching to abdominal fascia?
   A. Uterine suspension
   B. Pereyra procedure
   C. Perineoplasty
   D. Vaginofixation

8. Which anatomic approach means "through the cervix uteri"?
   A. Supracervical
   B. Transperineal
   C. Transuteri
   D. Transcervical

9. When is an antepartum visit billed using an E/M code?
   A. When it is part of the global obstetric package
   B. When a physician provides one to three antepartum visits
   C. When a physician provides seven or fewer antepartum visits
   D. Never

10. How would you code the following procedure? *A physician performed a repeat cesarean delivery after failed vaginal delivery and provided postpartum care.*
    A. 59410
    B. 59410
    C. 59622
    D. 59409, 59515

KEEP ON CODING

Instructions: Read the procedural statement, then use the appropriate Index and Tabular List to assign CPT procedure codes, quantities, and modifiers. Write the code(s) on the line provided.

Female Genital System

1. Laparoscopic fulguration of fallopian tubes. CPT Code(s) _____

2. D&C performed for a patient with dysfunctional bleeding. CPT Code(s) _____

3. Vaginal hysterectomy with salpingo-oophorectomy (uterus weight 250 g). CPT Code(s) _____

4. Biopsy of two lesions, one from labia minora and another from the vaginal orifice. CPT Code(s) _____

5. Incision and drainage of vaginal hematoma, post-trauma. CPT Code(s) _____

6. Endometrial cryoablation with ultrasonic guidance. CPT Code(s) _____

7. Vulvectomy, partial removal of skin and superficial subcutaneous tissues. CPT Code(s) _____

8. Retrieval of oocytes with ultrasound guidance. CPT Code(s) _____

9. Bilateral salpingo-oophorectomy, omentectomy for ovarian malignancy. CPT Code(s) _____

10. Radical abdominal hysterectomy with bladder aspiration and placement of suprapubic catheter. CPT Code(s) _____

11. Cold-knife conization of cervix. CPT Code(s) _____

12. Marsupialization of Bartholin's gland cyst. CPT Code(s) _____

13. Laparoscopic abdominal hysterectomy, 230-g uterus. CPT Code(s) _____

14. Uterine suspension. CPT Code(s) _____

15. Intrauterine in vitro fertilization. CPT Code(s) _____

Maternity Care and Delivery

16. Induced abortion with abortifacient. CPT Code(s) _____

17. Antepartum care only, 5 visits. CPT Code(s) _____

18. Vacuum-assisted vaginal delivery. CPT Code(s) _____

19. Fetal contraction stress test. CPT Code(s) _____

20. D&C for postpartum hemorrhage. CPT Code(s) _____

21. Cesarean delivery, delivery only, with total hysterectomy. CPT Code(s) _____

22. Repeat fetal scalp blood sampling by the same PA. CPT Code(s) _____

23. Repeat cesarean delivery after unsuccessful attempt at vaginal delivery. CPT Code(s) _____

24. Successful vaginal birth after cesarean delivery. CPT Code(s) _____

25. Ultrasound-guided amniocentesis. CPT Code(s) _____

CODING CHALLENGE

Instructions: Read the mini-medical-record of each patient's encounter, then abstract, assign, and arrange ICD-10-CM diagnosis codes and CPT procedure codes using the appropriate Index and Tabular List. Assign quantities and modifiers where needed. Write the code(s) on the line provided.

Female Genital System

1. OUTPATIENT SURGERY   Gender: F   Age: 27

Preprocedure diagnosis: Cervical dysplasia

Procedure: Loop electrical excision procedure (LEEP). Laser speculum inserted into vagina and colposcopic exam of the vagina and cervix performed. A loop electrical excision was done to remove all of the abnormal tissue on the posterior lip of the cervix consistent with moderate dysplasia. Procedure completed without incident.

1 ICD-10-CM Code _____

2 CPT Codes _____

2. INPATIENT HOSPITAL   Gender: F   Age: 62

Preprocedure diagnosis: Vault prolapse; previous hysterectomy

Procedure: Abdominosacrocolpopexy, lysis of adhesions. Significant adhesions encountered from previous surgeries and they were released. Mesh was attached to the vagina and lower part of the spine to pull the vagina into a normal position. Patient taken to PACU in stable condition.

Tip: A status code for the hysterectomy should not be used because the diagnosis code contains this information.

2 ICD-10-CM Codes _____

2 CPT Codes _____

3. INPATIENT HOSPITAL   Gender: F   Age: 56

Preprocedure diagnosis: Left anterior uterine wall fibroid, uterine descensus with cystocele and rectocele

Procedure: Hysteroscopy with D&C and endometrial ablation. The uterus and the cervix were sounded and measured 10 cm. Hysteroscopy completed with normal findings. Endocervical and endometrial curettage was carried out with copious curettings obtained. A NovaSure endometrial ablation procedure was then performed without difficulty. The follow-up hysteroscopy showed satisfactory ablation of the endometrium. Patient left the operating room in good condition.

(continued)

3. (continued)

Tip: Read the procedure description carefully to see what it includes.

2 ICD-10-CM Codes _____

_____

1 CPT Code _____

4. OUTPATIENT SURGERY   Gender: F   Age: 34

Preprocedure diagnosis: Infertility caused by adhesions

Procedure: Bilateral fimbrioplasty. An incision was made above the pubic hairline and fimbrial adhesions on both sides were lysed. Procedure tolerated well and patient sent to recovery.

2 ICD-10-CM Codes _____

1 CPT Code _____

5. OFFICE   Gender: F   Age: 32

Preprocedure diagnosis: Insertion of IUD for contraception

Procedure: IUD placement

Postprocedure diagnosis: Vaginal speculum placed, cervix prepped. Uterus was sounded to 6 cm and a Mirena IUD inserted. Threads were trimmed to 4 cm. Patient tolerated the procedure well.

1 ICD-10-CM Code _____

1 CPT Code _____

Maternity Care and Delivery

6. OUTPATIENT SURGERY   Gender: F   Age: 24

Gravida: 1   Para: 0   EGA: 19

Preprocedure diagnosis: Fetus at 19 weeks with posterior urethral valves resulting in bilateral urinary obstruction; progressive oligohydramnios.

Procedure: Vesicoamniotic shunt under spinal anesthesia using ultrasound for guidance. Fetus paralyzed using vecuronium. A vesicoamniotic shunt was placed low into the pelvis of the fetus. This was done in a single attempt, with good placement. Patient taken to recovery in stable condition.

Tip: Report a HCPCS Level II code for in utero surgical repair of the urinary tract obstruction in the fetus.

3 ICD-10-CM Codes _____

_____

1 CPT Code _____

1 HCPCS Code _____

(continued)

(continued from page 901)

---

7. INPATIENT HOSPITAL Gender: F Age: 33

Gravida: 3 Para: 2 EGA: 39 + 1

Preprocedure diagnosis: Intrauterine pregnancy at 39-1/7 weeks with breech/breech, dichorionic-diamniotic twin gestation. Patient desires primary low transverse cesarean delivery and bilateral tubal ligation for permanent sterilization.

Procedure: Low cervical cesarean delivery; bilateral tubal ligation. A low transverse incision was made in lower uterine segment. Baby A delivered without difficulty, as was Baby B. Cords clamped, infants suctioned and handed off to the pediatricians. Placenta delivered spontaneously. Uterus sutured. Attention turned to the tubal ligation. A 2-cm portion of each fallopian tube was removed and remaining ends cauterized. Uterus returned to the abdomen, fascia closed, skin closed, and patient and infants sent to recovery in stable condition.

Delivery: Cesarean delivery, Baby Boy A, complete breech, 4 lb. 7 oz; Baby Boy B, complete breech, 5 lb. 2 oz.

Tip: Remember to code outcome of delivery and weeks of gestation.

6 ICD-10-CM Codes _____

_____

2 CPT Codes _____

---

8. OFFICE Gender: F Age: 23

Preprocedure diagnosis: Suspected left ectopic pregnancy

Procedure: D&C, left salpingectomy. The cervix was dilated and uterus curetted. Tissue sent for immediate pathology, with no villi found. A laparotomy incision was made on the left. The ectopic pregnancy was excised from the proximal end of the tube and patency of the tube restored. After hemostasis was obtained, the fascia and skin were closed. Patient taken to the recovery room.

Postprocedure diagnosis: Ruptured left tubal pregnancy

1 ICD-10-CM Code _____

2 CPT Codes _____

---

9. INPATIENT HOSPITAL Gender: F Age: 27

Gravida: 4 Para: 2 EGA: 38 + 6

Preprocedure diagnosis: Postpartum hemorrhage

Procedure: Exam under anesthesia; removal of intrauterine clots 36 hours after an NSVD. I was able to remove the clots with my hand. Inspection of the uterus by hand revealed no retained placenta. Curettage was somewhat difficult due to contractions. Her hemoglobin was 9.1 and hematocrit 25.9 upon completion of the procedure.

Tip: Code only for this procedure. Because this procedure is occurring in the postoperative period, a modifier is needed.

1 ICD-10-CM Code _____

1 CPT Code _____

---

10. INPATIENT HOSPITAL Gender: F Age: 29

Gravida: 1 Para: 0 EGA: 38 + 4

Preprocedure diagnosis: Uterine fetal demise

Procedure: Normal spontaneous vaginal delivery of an intrauterine fetal demise. After induction of labor, patient was fully dilated and contracting. The female infant was delivered over a midline episiotomy. Apgars 0 and 0, weight 5 lb. 14 oz. Episiotomy repaired. Mother and father with infant. Physician has provided all routine obstetric care to this patient.

Tip: Use a HCPCS Level II code to report the induction of labor.

3 ICD-10-CM Codes _____

_____

1 CPT Code _____

1 HCPCS Code_____

Radiology Services (70010-79999)

Chapter 44

Learning Objectives

After completing this chapter, you should have the skills to:

44.1 Spell and define the key words, medical terms, and abbreviations related to radiology procedures. (Remember)

44.2 Summarize the types of radiology procedures. (Understand)

44.3 Adhere to CPT coding guidelines in the Radiology section. (Apply)

44.4 Examine and abstract procedural information from the medical record for coding Radiology section procedures. (Analyze)

44.5 Demonstrate how to assign codes for procedures in the Radiology section. (Apply)

44.6 Utilize guidelines for arranging (sequencing) codes for Radiology section procedures. (Apply)

Chapter Outline

- **Radiology Procedure Basics**
- **Coding Guidelines for Radiology Procedures**
- **Abstracting Radiology Procedures**
- **Assigning Codes for Radiology Procedures**
- **Arranging Codes for Radiology Procedures**

Key Terms and Abbreviations

contrast medium	interstitial	modality	radiopharmaceutical
diagnostic ultrasound	interventional radiologist	radiation oncologist	therapeutic ultrasound (radiologic)
endocavity	intra-articular	radiology technician	
gestational sac	intracavity	radiolucent	
imaging guidance	intrathecal	radiopaque	

In addition to the key terms listed here, students should know the terms defined within tables in this chapter.

INTRODUCTION

Digital imaging technology has transformed consumer photography from a complicated hobby that required film, processing, and printing to one that can conveniently capture and store images on a computer chip, where they can be accessed for manipulation, printing, and sharing. In the same way, radiology began as a film-based technology that today uses many forms of digital imaging to record the human body. In addition, radiology techniques are used to diagnose and treat a wide variety of conditions.

RADIOLOGY PROCEDURE BASICS

Radiology is a medical specialty that uses radiation, sound waves, magnetic fields, or radio fields to visualize internal body structures, such as arteries and bones. Radiological procedures can be noninvasive—such as an x-ray or MRI—or minimally invasive, such as fluoroscopy or angiography. Procedures can be performed to assist in diagnosing a condition, for imaging guidance (real-time visualization of body structures during a medical or surgical procedure), or for therapeutic (treatment) purposes.

A radiologist is a physician with specialized training in obtaining and interpreting radiological images to determine a patient's diagnosis and recommend additional testing or treatment. Radiologists can specialize in different areas of medicine, including diagnosing disorders of the cardiovascular system, gastrointestinal system, and breast. A radiation oncologist provides cancer treatment through radiation. An interventional radiologist performs minimally invasive, image-guided surgeries.

A radiology technician is a nonphysician staff member who is trained to operate and adjust imaging equipment, explain procedures to patients and answer questions, position patients for imaging, and ensure that the patient's exposure to radiation is limited. A radiology technician may also operate portable x-ray equipment to obtain images in the emergency room, operating room, or even at the patient's bedside. Both a registered radiologist assistant (RRA) and a radiology practitioner assistant (RPA) are radiological technologists with advanced education who perform more complex radiological procedures.

Radi/o is the combining form for x-ray. Radiology is the study of x-rays. Radiography is the process of recording x-rays. A radiograph is the image that results. x-rays or other radiographic images of specific body sites are often described by combining the word root for the anatomic site with the suffix *-graphy*, such as *mammography*, which means "making a recording of the breast." X-ray images, once recorded on traditional film, are now captured digitally and viewed on a computer screen.

The suffixes *-graph* and *-gram* can refer to other types of recordings besides x-rays and other radiological images. For example, an electrocardiogram is an electrical recording of the heart and a polysomnogram is a recording of multiple sleep parameters.

CODING CAUTION

Be alert for medical word roots that are spelled similarly and have different meanings.

dosi**metry** (*measurement of a dose*) and **densi**to**metry** (*measurement of density*)

anteroposterior (*from front to back*) and **postero**anterior (*from back to front*)

density (*mass or substance*) and **denti**stry (*the practice of a dentist*)

Refer to ■ TABLE 44-1 for a refresher on how to build medical terms related to Radiology.

Commonly performed radiology procedures are discussed next. Refer to detailed anatomic diagrams of specific parts of the digestive system when you need to refresh your memory of the relationship of organs and sites to each other.

Radiology Procedures

The field of radiology uses modalities (*methods of applying a therapeutic/physical treatment*) that employ distinct technology and equipment to obtain images. Radiological modalities include plain radiography, also called x-ray (■ FIGURE 44-1), ultrasound (US), computed tomography (CT) (■ FIGURE 44-2), nuclear medicine (NM), positron emission tomography (PET), and magnetic resonance imaging (MRI) (■ FIGURE 44-3). The physician who orders the procedure determines the modality to be used based on the information needed and the structure(s) to be examined. Some modalities provide clearer images of certain body structures; some are less invasive than others; and some are less costly.

Table 44-1   ■   **EXAMPLE OF CONSTRUCTING MEDICAL TERMS FOR RADIOLOGY PROCEDURES**

Combining Form	Suffix	Complete Medical Term
arthr/o (*joint*) **bronch/o** (*bronchus tube*) **sial/o** (*salivary duct, gland*) **tom/o** (*cut or slice*) **ur/o** (*urinary tract*)	**-graphy** (*process of recording*) **-gram** (*a record or picture*)	**arthro + graphy** (*process of recording a joint*) **broncho + graphy** (*process of recording the bronchus*) **sialo + graphy** (*process of recording the salivary duct*) **tomo + graphy** (*process of recording a slice*) **uro + graphy** (*process of recording the urinary tract*) **arthro + gram** (*a record or picture of a joint*) **broncho + gram** (*a record or picture of the bronchus*) **sialo + gram** (*a record or picture of the salivary duct*)

Source: © PB Resources, Inc. Used with permission.

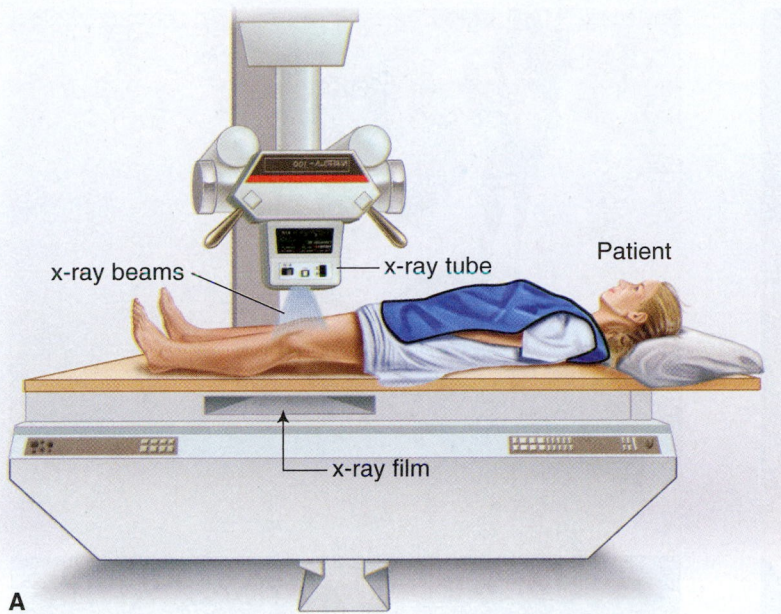

Image Receptor (film)

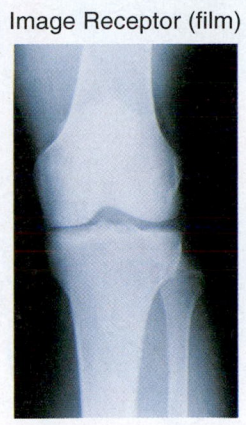

B   Knee x-ray

Figure 44-1 ■ X-ray of knee: (A) Procedure. (B) Image.

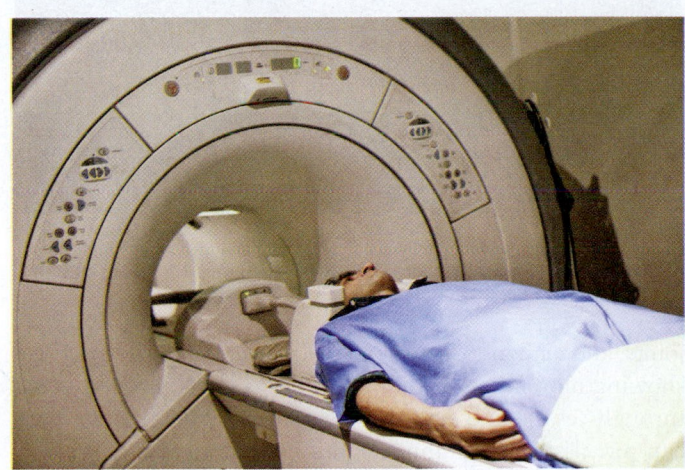

A

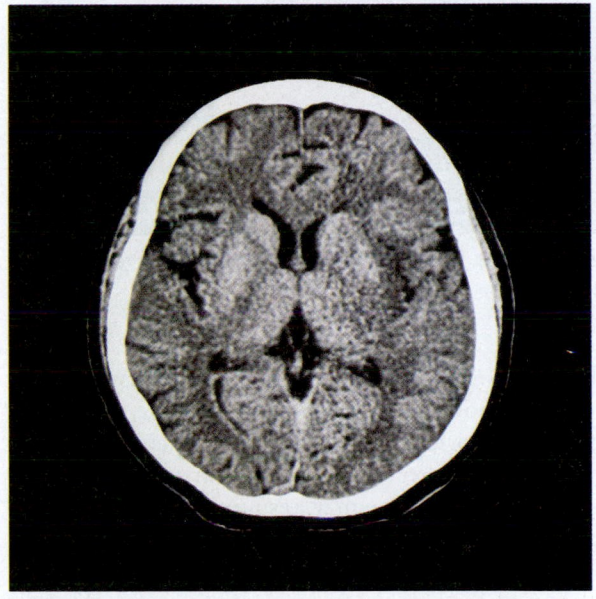

B

Figure 44-2 ■ CT scan of head: (A) Procedure. (B) Image.

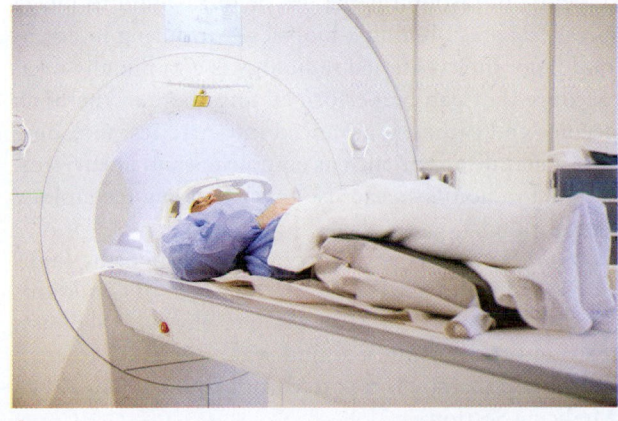

A

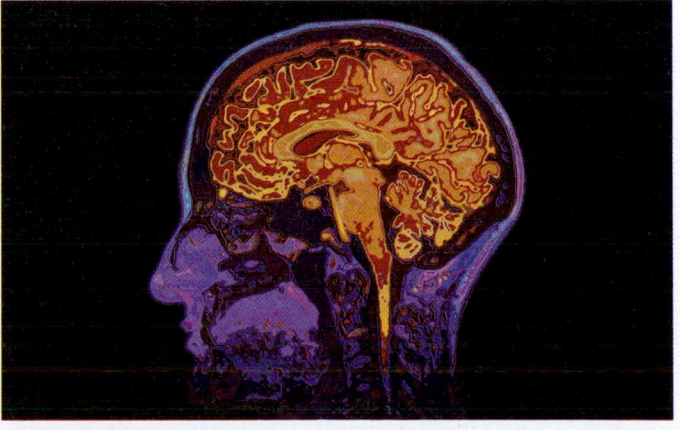

B

Figure 44-3 ■ MRI of head: (A) Procedure. (B) Image.

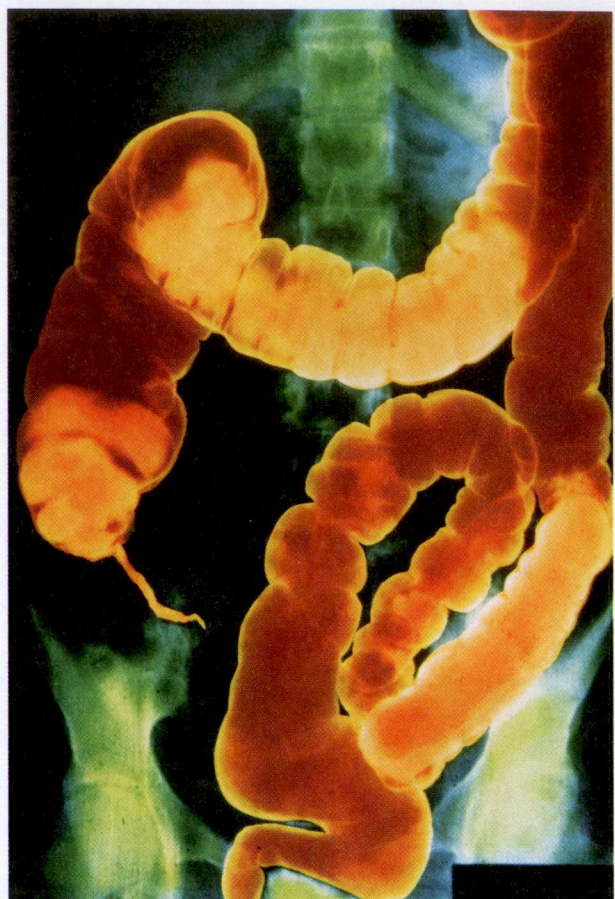

Figure 44-4 ■ X-ray image of the colon using contrast media (barium enema).

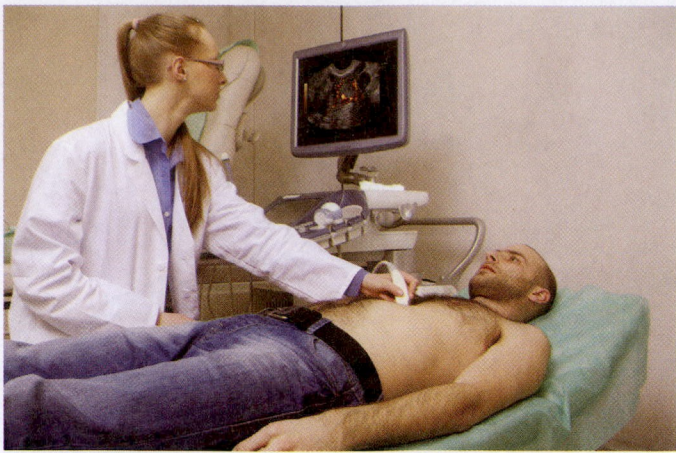

A

B

Figure 44-5 ■ Ultrasound of abdomen. (A) Procedure. (B) Image.

A **radiopaque** structure, such as a bone, allows few x-rays to pass through; it shows up as a light (white) image using plain radiography and provides a two-dimensional image of the surface. A **radiolucent** structure, such as the skin or lungs, permits x-rays to pass into and through it, resulting in a darker, shadowy image that shows layers within the structure. **Contrast medium** (*a radiopaque substance injected or swallowed*) can be used to help visualize other soft tissues that cannot otherwise be seen clearly in an x-ray by making them stand out from surrounding tissues (■ FIGURE 44-4).

Commonly performed radiology procedures are summarized in ■ TABLE 44-2. Ultrasound and nuclear medicine are discussed in detail next.

Ultrasound Imaging

Ultrasound literally means "beyond sound." Procedures use sound waves whose frequency is beyond human hearing to evaluate a patient's internal organs and structures. Ultrasound imaging can be used for diagnostic or therapeutic purposes within the field of radiology. Coders must be aware of the context and the type of ultrasound service to code it correctly.

Diagnostic ultrasound is a noninvasive imaging technology that captures an image of echoes from sound bouncing off structures such as the abdomen, pelvis, heart, vessels, muscles,

joints, and tendons. Ultrasound images are viewed in real time, showing movements within the body, such as blood flowing through vessels or a fetus moving in the womb. Ultrasounds can reveal structural abnormalities, show the presence of a lesion and whether it is solid or fluid-filled, monitor the growth of a fetus, and identify disorders of the arteries and veins, such as occlusions (■ FIGURE 44-5).

Therapeutic ultrasound is the use of ultrasound to image procedures—such as obtaining biopsies—or during interventional radiology. Interventional radiology is a minimally invasive procedure that can be performed anywhere in the body using needles and catheters advanced into arteries, including treating vascular disorders such as embolisms and aneurysms. Interventional radiologists can use other imaging technology besides ultrasound.

Ultrasound therapy is extracorporeal treatment by high-frequency sound waves used for direct treatment of conditions by non-radiologic providers. For example, physical therapists use ultrasound to transmit a sound wave vibration to treat pain. Ultrasound therapy is reported with codes **97605-97608** in the Medicine Section.

Table 44-2 ■ **COMMON RADIOLOGY PROCEDURES**

Procedure Name	Definition	Reason Performed
Cineradiography/ videoradiography	The process of making radiographs of moving objects in rapid sequence and quickly projecting them back to simulate a motion picture	Diagnose or evaluate heart or joint conditions
Clinical brachytherapy	Application of small, encapsulated radioactive elements implanted directly into or near a tumor	Malignant tumors
Computed tomography (CT)	Creation of a three-dimensional image of a body structure by computer, using a series of cross-sectional images	Infection, masses and tumors (including cancer), study blood vessels
Computer-aided detection (CAD)	Use of pattern recognition software to help identify suspicious features on a radiological image, to decrease false-negative readings	Mammography, chest CT, chest x-rays
Dual-energy x-ray absorptiometry (DXA/DEXA), bone density study	Measurement of the density or mass of a material is measured by comparing the amounts of material absorbed from x-ray beams of two different energies	Bone density study, osteoporosis screening
Fluoroscopy	Projection of a live x-ray image onto a fluorescent screen	Image-guided procedures, such as venous or arterial catheter placement
Hyperthermia, thermal therapy, thermotherapy	Exposing tissue to high temperatures (up to 113°F)	Damage or kill cancer cells in a localized area
Magnetic resonance angiography (MRA)	Use of a magnetic field and pulses of radio wave energy to visualize the heart, blood vessels, or blood flow in the circulatory system	Arterial aneurysm, aortic coarctation or dissection, carotid artery disease, atherosclerosis of the arms or legs
Magnetic resonance imaging (MRI)	Use of strong magnets and radio waves to produce computerized images of internal body tissues	Tumors, bleeding, infection, arthritis, soft-tissue damage, and many other conditions
Mammary ductogram, galactogram	Use of mammography and contrast material to view the inside of the breast's milk ducts	Lesions causing nipple discharge
Mammography—diagnostic	X-ray image of the male or female breast to determine whether a problem exists or to determine the nature of a problem	Signs or symptoms of breast disease, dense tissue, a personal history of breast cancer or benign breast disease, inconclusive screening mammogram results
Mammography—screening	X-ray image of the breast of a woman without signs or symptoms of breast disease	Early detection of breast cancer or other abnormalities
Proton beam treatment (PBT) delivery	Use of noninvasive electromagnetic radiation to treat both in situ benign and malignant tumors	Inoperable or radiation-resistant tumors
Positron emission tomography (PET)	Use of a positron-emitting radionuclide tracer to show how organs and tissues are working in real time	Check brain function, examine blood flow to the heart, diagnose cancer or metastases
Radiologic guidance/guided imaging	Use of a radiological modality to visualize access to an anatomic site in real time	Direct or guide the placement and/or removal of surgical objects
Radiosurgery	A form of radiation therapy that focuses high-power energy on a small area of the body (e.g., Cyberknife, Gamma Knife)	Treatment of tumors that lie too close to sensitive structures for traditional surgery; treatment of tumors in patients who are too high risk for traditional surgery
Single-photon emission computed tomography (SPECT)	Use of photons emitted by a radioactive tracer to create an image of lower quality than PET	Mapping brain function
Stereotactic imaging	Three-dimensional imaging to pinpoint a specific location	Biopsy of breast lesion
Ultrasound imaging	Use of sound waves to capture an image of echoes bouncing off structures showing real-time movements within the body	*Diagnostic*: structural abnormalities, show the presence of a lesion and if it is solid or fluid-filled, monitor the growth of a fetus, and identify disorders of the arteries and veins, such as occlusions *Therapeutic*: biopsies, interventional radiology, catheter placement

Table 44-3 ■ **TYPES OF ULTRASOUND MODALITIES**

Type of Ultrasound	Definition
A-mode (amplitude)	A one-dimensional ultrasonic measurement
M-mode (motion)	A one-dimensional ultrasonic measurement used to display movement of a structure
B-scan/gray-scale (brightness)	A two-dimensional ultrasonic scan that displays movement of tissues and organs
Real-time scan	A rapid succession of B-mode images producing a moving video; a two-dimensional ultrasonic scan, with displays of both two-dimensional structures and motion with time
3-D ultrasound	Taking and combining multiple two-dimensional scans using specialized computer software to form 3-D images
Doppler	Use of high-frequency sound to monitor a fetal heartbeat or assess the direction and velocity of blood flow

Source: © PB Resources, Inc. Used with permission.

There are various types of ultrasound scan modalities: one-, two-, or three-dimensional (3-D) or Doppler (■ TABLE 44-3). Three-dimensional ultrasound takes multiple two-dimensional scans and combines them using specialized computer software to form 3-D images. Doppler ultrasound uses high-frequency sound to monitor a fetal heartbeat or assess the direction and velocity (*speed*) of blood flow. Doppler ultrasound can be presented in black-and-white or color.

Nuclear Medicine

Nuclear medicine (NM) procedures use an extremely small amount of radioactive materials—called **radiopharmaceuticals**, radiotracers, or tracers—to image the body and to diagnose and treat diseases. Radioactive elements are administered to the patient through injection, swallowing, or inhalation. They are attracted to specific organs, bones, or tissues, which allows clinicians to image both structure and function of the anatomy. Not only can radiologists see what an organ looks like, they can also see how it functions. NM procedures are most often performed to image the thyroid, bone, heart, liver, brain, and lungs and help detect and treat a variety of diseases such as cancer, aneurysms, irregular or inadequate blood flow, and organ disorders (■ FIGURE 44-6).

Therapeutic NM can deliver palliative (*pain-relieving*) or therapeutic doses of radiation to specific tissues or body areas. Procedures help detect or locate tumor cells, kill the cancerous tissue, reduce the size of a tumor, or reduce pain. They can treat an overactive thyroid, thyroid cancer, blood disorders,

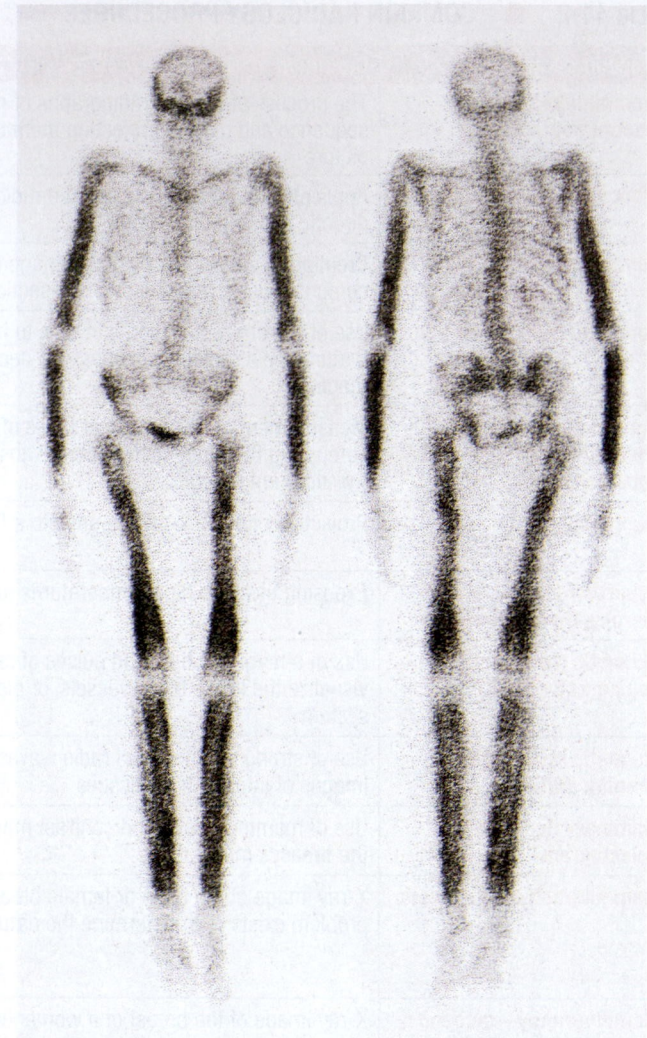

Figure 44-6 ■ Nuclear medicine bone scan image.

chronic inflammatory rheumatism, lymphoma, or certain metastatic bone lesions.

Examples of NM radiopharmaceuticals include:

- Sodium iodide I-123—For thyroid imaging
- Technetium-99m sestamibi—For various nuclear medicine procedures
- Thallium-201—For myocardial perfusion scans (heart functions)
- Strontium-89—For palliative treatment of pain from metastatic bone cancer

Radiology uses many techniques, equipment, and modalities that require detailed knowledge and are constantly changing because of advances in technology. This section provides a general reference to help understand the most common radiology procedures. Remember to keep standard reference books handy to locate additional information that may be needed for a specific situation.

CODING PRACTICE

Instructions: Use your medical terminology skills and resources to define the following procedures related to radiology, then identify the code(s) or code range listed in the CPT Index. Follow these steps:

- Use slash marks "/" to break down the underlined term into its root(s) and suffix.
- Define the meaning of the underlined word based on the meaning of each word part.
- Use the entire phrase to identify the code or code range shown in the CPT Index.

Example: laryngography laryngo/graphy   Meaning *making a recording of the larynx*   CPT Code *70373*

1. radiopharmaceutical therapy, oral   Meaning _____   CPT Code _____
2. x-ray, spine, thoracolumbar   Meaning _____   CPT Code _____
3. myelography, brain   Meaning _____   CPT Code _____
4. uterus, sonohysterography   Meaning _____   CPT Code _____
5. echoencephalography, intracranial   Meaning _____   CPT Code _____
6. spectroscopy, magnetic resonance   Meaning _____   CPT Code _____
7. hyperthermia treatment   Meaning _____   CPT Code _____
8. cholangiography, intraoperative   Meaning _____   CPT Code _____
9. pelvimetry   Meaning _____   CPT Code _____
10. mammography   Meaning _____   CPT Code _____

CODING GUIDELINES FOR RADIOLOGY PROCEDURES

Coders should understand the organization of this CPT section, section guidelines, and instructional notes in the Tabular List. This information is necessary for accurate coding. **Radiology (70010-79999)** is one of CPT's six major sections and contains seven subsections that are divided by modality (■ TABLE 44-4). Within the **Diagnostic Radiology** and **Diagnostic Ultrasound** subsections, categories are divided by anatomic region. In the **Diagnostic Radiology** categories, all modalities—radiography, CT, and MRI—appear sequentially within each anatomic category. CPT does not provide titles to separate these modalities in the Tabular List.

In other subsections, categories are divided by the type of procedure. Review the subheading and category names and code ranges listed in the Radiology section to become familiar with the content and organization.

This CPT section includes invasive and minimally invasive radiology procedures. Radiology section procedures must be supported by diagnosis codes that support the medical necessity of the procedure. Because radiology procedures are performed on every organ system and for many different reasons, diagnosis codes from any ICD-10-CM chapter might be used. The ordering physician provides the diagnosis code(s) with the order for the procedure.

CPT provides guidelines at the beginning of the Radiology section that apply to all codes in the section. In particular, coders need to understand radiological supervision and interpretation, administration of contrast materials, and written reports.

Supervision and Interpretation, Imaging Guidance

Most Radiology section codes, except those in the **Radiation Oncology** subsection, consist of a technical component and professional component. The technical component encompasses the costs of the facility, equipment, staff, and related expenses. Radiological supervision and interpretation (RS&I) describes the professional component of a radiological procedure that reports the physician's work. Supervision is the radiologist personally performing the procedure or overseeing radiology clinicians who perform the procedure. Interpretation is the radiologist's analysis of the image(s), or the findings, and writing of a report that documents the findings and provides a diagnosis. The report is sent to the referring physician, who considers the findings and radiological diagnosis, together with other clinical indicators and test results, to establish the patient's final diagnosis.

Many procedures in the CPT **Medicine** and **Surgery** sections have a radiology component for guided imaging. The guidelines, instructional notes, or code descriptors may state that imaging guidance is included in the CPT code and should not be reported separately. When this occurs, do not report separate Radiology section codes for imaging guidance or RS&I. When the imaging guidance is not bundled with the primary procedure code, assign a Radiology code.

Table 44-4   ■   **RADIOLOGY SUBHEADINGS**

Subheading	Code Range
Diagnostic Radiology (Diagnostic Imaging)	70010-76499
Diagnostic Ultrasound	76506-76999
Radiologic Guidance	77001-77022
Breast Mammography	77053-77067
Bone/Joint Studies	77071-77086
Radiation Oncology	77261-77799
Nuclear Medicine	78012-79999

All imaging guidance codes require documentation in the patient record and description of imaging guidance in the procedure report. All RS&I codes require documentation in the patient's permanent record and a procedure report or separate imaging report. The report must include written interpretation of information contained in the images and RS&I of the service.

Administration of Contrast Materials

Contrast materials, or contrast agents, are special dyes used to improve the visibility of structures or tissues. Radiation cannot penetrate body structures containing contrast, so contrast makes certain areas stand out more in an x-ray or other image. The patient receives contrast through various methods, such as through the rectum; by swallowing; or through injection into a vein, artery, or the subarachnoid space of the spinal cord. The guidelines identify when to report an additional code for the administration of contrast material, which is based on the route of administration:

- Intra-articular route—Assign an additional code for the joint injection.
- Intravascular route—A Radiology section code with the phrase **with contrast** includes the injection; do not assign a separate code.
- Intrathecal route—Assign **61055** or **62284** in addition to the Radiology code.
- Oral or rectal route—This does not qualify as a study with contrast.

Written Report

The physician who provides the RS&I must prepare and sign a report for each procedure. The written report, which can be electronic, typewritten, or handwritten, is a legal document outlining the reason for the procedure, the type of procedure, the physician's findings and discussion with the patient and/or family, and the definitive diagnosis. CPT guidelines define that radiographic "images" must contain anatomic information unique to each patient. "Images" can be acquired either via film or digitally. Do not assign a separate code for a written report because it is included in a radiology procedure or interpretation.

Additional Guidelines and Instructions

Special instructions at the beginning of many categories provide definitions and coding guidelines. Instructional notes appear throughout the Tabular List to alert coders to the need for modifiers, provide cross-references to codes for similar procedures on other sites, identify when additional codes for radiological services might be needed, alert you to other codes in CPT that you should not report with specific Radiology section codes, and highlight resequenced and recently deleted codes.

ABSTRACTING RADIOLOGY PROCEDURES

Plain radiographic procedures (x-rays) are described by the number and type of radiographic views—the angle and direction from which the image is taken. The view(s) also determines how the technician must position the patient. Refer to ■ FIGURE 44-7 for examples of common views and body positions. CT scans, MRIs, and other modalities are not described the same way

because cross-sectional views, real-time imaging, and functional mapping require different details in the physician orders.

The anatomic approach can refer to how a site is accessed—such as a transabdominal ultrasound—or how a substance or injection is administered, such as intracavity brachytherapy or intrathecal injection. Commonly used anatomic approaches include:

- **Endocavity**—Within a cavity
- **Interstitial**—Between tissues
- **Intra-articular**—Within a joint
- **Intracavity**—Within a cavity
- **Intrathecal**—Into the sheath (*outer covering*) of the spinal cord
- Transabdominal—Through the abdomen
- Transvaginal—Through the vagina

Refer to ■ TABLE 44-5 for guidance on how to abstract radiology procedures and ■ TABLE 44-6 for radiation oncology procedures, then work through the detailed example that follows. Remember that the abstracting questions are a guide and that not every question applies to, or can be answered for, every case. For example, the number of views is applicable to plain radiography procedures but not to MRIs or CT scans.

Table 44-5   ■   KEY CRITERIA FOR ABSTRACTING RADIOLOGY PROCEDURES

- ❏ What is the patient's age?
- ❏ What is the anatomic site?
- ❏ What is the type of radiology procedure?
- ❏ Is the procedure diagnostic or therapeutic?
- ❏ How many and what views are taken?
- ❏ What body positions are used?
- ❏ What is the anatomic approach?
- ❏ What is the laterality?
- ❏ Is contrast medium used?
- ❏ Is the service technical, professional, or global?
- ❏ Is imaging guidance used to assist in another procedure?
- ❏ What additional procedures are performed?

Source: © PB Resources, Inc. Used with permission.

Table 44-6   ■   KEY CRITERIA FOR ABSTRACTING RADIATION ONCOLOGY PROCEDURES

- ❏ Is the service treatment planning or treatment delivery?
- ❏ Is treatment planning clinical or simulation?
- ❏ What is the treatment delivery modality (radiation, proton beam, brachytherapy)?
- ❏ What anatomic site(s) is treated?
- ❏ How many distinct areas are treated?
- ❏ How many and what type of ports are used?
- ❏ How many and what type of blocks are used?
- ❏ What is the total radiation dose delivered?
- ❏ How many treatments are given in the period being reported?
- ❏ Is the service technical, professional, or global?

Source: © PB Resources, Inc. Used with permission.

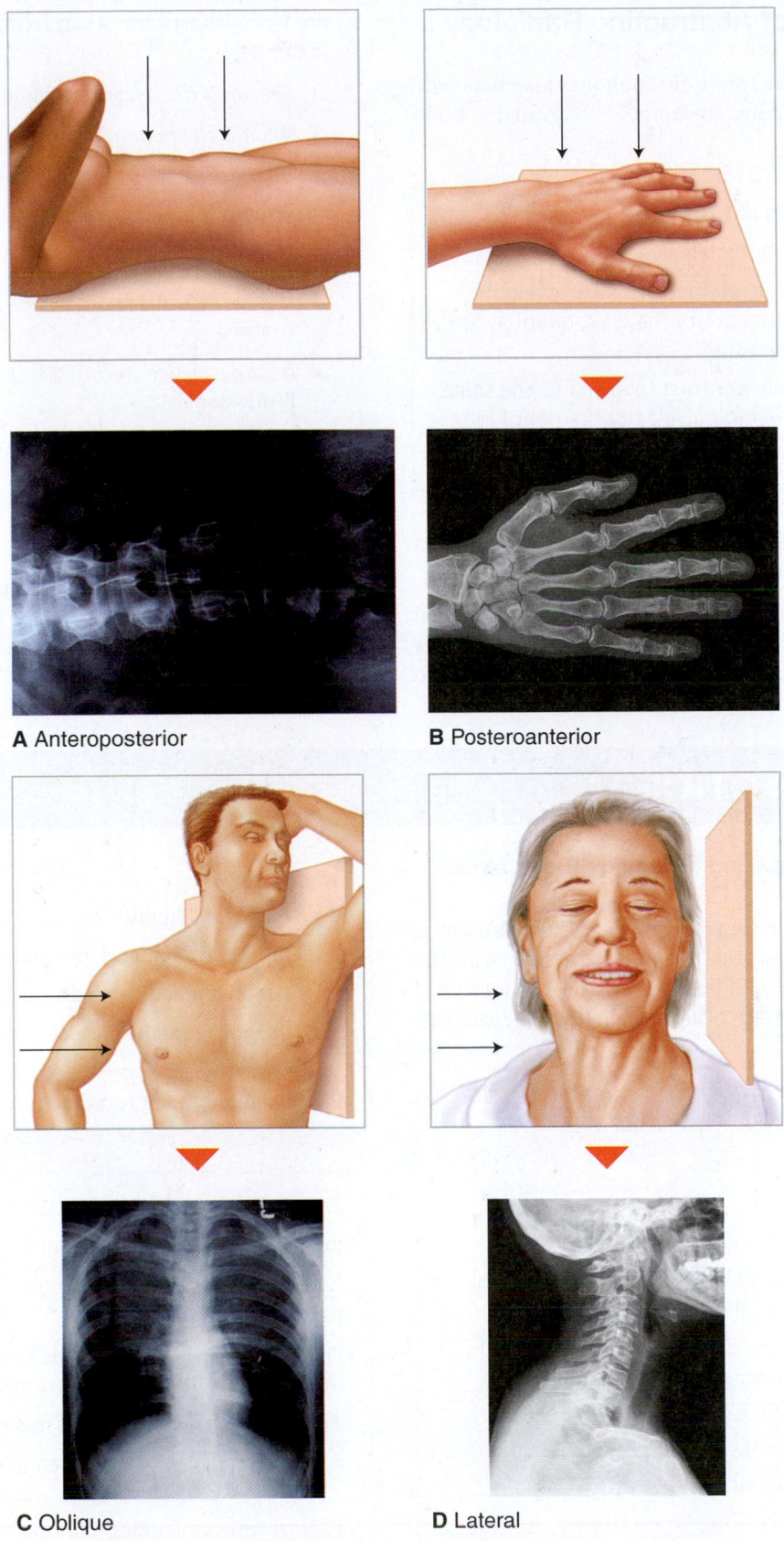

A Anteroposterior

B Posteroanterior

C Oblique

D Lateral

Figure 44-7 ■ Examples of common x-ray views (positions) and resulting images.

Guided Example of Abstracting Radiology Procedures

Refer to the following example throughout this chapter to practice skills for abstracting, assigning, and arranging Radiology section codes.

> OUTPATIENT HOSPITAL Gender: F Age: 52
>
> Referring physician: Cardiologist
>
> Referring diagnosis: Mitral valve prolapse, evaluate mitral regurgitation to quantify the leak, quantify left ventricular size and function
>
> Procedure: MRI without contrast followed by the same views with contrast, including velocity flow mapping
>
> *Note:* Code for the supervising radiologist.

Follow along as fictitious coder, Marcy Elwood, CCS, abstracts the procedure. Check off each step after you complete it.

▶ Marcy reads through the entire record, paying special attention to the reason for the encounter, the procedure performed, and the postoperative diagnosis. She refers to the Key Criteria for Abstracting Radiology Procedures (Table 44-5).

❑ *She notes the referring diagnosis:* Mitral value prolapse

❑ *What is the patient's age?* 52

❑ *What is the anatomic site?* Heart/mitral valve

❑ *What is the type of radiology procedure?* MRI

❑ *Is the procedure diagnostic or therapeutic?* Diagnostic

❑ *Is contrast medium used?* Yes, without and with contrast

❑ *Is the service technical, professional, or global?* Professional

❑ *Is imaging guidance used to assist in another procedure?* No

❑ *What additional procedures are performed?* Velocity flow mapping

▶ At this time, Marcy does not know which of these procedures may need to be coded, nor how many codes she will end up with. She will learn about this when she moves on to assigning codes.

CODING PRACTICE

Exercise 44.2   Abstracting Radiology Procedures

Instructions: Read the mini-medical-record of each patient's encounter and answer the abstracting questions. Write the answer on the line provided. Do not assign any codes. Read the tips with each exercise to help determine whether you are coding for a professional, technical, or global service.

> **1.** OUTPATIENT HOSPITAL   Gender: F
> Age: 16 months
>
> Referring physician: Pediatrician
>
> Referring diagnosis: Limping while walking
>
> Procedure: X-ray of the pelvis (AP), AP and bilateral frog-leg (lateral) view of the hips
>
> *Tip:* Code for the services of the hospital's radiology department only. The images were interpreted by a radiologist under contract with the hospital.
>
> a. What is the patient's age? _____
>
> b. What is the anatomic site? _____
>
> c. What is the type of radiology procedure? _____
>
> d. How many and what views are taken? _____
>
> e. What body positions are used? _____
>
> f. What is the anatomic approach? _____
>
> *(continued)*

> **1.** (continued)
> g. What is the laterality? _____
>
> h. Is the service technical, professional, or global? _____
>
> i. Is contrast medium used? _____
>
> j. Is imaging guidance used to assist in another procedure? _____
>
> k. What additional procedures are performed? _____

> **2.** OUTPATIENT HOSPITAL   Gender: F   Age: 46
>
> Referring physician: Oncologist
>
> Referring diagnosis: Status post-thyroidectomy due to thyroid cancer
>
> Procedure: One session, 3 MeV radiation treatment to the thyroid using a single port and simple block
>
> *Tip:* Code for the oncologist's services.
>
> a. Is the service treatment planning or treatment delivery? _____
>
> b. Is treatment planning clinical or simulation? _____
>
> c. What is the treatment delivery modality (radiation, proton beam, brachytherapy)? _____
>
> d. What anatomic site(s) is treated? _____
>
> *(continued)*

CODING PRACTICE *(continued)*

2. (continued)

e. How many distinct areas are treated? _____

f. How many and what type of ports are used? _____

g. How many and what type of blocks are used? _____

h. What is the total radiation dose delivered? _____

i. How many treatments are given in the period being reported? _____

j. Is the service technical, professional, or global? _____ _____

---

3. OUTPATIENT HOSPITAL   Gender: M   Age: 81

Referring physician: Pulmonologist

Referring diagnosis: SOB, mild chest pain, hemoptysis

Procedure: Ventilation-perfusion scan (V/Q scan)

Postprocedure diagnosis: Pulmonary artery thrombosis

Tip: Code for the technical services of the hospital's radiology department.

a. What is the patient's age? _____

b. What is the anatomic site? _____

c. What is the type of radiology procedure? _____

d. How many and what views are taken? _____

e. What body positions are used? _____

f. What is the anatomic approach? _____

g. What is the laterality? _____

h. Is the service technical, professional, or global? _____ _____

i. Is contrast medium used? _____

j. Is imaging guidance used to assist in another procedure? _____

k. What additional procedures are performed? _____

---

4. OUTPATIENT HOSPITAL   Gender: F   Age: 64

Referring physician: Pulmonologist

Referring diagnosis: Lifelong smoker, severe cough, hemoptysis

Procedure: AP and lateral chest x-ray, standing. A dense mass in the lower lobe of the left lung is noted. Patient's pulmonologist consents to performing a CT scan of the chest without contrast, which is done immediately.

Postprocedure diagnosis: Carcinoma of the left lower lobe

(continued)

---

4. (continued)

Tip: Code for the supervising radiologist.

a. What is the patient's age? _____

b. What is the anatomic site? _____

c. What is the type of radiology procedure? _____

d. How many and what views are taken? _____

e. What body positions are used? _____

f. What is the anatomic approach? _____

g. What is the laterality? _____

h. Is the service technical, professional, or global? _____

i. Is contrast medium used? _____

j. Is imaging guidance used to assist in another procedure? _____

k. What additional procedures are performed? _____

---

5. OFFICE   Gender: F   Age: 29

Performing physician: Obstetrician

Preprocedure diagnosis: Routine pregnancy, EGA 10 weeks

Procedure: Transabdominal ultrasound for fetal and maternal evaluation, supine

Postprocedure diagnosis: Twin fetuses

a. What is the patient's age? _____

b. What is the anatomic site? _____

c. What is the type of radiology procedure? _____

d. How many and what views are taken? _____

e. What body positions are used? _____

f. What is the anatomic approach? _____

g. What is the laterality? _____

h. Is the service technical, professional, or global? _____

i. Is contrast medium used? _____

j. Is imaging guidance used to assist in another procedure? _____

k. What additional procedures are performed? _____

---

6. OUTPATIENT HOSPITAL   Gender: M   Age: 55

Referring physician: Nephrologist

Diagnosis: ESRD, diabetic nephropathy

Procedure: Placed a central venous nontunneled catheter using fluoroscopic guidance for temporary dialysis access

(continued)

6. (continued)

Tip: Code for the service of the interventional radiologist.

a. What is the patient's age? _____

b. What is the anatomic site? _____

c. What is the type of radiology procedure? _____

d. How many and what views are taken? _____

e. What body positions are used? _____

f. What is the anatomic approach? _____

(continued)

6. (continued)

g. What is the laterality? _____

h. Is the service technical, professional, or global? _____
_____

i. Is contrast medium used? _____

j. Is imaging guidance used to assist in another procedure? _____

k. What additional procedures are performed? _____

ASSIGNING CODES FOR RADIOLOGY PROCEDURES

To assign codes for services in the Radiology section, search the Index for the Main Term of the modality, such as **X-ray**, **CT Scan**, **Ultrasound**, and so on. First-level modifying terms vary based on the modality, so review each Main Term entry carefully to understand how it is organized, then follow the necessary path to identify the anatomic site. For example, under the Main Term **X-ray**, first-level modifying terms identify the anatomic site. Under the Main Term **CT Scan**, most sites appear as second-level modifying terms under the first-level modifying terms **with contrast**, **without and with contrast**, and **without contrast**. Under the Main Term **Ultrasound**, most first-level modifying terms identify the anatomic site, but there are also first-level modifying terms for **3-D Rendering** and **Guidance**.

After locating the code range for the modality and anatomic site, refer to the Tabular List to select and verify the code based on the type of examination, number of views, and other details in the code descriptions. When searching a Main Term entry that has multiple levels of modifying terms, be sure to identify the correct first-level modifying term before selecting the anatomic site.

The following information gives examples of Radiology section coding for technical, professional, and global services; ultrasound; mammography; procedures using contrast; and radiation oncology.

Assigning Codes for Ultrasound

Ultrasound examinations of the pelvis are divided based on whether the procedure is obstetrical or nonobstetrical. Codes for obstetrical ultrasounds include the phrase **pregnant uterus**. Codes are further divided based on the age of fetus as younger than 14 weeks or 14 weeks and older (■ FIGURE 44-8). Codes are also divided for the first fetus, also called the gestational sac, and each additional fetus or gestational sac. To assign codes for a pelvic ultrasound procedure, search the Index for the Main Term **Ultrasound** and the first-level modifying term **Pelvis** for a nonobstetrical procedure or the first-level modifying term

Pregnant uterus for an obstetrical procedure. Refer to the Tabular List to select and verify the correct code based on the criteria contained in the code descriptions.

Assigning Codes for Mammography

CPT provides three codes for basic mammography, based on whether the procedure is for screening or diagnostic purposes. A screening mammogram is one performed for preventive reasons for a woman with no symptoms. By definition, a screening mammogram (code **77067**) is bilateral and does not require modifier **-50 Bilateral procedure**. A diagnostic mammogram is performed because of symptoms or a suspected problem and can be performed on both men and women. A diagnostic mammogram can be either unilateral (code **77065**) or bilateral (code **77066**). Append the appropriate laterality modifier **-RT Right side** or **-LT Left side** to code **77065** for a unilateral procedure, but do not report modifier **-50** with code **77066** because the code is defined as bilateral.

Screening and diagnostic mammography are supported by different ICD-10-CM diagnosis codes. In general, report **Z12.31** or **Z12.39** for a screening mammogram (■ FIGURE 44-9). For a diagnostic mammogram, use codes that describe the symptom(s) or condition(s) that caused the physician to order the procedure (■ FIGURE 44-10). Always check with payers for specific coding requirements.

Patient receives a transabdominal ultrasound examination with real-time image documentation and fetal and maternal evaluation. One gestational sac is identified with an estimated gestational age of 12 weeks.

76801 Ultrasound, pregnant uterus, real time with image documentation, fetal and maternal evaluation, first trimester (< 14 weeks 0 days), transabdominal approach; single or first gestation

Figure 44-8 ■ Example of coding obstetrical ultrasound.
Source: © PB Resources, Inc. Used with permission.

Patient was seen for a bilateral screening mammogram with 2 views of each breast.

Z12.31 Encounter for screening mammogram for malignant neoplasm of breast
77067 Screening mammography, bilateral (2-view study of each breast), including computer-aided detection (CAD) when performed

Figure 44-9 ■ Example of coding for a screening mammogram. *Source: © PB Resources, Inc. Used with permission. CPT codes only © American Medical Association.*

Patient was seen for a diagnostic mammogram of the right breast because of a suspicious lump.

N63.10 Unspecified lump in the right breast, unspecified quadrant
77065-RT Diagnostic mammography, including computer-aided detection (CAD) when performed; unilateral; -RT Right side

Figure 44-10 ■ Example of coding for a diagnostic mammogram. *Source: © PB Resources, Inc. Used with permission. CPT codes only © American Medical Association.*

Assigning Codes for with and without Contrast

A radiologist, radiologic technologist, or nurse may administer contrast media, subject to the requirements of state law. Radiology departments often provide physicians with a reference card that identifies the clinical circumstances under which imaging should be ordered without contrast, with contrast, or both. This enables physicians to obtain the most useful images possible while minimizing patient exposure to radiation or contrast medium. Overexposure to radiation can cause illness, gene mutation, and cancer. Contrast media can cause serious allergic reactions in some people.

The code description identifies whether and how contrast is used. The most common variations are discussed next.

With Contrast

When the Radiology section code descriptor includes the phrase **with contrast material(s)**, it means that clinicians performed the test using contrast. The code includes the radiological procedure and the contrast material(s).

A Radiology section code *usually* includes the injection procedure when contrast is administered by injection, but this is not *always* the case. Instructional notes may appear after the code descriptor for the primary procedure stating that a separate code for the injection can be reported. In this situation, assign a minimum of three codes:

- The primary procedure from the Surgery or Medicine section
- The injection procedure from the Surgery section
- The radiology procedure from the Radiology section

Contrast Supplies

Sometimes contrast is used but the Radiology code descriptor does not state **with contrast**. In this case, assign an additional code for the type of contrast administered, in addition to the procedure codes. Depending on the payer's requirements, report CPT code **99070 Supplies and materials** or a HCPCS code for the specific contrast agent.

Do not assign a code for oral or rectal contrast because these are bundled in the Radiology procedure code.

With or Without Contrast

Some radiology procedures can be performed either with contrast or without contrast, based on the judgment of the physician. These procedures may have two codes: one that states **with contrast** and a second that states **without contrast**. Select the appropriate code based on whether or not contrast was used.

Without Contrast Followed by With Contrast

In some cases, a radiology procedure might be performed twice at the same encounter: first *without* contrast and then again *with* contrast. This procedure is often done to evaluate tumors, metastases, infection, and hematuria. Different structures and tissues are visible without contrast than when using contrast. Both procedures are bundled into one code, so do not assign two Radiology section codes to report the two methods. Look for a code in which the description states **without contrast material(s), followed by contrast material(s)**.

Assigning Codes for Radiation Oncology

Radiation oncology, also called radiation therapy, is a form of cancer treatment that uses high-energy ionizing radiation to shrink or kill malignant neoplasms. It is also used to shrink benign neoplasms or stop their growth. Radiation is usually administered in a precise, calculated dose on a daily basis and over a period of several days to several weeks.

The radiation oncology treatment process is a complex, multidisciplinary service that involves a team of experts including a radiation oncologist physician, radiation therapist, physicist (*a scientist who plans resources and selects equipment to use*), medical dosimetrist (*a healthcare professional who measures and administers radiation*), nurse, and radiotherapy technician.

The **Radiation Oncology** subsection provides extensive special instructions regarding coding for the stages of radiation oncology treatment, which are summarized in ■ TABLE 44-7 (page 916). In many categories, codes are divided based on the complexity of the treatment. The special instructions define simple, intermediate, and complex services applicable to each category.

To locate codes for radiation oncology services, search the Index for the Main Term **Radiation Therapy**; the first-level modifying term for the type of service, such as **Treatment delivery** or **Dose plan**; and the second-level modifying term for the specific service provided. Refer to the Tabular List to

Table 44-7 ■ **SUMMARY OF RADIATION ONCOLOGY CODING**

Phase	Description	Coding Guidelines
Consultation and clinical management	Physician evaluation of patient's condition and recommendation of treatment options	Report codes from E/M, Medicine, and Surgery sections for the specific services provided.
Clinical treatment planning	The process of special testing and interpretation, tumor localization, treatment volume determination, treatment time/dosage determination, choice of treatment modality, determination of number and size of treatment ports, selection of appropriate treatment devices, and other procedures	Codes are divided by simple, intermediate, and complex planning based on the number of treatment areas and ports. Clinical treatment planning is reported once per patient for the entire course of treatment.
Simulation	Determination and testing of treatment field, location, and ports without administering any radiation	Codes are divided by simple, intermediate, and complex planning based on the number of treatment areas and ports. Simulation is usually reported once per patient for the entire course of treatment.
Isodose planning/dosimetry	Calculation and verification of the amount of radiation to be delivered	Codes are divided by the type and complexity of radiation delivery.
Treatment delivery	Technical-only services of providing radiation treatment according to the established plan	Codes are divided by the type of therapy; simple, intermediate, and complex; and volume of treatment. Treatment delivery is reported once per treatment session.
Treatment management	Physician supervision of the treatment process, including one physical examination and other specified services	Report one code (77427) per five treatments provided. If fewer than five treatments are given to finish out a course of treatment, report 77427 for three to five treatments. For one or two final treatments, do not report a code. CPT guidelines specify services to be provided. Additional codes report short-course treatments and stereotactic radiation therapy.

Source: © PB Resources, Inc. Used with permission.

Patient receives his final nine radiation treatment sessions to end his radiation therapy to treat esophageal cancer. Treatment is greater than 1 MeV, simple.

Facility services:
77402 × 9 Radiation treatment delivery, > than 1 MeV, simple
Physician services:
77427 × 2 Radiation treatment management, 5 treatments

Figure 44-11 ■ Example of coding for radiation oncology.
Source: © PB Resources, Inc. Used with permission. CPT codes only © American Medical Association.

review the guidelines and select the appropriate code based on the complexity of the service and other details of the code description. The CPT manual provides a table, "Radiation Management and Treatment Table" that summarizes how to use these codes.

Refer to ■ FIGURE 44-11 to learn more about coding for both facility and physician services for Radiation Oncology.

Guided Example of Assigning Radiology Procedure Codes

To practice skills for assigning codes for the Radiology section, continue with the example from earlier in the chapter about a patient who was seen for an MRI of the heart. Follow along

in your CPT manual as Marcy Elwood, CCS, assigns codes. Check off each step after you complete it.

▶ First, Marcy confirms the procedure: MRI without contrast followed by the same views with contrast, including velocity flow mapping.

▶ Marcy searches the Index for the Main Term **Magnetic Resonance Imaging (MRI)**.

❏ She locates the first-level modifying term **Heart**.

❏ She identifies the code range **75557-75565**.

▶ Marcy turns to the Tabular List to select and verify the codes. She notices that this code range comprises its own category, **Heart**, that has extensive special instructions, so she begins by studying the special instructions. She highlights several important points that may pertain to this case:

❏ Whereas traditional MRI produces static images, cardiac MRI provides a real-time **physiologic evaluation of cardiac function.**

❏ Some codes include contrast and others do not. Some codes include pharmacologic perfusion stress testing and others do not.

❏ Cardiac MRI for velocity flow mapping can be reported in conjunction with **75557, 75559, 75561, or 75563**.

❏ Only one add-on code for flow velocity can be reported per session.

❏ This information leads her to believe that she will probably need two codes: one for the MRI without and with contrast and one for the velocity flow mapping.

▶ Marcy reads the code descriptions to locate the code(s) she may need.

❏ Codes **75557** and **75559** are for without contrast, so they do not apply.

❏ Code **75561** describes **Cardiac magnetic resonance imaging for morphology and function without contrast material(s), followed by contrast material(s) and further sequences.** It identifies MRI as well as without and with contrast, so she makes a note of this code.

❏ Code **75563** is the same as **75561** with stress imaging added, but stress imaging was not performed.

❏ She reads the instructional note following code **75563** that states **(75558, 75560, 75564 have been deleted. To report flow velocity, use 75565).** She assumes that the codes listed as deleted must have been used for flow velocity previously, before the introduction of code **75565**.

❏ She reads the description for code **75565** and notes that it is the add-on code for **Cardiac magnetic resonance imaging for velocity flow mapping** discussed in the special instructions.

■ An instructional note following code **75565** states **(Use 75565 in conjunction with 75557, 75559, 75561, 75563),** which also concurs with the special instructions. She verifies that the MRI code she has tentatively selected, **75561**, appears in the list of allowed codes.

❏ The remaining codes in this category identify computed tomography, so they do not apply.

▶ Marcy reviews the procedure codes she has identified for this case and confirms that they accurately describe the procedures performed.

❏ **75565 Cardiac magnetic resonance imaging for velocity flow mapping**

❏ **75561 Cardiac magnetic resonance imaging for morphology and function without contrast material(s), followed by contrast material(s) and further sequences**

▶ Next, Marcy must determine how to sequence the codes.

CODING PRACTICE

Exercise 44.3   Assigning Codes for Radiology Procedures

Instructions: Read the mini-medical-record of each patient's encounter. Review the information abstracted in Exercise 44.2 for questions 1–3. For questions 4–6, abstract the case on your own. Read the tips with each exercise to help determine whether you are coding for a professional, technical, or global service. Assign CPT codes, quantities, and modifiers using the Index and Tabular List. Write the code(s) on the line provided.

---

1. OUTPATIENT HOSPITAL   Gender: F

Age: 16 months

Referring physician: Pediatrician

Referring diagnosis: Limping while walking

Procedure: X-ray of the pelvis (AP), AP and bilateral frog-leg (lateral) view of the hips

Tip: Code for the services of the hospital's radiology department only. The images were interpreted by a radiologist under contract with the hospital.

1 CPT Code _____

---

2. OUTPATIENT HOSPITAL   Gender: F   Age: 46

Performing physician: Oncologist

Preprocedure diagnosis: Status post-thyroidectomy due to thyroid cancer

Procedure: One session, 3 MeV radiation treatment to the thyroid, using a single port and simple block

Tip: Code for the oncologist's services.

1 CPT Code _____

---

3. OUTPATIENT HOSPITAL   Gender: M   Age: 81

Referring physician: Pulmonologist

Referring diagnosis: SOB, mild chest pain, hemoptysis

Procedure: Ventilation-perfusion scan (V/Q scan)

Impression: Pulmonary artery thrombosis

Tip: Code for the technical services of the hospital's radiology department.

1 CPT Code _____

(continued)

CODING PRACTICE (continued)

4. OFFICE Gender: F Age: 47

Referring physician: Primary care

Referring diagnosis: Recurring constipation

Procedure: Barium enema. Rectal tube inserted and barium instilled with fluoroscopy images of evacuation. Barium seemed to flow with no difficulty through the GI tract.

Impression: Normal barium enema

Tip: Code the professional and technical components.

1 CPT Code _____

5. OUTPATIENT HOSPITAL Gender: F Age: 29

Referring physician: Primary care

Referring diagnosis: Seizure disorder

Procedure: Noncontrast CT of head. No evidence of hemorrhage or infarction. No fluid indicating hydrocephalus. There is no midline shift.

(continued)

5. (continued)

Impression: Normal CT; no acute process seen.

Tip: Code only the professional component.

1 CPT Code _____

6. OFFICE Gender: M Age: 68

Performing physician: Cardiologist

Preprocedure diagnosis: CAD with ischemia

Procedure: Myocardial perfusion imaging. Following 4 minutes of exercise, the patient was injected with 3013 mCi of Cardiolite technetium-99m sestamibi. Perfusion images obtained to compare to resting images.

Impression: Abnormal perfusion imaging with a moderately large-sized defect consistent with anterior wall ischemia.

Tip: Code for the technical and professional components.

1 CPT Code _____

ARRANGING CODES FOR RADIOLOGY PROCEDURES

When multiple Radiology procedures are performed on the same date, sequence codes in descending RVU order. Be aware of how to report codes for radiologic guidance and how to apply modifiers correctly.

Multiple Coding for Radiologic Guidance

Radiologic guidance can be real time or static. Real-time guidance generates a live image of anatomic structures that the operating physician views on a screen to guide his movements. The combination of laparoscopic surgery and real-time imaging guidance makes minimally invasive procedures more readily available because open incisions to view and access the operative field are needed less often. In most cases, multiple coding is required: one code for the radiological imaging and one code for the surgical procedure. In some cases, a third code for the injection of the contrast medium is required. When the code for the surgical procedure specifies that a radiological procedure is being done at the same time, such as **with cholangiography**, the injection procedure is included in the CPT code for the surgical procedure. However, report the code for RS&I in addition to the surgical procedure code. When the Radiology code specifies **radiological supervision and interpretation**, the code identifies only the professional component, so modifier **-26 Professional component** is not required (■ FIGURE 44-12).

Static radiologic guidance involves the placement, usually during a biopsy, of a clip or wire to mark a site that must be treated or operated on at a later time. Multiple coding is required: one code for the placement of the clip or wire and one code for the surgical procedure.

Coders must always identify the physician they are coding for and the services provided by that physician. When a surgeon performs the surgical procedure and an interventional radiologist performs the imaging guidance, do not assign both codes for both providers. Assign codes for each physician codes based on the services personally performed respectively. When one physician performs both the surgery and the radiological guidance, assign both codes for the same physician.

A gastroenterologist performs a laparoscopic cholecystectomy with a cholangiogram as part of the procedure. The gastroenterologist also provides radiological supervision and interpretation.

47563 Laparoscopy, surgical; cholecystectomy with cholangiography

74300 Cholangiography and/or pancreatography; intraoperative, radiological supervision and interpretation

Figure 44-12 ■ Example of coding for real-time radiologic guidance. *Source: © PB Resources, Inc. Used with permission. CPT codes only © American Medical Association.*

Modifiers Used with Radiology

Modifiers that are frequently used with Radiology section codes include those that identify the professional and technical components, reduced services, and laterality. These are discussed next.

-26 Professional Component

Many service in the Radiology section consist of a professional component that includes physician supervision and interpretation and a technical component that includes space, equipment, and staff. When coding for a physician who provides only the professional component, append modifier **-26** to the Radiology code. The Medicare Physician Fee Schedule Database (MPFSDB) lists the total relative value units (RVUs), as well as the RVUs and pricing for both the professional and technical components. The allocation of cost between the professional and technical components varies by the complexity of a procedure and the amount of equipment and supplies required. Typically, the professional component ranges from 20–45% of the total procedure cost.

-TC Technical Component

When coding for a facility that provides only the technical component, append modifier **-TC** to the Radiology section code. Typically, the technical component ranges from 55–80% of the total procedure cost. Also apply modifier **-51** when multiple procedures with technical components are provided at the same time. When the same provider performs both the professional and technical components, code for a global service without any modifier.

In the workplace, coders have a clear understanding of whether they should code for the professional component, technical component, or global service based on the place of employment and organization of services. Consider the following examples:

- A coder who works for a radiology practice comprised of physicians who provide the RS&I component for a facility codes for the professional component only.

- A coder who works for a hospital outpatient department that provides the equipment, facility, and technicians but contracts out all professional services codes for the technical component only.

- A coder who works for a freestanding radiology facility that employs physicians and technical staff and owns all the equipment codes for a global service.

Refer to Chapter 27 of this text for more information and figures on the use of modifiers **-26** and **-TC**.

-52 Reduced Services

Sometimes more than one physician is involved in supervision and interpretation, with one physician supervising the procedure and another interpreting the results. Each physician reports the same procedure code and appends modifier **-52 Reduced services** to show that each physician did not perform a complete service. Submit a report with the claim to explain why the modifier is used. Also report modifier **-26** for codes that have both a technical and professional component.

Laterality

Report laterality modifiers with Radiology services on paired anatomic sites if laterality is not defined in the code. CPT provides two codes for some procedures: one defined as unilateral and one defined as bilateral. Report modifier **-RT** or **-LT** with the unilateral code, but do not report modifier **-50 Bilateral procedure** when the code description specifies that the procedure is bilateral.

-GG Same Day Screening and Diagnostic Mammograms for Medicare Patients

When a Medicare patient has a screening mammogram followed by a diagnostic mammogram *on the same day*, report codes for both procedures. Append HCPCS modifier **-GG Performance and payment of a screening mammogram and diagnostic mammogram on the same patient, same day** to the diagnostic mammogram code.

Guided Example of Arranging Radiology Procedure Codes

To practice skills for arranging codes for procedures in the Radiology section, continue with the example from earlier in the chapter about the patient who was seen for an MRI of the heart. Follow along in your CPT manual as Marcy Elwood, CCS, arranges the codes. Check off each step after you complete it.

▶ First, Marcy confirms the procedure in the medical record: MRI without contrast followed by the same views with contrast, including velocity flow mapping.

▶ Marcy arranges the codes in descending RVU order according to the MPFSDB. She uses the facility RVU because the procedure was performed at the hospital, not at the physician's office, and reviews the RVUs for the professional component (modifier **-26**).

❑ **75565 Cardiac magnetic resonance imaging for velocity flow mapping** Facility RVU = 1.55 (modifier -26 = 0.35/modifier –TC = 1.20)

❑ **75561 Cardiac magnetic resonance imaging for morphology and function without contrast material(s), followed by contrast material(s) and further sequences** Facility RVU = 12.00 (modifier -26 = 3.65/modifier -TC = 8.35)

▶ Marcy examines the need for modifiers. (Refer to Table 27-1, Key Criteria for Abstracting CPT Modifiers, or Appendix A in the CPT manual.)

❏ Code **75561** requires modifier **-26** because she is coding for the supervising radiologist, so only the professional component was provided.

❏ Code **75565** requires modifier **-26** because she is coding for the supervising radiologist, so only the professional component was provided.

▶ Marcy finalizes the procedure codes and sequencing for this case:

(1) **75561-26 Cardiac magnetic resonance imaging for morphology and function without contrast material(s), followed by contrast material(s) and further sequences; -26 Professional component**

(2) **75565-26 Cardiac magnetic resonance imaging for velocity flow mapping; -26 Professional component**

▶ Marcy also assigns and sequences the ICD-10-CM diagnosis codes that support the need for the service.

(1) **I34.1 Nonrheumatic mitral (valve) prolapse**

CODING PRACTICE

Exercise 44.4 Arranging Codes for Radiology Procedures

Instructions: Read the mini-medical-record of each patient's encounter. Review the information abstracted in Exercise 44.2 for questions 1–3. For questions 4–6, abstract the case on your own. Read the tips with each exercise to help determine whether you are coding for a professional, technical, or global service. Assign CPT codes, quantities, and modifiers using the Index and Tabular List, and arrange the codes in proper sequence. Write the code(s) on the line provided.

1. OUTPATIENT HOSPITAL   Gender: F   Age: 64

Referring physician: Pulmonologist

Referring diagnosis: Lifelong smoker, severe cough, hemoptysis

Procedure: AP and lateral chest x-ray, standing. A dense mass in the lower lobe of the left lung is noted. Patient's pulmonologist consents to performing a CT scan of the chest without contrast, which is done immediately.

Impression: Carcinoma of the left lower lobe

Tip: Code for the supervising radiologist.

2 CPT Codes_____

2. OFFICE   Gender: F   Age: 29

Performing physician: Obstetrician

Preprocedure diagnosis: Routine pregnancy, EGA 10 weeks

Procedure: Transabdominal ultrasound for fetal and maternal evaluation, supine

Impression: Twin fetuses

Tip: Read the Tabular List carefully to determine the second code.

2 CPT Codes _____

3. OUTPATIENT HOSPITAL   Gender: M   Age: 55

Referring physician: Nephrologist

Diagnosis: ESRD, diabetic nephropathy

Procedure: Placed a central venous nontunneled catheter using fluoroscopic guidance for temporary dialysis access

Tip: Code for the service of the interventional radiologist, who performs both the placement and the fluoroscopy.

2 CPT Codes _____

4. EMERGENCY ROOM   Gender: M   Age: 71

Referring physician: Emergency Medicine

Referring diagnosis: Pain in left hip s/p fall on ice

Procedure: AP pelvis and left hip radiograph performed. There is generalized demineralization of bone. There is an intertrochanteric fracture of the left hip with moderate angulation and displacement present.

Impression: Intertrochanteric fracture, left hip

Tip: Code only the technical component.

1 CPT Code _____

5. INPATIENT HOSPITAL   Gender: M   Age: 1 Day

Referring physician: Neonatologist

Preprocedure diagnosis: Facial mass

Procedure: MRI of orbit/face with and without contrast; MR angiography of the head with contrast. Multiplanar, multisequence images of the head and neck obtained without contrast followed by contrast. The origin of the mass could not be identified. MR angiography of the head with contrast was limited and suboptimal.

Impression: Hemangioma should be considered

Tip: Code only the professional component.

2 CPT Codes _____

CODING PRACTICE (continued)

---

6. OUTPATIENT HOSPITAL   Gender: F   Age: 10

Referring physician: Pediatrician

Referring diagnosis: Recurrent urinary tract infections

Procedure: Voiding cystogram. A Foley catheter was inserted through the urethra and the bladder filled

(continued)

---

6. (continued)

with contrast. The patient was instructed to void and x-ray images were obtained.

Impression: Vesicoureteral reflux

2 CPT Codes _____

CHAPTER SUMMARY

In this chapter you learned that:

- Radiology is a medical specialty that uses radiation, sound waves, magnetic fields, or radio fields to visualize internal body structures, such as arteries and bones; each type of technology is referred to as a modality.

- CPT provides guidelines at the beginning of the Radiology section that apply to all codes in the section; in particular, coders need to understand radiological supervision and interpretation, administration of contrast materials, and written reports.

- Plain radiographic procedures (x-rays) are described by the number and type of radiographic views—the angle and direction

from which the image is taken, which also determine how the technician must position the patient.

- To assign codes for Radiology section services, search the Index for the Main Term of the modality, then review how the first-level modifying terms are organized and follow the necessary path to identify the anatomic site.

- In most cases, multiple coding is required for radiological guidance: one code for the radiologic imaging and one code for the surgical procedure.

CONCEPT QUIZ

Take a moment to look back at the Radiology section and solidify your skills. Try to answer the questions from memory first, then refer to the discussion in this chapter if you need a little extra help.

Completion

Instructions: Write the term that completes each statement based on the information you learned in this chapter. Choose from the list below. Some choices may be used more than once and some choices may not be used at all.

A-mode

clinical brachytherapy

computed tomography

computer-aided detection

diagnostic

Doppler

DXA

fluoroscopy

hyperthermia

magnetic resonance angiography

magnetic resonance imaging

M-mode

PET

screening

stereotactic imaging

1. _____ is one form of an image-guided procedure using a live x-ray image on a fluorescent screen.

2. A(n) _____ ultrasound uses high-frequency sound to monitor a fetal heartbeat.

3. _____ is pattern recognition software used to decrease false-negative readings of images.

4. The purpose of _____ mammography is to determine the nature of a problem in the breast.

5. _____ may be used to pinpoint a specific location using 3-D imaging during a breast biopsy.

6. _____ is a one-dimensional ultrasonic measurement used to display movement of a structure.

7. _____ is the treatment of malignant tumors by implanting small, encapsulated radioactive elements in a tumor.

8. _____ shows the blood flow in the artery and helps determine a diagnosis of carotid artery disease.

9. _____ is a procedure used to expose tissue to high temperatures in order to damage cancer cells.

10. _____ is used to show how organs and tissues are working in real time using a positron-emitting radionuclide tracer.

(continued)

(continued from page 921)

Multiple Choice

Instructions: Circle the letter of the best answer to each question based on the information you learned in this chapter.

1. Which type of contrast media injection usually requires an additional code for the injection?
   A. Intra-articular
   B. Intravascular
   C. Intrathecal
   D. Rectal

2. Which service is included in RS&I?
   A. Injection
   B. Guided imaging
   C. Written report
   D. Department management

3. When might a physician order an image without contrast, followed by with contrast?
   A. Routine fracture
   B. Tumor
   C. Mammography
   D. Cholangiogram

4. What direction is an AP image taken from?
   A. Back to front
   B. Front to back
   C. Left to right
   D. Top to bottom

5. What anatomic approach means "within a joint"?
   A. Intra-articular
   B. Interstitial
   C. Intrathecal
   D. Intracavity

6. What second-level modifying term directs coders to obstetrical codes for an ultrasound of the pelvis?
   A. Pregnant uterus
   B. Maternity
   C. Obstetrical
   D. Fetus

7. What is the description of the type of structure that permits x-rays to pass into and through it, resulting in a darker, shadowy image that shows layers?
   A. Radiopaque
   B. Translucent
   C. Radiolucent
   D. Medium density

8. How would you code the following procedure? *A bilateral screening mammogram with 2 views of each breast was performed.*
   A. 77067
   B. 77067 x 2
   C. 77067-RT-LT
   D. 77067-50

9. How would you code the following procedure? *A physician provides radiation management services for a patient's final nine radiation treatment sessions for treatment of esophageal cancer.*
   A. 77427
   B. 77427 x 2
   C. 77427 x 5
   D. 77427 x 9

10. How would you code the following procedure? *A gastroenterologist performs a laparoscopic cholecystectomy with a cholangiogram as part of the procedure. The gastroenterologist also provides radiological supervision and interpretation.*
    A. 47563-26
    B. 74300
    C. 74300-26
    D. 47563, 74300

KEEP ON CODING

Instructions: Read the procedural statement, then use the appropriate Index and Tabular List to assign CPT procedure codes, quantities, and modifiers. Write the code(s) on the line provided.

1. CT of the abdomen and pelvis with oral contrast, professional component. CPT Code(s) _____

2. Bilateral screening mammogram, technical component. CPT Code(s) _____

3. Radiological supervision and interpretation of transvaginal and complete abdominal ultrasound with real-time imaging. CPT Code(s) ____

4. SPECT kidney imaging, technical component. CPT Code(s) _____

5. Radiological supervision and interpretation for ultrasonic guidance needle biopsy. CPT Code(s) _____

6. Simple simulation-aided field setting for prostate radiation treatment by radiation oncologist. CPT Code(s) _____

7. MRI of the upper abdomen with and without gadolinium, global component. CPT Code(s) _____

8. Thyroid uptake, single, technical component. CPT Code(s) _____

9. MUGA scan with right-ventricular ejection fraction by first-pass technique; global component. CPT Code(s) _____

10. Intraoperative cholangiopancreatography, radiologic supervision and interpretation. CPT Code(s) _____

11. Screening mammogram and ultrasound of breasts, global component. CPT Code(s) _____

12. Saline infusion hysterosonography with color flow Doppler, professional component. CPT Code(s) _____

13. Nuclear medicine lymphatic scan, global component. CPT Code(s) _____

14. IVP with KUB, global component. CPT Code(s) _____

15. Bilateral pulmonary angiogram, RS&I. CPT Code(s) _____

16. Voiding urethrocystography with contrast, professional component. CPT Code(s) _____

17. Testicular ultrasound, global component. CPT Code(s) _____

18. Lumbosacral myelogram, radiological supervision and interpretation. CPT Code(s) _____

19. Computed tomography, chest; without contrast material, followed by contrast material(s) and further sections, professional component. CPT Code(s) _____

20. X-ray lumbosacral spine, bending views only, 2 views, global component. CPT Code(s) _____

21. 3-D CT evaluation of the heart with contrast, technical component. CPT Code(s) _____

22. Radiation treatment delivery to four separate areas with a rotational beam at 4 MeV, global component. CPT Code(s) _____

23. Nuclear hepatic duct scan with contrast, technical component. CPT Code(s) _____

24. Ultrasound of the right upper and left upper quadrants of the abdomen, global component. CPT Code(s) _____

25. Review of dosimetry, dose delivery, and treatment parameters, five weekly treatments. CPT Code(s) _____

CODING CHALLENGE

Instructions: Read the mini-medical-record of each patient's encounter, then abstract, assign, and arrange ICD-10-CM diagnosis codes and CPT procedure codes using the appropriate Index and Tabular List. Assign quantities and modifiers where needed. Write the code(s) on the line provided.

1. OUTPATIENT HOSPITAL   Gender: M   Age: 65

Referring physician: Primary care

Referring diagnosis: Adenocarcinoma of the prostate, rule out bone metastasis

Procedure: Whole-body radionuclide bone scan. The skeleton was imaged in the anterior and posterior position after the IV administration of 26.5 mCi of technetium 99m MDP. The right parietal region of the skull showed abnormal activity. The uptake in the remainder of the skeleton is within normal limits.

Impression: Focus of abnormal increased tracer activity overlying the right parietal region of the skull. CT scanning or magnetic resonance imaging of the skull and brain could be done for further assessment if it is clinically indicated.

Tip: Code only for the professional component.

1 ICD-10-CM Code _____

1 CPT Code _____

2. OUTPATIENT SURGERY   Gender: M   Age: 59

Referring physician: Oncologist

Referring diagnosis: Pancreatic adenocarcinoma; procedure planned for typing and staging of pancreatic cancer

Procedure: Percutaneous biopsy of the pancreas guided by CT scan. Multiple biopsies taken. The scan shows a tumor of the head of the pancreas with invasion of the superior mesenteric artery, making it unresectable.

Impression: Stage III pancreatic cancer

1 ICD-10-CM Code _____

2 CPT Codes _____

3. OFFICE   Gender: F   Age: 23

Performing physician: Gynecologist

Preprocedure diagnosis: Pelvic pain

Procedure: Transvaginal ultrasound attempted. The patient fainted within the first 60 seconds of the procedure and it had to be discontinued. The procedure was not completed.

Impression: Procedure not completed

Tip: Assign ICD-10-codes for the condition requiring the procedure, the reason it was cancelled, and a Z-code to identify the cancellation itself. Use a modifier on the CPT code to report the procedure was discontinued.

3 ICD-10-CM Codes _____

_____

1 CPT Code _____

(continued)

(continued from page 923)

4. OFFICE Gender: M Age: 91

Performing physician: Gastroenterologist

Preprocedure diagnosis: Achalasia of the lower esophageal sphincter

Procedure: Balloon dilation of the esophagus with fluoroscopic guidance. Scope was passed under direct supervision. Webs were dilated with pneumatic 20-mm-diameter angioplasty balloons x2 for 10 seconds each across the LES. No complications.

Impression: The LES successfully dilated, with obliteration of the waist

Tip: Code the RS&I component for the fluoroscopic guidance by the gastroenterologist in addition to the primary procedure.

1 ICD-10-CM Code _____

2 CPT Codes _____

5. OFFICE Gender: F Age: 68

Performing physician: Primary care

Preprocedure diagnosis: Severe shoulder pain on the left

Procedure: X-ray of left shoulder, AP view

Findings: The bones of the glenohumeral and acromioclavicular joints showed normal alignment and normal bone density. No focal lytic or sclerotic lesion is detected in the visualized bones. Moderate to severe osteoarthritis of the acromioclavicular joint was identified. Normal soft tissues.

Impression: Moderate to severe osteoarthritis of the acromioclavicular joint.

Tip: Code both the professional component and technical component.

1 ICD-10-CM Code _____

1 CPT Code _____

6. OUTPATIENT HOSPITAL Gender: M Age: 63

Referring physician: Neurologist

Referring diagnosis: Impaired memory and apraxia, rule out Alzheimer's disease

Procedure: CT scan of the head without IV contrast

Findings: Revealed a diffuse, moderately large area of localized atrophy involving the superior-most portion of the left parietal region. There is no other significant abnormality.

Impression: Findings indicate early Alzheimer's disease.

Tip: Code only the technical component of the procedure.

2 ICD-10-CM Codes _____

1 CPT Code _____

7. INPATIENT HOSPITAL Gender: F Age: 58

Referring physician: Vascular surgeon

Referring diagnosis: Patient with HTN, hyperlipidemia, and leg pain who comes for arteriogram evaluation

Procedure: Magnetic resonance angiography of both lower extremities. One milliliter gadolinium-DTPA injected via cubital vein. On the left, the proximal anterior tibial artery has 90% atherosclerotic occlusion; the right proximal anterior tibial artery has 100% atherosclerotic occlusion.

Impression: Bilateral obstructive peripheral arterial disease (PAD)

Tip: Code only the professional component of the procedure.

4 ICD-10-CM Codes _____

_____

1 CPT Code _____

8. OUTPATIENT SURGERY Gender: M Age: 44

Performing physician: Anesthesiologist

Referring diagnosis: Chronic neck and back pain

Procedure: Epidural injection at L4-5 in a patient with chronic back and leg pain. Fluoroscopic guidance was used for needle placement. Contrast was injected, and it was confirmed that the needle tip was in the epidural space. Steroid injection was performed; the procedure was tolerated well.

3 ICD-10-CM Codes _____

_____

1 CPT Code _____

9. OFFICE   Gender: F   Age: 39

Reason for encounter: Right knee pain x2 weeks not relieved by NSAIDs. She reports the pain began shortly after her yoga class.

Assessment: Patient known to me is seen for complaint of severe knee pain, which is now interfering with activities of daily living. Exam of both knees showed limited movement on the right, normal on the left. Problem-focused history and examination was performed.

Procedure: Right knee x-ray, 2 views

Impression: X-ray shows tendinitis

Tip: Do not code the external cause of injury. Do assign an E/M code.

1 ICD-10-CM Code _____

2 CPT Codes _____

---

10. INPATIENT HOSPITAL   Gender: M   Age: 75

Referring physician: Neurologist

Referring diagnosis: MRI to rule out brain neoplasm; recurring confusion, increasing in duration over the past month; history of a stroke 10 years ago.

Procedure: MRI brain with and without contrast. Decreased T1 and increased T2 signal in the right temporal lobe. The lesion increased in size and enhances more greatly when compared with the previous MRI exam. There is also edema surrounding the affected area and associated mass effect.

Impression: MRI positive for astrocytoma, left temporal lobe

Tip: Code only the technical component for the procedure.

1 ICD-10-CM Code _____

1 CPT Code _____

Chapter 45

Pathology and Laboratory Services (80047-89398, 0001U and higher)

Chapter Outline

- **Pathology and Laboratory Procedure Basics**
- **Coding Guidelines for Pathology and Laboratory Procedures**
- **Abstracting Procedures for Pathology and Laboratory**
- **Assigning Codes for Pathology and Laboratory Procedures**
- **Arranging Codes for Pathology and Laboratory Procedures**

Learning Objectives

After completing this chapter, you should have the skills to:

45.1 Spell and define the key words, medical terms, and abbreviations related to pathology and laboratory procedures. (Remember)

45.2 Summarize the types of pathology and laboratory procedures. (Understand)

45.3 Adhere to CPT coding guidelines related in the Pathology and Laboratory section. (Apply)

45.4 Examine and abstract procedural information from the medical record for coding Pathology and Laboratory section procedures. (Analyze)

45.5 Demonstrate how to assign codes for procedures in the Pathology and Laboratory section. (Apply)

45.6 Utilize guidelines for arranging (sequencing) codes for Pathology and Laboratory section procedures. (Apply)

Key Terms and Abbreviations

analyte	clinical pathology	lab requisition	qualitative test
Bethesda System	conventional Pap smear	pathologist	quantitative test
Certificate of Compliance (COC)	definitive drug class testing	physician office laboratory (POL)	rapid strep test (RST)
Certificate of Waiver (COW)	direct optical observation	presumptive drug class screening	reference range
Clinical Laboratory Improvement Amendments (CLIA)	gross (examination)	provider-performed microscopy procedure (PPMP)	specimen
	lab report		therapeutic drug assay

In addition to the key terms listed here, students should know the terms defined within tables in this chapter.

INTRODUCTION

Any drugstore and many online outlets sell kits for at-home pregnancy testing, glucose testing, stool testing, and a variety of other simple laboratory tests. These tests provide preliminary results for patients. However, they are not a replacement for physician diagnosis and treatment or the detailed analysis and quality control of a professional laboratory.

This chapter discusses the services of a laboratory to process and interpret a test. Several components must be considered when laboratory services are provided. Physician examinations to determine the need for a test are usually included in the examination component of E/M codes or an appropriate procedure code if done as part of a procedure, such as a colonoscopy. Specimen collection is reported with the CPT code that describes the method of collection, such as venipuncture or a biopsy. Transfer of the specimen to the laboratory is reported with a separate CPT code. Physician review of the lab results, determination of the final diagnosis, and any other follow-up are included in the medical decision-making component of an E/M code.

PATHOLOGY AND LABORATORY PROCEDURE BASICS

Clinical pathology is a medical specialty that is concerned with the diagnosis of disease based on the laboratory analysis of bodily fluids and tissue. A **pathologist** is a physician who examines tissues, checks the accuracy of lab tests, and interprets the results. Recognized subspecialties include chemical pathology—also called clinical chemistry—clinical hematology, transfusion medicine, microbiology, cytogenetics, and molecular genetics. The patient's personal physician uses information from laboratory tests and pathology reports to determine the diagnosis and treatment plan.

Medical terms used for laboratory procedures utilize word parts from all body systems, with prefixes and suffixes that identify what action is being performed. Refer to ■ TABLE 45-1 for a refresher on how to build medical terms related to pathology and laboratory services.

The laboratory requisition, testing, and reporting process is discussed next, followed by a discussion of the Clinical

---

CODING CAUTION

Be alert for medical terms that are spelled similarly and have different meanings.

cyt/o (*cell*) and **cyst/o** (*bladder*)

antigen (*a foreign substance that evokes an immune response and possibly infection*) and **antibody** (*a protein in the blood that creates an immune response against an antigen or other invader*)

Laboratory Improvement Amendments (CLIA). The general types of laboratory procedures are discussed in the next section of this chapter, "Coding Guidelines for Pathology and Laboratory Procedures."

Overview of the Laboratory Testing Process

The most commonly performed pathology and laboratory services require a specimen to be collected and sent to a lab for processing. The physician must document in the patient's medical record the tests ordered and the medical necessity of each. The lab performs the test and sends a report back to the physician. The ordering physician reviews the test results and determines their implication for the patient's care, including documenting how the findings were used to determine a diagnosis and formulate a treatment plan.

A **specimen** is a sample of any bodily fluid or tissue. An **analyte** is the specific substance within the sample to be examined or tested for. For example, a blood specimen might be tested for a variety of analytes, such as glucose, sodium, or cholesterol.

Specimens can be acquired in the physician's office, during a medical procedure, by the patient at home, or at the lab. Physician offices that perform a limited number of laboratory tests in the office are called a **physician office laboratory (POL)**. Tests that cannot be processed in a physician's office are sent to a hospital or a reference laboratory for processing (■ TABLE 45-2, page 928).

Table 45-1 ■ **EXAMPLE OF CONSTRUCTING MEDICAL TERMS FOR PATHOLOGY AND LABORATORY PROCEDURES**

Combining Form	Prefix/Suffix	Complete Medical Term
hemat/o (*blood*) **bi/o** (*life*) **cyt/o** (*cell*) **path/o** (*abnormal*)	**micro-** (*small*)	**hemato + logy** (*study of the blood*) **patho + logy** (*study of the abnormal*) **cyto + patho + logy** (*study of abnormal cells*) **micro + bio + logy** (*study of small life*) **micro + scopy** (*visual examination of small things*)
	-scopy (*visual examination*) **-logy** (*study of*)	

Source: © PB Resources, Inc. Used with permission.

Table 45-2 ■ TYPES OF LABORATORY PROVIDERS

Type of Laboratory	Description
Physician Office Laboratory (POL)	Small laboratory in a physician office that performs a limited number of tests on site, eliminating the need to send them to an outside lab.
Hospital Laboratory	Laboratory located in a hospital facility, used to perform tests needed in emergency situations, tests where STAT results are needed rapidly for patient care, those done in high volume for both inpatients and outpatients.
Independent Clinical Lab/ Reference Lab	A Medicare-enrolled laboratory that receives a specimen performs the test(s) for a separate, referring laboratory.
Public Health Lab	Lab operated by state and local health departments to diagnose disease and protect the public from health threats, such as outbreaks of infectious diseases and environmental hazards.

Specimens that are sent out for processing must be accompanied by a lab requisition that describes the test(s) to be performed (■ FIGURE 45-1). A **lab requisition** typically lists the following information:

- Physician's name, address, and phone number
- Patient's name, date of birth, and medical record number
- Diagnosis to justify the lab test
- Type of test to perform
- Date and time the specimen was collected
- Any pertinent past medical history or past lab results that the lab needs to review
- Signature of the physician or clinician who ordered the test(s) (required by some payers)

A **lab report** provides the results of the test and other information useful to the physician in making a diagnosis. The lab report usually is electronic and typically contains:

- Patient name and identification number
- Name of laboratory

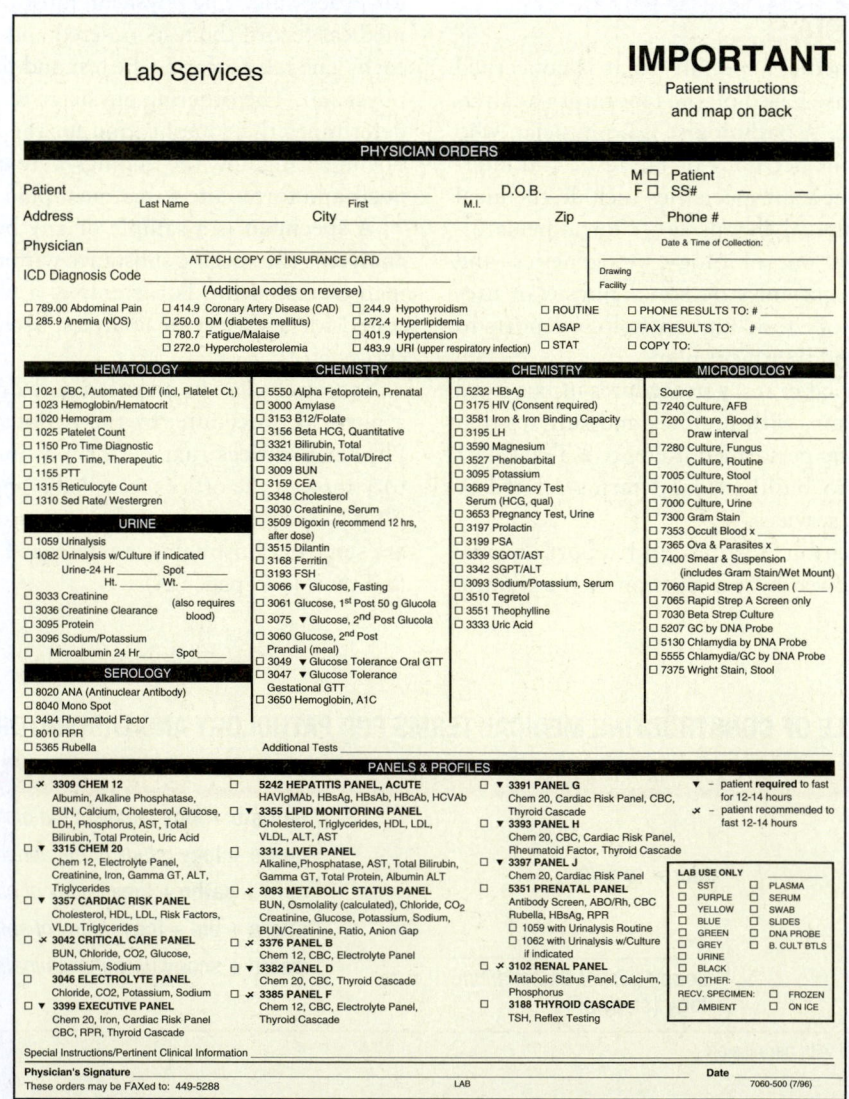

Figure 45-1 ■ Example of a laboratory requisition.

- Name of physician or practitioner ordering the test
- Date and time the specimen was collected and date and time of receipt
- Reason for an unsatisfactory specimen, if applicable
- Test or evaluation performed
- Result
- Date and time of report

The type of report or test results depends on the type of test performed. **Qualitative tests**—which include some chemistry and immunology tests—list a basic *Positive/Negative* or *Present/Absent* answer to questions such as *Is a particular substance* (such as a drug, virus, or bacteria) *present in the sample?*

Quantitative tests—which include most chemistry tests, drug assays, and some immunology tests—report the concentration of a substance in the sample, such as a glucose test that reports the concentration of glucose in blood plasma. Quantitative tests are usually accompanied by a **reference range**—a numeric range of typical results in the average population and the levels considered to be *High* or *Low*—determined by the statistical calculation of two standard deviations (■ FIGURE 45-2). Reference ranges are not universally standard for many analytes because they are specific to the equipment and testing methods used by the laboratory. Thus, each laboratory establishes its own reference ranges using data from its own equipment and methods. Physicians must evaluate whether the test result for a particular patient is considered normal, high, or low based on that patient's symptoms, medical history, and the reason the physician ordered the test. For some conditions, a physician may be concerned about a lab value that lies within the reference range because of the patient's particular situation. In other cases, a physician may not be concerned about a value flagged as high or low.

Results of microbiology cultures report the concentration and type of organism.

Surgical pathology reports provide a narrative description of the specimen and the pathologist's diagnosis.

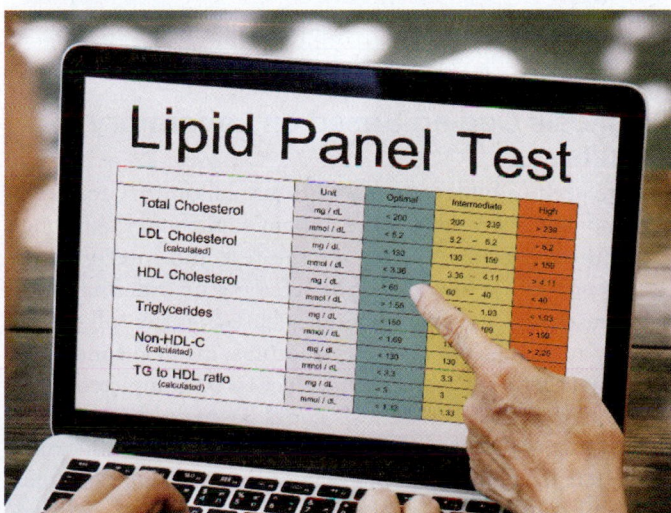

Figure 45-2 ■ Example of test results and reference ranges.

Clinical Laboratory Improvement Amendments

Congress passed the **Clinical Laboratory Improvement Amendments (CLIA)** in 1988 to establish quality standards for all laboratory testing to ensure the accuracy, reliability, and timeliness of patient test results regardless of where the test was performed. CLIA is administered by the Centers for Medicare and Medicaid Services (CMS), Survey and Certification Group, Division of Laboratory Services. CLIA requires all facilities that perform even one test for the diagnosis, prevention, or treatment of human disease, including waived tests, to meet certain federal requirements. If a facility performs tests for these purposes, it is considered a laboratory under CLIA and must apply and obtain from the CLIA program a certificate that corresponds to the complexity of tests performed. Five types of certificates are available under CLIA, with the most common being the Certificate of Compliance, Certificate of Waiver, and Certificate for Provider-Performed Microscopy Procedures.

Certificate of Compliance

A **Certificate of Compliance (COC)** is issued to a laboratory that performs nonwaived—moderate and high-complexity—testing. Each state's Department of Health conducts an inspection and determines that the laboratory is compliant with all applicable CLIA requirements. Labs with a CLIA COC are issued an individual CLIA number that identifies the lab.

Certificate of Waiver

Approximately 40 low-complexity lab tests are approved for a CLIA waiver. CLIA-waived lab tests do not require a trained lab technician or technologist to review and analyze them, such as a urine pregnancy test. If the lab or POL performs only waived tests, then it can obtain a CLIA **Certificate of Waiver (COW)** instead of a COC. The POL must complete an application and pay a Certificate of Waiver fee every two years.

The U.S. Department of Health and Human Services publishes the list of CLIA-waived tests on its website. For some waived tests, Medicare requires providers to append modifier **-QW CLIA-waived test** to the CPT or HCPCS code. There are a limited number of HCPCS codes for lab services—beginning with the letter **G**—which Medicare requires providers to submit instead of a CPT code. Refer to the CMS website, where you can find more information about waived tests, including those that require HCPCS codes and modifier **-QW**.

Certificate for Provider-Performed Microscopy Procedures

Provider-performed microscopy procedures (PPMPs) are moderate-complexity tests that require use of a microscope. The test must be performed during a patient visit on a specimen obtained from the provider's patient or a patient of the group practice. Examples include urinalysis with microscopy, pinworm examinations, semen analysis, and nasal smears for eosinophils.

CODING PRACTICE

Exercise 45.1 Pathology and Laboratory Procedure Basics

Instructions: Use your medical terminology skills and resources to define the following procedures, then identify the applicable code or code range. Follow these steps:

- Use slash marks "/" to break down the underlined term into its root(s) and suffix.
- Define the meaning of the underlined word based on the meaning of each word part.
- Look up the Main Term *Pathology and Laboratory* in the CPT Index.
- Use the entire phrase as the first- and second-level modifying terms and identify the code or code range shown in the CPT Index.

Example: flow <u>cytometry</u> cyto/metry   Meaning <u>*measurement of cells*</u>
(Look up the Main Term *Pathology and Laboratory*,
then the first-level modifying term *flow cytometry*.)   CPT Code <u>88182-88189</u>

1. <u>microorganism</u> identification, virus isolation   Meaning _____   CPT Code _____
2. <u>postmortem</u>   Meaning _____   CPT Code _____
3. <u>spectrometry</u>, mass, non-drug analytes   Meaning _____   CPT Code _____
4. surgical pathology, <u>decalcification</u> procedure   Meaning _____   CPT Code _____
5. chemistry, <u>chromatography</u>, sugars   Meaning _____   CPT Code _____
6. <u>radioimmunoassay</u>   Meaning _____   CPT Code _____
7. transfusion medicine, <u>leukocyte</u> transfusion   Meaning _____   CPT Code _____
8. sperm, <u>cryopreservation</u>   Meaning _____   CPT Code _____
9. white blood cell, <u>phagocytosis</u>   Meaning _____   CPT Code _____
10. surgical pathology, <u>immunocytochemistry</u>   Meaning _____   CPT Code _____

CODING GUIDELINES FOR PATHOLOGY AND LABORATORY PROCEDURES

Coders should understand the organization, guidelines, and instructional notes in the Tabular List of this CPT section. This information is necessary for accurate coding. The CPT section **Pathology and Laboratory Services (80047--89398, 0001U and higher)** contains 22 subsections that are divided by the type of procedure (■ TABLE 45-3). Review the subheading and category names and code ranges listed in the Pathology and Laboratory Services section to become familiar with the content and organization. Some editions of the CPT manual provide a summary list of the subheadings and categories at the beginning of the section and also displays an asterisk (*) next to categories that contain special coding instructions.

On claims, procedures represented by CPT codes in the Pathology and Laboratory section must be linked with diagnosis codes that support the medical necessity of the procedure. Diagnosis codes may come from any ICD-10-CM chapter.

CPT provides brief guidelines at the beginning of the Pathology and Laboratory section that discuss the provider of services, separate or multiple procedures, unlisted procedures, and special reports. Special instructions provide definitions and coding guidelines at the beginning of many subsections and categories.

The subsection **Proprietary Laboratory Analyses** (PLA) contains a different numbering sequence than the rest of the Pathology and Laboratory section. Codes begin with 00 and end with U, as in **0001U**. They are listed at the end of the Pathology and Laboratory section. Codes in this subsection identify privately owned lab analyses that labs or manufacturers want to identify their tests more specifically than other

codes do. Most of these codes are indexed under **Genomic Sequencing Procedure (GSP) and Other Molecular Multianalyte Assays**. The American Medical Association (AMA) publishes quarterly updates to PLA codes, so it is important to keep current with the changes by checking the AMA website and publications.

Instructional notes appear throughout the Tabular List to alert coders to the need for modifiers, provide cross-references to codes for similar procedures on other sites, identify when additional codes for radiological services might be needed, and highlight resequenced and recently deleted codes. Specific guidelines and instructional notes are discussed throughout this chapter of the text.

Diagnosis Coding Based on Laboratory Results

Coders need to understand how to use laboratory results to assign diagnosis codes for the patient's encounter. Although the pathologist who supervises the test and interprets the results provides a diagnosis, the referring or ordering physician must make the final diagnosis based on the full picture of the patient's health history, symptoms, medical conditions, and any other tests or procedures yet to be completed. Coders should not assign diagnosis codes based solely on the lab report, even when the results are clearly stated as abnormal. The referring or ordering physician must confirm the clinical significance of an abnormal result before it can be assigned as a diagnosis code (ICD-10-CM OGCR III.B).

Diagnosis coding rules differ between inpatient and outpatient. The Uniform Hospital Data Discharge Set (UHDDS)

Table 45-3   ■   **PATHOLOGY AND LABORATORY SUBHEADINGS**

Subsections	Code Range	Description
Organ or Disease-Oriented Panels	80047-80081	A group of tests performed at the same time for the same patient. All tests in the panel must be performed to report the code.
Drug Assay	80305-80377	Testing for the presence and amount of drugs through presumptive drug class screening (*identification of possible use or non-use of a drug class*) and definitive drug class testing (*identification of possible use or nonuse of a specific drug*), through qualitative or quantitative tests. Qualitative tests detect the presence of a substance in the specimen; quantitative tests are an analysis of the amount of a substance in the specimen. (These codes appear out of numerical sequence in the Tabular List, immediately after code 80076.)
Therapeutic Drug Assays	80150-80299	Quantitative tests for the amount of a prescribed drug present in the specimen.
Evocative/Suppression Testing	80400-80439	Administration of a pharmaceutical agent to test the body's response to the agent compared with normal bodily responses.
Consultations (Clinical Pathology)	80500-80502	Analysis of a specimen by a pathologist, based on a request by another physician, including a written report of the pathologist's medical interpretation of the findings.
Urinalysis	81000-81099	Tests on a urine specimen to identify abnormalities; may or may not include use of a microscope.
Molecular Pathology	81105-81408, 81479	Medical laboratory procedures involving analyses of nucleic acid to detect variants in genes that may be indicative of germline (e.g., constitutional disorders) or somatic (e.g., neoplasia) conditions, or to test for histocompatibility antigens. Genes are described using Human Genome Organization (HUGO)–approved gene names and are italicized in the code descriptors.
Genomic Sequencing Procedures (GSPs) and Other Molecular Multianalyte Assays	81410-81471	DNA or RNA sequence analysis methods that simultaneously assay multiple genes or genetic regions relevant to a clinical situation. They may target specific combinations of genes or genetic material or assay the exome or genome.
Multianalyte Assays with Algorithmic Analyses (MAAA)	81490-81599	Procedures that utilize multiple results from assays of various types, and possibly patient information, to perform algorithmic (*structured step-by-step*) analysis that is reported typically as a numeric score or probability about treatment options or disease outcomes.
Chemistry	82009-84999	Quantitative tests for numerous analytes on a wide variety of specimens; also includes a limited number of qualitative tests that are described as such.
Hematology and Coagulation	85002-85999	Tests to determine the number or behavior of various types of blood cells.
Immunology	86000-86849	Qualitative and quantitative tests on antigens, allergens, and antibodies.
Transfusion Medicine	86850-86999	Testing, treatment, and separation of blood products in preparation for a blood transfusion.
Microbiology	87003-87999	Testing for and identification of bacteria, fungi, parasites, and viruses in various types of specimens.
Anatomic Pathology	88000-88099	Autopsy; a postmortem examination of a cadaver to determine the cause of death, the victim's overall health at the time of death, circumstances surrounding the death, and whether medical treatment or neglect contributed to the death.
Cytopathology	88104-88199	Examination of cells from anywhere in the body to detect various conditions and determine whether neoplasms are benign or malignant.
Cytogenetic Studies	88230-88299	Tests involving the structure and function of cells, such as analysis of chromosomes, which carry genetic material and hereditary traits.
Surgical Pathology	88300-88399	Gross (*viewing with the naked eye*) and/or microscopic examination of a specimen removed from a patient during a procedure.
In Vivo (e.g., Transcutaneous) Laboratory Procedures	88720-88749	Tests to measure bilirubin and hemoglobin transcutaneously (*through unbroken skin*), most often performed on neonates to avoid painful blood draws.
Other Procedures	89049-89240	A miscellaneous group of tests not readily classified in other subsections, such as leukocyte assessment on a fecal specimen; nasal smear for eosinophils (*white blood cells*); sweat collection, to assess whether the patient has elevated chloride and sodium ions in the sweat, which indicates cystic fibrosis (CF); and meat fibers in feces, to determine whether the body properly digests food.
Reproductive Medicine Procedures	89250-89398	Testing and preparation for in vitro fertilization (IVF) or intrauterine insemination; testing on sperm, semen, oocytes, and embryos to identify disorders; and cryopreservation and thawing.
Proprietary Laboratory Analyses	0001U and higher	Proprietary clinical laboratory tests that the manufacturer or lab wants to identify in greater detail than other codes allow.

Source: © PB Resources, Inc. Used with permission. CPT codes only © American Medical Association.

defines the principal diagnosis for inpatient encounters as the one **established after study**, including after all test results are known (OGCR II). Inpatient coders must hold the patient's claim until lab results are released and confirmed to assign the diagnosis.

Outpatient coders can code the claim based on the information known at the time of billing. They can use the symptoms or ordering diagnosis on the claim if lab results are not available at the time of billing. They do not need to provide an update to the insurance company after lab results are available and confirmed (OGCR IV.K).

If there is reason to suspect that the claim could be denied or delayed by the payer pending lab results, it is best to wait until after lab results are available to send the outpatient claim. When a malignancy is suspected, outpatient coders should hold the claim until the malignancy is confirmed because some procedures—such as the excision of lesions—have separate CPT codes for malignant and benign lesions, with different payment rates.

When lab results are abnormal and confirmed as such by the ordering physician but a definitive diagnosis cannot be established, assign a code for abnormal test results. To locate the appropriate code, search the ICD-10-CM Index for the Main Term entry **Findings, abnormal, inconclusive, without diagnosis** and a subterm for the type of test or specimen, such as **Papanicolaou cervix** or **urine**. Locate any additional subterms needed to fully describe the result.

When the purpose of the encounter is a routine medical examination, such as those reported with ICD-10-CM categories **Z00** and **Z01**, separate codes for each type of examination are provided based on whether there are abnormal findings. An instructional note directs coders to **Use additional code to identify abnormal findings**.

ABSTRACTING PROCEDURES FOR PATHOLOGY AND LABORATORY

Abstracting for pathology and laboratory tests varies widely based on the type of test. In informal discussion, people make general references to tests such as a glucose test, strep test, or

Table 45-4 ■ KEY CRITERIA FOR ABSTRACTING PATHOLOGY AND LABORATORY PROCEDURES

- ❏ What is the referring or ordering diagnosis?
- ❏ What specimen is tested or examined?
- ❏ How many specimens are submitted?
- ❏ How many tests or examinations are performed?
- ❏ What type of test(s) or examination(s) is performed?
- ❏ Is the test qualitative or quantitative?
- ❏ What type of equipment is used (e.g., microscope, automated, nonautomated)?
- ❏ Are any panel tests performed? Are all tests in the code description performed?
- ❏ What testing method is used?
- ❏ What constituents or analytes are tested?
- ❏ Is only the professional component provided?
- ❏ Is the physician billing on behalf of an outside laboratory?
- ❏ Is the laboratory test repeated on the same day?
- ❏ Is the service a CLIA-waived test?

Source: © PB Resources, Inc. Used with permission.

urinalysis. Each of these has several distinct CPT codes based on the details of how it is performed. Refer to ■ TABLE 45-4 for guidance on how to abstract procedures in the Pathology and Laboratory section, then work through the detailed example that follows. Remember that the abstracting questions are a guide and that not every question applies to, or can be answered for, every case. For example, the type of equipment is not a factor for all tests.

Guided Example of Abstracting Pathology and Laboratory Procedures

Refer to the following example throughout this chapter to practice skills for abstracting, assigning, and arranging codes in the Pathology and Laboratory section.

HOSPITAL LABORATORY   Gender: M   Age: 62

Ordering diagnosis: Previous aldosterone /renin ratio (ARR) (*a test that calculates the ratio between aldosterone, a steroid hormone, and renin, an enzyme produced by the kidneys*) result was high at 30. Probable primary hyperaldosteronism (*overproduction of aldosterone*). Drug-resistant hypertension.

Ordering physician: Endocrinologist

Test ordered: Aldosterone suppression evaluation panel performed to confirm primary hyperaldosteronism as the cause for hypertension.

Hospital Lab: Patient was placed in a recumbent position. Specimen was acquired through venipuncture and aldosterone concentration and renin concentrations were performed. Two liters of saline were administered intravenously over 4 hours. A second specimen was acquired through venipuncture after 4 hours (*to determine whether the saline infusion lowered the aldosterone level to a normal level, which makes a diagnosis of primary hyperaldosteronism unlikely.*) BP and HR monitored throughout

Results: 0:00 hr aldosterone 22 ng/dL; 4:00 hr aldosterone 20 ng/dL; not a significant reduction

---

Follow along as fictitious coder Teresa Lee, CCS, abstracts the procedure. Check off each step after you complete it.

▶ Teresa reads through the entire record, paying special attention to the ordering diagnosis and the lab tests performed. She refers to the Key Criteria for Abstracting Pathology and Laboratory Procedures (Table 45-4).

- ❏ She determines that the referring diagnosis for the lab test is that the aldosterone/renin ratio (ARR) result was high. Although probable primary hyperaldosteronism is indicated as the reason the test is ordered, an uncertain or probable diagnosis cannot be used as the first-listed diagnosis on an outpatient claim.

- ❏ *What specimen is tested or examined?* Blood

- ❏ *How many specimens are obtained?* Two serum samples are obtained: one for a baseline and a second one after the infusion of the agent (saline)

❑ *How many tests or examinations are performed?* One panel

❑ *What type of test(s) or examination(s) is performed?* Aldosterone suppression evaluation panel

❑ *Are any panel tests performed? Yes. Are all tests in the code description performed?* Two aldosterone tests and two renin tests are performed. Teresa will need to compare the individual tests to the code description when assigning codes to determine whether all components of the panel were performed.

❑ *What constituents or analytes are tested?* Aldosterone and renin

❑ *Is only the professional component provided?* No

❑ *Is the physician billing on behalf of an outside laboratory?* No

▶ At this time, Teresa does not know which of these procedures may need to be coded, nor how many codes she will end up with. She will learn about this when she moves on to assigning codes.

CODING PRACTICE

Exercise 45.2 Abstracting Procedures for Pathology and Laboratory

Instructions: Read the mini-medical-record of each patient's encounter and answer the abstracting questions. Write the answer on the line provided. Do not assign any codes.

1. HOSPITAL LABORATORY Gender: F Age: 20

Ordering physician: Primary care

Referring diagnosis: Yellowish vaginal discharge with a foul odor

Specimen received: 2 slides with vaginal discharge

Tests: Chlamydia culture, Neisseria gonorrhea immunoassay with direct optical observation

Results: Positive for chlamydia, negative for gonorrhea

a. What is the referring or ordering diagnosis? _____

_____

b. What specimen is tested or examined? _____

_____

c. How many specimens are submitted? _____

_____

d. How many tests or examinations are performed?

_____

e. What type of test(s) or examination(s) is performed?

_____

f. What testing method is used? _____

_____

g. What constituents or analytes are tested? _____

_____

2. HOSPITAL LABORATORY Gender: F Age: 37

Ordering physician: Surgical oncologist

Referring diagnosis: Lung lesion, smoker, intraoperative frozen section, consultation requested

Specimen received: Lung, wedge biopsy right lower lobe

Gross description: 1-cm-diameter tissue

(continued)

2. (continued)

Microscopic description: Invasion of the overlying pleura with free resection margin

Results/findings: Adenocarcinoma, grade 2; called results up to operating suite

a. What is the referring or ordering diagnosis? _____

_____

b. What specimen is tested or examined? _____

_____

c. How many specimens are submitted? _____

_____

d. How many tests or examinations are performed?

_____

e. What type of test(s) or examination(s) is performed?

_____

f. What type of equipment is used? _____

3. HOSPITAL LABORATORY Gender: M Age: 68

Ordering physician: Cardiologist

Referring diagnosis: HTN, CHF

Specimen received: Venous blood

Tests: Therapeutic drug assay for total digoxin level

Results: Value: 0.4 Reference Range: 0.5–0.8 ng/mL Flag: Low

a. What is the referring or ordering diagnosis? _____

_____

b. What specimen is tested or examined? _____

_____

c. How many specimens are submitted? _____

_____

d. How many tests or examinations are performed?

_____

e. What type of test(s) or examination(s) is performed?

_____

(continued)

CODING PRACTICE (continued)

3. (continued)

f. Is the test qualitative or quantitative? _____
_____

g. What testing method is used? _____
_____

h. What constituents or analytes are tested? _____
_____

---

4. OFFICE   Gender: F   Age: 28

Gravida: 1   Para: 0   EGA: 10 weeks

Reason for encounter: Prenatal care

Assessment: Routine prenatal visit that will be part of the patient's total OB package

Office procedure: Venipuncture for OB panel (3 tubes)

Hospital lab procedure: CBC automated; automated differential WBC count; hepatitis B surface antigen (HBsAg); antibody rubella; syphilis test, nontreponemal antibody, qualitative; antibody screen, RBC; blood typing, ABO; blood typing, Rh (D)

a. What is the referring or ordering diagnosis? _____
_____

b. What specimen is tested or examined? _____
_____

c. How many specimens are submitted? _____
_____

d. How many tests or examinations are performed?
_____

e. What type of test(s) or examination(s) is performed?
_____

f. Are any panels performed? _____
Are all tests in the code description performed?

g. What antigens are tested for? _____
_____

h. What antibodies are tested for? _____
_____

i. Is the physician billing on behalf of an outside laboratory?_____

---

5. OFFICE   Gender: F   Age: 71

Diagnosis: Atrial fibrillation, long-term use of warfarin

Office procedure: Venipuncture for PT/PTT

Hospital lab procedure: Prothrombin time (PT); partial thromboplastin time (PTT) (1 tube)

(continued)

---

5. (continued)

Results: PT/INR: Value: 2.5 Reference Range: 2.0–3.0
INR Flag: None

PTT: Value: 60 Reference Range: 60–70 seconds Flag: None

a. What is the referring or ordering diagnosis? _____
_____

b. What specimen is tested or examined? _____
_____

c. How many specimens are submitted? _____
_____

d. How many tests or examinations are performed?
_____

e. What type of test(s) or examination(s) is performed?
_____

f. Is the physician billing on behalf of an outside laboratory? _____

---

6. OFFICE   Gender: F   Age: 25

Reason for encounter: Urinary frequency and dysuria

Assessment: Expanded problem-focused history, problem-focused examination, and low-complexity medical decision making

Office procedure: Urinalysis using the dip stick method, nonautomated, no microscopy

Finding: Leukocytes, nitrates, and a small amount of blood are present

Diagnosis: Urinary tract infection

a. What is the referring or ordering diagnosis? _____
_____

b. What specimen is tested or examined? _____
_____

c. How many specimens are submitted? _____
_____

d. How many tests or examinations are performed?
_____

e. What type of test(s) or examination(s) is performed?
_____

f. Is the test qualitative or quantitative? _____

g. What testing method is used? _____
_____

h. What equipment is used? _____
_____

i. Is the physician billing on behalf of an outside laboratory? _____

j. Was an E/M service provided at the same encounter?
_____

ASSIGNING CODES FOR PATHOLOGY AND LABORATORY PROCEDURES

Most laboratory procedures can be located in the CPT Index under the Main Term **Pathology and Laboratory**, then a first-level modifying term that corresponds to the Tabular List subsection, such as **Chemistry** or **Cytopathology**, then a second-level modifying term for the type of test. The Index provides numerous cross-references to other Main Terms, such as **Blood Test, Cell Count, See Blood Cell Count**. Many lab tests can also be located by searching the Index for one of the following types of Main Terms:

- Name of the test: blood test, blood cell count, occult blood, drug assay, urinalysis
- Analyte: substance tested for: glucose, lipoprotein, iron, insulin
- Type of specimen: bone marrow smear, tissue culture
- Method of testing: fine-needle aspiration, microbiology

When verifying codes in the Tabular List, confirm not only that the analyte is correct but also that the specimen and method of testing are accurate.

Assigning Codes for Specimen Collection

To assign codes for the collection of specimens, search the Index for the Main Term **Collection and Processing**, then select one of the following first-level modifying terms: **Brushings**, **Specimen**, **Stem Cells**, or **Washings**. Codes for blood specimens, sweat, sputum, tears, duodenum, and stomach appear under the first-level modifying term **Specimen**.

Most codes for specimen collection appear within the CPT Surgery section and the subsection for the body system. For example, codes for blood draws appear in the CPT Surgery section and the Cardiovascular subsection. A few codes for specimen collection, such as those for sputum and sweat, appear in the Pathology and Laboratory section. Codes for specimen collection can also be located by searching the Index for the Main Term of the anatomic site. ■ TABLE 45-5 shows alternative ways to locate codes for blood draws.

Some payers do not reimburse separately for a blood draw when a patient has an E/M service during the same encounter because they bundle the blood draw into the E/M service. To clarify that the blood draw is a separate and distinct service from the E/M service, append modifier **-25 Significant, separately identifiable evaluation and management service by the same physician or other qualified health care professional on the same day of the procedure or other service** to the E/M code.

Offices can also assign code **99000 Handling and/or conveyance of specimen for transfer from the physician's office to a laboratory** to show that they prepared and sent a blood specimen to an outside lab, including labeling and packaging. To locate this code, search the Index for the Main Term **Handling** and the first-level modifying term **Specimen transport**. Some payers do not pay separately for this service and may bundle it into other services the patient receives. Others pay for this service only when the specimen is blood.

Table 45-5 ■ **LOCATING CODES FOR COLLECTION OF BLOOD SPECIMENS**

Code	Description	Index Entry
36415	Collection of venous blood by venipuncture	Main Term: Venipuncture
		First-level modifying terms: Child/Adult, Infant, or Routine
36416	Collection of capillary blood specimen (e.g., finger, heel, ear stick)	Main Term: Finger
		First-level modifying term: Blood specimen, fingerstick
		Main Term: Heel
		First-level modifying term: Stick, for collection of blood
		Main Term: Ear
		First-level modifying term: Collection of blood
36600	Arterial puncture, withdrawal of blood for diagnosis	Main Term: Arterial Puncture
		First-level modifying term: For Diagnosis
		Main Term: Puncture
		Modifying terms: Artery, Diagnosis

Source: © PB Resources, Inc. Used with permission. CPT codes only © American Medical Association.

Assigning Codes for Urinalysis

To assign codes for urinalysis, search the Index for the Main Term **Urinalysis**, then select the appropriate first-level modifying term for the type of procedure. CPT provides four codes for **urinalysis by dipstick or tablet reagent (81000-81003)**. This type of procedure tests for any or all of the constituents bilirubin, glucose, hemoglobin, ketones, leukocytes, nitrite, pH, protein, specific gravity, and urobilinogen. In the Tabular List, these codes are divided based on whether the test is automated or nonautomated and whether microscopy is used. Code **81002** identifies **non-automated, without microscopy** and is often referred to as routine urinalysis.

Assigning Codes for Drug Assays

A drug assay determines the presence (qualitative) and amount (quantitative) of a drug in a specimen such as urine, blood, sputum, or hair. Drugs or classes of drugs may be commonly assayed first by a presumptive screening method followed by a definitive drug identification method. Procedures include presumptive drug class screening, definitive drug class testing, and therapeutic drug assays (TDAs). CPT provides extensive guidelines and definitions for these codes, which begin with **80305**. In the Tabular List, codes **80305-80377** appear out of numerical sequence, after code **80076**.

Presumptive drug class screening procedures are qualitative tests that identify the possible use or nonuse of a drug or drug class. Codes are divided by the testing methodology: direct visual observation **80305**, use of an instrument to assist in direct visual observation **80306**, and use of chemistry analyzer equipment **80307**. Special instructions appear at the beginning of this category in the Tabular List. After the presence of a drug or drug class has been identified with presumptive screening, definitive drug class testing can also be performed

The laboratory performed a presumptive drug class screening for oxycodone, using direct optical observation. The test gave a positive result for the presence of the drug, so then a quantitative definitive drug test was performed.

80305 Drug test(s), presumptive, any number of drug devices or procedures; capable of being read by direct optical observation only (eg, utilizing immunoassay [eg. dipsticks, cups, cards, cartridges]) includes sample validation when performed, per date of service

80365 Oxycodone

Figure 45-3 ■ Example of coding drug assays. *Source: © PB Resources, Inc. Used with permission. CPT codes only © American Medical Association.*

(■ FIGURE 45-3). The Tabular List provides a table, *Definitions and Acronym Conversion Listing*, to assist in identifying drug testing terms and acronyms.

Definitive drug testing identifies the individual drugs present in the sample using qualitative, quantitative, or semiquantitative methods. Codes are divided by drug class and the number of analytes reported. The Tabular List provides a table, *Definitive Drug Classes Listing*, which identifies the codes, classes, and individual drugs for each. Codes are reported once per date of service.

To locate codes for drug assays, search the Index for the Main Term **Drug Assay** and the first-level modifying term **Drug Procedure**. For presumptive drug class screening, select the third-level modifying term **Presumptive Drug Class**. For definitive drug testing, select the third-level modifying term **Definitive Drug Class** and the name of the drug class. Turn to the Tabular List to verify the code and make any additional code selections.

A therapeutic drug assay is performed to monitor a known, prescribed medication so the physician can evaluate how it is affecting the patient. Codes are divided by the name of the drug. To locate codes for therapeutic drug assays, search the Index for the Main Term **Therapeutic Drug Assay** and the first-level modifying term for the name of the drug. Verify the code in the Tabular List.

SUCCESS STEP

Always check for the annual code updates. The subsection **Drug Assays** is an example of a CPT subsection that was completely revised and updated in 2015. All existing codes were deleted; new codes with new organization and logic were added. New guidelines, tables, and definitions were added. Additional changes were made in 2017 and 2018. After such a drastic change, it can take physicians and payers a while to become clear and comfortable about how new codes and guidelines should be implemented.

Assigning Codes for Rapid Strep Tests

Physician offices often perform what is known as a **rapid strep test (RST)**, which produces results within 10–20 minutes. This is in contrast to a throat culture, which requires several days to produce a result. An RST detects the group A *Streptococcus*

(GAS) antigen from throat swabs and is used as an aid in the diagnosis of GAS infection, which typically causes strep throat, tonsillitis, and scarlet fever. Kits are supplied by several manufacturers. The clinician swabs the throat and tonsils to collect a sample of mucus from the infected area for testing. The mucus sample is then exposed to a reagent containing antibodies that bind specifically to a GAS antigen. Clinicians then use **direct optical observation** (*looking at the results with the naked eye*) to identify a specific feature—such as a color change—that indicates a positive result and the presence of the GAS bacteria. The test is typically reported with code **87880 Infectious agent antigen detection by immunoassay with direct optical observation; Streptococcus, group A**. Some offices may use other methods to perform a strep test, so always confirm the exact test that is being performed when the physician reports an RST.

Rapid stress test is not a Main Term in the CPT Index because it is an informal way of referring to a test and is not an official CPT code description. To locate the code for the procedure described as RST here, search the Index for the Main Term **Pathology and Laboratory**, the first-level modifying term **Streptococcus, Group A**, and the second-level modifying term **Direct optical observation**.

Assigning Codes for Surgical Pathology

Surgical pathology is the gross and microscopic examination of tissue specimens removed during surgery. The purpose is to identify any abnormalities or malignancies to aid in the diagnosis of disease. After examining the specimen, the pathologist writes a report describing the appearance of the tissue and the findings.

To assign codes for surgical pathology, search the Index for the Main Term **Pathology and Laboratory**, the first-level modifying term **Surgical pathology**, and the second-level modifying term **Gross and micro exam**. The third-level modifying terms list codes for **Level II** through **Level VI**. Refer to the second-level modifying term **Gross Exam, Level I, 88300** if the examination was gross, with no microscopic examination. Although experienced coders may know the level needed for a particular specimen, new coders and those coding for less common specimens may not know the level and must refer to the Tabular List to select the appropriate code.

The Tabular List organizes codes **88302-88309** for Level II through Level VI examinations based on the type of specimen, with the higher levels reflecting more difficult examinations. Under each code description, the names of the specimens appear in alphabetical order. Review the list of specimens under each code until you find the correct one. Some specimens appear under more than one level, with an indication of the purpose of the procedure. For example, an appendix from an incidental appendicectomy appears under code **88302 Level II**, whereas an appendix, other than incidental—such as an abscessed appendix—appears under code **88304 Level III**. Until coders are very familiar with the surgical pathology codes, they must review each specimen list under each code to be sure they have identified the correct level of examination.

■ FIGURE 45-4 provides an alphabetical crosswalk of specimens corresponding to the surgical pathology level. This tool

Specimen: Level

Abortion, induced: III

Abortion, spontaneous/ missed: IV

Abscess: III

Adrenal, resection: V

Aneurysm, arterial/ventricular: III

Anus, tag: III

Appendix incidental: II

Appendix, not incidental: III

Artery, atheromatous plaque: III

Artery, biopsy: IV

Bartholin's gland cyst: III

Bone, biopsy/curettings: V

Bone, exostosis: IV

Bone, fragment(s), other than pathologic fracture: III

Bone, fragment(s), pathologic fracture: V

Bone, marrow, biopsy: IV

Bone, resection: VI

Brain, biopsy: V

Brain/meninges, other than for tumor: IV

Brain/meninges, tumor: V

Breast, biopsy, not requiring microscopic evaluation of surgical margins: IV

Breast, excision of lesion, with microscopic evaluation of surgical margins: V

Breast, mastectomy, partial/simple: V

Breast, mastectomy, with regional lymph nodes: VI

Breast, reduction mammoplasty: IV

Bronchus, biopsy: IV

Bursa/synovial cyst: III

Carpal tunnel tissue: III

Cartilage, shavings: III

Cell block, any source: IV

Cervix, biopsy: IV

Cervix, conization: V

Cholesteatoma: III

Colon, biopsy: IV

Colon, colostomy stoma: III

Colon, segmental for tumor: VI

Colon, segmental resection, other than for tumor: V

Colon, total resection: VI

Conjunctiva, biopsy/ pterygium: III

Cornea: III

Diverticulum, esophagus/small intestine: III

Duodenum, biopsy: IV

Dupuytren contract tissue: III

Endocervix, curettings/biopsy: IV

Endometrium, curettings/ biopsy: IV

Esophagus, biopsy: IV

Esophagus, partial/total: VI

Extremity, amputation, non-traumatic: V

Extremity, amputation, traumatic: IV

Extremity, disarticulation: VI

Eye, enucleation: V

Fallopian tube, biopsy: IV

Fallopian tube, ectopic pregnancy: IV

Fallopian tube, sterilization: II

Femoral head, fracture: IV

Femoral head, other than fracture: III

Fetus, with dissection: VI

Fingers/toes, amputation, non-traumatic: IV

Fingers/toes, amputation, traumatic: II

Fissure/fistula: III

Foreskin, newborn: II

Foreskin, not newborn: III

Gallbladder: III

Ganglion cyst: III

Gingiva/oral mucosa, biopsy: IV

Heart valve: IV

Hematoma: III

Hemorrhoids: III

Hernia sac, any location: II

Hydatid of Morgagni: III

Hydrocele sac Nerve: II

Intervertebral disc: III

Joint, loose body: III

Joint, resection: IV

Kidney, biopsy: IV

Kidney, partial/total nephrectomy: V

Larynx, biopsy: IV

Larynx, partial/total, with regional lymph nodes: VI

Larynx, partial/total: V

Leiomyoma, uterine, myomec tomy, without uterus: IV

Lip, biopsy/wedge: IV

Liver, biopsy, needle/wedge: V

Liver, partial: V

Lung, total/lobe/segment: VI

Lung, transbronchial biopsy: IV

Lung, wedge biopsy: V

Lymph node, biopsy: IV

Lymph nodes, regional: V

Mediastinum, mass: V

Meniscus: III

Mucocele, salivary: III

Muscle, biopsy: IV

Myocardium, biopsy: V

Nasal mucosa, biopsy: IV

Nasopharynx/oropharynx, biopsy: IV

Nerve, biopsy: IV

Neuroma, Morton's/traumatic: III

Odontogenic tumor: V

Odontogenic/dental cyst: IV

Omentum, biopsy: IV

Ovary with or without tube, neoplastic: V

Ovary with or without tube, non-neoplastic: IV

Ovary, biopsy/wedge: IV

Pancreas, biopsy: V

Pancreas, total/subtotal: VI

Parathyroid gland: IV

Pericardium, biopsy/tissue: IV

Peritoneum, biopsy: IV

Pilonidal cyst/sinus: III

Pituitary tumor: IV

Placenta, other than third trimester: IV

Placenta, third trimester: V

Pleura, biopsy/tissue: IV

Polyp, cervical/endometrial: IV

Polyp, colorectal: IV

Polyp, stomach/small intest: IV

Polyps, inflammatory, nasal/ sinusoidal: III

Prostate, except radical: V

Prostate, needle biopsy: IV

Prostate, radical: VI

Prostate, TUR: IV

Salivary gland, biopsy: IV

Salivary gland: V

Sentinel lymph node: V

Sinus, paranasal biopsy: IV

Skin, debridement/cyst/tag: III

Skin, not debridement/cyst/ tag/plastic repair: IV

Skin, plastic repair: II

Small intestine, biopsy: IV

Small intestine, for tumor: VI

Small intestine, not tumor: V

Soft tissue, debridement: III

Soft tissue, lipoma: III

Soft tissue, mass (except lipoma) biopsy/simple excision: V

Soft tissue, other than tumor/ mass/ lipoma/debridement: IV

Soft tissue, tumor, extensive: VI

Spermatocele: III

Spleen: IV

Stomach, biopsy: IV

Stomach, subtotal/total for tumor: VI

Stomach, subtotal/total, not for tumor: V

Sympathetic ganglion: II

Synovium: IV

Tendon/tendon sheath: III

Testicular appendage: III

Testis, biopsy: V

Testis, castration: II

Testis, other than tumor/ biopsy/ castration: IV

Testis, tumor: VI

Thrombus or embolus: III

Thymus, tumor: V

Thyroglossal duct/brachial cleft cyst: IV

Thyroid, total/lobe: V

Tongue, biopsy: IV

Tongue/tonsil, for tumor: VI

Tonsil and/or adenoids: III

Tonsil, biopsy: IV

Trachea, biopsy: IV

Ureter, biopsy: IV

Ureter, resection: V

Urethra, biopsy: IV

Urinary bladder, biopsy: IV

Urinary bladder, partial/total: VI

Urinary bladder, TUR: V

Uterus, with or without tubes and ovaries, for prolapse: IV

Uterus, with or without tubes and ovaries, neoplastic: VI

Uterus, with or without tubes and ovaries, other than neoplastic/ prolapse: V

Vagina, biopsy: IV

Vaginal mucosa: Incidental: II

Varicocele: III

Vas deferens, other than sterilization: III

Vas deferens, sterilization: II

Vein: Varicosity: III

Vulva, total/subtotal: VI

Vulva/labia, biopsy: IV

Figure 45-4 ■ Crosswalk of specimens to surgical pathology levels. *Source: © PB Resources, Inc. Used with permission.*

is an aid to navigating these codes and understanding how they are organized, but all code choices should be verified in the Tabular List.

CPT also provides codes for a pathology consultation during surgery (**88329-88334**). The pathologist examines a specimen while the patient is still in surgery to determine whether the surgeon needs to perform additional procedures. The pathologist may be in the lab or be present in the operating room. The intraoperative consult can include the examination of tissue blocks and cytologic examination.

Pathology consults that involve examination of tissue specimens are coded based on the number of specimens or tissue blocks that are received. When a single specimen is frozen and multiple sections or slices are examined, code for one specimen. When multiple tissue blocks of the same or different sites are submitted, assign a code for each specimen. CPT provides add-on code **88332** to report each additional tissue block (**■ FIGURE 45-5**). Cytologic examinations are coded based on the number of sites examined, with code **88333** for the initial site and an add-on code (**88334**) for each additional site.

Assigning Codes for Pap Smears

CPT provides several series of codes for reporting Pap smears based on the type of screening and reporting performed. To locate codes for Pap smears, search the Index for the Main Term **Pap Smears**, then the first-level modifying term for the type of reporting system, to be discussed next.

Conventional Pap smears involve scraping cells from the cervix and fixing them on a slide to be evaluated by the lab. Codes are divided based on whether the screening is automated or manual and whether results are reported using the Bethesda System:

- **88147-88148** Automated screening and rescreening, regardless of reporting system

- **88150-88153** Conventional Pap smears using non-Bethesda reporting

- **88164-88167** Conventional Pap smears using the Bethesda System of reporting

Liquid-based Pap smears are reported using codes **88174-88175**.

The **Bethesda System** is a method of reporting findings from Pap tests that includes the following components:

- A statement of the adequacy of the specimen
- A general categorization of the specimen
- A descriptive diagnosis
- Interpretation of abnormalities using specific nomenclature (**■ TABLE 45-6**)
- A statement of review and any ancillary testing

Pap smear codes are technical services and describe screening for abnormalities. When the lab finds an abnormal Pap test, a pathologist interprets the slide and provides a diagnosis. Report the professional interpretation with code **88141 Cytopathology, cervical or vaginal (any reporting system), requiring interpretation by physician**.

Medicare and some other payers require the use of HCPCS codes to report Pap tests (**■ FIGURE 45-6**). Screening Paps are reported by different codes than diagnostic Paps. HCPCS provides multiple codes for professional interpretation, so the technical code must be linked to the appropriate professional code. Medicare has specific guidelines regarding the diagnoses that are acceptable to justify the need for the test, based on the frequency with which it is done and the risk level of a particular patient for developing cancer. Review Medicare billing guidelines to be sure you understand the rules.

SUCCESS STEP

Cytopathology codes for nongynecological procedures (**88104-88112** and **88160-88162**) include both the technical and professional service. Append modifier **-TC Technical component** or **-26 Professional component** to identify that a provider performed only one part of the service.

The pathologist receives two specimens that are sent to the lab during surgery. The first specimen is tissue from the right breast. The second specimen is the sentinel lymph node. The pathologist freezes both blocks and takes two sections from the breast tissue and one from the node. After examination, he determines that the breast tissue shows evidence of malignancy and the lymph node is clear. This suggests that the disease has not metastasized. The pathologist calls the operating room with the results and prepares a report.

88331 Pathology consultation during surgery; first tissue block, with frozen section(s), single specimen

88332 Pathology consultation during surgery; each additional tissue block with frozen section(s) (List separately in addition to code for primary procedure)

Figure 45-5 ■ Example of coding an intraoperative consultation. *Source: © PB Resources, Inc. Used with permission. CPT codes only © American Medical Association.*

Table 45-6 ■ BETHESDA SYSTEM CLASSIFICATION OF ABNORMAL PAP RESULTS

- ❏ Atypical squamous cells of undetermined significance (ASC-US)
- ❏ Atypical squamous cells—cannot exclude HSIL (ASC-H)
- ❏ Low-grade squamous intraepithelial lesion (LGSIL or LSIL)
- ❏ High-grade squamous intraepithelial lesion (HGSIL or HSIL)
- ❏ Squamous cell carcinoma
- ❏ Atypical glandular cells not otherwise specified (AGC-NOS)
- ❏ Atypical glandular cells, suspicious for AIS or cancer (AGC-neoplastic)
- ❏ Adenocarcinoma in situ (AIS)

HCPCS Code	Description	HCPCS Interpretation Code	Corresponding CPT Code	Key
P3000	Screening Papanicolaou smear, cervical or vaginal, up to three smears, by technician under physician supervision	P3001	88150	Technical service
P3001	Screening Papanicolaou smear, cervical or vaginal, up to three smears, requiring interpretation by physician		88141	Professional service
G0123	Screening cytopathology, cervical or vaginal (any reporting system), collected in preservative fluid, automated thin layer preparation, screening by cytotechnologist under physician supervision	G0124	88142	Screening method
G0124	Screening cytopathology, cervical or vaginal (any reporting system), collected in preservative fluid, automated thin layer preparation, requiring interpretation by physician		88141	
G0141	Screening cytopathology smears, cervical or vaginal, performed by automated system, with manual rescreening, requiring interpretation by physician		88141	
G0143	Screening cytopathology, cervical or vaginal (any reporting system), collected in preservative fluid, automated thin layer preparation, with manual screening and rescreening by cytotechnologist under physician supervision	G0124	88143	
G0144	Screening cytopathology, cervical or vaginal (any reporting system), collected in preservative fluid, automated thin layer preparation, with screening by automated system, under physician supervision	G0124	88174	
G0145	Screening cytopathology, cervical or vaginal (any reporting system), collected in preservative fluid, automated thin layer preparation, with screening by automated system and manual rescreening under physician supervision	G0124	88175	
G0147	Screening cytopathology smears, cervical or vaginal, performed by automated system under physician supervision	G0141	88147	
G0148	Screening cytopathology smears, cervical or vaginal, performed by automated system with manual rescreening	G0141	88148	

Figure 45-6 ■ HCPCS codes for pap smears. *Source: © PB Resources, Inc. Used with permission.*

Billing for Laboratory Tests

There are several types of providers involved in rendering laboratory-related services and several types of services that can potentially be billed. The physician's office may fulfill one of several roles related to laboratory testing:

- Collection of a specimen that is sent to a lab for testing
- Collection of a specimen that is tested in the office
- Collection of a specimen and billing for the lab services for a test performed by the lab

The physician's office bills for any specimen collection and specimen handling and conveyance. Specimen collection usually consists of venipuncture but could include other methods, such as a tissue biopsy or cell scraping. Collection of specimens by the patient, such as urine samples, are not billed. If an E/M service was provided in addition to the specimen collection, the physician's office also bills for that. When the physician orders the test but does not collect a specimen, bill only the E/M service. When the only service is specimen collection, do not bill an E/M service.

Always check with payer policies regarding the billing for specimen collection and handling and conveyance. Some payers disallow one or both of these services, especially when provided in conjunction with an E/M service.

The lab usually bills for performing the test when the physician's office sends a specimen to an outside lab for testing. Some payers—but not Medicare—allow the physician's office to bill for the lab test on behalf of the lab. This arrangement might be done as a convenience to the lab. The physician's office charges the payer the exact amount charged by the lab, then pays the lab that amount. No markup is allowed. The claim must be completed in a specific way to identify that the physician is billing for a test performed by an outside lab.

On the CMS-1500 complete Item 20 (■ FIGURE 45-7) by marking YES and entering the lab charge for the test in the "Charges" portion. In Item 24, enter the date of service, CPT code, charge, and other information normally required for a charge. In addition, enter charges for any services provided directly by the physician's office.

The same information must be provided when billing electronically using the 837P format. The screen layout and location of fields vary with the software program.

The lab bills for the venipuncture when it also collects the specimen, as occurs when the patient travels to a lab collection site for a blood draw.

When a POL collects the specimen and performs the test, it bills for both services. Enter the date of service, CPT code, charge, and other information in Item 24. Do not complete Item 20.

The supervising pathologist bills for professional supervision and interpretation and, in most cases, appends modifier **-26 Professional component** to the laboratory code.

Refer to ■ TABLE 45-7 for a summary of the services billed by various types of providers.

Guided Example of Assigning Pathology and Laboratory Procedure Codes

To practice skills for assigning codes for procedures in the and Laboratory section, continue with the example from earlier

Table 45-7 ■ **LABORATORY-RELATED SERVICES BILLED BY VARIOUS PROVIDER TYPES**

Provider Type	Services Billed
Physician office (not billing for an outside laboratory)	E/M service (when provided and separate from the lab draw)
	Venipuncture or other specimen collection
	Handling and conveyance
Physician office laboratory (POL)	E/M service (when provided and separate from the lab draw)
	Venipuncture or other specimen collection
	Conducting the test
Physician office billing for an outside laboratory	E/M service (when provided and separate from the lab draw)
	Venipuncture or other specimen collection
	Handling and conveyance
	Laboratory charges
Laboratory	Conducting the test
Pathologist	Supervision and interpretation of the laboratory test

Source: © PB Resources, Inc. Used with permission.

in the chapter about a patient who was seen for an aldosterone suppression evaluation panel. Follow along in your CPT manual as Teresa Lee, CCS, assigns codes. Check off each step after you complete it.

▶ First, Teresa confirms the procedure: aldosterone suppression evaluation panel.

▶ Teresa searches the Index for the Main Term **Aldosterone**.

❑ She locates the first-level modifying term **Suppression evaluation**.

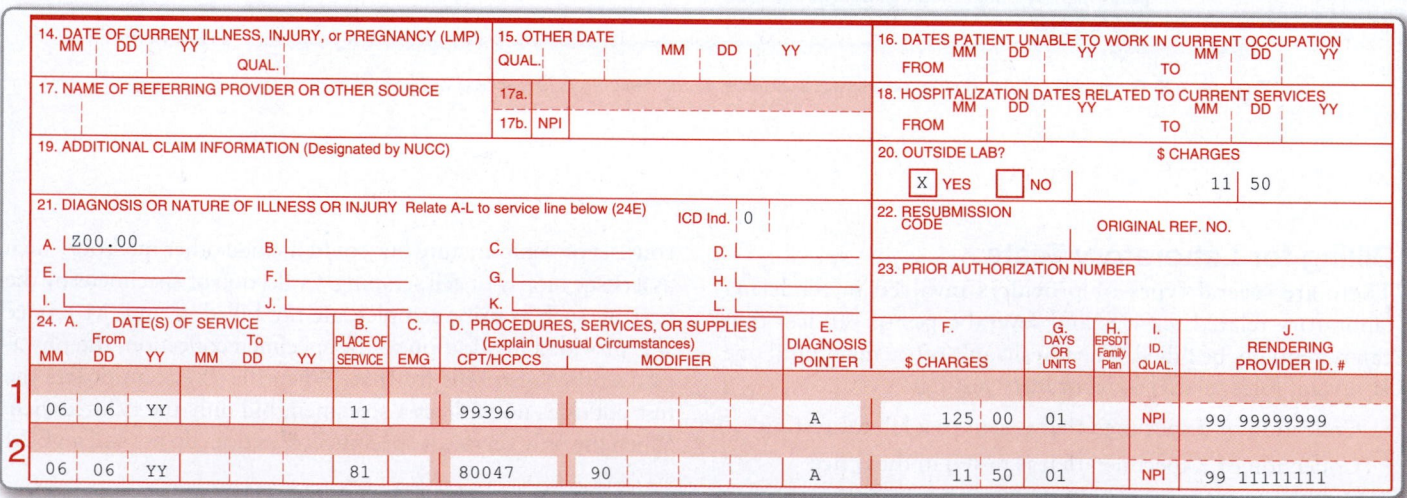

Figure 45-7 ■ Example of completing the CMS-1500 when physician office bills for the outside laboratory service.

❏ She identifies the code **80408**.

▶ Teresa verifies code **80408** in the Tabular List.

❏ She reads the code title for **80408: Aldosterone suppression evaluation panel (eg, saline infusion). This panel must include the following: Aldosterone (82088 × 2) Renin (84244 × 2)**.

❏ She identifies that the panel includes four tests, aldosterone ×2 and renin ×2. She confirms in the patient's record that all tests were performed. The first instance of each test was performed as a baseline. After administration of the saline suppression agent, both tests were administered a second time.

▶ Teresa checks for instructions in the Tabular List.

❏ She looks for instructional notes after the code entry and finds none.

❏ She cross-references the beginning of the subsection **Evocative/Suppression Testing** and reads the guidelines. She notices the instructions that state **For the administration of the evocative or suppressive agents, see Hydration, Therapeutic, Prophylactic, Diagnostic Injections and Infusions, and Chemotherapy and Other Highly Complex Drug or Highly Complex Biologic Agent Administration (eg, 96365, 96366, 96367, 96368, 96372, 96374, 96375, 96376)**.

❏ This information tells her that because the lab administered a saline infusion, she should code for that in addition to the test.

❏ She cross-references the beginning of the **Pathology and Laboratory** section and verifies that there are no additional guidelines that apply.

▶ Teresa turns to code **96365** in the Tabular List, as indicated in the subsection guidelines, to identify the code for the service of saline IV infusion, which was administered for four hours.

❏ She reads the description for code **96365 Intravenous infusion, for therapy, prophylaxis, or diagnosis (specify substance or drug); initial, up to 1 hour**.

❏ This seems to describe the service provided, but she notices that it reports only one hour, whereas the infusion was provided for four hours.

❏ She reads the description for code **96366**, which is an indented add-on code that reports **each additional hour** of IV infusion. She makes a note that she needs to report three occurrences of this code in addition to

one occurrence of code **96365** to report the full four hours of infusion.

❏ Codes **96367** and **96368** describe additional time and additional substances, so they do not apply.

❏ Codes **96369-96371** describe subcutaneous infusion, so they do not apply.

❏ Codes **96372-96376** describe injections, so they do not apply.

▶ Next, Teresa assigns a HCPCS code for the saline product.

❏ In the HCPCS manual, she turns to the *Table of Drugs and Biologicals*, then locates the entry for **Saline Solution, Sterile** in the first column.

❏ In the second column, she identifies the unit to be **500 ml** and in the third column, the route as **IV**. She confirms the amount documented in the patient's record to be two liters of saline. This means that four units were administered because one liter is 500 mL, so $500 \times 4 = 2000$ mL or two liters.

❏ She identifies the code listed in the fourth column of the table, **J7040**, and verifies it in the HCPCS Tabular List. The code description states **Infusion, normal saline solution, sterile (500 ml=1 unit)**.

▶ Finally, Teresa needs to code for the venipuncture procedures.

❏ She searches the Index for the Main Term **Venipuncture** and the first-level modifying term **Routine**.

❏ She identifies code **36415** and verifies it in the Tabular List. The code description states **Collection of venous blood by venipuncture**.

▶ Teresa reviews the procedure codes she has assigned for this case.

❏ **80408 Aldosterone suppression evaluation panel**

❏ **36415 Collection of venous blood by venipuncture**

❏ **J7040 Infusion, normal saline solution, sterile (500 ml=1 unit)**

❏ **96365 Intravenous infusion, for therapy, prophylaxis, or diagnosis (specify substance or drug); initial, up to 1 hour**

❏ **96366 Intravenous infusion, for therapy, prophylaxis, or diagnosis (specify substance or drug); each additional hour**

▶ Next, Teresa must determine how to sequence the codes.

CODING PRACTICE

Exercise 45.3 Assigning Codes for Pathology and Laboratory Procedures

Instructions: Read the mini-medical-record of each patient's encounter. Review the information abstracted in Exercise 45.2 for questions 1–3. For questions 4–6, abstract the case on your own. Assign CPT codes, quantities, and modifiers using the Index and Tabular List. Write the code(s) on the line provided.

---

1. HOSPITAL LABORATORY   Gender: F   Age: 20

Ordering physician: Primary care

Referring diagnosis: Yellowish vaginal discharge with a foul odor

Specimen received: 2 slides with vaginal discharge

Tests: Chlamydia culture, Neisseria gonorrhea immunoassay with direct optical observation

Results: Positive for chlamydia, negative for gonorrhea

Tip: The chlamydia culture is a higher-priced test than the *Neisseria* gonorrhea immunoassay.

2 CPT Codes _____

---

2. HOSPITAL LABORATORY   Gender: F   Age: 37

Ordering physician: Surgical oncologist

Referring diagnosis: Lung lesion, smoker, intraoperative frozen section, consultation requested

Specimen received: Lung, wedge biopsy right lower lobe

Gross description: 1-cm-diameter tissue

Microscopic description: Invasion of the overlying pleura with free resection margin

Results/findings: Adenocarcinoma, grade 2; called results up to operating suite

Tip: This service is surgical pathology.

1 CPT Code _____

---

3. HOSPITAL LABORATORY   Gender: M   Age: 68

Ordering physician: Cardiologist

Referring diagnosis: HTN, CHF

Specimen received: Blood

Tests: Therapeutic drug assay for total digoxin level

Results: Value: 0.4 Reference Range: 0.5–0.8 ng/mL Flag: Low

1 CPT Code _____

---

4. HOSPITAL LABORATORY   Gender: F   Age: 18

Ordering physician: Emergency medicine

Referring diagnosis: Intoxication

Specimen received: Blood

Tests: Blood alcohol level by chromatography

Results: Reportable at 0.020 g/dL (%)

1 CPT Code _____

---

5. HOSPITAL LABORATORY   Gender: F   Age: 39

Ordering physician: Gynecologist

Referring diagnosis: Vaginal chancres

Specimen received: Blood

Test: Syphilis, qualitative and quantitative

Results: Nonreactive

1 CPT Code _____

---

6. PATHOLOGY LABORATORY   Gender: F   Age: 62

Ordering physician: Dermatologist

Referring diagnosis: Grover disease

Specimen received: Skin of the chest, punch biopsy

Gross description: Specimen is 0.4 × 0.4 cm with a depth of 0.6 cm. Submitted in one cassette for microscopic examination.

Microscopic description: Focal areas of suprabasal clefting and a few acantholytic cells are seen

Results/findings: Corps ronds and grains are present, indicating Grover's disease.

Tip: Code for the pathologist service.

1 CPT Code _____

ARRANGING CODES FOR PATHOLOGY AND LABORATORY PROCEDURES

In general, codes for laboratory tests are sequenced in descending price or RVU order. Laboratory billing systems sequence codes automatically. When physician offices bill for laboratory tests they are sequenced after any E/M codes and other services because they are usually the lowest-priced service. Codes for lab tests should not be intermixed with codes that require modifier **-51 Multiple procedures** because the multiple procedure payment reduction does not apply. List the lab codes after any services that take modifier **-51** so that the payer does not accidentally apply a payment reduction.

Modifiers

Three unique modifiers are used only for laboratory services: **-90**, **-91**, and HCPCS modifier **-QW**. In addition, modifier **-26** for the professional component, modifier **-TC** for the technical component, and modifiers for separate procedures apply to lab services. Some modifiers are discussed earlier in this chapter, so the following information is a summary.

-90 Outside Laboratory

Report modifier **-90 Outside Laboratory** when a physician's office bills for services provided by an outside laboratory. Append this modifier to the codes for the lab tests performed by the lab. Do not apply it to any code other than a code for lab tests performed by an outside lab. Do not use this modifier when the physician's office collects the specimen, sends it to the lab, and the lab bills for the test or when the POL conducts the test.

Remember to complete Item 20 on the CMS-1500 when billing for outside lab services.

-91 Repeat Clinical Laboratory Test

Report modifier **-91 Repeat clinical laboratory test** when the physician orders that the same laboratory test be repeated on the same patient and same day to monitor or manage treatment (■ FIGURE 45-8). The key to using this modifier is the *clinical need* to repeat the test to obtain subsequent results as determined by the physician. Do not use modifier **-91** in the following situations:

- Tests rerun by the lab to confirm initial results
- Testing problems with specimens or equipment
- Any time a normal, one-time, reportable result is all that is required

> Patient presents to the Emergency Department with a headache, nausea and vomiting, and confusion. The physician diagnoses dehydration and orders electrolyte panel, which shows hyponatremia and hypokalemia. Fluids, as well as sodium and potassium, are administered. Later in the day, the physician orders a second electrolyte panel, which confirms that all components have returned to normal levels.
>
> **80051 × 1 Electrolyte panel**
> **80051-91 × 1 Electrolyte panel; -91 Repeat clinical laboratory test**

Figure 45-8 ■ Example of using modifier -91. *Source: © PB Resources, Inc. Used with permission. CPT codes only © American Medical Association.*

- Other codes describe a series of test results (e.g., glucose tolerance tests, evocative/suppression testing)

-92 Alternative Laboratory Platform Testing

Modifier **-92 Alternative laboratory platform testing** identifies the use of a kit or transportable instrument that employs a single-use, disposable analytical chamber. Use this modifier only with four codes for HIV testing: **86701**, **86702**, **86703**, and **87389**. Testing supplies can be hand carried or transported to the patient's location because the test does not require permanent dedicated space. The location of the testing does not determine the use of this modifier. Append the modifier to the laboratory procedure code.

-QW CLIA-Waived Test

When billing Medicare, physician offices with a COW must append modifier **-QW** to CLIA-waived tests, including PPM, performed in the office. Refer to the discussion on CLIA earlier in this chapter for details.

-26 Professional Component and -TC Technical Component

A limited number of lab codes, such as surgical pathology and some cytopathology codes, contain both professional and technical components. Append modifier **-26** or **-TC** to identify the component of the service provided by the billing entity. Codes for chemistry, drug assays, microbiology, immunology, evocation/suppression testing, and molecular pathology generally do not separate components. Refer to the Medicare Physician Fee Schedule Database (MPFSDB) to identify codes that accept these modifiers.

-XS Separate Structure and -XU Nonoverlapping Service

Modifier **-XS Separate structure** identifies the same laboratory procedure performed on more than one body site. Examples of this are wound cultures from separate parts of the body or skin biopsies from multiple sites.

Apply modifier **-XU Unusual non-overlapping service** when the same CPT code is used for separate procedures. For example, code **86003 Allergen specific IgE; quantitative or semiquantitative, crude allergen extract, each** reports allergen testing on multiple allergens. The code description specifies that each occurrence of the code reports one allergen. When multiple allergens are tested—for example, nuts, milk, eggs, and grass—report code **86003** once for each allergen and append modifier **-XU** to the second and subsequent tests.

Guided Example of Arranging Pathology and Laboratory Procedure Codes

To practice skills for arranging codes for procedures in the Pathology and Laboratory, section, continue with the example from earlier in the chapter about the patient who was seen for an aldosterone suppression evaluation panel. Follow along in your CPT manual as Teresa Lee, CCS, arranges the codes. Check off each step after you complete it.

▶ First, Teresa confirms the lab test performed: aldosterone suppression evaluation panel.

▶ Teresa reviews the procedure codes she has assigned for this case.

❏ **80408 Aldosterone suppression evaluation panel**

❏ **36415 Collection of venous blood by venipuncture**

❏ **J7040 Infusion, normal saline solution, sterile (500 ml=1 unit)**

❏ **96365 Intravenous infusion, for therapy, prophylaxis, or diagnosis (specify substance or drug); initial, up to 1 hour**

❏ **96366 Intravenous infusion, for therapy, prophylaxis, or diagnosis (specify substance or drug); each additional hour**

▶ Teresa determines the quantity for each code.

❏ Although four tests were performed, they are all bundled into one code for aldosterone suppression evaluation panel, so code **80408** is a quantity of 1.

❏ She notes that venipuncture was performed twice, so she assigns a quantity of 2 to code **36415**.

❏ One unit of code **J7040** is 500 mL, and 2 L were administered, so she reports a quantity of 4.

❏ Code **96365** identifies up to one hour of infusion, so the unit of reporting for this code is **1** because less than one hour was required.

▶ Teresa arranges the codes in descending price order according to the payer's fee schedule. No modifiers apply.

▶ Teresa finalizes the procedure codes and sequencing for this case:

(1) **80408 × 1 Aldosterone suppression evaluation panel**

(2) **96365 × 1 Intravenous infusion, for therapy, prophylaxis, or diagnosis (specify substance or drug); initial, up to 1 hour**

(3) **96366 × 3 Intravenous infusion, for therapy, prophylaxis, or diagnosis (specify substance or drug); each additional hour**

(4) **36415 × 2 Collection of venous blood by venipuncture**

(5) **J7040 × 4 Infusion, normal saline solution, sterile (500 ml=1 unit)**

▶ Teresa also assigns and sequences the ICD-10-CM diagnosis codes from the lab requisition that support the need for the service.

(1) **R79.89 Other specified abnormal findings of blood chemistry**

(2) **I10 Essential (primary) hypertension**

CODING PRACTICE

Exercise 45.4 Arranging Codes for Pathology and Laboratory Procedures

Instructions: Read the mini-medical-record of each patient's encounter. Review the information abstracted in Exercise 45.2 for questions 1–3. For questions 4–6, abstract the case on your own. Assign CPT codes, quantities, and modifiers using the Index and Tabular List, and arrange the codes in proper sequence. Write the code(s) on the line provided.

---

1. OFFICE   Gender: F   Age: 28

Gravida: 1   Para: 0   EGA: 10 weeks

Reason for encounter: Prenatal care

Assessment: Routine prenatal visit that will be part of the patient's total OB package

Office Procedure: Venipuncture for OB panel (3 tubes)

Hospital Lab Procedure: CBC automated; automated differential WBC count; hepatitis B surface antigen (HBsAg); antibody rubella; syphilis test, nontreponemal antibody, qualitative; antibody screen, RBC; blood typing, ABO; blood typing, Rh (D)

Tip: Assign codes for the physician's office and the laboratory.

Physician office: 2 CPT Codes _____

Laboratory: 1 CPT Code _____

---

2. OFFICE   Gender: F   Age: 71

Diagnosis: Atrial fibrillation, long-term use of warfarin

Office procedure: Venipuncture for PT/PTT (1 tube)

Hospital lab procedure: Prothrombin time (PT); partial thromboplastin time (PTT)

Results: PT/INR: Value: 2.5, Reference Range: 2.0–3.0, INR Flag: None

PTT: Value: 60, Reference Range: 60–70 seconds, Flag: None

Tip: Assign codes for the physician's office and the laboratory. The PTT test is a higher-priced code than the PT test.

Physician office: 2 CPT Codes _____

Laboratory: 2 CPT Codes _____

---

3. OFFICE   Gender: F   Age: 25

Reason for encounter: Urinary frequency and dysuria, established patient

Assessment: Expanded problem-focused history, problem-focused examination, and low-complexity medical decision making

(continued)

CODING PRACTICE (continued)

3. (continued)

Office procedure: Urinalysis using the dipstick method, nonautomated, no microscopy

Finding: Leukocytes, nitrates, and a small amount of blood are present

Diagnosis: Urinary tract infection

Tip: Assign an E/M code with the appropriate modifier to indicate that the E/M was provided on the same day as another service or procedure.

2 CPT Codes _____

4. HOSPITAL LABORATORY Gender: M Age: 2 weeks

Ordering physician: Pediatrician

Referring diagnosis: Positive newborn screen for cystic fibrosis

Specimen received: Sweat

Tests: Sweat stimulation, sweat collection by iontophoresis, and sweat chloride analysis

Results: Borderline results at 50 mEq/L

Tip: Sweat specimens are collected in duplicate from two different sites.

2 CPT Codes _____

5. HOSPITAL LABORATORY Gender: F Age: 24

Ordering physician: Neurologist

Referring diagnosis: Headache, neck stiffness, fever, and altered mental status. Workup for possible bacterial meningitis.

Specimen received: Cerebrospinal fluid

Tests: Cell count (and differential count) and culture

2 CPT Codes _____

6. OUTPATIENT LABORATORY Gender: F Age: 2

Ordering physician: Pediatrician

Referring diagnosis: Sickle cell trait

Specimen received: Blood

Tests: Hemoglobinopathy (Hb) electrophoresis, peripheral blood smear with manual differential

Results: HbA_1: 95%, HbA_2: 2%, HbF: <2%, HbC Absent, HbS Absent. Within normal limits.

2 CPT Codes _____

CHAPTER SUMMARY

In this chapter you learned that:

- Clinical pathology is a medical specialty that is concerned with the diagnosis of disease based on the laboratory analysis of bodily fluids and tissue.

- The subsections of *Pathology and Laboratory Services (80047-89398)* are divided by the type of procedure. CPT provides brief guidelines at the beginning of the Pathology and Laboratory section that address the provider of services, separate or multiple procedures, unlisted procedures, and special reports. Special instructions provide definitions and coding guidelines at the beginning of many subsections and categories.

- Abstracting for pathology and laboratory tests varies widely based on the type of test. In informal discussion, people make general references to tests such as a glucose test, strep test, or urinalysis; however, each of these has several distinct CPT codes based on the details of how it is performed.

- Most laboratory procedures can be located in the CPT Index under the Main Term *Pathology and Laboratory*, then a first-level modifying term that corresponds to the Tabular List subsection, such as *Chemistry* or *Cytopathology*, then a second-level modifying term for the type of test. Most procedures are also indexed by the name of the test, analyte, specimen, or testing method.

- Three unique modifiers are used only for laboratory services: *-90, -91,* and HCPC modifier *-QW*. In addition, modifiers for the professional and technical components, as well as separate procedures, apply to lab services.

CONCEPT QUIZ

Take a moment to look back at the Pathology and Laboratory section and solidify your skills. Try to answer the questions from memory first, then refer to the discussion in this chapter if you need a little extra help.

Completion

Instructions: Write the term that completes each statement based on the information you learned in this chapter. Choose from the list below. Some choices may be used more than once and some choices may not be used at all.

analyte	immunology
anatomic	in vivo
autopsy	microbiology
chemistry	microscope
cytogenic studies	molecular
cytopathology	qualitative
evocative/suppression testing	quantitative
gross	surgical

1. The _____ description of a pathology report is limited to what can be seen with the naked eye.

2. _____ pathology procedures involve the analysis of nucleic acid to detect variants in genes.

3. _____ is the administration of a pharmaceutical agent to test the body's response to the agent compared with normal bodily responses.

4. A(n) _____ may be used to identify abnormalities in a urine specimen.

5. The _____ subsection of CPT lists codes for tests for identification of bacteria.

6. The _____ portion of a drug assay detects the presence of a substance in the specimen.

7. A(n) _____ is another term for a postmortem exam to determine the cause of death.

8. _____ is the area of laboratory medicine that includes qualitative and quantitative tests on antigens.

9. _____ involves examination of cells from anywhere in the body to determine whether neoplasms are benign or malignant.

10. The _____ subsection of CPT lists codes for qualitative and quantitative tests on a wide variety of specimens.

Multiple Choice

Instructions: Circle the letter of the best answer to each question based on the information you learned in this chapter.

1. When should modifier -90 be reported?
   A. A lab test is performed in the office
   B. A specimen is sent to an outside lab
   C. A physician office bills for a test sent to an outside lab
   D. A specimen is collected by a lab

2. What type of lab is eligible for a COW?
   A. Labs that perform moderate- and high-complexity tests
   B. Labs that perform CLIA-waived tests only
   C. Labs that perform only microscopy
   D. Reference labs

3. What modifier should be appended to an E/M code when a venipuncture is performed during the encounter?
   A. -25
   B. -51
   C. -90
   D. -QW

4. How would you code the following procedure? *The laboratory performed a presumptive drug class screening for oxycodone, using direct optical observation. The test gave a positive result for the presence of the drug, so then a quantitative definitive drug test was performed.*
   A. 80305, 80365
   B. 80305, 80183
   C. 80306, 80365
   D. 80306, 80183

5. What Main Term in the CPT Index can be used to locate most lab tests?
   A. Pathology
   B. Laboratory
   C. Test
   D. Findings

6. What is the name for a qualitative test that identifies the possible use or nonuse of a drug or drug class?
   A. Therapeutic drug assay
   B. Presumptive drug class screening
   C. Cytopathology
   D. Definitive drug testing

7. How would you code the following procedure? *Results of an electrolyte panel performed on a patient in the Emergency Department show hyponatremia and hypokalemia. After treatment is provided, a second electrolyte panel is performed, which shows that all components have returned to normal levels.*
   A. 80051-51
   B. 80051-22
   C. 80051 x 2
   D. 80051, 80051-91

8. What is the Bethesda System?
   A. A format required by Medicare for reporting lab results
   B. A testing procedure for abnormal Pap smears
   C. A process for evocation/suppression testing
   D. A method of reporting findings from Pap tests

9. How would you code the following procedure? *A physician performed a gross and microscopic examination of an abscessed appendix specimen.*
   A. 88302
   B. 88304
   C. 88305
   D. 88307

10. How many tests must be performed to report code *80408 Aldosterone suppression evaluation panel*?
    A. 1
    B. 2
    C. 3
    D. 4

KEEP ON CODING

Instructions: Read the procedural statement, then use the appropriate Index and Tabular List to assign CPT procedure codes, quantities, and modifiers. Write the code(s) on the line provided.

1. Gross and microscopic examination of left mastectomy with regional lymph nodes. CPT Code(s) _____

2. Lipid panel: total serum cholesterol, HDL, and triglycerides; electrolyte panel: carbon dioxide, chloride, potassium, and sodium. CPT Code(s) _____

3. Nonautomated urinalysis (dipstick), without microscopy. CPT Code(s) _____

4. Quantitative screen for mercury and lead. CPT Code(s) _____

5. Hospital blood bank irradiates two units of leukoreduced red cells. CPT Code(s) _____

6. Physician orders part of a hepatic function panel: serum albumin, total bilirubin, and direct bilirubin. CPT Code(s) _____

7. Pathologist consultation and report on referred slides prepared elsewhere for evaluation of multiple myeloma. CPT Code(s) _____

8. Vancomycin assay for peak and trough levels. CPT Code(s) _____

9. Basic metabolic panel and renal function. CPT Code(s) _____

10. Urine culture, quantitative colony count. CPT Code(s) _____

11. Gross and microscopic examination of three transbronchial lung biopsy tissue samples. CPT Code(s) _____

12. Urine drug screen for cannabis. CPT Code(s) _____

13. Comprehensive metabolic panel. CPT Code(s) _____

14. PT with INR, PTT. CPT Code(s) _____

15. Automated CBC with differential WBC. CPT Code(s) _____

16. Patient underwent two lab tests to determine total bilirubin levels. The first specimen was obtained during the morning and the second in the afternoon on the same day. CPT Code(s) _____

17. Heelstick of newborn for thyroid-stimulating hormone (TSH). CPT Code(s) _____

18. Preoperative collection of blood for autotransfusion. CPT Code(s) _____

19. Thawing of cryopreserved embryos. CPT Code(s) _____

20. CRP (C-reactive protein test for systemic inflammation) and ANA (antinuclear antibodies). CPT Code(s) _____

21. Analysis of a Pap smear using the Bethesda System; manual screening under physician supervision was performed. CPT Code(s) _____

22. Amitriptyline level. CPT Code(s) _____

23. Interpretation of bone marrow smear. CPT Code(s) _____

24. Arterial blood gas analysis including pH, PCO_2, PO_2, O_2 saturation, base-excess, bicarbonate, total CO_2, and ventilation status. CPT Code(s) _____

25. Sperm count and motility. CPT Code(s) _____

CODING CHALLENGE

Instructions: Read the mini-medical-record of each patient's encounter, then abstract, assign, and arrange ICD-10-CM diagnosis codes, CPT procedure codes, and HCPCS codes using the appropriate Index and Tabular List. Assign quantities and modifiers where needed. Pay special attention to whether you are coding for the physician's office, the pathologist, or the laboratory facility. Write the code(s) on the line provided.

1. OFFICE   Gender: F   Age: 24

Reason for encounter: Routine prenatal visit of primipara at 26 weeks, 4 days

Assessment: Test performed at the office; results within normal limits

Office procedure: Glucose tolerance test, three specimens of blood drawn

2 ICD-10-CM Codes _____

1 CPT Code _____

2. OUTPATIENT LABORATORY   Gender: M   Age: 89

Ordering physician: Primary care

Referring diagnosis: Blood in urine; under treatment for prostate cancer with metastasis to the bladder and spine

Tests: Hemoglobin and hematocrit, microscopic urinalysis, coagulation profile (PT, PTT, INR)

Tip: Follow the outpatient coding guidelines for patients receiving diagnostic services only.

4 ICD-10-CM Codes _____

_____

5 CPT Codes _____

_____

3. OFFICE   Gender: M   Age: 70

Reason for encounter: Bloody stools, weight loss, constipation, and abdominal pain for the past two weeks. Patient is otherwise in good health for his age.

Assessment: Positive result for fecal occult blood. Referred to gastroenterologist for colonoscopy.

Office procedure: Stool guaiac test

4 ICD-10-CM Codes _____

_____

1 HCPCS Code _____

4. OFFICE   Gender: F   Age: 53

Reason for encounter: Complaint of vertigo/generalized dizziness for the past two weeks. This is not usually precipitated by change in position from supine to upright. History of hypertension and paroxysmal atrial fibrillation.

Office procedure: Blood drawn to be sent out for TSH level, lipid profile, LFTs, B12 level, and folic acid level

Outpatient laboratory procedure: TSH level, lipid profile, B12 level, and folic acid level

Plan: Obtain carotid ultrasound and refer to a neurologist

3 ICD-10-CM Codes _____

_____

Physician office: 2 CPT Codes _____

Laboratory: 4 CPT Codes _____

5. OUTPATIENT LABORATORY   Gender: M   Age: 21

Ordering physician: General surgeon

Referring diagnosis: Nonhealing surgical wound with abscess. The wound is malodorous and has purulent drainage.

Test(s): Wound culture to isolate bacteria; culture negative

1 ICD-10-CM Code _____

1 CPT Code _____

6. OUTPATIENT LABORATORY   Gender: F   Age: 39

Ordering physician: Rheumatologist

Referring diagnosis: Persistent pain and discomfort with swelling of joints of both hands/fingers. Maternal grandmother has rheumatoid arthritis.

Tests: Antinuclear antibody (ANA), rheumatoid factor, cyclic citrullinated peptide (CCP) antibodies, C-reactive protein (CRP), erythrocyte sedimentation rate, automated (ESR, or sed rate)

5 ICD-10-CM Codes _____

_____

5 CPT Codes _____

_____

7. PATHOLOGY LABORATORY   Gender: M   Age: 49

Clinical history: Low-density soft-tissue lesion at the nasolabial region seen on CT scan

Specimen received: Soft-tissue lesion

Gross description: Received in container labeled "nasolabial cyst" is an ovoid, yellowish cyst, measuring 1 cm × 1.8 cm in diameter

Microscopic description: Yellowish cyst consistent with an epidermal inclusion cyst

Diagnosis: Epidermal inclusion cyst of the nasolabial fold

Tip: Code for the pathologist service.

1 ICD-10-CM Code _____

1 CPT Code _____

---

8. PATHOLOGY LABORATORY   Gender: M   Age: 53

Clinical history: Patient has chronic hepatitis B. A liver biopsy is being done to determine the stage of fibrosis and grade of inflammation.

Specimen received: Liver biopsy

Gross description: The specimen is received in a container labeled "liver biopsy," retrieved with a percutaneous needle. The specimen is 1.5 cm in length and 1 mm in width.

Microscopic description: Hematoxylin stain shows stage 4 fibrosis (i.e., cirrhosis). Moderate portal inflammation and lymphocytic necrosis involving all portal tracts, with noticeable lobular inflammation and hepatocellular change consistent with grade 3 liver damage.

Diagnosis: Fibrosis (cirrhosis) of the liver due to chronic hepatitis B

Tip: Code for the pathologist service.

2 ICD-10-CM Codes _____

1 CPT Code _____

---

9. OFFICE   Gender: M   Age: 45

Reason for Encounter: New patient visit of a 45-year-old male for his annual wellness exam

Assessment: The patient states that he has had multiple sexual partners, both male and female. The rapid HIV test was negative.

Office procedure: Rapid HIV-1 immunoassay using a single-use disposable analytical chamber; venipuncture for CBC and BMP for transport to hospital outpatient laboratory

Laboratory procedure: CBC and BMP automated analysis

Tip: This is a new patient being seen for an initial comprehensive preventive medicine visit. Use the appropriate modifier to indicate that the E/M was provided on the same day as another service or procedure. Use of a kit for the immunoassay requires a modifier for alternative laboratory platform testing. Include the HCPCS code for the rapid HIV test kit.

3 ICD-10-CM Codes _____

_____

Physician office: 4 CPT Codes _____

_____

1 HCPCS Code: _____

Laboratory: 2 CPT Codes _____

---

10. OFFICE   Gender: F   Age: 45

Reason for encounter: Jaundiced appearance and complaint of sluggishness. The patient last seen one year ago.

Assessment: A problem-focused history with straightforward medical decision making and a problem-focused exam were completed

Office procedure: Blood specimen drawn and packaged for HBsAb (hepatitis B surface antibody) to be done at the hospital outpatient laboratory

Plan: Return to office in 2 weeks to review lab results

2 ICD-10-CM Codes _____

Physician office: 3 CPT Codes _____

_____

Laboratory: 1 CPT Code _____

SECTION FOUR

ICD-10-PCS Procedure Coding

Section Four: ICD-10-PCS Procedure Coding guides you through the steps of hospital procedure coding for each type of procedure. You learn the unique characteristics of ICD-10-PCS and how to apply the three skills of an "Ace" coder—abstract, assign, and arrange—for inpatient encounters.

PROFESSIONAL PROFILE

Rajinder Singh, RHIT
Pro-Fee Coder I
University of Washington Physicians

My associate degree in health information management gave me the knowledge about ICD-10-CM/PCS/CPT/HCPCS, abstracting data for E/M coding along with other health information management topics. My internship and volunteer experience at Multicare Health Systems gave me exposure to quality analysis of patient charts, release of information, and day-to-day operations. Apart from this, I also had 15 years of information technology experience in various positions such as instructor, programmer, and PC/LAN Admin Support.

I am responsible for coding evaluation and management (E/M) services for advanced registered nurse practitioners in the university inpatient and outpatient clinics. I enjoy being able to provide educational feedback to providers and to cross-train in other coding specialties to enhance my coding knowledge.

It can be challenging trying to understand and interpret various organizational policies and guidelines applicable to coding. We have a robust internal system for learning about new policies through a mix of internal online tutorials, roundtable sessions, and Q&A. All policies and supporting material are available through an internal website. Other staff—such as the lead coder, supervisor, manager, and director—are available to explain any questions regarding coding policies. We use encoder software to assign diagnosis and procedure codes, as well as look up National Correct Coding Initiative (NCCI) edits and verify Medicare local and national coverage determinations (LCD and NCD).

The registered health information technologist (RHIT) credential was extremely important in achieving the coding position with the organization and is required to maintain employment. The certification and required continuing education units (CEUs) help me to keep my knowledge up-to-date with healthcare regulations, guidelines, and coding updates. I am a member of the American Health Information Management Association (AHIMA) and often attend state and local chapter meetings to stay current with recent changes.

I encourage students to focus on abstracting of data from patient charts as beginners starting with E/M coding. To progress further into procedure coding, students should have thorough knowledge of anatomy and physiology and read the coding conventions carefully. Continuing education is very important to succeed in coding. Network and get involved with local and national organizations. Be a problem solver and you will be successful in any walk of life.

Chapter 46

Introduction to ICD-10-PCS Procedure Coding

Chapter Outline

- **Overview of ICD-10-PCS**
- **Organization of the ICD-10-PCS Coding Manual**
- **ICD-10-PCS Code Structure**
- **ICD-10-PCS Coding Guidelines**
- **Introduction to the Steps of ICD-10-PCS Procedure Coding**

Learning Objectives

After completing this chapter, you should have the skills to:

46.1 Spell and define the key words, medical terms, and abbreviations related to ICD-10-PCS coding. (Remember)

46.2 Summarize the history and purpose of ICD-10-PCS coding. (Understand)

46.3 Articulate the relationship between accurate ICD-10-PCS coding and reimbursement. (Apply)

46.4 Describe the organization of the ICD-10-PCS manual. (Understand)

46.5 Explain the ICD-10-PCS code structure. (Apply)

46.6 Adhere to the ICD-10-PCS Official Guidelines for Coding and Reporting. (Apply)

46.7 Identify the steps in the basic ICD-10-PCS procedure coding process. (Apply)

Key Terms and Abbreviations

approach	device	principal procedure	standardized terminology
body part	expandability	qualifier	structural integrity
body system	granular	revenue code	Table
character	ICD-10-PCS Official Guidelines for Coding and Reporting (PCS OGCR)	root operation	UB-04
charge capture		root type	unique definitions
charge description master (CDM)		section	value
completeness	multiaxial nature	significant procedure	

In addition to the key terms listed here, students should know the terms defined within tables in this chapter.

INTRODUCTION

When a new road is constructed that helps you reach your destination faster, it can be both exciting and confusing because you have to think about a trip that once was automatic. Coding is much the same way. ICD-10-PCS procedure coding is different from other coding systems, but you will appreciate its ease, consistency, and logic.

In this chapter, you learn about how ICD-10-PCS is structured and how to use it. Most importantly, you practice locating basic information in the ICD-10-PCS coding manual.

OVERVIEW OF ICD-10-PCS

The *International Classification of Diseases, 10th Revision, Procedure Coding System (ICD-10-PCS)* is used by hospitals for coding inpatient procedures. ICD-10-PCS, also referred to as PCS in this text, is a relatively new system designed from scratch and implemented in 2015. It was developed to overcome the limitations of other coding systems, with specific goals and usability criteria. All codes consist of seven alphanumeric characters, with each position of the code having a unique and defined purpose. The Health Insurance Portability and Accountability Act (HIPAA) mandates the use of ICD-10-PCS by all covered entities that handle electronic claims for inpatient hospital procedures. It is the standard for communication about inpatient hospital services among healthcare providers, regulators, and payers.

History of the ICD-10-PCS Code Set

In 1992 the Centers for Medicare and Medicaid Services (CMS) funded a project to design a complete replacement for the previous inpatient procedures coding system—ICD-9-CM Volume 3—that had been in place since 1979. The technology described in the previous system was out of date and there was limited room in the numbering format to add new codes. CMS awarded a contract to 3M Health Information Systems (3M) to develop a new inpatient procedure coding system, which was completed in 1998. ICD-10-PCS was developed by the United States solely for use in this country. After nearly two decades of testing and reporting of mortality data, ICD-10-PCS was implemented for daily use by inpatient hospitals on October 1, 2015.

Purpose of ICD-10-PCS Coding

ICD-10-PCS procedure codes identify billable procedures provided for hospital inpatients. Hospitals report PCS procedure codes on insurance claims—the UB-04 and its electronic equivalent, the 837I. Procedure codes are used to classify patients into diagnostic-related groups (DRGs) used for reimbursement by insurance companies and payers. Inpatient hospital reimbursement is discussed later in this chapter.

ICD-10-CM diagnosis codes are reported to identify the reason the procedures were performed. Coders must be certain to abstract and assign at least one ICD-10-CM diagnosis code for each procedure or service billed. The same diagnosis code can be used for more than one service, but coders cannot report a service that is not supported by a diagnosis.

Characteristics of ICD-10-PCS

A coding system that is internally consistent, logically constructed, and adaptable to new technology enables coders to use it more consistently, resulting in data that is more **granular** (*specific*), reliable (*reported in the same way by all users*), and valid (*accurately describes what it is intended to describe*). ICD-10-PCS was developed with six major attributes (*characteristics*) in mind:

- **Completeness**—There should be a unique code for every procedure that is significantly different in body part, approach, or method.

- **Unique definitions**—ICD-10-PCS codes are constructed of seven **characters**, or positions, each with a distinct purpose and meaning. New codes are created by adding a new value for at least one of the positions.

- **Expandability**—The structure of the code set allows new procedures to be easily incorporated.

- **Multiaxial nature**—Each position is defined with a specific meaning that should be used for all related codes and, to the extent possible, for all codes in the manual.

- **Standardized terminology**—ICD-10-PCS defines the specific meaning of each procedure so that all users apply it in the same way.

  - In general use, a composite medical term—such as *arthroplasty*—can refer to the repair of a joint, replacement of part of a joint, or replacement of the entire joint. ICD-10-PCS defines procedures in a specific way that must be applied by all users. For example, **Repair** is *restoring a body part to its normal structure*. **Replacement** is *putting in a device that replaces a body part*. Codes can be reported only for procedures that meet these definitions.

  - ICD-10-PCS eliminates the use of eponyms to describe procedures. For example, the Whipple procedure, a pancreaticoduodenectomy, is a complex surgical procedure that involves the pancreas, as well as portions of the stomach, duodenum, common bile duct, and gallbladder. The specific organs, and portions of the organs, removed depend on the patient's needs and the surgeon. Rather than providing only one code for this procedure, ICD-10-PCS breaks the procedure down into its component parts, with each organ receiving its own code, resulting in as many as five codes to report the procedure. Such detail provides accurate and consistent reporting.

  - ICD-10-PCS limits the use of combination codes, which describe two or more procedures with a single code. Instead, separate codes are reported for each separate procedure performed. This gives a full and accurate report of exactly what was done for each patient.

- **Structural integrity**—ICD-10-PCS can be expanded easily without disrupting the structure of the system because of the manner in which the seven characters of the code are defined.

ICD-10-PCS Compared with ICD-10-CM and CPT

Because coders learn and use several coding systems, they must understand the specific differences between them so they can use each system accurately. Just as you must learn to read new road signs when traveling in a different country, coders must learn the differences between code sets.

ICD-10-CM

Although ICD-10-CM and ICD-10-PCS both carry the name *ICD-10*, the two systems share *no* features or similarities. ICD-10-CM is used for diagnosis coding and is based on the World Health Organization's ICD-10, which is used internationally. ICD-10-PCS was developed by CMS for hospital inpatient procedure coding and is not based on another system. Both systems use alphanumeric codes, but each has a unique organization, code structure, and guidelines. Refer to ■ TABLE 46-1 for a summary of differences.

CPT

Although CPT and ICD-10-PCS are both procedure coding systems, they share *no* features or similarities. CPT was developed by the American Medical Association (AMA) for physician coding, whereas ICD-10-PCS was developed by CMS for hospital inpatient procedure coding. All procedures performed in an inpatient hospital setting are coded in both systems: physicians code and bill their services using CPT; hospitals code and bill their services related to the procedure using ICD-10-PCS. Each code set has a unique organization, code structure, terminology, and guidelines. Refer to ■ TABLE 46-2 for a summary of differences.

Table 46-1 ■ **COMPARISON OF ICD-10-PCS AND ICD-10-CM CODE SYSTEMS**

Characteristic	ICD-10-PCS	ICD-10-CM
Developed by	CMS/3M	WHO/CDC
Purpose	Procedures	Diagnoses
Used by	Inpatient hospitals	All HIPAA entities
Code length	Always 7 characters, no decimal	3 to 7 characters, decimal after 3rd character
7th character requirement	Always required	Sometimes required
Body system characters	Occupy 2nd position	Occupy 1st position
	Defined characters are unique to this system	First letters are unique to this system
	Example: Gastrointestinal = D	*Example*: Digestive = K
Laterality	Always reported	Sometimes reported
	Occupies 4th position	Occupies 5th or 6th position
Letters not used	O, I	U
Placeholder	Z	X
Combination codes	Not used	Many
Eponyms	Not used	Used

Source: © PB Resources, Inc. Used with permission.

Table 46-2 ■ **COMPARISON OF ICD-10-PCS AND CPT CODE SYSTEMS**

Characteristic	ICD-10-PCS	CPT
Developed by	CMS/3M	AMA
Purpose	Inpatient procedures	Outpatient procedures
Used by	Inpatient hospitals	Physicians, outpatient hospitals
Number of codes	78,000+	10,000+
Length	7 alphanumeric	5 digits (except F, T, and U codes which have 5 alphanumeric characters)
Modifiers	None	CPT, HCPCS modifiers
Body systems	31 defined systems subdivide traditional anatomic systems	Traditional anatomic organ systems
Laterality	4th character	Modifiers -RT, -LT, -50
Code structure	Multiaxial	Undefined
Resequenced codes	Not used	Yes
Combination codes	Not used	Yes
Eponyms	Not used	Yes
E/M codes	Not used	Yes
Indented (dependent) and add-on codes	Not used	Yes

Source: © PB Resources, Inc. Used with permission.

Physician Documentation for PCS

Inpatient hospital coding is based on physician documentation of the procedures performed. The accuracy of coding impacts the accuracy of reimbursement. This presents a unique challenge for hospitals because their reimbursement is ultimately based on documentation they do not generate. Physicians might not be accustomed to documenting the level of specificity needed for PCS coding such as laterality, anatomic site details, and certain procedural details. When physician documentation is incomplete, inpatient coders cannot assign codes with the specificity required by payers, or they need to spend significant amounts of time following up with and querying physicians regarding the necessary details of a procedure.

Inpatient Hospital Reimbursement

Hospitals use ICD-10-PCS procedure codes to identify the resources hospitals use in performing procedures when billing the patient's insurance. Hospital resources include:

- Hospital staff, such as nurses, surgical technicians, nurse aides, and ancillary personnel
- Space, equipment, and supplies, such as operating rooms; surgical instruments; x-ray, MRI, and CT equipment; surgical supplies; and linens
- Overhead, such as utilities, operating expenses, and general administration

Hospital resources do not include the physician. In most cases, physicians own their own practices or are members of a group practice. They are not employed by the hospital, even when the hospital owns the medical practice. The physician's practice bills the patient's insurance for the professional service performed by the physician. The hospital bills the patient's insurance for resources the hospital used.

Billing for inpatient hospital services requires more information and a different format than that used by physicians. The process is more complicated because charges must be collected from multiple departments for services that usually occur over a period of several days or longer. Charges are captured throughout the hospital stay; assigning the diagnosis and procedure codes is the final step that releases the bill to the payer. A summary of information about hospital charges, diagnosis-related groups, and claims follows. This provides an introduction to hospital billing. For more comprehensive information, refer to professional resource books and payer websites.

Principal Procedure

According to the Uniform Hospital Data Discharge Set (UHDDS), inpatient hospitals must report all **significant procedures**. Significant procedures are those that are surgical in nature, carry a procedural risk, carry an anesthetic risk, or require specialized training.

The **principal procedure** is one that was performed for definitive treatment, rather than one performed for diagnostic or exploratory purposes, or was necessary to take care of a complication. The principal procedure impacts the DRGs to which patients are assigned for reimbursement purposes. If there appear to be two procedures that meet the criteria for principal procedure, then the one most related to the principal diagnosis should be selected as the principal procedure. Recall that the principal diagnosis is the condition established after study to be chiefly responsible for occasioning the admission of the patient to the hospital for care, per the UHDDS. Refer to ICD-10-CM OGCR section II to review the guidelines for establishing the principal diagnosis.

The principal procedure is entered in FL 74 on the UB-04. Secondary procedures are entered in FL 74a–74e. The principal and additional diagnoses are entered in FL 67–67M (■ FIGURE 46-1).

Charge Capture

ICD-10-PCS codes report procedures performed, but not every supply item and resource used by the hospital. **Charge capture** is the process of entering the nonprocedural services provided throughout the patient stay. This is best done using a computer at the time the service is provided. For example, when a lab test is processed, the laboratory staff enter or scan an internal code that identifies the service provided. The services are listed in the facility's **charge description master (CDM)** and linked to the financial charge. For ancillary services such as laboratory and radiology, the service is also linked to the CPT or HCPCS code. The CDM assigns the charge to a **revenue code**, a four-digit code that identifies a general category of service, such as accommodation (*room charge*), type of ancillary service, pharmacy, or supplies. Revenue codes are used to summarize or "roll up" charges on the final inpatient bill. Refer to Chapter 2, "Coding and Reimbursement," of this text for more information about billing and reimbursement.

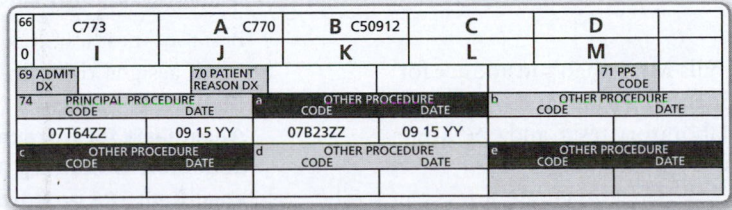

Figure 46-1 ■ Example of reporting the principal diagnosis and principal procedure on the UB-04 claim form. *Source: Annotations © PB Resources, Inc. Used with permission.*

Guided Example of Inpatient Hospital Coding

Refer to the following example throughout this chapter to learn about ICD-10-PCS codes.

Date of procedure: 8/26/yy   Location: Branton Medical Center   Surgeon: Tanya Schmitt, MD

Anesthesiologist: Reginald Pincus, MD

Patient: Michael Longo   Gender: M   Age: 52

Preprocedure diagnosis: Crohn's disease with abscess

Procedure description: Temporary loop ileostomy. Made incision in right abdominal wall. Opened anterior wall of ileum loop and brought through to the skin, then closed the wound around the exposed ileum. Patient tolerated px (procedure) well.

Postprocedure diagnosis: Crohn's disease of large intestine with abscess

---

Follow this patient's surgical procedure and bill through the hospital, physician's office, and anesthesiologist's office to understand the difference between inpatient procedure codes and physician procedure codes.

▶ Tanya Schmitt, MD, who is part of Branton Professional Group, uses the operating rooms, surgical instruments, equipment, supplies, and nursing staff at Branton Medical Center to perform the procedure.

▶ Reginald Pincus, MD, who is part of Branton Anesthesiology Providers, administers the anesthesia using Branton Medical Center's anesthesia equipment and supplies; monitors the patient during and after the procedure; and ensures that the patient wakes up without complications.

▶ After surgery, Mr. Longo is transferred to a medical-surgical floor. Dr. Schmitt checks on Mr. Longo each day and discharges him six days after surgery.

▶ Mr. Longo's insurance will receive three separate bills for services from the following organizations for the amounts listed:

1. Branton Medical Center, $12,500.00
2. Branton Professional Group, $1,027.00
3. Branton Anesthesiology Providers, $485.00

▶ Review the information outlined below to learn why there are three bills.

1. Branton Medical Center bills Mr. Longo's insurance for his entire length of stay, including room and board, the technical component of laboratory tests, and operating room resources. The cost is $12,500.00.

   • Branton Medical Center's coder, Marcy Elwood, CCS, assigns the ICD-10-CM diagnosis code **K50.114 Crohn's disease of large intestine with abscess** as the principal diagnosis. The coder

assigns an ICD-10-PCS procedure code, **0D1B0Z4 Bypass Ileum to Cutaneous, Open approach**, as the principal procedure. (You learn the details of how to assign PCS codes in the next chapter. ICD-10-CM coding for the digestive system is discussed in Chapter 8, "Diseases of the Digestive System," in this text.

   • The hospital's biller prepares the UB-04 form. The biller enters the principal diagnosis, ICD-10-CM code **K50.114** in FL 67; the principal procedure, ICD-10-PCS code **0D1B0Z4**, in the left side of FL 74; and the date of the procedure, 8/26/YY, in the right side of FL 74. In FL 77, the block for operating physician Dr. Schmitt's name and National Provider Identifier (NPI) are entered. Total charges are entered as $12,500.00 in FL 47, line 23. The facility is Branton Medical Center. Payment will be made to Branton Medical Center.

   • Refer to Chapter 2, (■ Figure 2-4), "Example of a completed UB-04 claim (with annotations)", in this text, to review the completed UB-04 for this case.

2. Branton Professional Group bills Mr. Longo's insurance for Dr. Schmitt's services, which include admitting him, performing the procedure, making the follow-up visits, and discharging him. The surgeon's fee is $1,027.00.

   • Branton Professional Group's coder, Chrystal Crago, CCA, assigns the same ICD-10-CM diagnosis code, **K50.114,** that the hospital did and assigns a CPT surgical code (**44310 Ileostomy or jejunostomy, non-tube**) for the procedure.

   • Branton Professional Group's biller prepares a claim on the CMS-1500 form (*the standard physician billing form*) or its electronic equivalent, the 837P. The biller lists the ICD-10-CM code **K50.114** in the diagnosis block (21), the date of the procedure, 8/26/YY, and CPT surgical code **44310** in the services block (24). The charge for the surgeon is $1,027.00. Branton Medical Center is listed as the service facility. The billing provider is Branton Professional Group. Payment will be made to Branton Professional Group. (CPT coding for the digestive system is discussed in Chapter 32, "Digestive System Procedures," in this text.)

3. Branton Anesthesiology Providers bills Mr. Longo's insurance for the anesthesia management by Dr. Pincus. The anesthesiologist's fee is $485.00.

   • Branton Anesthesiology Providers' coder, Lance Staiger, CPC, assigns the same ICD-10-CM diagnosis code, **K50.114**, but assigns a CPT anesthesia code (**00840-P1 Anesthesia for intraperitoneal procedures in lower abdomen including laparoscopy; not otherwise specified; -P1 a Normal healthy patient**) for the anesthesiologist's services.

   • The Branton Anesthesiology Providers' biller prepares a claim on the CMS-1500 form or its electronic equivalent. The biller enters the ICD-10-CM code **K50.114** as the diagnosis, the date of the procedure, 8/26/YY, and the CPT anesthesia code **00840-P1** in the services block. The charge for the anesthesiologist is $485.00. Branton Medical Center is listed as the service facility. The billing provider is Branton Anesthesiology Providers. Payment will be made to Branton Anesthesiology Providers. (CPT coding for anesthesia is discussed in Chapter 31, "Anesthesia Procedures," in this text.)

CODING PRACTICE

Exercise 46.1   The Purpose of ICD-10-PCS

Instructions: Fill in each blank with the correct term(s) from this section of the chapter.

1. Which attribute of ICD-10-PCS means that there should be a unique code for every procedure that is significantly different in body part, approach, or methods? _____
_____

2. Which attribute of ICD-10-PCS means that each position or character within a code number has a designated meaning or purpose and should be used for that meaning for all related codes? _____

3. Which attribute of ICD-10-PCS means that the code set includes definitions of the terminology it uses and each term must have only one meaning? _____
_____

4. How many characters appear in all ICD-10-PCS codes? _____
_____

5. What term describes procedures that are surgical in nature, carry a procedural risk, carry an anesthetic risk, or require specialized training? _____

6. What term describes a procedure that was performed for definitive treatment, rather than one performed for diagnostic or exploratory purposes or was necessary to take care of a complication? _____

7. What type of provider reports ICD-10-PCS codes? _____
_____

8. What are the three entities who submit bills after a patient has an inpatient hospital surgical procedure performed? _____
_____
_____
_____

9. Of the three entities listed in question 8, which one(s) bill using ICD-10-CM diagnosis codes? _____

10. Of the three entities listed in question 8, which one(s) bill using ICD-10-PCS procedure codes? _____

ORGANIZATION OF THE ICD-10-PCS CODING MANUAL

Coders need to be familiar with the organization of the PCS manual so that they can find needed information quickly. Not only do you need to understand where needed information is located, you also need to identify and interpret coding guidelines and conventions. The PCS manual is formatted differently than those of other code sets. Open the ICD-10-PCS manual and follow along with the information outlined next, which describes the overall organization of the manual.

Introduction

The Introduction describes the history of ICD-10-PCS and gives detailed instructions on how to use the manual. It provides reference material that lists the character definitions and values for each section of the manual. Some publishers include a list of new, revised, and deleted codes for the current code year.

Official Guidelines

ICD-10-PCS Official Guidelines for Coding and Reporting (PCS OGCR) provides the rules coders must apply for this code set. PCS OGCR contains several sections:

A. Conventions

B. Medical and Surgical Section Guidelines

C. Obstetrics Section Guidelines

D. New Technology Section Guidelines

Selection of Principal Procedure

Index

The Index is an alphabetical listing of procedures using the root operation or root type as the Main Term. A partial code in the Index identifies the correct reference table to use to build the code.

Tables

The Tables are reference grids used to build each ICD-10-PCS code (■ Figure 46-2, page 958). Tables appear in alphanumeric order based on the first three characters of the code.

Appendices

PCS contains several appendices with additional reference material. The naming, order, and content of the appendices can vary by publisher and from year to year. ■ Table 46-3 (page 958) lists the most common appendices. Coders should become familiar with the appendices because they contain valuable information that makes coding easier and more accurate.

Section	**0**	Medical and Surgical
Body System	**F**	Hepatobiliary System and Pancreas
Operation	**9**	Drainage Taking or letting out fluids and/or gases from a body part

Body Part Character 4	Approach Character 5	Device Character 6	Qualifier Character 7
0 Liver **1** Liver, Right Lobe **2** Liver, Left Lobe	**0** Open **3** Percutaneous **4** Percutaneous Endoscopic	**0** Drainage Device	**Z** No Qualifier
0 Liver **1** Liver, Right Lobe **2** Liver, Left Lobe	**0** Open **3** Percutaneous **4** Percutaneous Endoscopic	**Z** No Device	**X** Diagnostic **Z** No Qualifier
4 Gallbladder **G** Pancreas	**0** Open **3** Percutaneous **4** Percutaneous Endoscopic **8** Via Natural or Artificial Opening Endoscopic	**0** Drainage Device	**Z** No Qualifier
4 Gallbladder **G** Pancreas	**0** Open **3** Percutaneous **4** Percutaneous Endoscopic **8** Via Natural or Artificial Opening Endoscopic	**Z** No Device	**X** Diagnostic **Z** No Qualifier

Figure 46-2 ■ Example of a PCS Table.

Table 46-3 ■ ICD-10-PCS CODING MANUAL APPENDICES

Appendix Title	Contents	Use
Body Part Key	Crosswalk between anatomic terms and the PCS body part description.	Determine the body part value that corresponds with a specific anatomic site, such as a blood vessel, tendon, or nerve.
Comparison of Medical and Surgical Root Operations	Organizes Medical and Surgical root operations into nine groups with similar objectives.	Help determine the appropriate root operation.
Components of the Medical and Surgical Approach Definitions	Defines all approaches (Character 5) for the Medical and Surgical section.	Identify the official definition of surgical approaches.
Device Key and Aggregation Table	Device Key: Provides a crosswalk from device brand names and common names to the PCS device description (Character 6). Device Aggregation Table: Defines the operation, body system, and device value (Character 6) for each specific device.	Device Key: Determine the device value to use for a specific product. Device Aggregation Table: Determine the appropriate root operations, body systems, and PCS device value for each class of devices.
Root Operation Definitions	Defines all root operations in sections 0, Medical and Surgical, and sections 1 through 9, Medical and Surgical-Related. Organized by section.	Identify the official definition of root operations.
Sections B–H Character Definitions	Lists all possible values and meanings for Character 3 through Character 7 for Ancillary sections, B through H. Organized by character and section.	Interpret the meaning of codes already assigned.
Device Definitions	Lists specific types of devices included in each PCS value description (Character 6).	Identify the specific types of devices represented by a device value listed Character 6 Device in a PCS table.
Substance Key/Substance Definitions	Lists substances by trade name or synonym for PCS value descriptions in the Administration and New Technology sections.	Identify the specific substances represented by values in the Character 6 or Character 7 Substance in a PCS table.

ICD-10-PCS Reference Manual

CMS publishes a separate electronic *ICD-10-PCS Reference Manual* (■ Table 46-4) that is not part of the official coding manual. This document provides detailed background on ICD-10-PCS, explanations of all sections and root operations, tables of all character values, and many case examples. It was last updated in 2016 after the implementation of PCS, but still provides valuable reference material not found elsewhere. The *ICD-10-PCS Reference Manual* can be downloaded from the CMS website free of charge.

Table 46-4   ■   ICD-10-PCS REFERENCE MANUAL CONTENTS

Chapter	Title	Contents
1	Overview	Includes a general introduction to ICD-10-PCS, a brief history of its development, and a presentation of the code structure, organization, and characteristics.
2	Procedures in the Medical and Surgical Section	Provides reference material for each root operation in the Medical and Surgical section (0).
3	Procedures in the Medical and Surgical-Related Sections	Provides reference material for each of the Medical and Surgical-Related sections (1 through 9).
4	Procedures in the Ancillary Sections	Provides reference material for each of the ancillary sections (B through H).
Appendix A	ICD-10-PCS Definitions	Tables listing the full definitions of all root operations and approaches in the Medical and Surgical section.
Appendix B	ICD-10-PCS Device and Substance Classification	Discusses the distinguishing features of device, substance, and equipment as classified in ICD-10-PCS.

The *ICD-10-PCS Reference Manual* can be downloaded from **www.cms.gov**.

CODING PRACTICE

Exercise 46.2   ICD-10-PCS Coding Manual Organization

Instructions: Fill in each blank with the correct term(s) from this section of the chapter. Name the section or appendix of the ICD-10-PCS coding manual coders use to locate the following information.

1. Conventions _____

2. An alphabetical listing of procedures that identifies the correct reference table to use to build the code _____

3. Reference material that lists the character definitions and values for each section of the manual _____

4. Determine the body part value corresponds with a specific anatomic site _____

5. Determine the device value to use for a specific product _____

ICD-10-PCS CODE STRUCTURE

ICD-10-PCS codes have a logical, consistent structure that contains seven alphanumeric positions, called *characters*. An ICD-10-PCS code is best understood as the result of a process in which coders assign, or build, a code. The process consists of assigning values to each character based on specific characteristics of the procedure the physician performs. The ICD-10-PCS manual uses Tables, which are reference grids used to select the body part, operative approach, and other characteristics of the procedure.

ICD-10-PCS codes consist of seven positions or characters, each with a designated purpose, which creates consistency across codes. Coders select individual letters and numbers, called **values**, in a sequential order to occupy the seven characters of the code. Each character represents a specific aspect of the procedure and can have up to 34 different values. Values consist of the 10 digits—0–9—and 24 letters, A–H, J–N, and P–Z. Not every character uses all 34 values. For some sections and some characters, only a few values are used, whereas in others, most of the values are used. Each section of the manual designates how each character of the code is used within that section. The definition of each value, for example, **1** or **A**, is based on the position it occupies. Examples are provided in the discussion that follows.

The options and values for a character vary based on the first character of the code, which identifies the section. The largest section is Medical and Surgical, which is used as an example to introduce PCS codes in the remainder of this chapter. Characters in the Medical and Surgical section are defined as follows:

- Character 1 defines the section, or broad procedure category where the code is found.
- Character 2 defines the body system in which the procedure is performed.
- Character 3 defines the root operation, or the objective of the procedure.
- Character 4 defines the body part, or specific anatomic site where the physician performed the procedure.
- Character 5 defines the approach, or the surgical technique used to reach the procedure site.
- Character 6 defines the device left in place at the end of the procedure.
- Character 7 defines a qualifier for the code, which describes additional information about the procedure.

The Introduction in the ICD-10-PCS coding manual identifies the character meanings for each section.

The following discussion identifies the purpose of each character and gives examples of how it is used. The next several chapters of this text discuss how to use the Index and Tables to arrive at a code.

Character 1: Section

The first character in all PCS codes describes the section, or the broad procedure category, where the code is found (■ TABLE 46-5). The largest section is Medical and Surgical. Other sections classify medical and surgical-related procedures, such as obstetrics or chiropractic, ancillary services, such as nuclear medicine or mental health, and new technology.

Character 2: Body System

The second character in the Medical and Surgical section identifies the body system, the general physiological system or anatomic region involved, such as central nervous system or endocrine system. The Medical and Surgical section has 31 possible values for the body system. The body system values do not always correlate to commonly defined anatomic organ systems. Large anatomic systems may have multiple values in Character 2. For example, the skeletal system has five body system values, each referring to a specific component of the anatomic system (■ TABLE 46-6). Each PCS body system can use up to 34 values for body part, so codes can be more specific when large systems are divided into multiple values. This enables the skeletal system, for example, to have up to 170 body part values. If the skeletal system were defined with only one value, then the number of body part values would be limited to 34.

Many sections other than Medical and Surgical also use Character 2 to describe body system, but may also use it for

Table 46-5 ■ **CHARACTER 1: SECTION**

Value	Section Name
0	Medical and Surgical
Medical and Surgical-Related Procedures	
1	Obstetrics
2	Placement
3	Administration
4	Measurement and Monitoring
5	Extracorporeal and Systemic Assistance and Performance
6	Extracorporeal and Systemic Therapies
7	Osteopathic
8	Other Procedures
9	Chiropractic
Ancillary Procedures	
B	Imaging
C	Nuclear Medicine
D	Radiation Oncology
F	Physical Rehabilitation and Diagnostic Audiology
G	Mental Health
H	Substance Abuse Treatment
New Technology	
X	New Technology

Table 46-6 ■ **BODY SYSTEM VALUES FOR THE SKELETAL SYSTEM**

Value	Description
N	Head and Facial Bones
P	Upper Bones
Q	Lower Bones
R	Upper Joints
S	Lower Joints

other purposes. The Placement section (Section 2) uses Character 2 for Anatomical Orifice. The Physical Rehabilitation and Diagnostic Audiology section (Section F) uses Character 2 for Section Qualifier, which is a broad type of service such as Rehabilitation.

Character 3: Root Operation

The third character in the Medical and Surgical section, and most other sections, defines the root operation, which describes the objective of the procedure, such as excision, destruction, or extraction. The options and values for Character 3 vary from one section to the next and from one body part value to the next within a section. Root operations are Main Terms in the Index, so coders must be familiar with their names and definitions. The names and definitions of Character 3 appear at the top of each Table in the ICD-10-PCS manual. In addition, an appendix in most ICD-10-PCS manuals defines all the root operations for the Medical and Surgical section, provides expanded explanations, and gives examples.

For example, a composite medical term such as *gastrectomy* can mean removing all or part of the stomach. The definitions of the words *excision* and *resection* are sometimes used interchangeably in common medical usage, such as stomach excision or stomach resection, and can mean that either all of the stomach or part of the stomach is removed. Without referring to the operative report, the extent of the procedure is unclear. ICD-10-PCS defines these terms in specific ways. The root operation **Excision** is defined as *cutting off a portion of a body part without replacement* whereas the root operation **Resection** is defined as *cutting off all of a body part without replacement*. Therefore, cutting out a portion of the stomach is coded as the root operation **Excision** (value **B**), and cutting out all of the stomach is coded as the root operation **Resection** (value **T**).

The 31 Medical and Surgical root operations are organized into nine groups based on the overall objective of the procedure. An appendix in most ICD-10-PCS manuals provides a useful breakdown of the nine groups, which makes it easier to locate a desired root operation. The nine groups are not part of the final code—they are simply an organizational tool for coders.

> ## CODING CAUTION
>
> Coders are required to follow the definitions in the ICD-10-PCS manual, but physicians are not expected to change the words they use in documentation. Regardless of the word the physician uses to describe a procedure, coders are required to assign the root operation based on the official ICD-10-PCS definition (PCS OGCR A11).

Character 4: Body Part

The fourth character in the Medical and Surgical section identifies the body part, or specific anatomic site, where the physician performed the procedure. The body system (Character 2) provides a general indication of the procedure location. The body part and body system values together provide a precise description of the procedure site.

Most sections use Character 2 for body system and Character 4 for body part, but some sections use it for a different purpose. Sections that do not define body system in Character 2 may use Character 4 for body system.

The definition of each body part value in the Medical and Surgical section is unique to each body system table. For example, when the Body System (Character 2) value is **5 Upper veins**, the Body Part value **B** refers to the **right basilic vein**. When the Body System (Character 2) value is **7 Lymphatic and hemic systems**, the Body Part value **B** refers to the mesenteric lymphatic system. Review the appendix to see how the same value represents different information in different body system tables.

When selecting the body part for a particular root operation, coders must refer to the appropriate Table and identify how that Table defines body part. Some organs and anatomic areas are divided into multiple Body Parts for coding purposes. For example, the large intestine is a single organ, but ICD-10-PCS assigns multiple body part values (■ TABLE 46-7).

Coders should match the most specific body part value with the most specific root operation value. For example, when surgeons cut out the entire descending colon, they are taking out *part* of the organ, the large intestine, but *all* of the PCS Body Part value **M Descending Colon**. Therefore, coders select the root operation **T Resection**—defined as *cutting out, without replacement, all of a body part*—and match it with the Body Part value **M Descending Colon**. Do not assign the root operation **B Excision**—which is defined as *cutting out, without replacement, a portion of a body part*—and match it with the less specific Body Part value **E Large Intestine** (■ FIGURE 46-3).

Table 46-7 ■ EXAMPLE OF MULTIPLE BODY PART VALUES FOR A SINGLE ORGAN: THE LARGE INTESTINE

Value	Description
E	Large Intestine
F	Large Intestine, Right
G	Large Intestine, Left
H	Cecum
J	Appendix
K	Ascending Colon
L	Transverse Colon
M	Descending Colon
N	Sigmoid Colon
P	Rectum

From Table 0DB Excision, Gastrointestinal System: Character 4, Body Part.

Procedure description: Partial colectomy. Excised the entire descending colon.

CORRECT
Root Operation: **T - Resection,** *cutting out, without replacement, all of a body part*
Body Part: **M - Descending Colon**

INCORRECT
Root Operation: **B - Excision,** *cutting out, without replacement, a portion of a body part*
Body Part: **E - Large Intestine**
Explanation: Select the most specific Body Part value **(Descending Colon (M))** and match it with the most specific Root Operation **(Resection (T))**. Also notice that you should not select the Root Operation **Excision (B)** based on the physician's use of the word "excised." Select the Root Operation based on the PCS definition.

Figure 46-3 ■ Example of matching the root operation with the body part.

Character 5: Approach

The fifth character in the Medical and Surgical section defines the approach, or the surgical technique used to reach the procedure site, such as open, endoscopic, or external. Each Table in the ICD-10-PCS manual lists the acceptable approaches for each root operation value and Body Part value. Definitions for each approach appear in the PCS coding manual appendix and are discussed further in later chapters of this text.

Sections other than Medical and Surgical use Character 5 for a wide range of purposes. For example, the Extracorporeal and Systemic Therapies section (section value 6) uses Character 5 for **Duration**, whereas the Imaging section (section value **B**) uses Character 5 for **Contrast**.

Character 6: Device

The sixth character in the Medical and Surgical section identifies therapeutic material left in place at the end of the procedure. Devices includes grafts and prostheses, implants, simple or mechanical appliances, electronic appliances, stents, shunts, and clips. Each Table in the ICD-10-PCS manual lists the acceptable devices for each root operation value and device value. Many root operations do not use a device. When no device applies, the Table lists the value **Z No device** for Character 6.

Sections other than Medical and Surgical use Character 6 for a variety of purposes. For example, the Osteopathic section defines Character 6 as **Method**, which identifies the technique used. The Radiation Oncology section defines Character 6 as **Isotope**, which identifies the type of isotope used in the procedure. Review the Tables in each PCS section to identify how Character 6 is used.

SUCCESS STEP

When coding a specific procedure, you do not automatically know what information might be needed to code all the Characters. You have to look at the Table and review the information listed. You often need to check back and forth between the procedure description and the coding manual a few times to identify all the information needed for the code. This is especially true while learning.

Character 7: Qualifier

The seventh character in the Medical and Surgical section defines a qualifier for the code. A qualifier specifies additional attributes of the procedure. Examples of Medical and Surgical qualifiers are the type of adhesive used on a replacement joint—such as cemented or uncemented—and additional anatomic information, such as the ending site of a bypass procedure. The most commonly used qualifier identifies diagnostic procedures. Each Table in the ICD-10-PCS manual lists the acceptable qualifier values for each approach value. When no qualifier applies, the Table lists the value **Z No qualifier** for Character 7.

Other sections of PCS use Character 7 to identify a wide variety procedural details—such as a specific type of substance

used, the anatomic approach, and intraoperative treatments. You must refer to the PCS Table for the procedure to learn what information might be needed for Character 7. When Character 7 is not used in a section, the Table lists **Z None**, so you should code **Z** in the seventh position.

Guided Example of Building a PCS Code

Continue with the example of Michael Longo, who had an ileostomy, to learn the meaning of an ICD-10-PCS code.

Follow along as Marcy Elwood, CCS, the coder at Branton Medical Center, assigns the ICD-10-PCS code **0D1B0Z4**.

▶ Refer to ■ TABLE 46-8 to understand how a PCS code is structured. You learn how Marcy used the Index and Tables to arrive at this code in the following chapters of this text.

❑ The value **0** for Character 1 identifies that the procedure is from the Medical and Surgical section.

❑ The value **D** for Character 2 identifies that the body system is **Gastrointestinal**.

❑ The value **1** for Character 3 identifies that the root operation is **Bypass**. PCS defines **Bypass** as *altering the route of passage of the contents of a tubular body part*.

❑ The value **B** for Character 4 identifies that the Body Part is **Ileum**.

❑ The value **0** for Character 5 identifies that the approach is **Open**.

❑ The value **Z** for Character 6 identifies that the device is **No device** because the PCS Table does not provide any options for this character.

❑ The value **4** for Character 7 identifies that the qualifier is **Cutaneous** because in the root operation **Bypass**, PCS uses the qualifier to identify the end site of the bypass.

▶ Now you can see the entire meaning of the code **0D1B0Z4 Bypass Ileum to Cutaneous, Open approach**. You learn how to use the Index and Tables to arrive at this code in later chapters of this text.

Table 46-8 ■ **CODE 0D1B0Z4 BYPASS ILEUM TO CUTANEOUS, OPEN APPROACH**

Character (Position)	Name	Value	Description
1	Section	0	Medical and Surgical
2	Body System	D	Gastrointestinal
3	Root Operation	1	Bypass
4	Body Part	B	Ileum
5	Approach	0	Open
6	Device	Z	No Device
7	Qualifier	4	Cutaneous

CODING PRACTICE

Exercise 46.3 ICD-10-PCS Code Structure

Instructions: Fill in each blank with the correct term(s) from this section of the chapter.

Part A

1. _____ are reference grids used to select the body part, operative approach, and other characteristics of the procedure.

2. _____ are individual letters and numbers selected in a standard order to occupy the seven characters of the code.

3. ICD-10-PCS codes do not use the letters _____ and _____ to avoid confusion with numbers.

Part B

List the name of the following characters of a PCS code in the Medical and Surgical section.

4. _____: Character 1 has the value of 0 for all Medical and Surgical procedures.

5. _____: Character 2 identifies the general physiological system or anatomic region involved, such as central nervous system.

6. _____: Character 3 identifies the objective of the procedure, such as excision.

7. _____: Character 4 identifies the specific anatomic site where the physician performed the procedure, such as the right basilic vein.

8. _____: Character 5 identifies the technique used to reach the procedure site, such as open.

9. _____: Character 6 identifies therapeutic material left in place at the end of a procedure, such as a stent.

10. _____: Character 7 identifies various additional attributes of the root operation, such as the ending site of a bypass procedure.

ICD-10-PCS CODING GUIDELINES

ICD-10-PCS provides Official Guidelines for Coding and Reporting (OGCR) at the front of the ICD-10-PCS manual. OGCR is also available as a separate document that can be downloaded from **www.cms.gov** or **www.cdc.gov**. ICD-10-PCS OGCR is a separate document from ICD-10-CM OGCR. Guidelines are divided into five sections: A-Conventions; B-Medical and Surgical Section Guidelines; C-Obstetric Section Guidelines, D-New Technology Section Guidelines, and Selection of Principal Procedure. Throughout this text, information from the ICD-10-PCS OGCR is referenced as PCS OGCR, followed by the specific reference number, such as PCS OGCR A6 or PCS OGCR B3.6a. Follow along in the ICD-10-PCS manual to become acquainted with each section of the OGCR.

A—Conventions

Conventions describe how ICD-10-PCS codes are constructed and the basic rules of using ICD-10-PCS. Examples are presented for many specific guidelines. The most important guidelines to memorize while learning PCS include the following. This provides an overview. The details are discussed later in this chapter and other PCS chapters.

- A6—The purpose of the alphabetic index is to locate the appropriate table that contains all information necessary to construct a procedure code. The PCS tables should always be consulted to find the most appropriate valid code.

- A8—All seven characters must be specified to be a valid code. If the documentation is incomplete for coding purposes, query the physician for the necessary information.

- A9—Within a PCS table, valid codes include all combinations of choices in Characters 4 through 7 contained in the same row of the table.

- A11—Many of the terms used to construct PCS codes are defined within the system. It is the coder's responsibility to determine what the documentation in the medical record equates to in the PCS definitions.

B—Medical and Surgical Section Guidelines (Section 0)

Medical and Surgical section guidelines apply specifically to ICD-10-PCS in the Medical and Surgical section (value **0**). The organization of this section correlates with each character in the Medical and Surgical codes, as follows:

- B2 Body System
- B3 Root Operation
- B4 Body Part
- B5 Approach
- B6 Device
- B7 Qualifier

Each of these subsections contains *General guidelines*—which apply to the Medical and Surgical section as a whole—and also provides additional guidelines that apply to specific root operations, approaches, and other elements. Specific guidelines from this section are discussed in Chapters 47–53 of this text.

C—Obstetrics Section Guidelines (Section 1)

Obstetrics section Guidelines apply specifically to ICD-10-PCS in the Obstetrics section (value **1**). Obstetric codes are reported only for procedures on products of conception and procedures performed following a delivery or abortion. Procedures on the pregnant female or postpartum female not related to products of conception are coded from the Medical and Surgical section. Specific guidelines for Obstetrics (Section 1) are discussed in Chapter 54 of this text.

D—New Technology Section Guidelines (Section X)

New Technology Guidelines apply specifically to ICD-10-PCS in the New Technology section (value **X**). This section provides a place for codes that uniquely identify procedures requested via CMS's New Technology Application Process or that capture other new technologies that would overlap existing PCS codes in other sections. These are standalone codes that do not require another ICD-10-PCS code to be reported. Guidelines for New Technology (Section X) are discussed in Chapter 55 of this text.

Selection of Principal Procedure

Selection of Principal Procedure guidelines review the UHDDS coding criteria for selecting the inpatient principal procedure and clarification on the importance of the relation to the principal diagnosis when more than one procedure is performed. The principal diagnosis, as defined by the UHDDS, is "that condition established after study to be chiefly responsible for occasioning the admission of the patient to the hospital for care." Sequencing guidelines apply to all root operations. The general sequencing priorities for PCS codes are:

1. Definitive procedure related to principal diagnosis
2. Diagnostic procedure related to principal diagnosis
3. Definitive procedure related to secondary diagnosis
4. Diagnostic procedure related to secondary diagnosis

When more than one definitive procedure equally relates to the principal diagnosis, sequence the most extensive procedure as the principal procedure. Various types of procedure combinations are discussed in PCS OGCR and are summarized next.

- The principal procedure is the procedure performed for definitive treatment most related to principal diagnosis. Sequence procedures related to the secondary diagnoses as subsequent procedures (■ FIGURE 46-4).

- When a diagnostic procedure and a procedure for definitive treatment are performed for both the principal and secondary diagnoses, the principal procedure is the procedure performed for definitive treatment most related to the principal diagnosis. Diagnostic procedures related to the principal diagnosis are sequenced as secondary procedures. All procedures related to the secondary diagnoses are sequenced as secondary procedures (■ FIGURE 46-5).

- When a diagnostic procedure is performed for the principal diagnosis and definitive treatment is provided for the secondary diagnosis, the diagnostic procedure is the principal procedure because it is most related to the principal diagnosis (■ FIGURE 46-6).

Surgeon removed the descending colon due to cancer, using endoscopic access through the anus. A percutaneous biopsy was taken of the pelvic lymph nodes, which were positive for metastases, so a percutaneous endoscopic pelvic lymphadenectomy also was performed to remove several, but not all, nodes.

C18.6 Malignant neoplasm of descending colon
C77.5 Secondary and unspecified malignant neoplasm of intrapelvic lymph nodes
0DTM8ZZ Resection, Descending colon, Via natural or artificial opening endoscopic, No device, No qualifier
07BC4ZZ Excision, Lymphatic pelvis, Percutaneous endoscopic, No device, No qualifier
07BC3ZX Excision, Lymphatic pelvis, Percutaneous, No device, Diagnostic

Figure 46-4 ■ Example of sequencing procedures for the principal and secondary diagnoses. *Source:* © *PB Resources, Inc. Used with permission.*

Surgeon performs an endometrial biopsy using a speculum through the vaginal opening. The biopsy is found to be cancerous, so a vaginal hysterectomy is performed.

C54.1 Malignant neoplasm of endometrium
0UT97ZZ Resection, Uterus, Via natural or artificial opening, No device, No qualifier
0UDB7ZX Extraction, Endometrium, Via natural or artificial opening, No device, Diagnostic

Figure 46-5 ■ Example of sequencing definitive and diagnostic procedures. *Source:* © *PB Resources, Inc. Used with permission.*

Patient was admitted for alcoholic cirrhosis of the liver. An endoscopic excisional biopsy was performed of the left lobe of the liver. During additional workup, a rectal polyp was found which was removed endoscopically using fulguration.

K70.30 Alcoholic cirrhosis of liver without ascites
F10.188 Alcohol abuse with other alcohol-induced disorder
K62.1 Rectal polyp
0FB24ZX Excision, Liver left lobe, Percutaneous endoscopic, No device, Diagnostic
0D5P8ZZ Destruction, Rectum, Via natural or artificial opening endoscopic, No device, No qualifier

Figure 46-6 ■ Example of abstracting a root operation. *Source:* © *PB Resources, Inc. Used with permission.*

AHA Coding Clinic

The *AHA Coding Clinic* supplements the ICD-10-PCS Official Guidelines for Coding and Reporting to provide definitive guidance, clarification, and examples regarding inpatient coding issues. *AHA Coding Clinic* is published quarterly by the American Hospital Association (AHA) It is not a public domain document and is available for purchase from the AHA. Links to the content are included in many encoder software programs. Inpatient hospitals also develop internal coding guidelines to direct coders in specific situations.

- When the only procedure(s) performed relate to the secondary diagnosis, the principal procedure is the one performed for *definitive treatment* of the secondary diagnosis. Sequence *diagnostic* procedures related to the secondary diagnosis as secondary procedures. A procedure related to the secondary diagnosis must be the principal procedure when there are no procedures related to the principal diagnosis. (■ Figure 46-7).

- When no procedures are related to the principal diagnosis, sequence the principal procedure as the one for definitive treatment of the secondary diagnosis.

> Patient was admitted because of weakness due to hyponatremia and dehydration. Medical treatment was provided. During the admission, the patient developed a nosebleed, which was treated with electrocautery through the nasal opening.
>
> **E87.1 Hypo-osmolality and hyponatremia**
> **E86.0 Dehydration**
> **R04.0 Epistaxis**
> **095KXZZ Destruction, Ear nose sinus, Nose, External, No device, No qualifier**

Figure 46-7   ■   Example of sequencing a principal procedure for the secondary procedure. *Source: © PB Resources, Inc. Used with permission.*

CODING PRACTICE

Exercise 46.4   ICD-10-PCS Official Guidelines for Coding and Reporting

Instructions: Fill in each blank with the correct term(s) from this section of the chapter.

1. What part of the PCS OGCR describes how ICD-10-PCS codes are constructed and the basic rules of using ICD-10-PCS? _____

2. Which PCS OGCR states that all seven characters must be specified to be a valid code? _____

3. What section of the guidelines provides the UHDDS coding criteria for selecting the inpatient principal procedure? _____

4. Who is responsible to determine what the documentation in the medical record equates to in the PCS definitions? _____

5. What types of procedures are reported by codes in the Obstetrics section? _____

INTRODUCTION TO THE STEPS OF ICD-10-PCS PROCEDURE CODING

The three skills of an "Ace" coder apply to coding procedures, but the mechanics are unique to this code set. Follow these steps:

1. *Abstract* procedures from the medical record, beginning with PCS definitions of the root operation.

2. *Assign*, or build, the PCS code values using the Index and Tables.

3. *Arrange*, or sequence, PCS codes based on the definition of the principal procedure.

An overview of these skills is provided next. Chapters 47–55 of this text discuss these skills in detail and provide examples.

Abstract Procedures from the Medical Record

The key to accurate abstracting in PCS is to read the information provided in the procedure report and interpret it in a manner consistent with ICD-10-PCS definitions of the root operation or **root type** (*Character 3 of codes in the ancillary sections*). Abstracting involves reading the procedure report and identifying the objective of the procedure and how it was accomplished. Coders must identify the exact anatomic site, the surgical approach, and any devices left in the patient for therapeutic reasons. These details must be interpreted in light of the PCS root operation definitions to identify the accurate

root operation or root type. The root operation or root type functions as the Main Term in the Index and directs coders to the correct Table. **Root Operation** is used in the Medical and Surgical section **0** and Medical and Surgical-Related sections **1** through **9**. **Root Type** is used in the Ancillary sections **B** through **H** because the procedures in these sections are not operations. The *Introduction* of the ICD-10-PCS manual provides the definition for each root operation and root type, which are divided by section. Key criteria for abstracting each root operation are provided in the remaining chapters of this text and should be studied carefully.

Coders must read the procedure report and interpret what was done based on the definitions of the root operations or root types. Physicians are not required or expected to document using ICD-10-PCS definitions, but are allowed to document using the terminology they are most comfortable and familiar with. Coders will not find root operations described in the procedure report using the exact PCS terms (■ Figure 46-8, page 966). Even when physicians use words that are similar to root operations, such as *excision*, *resection*, or *removal*, the coder is obligated to interpret the physician's description in light of the PCS definitions. PCS OCGR A11 states the following:

> Many of the terms used to construct PCS codes are defined within the system. It is the coder's responsibility to determine what the documentation in the medical record equates to in the PCS definitions. The physician is

Procedure description: Appendectomy. Removed entire appendix laparoscopically.	
CORRECT Root Operation: **T - Resection** *cutting off all of a body part, without replacement*	
INCORRECT Root Operation: **P - Removal** *taking out or off a device from a body part*	
Explanation: Even though the documentation uses the word removed, do not use the Root Operation **Removal** because the PCS definition does not describe the procedure performed. The Root Operation **Removal** identifies taking devices out of the body. The Root Operation **Resection** describes cutting off a body part, such as the appendix.	

Figure 46-8 ■ Example of abstracting a root operation.

not expected to use the terms used in PCS code descriptions, nor is the coder required to query the physician when the correlation between the documentation and the defined PCS terms is clear.

Although you do not need to memorize specific codes or character values, you should plan to memorize the definitions of the most commonly used root operations and root types. While in the learning stage, always verify the definition of the root operation in the PCS manual.

Assign ICD-10-PCS Codes

Assigning PCS codes requires coders to locate the root operation in the Index then refer to a Table to build the code.

ICD-10-PCS Index

The Index uses two types of Main Terms for the Medical and Surgical section:

- The name of the root operation, such as **Excision**
- The composite medical term, such as *appendectomy*

Eponyms, such as *Nissan procedure*, do not appear as Main Terms.

When a composite medical term is listed, the Index provides a cross-reference to potential root operations. Coders cannot randomly choose the root operation; they must determine the specific root operations most appropriate for the case being coded.

Subterms that describe the anatomic sites or other variations of the root operation are indented under the Main Term. A partial code, which provides the first three to five characters of the code, is listed after the subterm. The first three characters of the partial code identify the appropriate Table to use.

ICD-10-PCS Tables

After locating the appropriate procedure in the Index and identifying the first three characters of the partial code, refer to the appropriate Table to build the rest of the code. Follow three steps to look up a PCS code in the tables:

1. Locate the Table using the first three characters of the partial code provided in the Index.

2. Build the code by locating the row in the Table that contains the appropriate body part value for Character 4. Then select the appropriate values for Characters 4, 5, 6, and 7 from within the same row of the Table.

3. Verify the character values by comparing each value to the documentation.

The ICD-10-PCS coding manual does not list a complete description for each full code because there are more than 78,000 codes. CMS offers a searchable electronic file with short and long code descriptions for all valid codes. Encoder software programs usually display the code description on the screen (■ Figure 46-9).

section	
	Medical and Surgical
body system	
	Gastrointestinal System
operations	
	Bypass: Altering the route of passage of the contents of a tubular body part
Code	
0D1B0Z4 ▾	Bypass Ileum to Cutaneous, Open Approach

Figure 46-9 ■ Example of a PCS code description in an encoder. *Source: SpeedeCoder, Reprinted with permission*

Arrange ICD-10-PCS Codes

Sequencing procedure codes is generally easier than sequencing diagnosis codes because there are fewer sequencing rules. When multiple procedures are performed, follow these general sequencing guidelines:

- Sequence as the first procedure the one most closely related to the principal diagnosis.
- When a procedure is required to care for a complication, sequence it before other related procedures.

- When a diagnostic or exploratory procedure is followed by a definitive treatment, and both procedures are related to the principal diagnosis, sequence the definitive procedure first and the diagnostic or exploratory procedure second.

ICD-10-PCS Medical and Surgical Section Guidelines provide guidance on coding multiple procedures (PCS OGCR B3.2). The PCS OGCR are discussed further in later chapters of this text.

CODING PRACTICE

Exercise 46.5   Introduction to the Steps of PCS Procedure Coding

Instructions: Fill in each blank with the correct term(s) from this section of the chapter.

1. What part of PCS functions as the Main Term in the Index and directs coders to the correct Table? _____

2. Which step in coding involves reading the procedure report and identifying the objective of the procedure and how it was accomplished? _____

3. In what part of the PCS Coding Manual can coders find the definitions of root operations and root types?_____

4. What part of PCS should coders plan to memorize? _____

5. What section of PCS OGCR provides guidelines on coding multiple procedures? _____

6. Are anatomic sites a Main Term or subterm in the Index? _____

7. What information do the first three characters of the partial code provide? _____

8. What is the third step of assigning PCS codes? _____

9. Which characters of the code are selected from the Table? _____

10. What information determines the first sequenced procedure? _____.

CHAPTER SUMMARY

In this chapter you learned that:

- ICD-10-PCS is a new coding system to be used by hospitals for coding inpatient procedures.

- The ICD-10-PCS manual contains the Introduction, ICD-10-PCS Official Guidelines for Coding and Reporting (OGCR), Index, Tables, and Appendices.

- ICD-10-PCS codes have a logical, consistent structure that contains seven alphanumeric positions, called characters.

- ICD-10-PCS OGCR are divided into five sections: Conventions, which are labeled beginning with the letter A; Medical and

Surgical Section Guidelines, which are labeled beginning with the letter B; Obstetric Section Guidelines, which are labeled beginning with the letter C, New Technology Section Guidelines, which are labeled beginning with the letter D, and Selection of the Principal Procedure.

- The three skills of an "Ace" coder—abstract, assign, and arrange—apply to coding procedures in ICD-10-PCS, but the mechanics are unique to this code set.

CONCEPT QUIZ

Take a moment to look back at your trip through ICD-10-PCS and solidify your skills. This is your opportunity to pull together everything you have learned.

Completion

Instructions: Write the term that completes each statement based on the information you learned in this chapter. Choose from the list below. Some choices may be used more than once and some choices may not be used at all. Refer to the discussion in this chapter and the Glossary at the end of this book if you need a little extra help.

approach(es)	multiaxial
body part(s)	qualifier(s)
body system(s)	root operation(s)
character(s)	section(s)
device(s)	standardized terminology
expandability	value(s)

1. ICD-10-PCS codes are constructed of seven _____ or positions, each with a distinct purpose and meaning.

2. _____ means that the structure of the code set allows new procedures to be easily incorporated.

3. _____ means that the code set includes definitions of the terminology it uses and each term must have only one meaning.

4. To build a PCS code, coders assign _____ to each character, based on specific characteristics of the procedure the physician performs.

5. Each section of the manual designates how each _____ of the code is used within that section.

6. The Medical and Surgical section has 31 possible values for the _____.

7. P, Upper Bones, is a(n) _____ value with the skeletal system.

8. The _____ describes the objective of the procedure.

9. Character 5 in the Medical and Surgical section provides definitions for the _____.

10. Assign value Z for Character 6 when there is no _____.

Multiple Choice

Instructions: Circle the letter of the best answer to each question based on the information you learned in this chapter. Refer to the discussion in this chapter and the Glossary at the end of this book if you need a little extra help.

1. What characteristic of PCS means that each position or character within a code number has a designated meaning or purpose?
   A. Completeness
   B. Standardized terminology
   C. Unique definitions
   D. Multiaxial nature

2. How many characters do all PCS codes have?
   A. 4
   B. 5
   C. 6
   D. 7

3. What services are billed using ICD-10-PCS?
   A. Physician services
   B. Hospital outpatient services
   C. Hospital inpatient services
   D. All of the above

4. Which characters of a code are used to identify a PCS Table?
   A. The first character
   B. The first two characters
   C. The first three characters
   D. The first four characters

5. What root operation is defined as *cutting off a portion of a body part without replacement*?
   A. Excision
   B. Resection
   C. Removal
   D. Bypass

6. What root operation is *ileostomy* an example of?
   A. Excision
   B. Resection
   C. Removal
   D. Bypass

7. What is the body part when coding an ileostomy?
   A. Gastrointestinal
   B. Small intestine
   C. Ilium
   D. Ileum

8. Which PCS Character functions as Main Terms in the Index?
   A. Body system
   B. Root operation
   C. Body part
   D. Approach

9. What part of the PCS manual is used to assign code values?
   A. Only the Index
   B. The Index and Tables
   C. The appendix
   D. Section descriptors

10. What resource supplements ICD-10-PCS Guidelines to provide direction for inpatient coding?
    A. AMA CPT Assistant
    B. ICD-10-PCS Supplement
    C. AHA Coding Clinic
    D. UB-04

KEEP ON CODING

Instructions: Using the PCS Index, look up the root operation and subterms listed. Write the partial code provided in the Index in the space provided.

Example: Alteration, Abdominal Wall. Partial Code *0W0F*

1. Alteration, Nasal Mucosa and Soft Tissue. Partial Code _____
2. Change device in, Diaphragm. Partial Code _____
3. Creation, Perineum, Male. Partial Code _____
4. Destruction, Cervix. Partial Code _____
5. Dilation, Esophagus. Partial Code _____
6. Extirpation, Anus. Partial Code _____
7. Fragmentation, Trachea. Partial Code _____
8. Inspection, Fallopian Tube. Partial Code _____
9. Map, Brain. Partial Code _____
10. Occlusion, Urethra. Partial Code _____
11. Reattachment, Tooth, Upper. Partial Code _____
12. Release, Nerve, Trigeminal. Partial Code _____
13. Repair, Jejunum. Partial Code _____
14. Supplement, Larynx. Partial Code _____
15. Transfer, Tendon, Head and Neck. Partial Code _____
16. Bypass, Duct, Hepatic, Left. Partial Code _____
17. Excision, Disc, Lumbosacral. Partial Code _____
18. Fusion, Metacarpophalangeal, Right. Partial Code _____
19. Release, Artery, Pulmonary Trunk. Partial Code _____
20. Supplement, Tendon, Foot, Left. Partial Code _____
21. Magnetic Resonance Imaging, Vein, Lower Extremity, Bilateral. Partial Code _____
22. Pharmacotherapy, for substance abuse, Naltrexone. Partial Code _____
23. Chiropractic Manipulation, Thoracic. Partial Code _____
24. Plain Radiography, Joint, Foot, Right. Partial Code _____
25. Change device in or on, Abdominal Wall. Partial Code _____

CODING CHALLENGE

Instructions: Look up the Table represented by the three-character partial code. Write out the values and names represented by the section, body system, and root operation.

Example: Table 021
Character 1, Section. Value: *0* Name: *Medical and Surgical*
Character 2, Body System. Value: *2* Name: *Heart and Great Vessels*
Character 3, Root Operation. Value: *1* Name: *Bypass*

1. Table B51

   Character 1, Section. Value: ___ Name: _____
   Character 2, Body System. Value: ___ Name: _____
   Character 3, Root Operation. Value: ___ Name: _____

2. Table 0H9

   Character 1, Section. Value: ___ Name: _____
   Character 2, Body System. Value: ___ Name: _____
   Character 3, Root Operation. Value: ___ Name: _____

3. Table 0KS

   Character 1, Section. Value: ___ Name: _____
   Character 2, Body System. Value: ___ Name: _____
   Character 3, Root Operation. Value: ___ Name: _____

4. Table 07L

   Character 1, Section. Value: ___ Name: _____
   Character 2, Body System. Value: ___ Name: _____
   Character 3, Root Operation. Value: ___ Name: _____

(*continued*)

(continued from page 969)

5. Table 04R

Character 1, Section. Value: ___ Name: _____

Character 2, Body System. Value: ___ Name: _____

Character 3, Root Operation. Value: ___ Name: _____

6. Table 10E

Character 1, Section. Value: ___ Name: _____

Character 2, Body System. Value: ___ Name: _____

Character 3, Root Operation. Value: ___ Name: _____

7. Table 2W3

Character 1, Section. Value: ___ Name: _____

Character 2, Anatomical Region. Value: ___ Name: _____

Character 3, Root Operation. Value: ___ Name: _____

8. Table BV2

Character 1, Section. Value: ___ Name: _____

Character 2, Body System. Value: ___ Name: _____

Character 3, Root Type. Value: ___ Name: _____

9. Table F07

Character 1, Section. Value: ___ Name: _____

Character 2, Section Qualifier. Value: ___ Name: _____

Character 3, Root Type. Value: ___ Name: _____

10. Table GZJ

Character 1, Section. Value: ___ Name: _____

Character 2, Body System. Value: ___ Name: _____

Character 3, Root Type. Value: ___ Name: _____

Abstracting for Medical and Surgical Procedures (Section 0)

Learning Objectives

After completing this chapter, you should have the skills to:

47.1 Spell and define the key words, medical terms, and abbreviations related to medical and surgical procedures. (Remember)

47.2 Adhere to PCS guidelines for Medical and Surgical procedures. (Apply)

47.3 Examine and abstract information from the medical record for each character of Medical and Surgical procedures. (Analyze)

Chapter Outline

- **Medical and Surgical Procedure Basics**
- **Coding Guidelines for Medical and Surgical Procedures**
- **Abstracting Medical and Surgical Procedures**

Key Terms and Abbreviations

diagnostic procedure
divided
External
Open

operative report
Percutaneous
Percutaneous Endoscopic
procedure report

therapeutic procedure
Via Natural or Artificial Opening
Via Natural or Artificial Opening Endoscopic

Via Natural or Artificial Opening Endoscopic with Percutaneous Endoscopic Assistance

In addition to the key terms listed here, students should know the terms defined within tables in this chapter.

INTRODUCTION

When you visit a new city, you might first go to the visitor's information center to gather some general information about the area before exploring individual attractions. Your introduction to the PCS Medical and Surgical Section is presented in two chapters. In this chapter, you become familiar with how the largest section in the PCS manual is structured and how to abstract information for each character of the code. Most importantly, you learn many of the definitions that are the cornerstone of ICD-10-PCS and are essential to accurate code assignment. Chapter 48 walks you through how to assign and arrange Medical and Surgical codes. Then, Chapters 49–53 discuss details about each root operation in this section of the coding manual.

MEDICAL AND SURGICAL PROCEDURE BASICS

Physicians perform a wide range of procedures on any body part. No coder can be familiar with every possible procedure, so it is important to apply medical terminology skills to combine familiar word roots, prefixes, and suffixes to define new procedural terms. Procedural terms combine the word root(s) for one or more body parts, such as *gastr/o*, with a suffix that describes the type of procedure, such as *-ectomy*. Refer to Table 25-1 in Chapter 25 to review procedural suffixes.

Although PCS establishes its own terminology and definitions of root operations, physicians will continue to use traditional Latin-based medical terms, such as *gastrectomy*, and eponyms, such as the Whipple procedure, which is one type of gastrectomy. Latin-based medical terms appear in the PCS Index and redirect coders to the most likely root operations. There is no direct correlation between medical terms and root operation definitions. Coders must read the operative report to determine exactly what was done and interpret this information in light of the root operations.

The surgical approach describes how the surgeon accessed the operative site. A variety of methods may be used for most procedures. The surgeon's decision is based on the reason the procedure is being done, the circumstances of the patient, the proven effectiveness of one approach over others, and other factors. In some cases, the surgeon may plan to use one approach then need to change to another approach due to complicating factors. For example, the surgeon may plan to perform an endoscopic cholecystectomy, but due to adhesions must change to an open approach. PCS definitions of the approach character are discussed in detail later in this chapter.

Procedure Reports

After completing a procedure, physicians prepare a **procedure report** or **operative report** that describes the details of what was done. The format varies with each physician or hospital but must include the following information:

- Date of procedure
- Name of procedure performed
- Names of the surgeon and all assistants
- Preprocedure or provisional diagnosis
- A detailed description of the procedure, including:
  - Patient preparation
  - Anesthesia
  - Instruments and supplies used
  - Incisions made
  - Visualized structures
  - Findings
  - Alterations performed
  - Tissue removed
  - Estimated blood loss
  - Closing process
  - Patient status
- Postprocedure diagnosis

The procedure report may be entered directly into an electronic health record (EHR) by the surgeon or be dictated, then transcribed. The procedure report is maintained in a designated section of the patient's overall medical record.

CODING PRACTICE

Exercise 47.1 Medical and Surgical Basics

Instructions: Use your medical terminology skills and resources to define the following terms, then look them up in the ICD-10-PCS Index.

Follow these steps:

- Use slash marks "/" to break down each term into its root(s) and suffix.
- Define the meaning of the word based on the meaning of each word part.
- Look up the term in the ICD-10-PCS Index, and write down the name(s) of root operation(s) the Index cross-references you to and the Table(s), if provided.
- Do not assign any codes.

CODING PRACTICE (continued)

Example: gastrectomy gastr/ectomy — Meaning *excision of the stomach* — Root Operation(s) *Excision, Resection*

1. angioplasty — Meaning _____ — Root Operation(s) _____
2. hysterectomy — Meaning _____ — Root Operation(s) _____
3. ovariocentesis — Meaning _____ — Root Operation(s) _____
4. arthrodesis — Meaning _____ — Root Operation(s) _____
5. herniorrhaphy — Meaning _____ — Root Operation(s) _____
6. adhesiolysis — Meaning _____ — Root Operation(s) _____
7. colostomy — Meaning _____ — Root Operation(s) _____
8. tracheotomy — Meaning _____ — Root Operation(s) _____
9. esophagoplication — Meaning _____ — Root Operation(s) _____
10. cholecystopexy — Meaning _____ — Root Operation(s) _____

CODING GUIDELINES FOR MEDICAL AND SURGICAL PROCEDURES

The Medical and Surgical Section is the largest Section of ICD-10-PCS, containing 31 body systems and 31 root operations, and comprising approximately 85% of PCS. ICD-10-PCS provides guidelines for Medical and Surgical codes in section B of the PCS OGCR. Five subdivisions of the guidelines, B2 through B6, correspond to each character within a Medical and Surgical code.

Characters of Medical and Surgical Procedures

The seven characters of Medical and Surgical PCS codes are summarized below. Information later in this chapter discusses in detail how to abstract needed information from the medical records.

- *Character 1: Section*—The Section value for Medical and Surgical is **0**. The characters of Medical and Surgical procedure codes are shown in ■ TABLE 47-1.

- *Character 2: Body System*—The second character in the Medical and Surgical Section defines the body system, general physiological system, or anatomic region. PCS divides most organ systems into multiple body system values in order to achieve a high level of granularity (*detail*). The Index is organized with the root operation as the Main Term with the first-level subterm often being the body system. Coders must select the most specific body system value available, which is often more specific than an anatomic system. Search for a subterm that identifies the specific body system—such as **Joint, Knee**—before selecting a subterm for the broader anatomic region, such as **Knee Region**.

- *Character 3: Root Operation*—The Medical and Surgical Section has 31 root operations, the most of any Section. Root operations are the core of PCS coding because they serve as Main Terms in the Index. Coders cannot assign a root operation based on the common meaning of a word such as "removal" or "excision;" they must apply the full definition that PCS provides in the Tables (PCS OGCR B3.1a). The PCS definition of all root operations appears in the appendix of most ICD-10-PCS coding manuals.

- *Character 4: Body Part*—The body part character identifies the specific anatomic site where the physician performed the procedure. In most cases, the Index directs coders not only to the correct Table, but also to the correct Character 4 value.

- *Character 5: Approach*—The approach character identifies how the surgeon accessed the operative site. Every code must be assigned an approach value from the PCS table. The Table lists only the approach values applicable to the root operation and body part. The seven values for approach in PCS are:

  - Open (0)
  - Percutaneous (3)
  - Percutaneous Endoscopic (4)
  - Via Natural or Artificial Opening (7)
  - Via Natural or Artificial Opening Endoscopic (8)
  - Via Natural or Artificial Opening Endoscopic with Percutaneous Endoscopic Assistance (F)
  - External (X)

- *Character 6: Device*—The device character identifies the type of material intentionally left in a patient for a

Table 47-1 ■ **SEVEN CHARACTERS OF MEDICAL AND SURGICAL PROCEDURES**

1	2	3	4	5	6	7
Section 0	Body System	Root Operation	Body Part	Approach	Device	Qualifier

therapeutic reason at the conclusion of a procedure. Medical equipment and supplies used to perform a procedure, as well as sutures, radiological markers, and temporary postoperative wound drains, *are not coded as devices* in PCS. Every code must be assigned a device value from the PCS table. The Table lists only the device values applicable to the root operation and body part. If a device is not left in the patient, select the value **Z No device** from the PCS table.

- *Character 7: Qualifier*—The qualifier character describes a wide range of additional attributes that may be applicable to a procedure. Every code must be assigned a qualifier value from the PCS table that corresponds to the root operation and body part. The Table lists only the qualifiers applicable to the root operation and body part. If there is no information to be reported for the qualifier, select the value **Z No qualifier** from the PCS table.

Official Guidelines for Coding and Reporting

PCS OGCR for Medical and Surgical procedures comprises section B of the guidelines, which is organized by character:

- B2 Body System
- B3 Root Operation
- B4 Body Part
- B5 Approach
- B6 Device
- No guidelines are provided for Character 7 Qualifier

PCS OGCR appears in most publishers' editions of the ICD-10-PCS coding manual and can be downloaded from the CMS website at **www.cms.gov**. Guidelines are updated annually on October 1.

Guidelines explain general coding rules and how to handle unusual exceptions. The following information highlights general guidelines for each section and summarizes additional detailed guidelines. PCS OGCR lists examples for each guideline that are not repeated here. Coders should become intimately familiar with the guidelines and example and review them frequently. If you are already familiar with CPT coding for physicians, be careful not to confuse CPT guidelines with PCS guidelines. The two are not comparable and are sometimes contradictory.

B2 Body System Guidelines

General guidelines for B2 Body System state that procedure codes in the general **Anatomical Regions** body systems can be used when the procedure is performed on an anatomic region rather than a specific body part. Body systems specified as *upper* (as in **Upper Arteries**) identify areas located above the diaphragm. Body systems specified as *lower* (as in **Lower Arteries**) identify areas located below the diaphragm.

B3 Root Operation Guidelines

General guidelines for B3 Root Operation emphasize that the full definition of a PCS root operation must be applied to determine the appropriate code. Components of a procedure specified in the root operation definition and explanation are not coded separately. Procedural steps necessary to reach the operative site and close the operative site, including anastomosis of a tubular body part, are not coded separately (PCS OGCR B3.1).

Multiple procedures are coded when (PCS OGCR B3.2):

- The same root operation is performed on different PCS body parts. Assign separate codes for the root operation on each body part.

- The same root operation is repeated in multiple anatomic sites that are classified into one PCS body part. Assign duplicate codes for the same root operation and same body part.

- Multiple root operations with distinct objectives are performed on the same PCS body part. Assign separate codes for the each root operation on the same body parts.

- The intended root operation is attempted using one approach, but is converted to a different approach. Assign separate codes for each approach on the same root operation and body part.

When a procedure is discontinued or incomplete (PCS OGCR B3.2), code the procedure to the root operation performed. If a procedure is discontinued before any other root operation is performed, code the root operation **Inspection** of the body part or anatomic region inspected.

Biopsy procedures (PCS OGCR B3.4) are coded using the root operations Excision, Extraction, or Drainage and the Character 7 Qualifier **Diagnostic**. If a diagnostic Excision, Extraction, or Drainage procedure (biopsy) is followed by a more definitive procedure at the same procedure site, such as Destruction, Excision, or Resection, code both the biopsy and the more definitive treatment. Code the biopsy using **Diagnostic** in Character 7. Code the definitive procedure using **No qualifier** or other appropriate value listed in the PCS Table for Character 7.

Code the body part that specifies the deepest layer reached when if the root operations Excision, Repair, or Inspection are performed on overlapping layers of the musculoskeletal system (PCS OGCR 3.5).

PCS OGCR B3 also provides guidelines on coding as many specific root operations. These guidelines are discussed in later chapters of this text where individual root operations are covered.

B4 Body Part Guidelines

General guidelines for B4 Body Part provide instructions on how to code the body part in situations where there might be confusion:

- If a procedure is performed on a portion of a body part that does not have a separate PCS body part value, code the next largest body part value.

- If the prefix *peri-* is combined with a body part name to identify the documented site of the procedure, and the site of the procedure is not further specified, then code to the most specific named PCS body part.

- If a procedure is performed on a continuous section of a tubular body part, code the body part value corresponding to the furthest anatomical site from the point of entry.

Guidelines B4.2 through B4.8 discuss branches of body parts; bilateral body part values, coronary arteries; tendons, ligaments, bursae, and fascia near a joint; skin, subcutaneous tissue and fascia overlying a joint; fingers and toes; and the upper and lower intestinal tract.

B5 Approach Guidelines

Guidelines for B4 Approach discuss details on how to assign certain approach values for unusual situations:

- Code the Open approach if open procedures use endoscopic assistance through the same access site.
- Code the External approach if procedures are performed within an orifice on structures that are visible without the aid of instrumentation such as an endoscope to visualize the site. This includes the mouth, tonsils, and visible portions of the ear, nose, anus, and vagina.
- Code the Percutaneous approach if procedures are performed percutaneously via a device placed for the procedure.

B6 Device Guidelines

A device is coded in Character 6 only if a device remains after the procedure is completed. In limited root operations, PCS provides Character 7 Qualifier values **Temporary** and **Intraoperative** for specific procedures where the purpose of the device is to be utilized for a brief duration during the procedure or current inpatient stay. Materials such as sutures, ligatures, radiological markers, and temporary post-operative wound drains are considered integral to performing a procedure and are not coded as PCS devices. Procedures performed on a device only and not on a body part are specified in the root operations Change, Irrigation, Removal, and Revision. A separate procedure to put in a drainage device is coded to the root operation Drainage.

SUCCESS STEP

PCS is unique among medical coding systems because it provides standard, official definitions for each character of the code. Although it may feel intimidating to memorize definitions, this feature makes the system user-friendly and logical.

ABSTRACTING MEDICAL AND SURGICAL PROCEDURES

Abstracting Medical and Surgical procedures requires abstracting unique information for each character. These criteria are discussed next. Separate Key Criteria for Abstracting tables are provided for each character of the PCS code.

Abstracting the Body System (Character 2)

Coders should be familiar with the PCS body systems and verify that the code they ultimately select is consistent with the correct body system value. PCS divides all anatomic systems except the endocrine system into multiple values (■ TABLE 47-2) for greater specificity. You must be able to identify the body system to locate the correct subterms when using the Index.

Table 47-2 ■ MEDICAL AND SURGICAL CHARACTER 2: BODY SYSTEM VALUES WITH ORGAN SYSTEM

Value	PCS Body System Description	Organ System
0	Central Nervous System	Nervous system
1	Peripheral Nervous System	
2	Heart and Great Vessels	
3	Upper Arteries	
4	Lower Arteries	Cardiovascular system
5	Upper Veins	
6	Lower Veins	
7	Lymphatic and Hemic System	Blood and immune system
8	Eye	Special senses
9	Ear, Nose, Sinus	Special senses (Ear) and Respiratory system
B	Respiratory System	
C	Mouth and Throat	
D	Gastrointestinal System	Digestive system
F	Hepatobiliary System and Pancreas	
G	Endocrine System	Endocrine system
H	Skin and Breast	
J	Subcutaneous Tissue and Fascia	Integumentary system
K	Muscles	
L	Tendons	Muscular system
M	Bursae and Ligaments	
N	Head and Facial Bones	
P	Upper Bones	
Q	Lower Bones	Skeletal system
R	Upper Joints	
S	Lower Joints	
T	Urinary System	
U	Female Reproductive System	Genitourinary system
V	Male Reproductive System	
W	Anatomical Regions, General	
X	Anatomical Regions, Upper Extremities	Body areas
Y	Anatomical Regions, Lower Extremities	

Source: Adapted from Department of Health and Human Services, Centers for Medicare and Medicaid Services, ICD-10-PCS Coding Manual.

For example, you should know that the median nerve is part of the nervous system, but you also need to identify whether it is part of the central or peripheral nervous systems because these are subdivided in PCS. Knowing the options PCS presents for a traditional anatomic system makes it easier to navigate the Index when you move on to the next step, assigning codes.

Body system values **W**, **X**, and **Y** describe Anatomic Regions, which are used when a procedure is performed on an area that is larger than a specific body part (PCS OGCR B2.1a). Do not use these body system values when a more specific value is available.

For example, for a procedure on the elbow, look up the Main Term for the root operation, then the subterm **Joint**, then the second-level subterm **Elbow**. Use the subterm **Elbow Region** only when an area larger than the joint is affected. Examples of situations in which an *Anatomic Region* should be used include the following types of procedures:

- Control of postprocedural bleeding in an extremity
- Amputation of all or part of an extremity
- Drainage of a body cavity

CODING PRACTICE

| Exercise 47.2 | Abstracting the Body System |

Instructions: Refer to Table 47-2, Medical and Surgical Character 2: Body System Values with Organ System. Using your knowledge of anatomy, identify the PCS body system each anatomic site belongs to. Refer to anatomic illustrations elsewhere in this text or in your own resources when needed. Write the character and name of the PCS body system on the lines provided.

1. Extraocular muscle. Character _____ Name _____

2. Left carotid artery. Character _____ Name _____

3. Thyroid gland. Character _____ Name _____

4. Right hip tendon. Character _____ Name _____

5. Cervical vertebral joint. Character _____ Name _____

Abstracting the Root Operation (Character 3)

Identifying the correct root operation is the basis of ICD-10-PCS coding, so coders must learn the differences between similar root operations. This enables them to abstract appropriately. Physicians are not expected to use PCS terminology when documenting. Coders must read what physicians document and equate it to the definitions provided by PCS (PCS OGCR A11). To assign a root operation, its full definition in the PCS manual must be applied (PCS OGCR B3.1a). If the full definition is not applicable, continue searching for another root operation.

Refer to PCS OGCR B3, which provides further details on root operations. Then, follow key criteria for abstracting Medical and Surgical procedures to identify the correct root operation.

To abstract for Medical and Surgical procedures, coders must read the procedure report, then use the resources in this chapter and the PCS coding manual to follow these steps:

1. Answer the questions in the general abstracting table (■ TABLE 47-3) to get a basic understanding of the procedure.

2. Refer to (■ TABLE 47-4) Key Criteria for Abstracting Root Operations. Answer the questions in the first column. One question should be answered *Yes*, the rest should be answered *No*.

3. For the Root Operation Question that was answered *Yes*, refer to the middle column to identify the root operations that could apply.

4. Identify the one root operation that matches the procedure documented using one of the following sources:

   - Refer to the right column of this table to locate the specific Key Criteria for Abstracting table from later chapters of this text. These abstracting tables guide you through the listed root operations in detail.

   - ■ Table 47-5 (page 978), Comparison of Medical and Surgical Root Operations, divides root operations into groups of procedures with similar objectives. Use this table as a resource to help quickly distinguish between similar root operations.

   - Look up the definition of each of the applicable root operations in the ICD-10-PCS coding manual appendix, "Root Operation Definitions" (■ TABLE 47-6, page 979).

5. Write down the root operation name because it will be the Main Term when you use the Index to assign the code, which is discussed in Chapter 48 of this text.

6. Repeat the abstracting process for each procedure that was performed.

PCS OGCR B3 provides several guidelines on how to code the root operation and how to code multiple procedures in situations where the choice might be unclear. These were summarized earlier in this chapter.

Abstracting criteria for Medical and Surgical-Related procedures and Ancillary procedures are presented in Chapters 54 and 55 of this text.

Table 47-3   ■   **KEY CRITERIA FOR ABSTRACTING MEDICAL AND SURGICAL PROCEDURES (GENERAL)**

❑ What is the stated procedure?
❑ What organ or body part is involved?
❑ How many sites are treated?
❑ What is the laterality (if applicable)?
❑ Is the procedure description what you would expect based on the name of the procedure?
❑ What surgical approach is used? (*Refer to Table 47-9, Key Criteria for Abstracting the Approach.*)
❑ Is a therapeutic device left in the patient after the procedure? (*Refer to Table 47-11, Key Criteria for Abstracting the Device.*)
❑ Was more than one procedure, or a combined procedure, performed?

Source: © PB Resources, Inc. Used with permission.

Table 47-4   ■   **KEY CRITERIA FOR ABSTRACTING ROOT OPERATIONS**

Root Operation Questions	Root Operation (Value)	Key Criteria for Abstracting (in this text)
❑ Did the procedure take out some or all of a body part without replacement?	Destruction (5) Detachment (6) Excision (B) Extraction (D) Resection (T)	See Table 49-9
❑ Did the procedure take out solids, fluids, or gases from a body part?	Drainage (9) Extirpation (C) Fragmentation (F)	See Table 52-8
❑ Did the procedure involve cutting or separation only, within or around a body part?	Division (8) Release (N)	See Table 52-11
❑ Did the procedure put in, put back, or move some or all of a body part?	Reattachment (M) Reposition (S) Transfer (X) Transplantation (Y)	See Table 50-7
❑ Did the procedure alter the diameter or route of a tubular body part?	Bypass (1) Dilation (7) Occlusion (L) Restriction (V)	See Table 51-7
❑ Did the procedure involve an external device left in place in, on, or in replacement of a body part?	Change (2) Insertion (H) Removal (P) Replacement (R) Revision (W) Supplement (U)	See Table 53-11
❑ Did the procedure involve examination only?	Inspection (J) Map (K)	See Table 52-14
Operations Involving Other Repairs ❑ Did the procedure stop or attempt to stop postprocedural or other acute bleeding? ❑ Did the procedure restore a body part to its normal structure?	Control (3) Repair (Q)	See Table 53-14
Operations Involving Other Objectives ❑ Did the procedure render a joint or articular body part immobile? ❑ Was the procedure for cosmetic purposes only, without affecting the function of the body part? ❑ Did the procedure use biological or synthetic material to form a new body part to replicate a missing body part?	Fusion (G) Alteration (0) Creation (4)	See Table 53-18

Source: © PB Resources, Inc. Used with permission.

Table 47-5 ■ **COMPARISON OF ROOT OPERATIONS**

Group: Root Operations That Take Out Some or All of a Body Part

Root Operation	Value	Objective of Procedure	Procedure Site	Example
Destruction	5	Eradicating without replacement	Some/all of a body part	Fulguration of endometrium
Detachment	6	Cutting out/off without replacement	Extremity only, any level	Amputation above elbow
Excision	B	Cutting out/off without replacement	Some of a body part	Breast lumpectomy
Extraction	D	Pulling out/off without replacement	Some/all of a body part	Suction D&C
Resection	T	Cutting out/off without replacement	All of a body part	Total mastectomy

Group: Root Operations That Take Out Solids/Fluids/Gases from a Body Part

Root Operation	Value	Objective of Procedure	Procedure Site	Example
Drainage	9	Taking/letting out	Fluids and/or gases from a body part	Incision and drainage
Extirpation	C	Taking/cutting out	Solid matter in a body part	Thrombectomy
Fragmentation	F	Breaking into pieces	Solid matter within a body part	Lithotripsy

Group: Root Operations Involving Cutting or Separation Only

Root Operation	Value	Objective of Procedure	Procedure Site	Example
Division	8	Cutting into/separating	Within a body part	Neurotomy
Release	N	Freeing a body part from constraint	Around a body part	Adhesiolysis

Group: Root Operations That Put In/Put Back or Move Some/All of a Body Part

Root Operation	Value	Objective of Procedure	Procedure Site	Example
Reattachment	M	Putting back a detached body part	Some/all of a body part	Reattach finger
Reposition	S	Moving a body part to normal or other suitable location	Some/all of a body part	Move undescended testicle
Transfer	X	Moving a body part to function for a similar body part	Some/all of a body part	Skin transfer flap
Transplantation	Y	Putting in a living body part from a person/animal	Some/all of a body part	Kidney transplant

Group: Root Operations That Alter the Diameter or Route of a Tubular Body Part

Root Operation	Value	Objective of Procedure	Procedure Site	Example
Bypass	1	Altering route of passage of contents	Tubular body part	Coronary artery bypass graft (CABG)
Dilation	7	Expanding naturally or artificially created orifice/lumen	Tubular body part	Percutaneous transluminal coronary angioplasty (PTCA)
Occlusion	L	Completely closing naturally or artificially created orifice/lumen	Tubular body part	Fallopian tube ligation
Restriction	V	Partially closing naturally or artificially created orifice/lumen	Tubular body part	Gastroesophageal fundoplication

Group: Root Operations That Always Involve Devices

Root Operation	Value	Objective of Procedure	Procedure Site	Example
Change	2	Exchanging device without cutting/puncturing	In/on a body part	Drainage tube change
Insertion	H	Putting in nonbiological device	In/on a body part	Central line insertion
Removal	P	Taking out device	In/on a body part	Central line removal
Replacement	R	Putting in device that replaces a body part	Some/all of a body part	Total hip replacement
Revision	W	Correcting a malfunctioning/displaced device	In/on a body part	Revision of pacemaker
Supplement	U	Putting in device that reinforces or augments a body part	In/on a body part	Abdominal wall herniorrhaphy using mesh

Table 47-5 ■ *(continued)*

Group: Root Operations Involving Examination Only			
Root Operation	**Value**	**Objective of Procedure**	**Procedure Site**	**Example**
Inspection	J	Visual/manual exploration	Some/all of a body part	Diagnostic cystoscopy
Map	K	Locating electrical impulses/functional areas	Brain/cardiac conduction mechanism	Cardiac electro-physiological study

Group: Root Operations That Define Other Repairs			
Root Operation	**Value**	**Objective of Procedure**	**Procedure Site**	**Example**
Control	3	Stopping/attempting to stop postprocedural or other acute bleeding	Anatomic region	Post-prostatectomy bleeding control, bleeding ulcer
Repair	Q	Restoring body part to its normal structure	Some/all of a body part	Suture laceration

Group: Root Operations That Define Other Objectives			
Root Operation	**Value**	**Objective of Procedure**	**Procedure Site**	**Example**
Alteration	0	Modifying body part for cosmetic purposes without affecting function	Some/all of a body part	Face lift
Creation	4	Using biological or synthetic material to form a new body part that replicates the anatomic structure or function of a missing body part	Perineum, valve	Sex change/artificial vagina/penis, atrioventricular valve creation
Fusion	G	Unification or immobilization	Joint or articular body part	Spinal fusion

Source: Department of Health and Human Services, Centers for Medicare and Medicaid Services, ICD-10-PCS Coding Manual.

Table 47-6 ■ **ROOT OPERATION DEFINITIONS IN ALPHABETICAL ORDER, WITH EXPLANATIONS AND EXAMPLES**

Value	Root Operation	Description
0	Alteration	**Definition:** Modifying the anatomic structure of a body part without affecting the function of the body part. **Explanation:** Principal purpose is to improve appearance. **Includes/Examples:** Face lift, breast augmentation
1	Bypass	**Definition:** Altering the route of passage of the contents of a tubular body part. **Explanation:** Rerouting contents of a body part to a downstream area of the normal route, to a similar route and body part, or to an abnormal route and dissimilar body part. Includes one or more anastomoses, with or without the use of a device. **Includes/Examples:** Coronary artery bypass, colostomy formation
2	Change	**Definition:** Taking out or off a device from a body part and putting back an identical or similar device in or on the same body part without cutting or puncturing the skin or a mucous membrane. **Explanation:** All Change procedures are coded using the approach External. **Includes/Examples:** Urinary catheter change, gastrostomy tube change
3	Control	**Definition:** Stopping, or attempting to stop, postprocedural or other acute bleeding. **Explanation:** The site of the bleeding is coded as an anatomic region and not to a specific body part. **Includes/Examples:** Control of post-prostatectomy hemorrhage, control of intracranial subdural hemorrhage, control of bleeding duodenal ulcer, control of retroperitoneal hemorrhage
4	Creation	**Definition:** Putting in or on biological or synthetic material to form a new body part that to the extent possible replicates the anatomic structure or function of an absent body part. **Explanation:** Used for gender reassignment surgery and corrective procedures in individuals with congenital anomalies. **Includes/Examples:** Creation of vagina in a male, creation of right and left atrioventricular valve from common atrioventricular valve
5	Destruction	**Definition:** Physical eradication of all or a portion of a body part by the direct use of energy, force, or a destructive agent. **Explanation:** None of the body part is physically taken out. **Includes/Examples:** Fulguration of rectal polyp, cautery of skin lesion

(continued)

Table 47-6   ■   (*continued*)

Value	Root Operation	Description
6	Detachment	**Definition:** Cutting off all or a portion of the upper or lower extremities. **Explanation:** The body part value is the site of the detachment, with a qualifier if applicable to further specify the level where the extremity was detached. **Includes/Examples:** Below-knee amputation, disarticulation of shoulder
7	Dilation	**Definition:** Expanding an orifice or the lumen of a tubular body part. **Explanation:** The orifice can be a natural orifice or an artificially created orifice. Accomplished by stretching a tubular body part using intraluminal pressure or by cutting part of the orifice or wall of the tubular body part. **Includes/Examples:** Percutaneous transluminal angioplasty, pyloromyotomy
8	Division	**Definition:** Cutting into a body part without draining fluids and/or gases from the body part in order to separate or transect a body part. **Explanation:** All or a portion of the body part is separated into two or more portions. **Includes/Examples:** Spinal cordotomy, osteotomy
9	Drainage	**Definition:** Taking or letting out fluids and/or gases from a body part. **Explanation:** The Diagnostic qualifier is used to identify drainage procedures that are biopsies. **Includes/Examples:** Thoracentesis, incision and drainage
B	Excision	**Definition:** Cutting out or off, without replacement, a portion of a body part. **Explanation:** The Diagnostic qualifier is used to identify excision procedures that are biopsies. **Includes/Examples:** Partial nephrectomy, liver biopsy
C	Extirpation	**Definition:** Taking or cutting out solid matter from a body part. **Explanation:** The solid matter may be an abnormal by-product of a biological function or a foreign body; it may be imbedded in a body part or in the lumen of a tubular body part. The solid matter may or may not have been previously broken into pieces. **Includes/Examples:** Thrombectomy, choledocholithotomy
D	Extraction	**Definition:** Pulling or stripping out or off all or a portion of a body part by the use of force. **Explanation:** The Diagnostic qualifier is used to identify extraction procedures that are biopsies. **Includes/Examples:** Dilation and curettage, vein stripping
F	Fragmentation	**Definition:** Breaking solid matter in a body part into pieces. **Explanation:** Physical force (e.g., manual, ultrasonic) applied directly or indirectly is used to break the solid matter into pieces. The solid matter may be an abnormal by-product of a biological function or a foreign body. The pieces of solid matter are not taken out. **Includes/Examples:** Extracorporeal shockwave lithotripsy, transurethral lithotripsy
G	Fusion	**Definition:** Joining together portions of an articular body part, rendering the articular body part immobile. **Explanation:** The body part is joined together by fixation device, bone graft, or other means. **Includes/Examples:** Spinal fusion, ankle arthrodesis
H	Insertion	**Definition:** Putting in a nonbiological appliance that monitors, assists, performs, or prevents a physiological function but does not physically take the place of a body part. **Includes/Examples:** Insertion of radioactive implant, insertion of central venous catheter
J	Inspection	**Definition:** Visually and/or manually exploring a body part. **Explanation:** Visual exploration may be performed with or without optical instrumentation. Manual exploration may be performed directly or through intervening body layers. **Includes/Examples:** Diagnostic arthroscopy, exploratory laparotomy
K	Map	**Definition:** Locating the route of passage of electrical impulses and/or locating functional areas in a body part. **Explanation:** Applicable only to the cardiac conduction mechanism and the central nervous system. **Includes/Examples:** Cardiac mapping, cortical mapping
L	Occlusion	**Definition:** Completely closing an orifice or the lumen of a tubular body part. **Explanation:** The orifice can be a natural orifice or an artificially created orifice. **Includes/Examples:** Fallopian tube ligation, ligation of inferior vena cava

Table 47-6   ■   (*continued*)

Value	Root Operation	Description
M	Reattachment	**Definition:** Putting back in or on all or a portion of a separated body part to its normal location or other suitable location. **Explanation:** Vascular circulation and nervous pathways may or may not be reestablished. **Includes/Examples:** Reattachment of hand, reattachment of avulsed kidney
N	Release	**Definition:** Freeing a body part from an abnormal physical constraint by cutting or by the use of force. **Explanation:** Some of the restraining tissue may be taken out, but none of the body part is taken out. **Includes/Examples:** Adhesiolysis, carpal tunnel release
P	Removal	**Definition:** Taking out or off a device from a body part. **Explanation:** If a device is taken out and a similar device put in without cutting or puncturing the skin or mucous membrane, the procedure is coded to the root operation Change. Otherwise, the procedure for taking out a device is coded to the root operation Removal. **Includes/Examples:** Drainage tube removal, cardiac pacemaker removal
Q	Repair	**Definition:** Restoring, to the extent possible, a body part to its normal anatomic structure and function. **Explanation:** Used only when the method to accomplish the repair is not one of the other root operations. **Includes/Examples:** Colostomy takedown, suture of laceration
R	Replacement	**Definition:** Putting in or on biological or synthetic material that physically takes the place and/or function of all or a portion of a body part. **Explanation:** The body part may have been taken out or replaced, or may be taken out, physically eradicated, or rendered nonfunctional during the Replacement procedure. A Removal procedure is coded for taking out the device used in a previous replacement procedure. **Includes/Examples:** Total hip replacement, bone graft, free skin graft
S	Reposition	**Definition:** Moving to its normal location, or other suitable location, all or a portion of a body part. **Explanation:** The body part is moved to a new location from an abnormal location or from a normal location where it is not functioning correctly. The body part may or may not be cut out or off to be moved to the new location. **Includes/Examples:** Reposition of undescended testicle, fracture reduction
T	Resection	**Definition:** Cutting out or off, without replacement, all of a body part. **Includes/Examples:** Total nephrectomy, total lobectomy of lung
V	Restriction	**Definition:** Partially closing an orifice or the lumen of a tubular body part. **Explanation:** The orifice can be a natural orifice or an artificially created orifice. **Includes/Examples:** Esophagogastric fundoplication, cervical cerclage
W	Revision	**Definition:** Correcting, to the extent possible, a portion of a malfunctioning device or the position of a displaced device. **Explanation:** Revision can include correcting a malfunctioning or displaced device by taking out or putting in components of the device, such as a screw or pin. **Includes/Examples:** Adjustment of position of pacemaker lead, recementing of hip prosthesis
U	Supplement	**Definition:** Putting in or on biological or synthetic material that physically reinforces and/or augments the function of a portion of a body part. **Explanation:** The biological material is nonliving or is living and from the same individual. The body part may have been previously replaced, and the Supplement procedure is performed to physically reinforce and/or augment the function of the replaced body part. **Includes/Examples:** Herniorrhaphy using mesh, free nerve graft, mitral valve ring annuloplasty, put a new acetabular liner in a previous hip replacement
X	Transfer	**Definition:** Moving, without taking out, all or a portion of a body part to another location to take over the function of all or a portion of a body part. **Explanation:** The body part transferred remains connected to its vascular and nervous supply. **Includes/Examples:** Tendon transfer, skin pedicle flap transfer
Y	Transplantation	**Definition:** Putting in or on all or a portion of a living body part taken from another individual or animal to physically take the place and/or function of all or a portion of a similar body part. **Explanation:** The native body part may or may not be taken out, and the transplanted body part may take over all or a portion of its function. **Includes/Examples:** Kidney transplant, heart transplant

Source: Department of Health and Human Services, Centers for Medicare and Medicaid Services, ICD-10-PCS Coding Manual.

CODING PRACTICE

Exercise 47.3 Abstracting the Root Operation

Instructions: Refer to Table 47-5, Comparison of Root Operations. Locate the name of the root operation in the first column of the table, then the value, objective, site, or example requested in the appropriate column. Write your answer to the question in the space provided.

1. What procedure is an example of the root operation Extirpation? _____

2. What is the objective of the procedure for the root operation Fragmentation? _____

3. What is the objective of the procedure for the root operation Restriction? _____

4. What is the objective of the procedure for the root operation Removal? _____

5. What is the procedure site for the root operation Fusion?
_____

6. What is the value for the root operation Transplantation?
_____

7. What procedure is an example of the root operation Map?
_____

8. What procedure is an example of the root operation Occlusion?
_____

9. What is the procedure site for the root operation Detachment?
_____

10. What is the value of the root operation Repair?
_____

Abstracting the Body Part (Character 4)

The PCS Body Part character identifies the anatomic site where the procedure is performed. The definition of each body part value in the Medical and Surgical Section is unique to each body system. For example, in body system **8 Eye**, the body part value **1** is **Left Eye**. In body system **L Tendons**, the body part value **1** is **Right Shoulder Tendon**. Body parts appear as first- or second-level subterms in the Index. Refer to ■ TABLE 47-7, Key Criteria for Abstracting the Body Part.

PCS subdivides some organs and other anatomic sites into multiple body part values to achieve greater specificity. For example, for some root operations the large intestine has multiple values. Coders must review the available body part values in a specific root operation table and choose the one applicable to the current procedure. The breakdown of body parts for the large intestine is as follows:

- Large Intestine—Use this value when the procedure is performed on the entire large intestine.

- Large Intestine, Right—Use this value when the procedure is performed on the right half of the intestine.

- Large Intestine, Left—Use this value when the procedure is performed on the left half of the intestine.

- Transverse Colon—Use this value when the procedure is performed only on the transverse segment of the large intestine.

- Descending Colon—Use this value when the procedure is performed only on the descending segment of the large intestine.

- Sigmoid Colon—Use this value when the procedure is performed only on the sigmoid segment of the large intestine.

The PCS Appendix, "Body Part Key," identifies the correct PCS body part value for many anatomic sites. For example, *acetabulofemoral joint* is classified to the PCS value **Hip Joint, Right** or **Hip Joint, Left**. Use of the "Body Part Key" is discussed in detail in Chapter 48, "Assigning Codes for Medical and Surgical Procedures."

PCS OGCR B4 provides several guidelines on how to code the body part in situations where the choice might be unclear. These were summarized earlier in this chapter.

Table 47-7 ■ KEY CRITERIA FOR ABSTRACTING THE BODY PART

- ❏ What organ or body part is involved?
- ❏ What body system is the site part of?
- ❏ How many sites are treated?
- ❏ What is the laterality (if applicable)?
- ❏ Does PCS subdivide the anatomic site into multiple segments or lobes for detailed body system or body part values?
  - If so, which segment applies to this procedure? (Refer to PCS coding manual Index, Tables, and Body Part Key.)

CODING PRACTICE

Exercise 47.4   Abstracting the Body Part

Instructions: Answer the abstracting questions about the following procedural statements. Do not assign any codes.

1. Closed reduction of nasal bone fracture

   a. What organ or body part is involved? _____

   b. What body system is the site part of? _____

   c. How many sites are treated? _____

   d. What is the laterality (if applicable)? _____

   e. Does PCS subdivide the anatomic site into multiple segments or lobes for detailed body system or body part values? If so, which segment applies to this procedure? _____

2. Banding of esophageal vein

   a. What organ or body part is involved? _____

   b. What body system is the site part of? _____

   c. How many sites are treated? _____

   d. What is the laterality (if applicable)? _____

   e. Does PCS subdivide the anatomic site into multiple segments or lobes for detailed body system or body part values? If so, which segment applies to this procedure? _____

3. Fine-needle aspiration of the upper lobe of the right lung

   a. What organ or body part is involved? _____

   b. What body system is the site part of? _____

   c. How many sites are treated? _____

   d. What is the laterality (if applicable)? _____

   e. Does PCS subdivide the anatomic site into multiple segments or lobes for detailed body system or body part values? If so, which segment applies to this procedure? _____

4. Exchange of a drainage tube from the right acetabulofemoral joint following a total hip replacement

   a. What organ or body part is involved? _____

   b. What body system is the site part of? _____

   c. How many sites are treated? _____

   d. What is the laterality (if applicable)? _____

   e. Does PCS subdivide the anatomic site into multiple segments or lobes for detailed body system or body part values? If so, which segment applies to this procedure? _____

5. Placement of a pacemaker lead in the left atrium

   a. What organ or body part is involved? _____

   b. What body system is the site part of? _____

   c. How many sites are treated? _____

   d. What is the laterality (if applicable)? _____

   e. Does PCS subdivide the anatomic site into multiple segments or lobes for detailed body system or body part values? If so, which segment applies to this procedure? _____

Abstracting the Approach (Character 5)

The Approach character identifies the surgical technique used to reach the site of the procedure. The Medical and Surgical section uses seven different values to define the approach (■ TABLE 47-8). An appendix in most ICD-10-PCS manuals defines each approach. PCS OGCR B5 discusses specific coding situations related to an open approach with percutaneous endoscopic assistance, the external approach, and percutaneous procedures performed with a device, such as fragmentation of kidney stones performed via percutaneous nephrostomy.

Every PCS code must contain a valid value for Character 5, Approach. *None* is never an option. The approach comprises three components: the access location, method, and type of instrumentation. Refer to ■ TABLE 47-9 for abstracting questions to ask about the surgical approach. These are discussed next.

The *access location*, also called the anatomic approach, refers to the anatomic site through which the target site for the procedure is reached. The two general types of access locations are the skin/mucous membranes and an external orifice. The skin or mucous membranes can be punctured or incised to reach the procedure site and is the access location for all percutaneous and open procedures. An external orifice may be natural—such as the nose, ears, mouth, urethra, anus, or vagina—or artificial, such as a colostomy stoma. An endoscopic procedure can be performed percutaneously or through an external orifice. The External approach identifies procedures performed directly on the skin or mucous membranes, such as the excision of a skin lesion, and those performed indirectly through the application of force, such as closed reduction of a fracture. Procedures performed in the mouth always use the External approach.

Table 47-8 ■ **MEDICAL AND SURGICAL APPROACH DEFINITIONS**

Value	Approach	Definition
0	Open	Cutting through the skin or mucous membrane and any other body layers necessary to visually expose the site of the procedure
3	Percutaneous	Entry, by puncture or minor incision, of instrumentation through the skin or mucous membrane and any other body layers necessary to reach the site of the procedure without visualization
4	Percutaneous Endoscopic	Entry, by puncture or minor incision, of instrumentation through the skin or mucous membrane and any other body layers necessary to reach and visualize the site of the procedure
7	Via Natural or Artificial Opening	Entry of instrumentation through a natural or artificial external opening to reach the site of the procedure
8	Via Natural or Artificial Opening Endoscopic	Entry of instrumentation through a natural or artificial external opening to reach and visualize the site of the procedure
F	Via Natural or Artificial Opening with Percutaneous Endoscopic Assistance	Entry of instrumentation through a natural or artificial external opening and entry, by puncture or minor incision, of instrumentation through the skin or mucous membrane and any other body layers necessary to aid in the performance of the procedure
X	External	Procedures performed directly on the skin or mucous membrane and procedures performed indirectly by the application of external force through the skin or mucous membrane

Source: Department of Health and Human Services, Centers for Medicare and Medicaid Services, ICD-10-PCS Coding Manual.

Table 47-9 ■ **KEY CRITERIA FOR ABSTRACTING THE APPROACH**

Key Criteria Questions	Method	PCS Approach
❑ Is a full incision made?	Skin and deeper layers are cut open to reach internal organs/sites.	Open (0)
❑ Is a needle or other puncture device used?	Skin is not cut open to expose deeper layers.	Percutaneous (3)
❑ Is an endoscope used?	Access is made through small incisions in the skin.	Percutaneous endoscopic (4)
	Access is made thorough a natural or pre-existing artificial opening.	Via natural or artificial opening endoscopic (8)
❑ Is a natural opening used for access to internal sites?	Direct entry access is made without endoscope.	Via natural or artificial opening (7)
	Access is made using an endoscope.	Via natural or artificial opening endoscopic (8)
❑ Is access made through a pre-existing artificial opening?	Direct entry access is made without endoscope.	Via natural or artificial opening (7)
	Access is made using an endoscope.	Via natural or artificial opening endoscopic (8)
❑ Is the procedure performed on the surface of the skin?	Skin is not cut open to reach deeper layers.	External (X)
❑ Is the procedure performed in the mouth or mucous membrane?	Site can be seen without use of an endoscope.	External (X)
❑ Is pressure applied to the skin?	Skin is not cut open. Direct or indirect force is applied, to move an internal structure.	External (X)
❑ Are there two access sites: one through a natural or artificial opening and a second through the skin with an endoscope?	Laparoscopically assisted vaginal hysterectomy Laparoscopically assisted anorectal pull-through procedure	Via natural or artificial opening with endoscopic assistance (F)

Source: © PB Resources, Inc. Used with permission.

Method identifies how the access location is entered to reach an internal body part. An open procedure involves cutting through the skin or mucous membrane and subcutaneous layers to reach the procedure site. The root operation Detachment always uses the open approach. When instrumentation, such as an endoscope, is used, the method identifies whether the instrumentation is introduced percutaneously or through an external orifice. The incisions during a percutaneous procedure are part of that method and are not identified or coded separately.

Instrumentation is specialized equipment used to reach an internal body part, such as an endoscope or needle. Use of a needle is classified as the Percutaneous approach in PCS. Endoscopy is a generic name for any procedure using a fiber-optic viewing scope. The procedure may also carry the name of the site accessed, such as colonoscopy, laparoscopy, or gastroscopy. Use of an endoscope can be classified as Percutaneous Endoscopic *or* Endoscopic Via Natural or Artificial Opening in PCS, depending whether the procedure site is accessed through the skin or through an opening. ■ Table 47-10 lists common types of endoscopy procedures and the approach used.

The seven PCS approach values are discussed next. These terms and definitions may differ slightly from those used in CPT. PCS OGCR B5 provides several guidelines on how to code the approach in situations where the choice might be unclear. These were summarized earlier in this chapter.

Open (0)

In a procedure using the **Open** approach, an incision is made through the skin and subcutaneous tissue to open the operative site to view (■ Figure 47-1A). Fascia and muscles are **divided** (*separated*) and the organ, body cavity, or region is directly visualized with the naked eye by the surgeon. All steps to access the procedure site, including the initial incision on the skin, subsequent divisions to reach the surgical site, and layered closure, are part of the procedure. An open approach is the most invasive and carries the highest risk to the patient. Surgeons will generally opt for a less invasive approach whenever possible. Code the Open approach when an open procedure is performed *with* percutaneous endoscopic assistance because PCS does not provide a unique value for these approaches used simultaneously. Examples of the open approach are an open appendectomy, abdominal hysterectomy, and open coronary artery bypass graft (CABG).

Percutaneous (3)

In the approach **Percutaneous**, the skin is punctured or a very small incision is made to access the site, but a full-length incision is not made (Figure 47-1B). An example is a needle biopsy of any joint or organ.

Percutaneous Endoscopic (4)

In the approach **Percutaneous Endoscopic**, the surgeon makes several—usually two to four—small incisions, approximately one-half to one inch in length. A fiber-optic camera

Table 47-10 ■ TYPES OF ENDOSCOPY PROCEDURES

Endoscopy Name	Procedure Site	Insertion Point	Type of Access
Anoscopy	Anus	Anus	Natural opening
Arthroscopy	Joint	Through a small incision in the skin	Percutaneous
Bronchoscopy	Lungs	Nose or mouth	Natural opening
Colonoscopy	Colon/large intestine	Anus	Natural opening
		Colostomy site	Artificial opening
Cystoscopy	Bladder	Urethra	Natural opening
		Cystostomy site	Artificial opening
Enteroscopy	Small intestine	Mouth or anus	Natural opening
		Ileostomy or jejunostomy site	Artificial opening
Esophagogastroduodenoscopy	Esophagus, stomach, and duodenum	Nose or mouth	Natural opening
Esophagoscopy	Esophagus	Nose or mouth	Natural opening
Gastroscopy	Stomach	Nose or mouth	Natural opening
Hysteroscopy	Uterus	Vagina	Natural opening
Laparoscopey	Abdominal or pelvic cavity	Through a small incision in the skin	Percutaneous
Laryngoscopy	Larynx (voice box)	Nose or mouth	Natural opening
		Tracheostomy site	Artificial opening
Proctoscopy	Anal cavity, rectum, or sigmoid colon	Anus	Natural opening
Rhinoscopy	Nose	Nose	Natural opening
Sigmoidoscopy	Sigmoid colon	Anus	Natural opening
Ureteroscopy	Ureter	Urethra	Natural opening

Source: © PB Resources, Inc. Used with permission.

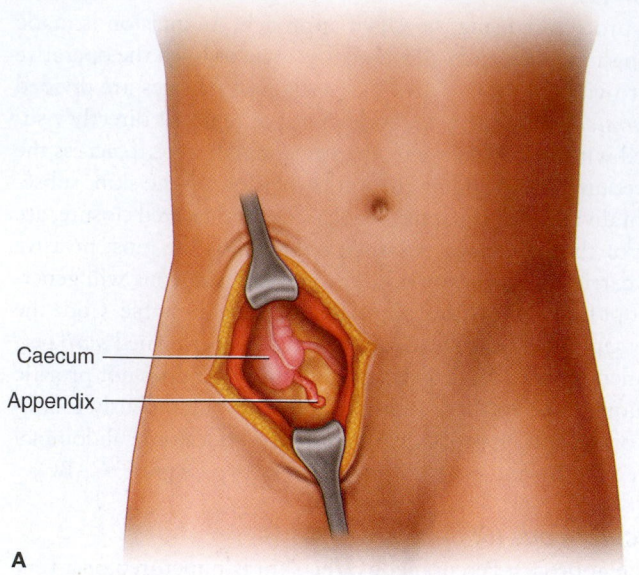

A

Approach: Open (0)
Example: Access through a major incision in the skin to perform an open appendectomy.

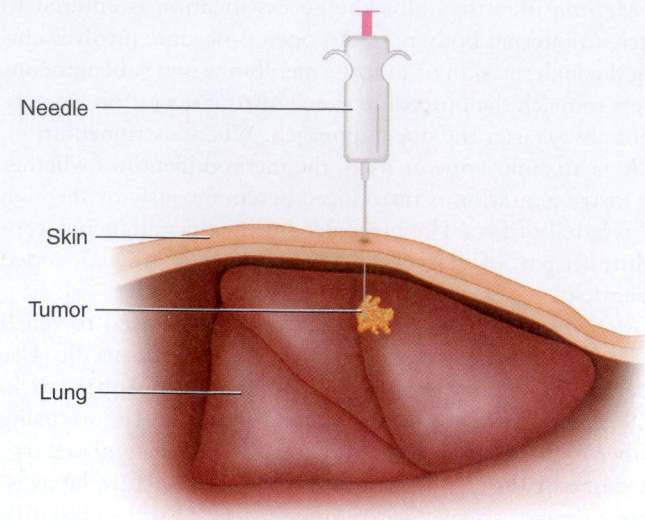

B

Approach: Percutaneous (3)
Example: Access through a puncture in skin during a needle biopsy of the lung.

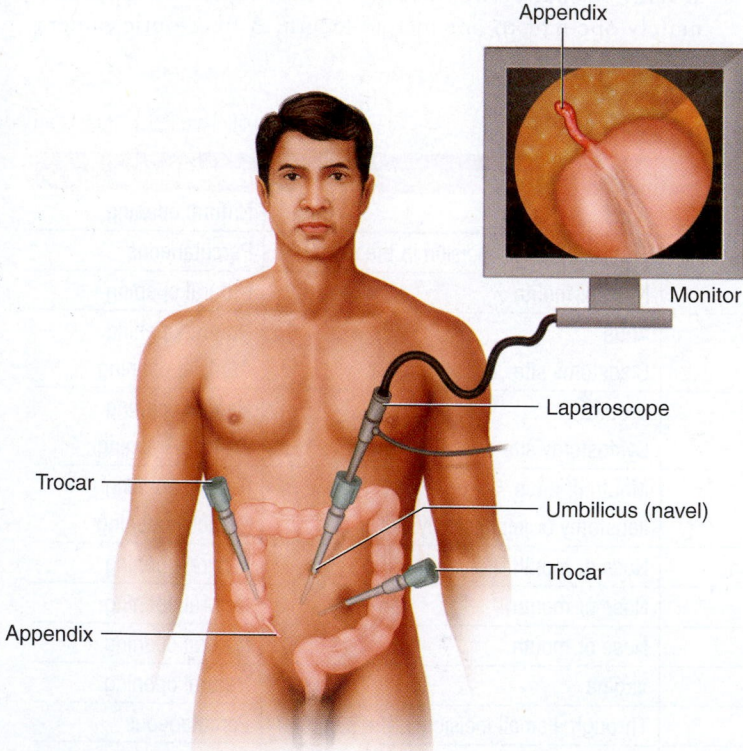

C

Approach: Percutaneous Endoscopic (4)
Example: Access through the skin with an endoscope during a laparoscopic appendectomy.

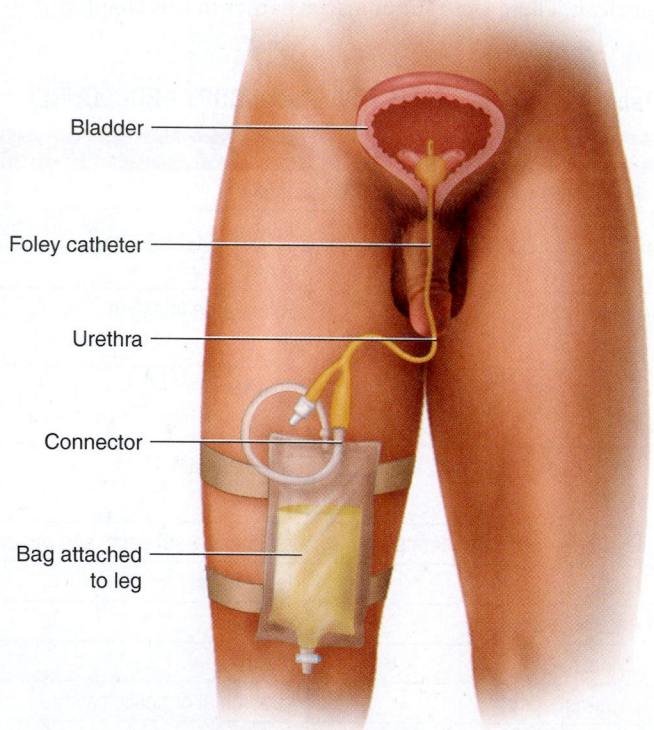

D

Approach: Via Natural or Artificial Opening (7)
Example: Access through a natural opening (urethra) for insertion of a Foley catheter.

Figure 47-1 ■ Examples of PCS approaches. *Source: © PB Resources, Inc. Used with permission.*

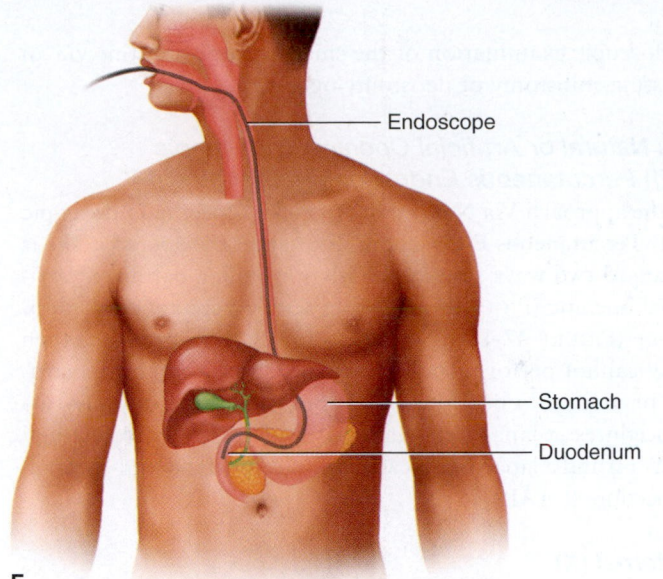

E

Approach: Via Natural or Artificial Opening Endoscopic (8)
Example: Access through a natural opening (oral cavity) during an esophagogastroduodenoscopy.

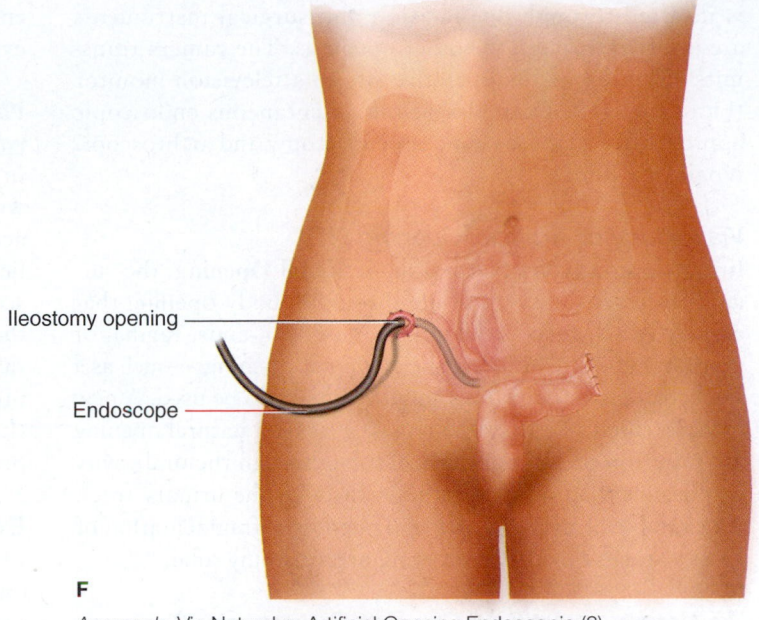

F

Approach: Via Natural or Artificial Opening Endoscopic (8)
Example: Access through an artifical opening (ileostomy opening) to examine the inside of the bowel.

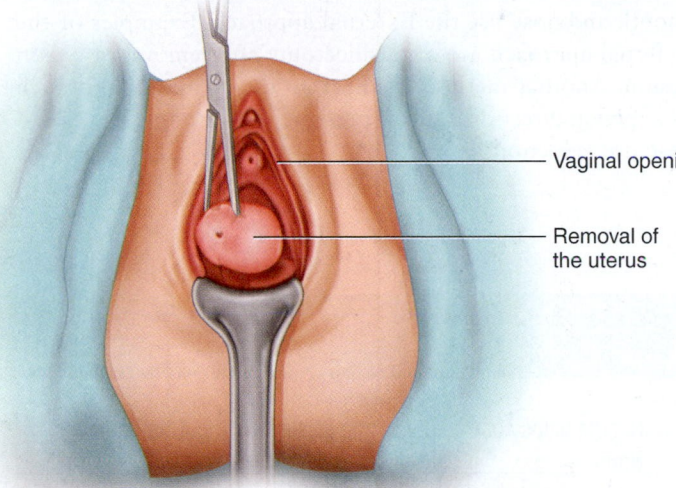

G

Approach: Via Natural or Artificial Opening with Percutaneous Endoscopic Assistance (F)
Example: Natural opening component of removing the uterus through the vagina during a laparoscopically assisted vaginal hysterectomy (LAVH).

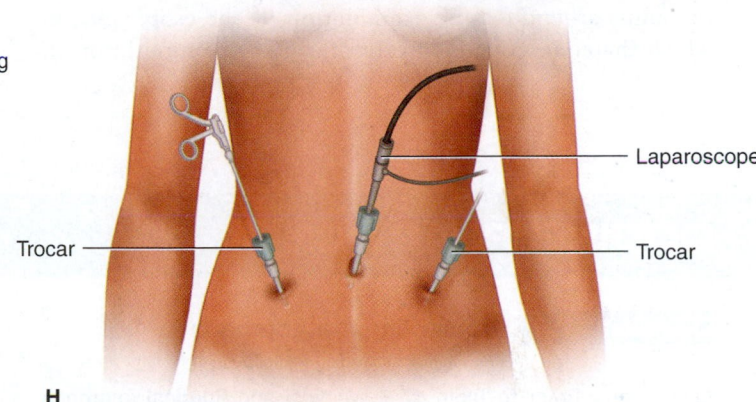

H

Approach: Via Natural or Artificial Opening with Percutaneous Endoscopic Assistance (F)
Example: Percutaneous endoscopic component with access through the abdomen during a laparoscopically assisted vaginal hysterectomy (LAVH).

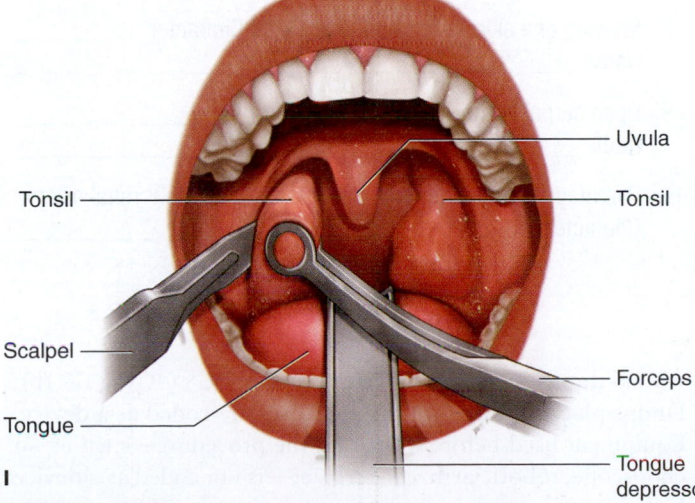

I

Approach: External (X)
Example: Tonsillectomy performed on the mucous membranes.

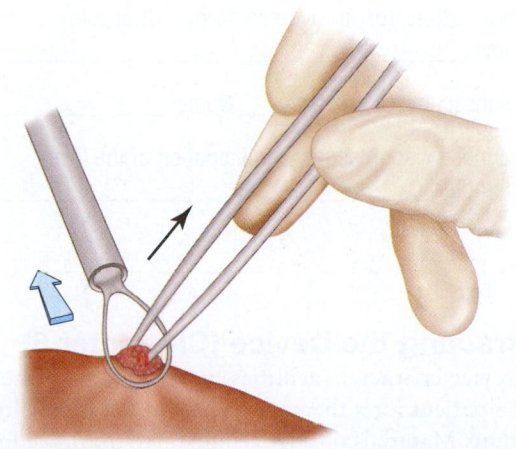

J

Approach: External (X)
Example: Removal of a skin lesion.

is inserted through one incision and surgical instruments are inserted through the other openings. The camera transmits an image of the operative site to a television monitor (FIGURE 47-1C). Examples of the percutaneous endoscopic approach are a laparoscopic appendectomy and arthroscopic repair of a joint.

Via Natural or Artificial Opening (7)

In the approach Via Natural or Artificial Opening, the surgeon accesses the surgical site through a body opening that already exists, such as the mouth, nose, ear, anus, vagina, or urethra (FIGURE 47-1D). Artificially made openings—such as a tracheostomy or colostomy mouth—may also be used. A new incision is not required. Examples of using a natural opening are insertion of an endotracheal tube through the oral cavity or placement of a Foley catheter through the urinary tract. An example of using an artificial opening is fragmentation of kidney stones through an existing nephrostomy tube.

Via Natural or Artificial Opening Endoscopic (8)

In the approach Via Natural or Artificial Opening Endoscopic, the surgeon inserts an endoscope through an existing natural (FIGURE 47-1E) or artificial (FIGURE 47-1F) opening. Examples are a colonoscopy, in which the endoscope is inserted through the anus; an endoscopic examination of the esophagus, in which the endoscope is inserted through the mouth; or an

endoscopic examination of the small or large intestine via an existing colostomy or ileostomy opening.

Via Natural or Artificial Opening Endoscopic with Percutaneous Endoscopic Assistance (F)

In the approach Via Natural or Artificial Opening Endoscopic with Percutaneous Endoscopic Assistance, the operative site is accessed two ways simultaneously: through a natural or artificial opening (FIGURE 47-1G) and with a percutaneous endoscope (FIGURE 47-1H). Surgeons choose this approach when they cannot perform the entire procedure through the natural or artificial opening. This approach is used on only two procedures: a laparoscopically assisted vaginal hysterectomy (LAVH) and a laparoscopically assisted anorectal pull-through procedure (LAAPP).

External (X)

In the External approach, the entire treatment is performed on the skin or mucous membranes. The operative site can be seen directly without the use of instrumentation (e.g., an endoscope) or an incision (FIGURE 47-1I and J). Procedures in the mouth and nose use the External approach. Examples of the external approach are a tonsillectomy and removal of a skin lesion. Another method used for an used external approach is applying direct or indirect pressure. An example is a closed fracture reduction.

CODING PRACTICE

Exercise 47.5   **Abstracting the Approach**

Instructions: Refer to Table 47-7, Medical and Surgical Approach Definitions, and Figure 47-1, Examples of PCS Approaches, and other information in this section. Read the procedural statements below and identify the PCS approach. Write the character and name of the approach on the lines provided.

1. The surgeon made a low transverse abdominal incision in preparation for a hysterectomy. Character _____ Name _____

2. Colonoscopy. Character _____ Name _____

3. Diagnostic laparoscopy with palpation of the liver. Character _____ Name _____

4. Needle biopsy of the lower lobe of the left lung. Character _____ Name _____

5. Tonsillectomy. Character _____ Name _____

6. Vaginal hysterectomy. Character _____ Name _____

7. Arthroscopic meniscectomy. Character _____ Name _____

8. Shaving of a skin lesion on the left arm. Character _____ Name _____

9. Open carpal tunnel release. Character _____ Name _____

10. Percutaneous transluminal angioplasty of the right renal artery. Character _____ Name _____

Abstracting the Device (Character 6)

The Device character identifies material that is intentionally left in a patient for a therapeutic reason at the conclusion of a procedure. Material considered integral to the procedure—such as sutures, radiological markers, and temporary postoperative

wound drains—are not coded as devices (PCS OGCR B6.1b). Drains placed for therapeutic purposes are coded as a device. Equipment used before or during the procedure—such as an endoscope, robotic arm, or sterilizer—is not coded as a device because it is not left in the patient.

Table 47-11 ■ KEY CRITERIA FOR ABSTRACTING THE DEVICE

- ❏ Was anything left in the patient to continue treating the condition?
- ❏ Was a therapeutic drain placed?
- ❏ Were clips placed around a vessel?
- ❏ Was a stent placed inside a vessel?
- ❏ Was an internal or external fixation device used to repair a fracture?
- ❏ Was a mechanical device, such as an infusion pump, placed in the patient?
- ❏ Was an electronic device, such as a pacemaker, placed in the patient?
- ❏ Was an artificial body part, such as a joint or limb, used to replace the natural part?
- ❏ Was a fusion device used?
- ❏ Was natural or artificial tissue used?
- ❏ Was an implant left in the patient?
- ❏ Was a shunt placed to move fluid from one area of the body to another?
- ❏ What material was used for the graft in a coronary artery bypass graft procedure?

Source: © PB Resources, Inc. Used with permission.

The coder's main task during abstracting is to identify potential devices listed in the medical record (■ Table 47-11). General types of devices include clips, bands, grafts, stents, shunts, prostheses, fixation devices, and electronic devices. Coders need to determine where the device is placed. They must identify whether the material for grafts and prostheses is obtained from the patient, from another human, from an animal, or synthetic. The type of synthetic material—such as metal, ceramic, and so on—needs to be identified for prostheses.

PCS classifies devices into more than 100 general categories rather than listing hundreds of individual devices. You can abstract the device based on the procedure description in the medical record. You will not always know how PCS classifies the device until you assign the code in the PCS table. Category choices are listed on the PCS table and are discussed under the section "Assigning Codes" for root operations in the chapters that follow. You need to cross-reference between the coding manual and the medical record to ensure that all devices are correctly identified and classified. Examples of devices, their description, and how PCS classifies them appear in ■ Table 47-12.

The majority of procedures do not require additional information in the device character, in which case the value **Z No device** is assigned to Character 6. PCS OGCR B6 provides several guidelines on how to code the device in situations where the choice might be unclear. These were summarized earlier in this chapter.

Table 47-12 ■ DEVICE EXAMPLES, DESCRIPTIONS, AND PCS CLASSIFICATION

Device	Description	PCS Classification
Blood glucose monitoring system Cardiac event recorder	An electronic device worn by the patient to monitor a physiological function	Monitoring device
Bone bank graft Cadaver tissue	Human tissue from a cadaver or live individual	Nonautologous tissue substitute
Metal occlusive clip Gastric band	A fixed ring or flexible strap placed around the outside of a vessel to narrow it or close it off	Extraluminal device
Cystostomy tube Foley catheter	A tube that continuously drains fluid to the outside of the body	Drainage device
Fixation device	Rods, pins, or screws applied to stabilize a bone	Internal or external fixation device
Gore-Tex graft	Artificial skin or tissue replacement	Synthetic substitute
Mesh	Material used for reinforcement of tissue or muscle	Synthetic substitute
Neuromuscular stimulator lead Carotid artery stimulator	A wire connected to an electronic device that emits impulses to encourage a physiological reaction	Stimulator lead
Pig heart valve Animal graft	Tissue taken from an animal	Zooplastic tissue substitute
Shunt	A tube or vein placed to move fluid to another site in the body where it can be reabsorbed	Autologous, nonautologous, or zooplastic substitute
Skin autograft Autologous vein graft	Tissue from another area of the patient's body	Autologous tissue substitute
Stent	A tube placed inside of a vessel for reinforcement; may or may not deliver medication	Intraluminal device Drug-eluting intraluminal device

Source: © PB Resources, Inc. Used with permission.

CODING PRACTICE

Instructions: Refer to Table 47-11, Key Criteria for Abstracting the Device, and Table 47-12, Device Examples, Descriptions, and PCS Classification. Identify the name of the device in the following procedural statements. Write the type of device on the line after the statement. If no device is mentioned, write *No Device*. Do not assign any codes.

1. Fallopian tube ligation using extraluminal clips. _____

2. Internal fixation of the tibia using screws and a rod. _____

3. Open drainage of a neck abscess. _____

4. Adjustment of a pacemaker lead in the left atrium. _____

5. Open right femoral-popliteal bypass using Gore-Tex graft. _____

6. Esophageal dilation using an endoscope. _____

7. Insertion of a drug-eluting stent in the carotid artery. _____

8. Total hip replacement with ceramic-on-ceramic prosthesis. _____

9. Endoscopic balloon dilation of the common bile duct _____

10. Insertion of a Foley catheter. _____

Abstracting the Qualifier (Character 7)

The qualifier character contains unique values for individual procedures. ■ TABLE 47-13 lists some of the most commonly used qualifiers and the key criteria for abstracting them. The coder must refer to the PCS table and cross-reference the choices in the table with the medical record to select the correct qualifier value. Qualifier choices for specific root operations are discussed in the "Assigning Codes" section of the chapters that follow. PCS uses hundreds of qualifier values, but many are used with only one body system and one root operation. Coders do not need to memorize qualifier values; they refer to the PCS table for the root operation and body system to identify the values for a particular clinical situation.

The most common qualifier identifies diagnostic procedures. Physicians may order procedures for either therapeutic or diagnostic purposes. A diagnostic procedure is performed to obtain information needed to make a diagnosis and treatment plan. Examples are performing a biopsy of a tumor in order to determine whether it is malignant or performing amniocentesis to determine whether a fetus has chromosomal abnormalities. Diagnostic procedures require the value **X Diagnostic** for the qualifier. A therapeutic procedure is performed in order to treat a disease or condition. Examples are a cholecystectomy due to gallbladder disease, a coronary artery bypass to treat atherosclerosis, or removal of a skin lesion that is cancerous. Procedures are assumed to be therapeutic unless stated to be diagnostic, so a specific qualifier is not required to identify the therapeutic nature of the procedure.

The majority of procedures do not require additional information in the qualifier character, in which case the value **Z No qualifier** is assigned to Character 7.

Table 47-13 ■ KEY CRITERIA FOR ABSTRACTING THE QUALIFIER

❏ Is the procedure a biopsy or otherwise diagnostic?

Bypass (Non-Coronary) Procedures
❏ What is the ending site of the bypass?

Coronary Bypass Procedures
❏ What vessel is bypassed from?

Amputation
❏ What is the exact anatomic site of the amputation?

Skin and Muscle Grafts
❏ To what depth is the procedure performed? Skin, subcutaneous tissue, fascia, partial thickness, full thickness
❏ What type of flap is created? Latissimus dorsi myocutaneous flap, transverse rectus abdominis myocutaneous flap, deep inferior epigastric artery perforator flap, superficial inferior epigastric artery flap, gluteal artery perforator flap

Spine Procedures
❏ What direction is the anatomic approach? Anterior (*incision/access from the front*) or posterior (*incision/access from the back*)?
❏ What part of the spinal column is treated? Anterior (*front side*) or posterior (*back side*)

Transplant and Replacement Procedures
❏ What type of tissue is used? Autologous, nonautologous, zooplastic, or synthetic

Source: © PB Resources, Inc. Used with permission.

CODING PRACTICE

Instructions: Read the following procedural statements and determine if each one is a diagnostic or therapeutic procedure. Circle the correct description following the statement.

1. Needle biopsy of the liver. Diagnostic   Therapeutic

2. Laparoscopic cholecystectomy for gallstones. Diagnostic   Therapeutic

3. Screening colonoscopy. Diagnostic   Therapeutic

4. Exploratory laparotomy of the peritoneum. Diagnostic   Therapeutic

5. Excision of malignant skin lesion. Diagnostic   Therapeutic

Abstracting for Multiple Procedures

General guidelines related to coding multiple procedures include the following. These guidelines apply to all root operations. Refer to the PCS OGCR for clinical examples of each.

■ TABLE 47-14 summarizes the criteria for identifying when multiple codes might be needed.

- Procedural components—The root operation definition includes all components of the procedure, which should not be coded separately. Procedural steps necessary to reach the operative site and close the operative site, including anastomosis of a tubular body part, are not coded separately (PCS OGCR B3.1b).

- Multiple body parts—When the same root operation is performed on different body part values defined in Character 4, assign separate codes for each body part value (PCS OGCR B3.2.a).

- Multiple anatomic sites—When the same root operation is repeated at different anatomic sites that are included in the same body part value, assign separate codes for each site using the same body part value (PCS OGCR B3.2.b).

- Multiple root operations—When multiple root operations with distinct objectives are performed on the same body part, assign separate codes for each root operation (PCS OGCR B3.2.c).

Table 47-14   ■   KEY CRITERIA FOR ABSTRACTING MULTIPLE PROCEDURES

- ❏ Which components are included in the root operation (Character 3) or procedural steps?
- ❏ Is the same root operation (Character 3) performed on multiple body parts (Character 4)?
- ❏ Is the same root operation (Character 3) performed on multiple anatomic sites with the same body part (Character 4) value?
- ❏ Are multiple root operations (Character 3) with distinct objectives performed on the same body part (Character 4)?
- ❏ Is a root operation (Character 3) attempted with one approach (Character 5) then converted to a different approach?
- ❏ Is the initial root operation (Character 3) discontinued or otherwise not completed and a different root operation completed?
- ❏ Are a biopsy and a definitive procedure performed at the same operative session?
- ❏ Is an autograft harvested from a distinct anatomic site?

Source: © PB Resources, Inc. Used with permission.

- Multiple approaches—When the intended root operation is attempted using one Approach (Character 5) but is converted to a different approach, assign separate codes for each approach value (PCS OGCR B3.2.d).

- Discontinued procedures—When the intended procedure is discontinued or otherwise not completed, assign one code for the root operation that is completed. If a procedure is discontinued and no other root operation is performed, code the root operation Inspection of the body part or Anatomical Region inspected (PCS OGCR B3.3). (*Note:* The root operation Inspection is discussed in Chapter 55 of this text.)

SUCCESS STEP

The PCS OGCR is not as extensive as the guidelines for ICD-10-CM or CPT, so you should try to memorize as many guidelines as possible. It is especially helpful to memorize the guidelines regarding multiple coding. Doing so will make the coding process faster and more accurate.

Guided Example of Abstracting PCS Procedures

The mini-medical-record used for procedure cases in this text provides a limited snapshot of the most pertinent information. Refer to ■ FIGURE 47-2 (page 992) to learn how to interpret the mini-medical-record used for procedure reports.

To practice skills for abstracting procedures, refer to the following example of Michael Longo, who had an ileostomy at Branton Medical Center, which is used throughout this chapter. Marcy Elwood, CCS, is the fictitious coder at the hospital who guides you through the coding process.

Follow along as Marcy Elwood, CCS, abstracts the root operation from the medical record. Check off each step after you complete it.

▶ Marcy reads through the procedure report, with special attention to the preprocedure diagnosis, the procedure name and description, and the postprocedure diagnosis.

▶ Marcy refers to Key Criteria for Abstracting Medical and Surgical Procedures (General) (Table 47-3).

  ❏ *What is the procedure?* Temporary loop ileostomy (■ FIGURE 47-3)

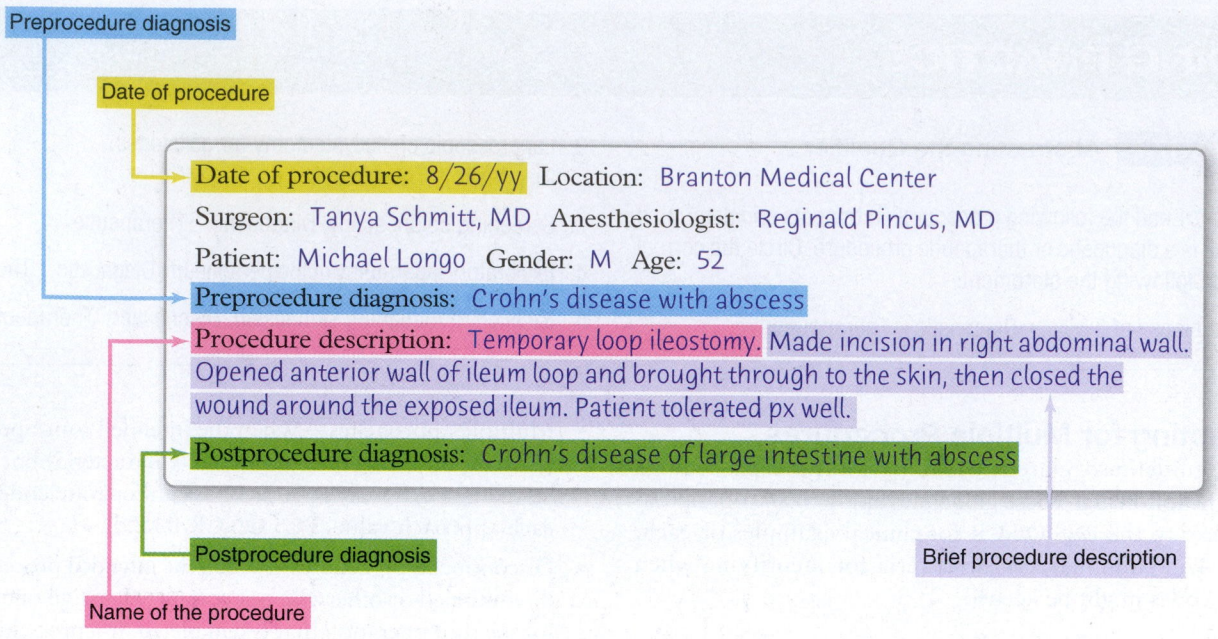

Preprocedure diagnosis

Date of procedure

Date of procedure: 8/26/yy Location: Branton Medical Center

Surgeon: Tanya Schmitt, MD Anesthesiologist: Reginald Pincus, MD

Patient: Michael Longo Gender: M Age: 52

Preprocedure diagnosis: Crohn's disease with abscess

Procedure description: Temporary loop ileostomy. Made incision in right abdominal wall. Opened anterior wall of ileum loop and brought through to the skin, then closed the wound around the exposed ileum. Patient tolerated px well.

Postprocedure diagnosis: Crohn's disease of large intestine with abscess

Postprocedure diagnosis

Name of the procedure

Brief procedure description

Figure 47-2 ■ Key to interpreting the procedure report mini-medical-record.

Date of procedure: 8/26/yy Location: Branton Medical Center Surgeon: Tanya Schmitt, MD

Anesthesiologist: Reginald Pincus, MD

Patient: Michael Longo Gender: M Age: 52

Preprocedure diagnosis: Crohn's disease with abscess

Procedure description: Temporary loop ileostomy. Made incision in right abdominal wall. Opened anterior wall of ileum loop and brought through to the skin, then closed the wound around the exposed ileum. Patient tolerated px (*procedure*) well.

Postprocedure diagnosis: Crohn's disease of large intestine with abscess

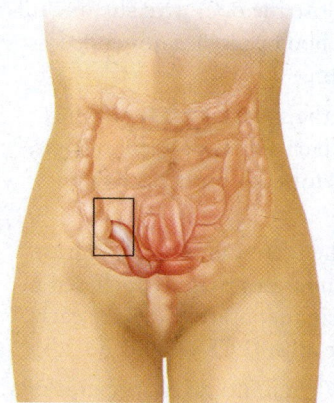
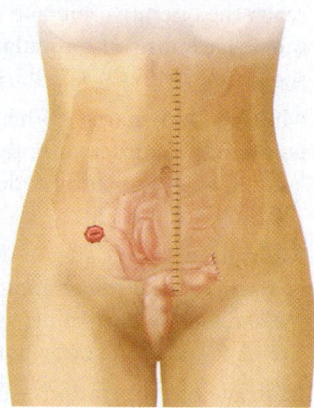

Figure 47-3 ■ A loop ileostomy reroutes the contents of the small intestine to bypass the large intestine.

❑ *What organ or body part is involved?* The ileum, which is the third section of the small intestine

❑ *Is the procedure description what you would expect based on the name of the procedure?* Yes, the ileum was divided and the free end was brought through the right abdominal wall to the skin. This created a new route to evacuate the contents of the small intestine so they would not pass through to the infected large intestine.

❑ *Was more than one procedure, or a combined procedure, performed?* No

❑ She refers to the table Key Criteria for Abstracting Root Operations and reads the abstracting questions that identify root operation groups. She answers "Yes" to the question, *Did the procedure alter the diameter or route of a tubular body part?*

▶ The Key Criteria for Abstracting Root Operations directs Marcy to review the definitions of four root operations.

▶ She turns to the appendix "Comparison of Medical and Surgical Root Operations" in the ICD-10-PCS coding manual. (This PCS appendix also appears in Table 47-5.)

   ❑ She locates the group titled Procedures That Alter the Diameter or Route of a Tubular Body Part and reads the definition of each root operation.

   ❑ After reading the definitions, she believes that **Bypass (1)** best describes the ileostomy.

▶ Next, Marcy turns to the appendix, "Root Operation Definitions," in the ICD-10-PCS manual. (This table also appears in Table 47-6.)

   ❑ She locates the entry for **1 Bypass**.

   ❑ She reads the Definition, Explanation, and Examples listed and concludes that **Bypass** is the correct root operation because this operation altered the route of a tubular body part, the ileum.

❑ *What surgical approach is used?* The approach is Open because an abdominal incision was made.

❑ The procedure is a bypass so Marcy must also identify the ending site of the bypass. The ending site is documented as *cutaneous*, which is the skin. This information is needed to assign the value for Character 7 Qualifier.

▶ At this time, Marcy has abstracted the procedure and determined that the root operation is **Bypass**. She also identified the approach and qualifier. Next, she will assign the PCS code, which is discussed in Chapter 48.

CHAPTER SUMMARY

In this chapter you learned that:

- Coders need to understand the difference between treatments and diagnostic procedures as well as the description of various surgical approaches.

- The Medical and Surgical Section is the largest Section of ICD-10-PCS, containing 31 body systems and 31 root operations.

- The seven characters of a Medical and Surgical procedure are (1) Section, (2) Body System, (3) Root Operation, (4) Body Part, (5) Approach, (6) Device, and (7) Qualifier.

- ICD-10-PCS provides guidelines for Medical and Surgical codes in section B of the PCS OGCR, which contains five subdivisions, corresponding to characters within a Medical and Surgical code. Coders should review the guidelines and examples frequently.

- Abstracting Medical and Surgical procedures requires abstracting unique information for each Character.

- Coders should be familiar with the PCS body systems and verify that the code they ultimately select is consistent with the correct body system value.

- Identifying the correct root operation is the basis of ICD-10-PCS coding, so coders must learn the differences between similar root operations.

- PCS subdivides some organs and other anatomic sites into multiple body part values to achieve greater specificity.

- PCS uses seven values to identify the approach, which is the surgical technique used to reach the procedure site.

- A device is material that is intentionally left in a patient for a therapeutic reason at the conclusion of a procedure.

- The qualifier character contains unique values for individual procedures. The coder must refer to the PCS table and cross-reference the choices in the table with the medical record to select the correct qualifier value.

CONCEPT QUIZ

Take a moment to look back at the abstracting for medical and surgical procedures and solidify your skills. Try to answer the questions from memory first, then refer to the discussion in this chapter if you need a little extra help.

Completion—Device

Instructions: Refer to Table 47-12, Device Examples, Descriptions, and PCS Classification. Identify the type of device described in each statement. Choose from the list below. Some choices may be used more than once and some choices may not be used at all. Write the answer on the line provided.

autologous tissue substitute
drainage device
drug-eluting intraluminal device
external fixation device
extraluminal device
internal fixation device

intraluminal device
monitoring device
nonautologous tissue substitute
stimulator lead
synthetic substitute
zooplastic tissue substitute

1. Gastric band. _____
2. Skin autograft. _____
3. Pig heart valve. _____
4. Foley catheter. _____

5. Stent that releases medication. _____
6. Rods inserted inside a bone to stabilize it. _____
7. Gore-Tex graft. _____
8. Bone bank graft. _____
9. Carotid artery stimulator. _____
10. Blood glucose monitoring system. _____

Multiple Choice

Instructions: Circle the letter of the best answer to each question based on the information you learned in this chapter. Refer to tables in the chapter for assistance.

1. What approach is used for a procedure in which an incision is made through the skin and subcutaneous tissue?
   A. Open
   B. Percutaneous
   C. Percutaneous Endoscopic
   D. External

2. What approach is used for a procedure in which the endoscope is inserted through the anus?
   A. Percutaneous Endoscopic
   B. Via Natural or Artificial Opening
   C. External
   D. Via Natural or Artificial Opening Endoscopic

(continued)

(continued from page 993)

3. Which of the following is a body system in ICD-10-PCS?
   A. Digestive System
   B. Skeletal System
   C. Upper Bones
   D. Cardiovascular System

4. Which root operation is lithotripsy an example of?
   A. Excision
   B. Destruction
   C. Fragmentation
   D. Removal

5. Which root operation is fallopian tube ligation an example of?
   A. Resection
   B. Occlusion
   C. Destruction
   D. Restriction

6. What root operation is used when the procedure involves cutting out the left upper lobe of the lung?
   A. Repair
   B. Resection
   C. Removal
   D. Excision

7. Which of the following is a valid qualifier value?
   A. T Therapeutic
   B. X Diagnostic
   C. 0 Open
   D. R Bilateral

8. What type of procedure is done when the surgeon leaves a drainage device in the patient?
   A. Therapeutic
   B. Diagnostic
   C. Exploratory
   D. Supplemental

9. How many PCS body systems are used for the muscular system?
   A. 1
   B. 2
   C. 3
   D. 5

10. Which of the following root operations always involves a device?
    A. Change
    B. Drainage
    C. Occlusion
    D. Reposition

KEEP ON CODING

Part A—Root Operation Examples

Instructions: Refer to Table 47-6, Root Operation Definitions in Alphabetical Order, with Explanations and Examples. Provide an example of each root operation.

Example: Change *Drainage tube change*

1. Supplement _____
2. Excision _____
3. Extraction _____
4. Restriction _____
5. Revision _____
6. Resection _____
7. Reposition _____
8. Release _____
9. Reattachment _____
10. Dilation _____

Part B—Root Operation Groups

Instructions: Refer to Table 47-5, Comparison of Root Operations. For each root operation group listed below, write down the names and character values of all root operations in the group.

Example: Root operations that define other objectives *Fusion G, Alteration 0, Creation 4*

11. Root operations involving examination only _____

_____

_____

12. Root operations that always involve a device _____
_____
_____

13. Root operations involving cutting or separation only _____
_____
_____

14. Root operations that put in/put back or move some/all of a body part _____
_____
_____

15. Root operations that take out solids/fluids/gases from a body part _____
_____
_____

Part C—Approach

Instructions: Refer to Table 47-8, Medical and Surgical Approach Definitions; Table 47-9, Key Criteria for Abstracting the Approach; and Figure 47-1, "Examples of PCS approaches." Read the procedural statements below and identify the PCS approach. Write the character and name of the approach on the lines provided. Do not assign any full codes.

16. Reduction of a fracture of the right ulna by applying pressure to the skin and bone. Approach value ____ Approach name _____

17. Transurethral (*through the urethra*) cystoscopy. Approach value ____ Approach name _____

18. Percutaneous insertion of neurostimulator lead in cervical spinal cord. Approach value ____ Approach name _____

19. Incision with removal of internal fixation device, left tibia. Approach value ____ Approach name _____

20. Percutaneous chest tube placement. Approach value ____ Approach name _____

21. Open retropubic prostatectomy. Approach value ____ Approach name _____

22. Cryotherapy (*freezing*) of a wart on the back. Approach value ____ Approach name _____

23. Cervical cerclage (*stitch*) with access through the vagina. Approach value ____ Approach name _____

24. Laparoscopy with lysis of abdominal adhesions. Approach value ____ Approach name _____

25. Tooth extraction with forceps. Approach value ____ Approach name _____

CODING CHALLENGE

Instructions: Refer to the abstracting tables in this chapter for each Character of the code. Read the mini-medical-record of each patient's encounter and answer the abstracting questions listed. Write the answer on the line provided. Do not assign any codes.

1. INPATIENT HOSPITAL   Gender: F   Age: 83

Preprocedure diagnosis: Pressure ulcer, left hip

Procedure description: Open excisional debridement of left hip. Used scissors to cut out necrosis and devitalized tissue, through full epidermis and subcutaneous tissue, 1 cm beyond the wound margin.

Postprocedure diagnosis: Healing stage III pressure ulcer, left hip

a. What is the stated procedure? _____

b. What organ or body part is involved? _____

(continued)

1. (continued)

c. Is the procedure description what you would expect based on the name of the procedure?

_____

d. Was more than one procedure, or a combined procedure, performed? _____

e. Review the Key Criteria for Abstracting Root Operations. To which question did you answer yes?

_____

f. Review the definitions of the root operations that answer this question. Which root operation correctly describes this procedure?

_____

g. Review the Key Criteria for Abstracting the Approach. What surgical approach is used?

_____

(continued)

(continued from page 995)

---

2. INPATIENT HOSPITAL   Gender: F   Age: 48

Preprocedure diagnosis: Mass in left breast

Procedure description: Needle biopsy. Using a needle, took out a tissue sample from the left breast that was previously marked with a wire.

Postprocedure diagnosis: Benign neoplasm, breast per pathology report

a. What is the stated procedure? _____

b. What organ or body part is involved? _____

c. Is the procedure description what you would expect based on the name of the procedure? _____

d. Was more than one procedure, or a combined procedure, performed? _____

e. Review the Key Criteria for Abstracting Root Operations. To which question did you answer yes?

_____

f. Review the definitions of the root operations that answer this question. Which root operation correctly describes this procedure? _____

g. Review the Key Criteria for Abstracting the Approach. What surgical approach is used? _____

h. Review the Key Criteria for Abstracting the Qualifier. Was the procedure diagnostic or therapeutic?

_____

---

3. INPATIENT HOSPITAL   Gender: M   Age: 15

Preprocedure assessment: Presented to ED with vomiting, acute abdominal pain, RLQ tenderness, T 101 degrees

Procedure description: Appendectomy. Made three small umbilical incisions and placed laparoscope. Expanded abdominal cavity with carbon dioxide to aid visualization. Grasped appendix and divided with stapler. Cauterized appendiceal stump. Removed appendix, irrigated and suctioned abdominal cavity. Removed instruments and closed incision. Patient tolerated procedure well, no complications.

Postprocedure diagnosis: Acute appendicitis with rupture

a. What is the stated procedure? _____

b. What organ or body part is involved? _____

(continued)

---

3. (continued)

c. Is the procedure description what you would expect based on the name of the procedure? _____

d. Was more than one procedure, or a combined procedure, performed? _____

e. Review the Key Criteria for Abstracting Root Operations. To which question did you answer yes?

_____

f. Review the definitions of the root operations that answer this question. Which root operation correctly describes this procedure? _____

g. Review the Key Criteria for Abstracting the Approach. What surgical approach is used? _____

---

4. INPATIENT HOSPITAL   Gender: F   Age: 61

Preprocedure diagnosis: Gangrene in left great toe due to nonhealing plantar (*sole of foot*) ulcer

Procedure description: Midlevel amputation of L great toe at interphalangeal joint

Postprocedure diagnosis: Diabetes with gangrene

a. What is the stated procedure? _____

b. What organ or body part is involved? _____

c. Is the procedure description what you would expect based on the name of the procedure? _____

d. Was more than one procedure, or a combined procedure, performed? _____

e. Review the Key Criteria for Abstracting Root Operations. To which question did you answer yes?

_____

f. Review the definitions of the root operations that answer this question. Which root operation correctly describes this procedure? _____

g. Review the Key Criteria for Abstracting the Approach. What surgical approach is used? _____

h. At what joint was the amputation performed?

_____

Is this site a low-, mid-, or high-level amputation? _____

5. INPATIENT HOSPITAL   Gender: F   Age: 23

Preprocedure: Hypermenorrhea

Procedure description: Transvaginal dilation and curettage. Inserted speculum to hold the vagina open. Progressively dilated cervix and uterus with os dilator. Inserted curette and scraped endometrial wall. Tissue sent to lab for analysis.

Postprocedure diagnosis: Hypermenorrhea

Tip: Curettage (*scraping*) is classified as removal by force.

a. What is the stated procedure? _____

b. What organ or body part is involved? _____

c. Is the procedure description what you would expect based on the name of the procedure? _____

d. Was more than one procedure, or a combined procedure, performed? _____

e. Review the Key Criteria for Abstracting Root Operations. To which question did you answer yes?

_____

f. Review the definitions of the root operations that answer this question. Which root operation correctly describes this procedure? _____

g. Review the Key Criteria for Abstracting the Approach. What surgical approach is used? _____

h. Review the Key Criteria for Abstracting the Qualifier. Was the procedure diagnostic or therapeutic?

_____

6. INPATIENT HOSPITAL   Gender: F   Age: 52

Preprocedure diagnosis: Endometriosis

Procedure description: Ablation of ovaries and endometrium. Inserted the endoscope through the vagina into the uterus to cauterize the endometrium (*lining of uterus*). When that was successfully completed, withdrew the scope, applied a new tip. Made three incisions on the lower abdomen and inserted endoscope to treat each ovary.

Postprocedure diagnosis: Endometriosis

Tip: Code multiple procedures when the same root operation is performed on different body parts as defined by distinct values of the body part character (PCS OGCR B3.2a).

a. What is the stated procedure? _____

b. What organ or body part is involved? _____

c. Is the procedure description what you would expect based on the name of the procedure? _____

(*continued*)

6. (continued)

d. Was more than one procedure, or a combined procedure, performed? _____

e. Review the Key Criteria for Abstracting Root Operations. To which question did you answer yes?

_____

f. Review the definitions of the root operations that answer this question. Which root operation correctly describes this procedure? _____

g. Review the Key Criteria for Abstracting the Approach. What surgical approach is used? _____

h. Repeat the abstracting process for each procedure that was performed. _____

7. INPATIENT HOSPITAL   Gender: F   Age: 52

Preprocedure diagnosis: Pain RUQ, T 102 degrees, vomiting, acute cholecystitis with calculi in the common bile duct, causing obstruction. Extensive known abdominal adhesions prevent a laparoscopic approach.

Procedure description: Cholecystectomy. Made subcostal incision and isolated gallbladder from surrounding structures with laparotomy packs. Excised entire gallbladder and common bile duct. Hemostasis was achieved. Closed operative wound. Patient tolerated procedure well.

Postprocedure diagnosis: Acute cholecystitis with calculi in the common bile duct, causing obstruction

Tip: Code multiple procedures when the same root operation is performed on different body parts as defined by distinct values of the body part character (PCS OGCR B3.2a).

a. What is the stated procedure? _____

b. What organ or body part is involved? _____

c. Is the procedure description what you would expect based on the name of the procedure? _____

d. Was more than one procedure, or a combined procedure, performed? _____

e. Review the Key Criteria for Abstracting Root Operations. To which question did you answer yes?

_____

f. Review the definitions of the root operations that answer this question. Which root operation correctly describes this procedure? _____

g. Review the Key Criteria for Abstracting the Approach. What surgical approach is used? _____

h. Repeat the abstracting process for each procedure that was performed. _____

(*continued*)

(continued from page 997)

---

8. INPATIENT HOSPITAL   Gender: M   Age: 43

Preprocedure diagnosis: Detached R retina

Procedure description: Trans pars plana vitrectomy (TPPV) with synthetic scleral buckle. Punctured the pars plana and used vitreous cutter to suction out all vitreous. Injected balanced saline solution (BSS) to replace vitreous. Sutured scleral buckle, which effectively closed the break. Pt tolerated px well.

Postprocedure diagnosis: Detached R retina

a. What is the stated procedure? _____

b. What organ or body part is involved? _____

c. Is the procedure description what you would expect based on the name of the procedure? _____

d. Was more than one procedure, or a combined procedure, performed? _____

e. Review the Key Criteria for Abstracting Root Operations. To which question did you answer yes?

_____

f. Review the definitions of the root operations that answer this question. Which root operation correctly describes this procedure? _____

g. Review the Key Criteria for Abstracting the Approach. What surgical approach is used? _____

h. Review the Key Criteria for Abstracting the Device. What device is used? _____

i. Repeat the abstracting process for each procedure that was performed. _____

---

9. INPATIENT HOSPITAL   Gender: M   Age: 75

Preprocedure diagnosis: Blepharoptosis obscuring vision

Procedure description: Bilateral upper blepharoplasty. Cut out a crescent of skin and subcutaneous tissue from fold of R eyelid, sutured to restore normal position of eyelid. Repeated on left side.

Postprocedure diagnosis: Blepharoptosis obscuring vision

a. What is the stated procedure? _____

b. What organ or body part is involved? _____

c. Is the procedure description what you would expect based on the name of the procedure? _____

(*continued*)

---

9. (continued)

d. Was more than one procedure, or a combined procedure, performed? _____

e. Review the Key Criteria for Abstracting Root Operations. To which question did you answer yes?

_____

f. Review the definitions of the root operations that answer this question. Which root operation correctly describes this procedure? _____

g. Review the Key Criteria for Abstracting the Approach. What surgical approach is used? _____

h. Repeat the abstracting process for each procedure that was performed. _____

---

10. INPATIENT HOSPITAL   Gender: F   Age: 23

Preprocedure diagnosis: Fractured R tibia and R humerus

Procedure description: Open reduction, R tibia with internal fixation device. Closed reduction, R humerus with percutaneous internal fixation. Applied cast to right humerus.

Postprocedure diagnosis: Fractured R tibia, fractured R humerus shaft

a. What is the stated procedure? _____

b. What organ or body part is involved? _____

c. Is the procedure description what you would expect based on the name of the procedure? _____

d. Was more than one procedure, or a combined procedure, performed? _____

e. Review the Key Criteria for Abstracting Root Operations. To which question did you answer yes?

_____

f. Review the definitions of the root operations that answer this question. Which root operation correctly describes this procedure? _____

g. Review the Key Criteria for Abstracting the Approach. What surgical approach is used? _____

h. Review the Key Criteria for Abstracting the Device. What device is used? _____

i. Repeat the abstracting process for each procedure that was performed. _____

Learning Objectives

After completing this chapter, you should have the skills to:

48.1 Spell and define the key words, medical terms, and abbreviations related to medical and surgical procedures. (Remember)

48.2 Demonstrate how to assign codes for Medical and Surgical procedures according to the ICD-10-PCS guidelines. (Apply)

48.3 Utilize guidelines for arranging (sequencing) codes for Medical and Surgical procedures. (Apply)

Key Terms and Abbreviations

Body Part Key
Device Aggregation Table
Device Definitions
Device Key

In addition to the key terms listed here, students should know the terms defined within tables in this chapter.

Chapter Outline

- **Assigning Medical and Surgical Procedure Codes**
- **Arranging Medical and Surgical Procedure Codes**

INTRODUCTION

After you get the lay of the land in a large sightseeing venue, you are better equipped to enjoy specific parts of it that are most appealing. In your continuing tour of the PCS Medical and Surgical section in this chapter, you have the opportunity to become more acquainted with the details. In the previous chapter you learned the basics of abstracting PCS codes. Now you learn the remaining skills of an "Ace" coder—assigning and arranging PCS Medical and Surgical codes.

ASSIGNING MEDICAL AND SURGICAL PROCEDURE CODES

Assigning PCS codes requires coders to locate the root operation in the Index, then refer to a Table to build the code. Follow the PCS OGCR in all aspects of assigning codes. PCS does not contain any modifiers. The Tables do not contain any instructional notes.

ICD-10-PCS Index

The Index is the first stop in the process of assigning PCS codes. The Index consists of Main Terms followed by a series of indented subterms. The Index uses two types of Main Terms for the Medical and Surgical Section:

- The name of the root operation
- The common procedure name

ICD-10-PCS does not use eponyms—such as the Whipple procedure or Bilroth procedure—as Main Terms or procedure names.

The most direct way to locate a code is to use the root operation. Chapter 47 of this text discussed in detail how to abstract the root operation. Chapters 49–55 discuss in detail how to abstract and assign codes for each root operation. Under the Main Term for the root operation, locate a first-level subterm for the body system, then a second-level subterm for the body part. A partial code is listed that identifies the correct PCS Table.

When the root operation is difficult to determine, locate a Main Term for the common procedure name, such as *colectomy*, then follow the cross-references to the appropriate Main Term(s) and Table(s) (■ FIGURE 48-1). The Index may provide more than one cross-reference because the common procedure names can be ambiguous. For example, a colectomy may involve any of the following procedures:

- Cutting out the entire colon, which is a **Resection**
- Cutting out one complete segment of the colon, which is also a **Resection**, because each segment has a separate Body Part value

Colectomy
see Excision, Gastrointestinal System 0DB
see Resection, Gastrointestinal System 0DT

Figure 48-1 ■ Example of Index entry for a common procedure name, with cross-references to multiple root operations.

- Cutting out a portion of one segment, which is an **Excision**, because a portion of a defined PCS body part is cut out

When the Index provides more than one cross-reference, it does *not* mean that you can randomly use any of the options listed for any procedure. It is the coder's responsibility to determine which specific root operation accurately describes the procedure you are coding. If you are unsure of which root operation to use, refer to the abstracting tables in Chapter 47 of this text. Also refer to Chapters 49–53, which discuss specific root operations in detail.

Following the subterm is the partial code, which provides the first three to five characters of the code. The first three characters of the partial code identify the appropriate Table to use.

Never assign a code based on the Index alone. You must always refer to the Table to build all seven characters of the code. The Index rarely lists more than three or four characters. Even when the Index provides a seven-character code, you must still verify the values using the Table to be certain it accurately describes the documented procedure.

ICD-10-PCS Tables

After locating the appropriate procedure in the Index and identifying the first three characters of the partial code, cross-reference the appropriate Table to build the rest of the code. Follow three steps to look up a PCS code in the tables:

1. Locate the Table.
2. Build the code.
3. Verify the character values.

Locate the Table

Locate the Table that matches the first *three* letters of the partial code. The Tables are organized in alphanumeric order by the Section, the first character of a code. Tables beginning with numbers **0** through **9** appear first, followed by Tables beginning with a letter, **B** through **Z**. Within each Section, Tables are sequentially arranged according to the value of the second character, body system.

For example, Tables that begin with **001** through **09Z** appear before Tables that begin with **0B1** through **0ZZ**. The first three letters of the code and the definition of each letter are listed at the top of the Table.

After you locate the Table, read the header at the top that identifies the body system and root operation. If the body system is not what you expect, return to the Index and rework your search.

EXAMPLE: *Extirpation of the axillary vein.* After conducting a search in the Index, you locate Table **03C Artery Extirpation**. You notice that you are in a Table for arteries rather than veins. This means that in the Index under the Main Term **Extirpation**, you selected the second-level subterm **axillary** from the first-level subterm **Artery**. You need to go back to the Index Main Term **Extirpation**, and look for first-level subterm **Vein**, then **axillary**, which leads to Table **05C**.

Build the Code

The three characters of the partial code that identify the Table are the first three characters of the code, representing the Section (**0** for Medical and Surgical), the body system, and the root operation. The Table consists of a grid that lists the available options for characters 4 through 7 (■ FIGURE 48-2). To build the rest of the code, select one value from each column to describe the procedure. The first column of the grid is for Body Part (Character 4); the second column is for Approach (Character 5); the third column is for Device (Character 6); and the final column is for Qualifier (Character 7). Select one, and only one, value from each column, staying within the same row. As you select the values for your code, write them down on a coding worksheet, such as the one shown in ■ TABLE 48-1.

Each row is mutually exclusive of other rows in the same Table. All values for a code must be taken from the *same* boxed row within the Table. Review the sample codes shown at the bottom of Figure 48-2 and note the following:

- Code **0F9130Z** is a valid code that is built from values in the first row of the table.

Table 48-1 ■ **CODING WORKSHEET FOR MEDICAL AND SURGICAL PROCEDURES**

Character (Position)	Name	Value	Description
1	Section	0	Medical and Surgical
2	Body System		
3	Root Operation		
4	Body Part		
5	Approach		
6	Device		
7	Qualifier		

Source: © PB Resources, Inc. Used with permission.

- Code **0F913ZX** is a valid code that is built from values in the second row of the table.

- Code **0F9130X** is *not* a valid code because it mixes a value from the first row for Character 6 with a value from the second row for Character 7.

The differences between the first and second rows of this Table are as follows:

- The first row contains a value for Character 6 for **0 Drainage device** and the second row does not.

- The second row contains a value for Character 7 for **X Diagnostic** and the first row does not.

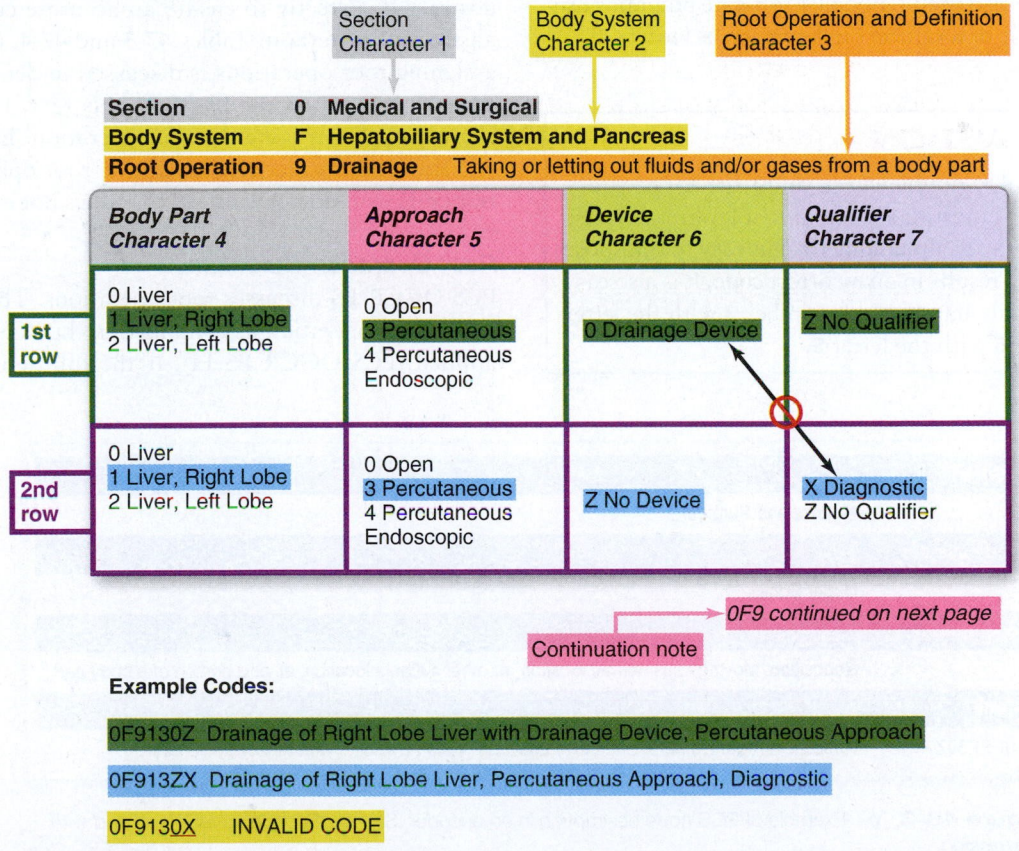

Figure 48-2 ■ Annotated PCS Table.

A procedure that leaves a drainage device in the patient is therapeutic by definition, not diagnostic. Therefore, the values for Character 6, Device, **0 Drainage**, and Character 7, qualifier, **X Diagnostic**, are mutually exclusive and cannot be used together. By choosing all character values from the same row of the Table, coders are able to construct valid codes.

If it seems that the row you are working from does not list the value choices you need, review the rest of the Table to see if another row applies. Only allowable combinations of the approach, device, and qualifier values appear in the same row. Sometimes, the values in the first column, Character 4, Body Part, are repeated in multiple rows, with other rows providing a different set of values for Characters 5 through 7. In the example Table **0F9**, Characters 4 and 5 are exactly the same in both rows, but Characters 6 and 7 are different.

Verify the Character Values

After building a valid code from values within the same row of the Table, review the final choices on your coding worksheet for accuracy. *Double-check the value of each character of the code to verify that it accurately describes the documented procedure.* Identify a statement in the documentation that supports each value chosen for the code.

The ICD-10-PCS coding manual does not list a complete description for each full code because there are more than 78,000 codes. CMS offers a searchable electronic file with short and long code descriptions for all valid codes. You can download the file from the ICD-10 page at **www.cms.gov**. The file name is Code Descriptions-Long and Abbreviated Titles. The associated README files are also useful. Encoder software programs usually display the code description on the screen (■ FIGURE 48-3).

CODING CAUTION

Always be careful to double-check your work for accuracy when writing or entering a code into software. Because ICD-10-PCS codes are alphanumeric, it is easy to transpose characters, which results in an incorrect code. It is also easy to confuse a hastily handwritten number **2** with the letter **Z** or the number **5** with the letter **S**.

Tips for Using Tables

Certain formatting and layout elements of a Table affect the ability to build an accurate code. Be alert for the following items:

- Pages may contain more than one grid. Be careful to select the grid that *exactly* matches the first three code characters listed in the Index.

- Tables may be subdivided into rows, which are separated with solid lines. To build a valid code, all values must come from the same row within the Table. Do not combine values from different rows or different Tables. Doing so will result in an invalid code.

- Body part values can be listed in more than one row of a table. If you cannot find the desired combination of approach, device, and qualifier in the first row you see with the body part, keep looking for additional rows. If you cannot find the desired combination in any row, that means that one of your choices is incorrect and you need to review the abstracting questions.

- Long Tables may span more than one page. If you cannot find what you need, even though you are confident that you have selected the correct three-character Table, look to see if it continues on the next page. When a Table is continued on the next page, a note stating *continued on next page* appears below the Table.

Assigning Character 3: Root Operation

The root operation is the basis of all PCS coding. It must be abstracted correctly to ensure an accurate code. Review the abstracting criteria in Tables 47-3 and 47-4. Abstracting and assigning root operations is discussed in detail for each root operation in Chapters 49–55 of this text. Exercises in this chapter explicitly state the root operation. In later chapters, you learn to abstract and assign the root operation that corresponds with documentation that does not explicitly state it.

Root Operation Guidelines

PCS OGCR B3 discusses root operations. The full definition of the root operation as contained in the PCS Tables must be applied (PCS OGCR B3.1a). If the full definition does not

---

section	
	Medical and Surgical
body system	
	Upper Bones
operations	
	Reposition: Moving to its normal location, or other suitable location, all or a portion of a body part
Code	
0PSF34Z ▾	Reposition Right Humeral Shaft with Internal Fixation Device, Percutaneous Approach

Figure 48-3 ■ Example of PCS code description in an encoder. *Source: SpeedeCoder, Reprinted with permission.*

apply, review the abstracting criteria and root operation definitions and examples to determine the correct one.

Components of a procedure specified in the root operation definition and explanation are not coded separately (PCS OGCR 3.1b). Procedural steps necessary to reach the operative site and close the operative site, including anastomosis of a tubular body part, are also not coded separately. For example, *resection* of a joint as part of a joint replacement procedure is included in the root operation definition of **Replacement** and is not coded separately. A laparotomy performed to reach the site of an open liver biopsy (**Excision**) is not coded separately. In a **Resection** of sigmoid colon with anastomosis of descending colon to rectum, the anastomosis is not coded separately.

Guidelines for multiple procedures are discussed later in this chapter. Guidelines for specific root operations are discussed in Chapters 49–55 of this text dedicated to the root operation.

Assigning Character 4: Body Part

The body part character identifies the specific anatomic site where the procedure was performed. Most of the work to identify the correct body part is done when using the Index. The body system is usually a first-level subterm in the Index with the body part a second-level subterm. Character 4 is almost always listed in the partial code. When the coder turns to the correct PCS table, the main task is to verify the body part value to be certain that the most specific value was selected. Also verify the laterality. Review Table 47-7, Key Criteria for Abstracting the Body Part.

Index Entries for the Body System and Body Part

Under the Main Term for each root operation in the Index are one to three levels of indented subterms that describe the body system or body part. It is absolutely essential to identify the correct first-level subterm for the body system before selecting the second-level subterm for the body part.

Coders must match the documented anatomic site to the most specific PCS body system and body part value. For example, under the root operation **Reposition**, PCS provides body system and body part values for the following sites in the upper arm:

- Muscles of the upper arm
- Tendons of the upper arm
- Head of the humerus
- Shaft of the humerus
- Acromioclavicular joint

Each of these is a separate Index entry (■ FIGURE 48-4) under root operation **Reposition (S)**. For sites in the musculoskeletal system, you must first identify the correct first-level subterm that identifies the body system as **Muscle**, **Tendon**, or **Joint**. Each of these has a second-level subterm for **upper arm**. The Index lists a first-level subterm for **Bone**, but only a few of the smaller bones that actually contain the word *bone* in their name are listed as second-level subterms, such as the **ethmoid** bone and **nasal** bone. Sites such as **Femur** and **Humeral head** are separate first-level subterms. If you cannot immediately

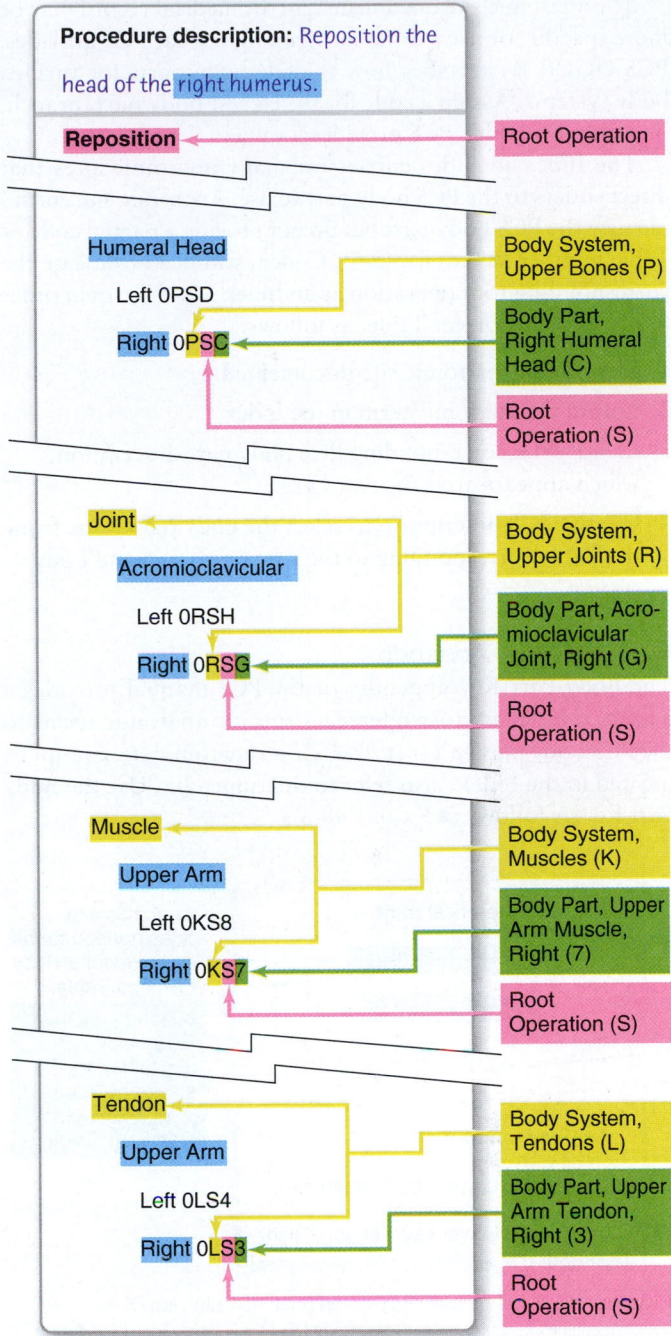

Figure 48-4 ■ Example of locating the correct body part in the Index. *Source:* © PB Resources, Inc. Used with permission.

find the site you are looking for, take time to look back carefully through all first-level subterms.

Sites in the circulatory system, such as those listed under the root operation **Bypass**, require the first-level subterm **Arteries** or **Veins**. The specific vessel is listed as a second-level subterm. You must identify whether it is an artery or vein first because the vessels can have similar names. For example, the second-level subterm **femoral** appears under first-level subterms for both **Artery** and **Vein**. When you find an entry such as femoral, always backtrack to identify the first-level subterm it is indented under to identify the *femoral artery* or *femoral vein*.

The anatomic site documented in the medical record may be more specific, or use a different term, than what PCS provides. PCS OGCR B4 specifies how to code body parts for various body systems. Assign a code for the closest body part, branch, or region for which PCS provides a value.

The Index includes entries for many anatomic sites that direct coders to the PCS body part to use. Anatomic site entries identify the PCS body part but do not provide a partial code or Table number (■ FIGURE 48-5). Coders still need to locate the corresponding root operation as an Index Main Term in order to identify the correct Table, as follows:

1. Identify the anatomic site documented.
2. Locate the anatomic term in the Index.
3. Identify the corresponding PCS body part description, which appears after the word *use*.
4. Use the PCS description to select the body part value from the Table corresponding to the root operation and body system.

Body Part Key Appendix

The **Body Part Key** appendix of the PCS manual provides a helpful table that cross-references specific anatomic terms to the PCS body part (■ TABLE 48-2). If an anatomic site cannot be located in the Index, also refer to this appendix. Use the Body Part Key as follows (■ FIGURE 48-6):

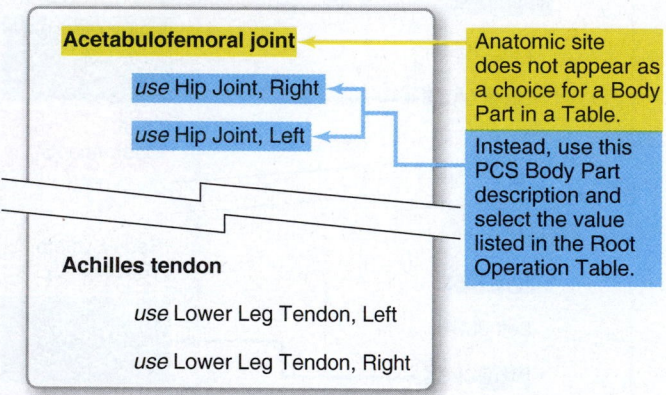

Figure 48-5 ■ Index entry for an anatomic site with cross-reference to PCS body part. *Source:* © PB Resources, Inc. Used with permission.

Table 48-2 ■ **EXCERPT FROM PCS BODY PART KEY APPENDIX**

Anatomic Term	PCS Description
Acetabulofemoral joint	Hip Joint, Right
	Hip Joint, Left
Achilles tendon	Lower Leg Tendon, Right
	Lower Leg Tendon, Left
Alveolar process of maxilla	Maxilla
Aortic intercostal artery	Upper Artery

Source: Department of Health and Human Services, Centers for Medicare and Medicaid Services, ICD-10-PCS Coding Manual.

1. Identify the anatomic site documented.
2. Locate the anatomic term in the first column.
3. Identify the corresponding PCS description in the second column.
4. Use the PCS description to locate a subterm in the Index, or select the body part value from the Table corresponding to the root operation and body system.

The same body part might be listed in more than one row of the table with unique values for the approach, device, and qualifier. Always check all rows of the Table to be sure that you have selected the correct combination of value for the procedure being coded.

Body Part Guidelines

PCS OGCR provides detailed guidance on how to assign body part values when a specific named anatomic site does not have a separate value. In general, code to the closest or next largest body part value available (PCS OGCR B4.1a). In anatomic areas that have parts of several systems, such as tendons, ligaments, bursae, and fascia near a joint, code to the specific body system that is the focus of the procedure, such as a ligament or the joint capsule itself.

Specific guidance is given for the following anatomic sites. Review these guidelines frequently and memorize them so you can assign codes accurately:

- Branches of body parts (PCS OGCR B4.2)
- Bilateral body part values (PCS OGCR B4.3)
- Coronary arteries (PCS OGCR B4.4)
- Tendons, ligaments, bursae and fascia, joints (PCS OGCR B4.5)
- Skin, subcutaneous tissue and fascia overlying a joint (PCS OGCR B4.6)
- Fingers and toes (PCS OGCR B4.7)
- Upper and lower intestinal tract (PCS OGCR B4.8)
- Upper and lower veins, arteries, joints, muscles, and tendons (PCS OGCR B2.1b)

Some root operations use the body part character in unique ways. These requirements are explained in the PCS OGCR but not in the tables for these root operations, so coders must be familiar with the protocol.

- **Control**, **Detachment**, **Drainage** of a body cavity: These root operations are often performed on a region rather than specific anatomic site. Use the body parts under the body system for anatomic regions (PCS OGCR B2.1a), such as:
  - **0W Anatomical Regions, General**
  - **0X Anatomical Regions, Upper Extremities**
  - **0Y Anatomical Regions, Lower Extremities**
- **Bypass**: Character 4 Body Part is used in a unique way for the root operation **Bypass (1)**. Identify both the site bypassed *from* and the site bypassed *to*. The Index Main Term is the root operation **Bypass**. The first- and

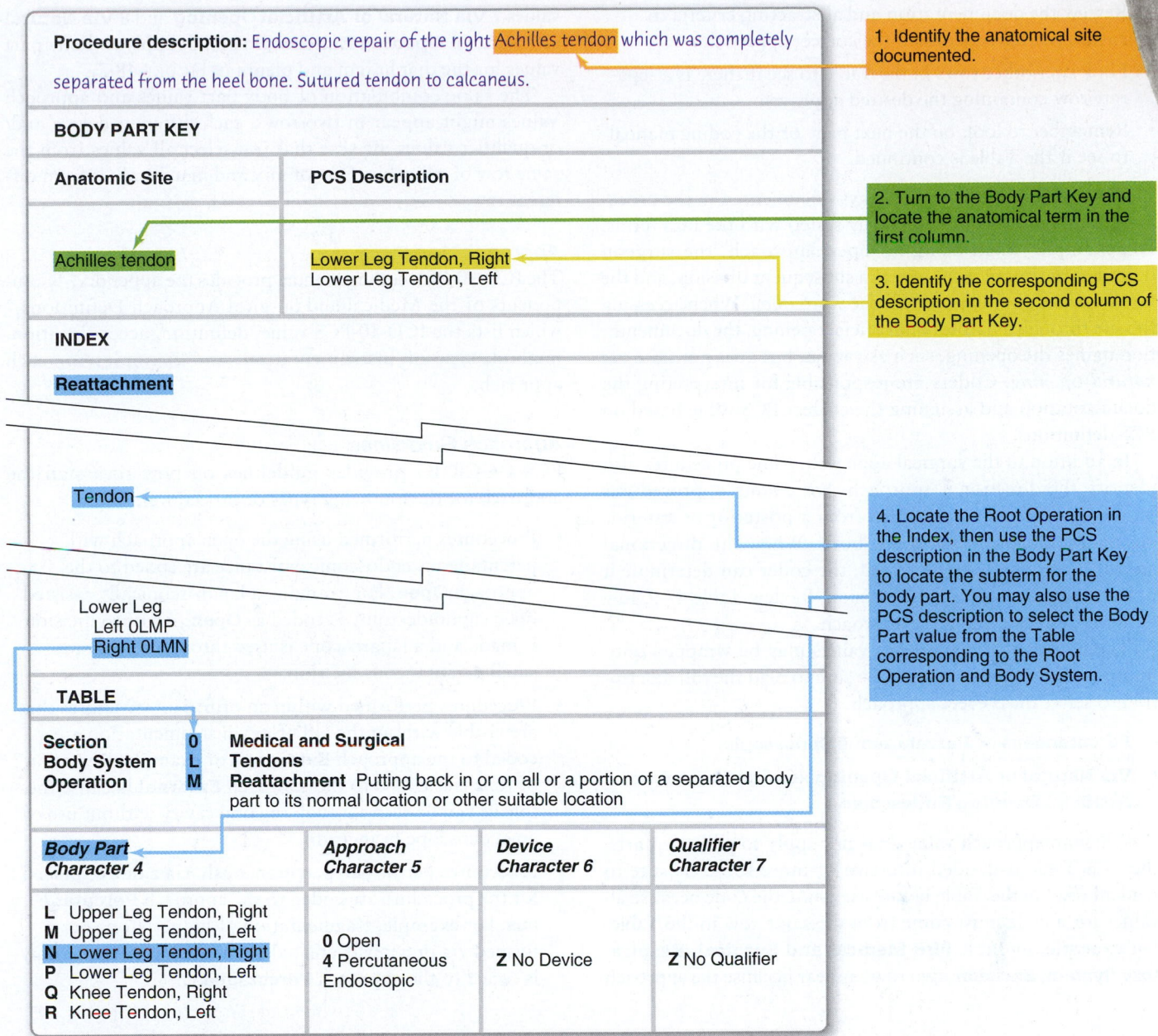

Figure 48-6 ■ Example of using the "Body Part Key" appendix to PCS body part.

second-level subterms identify the site bypassed *from*. The site bypassed *to* is identified in Character 7 Qualifier (PCS OGCR B3.6a).

- CABG: In a coronary artery bypass graft (CABG), Character 4 identifies the number of arteries bypassed *to* and Character 7 Qualifier identifies the vessel bypassed *from* (PCS OGCR B3.6b).

- **Release**: In the root operation **Release**, the body part value coded is the body part being freed and not the tissue being manipulated or cut to free the body part.

- **Transfer**: When the root operation **Transfer** is performed on a peripheral nerve, the nerve being transferred is

identified in Character 4 and the site it is transferred *to* is identified in Character 7 Qualifier.

These guidelines are discussed in detail in the chapters of this text that cover the specific root operation.

Assigning Character 5: Approach

The approach character identifies the surgical technique used to reach the procedure site. The PCS table lists the possible approach values for each body part and the root operation. If an expected approach value is not listed, double-check the following:

- Verify that you have selected the correct root operation and body system as listed at the top of the Table.

- Review the documentation and abstracting criteria to ensure you have identified the correct approach.

- Look over other rows in the Table to see if there is a separate row containing the desired approach.

- Remember to look on the next page of the coding manual to see if the Table is continued.

The surgical approach is always documented in the procedure note, but it is not necessarily stated with the PCS terms. For example, when using an open approach, the surgeon describes the initial incision, each subsequent division, and the layered closure but may not use the word *open*. When accessing the site through a natural or artificial opening, the documentation names the opening, such as vagina, but does not state *via natural opening*. Coders are responsible for interpreting the documentation and assigning the correct PCS value based on PCS definitions.

In addition to the surgical approach, some procedures also identify the directional approach. For example, procedures on the spine may be performed from a posterior or anterior approach and, in some cases, both. When the directional approach is not explicitly stated, the coder can determine it based on the location of the incision. Review Table 47-9, Key Criteria for Abstracting the approach.

The names of the approach values may be wrapped onto multiple lines in the PCS table. Be sure to read the full description to select the correct approach:

- **Percutaneous** or **Percutaneous Endoscopic**

- **Via Natural or Artificial Opening** and **Via Natural or Artificial Opening Endoscopic**

When an approach value does not apply to all body parts, the PCS Table is divided into two or more rows. Be sure to read all rows in the Table before assigning the code because all values for a code must come from the same row in the Table. For example, in Table **0BB Medical and Surgical, Respiratory System, Excision**, two rows appear because the approach values **7 Via Natural or Artificial Opening** and **8 Via Natural or Artificial Opening Endoscopic** do not apply to body part values for the diaphragm and pleura (■ Figure 48-7).

The same combination of body part values and approach Values might appear in two rows, each different device and/or qualifier values. Be sure that you select all values from the same row of the table. Do not mix and match values from different rows.

Approach Appendix

The ICD-10-PCS coding manual provides the appendix, "Components of the Medical and Surgical Approach Definitions," which lists the ICD-10-PCS value, definition, access location, method, type of instrumentation, and examples for each approach.

Approach Guidelines

PCS OGCR B5 provides guidelines on how to assign the approach for the following types of procedures:

- Procedures performed using the open approach with percutaneous endoscopic assistance are coded to the approach **Open**. For example, a laparoscopically assisted open sigmoidectomy is coded as **Open**. An open incision is made and a laparoscope is used through a separate small percutaneous incision.

- Procedures performed within an orifice on structures that are visible without the aid of any instrumentation are coded to the approach **External**. For example, Resection of tonsils is coded to the approach **External** because the tonsils can be seen through the oral cavity without use of an endoscope or incision.

- Procedures performed percutaneously via a device placed for the procedure are coded to the approach **Percutaneous**. For example, fragmentation of kidney stone performed via previously created percutaneous nephrostomy is coded to the approach **Percutaneous**.

Section	0	Medical and Surgical
Body System	C	Mouth and Throat
Operation	L	Occlusion: Completely closing an orifice or the lumen of a tubular body part

Body Part Character 4	Approach Character 5	Device Character 6	Qualifier Character 7
B Parotid Duct, Right C Parotid Duct, Left	0 Open 3 Percutaneous 4 Percutaneous Endoscopic	C Extraluminal Device D Intraluminal Device Z No Device	Z No Qualifier
B Parotid Duct, Right C Parotid Duct, Left	7 Via Natural or Artificial Opening 8 Via Natural or Artificial Opening Endoscopic	D Intraluminal Device Z No Device	Z No Qualifier

Figure 48-7 ■ Example of two rows in PCS table with different approach values.

Assigning Character 6: Device

The device character identifies material intentionally left in the patient after completion of the procedure for therapeutic purposes. Several general types of devices are used:

- Grafts and prostheses of biologic or synthetic material that reinforce or take the place of a body part
  - *Examples*: An artificial hip joint, mesh to reinforce a hernia repair, a stent that reinforces a vessel, a shunt that provides for transport of fluid from one body area to another
- Implants of therapeutic material that are not absorbed by the body
  - *Examples*: Subdermal progesterone implant, radioactive implant
- Simple or mechanical appliances that assist, replace, or prevent a physiological function
  - *Examples*: Intrauterine contraceptive device, orthopedic pins and screws, occlusive devices such as clips and rings
- Electronic appliances that assist, replace, or prevent a physiological function
  - *Examples*: Pacemaker, neurostimulator

Refer to the Character 6 column in the Table for a root operation to identify the device values that are available for each procedure. Review Table 47-11, Key Criteria for Abstracting the Device.

Device Guidelines

Device guidelines appear in PCS OGCR B6 and discuss the following situations.

A device is coded only if it remains after the procedure is completed. Frequently, no device is used. Assign **Z No device** when the documentation does not specify a device. Do not code a device that is not documented. For example, ligation refers to tying-off and can be done using cauterization, suture material, or an occlusive device such as clips. The procedure report identifies how the ligation is performed. If an occlusive device is not stated, then code **Z No device** (PCS OGCR 6.1a).

In limited root operations, the classification provides the qualifier values **Temporary** and **Intraoperative** for specific procedures involving clinically significant devices, where the purpose of the device is to be utilized for a brief duration during the procedure or current inpatient stay. If a device that is intended to remain has to be removed before the end of the procedure, assign separate codes for **Insertion** and **Removal** of the device. This can happen when a device is the wrong size or a complication occurs (PCS OGCR 6.1a).

Materials such as sutures, ligatures, radiological markers, and temporary post-operative wound drains are considered integral to the performance of a procedure and are not coded as devices (PCS OGCR 6.1b).

Procedures performed on a device only and not on a body part are specified in the root operations **Change**, **Irrigation**, **Removal**, and **Revision**, the group *Root operations that always involve a device*. Examples include insertion of a pacemaker and removal of a drainage tube (PCS OGCR 6.1c).

The root operation **Drainage** can be performed with or without putting in a drainage device. If a drainage device is not specified, code **Z No device**. This happens when the drainage is performed using an incision, suctioning, or a drain that is not left in the patient. When a therapeutic drain—such as a Jackson-Pratt drain—is left in, assign the value **Drainage device**. A separate procedure to put in a drainage device is coded to the root operation **Drainage** with the device value **Drainage device** (PCS OGCR B6.2.)

Devices unique to specific root operations are discussed in later chapters in the chapter subsection "Assigning Codes: Character 6 Device."

Device Appendices

The ICD-10-PCS coding manual contains useful appendices to assist in coding devices. These tables may comprise one, two, or three appendices depending on how the publisher organizes them. The purpose and use of these tables follows.

- **Device Key** appendix
  - *Purpose:* Provides a cross-walk that matches generic and brand-name devices with the appropriate PCS term.
  - *When to use this table:* You are unsure about how to code a specific device mentioned in the documentation.
  - *How to use this table:* Look up the brand or generic name of the device in the left column and identify the PCS value in the left column.
  - *Example:* The brand name *AFX® endovascular AAA system* is coded as **Intraluminal device** in PCS.
- **Device Aggregation Table** appendix
  - *Purpose:* Matches specific types of PCS device values used in specific root operations and body systems to the a more general PCS device value.
  - *When to use this table:* You are unsure about how to code a device when the root operation covers a wide range of body parts and the device characters identify a broader group of devices.
  - *How to use this table:* Look up the specific device in the left column, identify the specific root operation and body system(s) in the middle two columns, then identify the general device category in the right column.
  - *Example:* The value **External Fixation Device, Limb Lengthening (8)** is used in the root operation Insertion for the Lower Bones and Upper Bones. When the same device is used in other root operations, PCS classifies it as **External Fixation Device (5)**.
- **Device Definitions** appendix
  - *Purpose:* Identifies the types of generic and brand name devices coded to a specific PCS value. The table lists selected devices for which the classification might be unclear and is not all-inclusive.
  - *When to use this table:* You are unsure about exactly what devices might be included in a specific PCS value.

Section	0	Medical and Surgical
Body System	B	Respiratory System
Operation	B	Excision Cutting out off, without replacement, a portion of a body part

Body Part Character 4	Approach Character 5	Device Character 6	Qualifier Character 7
N Pleura, Right P Pleura, Left	0 Open 3 Percutaneous 4 Percutaneous Endoscopic 8 Via Natural or Artificial Opening Endoscopic	Z No Device	X Diagnostic Z No Qualifier

Figure 48-8 ■ Example of a diagnostic qualifier.

- *How to use this table:* Look up the PCS value in the left column, then identify the general types of devices included in that value in the left column.

- *Example:* The PCS value **Drainage device** includes a cystostomy tube, Foley catheter, percutaneous nephrostomy catheter, and a thoracostomy tube.

Assigning Character 7: Qualifier

The qualifier character describes a wide range of additional attributes that further describe a procedure. Qualifier values vary among procedures, depending on the information that needs to be reported. Coders need to review the qualifier options available and choose the one that matches the documentation. Review Table 47-13, Key Criteria for Abstracting the Qualifier.

Some procedures may be done either to help diagnose a disease or to treat it. One of the most common qualifier values is **X Diagnostic**, which identifies that the root operation **Excision**, **Extraction**, or **Drainage** was done for diagnostic purposes (■ FIGURE 48-8). This is generally indicated by use of the words *biopsy* or *diagnostic* in the documentation. For example, an *excisional biopsy* is coded as the root operation **Excision (B)** with the qualifier **Diagnostic (X)**. Excision may also be performed for treatment purposes, such as removal of a diseased organ. Assign qualifier value **Z No qualifier** when the purpose is therapeutic.

Many procedures have no applicable qualifier, in which case the value **Z No qualifier** is assigned.

Qualifier Guidelines

PCS OGCR does not provide a separate section for guidelines for the qualifier, but some root operation guidelines identify the qualifier purpose and use. PCS OGCR that discusses the qualifier include:

- Excision, Extraction, or Drainage biopsy procedures (PCS OGCR B3.4a)
- Bypass (non-coronary) procedures (PCS OGCR B3.6a)
- Coronary artery bypass procedures (PCS OGCR B3.6b-c)

In limited root operations, PCS provides the qualifier values **Temporary** and **Intraoperative**. These values are used for specific procedures involving clinically significant devices when the purpose of the device is to be utilized for a brief duration during the procedure or current inpatient stay. An example is temporary use of an intraluminal device during a procedure on the abdominal aorta, as in code **04L03DJ (Occlusion, Lower arteries, Abdominal aorta, Percutaneous, Intraluminal device, Temporary)** (PCS OGCR 6.1a).

Guided Example of Assigning Medical and Surgical Codes

To practice skills for building a code using the PCS Tables, continue with the example from earlier in the chapter of Michael Longo, who had an ileostomy at Branton Medical Center.

To practice skills for using the PCS Index, continue with the example from earlier in the chapter of Michael Longo, who had an ileostomy at Branton Medical Center.

Follow along as Marcy Elwood, CCS, searches the Index for the root operation. Check off each step after you complete it.

▶ First, Marcy confirms the procedure and root operation she abstracted.

❑ The root operation is **Bypass (1)**.

❑ The anatomic site is the ileum.

❑ The procedure is ileostomy.

▶ Marcy searches the Index for the Main Term **Bypass** and locates it (■ FIGURE 48-9).

❑ She locates the subterm **Ileum 0D1B**.

❑ She notes **0D1B** is the partial code.

❑ She determines that she needs Table **0D1**, which is the first three letters of the partial code.

▶ Marcy demonstrates an alternative way to locate the code, in case you are unsure of the root operation.

❑ She locates the Main Term **Ileostomy**.

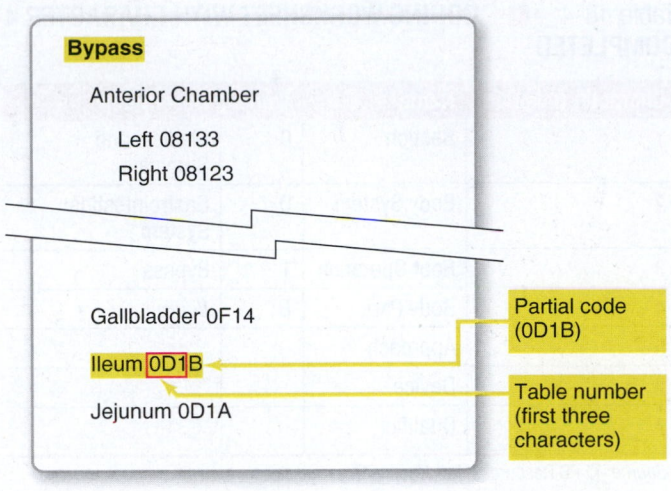

Bypass

  Anterior Chamber

    Left 08133

    Right 08123

  Gallbladder 0F14

  Ileum 0D1B ← Partial code (0D1B)

              ← Table number (first three characters)

  Jejunum 0D1A

Figure 48-9 ■ Index entry for Main Term "Bypass" and subterm "Ileum."

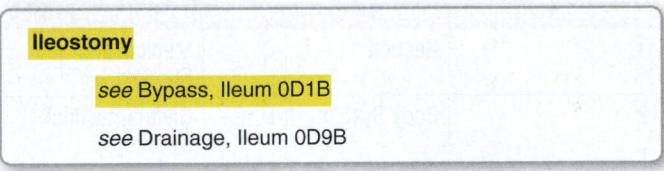

Ileostomy

    see Bypass, Ileum 0D1B

    see Drainage, Ileum 0D9B

Figure 48-10 ■ Index entry for the Main Term "Ileostomy".

❏ Under **Ileostomy**, the Index provides two subterm entries with cross-references to the root operations (■ FIGURE 48-10).

  ▪ **see Bypass, Ileum 0D1B**

  ▪ **see Drainage, Ileum 0D9B**

❏ These cross-references direct her to two possible root operations.

  ▪ She reviews the PCS definition of each root operation and determines that **Bypass** is the correct root operation based on the objective of the procedure.

▶ Next, Marcy will locate the Table and build the code.

❏ She creates a worksheet to help her track her progress while identifying each character of the code (Table 48-1).

▶ Marcy searches the Tables for Table **0D1** (■ FIGURE 48-11).

❏ She verifies the identifying information at the top of the Table to be certain she has the correct Table.

  ▪ Section **0 Medical and Surgical**

  ▪ Body system **D Gastrointestinal System**

  ▪ Operation **1 Bypass**: Altering the route of passage of the contents of a tubular body part

❏ She notes that **0D1** are the first three characters of the code and enters these characters into the worksheet (■ TABLE 48-3, page 1010).

Section	0	Medical and Surgical
Body System	D	Gastrointestinal System
Root Operation	1	**Bypass:** Altering the route of passage of the contents of a tubular body part

Body Part Character 4	Approach Character 5	Device Character 6	Qualifier Character 7
1 Esophagus, Upper 2 Esophagus, Middle 3 Esophagus, Lower 5 Esophagus	0 Open 4 Percutaneous Endoscopic 8 Via Natural or Artificial Opening Endoscopic	7 Autologous Tissue Substitute J Synthetic Substitute K Nonautologous Tissue Substitute Z No Device	4 Cutaneous 6 Stomach 9 Duodenum A Jejunum B Ileum
B Ileum	**0 Open** 4 Percutaneous Endoscopic 8 Via Natural or Artificial Opening Endoscopic	7 Autologous Tissue Substitute J Synthetic Substitute K Nonautologous Tissue Substitute **Z No Device**	**4 Cutaneous** B Ileum H Cecum K Ascending Colon L Transverse Colon M Descending Colon N Sigmoid Colon P Rectum Q Anus

Figure 48-11 ■ Table 0D1, code 0D1B0Z4.

Table 48-3 ■ CODING WORKSHEET WITH CHARACTERS 2 AND 3 COMPLETED

Character (Position)	Name	Value	Description
1	Section	0	Medical and Surgical
2	Body System	*D*	*Gastrointestinal System*
3	Root Operation	*1*	*Bypass*
4	Body Part		
5	Approach		
6	Device		
7	Qualifier		

Source: © PB Resources, Inc. Used with permission.

Table 48-4 ■ CODING WORKSHEET WITH CHARACTER 4 COMPLETED

Character (Position)	Name	Value	Description
1	Section	0	Medical and Surgical
2	Body System	D	Gastrointestinal System
3	Root Operation	1	Bypass
4	Body Part	*B*	*Ileum*
5	Approach		
6	Device		
7	Qualifier		

Source: © PB Resources, Inc. Used with permission.

► Marcy now needs to assign the value for Character 4, Body Part.

❏ She searches the first column of the Table until she locates the entry for **B Ileum**.

❏ **Ileum** occupies only one row of the Table, so she determines that this is the correct row to use.

❏ The value for Character 4 is **B**. She enters this character into the worksheet (■ TABLE 48-4).

❏ The code is now **0D1B**, which matches the partial code that was in the Index.

► Next, Marcy needs to assign the value for Character 5, Approach.

❏ She rereads the procedure description in the medical record and identifies that the surgeon used an open approach.

❏ In row **B Ileum** of the Table, she reads the values in the second column for approach.

❏ She locates the entry for **0 Open** and determines that it is consistent with the documentation because an incision was made in the abdominal wall.

❏ Marcy now has five characters in the code on her worksheet: **0D1B0** (■ TABLE 48-5).

► Next, Marcy needs to assign the value for Character 6, Device.

❏ She rereads the procedure description in the medical record and determines that no device was used.

❏ In row **B Ileum** of the Table, she reads the values in the third column for device.

❏ She locates the entry for **Z No device** and determines that it is consistent with the documentation.

❏ Marcy now has six characters in the code on her worksheet: **0D1B0Z** (■ TABLE 48-6).

Table 48-5 ■ CODING WORKSHEET WITH CHARACTER 5 COMPLETED

Character (Position)	Name	Value	Description
1	Section	0	Medical and Surgical
2	Body System	D	Gastrointestinal System
3	Root Operation	1	Bypass
4	Body Part	B	Ileum
5	Approach	*0*	*Open*
6	Device		
7	Qualifier		

Source: © PB Resources, Inc. Used with permission.

Table 48-6 ■ CODING WORKSHEET WITH CHARACTER 6 COMPLETED

Character (Position)	Name	Value	Description
1	Section	0	Medical and Surgical
2	Body System	D	Gastrointestinal System
3	Root Operation	1	Bypass
4	Body Part	B	Ileum
5	Approach	0	Open
6	Device	*Z*	*No Device*
7	Qualifier		

Source: © PB Resources, Inc. Used with permission.

► Finally, Marcy needs to assign the value for Character 7, Qualifier.

❏ She refers to PCS OGCR B3.6a, which states: **Bypass procedures are coded by identifying the body part bypassed 'from' and the body part bypassed 'to.' The fourth character body part specifies the body**

part bypassed from, and the qualifier specifies the body part bypassed to.

❏ She rereads the procedure description in the medical record and determines that the body part bypassed *to* was the skin.

❏ In row **B Ileum** of the Table, she reads the values in the fourth column for qualifier.

❏ She locates the entry for **4 Cutaneous** and determines that it is consistent with the documentation.

❏ Marcy now has all seven characters in the code on her worksheet: **0D1B0Z4** (■ TABLE 48-7). She cross-references the information on her worksheet with the coding manual to ensure that all characters match.

▶ Marcy double-checks each value in the code for accuracy.

❏ She compares each value of the code on her worksheet with the documentation and identifies the specific statement in the document to support each value.

- Gastrointestinal system: She confirms that the gastrointestinal system is the correct body system for a procedure on the ileum. She verifies that the value listed at the top of the PCS table is **D**.

- Bypass: She confirms that the root operation **Bypass** accurately describes the temporary loop ileostomy and that the value listed at the top of the PCS table is **1**.

- Body part: She confirms that the site bypassed from, per the PCS OGCR, is the ileum and the value listed in the PCS table is **B**.

Table 48-7   ■   **COMPLETED CODING WORKSHEET FOR CODE 0D1B0Z4**

Character (Position)	Name	Value	Description
1	Section	0	Medical and Surgical
2	Body System	D	Gastrointestinal
3	Root Operation	1	Bypass
4	Body Part	B	Ileum
5	Approach	0	Open
6	Device	Z	No Device
7	Qualifier	4	Cutaneous

Source: © PB Resources, Inc. Used with permission.

- Open: She confirms that the approach is **Open** because an incision was made in the abdominal wall and the value listed in the PCS table is **0**.

- Device: She confirms that no device is used for this procedure and value listed in the PCS table is **Z**.

- Cutaneous: She confirms per PCS PGCR that the qualifier identifies the site bypassed to, which is the skin. *Skin* is identified by **Cutaneous** in the PCS table and the value is **4**.

▶ Marcy's final code is **0D1B0Z4**, which means **Bypass Ileum to Cutaneous, Open approach**.

CODING PRACTICE

Exercise 48.1   **Assigning Medical and Surgical Procedure Codes**

Instructions: Make copies of the coding worksheet shown in Table 48-1, or create your own. Look up the following procedures in the Index and Tables. Follow the words in exactly the order listed in the exercise. Fill out the coding worksheet as you develop each code. Assign the code. Write the code on the line provided.

1. Excision, nerve, femoral, open approach, diagnostic. ICD-10-PCS Code _____

2. Fusion, lumbar vertebral joints, 2 or more, percutaneous endoscopic approach, nonautologous tissue substitute, posterior approach, posterior column. ICD-10-PCS Code _____

3. Insertion of device in, joint, ankle, left, percutaneous approach, infusion device. ICD-10-PCS Code_____

4. Map, cerebellum, percutaneous approach. ICD-10-PCS Code _____

5. Inspection, ear, inner left, via natural or artificial opening endoscopic. ICD-10-PCS Code _____

6. Bypass, vein, foot, right, percutaneous endoscopic, autologous venous tissue, lower vein. ICD-10-PCS Code _____

7. Drainage, hand, right, open, no device, diagnostic. ICD-10-PCS Code _____

8. Division, muscle, hip, right, percutaneous. ICD-10-PCS Code _____

9. Reattachment, tendon, lower leg, left, open. ICD-10-PCS Code _____

10. Bypass, artery, coronary, one artery, percutaneous endoscopic, autologous arterial tissue, aorta. ICD-10-PCS Code _____

ARRANGING MEDICAL AND SURGICAL PROCEDURE CODES

PCS OGCR B3.2 provides specific information about coding multiple procedures. Additional guidelines within B3 provide further direction relating to specific root operations. ICD-10-PCS does not use modifiers to indicate that multiple procedures were performed. A summary of multiple procedure guidelines follows.

Components of a Procedure

Do not assign separate codes to integral components of a root operation (PCS OGCR B3.1b). The procedural steps required to open the operative field, reach the operative site, and close the operative wound are included in the root operation and are not coded separately (■ FIGURE 48-12). A root operation definition that includes multiple steps should be assigned a single code (■ FIGURE 48-13).

Multiple Body Parts

When the same root operation is performed on different body parts with distinct values, assign separate codes for each body part character (PCS OGCR B3.2a). Sequence first the procedure most closely related to the principal diagnosis. If both procedures are equally related to the principal diagnosis, either may be sequenced first (■ FIGURE 48-14).

Separate Anatomic Sites with the Same Body Part Value

When the same root operation is performed on two different sites but they both share the same body part value, assign a separate code for each procedure (PCS OGCR B3.2b). Both codes will be exactly the same (■ FIGURE 48-15).

Multiple Root Operations on the Same Body Part

When more than one root operation, each with a distinct objective, is performed on the same body part, assign a separate code to each procedure. Use a separate root operation Table for each procedure (PCS OGCR B3.2c). For example, assign separate codes for **Destruction** of sigmoid lesion (Table **0D5**) and **Bypass** of sigmoid colon (Table **0D1**) performed at the same operative session.

Root Operation Is Converted

When an intended root operation is attempted using one approach but is converted to a different approach, assign separate codes for each approach (PCS OGCR B3.2d). For example, when a laparoscopic cholecystectomy is converted to an open cholecystectomy, code the laparoscopic approach as percutaneous endoscopic **Inspection (0FJ44ZZ)** because **Inspection** describes the first procedure that was performed using the percutaneous endoscopic approach. Code the open procedure as

open **Resection (0FT40ZZ)** because the cutting-out of the body part was performed using the open approach. Sequence the code for the approach that was converted *to* (**Resection**) first and the approach that was converted *from* (**Inspection**) second.

Discontinued Procedures

When the intended procedure is discontinued, code the procedure to the root operation performed (PCS OGCR B3.3). If a procedure is discontinued before any other root operation is performed, code the root operation **Inspection (J)** of the body part or anatomic region inspected. For example, a planned aortic valve replacement procedure is discontinued after the initial thoracotomy and before any incision is made in the heart muscle because the patient becomes hemodynamically unstable. This procedure is coded as an open **Inspection** of the mediastinum (**0WJC0ZZ**).

Biopsy Followed by More Definitive Treatment

Biopsies and therapeutic treatments may use the same root operations. When the procedure is stated to be diagnostic, assign Character 7 Qualifier as **X Diagnostic**. When a diagnostic **Excision (B)**, **Extraction (D)**, or **Drainage (9)** is followed by a definitive treatment, such as **Destruction (5)**, **Excision (B)**, or **Resection (T)** at the same procedure site, code *both* the biopsy and the definitive treatment (PCS OGCR B3.4b) (■ FIGURE 48-16). The definitive treatment is the procedure most closely related to the principal diagnosis, so sequence the definitive procedure first, followed by the diagnostic procedure.

Surgeon performed a laparotomy to reach the site of an open liver biopsy, excised tissue from the right lobe of the liver, and performed a layered closure

0FB10ZX   **Excision of Right Lobe Liver, Open Approach, Diagnostic**

Figure 48-12   ■   Example of a single code that includes the incision, excision, and layered closure.

Surgeon performed a laparoscopic repair of a left inguinal hernia and inserted a mesh panel for reinforcement.

0YU64JZ   **Supplement Left Inguinal Region with Synthetic Substitute, Percutaneous Endoscopic Approach**

Figure 48-13   ■   Example of a single code that includes multiple components.

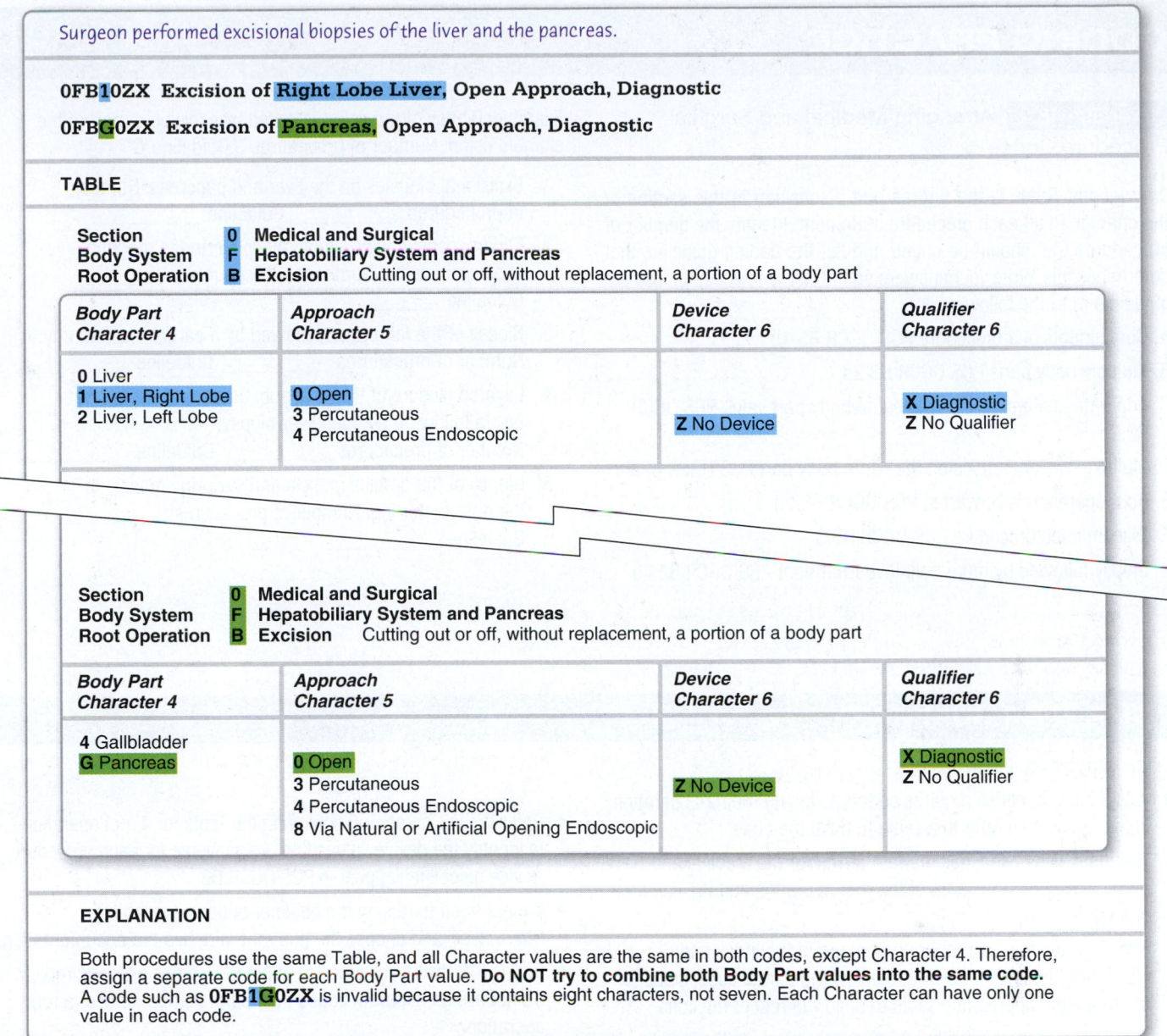

Surgeon performed excisional biopsies of the liver and the pancreas.

0FB10ZX Excision of Right Lobe Liver, Open Approach, Diagnostic

0FBG0ZX Excision of Pancreas, Open Approach, Diagnostic

TABLE

Section	0	Medical and Surgical
Body System	F	Hepatobiliary System and Pancreas
Root Operation	B	Excision Cutting out or off, without replacement, a portion of a body part

Body Part Character 4	Approach Character 5	Device Character 6	Qualifier Character 6
0 Liver 1 Liver, Right Lobe 2 Liver, Left Lobe	0 Open 3 Percutaneous 4 Percutaneous Endoscopic	Z No Device	X Diagnostic Z No Qualifier

Section	0	Medical and Surgical
Body System	F	Hepatobiliary System and Pancreas
Root Operation	B	Excision Cutting out or off, without replacement, a portion of a body part

Body Part Character 4	Approach Character 5	Device Character 6	Qualifier Character 6
4 Gallbladder G Pancreas	0 Open 3 Percutaneous 4 Percutaneous Endoscopic 8 Via Natural or Artificial Opening Endoscopic	Z No Device	X Diagnostic Z No Qualifier

EXPLANATION

Both procedures use the same Table, and all Character values are the same in both codes, except Character 4. Therefore, assign a separate code for each Body Part value. **Do NOT try to combine both Body Part values into the same code.** A code such as **0FB1G0ZX** is invalid because it contains eight characters, not seven. Each Character can have only one value in each code.

Figure 48-14 ■ Example of multiple coding of the same root operation and different body part values.

Surgeon performed percutaneous excisional biopsies on the sartorius muscle and gracilis muscle of the right leg.

BODY PART KEY

Anatomic Site	PCS Description
Gracilis muscle	Upper Leg Muscle, Right Upper Leg Muscle, Left
Sartorius muscle	Upper Leg Muscle, Right Upper Leg Muscle, Left

0KBQ3ZX Excision of Right Upper Leg Muscle, Percutaneous Approach, Diagnostic

0KBQ3ZX Excision of Right Upper Leg Muscle, Percutaneous Approach, Diagnostic

Figure 48-15 ■ Example of multiple coding for separate sites with the same body part value.

Surgeon performed a needle biopsy from a suspicious area of the left breast and sent to pathology for an intraoperative frozen section. The pathologist called back that the tissue was malignant, so an open partial mastectomy was performed.

(1) **0HBU0ZZ** Excision of Left Breast, Open Approach
(2) **0HBU3ZX** Excision of Left Breast, Percutaneous Approach, Diagnostic

Figure 48-16 ■ Example of sequencing biopsy followed by definitive treatment.

CODING PRACTICE

Exercise 48.2 Arranging Medical and Surgical Procedure Codes

Instructions: Refer to the figures and discussion in this section of the chapter. Read each procedure statement. Identify the number of procedures that should be coded and list the coding guideline that determines this. Write your answers on the lines provided. Choose the guideline from the following list:

A. Components of a procedure PCS OGCR B3.1b

B. Multiple body parts PCS OGCR B3.2a

C. Separate anatomic sites with same body part value PCS OGCR B3.2b

D. Multiple root operations on the same body part PCS OGCR B3.2c

E. Root operation is converted PCS OGCR B3.2d

F. Discontinued procedure PCS OGCR B3.3

G. Biopsy followed by more definitive treatment PCS OGCR B3.4b

Example: Biopsy of the colon followed by excision of part of the sigmoid colon. Number of procedures *2* Guideline *G*

1. Excisional biopsies on the liver and pancreas. Number of procedures _____ Guideline _____

2. Laparoscopic cholecystectomy converted to an open cholecystectomy. Number of procedures _____ Guideline _____

3. Biopsy of the left breast followed by a partial mastectomy. Number of procedures _____ Guideline _____

4. Layered closure of the skin, subcutaneous tissue, and fascia following an open liver biopsy. Number of procedures _____ Guideline _____

5. Biopsy of the gracilis muscle and sartorius muscle in the right upper leg. Number of procedures _____ Guideline _____

CHAPTER SUMMARY

In this chapter you learned that:

- Assigning PCS codes requires coders to locate the root operation in the Index, then refer to a Table to build the code.

- The Index uses two types of Main Terms for the Medical and Surgical section: the name of the root operation and the common procedure name.

- After locating the appropriate procedure in the Index and identifying the first three characters of the partial code, cross-reference the appropriate Table to build the rest of the code.

- The body system is usually a first-level subterm in the Index with the body part a second-level subterm.

- A PCS Table lists the possible approach values for each body part and the root operation.

- Refer to the Character 6 column in the Table for a root operation to identify the device values that are available for each procedure. Device guidelines appear in PCS OGCR B6.

- Coders need to review the qualifier options available for Character 7 and choose the one that matches the documentation.

- PCS OGCR discusses when multiple PCS codes are required. Do not assign separate codes to integral components of a root operation.

- PCS OGCR discusses how to code for multiple body parts, separate anatomic sites, multiple root operations on the same body part, procedures converted from one root operation to a different one, discontinued procedures, and biopsies.

CONCEPT QUIZ

Take a moment to look back at your trip through assigning and arranging Medical and Surgical procedure codes and solidify your skills. This is your opportunity to pull together everything you have learned.

Completion

Instructions: Write the term that completes each statement based on the information you learned in this chapter. Choose from words in parentheses in each statement. Refer to the discussion in this chapter if you need a little extra help.

1. When coding an ileostomy, Character 7 identifies the site bypassed (to/from) _____.

2. When a diagnostic procedure is followed by a definitive treatment at the same procedure site, assign (one/two) _____ code(s).

3. ICD-10-PCS (does/does not) _____ require modifiers to indicate that multiple procedures were performed.

4. When coding CABG, Character 7 identifies the site bypassed (to/from) _____.

5. When dilation is a procedural step necessary to reach the operative site, it (does/does not) _____ get a separate code.

6. Endoscopic ablation of endometriosis in the endometrium and ovaries is assigned (one/two) _____ code(s).

7. When the root operation Transfer is performed on a peripheral nerve, the site it is transferred *to* is identified in Character (4/7) _____.

8. A PCS Table (does/does not) _____ contain instructional notes.

9. When coding a colostomy, Character 4 identifies the site bypassed (to/from) _____.

10. When the Index provides more than one cross-reference, it (does/does not) _____ mean that you can choose any of the options listed for any procedure.

Multiple Choice

Instructions: Circle the letter of the best answer to each question based on the information you learned in this chapter. Refer to the discussion in this chapter and the Glossary at the end of this book if you need a little extra help.

1. Where should coders look to find a full description of PCS codes?
   A. PCS Table
   B. PCS appendix
   C. PCS Index
   D. CMS website

2. Which PCS code Character identifies the surgical approach?
   A. Character 4
   B. Character 5
   C. Character 6
   D. Character 7

3. How is a biopsy identified in a PCS code?
   A. Qualifier X Diagnostic
   B. Qualifier B Biopsy
   C. Qualifier T Therapeutic
   D. Root operation B Biopsy

4. Which PCS OGCR for multiple procedures applies to this procedure? *A planned aortic valve replacement procedure is discontinued after the initial thoracotomy when the patient becomes unstable.*
   A. Components of a procedure PCS OGCR B3.1b
   B. Multiple root operations on the same body part PCS OGCR B3.2c
   C. Root operation is converted PCS OGCR B3.2d
   D. Discontinued procedure PCS OGCR B3.3

5. Which PCS appendix provides a cross-walk that matches generic and brand-name devices with the appropriate PCS term?
   A. Device Aggregation Table
   B. Device Key
   C. Device Crosswalk
   D. Device Definitions

6. Which Character identifies the site bypassed *to* in a noncoronary bypass?
   A. Character 4
   B. Character 5
   C. Character 6
   D. Character 7

7. Which PCS appendix cross-references specific anatomic terms to the PCS body part?
   A. Body Part Definitions
   B. Body Part Aggregation Table
   C. Body Part Cross-Reference
   D. Body Part Key

8. Which of the following Tables appears first in the ICD-10-PCS manual?
   A. 09Z
   B. 0D1
   C. 102
   D. B00

9. Which of the following is a characteristic of PCS Tables?
   A. Each page contains one Table.
   B. Tables may contain more than one root operation.
   C. Tables may be subdivided into rows.
   D. No Table is longer than one page.

10. What root operation(s) should be reported for a laparoscopic cholecystectomy converted to an open cholecystectomy?
    A. Assign the root operation Conversion to report both procedures.
    B. Assign the root operation Inspection for the laparoscopic cholecystectomy and the root operation Resection for the open procedure.
    C. Assign the root operation Resection to report the open procedure only.
    D. Assign the root operation Removal to report both procedures.

KEEP ON CODING

Instructions: Make copies of the coding worksheet shown in Table 48-1 or create your own. Read the procedural statement. The root operation is stated, but words are not listed in the exactly same order as in the coding manual. Look up root operation in the Index, identify the body system and/or body part subterms. Refer to the Table listed and complete the code using the coding worksheet. Write the code on the line provided.

Example: Resection of the gallbladder, percutaneous endoscopic approach. ICD-10-PCS Code(s) *OFT44ZZ*

1. Extirpation of a tumor from the brain, open approach. ICD-10-PCS Code(s) _____

2. Excision of the lower lobe of the left bronchus, via the oral cavity endoscopic, biopsy. ICD-10-PCS Code(s) _____

3. Repair of the left nipple, external approach. ICD-10-PCS Code(s) _____

4. Insertion of a limb-lengthening external fixation device on the left fibula, percutaneous approach. ICD-10-PCS Code(s) _____

5. Dilation of both ureters using an intraluminal device, percutaneous endoscopic approach. ICD-10-PCS Code(s) _____

6. Bypass to two coronary arteries from a coronary vein using an intraluminal drug-eluting device. ICD-10-PCS Code(s) _____

7. Insertion of a stimulator lead into the trapezius muscle, percutaneous approach. ICD-10-PCS Code(s) _____

8. Occlusion of the vagina using an intraluminal device, via the vaginal opening. ICD-10-PCS Code(s) _____

9. Supplement of the ileocecal valve with a synthetic substitute, percutaneous endoscopic approach. ICD-10-PCS Code(s) _____

10. Drainage of the bursa of a rib with placement of a drainage device, percutaneous endoscopic approach. ICD-10-PCS Code(s) _____

11. Excision of the vitreous of the left eye, percutaneous approach, diagnostic. ICD-10-PCS Code(s) _____

12. Resection of the appendix, percutaneous laparoscopic approach. ICD-10-PCS Code(s) _____

13. Detachment (amputation) of the left thumb, open approach, high level. ICD-10-PCS Code(s) _____

14. Destruction of the endometrium using an endoscope through the vagina. ICD-10-PCS Code(s) _____

15. Excision from the right lobe of the liver for a biopsy, percutaneous (needle) approach. ICD-10-PCS Code(s) _____

16. Reposition of the right tibia, external approach. ICD-10-PCS Code(s) _____

17. Transplantation of the left kidney, open approach, using a live donor organ (allogenic). ICD-10-PCS Code(s) _____

18. Drainage of an abscess on the skin of the right upper arm, external approach, no device. ICD-10-PCS Code(s) _____

19. Replacement of the right hip joint with a metal on polyethylene synthetic substitute, uncemented bone, open approach. ICD-10-PCS Code(s) _____

20. Bypass of the right ureter to the bladder using a nonautologous tissue substitute, percutaneous endoscopic approach. ICD-10-PCS Code(s) _____

21. Removal of an external fixation device from the left ankle joint using the external approach. ICD-10-PCS Code(s) _____

22. Supplement of a right upper leg muscle with synthetic mesh using the percutaneous endoscopic approach. ICD-10-PCS Code(s) _____

23. Extirpation of the left saphenous vein, percutaneous endoscopic approach. ICD-10-PCS Code(s) _____

24. Transfer of the radial nerve to the median nerve, open approach. ICD-10-PCS Code(s) _____

25. Restriction of the stomach pylorus with an extraluminal device, percutaneous endoscopic approach. ICD-10-PCS Code(s) _____

CODING CHALLENGE

Instructions: Read the mini-medical-record of each patient's encounter. Review the information abstracted in the Coding Challenge in Chapter 47, then assign Assign ICD-10-PCS procedure codes using the Index and Tables, and arrange them correctly.

1. INPATIENT HOSPITAL   Gender: F   Age: 83

Preprocedure diagnosis: Pressure ulcer, left hip

Procedure description: Open excisional debridement of left hip. Used scissors to cut out necrosis and devitalized tissue, through full epidermis and subcutaneous tissue, 1 cm beyond the wound margin.

Postprocedure diagnosis: Healing stage III pressure ulcer, left hip

Tip: Use the "Body Part Key" appendix of the ICD-10-PCS manual to determine how to classify the hip.

1 PCS Code _____

2. INPATIENT HOSPITAL   Gender: F   Age: 48

Preprocedure diagnosis: Mass in left breast

Procedure description: Needle biopsy. Using a needle, took out a tissue sample from the left breast that was previously marked with a wire.

Postprocedure diagnosis: Benign neoplasm, left breast per pathology report

1 PCS Code _____

3. INPATIENT HOSPITAL   Gender: M   Age: 15

Preprocedure assessment: Presented to ED with vomiting, acute abdominal pain, RLQ tenderness, T 101 degrees

Procedure description: Appendectomy. Made three small umbilical incisions and placed laparoscope. Expanded abdominal cavity with carbon dioxide to aid visualization. Grasped appendix and divided with stapler. Cauterized appendiceal stump. Removed appendix, irrigated and suctioned abdominal cavity. Removed instruments and closed incision. Patient tolerated procedure well, no complications.

Postprocedure diagnosis: Acute appendicitis with rupture

1 PCS _____

4. INPATIENT HOSPITAL   Gender: F   Age: 61

Preprocedure diagnosis: Gangrene in left great toe, due to nonhealing plantar (*sole of foot*) ulcer

Procedure description: Midlevel amputation of L great toe at interphalangeal joint

Postprocedure diagnosis: Diabetes with gangrene

1 PCS Code _____

5. INPATIENT HOSPITAL   Gender: F   Age: 23

Preprocedure: Hypermenorrhea

Procedure description: Transvaginal dilation and curettage. Inserted speculum to hold the vagina open. Progressively dilated cervix and uterus with os dilator. Inserted curette and scraped endometrial wall. Tissue sent to lab for analysis.

Postprocedure diagnosis: Hypermenorrhea

Tip: Hypermenorrhea is abnormally heavy menstrual flow. Dilation is a procedural step necessary to reach the operative site (uterus), so it does not get a separate code (PCS OGCR B3.1b).

1 PCS Code _____

6. INPATIENT HOSPITAL   Gender: F   Age: 52

Preprocedure diagnosis: Endometriosis

Procedure description: Ablation of ovaries and endometrium. Inserted the endoscope through the vagina into the uterus to cauterize the endometrium (*lining of uterus*). When that was successfully completed, withdrew the scope, applied a new tip. Made three incisions on the lower abdomen and inserted endoscope to treat each ovary.

Postprocedure diagnosis: Endometriosis

Tip: This procedure describes endoscopic ablation of endometriosis in the endometrium and ovaries. Assign one code for each site.

2 PCS Codes _____

(continued from page 1017)

---

7. INPATIENT HOSPITAL Gender: F Age: 52

Preprocedure diagnosis: Pain RUQ, T 102 degrees, vomiting, acute cholecystitis with calculi in the common bile duct causing obstruction. Extensive known abdominal adhesions prevent a laparoscopic approach.

Procedure description: Cholecystectomy. Made subcostal incision and isolated gallbladder from surrounding structures with laparotomy packs. Excised entire gallbladder and common bile duct. Hemostasis was achieved. Closed operative wound. Patient tolerated procedure well.

Postprocedure diagnosis: Acute cholecystitis with calculi in the common bile duct causing obstruction

2 PCS Codes _____

---

8. INPATIENT HOSPITAL Gender: M Age: 43

Preprocedure diagnosis: Detached R retina

Procedure description: Trans pars plana vitrectomy (TPPV) with synthetic scleral buckle. Made incision in pars plana and used vitreous cutter to suction out all vitreous. Injected balanced saline solution (BSS) to replace vitreous. Sutured scleral buckle, which effectively closed the break. Pt tolerated px well.

Postprocedure diagnosis: Detached R retina

2 PCS Codes _____

---

9. INPATIENT HOSPITAL Gender: M Age: 75

Preprocedure diagnosis: Blepharoptosis obscuring vision

Procedure description: Bilateral upper blepharoplasty. Cut out a crescent of skin and subcutaneous tissue from fold of R eyelid, sutured to restore normal position of eyelid. Repeated on left side.

Postprocedure diagnosis: Blepharoptosis obscuring vision

2 PCS Codes _____

---

10. INPATIENT HOSPITAL Gender: F Age: 23

Preprocedure diagnosis: Fractured R tibia and R humerus

Procedure description: Open reduction, R tibia with internal fixation device. Closed reduction, R humerus with percutaneous internal fixation. Applied cast to right humerus.

Postprocedure diagnosis: Fractured R tibia, fractured R humerus shaft

Tip: Refer to PCS OGCR B3.15.

2 PCS Codes _____

Section 0: Root Operations 5, 6, B, D, T

Destruction • Detachment • Excision • Extraction • Resection

Chapter
49

Learning Objectives

After completing this chapter, you should have the skills to:

49.1 Spell and define the key words, medical terms, and abbreviations related to procedures that take out some or all of a body part. (Remember)

49.2 Identify the types of procedures performed for the root operations Destruction, Detachment, Excision, Extraction, and Resection. (Apply)

49.3 Adhere to ICD-10-PCS coding guidelines related to root operations 5, 6, B, D, and T. (Apply)

49.4 Examine and abstract procedural information from the medical record for coding for the root operations 5, 6, B, D, and T. (Analyze)

49.5 Demonstrate how to assign codes for the root operations 5, 6, B, D, and T. (Apply)

49.6 Utilize guidelines for arranging (sequencing) codes for root operations 5, 6, B, D, and T. (Apply)

Chapter Outline

- **Basics of Procedures That Take Out Some or All of a Body Part**
- **Coding Guidelines for Root Operations 5, 6, B, D, and T**
- **Abstracting for Root Operations 5, 6, B, D, and T**
- **Assigning Characters 4–7 for Root Operations 5, 6, B, D, and T**
- **Arranging Codes for Root Operations 5, 6, B, D, and T**

Key Terms and Abbreviations

biopsy
definitive treatment
dilation and curettage (D&C)
principal procedure
phacoemulsification

In addition to the key terms listed here, students should know the terms defined within tables in this chapter.

INTRODUCTION

Traveling in an unfamiliar place or a new country can be challenging because you need to learn new names, new terms, and new customs. However, as you take small steps and become familiar with one thing at a time, you quickly become oriented and comfortable in your new surroundings. By approaching new coding material in an organized manner, you will adapt to—and even enjoy—the new environment.

This chapter discusses the five Medical and Surgical root operations in the group *Procedures that take out some or all of a body part*: Destruction, Detachment, Excision, Extraction, and Resection. Although the root operations share a common purpose—taking out some or all of a body part—each has a unique aspect that makes it different from the other procedures in this group. Pay careful attention to the differences between each root operation so that you can use each confidently and accurately.

BASICS OF PROCEDURES THAT TAKE OUT SOME OR ALL OF A BODY PART

The root operation group *Procedures that take out some or all of a body part* includes five root operations. ■ TABLE 49-1 provides the definitions and values of root operations in this group and identifies procedural terms frequently associated with each. Some commonly used terms, such as *excision* and *removal*, can be associated with more than one root operation. There is not a direct match between a specific procedural term and a root operation because some medical terms, such as excision and removal, can be associated with more than one root operation.

PCS definitions that include cutting allow for the use of a variety of sharp instruments such as a scalpel, wire, scissors, bone saw, or electrocautery tip. The instrument(s) point the coder in the direction of certain root operations, but there is not a requirement or direct match between most root operations and the instruments used.

Root operations are assigned based on the content of the operative report regarding what was actually performed, not on the terms used by the physician in documentation. Details of the differences between the root operations are discussed in the "Abstracting Procedures" and "Assigning Codes" sections of this chapter.

Refer to detailed anatomic diagrams of specific organ systems in Chapters 8–43 of this text, or in external references, when you need to refresh your memory of human anatomy.

Refer to ■ TABLE 49-2 for a refresher on how to build medical terms related to procedures that take out some or all of a body part.

> ## CODING CAUTION
>
> Be alert for root operations that have similar English meanings but different PCS definitions.
>
> **Excision** (B) (*cutting out or off, without replacement, a portion of a PCS body part*) and **Resection** (T) (*cutting out or off, without replacement, all of a PCS body part*)
>
> **Destruction** (5) (*physical eradication of all or a portion of a body part or abnormal tissue by the direct use of energy, force, or a destructive agent without removing it from the body*) and **Fragmentation** (F) (*breaking abnormal solid matter in a body part into pieces*)

Table 49-1 ■ **ROOT OPERATIONS THAT TAKE OUT SOME OR ALL OF A BODY PART**

Root Operation	Value	Definition	Terms
Destruction	5	Physical eradication of all or a portion of a body part by the direct use of energy, force, or a destructive agent	Ablation, cautery, electrosurgery, coagulation, cryosurgery, laser surgery, fulguration, thermotherapy, electrodessication, photocoagulation
Detachment	6	Cutting off all or a portion of the upper or lower extremities	Amputation, disarticulation, removal
Excision	B	Cutting out or off, without replacement, a portion of a PCS body part	Excision, removal, cutting, biopsy
Extraction	D	Pulling or stripping out or off all or a portion of a body part by the use of force	Ligation, microincision, suction, curettage
Resection	T	Cutting out or off, without replacement, all of a PCS body part	Excision, removal, cutting

Table 49-2 ■ **EXAMPLE OF CONSTRUCTING MEDICAL TERMS FOR PROCEDURES THAT TAKE OUT SOME OR ALL OF A BODY PART**

Combining Form	Prefix/Suffix	Complete Medical Term
neur/o (*nerve*)		**cryo + surgery** (*surgery using cold*)
	cryo- (prefix; *cold*)	**electro + surgery** (*surgery using electrical energy*)
	-ectomy (suffix; *surgical excision*)	**electro + desiccation** (*destruction using electrical energy*)
gastr/o (*stomach*)		**neur + ectomy** (*excision of a nerve*)
	-desiccation (suffix; *destruction*)	**gastr + ectomy** (*excision of the stomach*)
electr/o (*electrical energy*)		

Source: © PB Resources, Inc. Used with permission.

CODING PRACTICE

Exercise 49.1 Basics of Procedures That Take Out Some or All of a Body Part

Instructions: Use your medical terminology skills and resources to define the following procedures that take out some or all of a body part, then identify the code(s) or code range listed in the ICD-10-PCS Index. Follow these steps:

- Use slash marks "/" to break down each underlined term into its root(s) and suffix.
- Define the meaning of the underlined word based on the meaning of each word part.
- Look up the phrase in the ICD-10-PCS Index, and write down the name(s) of root operation(s) the Index cross-references you to and the Table(s), if provided.
- Do not assign any codes.

Example: <u>fasciectomy</u> fasci/ectomy   Meaning *excision of the fascia*   PCS Root Operation(s)/Table(s) *Excision 0JB*

1. <u>cryoablation</u>   Meaning _____   PCS Root Operation(s)/Table(s) _____
2. <u>phacoemulsification</u>, lens   Meaning _____   PCS Root Operation(s)/Table(s) _____
3. <u>polypectomy</u>, gastrointestinal   Meaning _____   PCS Root Operation(s)/Table(s) _____
4. <u>electrocautery</u>   Meaning _____   PCS Root Operation(s)/Table(s) _____
5. <u>phlebectomy</u>   Meaning _____   PCS Root Operation(s)/Table(s) _____
6. <u>adenoidectomy</u>   Meaning _____   PCS Root Operation(s)/Table(s) _____
7. <u>disarticulation</u>   Meaning _____   PCS Root Operation(s)/Table(s) _____
8. <u>chondrectomy</u>   Meaning _____   PCS Root Operation(s)/Table(s) _____
9. <u>phrenicoexeresis</u>   Meaning _____   PCS Root Operation(s)/Table(s) _____
10. <u>arteriectomy</u>   Meaning _____   PCS Root Operation(s)/Table(s) _____

CODING GUIDELINES FOR ROOT OPERATIONS 5, 6, B, D, AND T

Coders should understand the guidelines for the Medical and Surgical section (0). PCS OGCR section B is organized by the characters of the PCS code:

- B2 Body System
- B3 Root Operation
- B4 Body Part
- B5 Approach
- B6 Device

Within the guidelines for each character, general guidelines appear first, followed by those for specific root operations. Information about specific qualifiers appears throughout the guidelines, but there is not a separate section with guidelines for Character 7, Qualifier.

Guidelines specific to the root operations 5, 6, B, D, and T include the following. Refer to the PCS OGCR for clinical examples of each guideline.

- **Biopsy** procedures—Code biopsy procedures—those done to determine a diagnosis— using the root operations Excision, Extraction, or Drainage and the qualifier Diagnostic

(X) (PCS OGCR B3.4a). (*Note:* The root operation Drainage is discussed in Chapter 52 of this text.)

- Biopsy followed by more **definitive treatment**—When biopsy is followed by a more definitive procedure, such as Excision or Resection, at the same procedure site, code both the biopsy and the more definitive treatment (PCS OGCR B3.4b). PCS uses the term *definitive treatment* similarly to therapeutic treatment—a treatment intended to cure, eliminate, improve, or reduce the effects of a condition.

- Excision and Resection—Use the most specific body part to assign the root operation. Assign Resection of the specific body part whenever all of the body part is cut out or off, rather than coding Excision of a less specific body part (PCS OGCR B3.8).

- Excision for graft—When an autograft is harvested from a different procedure site to complete the objective of the procedure, assign separate codes for harvesting the graft and performing the primary procedure (PCS OGCR B3.9).

Specific guidelines and instructions are discussed throughout this chapter of the text.

ABSTRACTING FOR ROOT OPERATIONS 5, 6, B, D, AND T

Abstracting for PCS focuses on identifying the correct root operation, which involves reading the operative report and interpreting it in light of root operation definitions. When reading the operative report, remember to focus on the objective of the procedure and the activities performed, not just the specific medical terms the surgeon uses to describe the procedure. Many times the root operation can be determined conclusively during abstracting. Other times, the root operation can be narrowed down to two options, which must be differentiated based on other characters that are assigned from the PCS Tables. This occurs frequently with the root operations Excision and Resection. The root operation definition is a combination of the functional objective of the procedure and the anatomic site. The following information summarizes the objective, definition, unique features, and examples of root operations 5, 6, B, D, and T.

Abstracting for Destruction (5)

The objective of the root operation Destruction is eradicating without replacement. The site of the procedure is some or all of a body part. There is not a distinction between eradicating some of a body part compared with all of a body part. Physical eradication involves the direct use of energy, force, or a destructive agent on an anatomic body part. None of the body part is physically removed.

Destruction "takes out" a body part in the sense that it obliterates the body part so it is no longer there. This root operation defines a broad range of common procedures and can be used anywhere in the body to treat a variety of conditions, including warts, polyps, lesions, and varices.

Assign the root operation Destruction only when the body part is not replaced, supplemented, reinforced, moved, repaired, or performed as part of a procedure with a more specific objective. Examples of Destruction are fulguration of a rectal polyp and cautery of a skin lesion.

Destruction can be confused with the root operation Fragmentation (F), which is discussed in Chapter 52 of this text. Fragmentation is breaking solid matter in a body part, such as a foreign body or an abnormal by-product, into pieces, whereas Destruction is the eradication of the body part itself or abnormal tissue in the body part (■ TABLE 49-3).

Abstracting for Detachment (6)

The objective of the root operation Detachment is cutting out or off without replacement. The site of the procedure is all or part of any extremity—arms, legs, hands, feet, fingers, or toes. Assign the root operation Detachment only when the body part is not replaced, supplemented, reinforced, moved, repaired, or performed as part of a procedure with a more specific objective. Examples of Detachment are amputation of the foot or part of a finger (■ TABLE 49-4).

Abstracting for Excision (B)

The objective of the root operation Excision is cutting out or off without replacement. The site of the procedure is

Table 49-3 ■ **EXAMPLES OF THE ROOT OPERATION DESTRUCTION (5)**

Organ System	Procedural Examples
Cardiovascular	Vein stripping, ablation of arrhythmogenic focus
Digestive	Fulguration of rectal polyp
Endocrine	Radioablation of parathyroid gland
Genitourinary	Fulguration of endometrium, conization of cervix by cryotherapy
Hepatobiliary	Ablation of tumor in cystic duct
Integumentary	Cautery of skin lesion, cryotherapy of wart
Nervous	Sclerotherapy of nerve lesion, radiofrequency destruction of a nerve
Respiratory	Cautery of nosebleed
Special Senses (Ear, Eye)	Laser coagulation of retinal hemorrhage

Source: © PB Resources, Inc. Used with permission.

Table 49-4 ■ **EXAMPLES OF THE ROOT OPERATION DETACHMENT (6)**

Organ System	Procedural Examples
Musculoskeletal	Amputation above elbow, disarticulation of shoulder, below-knee amputation

Source: © PB Resources, Inc. Used with permission.

some of a body part as defined by PCS. The body part definition may be more or less specific than the physical structure. For example, PCS divides the colon into 10 body part values for the root operation Excision but only one body part value for the root operation Revision. Therefore, when abstracting the root operation, you may be able to narrow it down to only two options—Excision or Resection—until you refer to the Table to identify how body parts are divided. This process is discussed later in this chapter in the section "Assigning Characters 4–7 for root operations 5, 6, B, D, and T."

Assign the root operation Excision only when the body part is not replaced, supplemented, reinforced, moved, repaired, or performed as part of a procedure with a more specific objective. Biopsies obtained through cutting are coded to the root operation Excision, but biopsies obtained through other methods are coded to the root operation that describes the method used, such as Drainage, used for needle aspiration, or Extraction, used for pulling or scraping. Examples of Excision are a breast lumpectomy—in which a tumor and surrounding tissue is cut out of the breast—or excision of a single lymph node (■ TABLE 49-5).

Abstracting for Extraction (D)

The objective of the root operation Extraction is pulling out or off without replacement. The site of the procedure is some or all of a body part. There is not a distinction between pulling

Table 49-5 ■ EXAMPLES OF THE ROOT OPERATION EXCISION (B)

Organ System	Procedural Examples
Blood and Immune	Harvesting of saphenous vein for grafting, lymph node excision
Cardiovascular	Open endarterectomy of an artery
Digestive	EGD with biopsy
Endocrine	Thyroid biopsy
Genitourinary	Partial nephrectomy
Hepatobiliary	Liver biopsy, excision of tail of pancreas
Integumentary	Breast lumpectomy, excision of cyst or lesion
Lymphatic and Hemic	Excision of a single lymph node
Musculoskeletal	Muscle biopsy, partial discectomy (*removal of disc fragments*)
Nervous	Brain biopsy
Respiratory	Biopsy of lung, excision of partial lobe of lung
Special Senses (Ear, Eye)	Biopsy of eye

Source: © PB Resources, Inc. Used with permission.

Table 49-6 ■ EXAMPLES OF THE ROOT OPERATION EXTRACTION (D)

Organ System	Procedural Examples
Cardiovascular	Microincisional phlebectomy of varicose veins, vein stripping, and ligation
Digestive	Tooth extraction
Genitourinary	Suction dilation and curettage, endometrial biopsy
Integumentary	Nail removal, liposuction for medical reasons
Musculoskeletal	Bone marrow biopsy
Nervous	Extraction of hypoglossal nerve
Respiratory	Extraction of the pleura
Special Senses (Ear, Eye)	Cataract phacoemulsification without intraocular lens implant

Source: © PB Resources, Inc. Used with permission.

Table 49-7 ■ EXAMPLES OF THE ROOT OPERATION RESECTION (T)

Organ System	Procedural Examples
Blood and Immune	Lymph chain excision
Digestive	Sigmoidectomy
Endocrine	Total excision of left lobe of thyroid
Genitourinary	Total nephrectomy, vaginal hysterectomy
Hepatobiliary	Cholecystectomy
Integumentary	Total mastectomy
Lymphatic and Hemic	Excision of an entire lymph chain
Musculoskeletal	Excision of entire disc
Respiratory	Excision of entire lobe of lung
Special Senses (Ear, Eye)	Enucleation of eyeball

Source: © PB Resources, Inc. Used with permission.

out or off some of a body part compared with all of a body part. Extraction is coded when the method used to take out the body part is pulling or stripping. Minor cutting, such as that used in vein stripping procedures, is included in Extraction and is not coded separately if the objective of the procedure is met by pulling or stripping. When a biopsy is obtained through pulling or stripping, as occurs with an endometrial biopsy, the root operation is Extraction.

Assign the root operation Extraction only when the body part is not replaced, supplemented, reinforced, moved, repaired, or performed as part of a procedure with a more specific objective. Examples of Extraction are a suction dilation and curettage (D&C)—in which the cervix is dilated and the endometrium (*lining of the uterus*) is scraped away—and phacoemulsification (*use of ultrasonic vibrations to reduce the lens of the eye to a liquid, followed by draining out the liquid*) without implantation of an intraocular lens (■ TABLE 49-6).

Abstracting for Resection (T)

The objective of the root operation Resection is cutting out or off without replacement. The site of the procedure is all of a body part as defined by PCS. The only difference between the root operations Excision and Resection is whether the PCS body part is partially or completely removed. This determination can be made only after consulting the PCS Table. As you become more proficient with PCS coding, you will learn how body parts are defined for various organ systems, and determining which root operation is applicable in a given situation will be easier.

As with Excision, assign the root operation Resection only when the body part is not replaced, supplemented, reinforced,

moved, repaired, or performed as part of a procedure with a more specific objective. Examples of Resection are a total mastectomy—in which the entire breast tissue is cut out—or excision of an entire lymph chain (■ TABLE 49-7).

Key Criteria for Abstracting

Refer to Table 47-2 and 47-3 for general guidance on abstracting PCS procedures and root operation groups. Then refer to ■ TABLE 49-8, (page 1024) for more specific guidance on how to abstract and distinguish among procedures in the root operation group *Procedures that take out some or all of a body part.* Answer the questions in the left-hand column, then refer to the suggested root operation(s) in the right-hand column. The first three questions help verify that you have identified the correct root operation Groups. The remaining questions help identify the correct root operation within the group.

Coders must use good judgment and critical thinking when answering the questions and applying root operation

Table 49-8 ■ **KEY CRITERIA FOR ABSTRACTING ROOT OPERATIONS THAT TAKE OUT SOME OR ALL OF A BODY PART**

Question	Root Operation (Value)
❏ Was a body part or abnormal tissue growth (such as a lesion or tumor) removed?	If *Yes*, continue below to root operations 5, 6, B, D, and T.
❏ Was a foreign object or abnormal material (such as calculus) removed?	If *Yes*, do not use root operations 5, 6, B, D, and T.
❏ Was the body part replaced with a natural or synthetic substitute?	If *Yes*, do not use root operations 5, 6, B, D, and T.
Answer the following questions to help distinguish Root Operations 5, 6, B, D, and T	
❏ Was removal performed by cutting?	Excision (B)
	Resection (T)
❏ Was removal performed through physical eradication, such as energy, force, or a destructive agent?	Destruction (5)
❏ Was an extremity cut off?	Detachment (6)
❏ Was removal performed through the use of force, such as pulling or stripping?	Extraction (D)

Source: © PB Resources, Inc. Used with permission.

definitions. There may be overlap between some questions, in which case you must refer to the root operation definitions to determine the correct procedure. For example, when an amputation is performed, two questions are answered *Yes*:

- Was removal performed by cutting?
- Was an extremity removed?

The only correct root operation for an amputation is Detachment (D)—cutting off all or a portion of the upper or lower extremities—because it is more specific than Excision (B) or Resection (T).

Cutting might be performed as a component of the surgical process and followed by another method, such as stripping or suction. In this situation, cutting is not coded because it is integral to the root operation. Use only the stripping or suction method to determine the root operation.

In some cases you may not be able to determine the final root operation during abstracting. For example, you may not be able to distinguish between Excision and Resection until you refer to PCS Tables when assigning codes. A guided example of abstracting for the root operations Excision and Resection follows.

Guided Example of Abstracting for Excision and Resection

Refer to the following example throughout this chapter to practice skills for abstracting, assigning, and arranging codes for the root operations Excision and Resection. Similar principles apply to working with other root operations that take out some or all of a body part.

INPATIENT HOSPITAL   Gender: F   Age: 48

Preoperative diagnosis: Metastatic breast cancer

Procedure: Lymphadenectomy. Open left lymphadenectomy of entire axillary chain and percutaneous left cervical lymphadenectomy of the first node only.

Postoperative diagnosis: Left breast cancer with metastasis to lymph nodes

---

Follow along as fictitious coder Marcy Elwood, CCS, abstracts the procedure. Check off each step after you complete it.

▶ Marcy reads through the entire record, paying special attention to the reason for the encounter, the procedure performed, and the postoperative diagnosis. She refers to the Key Criteria for Abstracting Root Operations that Take Out Some or All of a Body Part (Table 49-8) and Key Criteria for Abstracting Multiple Procedures (Table 47-14).

❏ She notes the preoperative diagnosis: Metastatic breast cancer.

❏ *What is the stated procedure?* Lymphadenectomy

❏ *What organ or body part is involved?* Axillary chain for the first procedure; left cervical node for the second procedure

❏ *Is the procedure description what you would expect based on the name of the procedure?* Yes

❏ *What surgical approach(es) is used?* Open for the first procedure; percutaneous for the second procedure

❏ *Was more than one procedure, or a combined procedure, performed?* Yes, the first procedure is open left lymphadenectomy of entire axillary chain; the second procedure is percutaneous left cervical lymphadenectomy of the first node

❏ *Did the procedure take out some or all of a body part without replacement?* Yes

❏ *Was a body part or abnormal tissue growth (such as a lesion or tumor) removed?* Yes, a cancerous tumor or lesion was removed

❏ *Was a foreign object or abnormal material (such as calculus) removed?* No

❏ *Was the body part replaced with a natural or synthetic substitute?* No

❏ *Was removal performed by cutting?* Yes

❏ *Was removal performed through physical eradication, such as energy, force, or a destructive agent?* No

❏ *Was an extremity removed?* No

❏ *Was removal performed through the use of force, such as pulling or stripping?* No

▶ At this time, Marcy believes that she will use the root operations Excision and/or Resection and anticipates that she will need two codes, one for each procedure. She will verify this information when she refers to the PCS Tables to assign codes.

CODING PRACTICE

Exercise 49.2 Abstracting for Root Operations 5, 6, B, D, and T

Instructions: Read the mini-medical-record of each patient's encounter and answer the abstracting questions. Write the answer on the line provided. Do not assign any codes.

---

1. INPATIENT HOSPITAL   Gender: F   Age: 26

Preprocedure diagnosis: Polycystic ovaries

Procedure: Oophorectomy. Approached transvaginally with laparoscopic assistance. Located and removed entirety of both ovaries.

Postprocedure diagnosis: Polycystic ovaries

a. What is the stated procedure? _____

b. What organ or body part is involved? _____

c. What is the laterality? _____

d. Is the procedure description what you would expect based on the name of the procedure? _____

e. What surgical approach is used? _____

f. Was more than one procedure, or a combined procedure, performed? _____

g. Did the procedure take out some or all of a body part without replacement? _____

h. Was a body part or abnormal tissue growth (such as a lesion or tumor) removed? _____

i. Was a foreign object or abnormal material (such as calculus) removed? _____

j. Was the body part replaced with a natural or synthetic substitute? _____

k. Was removal performed by cutting? _____

l. Was removal performed through physical eradication, such as energy, force, or a destructive agent? _____ _____

m. Was an extremity removed? _____

n. Was removal performed through the use of force, such as pulling or stripping? _____

o. Which root operation(s) should be considered for this procedure? _____
Why? _____

---

2. INPATIENT HOSPITAL   Gender: F   Age: 47

Preprocedure diagnosis: Star cataract, right eye

Procedure: Extracapsular cataract phacoemulsification without intraocular lens implantation, right eye. Performed phacoemulsification using hydrodissection to separate the lens nucleus by injecting fluid into the capsule (percutaneously), then suctioned out the lens and fluid.

Postprocedure diagnosis: Star cataract, right eye

a. What is the stated procedure? _____

b. What organ or body part is involved? _____

c. What is the laterality? _____

d. Is the procedure description what you would expect based on the name of the procedure? _____

e. What surgical approach is used? _____

f. Was more than one procedure, or a combined procedure, performed? _____

g. Did the procedure take out some or all of a body part without replacement? _____

h. Was a body part or abnormal tissue growth (such as a lesion or tumor) removed? _____

i. Was a foreign object or abnormal material (such as calculus) removed? _____

j. Was the body part replaced with a natural or synthetic substitute? _____

k. Was removal performed by cutting? _____

l. Was removal performed through physical eradication, such as energy, force, or a destructive agent? _____ _____

m. Was an extremity removed? _____

n. Was removal performed through the use of force, such as pulling or stripping? _____

o. Which root operation(s) should be considered for this procedure? _____
Why? _____

(continued)

CODING PRACTICE (continued)

3. INPATIENT HOSPITAL Gender: F Age: 36

Preprocedure diagnosis: Varicose veins

Procedure: Vein stripping of left greater saphenous vein to the level of the knee. Small incisions were made in the groin area and below the vein, then a wire was threaded up the vein to the first incision, and the vein was grasped and removed.

Postprocedure diagnosis: Varicose veins

Tip: Stripping is the removal of the vein through incisions. In a percutaneous approach, small incisions are made through which instruments are inserted. In an open approach, the entire operative field is opened up with a large incision.

a. What is the stated procedure? _____

b. What organ or body part is involved? _____

c. What is the laterality? _____

d. Is the procedure description what you would expect based on the name of the procedure? _____

e. What surgical approach is used? _____

f. Was more than one procedure, or a combined procedure, performed? _____

g. Did the procedure take out some or all of a body part without replacement? _____

h. Was a body part or abnormal tissue growth (such as a lesion or tumor) removed? _____

i. Was a foreign object or abnormal material (such as calculus) removed? _____

j. Was the body part replaced with a natural or synthetic substitute? _____

k. Was removal performed by cutting? _____

l. Was removal performed through physical eradication, such as energy, force, or a destructive agent? _____ _____

m. Was an extremity removed? _____

n. Was removal performed through the use of force, such as pulling or stripping? _____

o. Which root operation(s) should be considered for this procedure? _____ Why? _____

4. INPATIENT HOSPITAL Gender: M Age: 18

Preprocedure diagnosis: Spinal cord lesions

Procedure: Electrocauterization. Made two 1.5-cm incisions at T7 and inserted endoscope and electrocautery device. Cauterized single lesion. Withdrew instruments and closed wounds. Proceeded to make two 1.5-cm incisions at L3 and inserted endoscope and electrocautery device. Cauterized two lesions. Withdrew instruments and closed wounds.

Postprocedure diagnosis: Benign neoplasm, spinal cord, lumbar and thoracic

a. What is the stated procedure? _____

b. What organ or body part is involved? _____

c. How many and which sites are treated? _____

d. Is the procedure description what you would expect based on the name of the procedure? _____

e. What surgical approach is used? _____

f. Did the procedure take out some or all of a body part without replacement? _____

g. Was a body part or abnormal tissue growth (such as a lesion or tumor) removed? _____

h. Was a foreign object or abnormal material (such as calculus) removed? _____

i. Was the body part replaced with a natural or synthetic substitute? _____

j. Was removal performed by cutting? _____

k. Was removal performed through physical eradication, such as energy, force, or a destructive agent? _____ _____

l. Was an extremity removed? _____

m. Was removal performed through the use of force, such as pulling or stripping? _____

n. Which root operation(s) should be considered for this procedure? _____ Why? _____

5. INPATIENT HOSPITAL Gender: M Age: 61

Preprocedure diagnosis: Cholecystitis with gallstones

Procedure: Laparoscopic cholecystectomy and CBD removal; wedge biopsy, liver. Created 3 ports to access RUQ and examined the area with laparoscope. Identified gallbladder inflammation and gall stones in the common bile duct. Dissected the gallbladder and common bile duct. Visualized a nodule on the right

(continued)

CODING PRACTICE (continued)

5. (continued)

lobe of liver and obtained a wedge biopsy that was sent to pathology with the gallbladder.

Postprocedure diagnosis: Acute cholecystitis with cholelithiasis, adenoma of liver

a. What is the stated procedure? _____

b. What organ or body part is involved? _____

c. What is the laterality? _____

d. Is the procedure description what you would expect based on the name of the procedure? _____

e. What surgical approach is used? _____

f. Was more than one procedure, or a combined procedure, performed? _____

g. Did the procedure take out some or all of a body part without replacement? _____

h. Was a body part or abnormal tissue growth (such as a lesion or tumor) removed? _____

i. Was a foreign object or abnormal material (such as calculus) removed? _____

j. Was the body part replaced with a natural or synthetic substitute? _____

k. Was removal performed by cutting? _____

l. Was removal performed through physical eradication, such as energy, force, or a destructive agent? _____ _____

m. Was an extremity removed? _____

n. Was removal performed through the use of force, such as pulling or stripping? _____

o. Which root operation(s) should be considered for this procedure? _____ Why? _____

6. INPATIENT HOSPITAL   Gender: M   Age: 26

Preprocedure diagnosis: Necrosis and spreading infection after injury 1 month ago, with potential for sepsis

Procedure: Amputation. Removed 4th phalanx and entire metacarpal, right hand, and 5th phalanx at the proximal interphalangeal joint, right hand

Postprocedure diagnosis: Infection, subcutaneous tissue, right hand, organism unknown

a. What is the stated procedure? _____

b. What organ or body part is involved? _____

c. How many sites are treated? _____

d. What is the laterality? _____

e. Is the procedure description what you would expect based on the name of the procedure? _____

f. What surgical approach is used? _____

g. Was more than one procedure, or a combined procedure, performed? _____

h. Did the procedure take out some or all of a body part without replacement? _____

i. Was a body part or abnormal tissue growth (such as a lesion or tumor) removed? _____

j. Was a foreign object or abnormal material (such as calculus) removed? _____

k. Was the body part replaced with a natural or synthetic substitute? _____

l. Was removal performed by cutting? _____

m. Was removal performed through physical eradication, such as energy, force, or a destructive agent? _____ _____

n. Was an extremity removed? _____

o. Was removal performed through the use of force, such as pulling or stripping? _____

p. Which root operation(s) should be considered for this procedure? _____ Why? _____

ASSIGNING CHARACTERS 4–7 FOR ROOT OPERATIONS 5, 6, B, D, AND T

To assign codes after the root operation is determined, search the PCS Index for the name of the root operation as the Main Term. Locate the subterm(s) for the correct anatomic site and identify the PCS Table. When you locate the PCS Table, verify the first three characters of the code, then locate the row with the body part. Assign the remaining characters from each respective column of the Table. The following information

summarizes and highlights unique information for working with the Tables for each root operation 5, 6, B, D, and T. Each root operation has one Table in each applicable PCS body system. Because of the differences between organ systems, Table details vary.

Character 4: Body Part

Every PCS code must contain a valid value for Character 4, Body Part. *None* is never an option. PCS lists the body part values separately for each body system value and each root operation. A body system might not contain the same body part values for each root operation, so refer to the appropriate PCS Table to identify the body part options for the combination of the applicable body system and root operation.

For example, in Table **09B** (Ear, Nose, Sinus Excision) the body part values include **0 External Ear, Right**, **1 External Ear, Left**, and **K Nose**. In Table **09D** (Ear, Nose, Sinus Extraction), the body part values do not include the external ear or nose because the root operation Extraction does not apply to these sites.

Body Parts for Excision and Resection

The body part value(s) must be identified to distinguish between the root operations Excision and Resection. The root operation cannot be assigned until the level of specificity of the body part values is known. Resection is cutting off all of a body part and Excision is cutting off only a portion of a body part. The coder often needs to review both the Table for Excision and the Table for Resection to identify how the body part value is defined, so they can determine whether all or only a portion *of* the body part is cut off (PCS OGCR B3.8). The PCS body part value may identify all of an organ—such as the appendix—or may assign separate body part values for segments of an organ, such as the sigmoid and ascending sections of the colon.

Sometimes body part values overlap, in which case you need to select the most specific body part value applicable to the procedure. Assign the root operation Excision only when a portion of a body part, as identified by the smallest body part value, is removed.

PCS provides nine overlapping body part values for lungs, with various levels of specificity. Body part values range from the most general—**M Lungs, Bilateral**—to each side right (**K**) and left (**L**), and then to each lobe and the lingula (*a tongue-like projection of the upper left lobe*). Select the most specific body part value applicable to the root operation Resection. When one entire lobe is cut out, use Resection to identify that the entire lobe was removed. Do not use Excision to describe that a portion of the entire organ (such as the lung) was removed when a more specific body part is provided (■ FIGURE 49-1). When a portion of a lobe is removed, code the root operation Excision because no smaller body part value is available.

By contrast, the stomach has only two PCS body part values: Stomach, **Pylorus (7)** and **Stomach (6)**. When the pylorus or the entire stomach is removed, code Resection. When any portion of the stomach is removed, code Excision.

The body part value for Lymphatic identifies an entire lymph chain. Assign the root operation Resection when an entire lymph chain is cut out. Assign the root operation Excision when one or more lymph nodes are cut out (*ICD-10-PCS Reference Manual*). Lymph chains are divided by anatomic site and laterality.

SUCCESS STEP

When a colectomy is performed, PCS requires only the root operation Excision or Resection. The type of anastomosis—such as end-to-side or side-to-side—is not reported with a character value or a separate code.

Surgeon performed an open procedure to remove the upper lobe of the left lung.

0BTG0ZZ Resection of Left Upper Lung Lobe, Open Approach

Section	**0**	**Medical and Surgical**
Body System	**B**	**Respiratory System**
Operation	**T**	**Resection** Cutting out or off, without replacement, all of a body part

Body Part Character 4	Approach Character 5	Device Character 6	Qualifier Character 7
8 Upper Lobe Bronchus, Left 9 Lingula Bronchus B Lower Lobe Bronchus, Left C Upper Lung Lobe, Right D Middle Lung Lobe, Right F Lower Lung Lobe, Right G Upper Lung Lobe, Left H Lung Lingula J Lower Lung Lobe, Left K Lung, Right L Lung, Left M Lungs, Bilateral	0 Open 4 Percutaneous Endoscopic	Z No Device	Z No Qualifier

Figure 49-1 ■ Example of coding resection for one lobe of the lung.

Body Parts for Detachment

The root operation Detachment appears only for the body system values **X Anatomical Regions, Upper Extremities** and **Y Anatomical Regions, Lower Extremities**. Refer to Tables **0X6** and **0Y6**. An amputation is performed on a region that includes multiple body systems—such as bones, skin, veins, arteries, muscles, tendons, and so on. For this reason, Detachment does not apply to anatomic systems and the PCS values for an **Anatomical Region** are used. For example, amputation of the foot involves all the anatomic structures in the foot, not only the bones or muscles.

Character 5: Approach

All PCS approach values are used with the root operations in this group. Each PCS table lists the approach values valid for a root operation/body system combination.

The root operation Detachment always uses the **Open (4)** approach.

Excision procedures in the oral cavity, including those performed on the teeth, gums, and tonsils, use the **External (X)** approach because the procedure site is viewed without the aid of any instruments (PCS OGCR B5.3a).

Procedures performed that use the **Open** approach also include percutaneous endoscopic assistance. PCS does not provide a unique value that reports simultaneous use of both techniques (PCS OGCR B5.2).

The approach **Via Natural or Artificial Opening With Percutaneous Endoscopic Assistance (F)** is used only with the root operations Excision and Resection in the Gastrointestinal System (D) and Female Reproductive System (U). It is not used for any other PCS procedures.

The approach **Via Natural or Artificial Opening With Percutaneous Endoscopic Assistance (F)** is used for an anorectal pull-through procedure in the Gastrointestinal System (D). The procedure—performed to correct a congenital malformation—is sometimes referred to as laparoscopically assisted anorectal pull-through (LAARP). The primary portion of the procedure is performed through the anus, a natural opening. An endoscopic is used percutaneously to assist with manipulation the structures. Use of the endoscope minimizes the risk of perforating the colon during the procedure. This approach is listed in Table **0DB** with body part values for segments of the colon.

This approach also is used for laparoscopically-assisted vaginal hysterectomy (LAVH) (see Figure 47-1G and 47-1H, Examples of PCS Approaches). Most commonly, the uterus is excised through the vaginal opening and the ovaries and fallopian tubes are accessed laparoscopically. The root operation Resection is assigned because the entire body part(s) are cut out.

Character 6: Device

None of the root operations in this group, *Procedures that take out some or all of a body part*, use Character 6, Device. The value is always **Z No device**. Temporary devices such as postoperative drains are considered part of the procedure and are not coded separately. When a permanent device is put in place, a different root operation is required.

Character 7: Qualifier

Character 7, Qualifier, is used for root operations in this group primarily to identify biopsies in the root operations Excision and Extraction, the level of an amputation in the root operation Detachment, and the number of teeth removed. When no qualifier applies, assign **Z No qualifier**.

Biopsy Qualifiers

A biopsy is performed for diagnostic reasons as opposed to therapeutic or treatment reasons. Biopsies take out only a portion of an organ or structure and are reported only with the root operations **Excision**, **Drainage**, and **Extraction**. Biopsies involving cutting are coded to Excision (B). Biopsies such as needle aspiration are coded to the root operation **Drainage**. Biopsies involving pulling or scraping—such as a diagnostic dilation and curettage—are coded to the root operation **Extraction**. When a biopsy is performed, assign the Character 7, Qualifier value **X Diagnostic**.

Qualifiers for Detachment

Qualifier values for the root operation **Detachment (6)** identify the anatomic level at which an amputation is performed and vary based on the body part value in the upper- and lower-extremity body systems. ■ TABLE 49-9, (page 1030) defines the meaning of the qualifiers used in both the upper and lower extremities. ■ FIGURE 49-2, (page 1030) provide an anatomic illustration of the hand and identifies the bones, joints, and how PCS identifies the level of amputation.

Qualifiers for the Teeth

The qualifier identifies the number of teeth removed in Extraction (D), Extirpation (C), and Resection (T) procedures. The body parts Upper Tooth (W) and Lower Tooth (X) use one of the following qualifier values.

- **0 Single**
- **1 Multiple**
- **2 All**

Other Qualifiers

Unique values appear in the qualifier column for selected procedures when further information is required about an anatomic site. These qualifiers are rare and are not explained in the PCS OGCR or other instructions. They appear only in the Character 7 column of the Table with no instructions. Coders must be alert to their presence and interpret their application based on the scenario being coded. Examples include:

- A supracervical hysterectomy is assigned the same code as a full hysterectomy, with the exception of the qualifier **L Supracervical**:
  - **0UT98ZL Resection of Uterus, Via Natural or Artificial Opening Endoscopic, Supracervical**

- Destruction of the left atrial appendage in the left atrium of the heart is coded to the body part Left Atrium and the qualifier **K Left Atrial Appendage**:
  - **02574ZK Destruction, Atrium left, Percutaneous Endoscopic Approach, Left Atrial Appendage**

Table 49-9 ■ **CHARACTER 7 QUALIFIER VALUES FOR THE ROOT OPERATION DETACHMENT**

Value	Meaning	Definition
Arm and Leg		
1	High	Amputation at the proximal portion of the shaft (ARM, Upper: humerus; Lower: radius/ulna. LEG, Upper: femur; Lower: tibia/fibula)
2	Mid	Amputation at the middle portion of the shaft (ARM, Upper: humerus; Lower: radius/ulna. LEG, Upper: femur; Lower: tibia/fibula)
3	Low	Amputation at the distal portion of the shaft (ARM, Upper: humerus; Lower: radius/ulna. LEG, Upper: femur; Lower: tibia/fibula)
Hand and Foot		
0	Complete	Complete: Amputation through the carpometacarpal joint of the hand or through the tarsal-metatarsal joint of the foot
4	Complete 1st Ray	
5	Complete 2nd Ray	
6	Complete 3rd Ray	
7	Complete 4th Ray	
8	Complete 5th Ray	
9	Partial 1st Ray	Partial: Amputation anywhere along the shaft or head of the metacarpal bone of the hand or of the metatarsal bone of the foot
B	Partial 2nd Ray	
C	Partial 3rd Ray	
D	Partial 4th Ray	
F	Partial 5th Ray	
Thumb, Finger, or Toe		
0	Complete	Amputation at the metacarpophalangeal/metatarsal–phalangeal joint
1	High	Amputation anywhere along the proximal phalanx
2	Mid	Amputation through the proximal interphalangeal joint or anywhere along the middle phalanx
3	Low	Amputation through the distal interphalangeal joint or anywhere along the distal phalanx

Source: © PB Resources, Inc. Used with permission.

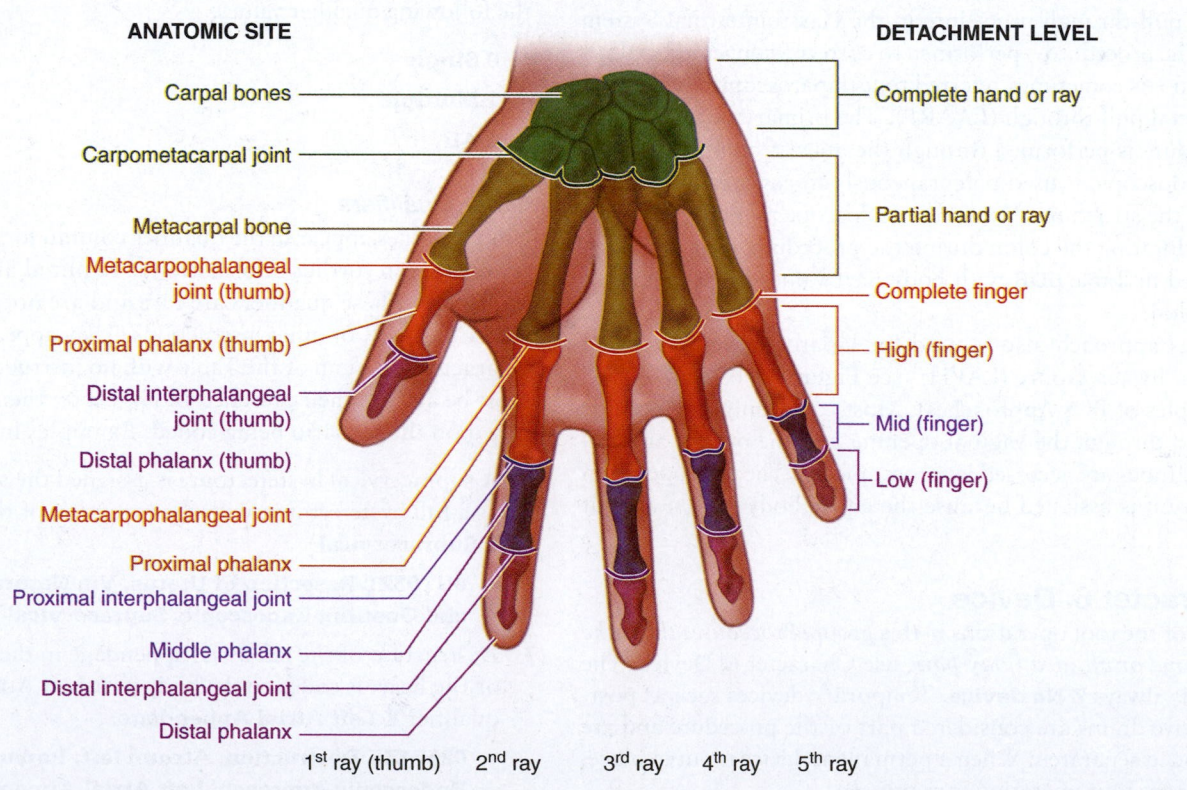

Figure 49-2 ■ Detachment levels for the hand.

Guided Example of Assigning Characters 4–7 for Excision and Resection

To practice skills for assigning codes for Excision and Resection, continue with the example from earlier in the chapter about a patient who was seen for a lymphadenectomy. Follow along in your ICD-10-PCS manual as Marcy Elwood, CCS, assigns codes. Check off each step after you complete it.

▶ First, Marcy confirms the procedures: open left lymphadenectomy of entire axillary chain and percutaneous left cervical lymphadenectomy of the first node only.

   ❏ She confirms that the root operations are Excision and/or Resection, depending on how body part values are identified in the PCS Table.

▶ Marcy searches the Index for the Main Term **Excision**.

   ❏ She locates the first-level subterm **Lymphatic**.

   ❏ She locates the second-level subterm **Axillary**.

   ❏ She locates the third-level subterm **Left**.

   ❏ She identifies the Table: **07B6**.

   ❏ She then locates another second-level subterm **Neck** for the cervical lymph node.

   ❏ She locates the third-level subterm **Left**.

   ❏ She identifies the Table: **07B2**.

   ❏ The first three letters of each partial code, **07B**, refer her to the PCS Table for the Lymphatic system, root operation Excision. The fourth character identifies the body part.

▶ Then, Marcy searches the Index for the Main Term **Resection** to cross-reference the values with **Excision**.

   ❏ She locates the first-level subterm **Lymphatic**.

   ❏ She locates the second-level subterm **Axillary**.

   ❏ She locates the third-level subterm **Left**.

   ❏ She identifies the Table: **07T6**.

   ❏ She then locates another second-level subterm **Neck** for the cervical lymph node.

   ❏ She locates the third-level subterm **Left**.

   ❏ She identifies the Table: **07T2**.

   ❏ The first three letters of each partial code, **07T**, refer her to the PCS Table for the Lymphatic system, root operation Resection. The fourth character identifies the body part.

▶ To confirm her choices, Marcy searches the Index for the Main Term **Lymphadenectomy**. She reads the cross-reference notes that appear below the Main Term.

   ❏ **see Excision, Lymphatic and Hemic Systems 07B**

   ❏ **see Resection, Lymphatic and Hemic Systems 07T**

▶ Marcy turns to Table **07B** for the root operation Excision.

   ❏ She reads the Table title **07B, Section 0 Medical and Surgical**, body system **7 Lymphatic and Hemic Systems**, root operation **B Excision** and confirms that this accurately describes the body system and root operation.

She reads the root operation definition **Cutting out or off, without replacement, a portion of a body part** and confirms that the definition is what she expected.

▶ Marcy reads the values for Character 4, Body Part, to identify how the body parts are defined.

   ❏ The value **6** identifies **Lymphatic, Left Axillary**, referring to the entire lymph chain. The *entire* left axillary chain was removed, so the root operation Excision does not apply because Excision describes removing only a portion of the body part. She will need to refer to the root operation Resection for removal of the entire lymph chain.

   ❏ The value **2** identifies **Lymphatic, Left Neck** and does not specify individual lymph nodes. Because only one cervical lymph node was removed, the root operation Excision applies because a *portion* of the lymph chain—a single node—was removed. She will assign the remainder of the code for the cervical lymph node removal from the Excision Table.

▶ Marcy assigns the value for Character 5, Approach.

   ❏ She refers to the operative report, which documents percutaneous left cervical lymphadenectomy.

   ❏ She assigns the value **3 Percutaneous** for the approach.

▶ Marcy assigns the value for Character 6, Device.

   ❏ The Table provides only one option: **Z No device**.

▶ Marcy assigns the value for Character 7, Qualifier.

   ❏ She refers to the operative report and confirms that the procedure was not a biopsy.

   ❏ She assigns the value **Z No qualifier**.

   ❏ She reviews the code she has assigned for the percutaneous left cervical lymphadenectomy: **07B23ZZ** (■ FIGURE 49-3, page 1032).

▶ Next, Marcy turns to Table **07T** for the root operation Resection to assign the code for open left lymphadenectomy of entire axillary chain.

   ❏ She reads the Table title **07T, Section 0 Medical and Surgical**, body system **7 Lymphatic and Hemic Systems**, root operation **T Resection** and confirms that this accurately describes the body system and root operation. She reads the root operation definition **Cutting out or off, without replacement, all of a body part** and confirms that the definition is what she expected.

▶ Marcy reads the values for Character 4, Body Part.

   ❏ The value **6** identifies **Lymphatic Left Axillary**, referring to the entire lymph chain. The entire left axillary chain was removed, so the root operation Resection applies.

▶ Marcy assigns the value for Character 5, Approach.

   ❏ She refers to the operative report, which documents open left lymphadenectomy.

   ❏ She assigns the value **0 Open** for the approach.

▶ Marcy assigns the value for Character 6, Device.

❑ The Table provides only one option: **Z No device.**

▶ Marcy assigns the value for Character 7, Qualifier.

❑ The Table provides only one option: **Z No qualifier.**

❑ She reviews the code she has assigned for the open left lymphadenectomy of entire axillary chain: **07T60ZZ** (■ FIGURE 49-4).

▶ Next, Marcy must determine how to sequence the codes.

Section	0	Medical and Surgical
Body System	7	Lymphatic and Hemic Systems
Operation	B	Excision: Cutting out or off, without replacement, a portion of a body part

Body Part Character 4	Approach Character 5	Device Character 6	Qualifier Character 7
0 Lymphatic, Head **1** Lymphatic, Right Neck **2** Lymphatic, Left Neck **3** Lymphatic, Right Upper Extremity **4** Lymphatic, Left Upper Extremity	**0** Open **3** Percutaneous **4** Percutaneous Endoscopic	**Z** No Device	**X** Diagnostic **Z** No Qualifier

Figure 49-3 ■ Assigning code 07B23ZZ. *Source: Annotation © PB Resources, Inc. Used with permission.*

Section	0	Medical and Surgical
Body System	7	Lymphatic and Hemic Systems
Operation	T	Resection: Cutting out or off, without replacement, all of a body part

Body Part Character 4	Approach Character 5	Device Character 6	Qualifier Character 7
0 Lymphatic, Head **1** Lymphatic, Right Neck **2** Lymphatic, Left Neck **3** Lymphatic, Right Upper Extremity **4** Lymphatic, Left Upper Extremity **5** Lymphatic, Right Axillary **6** Lymphatic, Left Axillary **7** Lymphatic, Thorax	**0** Open **4** Percutaneous Endoscopic	**Z** No Device	**Z** No Qualifier

Figure 49-4 ■ Assigning code 07T60ZZ. *Source: Annotation © PB Resources, Inc. Used with permission.*

CODING PRACTICE

Exercise 49.3 Assigning Characters 4–7 for Root Operations 5, 6, B, D, and T

Instructions: Read the mini-medical-record of each patient's encounter. Review the information abstracted in Exercise 49.2 for questions 1–3. For questions 4–6, abstract the case on your own. Assign PCS codes using the Index and Tables. Write the code(s) on the line provided.

1. INPATIENT HOSPITAL   Gender: F   Age: 26

Preprocedure diagnosis: Polycystic ovaries

Procedure: Oophorectomy. Approached transvaginally with laparoscopic assistance. Located and removed entirety of both ovaries.

Postprocedure diagnosis: Polycystic ovaries

Tip: Ovary is defined as a distinct body part. All of the ovary was removed.

1 PCS Code _____

CODING PRACTICE (continued)

2. INPATIENT HOSPITAL   Gender: F   Age: 47

Preprocedure diagnosis: Star cataract, right eye

Procedure: Extracapsular cataract phacoemulsification without intraocular lens implantation, right eye. Performed phacoemulsification using hydrodissection to separate the lens nucleus by injecting fluid into the capsule, then suctioned out the lens and fluid.

Postprocedure diagnosis: Star cataract, right eye

1 PCS Code _____

3. INPATIENT HOSPITAL   Gender: F   Age: 36

Preprocedure diagnosis: Varicose veins

Procedure: Vein stripping of left greater saphenous vein to the level of the knee. Small incisions were made in the groin area and below the vein, then a wire was threaded up the vein to the first incision, and the vein was grasped and removed.

Postprocedure diagnosis: Varicose veins

Tip: Stripping is the removal of the vein through incisions. In a percutaneous approach, small incisions are made through which instruments are inserted. In an open approach, the entire operative field is opened up with a large incision.

1 PCS Code _____

4. INPATIENT HOSPITAL   Gender: F   Age: 62

Preprocedure diagnosis: Hallux abductovalgus with bunion deformity

Procedure: Keller bunionectomy, right. Incision made over 1st metatarsal head. Exostosis removed and head remodeled. Excellent capillary refill after tourniquet release.

(continued)

4. (continued)

Postprocedure diagnosis: Hallux abductovalgus with bunion deformity

Tip: A bunion is an enlargement of the joint at the base of the big toe composed of bone and soft tissue.

1 PCS Code _____

5. INPATIENT HOSPITAL   Gender: M   Age: 44

Preprocedure diagnosis: Myasthenia gravis, thymoma

Procedure: Transthoracic thymectomy. Made a lengthwise incision in the chest slightly left of the midline. Explored the chest and excised the entire thymus gland. No adjacent structures were disturbed. Inspected the surgical field to ensure no residual thymic tissue. Closed surgical wound and transferred patient to the postoperative area in stable condition.

Postprocedure diagnosis: Thymoma

Tip: The entire thymus (body part) was removed.

1 PCS Code _____

6. INPATIENT HOSPITAL   Gender: M   Age: 28

Preprocedure diagnosis: Uncontrolled bilateral epistaxis

Procedure: Limited cautery of nasal hemorrhage. Used nasal speculum to locate site of bleeding in the right anterior nasal passage, cleaned, and applied silver nitrate stick to cauterize. Repeated on the left anterior passage. Hemostasis was achieved.

Postprocedure diagnosis: Epistaxis

Tip: Read the definitions for destruction and repair carefully.

1 PCS Code _____

ARRANGING CODES FOR ROOT OPERATIONS 5, 6, B, D, AND T

Procedures assigned to Destruction, Detachment, Excision, Extraction, and Resection can be performed in connection with each other or with other root operations. Hospitals must determine the **principal procedure** during an inpatient admission. Selection of the principal procedure is directly related to the principal diagnosis. Sequence a definitive procedure for the principal diagnosis before a diagnostic procedure for the principal diagnosis. A definitive procedure is one that treats the diagnosis. A diagnostic procedure is one that seeks to establish

a diagnosis. If no procedures are related to the principal diagnosis, sequence the definitive procedure for the secondary diagnosis before a diagnostic procedure for the secondary diagnosis. Refer to Chapter 46 of this text and the PCS OGCR section "Selection of the Principal Procedure" for details and examples.

A single operative procedure may require multiple PCS codes when multiple PCS body parts are removed or destroyed.

EXAMPLE: *Percutaneous endoscopic excision of bilateral cervical lymph nodes.*

07B14ZZ Excision, Lymphatic, Right Neck, Percutaneous endoscopic

07B24ZZ Excision, Lymphatic, Left Neck, Percutaneous endoscopic

A single operative procedure may require multiple codes when multiple sites within a single body part value are treated.

EXAMPLE: *Destruction of two polyps in the ascending colon during a colonoscopy.*

0D5K8ZZ Destruction, Colon, Ascending Via Natural or Artificial Opening Endoscopic

0D5K8ZZ Destruction, Colon, Ascending Via Natural or Artificial Opening Endoscopic

Guided Example of Arranging Codes for Excision and Resection

To practice skills for arranging codes for procedures of the root operations **Excision** and **Resection**, continue with the example from earlier in the chapter about the patient who was seen for a lymphadenectomy. Follow along in your ICD-10-PCS manual as Marcy Elwood, CCS, arranges the codes. Check off each step after you complete it.

▶ First, Marcy confirms the codes she assigned:

❏ **07B23ZZ Excision, Lymphatic left neck, Percutaneous, No device, No qualifier**

❏ **07T60ZZ Resection, Lymphatic left axillary, Open, No device, No qualifier**

▶ Marcy reviews the diagnoses for this case: left breast cancer with metastasis to lymph nodes.

❏ Metastasis to the lymph nodes is the reason for the hospital admission and the services provided.

❏ In the ICD-10-CM Table of Neoplasms, diagnosis codes for lymph node metastases are divided by site.

Both the cervical node and axillary chain equally meet the criteria for principal diagnosis.

- Marcy sequences the axillary chain as the principal diagnosis because it is the predominant, or larger, site.
- Marcy sequences metastasis to the single cervical node as a secondary diagnosis.

❏ Marcy sequences left breast cancer as a secondary diagnosis because it was not treated during this admission.

▶ Next, Marcy arranges the procedure codes.

❏ Resection of the left axillary lymph chain is a definitive procedure related to the principal diagnosis, so she sequences it as the principal procedure.

❏ Excision of the cervical lymph node is a definitive procedure related to a secondary diagnosis, so she sequences it as a secondary procedure.

▶ Marcy finalizes the procedure codes and sequencing for this case:

(1) **07T60ZZ Resection, Lymphatic left axillary, Open, No device, No qualifier**

(2) **07B23ZZ Excision, Lymphatic left neck, Percutaneous, No device, No qualifier**

▶ Marcy also assigns and sequences the ICD-10-CM diagnosis codes that support the need for the service.

(1) **C77.3 Secondary and unspecified malignant neoplasm of axilla and upper limb lymph nodes**

(2) **C77.0 Secondary and unspecified malignant neoplasm of lymph nodes of head, face and neck**

(3) **C50.912 Malignant neoplasm of unspecified site of left female breast**

CODING PRACTICE

Exercise 49.4 Arranging Codes for Root Operations 5, 6, B, D, and T

Instructions: Read the mini-medical-record of each patient's encounter. Review the information abstracted in Exercise 49.2 for questions 1–3. For questions 4–6, abstract the case on your own. Assign PCS codes using the Index and Tables, and arrange the codes in proper sequence. Write the code(s) on the line provided.

1. INPATIENT HOSPITAL Gender: M Age: 18

Preprocedure diagnosis: Spinal cord lesions

Procedure: Electrocauterization. Made two 1.5-cm incisions at T7 and inserted endoscope and electrocautery device. Cauterized single lesion. Withdrew instruments and closed wounds. Proceeded to make two 1.5-cm incisions at L3 and inserted endoscope and electrocautery device. Cauterized two lesions. Withdrew instruments and closed wounds.

Postprocedure diagnosis: Benign neoplasm, spinal cord, lumbar and thoracic

Tip: When the same root operation is performed at two distinct body part sites, assign separate codes (PCS OGCR B3.2a).

2 PCS Codes _____

CODING PRACTICE (continued)

2. INPATIENT HOSPITAL   Gender: M   Age: 61

Preprocedure diagnosis: Cholecystitis with gallstones

Procedure: Laparoscopic cholecystectomy and CBD removal; wedge biopsy, liver. Created 3 ports to access RUQ and examined the area with laparoscope. Identified gallbladder inflammation and gall stones in the common bile duct. Dissected the gallbladder and common bile duct. Visualized a nodule on the right lobe of liver and obtained a wedge biopsy that was sent to pathology with the gallbladder.

Postprocedure diagnosis: Acute cholecystitis with cholelithiasis, adenoma of liver

Tip: A biopsy is diagnostic.

3 PCS Codes _____

_____

_____

3. INPATIENT HOSPITAL   Gender: M   Age: 26

Preprocedure diagnosis: Necrosis and spreading infection after injury 1 month ago, with potential for sepsis

Procedure: Amputation. Removed 4th phalanx and entire metacarpal, right hand, and 5th phalanx at the proximal interphalangeal joint, right hand

Postprocedure diagnosis: Infection, subcutaneous tissue, right hand, organism unknown

Tip: Assign the qualifier based on the extent of the amputation. Refer to Table 49-9 and Figure 49-2.

2 PCS Codes _____

4. INPATIENT HOSPITAL   Gender: M   Age: 56

Preprocedure diagnosis: Multi-invasive bladder cancer

Procedure: Laparoscopic radical cystectomy with bilateral pelvic lymph node dissections and orthotopic neobladder. After port placement, the bladder was meticulously dissected free and removed. Right and

(continued)

4. (continued)

left obturator and pelvic lymph nodes were dissected next. The continent urinary diversion was performed by another surgeon and is reported separately.

Tip: Code only the procedures for the primary surgeon.

2 PCS Codes _____

5. INPATIENT HOSPITAL   Gender: F   Age: 34

Preprocedure diagnosis: Painful enlarged navicula, right foot; osteochondroma of right fifth metatarsal

Procedure: Partial tarsectomy navicular and partial metatarsectomy, fifth metatarsal right foot. The enlarged portion of the navicular bone was removed. Osteochondroma removed from the fifth metatarsal neck. Tourniquet released with good capillary refill.

Tip: A portion of the tarsal and metatarsal bones were removed on the same foot.

2 PCS Codes _____

6. INPATIENT HOSPITAL   Gender: M   Age: 63

Preprocedure diagnosis: Carious teeth and periodontal disease affecting all remaining teeth

Procedure: Extraction of remaining teeth numbers 2, 3, 4, 5, 7, 8, 9, 10, 11, 12, 13, 14, 15, 16, 17, 18, 19, 20, 21, 22, 23, 24, 25, 26, 27, 28, 29, 30, 31, and 32. Routine forceps extraction of teeth was begun on the upper left quadrant followed by the lower left quadrant. Attention turned to extraction of teeth on the upper right quadrant and right lower quadrant.

Postprocedure diagnosis: Carious teeth and periodontal disease

Tip: Report the number of teeth removed using the qualifier.

2 PCS Codes _____

CHAPTER SUMMARY

In this chapter you learned that:

- The root operation group *Procedures that take out some or all of a body part* includes five root operations: Destruction (5), Detachment (6), Excision (B), Extraction (D), and Resection (T).

- The root operation Destruction (5) is physical eradication of all or a portion of a body part by the direct use of energy, force, or a destructive agent.

- The root operation Detachment (6) is cutting off all or a portion of the upper or lower extremities.

- The root operation Excision (B) is cutting out or off, without replacement, a portion of a PCS body part.

- The root operation Extraction (D) is pulling or stripping out or off all or a portion of a body part by the use of force.

- The root operation Resection (T) is cutting out or off, without replacement, all of a PCS body part.

- PCS OGCR section B provides guidelines for the Medical and Surgical Section (0), organized by the characters of the PCS code.

- Specific guidelines are provided for biopsy procedures, biopsy followed by more definitive treatment, comparison of Excision and Resection, and Excision for a graft.

- Abstracting for PCS focuses on identifying the correct root operation, which involves reading the operative report and interpreting it in light of root operation definitions.

- Identifying the PCS body part values is the key to distinguishing between the root operations Excision and Resection.

- When an approach value does not apply to all body parts, the PCS Table is divided into two or more rows.

- None of the root operations in this group use Character 6, Device.

- Character 7, Qualifier, is used for root operations in this group primarily to identify biopsies, the level of an amputation, and the number of teeth extracted.

CONCEPT QUIZ

Take a moment to look back at root operations that take out some or all of a body part and solidify your skills. Try to answer the questions from memory first, then refer to the discussion in this chapter if you need a little extra help.

Completion

Instructions: Write the term that completes each statement based on the information you learned in this chapter. Choose from the list below. Some choices may be used more than once and some choices may not be used at all.

Destruction	Extraction
Detachment	Resection
Excision	

1. The root operation for traumatic amputation of the hand is _____.

2. The Main Term for a nonobstetric suction curettage is _____.

3. To code enucleation of the eyeball, search for the Main Term _____.

4. An amputation of the leg above the knee is the root operation _____.

5. A biopsy can be found under the Main Term, Drainage, _____, or _____.

6. A cholecystectomy is indexed under the root operations _____ or _____.

7. Cautery of a nosebleed is an example of the root operation _____.

8. To find the root operation for a bone marrow biopsy, search for the Main Term _____.

9. The root operation for cryotherapy of a wart is _____.

10. A partial discectomy is indexed under the root operation _____.

Multiple Choice

Instructions: Circle the letter of the best answer to each question based on the information you learned in this chapter.

1. How would you code the following procedure? *A physician performs destruction of two polyps in the ascending colon during a colonoscopy.*
   A. 0D5K8ZZ
   B. 0D5K8ZZ, 0D5K8ZZ
   C. 0D5K8ZZ-51
   D. 0D5K8ZX

2. What qualifier is used to report an amputation anywhere along the proximal phalanx?
   A. Complete
   B. High
   C. Mid
   D. Low

3. Which of the following is coded to the root operation Excision?
   A. Fine-needle aspiration biopsy of the lung
   B. Bone marrow biopsy
   C. Lymph node sampling with biopsy
   D. Endometrial biopsy

4. How would you code the following procedure? *A physician performs a partial resection of the descending colon, percutaneous endoscopic approach.*
   A. 0DTM4ZX
   B. 0DTM4ZZ
   C. 0DBM4ZX
   D. 0DBM4ZZ

5. What approach is always used for Excision procedures in the oral cavity in which the operative site can be seen without instrumentation?
   A. External
   B. Open
   C. Percutaneous
   D. Percutaneous Endoscopic

6. What approach is reported for a laparoscopically assisted anorectal pull-through (LAARP) procedure?
   A. Percutaneous Endoscopic (4)
   B. Via Natural or Artificial Opening (7)
   C. Via Natural or Artificial Opening (8)
   D. Via Natural or Artificial Opening Endoscopic with Percutaneous Endoscopic Assistance (F)

7. Which root operation is used for cutting out of a lymph node?
   A. Extraction
   B. Detachment
   C. Resection
   D. Excision

8. When should the Character 7, Qualifier X be used?
   A. To identify the External approach
   B. To identify a biopsy or diagnostic procedure
   C. To report *No qualifier*
   D. To identify a multiple procedure modifier

9. How would you code the following procedure? *A physician performs a partial discectomy, T1-T2 disc, percutaneous.*
   A. 0RB93ZZ
   B. 0RT93ZZ
   C. 0R593ZZ
   D. 0PD40ZZ

10. Which character value must be identified to determine whether the root operation Excision or Resection should be used?
    A. Approach
    B. Device
    C. Body Part
    D. Qualifier

KEEP ON CODING

Instructions: Read the procedural statement, abstract the root operation, then use the appropriate Index and Tables to assign PCS procedure codes. Assign only the root operations discussed in this chapter. Write the code(s) on the line provided.

1. Open excisional biopsy of left extraocular muscle. ICD-10-PCS Code(s) _____

2. Laparoscopic excision of all of the sigmoid colon through the anus and rectum. ICD-10-PCS Code(s) _____

3. Amputation of the left first toe, complete, open approach. ICD-10-PCS Code(s) _____

4. Destroyed a wart from epidermis of the right hand using nitrous oxide. ICD-10-PCS Code(s) _____

5. Diagnostic dilation and curettage (D&C). ICD-10-PCS Code(s) _____

6. Percutaneous endoscopic polypectomy excision, nasal mucosa in the right internal naris (*internal nostril in the posterior nasal cavity*). ICD-10-PCS Code(s) _____

7. Complete thyroidectomy of the right lobe, open approach. ICD-10-PCS Code(s) _____

8. Cataract extraction, lens of right eye, percutaneous. ICD-10-PCS Code(s) _____

9. Amputation of left thumb at the distal interphalangeal joint, open approach. ICD-10-PCS Code(s) _____

10. Fulguration of bladder polyp using a cystoscope. ICD-10-PCS Code(s) _____

11. Upper gingivectomy (cutting out of the gum). ICD-10-PCS Code(s) _____

12. Nephrectomy, entire left kidney, open approach. ICD-10-PCS Code(s) _____

13. Percutaneous extraction of bone marrow of the iliac crest for biopsy. ICD-10-PCS Code(s) _____

14. Complete amputation of little right toe, open approach. ICD-10-PCS Code(s) _____

15. Cauterization with electrocautery of skin of right upper leg. ICD-10-PCS Code(s) _____

16. Left breast percutaneous lumpectomy, partial. ICD-10-PCS Code(s) _____

17. Total excision of pituitary gland, open approach. ICD-10-PCS Code(s) _____

18. Phacoemulsification of left eye lens without intraocular implant. ICD-10-PCS Code(s) _____

19. Midlevel BKA (below-knee amputation), right leg, open approach. ICD-10-PCS Code(s) _____

20. Percutaneous partial sialectomy (cutting out of the salivary gland), left sublingual gland. ICD-10-PCS Code(s) _____

21. Endoscopic cauterization of esophageal varices. ICD-10-PCS Code(s) _____

22. Total splenectomy, open approach. ICD-10-PCS Code(s) _____

23. Percutaneous stripping, lesser saphenous vein, left leg. ICD-10-PCS Code(s) _____

24. Cryoablation of cervix. ICD-10-PCS Code(s) _____

25. Transmetacarpal amputation of left hand at index finger, open approach. ICD-10-PCS Code(s) _____

CODING CHALLENGE

Instructions: Read the mini-medical-record of each patient's encounter, then abstract, assign, and arrange ICD-10-CM diagnosis codes and PCS procedure codes using the appropriate Index and Tables. Write the code(s) on the line provided.

---

1. INPATIENT HOSPITAL Gender: F Age: 26

Preprocedure diagnosis: Menorrhagia

Procedure: Endometrial ablation. Uterus dilated to 10 cm and a NovaSure balloon inserted into the uterine cavity. Full cycle of 8 minutes with pressure of 170 completed. Balloon deflated and withdrawn.

Postprocedure diagnosis: Menorrhagia

Tip: Ablation is removal of material from the surface of an object by vaporization, chipping, or other erosive processes.

1 ICD-10-CM Code _____

1 ICD-10-PCS Code _____

---

2. INPATIENT HOSPITAL Gender: M Age: 6

Preprocedure diagnosis: Multiple warts on the left foot

Procedure: Cryotherapy of 2 warts on left great toe and 3 warts on left heel. Using a cotton swab, liquid nitrogen was applied to the warts until a white margin was evident, approximately 60 seconds.

Postprocedure diagnosis: Verruca plantaris of left great toe and left heel

Tip: If a body system does not contain a separate body part value for toes, procedures performed on the toes are coded to the body part value for the foot.

1 ICD-10-CM Code _____

1 ICD-10-PCS Code _____

---

3. INPATIENT HOSPITAL Gender: M Age: 18

Preprocedure diagnosis: Chronic ethmoidal sinusitis, nasal polyposis

Procedure: Percutaneous endoscopic sinus surgery, bilateral total ethmoidectomy, bilateral ethmoid polypectomy. Sinus endoscopy confirmed gross ethmoidal polypoid disease. The tissue of the anterior ethmoid was very thickened and polypoid.

2 ICD-10-CM Codes _____

4 ICD-10-PCS Codes _____

_____

---

4. INPATIENT HOSPITAL Gender: F Age: 56

Preprocedure diagnosis: Submucous leiomyoma of the uterus, postmenopausal bleeding

Procedure: Open total abdominal hysterectomy and open bilateral salpingo-oophorectomy. Upon entering the peritoneal cavity the uterus and bilateral tubes and ovaries were freed and removed from the cavity. Fascia and skin were closed. Patient tolerated the procedure well.

Tip: Three procedure codes are required, one for each body part. There are bilateral values for the tubes and ovaries.

2 ICD-10-CM Codes _____

3 ICD-10- PCS Codes _____

_____

---

5. INPATIENT HOSPITAL Gender: M Age: 56

Preprocedure diagnosis: Squamous cell carcinoma of the supraglottis; 2 pack per day cigarette smoker

Procedure: Total open laryngectomy; bilateral modified radical neck dissection of lymph chains. A hemi-apron incision was made and a level 2, 3, 4 lymphatic neck dissection was performed. A partial laryngectomy could not be performed due to invasion of the tumor into the cricoid cartilage.

Postprocedure diagnosis: Squamous cell carcinoma of the supraglottis with invasion to the cricoid cartilage; cervical lymphatic metastases

Tip: Follow the instruction at the diagnosis category in the ICD-10-CM Tabular List to identify one of the diagnosis codes.

4 ICD-10-CM Codes _____

_____

3 ICD-10-PCS Codes _____

_____

6. INPATIENT HOSPITAL   Gender: M   Age: 48

Preprocedure diagnosis: Normal-volume azoospermia (*absence of viable sperm*)

Procedure: Bilateral testis biopsies. Percutaneous testis biopsy on the left positive for motile sperm. The same procedure was performed on the right testis; however, the biopsy was negative for motile sperm. The patient tolerated the procedure well.

Postprocedure diagnosis: Azoospermia

1 ICD-10-CM Code _____

1 ICD-10-PCS Code _____

7. INPATIENT HOSPITAL   Gender: F   Age: 20

Preprocedure diagnosis: Increasing fatigue and lethargy

Procedure: Bone marrow biopsy. After making percutaneous access, an 11-gauge Jamshidi biopsy needle was used to obtain a core bone marrow biopsy sample from the right posterior iliac crest.

Postprocedure diagnosis: Acute lymphoblastic leukemia

1 ICD-10-CM Code _____

1 ICD-10-PCS Code _____

8. INPATIENT HOSPITAL   Gender: F   Age: 17

Preprocedure diagnosis: Hyperhidrosis involving the soles of the feet, hands, and underarms

Procedure: Bilateral endoscopic thoracic sympathectomy under general anesthesia. After making small incisions under the armpit for percutaneous access, the endoscope was inserted. Sympathetic nerves were partially excised and the instrument withdrawn. No drains left in place.

Postprocedure diagnosis: Hyperhidrosis involving the soles of the feet, hands, and underarms

3 ICD-10-CM Codes _____

_____

1 ICD-10-PCS Code _____

9. INPATIENT HOSPITAL   Gender: F   Age: 28

Preprocedure diagnosis: Moderately atypical melanocytic nevus, abdomen

Procedure: Excision of atypical melanocytic nevus, abdomen, and complex repair approximately 3 cm. A 15 blade was used to excise a specimen through skin and superficial subcutaneous tissue.

Postprocedure diagnosis: Moderately atypical melanocytic nevus proliferation, abdomen

1 ICD-10-CM Code _____

1 ICD-10-PCS Code _____

10. INPATIENT HOSPITAL   Gender: M   Age: 66

Preprocedure diagnosis: Chronic diabetic ulcer of left midfoot with muscle necrosis

Procedure: Below-the-knee amputation at the distal portion, left leg. After inflation of the tourniquet, skin incised. The tibia and fibula were divided using an oscillating saw and hand-held bone cutter. An amputation knife was used to complete the amputation. Bleeding controlled with cautery.

Postprocedure diagnosis: Diabetic ulcer of plantar surface of the left midfoot with muscle necrosis

2 ICD-10-CM Codes _____

1 ICD-10-PCS Code _____

Chapter 50

Section 0: Root Operations M, S, X, Y

Reattachment • Reposition • Transfer • Transplantation

Chapter Outline

- **Basics of Procedures That Put in/Put Back or Move Some/All of a Body Part**
- **Coding Guidelines for Root Operations M, S, X, and Y**
- **Abstracting for Root Operations M, S, X, and Y**
- **Assigning Characters 4–7 for Root Operations M, S, X, and Y**
- **Arranging Codes for Root Operations M, S, X, and Y**

Learning Objectives

After completing this chapter, you should have the skills to:

50.1 Spell and define the key words, medical terms, and abbreviations related to procedures that put in/put back or move some/all of a body part. (Remember)

50.2 Identify the types of procedures performed for the root operations Reattachment, Reposition, Transfer, and Transplantation. (Apply)

50.3 Adhere to ICD-10-PCS coding guidelines related to the root operations M, S, X, and Y. (Apply)

50.4 Examine and abstract procedural information from the medical record for coding for the root operations M, S, X, and Y. (Analyze)

50.5 Demonstrate how to assign codes for the root operations M, S, X, and Y. (Apply)

50.6 Utilize guidelines for arranging (sequencing) codes for root operations M, S, X, and Y. (Apply)

Key Terms and Abbreviations

avulsed	free flap	pedicle flap	United Network for Organ Sharing
forequarter	musculocutaneous	transposition	(UNOS)

In addition to the key terms listed here, students should know the terms defined within tables in this chapter.

INTRODUCTION

Traffic engineers sometimes need to reconfigure an intersection to make traffic flow more smoothly. This might involve reinstalling detached lines or cables to a traffic signal, replacing a malfunctioning traffic signal, or moving an exit ramp to a new location. Surgeons might need to perform similar procedures for malfunctioning body parts.

This chapter discusses the Medical and Surgical root operations in the group *Procedures that put in/put back or move some/all of a body part*: Reattachment, Reposition, Transfer, and Transplantation. Although the root operations share a common purpose—putting back or moving some or all of a body part—each has a unique aspect that makes it different from the other procedures in this group. Pay careful attention to the differences between each root operation so that you can use each confidently and accurately.

BASICS OF PROCEDURES THAT PUT IN/PUT BACK OR MOVE SOME/ALL OF A BODY PART

The group *Procedures that put in/put back or move some/all of a body part* includes four root operations. ■ TABLE 50-1 provides the definitions and values of root operations in this group and identifies procedural terms frequently associated with each. Some procedural terms, such as *transfer* or *reposition*, can be associated with more than one root operation. There is not a direct match between a specific procedural term and a root operation because some medical terms can be associated with more than one root operation. For example, the suffix *-plasty* can be used for several root operations, including Repair, Replacement, Reposition, and Supplement. Root operations are assigned based on the content of the operative report regarding what was actually performed, not on the terms used by the physician in documentation. Refer to ■ TABLE 50-2 for a refresher on how to build medical terms related to *Procedures that put in/put back or move some/all of a body part*.

Refer to detailed anatomic diagrams of specific organ systems in Chapters 8–43 of this text, or in external references, when you need to refresh your memory of human anatomy.

Table 50-1   ■   **ROOT OPERATIONS THAT PUT IN/PUT BACK OR MOVE SOME/ALL OF A BODY PART**

Root Operation	Value	Definition	Terms
Reattachment	M	Putting back in or on all or a portion of a separated body part to its normal location or other suitable location	Reattachment, replantation
Reposition	S	Moving to its normal location, or other suitable location, all or a portion of a body part	Reposition, reduction, move, relocate, transposition
Transfer	X	Moving, without taking out, all or a portion of a body part to another location to take over the function of all or a portion of a body part	Transfer, move
Transplantation	Y	Putting in or on all or a portion of a living body part taken from another individual or animal to physically take the place and/or function of all or a portion of a similar body part	Transplant

CODING CAUTION

Be alert for root operations that have similar English meanings but different PCS definitions.

Transfer (X) (*Moving, without taking out, all or a portion of a body part to <u>another location to take over the function</u> of all or a portion of a body part*) and **Reposition (S)** (*Moving <u>to its normal location</u>, or other suitable location, all or a portion of a body part*)

Reattachment (M) (*Putting back in or on all or a portion of a <u>separated body part</u> to its normal location or other suitable location*) and **Fusion (G)** (*Joining together <u>portions of an articular body</u> part rendering the articular body part <u>immobile</u>*)

Table 50-2   ■   **EXAMPLE OF CONSTRUCTING MEDICAL TERMS FOR PROCEDURES THAT PUT IN/PUT BACK OR MOVE SOME/ALL OF A BODY PART**

Combining Form	Suffix	Complete Medical Term
col/o (*colon*)		
colp/o (*vagina*)	**-pexy** (*surgical fixation*) **-plasty** (*repair*)	**colo + pexy** (*surgical fixation of the colon*) **colpo + pexy** (*surgical fixation of the vagina*)
choledoch/o (*common bile duct*)		**choledocho + plasty** (*repair of the common bile duct*) **conjunctivo + plasty** (*repair of the conjunctiva*)
conjunctiv/o (*conjunctiva*)		

Source: © PB Resources, Inc. Used with permission.

CODING PRACTICE

Exercise 50.1 Basics of Procedures That Put in/Put Back or Move Some/All of a Body Part

Instructions: Use your medical terminology skills and resources to define the following procedures that take out some or all of a body part, then identify the code(s) or code range listed in the ICD-10-PCS Index. Follow these steps:

- Use slash marks "/" to break down each term into its root(s) and suffix.
- Define the meaning of the underlined word based on the meaning of each word part.
- Look up the term in the ICD-10-PCS Index, and write down the name(s) of root operation(s) the Index cross-references you to and the Table(s), if provided.
- Do not assign any codes.

Example: <u>pneumonopexy</u> pneumono/pexy   Meaning *fixation of the lung*   PCS Root Operation(s)/Table(s) *Repair 0BQ, Reposition 0BS*

1. <u>arthropexy</u>   Meaning _____   PCS Root Operation(s)/Table(s) _____
2. <u>transposition</u>   Meaning _____   PCS Root Operation(s)/Table(s) _____
3. <u>patellapexy</u>   Meaning _____   PCS Root Operation(s)/Table(s) _____
4. <u>blepharoplasty</u>   Meaning _____   PCS Root Operation(s)/Table(s) _____
5. <u>reimplantation</u>   Meaning _____   PCS Root Operation(s)/Table(s) _____
6. <u>ileopexy</u>   Meaning _____   PCS Root Operation(s)/Table(s) _____
7. <u>cecopexy</u>   Meaning _____   PCS Root Operation(s)/Table(s) _____
8. <u>autotransplant</u>   Meaning _____   PCS Root Operation(s)/Table(s) _____
9. <u>detorsion</u>   Meaning _____   PCS Root Operation(s)/Table(s) _____
10. pedicled TRAM (transverse rectus abdominis <u>myocutaneous</u>) flap reconstruction   Meaning _____   PCS Root Operation(s)/Table(s) _____

CODING GUIDELINES FOR ROOT OPERATIONS M, S, X, AND Y

Root operations in this group involve putting in, putting back, or moving some or all of a body part. These procedures do not include repair or removal of a body part.

Coders should understand the guidelines specific to the root operations M, S, X, and Y. Refer to the PCS OGCR for clinical examples of each guideline.

- Reposition for fracture treatment—Reduction of a displaced fracture is coded to the root operation Reposition (S) (PCS OGCR B3.15). The application of a cast or splint in conjunction with the Reposition procedure is not coded separately. For example, reduction and casting of a displaced fracture is coded to the root operation Reposition. Treatment of a nondisplaced fracture is coded to the procedure performed. For example, casting of a nondisplaced fracture is coded to the root operation Immobilization (3) in the Placement (2) section.

- Transfer—The root operation Transfer can involve transfer of multiple tissue layers—such as the skin, subcutaneous tissue, fascia, or muscle. Character 4, Body Part, identifies the deepest tissue layer in the flap. Character 7, Qualifier, identifies the intermediate layers in the transfer flap (PCS OGCR 3.17).

- Transplantation versus Administration—The root operation Transplantation (Y) is putting in a mature and functioning living body part taken from another individual or animal (PCS OGCR 3.16), such as transplantation of a kidney or lung. Root operations in the Administration (3) section report putting in autologous or nonautologous cells. For example, putting in autologous or nonautologous bone marrow, pancreatic islet cells, or stem cells is coded to the root operation Transfusion (2). Procedures in the Administration section are discussed in Chapter 54 of this text.

- Devices—A device is coded only if a device remains after the procedure is completed. If no device remains, the value **No device (Z)** is coded (PCS OGCR B6.1a). The root operation Reposition uses Character 6, Device, to identify the type of internal or external fixation devices left in place.

Specific guidelines and instructions are discussed throughout this chapter of the text.

ABSTRACTING FOR ROOT OPERATIONS M, S, X, AND Y

The root operation definition reflects the functional objective of the procedure. The functional objective identifies what the surgeon's goal is for the procedure. The following information summarizes the objectives, definitions, unique features, and examples of root operations M, S, X, and Y.

Abstracting for Reattachment (M)

The objective of the root operation Reattachment is putting back a detached body part. The site of the procedure is some or all of a body part.

Procedures coded to Reattachment include putting back a body part that has been cut off or **avulsed** (*ripped or torn away*). Nerves and blood vessels may or may not be reconnected in a Reattachment procedure. If these are reconnected, the reconnection is included in the Reattachment procedure and is not coded separately.

Examples of Reattachment are reattachment of the hand that perhaps was torn off in an accident and reattachment of an avulsed kidney that became detached in an accident (■ TABLE 50-3).

Abstracting for Reposition (S)

The objective of the root operation Reposition is moving a body part to its normal or another suitable location. The site of the procedure is some or all of a body part.

The body part is moved to a new location from an abnormal location to its normal location or from a normal location where it is not functioning correctly to a new location to enhance its ability to function. The body part may or may not be cut out or off to be moved to the new location.

In medical documentation, physicians often use the term **transposition** to identify when an anatomic structure is moved but not reconfigured or reconnected. This procedure typically meets the criteria for the PCS root operation Reposition. For example, in a nerve transposition, the nerve might

Table 50-3   ■   EXAMPLES OF THE ROOT OPERATION REATTACHMENT (M)

Organ System	Procedural Examples
Digestive	Replantation of avulsed teeth, tongue, lip, intestine
Endocrine	Reattachment of thyroid, parathyroid, or adrenal gland(s)
Genitourinary	Reattachment of severed testes, kidney, ureter, bladder, ovary, vulva
Hepatobiliary	Replantation of liver or pancreas
Integumentary	Replantation of avulsed scalp, skin from any location, or breast
Musculoskeletal	Reattachment of muscle, tendon, or ligament avulsion; reattachment of severed extremity
Respiratory	Replantation of lung, bronchus, or trachea
Special Senses (Ear, Eye)	Reattachment of severed ear or eyelid

Source: © PB Resources, Inc. Used with permission.

Table 50-4   ■   EXAMPLES OF THE ROOT OPERATION REPOSITION (S)

Organ System	Procedural Examples
Blood and Immune	Reposition of thymus or spleen
Cardiovascular	Reposition of thoracic aorta, pulmonary artery, pulmonary vein, or peripheral arteries or veins
Digestive	Gastropexy for malrotation; reposition of a portion of the large or small intestine
Endocrine	Reposition of thyroid, parathyroid, or adrenal glands
Genitourinary	Orchiopexy; reposition of kidney, ureter, bladder, or urethra, ovary, uterus, vagina
Hepatobiliary	Reposition of the liver, gallbladder, pancreas, or related duct(s)
Integumentary	Reposition of hair, breast, or nipple
Musculoskeletal	Reposition of muscle, tendon, ligament, or bone; fracture reduction (open or closed, with or without fixation device)
Nervous	Transposition of nerve
Respiratory	Reposition of bronchus, lung, diaphragm
Special Senses (Ear, Eye)	Reposition of ocular muscles, vessels, or eyelid; reposition of external ear, nose, nasal septum, tympanic membrane

Source: © PB Resources, Inc. Used with permission.

be moved away from a structure where it is constricted or "pinched" but is not cut and reconnected. It still serves its original function.

Examples of Reposition are the reposition of an undescended testicle (*moving a congenitally misplaced testicle from the abdomen into the scrotum*) and fracture reduction, in which pressure applied to the bone moves the displaced segments back into alignment. (■ TABLE 50-4).

Abstracting for Transfer (X)

The objective of the root operation Transfer is moving a body part to function for a similar body part. The site of the procedure is some or all of a body part.

The body part transferred remains connected to its vascular and nervous supply. The root operation Transfer is used to identify procedures where a body part is moved to another location without disrupting its vascular and nervous supply. In the body systems that classify the subcutaneous tissue, fascia, and muscle body parts, Character 7, Qualifier, can be used to specify when more than one tissue layer was used in the transfer procedure, such as a **musculocutaneous** (*pertaining to both muscles and skin*) flap transfer.

Transfer of a nerve, tendon, or other part differs from the root operation Reposition in the following ways:

- In Transfer the body part is moved to take over the function of another body part, whereas in Reposition the goal is to improve the function of the body part moved.

- In Transfer, the body part moved remains connected to its original nerve and vascular supply, so one aspect, not all, of the structure may be disconnected then reconnected

Table 50-5 ■ **EXAMPLES OF THE ROOT OPERATION TRANSFER (X)**

Organ System	Procedural Examples
Digestive	Lip, gingiva, stomach, small or large intestine
Integumentary	Pedicle flap
Musculoskeletal	Muscle, tendon, or ligament transfer
Nervous	Nerve transfer
Special Senses (Ear, Eye)	Extraocular muscle transfer

Source: © PB Resources, Inc. Used with permission.

to a different site. In Reposition, the body part moved may remain completely attached to its original supply or partially or completely disconnected.

Examples of Transfer are a nerve transfer—in which one end of a nerve is moved to take over the function of another nerve that is not working properly—and **pedicle flap** transfer, in which a flap of skin and subcutaneous tissue is separated and moved to cover a nearby damaged area while the original blood vessels and nerves remain connected to the original site (■ TABLE 50-5). In contrast, in a **free flap** the blood vessels and nerves are completely disconnected from the original site and reconnected to vessels and nerves at the new site. A free flap is coded to the root operation Replacement and the device value autologous tissue substitute.

Abstracting for Transplantation (Y)

The objective of the root operation Transplantation is putting in a living body part from a person or animal. The site of the procedure is some or all of a body part. The body part can be an organ, part of an organ, or tissue.

Transplantation includes a small number of procedures because a limited number of organs can be transplanted. The root operation includes only the procedure on the body part(s) being transplanted. The native organ may or may not be taken out, and the transplanted organ may take over all or a portion of its function. Harvesting of the donor organ and any other procedures necessary to complete the transplant, such as cardiopulmonary bypass, are coded separately.

Examples of Transplantation are a kidney transplant and heart transplant, in which new organs are placed into a person to replace severely damaged or diseased organs (■ TABLE 50-6).

CODING CAUTION

Bone marrow transplant procedures are coded with the root operation Transfusion (3), which is part of PCS section 3, Administration, because replacement bone marrow is administered or transfused into the patient.

The **United Network for Organ Sharing (UNOS)** is a nonprofit organization that administers the United States' Organ Procurement and Transplantation Network, including the organ transplant waiting list. UNOS deals with six major organs: the heart, kidney, lung, pancreas, liver, and intestine.

Table 50-6 ■ **EXAMPLES OF THE ROOT OPERATION TRANSPLANTATION (Y)**

Organ System	Procedural Examples
Cardiovascular	Heart transplant
Digestive	Stomach, esophagus, intestine transplant
Endocrine	Thymus, spleen transplant
Genitourinary	Kidney, ovary transplant
Hepatobiliary	Liver, pancreas transplant
Respiratory	Lung transplant
Special Senses (Ear, Eye)	Cornea transplant

Source: © PB Resources, Inc. Used with permission.

The kidney is the most commonly transplanted single organ, and the least common is the intestine. A double transplant is the transplantation of two related organs, such as the heart and lung or kidney and pancreas.

Key Criteria for Abstracting

Refer to Table 47-2 and 47-3 for general guidance on abstracting PCS procedures and root operation groups. Then refer to ■ TABLE 50-7 for more specific guidance on how to abstract procedures that *Put in/put back or move some/all of a body part* and distinguish among root operations in this group. A guided example of abstracting for the root operation Reposition follows.

Table 50-7 ■ **KEY CRITERIA FOR ABSTRACTING ROOT OPERATIONS THAT PUT IN/PUT BACK OR MOVE SOME/ALL OF A BODY PART**

Question	Root Operation (Value)
❏ Was a body part reattached, replaced, or moved? ❏ Was a body part replaced with a human or animal substitute?	If *Yes*, continue below to root operations M, S, X, and Y.
❏ Was a body part replaced with a synthetic substitute?	Do not use root operations M, S, X, or Y.
Answer *Yes* to one of the following questions to help distinguish root operations M, S, X, and Y	
❏ Was a severed or avulsed body part or extremity reattached?	Reattachment (M)
❏ Was a body part moved to a new location from an abnormal location to improve its function, with or without detaching it? ❏ Was a body part moved to a new location from its normal location where it was not functioning properly to improve its function, with or without detaching it?	Reposition (S)
❏ Was a body part moved, without disrupting its nervous or blood supply, to serve a similar function in a new location?	Transfer (X)
❏ Was an organ or part of an organ replaced (transplanted) with a human or animal substitute?	Transplantation (Y)

Source: © PB Resources, Inc. Used with permission.

Remember that the abstracting questions are a guide and that not every question applies to, or can be answered for, every case.

Guided Example of Abstracting for Reposition

Refer to the following example throughout this chapter to practice skills for abstracting, assigning, and arranging codes for the root operation Reposition. Similar principles apply to working with other root operations that put in/put back or move some/all of a body part.

INPATIENT HOSPITAL   Gender: F   Age: 23

Preoperative diagnosis: Fractured R tibia and R humerus

Procedure: Open reduction, R tibia, with internal fixation device. Closed reduction, R humerus, percutaneous external fixation using a monoplanar device.

Postoperative diagnosis: Displaced fracture R tibia, displaced fracture R humerus shaft

---

Follow along as fictitious coder Marcy Elwood, CCS, abstracts the procedure. Check off each step after you complete it.

▶ Marcy reads through the entire record, paying special attention to the reason for the encounter, the procedure performed, and the postoperative diagnosis. She refers to the Key Criteria for Abstracting (Table 50-7).

❏ She notes the preoperative diagnosis: displaced fracture R tibia and R humerus.

❏ *What are the stated procedures?* Reduction of two fractures

❏ *What organ or body part(s) is involved?* R tibia, R humerus

❏ *Is the procedure description what you would expect based on the name of the procedure?* Yes

❏ *What surgical approach is used for the first procedure (right tibia)?* Open

❏ *Was more than one procedure, or a combined procedure, performed?* Yes, internal fixation was used

❏ *What surgical approach is used for the second procedure (right humerus)?* Closed

❏ *Was more than one procedure, or a combined procedure, performed?* Yes, external fixation was used

❏ *Did the procedure put in/put back or move some/all of a body part?* Yes

❏ *Was a body part reattached, replaced, or moved?* Yes, both body parts were moved

❏ *Was a body part replaced with a human or animal substitute?* No

❏ *Was a body part replaced with a synthetic substitute?* No

❏ *Was an organ or part of an organ replaced with a human or animal substitute?* No

❏ *Was a severed or avulsed body part or extremity reattached?* No

❏ *Was a body part moved, without disrupting its nervous or blood supply, to serve a similar function in a new location?* No

❏ *Was a body part moved to a new location from an abnormal location to improve its function, with or without detaching it?* Yes

❏ *Was a body part moved to a new location from its normal location where it was not functioning properly to improve its function, with or without detaching it?* No

▶ At this time, Marcy believes that she will use the root operation Reposition (PCS OGCR B3.15). She anticipates that she will need two codes because the same root operation was performed on two distinct sites (PCS OGCR B3.2a). She will verify this information when she refers to the PCS Tables to assign codes.

CODING PRACTICE

Exercise 50.2 Abstracting for Root Operations M, S, X, and Y

Instructions: Read the mini-medical-record of each patient's encounter and answer the abstracting questions. Write the answer on the line provided. Do not assign any codes.

---

1. INPATIENT HOSPITAL   Gender: M

Age: 15 months

Preprocedure diagnosis: Undescended testicles in inguinal canal

(continued)

---

1. (continued)

Procedure: Orchiopexy; an inguinal incision was made in the left groin and carried through the subcutaneous tissues to the anterior fascia. The fascia was opened, exposing the testicle, which lay high in the canal. The testicle was located in a superficial pouch of the inguinal canal and there was adequate length on the spermatic cord to reposition it without problem. The testicle was freed with dissection and moved to its normal location. Procedure was repeated on right side. Patient tolerated procedure well. No other abnormalities were found.

Postprocedure diagnosis: Bilateral undescended testicles

(continued)

CODING PRACTICE (continued)

1. (continued)

a. What is the stated procedure? _____

b. What organ or body part is involved? _____

c. What is the laterality? _____

d. Is the procedure description what you would expect based on the name of the procedure? _____

e. What surgical approach is used? _____

f. Was more than one procedure, or a combined procedure, performed? _____

g. Was a body part reattached, replaced, or moved? _____

h. Was a body part replaced with a human or animal substitute? _____

i. Was a body part replaced with a synthetic substitute? _____

j. Was an organ or part of an organ replaced (transplanted) with a human or animal substitute? _____

k. Was a severed or avulsed body part or extremity reattached? _____

l. Was a body part moved, without disrupting its nervous or blood supply, to serve a similar function in a new location? _____

m. Was a body part moved to a new location from an abnormal location to improve its function, with or without detaching it? _____

n. Was a body part moved to a new location from its normal location where it was not functioning properly to improve its function, with or without detaching it? _____

o. What is the root operation? _____

---

2. INPATIENT HOSPITAL   Gender: F   Age: 52

Preprocedure diagnosis: Hyperparathyroidism

Procedure: Parathyroid autotransplantation; endoscopic transthoracic parathyroidectomy ×4 with mediastinal exploration and parathyroid autotransplantation to left forearm

a. What is the stated procedure? _____

b. What organ or body part is involved? _____

c. What is the laterality? _____

d. Is the procedure description what you would expect based on the name of the procedure? _____

e. What surgical approach is used? _____

---

2. (continued)

f. Was more than one procedure, or a combined procedure, performed? _____

g. Was a body part reattached, replaced, or moved? _____

h. Was a body part replaced with a human or animal substitute? _____

i. Was a body part replaced with a synthetic substitute? _____

j. Was an organ or part of an organ replaced (transplanted) with a human or animal substitute? _____ _____

k. Was a severed or avulsed body part or extremity reattached? _____

l. Was a body part moved, without disrupting its nervous or blood supply, to serve a similar function in a new location? _____

m. Was a body part moved to a new location from an abnormal location to improve its function, with or without detaching it? _____

n. Was a body part moved to a new location from its normal location where it was not functioning properly to improve its function, with or without detaching it? _____

o. What is the root operation? _____

---

3. INPATIENT HOSPITAL   Gender: F   Age: 23

Preprocedure diagnosis: Fractured R ulna

Procedure: Open reduction, R ulna with clamp and rod internal fixation (CRIF)

a. What is the stated procedure? _____

b. What organ or body part is involved? _____

c. What is the laterality? _____

d. Is the procedure description what you would expect based on the name of the procedure? _____

e. What surgical approach is used? _____

f. Was more than one procedure, or a combined procedure, performed? _____

g. Was a body part reattached, replaced, or moved? _____

h. Was a body part replaced with a human or animal substitute? _____

(continued)

CODING PRACTICE *(continued)*

3. *(continued)*

i. Was a body part replaced with a synthetic substitute? _____

j. Was an organ or part of an organ replaced (transplanted) with a human or animal substitute? _____

k. Was a severed or avulsed body part or extremity reattached? _____

l. Was a body part moved, without disrupting its nervous or blood supply, to serve a similar function in a new location? _____

m. Was a body part moved to a new location from an abnormal location to improve its function, with or without detaching it? _____

n. Was a body part moved to a new location from its normal location where it was not functioning properly to improve its function, with or without detaching it? _____

o. What is the root operation? _____

4. INPATIENT HOSPITAL   Gender: M   Age: 27

Preprocedure diagnosis: Traumatic amputation of distal segment of little finger and two segments of the ring finger on left hand while using a table saw in home workshop

Procedure: Replantation of distal segments of the little finger and ring finger on the left hand

a. What is the stated procedure? _____

b. What organ or body part is involved? _____

c. What is the laterality? _____

d. Is the procedure description what you would expect based on the name of the procedure? _____

e. What surgical approach is used? _____

f. Was more than one procedure, or a combined procedure, performed? _____

g. Was a body part reattached, replaced, or moved? _____

h. Was a body part replaced with a human or animal substitute? _____

i. Was a body part replaced with a synthetic substitute? _____

j. Was an organ or part of an organ replaced (transplanted) with a human or animal substitute? _____

(continued)

4. *(continued)*

k. Was a severed or avulsed body part or extremity reattached? _____

l. Was a body part moved, without disrupting its nervous or blood supply, to serve a similar function in a new location? _____

m. Was a body part moved to a new location from an abnormal location to improve its function, with or without detaching it? _____

n. Was a body part moved to a new location from its normal location where it was not functioning properly to improve its function, with or without detaching it? _____

o. What is the root operation? _____

5. INPATIENT HOSPITAL   Gender: F   Age: 36

Preprocedure diagnosis: Type 1 diabetes mellitus, unresponsive to treatment

Procedure: Simultaneous kidney-pancreas transplantation. The donor kidney came from the patient's identical twin. The donor pancreas came from a cadaver. Patient's left kidney was removed and replaced.

a. What is the stated procedure? _____

b. What organ or body part is involved? _____

c. What is the laterality? _____

d. Is the procedure description what you would expect based on the name of the procedure? _____

e. What surgical approach is used? _____

f. Was more than one procedure, or a combined procedure, performed? _____

g. Was a body part reattached, replaced, or moved? _____

h. Was a body part replaced with a human or animal substitute? _____

i. Was a body part replaced with a synthetic substitute? _____

j. Was an organ or part of an organ replaced (transplanted) with a human or animal substitute? _____

k. Was a severed or avulsed body part or extremity reattached? _____

l. Was a body part moved, without disrupting its nervous or blood supply, to serve a similar function in a new location? _____

(continued)

5. (continued)

m. Was a body part moved to a new location from an abnormal location to improve its function, with or without detaching it? _____

n. Was a body part moved to a new location from its normal location where it was not functioning properly to improve its function, with or without detaching it? _____

o. What is the root operation? _____

6. INPATIENT HOSPITAL Gender: F Age: 43

Preprocedure diagnosis: Low radial nerve palsy, right arm

Procedure: Tendon transfer, open. Rerouted the belly and insertion point of palmaris longus tendon to the extensor pollicis longus (EPL) muscle, leaving the blood and nerve supply intact. Rerouted belly and insertion point of the pronator teres tendon to the abductor pollicis longus (APL) muscle, leaving the blood and nerve supply intact.

a. What is the stated procedure? _____

b. What organ or body part is involved? _____

c. What is the laterality? _____

d. Is the procedure description what you would expect based on the name of the procedure? _____

e. What surgical approach is used? _____

6. (continued)

f. Was more than one procedure, or a combined procedure, performed? _____

g. Was a body part reattached, replaced, or moved? _____

h. Was a body part replaced with a human or animal substitute? _____

i. Was a body part replaced with a synthetic substitute? _____

j. Was an organ or part of an organ replaced (transplanted) with a human or animal substitute? _____

k. Was a severed or avulsed body part or extremity reattached? _____

l. Was a body part moved, without disrupting its nervous or blood supply, to serve a similar function in a new location? _____

m. Was a body part moved to a new location from an abnormal location to improve its function, with or without detaching it? _____

n. Was a body part moved to a new location from its normal location where it was not functioning properly to improve its function, with or without detaching it? _____

o. What is the root operation? _____

ASSIGNING CHARACTERS 4–7 FOR ROOT OPERATIONS M, S, X, AND Y

To assign codes after the root operation is determined, search the PCS Index for the name of the root operation as the Main Term. Locate the subterm(s) for the correct anatomic site and identify the PCS Table. When you locate the PCS Table, verify the first three characters of the code, then locate the row with the body part needed. Assign the remaining characters from each respective column of the Table. If more than one row contains the desired body part, compare the combinations of body part, approach, device, and qualifier to build the correct code. All values must be chosen from the same row in the table. The following information summarizes and highlights unique information for working with the Tables for each root operation M, S, X, and Y. Each root operation has one Table in each applicable PCS body system. Because of the differences between organ systems, Table details vary.

Character 4: Body Part

The body part identifies the anatomic site treated in the root operation, such as the organ transplanted and the structure reattached, transferred, or repositioned. Use the most specific body part value provided in the Table being used. For example, in Table 0BY, Respiratory System Transplantation, select the most specific part of the lung applicable. When only one lobe of the lung is transplanted, select the body part value for the appropriate lobe. When the entire lung is transplanted, assign **K Lung, Right** or **L Lung, Left**. When both lungs are transplanted, assign **M Lungs, Bilateral**.

In the root operation Transfer, Character 4, Body Part, identifies the *deepest* layer of tissue moved. In Reposition, Character 4 identifies the site that is moved.

Reattachment of the extremities is reported with the body system Anatomical Regions, because the entire limb is reattached. Do not code **Upper Bones** or **Lower Bones** because more body systems than the bones are treated. The body part values identify various segments and the laterality of each extremity (■ TABLE 50-8).

The body part **forequarter** refers to the extremity and all or part of the adjoining structure, such as the arm, shoulder joint, and all or part of the scapula and clavicle or the leg, hip joint, and all or part of the pelvic girdle.

Table 50-8 ■ **CHARACTER 4, BODY PART VALUES FOR TABLE 0XM: BODY SYSTEM ANATOMICAL REGIONS, UPPER EXTREMITIES (X) AND ROOT OPERATION REATTACHMENT (M)**

Value	Body Part
0	Forequarter, Right
1	Forequarter, Left
2	Shoulder Region, Right
3	Shoulder Region, Left
4	Axilla, Right
5	Axilla, Left
6	Upper Extremity, Right
7	Upper Extremity, Left
8	Upper Arm, Right
9	Upper Arm, Left
B	Elbow Region, Right
C	Elbow Region, Left
D	Lower Arm, Right
F	Lower Arm, Left
G	Wrist Region, Right
H	Wrist Region, Left
J	Hand, Right
K	Hand, Left
L	Thumb, Right
M	Thumb, Left
N	Index Finger, Right
P	Index Finger, Left
Q	Middle Finger, Right
R	Middle Finger, Left
S	Ring Finger, Right
T	Ring Finger, Left
V	Little Finger, Right
W	Little Finger, Left

Character 5: Approach

Refer to the Tables for each root operation/body system combination to identify the valid approach for a particular procedure. In particular, note:

- Transplantation: The approach is always Open.
- Reattachment: The approach is Open, Percutaneous Endoscopic, or External.
- Reposition: All approaches are used except Via Natural or Artificial Opening with Percutaneous Endoscopic Assistance.
- Skin and Breast: The approach for procedures coded to Reattachment, Transfer, and Reposition is always External.

Character 6: Device

The root operation Reposition uses the device character to identify the type of internal or external skeletal fixation device applied (■ TABLE 50-9 and ■ FIGURE 50-1). PCS provides specific values for fixation devices based on the body systems and body part because

Table 50-9 ■ **TYPES OF SKELETAL FIXATION DEVICES**

External Fixation Devices
- ❏ Delta frame external fixator
- ❏ Ilizarov external fixator
- ❏ Monoplanar (uniplanar) external fixator
- ❏ Sheffield hybrid external fixator
- ❏ Sheffield ring external fixator

Internal Fixation Devices
- ❏ Bone screw (interlocking, lag, pedicle, recessed)
- ❏ Clamp and rod internal fixation (CRIF) system
- ❏ Fusion screw (compression, lag, locking)
- ❏ Intramedullary (IM) rod (nail)
- ❏ Intramedullary skeletal kinetic distractor (ISKD)
- ❏ Joint fixation plate
- ❏ Kirschner wire (K-wire)
- ❏ Kuntscher nail
- ❏ Neutralization plate
- ❏ Titanium sternal fixation system (TSFS)

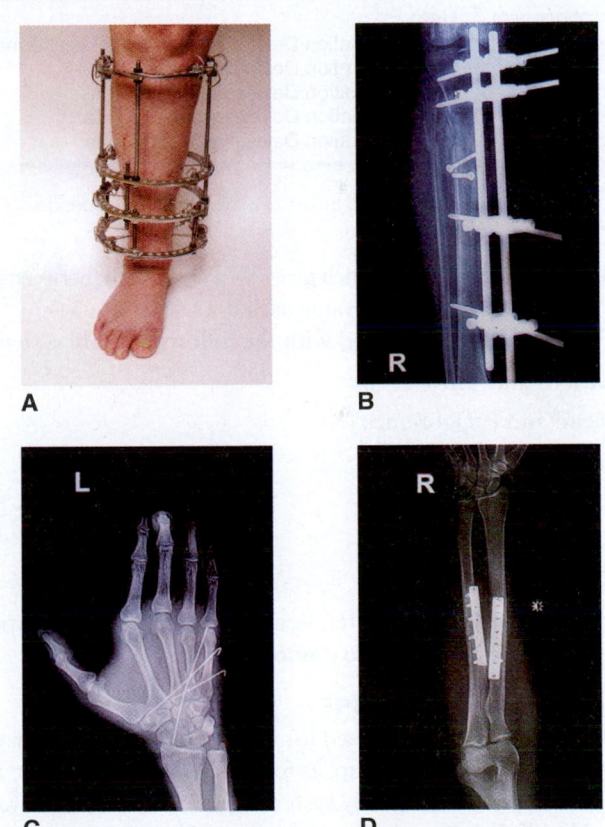

A   **B**   **C**   **D**

Figure 50-1 ■ Images of fixation devices. (A) Ilizarov ring external fixation *(Source: Sima/Shutterstock)*. (B) Monoplanar external fixation *(Source: Praisaeng/Shutterstock)*. (C) Kirschner wire (K-wire) Internal fixation *(Source: Praisaeng/Shutterstock)*. (D) Plate and screw internal fixation *(Source: Praisaeng/Shutterstock)*.

not all fixation devices are used on all anatomic sites (■ FIGURE 50-2, page 1050). The type of fixation is documented in the operative report, so the coder must identify the specific device used and convert it to the appropriate PCS value. If the correct PCS value is not immediately obvious, refer to the Device Key Appendix in

Section	0	Medical and Surgical
Body System	P	Upper Bones
Operation	S	Reposition: Moving to its normal location, or other suitable location, all or a portion of a body part

Body Part Character 4	Approach Character 5	Device Character 6	Qualifier Character 7
C Humeral Head, Right D Humeral Head, Left F Humeral Shaft, Right G Humeral Shaft, Left H Radius, Right J Radius, Left K Ulna, Right L Ulna, Left	0 Open 3 Percutaneous 4 Percutaneous Endoscopic	4 Internal Fixation Device 5 External Fixation Device 6 Internal Fixation Device, Intramedullary B External Fixation Device, Monoplanar C External Fixation Device, Ring D External Fixation Device, Hybrid Z No Device	Z No Qualifier

Figure 50-2 ■ Example of Character 6, Device values for skeletal fixation devices.

Term	ICD-10-PCS Value
Joint fixation plate	**Use:** Internal Fixation Device in Upper Joints Internal Fixation Device in Lower Joints
Kirschner wire (K-wire)	**Use:** Internal Fixation Device in Head and Facial Bones Internal Fixation Device in Upper Bones Internal Fixation Device in Lower Bones Internal Fixation Device in Upper Joints Internal Fixation Device in Lower Joints

Figure 50-3 ■ Example of the PCS coding manual appendix "Device Key."

the ICD-10-PCS manual, which provides a cross-walk between the specific device and the PCS value (■ FIGURE 50-3).

Fixation devices are used with the following body systems:

- Mouth and Throat (C)
- Head and Facial Bones (N)
- Upper Bones (P)
- Lower Bones (Q)
- Upper Joints (R)
- Lower Joints (S)

The root operations Transfer, Reattachment, Transplantation always have a value of **Z No device**.

Character 7: Qualifier

Character 7, Qualifier, is used for a variety of purposes for the root operations in this group, as follows. Refer to the Table for the root operation and body system to verify the options available. Highlights of each root operation follow.

Reposition and Reattachment

In the root operation Reposition, the qualifier identifies the location to which the body part is moved. The qualifier also identifies the number of teeth being repositioned or reattached for the root operations Reposition and Reattachment and the body system **C Mouth and Throat**. Refer to PCS Table **0CS**. For all other procedures, the value is always **Z No qualifier**.

Transplantation

Qualifier values specify the genetic compatibility of the body part transplanted for the root operation Transplantation:

- **0 Allogeneic** (*from another member of the same species, such as another person*)
- **1 Syngeneic** (*from an genetically identical species, such as an identical twin*)
- **2 Zooplastic** (*from an animal*)

Transfer

For the root operation Transfer, the qualifier provides additional details about the procedure. For procedures involving transfer of tissue layers such as skin, fascia, and muscle, the qualifier identifies the intermediate tissue layers being transferred when the tissue transferred is composed of more than one tissue layer (■ FIGURE 50-4). The body system value identifies the deepest tissue layer in the flap. Assign **Z No qualifier** when only one tissue layer is transferred.

For Transfer procedures classified to other body systems, such as the peripheral nervous system, the qualifier identifies the destination site of the transfer (*to*) (■ FIGURE 50-5). The body part specifies the source site of the transfer (*from*).

Surgeon performed an open fasciocutaneous flap closure of left thigh.

0JXM0ZC Medical and Surgical, Subcutaneous tissue and fascia, Transfer, Subcutaneous tissue and fascia left upper leg, Open, No device, Skin subcutaneous tissue and fascia

Figure 50-4 ■ Example of coding a tissue flap transfer. *Source:* © PB Resources, Inc. Used with permission.

Surgeon performed a percutaneous endoscopic transfer of the trigeminal nerve to the facial nerve.

00XK4ZM Medical and Surgical, Central nervous system, Transfer, Trigeminal nerve, Percutaneous endoscopic, No device, Facial nerve

Figure 50-5 ■ Example of coding a nerve transfer. *Source:* © PB Resources, Inc. Used with permission.

Guided Example of Assigning Characters 4–7 for Reposition

To practice skills for assigning codes for the root operation Reposition, continue with the example from earlier in the chapter about a patient who was seen for fracture reduction and fixation. Follow along in your ICD-10-PCS manual as Marcy Elwood, CCS, assigns codes. Check off each step after you complete it.

▶ First, Marcy confirms the procedures.

- ❏ The root operation for the first procedure, open reduction of the right tibia, is Reposition.

- ❏ The root operation for the second procedure, closed reduction of the right humerus, is Reposition.

▶ Marcy searches the Index for the Main Term **Reposition**.

- ❏ She locates the first-level subterm **Tibia**.

- ❏ She locates the second-level subterm **Right**.

- ❏ She identifies the Table **0QS** for reduction of the right tibia.

▶ Under the same Main Term for **Reposition** she searches for the entry for the humerus. She notices there are two subterms: **Humeral head** and **Humeral shaft**. She refers to the documentation to confirm the site as R humerus shaft.

- ❏ She locates the second-level subterm **Humeral shaft** and the third-level subterm **Right**.

- ❏ She identifies the Table **0PS** for reduction of the right humerus.

▶ Marcy turns to Table **0QS** to assign the code for reduction of the right tibia.

- ❏ She reads the Table title **0QS, Medical and Surgical, Lower Bones, Reposition** and confirms that this accurately describes the body system and root operation.

▶ Marcy assigns the value for Character 4, Body Part.

- ❏ She notices that Table **0QS** contains several rows and searches for the one that contains the tibia.

- ❏ She locates tibia and notices there are two rows that contain a value for the tibia. She reads the entire row and identifies that one row provides multiple options for Character 5, Approach, and Character 6, Device. The other row provides only one option, **X External**, for Character 5, Approach, and only one option, **Z No device**, for Character 6, Device. Because a fixation device was used, she selects the row that provides multiple options for Character 6, Device.

- ❏ She returns to the column for Character 4, Body Part, and selects **G Tibia, Right**. This value is consistent with the partial code 0QSG provided in the Index.

▶ Marcy assigns the value for Character 5, Approach.

- ❏ She refers to the documentation and confirms the approach is open reduction.

- ❏ She selects **0 Open** for the approach value.

▶ Marcy assigns the value for Character 6, Device.

- ❏ She refers to the documentation and confirms the device is internal fixation.

- ❏ She selects **4 Internal Fixation Device** for the device value.

▶ Marcy assigns the value for Character 7, Qualifier.

- ❏ The Table provides only one option, **Z No qualifier**.

▶ She reviews the code she has assigned for the open reduction, R tibia with internal fixation device: **0QSG04Z** (■ FIGURE 50-6).

▶ Marcy turns to Table **0PS** to assign the code for reduction of the right humerus.

- ❏ She reads the Table title **0PS, Medical and Surgical, Upper Bones, Reposition** and confirms that this accurately describes the body system and root operation for reduction of the humerus.

Section	0	Medical and Surgical
Body System	Q	Lower Bones
Operation	S	Reposition: Moving to its normal location, or other suitable location, all or a portion of a body part

Body Part Character 4	Approach Character 5	Device Character 6	Qualifier Character 7
6 Upper Femur, Right 7 Upper Femur, Left 8 Femoral Shaft, Right 9 Femoral Shaft, Left B Lower Femur, Right C Lower Femur, Left G Tibia, Right H Tibia, Left J Fibula, Right K Fibula, Left	0 Open 3 Percutaneous 4 Percutaneous Endoscopic	4 Internal Fixation Device 5 External Fixation Device 6 Fixation Device, Intramedullary B External Fixation Device, Monoplanar C External Fixation Device, Ring D External Fixation Device, Hybrid Z No Device	Z No Qualifier

Figure 50-6 ■ Assigning code 0QSG04Z. *Source:* Annotation © PB Resources, Inc. Used with permission.

Section	0	**Medical and Surgical**
Body System	P	**Upper Bones**
Operation	S	**Reposition:** Moving to its normal location, or other suitable location, all or a portion of a body part

Body Part Character 4	Approach Character 5	Device Character 6	Qualifier Character 7
C Humeral Head, Right D Humeral Head, Left **F Humeral Shaft, Right** G Humeral Shaft, Left H Radius, Right J Radius, Left K Ulna, Right L Ulna, Left	0 Open **3 Percutaneous** 4 Percutaneous Endoscopic	4 Internal Fixation Device 5 External Fixation Device 6 Internal Fixation Device, Intramedullary **B External Fixation Device, Monoplanar** C External Fixation Device, Ring D External Fixation Device, Hybrid Z No Device	**Z No Qualifier**

Figure 50-7 ■ Assigning code 0PSF3BZ. *Source: Annotation © PB Resources, Inc. Used with permission.*

▶ Marcy assigns the value for Character 4, Body Part.

❏ She locates the row of the table that contains body part values for the humerus.

❏ She notices that she must select either **Humeral head** or **Humeral shaft**, so she refers to the documentation and confirms that the humeral shaft was involved.

❏ She also must select laterality and identifies body part value **F Humeral shaft, right**.

▶ Marcy assigns the value for Character 5, Approach.

❏ She refers to the documentation and confirms the approach is closed reduction, percutaneous external fixation.

❏ She selects **3 Percutaneous** for the approach value.

▶ Marcy assigns the value for Character 6, Device.

❏ She notices that there are several options for an external fixation device. She refers to the documentation to confirm that the type of device is monoplanar.

❏ She assigns **B External Fixation device, Monoplanar.**

▶ Marcy assigns the value for Character 7, Qualifier.

❏ She assigns the only choice, **Z No qualifier.**

▶ Marcy reviews the code she assigned for closed reduction, R humerus, percutaneous external fixation using a monoplanar device: **0PSF3BZ** (■ Figure 50-7).

▶ Marcy reviews the procedure codes she has assigned for this case.

❏ **0QSG04Z** Reposition, Lower Bones, Tibia Right, Open, Internal Fixation device, No qualifier

❏ **0PSF3BZ** Reposition, Upper Bones, Humeral Shaft Right, Percutaneous, External Fixation Device, Monoplanar, No qualifier

▶ Next, Marcy must determine how to sequence the codes.

CODING PRACTICE

Exercise 50.3 Assigning Characters 4–7 for Root Operations M, S, X, and Y

Instructions: Read the mini-medical-record of each patient's encounter. Review the information abstracted in Exercise 50.2 for questions 1–3. For questions 4–6, abstract the case on your own. Assign PCS codes using the Index and Tables. Write the code(s) on the line provided.

1. INPATIENT HOSPITAL Gender: M Age: 15 months

Preprocedure diagnosis: Undescended testicles in inguinal canal

Procedure: Orchiopexy; an inguinal incision was made in the left groin and carried through the subcutaneous
(continued)

1. (continued)

tissues to the anterior fascia. The fascia was opened, exposing the testicle, which lay high in the canal. The testicle was located in a superficial pouch of the inguinal canal and there was adequate length on the spermatic cord to reposition it without problem. The testicle was freed with dissection and moved to its normal location. Procedure was repeated on right side. Patient tolerated procedure well. No other abnormalities were found.

Postprocedure diagnosis: Bilateral undescended testicles

1 PCS Code _____

CODING PRACTICE (continued)

2. INPATIENT HOSPITAL   Gender: F   Age: 52

Preprocedure diagnosis: Hyperparathyroidism

Procedure: Parathyroid autotransplantation;
endoscopic transthoracic parathyroidectomy
× 4 with mediastinal exploration and parathyroid
autotransplantation to left forearm

1 PCS Code _____

3. INPATIENT HOSPITAL   Gender: F   Age: 23

Preprocedure diagnosis: Fractured R ulna

Procedure: Open reduction, R ulna with clamp and rod
internal fixation (CRIF)

1 PCS Code _____

4. INPATIENT HOSPITAL   Gender: F   Age: 34

Preprocedure diagnosis: Complete tear of the patellar
tendon, right knee

Procedure: Arthroscopic repair of the patellar tendon.
Using three suture anchors, the tendon was sewn
to the bottom of the patella. Fixation was tested and
no pull-out occurred. Hemostasis was obtained with
electrocautery.

1 PCS Code _____

5. INPATIENT HOSPITAL   Gender: M   Age: 44

Preprocedure diagnosis: Deltoid muscle paralysis, left
shoulder

Procedure: Trapezius muscle transfer. Fascia over
trapezius muscle incised and trapezius detached from
insertion. Deltoid muscle was exposed. The detached
trapezius muscle was transferred and sutured as
close as possible to the insertion of the deltoid
muscle. Highest possible tension was achieved in the
transferred muscle.

1 PCS Code _____

6. INPATIENT HOSPITAL   Gender: F   Age: 34

Preprocedure diagnosis: Previous bilateral tubal
ligation desiring reversal

Procedure: Endoscopic tubal reanastomosis. Using the
laparoscope, we obtained access to the fallopian tubes.
The ends of the left fallopian tube were incised to open
the lumen and reattached with use of the operating
microscope. The procedure was repeated on the right.
Methylene blue was used to ensure tubal patency.

Tip: If the identical procedure is performed on
contralateral body parts, and a bilateral body part value
exists for that body part, a single procedure is coded
using the bilateral body part value. PCS OGCR B4.3.

1 PCS Code _____

ARRANGING CODES FOR ROOT OPERATIONS M, S, X, AND Y

Multiple coding is required with PCS. Refer to PCS OGCR and Chapters 47 and 48 of this text for guidance on situations when multiple coding may be required. In addition to this general guidance, specific situations for root operations M, S, X, and Y that require multiple coding include:

- Transplantation: Root operation Y identifies only transplantation of the organ or tissue. Assign separate codes for harvesting of the donor organ and any other procedures necessary to complete the transplant, such as cardiopulmonary bypass. The organ transplant should be sequenced as the principal procedure and the associated procedures should be sequenced as secondary. Assign separate codes for each organ transplanted when more than one organ is transplanted during the same procedure.

- Laterality: Most body part values associated with Transfer, Reposition, and Reattachment procedures are unilateral because the procedures are typically performed unilaterally. When the procedure is performed bilaterally, assign separate codes for each side if no bilateral body part value is available. Typically, either side can be sequenced as the principal procedure.

Guided Example of Arranging Codes for Reposition

To practice skills for arranging codes for procedures of the root operation Reposition, continue with the example from earlier in the chapter about the patient who was seen for fracture reduction and fixation. Follow along in your ICD-10-PCS manual as Marcy Elwood, CCS, arranges the codes. Check off each step after you complete it.

▶ First, Marcy confirms the procedures: open reduction of the right tibia and closed reduction of the right humerus.

▶ Marcy reviews the codes she assigned:

❏ **0QSG04Z Reposition, Lower Bones, Tibia Right, Open, Internal Fixation Device, No qualifier**

❏ **0PSF3BZ Reposition, Upper Bones, Humeral Shaft Right, Percutaneous, External Fixation Device, Monoplanar, No qualifier**

▶ Both procedures equally meet the PCS OGCR criteria for the principal procedure:

❏ **Sequence procedure performed for definitive treatment most related to principal diagnosis as principal procedure.**

❏ She chooses to sequence the open reduction of the right tibia first because it is the more extensive procedure.

▶ Marcy finalizes the procedure codes and sequencing for this case:

(1) **0QSG04Z Reposition, Lower bones, Tibia right, Open, Internal fixation Device, No qualifier**

(2) **0PSF3BZ Reposition, Upper bones, Humeral shaft right, Percutaneous, External fixation device, monoplanar, No qualifier**

▶ Marcy also assigns and sequences the ICD-10-CM diagnosis codes that support the need for the service.

(1) **S82.201A Unspecified fracture of shaft of right tibia, initial encounter for closed fracture**

(2) **S42.301A Unspecified fracture of shaft of humerus, right arm, initial encounter for closed fracture**

▶ ICD-10-CM codes for the external cause of injury, if known, can also be assigned.

CODING PRACTICE

Exercise 50.4 **Arranging Codes for Root Operations M, S, X, and Y**

Instructions: Read the mini-medical-record of each patient's encounter. Review the information abstracted in Exercise 50.2 for questions 1–3. For questions 4–6, abstract the case on your own. Assign PCS codes using the Index and Tables, and arrange the codes in proper sequence. Write the code(s) on the line provided.

---

1. INPATIENT HOSPITAL Gender: M Age: 27

Preprocedure diagnosis: Traumatic amputation of distal segment of little finger and two segments of the ring finger on left hand while using a table saw in home workshop

Procedure: Replantation of distal segments of the little finger and ring finger on the left hand

2 PCS Codes _____

---

2. INPATIENT HOSPITAL Gender: F Age: 36

Preprocedure diagnosis: Type 1 diabetes mellitus, unresponsive to treatment

Procedure: Simultaneous kidney–pancreas transplantation. The donor kidney came from the patient's identical twin. The donor pancreas came from a cadaver. Patient's left kidney was removed and replaced.

2 PCS Codes _____

---

3. INPATIENT HOSPITAL Gender: F Age: 43

Preprocedure diagnosis: Low radial nerve palsy, right arm

Procedure: Tendon transfer, open. Rerouted the palmaris longus tendon to the extensor pollicis longus (EPL) muscle. Rerouted the pronator teres tendon to the abductor pollicis longus (APL) muscle.

Tip: Refer to PCS OGCR B3.2.b Multiple Procedures.

2 PCS Codes _____

---

4. INPATIENT HOSPITAL Gender: M Age: 44

Preprocedure diagnosis: Left angle and right body mandible fractures

Procedure: Closed reduction of mandible fractures with Erich arch bars and elastic fixation. Arch bars placed on the maxillary and mandibular dentition and secured with 25-gauge wire. Elastic fixation was placed on the arch bars; patient awakened

Tip: If no bilateral body part value exists, each procedure is coded separately using the appropriate body part value. PCS OGCR B4.3.

2 PCS Codes _____

CODING PRACTICE (continued)

5. INPATIENT HOSPITAL   Gender: M   Age: 54

Preprocedure diagnosis: Right tibiotalar subluxation; right distal tibiofibular fracture

Procedure: Application of spanning external fixator to reduce tibiotalar subluxation; open reduction and internal fixation with arthroscopic-assisted fixation of the distal tibia. A series of 0.062 K-wires and 2-mm K-wires were used to reduce the posterior impaction. Medial malleolar fixation was then performed with two medial malleolar screws, inserting and reducing the medial malleolar articular surface.

Tip: The spanning external fixator is used to prevent ankle dislocation. The distal tibiofibular joint is formed by the convex distal aspect of the fibula and the concave lateral aspect of the distal end of the tibia.

2 PCS Codes _____

6. INPATIENT HOSPITAL   Gender: M   Age: 44

Preprocedure diagnosis: Blepharoptosis, both eyes, obstructing the field of vision

Procedure: Levator aponeurosis resection and advancement of both upper eyelids using an Open approach. The desired level of lid elevation achieved by advancing the superior aspect of the tarsus to the inferior margin of the tarsus. Careful hemostasis obtained and skin closed with 6-0 Prolene.

2 PCS Codes _____

CHAPTER SUMMARY

In this chapter you learned that:

- The Medical and Surgical root operations in the group *Procedures that put in/put back or move some/all of a body part*: Reattachment (M), Reposition (S), Transfer (X), and Transplantation (Y).

- The root operation Reattachment (M) is putting back in or on all or a portion of a separated body part to its normal location or other suitable location.

- The root operation Reposition (S) is moving to its normal location, or another suitable location, all or a portion of a body part.

- The root operation Transfer (X) is moving, without taking out, all or a portion of a body part to another location to take over the function of all or a portion of a body part.

- The root operation Transplantation (Y) is putting in or on all or a portion of a living body part taken from another individual or animal to physically take the place and/or function of all or a portion of a similar body part.

- PCS provides guidelines for Reposition of a fracture and the use of the root operations Transplantation and Administration.

- The root operation definition is a combination of the functional objective of the procedure and the anatomic site.

- For the root operations Transfer and Reposition, identify the site that is moved, not the location to which it is moved.

- The root operation Reposition uses the device character to identify the type of internal or external skeletal fixation device applied.

- For the root operation Transfer, the qualifier can identify the deepest tissue layer in a flap or the site that is the destination of the transfer.

- The root operation Transplantation uses the qualifier to identify the genetic compatibility of the transplanted tissue.

- When a Transfer, Reposition, or Reattachment procedure is performed bilaterally, assign separate codes for each side if no bilateral body part value is available.

CONCEPT QUIZ

Take a moment to look back at root operations that put in/put back or move some or all of a body part (M, S, X, and Y) and solidify your skills. Try to answer the questions from memory first, then refer to the discussion in this chapter if you need a little extra help.

Completion

Instructions: Write the term that completes each statement based on the information you learned in this chapter. Choose from the list that follows. Some choices may be used more than once and some choices may not be used at all.

allogeneic
animal
autologous
external
fixation
internal
kidney
lung
open

orchiopexy
Reattachment
Reposition
syngeneic
synthetic
Transfer
Transplantation
zooplastic

(continued)

(continued from page 1055)

1. The root operation _____ is reported for closed reduction of a dislocated shoulder.

2. The _____ is the most commonly transplanted organ.

3. The root operation _____ is reported for a pedicle graft.

4. A(n) procedure for the root operation _____ may or may not include reconnection of nerves and blood vessels.

5. The root operation _____ is reported for a replantation.

6. A K-wire is an example of a(n) _____ fixation device.

7. _____ refers to a tissue substitute from an animal.

8. There are a small number of procedures in the root operation _____.

9. The 6th character of code 0SSGX5Z indicates a(n) _____ fixation device.

10. _____ refers to a tissue substitute from another human.

Multiple Choice

Instructions: Circle the letter of the best answer to each question based on the information you learned in this chapter.

1. Which root operation is used to report reduction of a fracture?
   A. Transplantation
   B. Reattachment
   C. Transfer
   D. Reposition

2. How would you code the following procedure? *A physician performs an open right kidney transplant from a human organ donor.*
   A. 0TY00Z0
   B. 0TY00Z1
   C. 0TY00Z2
   D. 0TR307Z

3. What root operation reports a body part that may or may not be cut out or off to be moved to the new location?
   A. Transplantation
   B. Reattachment
   C. Transfer
   D. Reposition

4. What body part is identified in ICD-10-PCS code 0LX80ZZ?
   A. Tendons
   B. Left hand tendon
   C. Upper tendon
   D. Lower tendon

5. How would you code the following procedure? *A physician performs a percutaneous endoscopic gastropexy.*
   A. 0DS64ZZ
   B. 0DY60Z0
   C. 0DM64ZZ
   D. 0DX64Z5

6. How would you code the following procedure? *A physician performs a reduction of fracture of the nasal septum, percutaneous endoscopic approach.*
   A. 09MMXZZ
   B. 09MKXZZ
   C. 09SK4ZZ
   D. 09SM4ZZ

7. What is the root operation for the procedure to treat an avulsed kidney?
   A. Transplantation
   B. Reattachment
   C. Transfer
   D. Reposition

8. Which root operation does the medical term *transposition* translate to?
   A. Transfer
   B. Reattachment
   C. Transplantation
   D. Reposition

9. What qualifier is identified in ICD-10-PCS code 0JX00ZC?
   A. No qualifier
   B. Skin and subcutaneous tissue
   C. Skin and fascia
   D. Skin, subcutaneous tissue, and fascia

10. What is the approach for all transplants?
    A. Closed
    B. External
    C. Open
    D. Percutaneous

KEEP ON CODING

Instructions: Read the procedural statement, abstract the root operation, then use the appropriate Index and Tables to assign PCS procedure codes. Assign only the root operations discussed in this chapter. Write the code(s) on the line provided.

1. Open pancreas transplant from human organ donation. ICD-10-PCS Code(s) _____

2. Reattachment of right index finger, open approach. ICD-10-PCS Code(s) _____

3. Endoscopic facial nerve transfer. ICD-10-PCS Code(s) _____

4. Open reduction internal fixation (ORIF) of left humeral head. ICD-10-PCS Code(s) _____

5. Open heart transplantation from human organ donation. ICD-10-PCS Code(s) _____

6. Reattachment of the tip of the nose (nasal mucosa and soft tissue), external approach. ICD-10-PCS Code(s) _____

7. Open transfer of the radial nerve to the median nerve. ICD-10-PCS Code(s) _____

8. Reposition of left extraocular muscle, percutaneous approach. ICD-10-PCS Code(s) _____

9. Glossopexy of tongue, external approach. ICD-10-PCS Code(s) _____

10. Transplantation of right kidney from human organ donation, open approach. ICD-10-PCS Code(s) _____

11. Reattachment of left thumb, open approach. ICD-10-PCS Code(s) _____

12. Adjacent skin transfer of forehead, external approach. ICD-10-PCS Code(s) _____

13. Orchiopexy of left undescended testicle via endoscopy. ICD-10-PCS Code(s) _____

14. Transfer of subcutaneous tissue of anterior neck, right side, open approach. ICD-10-PCS Code(s) _____

15. Liver transplantation from human organ donation. ICD-10-PCS Code(s) _____

16. Open reduction internal fixation (ORIF) of tibial fracture of left leg. ICD-10-PCS Code(s) _____

17. Endoscopic colpopexy of vagina. ICD-10-PCS Code(s) _____

18. Reattachment of 5th left toe, open approach. ICD-10-PCS Code(s) _____

19. Percutaneous endoscopic reattachment of the right tunica vaginalis. ICD-10-PCS Code(s) _____

20. Open detorsion of transverse colon. ICD-10-PCS Code(s) _____

21. Reattachment of left testicle, open approach. ICD-10-PCS Code(s) _____

22. Bilateral percutaneous endoscopic salpingopexy. ICD-10-PCS Code(s) _____

23. Left lung transplantation from organ donation. ICD-10-PCS Code(s) _____

24. Pedicle flap of scalp to repair 3 sq cm, external approach. ICD-10-PCS Code(s) _____

25. Percutaneous endoscopic reposition of left kidney. ICD-10-PCS Code(s) _____

CODING CHALLENGE

Instructions: Read the mini-medical-record of each patient's encounter, then abstract, assign, and arrange ICD-10-CM diagnosis codes and PCS procedure codes using the appropriate Index and Tables. Write the code(s) on the line provided.

1. INPATIENT HOSPITAL   Gender: M   Age: 38

Preprocedure diagnosis: Right shoulder, rotator cuff repair

Procedure: Rotator cuff repair. Complete tear of rotator cuff repaired by arthroscopic reattachment of the tendon. A synovectomy of the shoulder was also done through the arthroscope due to significant tenosynovitis.

Postprocedure diagnosis: Complete tear of right shoulder rotator cuff, tenosynovitis

2 ICD-10-CM Codes _____

2 ICD-10-PCS Codes _____

2. INPATIENT HOSPITAL   Gender: M   Age: 26

Preprocedure diagnosis: Cubital tunnel syndrome, left arm

Procedure: Subcutaneous left ulnar nerve transposition. The nerve was transposed anteriorly to the medial epicondyle, lying under the skin and fat but

(continued)

2. continued

on top of the muscle. Flexor-pronator fascia was used to prevent the nerve from relocating.

Tip: Refer to the definitions to select the correct approach character.

1 ICD-10-CM Code _____

1 ICD-10-PCS Code _____

3. INPATIENT HOSPITAL   Gender: F   Age: 17

Preprocedure diagnosis: Acute traumatic nasal bone fracture with obstruction as a result of being hit with a baseball; severe orbital bruising, bilateral

Procedure: Closed reduction of nasal bone fracture with stabilization. The nose was manually refractured and repositioned to its normal anatomic position. A thermoplastic cast was placed externally to stabilize the fracture.

Tip: Application of a cast or splint in conjunction with the reposition procedure is not coded separately. PCS OGCR B3.15.

3 ICD-10-CM Codes _____

1 ICD-10-PCS Code _____

(continued)

(continued from page 1057)

4. INPATIENT HOSPITAL   Gender: F   Age: 21

Preprocedure diagnosis: Right ear was torn off during pit bull attack

Procedure: Severed pinna of right ear reattached. Using a microscope and extremely delicate tools the ear was reattached. I found a tiny artery only 0.3 millimeters in diameter and reattached the vessel to the woman's blood supply with three microscopic stitches. We were unable to find any viable veins and will use leech therapy to allow the veins to regenerate.

Tip: Assign an ICD-10-CM external cause code.

2 ICD-10-CM Codes _____

1 ICD-10-PCS Code _____

5. INPATIENT HOSPITAL   Gender: F   Age: 55

Preprocedure diagnosis: Prolapse of vaginal vault status post hysterectomy 6 years prior

Procedure: Da Vinci laparoscopic sacrocolpopexy. After ports were placed the robot was docked. The posterior and anterior vaginal walls were dissected from the peritoneum. GyneMesh was used to lift the vagina into the pelvic cavity and secured with Gore-Tex suture. All instruments were removed; excellent hemostasis.

Tip: In addition to the procedure code, assign a code for the robotic procedure. Search for Index entry *Robotic assisted procedure, trunk region.*

1 ICD-10-CM Code _____

2 ICD-10-PCS Codes _____

6. INPATIENT HOSPITAL   Gender: M   Age: 64

Preprocedure diagnosis: End-stage renal disease with need for a long-term hemodialysis access.

Procedure: Right basilic vein transposition. Incision made along the medial aspect of the arm to expose the vein. Sharp dissection used to free the entire vein. Excellent flow through the vein with a palpable thrill.

Tip: End-stage renal disease (kidney failure) is when your kidneys stop working well enough for you to live without dialysis or a kidney transplant.

2 ICD-10-CM Codes _____

1 ICD-10-PCS Code _____

7. INPATIENT HOSPITAL   Gender: F   Age: 49

Preprocedure diagnosis: Right hamstring avulsion

Procedure: Reattachment of right hamstring to the ischial tuberosity. A vertical incision was made under the gluteal fold, and after identification and neurolysis of the sciatic nerve, transosseous tendon reinsertion to the pelvis was performed with four resorbable suture anchors.

Tip: The hamstring is a group of three muscles that run along the back of the thigh.

1 ICD-10-CM Code _____

1 ICD-10-PCS Code _____

8. INPATIENT HOSPITAL   Gender: M   Age: 16

Preprocedure diagnosis: Involved in a fist fight; the lateral and central incisors of the lower jaw were knocked out

Procedure: Closed replantation of two avulsed permanent teeth, lower jaw

Postprocedure diagnosis: Under local anesthesia, the lateral incisor alveolar socket was irrigated with saline solution. Using slight digital pressure, the tooth was slowly replanted. This was repeated for the central incisor. X-ray confirmed normal position of teeth. A flexible splint was applied to be worn for two weeks.

Tip: Assign an ICD-10-CM external cause code.

2 ICD-10-CM Codes _____

1 ICD-10-PCS Code _____

9. INPATIENT HOSPITAL   Gender: F   Age: 8

Preprocedure diagnosis: Right elbow fracture

Procedure: Closed reduction of oblique fracture of the right distal humerus. Using conscious sedation, gentle traction applied to distal elbow and force applied to the olecranon to reduce the fracture. Long-arm fiberglass splint applied.

1 ICD-10-CM Code _____

1 ICD-10-PCS Code _____

10. INPATIENT HOSPITAL   Gender: M   Age: 73

Preprocedure diagnosis: Acquired defect of left nose following Mohs procedure yesterday for basal cell carcinoma

Procedure: Local cheek advancement and full-thickness skin graft measuring 1 cm × 3 cm. The area on the nose was debrided to remove necrotic tissue. A subcutaneous incision was made over the cheek and the flap advanced to the defect of the nose. Flap secured and a tie-over bolster used to secure the graft.

1 ICD-10-CM Code _____

2 ICD-10-PCS Codes _____

Chapter

51

Learning Objectives

After completing this chapter, you should have the skills to:

51.1 Spell and define the key words, medical terms, and abbreviations related to procedures that alter the diameter or route of a tubular body part. (Remember)

51.2 Identify the types of procedures that alter the diameter or route of a tubular body part. (Apply)

51.3 Adhere to ICD-10-PCS coding guidelines related to root operations Bypass, Dilation, Occlusion, and Restriction. (Apply)

51.4 Examine and abstract procedural information from the medical record for coding for root operations 1, 7, L, and V. (Analyze)

51.5 Demonstrate how to assign codes for root operations 1, 7, L, and V. (Apply)

51.6 Utilize guidelines for arranging (sequencing) codes for root operations 1, 7, L, and V. (Apply)

Chapter Outline

- **Basics of Procedures That Alter the Diameter or Route of a Tubular Body Part**
- **Coding Guidelines for Root Operations 1, 7, L, and V**
- **Abstracting for Root Operations 1, 7, L, and V**
- **Assigning Characters 4–7 for Root Operations 1, 7, L, and V**
- **Arranging Codes for Root Operations 1, 7, L, and V**

Key Terms and Abbreviations

extraluminal
intraluminal
ligation
orifice

In addition to the key terms listed here, students should know the terms defined within tables in this chapter.

INTRODUCTION

Most urban areas have one or more bypass highways that reroute traffic around a congested area to improve traffic flow. The PCS root operation Bypass reroutes the contents of a tubular body part around a problem area of the anatomy to improve functioning.

This chapter discusses the four Medical and Surgical root operations in the group *Procedures that alter the diameter or route of a tubular body part*: Bypass, Dilation, Occlusion, and Restriction. Although the root operations share a common purpose—altering the diameter or route of a body part—each has a unique aspect that makes it different from the other procedures in this group. Pay careful attention to the differences between each root operation so that you can use each confidently and accurately.

BASICS OF PROCEDURES THAT ALTER THE DIAMETER OR ROUTE OF A TUBULAR BODY PART

■ TABLE 51-1 defines root operations in this group and identifies procedural terms frequently associated with each. Some terms, such as *embolization*, can be associated with more than one root operation. There is no direct match between a specific procedural term and a root operation because some medical terms, such as *embolization*, can be associated with more than one root operation. Root operations are assigned based on the content of the operative report regarding what was actually performed, not on the specific words used by the physician in documentation.

Refer to detailed anatomic diagrams of specific organ systems in Chapters 8–43 of this text, or in external references, when you need to refresh your memory of human anatomy.

Examples of root operations that alter the diameter or route of a tubular body part appear later in this chapter in Table 51-3 through Table 51-6. This section provides a general reference to help understand the most common procedures that alter the diameter or route of a tubular body part. Remember to keep standard reference books handy in case you get stuck.

Refer to ■ TABLE 51-2 for a refresher on how to build medical terms related to procedures that alter the diameter or route of a tubular body part. Medical terms for these procedures sometimes use a separate term—such as *bypass* or *dilation*—rather than a word part to describe the procedure.

> ## CODING CAUTION
>
> Be alert for root operations that have similar English meanings but different PCS definitions.
>
> **Restriction (V)** (*Partially* closing a tubular PCS body part) and **Occlusion (L)** (*Completely* closing a tubular PCS body part)
>
> **Bypass (1)** (*Rerouting* the contents of a tubular PCS body part) and **Transfer (F)** (*Moving, without taking out*, all or a portion of a body part *to another location to take over the function* of all or a portion of a body part)

Table 51-1 ■ **ROOT OPERATIONS THAT ALTER THE DIAMETER OR ROUTE OF A TUBULAR BODY PART**

Root Operation	Value	Definition	Terms
Bypass	1	Altering the route of passage of the contents of a tubular body part	Bypass, shunt, stoma, diversion
Dilation	7	Expanding an orifice or the lumen of a tubular body part	Dilation, balloon dilation, intraluminal dilation, angioplasty
Occlusion	L	Completely closing an orifice or the lumen of a tubular body part	Occlusion, ligation, embolization
Restriction	V	Partially closing an orifice or the lumen of a tubular body part	Restriction, cerclage, banding, clipping, embolization

Source: © PB Resources, Inc. Used with permission.

Table 51-2 ■ **EXAMPLE OF CONSTRUCTING MEDICAL TERMS FOR PROCEDURES THAT ALTER THE DIAMETER OR ROUTE OF A TUBULAR BODY PART**

Combining Form	Suffix	Complete Medical Term
trache/o (*trachea*)	**-stomy** (*new opening/mouth*)	**tracheo + stomy** (*creation of a new opening in the trachea*)
gastr/o (*stomach*)	**-plication** (*folding*) **-plasty** (*repair*)	**gastro + plication** (*folding of the stomach*)
angi/o (*vessel*)		**angio + plasty** (*repair of a vessel*)

Source: © PB Resources, Inc. Used with permission.

CODING PRACTICE

Exercise 51.1 Basics of Procedures That Alter the Diameter or Route of a Tubular Body Part

Instructions: Use your medical terminology skills and resources to define the following procedures that alter the diameter or route of a tubular body part , then identify the code(s) or code range listed in the ICD-10-PCS Index. Follow these steps:

- Use slash marks "/" to break down each underlined term into its root(s) and suffix.
- Define the meaning of the underlined word based on the meaning of each word part.
- Look up the term in the ICD-10-PCS Index, and write down the name(s) of root operation(s) the Index cross-references you to and the Table(s), if provided.
- Do not assign any codes.

Example: <u>angioplasty</u> angio/plasty   Meaning <u>*repair of a vessel*</u>   PCS Root Operation(s)/Table(s) <u>*Dilation 027, 047, 037*</u>

1. <u>pyelostomy</u>   Meaning _____   PCS Root Operation(s)/Table(s) _____
2. <u>ligation</u>, hemorrhoid   Meaning _____   PCS Root Operation(s)/Table(s) _____
3. <u>cannulation</u>   Meaning _____   PCS Root Operation(s)/Table(s) _____
4. <u>catheterization</u>   Meaning _____   PCS Root Operation(s)/Table(s) _____
5. <u>embolization</u>   Meaning _____   PCS Root Operation(s)/Table(s) _____
6. <u>anastomosis</u>   Meaning _____   PCS Root Operation(s)/Table(s) _____
7. <u>vasoligation</u>   Meaning _____   PCS Root Operation(s)/Table(s) _____
8. <u>cecocolostomy</u>   Meaning _____   PCS Root Operation(s)/Table(s) _____
9. <u>pylorodiosis</u>   Meaning _____   PCS Root Operation(s)/Table(s) _____
10. <u>ureteroplication</u>   Meaning _____   PCS Root Operation(s)/Table(s) _____

CODING GUIDELINES FOR ROOT OPERATIONS 1, 7, L, AND V

Coders should understand the guidelines specific to the root operations 1, 7, L, and V. PCS OGCR clarifies the difference between the root operations Occlusion and Restriction and discusses the use of Character 4 and Character 7 with the root operation Bypass. These are discussed next. Refer to the PCS OGCR for additional details and clinical examples of each guideline.

Bypass

Bypass procedures identify the body part bypassed *from* and the body part bypassed *to*. In noncoronary artery bypass procedures Character 4, Body Part, specifies the body part bypassed *from*, and Character 7, Qualifier, specifies the body part bypassed *to* (PCS OGCR B3.6a) (■ FIGURE 51-1).

Coronary artery bypass procedures are coded differently than other bypass procedures. Coronary arteries are classified by the number of sites bypassed, rather than the anatomic name of a coronary artery. Character 4, Body Part, identifies the *number* of coronary arteries bypassed *to*, and Character 7, Qualifier, specifies the *vessel* bypassed *from* (PCS OGCR B3.6b) (■ FIGURE 51-2).

Surgeon performs a percutaneous endoscopic bypass from the stomach to the jejunum, using autologous tissue.

0D1647A Medical and Surgical, Gastrointestinal, Stomach, Percutaneous Endoscopic, Autologous Tissue Substitute, Jejunum

Figure 51-1 ■ Example of guideline for coding a noncoronary bypass procedure.
Source: © PB Resources, Inc. Used with permission.

Surgeon performs an aortocoronary artery bypass of the left anterior descending coronary artery and the obtuse marginal coronary artery. The greater saphenous vein was used for both arteries.

021109W Medical and Surgical, Heart and Great Vessels, Bypass, Coronary artery two arteries, Open, Autologous venous tissue, Aorta

Figure 51-2 ■ Example of guideline for coding coronary artery bypass. *Source: © PB Resources, Inc. Used with permission.*

When multiple coronary arteries are bypassed, code a separate procedure for each coronary artery that uses a different device and/or qualifier value (PCS OGCR B3.6c). For example, when both an aortocoronary artery bypass and internal mammary coronary artery bypass are performed, assign two codes.

It is helpful to memorize PCS OGCR B3.6a–c about the root operation Bypass. PCS Tables list the body part and qualifier values, but do not provide instructions on how to assign the values.

Occlusion and Restriction

A vessel embolization procedure might be performed to completely close a vessel—as is done with a tumor embolization to cut off blood supply to the tumor—or to narrow the diameter but not completely close it, as is done with an aneurysm to minimize the expansion of the vessel. When the objective is to completely close the vessel, code the root operation Occlusion. When the objective is to narrow it, code the root operation Restriction (PCS OGCR B3.12). Physicians do not necessarily document using the PCS root operation names, so the coder must identify the objective of the procedure to assign the correct root operation.

ABSTRACTING FOR ROOT OPERATIONS 1, 7, L, AND V

Abstracting for PCS focuses on identifying the correct root operation, which involves reading the operative report and interpreting it in light of root operation definitions. When reading the operative report, remember to focus on the objective of the procedure and the activities performed, not the specific medical terms the surgeon uses to describe the procedure. Many times the root operation can be determined conclusively during abstracting. Other times, the root operation can be narrowed down to two options, which must be differentiated based on other Characters that are assigned from the PCS Tables. The root operation definition is a combination of the functional objective of the procedure and the anatomic site. The following information summarizes the objectives, definitions, unique features, and examples of root operations 1, 7, L, and V.

Root operations in this group treat a tubular body part. Examples of tubular body parts include the following:

- Cardiovascular system: arteries, veins, and vessels
- Digestive system: esophagus, stomach, small intestine, and large intestine
- Female reproductive system: vagina, uterus, fallopian tubes
- Male reproductive system: vas deferens; and many others
- Respiratory system: trachea, bronchus
- Urinary system: urethra, ureters, kidney pelvis, bladder, bladder neck

These root operations are also used on various ducts throughout the body, such as the common bile duct, lacrimal ducts, and lymphatic ducts. Body systems—such as the integumentary and musculoskeletal systems—that do not contain tubular body parts do not use root operations in this group.

Abstracting for Bypass (1)

The objective of the root operation Bypass is altering route of passage. The site of the procedure is a tubular body part.

Contents of a body part are rerouted to a downstream area of the normal route, to a similar route and body part, or to an abnormal route and dissimilar body part. The procedure includes one or more anastomoses, with or without the use of a device.

Examples of Bypass are coronary artery bypass graft (CABG) and colostomy formation (*rerouting of the colon to the abdominal wall*) (■ TABLE 51-3).

Abstracting for Dilation (7)

The objective of the root operation Dilation is expanding an orifice/lumen. The site of the procedure is a tubular body part.

The root operation Dilation is coded when the objective of the procedure is to enlarge the diameter of a tubular body part or orifice. The orifice can be a natural orifice or artificially created. Dilation is accomplished by stretching a tubular body part using intraluminal pressure or by cutting part of the orifice or wall of the tubular body part and includes both intraluminal and extraluminal methods of enlarging the diameter. A device that is placed to maintain the new diameter is an integral part of the Dilation procedure and is coded to Character 6, Device.

Examples of Dilation are percutaneous transluminal coronary angioplasty (PTCA) and dilation of the bladder neck (■ TABLE 51-4).

Abstracting for Occlusion (L)

The objective of the root operation Occlusion is completely closing an orifice/lumen. The site of the procedure is a tubular body part.

The root operation Occlusion is coded when the objective of the procedure is to close off a tubular body part or orifice. Division of the tubular body part before closing it is an

Table 51-3 ■ **EXAMPLES OF THE ROOT OPERATION BYPASS (1)**

Organ System	Procedural Examples
Cardiovascular	Femoral–popliteal artery bypass
Digestive	Gastric bypass, colostomy formation
Genitourinary	Urinary diversion
Nervous	Placement of ventriculoperitoneal shunt
Respiratory	Tracheostomy formation with tracheostomy tube placement

Source: © PB Resources, Inc. Used with permission.

Table 51-4 ■ **EXAMPLES OF THE ROOT OPERATION DILATION (7)**

Organ System	Procedural Examples
Cardiovascular	Percutaneous transluminal coronary angioplasty (PTCA), dilation of old anastomosis
Digestive	Pyloromyotomy, balloon dilation of common bile duct, dilation of upper esophageal stricture
Genitourinary	Intraluminal dilation of bladder neck stricture, balloon dilation of fallopian tubes, internal urethrotomy
Respiratory	Dilation of tracheal stenosis
Special Senses (Ear, Eye)	Transnasal dilation and stent placement in right lacrimal duct

Source: © PB Resources, Inc. Used with permission.

integral part of the Occlusion procedure. Occlusion includes both intraluminal or extraluminal methods of closing off the body part, such as a clip either inside or outside of the vessel. Coders must read the operative report to determine the method used because different occlusive methods are reported with different device values in Character 6.

Ligation means tying or closing off. The term *ligation* might be used to describe a procedure coded to Occlusion or Destruction. The method of ligation affects the choice of root operation and must be determined from the operative report. Ligation performed with clips, sutures, or rings is coded as Occlusion, but ligation performed with cauterization or electrocoagulation is coded to the root operation Destruction (5) (■ Figure 51-3). The root operation Destruction is discussed in Chapter 49 of this text.

Examples of Occlusion are fallopian tube ligation for sterilization and uterine artery embolization to cut off the blood supply to a fibroid (■ TABLE 51-5).

Abstracting for Restriction (V)

The objective of the root operation Restriction is partially closing an **orifice** (*opening*) or lumen. The site of the procedure is a tubular body part. The orifice can be a natural orifice or an artificially created orifice such as a stoma. The root operation Restriction is coded when the objective of the procedure is to narrow the diameter of a tubular body part or orifice to leave it partially open. Restriction includes both **intraluminal** (*from within the vessel*) or **extraluminal** (*from outside the vessel*) methods for narrowing the diameter.

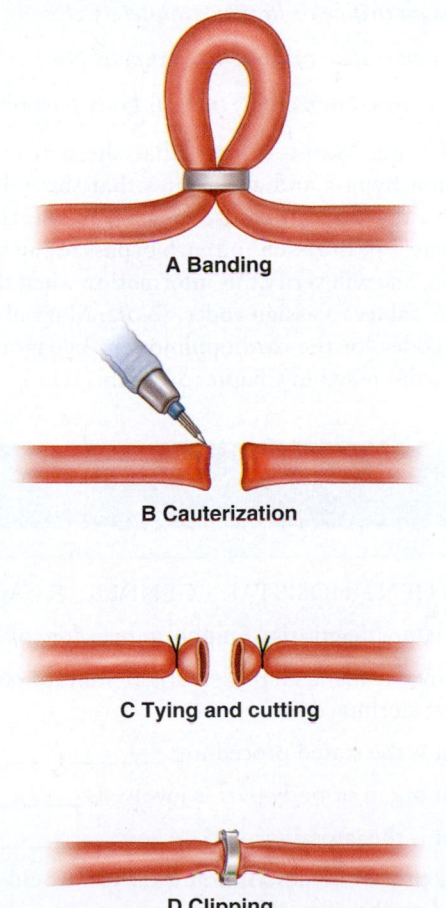

A Banding

B Cauterization

C Tying and cutting

D Clipping

Figure 51-3 ■ Methods of ligation.

Table 51-5 ■ **EXAMPLES OF THE ROOT OPERATION OCCLUSION (L)**

Organ System	Procedural Examples
Cardiovascular	Ligation of a vein, suture ligation of failed arteriovenous graft
Genitourinary	Uterine artery embolization, fallopian tube ligation (clipping), vasectomy (clipping or sealing)

Source: © PB Resources, Inc. Used with permission.

Examples of Restriction are esophagogastric fundoplication (*wrapping part of the fundus stomach around the lower esophagus*) to treat gastroesophageal reflux and cervical cerclage (*suturing to temporarily close or reinforce the cervix*) to treat cervical insufficiency during pregnancy (■ TABLE 51-6).

Key Criteria for Abstracting

Refer to Tables 47-2 and 47-3 for general guidance on abstracting PCS procedures and root operation groups. Then refer to ■ TABLE 51-7 for more specific guidance on how to abstract procedures that alter the diameter or route of a tubular body part and distinguish among root operations in this group. A guided example of abstracting for the root operation Bypass follows. Remember that the abstracting questions are a guide and that not every question applies to, or can be answered for, every case.

Table 51-6 ■ **EXAMPLES OF THE ROOT OPERATION RESTRICTION (V)**

Organ System	Procedural Examples
Blood and Immune	Restriction of thoracic lymphatic duct
Cardiovascular	Banding of pulmonary artery, clipping of cerebral aneurysm
Digestive	Esophagogastric fundoplication
Genitourinary	Cervical cerclage
Special Senses (Ear, Eye)	Stent placement in right lacrimal duct

Source: © PB Resources, Inc. Used with permission.

Table 51-7 ■ **KEY CRITERIA FOR ABSTRACTING ROOT OPERATIONS THAT ALTER THE DIAMETER OR ROUTE OF A TUBULAR BODY PART**

Question	Root Operation (Value)
❏ What tubular body part was treated?	If a tubular body part was not treated, do not use root operations 1, 7, L, or V.
Answer *Yes* to one of the following questions to help distinguish Root Operations 1, 7, L, and V	
❏ Were the contents of a tubular body part rerouted?	Bypass (1)
❏ Was an orifice or lumen expanded?	Dilation (7)
❏ Was an orifice or lumen completely closed?	Occlusion (L)
❏ Was an orifice or lumen partially closed?	Restriction (V)

Source: © PB Resources, Inc. Used with permission.

Guided Example of Abstracting for Bypass

Refer to the following example throughout this chapter to practice skills for abstracting, assigning, and arranging codes for the root operation Bypass. Similar principles apply to working with other root operations that alter the diameter or route of a tubular body part.

INPATIENT HOSPITAL   Gender: M   Age: 67

Preoperative diagnosis: Chronic unstable angina, acute STEMI involving the anterior wall and left anterior descending (LAD) coronary artery

Procedure: Coronary artery bypass grafting (CABG) ×2. The sternotomy was performed, the heart was physically stabilized, and the pericardium was entered. Total cardiopulmonary bypass (CPB) was initiated. Used the left internal mammary artery (LIMA) to LAD. The LIMA was clipped distally, divided, and spatulated (*spread open*) for anastomosis. The LAD was identified and opened. End-to-side anastomosis was performed through the LIMA. The right greater saphenous vein (GSV) was harvested laparoscopically and grafted from the aorta to the obtuse marginal (OM) coronary artery. The OM was identified, opened, and anastomosed in an end-to-side fashion to the reversed autologous GSV. An aortotomy was made and the vein was cut to fit and sutured in place. The patient was fully warmed and weaned from CPB. Good hemostasis was noted. A single mediastinal and left pleural chest tube was placed. The sternum was closed with interrupted wire, and the linea alba, sternal fascia, and subcutaneous tissue were closed. The patient tolerated the procedure well and was transferred to PACU in stable condition.

Postoperative diagnosis: Acute STEMI LAD; atherosclerotic heart disease with 90% blockage in LAD and 80% blockage in the OM. Unstable angina due to 50 years' continuous cigarette nicotine dependence.

Follow along as fictitious coder Marcy Elwood, CCS, abstracts the procedure. Check off each step after you complete it.

► Marcy reads through the entire record, paying special attention to the reason for the encounter, the procedure performed, and the postoperative diagnosis. She refers to the Key Criteria for Abstracting Root Operations That Alter the Diameter or Route of a Tubular Body Part (Table 51-7).

❏ She notes preoperative diagnosis: chronic unstable angina, acute STEMI.

❏ *What is the stated procedure?* Coronary artery bypass grafting (CABG) ×2

❏ *What organ or body part is involved?* Coronary arteries (LAD and OM)

❏ *Is the procedure description what you would expect based on the name of the procedure?* Yes

❏ *What surgical approach is used?* Open

❏ *Was more than one procedure, or a combined procedure, performed?* Two arteries were bypassed using different tissue substitutes. Cardiopulmonary bypass equipment was also used.

❏ *Did the procedure alter the diameter or route of a tubular body part?* Yes

❏ *What tubular body part was treated?* Coronary arteries

❏ *Was an orifice or lumen partially closed?* No

❏ *Was an orifice or lumen completely closed?* No

❏ *Was an orifice or lumen expanded?* No

❏ *Were the contents of a tubular body part rerouted?* Yes

► At this time, Marcy believes that she will use the root operation Bypass and anticipates that she will need two codes for the CABG because each artery was treated with a separate type of tissue and each bypass began in a distinct location. She will verify this information when she refers to the PCS Tables to assign codes. (*Note:* Mary also needs to assign codes for the cardiopulmonary bypass equipment, which is discussed in Chapter 54 of this text.)

CODING PRACTICE

Exercise 51.2   Abstracting for Root Operations 1, 7, L, and V

Instructions: Read the mini-medical-record of each patient's encounter and answer the abstracting questions. Write the answer on the line provided. Do not assign any codes.

---

1. INPATIENT HOSPITAL   GENDER: F   Age: 55

Preprocedure diagnosis: Epiphora (*overflow of tears*)

Procedure: Transnasal placement of stent to partially close left lacrimal duct

a. What is the stated procedure? _____

b. What organ or body part is involved? _____

c. What is the laterality? _____

d. Is the procedure description what you would expect based on the name of the procedure? _____

(continued)

CODING PRACTICE (continued)

1. (continued)

e. What surgical approach is used? _____

f. Was more than one procedure, or a combined procedure, performed? _____

g. What tubular body part was treated? _____

h. Was an orifice or lumen partially closed? _____

i. Was an orifice or lumen completely closed? _____

j. Was an orifice or lumen expanded? _____

k. Were the contents of a tubular body part rerouted? _____

l. What is the root operation(s)? _____

---

2. INPATIENT HOSPITAL   Gender: M   Age: 61

Preprocedure diagnosis: Esophageal varices, portal hypertension due to cirrhosis

Procedure: Ligation of esophageal vein. Passed endoscope through the mouth down the esophagus and visualized the varices. Snared the varices and placed extraluminal rubber bands around the veins to tie them off. Patient tolerated procedure well.

a. What is the stated procedure? _____

b. What organ or body part is involved? _____

c. What is the laterality? _____

d. Is the procedure description what you would expect based on the name of the procedure? _____

e. What surgical approach is used? _____

f. Was more than one procedure, or a combined procedure, performed? _____

g. What tubular body part was treated? _____

h. Was an orifice or lumen partially closed? _____

i. Was an orifice or lumen completely closed? _____

j. Was an orifice or lumen expanded? _____

k. Were the contents of a tubular body part rerouted? _____

l. What is the root operation(s)? _____

---

3. INPATIENT HOSPITAL   Gender: F   Age: 57

Preprocedure diagnosis: Occlusive disease, right iliac artery

Procedure: Fem-fem bypass from left femoral artery to right femoral artery due to a blocked right iliac artery.

(continued)

---

3. (continued)

Made bilateral longitudinal incisions to expose both femoral arteries. Carried out subcutaneous tunneling, paying careful attention to the geometry of the graft to avoid kinking. Passed the Dacron graft through the tunnel in a C shape and completed end-to-side anastomoses on both sides.

a. What is the stated procedure? _____

b. What organ or body part is involved? _____

c. What is the laterality? _____

d. Is the procedure description what you would expect based on the name of the procedure? _____

e. What surgical approach is used? _____

f. Was more than one procedure, or a combined procedure, performed? _____

g. What tubular body part was treated? _____

h. Was an orifice or lumen partially closed? _____

i. Was an orifice or lumen completely closed? _____

j. Was an orifice or lumen expanded? _____

k. Were the contents of a tubular body part rerouted? _____

l. What is the root operation(s)? _____

---

4. INPATIENT HOSPITAL   Gender: M   Age: 66

Preprocedure diagnosis: Atherosclerosis with 50% blockage of LAD and 30% blockage of RCA

Procedure: PTCA of two coronary arteries, LAD with stent placement, RCA with no stent

a. What is the stated procedure? _____

b. What organ or body part is involved? _____

c. What is the laterality? _____

d. Is the procedure description what you would expect based on the name of the procedure? _____

e. What surgical approach is used? _____

f. Was more than one procedure, or a combined procedure, performed? _____

g. What tubular body part was treated? _____

h. Was an orifice or lumen partially closed? _____

i. Was an orifice or lumen completely closed? _____

j. Was an orifice or lumen expanded? _____

k. Were the contents of a tubular body part rerouted? _____

l. What is the root operation(s)? _____

(continued)

CODING PRACTICE (continued)

5. INPATIENT HOSPITAL   Gender: F   Age: 43

Preprocedure diagnosis: Uterine fibroids

Procedure: Uterine artery embolization using intraluminal coils. Accessed the right internal iliac artery with a needle puncture. Introduced sheath and guide wire into the artery and guided it to the right uterine artery under fluoroscopic guidance. Placed coil within the vessel. Then accessed the left internal iliac artery in the same manner and placed a coil in the left uterine artery.

a. What is the stated procedure? _____

b. What organ or body part is involved? _____

c. What is the laterality? _____

d. Is the procedure description what you would expect based on the name of the procedure? _____

e. What surgical approach is used? _____

f. Was more than one procedure, or a combined procedure, performed? _____

g. What tubular body part was treated? _____

h. Was an orifice or lumen partially closed? _____

i. Was an orifice or lumen completely closed? _____

j. Was an orifice or lumen expanded? _____

k. Were the contents of a tubular body part rerouted? _____

l. What is the root operation(s)? _____

6. INPATIENT HOSPITAL   Gender: M   Age: 72

Preprocedure diagnosis: Intracranial cerebral aneurysm, left internal carotid aneurysm

Procedure: Craniotomy with clipping of cerebral aneurysm in an intracranial artery. A clip was placed lengthwise around the outside of the widened portion of the vessel. Using a percutaneous approach, placed an intraluminal bioactive stent in the left internal carotid artery.

a. What is the stated procedure? _____

b. What organ or body part is involved? _____

c. What is the laterality? _____

d. Is the procedure description what you would expect based on the name of the procedure? _____

e. What surgical approach is used? _____

f. Was more than one procedure, or a combined procedure, performed? _____

g. What tubular body part was treated? _____

h. Was an orifice or lumen partially closed? _____

i. Was an orifice or lumen completely closed? _____

j. Was an orifice or lumen expanded? _____

k. Were the contents of a tubular body part rerouted? _____

l. What is the root operation(s)? _____

ASSIGNING CHARACTERS 4–7 FOR ROOT OPERATIONS 1, 7, L, AND V

To assign codes after the root operation is determined, search the PCS Index for the name of the root operation as the Main Term. Locate the subterm(s) for the correct anatomic site and identify the PCS Table. When you locate the PCS Table, verify the first three characters of the code, then locate the row with the body part needed. Assign the remaining characters from each respective column of the table. The following information summarizes and highlights unique information for working with the Tables for each root operation 1, 7, L, and V. Each root operation has one table in each applicable PCS body system. Because of the differences between organ systems, table details vary.

Character 4: Body Part

As discussed earlier in this chapter, the root operation Bypass uses body part to identify the site bypassed from. In a coronary artery bypass, Character 4 identifies the number of arteries bypassed to.

PCS classifies the coronary arteries as a single body part and uses Character 4 to identify the number of arteries bypassed to. When searching the Index, the Main Term is the root operation and the subterms are Character 4, Body Part values. Under the Main Term Bypass, the subterm for a coronary artery procedure is the number of arteries bypassed to, whereas the subterm for other bypass procedures is the body part bypassed from. Separate body part values identify the number of arteries bypassed to, such as one, two, three, or four arteries, when the same procedure is performed on multiple coronary arteries including the same device and qualifier values (PCS OGCR B4.4) (■ Figure 51-4). When multiple sites on one artery are treated with separate grafts or stents, report each site separately and use different device values.

PCS provides no body part value and no modifiers to identify the names of the coronary arteries treated. When reporting Bypass or Dilation of other arteries and veins, the body part value identifies the name and laterality of the vessel.

Surgeon performs percutaneous angioplasty of two distinct sites in the left anterior descending coronary artery, one with an intraluminal stent and one without.

> **02704DZ** Medical and Surgical, Heart and great vessels, Dilation, Coronary artery one artery, Percutaneous endoscopic, Intraluminal Device, No qualifier
>
> **02704ZZ** Medical and Surgical, Heart and great vessels, Dilation, Coronary artery one artery, Percutaneous endoscopic, No device, No qualifier

Figure 51-4 ■ Example of coding angioplasty on coronary arteries. *Source: © PB Resources, Inc. Used with permission.*

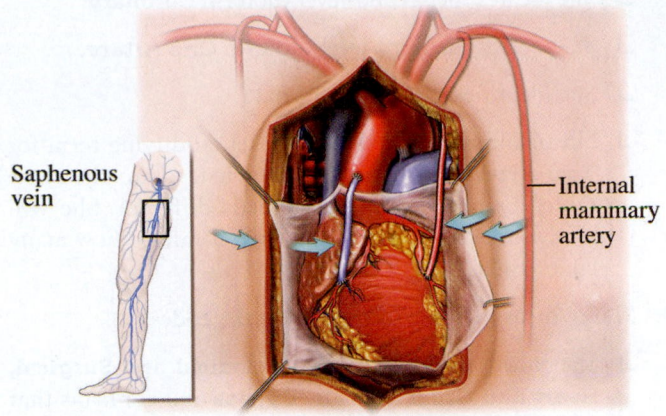

Figure 51-5 ■ Use of the internal mammary artery and greater saphenous vein for coronary artery bypass. *Source: Nucleus Medical Media Inc/Alamy Stock Photo.*

Character 5: Approach

All approaches are used for root operations in this group except **External (X)** and **Via Natural or Artificial Opening With Percutaneous Endoscopic Assistance (F)**. Restriction, Occlusion, and Dilation procedures on vessels are often performed using the Percutaneous or Percutaneous Endoscopic approach. Procedures on the Gastrointestinal and Respiratory systems might be performed Via Natural or Artificial Opening or Via Natural or Artificial Opening Endoscopic. The natural openings used to access the gastrointestinal system are the nose, mouth, and anus. Bypass procedures are more likely to use an Open approach but can also use a Percutaneous or Percutaneous Endoscopic approach. Read the documentation carefully to identify the correct approach.

Character 6: Device

The root operations Restriction, Occlusion, and Dilation use Character 6, Device to identify the type of device left in place. Options vary by procedure and can include intraluminal, extraluminal, drug-eluting, radioactive, or other characteristics of the stent.

The root operation Bypass uses the device to identify the type of tissue or tissue substitute used for the bypass procedure. It also identifies any intraluminal device left in place and whether it is drug-eluting.

Coronary artery bypass procedures often use the internal mammary artery (IMA) for the bypass. The right and left IMAs—also called internal thoracic arteries—begin at the subclavian artery and run to the anterior thoracic wall and breasts. Because of the location of the IMA, the vessel does not need to be harvested as do those from distant sites, such as the saphenous vein. Instead, the proximal end of the IMA remains connected to the subclavian artery and the distal end is freed and grafted to the destination site on a coronary artery (■ FIGURE 51-5). Therefore, use of the IMA is coded as **Z No device** because no tissue substitute is used. The IMA is identified in Character 7 as the vessel bypassed from.

When an autologous vein such as the saphenous vein is harvested and used for the graft, select device value **9 Autologous**

Venous Tissue. When an autologous artery such as the radial artery is harvested and used for the graft, select device value **A Autologous Arterial Tissue**. Select other device values for Synthetic (J) or Nonautologous Tissue (K) substitutes as appropriate.

Character 7: Qualifier

Coronary artery bypass procedures use Character 7 to identify the vessel bypassed from. This includes the IMA when used:

- **8 Internal Mammary, Right**
- **9 Internal Mammary, Left**

Noncoronary artery bypass procedures identify the ending site of the Bypass in Character 7.

The root operation Occlusion uses the qualifier for the body system Heart and Great Vessels (Table 02L) to identify the Left Atrial Appendage (K) and Ductus Arteriosus (T).

The root operation Restriction uses the qualifier to identify a temporary procedure for the Abdominal Aorta (Table 04V).

Guided Example of Assigning Characters 4–7 for Bypass

To practice skills for assigning codes for the root operation Bypass, continue with the example from earlier in the chapter about a patient who was seen for CABG ×2. Follow along in your ICD-10-PCS manual as Marcy Elwood, CCS, assigns codes. Check off each step after you complete it.

▶ First, Marcy confirms the procedure CABG ×2, LIMA to LAD and aorta to OM.

    ❑ The root operation for both procedures is Bypass, but separate codes are assigned because each artery was treated with a separate type of tissue and each bypass began in a distinct location.

▶ Marcy searches the Index for the Main Term **Bypass**.

    ❑ She locates the first-level subterm **Artery**.

❏ She locates the second-level subterm **Coronary**.

❏ She locates the third-level subterm **One Artery**.

❏ She identifies the PCS Table: **021**.

❏ She also reviews the second-level modifying term for **Two Arteries** and notices that it leads to the same table, but the fourth character is different. She will refer to the Table to determine the details of how many codes are needed.

▶ Marcy turns to Table **021** to assign the codes.

❏ She reads the Table title **021 Medical and Surgical, Heart and Great Vessels, Bypass** and confirms that this accurately describes the body system and root operation.

▶ Marcy assigns the value for Character 4, Body Part for the bypass of the LIMA to the LAD.

❏ She selects **0 Coronary Artery, One Artery**.

❏ The Table contains several rows with this body part value. She notices that Characters 5–7 provide different values in each row.

▶ Marcy assigns the value for Character 5, Approach.

❏ She knows the approach is **0 Open** because the operative report identifies that a sternotomy was performed.

❏ The Table provides two rows that contain the value **0 Open** for approach. Marcy will need to determine which row to use as she continues through each character of the code.

▶ Marcy assigns the value for Character 6, Device.

❏ Because the LIMA was used, the vessel was not harvested. The proximal end of the LIMA was freed and reconnected to the LDA, and the distal end remained intact.

❏ She selects the row that contains **Z No device** because no tissue substitute was used.

▶ Marcy assigns the value for Character 7, Qualifier.

❏ For Bypass procedures, Character 7 identifies the site bypassed from.

❏ She selects **9 Internal Mammary, Left**.

▶ She reviews the code she has assigned for the CABG LIMA to LAD: **02100Z9** (■ Figure 51-6).

▶ Marcy remains in Table 021 to assign the code for CABG aorta to OM using the GSV.

▶ Marcy assigns the value for Character 4, Body Part.

❏ She selects **0 Coronary Artery, One Artery**.

▶ Marcy assigns the value for Character 5, Approach.

❏ The approach is the same as for the previous procedure, **0 Open**.

▶ Marcy assigns the value for Character 6, Device.

❏ The GSV is **9 Autologous Venous Tissue**.

❏ The value for the device is in a different row of the Table than the one used for the previous procedure, so this is the reason she needs two codes, each with the body part value **0 Coronary Artery, One Artery**.

▶ Marcy assigns the value for Character 7, Qualifier.

❏ She selects **W Aorta** as the site bypassed from.

▶ She reviews the code she has assigned for the CABG aorta to OM using the GSV: **021009W** (■ Figure 51-7).

▶ Marcy reviews the procedure codes she has assigned for this case.

❏ **02100Z9** Medical and Surgical, Heart and great vessels, Bypass, Coronary artery one artery, Open, No device, Internal mammary left

❏ **021009W** Medical and Surgical, Heart and great vessels, Bypass, Coronary artery one artery, Open, Autologous venous tissue, Aorta

▶ Next, Marcy must determine how to sequence the codes.

Section	0	Medical and Surgical
Body System	2	Heart and Great Vessels
Operation	1	Bypass: Altering the route of passage of the contents of a tubular body part

Body Part Character 4	Approach Character 5	Device Character 6	Qualifier Character 7
0 Coronary Artery, One Artery 1 Coronary Artery, Two Arteries 2 Coronary Artery, Three Arteries 3 Coronary Artery, Four or More Arteries	**0 Open**	**Z No Device**	3 Coronary Artery 8 Internal Mammary, Right **9 Internal Mammary, Left** C Thoracic Artery F Abdominal Artery

Figure 51-6 ■ Assigning code 02100Z9. *Source: Annotation © PB Resources, Inc. Used with permission.*

Section	0	Medical and Surgical
Body System	2	Heart and Great Vessels
Operation	1	**Bypass:** Altering the route of passage of the contents of a tubular body part

Body Part Character 4	Approach Character 5	Device Character 6	Qualifier Character 7
0 Coronary Artery, One Artery 1 Coronary Artery, Two Arteries 2 Coronary Artery, Three Arteries 3 Coronary Artery, Four or More Arteries	**0 Open**	8 Zooplastic Tissue **9 Autologous Venous Tissue** A Autologous Arterial Tissue J Synthetic Substitute K Nonautologous Tissue Substitute	3 Coronary Artery 8 Internal Mammary, Right 9 Internal Mammary, Left C Thoracic Artery F Abdominal Artery **W Aorta**

Figure 51-7 ■ Assigning code 021009W. *Source: Annotation © PB Resources, Inc. Used with permission.*

CODING PRACTICE

Exercise 51.3   Assigning Characters 4–7 for Root Operations 1, 7, L, and V

Instructions: Read the mini-medical-record of each patient's encounter. Review the information abstracted in Exercise 51.2 for questions 1–3. For questions 4–6, abstract the case on your own. Assign PCS codes using the Index and Tables. Write the code(s) on the line provided.

1. INPATIENT HOSPITAL   Gender: F   Age: 55

Preprocedure diagnosis: Epiphora (*overflow of tears*)

Procedure: Transnasal placement of stent to partially close left lacrimal duct

1 PCS Code _____

2. INPATIENT HOSPITAL   Gender: M   Age: 61

Preprocedure diagnosis: Esophageal varices, portal hypertension due to cirrhosis

Procedure: Ligation of esophageal vein. Passed endoscope through the mouth down the esophagus and visualized the varices. Snared the varices and placed extraluminal rubber bands around the veins to tie them off. Patient tolerated procedure well.

1 PCS Code _____

3. INPATIENT HOSPITAL   Gender: F   Age: 57

Preprocedure diagnosis: Occlusive disease, right iliac artery

Procedure: Fem-fem bypass from left femoral artery to right femoral artery due to a blocked right iliac artery. Made bilateral longitudinal incisions to expose both femoral arteries. Carried out subcutaneous tunneling, paying careful attention to the geometry of the graft to avoid kinking. Passed the Dacron graft through the tunnel in a C shape and completed end-to-side anastomoses on both sides.

Tip: Refer to PCS OGCR B3.6a to identify the use of Characters 4 and 7.

1 PCS Code _____

4. INPATIENT HOSPITAL   Gender: F   Age: 50

Preprocedure diagnosis: GERD

Procedure: Nissen fundoplication. Entrance to the abdomen gained via laparoscope. The fundus of the stomach was wrapped around the esophagus and sewn into place. The lower portion of the esophagus was passed through a stomach muscle tunnel to strengthen the lower esophageal sphincter. Patient tolerated the procedure well with no complications.

1 PCS Code _____

(continued)

CODING PRACTICE (continued)

5. INPATIENT HOSPITAL Gender: M Age: 44

Preprocedure diagnosis: Right subclavian artery steal syndrome

Procedure: Right common carotid artery to subclavian artery bypass. The common carotid artery was exposed and dissected free. The right subclavian artery was exposed. An arteriotomy incision was made and a Dacron 8-mm graft used for the bypass in an end-to-end fashion.

1 PCS Code _____

6. INPATIENT HOSPITAL Gender: F Age: 2 weeks

Preprocedure diagnosis: Patent ductus arteriosus, severe prematurity, operative weight less than 4 kg (600 grams)

Procedure: Ligation (*clip interruption*) of patent ductus arteriosus. A posterolateral thoracotomy incision was performed and the ductus arteriosus was interrupted with a medium titanium clip. There was good pulsatile flow and palpable bilateral femoral pulses were noted.

1 PCS Code _____

ARRANGING CODES FOR ROOT OPERATIONS 1, 7, L, AND V

In addition to general guidance provided by PCS OGCR on assigning and sequencing multiple codes, specific situations for root operations 1, 7, L, and V may require multiple coding.

The body part values for the coronary arteries are identified by the number of arteries treated for the root operations Bypass and Dilation, so that multiple arteries can be reported with a single code. However, separate codes must be assigned for each site with a unique combination of device (Character 6) and qualifier (Character 7). For example, if three arteries are treated but there are multiple device or qualifier values, do not use body part value **2 Coronary Artery, Three Arteries**. Instead, assign separate codes for each combination of values (■ FIGURE 51-8).

CABG procedures require multiple codes for different treatments of multiple arteries, graft harvesting, cardiopulmonary bypass, catheterization, and so on.

Cardiologist performed percutaneous transluminal coronary angioplasty on three arteries. An intraluminal drug-eluting stent was inserted into the LAD and non-drug eluting stents were inserted into the RCA and OM of the left circumflex artery.

027034Z Medical and Surgical, Heart and great vessels, Dilation, Coronary artery one artery, Percutaneous, Intraluminal device drug-eluting, No qualifier

02713DZ Medical and Surgical, Heart and great vessels, Dilation, Coronary artery two arteries, Percutaneous, Intraluminal device, No qualifier

Figure 51-8 ■ Example of multiple coding for coronary arteries.
Source: © PB Resources, Inc. Used with permission.

Guided Example of Arranging Codes for Bypass

To practice skills for arranging codes for procedures of the root operation Bypass, continue with the example from earlier in the chapter about the patient who was seen for CABG ×2. Follow along in your ICD-10-PCS manual as Marcy Elwood, CCS, arranges the codes. Check off each step after you complete it.

▶ First, Marcy confirms the procedure CABG ×2, LIMA to LAD and aorta to OM.

▶ Marcy reviews the procedure codes she has assigned for this case.

❑ **02100Z9 Medical and Surgical, Heart and great vessels, Bypass, Coronary artery one artery, Open, No device, Internal mammary left**

❑ **021009W Medical and Surgical, Heart and great vessels, Bypass, Coronary artery one artery, Open, Autologous venous tissue, Aorta**

▶ Marcy arranges the codes following the definition of the principal procedure contained in PCS OGCR and the Uniform Hospital Data Discharge Set (UHDDS).

❑ The principal diagnosis is acute STEMI LAD.

❑ CABG of the LIMA to LAD is the procedure most directly related to the principal diagnosis, so she sequences code **02100Z9** first.

▶ Marcy finalizes the procedure codes and sequencing for this case:

(1) **02100Z9 Medical and Surgical, Heart and great vessels, Bypass, Coronary artery one artery, Open approach, No device, Internal mammary artery left**

(2) **021009W Medical and Surgical, Heart and great vessels, Bypass, Coronary artery one artery, Open, Autologous venous tissue, Aorta**

▶ A separate code is assigned for harvesting of the GSV.

(3) **06BP4ZZ Medical and Surgical, Lower veins, Excision, Saphenous vein right, Percutaneous endoscopic approach, No device, No qualifier**

▶ The code for use of cardiopulmonary bypass equipment is assigned from PCS Section 5, Extracorporeal Assistance and Performance. These codes are discussed in Chapter 54 of this text.

(4) **5A1221Z Extracorporeal assistance and performance, Physiological Systems, Performance, Cardiac, continuous, Output, No qualifier**

▶ Marcy also assigns and sequences the ICD-10-CM diagnosis codes that support the need for the service.

(1) **I21.02 ST elevation (STEMI) myocardial infarction involving left anterior descending coronary artery**

(2) **I25.110 Atherosclerotic heart disease of native coronary artery with unstable angina pectoris**

(3) **F17.218 Nicotine dependence, cigarettes, with other nicotine-induced disorders**

CODING PRACTICE

Exercise 51.4 Arranging Codes for Root Operations 1, 7, L, and V

Instructions: Read the mini-medical-record of each patient's encounter. Review the information abstracted in Exercise 51.2 for questions 1–3. For questions 4–6, abstract the case on your own. Assign PCS codes using the Index and Tables, and arrange the codes in proper sequence. Write the code(s) on the line provided.

---

1. INPATIENT HOSPITAL Gender: M Age: 66

Preprocedure diagnosis: Atherosclerosis with 50% blockage of LAD and 30% blockage RCA

Procedure: PTCA of two coronary arteries, LAD with stent placement, RCA with no stent

2 PCS Codes _____

---

2. INPATIENT HOSPITAL Gender: F Age: 43

Preprocedure diagnosis: Uterine fibroids

Procedure: Uterine artery embolization using intraluminal coils. Accessed the right internal iliac artery with a needle puncture. Introduced sheath and guide wire into the artery and guided it to the right uterine artery under fluoroscopic guidance. Placed coil within the vessel. Then accessed the left internal iliac artery in the same manner and placed a coil in the left uterine artery.

Tip: Do not code the fluoroscopy for this exercise.

2 PCS Codes _____

---

3. INPATIENT HOSPITAL Gender: M Age: 72

Preprocedure diagnosis: Intracranial cerebral aneurysm, left internal carotid aneurysm

Procedure: Open craniotomy with clipping of cerebral aneurysm in an intracranial artery. A clip was placed lengthwise around the outside of the widened portion of the vessel. Using a percutaneous approach, placed an intraluminal bioactive stent in the left internal carotid artery.

2 PCS Codes _____

---

4. INPATIENT HOSPITAL Gender: F Age: 59

Preprocedure diagnosis: Angina, coronary artery bypass graft one year ago

Procedure: Left heart catheterization; percutaneous transluminal coronary angioplasty and stenting with Cypher drug-eluting stent. Using the right femoral artery, catheters were used for left ventriculography and selective coronary angiography. The LAD was 60% stenosed in the mid vessel and a balloon was deployed with minimal pressure ×2 with reduction to 0% stenosis. The proximal RCA was 80% occluded and a Cypher drug-eluting stent was deployed with reduction to 0%.

Tip: Refer to PCS OGCR B4.4.

2 PCS Codes _____

(continued)

CODING PRACTICE (continued)

5. INPATIENT HOSPITAL Gender: M Age: 51

Preprocedure diagnosis: Ureteropelvic obstruction, bilateral

Procedure: Endoscopic ureteral stent on the right and balloon dilation on the left. Cystoscope was passed though urethra without difficulty. A small incision was made at the blocked portion of the right ureter and a stent was inserted. We then turned our attention to the left ureter, where we deployed a balloon. With minimal pressure, the ureter opened nicely and the balloon was removed. There was good flow of urine upon completion.

Tip: Refer to the PCS OGCR B3.2.

2 PCS Codes _____

6. INPATIENT HOSPITAL Gender: M Age: 3 weeks

Preprocedure diagnosis: Infantile hypertrophic pyloric stenosis

Procedure: Laparoscopic pyloromyotomy converted to open. Using the laparoscope we attempted a 1.5-cm incision in the pylorus. Because of the pyloric thickness I wasn't confident of the depth of the incision and elected to open the patient with a right semicircular umbilical incision. As suspected, the incision was incomplete, which I corrected and enlarged to a 2-cm incision.

Tip: Refer to PCS OGCR B3.2. Code the laparoscopic procedure using the root operation Inspection because the laparoscopic procedure was converted to an open procedure. The root operation Inspection is discussed in Chapter 52 of this text.

2 PCS Codes _____

CHAPTER SUMMARY

In this chapter you learned that:

- The Medical and Surgical root operations in the group *Procedures that alter the diameter or route of a tubular body part* are Bypass, Dilation, Occlusion, and Restriction.

- The root operation Bypass (1) is altering the route of passage of the contents of a tubular body part.

- The root operation Dilation (7) is expanding an orifice or the lumen of a tubular body part.

- The root operation Occlusion (L) is completely closing an orifice or the lumen of a tubular body part.

- The root operation Restriction (V) is partially closing an orifice or the lumen of a tubular body part.

- PCS provides guidelines for Bypass and for distinguishing Occlusion from Restriction.

- Root operations in this group treat a tubular body part, such as arteries, veins, and vessels; organs of the digestive system; urethra and ureters; and many others.

- The Root operation Bypass uses Character 4, Body Part, to identify the site bypassed from. In a coronary artery bypass, Character 4 identifies the number of arteries bypassed to.

- The Root operations Restriction, Occlusion, and Dilation use Character 6, Device, to identify the type of device left in place.

- Character 7, Qualifier, is used for limited purposes in this group except for the root operation Bypass, which uses it to identify the site bypassed to or, for coronary artery bypass, the vessel bypassed from.

CONCEPT QUIZ

Take a moment to look back at root operations that alter the diameter or route of a tubular body part (1, 7, L, and V) and solidify your skills. Try to answer the questions from memory first, then refer to the discussion in this chapter if you need a little extra help.

Completion

Instructions: Write the term that completes each statement based on the information you learned in this chapter. Choose from the list that follows. Some choices may be used more than once and some choices may not be used at all.

Bypass   Occlusion

Dilation   Restriction

1. Balloon angioplasty is an example of the root operation _____.

2. The root operation _____ is altering the route of passage of the contents of a tubular body part.

3. Vasectomy using clips is an example of the root operation _____.

4. _____ is partially closing an orifice or the lumen of a tubular body part.

5. Urinary diversion is an example of the root operation _____.

6. The root operation _____ is completely closing an orifice or the lumen of a tubular body part.

7. Esophagogastric fundoplication is an example of the root operation _____.

8. The root operation _____ is expanding an orifice or the lumen of a tubular body part.

9. Placement of a ventriculoperitoneal shunt is an example of the root operation _____.

10. Clipping of cerebral aneurysm is an example of the root operation _____.

Multiple Choice

Instructions: Circle the letter of the best answer to each question based on the information you learned in this chapter.

1. What is the criterion for assigning the body part value for Coronary Artery?
   A. The name of the artery
   B. The number of arteries treated
   C. The number of sites treated
   D. The number of branches treated

2. How would you code the following procedure? *A physician performs bypass of two coronary arteries from the aorta using the saphenous vein.*
   A. 02100A3
   B. 02100KW, 021009W
   C. 021109W
   D. 0210093

3. What does Character 4 identify in a noncoronary Bypass procedure?
   A. The site bypassed from
   B. The site bypassed to
   C. The approach
   D. The type of anastomosis

4. What device value for Character 6 is used to identify the internal mammary artery in a coronary artery bypass?
   A. Autologous arterial tissue
   B. Autologous venous tissue
   C. Native artery
   D. No device

5. Which body system is most likely to use the approach Via Natural or Artificial Opening Endoscopic?
   A. Heart and Great Vessels
   B. Endocrine
   C. Nervous
   D. Gastrointestinal

6. What is the term for a device placed around the outside of a body part?
   A. Extraluminal
   B. External
   C. Intraluminal
   D. Internal

7. What does Character 7 identify in a coronary bypass procedure?
   A. The number of sites treated
   B. The vessel bypassed from
   C. The vessel bypassed to
   D. The type of stent

8. How would you code the following procedure? *A physician performs dilation of the urethra using a stent inserted endoscopically into the urethra.*
   A. 0T7D8DZ
   B. 0T784DZ
   C. 0T7D4ZZ
   D. 0T748ZZ

9. How would you code the following procedure? *A physician performs laparoscopic bilateral fallopian tube ligation using cauterization.*
   A. 0UL74CZ
   B. 0UL74ZZ
   C. 0UL74DZ
   D. 0UL73ZZ

10. Which procedure should be coded separately when a CABG is performed?
    A. Sternotomy
    B. Harvesting of the graft
    C. STEMI
    D. Anastomosis

KEEP ON CODING

Instructions: Read the procedural statement, abstract the root operation, then use the appropriate Index and Tables to assign PCS procedure codes. Assign only the Root Operations discussed in this chapter. Write the code(s) on the line provided. *Tip:* Terms indicating a device are underlined.

1. Open <u>clipping</u> to completely close off an aneurysm of the right vertebral artery, extraluminal. ICD-10-PCS Code(s) _____

2. Endoscopic bilateral vasectomy with extraluminal <u>clips</u>. ICD-10-PCS Code(s) _____

3. Endoscopic dilation of ileocecal valve. ICD-10-PCS Code(s) _____

4. Bypass ileum to skin, open. ICD-10-PCS Code(s) _____

5. Dilation of urethral stricture by passage of urethral dilator via the urethra without visualization. ICD-10-PCS Code(s) _____

(continued)

(continued from page 1073)

6. Open bypass using a Gore-Tex <u>graft</u>, venous, right femoral-popliteal. ICD-10-PCS Code(s) _____

7. Percutaneous tumor embolization of right temporal artery. ICD-10-PCS Code(s) _____

8. Percutaneous revascularization of the left anterior descending artery using XIENCE Alpine Everolimus Eluting Coronary <u>Stent</u>. ICD-10-PCS Code(s) _____

9. Percutaneous endoscopic ligation of esophageal varices (*abnormal, enlarged veins*) using cautery. ICD-10-PCS Code(s) _____

10. Percutaneous embolization of a bleeding maxillary arteriovenous malformation in the face. ICD-10-PCS Code(s) _____

11. Open splenorenal shunt using splenic vein to right renal vein. ICD-10-PCS Code(s) _____

12. Open suture ligation of failed arteriovenous hemodialysis graft, left brachial artery. ICD-10-PCS Code(s) _____

13. Laparoscopic bilateral tubal ligation using extraluminal <u>clips</u>. ICD-10-PCS Code(s) _____

14. Ventriculoperitoneal <u>shunting</u> with synthetic substitute to peritoneal cavity, open. ICD-10-PCS Code(s) _____

15. Hysteroscopy with dilation of fallopian tubes, bilateral. ICD-10-PCS Code(s) _____

16. Open occlusion of left atrial appendage (*a small, ear-shaped sac in the muscle wall of the left atrium*), using extraluminal pressure <u>clips</u>. ICD-10-PCS Code(s) _____

17. Percutaneous revascularization of the left common iliac artery using the Absolute Pro Vascular Self-Expanding <u>Stent</u>. ICD-10-PCS Code(s) _____

18. Endoscopic placement of restrictive <u>stent</u> in left parotid duct. ICD-10-PCS Code(s) _____

19. Percutaneous endoscopic ligation of portal vein. ICD-10-PCS Code(s) _____

20. Percutaneous transluminal coronary angioplasty (PTCA) of left anterior descending artery with placement of two drug-eluting <u>stents</u>. ICD-10-PCS Code(s) _____

21. Percutaneous transjugular intrahepatic portosystemic <u>shunt</u> (TIPS) from portal vein to hepatic vein with synthetic substitute. ICD-10-PCS Code(s) _____

22. Percutaneous ligation of left brachial artery. ICD-10-PCS Code(s) _____

23. Percutaneous endoscopic occlusion of mesenteric lymphatic duct. ICD-10-PCS Code(s) _____

24. Open gastric bypass with Roux-en-Y limb to ileum. ICD-10-PCS Code(s) _____

25. Percutaneous transluminal angioplasty, left renal artery. ICD-10-PCS Code(s) _____

CODING CHALLENGE

Instructions: Read the mini-medical-record of each patient's encounter, then abstract, assign, and arrange ICD-10-CM diagnosis codes and PCS procedure codes using the appropriate Index and Tables. Write the code(s) on the line provided.

1. INPATIENT HOSPITAL   Gender: F   Age: 59

Preprocedure diagnosis: Elevated liver function study; dilated CBD on ultrasound

Procedure: ERCP with balloon dilation of common bile duct. The endoscope was inserted in the esophagus and advanced into the descending duodenum. Cholangiogram showed filling defects and so a balloon was advanced and dragged through the common bile duct, removing sludge but no stones. No strictures seen and the scope was withdrawn.

Tip: Only code the dilation.

2 ICD-10-CM Codes _____

1 ICD-10-PCS Code _____

2. INPATIENT HOSPITAL   Gender: F   Age: 59

Preprocedure diagnosis: Peripheral arterial disease, left leg, with disabling intermittent claudication, ASHD

Procedure: Femoral-tibial bypass with a polytetrafluoroethylene (PTFE) graft. An incision was made in the groin and thigh to expose the affected artery above the blockage and another incision to expose the artery below the blockage. The arteries were blocked off with vascular clamps. The PTFE graft was sutured into an opening in the side of the femoral artery and then into the side of the posterior tibial artery. The clamps were removed, with good blood flow through the bypass.

2 ICD-10-CM Codes _____

1 ICD-10-PCS Code _____

3. INPATIENT HOSPITAL   Gender: M   Age: 19

Preprocedure diagnosis: Recurrent stenosis of left arteriovenous fistula, end-stage renal disease, on dialysis

Procedure: Left arm fistula/cephalic vein balloon angioplasty. Fistulogram showed a stenosis of about 75% at the arterial anastomosis. The fistula was accessed percutaneously with guide wire threaded toward the wrist. Balloon angioplasty was completed with a 6–mm-diameter × 4-cm balloon up to 8 atmospheres for two minutes. Fistulogram showed the vein now well dilated.

Tip: Only code the angioplasty.

3 ICD-10-CM Codes _____

_____

1 ICD-10-PCS Code _____

4. INPATIENT HOSPITAL   Gender: F   Age: 41

Preprocedure diagnosis: Grade II bleeding internal hemorrhoids

Procedure: Endoscopic band ligation of two prolapsed internal rectal hemorrhoids. After inserting the anoscope into the anus, the right posterior hemorrhoid was grasped and a rubber band placed tightly around the base of it. The same procedure was repeated for the right anterior hemorrhoid.

Tip: Code the rubber band as a device.

1 ICD-10-CM Code _____

1 ICD-10-PCS Code _____

5. INPATIENT HOSPITAL   Gender: M   Age: 70

Preprocedure diagnosis: Severe segmental arteriosclerotic stenosis of the distal abdominal aorta, COPD, alcoholic cirrhosis

Procedure: Aortobifemoral bypass graft using 19 × 8 Gelsoft Vascutek bifurcated graft. Both groins and the retroperitoneum were opened. The bifurcated graft from the aorta was tunneled down to the groin and the graft sutured to the right and then the left femoral artery. Flow was restored to both lower extremities and there were palpable femoral and dorsalis pedis pulses bilaterally.

3 ICD-10-CM Codes _____

_____

1 ICD-10-PCS Code _____

6. INPATIENT HOSPITAL   Gender: M   Age: 63

Preprocedure diagnosis: Esophageal stricture from reflux of stomach acid, dysphagia

Procedure: Esophageal dilation. The endoscope was passed through the mouth and into the esophagus. A 15- to 18-mm balloon was used to dilate the mild ring at the lower esophageal sphincter. The patient tolerated the procedure well.

2 ICD-10-CM Codes _____

1 ICD-10-PCS Code _____

7. INPATIENT HOSPITAL   Gender: F   Age: 29

Preprocedure diagnosis: Two second-trimester miscarriages, high risk for premature birth, cervical incompetence at 12 weeks

Procedure: Transvaginal intraluminal cervical cerclage using the Shirodkar technique. The cervix was exposed at the level of the internal os and a curved Allis clamp was used to grasp the lateral edges of the anterior and posterior aspects of the transverse incisions and some paracervical tissue. A suture was then placed anteriorly and tied posteriorly using a 5-mm tape suture with a double blunt needle at each end.

3 ICD-10-CM Codes _____

_____

1 ICD-10-PCS Code _____

8. INPATIENT HOSPITAL   Gender: F   Age: 46

Preprocedure diagnosis: Clotted arteriovenous graft of left upper arm, end-stage renal disease on dialysis

Procedure: Removal of AV graft, left upper arm, and repair of brachial artery with end-to-end anastomosis. Old arterial incision opened and the graft artery anastomosis was excised, leaving an end-to-end portion of the artery for reanastomosis, which was done without difficulty. Wounds closed with a mid-portion of the graft left open for drainage.

3 ICD-10-CM Codes _____

_____

1 ICD-10-PCS Code _____

(*continued*)

(continued from page 1075)

9. INPATIENT HOSPITAL   Gender: M   Age: 66

Preprocedure diagnosis: Subglottic upper tracheal stenosis, former 2 ppd smoker ten years ago

Procedure: Direct laryngoscopy, rigid bronchoscopy, and dilation of subglottic upper tracheal stenosis. A rigid bronchoscope showed a narrowing in the upper trachea. The area was dilated and the remainder of the bronchi evaluated. A bronchoscope was then used for further dilation. Tolerated well without complication.

2 ICD-10-CM Codes _____

1 ICD-10-PCS Code _____

10. INPATIENT HOSPITAL   Gender: F   Age: 50

Preprocedure diagnosis: Cerebral aneurysm, hypertension

Procedure: Craniotomy with clipping of a cerebral aneurysm. Small burr holes were made and, using a microscope, the right middle cerebral artery was isolated. The clip was placed on the neck of the aneurysm, effectively stopping any flow.

Tip: Clips are made of titanium and remain on the artery permanently.

2 ICD-10-CM Codes _____

1 ICD-10-PCS Code _____

Section 0: Root Operations 8, 9, C, F, J, K, N

Division • Drainage • Extirpation • Fragmentation • Inspection • Map • Release

Learning Objectives

After completing this chapter, you should have the skills to:

52.1 Spell and define the key words, medical terms, and abbreviations related to procedures that take out solids, fluids, or gases from a body part, involving cutting or separation only, or involving examination only. (Remember)

52.2 Identify the types of procedures that take out solids, fluids, or gases from a body part; involving cutting or separation only; or involving examination only. (Apply)

52.3 Adhere to ICD-10-PCS coding guidelines related to root operations Drainage, Extirpation, Fragmentation, Release, Division, Inspection, and Map. (Apply)

52.4 Examine and abstract procedural information from the medical record for coding for the root operations 8, 9, C, F, J, K, and N. (Analyze)

52.5 Demonstrate how to assign codes for the root operations 8, 9, C, F, J, K, and N. (Apply)

52.6 Utilize guidelines for arranging (sequencing) codes for root operations 8, 9, C, F, J, K, and N. (Apply)

Chapter Outline

- **Basics of Procedures 8, 9, C, F, J, K, and N**
- **Coding Guidelines for Root Operations 8, 9, C, F, J, K, and N**
- **Abstracting for Root Operations 8, 9, C, F, J, K, and N**
- **Assigning Characters 4–7 for Root Operations 8, 9, C, F, J, K, and N**
- **Arranging Codes for Root Operations 8, 9, C, F, J, K, and N**

Key Terms and Abbreviations

rhizotomy
solid matter (PCS)

In addition to the key terms listed here, students should know the terms defined within tables in this chapter.

INTRODUCTION

An electronic or paper map shows common features as well as highlights and hazards you might want to be aware of during your trip. PCS provides the root operation Map to identify procedures that generate electronic images of the brain or conduction system. The root operation Map is one of two root operations involving examination only.

This chapter discusses three groups of Medical and Surgical root operations:

- Procedures that take out solids, fluids, or gases from a body part (9, C, F)
- Procedures involving cutting or separation only (8, N)
- Procedures involving examination only (J, K)

Although the root operations in each group share a common purpose, each has a unique aspect that makes it different from the other procedures in this group. Sometimes only a few words distinguish one root operation from a similar one. Pay careful attention to the differences between root operations so that you can use each confidently and accurately.

BASICS OF PROCEDURES 8, 9, C, F, J, K, AND N

This section introduces each root operation group and provides definitions and examples of each root operation. Details are discussed as you progress through this chapter.

Basics of Procedures That Take Out Solids, Fluids, or Gases from a Body Part (9, C, F)

Procedures that take out solids, fluids, or gases from a body part include root operations **9 Drainage**, **C Extirpation**, and **F Fragmentation**. These procedures focus on the removal of the unwanted substance and not on removal of the body part itself. **Solid matter** refers to a non-native solid that may result from biological processes, such as calculi or a clot, or may be a nonbiological solid, such as a foreign body. Fluids can include any bodily fluid such as urine, blood, water, or a nonnative fluid introduced into the body. Air is the most common gas treated. Refer to ■ TABLE 52-1 for the definitions, values, and terms commonly used with the root operations Drainage (9), Extirpation (C), and Fragmentation (F).

Basics of Procedures Involving Cutting or Separation Only (8, N)

Procedures involving cutting or separation include the root operations **8 Division** and **N Release**. These procedures focus only on separating, transecting, or freeing a body part without removing the body part itself and without draining fluids or gases from the body part. Separation can be accomplished through cutting or other use of force. Refer to ■ TABLE 52-2 for the definitions, values, and terms commonly used with the root operations Division (8) and Release (N).

Basics of Procedures Involving Examination Only (J, K)

Procedures involving examination only include the root operations **J Inspection** and **K Map**. These procedures focus on visualizing, exploring, or mapping a body part for diagnostic purposes. The body part is *not treated* in these root operations. When the body part is treated, assign the appropriate root operation that describes the work done. Refer to ■ TABLE 52-3 for the definitions, values, and terms commonly used with the root operations Inspection (J) and Map (K).

■ TABLE 52-4 (page 1079) provides a refresher on how to build medical terms related to procedures that are discussed in this chapter. Some suffixes, such as *-ectomy*, *-tomy*, and *-scopy*,

Table 52-1 ■ ROOT OPERATIONS THAT TAKE OUT SOLIDS, FLUIDS, OR GASES FROM A BODY PART

Root Operation	Value	Definition	Terms
Drainage	9	Taking or letting out fluids and/or gases from a body part	Drainage, centesis, placement, aspiration
Extirpation	C	Taking or cutting out solid matter from a body part	Removal, excision
Fragmentation	F	Breaking solid matter in a body part into pieces	Lithotripsy, crushing, fragmentation

Table 52-2 ■ ROOT OPERATIONS INVOLVING CUTTING OR SEPARATION ONLY

Root Operation	Value	Definition	Terms
Division	8	Cutting into a body part, without draining fluids and/or gases from the body part, to separate or transect a body part	Separation, division
Release	N	Freeing a body part from an abnormal physical constraint by cutting or by the use of force	Lysis, release, freeing

Table 52-3 ■ ROOT OPERATIONS INVOLVING EXAMINATION ONLY

Root Operation	Value	Definition	Terms
Inspection	J	Visually and/or manually exploring a body part	Endoscopy, laparoscopy, diagnostic, exploration
Map	K	Locating the route of passage of electrical impulses and/or locating functional areas in a body part	Mapping

Table 52-4 ■ **EXAMPLE OF CONSTRUCTING MEDICAL TERMS FOR PROCEDURES 8, 9, C, F, J, K, AND N**

Combining Form	Suffix	Complete Medical Term
esophag/o (*esophagus*)	**-scopy** (*visual examination*) **-ectomy** (*excision*)	**esophago + gastro + duodeno + scopy** (*visual examination of the esophagus, stomach, and duodenum*)
gastr/o (*stomach*)		**esophag + ectomy** (*excision of the esophagus*) **gastr + ectomy** (*excision of the stomach*)
duoden/o (*duodenum*)		**duoden + ectomy** (*excision of the duodenum*)

Source: © PB Resources, Inc. Used with permission.

can be associated with more than one root operation. There is no direct match between a specific procedural term and a root operation because some medical terms, such as excision and endoscopy, can be associated with more than one root operation. Root operations are assigned based on the content of the operative report regarding what was actually performed, not on the terms used by the physician in documentation or by the surgical approach.

Refer to detailed anatomic diagrams of specific organ systems in Chapters 8–43 of this text, or in external references, when you need to refresh your memory of human anatomy.

CODING CAUTION

Be alert for root operations that have similar English meanings but different PCS definitions.

Extirpation (C) (*Taking or cutting out __abnormal solid matter from__ within a PCS body part*) and **Extraction (D)** (*Pulling out or off without replacement a __portion of__ a PCS body part*)

Release (N) (*__Freeing__ a body part from an __abnormal physical constraint__ by cutting or by the use of force*) and **Detachment (6)** (*__Cutting an extremity out/off__ without replacement*)

CODING PRACTICE

Exercise 52.1   Basics of Procedures 8, 9, C, F, J, K, and N

Instructions: Use your medical terminology skills and resources to define the 8, 9, C, F, J, K, and N procedures, then identify the code(s) or code range listed in the PCS Index. Follow these steps:

- Use slash marks "/" to break down each term into its root(s) and suffix.
- Define the meaning of the word based on the meaning of each word part.
- Look up the term in the ICD-10-PCS Index, and write down the name(s) of the root operation(s) the Index cross-references you to and the Table(s), if provided.
- Do not assign any codes.

Example: thoracotomy thoraco/tomy Meaning *incision into the chest*   PCS Root Operation(s)/Table(s) *Drainage 0W9*

1. oophorotomy   Meaning _____   PCS Root Operation(s)/Table(s) _____
2. cholecystostomy   Meaning _____   PCS Root Operation(s)/Table(s) _____
3. lithotripsy   Meaning _____   PCS Root Operation(s)/Table(s) _____
4. colopuncture   Meaning _____   PCS Root Operation(s)/Table(s) _____
5. laminotomy   Meaning _____   PCS Root Operation(s)/Table(s) _____
6. arthrolysis   Meaning _____   PCS Root Operation(s)/Table(s) _____
7. thrombectomy   Meaning _____   PCS Root Operation(s)/Table(s) _____
8. laparoscopy   Meaning _____   PCS Root Operation(s)/Table(s) _____
9. thoracocentesis   Meaning _____   PCS Root Operation(s)/Table(s) _____
10. lobotomy   Meaning _____   PCS Root Operation(s)/Table(s) _____

CODING GUIDELINES FOR ROOT OPERATIONS 8, 9, C, F, J, K, AND N

Coders need to understand the guidelines for root operations in the procedure groups discussed in this chapter. PCS OGCR provides several criteria for the root operation Inspection. General guidelines related to coding multiple procedures using Inspection are discussed below, and those specific to Characters 4–7 are discussed later in this chapter. PCS OGCR provides a guideline regarding coding biopsies using the root operation Drainage and also clarify the difference between the root operation Release and Division. These are discussed next. Refer to the PCS OGCR for additional details and clinical examples of each guideline.

Guidelines for Inspection

Sometimes a procedure is begun but cannot be completed using the intended approach, so a different approach is used. Assign separate procedure codes for each approach when the intended root operation is attempted using one approach but is converted to a different approach. A laparoscopic procedure converted to an open procedure is coded as a percutaneous endoscopic Inspection; the open procedure is coded as an Excision or Resection (PCS OGCR B3.2.d) (■ FIGURE 52-1).

When a procedure is begun but discontinued or not completed before any other root operation is performed, code the root operation Inspection to the body part or anatomic region inspected (PCS OGCR B3.3) (■ FIGURE 52-2). A second code is not required because no other procedure was performed.

Surgeon made 4 abdominal incisions for a laparoscopic cholecystectomy. Due to the level of inflammation, the procedure was converted to an open approach and completed.

0FT40ZZ Medical and Surgical, Hepatobiliary System and Pancreas, Resection, Gallbladder, Open, No device, No qualifier
0FJ44ZZ Medical and Surgical, Hepatobiliary System and Pancreas, Inspection, Gallbladder, Percutaneous endoscopic, No device, No qualifier

---

Figure 52-1 ■ Example of coding a laparoscopic procedure converted to open approach. *Source: © PB Resources, Inc. Used with permission.*

Surgeon made the initial thoracotomy incision for aortic valve replacement procedure. The patient became hemodynamically unstable so the procedure was discontinued before the heart muscle was incised.

0WJC0ZZ Medical and Surgical, Anatomical regions general, Inspection, Mediastinum, Open, No device, No qualifier

---

Figure 52-2 ■ Example of coding the root operation Inspection for a discontinued procedure. *Source: © PB Resources, Inc. Used with permission.*

Guidelines for Drainage

Drainage procedures can be done for diagnostic or therapeutic purposes. A physician may aspirate fluid to sample it and determine a diagnosis before creating a treatment plan. When a diagnostic Drainage, Excision, or Resection procedure (biopsy) is followed by a more definitive procedure, such as Destruction, Excision, or Resection, at the same procedure site, code both the biopsy and the more definitive treatment (PCS OGCR B3.4b).

Guidelines for Release and Division

Use the root operation Release when the sole objective of the procedure is freeing a body part without cutting the body part. Use the root operation Division when the sole objective of the procedure is separating or transecting a body part (PCS OGCR B3.14). For example, freeing a nerve root from surrounding scar tissue to relieve pain is coded to the root operation Release. Severing a nerve root to relieve pain is coded to the root operation Division.

ABSTRACTING FOR ROOT OPERATIONS 8, 9, C, F, J, K, AND N

Abstracting for PCS focuses on identifying the correct root operation, which involves reading the operative report and interpreting it in light of root operation definitions. When reading the operative report, remember to focus on the objective of the procedure and the activities performed, not the specific medical terms the surgeon uses to describe the procedure. Many times the root operation can be determined conclusively during abstracting. Other times the root operation can be narrowed down to two options, which must be differentiated based on other characters that are assigned from the PCS Tables. The following information summarizes the root operations in each of the groups discussed in this chapter. Refer to Tables 47-2 and 47-3 for general guidance on abstracting PCS procedures and root operation groups, then refer to the Key Criteria for Abstracting Root Operations in each of the following sections. This information is followed by a Guided Example of Abstracting Inspection, Release, and Resection.

Abstracting for Procedures That Take Out Solids, Fluids, or Gases from a Body Part

The following information summarizes the objective, definition, unique features, examples, and Key Criteria for Abstracting root operations for procedures that take out solids, fluids, or gases from a body part.

Abstracting for Drainage (9)

The objective of the root operation Drainage is taking or letting out. The site of the procedure is fluids or gases from a body part.

The root operation Drainage is coded for both diagnostic and therapeutic drainage procedures. When drainage is accomplished by putting in a catheter, assign the value **Drainage device (0)** for Character 6, Device. When the purpose is diagnostic, assign the value **Diagnostic (X)** for Character 7, Qualifier.

Examples of Drainage are thoracentesis—in which fluid is removed from the space between pleura and the wall of the chest—and incision and drainage (I&D), which is performed in multiple body systems (■ TABLE 52-5).

Table 52-5 ■ **EXAMPLES OF THE ROOT OPERATION DRAINAGE (9)**

Organ System	Procedural Examples
Cardiovascular	Thoracentesis
Digestive	Incision and drainage of external perianal abscess, percutaneous drainage of ascites
Genitourinary	Urinary nephrostomy catheter placement, routine Foley catheter placement, ovarian cystotomy and drainage
Hepatobiliary	Drain placement for liver abscess
Musculoskeletal	Arthrotomy with drain placement
Nervous	Ventricular CSF drainage catheter placement
Respiratory	Chest tube placement for right pneumothorax, sinus drainage, pleurocentesis

Source: © PB Resources, Inc. Used with permission.

Abstracting for Extirpation (C)

The objective of the root operation Extirpation is taking or cutting out. The site of the procedure is solid matter in a body part.

Extirpation represents a range of procedures where the body part itself is not the focus of the procedure. Instead, the objective is to remove non-native solid matter such as a foreign body, thrombus, or calculus from the body part. The solid matter may be an abnormal by-product of a biological function and it may be imbedded in a body part or in the lumen of a tubular body part. The solid matter may or may not have been previously broken into pieces. Extirpation is not used to identify removal of the body part itself.

Examples of Extirpation are a thrombectomy (*removal of a blood clot*) and choledocholithotomy, in which the common bile duct is cut into to remove a gallstone (■ TABLE 52-6).

Table 52-6 ■ **EXAMPLES OF THE ROOT OPERATION EXTIRPATION (C)**

Organ System	Procedural Examples
Cardiovascular	Declotting of AV dialysis graft, mechanical thrombectomy, endarterectomy
Digestive	Removal of bezoar from stomach
Genitourinary	Removal of bladder stone
Integumentary	Foreign body removal, skin of left thumb
Respiratory	Removal of foreign body in right nostril
Special Senses (Ear, Eye)	Removal of foreign body from cornea

Source: © PB Resources, Inc. Used with permission.

> ### CODING CAUTION
> Removal of a tumor or lesion is coded to the root operation Excision, which was discussed in Chapter 49 of this text.

Abstracting for Fragmentation (F)

The objective of the root operation Fragmentation is breaking into pieces. The site of the procedure is solid matter within a body part. The solid matter is non-native material such as calculus.

Physical force, including manual and ultrasonic, is applied directly or indirectly to break the solid matter into pieces. The solid matter may be an abnormal by-product of a biological function or a foreign body. The pieces of solid matter are not taken out. Fragmentation is coded for procedures to break up, but not remove, solid material such as a calculus or foreign body. This root operation includes both direct and extracorporeal Fragmentation procedures (■ FIGURE 52-3).

LITHOTRIPSY

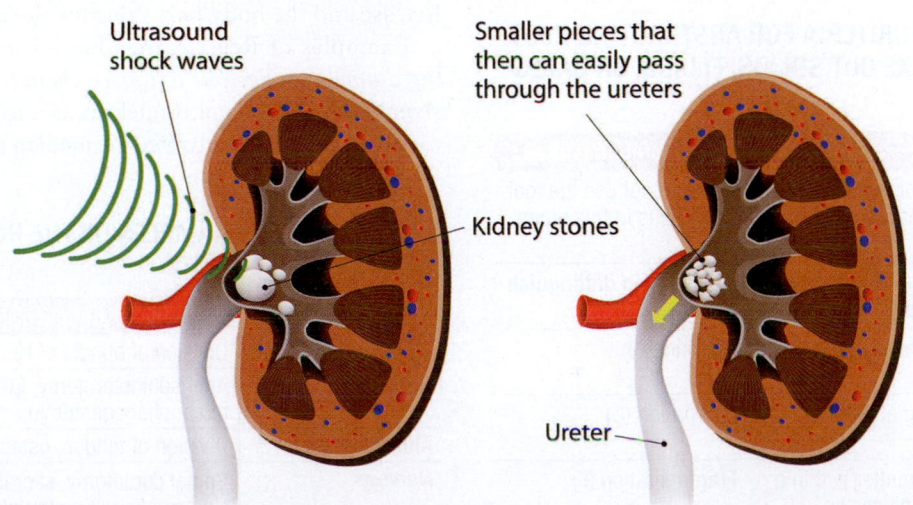

Figure 52-3 ■ Extracorporeal shockwave lithotripsy (ESWL) for kidney stones.

Table 52-7 ■ EXAMPLES OF THE ROOT OPERATION FRAGMENTATION (F)

Organ System	Procedural Examples
Cardiovascular	Thoracotomy with crushing of pericardial calcifications
Genitourinary	Extracorporeal shockwave lithotripsy (ESWL) of kidney, intraluminal lithotripsy of fallopian tube calcification
Hepatobiliary	Endoscopic retrograde cholangiopancreatography (ERCP) with lithotripsy of common bile duct stone

Source: © PB Resources, Inc. Used with permission.

Fragmentation differs from the root operation Destruction (5), which was discussed in Chapter 49 of this text. The focus of Fragmentation is non-native solid matter, whereas the focus of Destruction is the body part itself, such as fulguration of a polyp or cauterization of a skin lesion.

The most common example of Fragmentation is destruction of calculus, which can be accomplished using a number of different methods, such as ultrasound, a laser beam, and extracorporeal shock wave technology (■ TABLE 52-7).

CODING CAUTION

Fragmentation and Extirpation should not be used together for the same procedure. When solid matter is broken up, then removed by force, assign only the root operation Extirpation. Extirpation includes removal of the fragments. When the solid matter is broken up but not removed, assign the root operation Fragmentation.

Key Criteria for Abstracting Root Operations 9, C, and F

Refer to ■ TABLE 52-8 for more specific guidance on how to abstract *Procedures that take out solids, fluids, or gases* from a body part and distinguish among root operations in this group.

Table 52-8 ■ KEY CRITERIA FOR ABSTRACTING ROOT OPERATIONS THAT TAKE OUT SOLIDS, FLUIDS, OR GASES FROM A BODY PART

Question	Root Operation (Value)
❏ Did the procedure involve taking out gases, fluids, or non-native solid matter?	If *No*, do not use the root operations in this group.
Answer *Yes* to one of the following questions to help distinguish root operations 9, C, and F	
❏ Were gases or fluids let out from within a body part?	Drainage (9)
❏ Was non-native solid matter taken out of a body part?	Extirpation (C)
❏ Was non-native solid matter within a body part broken into pieces?	Fragmentation (F)

Source: © PB Resources, Inc. Used with permission.

Abstracting for Procedures Involving Cutting or Separation Only

The following information summarizes the objective, definition, unique features, examples, and Key Criteria for Abstracting root operations for procedures involving cutting or separation only.

Abstracting for Division (8)

The objective of the root operation Division is cutting into or separating a body part. The site of the procedure is within a body part. All or a portion of the body part is separated into two or more portions. The root operation Division is coded when the objective of the procedure is to cut into, transect, or otherwise separate all or a portion of a body part. If the body part itself is not cut or separated into portions, do not assign this root operation.

Examples of Division are a spinal cordotomy—in which nerves in the spinal cord are cut to relieve pain—and an osteotomy, in which a bone is cut to change its length or alignment (■ TABLE 52-9).

Abstracting for Release (N)

The objective of the root operation Release is freeing a body part from constraint. The site of the procedure is around a body part.

The objective of procedures represented in the root operation Release is to free a body part from abnormal constraint. Release procedures are coded to the body part being freed, not sites causing the constraint that might be cut as part of the procedure. The procedure can be performed on the area around a body part, on the attachments to a body part, or between subdivisions of a body part that are causing the abnormal constraint. Assign Release when the objective is to cut or separate the area around a body part, the attachments to a body part, or between subdivisions of a body part that are causing abnormal constraint. Some of the restraining tissue may be taken out but none of the body part is taken out.

Keep the ultimate objective of the procedure in mind. When one body part is cut to free another body part being constrained, the ultimate objective is freeing of the second body part. For example, in the procedure commonly referred to as carpal tunnel release, the transverse carpal ligament is cut to release pressure on the median nerve. Assign the root operation Release and the body part value for the median nerve.

Examples of Release are adhesiolysis (*dividing or breaking down of adhesions to loosen them from normal anatomic structures*) and carpal tunnel release, in which the transverse carpal ligament is cut to free the median nerve (■ TABLE 52-10).

Table 52-9 ■ EXAMPLES OF THE ROOT OPERATION DIVISION (8)

Organ System	Procedural Examples
Cardiovascular	Division of bundle of His
Digestive	Anal sphincterotomy, EGD with esophagotomy of esophagogastric junction
Musculoskeletal	Division of tendon, osteotomy
Nervous	Spinal cordotomy, sacral nerve rhizotomy (*interruption of a cranial or spinal nerve root*)

Source: © PB Resources, Inc. Used with permission.

Table 52-10 ■ EXAMPLES OF THE ROOT OPERATION RELEASE (N)

Organ System	Procedural Examples
Cardiovascular	Mitral valvulotomy for release of fused leaflets
Digestive	Frenulotomy, lysis of peritoneal adhesions
Genitourinary	Adhesiolysis of ureter
Integumentary	Incision of scar contracture
Musculoskeletal	Ligament release, tendon release
Nervous	Carpal tunnel release

Source: © PB Resources, Inc. Used with permission.

Key Criteria for Abstracting Root Operations 8 and N

Refer to ■ TABLE 52-11 for more specific guidance on how to abstract *Procedures involving cutting or separation only* and distinguish among root operations in this group.

Abstracting for Procedures Involving Examination Only

The following information summarizes the objective, definition, unique features, examples, and Key Criteria for Abstracting root operations for procedures involving examination only.

Abstracting for Inspection (J)

The objective of the root operation Inspection is visual or manual exploration. The site of the procedure is some or all of a body part.

Visual exploration may be performed with or without optical instrumentation. Manual exploration may be performed directly or through intervening body layers. The root operation Inspection represents procedures where the sole objective is to examine a body part. When examination is integral to a more definitive procedure, code only the more definitive procedure. Procedures that are discontinued without any other root operation being performed are also coded to Inspection.

Examples of Inspection are a diagnostic arthroscopy (*endoscopic examination of a joint*) or exploratory laparotomy, in which an incision is made into the abdomen to diagnose a problem (■ TABLE 52-12).

Table 52-11 ■ KEY CRITERIA FOR ABSTRACTING ROOT OPERATIONS INVOLVING CUTTING OR SEPARATION ONLY

Question	Root Operation (Value)
❏ Did the procedure involve cutting or separation only, with no other objective intended?	If *No*, do not use the root operations in this group.
Answer *Yes* to one of the following questions to help distinguish root operations 8 and N	
❏ Was a body part cut into to separate or transect it, without draining fluids and/or gases?	Division (8)
❏ Was a body part freed of abnormal constraint by loosening or removing an attachment or constraint around the body part?	Release (N)

Source: © PB Resources, Inc. Used with permission.

Table 52-12 ■ EXAMPLES OF THE ROOT OPERATION INSPECTION (J)

Organ System	Procedural Examples
Digestive	Colonoscopy, esophagogastroduodenoscopy (EGD), digital rectal exam (DRE)
Genitourinary	Colposcopy, transurethral diagnostic cystoscopy
Hepatobiliary	Laparotomy with palpation of liver
Musculoskeletal	Exploratory arthrotomy
Respiratory	Diagnostic laryngoscopy, sinus endoscopy

Source: © PB Resources, Inc. Used with permission.

Abstracting for Map (K)

The objective of the root operation Map is locating electrical impulses and/or functional areas. The site of the procedure is the brain or cardiac conduction mechanism.

Map represents a very narrow range of procedures that involve placement of electrodes or other sensors on areas of the brain or heart to receive impulses and create an image of electrophysiological activity. The root operation Map is applicable only to the cardiac conduction mechanism and the central nervous system.

Examples of Map are cardiac mapping and cortical mapping (*mapping of the cerebral cortex in the brain*) (■ TABLE 52-13).

Key Criteria for Abstracting Root Operations J and K

Refer to ■ TABLE 52-14 for more specific guidance on how to abstract *Procedures involving examination only* and distinguish among root operations in this group.

Table 52-13 ■ EXAMPLES OF THE ROOT OPERATION MAP (K)

Organ System	Procedural Examples
Cardiovascular	Cardiac mapping during heart catheterization or open heart surgery
Nervous	Cortical mapping, mapping of basal ganglia, intraoperative whole-brain mapping

Source: © PB Resources, Inc. Used with permission.

Table 52-14 ■ KEY CRITERIA FOR ABSTRACTING ROOT OPERATIONS INVOLVING EXAMINATION ONLY

Question	Root Operation (Value)
❏ Was a body part examined but not treated?	If *No*, do not use the root operations in this group.
Answer *Yes* to one of the following questions to help distinguish root operations J and K	
❏ Was some or all of a body part visually or manually examined or explored?	Inspection (J)
❏ Was a brain or cardiac conduction mechanism mapped to locate electrical impulses or functional areas?	Map (K)

Source: © PB Resources, Inc. Used with permission.

Guided Example of Abstracting or Inspection, Release, and Resection

Refer to the following example throughout this chapter to practice skills for abstracting, assigning, and arranging codes for multiple root operations from different groups. In this example, two root operations discussed in this chapter are used and one root operation from Chapter 49 is used.

INPATIENT HOSPITAL Gender: F Age: 37

Preoperative diagnosis: Acute appendicitis

Procedure: Laparoscopic appendectomy converted to open due to extensive adhesions in abdominal cavity, requiring an additional 30 minutes to lyse. A periumbilical incision was made and the fascia was incised. The peritoneal cavity entered bluntly. A 10-mm trocar and scope was passed. Peritoneal cavity was insufflated. Five-millimeter ports placed in left lower and hypogastric areas. We were unable to visualize the appendix or most of the right lower quadrant because of extensive adhesions to the colon and peritoneum. These are likely the result of scarring after multiple surgeries 10 years ago following an automobile accident. We worked on freeing the adhesions laparoscopically until we made no further progress, then, after careful consideration, converted to an open procedure. After making a McBurney incision, we spent another 30 minutes dissecting the adhesions from the peritoneum and the right side of the large intestine until we were able to visualize and access the appendix. We proceeded to take the mesoappendix down to the base, and once the base was free, we performed simple ligation with 2-0 plain Vicryl, tying off the base twice, and removed the appendix through the wound. The wound was copiously irrigated and a layered closure was performed. Patient tolerated procedure well.

Postoperative diagnosis: Acute appendicitis, peritoneal and intestinal adhesions

---

Follow along as fictitious coder Marcy Elwood, CCS, abstracts the procedure. Check off each step after you complete it.

▶ Marcy reads through the entire record, paying special attention to the reason for the encounter, the procedure performed, and the postoperative diagnosis. She refers to several tables of Key Criteria for Abstracting because multiple procedures are performed.

  ❑ She notes a preoperative diagnosis of acute appendicitis.

  ❑ *What is the stated procedure?* Appendectomy

  ❑ *What organ or body part is involved?* Appendix

❑ *Is the procedure description what you would expect based on the name of the procedure?* Yes

❑ *What surgical approach is used?* Laparoscopic converted to open

❑ *Was more than one procedure, or a combined procedure, performed?* Yes, laparoscopic access, open appendectomy, and extensive lysis of adhesions

❑ First, Marcy abstracts for the open appendectomy (Table 49-9).

  ▪ *Did the procedure take out some or all of a body part without replacement?* Yes

  ▪ *Was removal performed by cutting?* Yes

  ▪ *Was all of a body part or only a portion of a body part removed?* The entire appendix was removed, and Marcy believes this will equate to all of a PCS body part. She will need to verify this when she refers to the PCS Tables.

  ▪ *What is the most likely root operation?* Resection. (Refer to Chapter 49 of this text for more information on Resection procedures.)

❑ Next, Marcy abstracts for the lysis of adhesions (Table 52-11). She believes that she can code for this procedure in addition to the appendectomy because it required substantial additional time, documented as an additional 30 minutes, and was the reason that conversion to an open procedure was necessary.

  ▪ *Did the procedure involve cutting or separation only?* Yes

  ▪ *Was a body part cut into to separate or transect it, without draining fluids and/or gases?* No

  ▪ *Was a body part freed of abnormal constraint by loosening or removing an attachment or constraint around the body part?* Yes

  ▪ *What is the most likely root operation?* Release

❑ Marcy is unsure how to code for the initial laparoscopic procedure, or whether it should be coded at all. She refers to PCS OGCR B3.2.d, which confirms that a laparoscopic procedure converted to an open procedure is coded as a percutaneous endoscopic Inspection. She verifies that this is consistent with the abstracting question for Inspection (Table 52-14).

  ▪ *Was some or all of a body part visually or manually examined or explored?* Yes, the peritoneal cavity was examined laparoscopically

▶ At this time, Marcy believes that she will need three codes and uses the root operations Inspection, Release, and Resection. She will verify this information when she refers to the PCS Tables to assign codes.

CODING PRACTICE

Exercise 52.2 **Abstracting for Root Operations 8, 9, C, F, J, K, and N**

Instructions: Read the mini-medical-record of each patient's encounter and answer the abstracting questions. Write the answer on the line provided. Do not assign any codes.

---

1. INPATIENT HOSPITAL   Gender: F   Age: 62

Preprocedure diagnosis: Acute urinary retention

Procedure: Inserted Foley catheter to drain urine. After prepping the patient, we identified the urinary meatus and guided the tube until urine was observed. We inflated the balloon and connected the catheter to the drainage system.

a. What is the stated procedure? _____

b. What organ or body part is involved? _____

c. What is the laterality? _____

d. Is the procedure description what you would expect based on the name of the procedure? _____

e. What surgical approach is used? _____

f. Was more than one procedure, or a combined procedure, performed? _____

g. Were gases or fluids let out from within a body part? _____

h. Was non-native solid matter taken out of a body part? _____

i. Was non-native solid matter within a body part broken into pieces? _____

j. What is the root operation? _____

---

2. INPATIENT HOSPITAL   Gender: M   Age: 48

Preprocedure diagnosis: Clotted AV graft

Procedure: Embolectomy. Made a transverse incision 1 cm below the elbow crease on the right arm. The venous limb of the graft was dissected free up to the venous anastomosis.

A small incision on the graft was performed. Then a catheter was passed on the venous side. The cephalic vein was found to be obstructed about 4 cm proximal to the anastomosis. A large number of clots were extracted. After the embolectomy a good back flow from the venous side was obtained. Then the embolectomy was performed throughout the limb on the arterial side of the cephalic vein. More clots were extracted and a good arterial flow was obtained.

(continued)

---

2. (continued)

a. What is the stated procedure? _____

b. What organ or body part is involved? _____

c. What is the laterality? _____

d. Is the procedure description what you would expect based on the name of the procedure? _____

e. What surgical approach is used? _____

f. Was more than one procedure, or a combined procedure, performed? _____

g. Were gases or fluids let out from within a body part? _____

h. Was non-native solid matter taken out of a body part? _____

i. Was non-native solid matter within a body part broken into pieces? _____

j. What is the root operation? _____

---

3. INPATIENT HOSPITAL   Gender: F   Age: 33

Preprocedure diagnosis: Carpal tunnel syndrome

Procedure: Carpal tunnel release. A small incision was made over the right palm and wrist. We cut through the palmar fascia and exposed the carpal ligament. The ligament was surgically divided to release pressure on the median nerve. Care was taken to ensure safety of the median nerve and the tendons surrounding it. A layered closure was performed.

a. What is the stated procedure? _____

b. What organ or body part is involved? _____

c. What is the laterality? _____

d. Is the procedure description what you would expect based on the name of the procedure? _____

e. What surgical approach is used? _____

f. Was more than one procedure, or a combined procedure, performed? _____

g. Was a body part cut into in order to separate or transect it, without draining fluids and/or gases? _____

h. Was a body part freed of abnormal constraint by loosening or removing an attachment or constraint around the body part? _____

i. What is the root operation? _____

(continued)

CODING PRACTICE (continued)

4. INPATIENT HOSPITAL Gender: M Age: 68

Preprocedure diagnosis: Atrial arrhythmia

Procedure: During open heart surgery, divided the bundle of His using sharp division of the atrial septum at its attachment to the right fibrous trigone. Also performed intraoperative cardiac mapping.

a. What is the stated procedure? _____

b. What organ or body part is involved? _____

c. What is the laterality? _____

d. Is the procedure description what you would expect based on the name of the procedure? _____

e. What surgical approach is used? _____

f. Was more than one procedure, or a combined procedure, performed? _____

g. Was some or all of a body part visually or manually examined or explored? _____

h. Was a brain or cardiac conduction mechanism mapped to locate electrical impulses or functional areas? _____

i. Was a body part cut into in order to separate or transect it, without draining fluids and/or gases? ____

j. Was a body part freed of abnormal constraint by loosening or removing an attachment or constraint around the body part? _____

k. What are the root operations? _____

5. INPATIENT HOSPITAL Gender: M Age: 52

Preprocedure diagnosis: Renal calculi

Procedure: ESWL. The patient was placed on a fluid-filled cushion on the treatment table. Located the calculi in both the left and right renal pelvis using fluoroscopic guidance. Directed ultrasound shock waves at the stones through the water medium, breaking up the calculi into small fragments. Patient tolerated procedure well.

a. What is the stated procedure? _____

b. What organ or body part is involved? _____

c. What is the laterality? _____

d. Is the procedure description what you would expect based on the name of the procedure? _____

e. What surgical approach is used? _____

f. Was more than one procedure, or a combined procedure, performed? _____

(continued)

5. (continued)

g. Were gases or fluids let out from within a body part? _____

h. Was non-native solid matter taken out of a body part? _____

i. Was non-native solid matter within a body part broken into pieces? _____

j. What is the root operation? _____

6. INPATIENT HOSPITAL Gender: F Age: 41

Preprocedure diagnosis: Mass in liver

Procedure: Diagnostic laparoscopy with palpation of liver, followed by open procedure to cut out a tumor from right lobe.

Postprocedure diagnosis: Focal nodular hyperplasia (FNH)

a. What is the stated procedure? _____

b. What organ or body part is involved? _____

c. What is the laterality? _____

d. Is the procedure description what you would expect based on the name of the procedure? _____

e. What surgical approach is used? _____

f. Was more than one procedure, or a combined procedure, performed? _____

g. Was some or all of a body part visually or manually examined or explored? _____

h. Was a brain or cardiac conduction mechanism mapped to locate electrical impulses or functional areas? _____

i. Were gases or fluids let out from within a body part? _____

j. Was non-native solid matter taken out of a body part? _____

k. Was non-native solid matter within a body part broken into pieces? _____

l. Did the procedure take out some or all of a body part without replacement? _____

m. Was removal performed by cutting? _____

n. Was all of body part or only a portion of a body part removed? _____

o. What are the root operations? _____

Tip: This scenario requires a root operation discussed in a previous chapter of this text.

ASSIGNING CHARACTERS 4–7 FOR ROOT OPERATIONS 8, 9, C, F, J, K, AND N

To assign codes after the root operation is determined, search the PCS Index for the name of the root operation as the Main Term. Locate the subterm(s) for the correct body system and/or anatomic site and identify the PCS Table. When you locate the PCS Table, verify the first three characters of the code, then locate the row with the appropriate body part. Assign the remaining characters from each respective column of the Table. The following information summarizes and highlights unique information for working with the Tables for the root operations discussed in this chapter. Each root operation has one Table in each applicable PCS body system. Because of the differences between organ systems, Table details vary.

Character 4: Body Part

Character 4, Body Part is usually identified in the Index, but it is important to verify it in the PCS Table as well. PCS OGCR provide guidelines for reporting of the body part for the root operations Inspection, Release, and Division. Some body parts may appear in more than one row of a Table, in which case Characters 5–7 must also be reviewed to select the correct row. For example, in some Tables, certain combinations of Character 6 and Character 7 cannot be used in the same code, so the valid combinations for these characters appear in different rows, but with the same body part values for Character 4. This occurs with the root operation Drainage because a drainage procedure can have a drainage device (Character 6) or be diagnostic in nature (Character 7), but one procedure cannot meet both criteria. (Refer back to Figure 48-2 for an example.)

Drainage Procedures

The procedure codes in the general body systems for Anatomical Regions can be used when the procedure is performed on an anatomical region rather than a specific body part, such as the root operation Drainage performed on a body cavity.

> EXAMPLE: *Percutaneous placement of chest tube to drain the right pleural cavity*
> 0W993ZZ Drainage, Pleural cavity right, Percutaneous approach, No device, No qualifier

Inspection Procedures

When the root operations Inspection, Excision, or Repair are performed on overlapping layers of the musculoskeletal system, code the body part that identifies the deepest layer (PCS OGCR B3.5).

When a body part is inspected as part of a larger procedure with a specific objective, the inspection—usually endoscopy—is included in the broader procedure and is not coded separately (PCS OGCR B3.11a). For example, when fiber-optic bronchoscopy is performed for irrigation of bronchus, code only the irrigation procedure with the approach value **Via natural or artificial opening endoscopic**. Do not assign a separate code for the root operation Inspection.

When multiple tubular body parts are inspected, code the most distal body part inspected (PCS OGCR B3.11b). For example, a cystoureteroscopy with inspection of bladder and ureters is coded to the body part value for the ureter. This requires anatomic knowledge of the relationship of the bladder and ureters. When multiple nontubular body parts in a region are inspected, code the body part that specifies the entire area inspected. This may require use of the one of the body system values for **Anatomical Regions (W, X, or Y)**, rather than a specific organ system.

Assign a general body part value when the specific body part value is not in the Table (PCS OGCR B4.8). For example, when coding for Inspection of the esophagus, assign body part **0 Upper Intestinal Tract** because Table 0DJ does not provide a specific value for the esophagus.

An exploratory laparotomy with examination of the general abdominal contents is coded to the root operation Inspection and the body part value Peritoneal Cavity (G). This body part belongs to the body system Anatomical Regions, General (W).

Release Procedures

In the root operation Release, assign the body part value for the body part being freed, not the tissue being manipulated or cut to free the body part (PCS OGCR B3.13). For example, lysis of intestinal adhesions uses the body part value for the intestine. Carpal tunnel release in which the median nerve is released is coded as the root operation Release and the body part median nerve.

Character 5: Approach

PCS OGCR provides guidelines for using Character 5, Approach with root operations in this chapter.

- Procedures performed percutaneously via a device placed for the procedure are coded to the approach Percutaneous (PCS OGCR B5.4) (■ FIGURE 52-4).

- Both an Inspection procedure and another procedure might be performed on the same body part during the same operative episode. Code the Inspection procedure separately when it is performed using a different approach than the other procedure (PCS OGCR B3.11c) (■ FIGURE 52-5, page 1088).

Procedures performed on the skin and mucous membranes with direct visualization—such as a frenulotomy—always use the External approach.

ESWL is performed from outside of the body, so the approach is External.

> Surgeon places a percutaneous nephrostomy tube into the left kidney to crush calculi.
>
> **0TF43ZZ Medical and Surgical, Urinary System, Fragmentation, Kidney pelvis left, Percutaneous, No device, No qualifier**

Figure 52-4 ■ Example of coding percutaneous device placement.
Source: © PB Resources, Inc. Used with permission.

Surgeon performs a duodenoscopy through the oral cavity followed by an open excision of a portion of the duodenum.

0DB90ZZ Medical and Surgical, Gastrointestinal System, Excision, Duodenum, Open, No device, No qualifier

0WJP8ZZ Medical and Surgical, Anatomical Regions General, Inspection, Gastrointestinal tract, Via natural or artificial opening endoscopic, No device, No qualifier

Figure 52-5 ■ Example of coding inspection followed by excision. *Source: © PB Resources, Inc. Used with permission.*

Character 6: Device

When a separate procedure is performed to put in a drainage device, assign the root operation Drainage with the value **0 Drainage device** for Character 6 (PCS OGCR B6.2). A Drainage procedure can have a **Drainage Device (0)** for Character 6 or a **Diagnostic (X)** qualifier for Character 7, but not both. These values appear in separate rows of the PCS Table, so be sure to locate the correct row.

The root operations Division, Release, Map, Inspection, Extirpation, and Fragmentation do not use Character 6, Device. Assign the value **Z No device**.

Character 7: Qualifier

The root operations Release and Extirpation use the qualifier with the body system **Mouth and Throat** to identify the number of teeth treated.

The root operation Drainage uses the qualifier **Diagnostic (X)** to identify Drainage procedures that are biopsies (PCS OGCR B3.4a) (■ FIGURE 52-6).

The root operations Division, Map, Inspection, and Fragmentation do not use Character 7, Qualifier. Assign the value **Z No qualifier**.

Guided Example of Assigning Characters 4–7 for Inspection, Release, and Resection

To practice skills for assigning codes for the root operations Inspection, Release, and Resection, continue with the example from earlier in the chapter about the patient who was seen for an appendectomy. Follow along in your ICD-10-PCS manual as Marcy Elwood, CCS, assigns codes. Check off each step after you complete it.

▶ First, Marcy confirms the procedure: laparoscopic appendectomy converted to open due to extensive adhesions.

❏ The root operation for the laparoscopic access is Inspection.

Surgeon performs a diagnostic fine needle aspiration of the upper lobe of the right lung.

0B9C3ZX Medical and Surgical, Respiratory System, Drainage, Upper lung lobe right, Percutaneous, No device, Diagnostic

Figure 52-6 ■ Example of coding a diagnostic drainage procedure. *Source: © PB Resources, Inc. Used with permission.*

❏ The root operation for the adhesiolysis is Release.

❏ The root operation for the open appendectomy is Resection. If only a portion of a PCS body part was removed, she would use the root operation Excision.

▶ Marcy searches the Index for the Main Term **Inspection** for the laparoscopic access.

❏ She locates a first-level subterm for **Abdominal Wall** but not *abdominal cavity*. The site inspected is not the abdominal wall, so she searches further and locates a first-level subterm for **Peritoneal Cavity**.

❏ She identifies the Table **0WJ** and partial code **0WJG**.

▶ Marcy turns to Table **0WJ** to assign the code for Inspection of the peritoneal cavity.

❏ She reads the Table title **0WJ, Medical and Surgical, Anatomical Regions General, Inspection** and confirms that this accurately describes the body system and root operation.

❏ Marcy assigns the value for Character 4, Body Part.
  ▪ She reviews the values provided and confirms that **G Peritoneal cavity**, which was part of the partial code **0WJG** provided in the Index, is correct.

❏ Marcy assigns the value for Character 5, Approach.
  ▪ The root operation Inspection is used to identify the initial laparoscopic approach that was discontinued, so she assigns **4 Percutaneous endoscopic**.

❏ Marcy assigns the value **Z No device** for Character 6, Device.

❏ Marcy assigns the value **Z No qualifier** for Character 7, Qualifier.

❏ She reviews the code she has assigned for the discontinued laparoscopy that was converted: **0WJG4ZZ** (■ FIGURE 52-7).

▶ Marcy searches the Index for the Main Term **Release** for adhesiolysis.

❏ She refers to the documentation to confirm that two sites were documented for the adhesions, extensive adhesions to the right side of the colon and peritoneum, so she will need to locate subterms and assign codes for each site. If the adhesions had been documented as adhered to the appendix only, she would have selected a subterm for the appendix.

❏ She locates the first-level subterm **Peritoneum**.

❏ She identifies the Table **0DN** and partial code **0DNW**.

❏ She locates the first-level subterm **Large Intestine, Right**.

❏ She identifies the Table **0DN** and partial code **0DNF**.

Section	0	Medical and Surgical
Body System	W	Anatomical Regions, General
Operation	J	Inspection: Visually and/or manually exploring a Body Part

Body Part Character 4	Approach Character 5	Device Character 6	Qualifier Character 7
1 Cranial Cavity 9 Pleural Cavity, Right B Pleural Cavity, Left C Mediastinum D Pericardial Cavity G Peritoneal Cavity H Retroperitoneum J Pelvic Cavity	0 Open 3 Percutaneous 4 Percutaneous Endoscopic	Z No Device	Z No Qualifier

Figure 52-7 ■ Assigning code 0WJG4ZZ. *Source: Annotation © PB Resources, Inc. Used with permission.*

► Marcy turns to Table **0DN** to assign the code for adhesiolysis.

❏ She reads the Table title **0DN, Medical and Surgical, Gastrointestinal System, Release: Freeing a body part from an abnormal physical constraint by cutting or by the use of force** and confirms that this accurately describes the body system and root operation.

❏ She assigns the value **W Peritoneum** for Character 4, Body Part, which is consistent with the partial code **0DNW** provided in the Index.

❏ She assigns the value **0 Open** for Character 5, Approach. Although some lysis was performed laparoscopically, the significant portion was performed after the open procedure was initiated.

❏ She assigns the value **Z No device** for Character 6, Device.

❏ She assigns the value **Z No qualifier** for Character 7, Qualifier.

❏ She reviews the code she has assigned for adhesiolysis of the peritoneum: **0DNW0ZZ** ■ Figure 52-8, lower row (page 1090).

► Marcy uses the same table to assign the code for lysis of the intestinal adhesions.

❏ She assigns the value **F Large Intestine, Right** for Character 4, Body Part, which is consistent with the partial code **0DNF** provided in the Index.

■ She notices that this body part value appears in a different row of the Table than the value for the peritoneum. She determines this is because the procedures for the body parts in this row can be performed by approaches not available in the row with the peritoneum. Specifically, the body parts in this row can be accessed using Via Natural or Artificial Opening (7) or Via Natural or Artificial Opening Endoscopic (8).

❏ The other values of the code are the same as those for the peritoneal adhesiolysis:

■ **0 Open** for Character 5, Approach

■ **Z No device** for Character 6, Device

■ **Z No qualifier** for Character 7, Qualifier

❏ She reviews the code she has assigned for adhesiolysis of the large intestine, **0DNF0ZZ** (Figure 52-8, upper row).

► Marcy searches the Index for the Main Term **Resection** for the open appendectomy.

❏ She locates the first-level subterm **Appendix**.

❏ She identifies the Table **0DT** and partial code **0DTJ**.

► Marcy turns to Table **0DT** to assign the code for the open appendectomy.

❏ She reads the Table title **0DT, Medical and Surgical, Gastrointestinal System, Resection: Cutting out or off, without replacement, all of a body part** and confirms that this accurately describes the body system and root operation.

❏ Marcy assigns the value **J Appendix** for Character 4, Body Part.

■ If only a portion of a body part had been removed, she would need to use the root operation Excision. However, the entire appendix was removed and it would be extremely rare for only part of the appendix to be removed.

❏ Marcy assigns the value **0 Open** for Character 5, Approach because the Resection was performed after the procedure was converted to an open approach.

❏ Marcy assigns the value **Z No device** for Character 6, Device.

❏ Marcy assigns the value **Z No qualifier** for Character 7, Qualifier.

Section	0	Medical and Surgical
Body System	D	Gastrointestinal System
Operation	N	Release: Freeing a Body Part from an abnormal physical constraint by cutting or by the use of force

Body Part Character 4	Approach Character 5	Device Character 6	Qualifier Character 7
C Ileocecal Valve E Large Intestine F Large Intestine, Right G Large Intestine, Left H Cecum J Appendix	0 Open 3 Percutaneous 4 Percutaneous Endoscopic 7 Via Natural or Artificial Opening 8 Via Natural or Artificial Opening Endoscopic	Z No Device	Z No Qualifier
R Anal Sphincter U Omentum V Mesentery W Peritoneum	0 Open 3 Percutaneous 4 Percutaneous Endoscopic	Z No Device	Z No Qualifier

Figure 52-8 ■ Assigning codes 0DNF0ZZ and 0DNW0ZZ. *Source: Annotation © PB Resources, Inc. Used with permission.*

Section	0	Medical and Surgical
Body System	D	Gastrointestinal System
Operation	T	Resection: Cutting out or off, without replacement, all of a Body Part

Body Part Character 4	Approach Character 5	Device Character 6	Qualifier Character 7
F Large Intestine, Right G Large Intestine, Left H Cecum J Appendix K Ascending Colon P Rectum Q Anus	0 Open 4 Percutaneous Endoscopic 7 Via Natural or Artificial Opening 8 Via Natural or Artificial Opening Endoscopic	Z No Device	Z No Qualifier

Figure 52-9 ■ Assigning code 0DTJ0ZZ. *Source: Annotation © PB Resources, Inc. Used with permission.*

❏ She reviews the code she has assigned for the open appendectomy, **0DTJ0ZZ** (■ Figure 52-9).

▶ Marcy reviews the procedure codes she has assigned for this case.

❏ **0DNW0ZZ** Medical and Surgical, Gastrointestinal system, Release, Peritoneum, Open, No device, No qualifier

❏ **0DNF0ZZ** Medical and Surgical, Gastrointestinal system, Release, Large intestine right, Open, No device, No qualifier

❏ **0WJG4ZZ** Medical and Surgical, Anatomical regions, General, Inspection, Peritoneal cavity, Percutaneous endoscopic, No device, No qualifier

❏ **0DTJ0ZZ** Medical and Surgical, Gastrointestinal system, Resection, Appendix, Open, No device, No qualifier

▶ Next, Marcy must determine how to sequence the codes.

CODING PRACTICE

Exercise 52.3 Assigning Characters 4–7 for Root Operations 8, 9, C, F, J, K, and N

Instructions: Read the mini-medical-record of each patient's encounter. Review the information abstracted in Exercise 52.2 for questions 1–3. For questions 4–6, abstract the case on your own. Assign PCS codes using the Index and Tables. Write the code(s) on the line provided.

---

1. INPATIENT HOSPITAL   Gender: F   Age: 62

Preprocedure diagnosis: Acute urinary retention

Procedure: Inserted Foley catheter to drain urine from the bladder. After prepping the patient, we identified the urinary meatus and guided the tube until urine was observed. We inflated the balloon and connected the catheter to the drainage system.

1 PCS Code _____

---

2. INPATIENT HOSPITAL   Gender: M   Age: 48

Preprocedure diagnosis: Clotted AV graft

Procedure: Embolectomy. Made a transverse incision 1 cm below the elbow crease on the right arm. The venous limb of the graft was dissected free up to the venous anastomosis.

A small incision on the graft was performed. Then a catheter was passed on the venous side. The cephalic vein was found obstructed about 4 cm proximal to the anastomosis. A large number of clots were extracted. After the embolectomy a good back flow from the venous side was obtained. Then the embolectomy was performed throughout the limb on the arterial side of the cephalic vein. More clots were extracted and a good arterial flow was obtained.

1 PCS Code _____

---

3. INPATIENT HOSPITAL   Gender: F   Age: 33

Preprocedure diagnosis: Carpal tunnel syndrome

Procedure: Carpal tunnel release. A small incision was made over the right palm and wrist. We cut through the palmar fascia and exposed the carpal ligament. The ligament was surgically divided to release pressure on the median nerve. Care was taken to ensure safety of the median nerve and the tendons surrounding it. A layered closure was performed.

Tip: The body part value identifies the structure released, not the structure cut to obtain the release.

1 PCS Code _____

---

4. INPATIENT HOSPITAL   Gender: F   Age: 54

Preprocedure diagnosis: Chronic plantar fasciitis

Procedure: Open plantar fasciotomy, right foot. Blunt dissection was carried out to expose the deep fascia and the medial plantar fascial band. Transection of the medial two-thirds of the plantar fascia band began at the junction of the deep fascia of the abductor hallucis muscle belly and medial plantar fascial band, extending to the lateral two-thirds of the band. Visualization and finger probe confirmed adequate transection.

1 PCS Code _____

---

5. INPATIENT HOSPITAL   Gender: F   Age: 4

Preprocedure diagnosis: Father noticed child placing an object into her nose

Procedure: Removal of foreign body in right nostril. Under mild sedation, a pebble was removed from her nasal passage (nasal mucosa and soft tissue) with forceps.

1 PCS Code _____

---

6. INPATIENT HOSPITAL   Gender: F   Age: 34

Preprocedure diagnosis: Recurrent right lower extremity soft-tissue infection, diabetes

Procedure: Incision and drainage of right lower extremity soft-tissue abscess. The old incision was elongated. Loculations of fibrous tissue were broken up. Seropurulent, somewhat bloody fluid was noted. The infection appeared contained to a golf ball–sized area in the subcutaneous tissues above the fascia. The area was cleaned and the wound packed.

1 PCS Code _____

ARRANGING CODES FOR ROOT OPERATIONS 8, 9, C, F, J, K, AND N

Sequence PCS codes based on the Uniform Hospital Data Discharge Set (UHDDS) definition of the principal procedure. Do not sequence codes based only on the order in which the procedures were performed. Consider the following situations discussed earlier in this chapter:

- When a laparoscopic procedure is converted to an open procedure, sequence the open procedure first because it is most directly related to the principal diagnosis.

- When multiple procedures are performed at the same operative session, sequence the principal procedure as the one most related to the principal diagnosis. In this chapter, procedures such as those classified by the root operation Map might be secondary procedures in addition to a definitive procedure. Sequence the definitive procedure as the principal procedure.

- Division of the bundle of His during open heart surgery could be a principal or secondary procedure, depending on the principal diagnosis and reason the open heart surgery is performed. However, it is unlikely that open heart surgery is performed primarily to divide the bundle of His because it can also be done using a percutaneous endoscopic approach.

- When a biopsy is followed by a more definitive procedure, sequence the definitive treatment as the principal procedure.

- Adhesiolysis is often performed to reach an organ for a definitive procedure, so when this occurs, sequence adhesiolysis as a secondary procedure.

Also keep in mind when multiple procedures should not be coded:

- A procedure, such as endoscopy, is done as part of the objective of a more definitive procedure.

- Fragmentation and Extirpation of the same solid matter should not be coded together because they are mutually exclusive. For example, if calculi are crushed, then extracted, code only Extirpation, not Fragmentation. Code Fragmentation only when the solid matter remains in the body after the procedure.

- Code only the deepest tissue layer when multiple layers are accessed in one operation.

Guided Example of Arranging Codes for Inspection, Release, and Resection

To practice skills for arranging codes for the root operations Inspection, Release, and Resection, continue with the example from earlier in the chapter about the patient who was seen for an appendectomy. Follow along in your ICD-10-PCS manual as Marcy Elwood, CCS, arranges the codes. Check off each step after you complete it.

▶ First, Marcy confirms laparoscopic appendectomy converted to open due to extensive adhesions and reviews the codes she has assigned.

❑ **0DNW0ZZ** Medical and Surgical, Gastrointestinal system, Release, Peritoneum, Open, No device, No qualifier

❑ **0DNF0ZZ** Medical and Surgical, Gastrointestinal system, Release, Large intestine right, Open, No device, No qualifier

❑ **0WJG4ZZ** Medical and Surgical, Anatomical regions, General, Inspection, Peritoneal cavity, Percutaneous endoscopic, No device, No qualifier

❑ **0DTJ0ZZ** Medical and Surgical, Gastrointestinal system, Resection, Appendix, Open, No device, No qualifier

▶ The principal procedure must be the one most closely related to the principal diagnosis—acute appendicitis—so Marcy sequences code **0DTJ0ZZ** for Resection of the appendix first.

▶ Marcy sequences codes **0DNW0ZZ** and **0DNF0ZZ** for Release of the adhesions second and third because they are related to the secondary diagnosis and are the reason the procedure was converted from laparoscopic to open. The order of these two codes does not matter.

▶ Marcy sequences code **0WJG4ZZ** for Inspection of the peritoneal cavity fourth.

▶ Marcy finalizes the procedure codes and sequencing for this case:

(1) **0DTJ0ZZ** Medical and Surgical, Gastrointestinal system, Resection, Appendix, Open, No device, No qualifier

(2) **0DNW0ZZ** Medical and Surgical, Gastrointestinal system, Release, Peritoneum, Open, No device, No qualifier

(3) **0DNF0ZZ** Medical and Surgical, Gastrointestinal system, Release, Large intestine right, Open, No device, No qualifier

(4) **0WJG4ZZ** Medical and Surgical, Anatomical regions, General, Inspection, Peritoneal cavity, Percutaneous endoscopic, No device, No qualifier

▶ Marcy also assigns and sequences the ICD-10-CM diagnosis codes that support the need for the service.

(1) **K35.80 Unspecified acute appendicitis**

(2) **K66.0 Peritoneal adhesions (postprocedural) (postinfection)**

CODING PRACTICE

Exercise 52.4 Arranging Codes for Root Operations 8, 9, C, F, J, K, and N

Instructions: Read the mini-medical-record of each patient's encounter. Review the information abstracted in Exercise 52.2 for questions 1–3. For questions 4–6, abstract the case on your own. Assign PCS codes using the Index and Tables, and arrange the codes in proper sequence. Write the code(s) on the line provided.

---

1. INPATIENT HOSPITAL   Gender: M   Age: 68

Preprocedure diagnosis: Atrial arrhythmia

Procedure: During open heart surgery, divided the bundle of His using sharp division of the atrial septum at its attachment to the right fibrous trigone. Also performed intraoperative cardiac mapping.

Tip: The bundle of His is a conduction mechanism.

2 PCS Codes _____

---

2. INPATIENT HOSPITAL   Gender: M   Age: 52

Preprocedure diagnosis: Renal calculi

Procedure: ESWL. The patient was placed on a fluid–filled cushion on the treatment table. Located the calculi in both the left and right renal pelvis using fluoroscopic guidance. Directed ultrasound shock waves at the stones through the water medium, breaking up the calculi into small fragments. Patient tolerated procedure well.

2 PCS Codes _____

---

3. INPATIENT HOSPITAL   Gender: F   Age: 41

Preprocedure diagnosis: Mass in liver

Procedure: Diagnostic laparoscopy with palpation of liver, followed by open procedure to cut out a tumor from right lobe.

Postprocedure diagnosis: Focal nodular hyperplasia (FNH)

2 PCS Codes _____

---

4. INPATIENT HOSPITAL   Gender: M   Age: 44

Preprocedure diagnosis: Chronic subcutaneous abscess of a midline wound, large left thigh lipoma.

Procedure: Excision of chronic abscess pocket in the subxiphoid region of the epigastrium; excision of left thigh lipoma. Incision was made at the level of the skin around the chronic abscess cavity. Dissection was carried down to the subcutaneous tissue. The abscess cavity appeared to have been excised in its entirety. We decided to leave a drain in this time to see if it would prevent recurrence. Following this a skin incision was made overlying the lipoma. Dissection was carried down the subcutaneous tissue and the lipoma excised intact.

2 PCS Codes _____

---

5. INPATIENT HOSPITAL   Gender: M   Age: 54

Preprocedure diagnosis: Proximal interphalangeal (PIP) joint flexion contracture of 30°, right little finger; metacarpophalangeal (MCP) joint contracture of 50°, right ring finger.

Procedure: PIP joint release, right little finger, followed by MCP joint release, right ring finger. The palmar fascia was exposed and carefully separated from nerves, arteries, and tendons. Special care was taken not to damage the nearby nerves and blood vessels. The fibrous tissue was dissected free at the PIP joint of the little finger and the MCP joint of the ring finger.

2 PCS Codes _____

---

6. INPATIENT HOSPITAL   Gender: M   Age: 44

Preprocedure diagnosis: Ureteral calculi, bilateral

Procedure: ESWL bilateral ureters. The patient was treated at a power setting of 7 and 8 for total of 2500 shocks delivered to all areas of the stone in the right ureter. The procedure was repeated on the left. There appeared to be good fragmentation of the stone.

Tip: Refer to PCS OGCR B3.2, multiple procedures, for guidance.

2 PCS Codes _____

CHAPTER SUMMARY

In this chapter you learned that:

- The Medical and Surgical root operations in the group *Procedures that take out solids, fluids, or gases from a body part* are root operations Drainage (9), Extirpation (C), and Fragmentation (F).

- The root operation Drainage (9) is taking or letting out fluids and/or gases from a body part.

- The root operation Extirpation (C) is taking or cutting out solid matter from a body part.

- The root operation Fragmentation (F) is breaking solid matter in a body part into pieces.

- The Medical and Surgical root operations in the group *Procedures involving cutting or separation only* are Division (8) and Release (N).

- The root operation Division (8) is cutting into a body part, without draining fluids and/or gases from the body part, in order to separate or transect a body part.

- The root operation Release (N) is freeing a body part from an abnormal physical constraint by cutting or by the use of force.

- The Medical and Surgical root operations in the group *Procedures involving examination only* are Inspection (J) and Map (K).

- The root operation Inspection (J) is visually and/or manually exploring a body part.

- The root operation Map (K) is locating the route of passage of electrical impulses and/or locating functional areas in a body part.

- PCS provides guidelines regarding coding biopsies using the root operation Drainage and also clarifies the difference between the root operation Release and Division. Other references to root operation in this chapter appear throughout PCS OGCR.

- When a body part is inspected as part of a larger procedure with a specific objective, the inspection is included in the broader procedure and is not coded separately.

- In the root operation Release, assign the body part value for the body part being freed, not the tissue being manipulated or cut.

- When an Inspection procedure and another procedure are performed on the same body part during the same operative episode, assign a separate code for the Inspection procedure when it is performed using a different approach.

CONCEPT QUIZ

Take a moment to look back at root operations 9, C, F, N, 8, J, and K and solidify your skills. Try to answer the questions from memory first, then refer to the discussion in this chapter if you need a little extra help.

Completion

Instructions: Write the term that completes each statement based on the information you learned in this chapter. Choose from the list below. Some choices may be used more than once and some choices may not be used at all.

Division	Inspection
Drainage	Map
Extirpation	Release
Fragmentation	

1. The root operation _____ is taking or letting out fluids and/or gases from a body part.

2. The root operation _____ is visually and/or manually exploring a body part.

3. The root operation _____ is cutting into a body part, without draining fluids and/or gases from the body part, in order to separate or transect a body part.

4. The root operation _____ is sometimes described by the suffix *-lysis*.

5. The root operation _____ is taking or cutting out solid matter from a body part.

6. The root operation _____ is sometimes described by the suffix *-centesis*.

7. The root operation _____ is sometimes described by the medical term *lithotripsy*.

8. The root operation _____ is breaking solid matter in a body part into pieces.

9. The root operation _____ is locating the route of passage of electrical impulses and/or locating functional areas in a body part.

10. The root operation _____ is freeing a body part from an abnormal physical constraint by cutting or by the use of force.

Multiple Choice

Instructions: Circle the letter of the best answer to each question based on the information you learned in this chapter.

1. Which root operation discussed in this chapter uses the qualifier Diagnostic (X) for biopsies?
   A. Drainage
   B. Inspection
   C. Extirpation
   D. Release

2. What code(s) should be assigned when the intended root operation is attempted using one approach but is discontinued and converted to a different approach?
   A. Assign only a code for the procedure completed.
   B. Assign only a code for the procedure intended.
   C. Assign separate procedure codes for each approach.
   D. Assign a code for the procedure completed and Character 7, Qualifier to identify the discontinued procedure.

3. What body part value is assigned for an exploratory laparotomy with examination of the general abdominal contents?
   A. Abdominal wall
   B. Peritoneal cavity
   C. Thoracic cavity
   D. Abdominal cavity

4. Which root operation discussed in this chapter uses Character 6, Device?
   A. Fragmentation
   B. Drainage
   C. Extirpation
   D. Inspection

5. Which root operation discussed in this chapter uses the qualifier with the body system Mouth and Throat to identify the number of teeth treated?
   A. Extirpation
   B. Fragmentation
   C. Inspection
   D. Division

6. How should you code the following procedure? *Aortic valve replacement procedure was discontinued after the initial thoracotomy incision when the patient became hemodynamically unstable.*
   A. 02RF07Z
   B. 0J960ZZ
   C. 02K80ZZ
   D. 0WJC0ZZ

7. What anatomic site determines the body part value in the root operation Release?
   A. The site removed
   B. The site causing constraint
   C. The site cut or transected
   D. The site being freed

8. How should you code the following procedure? *A physician performs a percutaneous placement of chest tube to drain the pleural cavity bilaterally.*
   A. 0W983ZZ
   B. 0W9930Z, 0W9B30Z
   C. 0B9M3ZZ
   D. 0B9N30Z, 0B9P30Z

9. How should you code the following procedure? *A physician performs a percutaneous endoscopic thrombectomy of the left saphenous vein.*
   A. 06CQ4ZZ
   B. 069Q4ZZ
   C. 06FQ4ZZ
   D. 06NQ4ZZ

10. What body part value should be assigned when the root operation Inspection is performed on overlapping layers of the musculoskeletal system?
    A. Assign a body part value for multiple sites.
    B. Assign separate codes with different body part values for each layer accessed.
    C. Assign a body part value for the first layer accessed.
    D. Assign a body part value for the deepest layer reached.

KEEP ON CODING

Instructions: Read the procedural statement, abstract the root operation, then use the appropriate Index and Tables to assign PCS procedure codes. Assign only the root operations discussed in this chapter. Write the code(s) on the line provided.

1. Drainage of right knee fluid, percutaneous. ICD-10-PCS Code(s) _____

2. Endoscopic left internal carotid endarterectomy. ICD-10-PCS Code(s) _____

3. Extracorporeal shockwave lithotripsy (ESWL) of calculus in right ureter. ICD-10-PCS Code(s) _____

4. Release of the right tibial nerve, endoscopic. ICD-10-PCS Code(s) _____

5. Open trigeminal neurotomy. ICD-10-PCS Code(s) _____

6. Arthroscopic examination of left ankle. ICD-10-PCS Code(s) _____

7. Craniotomy with brain mapping, open approach. ICD-10-PCS Code(s) _____

8. Percutaneous drainage of left knee bursa. ICD-10-PCS Code(s) _____

9. Cystoscopy through the urethra with left ureteral stone basketing of ureteral calculi. ICD-10-PCS Code(s) _____

10. Endoscopic lithotripsy of common bile duct stone with access through oral cavity into the upper GI tract. ICD-10-PCS Code(s) _____

11. Frenulotomy to release buccal mucosa in the oral cavity. ICD-10-PCS Code(s) _____

12. Open division of median nerve. ICD-10-PCS Code(s) _____

13. Exploratory laparotomy of the retroperitoneum. ICD-10-PCS Code(s) _____

14. Bundle of His Mapping (conduction mechanism), percutaneous. ICD-10-PCS Code(s) _____

(*continued*)

(continued from page 1095)

15. Drainage of peritoneum via percutaneous Jackson-Pratt drain. ICD-10-PCS Code(s) _____

16. Removal of rusted nail from sole of left foot using forceps. ICD-10-PCS Code(s) _____

17. Percutaneous fragmentation of calculus of right parotid duct. ICD-10-PCS Code(s) _____

18. Percutaneous endoscopic release of the right median nerve. ICD-10-PCS Code(s) _____

19. Drainage of neck abscess, open approach. ICD-10-PCS Code(s) _____

20. Percutaneous endoscopic hemilaminotomy of phrenic nerve. ICD-10-PCS Code(s) _____

21. Arthroscopy of right shoulder joint. ICD-10-PCS Code(s) _____

22. Division of chordae tendineae, percutaneous endoscopic. ICD-10-PCS Code(s) _____

23. Removal of popcorn kernel from right nostril (nasal mucosa and soft tissue) using forceps. ICD-10-PCS Code(s) _____

24. Arthroscopy of left knee joint. ICD-10-PCS Code(s) _____

25. Gastrolysis, open release of the stomach. ICD-10-PCS Code(s) _____

CODING CHALLENGE

Instructions: Read the mini-medical-record of each patient's encounter, then abstract, assign, and arrange ICD-10-CM diagnosis codes and PCS procedure codes using the appropriate Index and Tables. Write the code(s) on the line provided.

1. INPATIENT HOSPITAL   Gender: M   Age: 52

Preprocedure diagnosis: Left patellar chondromalacia, bilateral osteoarthritis of hips

Procedure: Left knee arthroscopy with lateral capsular release. After inflation of the tourniquet, ports were placed. Visualization of patellofemoral joint revealed type 2 chondromalacia with slight lateral subluxation. The anteromedial portal was used to identify the lateral capsule and it was released using the Excise PDW Plasma Wand. Instruments were removed, portals closed, and the tourniquet released.

2 ICD-10-CM Codes _____

1 ICD-10-PCS Code _____

2. INPATIENT HOSPITAL   Gender: F   Age: 74

Preprocedure diagnosis: Left malignant pleural effusion secondary to a left lung adenocarcinoma

Procedure: Thoracentesis at bedside. After infiltrating the skin with an anesthetic, an incision was made below the 6th rib and meticulously dissected to the pleural space. A serosanguineous effusion was encountered and a Yankauer suction tip used to drain the fluid. A portable chest x-ray showed a significant decrease in the effusion.

2 ICD-10-CM Codes _____

1 ICD-10-PCS Code _____

3. INPATIENT HOSPITAL   Gender: F   Age: 59

Preprocedure diagnosis: Streptococcal cellulitis, left foot, status post left foot incision and drainage, status post left foot Austin bunionectomy

Procedure: Left foot, incision and drainage and delayed primary closure. The two sutures at the previous incision site were removed and the site opened. The incision was deepened and frank purulence noted at the fascia level. This was drained and the incision irrigated. We decided to leave the wound open to try clear this infection up.

3 ICD-10-CM Codes _____

_____

1 ICD-10-PCS Code _____

4. INPATIENT HOSPITAL   Gender: M   Age: 70

Preprocedure diagnosis: Carotid artery stenosis, 80% on right and 50% on left, ASHD, hypertension

Procedure: Right common carotid artery endarterectomy. Incision made on the right side of the neck to expose the carotid artery. The artery was clamped above the blocked area and the area incised. The plaque was removed from the artery and the artery closed. Clamp released, showing excellent flow. The neck incision was closed and the patient taken to the recovery room.

3 ICD-10-CM Codes _____

_____

1 ICD-10-PCS Code _____

5. INPATIENT HOSPITAL   Gender: F   Age: 53

Preprocedure diagnosis: Surveillance EGD for history of esophageal cancer, surveillance colonoscopy for history of adenomatous colonic polyps

Procedure: Esophagogastroduodenoscopy, colonoscopy with polypectomy. The endoscope was passed through the oral cavity under direct visualization and advanced to the second portion of the duodenum. Findings are consistent with esophagectomy colonic transposition. The patient was turned and an Olympus colonoscope was passed through the anal verge under direct visualization. Cecum, ascending and descending colon revealed melanosis coli. Two sessile polyps of the transverse colon were removed by cold forceps and sent to pathology.

Postprocedure diagnosis: Diffuse melanosis coli, transverse colon polyps, no abnormal findings on EGD

Tip: Select the principal procedure using the PCS OGCR D.

5 ICD-10-CM Codes _____

_____

2 ICD-10-PCS Codes _____

6. INPATIENT HOSPITAL   Gender: F   Age: 9

Preprocedure diagnosis: Chronic adenotonsillitis and ankyloglossia

Procedure: Adenoidectomy and tonsillectomy, lingual frenotomy. Metzenbaum scissors were used to free the lingual frenulum. The right tonsil was freed from the anterior pillar and posterior pillar and amputated at the same plane as the tongue base. An adenoid curet was used to remove the adenoid tissue. The same procedure was repeated on the left. Hemostasis was achieved and patient was extubated.

Tip: Each procedure is coded separately.

2 ICD-10-CM Codes _____

3 ICD-10-PCS Codes _____

_____

7. INPATIENT HOSPITAL   Gender: F   Age: 60

Preprocedure diagnosis: Acquired chronic subglottic stenosis from endotracheal intubation

Procedure: Fiber optic bronchoscopy. The bronchoscope was inserted orally and we could see scar tissue and narrowing of the upper trachea just below the vocal cords in the subglottic area. No abnormalities seen of the carina, right upper, middle, and lower lobe bronchi; left main stem bronchus and upper and lower lobe bronchi. No specimens were collected. Patient tolerated the procedure well.

1 ICD-10-CM Code _____

1 ICD-10-PCS Code _____

8. INPATIENT HOSPITAL   Gender: F   Age: 27

Preprocedure diagnosis: Chronic anal fissure with persistent pain and bleeding, old anal sphincter tear

Procedure: Lateral internal sphincterotomy. A linear incision was made from the dentate line to just beyond the anal verge. The dissection was carried out until the internal sphincter and a few fibers of the external sphincter were exposed. Under direct vision, the full thickness of the internal sphincter was divided from the level of the dentate line distally. The incision was closed with a 3-0 chromic catgut suture.

2 ICD-10-CM Codes _____

1 ICD-10-PCS Code _____

9. INPATIENT HOSPITAL   Gender: M   Age: 8

Preprocedure diagnosis: Spastic cerebral palsy, dysarthria

Procedure: Selective dorsal rhizotomy. The spinous processes and a portion of the lamina were removed to expose the spinal cord and spinal nerves at L1. The sensory nerves were exposed and tested with EMG. The severely abnormal roots were cut between L1 and S1/S2. The dura was closed and tissue layers closed up to the skin, which was closed with glue.

Tip: Procedural steps necessary to reach the operative site are not coded separately (PCS OGCR B3.1b).

2 ICD-10-CM Codes _____

1 ICD-10-PCS Code _____

10. INPATIENT HOSPITAL   Gender: M   Age: 3

Preprocedure diagnosis: Esophageal foreign body; patient swallowed a quarter, which lodged in his esophagus, and is having difficulty breathing

Procedure: Esophagoscopy with removal of foreign body. A flexible EGD was performed under general anesthesia. The quarter was seen at the mid esophagus and removed with a grasper. The patient tolerated the procedure well.

1 ICD-10-CM Code _____

1 ICD-10-PCS Code _____

Chapter 53

Section 0: Root Operations 0, 2, 3, 4, G, H, P, Q, R, U, W

Alteration • Change • Control • Creation • Fusion • Insertion • Removal • Repair • Replacement • Supplement • Revision

Chapter Outline

- **Basics of Procedures 0, 2, 3, 4, G, H, P, Q, R, U, and W**
- **Coding Overview of Root Operations 0, 2, 3, 4, G, H, P, Q, R, U, and W**
- **Abstracting for Root Operations 0, 2, 3, 4, G, H, P, Q, R, U, and W**
- **Assigning Characters 4–7 for Root Operations 0, 2, 3, 4, G, H, P, Q, R, U, and W**
- **Arranging Codes for Root Operations 0, 2, 3, 4, G, H, P, Q, R, U, and W**

Learning Objectives

After completing this chapter, you should have the skills to:

53.1 Spell and define the key words, medical terms, and abbreviations related to procedures 0, 2, 3, 4, G, H, P, Q, R, U, and W. (Remember)

53.2 Identify the types of procedures that always involve a device, that define other repairs, and that define other objectives. (Apply)

53.3 Adhere to ICD-10-PCS coding guidelines related to root operations Alteration, Change, Control, Creation, Fusion, Insertion, Removal, Repair, Replacement, Supplement, and Revision. (Apply)

53.4 Examine and abstract procedural information from the medical record for coding for the root operations 0, 2, 3, 4, G, H, P, Q, R, U, and W. (Analyze)

53.5 Demonstrate how to assign codes for the root operations 0, 2, 3, 4, G, H, P, Q, R, U, and W. (Apply)

53.6 Utilize guidelines for arranging (sequencing) codes for root operations 0, 2, 3, 4, G, H, P, Q, R, U, and W. (Apply)

Key Term and Abbreviation

cervical
free skin graft
postprocedural bleeding

In addition to the key term listed here, students should know the terms defined within tables in this chapter.

INTRODUCTION

When repairing a car, sometimes a part must be removed and replaced with an identical one, and other times modifications or repairs can be made to the original part so it functions properly. Mechanical devices are frequently used to take the place of or augment a body part. The root operations discussed in this chapter include procedures that always involve a device.

This chapter discusses three groups of Medical and Surgical root operations:

- Procedures That Always Involve a Device (2, H, P, R, U, W)
- Procedures That Define Other Repairs (3, Q)
- Procedures That Define Other Objectives (0, 4, G)

Although the root operations within each group share a common purpose, each has a unique aspect that makes it different from the other procedures in the same group. Pay careful attention to the differences between each root operation so that you can use each confidently and accurately.

BASICS OF PROCEDURES 0, 2, 3, 4, G, H, P, Q, R, U, AND W

This section introduces each root operation group and provides definitions and examples of each root operation. Details are discussed as you progress through this chapter. Some terms, such as *removal* and *repair*, can be associated with more than one root operation. There is no direct match between a specific procedural term and a root operation. Some medical terms, such as *excision* and *removal*, can be associated with more than one root operation. Root operations are assigned based on the content of the operative report regarding what was actually performed, not on the terms used by the physician in documentation. Physicians are not required to document using PCS terminology. Coders must read the medical record and interpret it using official PCS definitions.

Refer to detailed anatomic diagrams of specific organ systems in Chapters 8–43 of this text, or in external references, when you need to refresh your memory of human anatomy.

Basics of Procedures That Always Involve a Device

Procedures that always involve a medical device in or on a body part do not involve changes to the body part itself. Assign an additional code to identify the type of treatment to the body part if it is treated in addition to the procedure related to the device. The root operations in this group always involve a device, by definition. This differs from the use of Character 6, Device with other root operations in that other root operations do not always involve a device. For example, insertion, replacement, or repair of a pacemaker, by definition, always involves a device—a pacemaker. The reduction of a fracture might or might not involve a fixation device.

Refer to ■ TABLE 53-1 for the definitions, values, and procedural terms commonly used with the root operations Change (2), Insertion (H), Replacement (R), Removal (P), Supplement (U), and Revision (W).

Table 53-1 ■ **ROOT OPERATIONS THAT ALWAYS INVOLVE A DEVICE**

Root Operation	Value	Definition	Terms
Change	2	Taking out or off a device from a body part and putting back an identical or similar device in or on the same body part without cutting or puncturing the skin or a mucous membrane	Replace, exchange
Insertion	H	Putting in a nonbiological appliance that monitors, assists, performs, or prevents a physiological function but does not physically take the place of a body part	Insert, install, place
Removal	P	Taking out or off a device from a body part	Remove, take out
Replacement	R	Putting in or on biological or synthetic material that physically takes the place and/or function of all or a portion of a body part	Joint replacement, arthroplasty, replace, exchange
Supplement	U	Putting in or on biological or synthetic material that physically reinforces and/or augments the function of a portion of a body part	Reinforce, supplement
Revision	W	Correcting, to the extent possible, a portion of a malfunctioning device or the position of a displaced device	Revise, correct, replace

Source: © PB Resources, Inc. Used with permission.

Basics of Procedures That Define Other Repairs

Two root operations in the group *Procedures that define other repairs* identify unrelated repair procedures that are not described by other root operation groups (■ TABLE 53-2).

Table 53-2 ■ **ROOT OPERATIONS THAT DEFINE OTHER REPAIRS**

Root Operation	Value	Definition	Terms
Control	3	Stopping, or attempting to stop, postprocedural or other acute bleeding	Control
Repair	Q	Restoring, to the extent possible, a body part to its normal anatomic structure and function	Repair, suture

Source: © PB Resources, Inc. Used with permission.

Basics of Procedures That Define Other Objectives

Three root operations in the group *Procedures that define other objectives* identify unrelated procedures that are not described by the objectives of other root operation groups (■ TABLE 53-3).

When reading medical terms related to procedures in this chapter, remember that the same suffix can describe a wide variety of procedures and multiple root operations. Although terms ending with *-ectomy* most often identify procedures coded with the root operation Excision or Resection, they could also identify procedures coded with Extirpation, Extraction, Destruction, or Alteration. The suffix *-plasty* can identify procedures coded with the root operations Repair, Replacement, Supplement, Reposition, Alteration, and Excision. Refer to ■ TABLE 53-4 for a refresher on how to build medical terms related to procedures discussed in this chapter.

This section provides a general reference to help understand the most common procedures that always involve a device, as well as procedures that define other repairs and other objectives. Remember to keep standard reference books handy in case you get stuck.

Table 53-3 ■ ROOT OPERATIONS THAT DEFINE OTHER OBJECTIVES

Root Operation	Value	Definition	Terms
Alteration	0	Modifying the anatomic structure of a body part without affecting the function of the body part	Liposuction, face lift
Creation	4	Putting in or on biological or synthetic material to form a new body part that to the extent possible replicates the anatomic structure or function of an absent body part	Transgender operation, valve creation
Fusion	G	Joining together portions of an articular body part, rendering the articular body part immobile	Arthrodesis, fusion

Source: © PB Resources, Inc. Used with permission.

CODING CAUTION

Be alert for root operations that have similar English meanings but different PCS definitions.

Insertion (H) (*Putting in a nonbiological appliance that* <u>*monitors, assists, performs, or prevents*</u> *a physiological function but does not physically take the place of a body part*) and **Supplement (U)** (*Putting in or on biological or synthetic material that* <u>*physically reinforces and/ or augments*</u> *the function of a portion of a body part*)

Removal (P) (*Taking out or off* <u>*a device from*</u> *a body part*) and **Resection (T)** (*Cutting out or off without replacement* <u>*all of a body part*</u>)

Table 53-4 ■ EXAMPLE OF CONSTRUCTING MEDICAL TERMS FOR PROCEDURES 0, 2, 3, 4, G, H, P, Q, R, U, AND W

Combining Form	Suffix	Complete Medical Term
stomat/o (*mouth*)	-rrhaphy (*suturing*) -plasty (*surgical repair*)	stomato + rrhaphy (*suturing of the mouth*) tendono + rrhaphy (*suturing of a tendon*) spleno + rrhaphy (*suturing of the spleen*)
tendon /o (*tendon*)		stomato + plasty (*surgical repair of the mouth*) tendono + plasty (*surgical repair of a tendon*) spleno + plasty (*surgical repair of the spleen*)
splen/o (*spleen*)		

Source: © PB Resources, Inc. Used with permission.

CODING PRACTICE

Exercise 53.1 Basics of Procedures 0, 2, 3, 4, G, H, P, Q, R, U, and W

Instructions: Use your medical terminology skills and resources to define the following procedures, then identify the code(s) or code range listed in the PCS Index. Follow these steps:

- Use slash marks "/" to break down the underlined term into its root(s) and suffix.
- Define the meaning of the word based on the meaning of each word part.
- Look up the phrase in the ICD-10-PCS Index, and write down the name(s) of the root operation(s) the Index cross-references you to and the Table(s), if provided.
- Do not assign any codes.

CODING PRACTICE (continued)

Example: conjunctivoplasty conjunctivo/plasty	Meaning *surgical repair of the lining of the eyelids*	PCS Root Operation(s)/Table(s) *Repair 08Q, Replacement 08R*
1. epididymorrhaphy	Meaning _____	PCS Root Operation(s)/Table(s) _____
2. acromioplasty	Meaning _____	PCS Root Operation(s)/Table(s) _____
3. diaphragmatic pacemaker lead	Meaning _____	PCS Root Operation(s)/Table(s) _____
4. neurostimulator generator	Meaning _____	PCS Root Operation(s)/Table(s) _____
5. epiphysiodesis	Meaning _____	PCS Root Operation(s)/Table(s) _____
6. genioplasty	Meaning _____	PCS Root Operation(s)/Table(s) _____
7. canthorrhaphy	Meaning _____	PCS Root Operation(s)/Table(s) _____
8. costosternoplasty	Meaning _____	PCS Root Operation(s)/Table(s) _____
9. esophagocoloplasty	Meaning _____	PCS Root Operation(s)/Table(s) _____
10. intraluminal device, endotracheal airway	Meaning _____	PCS Root Operation(s)/Table(s) _____

CODING GUIDELINES FOR ROOT OPERATIONS 0, 2, 3, 4, G, H, P, Q, R, U, AND W

The PCS OGCR provide several guidelines specific to the root operations discussed in this chapter. A general guideline related to the root operation Control is discussed below. Guidelines specific to Characters 4–7 are discussed later in this chapter. Refer to the PCS OGCR for additional details and clinical examples of each guideline.

The definition of the root operation Control is *stopping, or attempting to stop, postprocedural or other acute bleeding*. Postprocedural bleeding, also called postoperative bleeding or hemorrhage, is bleeding that occurs after a surgical procedure. It may occur immediately or be delayed. Common causes are a deficient clotting mechanism in the blood or loose clips or ties around blood vessels. An initial attempt to control postoperative bleeding might be unsuccessful and require that a more definitive root operation—such as Bypass, Detachment, Excision, Extraction, Reposition, Replacement, or Resection—be performed. In this situation, code only the more definitive root operation. Assign the root operation Control only when a more definitive procedure is not performed (PCS OGCR B3.7).

The procedure codes in the general Anatomical Regions body systems (**W, X, Y**) can be used when the procedure is performed on an anatomical region rather than a specific body part. The root operation **Control** is coded to an Anatomical Region rather than a specific anatomic site OPCS OGCR B2.1a).

ABSTRACTING FOR ROOT OPERATIONS 0, 2, 3, 4, G, H, P, Q, R, U, AND W

Abstracting for PCS focuses on identifying the correct root operation, which involves reading the operative report and interpreting it in light of root operation definitions. When reading the operative report, remember to focus on the objective of the procedure and the activities performed, not specific medical terms.

Many times the root operation can be determined conclusively during abstracting. Other times the root operation can be narrowed down to two options, which must be differentiated based on other characters that are assigned from the PCS Tables. The root operation identifies the functional objective of the procedure and may be influenced by the anatomic site. The following information summarizes the objectives, definitions, unique features, and examples of root operations discussed in this chapter.

A table that outlines the Key Criteria to Abstracting Root Operations appears for each root operation group to help distinguish among procedures in the group. Refer to Tables 47-2 and 47-3 for general guidance on abstracting PCS procedures and root operation groups. A guided example of abstracting for the root operations Fusion, Insertion, and Resection is presented. Refer to Chapter 49 of this text for a refresher on the root operation Resection.

Abstracting for Procedures That Always Involve a Device

The following information summarizes the objectives, definitions, unique features, examples, and Key Criteria for Abstracting Root Operations for *Procedures that always involve a device*. Differences among root operations in this group include whether the device is put in, taken out, or repaired. Root operations are also distinguished based on whether the device augments the function of a body part or replaces it entirely.

Abstracting for Change (2)

The objective of the root operation Change is exchanging a device without cutting or puncturing. The site of the procedure is in or on a body part. The approach is always External. When any other approach is used, assign a root operation that identifies what was done. For example, when the skin is cut or punctured to take out a device and put in a new one, assign two root operations—Removal and Replacement.

Examples of Change are urinary catheter change, in which a catheter is removed from the urethra and a different one put

Table 53-5 ■ EXAMPLES OF THE ROOT OPERATION CHANGE (2)

Organ System	Procedural Examples
Digestive	Gastrostomy tube change
Genitourinary	Foley catheter exchange
Musculoskeletal	Exchange of drainage tube in a joint
Respiratory	Tracheostomy tube exchange, change chest tube for left pneumothorax

Source: © PB Resources, Inc. Used with permission.

in, and drainage tube change, in which a drainage tube is pulled out and a different one put into the existing access site without cutting or puncturing the skin (■ TABLE 53-5).

Abstracting for Insertion (H)

The objective of the root operation Insertion is putting in a non-biological device. The site of the procedure is in or on a body part.

The root operation Insertion represents those procedures where the sole objective is to put in a device without doing anything else to a body part. Procedures typical of those coded to Insertion include putting in a vascular catheter, a pacemaker lead, or a tissue expander. Imaging guidance done to assist in the performance of a procedure can be coded separately in the Imaging section (Section B).

Examples of Insertion are insertion of radioactive implant—in which radioactive seeds are implanted into a body part, usually to treat cancer—or insertion of a central venous catheter, in which a tube is inserted into a large vein in the arm or chest to deliver medicines, fluids, nutrients, or blood products over a long period of time (■ TABLE 53-6).

Abstracting for Removal (P)

The objective of the root operation Removal is taking out a device. The site of the procedure is in or on a body part. When the device is taken out by cutting or puncturing the skin, or

Table 53-6 ■ EXAMPLES OF THE ROOT OPERATION INSERTION (H)

Organ System	Procedural Examples
Cardiovascular	Insertion of central venous catheter, pacemaker insertion, percutaneous replacement of broken pacemaker lead in left atrium
Genitourinary	Insertion of urinary catheter, placement of brachytherapy seeds in prostate gland
Integumentary	Percutaneous placement of intrathecal infusion pump in the subcutaneous tissue of the back for pain management
Musculoskeletal	Placement of bone growth stimulator
Nervous	Insertion of spinal neurostimulator generator to replace old neurostimulator
Respiratory	Insertion of brachytherapy seeds in bronchus
Special Senses (Ear, Eye)	Insertion of multiple-channel cochlear implant

Source: © PB Resources, Inc. Used with permission.

Table 53-7 ■ EXAMPLES OF THE ROOT OPERATION REMOVAL (P)

Organ System	Procedural Examples
Cardiovascular	Removal of a broken pacemaker lead, removal of cardiac pacemaker, nonincisional removal of Swan-Ganz catheter
Digestive	Nonincisional PEG tube removal
Genitourinary	Transvaginal removal of brachytherapy seeds, endoscopic retrieval of ureteral stent
Musculoskeletal	Removal of arm or leg external fixation device, incision with removal of K-wire fixation
Nervous	Removal of an old neurostimulator generator
Respiratory	Extubation of endotracheal tube, removal of nasogastric drainage tube

Source: © PB Resources, Inc. Used with permission.

taken out and not replaced, assign the root operation Removal. Distinguish Removal from similar root operations as follows:

- Replacement: Assign this root operation when the device is replaced.
- Change: Assign this root operation when a device is taken out and a similar device put in without cutting or puncturing the skin or mucous membrane.

Examples of Removal are drainage tube removal and cardiac pacemaker removal (■ TABLE 53-7).

Abstracting for Replacement (R)

The objective of the root operation Replacement is putting in a device that replaces a body part. The site of the procedure is some or all of a body part. The body part may have been taken out or replaced previously, or may be taken out, physically eradicated, or rendered nonfunctional during the Replacement procedure. When a device that was put in during a previous encounter is taken out, assign the root operation Removal.

Replacement encompasses a wide range of procedures, from joint replacements to grafts of all kinds. Examples of Replacement are a total hip replacement—in which all or part of the native acetabulofemoral joint (*the joint between the ball of the femur [thigh] and acetabulum [hip socket]*) is replaced with synthetic substitutes—or a **free skin graft**, in which a section of skin is replaced with skin from another area of the body, donor skin, or a synthetic substitute (■ TABLE 53-8).

Table 53-8 ■ EXAMPLES OF THE ROOT OPERATION REPLACEMENT (R)

Organ System	Procedural Examples
Cardiovascular	Excision of abdominal aorta with Gore-Tex graft replacement, mitral valve replacement
Integumentary	Free skin graft, mastectomy with insertion of saline breast implants, mastectomy with free TRAM flap reconstruction
Musculoskeletal	Joint replacement, excision of diseased bone with bone graft
Special Senses (Ear, Eye)	Prosthetic lens implantation

Source: © PB Resources, Inc. Used with permission.

A free skin differs from a pedicle graft, which is coded to the root operation Transfer because the vascular and nervous supply remains intact.

Abstracting for Supplement (U)

The objective of the root operation Supplement is putting in a device that reinforces or augments a body part. The site of the procedure is in or on a body part.

The biological material is nonliving or is living and from the same individual. The body part may have been previously replaced, with the Supplement procedure being performed to physically reinforce or augment the function of the replaced body part.

Examples of Supplement are a herniorrhaphy using mesh—in which a displaced or defective muscle is repositioned and reinforced with a mesh patch—and putting a new acetabular liner in a previous hip replacement, in which a new liner is put in to update a liner from a previous hip replacement procedure (■ TABLE 53-9). Replacing the acetabular liner is not coded to Replacement because Replacement identifies the replacement of a body part. It is not coded to the root operation Change because Change is used only when no cutting is performed, but an incision must be made to replace the joint liner. It is not coded to Revision because no adjustments are made to the existing liner.

Abstracting for Revision (W)

The objective of the root operation Revision is correcting a malfunctioning or displaced device. The site of the procedure is in or on a body part.

Revision can include correcting a malfunctioning or displaced device by taking out or putting in components of the device such as a screw or pin.

Examples of Revision are adjusting the position of pacemaker lead and recementing of a hip prosthesis (■ TABLE 53-10).

Table 53-9   ■   EXAMPLES OF THE ROOT OPERATION SUPPLEMENT (U)

Organ System	Procedural Examples
Cardiovascular	Mitral valve ring annuloplasty
Genitourinary	Colporrhaphy with Gynemesh
Musculoskeletal	Hernia with Marlex plug, resurfacing procedure on femoral head, replacement of joint liner in previous joint replacement
Nervous	Free nerve graft

Source: © PB Resources, Inc. Used with permission.

Table 53-10   ■   EXAMPLES OF THE ROOT OPERATION REVISION (W)

Organ System	Procedural Examples
Cardiovascular	Adjusting the position of pacemaker lead, repositioning of Swan-Ganz catheter
Musculoskeletal	Recementing of joint prosthesis, replacement of screw in a fracture plate

Source: © PB Resources, Inc. Used with permission.

Table 53-11   ■   KEY CRITERIA FOR ABSTRACTING ROOT OPERATIONS THAT ALWAYS INVOLVE A DEVICE

Question	Root Operation (Value)
❏ Did the procedure involve an external device left in place in, on, or in replacement of a body part?	If *No*, do not use the root operations in this group.
Answer *Yes* to one of the following questions to help distinguish root operations 2, H, P, R, U, and W	
❏ Was a device exchanged without cutting or puncturing the skin?	Change (2)
❏ Was a nonbiological device put in or on a body part?	Insertion (H)
❏ Was a device taken out and not replaced?	Removal (P)
❏ Was a device taken out by cutting or puncturing the skin?	
❏ Was a device put in to replace a body part?	Replacement (R)
❏ Was a device put in to reinforce or augment a body part?	Supplement (U)
❏ Was a malfunctioning or displaced device corrected?	Revision (W)

Source: © PB Resources, Inc. Used with permission.

Key Criteria for Abstracting Root Operations 2, H, P, R, U, and W

Refer to ■ TABLE 53-11 for more specific guidance on how to abstract *Procedures that always take out a device* and distinguish among root operations in this group.

Abstracting for Procedures That Define Other Repairs

The root operation group *Procedures that define other repairs* consists of procedures that do not fit in any of the other root operation groups. The root operation Control is very specific and is used in a narrow range of circumstances. The other root operation in this group, Repair, is very general and is used to code for procedures not classified by other root operations.

Abstracting for Control (3)

The objective of the root operation Control is stopping or attempting to stop postprocedural or other acute bleeding. The site of the procedure is an anatomic region rather than a specific body part. Control is used to represent a small range of procedures and is not coded separately when a more definitive root operation—such as Bypass, Detachment, Excision, Extraction, Reposition, Replacement, or Resection—is performed to stop the bleeding.

> EXAMPLE: *Percutaneous endoscopic resection of the spleen to stop acute bleeding*
> 07TP4ZZ Resection, Spleen, Percutaneous endoscopic approach

An example using the root operation Control for postprocedural bleeding is control of postprostatectomy hemorrhage.

Table 53-12 ■ EXAMPLES OF THE ROOT OPERATION CONTROL (3)

Organ System	Procedural Examples
Cardiovascular	Control of postop hemopericardium
Digestive	Control of bleeding duodenal ulcer
Genitourinary	Control of postprostatectomy hemorrhage, cautery of posthysterectomy oozing and evacuation of clot
Musculoskeletal	Exploration and ligation of postop arterial bleeder in arm, drainage of hemarthrosis at previous operative site
Nervous	Control of intracranial subdural hemorrhage

Source: © PB Resources, Inc. Used with permission.

An example of using the root operation Control for other acute bleeding is control of a bleeding duodenal ulcer (■ TABLE 53-12). Examples given in this text are listed by the organ system in which the original procedure was performed. The root operation Control is always coded to one of the PCS body systems labeled Anatomical Regions. Use procedure codes in body systems for general Anatomical Regions (**W**, **X**, or **Y**) when the procedure is performed on an anatomic region rather than a specific body part or on the rare occasion when no information is available to support assignment of a code to a specific body part (PCS OGCR B2.1a).

Abstracting for Repair (Q)

The objective of the root operation Repair is restoring a body part to its normal structure. The site of the procedure is some or all of a body part.

Use the root operation Repair only when the method to accomplish the repair is not defined by another root operation. The root operation Repair represents a broad range of procedures for restoring the anatomic structure of a body part, such as suture of lacerations. Repair also functions as a general root operation, to be used when the procedure performed does not meet the definition of one of the other root operations.

Examples of Repair are a herniorrhaphy—in which a hernia sac is opened and the contents returned to their normal position and sutured into place without mesh or other supplement—and suture of a laceration (■ TABLE 53-13).

Table 53-13 ■ EXAMPLES OF THE ROOT OPERATION REPAIR (Q)

Organ System	Procedural Examples
Digestive	Colostomy takedown
Genitourinary	Perineoplasty with repair of old obstetric laceration
Musculoskeletal	Suture repair of right biceps tendon laceration, closure of abdominal wall stab wound, herniorrhaphy
Nervous	Repair of nerve laceration

Source: © PB Resources, Inc. Used with permission.

Table 53-14 ■ KEY CRITERIA FOR ABSTRACTING ROOT OPERATIONS THAT DEFINE OTHER REPAIRS

Question	Root Operation (Value)
Answer *Yes* to one of the following questions to help distinguish root operations 3 and Q	
❏ Did the procedure stop or attempt to stop postprocedural or other acute bleeding?	Control (3)
❏ Was another root operation performed to stop postprocedural or other acute bleeding?	Assign a root operation that describes the procedure performed.
❏ Did the procedure restore a body part to its normal structure?	Repair (Q)
❏ Is the procedure more specifically identified by another root operation?	Assign a root operation other than Repair.

Source: © PB Resources, Inc. Used with permission.

Key Criteria for Abstracting Root Operations 3 and Q

Refer to ■ TABLE 53-14 for more specific guidance on how to abstract *Procedures that define other repairs* and distinguish among root operations in this group.

Abstracting for Procedures That Define Other Objectives

The root operation group *Procedures that define other objectives* is a collection of three root operations that are not related to each other. Each root operation is used in very limited and specific situations.

Abstracting for Alteration (0)

The objective of the root operation Alteration is modifying a body part for cosmetic purposes without affecting function. The site of the procedure is some or all of a body part.

The principal purpose is to improve appearance. Alteration is coded for all procedures performed solely to improve appearance. All methods, approaches, and devices used for the objective of improving appearance are coded here. Because some surgical procedures can be performed for either medical or cosmetic purposes, coding for Alteration requires confirmation of the diagnosis to verify that the surgery is performed to improve appearance.

Examples of Alteration are cosmetic face lift and cosmetic breast augmentation (■ TABLE 53-15). Do not use Alteration when these procedures are done for therapeutic rather than cosmetic reasons.

Table 53-15 ■ EXAMPLES OF THE ROOT OPERATION ALTERATION (0)

Organ System	Procedural Examples
Integumentary	Cosmetic liposuction, breast augmentation, face lift
Respiratory	Cosmetic rhinoplasty
Special Senses (Ear, Eye)	Cosmetic blepharoplasty

Source: © PB Resources, Inc. Used with permission.

Table 53-16 ■ EXAMPLES OF THE ROOT OPERATION CREATION (4)

Organ System	Procedural Examples
Cardiovascular	Creation of a congenitally absent atrioventricular valve
Genitourinary	Creation of vagina in a male, creation of penis in a female

Source: © PB Resources, Inc. Used with permission.

Abstracting for Creation (4)

The objective of the root operation Creation is using biologic or synthetic material to form a new body part that replicates the anatomic structure or function of a missing body part. The site of the procedure is either the perineum or a heart valve. No other anatomic sites are used. This root operation is used for gender reassignment surgery and corrective procedures in individuals with congenital anomalies. When a separate procedure is performed to harvest autograft tissue, assign a secondary code for the root operation for the harvesting that describes the work performed, which often is Excision. This code is in addition to the primary procedure for the sex change or valve creation operation.

Examples of Creation are creation of a vagina in a male, creation of a penis in a female, and creation of a congenitally absent missing heart valve (■ TABLE 53-16).

Abstracting for Fusion (G)

The objective of the root operation Fusion is unification or immobilization. The site of the procedure is a joint or other articular body part. No other anatomic sites are used.

The body part is joined together by fixation device, bone graft, or other means. A limited range of procedures is represented in the root operation Fusion because fusion procedures, by definition, are performed only on the joints.

Examples of Fusion are spinal fusion—in which two or more vertebra are joined using hardware or grafts to stabilize them—and ankle arthrodesis, in which the distal tibia, talus, and/or fibula are joined using hardware or grafts (■ TABLE 53-17).

Key Criteria for Abstracting Root Operations G, 0, and 4

Refer to ■ TABLE 53-18 for more specific guidance on how to abstract *Procedures that define other objectives* and distinguish among root operations in this group.

Guided Example of Abstracting for Fusion and Resection

Refer to the following example throughout this chapter to practice skills for abstracting, assigning, and arranging codes for the root operations Fusion, Insertion, and Resection. Similar principles apply to working with other root operations that always involve a device, define other repairs, or define other objectives.

Table 53-17 ■ EXAMPLES OF THE ROOT OPERATION FUSION (G)

Organ System	Procedural Examples
Musculoskeletal	Vertebral fusion, hand fusion, interphalangeal fusion

Source: © PB Resources, Inc. Used with permission.

Table 53-18 ■ KEY CRITERIA FOR ABSTRACTING ROOT OPERATIONS THAT DEFINE OTHER OBJECTIVES

Question	Root Operation (Value)
Answer *Yes* to one of the following questions to help distinguish root operations 0, 4, and G	
❏ Was the procedure for cosmetic purposes only, without affecting the function of a body part?	Alteration (0)
❏ Did the procedure create a new body part that previously did not exist?	Creation (4)
❏ Did the procedure render a joint immobile?	Fusion (G)

Source: © PB Resources, Inc. Used with permission.

INPATIENT HOSPITAL   Gender: M   Age: 27

Preoperative diagnosis: Degenerative disc disease

Procedure: Discectomy with spinal arthrodesis. A vertical incision 11 cm in length was made over L4-L5. The interspace was visualized. All disc material was excised and the area was irrigated. Applied a synthetic bone substitute to the posterior column using the same incision. Fixation plate and screws also were installed through the same incision. Hemostasis was achieved and the incision was closed. Patient was transferred to PACU in stable condition.

Follow along as fictitious coder Marcy Elwood, CCS, abstracts the procedure. Check off each step after you complete it.

▶ Marcy reads through the entire record, paying special attention to the reason for the encounter, the procedure performed, and the postoperative diagnosis.

❏ She notes the preoperative diagnosis of degenerative disc disease.

❏ *What is the stated procedure?* Discectomy with spinal arthrodesis

❏ *What organ or body part is involved?* L4-L5 disc

❏ *Is the procedure description what you would expect based on the name of the procedure?* Yes

❏ *What surgical approach is used?* Open

❏ *Was more than one procedure, or a combined procedure, performed?* Yes, discectomy, arthrodesis, and insertion of fixation device

❏ First, Marcy abstracts for the arthrodesis (■ Table 53-18).

  ▪ *Did the procedure render a joint immobile?* Yes

  ▪ *Was the procedure for cosmetic purposes only, without affecting the function of a body part?* No

  ▪ Insertion of a fixation device is an integral component to arthrodesis, so it will not be coded separately.

❑ Next, Marcy abstracts for the discectomy (Table 49-9).

- *Did the procedure take out some or all of a body part without replacement?* Yes

- *Was removal performed by cutting?* Yes

- *Was all of a body part or only a portion of a body part removed?* The entire disc was removed, and Marcy believes this will equate to all of a PCS body part. She will need to verify this when she refers to the PCS Tables.

- *What is the most likely root operation?* Resection

▶ At this time, Marcy believes that she will use the root operations Fusion and Resection and/or Excision and anticipates that she will need three codes. She will verify this information when she refers to the PCS Tables to assign codes.

CODING PRACTICE

Exercise 53.2 Abstracting for Root Operations 0, 2, 3, 4, G, H, P, Q, R, U, and W

Instructions: Read the mini-medical-record of each patient's encounter and answer the abstracting questions. Write the answer on the line provided. Do not assign any codes.

1. INPATIENT HOSPITAL Gender: F **Age:** 81

Preprocedure diagnosis: Status post-arthroplasty

Procedure: Exchange of drainage tube from right hip joint following total hip replacement

a. What is the stated procedure? _____

b. What body part is involved? _____

c. What is the laterality? _____

d. Is the procedure description what you would expect based on the name of the procedure? _____

e. What surgical approach is used? _____

f. Was more than one procedure, or a combined procedure, performed? _____

g. Did the procedure involve an external device left in place in, on, or in replacement of a body part? _____

h. Was a nonbiological device put in or on a body part? _____

i. Was a device put in to replace a body part? _____

j. Was a device put in to reinforce or augment a body part? _____

k. Was a device exchanged without cutting or puncturing the skin? _____

l. Was a device taken out and not replaced? _____

m. Was a device taken out by cutting or puncturing the skin? _____

n. Was a malfunctioning or displaced device corrected? _____

o. Which root operation(s) should be considered for this procedure? _____ Why? _____

2. INPATIENT HOSPITAL Gender: M Age: 75

Preprocedure diagnosis: Sick sinus syndrome, displaced pacemaker lead

Procedure: Percutaneous adjustment of position of left pacemaker lead in left atrium

a. What is the stated procedure? _____

b. What body part is involved? _____

c. What is the laterality? _____

d. Is the procedure description what you would expect based on the name of the procedure? _____

e. What surgical approach is used? _____

f. Was more than one procedure, or a combined procedure, performed? _____

g. Did the procedure involve an external device left in place in, on, or in replacement of a body part? _____

h. Was a nonbiological device put in or on a body part? _____

i. Was a device put in to replace a body part? _____

j. Was a device put in to reinforce or augment a body part? _____

k. Was a device exchanged without cutting or puncturing the skin? _____

l. Was a device taken out and not replaced? _____

m. Was a device taken out by cutting or puncturing the skin? _____

n. Was a malfunctioning or displaced device corrected? _____

o. Which root operation(s) should be considered for this procedure? _____ Why? _____

CODING PRACTICE (continued)

3. INPATIENT HOSPITAL Gender: F Age: 36

Preprocedure diagnosis: Drooping right upper eyelid affects patient's perception of appearance but does not interfere with vision

Procedure: Cosmetic blepharoplasty. Cut out a crescent of skin and subcutaneous tissue from fold of R eyelid, sutured to restore normal position of eyelid.

a. What is the stated procedure? _____

b. What body part is involved? _____

c. What is the laterality? _____

d. Is the procedure description what you would expect based on the name of the procedure? _____

e. What surgical approach is used? _____

f. Was more than one procedure, or a combined procedure, performed? _____

g. Was the procedure for cosmetic purposes only, without affecting the function of a body part? _____

h. Which root operation(s) should be considered for this procedure? _____ Why? _____

4. INPATIENT HOSPITAL Gender: M Age: 72

Preprocedure diagnosis: Blepharoptosis obscuring vision

Procedure: Bilateral upper blepharoplasty. Cut out a crescent of skin and subcutaneous tissue from fold of R eyelid, sutured to restore normal position of eyelid. Repeated on left side.

a. What is the stated procedure? _____

b. What body part is involved? _____

c. What is the laterality? _____

d. Is the procedure description what you would expect based on the name of the procedure? _____

e. What surgical approach is used? _____

f. Was more than one procedure, or a combined procedure, performed? _____

g. Did the procedure restore a body part to its normal structure? _____

h. Is the procedure more specifically identified by another root operation? _____

i. Which root operation(s) should be considered for this procedure? _____ Why? _____

5. INPATIENT HOSPITAL Gender: M Age: 53

Preprocedure diagnosis: Detached R retina

Procedure: Trans pars plana vitrectomy (TPPV) with synthetic scleral buckle. Made incision in pars plana and used vitreous cutter to remove all vitreous. Injected balanced saline solution (BSS) to replace vitreous. Sutured scleral buckle, which effectively closed the retinal break. Pt tolerated px well.

a. What is the stated procedure? _____

b. What body part is involved? _____

c. What is the laterality? _____

d. Is the procedure description what you would expect based on the name of the procedure? _____

e. What surgical approach is used? _____

f. Was more than one procedure, or a combined procedure, performed? _____

g. Did the first procedure (vitrectomy) take out some or all of a body part without replacement? _____

h. Was a body part or abnormal tissue growth (such as a lesion or tumor) removed? _____

i. Was a foreign object or abnormal material (such as calculus) removed? _____

j. Was the body part replaced with a natural or synthetic substitute? _____

k. Was removal performed by cutting? _____

l. Was removal performed through physical eradication, such as energy, force, or a destructive agent? _____

m. Was removal performed through the use of force, such as pulling or stripping? _____

n. Which root operation(s) should be considered for the first procedure? _____ Why? _____

o. Did the second procedure (application of scleral buckle) involve an external device left in place in, on, or in replacement of a body part? _____

p. Was a nonbiological device put in or on a body part? _____

q. Was a device put in to replace a body part? _____

r. Was a device put in to reinforce or augment a body part? _____

s. Was a device exchanged without cutting or puncturing the skin? _____

t. Was a device taken out and not replaced? _____

(continued)

CODING PRACTICE (continued)

5. (continued)

u. Was a device taken out by cutting or puncturing the skin? _____

v. Was a malfunctioning or displaced device corrected? _____

w. Which root operation(s) should be considered for the second procedure? _____ Why? _____

---

6. INPATIENT HOSPITAL   Gender: F   Age: 68

Preprocedure diagnosis: Bradycardia, malfunctioning pacemaker lead

Procedure: Percutaneous exchange of a malfunctioning pacemaker lead in the left atrium with a new one

a. What is the stated procedure? _____

b. What body part is involved? _____

c. What is the laterality? _____

d. Is the procedure description what you would expect based on the name of the procedure? _____

(continued)

6. (continued)

e. What surgical approach is used? _____

f. Was more than one procedure, or a combined procedure, performed? _____

g. Did the procedure involve an external device left in place in, on, or in replacement of a body part? _____

h. Was a nonbiological device put in or on a body part? _____

i. Was a device put in to replace a body part? _____

j. Was a device put in to reinforce or augment a body part? _____

k. Was a device exchanged without cutting or puncturing the skin? _____

l. Was a device taken out and not replaced? _____

m. Was a device taken out by cutting or puncturing the skin? _____

n. Was a malfunctioning or displaced device corrected? _____

o. Which root operation(s) should be considered for this procedure? _____ Why? _____

ASSIGNING CHARACTERS 4–7 FOR ROOT OPERATIONS 0, 2, 3, 4, G, H, P, Q, R, U, AND W

To assign codes after the root operation is determined, search the PCS Index for the name of the root operation as the Main Term. Locate the subterm(s) for the correct anatomic site and identify the PCS Table. When you locate the PCS Table, verify the first three characters of the code, then locate the row with the body part needed. Assign the remaining characters from each respective column of the Table. The following information summarizes and highlights unique information for working with the Tables for each root operation 0, 2, 3, 4, G, H, P, Q, R, U, and W. Each root operation has one Table in each applicable PCS body system. Because of the differences between organ systems, Table details vary.

In the Index, the Main Term entries for the root operations **Change, Insertion, Removal,** and **Revision** include the phrase **of device in** or **of device from** to clarify that the procedure is performed on a device rather than a body part. Coders must distinguish between Index entries for **Removal** procedures in the Medical and Surgical section (0) and those in the Placement section (2). Medical and Surgical procedures are indexed under the entry **Removal of device from,** whereas procedures in the Placement section use the Main Term

Removal. These entries lead to root operations with different definitions (■ FIGURE 53-1). When coding for the removal of a device from a body part, be certain to select the entry from the Medical and Surgical section, with codes beginning with **0.** Codes from the Placement section begin with **2** and are discussed in Chapter 54 of this text.

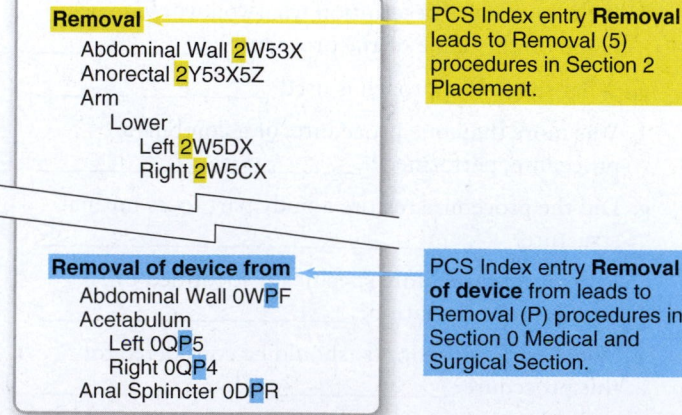

Figure 53-1 ■ PCS Index entries for removal procedures. *Source:* © PB Resources, Inc. Used with permission.

Character 4: Body Part

PCS OGCR provide guidelines for assigning body part values when coding the root operations Control, Change/Revision/ Removal, and Fusion. These are discussed next.

Control Procedures

Control procedures are indexed as **Control of bleeding in** with subterms for the anatomic region. The site of the bleeding is coded using a region within the Anatomical Regions body systems (**W, X, Y**).

Change, Insertion, Revision, and Removal Procedures

A PCS Table might not always provide a specific body part value for the anatomic site treated. Assign a general body part value when the specific body part value is not in the Table. For example, in the Gastrointestinal (D) body system, the general body part values **Upper Intestinal Tract** and **Lower Intestinal Tract** are provided as options for the root operations Change, Insertion, Removal, and Revision. The upper intestinal tract includes from the esophagus down to and including the duodenum. The lower intestinal tract includes from the jejunum down to and including the rectum and anus (PCS OGCR B4.8). ■ FIGURE 53-2 demonstrates how to code the general body part value **0 Upper Intestinal Tract** because Table 0D2 does not provide a specific value for the stomach.

Fusion Procedures

In documentation, a vertebral joint is named based on the vertebra joined, such as C4-C5 for the fusion of the fourth and fifth cervical (*pertaining to the neck*) vertebrae. PCS Tables for the root operation Fusion do not identify the specific vertebral segments but, rather, the overall level of the spine: cervical, thoracic, lumbar, and sacral. Follow these PCS OGCR when assigning body part values for Fusion procedures.

- Assign the body part value that identifies the level of the spine rendered immobile (PCS OGCR B3.10a). PCS Tables provide distinct body part values for a single vertebral joint and multiple vertebral joints at each spinal level. Tables also provide values for joints that link sections of the spine, such as cervicothoracic and sacrococcygeal.

- When multiple vertebral joints are fused, a separate procedure is coded for each vertebral joint at the same level that uses a different device or qualifier (PCS OGCR B3.10b). For example, when two joints are fused, one using posterior approach, anterior column and one using posterior approach, posterior column, assign two codes. In ■ FIGURE 53-3, although two cervical joints

Surgeon removed a feeding gastrostomy tube and replaced it with a new one using the existing stoma in the stomach.

0D20XUZ Medical and Surgical, Gastrointestinal System, Change device in, Upper intestinal tract, External, Feeding device, No qualifier

Figure 53-2 ■ Example of assigning a general body part value. *Source: © PB Resources, Inc. Used with permission.*

Surgeon performed spinal fusion on C3-C4 using an open posterior approach, anterior column and C4-C5 using an open posterior approach, posterior column. Autologous tissue was used for both procedures.

0RG107J Medical and Surgical, Upper Joints, Fusion, Cervical Vertebral Joint, Open, Autologous tissue substitute, Posterior approach, anterior column
0RG1071 Medical and Surgical, Upper Joints, Fusion, Cervical Vertebral Joint, Open, Autologous tissue substitute, Posterior approach, posterior column

Figure 53-3 ■ Example of coding multiple fusion procedures at the same level. *Source: © PB Resources, Inc. Used with permission.*

are treated, the body part value for each code is **Cervical Vertebral Joint**, not **Cervical Vertebral Joints, 2 or more**. Each code describes the procedure on only one joint. Likewise, when different values are used for Character 5, Approach or Character 6, Device assign separate codes.

Character 5: Approach

The root operations Change and Fusion have special considerations regarding Character 5.

The root operation Change always uses the approach External because the definition of the procedure is **Taking out or off a device from a body part and putting back an identical or similar device in or on the same body part without cutting or puncturing the skin or a mucous membrane**. When the exchange of a device requires cutting or puncturing, assign two root operations: Removal and Insertion.

In the root operation Fusion, Character 5 describes the surgical approach as open, percutaneous, and so on, as it does in other PCS codes. Character 7, Qualifier describes the directional approach—from the back, a posterior approach, or from the front, an anterior approach—and the anatomic site on the spinal column, that is, the posterior or anterior side of the vertebra. Refer to Chapter 35 of this text for a refresher on the approaches for spinal procedures.

Character 6: Device

Six of the root operations discussed in this chapter always involve a device, so Character 6 is frequently used to identify the specific device or type of device involved (■ TABLE 53-19 page 1110).

The root operations Change, Removal, and Revision describe procedures performed on a device only and not on a body part. Code the procedure on the device to the appropriate root operation based on the definition of each root operation (PCS OGCR B6.1c).

Occasionally, a device is inserted and intended to remain after the procedure is completed, but requires immediate removal before the end of the operative episode. For example, a device might be removed immediately if it is the wrong size or a complication occurs. When this happens, assign two codes, one for the root operation Insertion and a second code for the root operation Removal to describe the entire process.

Table 53-19 ■ **EXAMPLES OF DEVICES IDENTIFIED BY CHARACTER 6**

- ❏ Artificial sphincter
- ❏ Autologous tissue substitute
- ❏ Contraceptive device
- ❏ Feeding device
- ❏ Hearing device, single-channel cochlear prosthesis
- ❏ Infusion device
- ❏ Internal fixation device
- ❏ Intraluminal device, pessary
- ❏ Monitoring device
- ❏ Monitoring electrode
- ❏ Neurostimulator lead
- ❏ Pacemaker, single-chamber rate responsive
- ❏ Radioactive element
- ❏ Spacer
- ❏ Spinal stabilization device, interspinous process
- ❏ Tissue expander
- ❏ Tracheostomy device

Source: © PB Resources, Inc. Used with permission.

CODING CAUTION

Character values, including device values, can vary among PCS Tables for different root operations and body systems. Although many letter and number values have consistent meanings across most Tables in the Medical and Surgical section, they can have different meanings in different tables. For example, the value **4** for Character 6, Device identifies a single chamber pacemaker in Table 0JH, a bone conduction hearing device in Table 09H, and an autologous tissue substitute in Table 0QP.

The root operation Creation uses Character 6 to identify the type of material used to create the new anatomic structure as autologous tissue, nonautologous tissue, zooplastic tissue, or synthetic substitute.

Fusion Devices

The root operation Fusion uses Character 6 to identify the type of tissue or tissue substitute used to render a vertebral joint immobile. PCS OGCR B3.10c provides the following guidance regarding how to assign Character 6 when combinations of devices and materials are used on the same vertebral joint:

- Interbody fusion device—When an interbody fusion device is used to render the joint immobile, alone or in combination with another material such as a bone graft, use the device value **Interbody Fusion Device**.
- Bone graft—When bone graft is the only device used to render the joint immobile, assign device value **Nonautologous Tissue Substitute** or **Autologous Tissue Substitute** as appropriate.

- Mixture of tissue substitutes—Code a combination of autologous and nonautologous bone graft used to render the joint immobile with the device value **Autologous Tissue Substitute**. Code the use of both autologous bone graft and bone bank bone graft with the device value **Autologous Tissue Substitute**.
- Bone dowel interbody fusion device—Code fusion of a vertebral joint using a bone dowel interbody fusion device made of cadaver bone and packed with a mixture of local morsellized bone and demineralized bone matrix with the device value **Interbody Fusion Device**.

Insertion of a fixation device is an integral component to a fusion procedure, so it is not coded separately (PCS OGCR B3.1b). Code only the Fusion procedure when a fixation device is used in addition to another means of fixation, such as a bone graft.

Insertion, Reposition, and Replacement Devices

Although some PCS device values are very specific, in other cases they are more general, representing an entire family of devices. A device can have a specific value in a Table for one root operation and body system and a more general value in the Table for another root operation or body system. For example, in PCS Table 02P, a cardiac pacemaker lead has the device value **J** and a cardiac defibrillator lead has the Device value **K**. However, in PCS Table 02H, the device value **M Cardiac Lead** identifies any type of cardiac lead, including both a pacemaker lead and a defibrillator lead. The Device Aggregation Table, located in the PCS coding manual appendix, identifies when this situation occurs. It provides a cross-walk of the specific device type to the more general Character 6, Device value needed in some PCS Tables (■ Figure 53-4).

When the documentation specifies a brand name device that you are uncertain how to code, you often can look up the brand name in the Index to obtain a cross-reference to the correct Character 6, Device value. The PCS coding manual provides several tables in the appendix to help identify devices: the Device Key, Device Aggregation Table, and Device Definitions.

Character 7: Qualifier

As discussed earlier in this chapter, the root operation Fusion uses Character 7 to specify whether a vertebral joint fusion uses an anterior or posterior approach and whether the anterior or posterior column of the spine is fused. Other uses of the qualifier with root operations discussed in this chapter include:

- Identify the source of autologous tissue in a graft or fusion procedure (■ Figure 53-5)
- Distinguish whether a prosthetic joint is cemented or uncemented
- Indicate the use of a partial- or full-thickness graft in skin graft procedures
- Specify the structure involved in the creation of a new body part
- Provide greater specificity of the anatomic site

Guided Example of Assigning Characters 4–7 for Fusion and Resection

To practice skills for assigning codes for the root operations Fusion and Resection, continue with the example from earlier in the chapter about a patient who was seen for a lumbar discectomy and spinal fusion. Follow along in your ICD-10-PCS manual as Marcy Elwood, CCS, assigns codes. Check off each step after you complete it.

▶ First, Marcy confirms the procedures: discectomy with spinal arthrodesis and internal fixation device.

❏ The root operation for the arthrodesis is Fusion.

❏ The root operation for the discectomy is Resection or Excision.

▶ Marcy searches the Index for the Main Term **Fusion** for the arthrodesis.

❏ She locates the first-level subterm **Lumbar vertebral**.

❏ She identifies the Table **0SG** and partial code **0SG0**.

▶ Marcy turns to Table **0SG** to assign the code for arthrodesis.

❏ She reads the Table title **0SG, Medical and Surgical, Lower Joints, Fusion** and confirms that this accurately describes the body system and root operation.

❏ Marcy assigns the value for Character 4, Body Part.

  ▪ She reviews the values provided and confirms that **0 Lumbar vertebral**, which was part of the partial code **0SG0** provided in the Index, is correct.

Specific Device	for Operation	in Body System	General Device
Cardiac Lead, Defibrillator	Insertion	Heart and Great Vessels	M Cardiac Lead
Cardiac Lead, Pacemaker	Insertion	Heart and Great Vessels	M Cardiac Lead
Cardiac Resynchronization Defibrillator Pulse Generator	Insertion	Subcutaneous Tissue and Fascia	P Cardiac Rhythm Related Device
Cardiac Resynchronization Pacemaker Pulse Generator	Insertion	Subcutaneous Tissue and Fascia	P Cardiac Rhythm Related Device

One general Device value in a PCS Table might be used to report several different types of specific devices.

Figure 53-4 ■ Example of PCS coding manual appendix "Device Aggregation Table". *Source: Annotations © PB Resources, Inc. Used with permission.*

Section	0	Medical and Surgical
Body System	H	Skin and Breast
Operation	R	Replacement: Putting in or on biological or synthetic material that physically takes the place and/or function of all or a portion of a Body Part

Body Part Character 4	Approach Character 5	Device Character 6	Qualifier Character 7
T Breast, Right U Breast, Left V Breast, Bilateral	0 Open	7 Autologous Tissue Substitute	5 Latissimus Dorsi Myocutaneous Flap 6 Transverse Rectus Abdominis Myocutaneous Flap 7 Deep Inferior Epigastric Artery Perforator Flap 8 Superficial Inferior Epigastric Artery Flap 9 Gluteal Artery Perforator Flap Z No Qualifier

Figure 53-5 ■ Example of using Character 7 to identify the source of autologous tissue.

- The second value for the lumbar spine is **Lumbar vertebral joints, 2 or more.** L4 and L5 comprise one joint, which is the joint being fused. If the fusion was L4-L5 and L5-L6, the value for two or more joints would be used.

- There is also an option for Lumbosacral joint, which does not apply to this case.

❏ Marcy assigns the value **0 Open** for Character 5, Approach because an incision was made and there is no documentation of a percutaneous or endoscopic procedure.

❏ Marcy assigns the value for Character 6, Device.
  - She checks the documentation and identifies that a synthetic bone substitute was used.
  - She selects **J Synthetic Substitute** as the device.

❏ Marcy assigns the value for Character 7, Qualifier.
  - She checks the documentation and identifies that a posterior approach was used because an 11-cm incision was made directly over L4-L5.
  - She checks the documentation and identifies that the posterior column was treated.
  - She selects **1 Posterior Approach, Posterior Column** as the qualifier.

❏ She reviews the code she has assigned for the spinal arthrodesis: **0SG00J1** (■ FIGURE 53-6).

▶ Marcy searches the Index for the Main Term **Resection** for the discectomy. Because the documentation specifies all disc material, and not just a portion of the disc, was removed, she can use the root operation **Resection** rather than **Excision.**

❏ She locates the first-level subterm **Disc.**

❏ She locates the second-level subterm **Lumbar Vertebral.**

❏ She identifies Table **0ST** and partial code **0ST20ZZ.** Although this appears to be a complete seven-character code, she knows she cannot assign the code from the Index and must refer to the PCS Table to verify all the characters.

▶ Marcy turns to Table **0ST** to assign the code for the discectomy.

❏ She reads the Table title **0ST, Medical and Surgical, Lower Joints, Resection** and confirms that this accurately describes the body system and root operation.

❏ Marcy assigns the value **2 Lumbar Vertebral Disc** for Character 4, Body Part.

❏ Marcy assigns the value **0 Open** for Character 5, Approach, which is the only choice.

❏ Marcy assigns the value **Z No device** for Character 6, Device, which is the only choice.

❏ Marcy assigns the value **Z No qualifier** for Character 7, Qualifier, which is the only choice.

❏ She reviews the code she has assigned for the discectomy: **0ST20ZZ** (■ FIGURE 53-7).

▶ Marcy reviews the procedure codes she has assigned for this case:

❏ **0SG00J1** Fusion, Lumbar vertebral joint, Open, Synthetic substitute, Posterior approach posterior column

❏ **0ST20ZZ** Resection, Lumbar vertebral disc, Open, No device, No qualifier

▶ Next, Marcy must determine how to sequence the codes.

Section	0	Medical and Surgical
Body System	S	Lower Joints
Operation	G	Fusion: Joining together portions of an articular Body Part rendering the articular Body Part immobile

Body Part Character 4	Approach Character 5	Device Character 6	Qualifier Character 7
0 Lumbar Vertebral Joint 1 Lumbar Vertebral Joints, 2 or more 3 Lumbosacral Joint	0 Open 3 Percutaneous 4 Percutaneous Endoscopic	7 Autologous Tissue Substitute J Synthetic Substitute K Nonautologous Tissue Substitute	0 Anterior Approach, Anterior Column 1 Posterior Approach, Posterior Column J Posterior Approach, Anterior Column

Figure 53-6 ■ Assigning code 0SG00J1. *Source: Annotation © PB Resources, Inc. Used with permission.*

Section	0	Medical and Surgical
Body System	S	Lower Joints
Operation	T	Resection: Cutting out or off, without replacement, all of a Body Part

Body Part Character 4	Approach Character 5	Device Character 6	Qualifier Character 7
2 Lumbar Vertebral Disc	0 Open	Z No Device	Z No Qualifier
4 Lumbosacral Disc			
5 Sacrococcygeal Joint			
6 Coccygeal Joint			
7 Sacroiliac Joint, Right			
8 Sacroiliac Joint, Left			

Figure 53-7 ■ Assigning code 0ST20ZZ. *Source: Annotation © PB Resources, Inc. Used with permission.*

CODING PRACTICE

Exercise 53.3 **Assigning Characters 4–7 for Root Operations 0, 2, 3, 4, G, H, P, Q, R, U, and W**

Instructions: Read the mini-medical-record of each patient's encounter. Review the information abstracted in Exercise 53.2 for questions 1–3. For questions 4–6, abstract the case on your own. Assign PCS codes using the Index and Tables. Write the code(s) on the line provided.

1. INPATIENT HOSPITAL   Gender: F   Age: 81

Preprocedure diagnosis: Status post-arthroplasty

Procedure: Exchange of drainage tube from right hip joint following total hip replacement

Tip: The skin was not pierced to replace the drainage tube.

1 PCS Code _____

2. INPATIENT HOSPITAL   Gender: M   Age: 75

Preprocedure diagnosis: Sick sinus syndrome, displaced pacemaker lead

Procedure: Percutaneous adjustment of position of left pacemaker lead in left atrium

1 PCS Code _____

3. INPATIENT HOSPITAL   Gender: F   Age: 36

Preprocedure diagnosis: Drooping right upper eyelid affects patient's perception of appearance but does not interfere with vision

Procedure: Cosmetic blepharoplasty. Cut out a crescent of skin and subcutaneous tissue from fold of R eyelid, sutured to restore normal position of eyelid.

(continued)

3. (continued)

Tip: Review the purpose of the procedure to determine the root operation.

1 PCS Code _____

4. INPATIENT HOSPITAL   Gender: M   Age: 25

Preprocedure diagnosis: Puncture wound from knife, left lower arm surface

Procedure: Suture of 2-cm laceration, depth of 0.6 cm into the dermis. Wound irrigated. Deep sutures 4/0 PDS with 5-0 nylon running suture used to realign the skin. Antibiotic ointment and compression bandage applied.

Tip: Lacerations most often affect the skin, but any tissue may be lacerated, including subcutaneous tissue, tendon, muscle, or bone.

1 PCS Code _____

5. INPATIENT HOSPITAL   Gender: F   Age: 35

Preprocedure diagnosis: Central venous pressure measurement, septic shock

Procedure: Emergency internal jugular central venous catheter insertion, left side. An 8.5 French CV quad-lumen catheter was advanced into the internal jugular vein and secured in place with the tip of the catheter in the superior vena cava.

Tip: The CVP is inserted for hemodynamic monitoring.

1 PCS Code _____

(continued)

CODING PRACTICE (continued)

6. INPATIENT HOSPITAL   Gender: **F**   Age: **42**

Preprocedure diagnosis: Bleeding postop hysterectomy

Procedure: Control of postop hemorrhage and evacuation of clot via hysteroscope. Bleeders cauterized and blood clot evacuated. No further bleeding noted.

(continued)

6. (continued)

Tip: The only objective of the procedure is to stop hemorrhaging after the procedure.

1 PCS Code _____

ARRANGING CODES FOR ROOT OPERATIONS 0, 2, 3, 4, G, H, P, Q, R, U, AND W

Coders should be alert for specific situations related to the root operations discussed in this chapter when multiple coding might be required. Also be familiar with the general PCS OGCR for multiple coding,

Multiple codes with multiple root operations are required with Insertion procedures when:

- A device is placed during a procedure and the more definitive procedure does not provide a Character 6, Device value. Sequence the more definitive procedure as the principal procedure because it is most related to the principal diagnosis.

- An existing device is taken out and replaced with a new one, requiring an approach other than External. Code the root operation Insertion for placement of the new device. Recall that the root operation Change is used for an exchange procedure only when the skin or mucous membrane is not punctured or cut.

Multiple codes with multiple root operations are required with Removal procedures when:

- An existing device is taken out and replaced with a new one, requiring an approach other than External. Code the root operation Removal for taking out the existing device.

Multiple codes using the root operation Fusion are required when:

- Multiple vertebral segments within the same spinal region use different surgical approaches, anatomic approaches, or devices.

Guided Example of Arranging Codes for Fusion and Resection

To practice skills for arranging codes for the root operations Fusion and Resection, continue with the example from earlier

in the chapter about a patient who was seen for a lumbar discectomy and spinal fusion. Follow along in your ICD-10-PCS manual as Marcy Elwood, CCS, arranges the codes. Check off each step after you complete it.

▶ First, Marcy confirms the procedures discectomy with spinal arthrodesis and fixation plate and screws and reviews the codes she has assigned.

❏ **0SG00J1 Fusion, Lumbar vertebral joint, Open, Synthetic substitute, Posterior approach posterior column**

❏ **0ST20ZZ Resection, Lumbar vertebral disc, Open, No device, No qualifier**

▶ The principal procedure must be the one most closely related to the principal diagnosis, degenerative disc disease. All the procedures are directly related to the principal diagnosis, so because there was a specific problem with the L4-L5 disc, she sequences code **0ST20ZZ** for Resection of the disc first.

▶ Marcy sequences code **0SG00J1** for the arthrodesis second.

▶ Marcy finalizes the procedure codes and sequencing for this case:

(1) **0ST20ZZ Resection, Lumbar vertebral disc, Open, No device, No qualifier**

(2) **0SG00J1 Fusion, Lumbar vertebral joint, Open, Synthetic substitute, Posterior approach posterior column**

▶ Marcy also assigns and sequences the ICD-10-CM diagnosis code that supports the need for the service.

(1) **M51.36 Other intervertebral disc degeneration, lumbar region**

CODING PRACTICE

Exercise 53.4   Arranging Codes for Root Operations 0, 2, 3, 4, G, H, P, Q, R, U, and W

Instructions: Read the mini-medical-record of each patient's encounter. Review the information abstracted in Exercise 53.2 for questions 1–3. For questions 4–6, abstract the case on your own. Assign PCS codes using the Index and Tables, and arrange the codes in proper sequence. Write the code(s) on the line provided.

---

1. INPATIENT HOSPITAL   Gender: M   Age: 72

Preprocedure diagnosis: Blepharoptosis obscuring vision

Procedure: Bilateral upper blepharoplasty. Cut out a crescent of skin and subcutaneous tissue from fold of R eyelid, sutured to restore normal position of eyelid. Repeated on left side.

Tip: Review the purpose of the procedure to determine the root operation.

2 PCS Codes _____

---

2. INPATIENT HOSPITAL   Gender: M   Age: 53

Preprocedure diagnosis: Detached R retina

Procedure: Trans pars plana vitrectomy (TPPV) with synthetic scleral buckle. Made incision in pars plana and used vitreous cutter to remove all vitreous. Injected balanced saline solution (BSS) to replace vitreous. Sutured scleral buckle, which effectively closed the retinal break. Pt tolerated px well.

Tip: Injection of BSS is part of the procedure and is not coded separately.

2 PCS Codes _____

---

3. INPATIENT HOSPITAL   Gender: F   Age: 68

Preprocedure diagnosis: Bradycardia, malfunctioning pacemaker lead

Procedure: Percutaneous exchange of a malfunctioning pacemaker lead in the left atrium with a new one

Tip: The PCS Tables for each root operation provide different body part and device values.

2 PCS Codes _____

---

4. INPATIENT HOSPITAL   Gender: F   Age: 59

Preprocedure diagnosis: Adenocarcinoma of the right breast

Procedure: Right modified radical mastectomy with immediate breast reconstruction with tissue expander. The breast was removed, including the skin, breast tissue, areola, and nipple, and most of the lymph nodes under the arm. The pectoralis major muscle was spared for reconstruction. The expander was placed and the pectoralis muscle reapproximated for total muscle coverage. Wounds were closed and skin flap appeared healthy.

2 PCS Codes _____

---

5. INPATIENT HOSPITAL   Gender: M   Age: 57

Preprocedure diagnosis: Metastatic glossal carcinoma, needing chemotherapy and a port

Procedure: Open exploration of the left subclavian/axillary vein; insertion of a double lumen port through the left femoral vein, radiological guidance. The subclavian vein was identified and we were unable to subcutaneously cannulate it due to sclerosis. Decision was made to insert the port through the left femoral vein. Femoral vein cannulated without difficulty and double lumen port inserted.

Tip: If the intended procedure is discontinued, code the procedure to the root operation performed, PCS OGCR B3.3.

2 PCS Codes _____

---

6. INPATIENT HOSPITAL   Gender: M   Age: 13 months

Preprocedure diagnosis: Involutional entropion, right and left lower eyelids

Procedure: Tightening of the eyelid was achieved via the lateral tarsal strip procedure. The tarsal plate (*cartilage in the lower lid*) was shortened and used as the tendon to suspend to the orbital bone. The procedure was performed on both sides.

2 PCS Codes _____

CHAPTER SUMMARY

In this chapter you learned that:

- The Medical and Surgical root operations in the group *Procedures that always involve a device* are Change (2), Insertion (H), Removal (P), Replacement (R), Supplement (U), and Revision (W).

- The root operation Change (2) is taking out or off a device from a body part and putting back an identical or similar device in or on the same body part without cutting or puncturing the skin or a mucous membrane.

- The root operation Insertion (H) is putting in a nonbiological appliance that monitors, assists, performs, or prevents a physiological function but does not physically take the place of a body part.

- The root operation Removal (P) is taking out or off a device from a body part.

- The root operation Replacement (R) is putting in or on biological or synthetic material that physically takes the place and/or function of all or a portion of a body part.

- The root operation Supplement (U) is putting in or on biological or synthetic material that physically reinforces and/or augments the function of a portion of a body part.

- The root operation Revision (W) is correcting, to the extent possible, a portion of a malfunctioning device or the position of a displaced device.

- The Medical and Surgical root operations in the group *Procedures that define other repairs* are Control (3) and Repair (Q).

- The root operation Control (3) is stopping, or attempting to stop, postprocedural or other acute bleeding.

- The root operation Repair (Q) is restoring, to the extent possible, a body part to its normal anatomic structure and function.

- The Medical and Surgical root operations in the group *Procedures that define other objectives* are Alteration (0), Creation (4), and Fusion (G).

- The root operation Alteration (0) is modifying the anatomic structure of a body part without affecting the function of the body part.

- The root operation Creation (4) is putting in or on biological or synthetic material to form a new body part that to the extent possible replicates the anatomic structure or function of an absent body part.

- The root operation Fusion (G) is joining together portions of an articular body part, rendering the articular body part immobile.

- PCS provides guidelines related to the root operations Change, Control, and Fusion. It also provides guidance regarding the use of Character 4, Body Part and Character 6, Device related to root operations discussed in this chapter.

- When a PCS Table does not provide a specific body part value for the anatomic site treated, assign a more general body part value.

- PCS Tables for the root operation Fusion do not identify the specific vertebral segments but, rather, the overall level of the spine: cervical, thoracic, lumbar, and sacral.

- The root operation Change always uses the approach External.

- The root operation Fusion uses Character 6 to identify the type of tissue or tissue substitute used to render a vertebral joint immobile.

- The "Device Aggregation Table," located in the PCS coding manual appendix, provides a cross-walk of a specific device type to a more general Character 6, Device value needed in some PCS Tables.

CONCEPT QUIZ

Take a moment to look back at root operations discussed in this chapter and solidify your skills. Try to answer the questions from memory first, then refer to the discussion in this chapter if you need a little extra help.

Completion

Instructions: Write the term that completes each statement based on the information you learned in this chapter. Choose from the list below. Some choices may be used more than once and some choices may not be used at all.

Alteration	Removal
Change	Repair
Control	Replacement
Creation	Revision
Fusion	Supplement
Insertion	

1. The root operation _____ is joining together portions of an articular body part, rendering the articular body part immobile.

2. The root operation _____ is putting in or on biological or synthetic material to form a new body part that to the extent possible replicates the anatomic structure or function of an absent body part.

3. The root operation _____ is restoring, to the extent possible, a body part to its normal anatomic structure and function.

4. The root operation _____ is putting in or on biological or synthetic material that physically takes the place and/or function of all or a portion of a body part.

5. The root operation _____ is putting in or on biological or synthetic material that physically reinforces and/or augments the function of a portion of a body part.

6. The root operation _____ is modifying the anatomic structure of a body part without affecting the function of the body part.

7. The root operation _____ is putting in a nonbiological appliance that monitors, assists, performs, or prevents a physiological function but does not physically take the place of a body part.

8. The root operation _____ is correcting, to the extent possible, a portion of a malfunctioning device or the position of a displaced device.

9. The root operation _____ is taking out or off a device from a body part and putting back an identical or similar device in or on the same body part without cutting or puncturing the skin or a mucous membrane.

10. The root operation _____ is taking out or off a device from a body part.

Multiple Choice

Instructions: Circle the letter of the best answer to each question based on the information you learned in this chapter.

1. What root operation always uses the approach External?
   A. Removal (P)
   B. Control (3)
   C. Alteration (0)
   D. Change (2)

2. Which procedure is an example of the root operation Supplement (U)?
   A. Prosthetic lens implantation
   B. Placement of bone growth stimulator
   C. Mitral valve ring annuloplasty
   D. Vertebral arthrodesis

3. What feature in the PCS coding manual appendix provides a cross-walk of a specific device type to a more general Character 6, Device value needed in some PCS Tables?
   A. Device Combination Crosswalk
   B. Device Conversion Guide
   C. Device Key
   D. Device Aggregation Table

4. What root operation uses Character 6 to identify the type of tissue or tissue substitute used to render a vertebral joint immobile?
   A. Fusion (G)
   B. Control (3)
   C. Repair (Q)
   D. Revision (W)

5. How would you code the following procedure? *A physician performs an open cosmetic rhinoplasty.*
   A. 09UK07Z
   B. 090K0ZZ
   C. 09WK07Z
   D. 09QK0ZZ

6. How would you code the following procedure? *A physician puts in a multiple-channel cochlear implant, right ear, percutaneous endoscopic approach.*
   A. 09UD8JZ
   B. 09RD0JZ
   C. 09HD46Z
   D. 09HD35Z

7. Which of the following situations requires multiple codes?
   A. Multiple vertebral segments within the same spinal region use different devices.
   B. An attempt to control postprocedural bleeding is unsuccessful, so a resection procedure must be performed.
   C. An existing device is taken out and replaced with a new one using the external approach.
   D. A combination of autologous and nonautologous bone graft tissue is used to render a joint immobile.

8. Which PCS character is used to distinguish whether a prosthetic joint is cemented or uncemented?
   A. 4
   B. 5
   C. 6
   D. 7

9. Which root operation is used for sex change operations?
   A. Change (2)
   B. Creation (4)
   C. Revision (W)
   D. Replacement (R)

10. How would you code the following procedure? *A physician exchanges a feeding gastrostomy tube with a new one through an existing stoma in the stomach.*
   A. 0D20XUZ
   B. 0DH67UZ
   C. 0DW0XUZ
   D. 0DS67ZZ

KEEP ON CODING

Instructions: Read the procedural statement, abstract the root operation, then use the appropriate Index and Tables to assign PCS procedure codes. Assign only the root operations discussed in this chapter. Write the code(s) on the line provided. *Tip:* Terms indicating the presence of a device are underlined.

1. Central line insertion, percutaneous, right subclavian vein for infusion therapy. ICD-10-PCS Code(s) _____

2. Open right total knee replacement with cemented implant. ICD-10-PCS Code(s) _____

3. Open right inguinal herniorrhaphy with mesh. ICD-10-PCS Code(s) _____

4. PEG (feeding) tube change, external approach. ICD-10-PCS Code(s) _____

(continued)

(continued from page 1117)

5. External removal (pulling out) of <u>drainage tube</u> from gallbladder. ICD-10-PCS Code(s) _____

6. Open revision of left hip replacement <u>liner</u>. ICD-10-PCS Code(s) _____

7. Control acute bleeding of an intracranial hemorrhage, percutaneous endoscopic approach. ICD-10-PCS Code(s) _____

8. Suture of laceration of skin of back, external approach. ICD-10-PCS Code(s) _____

9. Open fusion of right finger phalangeal joint with <u>internal fixation</u>. ICD-10-PCS Code(s) _____

10. Bilateral breast augmentation with Corning silicone <u>implants</u>, open approach. ICD-10-PCS Code(s) _____

11. Gender alteration of male with creation of vagina using <u>synthetic material</u>, open approach. ICD-10-PCS Code(s) _____

12. Insertion of Vaxcel Plus dialysis <u>catheter</u> in the right internal jugular vein, percutaneous. ICD-10-PCS Code(s) _____

13. Aortic valve replacement with <u>Medtronic mechanical valve</u>, open approach. ICD-10-PCS Code(s) _____

14. Remove subclavian cardiac output monitoring <u>central line</u>, external approach. ICD-10-PCS Code(s) _____

15. <u>Percutaneous Vaxcel port</u> implantation for central access chemotherapy infusion via the left internal jugular (LIJ). ICD-10-PCS Code(s) _____

16. Placement (insertion) of <u>brachytherapy seeds</u> (radioactive) in prostate gland via cystoscopy. ICD-10-PCS Code(s) _____

17. Creation of mitral value from the common atrioventricular valve using <u>donor tissue</u>, open approach. ICD-10-PCS Code(s) _____

18. Change <u>chest tube</u> in pleural cavity for right hemothorax, external approach. ICD-10-PCS Code(s) _____

19. Anterior spinal fusion of C3-C4 with cadaver bone <u>graft</u>, open approach. ICD-10-PCS Code(s) _____

20. Percutaneous revision of <u>internal fixation device</u> in left tibia by removing loose screw and inserting a larger one. ICD-10-PCS Code(s) _____

21. Laparoscopic control of perineum bleeding, posthysterectomy. ICD-10-PCS Code(s) _____

22. Percutaneous endoscopic tympanoplasty, or right ruptured tympanic membrane. ICD-10-PCS Code(s) _____

23. Endoscopic posterior spinal fusion L3-L4, posterior column, using cadaver bone <u>graft</u>. ICD-10-PCS Code(s) _____

24. <u>PICC (peripherally inserted central catheter)</u> into the left cephalic vein for antibiotic infusion therapy, percutaneous approach. ICD-10-PCS Code(s) _____

25. Percutaneous revision of left breast <u>tissue expander</u>. ICD-10-PCS Code(s) _____

CODING CHALLENGE

Instructions: Read the mini-medical-record of each patient's encounter, then abstract, assign, and arrange ICD-10-CM diagnosis codes and PCS procedure codes using the appropriate Index and Tables. Write the code(s) on the line provided.

1. INPATIENT HOSPITAL   Gender: F   Age: 68

Preprocedure diagnosis: Primary degenerative osteoarthritis localized to the knee, extreme difficulty walking

Procedure: Total L knee replacement. Made midline incision 10 cm above L patella, entered joint capsule medially, and exposed tibiofemoral joint. Resected tibia and femur, then sized for prosthetic. Inserted synthetic knee prosthesis, cemented in place, and closed operative wound. Minimal blood loss. Patient tolerated procedure well.

1 ICD-10-CM Code _____

1 ICD-10-PCS Code _____

2. INPATIENT HOSPITAL   Gender: F   Age: 74

Preprocedure diagnosis: Macular edema, right eye

Procedure: Insertion of radioactive plaque, right eye with lateral canthotomy. The plaque was positioned on the scleral surface immediately behind the macula and secured with two sutures of 5-0 Dacron. The placement was confirmed with indirect ophthalmoscopy.

1 ICD-10-CM Code _____

1 ICD-10-PCS Code _____

3. INPATIENT HOSPITAL   Gender: M   Age: 26

Preprocedure diagnosis: Left ventral hernia

Procedure: Left ventral hernia repair with Marlex mesh via laparoscope. Ports placed in the abdomen and a stab incision made overlying the skin and hernia. Marlex mesh introduced and secured in position overlying the hernia. Ports removed and incisions closed.

1 ICD-10-CM Code _____

1 ICD-10-PCS Code _____

4. INPATIENT HOSPITAL   Gender: F   Age: 68

Preprocedure diagnosis: Abdominal aortic aneurysm (AAA)

Procedure: EVAR (endovascular aneurysm repair) with synthetic graft. Made incision into the femoral artery. With fluoroscopic guidance, guided delivery catheter with compressed graft into abdominal aorta to site of aneurysm. Inflated balloon to expand graft and affix it to vessel wall. Withdrew catheter and closed incision.

Tip: An endovascular graft is placed inside the vessel and physically takes over the function, rendering the original vessel nonfunctional. Do not assign an additional code for the fluoroscopy portion because it is not a Medical and Surgical procedure from Section 0.

1 ICD-10-CM Code _____

1 ICD-10-PCS Code _____

5. INPATIENT HOSPITAL   Gender: F   Age: 17

Preprocedure diagnosis: Second debridement for extensive burns on both arms

Procedure: Excisional debridement and graft. Cut out necrotic subcutaneous tissue and fascia and applied autologous skin substitute on both lower arms and nonautologous tissue substitute on both upper arms.

Postprocedure diagnosis: Second- and third-degree burns to anterior and posterior of right and left upper and lower arms, 18% TBSA (total body surface area) with burns, 9% TBSA third-degree burns.

Tip: Each portion (upper and lower) of each arm is coded as a separate body area for the diagnosis and procedure. Refer to OGCR I.C.19.a to review the use of ICD-10-CM code extensions. Do not code external cause, source, or intent of burns.

5 ICD-10-CM Codes _____

_____

4 ICD-10-PCS Codes _____

_____

(continued)

(continued from page 1119)

6. INPATIENT HOSPITAL   Gender: F   Age: 6

Preprocedure diagnosis: Congenital cleft earlobe defect, left ear

Procedure: Open cosmetic plastic repair of deformed left ear lobe. The skin of the cleft was completely excised and a flap along the cleft made at the posterior side of the lobe. The wound was closed with simple stitches on both anterior and posterior sides of the lobe.

1 ICD-10-CM Code _____

1 ICD-10-PCS Code _____

7. INPATIENT HOSPITAL   Gender: M   Age: 4

Preprocedure diagnosis: Congenital myotonic muscular dystrophy with bilateral planovalgus feet

Procedure: Bilateral Crawford subtalar arthrodesis with open Achilles Z-lengthening and bilateral long-leg cast. Incision was made over the left lateral aspect of the hind foot. A 7/8-inch staple was placed across the sinus tarsi to maintain the desired reduction. The incision was extended posteriorly to allow for visualization of the Achilles, which was Z-lengthened with the release of the lateral distal half. Wounds closed and dressing applied. The procedure was performed on both the right and left side without complication.

2 ICD-10-CM Codes _____

4 ICD-10-PCS Codes _____

_____

8. INPATIENT HOSPITAL   Gender: M   Age: 22

Preprocedure diagnosis: Epistaxis, left nasal passage, following sinus endoscopy six hours prior

Procedure: Endoscopic left anterior ethmoid artery cauterization, sphenopalatine artery cauterization. No obvious bleeding site seen endoscopically. Incision carried down to ethmoid artery, which was cauterized, and incision closed. Attention turned to the nose; the sphenopalatine artery identified and cauterized using suction cautery. Hemostasis obtained and the area packed with Metrogel.

2 ICD-10-CM Codes _____

1 ICD-10-PCS Code _____

9. INPATIENT HOSPITAL   Gender: F   Age: 10

Preprocedure diagnosis: Dislodged G tube, inserted 12 hours prior; spastic cerebral palsy

Procedure: Gastrostomy tube change. The G tube inserted earlier today was removed. The tract was assessed; new G tube lubricated and slid easily into the tract. Tube secured and placement verified by x-ray.

Tip: The device was removed and a similar device immediately inserted without making an incision or puncturing the skin or mucous membrane.

2 ICD-10-CM Codes _____

1 ICD-10-PCS Code _____

10. INPATIENT HOSPITAL   Gender: F   Age: 25

Preprocedure diagnosis: Menorrhagia; dyspareunia

Procedure: Intrauterine device extraction. IUD strings identified and grasped with the ring forceps. Steady gentle outward traction was applied and the IUD easily appeared in the vagina and was removed.

2 ICD-10-CM Codes _____

1 ICD-10-PCS Code _____

Sections 1–9: Medical and Surgical-Related Procedures

Obstetrics • Placement • Administration • Measurement and Monitoring • Extracorporeal or Systemic Assistance, Performance, and Therapies • Osteopathic • Chiropractic • Other Procedures

Chapter 54

Learning Objectives

After completing this chapter, you should have the skills to:

54.1 Spell and define the key words, medical terms, and abbreviations used with medical and surgical–related procedures. (Remember)

54.2 Identify the types of procedures covered by medical and surgical–related procedures. (Apply)

54.3 Adhere to ICD-10-PCS coding guidelines associated with medical and surgical–related procedures. (Apply)

54.4 Examine and abstract procedural information from the medical record for coding for medical and surgical–related procedures. (Analyze)

54.5 Demonstrate how to assign codes for the root operations for medical and surgical–related procedures. (Apply)

54.6 Utilize guidelines for arranging (sequencing) codes for root operations for medical and surgical–related procedures. (Apply)

Chapter Outline

- **Basics of Medical and Surgical-Related Procedures**
- **Coding Guidelines for Medical and Surgical-Related Procedures**
- **Abstracting for Medical and Surgical-Related Procedures**
- **Assigning Characters 4–7 for Medical and Surgical-Related Procedures**
- **Arranging Codes for Medical and Surgical-Related Procedures**

Key Terms and Abbreviations

abortifacient	cardiopulmonary bypass (CPB)	doctor of osteopathy (DO)	hyperbaric oxygen treatment (HBOT)
allopathic	chiropractic manipulation	extracorporeal	products of conception

In addition to the key terms listed here, students should know the terms defined within tables in this chapter.

INTRODUCTION

If you are an avid traveler, going to new places does not intimidate you. After you learn how to get around a few towns or even a few backcountry areas, you learn certain strategies and techniques that you can use anywhere you go. Thus you are able to quickly adapt to a new environment and begin seeing what it has to offer. PCS coding is similar. After you understand the structure of a PCS code and develop the skills for navigating the Medical and Surgical section, you can apply those skills to learn how to code procedures in other sections.

This chapter discusses PCS Sections 1–9, referred to as medical and surgical-related procedures. Note the presence of the word *related* in the section title to avoid potential confusion with PCS Section 0, Medical and Surgical procedures. You learn how codes in these sections are structured, how root operations are defined, and other unique characteristics. As with the Medical and Surgical section, pay careful attention to the differences between each root operation so that you can use each confidently and accurately.

BASICS OF MEDICAL AND SURGICAL-RELATED PROCEDURES

Medical and surgical-related procedures is a descriptive title that summarizes nine PCS sections, but it does not occupy a character within the code itself. ■ Table 54-1 summarizes the value, name, and purpose of each section. This part of PCS has many sections and some new root operations. Medical and surgical-related sections contain approximately 3,200 codes, or 4% of PCS, compared with over 68,000 codes (87%) in the Medical and Surgical (0) section.

Medical and surgical-related procedure codes have seven characters, but in some sections the purpose of a character is different than in the Medical and Surgical (0) section (■ Table 54-2). In the Obstetrics (1) and Placement (2) sections, all seven characters are defined in the same way as they are in

Table 54-1 ■ CHARACTER 1: SECTION NAMES AND PURPOSE OF MEDICAL AND SURGICAL-RELATED PROCEDURES

Value	Section Name	Purpose
1	Obstetrics	Procedures on an embryo, fetus, or unborn child
2	Placement	Procedures involving devices and materials that are performed without making an incision or a puncture
3	Administration	Procedures in which a diagnostic or therapeutic substance is given to the patient
4	Measurement and Monitoring	Procedures that take a single or series of readings of physiologic levels, such as temperature or heart rate
5	Extracorporeal or Systemic Assistance and Performance	Procedures in which equipment outside the body is used to assist or perform a physiological function
6	Extracorporeal or Systemic Therapies	Use of equipment outside the body for a therapeutic purpose that does not involve the assistance or performance of a physiological function
7	Osteopathic	Osteopathic manipulation procedures
8	Other Procedures	Miscellaneous procedures not included in other medical and surgical-related sections
9	Chiropractic	Chiropractic manipulation procedures

Table 54-2 ■ SEVEN CHARACTERS OF MEDICAL AND SURGICAL-RELATED PROCEDURES

	Character					
1 Section	**2**	**3**	**4**	**5**	**6**	**7**
Obstetrics (1)	Body System	Root Operation	Body Part	Approach	Device	Qualifier
Placement (2)	Body System	Root Operation	Body Region	Approach	Device	Qualifier
Administration (3)	Body System	Root Operation	Body System/Region	Approach	Substance	Qualifier
Measurement and Monitoring (4)	Body System	Root Operation	Body System	Approach	Function/Device	Qualifier
Extracorporeal or Systemic Assistance and Performance (5)	Body System	Root Operation	Body System	Duration	Function	Qualifier
Extracorporeal or Systemic Therapies (6)	Body System	Root Operation	Body System	Duration	Qualifier	Qualifier
Osteopathic (7)	Body System	Root Operation	Body Region	Approach	Method	Qualifier
Other Procedures (8)	Body System	Root Operation	Body Region	Approach	Method	Qualifier
Chiropractic (9)	Body System	Root Operation	Body Region	Approach	Method	Qualifier

Table 54-3   ■   **EXAMPLE OF CONSTRUCTING MEDICAL TERMS FOR MEDICAL AND SURGICAL-RELATED PROCEDURES**

Combining Form	Suffix	Complete Medical Term
amni/o (*amnion [sac surrounding the embryo]*)	**-scopy** (*visual examination*) **-centesis** (*surgical puncture to remove fluid*) **-tomy** (*incision into*) **-infusion** (*introducing a substance*)	**amnio + scopy** (*visual examination of the amnion*) **amnio + centesis** (*surgical puncture to remove fluid from the amnion*) **amnio + tomy** (*incision into the amnion*) **amnio + infusion** (*introducing a substance into the amnion*)
electr/o (*electrical*) **cardi/o** (*heart*) **encephal/o** (*brain*) **cyst/o** (*bladder*) **metr/o** (*measurement*)	**-graphy** (*the process of making a recording*) **-gram** (*a visual record or recording*)	**electro + cardio + graphy** (*the process of making a recording of the electrical activity of the heart*) **electro + encephalo + graphy** (*the process of making a recording of the electrical activity of the brain*) **cysto + metro + gram** (*a visual record or recording of measurement [of pressure] in the bladder*)

Source: © PB Resources, Inc. Used with permission.

the Medical and Surgical section. In Sections 3–9, Character 6 is used for new purposes as follows:

- Section **3 Administration** defines Character 6 as **Substance**.
- Section **4 Measurement and Monitoring** and **5 Extracorporeal or Systemic Assistance and Performance** define Character 6 as **Function**.
- Sections **7 Osteopathic**, **8 Other Procedures**, and **9 Chiropractic** define Character 6 as **Method**.

Details of how to abstract, assign, and arrange codes for each section are discussed in the remainder of this chapter.

Medical terms for medical and surgical-related procedures sometimes use different suffixes than those in the Medical and Surgical section. Familiar suffixes such as *-ectomy* and *-plasty* do not appear because procedures in these sections do not cut out or repair body parts. The exception is the Obstetrics (1) section, which does classify invasive procedures. Some procedure names do not use Latin forms at all. There is no direct match between a specific procedural term and a root operation. Root operations are assigned based on the content of

the operative report regarding what was actually performed, not on specific words used by the physician in documentation. Refer to ■ Table 54-3 for a refresher on how to build terms related to medical and surgical-related procedures.

CODING CAUTION

Be alert for root operations that have similar English meanings but different PCS definitions.

Immobilization (3) (*Limiting or preventing motion of a body region by external methods and devices*) and **Fusion** (G) (*Joining together portions of an articular body part, rendering the articular body part immobile*)

Introduction (5) (*Putting in or on a therapeutic, diagnostic, nutritional, physiological, or prophylactic substance except blood or blood products*) and **Insertion** (H) (*Putting in a nonbiological appliance that monitors, assists, performs, or prevents a physiological function but does not physically take the place of a body part*)

CODING PRACTICE

Exercise 54.1   Basics of Medical and Surgical-Related Procedures

Instructions: Use your medical erminology skills and resources to define the following medical and surgical-related procedures, then identify the code(s) or code range listed in the PCS Index. Follow these steps:

- Use slash marks "/" to break down the underlined term into its root(s) and suffix.
- Do not attempt to break down abbreviations in questions 9 and 10.
- Define the meaning of the word based on the meaning of each word part or letter in the abbreviation.
- Look up the phrase in the ICD-10-PCS Index, and write down the name(s) of Root Operation(s) the Index cross-references you to and the Table(s), if provided. If the Index lists only a code and not the root operation, list only the Table characters.
- Do not assign any codes.

(continued)

CODING PRACTICE (continued)

Example: <u>peritoneal</u> dialysis peritone/al   Meaning <u>*pertaining to the peritoneum*</u>   PCS Root Operation(s)/Table(s) <u>*3E1*</u>

1. <u>chemoembolization</u>   Meaning _____   PCS Root Operation(s)/Table(s) _____

2. <u>electromyogram</u>   Meaning _____   PCS Root Operation(s)/Table(s) _____

3. <u>leukopheresis</u>, therapeutic   Meaning _____   PCS Root Operation(s)/Table(s) _____

4. measurement, <u>olfactory</u> acuity   Meaning _____   PCS Root Operation(s)/Table(s) _____

5. <u>pleurodesis</u>   Meaning _____   PCS Root Operation(s)/Table(s) _____

6. near-infrared <u>spectroscopy</u>, circulatory system   Meaning _____   PCS Root Operation(s)/Table(s) _____

7. <u>oximetry</u>, fetal pulse   Meaning _____   PCS Root Operation(s)/Table(s) _____

8. <u>neurophysiologic</u> monitoring   Meaning _____   PCS Root Operation(s)/Table(s) _____

9. ECMO   Meaning _____   PCS Root Operation(s)/Table(s) _____

10. IPPB   Meaning _____   PCS Root Operation(s)/Table(s) _____

CODING GUIDELINES FOR MEDICAL AND SURGICAL-RELATED PROCEDURES

Coders need to understand and refer to the official coding guidelines. Obstetrics is the only medical and surgical-related section that has guidelines. Obstetrics guidelines, which appear in section C of the PCS OGCR, help clarify the types of procedures to be coded from the Obstetrics (1) section and those to be coded from the Medical and Surgical (0) section.

- The Obstetrics section classifies procedures performed on the body part Products of Conception only (PCS OGCR C1). For example, therapeutic amniocentesis is coded using the root operation Drainage and the body part Products of Conception in the Obstetrics section, resulting in the code **10903ZC**.

- Procedures performed on the pregnant female, other than the products of conception, are coded with the appropriate root operation in the Medical and Surgical section. For example, repair of an obstetric urethral laceration is coded using the root operation Repair and the body part Urethra in the Medical and Surgical section, resulting in a code such as **0TQD8ZZ**, depending on the approach.

- Procedures performed following a delivery or abortion for curettage of the endometrium or evacuation of retained products of conception are coded in the Obstetrics section (PCS OGCR C2). Assign the root operation Extraction and the body part Products of Conception, Retained, resulting in a code such as **10D18ZZ**, depending on the approach.

- Diagnostic or therapeutic dilation and curettage performed during times other than the postpartum or postabortion period are coded in the Medical and Surgical section using the root operation Extraction and the body part Endometrium, resulting in a code such as **0UDB7ZZ**, depending on the approach and purpose of the procedure.

ABSTRACTING FOR MEDICAL AND SURGICAL-RELATED PROCEDURES

Medical and surgical-related procedures in Sections 1–9 are usually performed in conjunction with Medical and Surgical (Section 0) procedures but are not operative procedures in and of themselves. Abstracting for medical and surgical-related procedures is similar to abstracting Medical and Surgical (0) procedures and focuses on reading the procedure report and interpreting it in light of root operation definitions. Remember to focus on the objective of the procedure and the activities performed, not the specific medical terms used to describe the procedure.

The following information highlights the definitions and unique criteria for Sections 1–9 and provides a Key Criteria for Abstracting table to identify the root operations in each section. After reading the procedure report, use the abstracting table as follows:

1. Answer the General Questions to get a basic understanding of the procedure (■ TABLE 54-4).

2. Answer the Root Operation Questions. One question should be answered *Yes*; the rest should be answered *No*.

3. For the Root Operation Question that was answered *Yes*, refer to the section identified in the second column and review the root operations available in that section. Refer to the tables for Key Criteria for Abstracting each section that appear in this chapter.

4. Look up the definition of each of the applicable root operations in the appendix of the ICD-10-PCS coding manual.

5. Identify the one root operation that matches the procedure documented. This root operation is the Main Term when you use the Index.

6. Repeat the abstracting process for each procedure that was performed.

Table 54-4 ■ **KEY CRITERIA FOR ABSTRACTING MEDICAL AND SURGICAL-RELATED SECTIONS**

General Questions
❏ What is the stated procedure?
❏ What body region or body part is involved?
❏ How many sites are treated?
❏ What is the laterality (if applicable)?
❏ What approach is used?
❏ Is the procedure description what you would expect based on the name of the procedure?
❏ Was more than one procedure, or a combined procedure, performed?

Section Questions (Answer *Yes* to one question)	Refer to Root Operations in This Section
❏ Does the procedure involve a fetus?	Section 1 Obstetrics
❏ Does the procedure place an object in or on the patient without cutting or puncturing the skin or mucous membrane?	Section 2 Placement
❏ Is a diagnostic or therapeutic substance given to the patient?	Section 3 Administration
❏ Does the procedure involve measurement or monitoring?	Section 4 Measurement and Monitoring
❏ Does the procedure use equipment outside the body to assist or perform a physiological function?	Section 5 Extracorporeal or Systemic Assistance and Performance
❏ Does the procedure use equipment outside the body for a therapeutic purpose that does not involve the assistance or performance of a physiological function?	Section 6 Extracorporeal or Systemic Therapies
❏ Is osteopathic or chiropractic manipulation provided?	Section 7 Osteopathic or Section 9 Chiropractic
❏ Does the procedure involve another methodology in an attempt to remediate or cure a disorder or disease?	Section 8 Other Procedures

Source: © PB Resources, Inc. Used with permission.

Because some of these sections are relatively short with few codes, brief information on assigning codes is presented with selected sections or root operations discussed next. There are no separate sections for each root operation. Procedures with more extensive information about assigning codes are discussed later in the chapter under the topic "Assigning Characters 4–7 for Medical and Surgical-Related Procedures."

> ### CODING CAUTION
>
> Root operation values are independent between sections, so the same alphanumeric value can be reused for root operations in different sections. For example, you will find that several sections use the values 0, 1, 2, and so on for different root operations. Always refer to the values listed in a specific PCS Table to determine the meaning of an alphanumeric character.

Abstracting for Obstetrics (Section 1)

The Obstetrics section classifies procedures performed on the **products of conception**, which encompasses all components of pregnancy, including the embryo, fetus, amnion, placenta, and umbilical cord. Examples of procedures are vaginal and cesarean delivery, abortion, amniocentesis, and transfusions. Procedures performed on the pregnant female are coded with the appropriate root operation from the Medical and Surgical or other PCS sections.

The only value for Character 2, Body System in the Obstetrics section is Pregnancy (0). This section has only three Character 4 Body Part values:

- Products of Conception (0)
- Products of Conception, Retained (1)
- Products of Conception, Ectopic (2)

The Obstetrics section has 12 root operations. Ten of these are also used in the Medical and Surgical (0) section and carry the same values and definitions in this section. Two root operations are unique to Obstetrics and are defined in ■ TABLE 54-5. The root operations in the Obstetrics section are:

- Change (2)
- Drainage (9)

Table 54-5 ■ **UNIQUE ROOT OPERATIONS IN THE OBSTETRICS SECTION**

Root Operation	Value	Definition	Examples
Abortion	A	Artificially terminating a pregnancy	Mechanical abortion, surgical abortion, use of **abortifacient** (*an agent that causes abortion*)
Delivery	E	Assisting the passage of the Products of Conception from the genital canal	Vaginal delivery, manually assisted delivery, spontaneous delivery

Source: © PB Resources, Inc. Used with permission.

- Abortion (A)
- Extraction (D)
- Delivery (E)
- Insertion (H)
- Inspection (J)
- Removal (P)
- Repair (Q)
- Reposition (S)
- Resection (T)
- Transplantation (Y)

To abstract for Obstetrics procedures, first identify that the procedure is performed on the Products of Conception, then apply abstracting questions for each potential root operation. Abstracting criteria for root operations shared with the Medical and Surgical section are the same as those presented in previous chapters of this text, with the added specificity that the procedure is performed on the Products of Conception (■ Table 54-6).

Cesarean delivery and forceps-assisted vaginal delivery are coded to the root operation **Extraction (D)** because force is used in these procedures. The root operation **Delivery (E)** is not used for these types of assisted deliveries.

Some procedures on the Products of Conception are coded from sections other than Obstetrics. For example, fetal heart rate monitoring is coded from Section 4, Measurement and Monitoring. Follow the guidance in the Index when coding such procedures.

SUCCESS STEP

When coding procedures performed for pregnant women, use ICD-10-PCS procedure codes from any section of the manual, based on the root operation performed. This differs from coding diagnoses for pregnant women because you must always assign a code from the ICD-10-CM obstetrics chapter, even if the condition was not caused by the pregnancy, such as preexisting diabetes or hypertension. You then assign additional diagnosis codes from other ICD-10-CM chapters when needed to fully describe the condition.

Abstracting for the Placement (2), Administration (3), and Measurement and Monitoring (4) Sections

The next three sections are Placement (2), Administration (3), and Measurement and Monitoring (4). Each section has separate purposes and separate root operations.

Table 54-6 ■ KEY CRITERIA FOR ABSTRACTING OBSTETRICS PROCEDURES

Section Question	
❑ Is the procedure performed on the products of conception?	If *No*, do not use Obstetrics codes.
Root Operation Questions	**Root Operation (Value)**
Answer *Yes* to one of the following questions to help distinguish Root Operations in the Obstetrics (1) section	
❑ Does the procedure take a device out or off from a body part on the fetus and put back an identical or similar device in or on the same body part without cutting or puncturing the skin or a mucous membrane?	Change (2)
❑ Does the procedure take or let fluids and/or gases from a body part on the fetus?	Drainage (9)
❑ Is a pregnancy artificially terminated?	Abortion (A)
❑ Does the procedure pull or strip out or off all or a portion of a body part on the fetus by the use of force?	Extraction (D)
❑ Is a cesarean section delivery performed?	
❑ Are forceps used to assist a vaginal delivery?	
❑ Does the procedure assist a fetus, embryo, or unborn child to pass through the genital canal?	Delivery (E)
❑ Was a nonbiological appliance put in the fetus that monitors, assists, performs, or prevents a physiological function but does not physically take the place of a body part?	Insertion (H)
❑ Is all or part of a body part of the fetus visually and/or manually explored?	Inspection (J)
❑ Is a device taken off from a body part, region, or orifice on the fetus?	Removal (P)
❑ Is a body part of the fetus restored to its normal anatomic structure and function to the extent possible?	Repair (Q)
❑ Is all or a portion of a body part of the fetus moved to its normal location, or other suitable location?	Reposition (S)
❑ Is a body part of the fetus cut out or off, without replacement?	Resection (T)
❑ Does the procedure put in or on all or a portion of a living body part taken from another individual or animal to physically take the place and/or function of all or a portion of a similar body part on the fetus?	Transplantation (Y)

Source: © PB Resources, Inc. Used with permission.

Table 54-7 ■ UNIQUE ROOT OPERATIONS IN THE PLACEMENT SECTION

Root Operation	Value	Definition	Examples
Compression	1	Putting pressure on a body region	Placement of intermittent pressure device
Dressing	2	Putting material on a body region for protection	Application of sterile dressing to wound
Immobilization	3	Limiting or preventing motion of a body region	Neck brace, arm cast
Packing	4	Putting material in a body region or orifice	Nasal packing, packing of wound
Traction	6	Exerting a pulling force on a body region in a distal direction	Mechanical traction of arm or leg

Source: © PB Resources, Inc. Used with permission.

Placement (Section 2) Root Operations

The Placement section has seven root operations. Two of these, Change and Removal, are also used in the Medical and Surgical (0) section and carry the same definitions but have different values for the root operations in Character 3. Five root operations are unique to Placement and are defined in ■ TABLE 54-7. The root operations in the Placement section are:

- Change (0)
- Removal (5)
- Compression (1)
- Dressing (2)
- Immobilization (3)
- Packing (4)
- Traction (6)

Placement section procedures use two values for Character 2, Body System:

- Anatomical Regions (W)
- Anatomical Orifices (Y)

To abstract for Placement procedures, apply abstracting questions for each potential root operation (■ TABLE 54-8). Abstracting criteria for root operations shared with the Medical and Surgical section are the same as those presented in previous chapters of this text.

Coders need to make distinctions between certain procedures in Section 2, Placement compared to Section F, Physical Rehabilitation and Diagnostic Audiology. The root operation Immobilization (3) in the Placement section applies to the fitting of devices, such as splints and braces, in inpatient settings other than rehabilitation (■ FIGURE 54-1). When these services are provided in a rehabilitation setting, use the root operation

Table 54-8 ■ KEY CRITERIA FOR ABSTRACTING PLACEMENT PROCEDURES

Section Question	
❏ Is the procedure performed on an anatomic region or natural orifice without making an incision or puncture?	If *No*, do not use Placement codes.

Root Operation Questions	Root Operation (Value)
Answer *Yes* to one of the following questions to help distinguish Root Operations in the Placement (2) section	
❏ Does the procedure take a device out or off of a body part and put back an identical or similar device in or on the same body part without cutting or puncturing the skin or a mucous membrane?	Change (0)
❏ Is pressure applied on a body region?	Compression (1)
❏ Is material put on a body region for protection?	Dressing (2)
❏ Does the procedure limit or prevent the movement of a body region?	Immobilization (3)
❏ Is material put in a body region or orifice?	Packing (4)
❏ Is a device taken off from a body part, region, or orifice?	Removal (5)
❏ Is a force pulling in a distal direction exerted on a body region?	Traction (6)

Source: © PB Resources, Inc. Used with permission.

Device Fitting (D) in Section F, Physical Rehabilitation and Diagnostic Audiology. Section F is part of ancillary procedures, discussed in Chapter 55 of this text.

The root operation Traction (6) in the Placement section applies to the use of a mechanical traction apparatus. When manual traction is performed by a physical therapist or physician, use Section F, Physical Rehabilitation and Diagnostic Audiology, root type Motor Treatment (7), and the type qualifier Manual Therapy Techniques (7) (■ FIGURE 54-2, page 1128).

Devices coded in Section 2 are manufactured and ready to use without extensive fabrication or fitting. Custom-fabricated devices or those requiring extensive fitting are coded in Section F of ancillary procedures, Physical Rehabilitation and Diagnostic Audiology.

> Physician places a cast on the left forearm of a hospital inpatient.
>
> **2W3DX2Z Placement, Anatomical Regions, Immobilization, Lower arm left, External, Cast, No qualifier**

Figure 54-1 ■ Example of coding from the Placement Section for a hospital inpatient. *Source:* © PB Resources, Inc. Used with permission.

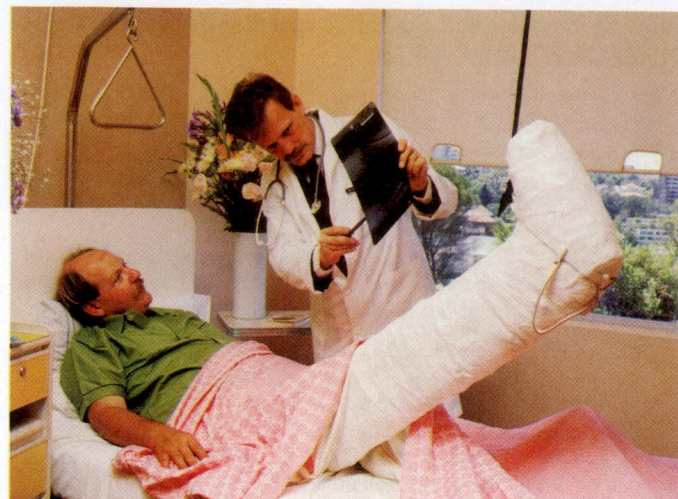

A Mechanical traction

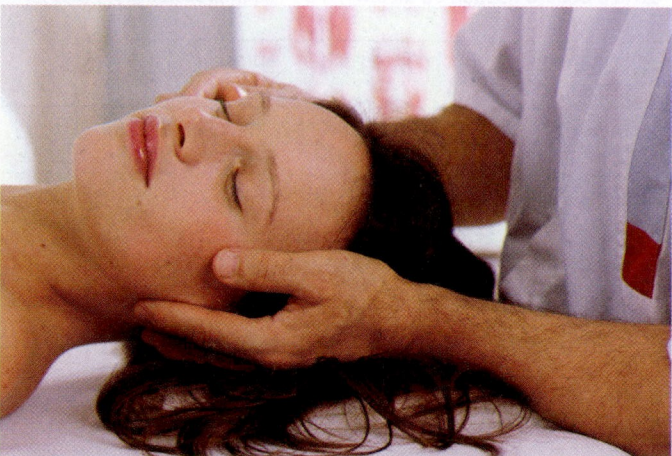

B Manual traction

Figure 54-2 ■ Types of traction. (A) Mechanical traction uses equipment to apply a pulling force *Source: Camerique/ClassicStock/Alamy Stock Photo.* (B) Manual traction is performed with the hands. *Source: BSIP/Universal Images Group/Getty Images.*

Table 54-9 ■ UNIQUE ROOT OPERATIONS IN THE ADMINISTRATION SECTION

Root Operation	Value	Definition	Examples
Introduction	0	Putting in or on a therapeutic, diagnostic, nutritional, physiological, or prophylactic substance except blood or blood products	Nerve block injection, transabdominal in vitro fertilization
Irrigation	1	Putting in or on a cleansing substance	Flushing of the eye, peritoneal dialysis using indwelling catheter
Transfusion	2	Putting in blood or blood products	Blood transfusion, bone marrow transplant

Source: © PB Resources, Inc. Used with permission.

Table 54-10 ■ KEY CRITERIA FOR ABSTRACTING ADMINISTRATION PROCEDURES

Section Question	
❏ Is a diagnostic or therapeutic substance given to the patient?	If *No*, do not use Administration codes.
Root Operation Questions	**Root Operation (Value)**
Answer *Yes* to one of the following questions to help distinguish Root Operations in the Administration (3) section	
❏ Is a cleansing substance put in or administered to the patient?	Irrigation (1)
❏ Is blood or blood products put in or administered to the patient?	Transfusion (2)
❏ Is a therapeutic, diagnostic, nutritional, physiological, or prophylactic substance except blood or blood products put in or administered to the patient?	Introduction (0)

Source: © PB Resources, Inc. Used with permission.

Administration (Section 3) Root Operations

The Administration section classifies procedures in which a therapeutic, prophylactic, protective, diagnostic, nutritional, or physiological substance is given to the patient. It includes infusions, injections, and transfusions, as well as other related procedures, such as irrigation and tattooing.

The Administration section has three root operations, all unique to this section, which are classified according to the broad category of substance administered (■ TABLE 54-9). Use the root operation Transfusion when a blood product is given. Use the root operation Irrigation when a cleansing substance is administered. Use the root operation Introduction for all other substances administered, such as antineoplastic substances.

Character 2, Body System uses three values:

- Circulatory (0)
- Indwelling Device (C)
- Physiological Systems and Anatomical Regions (E)

Character 5, Approach uses values from the Medical and Surgical section. Assign the approach Percutaneous (3) for all injections, regardless of whether they are administered using an intradermal, subcutaneous, or intramuscular route.

To abstract for Administration section procedures, apply abstracting questions for each potential root operation (■ TABLE 54-10). Abstracting criteria for root operations shared with the Medical and Surgical section are the same as those presented in previous chapters of this text.

Measurement and Monitoring (Section 4) Root Operations

The Measurement and Monitoring section classifies procedures that measure the level of a physiological or

Table 54-11 ■ UNIQUE ROOT OPERATIONS IN THE MEASUREMENT AND MONITORING SECTION

Root Operation	Value	Definition	Examples
Measurement	0	Determining the level of a physiological or physical function at a point in time	Routine ECG, venous pulse single measurement
Monitoring	1	Determining the level of a physiological or physical function repetitively over a period of time	Holter monitoring, fetal heart monitoring

Source: © PB Resources, Inc. Used with permission.

physical function, such as temperature, visual mobility, or urinary pressure. This section has two root operations, Measurement (0) and Monitoring (1), both unique to this section (■ TABLE 54-11).

Be aware that overlap exists between the name of the section and the names of the two root operations. The section Measurement and Monitoring has a Character 1 value of **4**. The root operation Measurement has a Character 3 value of **0**, and the root operation Monitoring has a Character 3 value of **1**.

Character 2, Body System uses two values:

- Physiological Systems (A), used with the root operation Measurement and Monitoring
- Physiological Devices (B), used with the root operation Measurement

When abstracting for procedures in this section, keep in mind the definitions of the root operations. The root operations Measurement and Monitoring both record levels of the same physiological and physical functions. The root operation Measurement takes a single reading at a point in time, whereas the root operation Monitoring takes multiple readings at intervals over a period of time. The number of measurements is the only criterion that distinguishes between these two root operations (■ TABLE 54-12).

Table 54-12 ■ KEY CRITERIA FOR ABSTRACTING MEASUREMENT AND MONITORING PROCEDURES

Section Question	
❏ Does the procedure measure the level of a physiological or physical function?	If *No*, do not use Measurement and Monitoring codes.
Root Operation Questions	**Root Operation (Value)**
Answer *Yes* to one of the following questions to help distinguish Root Operations in the Measurement and Monitoring (4) section	
❏ Does the procedure take a single reading at a point in time?	Measurement (0)
❏ Are multiple readings of the same function taken repetitively over a period of time?	Monitoring (1)

Source: © PB Resources, Inc. Used with permission.

Character 6, Function/Device identifies the physiological function being tested, such as conductivity, pressure, or temperature.

Abstracting for the Extracorporeal or Systemic (5, 6) Procedures Sections

PCS provides two sections of root operations for **extracorporeal** procedures and processes, which are those that take place outside of the body. Each of these sections is discussed next.

Extracorporeal or Systemic Assistance and Performance (Section 5) Root Operations

Procedures in the section Extracorporeal or Systemic Assistance and Performance (5) use equipment to support a physiological function, such as breathing, circulating the blood, or restoring the natural rhythm of the heart. Procedures include those performed in a critical care setting but are not restricted to a designated critical care unit. An operating room or emergency department also qualifies as a critical care setting. Examples of critical care procedures are mechanical ventilation and cardioversion. Other procedures in this section are hemodialysis and **hyperbaric oxygen treatment** (**HBOT**) (*breathing 100% oxygen under increased atmospheric pressure*).

The section Extracorporeal or Systemic Assistance and Performance has three root operations, all of which are unique to this section (■ TABLE 54-13). The root operations Assistance (0) and Performance (1) describe similar types of procedures. They vary only in the degree of control exercised over the physiological function. Assistance classifies procedures that *support* a physiological function but do not take complete control of it, such as an intra-aortic balloon pump used to support cardiac output and hyperbaric oxygen

Table 54-13 ■ UNIQUE ROOT OPERATIONS IN THE EXTRACORPOREAL OR SYSTEMIC ASSISTANCE AND PERFORMANCE SECTION

Root Operation	Value	Definition	Examples
Assistance	0	Taking over a portion of a physiological function by extracorporeal means	Hyperbaric oxygenation of wound, continuous intra-aortic balloon pump (IABP)
Performance	1	Completely taking over a physiological function by extracorporeal means	Cardiopulmonary bypass, hemodialysis encounter, continuous mechanical ventilation
Restoration	2	Returning, or attempting to return, a physiological function to its original state by extracorporeal means	External cardioversion, defibrillation

Source: © PB Resources, Inc. Used with permission.

treatment. Performance classifies procedures where *complete control* is exercised over a physiological function, such as total mechanical ventilation, cardiac pacing, and cardiopulmonary bypass.

Characters 5 and 6 are used differently than in the Medical and Surgical (0) section. Character 5 is Duration, which describes the duration of the procedure. Character 6 is Function, which identifies the body function being acted on.

Extracorporeal or Systemic Therapies (Section 6) Root Operations

The section Extracorporeal or Systemic Therapies describes other extracorporeal procedures that are not defined by Section 5, Assistance and Performance. Examples are Bili-lite phototherapy, apheresis, and whole-body hypothermia.

The Extracorporeal or Systemic Therapies section has 11 root operations, all unique to this section (■ TABLE 54-14).

Character 2, Body System provides one choice, Physiological Systems. Character 6 is defined as a qualifier but contains no specific qualifier values. Character 7, Qualifier identifies various blood components separated out in pheresis procedures.

Refer to ■ TABLE 54-15 for assistance in abstracting Extracorporeal or Systemic procedures. The table encompasses both Sections 5 and 6. To avoid redundancy, the definitions of Section 6 root operations are not repeated in the abstracting table.

The definitions of most root operations in this section are consistent with terms used in the medical community, but

Table 54-14 ■ UNIQUE ROOT OPERATIONS IN THE EXTRACORPOREAL OR SYSTEMIC THERAPIES SECTION

Root Operation	Value	Definition
Atmospheric Control	0	Extracorporeal control of atmospheric pressure and composition
Decompression	1	Extracorporeal elimination of undissolved gas from body fluids
Electromagnetic Therapy	2	Extracorporeal treatment by electromagnetic rays
Hyperthermia	3	Extracorporeal raising of body temperature
Hypothermia	4	Extracorporeal lowering of body temperature
Pheresis	5	Extracorporeal separation of blood products
Phototherapy	6	Extracorporeal treatment by light rays
Ultrasound Therapy	7	Extracorporeal treatment by ultrasound
Ultraviolet Light Therapy	8	Extracorporeal treatment by ultraviolet light
Shock Wave Therapy	9	Extracorporeal treatment by shock waves
Perfusion	B	Extracorporeal treatment by diffusion of therapeutic fluid

Source: © PB Resources, Inc. Used with permission.

Table 54-15 ■ KEY CRITERIA FOR ABSTRACTING EXTRACORPOREAL OR SYSTEMIC PROCEDURES

Section Question	
❏ Does the procedure use equipment to support a physiological function?	If *No*, do not use Extracorporeal or Systemic Assistance and Performance codes.

Root Operation Questions	Root Operation (Value)
Answer *Yes* to one of the following questions to help distinguish Root Operations in the Extracorporeal or Systemic Assistance and Performance (5) section	
❏ Does the procedure take over a portion of a physiological function by extracorporeal or systemic means?	Assistance (0)
❏ Does the procedure completely take over a portion of a physiological function by extracorporeal or systemic means?	Performance (1)
❏ Does the procedure return, or attempt to return, a failed physiological function to its original state by extracorporeal or systemic means?	Restoration (2)
❏ Does the procedure use other methods, such as light, heat, cold, electromagnetic force, diffusion of fluid, or similar, to support a physiological function?	Review and select the appropriate root operation from Section 6, Extracorporeal or Systemic Therapies.

Source: © PB Resources, Inc. Used with permission.

coders should still refer to the PCS definition of each procedure. For example, the root operations Decompression (1) and Hyperthermia (4) have more specialized meanings in PCS than in the medical community in general. Decompression describes treatment for decompression sickness (the bends) in a hyperbaric chamber. Hyperthermia is the intentional lowering of body temperature to treat temperature imbalance.

Pheresis is used to treat diseases where too much of a blood component is produced, such as leukemia, or to remove a blood product such as platelets from a donor for transfusion into a patient who needs them.

Phototherapy to the circulatory system means exposing the blood to light rays outside the body, using a machine that recirculates the blood and returns it to the body after phototherapy.

Perfusion reports the great amount of time, effort, and equipment needed to supply blood to and assess a donor organ. These services are not included in the codes to perform the transplant.

Abstracting for the Osteopathic (7), Chiropractic (9), and Other Procedures (8) Sections

The final three sections of medical and surgical-related procedures are the short sections for osteopathic and chiropractic services and a grouping of miscellaneous procedures not classified in other sections. Refer to Table 54-4 to abstract for procedures in these sections.

Table 54-16 ■ UNIQUE ROOT OPERATIONS IN THE OSTEOPATHIC SECTION

Root Operation	Value	Definition
Treatment	0	Manual treatment to eliminate or alleviate somatic dysfunction and related disorders

Source: © PB Resources, Inc. Used with permission.

Osteopathic (Section 7) Root Operations

Section 7, Osteopathic, consists of a single body system, Anatomical Regions, and a single root operation, Treatment, which is unique to this section (■ TABLE 54-16). Osteopathic manipulative treatment (OMT) uses the hands to diagnose, treat, and prevent illness or injury. The physician moves muscles and joints using techniques such as stretching, gentle pressure, and resistance. A doctor of osteopathy (DO) is a licensed physician who has the same licensing, training, and qualifications as a doctor of medicine (MD), also called allopathic physicians. Osteopathic physicians receive an additional 300–500 hours in the study of the musculoskeletal system and hands-on manual manipulation. The codes in this section are specifically for osteopathic manual manipulation. Assign codes from any PCS section for other services provided by an osteopath.

Character 4, Body Region identifies the regions of the spine, extremities, and trunk. Character 5, Approach is always **X External**. Character 6 is method of treatment, such as Lymphatic Pump and Fascial Release. The definitions of methods rely on the standard definitions as used in this specialty and are not explicitly defined in PCS. ■ TABLE 54-17 provides a summary of commonly used osteopathic methods. Character 7, Qualifier is always **Z None**.

Table 54-17 ■ OSTEOPATHIC TREATMENT METHODS

Method	Description
Articulatory-raising	Rotation of rib heads through direct application of force
Counterstrain or indirect	Positioning of a patient to passively release tenderness on a specific point
General mobilization	Movement of joints and tissues to release tension
High velocity–low amplitude (HVLA) or thrust technique	Use of a brief, rapid force that engages and releases a restrictive barrier within a joint's anatomic range of motion
Low velocity–high amplitude	Large-scale mobilization to relieve tension
Lymphatic pump treatment (LPT)	Application of manual force to the thoracic cage, abdomen, pelvis, and other areas to stimulate lymph flow
Muscle energy—isotonic	Application of resistance against the patient's motion
Muscle energy—isometric	Application of equal force against the patient's motion
Myofascial release or fascial release	Application of manual pressure to trigger points to relax contracted muscles, stimulate the stretch reflex, and increase circulation and lymphatic drainage

Source: © PB Resources, Inc. Used with permission.

Table 54-18 ■ UNIQUE ROOT OPERATIONS IN THE CHIROPRACTIC SECTION

Root Operation	Value	Definition
Manipulation	B	Manual procedure that involves a directed thrust to move a joint past the physiological range of motion, without exceeding the anatomic limit

Source: © PB Resources, Inc. Used with permission.

Chiropractic (Section 9) Root Operations

The Chiropractic section consists of a single body system, Anatomical Regions, and a single root operation, Manipulation (■ TABLE 54-18).

Chiropractic focuses on disorders of the musculoskeletal and nervous system and the effects of these disorders on general health. Chiropractic manipulation or adjustment uses direct manual force or an instrument to manipulate the joints of the body, most commonly the spine, to restore or enhance joint function. Treatment focuses on neuromusculoskeletal complaints, such as pain in the back, neck, and joints, and headaches. Doctors of Chiropractic (DCs) are trained in chiropractic colleges and have broad diagnostic skills. They are also qualified to recommend therapeutic and rehabilitative exercises, as well as to provide nutritional, dietary, and lifestyle counseling.

Character 4, body region identifies the regions of the spine, extremities, and trunk. Character 5, Approach is always **X External**. Character 6 is method of treatment, such as non-manual and mechanically assisted. The definitions of methods rely on the standard usage in the chiropractic specialty and are not explicitly defined in PCS. ■ TABLE 54-19 provides a summary of commonly used chiropractic methods. Character 7, Qualifier is always **Z None**.

Table 54-19 ■ CHIROPRACTIC TREATMENT METHODS

Method	Description
Direct visceral	Treatment of internal organ dysfunction, adhesions, or tension by direct pressure to mobilize the organ
Extra-articular	Manipulation of areas other than joints
Indirect visceral	Treatment of internal organ dysfunction by stretching or mobilizing areas adjacent to the organ
Long- and short-lever-specific contact	A combination of direct spinal thrusts and long lever contact (femur, head, or pelvis)
Long-lever-specific contact	Manipulation of the femur, head, or pelvis to adjust the spine
Mechanically assisted	Use of an instrument to aid in manipulation
Nonmanual	Heat, ice, ultrasound, electrical stimulation, therapeutic exercise
Short-lever-specific contact	Direct thrusts applied to the spine

Source: © PB Resources, Inc. Used with permission.

Table 54-20 ■ UNIQUE ROOT OPERATIONS IN THE OTHER PROCEDURES SECTION

Root Operation	Value	Definition
Other Procedures	0	Methodologies that attempt to remediate or cure a disorder or disease

Source: © PB Resources, Inc. Used with permission.

Other Procedures (Section 8) Root Operations

The Other Procedures section contains codes for procedures not included in the other medical and surgical-related sections. This section has one root operation, Other Procedures (0) (■ TABLE 54-20). Character 2, body system, has two values:

- Indwelling Device (C)
- Physiological Systems and Anatomical Regions (E)

There are relatively few procedure codes in this section for non-traditional, whole-body therapies including acupuncture and meditation. There is also a code for the fertilization portion of an in vitro fertilization procedure.

Character 6 is method and identifies the method or technique used in the procedure. Examples include Robotic Assisted Procedure (C), Computer Assisted Procedure (B), Acupuncture (0), and Therapeutic Massage (1). Codes for robotic and computer assisted procedures report only the additional assistance, not the definitive procedure. These should be assigned in addition to a code(s) from the medical and surgical section.

Guided Example of Abstracting for Medical and Surgical-Related Procedures

Refer to the following example throughout this chapter to practice skills for abstracting, assigning, and arranging codes for medical and surgical-related procedures. Two services use root operations in medical and surgical-related sections. Three services are coded from the Medical and Surgical (0) section and were discussed in the Guided Example in Chapter 51 of this text. Refer to Chapter 51 for details of abstracting and assigning codes for these procedures.

INPATIENT HOSPITAL   Gender: M   Age: 72

Reason for admission: Angina, SOB

Procedures: Cardiac stress test of total activity, single measurement. CABG x2 with CP bypass, LIMA to LAD, OM with GSV.

Discharge diagnosis: Atherosclerotic heart disease with 90% blockage in LAD and 80% blockage in the OM with unstable angina pectoris

Follow along as fictitious coder Marcy Elwood, CCS, abstracts the procedure. Check off each step after you complete it.

▶ Marcy reads through the entire record, paying special attention to the reason for admission, the procedure performed, and the principal diagnosis. She refers to the Key Criteria for Abstracting Medical and Surgical-Related sections (Table 54-4).

❑ She notes the reason for admission: angina, SOB.

❑ She also notes the discharge diagnosis: atherosclerotic heart disease with 90% blockage in LAD and 80% blockage in the OM with unstable angina pectoris.

❑ *What services were provided during the inpatient stay?*
  - Cardiac stress test
  - CABG ×2
  - CP bypass

▶ First, Marcy abstracts for the cardiac stress test. She refers to Table 54-4, Key Criteria for Abstracting Medical and Surgical-Related Sections.

❑ *What is the stated procedure?* Cardiac stress test

❑ *What body region or body part is involved?* Heart

❑ She reviews the abstracting questions and answers *Yes* to one question:
  - *Does the procedure involve measurement or monitoring?* Refer to the Measurement and Monitoring (4) section

❑ Marcy reviews the root types for the Measurement and Monitoring section. To select the root operation she must determine whether the measurement was taken at a point in time or was a series of readings over a period of time.
  - The documentation states single measurement, so she selects the definition that describes the procedure: **Measurement (0): Determining the level of a physiological or physical function at a point in time.**

▶ Next, Marcy abstracts for CP bypass. She again refers to Table 54-4.

❑ *What is the stated procedure?* Cardiopulmonary bypass during open heart surgery

❑ *What body region or body part is involved?* Heart and lungs

❑ She reviews the abstracting questions and answers *Yes* to one question:
  - *Is a procedure performed in a critical care setting to support a physiological function(s)?* Refer to the Extracorporeal or Systemic Assistance and Performance (5) section.

❑ Marcy reviews the root types for the Extracorporeal or Systemic Assistance and Performance section and selects the one definition that describes the procedure:
  - **Performance (1): Completely taking over a physiological function by extracorporeal means.**

▶ At this time, Marcy believes that she will need five codes: two for the CABG (abstracted in Chapter 51 of this text), one for harvesting the GSV (also abstracted in Chapter 51), one for the cardiac stress test, and one for cardiopulmonary bypass. She believes that she will use the root operation Measurement for the cardiac stress test and the root operation Performance for cardiopulmonary bypass. She will verify this information when she refers to the PCS Tables to assign codes.

CODING PRACTICE

Exercise 54.2 Abstracting for Medical and Surgical-Related Procedures

Instructions: Read the mini-medical-record of each patient's encounter and answer the abstracting questions. Write the answer on the line provided. Do not assign any codes.

1. INPATIENT HOSPITAL Gender: F Age: 22

Gravida: 2 Para: 2 EGA: 33 + 2

Reason for admission: Premature rupture of membranes

Assessment: Severe preeclampsia requires C/S

Delivery: Low C/S, PTBLC, 1 girl

Tip: PTBLC (Preterm birth, live child)

a. What is the stated procedure? _____

b. What body region or body part is involved? _____

c. What approach is used? _____

d. Was more than one procedure, or a combined procedure, performed? _____

e. Does the procedure involve a fetus? _____

f. Does the procedure place an object in or on the patient without cutting or puncturing the skin or a mucous membrane? _____

g. Is a diagnostic or therapeutic substance given to the patient? _____

h. Does the procedure involve measurement or monitoring? _____

i. Does the procedure use equipment outside the body to assist or perform a physiological function?

_____

j. Does the procedure use equipment outside the body for a therapeutic purpose that does not involve the assistance or performance of a physiological function? _____

k. Is osteopathic or chiropractic manipulation provided? _____

l. What PCS section should be used? _____

m. Review the root operations in the section selected. What is the most likely root operation? _____

2. INPATIENT HOSPITAL Gender: M Age: 32

Preprocedure diagnosis: Peripheral neuritis, left arm

Procedure: Nerve block injection to the median nerve using an anesthetic agent

a. What is the stated procedure? _____

b. What body region or body part is involved? _____

c. What approach is used? _____

d. Was more than one procedure, or a combined procedure, performed? _____

e. Does the procedure involve a fetus? _____

f. Does the procedure place an object in or on the patient without cutting or puncturing the skin or a mucous membrane? _____

g. Is a diagnostic or therapeutic substance given to the patient? _____

h. Does the procedure involve measurement or monitoring?

_____

i. Does the procedure use equipment outside the body to assist or perform a physiological function? _____

j. Does the procedure use equipment outside the body for a therapeutic purpose that does not involve the assistance or performance of a physiological function? _____

k. Is osteopathic or chiropractic manipulation provided?

_____

l. What PCS section should be used? _____

m. Review the root operations in the section selected. What is the most likely root operation? _____

3. INPATIENT HOSPITAL Gender: M Age: 17

Preprocedure diagnosis: Aplastic anemia

Procedure: Bone marrow transplant via central venous line using donor marrow from his identical twin

a. What is the stated procedure? _____

b. What body region or body part is involved? _____

c. What approach is used? _____

d. Was more than one procedure, or a combined procedure, performed? _____

e. Does the procedure involve a fetus? _____

f. Does the procedure place an object in or on the patient without cutting or puncturing the skin or a mucous membrane? _____

(continued)

CODING PRACTICE (continued)

3. (continued)

g. Is a diagnostic or therapeutic substance given to the patient? _____

h. Does the procedure involve measurement or monitoring? _____

i. Does the procedure use equipment outside the body to assist or perform a physiological function? _____

j. Does the procedure use equipment outside the body for a therapeutic purpose that does not involve the assistance or performance of a physiological function? _____

k. Is osteopathic or chiropractic manipulation provided? _____

l. What PCS section should be used? _____

m. Review the root operations in the section selected. What is the most likely root operation? _____

---

4. INPATIENT HOSPITAL   Gender: F   Age: 15

Preprocedure diagnosis: Displaced fracture R tibia

Procedure: Closed reduction of fracture with percutaneous insertion of internal fixation device. Applied leg cast and initiated mechanical traction of lower R leg

a. What is the stated procedure? _____

b. What body region or body part is involved? _____

c. What approach is used? _____

d. Was more than one procedure, or a combined procedure, performed? _____

e. Does the procedure involve a fetus? _____

f. Does the procedure place an object in or on the patient without cutting or puncturing the skin or a mucous membrane? _____

g. Is a diagnostic or therapeutic substance given to the patient? _____

h. Does the procedure involve measurement or monitoring? _____

i. Does the procedure use equipment outside the body to assist or perform a physiological function? _____

j. Does the procedure use equipment outside the body for a therapeutic purpose that does not involve the assistance or performance of a physiological function? _____

---

4. (continued)

k. Is osteopathic or chiropractic manipulation provided? _____

l. What PCS section(s) should be used? _____

m. Review the root operations in the section selected. What is the most likely root operation(s)? _____

---

5. INPATIENT HOSPITAL   Gender: F   Age: 33

Gravida: 2   Para: 2   EGA: 39 + 1

Assessment: Fetal bradycardia

Procedure: Mid forceps delivery with repair of perineal laceration

Delivery: TBLC, 1 girl

Tip: TBLC (Term birth, live child)

a. What is the stated procedure? _____

b. What body region or body part is involved? _____

c. What approach is used? _____

d. Was more than one procedure, or a combined procedure, performed? _____

e. Does the procedure involve a fetus? _____

f. Does the procedure place an object in or on the patient without cutting or puncturing the skin or a mucous membrane? _____

g. Is a diagnostic or therapeutic substance given to the patient? _____

h. Does the procedure involve measurement or monitoring? _____

i. Does the procedure use equipment outside the body to assist or perform a physiological function?

_____

j. Does the procedure use equipment outside the body for a therapeutic purpose that does not involve the assistance or performance of a physiological function? _____

k. Is osteopathic or chiropractic manipulation provided? _____

l. What PCS section(s) should be used? _____

m. Review the root operations in the section selected. What is the most likely root operation(s)?

_____

(continued)

CODING PRACTICE (continued)

6. INPATIENT HOSPITAL Gender: F Age: 75

Preprocedure diagnosis: Cardiac arrhythmia

Procedure: 24-hour ambulatory Holter monitoring followed by external measurement of cardiac output

a. What is the stated procedure? _____

b. What body region or body part is involved? _____

c. What approach is used? _____

d. Was more than one procedure, or a combined procedure, performed? _____

e. Does the procedure involve a fetus? _____

f. Does the procedure place an object in or on the patient without cutting or puncturing the skin or a mucous membrane? _____

g. Is a diagnostic or therapeutic substance given to the patient? _____

6. (continued)

h. Does the procedure involve measurement or monitoring? _____

i. Does the procedure use equipment outside the body to assist or perform a physiological function? _____

j. Does the procedure use equipment outside the body for a therapeutic purpose that does not involve the assistance or performance of a physiological function? _____

k. Is osteopathic or chiropractic manipulation provided? _____

l. What PCS section(s) should be used? _____

m. Review the root operations in the section selected. What is the most likely root operation(s)? _____

ASSIGNING CHARACTERS 4–7 FOR MEDICAL AND SURGICAL-RELATED PROCEDURES

To assign codes after the root operation is determined, search the PCS Index for the name of the root operation as the Main Term. Locate the subterm(s) for the correct anatomic site and identify the PCS Table. When you locate the PCS Table, verify the first three characters of the code, then locate the row with the body part needed. Assign the remaining characters from each respective column of the Table. Never code directly from the Index even when a full code is listed. You must refer to the PCS Table to verify the code.

For many procedures, you can also look up the common name of the procedure, such as **Cardioversion**, or an abbreviation, such as **EEG**, in the Index. This method might give you a partial or full code. Other times, the Index lists an instruction that cross-references you to one or more possible root operations. If you have difficulty locating a code using one Main Term or method, try a different one.

As discussed earlier in this chapter, the meaning of Characters 4–7 varies based on the section, so it is important to review the character meanings in each PCS Table. Special considerations for the use of Characters 4–7 were discussed with the individual sections or root operations in the "Abstracting" section of this chapter.

In the root operation Introduction (0), Character 4, Body Part identifies the site where the procedure occurs, although the substance introduced might affect a different site. Character 6 identifies the substance introduced. Character 7, Qualifier identifies additional details about the substance.

EXAMPLE: *Introduction of the hormone human B-type natriuretic peptide into a peripheral vein, open approach* 3E030VH Introduction, Peripheral Vein, Open approach, Hormone, Human B-type Natriuretic Peptide

In the root operation Irrigation (1), Character 4, body part identifies the site that is irrigated.

Additional information regarding Obstetrics procedures is discussed next.

Assigning Codes for Obstetrics (1)

The type of delivery is described by Character 3, root operation as follows:

• Use the root operation Extraction (D) for cesarean section deliveries and forceps-assisted vaginal deliveries (■ FIGURE 54-3).

• Use the root operation Delivery (E) for manually assisted vaginal deliveries.

For procedures performed following a delivery or abortion involving curettage of the endometrium or evacuation of

---

Surgeon delivers one liveborn infant with a low cesarean delivery.

10D00Z1 Medical and Surgical-Related, Obstetrics, Extraction, Products of conception, Open, No device, Low

Figure 54-3 ■ Example of coding for the Obstetrics Section, root operation Extraction. *Source: © PB Resources, Inc. Used with permission.*

retained products of conception, use the root operation Extraction (D) and the body part Products of Conception, Retained (0).

For diagnostic or therapeutic dilation and curettage performed during times *other* than the postpartum or postabortion period, use Section 0, Medical and Surgical, root operation D Extraction, and the body part B Endometrium (PCS OGCR C2).

For the root operation Abortion (Table **10A**), qualifier values identify whether an additional device such as a laminaria or abortifacient is used, or whether the abortion is performed by mechanical means. When a laminaria or abortifacient is used, the approach is Via Natural or Artificial Opening and the qualifier identifies the method or device. All other abortion procedures are performed by mechanical means because the products of conception are physically removed using instrumentation. Mechanical abortions are coded from a separate row in Table **10A**. A choice of approaches is provided; device is always **No device (Z)**; qualifier is always **No qualifier (Z)**.

Guided Example of Assigning Characters 4–7 for Medical and Surgical-Related Procedures

To practice skills for assigning codes for medical and surgical-related procedures, continue with the example from earlier in the chapter about a patient who was seen for a cardiac stress test and CABG. Follow along in your ICD-10-PCS manual as Marcy Elwood, CCS, assigns codes. Check off each step after you complete it.

▶ First, Marcy confirms the services provided and the root operations she abstracted:

❏ The root operation for the cardiac stress test of total activity, single measurement, is Measurement (0) from the Measurement and Monitoring (4) section.

❏ The root operation for CP bypass is Performance (1) from the Extracorporeal or Systemic Assistance and Performance (5) section.

▶ Marcy searches the Index for the Main Term **Stress** for the cardiac stress test.

❏ She locates two codes, **4A02XM4** and **4A12XM4**.

❏ She recognizes that the codes are exactly the same except for Character 3, root operation.

❏ She identifies that she must consult and compare two Tables: **4A0** and **4A1**.

❏ Alternatively, Marcy could search the Index for the Main Term of the root operation **Measurement** and the subterms **Cardiac** and **Total Activity**. This path also leads to code **4A02XM4**, Table **4A0**.

▶ Marcy turns to Table **4A0** to assign the code for the cardiac stress test.

❏ She reads the Table title **4A0, Measurement and Monitoring, Physiological Systems, Measurement** and confirms that this accurately describes the body system and root operation Measurement.

❏ As a confirmation, she also checks Table **4A1, Measurement and Monitoring, Physiological Systems, Monitoring**. She determines this Table is not correct because the procedure was a single measurement, not monitoring.

❏ Marcy verifies the value for Character 4, Body System: **2 Cardiac**.

❏ Marcy verifies the value for Character 5, Approach: **X External**.

❏ Marcy assigns the value for Character 6, Function/Device: **M Total Activity**.

❏ Marcy assigns the value for Character 7, Qualifier: **4 Stress**.

❏ She reviews the code she has assigned for the cardiac stress test, single measurement: **4A02XM4** (■ Figure 54-4).

❏ **4A02XM4 Measurement and monitoring, Physiological systems, Measurement, Cardiac, External, Total activity, Stress**

▶ Marcy searches the Index for the Main Term **Performance** for cardiopulmonary bypass. She does not use the Main Term Bypass because it would lead to Tables for the root operation Bypass (1) in the Medical and Surgical (0) section,

Section	4	Measurement and Monitoring
Body System	A	Physiological Systems
Operation	0	Measurement: Determining the level of a physiological or physical function at a point in time

Body System Character 4	Approach Character 5	Function/Device Character 6	Qualifier Character 7
2 Cardiac	X External	M Total Activity	4 Stress

Figure 54-4 ■ Assigning Code 4A02XM4. *Source: Annotation © PB Resources, Inc. Used with permission.*

Section   **5** **Extracorporeal Assistance and Performance**
Body System **A** **Physiological Systems**
Operation   **1** **Performance:** Completely taking over a physiological function by extracorporeal means

Body System Character 4	Duration Character 5	Function Character 6	Qualifier Character 7
2 Cardiac	2 Continuous	1 Output 3 Pacing	Z No Qualifier

Figure 54-5 ■ Assigning Code 5A1221Z. *Source: Annotation © PB Resources, Inc. Used with permission.*

defined as *Altering the route of passage of the contents of a tubular body part.* **Cardiopulmonary bypass (CPB)** refers to the equipment that takes over the function of the heart and lungs, maintaining the circulation of blood and the oxygen content of the body.

❑ She locates the first-level subterm **Cardiac.**

❑ She locates the second-level subterm **Continuous.**

❑ She locates the third-level subterm **Output.**

❑ She identifies Table **5A1** and code **5A1221Z.**

❑ Although a full seven-character code is listed, Marcy knows that she cannot assign a code from the Index and must verify the code in the PCS Table.

▶ Marcy turns to Table **5A1** to assign the code for the cardiopulmonary bypass.

❑ She reads the Table title **5A1, Extracorporeal or Systemic Assistance and Performance, Physiological Systems, Performance** and confirms that this accurately describes the body system and root operation.

❑ Marcy verifies the value for Character 4, Body System: **2 Cardiac.**

❑ Marcy verifies the value for Character 5, Duration: **2 Continuous.**

❑ Marcy verifies the value for Character 6, Function: **1 Output.**

❑ Marcy verifies the value for Character 7, Qualifier: **Z No qualifier.**

❑ She reviews the code she has assigned for the cardiopulmonary bypass: **5A1221Z** (■ Figure 54-5).

❑ **5A1221Z** Extracorporeal or systemic assistance and performance, Physiological systems, Performance, Cardiac, Continuous, Output, No qualifier

▶ Marcy reviews the procedure codes she has assigned for this case.

❑ **4A02XM4** Measurement and monitoring, Physiological systems, Measurement, Cardiac, External, Total activity, Stress

❑ **5A1221Z** Extracorporeal or systemic assistance and performance, Physiological systems, Performance, Cardiac, Continuous, Output, No qualifier

▶ Next, Marcy must determine how to sequence the codes.

CODING PRACTICE

Exercise 54.3   Assigning Characters 4–7 for Medical and Surgical-Related Procedures

Instructions: Read the mini-medical-record of each patient's encounter. Review the information abstracted in Exercise 54.2 for questions 1–3. For questions 4–6, abstract the case on your own. Assign PCS codes using the Index and Tables. Write the code(s) on the line provided.

1. INPATIENT HOSPITAL   Gender: F   Age: 22
Gravida: 2   Para: 2   EGA: 33 + 2
Reason for admission: Premature rupture of membranes
Assessment: Severe preeclampsia requires C/S
Delivery: Low C/S, PTBLC, 1 girl
Tip: PTBLC (Preterm birth, live child)
1 PCS Code _____

(continued)

CODING PRACTICE (continued)

2. INPATIENT HOSPITAL Gender: M Age: 32

Preprocedure diagnosis: Peripheral neuritis, left arm

Procedure: Nerve block injection to the median nerve using an anesthetic agent

Tip: The median nerve is in the arm.

1 PCS Code _____

3. INPATIENT HOSPITAL Gender: M Age: 17

Preprocedure diagnosis: Aplastic anemia

Procedure: Bone marrow transplant via central venous line using donor marrow from his identical twin

1 PCS Code _____

4. INPATIENT HOSPITAL Gender: F Age: 15

Preprocedure diagnosis: Fractured R radius

Procedure: Application of three layers of fiberglass short arm cast. Cast was molded to arm.

Tip: The root operation Immobilization (3) in Section 2, Placement applies to the fitting of devices in inpatient settings other than rehabilitation.

1 PCS Code _____

5. INPATIENT HOSPITAL Gender: F Age: 19

Preprocedure diagnosis: 3rd-degree burn to left groin

Procedure: Sterile dressing placement to left groin region. The old dressing was removed and the burned area was washed with mild soap and water. A clean sterile dressing was applied and held in place by wrapping a sterile gauze roll over the dressings, securing the ends with tape.

1 PCS Code _____

6. INPATIENT HOSPITAL Gender: M Age: 53

Preprocedure diagnosis: Achalasia

Procedure: Esophagogastroscopy with Botox injection into esophageal sphincter. Under endoscopic guidance, I injected 20 units BT-A, diluted in 1 mL of saline, in each of the 4 lower esophageal sphincter quadrants approximately 1 cm above the Z-line into the bulging muscle.

Tip: Botulinum toxin is a paralyzing agent with temporary effects; it does not sclerose or destroy the nerve.

1 PCS Code _____

ARRANGING CODES FOR MEDICAL AND SURGICAL-RELATED PROCEDURES

Procedures from the Obstetrics section are usually sequenced as the principal procedure because delivery is commonly the reason for admission and the services provided during the inpatient admission. By contrast, many medical and surgical-related procedures are not sequenced as the principal procedure because they are performed in addition to a more definitive procedure. Refer to ■ FIGURE 54-6 for an example in which the root operation Reposition (S) from the Medical and Surgical (0) section is sequenced as the principal diagnosis, followed by the root operations Immobilization (3) and Traction (6) from the Placement (2) section. In this example, Reposition is the definitive procedure.

SUCCESS STEP

Many procedures in the medical and surgical-related section are also performed as standalone outpatient procedures, Outpatient services are reported with CPT codes. PCS is used only by inpatient facilities.

Patient was admitted with a displaced fracture of the left femoral shaft and a fractured left radius. Open reduction with internal fixation was performed on the femur and a short arm cast was applied. Following surgery, the femur was placed in mechanical traction.

0QS904Z Medical and surgical, Lower bones, Reposition, Femoral shaft left, Open, Internal fixation device, No qualifier
2W3DX2Z Medical and surgical, Anatomical regions, Immobilization, Lower arm left, External, Cast, No qualifier
2W6PX0Z Medical and surgical, Anatomical regions, Traction, Upper leg left, External, Traction apparatus, No qualifier

Figure 54-6 ■ Example of arranging medical and surgical-related procedure codes. *Source:* © PB Resources, Inc. Used with permission.

Guided Example of Arranging Codes for Medical and Surgical-Related Procedures

To practice skills for arranging codes for medical and surgical-related procedures, continue with the example from earlier in the chapter about the patient who was seen for a cardiac stress test and CABG. Follow along in your ICD-10-PCS manual as Marcy Elwood, CCS, arranges the codes. Check off each step after you complete it.

▶ First, Marcy confirms the procedures performed:

❏ Cardiac stress test

❏ Cardiopulmonary bypass

❏ CABG × 2 of LIMA to LAD, OM with GSV

❏ Harvesting of the GSV

▶ Marcy reviews the diagnoses and determines the principal diagnosis:

❏ Atherosclerotic heart disease with 90% blockage in LAD and 80% blockage in the OM with unstable angina pectoris

❏ She also identifies the definitive procedure as the CABG.

▶ Marcy reviews the procedure codes assigned:

❏ **4A02XM4 Measurement and monitoring, Physiological systems, Measurement, Cardiac, External, Total activity, Stress**

❏ **5A1221Z Extracorporeal or systemic assistance and performance, Physiological systems, Performance, Cardiac, Continuous, Output, No qualifier**

❏ **0210093 Medical and surgical, Heart and great vessels, Bypass, Coronary artery one artery, Open approach, Autologous venous tissue, Coronary artery** (Chapter 51)

❏ **02100Z9 Medical and surgical, Heart and great vessel, Bypass, Coronary artery one artery, Open approach, No device, Internal mammary artery left** (Chapter 51)

❏ **06BP4ZZ Medical and surgical, Lower veins, Excision, Saphenous vein right, Percutaneous endoscopic approach, No device, No qualifier** (Chapter 51)

▶ Marcy determines that the principal procedure is the CABG. The principal diagnosis determines the sequencing order because the principal procedure must be the one most closely related to the principal diagnosis. The CABG is the definitive procedure, so the codes for Bypass are sequenced first.

▶ Marcy finalizes the procedure codes and sequencing for this case:

(1) **0210093 Medical and surgical, Heart and great vessels, Bypass, Coronary artery one artery, Open approach, Autologous venous tissue, Coronary artery**

(2) **02100Z9 Medical and surgical, Heart and great vessels, Bypass, Coronary artery one artery, Open approach, No device, Internal mammary artery left**

(3) **06BP4ZZ Medical and surgical, Lower veins, Excision, Saphenous vein right, Percutaneous endoscopic approach, No device, No qualifier**

(4) **5A1221Z Extracorporeal or systemic assistance and performance, Physiological systems, Performance, Cardiac, Continuous, Output, No qualifier**

(5) **4A02XM4 Measurement and monitoring, Physiological systems, Measurement, Cardiac, External, Total activity, Stress**

▶ Marcy also assigns the ICD-10-CM diagnosis code that supports the need for the service.

(1) **I25.110 Atherosclerotic heart disease of native coronary artery with unstable angina pectoris**

CODING PRACTICE

Exercise 54.4 Arranging Codes for Medical and Surgical-Related Procedures

Instructions: Read the mini-medical-record of each patient's encounter. Review the information abstracted in Exercise 54.2 for questions 1–3. For questions 4–6, abstract the case on your own. Assign PCS codes using the Index and Tables, and arrange the codes in proper sequence. Write the code(s) on the line provided.

---

1. INPATIENT HOSPITAL   Gender: F   Age: 15

Preprocedure diagnosis: Displaced fracture, R tibia

Procedure: Closed reduction of fracture with percutaneous insertion of internal fixation device. Applied leg cast and initiated mechanical traction of lower R leg

Tip: The root operation Immobilization (3) in Section 2, Placement applies to the fitting of devices in inpatient settings other than rehabilitation.

3 PCS Codes _____

(continued)

CODING PRACTICE (continued)

---

2. INPATIENT HOSPITAL Gender: F Age: 33

Gravida: 2 Para: 2 EGA: 39 + 1

Assessment: Fetal bradycardia

Procedure: Mid forceps delivery with repair of perineal laceration

Delivery: TBLC, 1 girl

Tip: TBLC (Term birth, live child)

2 PCS Codes _____

---

3. INPATIENT HOSPITAL Gender: F Age: 75

Preprocedure diagnosis: Cardiac arrhythmia

Procedure: 24-hour ambulatory Holter monitoring followed by external measurement of cardiac output

2 PCS Codes _____

---

4. INPATIENT HOSPITAL Gender: F Age: 78

Preprocedure diagnosis: Left hip fracture following a fall

Procedure: Placement of intermittent pneumatic compression (IPC) device covering both calves to prevent deep venous thrombosis (DVT)

2 PCS Codes _____

---

5. INPATIENT HOSPITAL Gender: F Age: 39

Preprocedure diagnosis: Primigravida at term, 39 weeks 4 days, in labor

Procedure: NSVD of term newborn; fetal heart rate monitoring, transvaginal. Patient in active labor, fetal heart monitor applied to monitor any variability. Patient delivered a healthy 7 lb. 2 oz female via manually assisted delivery.

Tip: For internal monitoring, a sensor is attached to the thigh of the mother. An electrode from the sensor is inserted transvaginally into the uterus and the electrode is attached to the baby's scalp.

2 PCS Codes _____

---

6. INPATIENT HOSPITAL Gender: M Age: 62

Preprocedure diagnosis: Angina

Procedure: Cardiac exercise stress test, Bruce protocol; cardiac countershock. At the conclusion of the stress portion of the test, the patient went into cardiac arrest. He was successfully converted to sinus rhythm.

2 PCS Codes _____

CHAPTER SUMMARY

In this chapter you learned that:

- The medical and surgical-related sections are Obstetrics (1), Placement (2), Administration (3), Measurement and Monitoring (4), Extracorporeal or Systemic Assistance and Performance (5), Extracorporeal or Systemic Therapies (6), Osteopathic (7), Other Procedures (8), and Chiropractic (9).

- The section Obstetrics (1) is procedures on an embryo, fetus, or unborn child and has 12 root operations, two of which are unique to this section.

- The section Placement (2) is procedures involving devices and materials that are performed without making an incision or a puncture and has seven root operations, five of which are unique to this section.

- The section Administration (3) is procedures in which a diagnostic or therapeutic substance is given to the patient and has three root operations, all unique to this section.

- The section Measurement and Monitoring (4) is procedures that take a single or series of readings of physiologic levels, such as temperature or heart rate, and has two root operations, both unique to this section.

- The section Extracorporeal or Systemic Assistance and Performance (5) is procedures performed in a critical care setting to support physiologic functions and has three root operations, all unique to this section.

- The section Extracorporeal or Systemic Therapies (6) is other extracorporeal procedures not described in Section 5 and has 10 root operations, all unique to this Section.
- The section Osteopathic (7) is osteopathic manipulation procedures and has one root operation, which is unique to this Section.
- The section Other Procedures (8) is miscellaneous procedures not included in other medical and surgical-related sections and has one root operation, which is unique to this section.
- The section Chiropractic (9) is chiropractic manipulation procedures and has one root operation, which is unique to this section.

- The meaning of Characters 4–7 varies based on the section, so it is important to review the character meanings in each PCS Table.
- Many medical and surgical-related procedures are not sequenced as the principal procedure because they are performed in addition to a more definitive procedure.
- PCS provides guidelines for the Obstetrics section, which clarify the types of procedures to be coded from the Obstetrics section and those to be coded from the Medical and Surgical (0) section.

CONCEPT QUIZ

Take a moment to look back at medical and surgical-related procedures and solidify your skills. Try to answer the questions from memory first, then refer to the discussion in this chapter if you need a little extra help.

Completion

Instructions: Write the root operation that matches the definition based on the information you learned in this chapter. Choose from the list below. Some choices may be used more than once and some choices may not be used at all.

Assistance (0)	Monitoring (1)
Dressing (2)	Other Procedures (8)
Hyperthermia (3)	Packing (4)
Hypothermia (4)	Pheresis (5)
Immobilization (3)	Restoration (2)
Introduction (0)	Traction (6)
Irrigation (1)	Treatment (0)

1. The root operation _____ from the Administration (3) section is putting in or on a cleansing substance.

2. The root operation _____ from the Extracorporeal or Systemic Assistance and Performance (5) section is returning, or attempting to return, a physiological function to its original state by extracorporeal means.

3. The root operation _____ from the Placement (2) section is limiting or preventing motion of a body region.

4. The root operation _____ from the Administration (3) section is putting in or on a therapeutic, diagnostic, nutritional, physiological, or prophylactic substance except blood or blood products.

5. The root operation _____ from the Measurement and Monitoring (4) section is determining the level of a physiological or physical function repetitively over a period of time.

6. The root operation _____ from the Extracorporeal or Systemic Therapies (6) section is extracorporeal separation of blood products

7. The root operation _____ from the Osteopathic (7) section is manual treatment to eliminate or alleviate somatic dysfunction and related disorders.

8. The root operation _____ from the Placement (2) section is putting material on a body region for protection.

9. The root operation _____ from the Extracorporeal or Systemic Assistance and Performance (5) section is taking over a portion of a physiological function by extracorporeal means.

10. The root operation _____ from the Extracorporeal or Systemic Therapies (6) section is extracorporeal raising of body temperature.

Multiple Choice

Instructions: Circle the letter of the best answer to each question based on the information you learned in this chapter.

1. Which section classifies procedures in which a diagnostic or therapeutic substance is given to the patient?
   A. Placement (2)
   B. Extracorporeal or Systemic Therapies (6)
   C. Other Procedures (8)
   D. Administration (3)

2. Which root operation is unique to the Placement (2) section?
   A. Change
   B. Compression
   C. Treatment
   D. Removal

3. What section defines Character 6 as Substance?
   A. Extracorporeal or Systemic Therapies (6)
   B. Obstetrics (1)
   C. Other Procedures (8)
   D. Administration (3)

4. How would you code the following procedure? *A patient was placed on CPB during open heart surgery*.
   A. 5A1221Z
   B. 5A1223Z
   C. 02100KW
   D. 02100Z3

5. Which medical and surgical-related section has guidelines in PCS OGCR?
   A. Obstetrics (1)
   B. Placement (2)
   C. Administration (3)
   D. Extracorporeal or Systemic Therapies (6)

(continued)

(continued from page 1141)

6. How would you code the following procedure? *A physician performs mechanical traction of the femur following open reduction internal fixation on the left femur.*
   A. 2W6RXZZ
   B. 2W6RXZZ
   C. 2W6RX0Z
   D. 2W6PX0Z

7. Which section classifies procedures that use equipment to support a physiological function in a critical care setting?
   A. Administration (3)
   B. Extracorporeal or Systemic Assistance and Performance (5)
   C. Placement (2)
   D. Measurement and Monitoring (4)

8. What is the only body part value in the Obstetrics (1) section?
   A. Products of Conception
   B. Fetus
   C. Uterus
   D. Birth Canal

9. What section uses the Character 2, body system value Indwelling Device (C)?
   A. Placement (2)
   B. Measurement and Monitoring (4)
   C. Extracorporeal or Systemic Assistance and Performance (5)
   D. Other Procedures (8)

10. How would you code the following procedure? *A physician performs chiropractic manipulation of the neck using direct visceral method.*
   A. 9WB7XCZ
   B. 9WB5XBZ
   C. 9WB1XFZ
   D. 9WB0XFZ

KEEP ON CODING

Instructions: Read the procedural statement , abstract the root operation, then use the appropriate Index and Tables to assign PCS procedure codes. Assign only the root operations discussed in this chapter. Write the code(s) on the line provided.

1. Abortion using laminaria. ICD-10-PCS Code(s) _____

2. Pain nerve block injection of an anesthetic agent in the spine. ICD-10-PCS Code(s) _____

3. Traction for fracture of right upper leg. ICD-10-PCS Code(s) _____

4. Esophageal motility study consisting of multiple readings over a period of time, via endoscope. ICD-10-PCS Code(s) _____

5. Splinting of left hand. ICD-10-PCS -10-PCS Code(s) _____

6. Cesarean delivery, high. ICD-10-PCS Code(s) _____

7. Transfusion (percutaneous) of nonautologous frozen red blood cells via peripheral vein. ICD-10-PCS Code(s) _____

8. Electroencephalogram (EEG). ICD-10-PCS Code(s) _____

9. Intermittent positive airway pressure (IPAP) respiratory ventilation for 36 hours. ICD-10-PCS Code(s) _____

10. Measurement of basal metabolic rate (BMR). ICD-10-PCS Code(s) _____

11. Transfusion (percutaneous) of 2 units of fresh RBCs via peripheral vein, nonautologous. ICD-10-PCS Code(s) _____

12. Osteopathic treatment of the neck using general mobilization. ICD-10-PCS Code(s) _____

13. Collection of sperm for fertility study. ICD-10-PCS Code(s) _____

14. Chiropractic manipulation of the lumbar spine using mechanically assisted technique. ICD-10-PCS Code(s) _____

15. Continuous hyperbaric oxygen treatment for nonhealing ulcer, left ankle. ICD-10-PCS Code(s) _____

16. Peritoneal dialysis using dialysate via Port-a-Cath. ICD-10-PCS Code(s) _____

17. Saline irrigation of nasopharynx via nose. ICD-10-PCS Code(s) _____

18. Cortisone injection in right ankle joint. ICD-10-PCS Code(s) _____

19. Robotic-assisted endoscopic right knee arthroplasty. ICD-10-PCS Code(s) _____

20. Whole-body hyperthermia. ICD-10-PCS Code(s) _____

21. Musculoskeletal shock wave therapy, multiple. ICD-10-PCS Code(s) _____

22. Sandbag compression (pressure dressing) for hematoma at right femoral catheter insertion site. ICD-10-PCS Code(s) _____

23. Manually assisted vaginal delivery. ICD-10-PCS Code(s) _____

24. Perfusion of one donor kidney before transplantation. ICD-10-PCS Code(s) _____

25. Hemodialysis, single session. ICD-10-PCS Code(s) _____

CODING CHALLENGE

Instructions: Read the mini-medical-record of each patient's encounter, then abstract, assign, and arrange ICD-10-CM diagnosis codes and PCS procedure codes using the appropriate Index and Tables. Write the code(s) on the line provided.

---

1. INPATIENT HOSPITAL   Gender: F   Age: 42

Preprocedure diagnosis: Nosebleed, status post rhinoplasty 30 days prior

Procedure: Both nostrils packed with a 7.5-cm Rhino Rocket. During this procedure the patient became unresponsive for about 45 seconds and was resuscitated with a liter bolus of normal saline intravenously.

Postprocedure diagnosis: Epistaxis, transient loss of consciousness

Tip: Patient had a loss of consciousness but not a loss of cardiac or respiratory function.

2 ICD-10-CM Codes _____

2 ICD-10-PCS Codes _____

---

2. INPATIENT HOSPITAL   Gender: F   Age: 50

Preprocedure diagnosis: Suspected ventricular tachycardia following an episode of syncope. Transient heart arrhythmias and transient cardiac ischemia.

Procedure: 24-hour Holter monitor

Postprocedure diagnosis: Ventricular tachycardia confirmed

1 ICD-10-CM Code _____

1 ICD-10-PCS Code _____

---

3. INPATIENT HOSPITAL   Gender: F   Age: 37

Preprocedure diagnosis: Plantar fasciitis, right and left foot

Procedure: Extracorporeal shock wave therapy directed at the plantar fascia on the right and left. Patient tolerated the procedure with minimal discomfort.

Tip: Identify the repeated nature of this procedure in Character 5, Duration with the value Multiple.

1 ICD-10-CM Code _____

1 ICD-10-PCS Code _____

---

4. INPATIENT HOSPITAL   Gender: F   Age: 25

Preprocedure diagnosis: Active labor, 40 weeks, 3 days

Procedure: Placement of epidural catheter with continuous infusion of 0.2% ropivacaine with 1.5 mL of fentanyl at 10 mL per hour. The catheter was placed at the level of L3–L4 without incident. Patient experienced immediate pain relief.

Tip: An epidural catheter is a plastic catheter placed through the skin into the epidural space within the spinal canal.

2 ICD-10-CM Codes _____

2 ICD-10-PCS Codes _____

---

5. INPATIENT HOSPITAL   Gender: F   Age: 27

Preprocedure diagnosis: Full-term labor, EGA 37 + 5

Procedure: Spontaneous vaginal delivery of one liveborn female

3 ICD-10-CM Codes _____

_____

_____

1 ICD-10-PCS Code _____

(continued)

(continued from page 1143)

---

6. INPATIENT HOSPITAL   Gender: M   Age: 31

Preprocedure diagnosis: Postpolio syndrome (PPS). Severe neck pain and weakness. Had polio at age 5 when living overseas.

Procedure: Osteopathic myofascial release of the neck. Pressure was applied to release the trigger points of the cervical area.

2 ICD-10-CM Codes _____

1 ICD-10-PCS Code _____

---

7. INPATIENT HOSPITAL   Gender: F   Age: 40

Preprocedure diagnosis: Cervical spinal stenosis status post decompression, opioid dependence, long-standing low-back pain radiating into the right leg.

Procedure: Needle EMG, nerve conduction study. Needle EMG was performed on the right leg and lumbosacral paraspinal muscles using a disposable concentric needle. It revealed the spontaneous activity in right peroneus longus and gastrocnemius medialis muscles as well as the right lower lumbosacral paraspinal muscles. There is evidence of denervation in right gastrocnemius medialis muscle.

Postprocedure diagnosis: No evidence of left lower extremity radiculopathy, peripheral neuropathy, or entrapment neuropathy.

Tip: Refer to ICD-10-CM OGCR I.C.6.b.(ii) for diagnosis sequencing instructions. Two codes for the EMG procedure are needed: one for the nervous system and one for the musculoskeletal system.

4 ICD-10-CM Codes _____

_____

2 ICD-10-PCS Codes _____

---

8. INPATIENT HOSPITAL   Gender: F   Age: 32

Preprocedure diagnosis: Intrauterine fetal demise at 34 weeks' gestation

Procedure: Preterm induced vaginal delivery of intrauterine fetal demise. IV Pitocin initiated and labor progressed to complete dilation after AROM. A stillborn fetus was delivered vaginally without incident.

Tip: Products of conception refer to all components of pregnancy, including the fetus, embryo, amnion, umbilical cord, and placenta.

3 ICD-10-CM Codes _____

_____

3 ICD-10-PCS Codes _____

_____

---

9. INPATIENT HOSPITAL   Gender: M   Age: 3 days

Preprocedure diagnosis: NSVD of newborn now with jaundice and hyperbilirubinemia

Procedure: Phototherapy with Bili light x2 days. Baby was placed under the Bili light with soft eye patches and a diaper. After two days of therapy bilirubin returned to normal.

2 ICD-10-CM Codes _____

1 ICD-10-PCS Code _____

---

10. INPATIENT HOSPITAL   Gender: M   Age: 57

Preprocedure diagnosis: Angina pectoris

Procedure: Cardiac stress test to measure total activity, single measurement, followed by catheterization of left and right heart to obtain sampling and pressure.

Tip: Heart catheterization by definition uses a percutaneous approach.

1 ICD-10-CM Code _____

2 ICD-10-PCS Codes _____

Learning Objectives

After completing this chapter, you should have the skills to:

55.1 Spell and define the key words, medical terms, and abbreviations related to ancillary and new technology procedures. (Remember)

55.2 Identify the types of procedures in the ancillary sections. (Apply)

55.3 Adhere to ICD-10-PCS coding guidelines related to the ancillary sections. (Apply)

55.4 Examine and abstract information from the medical record for coding procedures in the ancillary sections. (Analyze)

55.5 Demonstrate how to assign codes for the root types for procedures in the ancillary sections. (Apply)

55.6 Utilize guidelines for arranging (sequencing) codes for root types for procedures in the ancillary section. (Apply)

55.7 Adhere to ICD-10-PCS coding guidelines related to the New Technology section. (Apply)

55.8 Demonstrate how to abstract and assign codes for procedures in the New Technology section. (Apply)

Chapter Outline

- **Basics of Ancillary Procedures**
- **Coding Guidelines for Ancillary Procedures**
- **Abstracting for Ancillary Procedures**
- **Assigning Characters 4–7 for Ancillary Procedures**
- **Arranging Codes for Ancillary Procedures**
- **New Technology (Section X)**

Key Terms and Abbreviations

activities of daily living (ADLs)	assessment (PCS Section F)	orthosis	radiopharmaceutical
anatomic imaging	functional imaging	prosthesis	treatment (PCS Section F)

In addition to the key terms listed here, students should know the terms defined within tables in this chapter.

INTRODUCTION

Visual images of a trip can be either still or motion. Likewise, physicians use a variety of imaging technologies to better understand the human body. Radiographic imaging is one of several types of procedures classified in the PCS ancillary sections.

This chapter discusses PCS sections B, C, D, F, G, and H, referred to as ancillary procedures and section X, New Technology. (There is no section E.) You learn how codes in these sections are structured, how root types are defined, and other unique characteristics. As with other PCS sections, pay careful attention to the differences between each root type so that you can use each confidently and accurately.

BASICS OF ANCILLARY PROCEDURES

"Ancillary procedures" is a descriptive title that summarizes nine PCS sections, but it does not occupy a character within the code itself. ■ TABLE 55-1 summarizes the value, name, and purpose of each section. Ancillary sections contain approximately 6,800 codes and represent 9% of PCS. All root types are unique to sections in this portion of PCS.

Ancillary procedure codes have seven characters, but the purpose of many characters is different than in the Medical and Surgical (0) section (■ TABLE 55-2). Character names and values used in ancillary procedures are frequently unique to a particular Table, so take time to review the character definitions when coding from this portion of PCS to avoid confusion. Some of the differences include:

- In the section Physical Rehabilitation and Diagnostic Audiology (F), Character 2 is the Section Qualifier that distinguishes between the two types of service reported in this section: Physical Rehabilitation (0) or Diagnostic Audiology (1).

- All sections except Radiation Therapy (D) define Character 3 as root type rather than root operation because no operations are performed. Radiation Therapy defines Character 3 as Modality.

- The Imaging (B) section defines Character 5 as Contrast and Character 6 as Qualifier.

- The Nuclear Medicine (C) section defines Character 5 as Radionuclide.

- The Radiation Therapy (D) section defines Character 4 as Treatment Site, Character 5 as Modality Qualifier, and Character 6 as Isotope.

Table 55-1 ■ **CHARACTER 1: SECTION NAMES AND PURPOSE FOR ANCILLARY PROCEDURES**

Value	Section Name	Purpose
B	Imaging	Creating a visual representation of internal body structures to diagnose conditions
C	Nuclear Medicine	Introduction of radioactive materials into the body to capture images, diagnose diseases, or treat abnormalities
D	Radiation Therapy	Use of radiation to treat malignancies
F	Physical Rehabilitation and Diagnostic Audiology	Procedures and therapy to help patients regain body functions lost due to medical conditions or injury; procedures to diagnose hearing-related conditions
G	Mental Health	A variety of methods to diagnose and treat psychiatric and mental disorders
H	Substance Abuse Treatment	Procedures to treat disorders related to substance abuse

CODING CAUTION

Be alert for root types that are spelled similarly but have different PCS definitions.

Computerized Tomography (2) (Section B) (*Computer-reformatted digital display* of multiplanar images developed from the capture of multiple exposures of *external ionizing radiation*) and **Tomographic (Tomo) Nuclear Medicine Imaging (2) (Section C)** (*Introduction of radioactive materials into the body* for three-dimensional display of images developed from the capture of radioactive emissions)

Ultrasonography (4) (Section B) (*Real-time display of images* of anatomy or flow information developed from the capture of reflected and attenuated high-frequency sound waves) and **Ultrasound Therapy (7) (Section F)** (*Extracorporeal treatment* by high-frequency sound waves [ultrasound])

Table 55-2 ■ **SEVEN CHARACTERS OF ANCILLARY PROCEDURES**

1 Section	2	3	4	5	6	7
Imaging B	Body System	Root Type	Body Part	Contrast	Qualifier	Qualifier
Nuclear Medicine C	Body System	Root Type	Body Part	Radionuclide	Qualifier	Qualifier
Radiation Therapy D	Body System	Modality	Treatment Site	Modality Qualifier	Isotope	Qualifier
Physical Rehabilitation and Diagnostic Audiology F	Section Qualifier	Root Type	Body System/Region	Type Qualifier	Equipment	Qualifier
Mental Health G	Body System	Root Type	Type Qualifier	Qualifier	Qualifier	Qualifier
Substance Abuse Treatment H	Body System	Root Type	Type Qualifier	Qualifier	Qualifier	Qualifier

Table 55-3   ■   **EXAMPLE OF CONSTRUCTING MEDICAL TERMS FOR ANCILLARY PROCEDURES**

Combining Form	Suffix	Complete Medical Term
radi/o (*radiation*) son/o (*sound*) tom/o (*cut, slice*)	-graph/-gram (*record*) -therapy (*treatment*)	**radio + graph** (*a record made with radiation*) **sono + gram** (*a record made with sound*) **tomo + graph** (*a record made with [visual] slices*)
psych/o (*mind*) ultra/sound (*high-frequency sound*)		**radio + therapy** (*treatment with radiation*) **ultrasound + therapy** (*treatment with high-frequency sound waves*) **psycho + therapy** (*treatment of the mind*)

Source: © PB Resources, Inc. Used with permission.

- Physical Rehabilitation and Diagnostic Audiology defines Character 4 as body system and region. It defines Character 5 as type qualifier and Character 6 as equipment.
- The Mental Health (G) and Substance Abuse Treatment (H) sections define Characters 4–7 as Qualifier. These characters always have the value None (Z).

Medical terms for ancillary procedures often contain a suffix that describes the type of procedure performed, such as making a recording (*-graphy*) or providing therapy (*-therapy*), and a root that identifies the specific method, such as radiation (*radi/o*) or sound waves (*son/o*). Procedure names can combine the medical term for the procedure with additional terms for the anatomic site and isotope, contrast agent, or other pharmaceutical used. Be sure to review documentation thoroughly to locate all modifying terms that describe the procedure. Refer to ■ TABLE 55-3 for a refresher on how to build medical terms related to ancillary procedures. Refer to detailed anatomic diagrams of specific organ systems in Chapters 8–43 of this text, or in external references, when you need to refresh your memory of human anatomy.

CODING PRACTICE

Exercise 55.1	Basics of Ancillary Procedures

Instructions: Use your medical terminology skills and resources to define the following ancillary procedures, then identify the code(s) or code range listed in the PCS Index. Follow these steps:

- Use slash marks "/" to break down the underlined term into its root(s) and suffix.
- Do not attempt to break down abbreviations.
- Define the meaning of the underlined term based on the meaning of each word part or each letter of an abbreviation.
- Look up the phrase in the ICD-10-PCS Index, and write down the name(s) and Root Type(s) or Modality(ies) the Index cross-references you to and the Table(s), if provided.
- Do not assign any codes.

Example: discography, bones
disco/graphy   Meaning: *make a recording of an intervertebral disc* PCS Root Type(s)/Table(s): *Plain Radiography BR0*

1. audiometry   Meaning _____ PCS Root Type(s)/Table(s) _____
2. pyelography   Meaning _____ PCS Root Type(s)/Table(s) _____
3. pharmacotherapy for   Meaning _____ PCS Root Type(s)/Table(s) _____
   substance abuse
4. tonometry   Meaning _____ PCS Root Type(s)/Table(s) _____
5. cholangiogram   Meaning _____ PCS Root Type(s)/Table(s) _____
6. KUB x-ray   Meaning _____ PCS Root Type(s)/Table(s) _____
7. myelogram   Meaning _____ PCS Root Type(s)/Table(s) _____
8. electroconvulsive therapy   Meaning _____ PCS Root Type(s)/Table(s) _____
9. venography   Meaning _____ PCS Root Type(s)/Table(s) _____
10. laser interstitial thermal ther-   Meaning _____ PCS Root Type(s)/Table(s) _____
    apy, brainstem

CODING GUIDELINES FOR ANCILLARY PROCEDURES

PCS OGCR provides no guidelines for ancillary procedures. The appendix in the PCS coding manual "Type and Type Qualifier Definitions, Sections B–H" provides official definitions of many of the terms used in the ancillary sections (■ FIGURE 55-1). The sections and characters for which definitions are provided are as follows:

- Section B, Imaging
  - Character 3, Root Type
- Section C, Nuclear Medicine
  - Character 3, Root Type
- Section F, Physical Rehabilitation and Diagnostic Audiology
  - Character 3, Root Type
  - Character 5, Type Qualifier
- Section G, Mental Health
  - Character 3, Root Type
  - Character 4, Type Qualifier
- Section H, Substance Abuse
  - Character 3, Root Type

Use the appendix as follows when assigning codes in PCS sections B–H:

1. Locate the desired section name in the appendix.
2. Confirm the character position and name.
3. If the section defines values for more than one character, locate the segment for the correct character.
4. Locate the character value(s) needed, read the definition, and confirm whether it accurately describes the service to be coded.
5. If the definition is not accurate, review other definitions to find the appropriate one.

ABSTRACTING FOR ANCILLARY PROCEDURES

The following information highlights the definitions and unique criteria for sections B, C, D, F, G, and H. Because of the brief and specialized nature of these sections, guidance about Characters 4–7 is incorporated into the following discussion. General information about assigning codes is presented in the "Assigning" section of this chapter. A Key Criteria for Abstracting table helps determine the appropriate PCS section. Individual abstracting tables for each section are not provided because the appropriate root types can generally be determined by reviewing the PCS definitions.

Key Criteria for Abstracting Ancillary Procedures

Key abstracting criteria aid in identifying the section that should be used to identify the correct root type (■ TABLE 55-4). After reading the procedure report, use the abstracting table as follows:

1. Answer the General Questions to get a basic understanding of the procedure.
2. Answer the Section Questions. One question should be answered *Yes*; the rest should be answered *No*.
3. For the Section Question that was answered *Yes*, refer to the section identified to review the root types that could apply.
4. Look up the definition of each of the applicable root types in the appendix of the ICD-10-PCS coding manual.
5. Identify the one root type or modality that matches the procedure documented. This will be the Main Term when you use the Index.
6. Repeat the abstracting process for each procedure performed.

Section F: Physical Rehabilitation and Diagnostic Audiology Character 3: Root Type	
Value	Definition
Activities of Daily Living Assessment	Measurement of functional level for activities of daily living
Activities of Daily Living Treatment	Exercise or activities to facilitate functional competence for activities of daily living
Caregiver Training	Training in activities to support patient's optimal level of function
Cochlear Implant Treatment	Application of techniques to improve the communication abilities of individuals with cochlear implant

Figure 55-1 ■ Example of PCS appendix, "Type and Type Qualifier Definitions, Sections B–H."

Table 55-4 ■ **KEY CRITERIA FOR ABSTRACTING ANCILLARY PROCEDURES**

General Questions
❏ What is the stated procedure?
❏ What body region or body part is involved?
❏ What method is used?
❏ Is the procedure description what you would expect based on the name of the procedure?
❏ Was more than one procedure, or a combined procedure, performed?

Section Questions (Answer *Yes* to one question)	Refer to Root Types in This Section
❏ Does the procedure involve imaging/radiography?	Section B Imaging
❏ Does the procedure involve nuclear medicine?	Section C Nuclear Medicine
❏ Does the procedure involve radiation treatment for a malignancy?	Section D Radiation Therapy
❏ Does the procedure involve physical rehabilitation or diagnostic audiology?	Section F Physical Rehabilitation and Diagnostic Audiology
❏ Are mental health services provided?	Section G Mental Health
❏ Is substance abuse treatment provided?	Section 6 Substance Abuse Treatment

Source: © PB Resources, Inc. Used with permission.

Abstracting for Radiology Procedures (Sections B, C, and D)

Ancillary procedures include three classes of radiology procedures, each with a separate PCS section: Imaging (B), Nuclear Medicine (C), and Radiation Therapy (D). The root types within each section identify various techniques and modalities.

Imaging (Section B) Root Types

The Imaging (B) section includes diagnostic radiology and its branches, each of which is a root type (■ TABLE 55-5), for

Table 55-5 ■ **ROOT TYPES IN THE IMAGING (B) SECTION**

Value	Description	Definition
0	Plain Radiography	Planar (*flat, single plane*) display of an image developed from the capture of external ionizing radiation on photographic or photoconductive plate
1	Fluoroscopy	Single plane or biplane real-time display of an image developed from the capture of external ionizing radiation on a fluorescent screen; may also be stored by either digital or analog means
2	Computerized Tomography (CT scan)	Computer-reformatted digital display of multiplanar images developed from the capture of multiple exposures of external ionizing radiation
3	Magnetic Resonance Imaging (MRI)	Computer-reformatted digital display of multiplanar images developed from the capture of radiofrequency signals emitted by nuclei in a body site excited within a magnetic field
4	Ultrasonography	Real-time display of images of anatomy or flow information developed from the capture of reflected and attenuated high-frequency sound waves

a total of five root types. This section classifies **anatomic imaging**, which captures a static image of an anatomic part. ■ FIGURE 55-2 (page 1150) shows images created by various imaging methods. Characters are defined as follows:

- Character 4, Body System provides values for the major body systems, as well as Anatomical Regions (W) and Fetus and Obstetrical (Y). The skeletal system is identified by the following values, which differ from the classical divisions of axial skeleton and appendicular skeleton:
  - Skull and Facial Bones (N)
  - Axial Skeletal System, Except Skull and Facial Bones (R), which includes the vertebral column, pelvis, and sternum
  - Non-axial Upper Bones (P), which includes the shoulders, ribs, arms, and hands
  - Non-axial Lower Bones (Q), which includes the legs and feet
- Character 5, Contrast identifies the type of contrast medium used, if any. Because x-ray beams pass through soft tissue, the use of a contrast dye makes soft structures more readily visible. Examples of Contrast values are High Osmolar and Low Osmolar.
- Character 6, Qualifier, Unenhanced and Enhanced (0) identifies an image taken without contrast followed by one with contrast. When no contrast medium is used, assign the value None (Z).
- Character 7, Qualifier has only one value, None (Z), which should be assigned for all codes.

The root type Plain Radiography (0) includes traditional x-ray and mammography.

Operative procedures sometimes use imaging guidance to assist in visualizing the procedure with the use of fluoroscopy or ultrasound. Code the operative procedure as the definitive procedure, usually from the Medical and Surgical (0) section, then assign an additional code from the Imaging section for the imaging guidance. Use the Character 7, Qualifier value for Guidance (A) (■ FIGURE 55-3, page 1150).

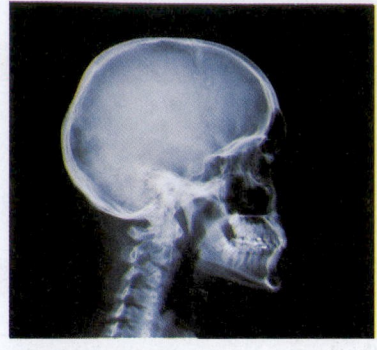

A Plain radiography

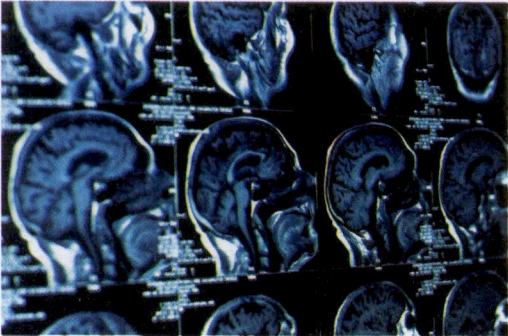

B Computed tomography (CT)

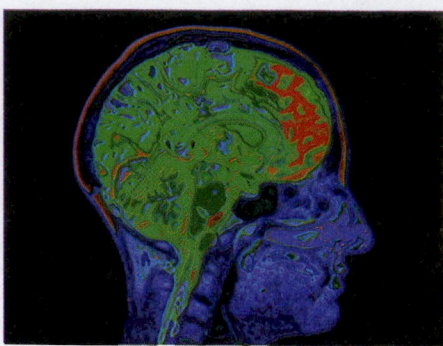

C Magnetic resonance imaging (MRI)

Figure 55-2 ■ Examples of imaging methods. (A) Plain radiography. *Source: Itsmejust/Shutterstock.* (B) Computed tomography (CT). *Source: SvedOliver/Shutterstock.* (C) Magnetic resonance imaging (MRI). *Source: SpeedKingz/Shutterstock.*

Radiologist provided fluoroscopic guidance with high osmolar contrast for a percutaneous thrombectomy in the right popliteal vein.

06CY3ZZ Medical and surgical, Lower veins, Extirpation, Lower vein, Percutaneous, No device, No qualifier
B51B0ZA Imaging, Veins, Fluoroscopic, Lower extremity veins right, High osmolar, None, Guidance

Figure 55-3 ■ Example of coding for imaging guidance. *Source: © PB Resources, Inc. Used with permission.*

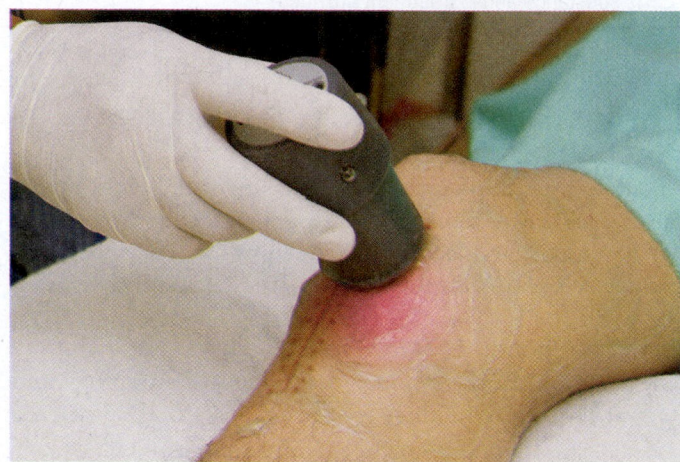

A Ultrasound therapy

Ultrasound is energy created by high-frequency sound waves, which can be used for therapy—such as stimulating muscle and nerve tissue—or for imaging purposes. In ultrasound imaging—also called ultrasonography or sonogram—sounds waves are bounced off a structure in the body to create an image. Ultrasound therapy works by driving sound waves into the tissue to help alleviate pain, inflammation, and muscle spasms while increasing range of motion. Ultrasound imaging is performed at a different frequency than ultrasound therapy. When you see a reference to ultrasound, identify whether it is ultrasound imaging or therapeutic ultrasound so you can select the correct root type (■ FIGURE 55-4).

EXAMPLE: *An transesophageal ultrasound image was made of the right heart to diagnose abnormalities.*

B244ZZ4 Ultrasonography, heart, right, transesophageal

EXAMPLE: *Ultrasound therapy was performed on the heart to treat ischemia, single session.*

6A750Z5 Ultrasound therapy, heart, circulatory, single, no qualifier, heart

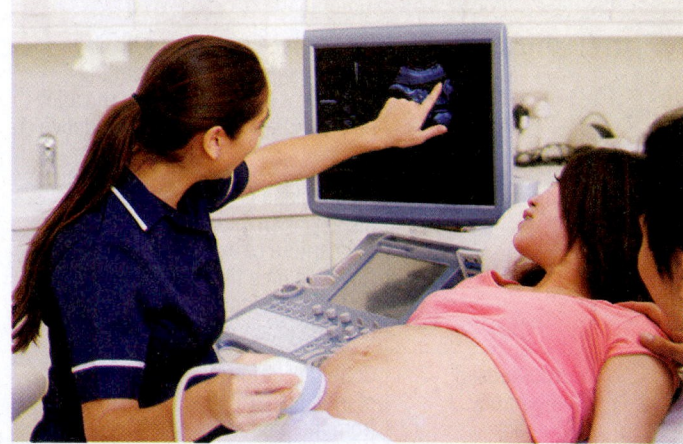

B Ultrasound imaging

Figure 55-4 ■ (A) Ultrasound therapy uses sound waves to stimulate tissue. *Source: Praisaeng/Shutterstock.* (B) Ultrasound imaging (ultrasonography) uses sound waves to create an image. *Source: Monkey Business Images/Shutterstock.*

Nuclear Medicine (Section C) Root Types

Root types for Nuclear Medicine (C) identify the methods used (■ TABLE 55-6). Nuclear medicine is a specialized branch of radiology that provides **functional imaging**, which allows the physician to observe organ function in real time. Patients take a very small amount of radioactive material, also called a **radiopharmaceutical**, internally. The radiopharmaceutical substance emits gamma rays that are detected by equipment to create an image.

Table 55-6 ■ ROOT TYPES IN THE NUCLEAR MEDICINE (C) SECTION

Value	Description	Definition
1	Planar Nuclear Medicine Imaging	Introduction of radioactive materials into the body for single-plane display of images developed from the capture of radioactive emissions
2	Tomographic (Tomo) Nuclear Medicine Imaging	Introduction of radioactive materials into the body for three-dimensional display of images developed from the capture of radioactive emissions
3	Positron Emission Tomography (PET)	Introduction of radioactive materials into the body for three-dimensional display of images developed from the simultaneous capture, 180 degrees apart, of radioactive emissions
4	Nonimaging Nuclear Medicine Uptake	Introduction of radioactive materials into the body for measurements of organ function from the detection of radioactive emissions
5	Nonimaging Nuclear Medicine Probe	Introduction of radioactive materials into the body for the study of distribution and fate of certain substances by the detection of radioactive emissions from an external source
6	Nonimaging Nuclear Medicine Assay	Introduction of radioactive materials into the body for the study of body fluids and blood elements by the detection of radioactive emissions
7	Systemic Nuclear Medicine Therapy	Introduction of unsealed radioactive materials into the body for treatment

The Nuclear Medicine section uses Characters 5–7 as follows:

- Character 5, Radionuclide, identifies the radiation source used in the procedure. Choices are dependent on the procedure described by the root type. Examples are Carbon 11 and Fluorine.

- Character 6, Qualifier, and Character 7, Qualifier, have only one value, None (Z), which should be assigned in both positions for all codes.

Radiation Therapy (Section D) Modalities

The Radiation Therapy (D) section contains therapeutic radiology procedures performed for cancer treatment. Character meanings are described below.

- Character 3 is Modality rather than root type. Modality definitions are based on standard usage within the specialty (■ TABLE 55-7) and are not provided within the PCS system.

- Character 4, Treatment Site, is the site targeted by the radiation treatment.

- Character 5, Modality Qualifier, further specifies treatment modality, such as the type or dose of radiation.

Table 55-7 ■ MODALITIES IN THE RADIATION THERAPY (D) SECTION

Value	Description	Definition
0	Beam radiation	Aiming radiation beams at a small target area to destroy tissue
1	Brachytherapy	Insertion of radioactive implants directly into body tissue
2	Stereotactic radiosurgery	Delivery of high doses of radiation to a target area with minimal exposure to the surrounding healthy tissue
V	Other radiation	Modalities not identified by other values

Source: © PB Resources, Inc. Used with permission.

Examples for Beam Radiation (0) are Photons <1 MeV, Photons 1–10 MeV, and so on. Values for Brachytherapy (1) are High Dose Rate and Low Dose Rate.

- Character 6, Isotope, defines the radioactive isotope used, if applicable. This character is used in Brachytherapy (1). Examples are Cesium 137 and Iridium 192.

- Character 7, Qualifier, has only one value, None (Z), which is assigned for all codes.

Abstracting for Sections F, G, and H

The remaining ancillary sections classify physical rehabilitation, diagnostic audiology, mental health, and substance abuse. These are discussed next.

Physical Rehabilitation and Diagnostic Audiology (Section F) Root Types

This section classifies two general types of procedures that are not related: physical rehabilitation and diagnostic audiology. Physical rehabilitation includes physical, occupational, and speech therapy services. Diagnostic audiology includes services to diagnose hearing conditions. Character 2, Section Qualifier distinguishes between these two types of services. Values for Characters 3–7 are dependent on the Character 2 value.

The character definitions in this section are distinct from other PCS sections as follows:

Character 2 is Section Qualifier, rather than body system, and specifies whether the procedure is Rehabilitation (0) or Diagnostic Audiology (1).

- Character 3, Root Type defines the general type of procedure (■ TABLE 55-8, page 1152).

- Character 4, Body System and Region defines the body system and body region combined, where applicable.

- Character 5, Type Qualifier further specifies the procedure type beyond what is specified in Character 3.

- Character 6, Equipment specifies the equipment used, if any.

- Character 7, Qualifier has only one value, None (Z), which should be assigned for all codes.

Table 55-8 ■ **ROOT TYPES IN THE PHYSICAL REHABILITATION AND DIAGNOSTIC AUDIOLOGY (F) SECTION**

Value	Description	Definition
0	Speech Assessment	Measurement of speech and related functions
1	Motor and/or Nerve Function Assessment	Measurement of motor, nerve, and related functions
2	Activities of Daily Living Assessment	Measurement of functional level for activities of daily living
3	Hearing Assessment	Measurement of hearing and related functions
4	Hearing Aid Assessment	Measurement of the appropriateness and/or effectiveness of a hearing device
5	Vestibular Assessment	Measurement of the vestibular system and related functions
6	Speech Treatment	Application of techniques to improve, augment, or compensate for speech and related functional impairment
7	Motor Treatment	Exercise or activities to increase or facilitate motor function
8	Activities of Daily Living Treatment	Exercise or activities to facilitate functional competence for activities of daily living
9	Hearing Treatment	Application of techniques to improve, augment, or compensate for hearing and related functional impairment
B	Hearing Aid Treatment	Application of techniques to improve the communication abilities of individuals with cochlear implant
C	Vestibular Treatment	Application of techniques to improve, augment, or compensate for vestibular and related functional impairment
D	Device Fitting	Fitting of a device designed to facilitate or support achievement of a higher level of function
F	Caregiver Training	Training in activities to support patient's optimal level of function

In this section, the term **treatment** classifies a wide variety of activities typically associated with rehabilitation, such as swallowing-dysfunction exercises, bathing and showering techniques, wound management, and gait training. **Assessments** are procedures to diagnose a condition and are classified into more than 100 tests and methods. The majority of these focus on hearing and speech, but others focus on various aspects of body function and on the patient's quality of life, such as muscle performance, neuromotor development, and reintegration skills.

Character 5 of the root type Device Fitting (D) describes the device being fitted, not the method used to fit the device. PCS provides definitions for some devices, located in the definitions appendix of the PCS coding manual, under section F, Character 5. For example, in the root type Vestibular Treatment (C), the type qualifier identifies the type of treatment, such as Postural Control (3), Vestibular (0), Perceptual Processing (1), or Visual Motor Integration (2). This root type is for use by inpatient rehabilitation facilities only and can include highly customized devices (■ FIGURE 55-5). All other inpatient facilities should assign codes for the root operation Immobilization (3) from the Placement (2) section.

The root type Caregiver Training (F) is divided into several broad subjects taught to help a caregiver provide proper patient care. Character 5, Type Qualifier identifies the specific type of training. Character 6, Equipment identifies any equipment used (■ FIGURE 55-6).

The root type Motor Treatment includes a wide variety of activities typically associated with physical therapy, such as therapeutic exercise, wheelchair training, and gait training.

Coders must use their knowledge of medical equipment to select the correct value for Character 6, Equipment because PCS does not provide official definitions. The value can be specific, such as Audiometer (1), or general, such as Assistive, Adaptive, Supportive, or Protective (F). An **orthosis** is an orthopedic appliance or apparatus used to support, align, prevent, or correct deformities or to improve the function of movable parts of the body. A **prosthesis** is an artificial substitute for a missing body part. An assistive, adaptive, supportive, or protective device aids or protects a patient while performing **activities of daily living (ADLs)** (*daily self-care activities such as bathing, dressing, grooming, eating, and leisure*). Examples of such devices are wheelchairs, walkers, bath chairs, and special beds, chairs, and tables.

Mental Health (Section G) Root Types

Section G Mental Health uses Character 3, Root Type (■ TABLE 55-9) and Character 4, Type Qualifier. Characters 2, 5, 6, and 7 are placeholders only and are assigned the value None (Z) for all codes.

> Physician places a static orthosis on the left forearm of an inpatient in a rehabilitation facility.
>
> **F0DZ7EZ Physical rehabilitation and diagnostic audiology, Rehabilitation, Device fitting, None, Static orthosis, Orthosis, None**

Figure 55-5 ■ Example of coding the root type Device Fitting (3) for a rehabilitation facility patient. *Source: © PB Resources, Inc. Used with permission.*

> The mother of a child with club foot was trained how to apply a solid bar abduction brace.
>
> **F0FZFEZ Physical Rehabilitation and Diagnostic Audiology, Rehabilitation, Caregiver training, None, Application proper use and care of orthoses, Orthoses, None**

Figure 55-6 ■ Example of coding for root type Caregiver Training. *Source: © PB Resources, Inc. Used with permission.*

Table 55-9 ■ ROOT TYPES IN THE MENTAL HEALTH (G) SECTION

Value	Description	Definition
1	Psychological Tests	The administration and interpretation of standardized psychological tests and measurement instruments for the assessment of psychological function
2	Crisis Intervention	Treatment of a traumatized, acutely disturbed, or distressed individual for the purpose of short-term stabilization
3	Medication Management	Monitoring and adjusting the use of medications for the treatment of a mental health disorder
5	Individual Psychotherapy	Treatment of an individual with a mental health disorder by behavioral, cognitive, psychoanalytic, psychodynamic, or psychophysiological means to improve functioning or well-being
6	Counseling	The application of psychological methods to treat an individual with normal developmental issues and psychological problems in order to increase function, improve well-being, alleviate distress, address maladjustment, or resolve crises
7	Family Psychotherapy	Treatment that includes one or more family members of an individual with a mental health disorder by behavioral, cognitive, psychoanalytic, psychodynamic, or psychophysiological means to improve functioning or well-being
B	Electroconvulsive Therapy	The application of controlled electrical voltages to treat a mental health disorder
C	Biofeedback	Provision of information from the monitoring and regulating of physiological processes in conjunction with cognitive-behavioral techniques to improve patient functioning or well-being
F	Hypnosis	Induction of a state of heightened suggestibility by auditory, visual, and tactile techniques to elicit an emotional or behavioral response
G	Narcosynthesis	Administration of intravenous barbiturates in order to release suppressed or repressed thoughts
H	Group Therapy	Treatment of two or more individuals with a mental health disorder by behavioral, cognitive, psychoanalytic, psychodynamic, or psychophysiological means to improve functioning or well-being
J	Light Therapy	Application of specialized light treatments to improve functioning or well-being

Table 55-10 ■ ROOT TYPES IN THE SUBSTANCE ABUSE TREATMENT (H) SECTION

Value	Description	Definition
2	Detoxification Services	Detoxification from alcohol and/or drugs
3	Individual Counseling	The application of psychological methods to treat an individual with addictive behavior
4	Group Counseling	The application of psychological methods to treat two or more individuals with addictive behavior
5	Individual Psychotherapy	Treatment of an individual with addictive behavior by behavioral, cognitive, psychoanalytic, psychodynamic, or psychophysiological means
6	Family Counseling	The application of psychological methods that includes one or more family members to treat an individual with addictive behavior
8	Medication Management	Monitoring and adjusting the use of replacement medications for the treatment of addiction
9	Pharmacotherapy	The use of replacement medications for the treatment of addiction

Root types Medication Management (8) and Pharmacotherapy (9) use Character 4 to identify the medication. The root type Medication Management appears both in this section with the value **8** and in the Mental Health (G) section with the value **3** and a different definition.

Guided Example of Abstracting for Ancillary Procedures

Refer to the following example throughout this chapter to practice skills for abstracting, assigning, and arranging codes for procedures in the ancillary sections. The Guided Example uses two root types from the ancillary sections and one root operation from the Medical and Surgical section (0). The principles discussed here also apply to other ancillary root types.

Substance Abuse Treatment (Section H) Root Types

The Substance Abuse Treatment (H) section is organized similar to Mental Health and has seven root types (■ Table 55-10). The root type Detoxification Services (2) does not provide values for Characters 4–7. Root types 3–6 use Character 4 for Type Qualifier, which describes the type of counseling provided.

INPATIENT HOSPITAL Gender: M Age: 84

Reason for admission: Hip pain and inability to bear weight following fall on the stairs in her single-family home

Procedures performed: X-ray of the acetabulofemoral joint with low osmolar contrast medium, total left hip arthroplasty with an uncemented metal on polyethylene prosthesis, gait training with walker

Discharge diagnosis: Fractured left hip at the base of the femoral neck

Follow along as fictitious coder Marcy Elwood, CCS, abstracts the procedure. Check off each step after you complete it.

▶ Marcy reads through the entire record, paying special attention to the reason for the admission, the procedures performed, and the final diagnosis.

   ❏ She notes the reason for admission: hip pain and inability to bear weight following fall on the stairs in her single-family home.

   ❏ She also notes the discharge diagnosis: fractured left hip at the base of the femoral neck.

   ❏ *What services were provided during the inpatient stay?*
      ▪ X-ray of the acetabulofemoral joint
      ▪ Total left hip arthroplasty
      ▪ Gait training with walker

▶ First, Marcy abstracts for the surgical procedure, total left hip arthroplasty. She refers to Table 47-3, Key Criteria for Abstracting Medical and Surgical Procedures, and Table 47-4, Key Criteria for Abstracting Root Operations.

   ❏ *What organ or body part is involved?* Left hip

   ❏ *Did the procedure involve an external device left in place in, on, or in replacement of a body part?* Yes. The abstracting table refers the coder to the root operations Change (2), Insertion (H), Removal (P), Replacement (R), Revision (W), and Supplement (U).

   ❏ To abstract the correct root operation, Marcy refers to Table 53-11, Key Criteria for Abstracting Root Operations That Always Involve a Device. Marcy abstracts the root operation.

      ▪ She reviews the abstracting questions and answers *Yes* to one question: *Was a device put in to replace a Body Part?* Refer to the root operation Replacement (R)

▶ Next, Marcy abstracts for x-ray of the acetabulofemoral joint. She refers to the Key Criteria for Abstracting Ancillary Procedures (Table 55-4).

   ❏ *What is the stated procedure?* X-ray

   ❏ *What body region or body part is involved?* Acetabulofemoral joint

   ❏ *What method is used?* Low osmolar contrast medium

   ❏ She reviews the abstracting questions and answers *Yes* to one question: *Does the procedure involve imaging/radiography?* Refer to the Imaging (B) section.

   ❏ Marcy reviews the root types for the Imaging section and selects the one definition that describes the procedure:

      ▪ Plain Radiography (0): Planar display of an image developed from the capture of external ionizing radiation on photographic or photoconductive plate.

▶ Next, Marcy abstracts for gait training with walker. She again refers to Table 55-4.

   ❏ *What is the stated procedure?* Gait training

   ❏ *What equipment is used?* Walker

   ❏ She reviews the abstracting questions and answers *Yes* to one question: *Does the procedure involve physical rehabilitation or diagnostic audiology?* Refer to the section Physical Rehabilitation and Diagnostic Audiology (F)

   ❏ Marcy reviews the root types for the Physical Rehabilitation and Diagnostic Audiology section and selects the one definition that describes the procedure:

      ▪ Motor Treatment (7): Exercise or activities to increase or facilitate motor function.

▶ At this time, Marcy anticipates that she will need three codes, one for each service. She believes that she will use the root operation Replacement for the hip arthroplasty, the root type Plain Radiography for the x-ray, and the root type Motor Training for the gait training. She will verify this information when she refers to the PCS Tables to assign codes.

CODING PRACTICE

Exercise 55.2   **Abstracting for Ancillary Procedures**

Instructions: Read the mini-medical-record of each patient's encounter and answer the abstracting questions. Write the answer on the line provided. Do not assign any codes.

1. INPATIENT HOSPITAL   Gender: M   Age: 57

Preprocedure diagnosis: Cirrhosis, rule out hepatocellular carcinoma

Procedure: CT scan of liver with and without contrast (high osmolar)

Findings: Enlarged liver as expected but no tumors identified

a. What is the stated procedure? _____

(continued)

CODING PRACTICE (continued)

1. (continued)

b. What body region or body part is involved? _____

c. What method is used? _____

d. Was more than one procedure, or a combined procedure, performed? _____

e. Does the procedure involve imaging/radiography? _____

f. Does the procedure involve nuclear medicine? _____ _____

g. Does the procedure involve radiation treatment for a malignancy? _____

h. Does the procedure involve physical rehabilitation or diagnostic audiology? _____

i. Are mental health services provided? _____

j. Is substance abuse treatment provided? _____

k. What PCS section should be used? _____

l. Review the root types in the section selected. What is the most likely root type? _____

---

2. INPATIENT HOSPITAL   Gender: M   Age: 61

Preprocedure diagnosis: Prostate cancer

Procedure: Low dose rate (LDR) brachytherapy of prostate using Iridium 192

a. What is the stated procedure? _____

b. What body region or body part is involved? _____

c. What method is used? _____

d. Was more than one procedure, or a combined procedure, performed? _____

e. Does the procedure involve imaging/radiography? _____

f. Does the procedure involve nuclear medicine? _____

g. Does the procedure involve radiation treatment for a malignancy? _____

h. Does the procedure involve physical rehabilitation or diagnostic audiology? _____

i. Are mental health services provided? _____

j. Is substance abuse treatment provided? _____

k. What PCS section should be used? _____

l. Review the root types or modalities in the section selected. What is the most likely root type or modality? _____

---

3. INPATIENT HOSPITAL   Gender: F   Age: 81

Preprocedure diagnosis: Status post–hip replacement, left hip

Procedure: Range of motion and joint mobility exercises for the left hip with walker

a. What is the stated procedure? _____

b. What body region or body part is involved? _____

c. What method or equipment is used? _____

d. Was more than one procedure, or a combined procedure, performed? _____

e. Does the procedure involve imaging/radiography? _____

f. Does the procedure involve nuclear medicine? _____ _____

g. Does the procedure involve radiation treatment for a malignancy? _____

h. Does the procedure involve physical rehabilitation or diagnostic audiology? _____

i. Are mental health services provided? _____

j. Is substance abuse treatment provided? _____

k. What PCS section should be used? _____

l. Review the root types or modalities in the section selected. What is the most likely root type or modality? _____

---

4. INPATIENT HOSPITAL   Gender: M   Age: 18

Preprocedure diagnosis: Injured left leg, multiple sites

Procedure: X-ray of left femur, tibia, and fibula, MRI pelvis unenhanced and enhanced with contrast

Postprocedure diagnosis: Fractures of the left femur, tibia, and pelvis

a. What is the stated procedure? _____

b. What body region or body part is involved? _____

c. What method is used? _____

d. Was more than one procedure, or a combined procedure, performed? _____

e. Does the procedure involve imaging/radiography? _____

f. Does the procedure involve nuclear medicine? _____ _____

g. Does the procedure involve radiation treatment for a malignancy? _____

(continued)

(continued)

CODING PRACTICE (continued)

4. (continued)

h. Does the procedure involve physical rehabilitation or diagnostic audiology? _____

i. Are mental health services provided? _____

j. Is substance abuse treatment provided? _____

k. What PCS section should be used? _____

l. Review the root types in the section selected. What is the most likely root type? _____

5. INPATIENT HOSPITAL   Gender: M   Age: 47

Preprocedure diagnosis: Peripheral artery disease

Procedure: Intraoperative percutaneous transluminal angioplasty (PTA) of left common femoral artery with laser fluoroscopic guidance, low osmolar contrast. Placed an intraluminal drug-eluting stent.

a. What is the stated procedure? _____

b. What body region or body part is involved? _____

c. What method is used? _____

d. Was more than one procedure, or a combined procedure, performed? _____

e. Does the procedure involve imaging/radiography? _____

f. Does the procedure involve nuclear medicine? _____

g. Does the procedure involve radiation treatment for a malignancy? _____

h. Does the procedure involve physical rehabilitation or diagnostic audiology? _____

i. Are mental health services provided? _____

5. (continued)

j. Is substance abuse treatment provided? _____

k. What PCS section(s) should be used? _____

l. Review the root operation(s) and root type(s) in the section(s) selected. What are the most likely root operation(s) and root type(s)? _____

6. INPATIENT HOSPITAL   Gender: M   Age: 47

Preprocedure diagnosis: Angina pectoris

Procedure: Cardiac stress test to measure total activity, single measurement, followed by ECC of the right and left heart

a. What is the stated procedure? _____

b. What body region or body part is involved? _____

c. What method is used? _____

d. Was more than one procedure, or a combined procedure, performed? _____

e. Does the procedure involve imaging/radiography? _____

f. Does the procedure involve nuclear medicine? _____

g. Does the procedure involve radiation treatment for a malignancy? _____

h. Does the procedure involve physical rehabilitation or diagnostic audiology? _____

i. Are mental health services provided? _____

j. Is substance abuse treatment provided? _____

k. What PCS section(s) should be used? _____

l. Review the root operation(s) and root type(s) in the section selected. What is the most likely root operation(s) and root type(s)? _____

ASSIGNING CHARACTERS 4–7 FOR ANCILLARY PROCEDURES

To assign codes after the root type is determined, search the PCS Index for the name of the root type as the Main Term. Locate the subterm(s) for the correct anatomic site and identify the PCS Table. For many ancillary procedures, the root type is also the common name of the procedure, such as **Fluoroscopy**, or a slight variation of the common name, such as speech therapy, which is classified under the root type and Main Term **Speech Treatment**. Other times, the Index lists an instruction that cross-references you to one or more possible root types. If you have difficulty locating a code using one Main Term or method, try a different one.

When you locate the PCS Table, verify the first three characters of the code, then locate the row with the Body Part needed. Assign the remaining characters from each respective column of the Table.

Each section of ancillary procedures introduces characters and definitions unique to its procedures. When a particular character is not used for a specific purpose, it is labeled as a qualifier with the default value **Z None**. All codes must contain seven characters. Refer to the PCS coding manual appendix, "Type and Type Qualifier Definitions, Sections B–H," for detailed definitions used in these sections.

Guided Example of Assigning Characters 4–7 for Ancillary Procedures

To practice skills for assigning codes for procedures in the ancillary sections, continue with the example from earlier in the chapter about the patient who was seen for a total hip replacement, with x-ray and gait training. Follow along in your ICD-10-PCS manual as Marcy Elwood, CCS, assigns codes. Check off each step after you complete it.

▶ First, Marcy confirms the services provided and the root operations and root types she abstracted.

❑ The root operation for the total left hip arthroplasty is Replacement (R) in the Medical and Surgical (0) section.

❑ The root type for x-ray of the acetabulofemoral joint is Plain Radiography (0) in the Imaging (B) section.

❑ The root type for gait training is Motor Training (7) in the Physical Rehabilitation and Diagnostic Audiology (F) section.

▶ Marcy assigns the code for the total hip arthroplasty procedure (■ Figure 55-7). Refer to Chapter 53 of this text for more information about assigning codes for the root operation Replacement.

❑ **0SRB02A Medical and Surgical, Lower Joints, Replacement, Synthetic Substitute, Metal on Polyethylene, Uncemented, Open approach**

▶ Marcy assigns the code for x-ray of the acetabulofemoral joint.

❑ She searches the Index for the Main Term for the root type **Plain Radiography**.

❑ She does not locate a subterm for acetabulofemoral joint and is unsure whether it should be coded to the hip, the femur, or another value.

- She refers to the Body Part Key in the Appendix of the PCS coding manual.

- She locates an entry for **Acetabulofemoral joint**, which refers her to the PCS Body Part **Hip Joint**.

❑ In the Index, she locates the first-level subterm **Hip** under the Main Term **Plain Radiography**.

❑ She verifies the laterality in the documentation and locates the second-level subterm **Left**.

❑ She sees a third-level subterm **Densitometry**, but this is not the procedure performed, so she does not use it.

❑ She identifies the Table **BQ0** and partial code **BQ01**.

▶ Marcy turns to Table **BQ0** to assign the code for the x-ray.

❑ She reads the Table title **BQ0, Imaging, Non-Axial Lower Bones, Plain Radiography** and confirms that this accurately describes the body system and root type.

❑ Marcy assigns the value for Character 4, Body Part.

- She verifies the laterality in the documentation and assigns **1 Hip, Left**.

❑ Marcy assigns the value for Character 5, Contrast.

- She verifies the type of contrast in the documentation and assigns **1 Low Osmolar**.

❑ Marcy assigns the value for Character 6, Qualifier, **Z None**.

Section	0	Medical and Surgical
Body System	S	Lower Joints
Operation	R	Replacement: Putting in or on biological or synthetic material that physically takes the place and/or function of all or a portion of a body part

Body Part Character 4	Approach Character 5	Device Character 6	Qualifier Character 7
9 Hip Joint, Right **B** Hip Joint, Left	**0** Open	**1** Synthetic Substitute, Metal **2** Synthetic Substitute, Metal on Polyethylene **3** Synthetic Substitute, Ceramic **4** Synthetic Substitute, Ceramic on Polyethylene **6** Synthetic Substitute, Oxidized Zirconium on Polyethylene **J** Synthetic Substitute	**9** Cemented **A** Uncemented **Z** No Qualifier

Figure 55-7 ■ Assigning code 0SRB02A. *Source: Annotation © PB Resources, Inc. Used with permission.*

❑ Marcy assigns the value for Character 7, Qualifier, **Z None**.

❑ She reviews the code she has assigned for the x-ray of the acetabulofemoral joint: **BQ011ZZ** (■ FIGURE 55-8)

- **BQ011ZZ Imaging, Non-Axial Lower Bones, Plain radiography, Hip left, Low osmolar, None, None**

▶ Marcy searches the Index for the Main Term **Gait Training** for gait training with walker.

❑ She reads the instructional note with a cross-reference that states **see Motor Treatment, Rehabilitation F07**.

▶ Marcy turns to Table **F07** to assign the code for gait training.

❑ She reads the Table title **F07, Physical Rehabilitation and Diagnostic Audiology, Rehabilitation, Motor Treatment** and confirms that this accurately describes the body system and root type.

❑ Marcy assigns the value for Character 4, Body System/Region, **Z None**.

❑ Marcy assigns the value for Character 5, Type Qualifier.

- She must search through several rows of the Table to locate the entry for gait training and assigns the only value, **9 Gait Training/Functional Ambulation**.

❑ Marcy assigns the value for Character 6, Equipment.

- A walker is assistive equipment, so she assigns **F Assistive, Adaptive, Supportive or Protective**.

❑ Marcy assigns the value for Character 7, Qualifier, **Z None**.

❑ She reviews the code she has assigned for gait training with walker: **F07Z9FZ** (■ FIGURE 55-9).

- **F07Z9FZ Physical Rehabilitation and Diagnostic Audiology, Rehabilitation, Motor treatment, None, Gait training/functional ambulation, Assistive adaptive supportive or protective, None**

▶ Marcy reviews all the procedure codes she has assigned for this case.

❑ **0SRB02A Medical and surgical, Lower joints, Replacement, Synthetic substitute metal on polyethylene, Uncemented, Open approach**

❑ **BQ011ZZ Imaging, Non-axial lower bones, Plain radiography, Hip left, Low osmolar, None, None**

❑ **F07Z9FZ Physical rehabilitation and diagnostic audiology, rehabilitation, Motor treatment, None, Gait training/functional ambulation, Assistive adaptive supportive or protective, None**

▶ Next, Marcy must determine how to sequence the codes.

Section	B	Imaging
Body System	Q	Non-Axial Lower Bones
Type	0	Plain Radiography: Planar display of an image developed from the capture of external ionizing radiation on photographic or photoconductive plate

Body Part Character 4	Contrast Character 5	Qualifier Character 6	Qualifier Character 7
0 Hip, Right 1 Hip, Left	0 High Osmolar 1 Low Osmolar Y Other Contrast	Z None	Z None

Figure 55-8 ■ Assigning code BQ011ZZ. *Source: Annotation © PB Resources, Inc. Used with permission.*

Section	F	Physical Rehabilitation and Diagnostic Audiology	
Section Qualifier	0	Rehabilitation	
Type	7	**Motor Treatment:** Exercise or activities to increase or facilitate motor function	

Body System/Region Character 4	Type Qualifier Character 5	Equipment Character 6	Qualifier Character 7
Z None	**9** Gait Training/ Functional Ambulation	**C** Mechanical **D** Electrotherapeutic **E** Orthosis **F** Assistive, Adaptive, Supportive or Protective **G** Aerobic Endurance and Conditioning **U** Prosthesis **Y** Other Equipment **Z** None	**Z** None

Figure 55-9 ■ Assigning code F07Z9FZ. *Source: Annotation © PB Resources, Inc. Used with permission.*

CODING PRACTICE

Exercise 55.3   Assigning Characters 4–7 for Ancillary Procedures

Instructions: Read the mini-medical-record of each patient's encounter. Review the information abstracted in Exercise 55.2 for questions 1–3. For questions 4–6, abstract the case on your own. Assign PCS codes using the Index and Tables. Write the code(s) on the line provided.

1. INPATIENT HOSPITAL   Gender: M   Age: 57

Preprocedure diagnosis: Cirrhosis, rule out hepatocellular carcinoma

Procedure: CT scan of liver with and without contrast (high osmolar)

Findings: Enlarged liver as expected but no tumors identified

1 PCS Code _____

2. INPATIENT HOSPITAL   Gender: M   Age: 61

Preprocedure diagnosis: Prostate cancer

Procedure: Low dose rate (LDR) brachytherapy of prostate using Iridium 192

Tip: Iridium 192 is the isotope used.

1 PCS Code _____

3. INPATIENT HOSPITAL   Gender: F   Age: 81

Preprocedure diagnosis: Status post–hip replacement, left hip

Procedure: Range of motion and joint mobility exercises for the left hip with walker

Tip: A walker is assistive equipment.

1 PCS Code _____

4. INPATIENT HOSPITAL   Gender: M   Age: 26

Preprocedure diagnosis: Severe depression

Procedure: Electroconvulsive therapy (ECT) bilateral, single seizure, done under general anesthesia

Tip: The aim of ECT is to induce a therapeutic seizure in which the person loses consciousness and has convulsions lasting for at least 15 seconds.

1 PCS Code _____

(continued)

CODING PRACTICE *(continued)*

---

5. INPATIENT HOSPITAL Gender: M Age: 46

Preprocedure diagnosis: Bladder cancer; previously removed the bladder and created an ileal conduit *(use of a segment of the ileum to connect the ureters to a stoma on the abdominal wall)*

Procedure: Ureteropyelography; injected high osmolar contrast medium through the existing stoma to view the ureters and ileal conduit. Ileal conduit was visualized to be functioning properly.

1 PCS Code _____

---

6. INPATIENT HOSPITAL Gender: M Age: 57

Preprocedure diagnosis: Cirrhosis, r/o hepatocellular carcinoma

Procedure: CT scan of pelvis, without contrast and with nonionic low osmolar contrast.

Postprocedure diagnosis: Enlarged liver as expected but no tumors identified

Tip: Contrast dye is used to help certain areas show up better.

1 PCS Code _____

ARRANGING CODES FOR ANCILLARY PROCEDURES

Ancillary procedures are often performed in addition to a more definitive procedure while a patient is hospitalized, so they might not qualify as a principal procedure. Be sure to review the documentation carefully to ensure that all services are identified and coded. Failure to code and report ancillary services can result in revenue loss to the hospital. When services reported in the ancillary sections are performed as stand-alone outpatient procedures, they are reported with CPT codes because PCS is used only by inpatient facilities.

Guided Example of Arranging Codes for Ancillary Procedures

To practice skills for arranging codes for ancillary procedures, continue with the example from earlier in the chapter about the patient who was seen for a total hip replacement, with x-ray and gait training. Follow along in your ICD-10-PCS manual as Marcy Elwood, CCS, arranges the codes. Check off each step after you complete it.

▶ First, Marcy confirms the procedures performed:

❑ X-ray of the acetabulofemoral joint

❑ Total left hip arthroplasty

❑ Gait training with walker

▶ Marcy reviews the diagnoses and determines the principal diagnosis. The Uniform Hospital Discharge Data Set (UHDDS) defines the principal diagnosis as "that condition established after study to be chiefly responsible for occasioning the admission of the patient to the hospital for care."

❑ Fractured left hip at the base of the femoral neck

▶ Marcy reviews the procedure codes assigned:

❑ **0SRB02A Medical and surgical, Lower joints, Replacement, Synthetic substitute metal on poly-ethylene, Uncemented, Open approach**

❑ **BQ011ZZ Imaging, Non-axial lower bones, Plain radiography, Hip left, Low osmolar, None, None**

❑ **F07Z9FZ Physical rehabilitation and diagnostic audiology, Rehabilitation, Motor treatment, Non, Gait training/functional ambulation, Assistive adaptive supportive or protective, None**

▶ Marcy determines that the principal procedure is the surgical procedure of the hip replacement. The principal diagnosis determines the sequencing order because the principal procedure must be the one most closely related to the principal diagnosis.

▶ Marcy finalizes the procedure codes and sequencing for this case:

(1) **0SRB02A Medical and surgical, Lower joints, Replacement, Synthetic substitute metal on poly-ethylene, Uncemented, Open approach**

(2) **BQ011ZZ Imaging, Non-axial lower bones, Plain radiography, Hip left, Low osmolar, None, None**

(3) **F07Z9FZ Physical rehabilitation and diagnostic audiology, Rehabilitation, Motor treatment, Non, Gait training/functional ambulation, Assistive adaptive supportive or protective, None**

▶ Marcy also assigns and sequences the ICD-10-CM diagnosis codes that support the need for the services.

(1) **S72.042A Displaced fracture of base of neck of left femur, initial encounter for closed fracture**

(2) **W10.9XXA Fall (on) (from) unspecified stairs and steps, initial encounter**

(3) **Y92.019 Unspecified place in single-family (private) house as the place of occurrence of the external cause**

CODING PRACTICE

Exercise 55.4   Arranging Codes for Ancillary Procedures

Instructions: Read the mini-medical-record of each patient's encounter. Review the information abstracted in Exercise 55.2 for questions 1–3. For questions 4–6, abstract the case on your own. Assign PCS codes using the Index and Tables, and arrange the codes in proper sequence. Write the code(s) on the line provided.

---

1. INPATIENT HOSPITAL   Gender: M   Age: 18

Preprocedure diagnosis: Injured left leg, multiple sites

Procedure: X-ray of left femur, tibia, and fibula, MRI pelvis unenhanced and enhanced with contrast

Postprocedure diagnosis: Fractures of the left femur, tibia, and pelvis

2 PCS Codes _____

---

2. INPATIENT HOSPITAL   Gender: M   Age: 47

Preprocedure diagnosis: Peripheral artery disease

Procedure: Intraoperative percutaneous transluminal angioplasty (PTA) of left common femoral artery with laser fluoroscopic guidance, low osmolar contrast. Placed an intraluminal drug-eluting stent.

2 PCS Codes _____

---

3. INPATIENT HOSPITAL   Gender: M   Age: 47

Preprocedure diagnosis: Angina pectoris

Procedure: Cardiac stress test to measure total activity, single measurement, followed by ECC of the right and left heart

2 PCS Codes _____

---

4. INPATIENT HOSPITAL   Gender: F   Age: 68

Preprocedure diagnosis: Locally advanced colorectal carcinoma

Procedure: Sigmoid colectomy with IORT (intraoperative radiation therapy) of colon, 3 ports. A midline incision was made and the colon wall divided with a stapler. Dissection continued to the distal margin, where the colon was resected. Following removal of the sigmoid colon, a single IORT dose of 20.0 Gy was delivered to the excised tumor area.

2 PCS Codes _____

---

5. INPATIENT HOSPITAL   Gender: M   Age: 46

Preprocedure diagnosis: Carotid artery occlusive disease; peripheral vascular disease

Procedure: Bilateral internal carotid artery angiogram; right femoral-popliteal angiogram. The right carotid artery showed no significant disease. The intracranial portion of the left carotid artery showed a 40–50% stenosis. Visualization of the right lower extremity femoral and popliteal arteries under fluoroscopic guidance showed no significant disease.

2 PCS Codes _____

---

6. INPATIENT HOSPITAL   Gender: F   Age: 54

Preprocedure diagnosis: Alcohol withdrawal and dependence; marital and family conflict due to alcohol dependence

Procedure: Group counseling through Alcoholics Anonymous; marital counseling

2 PCS Codes _____

NEW TECHNOLOGY (SECTION X)

Section **X, New Technology**, classifies selected new technology procedures that need to be distinguished from existing codes. Section X identifies procedures requested through the Centers for Medicare and Medicaid Services' (CMS) new technology application process, as well as new technologies not otherwise classified in PCS. CMS' new technology application process allows hospitals to request add-on payments for certain new medical services and technologies.

Codes identify a broad range of new technology procedures including medical and surgical, medical and surgical–related, and ancillary. Examples are infusion of new technology drugs, orbital atherectomy technology used to treat coronary artery disease, and an intraoperative knee replacement sensor used for soft tissue balancing in total knee arthroplasty.

Structure of New Technology Codes

The section value for New Technology is **X**. The characters of New Technology codes are summarized as follows (■ TABLE 55-11, page 1162):

• Character 2: Body System—Character 2 combines the uses of body system, body region, and physiological system as specified in other PCS sections, resulting in broader values than elsewhere in the code set. Body part

Table 55-11   ■   SEVEN CHARACTERS OF NEW TECHNOLOGY PROCEDURES

1	2	3	4	5	6	7
Section X	Body System	Root Operation	Body Part	Approach	Device/Substance/Technology	Qualifier

values are as general or specific needed for any specific new technology.

- Character 3: Root Operation—Root operations use the same values and same definitions as in other PCS sections.

- Character 4: Body Part—Body parts use the same values as their closest counterparts in other PCS sections.

- Character 5: Approach—Approach uses the same values and definitions as in other PCS sections.

- Character 6: Device/Substance/Technology—Character 6 provides a general description of the key feature of the new technology, such as the name of the drug.

- Character 7: Qualifier—Character 7 identifies the New Technology Group, a value that is updated each year. For example, Section X codes added in 2016—the first year PCS was implemented—have the seventh character value **1 New Technology Group 1**, and codes added in 2017 have the seventh character value **2 New Technology Group 2**, and so on. The updating of the seventh character each year allows the PCS system to reuse values in Characters 3, 4, and 5 as needed and still retain unique codes for each procedure. This process maximizes the flexibility of Section X, allowing it evolve as medical technology evolves and not run out of codes.

Coding Guidelines for New Technology Procedures

PCS OGCR D discusses the use of Section X codes and clarifies that they are standalone codes. When a Section X code fully describes the procedure being done, it is not necessary to report an additional less specific code from another PCS section.

Assigning New Technology Codes

New Technology codes can be somewhat challenging to locate in the Index. It is helpful when coders are aware they are coding a procedure that has been approved under the CMS new technology criteria. Fortunately, there are only a few procedures in this section and facilities know they are using them. Locate procedures in the Index in the following ways:

1. Search for the Main Term **New Technology** and a subterm for the name of the technology, such as **Ceftazidime-Avibactam Anti-infective**.

2. Search for the name of the technology as the Main Term, such as **Ceftazidime-Avibactam Anti-infective**.

3. Search for the root operation as the Main Term, such as **Introduction** and a subterm for the technology. PCS does not use this indexing method consistently.

Any particular New Technology procedure may be indexed under only one or two of these methods. If you cannot find it under the first Main Term chosen, try another one. Regardless of the Main Term selected, always identify the Table listed in the Index, then refer to the Table to assign and verify all characters of the code (■ TABLE 55-12).

Table 55-12   ■   CODE XW03321 INFUSION OF CEFTAZIDIME VIA PERIPHERAL VENOUS CATHETER

Character	Name	Value	Description
1	Section	X	New Technology
2	Body System	W	Anatomical Regions
3	Root Operation	0	Introduction
4	Body Part	3	Peripheral Vein
5	Approach	3	Percutaneous
6	Device/Substance/Technology	2	Ceftazidime-Avibactam Anti-infective
7	Qualifier	1	New Technology Group 1

CODING PRACTICE

Exercise 55.5   New Technology (Section X)

Instructions: Read the procedural statement, then use the Index and Tables to assign the PCS procedure code from the New Technology section. Write the code on the line provided.

1. Infusion of blinatumomab antineoplastic immunotherapy via central catheter. 1 ICD-10-PCS Code _____

2. Monitoring of soft tissue balancing during a total left knee arthroplasty using an intraoperative knee replacement sensor. 1 ICD-10-PCS Code _____

3. Use of an orbital atherectomy system to clear a severely calcified lesion in the RCA. 1 ICD-10-PCS Code _____

4. Intramuscular injection of concentrated bone marrow aspirate (CBNA) to treat critical limb ischemia of the right leg. 1 ICD-10-PCS Code _____

5. Open insertion of a magnetically controlled growth rod into L4-L5-L6. 1 ICD-10-PCS Code _____

6. Endoscopic robotic waterjet ablation of the prostate via urethra. 1 ICD-10-PCS Code _____

CHAPTER SUMMARY

In this chapter you learned that:

- The ancillary sections are Imaging (B), Nuclear Medicine (C), Radiation Therapy (D), Physical Rehabilitation and Diagnostic Audiology (F), Mental Health (G), and Substance Abuse Treatment (H).

- PCS does not provide guidelines for ancillary procedures. New Technology section guidelines appear in PCS OGCR D.

- The section Imaging (B) is creating a visual representation of internal body structures to diagnose conditions and has five root types.

- The section Nuclear Medicine (C) is the introduction of radioactive materials into the body to capture images, diagnose diseases, or treat abnormalities and has seven root types.

- The section Radiation Therapy (D) is the use of radiation to treat malignancies and has four root types.

- The section Physical Rehabilitation and Diagnostic Audiology (F) is procedures and therapy to help patients regain body functions lost due to medical conditions or injury and to diagnose hearing-related conditions. It has 14 root types.

- The section Mental Health (G) consists of a variety of methods to diagnose and treat psychiatric and mental disorders and has 13 root types.

- The section Substance Abuse Treatment (H) is procedures to treat disorders related to substance abuse and has eight root types.

- The meaning of Characters 4–7 varies based on the section, so it is important to review the character meanings in each PCS Table .

- Many ancillary procedures are not sequenced as the principal procedure because they are performed in addition to a more definitive procedure root type.

- Section X New Technology, classifies procedures requested through the Centers for Medicare and Medicaid Services (CMS) new technology application process, as well as new technologies not otherwise classified in PCS.

CONCEPT QUIZ

Take a moment to look back at ancillary procedures and solidify your skills. Try to answer the questions from memory first, then refer to the discussion in this chapter if you need a little extra help.

Completion

Instructions: Write the term that completes each statement based on the information you learned in this chapter. Choose from the list below. Some choices may be used more than once and some choices may not be used at all.

Beam Radiation (0)	Pharmacotherapy (9)
Brachytherapy (1)	Plain Radiography (0)
Computerized Tomography (2)	Positron Emission Tomography (PET) (3)
Fluoroscopy (1)	
Medication Management (8)	Speech Assessment (0)
Motor and/or Nerve Function Assessment (1)	Speech Treatment (6)
Motor Treatment (7)	Systemic Nuclear Medicine Therapy (7)
Narcosynthesis (G)	Tomographic Nuclear Medicine Imaging (2)
Nonimaging Nuclear Medicine Uptake (4)	

1. The root type _____ from the Nuclear Medicine (C) section is the introduction of unsealed radioactive materials into the body for treatment.

2. The root type _____ from the Physical Rehabilitation and Diagnostic Audiology (F) section is exercises or activities to increase or facilitate motor function.

3. The root type _____ from the Imaging (B) section is the computer-reformatted digital display of multiplanar images developed from the capture of multiple exposures of external ionizing radiation.

4. The root type _____ from the Nuclear Medicine (C) section is the introduction of radioactive materials into the body for three-dimensional display of images developed from the capture of radioactive emissions.

5. The root type _____ from the Physical Rehabilitation and Diagnostic Audiology (F) section is the application of techniques to improve, augment, or compensate for speech and related functional impairment.

6. The root type _____ from the Imaging (B) section is the planar display of an image developed from the capture of external ionizing radiation on a photographic or photoconductive plate.

7. The root type _____ from the Imaging (B) section is the single plane or biplane real-time display of an image developed from the capture of external ionizing radiation on a fluorescent screen.

8. The modality _____ from the Radiation Therapy (D) section is the insertion of radioactive implants directly into body tissue.

9. The root type _____ from the Mental Health (G) section is the administration of intravenous barbiturates in order to release suppressed or repressed thoughts.

10. The root type _____ from the Substance Abuse Treatment (H) section is monitoring and adjusting the use of replacement medications for the treatment of addiction.

(continued)

(continued from page 1163)

Multiple Choice

Instructions: Circle the letter of the best answer to each question based on the information you learned in this chapter.

1. What type of service is classified in the Nuclear Medicine (C) section?
   A. Functional imaging
   B. Planar imaging
   C. Anatomic imaging
   D. Radioactive implant imaging

2. What is the value Cesium 137 an example of?
   A. Modality
   B. Modality Qualifier
   C. Isotope
   D. Radionuclide

3. How would you code the following procedure? *Placement of a static orthosis on the left forearm for a patient in an inpatient rehabilitation facility.*
   A. F0DZ7FZ
   B. F0DZ7EZ
   C. F0DZ8EZ
   D. F0DZ8UZ

4. Which character in section F identifies whether the procedure is Rehabilitation or Diagnostic Audiology?
   A. Character 2, Section Qualifier
   B. Character 3, Root Type
   C. Character 4, Body System
   D. Character 5, Qualifier

5. What information is identified by Character 5 in the Imaging (B) section?
   A. Isotope
   B. Contrast
   C. Approach
   D. Type qualifier

6. What is an orthopedic appliance or apparatus used to support, align, prevent, or correct deformities or to improve the function of movable parts of the body?
   A. Orthopedic
   B. Arthrodesis
   C. Prosthesis
   D. Orthosis

7. How would you code the following procedure? *Fluoroscopic guidance with high osmolar contrast in the right popliteal vein.*
   A. B51B1ZA
   B. B51B0ZA
   C. B51BZZA
   D. B51B0ZZ

8. What Character 6, Qualifier value identifies an image taken without contrast followed by one with contrast in the Imaging (B) section?
   A. Contrast
   B. Both
   C. With and Without
   D. Unenhanced and Enhanced

9. What character in the Nuclear Medicine (C) section identifies the radiation source used in the procedure?
   A. Character 4, Source
   B. Character 5, Radionuclide
   C. Character 6, Isotope
   D. Character 7, Qualifier

10. How would you code the following procedure? *Transesophageal ultrasound imaging of the heart.*
    A. BY49ZZZ
    B. 10J08ZZ
    C. 6A750Z5
    D. B244ZZ4

KEEP ON CODING

Instructions: Read the procedural statement, abstract the root type or procedure, then use the appropriate Index and Tables to assign PCS procedure codes. Assign only the root operations discussed in this chapter. Write the code(s) on the line provided.

1. Magnetic resonance imaging (MRI) of the brain without contrast. ICD-10-PCS Code(s) _____

2. Positron emission tomography (PET) scan of heart. ICD-10-PCS Code(s) _____

3. Stereotactic radiosurgery of the prostate using gamma beam. ICD-10-PCS Code(s) _____

4. Fitting of left prosthetic leg. ICD-10-PCS Code(s) _____

5. Fusion of T4-T5-T6-T7 using a radiolucent porous interbody fusion device, eligible for new technology payments. ICD-10-PCS Code(s) _____

6. Ultrasound imaging of the gallbladder. ICD-10-PCS Code(s) _____

7. Alcohol detoxification. ICD-10-PCS Code(s) _____

8. Fluoroscopic imaging of right internal mammary bypass graft, low osmolar. ICD-10-PCS Code(s) _____

9. Individual interpersonal mental health services. ICD-10-PCS Code(s) _____

10. Hearing screening assessment in a sound booth. ICD-10-PCS Code(s) _____

11. Individual interactive mental health psychotherapy services. ICD-10-PCS Code(s) _____

12. Pharmacotherapy, methadone maintenance for heroin addiction. ICD-10-PCS Code(s) _____

13. Technetium 99m myocardial nuclear imaging. ICD-10-PCS Code(s) _____

14. Intraoperative 6-MeV photonic beam radiation of the thymus. ICD-10-PCS Code(s) _____

15. Mobility training using a wheelchair. ICD-10-PCS Code(s) _____

16. Technetium 99m nuclear imaging (planar) of the thyroid gland. ICD-10-PCS Code(s) _____

17. Electroconvulsive therapy (ECT), bilateral–multiple seizures. ICD-10-PCS Code(s) _____

18. Group 12-step substance abuse counseling. ICD-10-PCS Code(s) _____

19. Annual hearing screening of a commercial airline pilot. ICD-10-PCS Code(s) _____

20. Chest wall radiation therapy, 8 MeV. ICD-10-PCS Code(s) _____

21. Positron emission tomographic (PET) imaging of myocardium using Fluorine 18. ICD-10-PCS Code(s) _____

22. High-dose Cesium 137 brachytherapy of the bladder. ICD-10-PCS Code(s) _____

23. Electrophysiologic motor function test of facial nerves. ICD-10-PCS Code(s) _____

24. Clonidine management for substance abuse. ICD-10-PCS Code(s) _____

25. Light therapy. ICD-10-PCS Code(s) _____

CODING CHALLENGE

Instructions: Read the mini-medical-record of each patient's encounter, then abstract, assign, and arrange ICD-10-CM diagnosis codes and PCS procedure codes using the appropriate Index and Tables. Write the code(s) on the line provided.

1. INPATIENT HOSPITAL   Gender: F   Age: 4 weeks

Diagnosis: Congenital biliary atresia

Procedure: Cholangiogram and laparoscopic cholecystojejunostomy. Infant was admitted with obstructive jaundice due to biliary atresia. A cholangiocatheter was threaded to the gallbladder, bile ducts, and pancreatic ducts. Low osmolar contrast was injected and fluoroscopic images obtained. After that, a hepatobiliary-pancreatic bypass was performed and anastomosis of the gallbladder and jejunum was performed.

1 ICD-10-CM Code _____

2 ICD-10-PCS Codes _____

2. INPATIENT HOSPITAL   Gender: F   Age: 18

Preprocedure diagnosis: AAA

Procedure: EVAR (endovascular aneurysm repair) with synthetic graft. Made incision into femoral artery. With low osmolar fluoroscopic guidance, guided delivery catheter with compressed graft into abdominal aorta to site of aneurysm. Inflated balloon to expand graft and affix it to vessel wall. Withdrew catheter and closed incision.

Tip: You coded the repair and the graft in another chapter. Now code the entire procedure, including the fluoroscopy.

1 ICD-10-CM Code _____

2 ICD-10-PCS Codes _____

3. INPATIENT HOSPITAL   Gender: M   Age: 52

Diagnosis: Unabated angina; left ventricular failure

Procedure: PET scan of myocardium using Fluorine 18 to assess myocardial viability and patient's capacity for a revascularization procedure.

Findings: Viable heart muscle. Schedule transmyocardial revascularization (TMR) using laser to produce channels directly into the heart muscle.

1 ICD-10-CM Code _____

1 ICD-10-PCS Code _____

4. INPATIENT HOSPITAL   Gender: F   Age: 48

Diagnosis: Pancreatic cancer with liver metastases

Procedure: Photon beam radiation >10 MeV treatment of pancreas and heavy-particle radiation treatment of liver

Tip: "10 MeV" describes the strength of the radiation.

2 ICD-10-CM Codes _____

2 ICD-10-PCS Codes _____

(continued)

(continued from page 1165)

5. INPATIENT HOSPITAL Gender: M Age: 25

Diagnosis: Patient found running naked down the street in the night. Previously diagnosed with bipolar personality disorder. Parents report that he recently stopped his meds because he felt "cured."

Procedure: Crisis intervention. Placed on 72-hour hold, lithium (gluconate) resumed plus antipsychotic meds.

Plan: Begin psychotherapy and medication regimen to stabilize patient. Family session scheduled to discuss OP tx plan and medication review.

Tip: Assign external cause codes related to stopping the medications using the Table of Drugs and Chemicals.

3 ICD-10-CM Codes _____

_____

1 ICD-10-PCS Code _____

6. INPATIENT HOSPITAL Gender: M Age: 57

Diagnosis: Alcohol addiction with delirium tremens

Procedure: Antabuse therapy

Plan: Continue detox with a stimulus-free environment, liver function tests. Admit to inpatient alcohol rehab.

1 ICD-10-CM Code _____

1 ICD-10-PCS Code _____

7. INPATIENT HOSPITAL Gender: F Age: 35

Reason for encounter: Multigravida with twin gestation of 16 weeks, 2 days; spotting

Procedure: Fetal ultrasound, twin gestation

Findings: Fetal movement recorded, fetus A: 12 oz, fetus B: 11.5 oz, cardiac heart rate noted. Mother on bedrest; monitor cervix with vaginal ultrasound.

4 ICD-10-CM Codes _____

_____

1 ICD-10-PCS Code _____

8. INPATIENT HOSPITAL Gender: F Age: 32

Diagnosis: Traumatic brain injury, cervical musculoskeletal strain

Procedure: Neuromuscular reeducation including therapeutic conditioning exercise to improve range of motion, strength, and coordination; home management

Plan: Patient did not reach goal because he has been admitted to inpatient rehabilitation

2 ICD-10-CM Codes _____

2 ICD-10-PCS Codes _____

9. INPATIENT HOSPITAL Gender: M Age: 59

Diagnosis: Atrial fibrillation, persistent, with rapid ventricular rate

Procedure: Transesophageal echocardiogram (TEE) and direct current cardioversion. Transesophageal probe was placed in the esophagus, and views of the right and left heart were then obtained. Following this, direct current cardioversion performed. Unsuccessful conversion to sinus rhythm; remained in atrial fibrillation.

Findings: Preserved left ventricular systolic function; dilated left atrium; moderate mitral regurgitation; aortic valve sclerosis with mild to moderate aortic insufficiency; left atrial appendage is free of clots.

2 ICD-10-CM Codes _____

2 ICD-10-PCS Codes _____

10. INPATIENT HOSPITAL Gender: F Age: 76

Diagnosis: Dementia of Alzheimer type with primary parietooccipital involvement

Procedure: MRI brain showed mild generalized atrophy, more severe in the occipital-parietal regions. An FDG-PET scan revealed decreased uptake in the right posterior temporal-parietal and lateral occipital regions.

Findings: Unchanged from MRI and PET scan 12 months ago

Tip: Fluorodeoxyglucose (FDG) is the most commonly used radioactive drug (tracer) used in PET scanning.

2 ICD-10-CM Codes _____

2 ICD-10-PCS Codes _____

Putting It All Together

Section Five: Putting It All Together consolidates what you have learned and launches you toward the next steps in your coding career. You learn how to make the transition to coding from full chart notes and operative reports similar to what you will encounter in the workplace. You continue to use the three skills of an "Ace" coder—abstract, assign, and arrange (sequence)—within the context of more detailed instructions. You also learn how skills in professionalism will help enhance your coding career.

PROFESSIONAL PROFILE

Ruth Berger, RHIA
Health Information Technology Program Director, Florida Gateway College

My education and health information management (HIM) credentials have been essential to my successful and varied career. I started with an associate degree in HIM. The associate degree led me to an interest in the coding profession where there is always something new to learn. I was hired by the hospital where I completed my clinical internship. I started out as an accredited record technician (ART) credential, which is now registered health information technician (RHIT).

As I moved into a supervisory position, I decided to complete a bachelor of science degree in healthcare management. This enabled me to earn the registered health information administrator (RHIA) credential. At the hospital I had many opportunities to host students for a professional practice experience (PPE) site

and really enjoyed this. When an opportunity to teach appeared, I decided to become an educator. As a full-time educator, I felt it was appropriate to complete a master degree in education to ensure that I was giving students the best learning experience.

I am currently a member of AHIMA, FHIMA, and NEFHIMA and have served on many committees over the years. In my job as program director, I coordinate all aspects of the associate degree program and coding certificate programs. I also teach HIM courses and medical terminology. I teach students how to use an encoder to reach the correct code. There is always something new to learn, a new procedure or condition. It can be challenging to keep up with annual changes to the code sets and ensure students understand the importance of coding.

My advice to students is to research any disease, condition, or procedure that you are unfamiliar with. Ask questions. Keep current by reading articles and notices from the Centers for Medicare and Medicaid Services (CMS) and professional organizations.

Chapter 56

Advanced Coding Skills

Chapter Outline

- **Coding from Chart Notes**
- **Coding from Operative Reports**

Learning Objectives

After completing this chapter, you should have the skills to:

56.1 Spell and define the key words, medical terms, and abbreviations related to chart notes and operative reports. (Remember)

56.2 Demonstrate how to abstract, assign, and arrange codes using chart notes. (Apply)

56.3 Demonstrate how to abstract, assign, and arrange codes using operative reports. (Apply)

Key Terms and Abbreviations

assessment	Mayo-Hegar	physical examination (PE or PX)
chief complaint (CC)	Metzenbaum	plan
history of present illness (HPI)	past medical history (PMH)	recommendation

In addition to the key terms listed here, students should know the terms defined within tables in this chapter.

INTRODUCTION

When you return home after an extended road trip, it is fun to look back through all the maps, brochures, souvenirs, and photographs you collected along the way. At the same time, you are already planning your next trip: where you will go, who will go with you, and what new experiences you anticipate.

In this chapter you preview advanced coding skills—the next step of your coding career. Depending on your work setting, you will be coding from chart notes and/or operative reports. Continue to use the three skills of an "Ace" coder—abstract, assign, and arrange. Refer to all the chapters in this textbook for details on each code set and body system. Refer to the end of this textbook to view Key Criteria to Abstracting tables for all body systems and all code sets in one place.

CODING FROM CHART NOTES

Physicians document each patient encounter in a chart note or progress note. Coders must read through all the details of the encounter, abstract the relevant information, then assign and sequence codes. A variety of documentation formats are used, depending on physician preference, organizational protocols, and electronic health record (EHR) systems in use, but in all cases, coders need to read, locate, and interpret information in order to assign codes. The mini-medical-record used in this text encapsulates the essential nuggets from documentation. After coders master basic coding, they continue to learn in order to develop advanced skills in sorting through all of the information contained in a piece of documentation.

To abstract from chart notes, coders must become familiar with their organization and headings. These may vary across electronic health record systems and among physicians. In general, chart notes contain sections with headings similar to the following:

- **Chief complaint (CC)**/Reason for encounter/Consultation—The patient's stated reason for the visit or, for consultations, the reason stated in the referral request for the specialist to examine the patient.

- **History of present illness (HPI)**—A statement of how the patient's current condition began and how it has progressed.

- **Past medical history (PMH)**—A review of the patient's past conditions, which may or may not be resolved, and past surgical procedures. It also includes any current problems that are not included in the reason for the encounter or referral.

- **Physical examination (PE or PX)**—The physician's examination and factual findings and results of tests performed or reviewed.

- **Assessment**—The physician's diagnostic statement.

- **Plan/Recommendations**—Planned treatments, prescriptions, patient instructions, and recommended treatments.

After locating this information, coders should also refer to the Key Criteria for Abstracting table(s) for the relevant body system(s), diagnoses, and procedures.

Annotated Example of Coding from Chart Notes

When coding from an actual chart note, coders must read the documentation several times and aggregate details from various sections of the report in order to form a complete picture of the encounter and determine the diagnoses to code. The entire chart note must be analyzed for the needed information. Do not rely on a few isolated statements to arrive at the code(s). Remember to refer to the abstracting table(s) for the body system(s) and condition(s) being treated. To code diagnoses from a chart note, follow these steps and cross-reference the examples of each in ■ FIGURE 56-1 (page 1170) using the numbers provided in parentheses:

- Read the patient's chief complaint (1) and the physician's assessment (5). Determine whether these are consistent with each other and/or add any details that may be required.

- Refer to the key criteria for abstracting for the body system(s) related to the diagnostic statement. Read through the entire record, noting what items support or modify the stated diagnosis.

- Identify the symptoms (2) and signs (4). Determine whether they are consistent with the assessment (5) and/or add any details that may be required by the codes.

- Identify any statement of personal disease history (3a), family disease history (3b), or risk factors (3c) that may contribute information to the diagnosis.

- Review the examination findings (4) and identify any additional risk factors or findings that contribute to the diagnosis.

- Review the plan (6) to identify any additional risk factors or symptoms the physician considers significant and to identify all conditions treated during the encounter.

- Reread the assessment (5) and assign all required diagnosis codes. Identify all confirmed diagnoses. Compare the diagnoses to the symptoms identified earlier (2) to determine which are integral to the condition and which may not be. In the outpatient setting, do not assign codes for uncertain or rule-out diagnoses (OGCR IV.D and H). Do not assign diagnosis codes for conditions not managed or not stated as significant to the current problem.

- Do not assign codes for scheduled treatments (6) because they were not provided during the encounter.

- Arrange (sequence) the diagnoses according to the problem chiefly responsible for the services provided (OGCR IV.G).

Physician encounters also require that CPT codes be assigned to identify the services provided. Typically this includes an evaluation and management (E/M) code and codes for any additional services provided. Refer to Chapters 28–43 of this text for instructions and examples of assigning E/M codes from chart notes.

CODING CAUTION

Do not assign diagnosis codes solely from the Chief Complaint or Assessment sections of the chart note. You need to read the entire chart note to identify any additional details or variations.

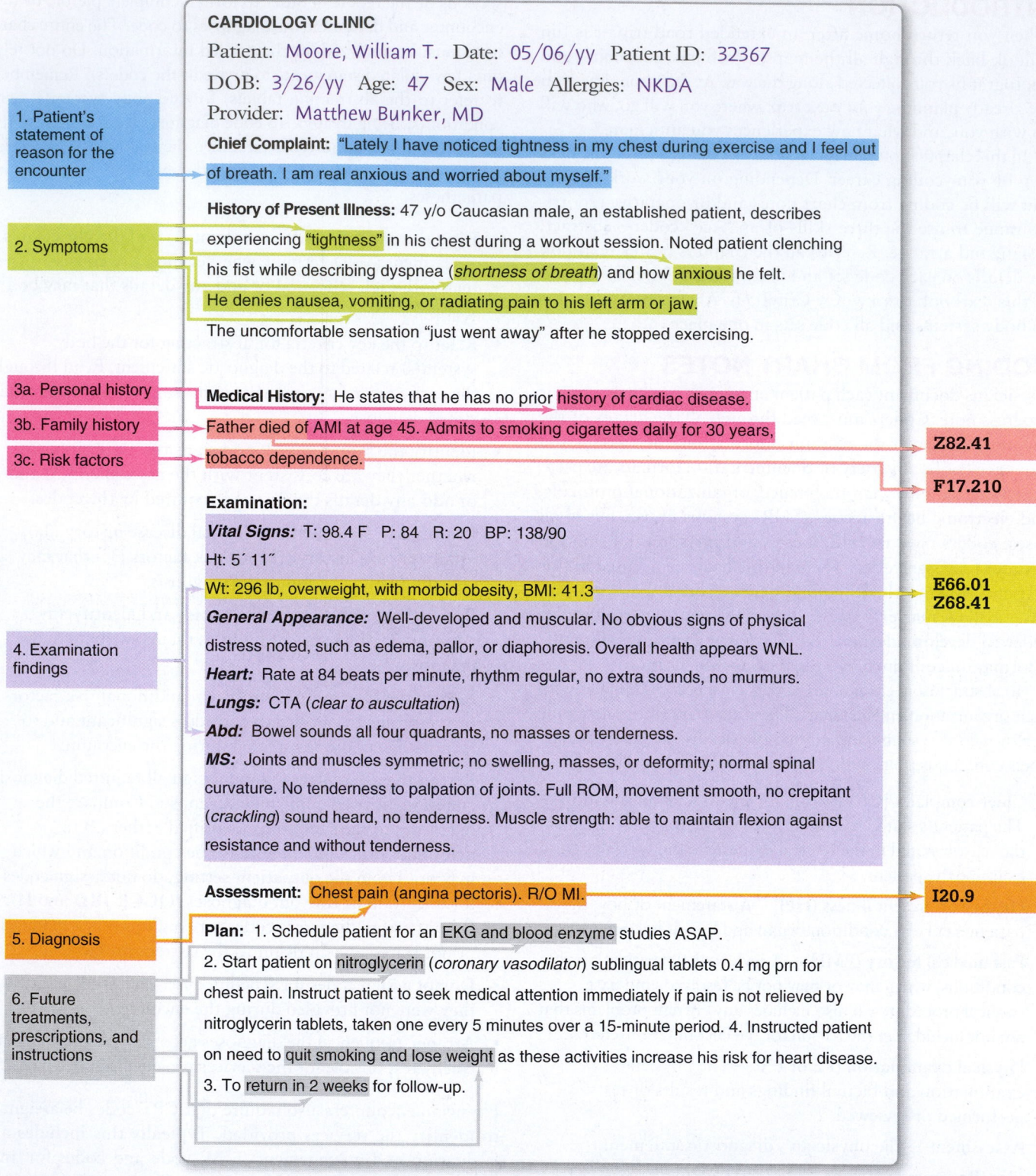

1. Patient's statement of reason for the encounter

2. Symptoms

3a. Personal history

3b. Family history

3c. Risk factors

4. Examination findings

5. Diagnosis

6. Future treatments, prescriptions, and instructions

CARDIOLOGY CLINIC

Patient: Moore, William T.   Date: 05/06/yy   Patient ID: 32367

DOB: 3/26/yy   Age: 47   Sex: Male   Allergies: NKDA

Provider: Matthew Bunker, MD

Chief Complaint: "Lately I have noticed tightness in my chest during exercise and I feel out of breath. I am real anxious and worried about myself."

History of Present Illness: 47 y/o Caucasian male, an established patient, describes experiencing "tightness" in his chest during a workout session. Noted patient clenching his fist while describing dyspnea (*shortness of breath*) and how anxious he felt. He denies nausea, vomiting, or radiating pain to his left arm or jaw. The uncomfortable sensation "just went away" after he stopped exercising.

Medical History: He states that he has no prior history of cardiac disease. Father died of AMI at age 45. Admits to smoking cigarettes daily for 30 years, tobacco dependence.

Z82.41

F17.210

Examination:

Vital Signs: T: 98.4 F   P: 84   R: 20   BP: 138/90

Ht: 5´ 11˝

Wt: 296 lb, overweight, with morbid obesity, BMI: 41.3

E66.01
Z68.41

General Appearance: Well-developed and muscular. No obvious signs of physical distress noted, such as edema, pallor, or diaphoresis. Overall health appears WNL.

Heart: Rate at 84 beats per minute, rhythm regular, no extra sounds, no murmurs.

Lungs: CTA (*clear to auscultation*)

Abd: Bowel sounds all four quadrants, no masses or tenderness.

MS: Joints and muscles symmetric; no swelling, masses, or deformity; normal spinal curvature. No tenderness to palpation of joints. Full ROM, movement smooth, no crepitant (*crackling*) sound heard, no tenderness. Muscle strength: able to maintain flexion against resistance and without tenderness.

Assessment: Chest pain (angina pectoris). R/O MI.

I20.9

Plan: 1. Schedule patient for an EKG and blood enzyme studies ASAP.

2. Start patient on nitroglycerin (*coronary vasodilator*) sublingual tablets 0.4 mg prn for chest pain. Instruct patient to seek medical attention immediately if pain is not relieved by nitroglycerin tablets, taken one every 5 minutes over a 15-minute period. 4. Instructed patient on need to quit smoking and lose weight as these activities increase his risk for heart disease.

3. To return in 2 weeks for follow-up.

A

Figure 56-1 ■ (A) Example of a cardiology chart note. *Source: Adapted from Rice, Jane,* Medical Terminology: A Word-Building Approach, *6th Ed., © 2008. Reprinted and electronically reproduced by permission of Pearson Education, Inc., Upper Saddle River, New Jersey.*

ICD-10-CM Codes:

(1) **I20.9 Angina pectoris**

(2) **F17.210 Nicotine dependence, cigarettes, uncomplicated**

(3) **Z82.41 Family history of sudden cardiac death**

(4) **E66.01 Morbid (severe) obesity due to excess calories**

(5) **Z68.41 Body mass index (BMI) 40.0-44.9, adult**

CPT Code:
- **99215** (2/3 key criteria must be met)
- Established patient, outpatient
- Detailed history (extended HPI, extended ROS, complete PFSH)
- Comprehensive examination (1995 Documentation Guidelines)
- High-complexity medical decision making (high management options, minimal data, high risk)

B

Figure 56-1 ■ (B) Coding for cardiology chart note.

CODING PRACTICE

| Exercise 56.1 | Coding from Chart Notes |

Instructions: Write the abbreviation(s) that complete(s) each statement based on the information you learned in this section. Choose from the list below.

| assessment | HPI | plan |
| CC | PE | PMH |

1. The _____ is a statement of how the patient's current condition began and how it has progressed.

2. The _____ is a review of the patient's past conditions, which may or may not be resolved, and past surgical procedures.

3. Review the _____ to identify any additional risk factors or symptoms the physician considers significant and to identify all conditions treated during the encounter.

4. The _____ is the physician's diagnostic statement.

5. Do not code for future treatments, which appear in the _____.

CODING FROM OPERATIVE REPORTS

Physicians document surgical operations and procedures with operative reports, which provide the details of exactly how the procedure was performed. Coders must read through all the details of the procedure, abstract the relevant information, then assign and sequence codes. This can be challenging and overwhelming because many of the details reported—such as the anesthetic, instruments, sutures, and other supplies—are not required in order to assign diagnosis and procedure codes. All of the information for a code is not concisely listed in one spot. Coders must read the report several times until they have identified all the details necessary to assign codes. Do not rely on just a few isolated statements to determine the procedure code.

The mini-medical-record used in this text encapsulates the essential nuggets from operative reports. After coders master the basic mechanics of coding, they need to develop advanced analytical skills to sort through all of the details in an operative report in order to locate the essential coding information.

To abstract from operative reports, coders must become familiar with their organization and headings. These may vary across electronic health record systems, facilities, and surgeons.

A typical operative report contains sections with headings similar to the following. The format varies with each physician or hospital but must include the following information:

- Date of procedure
- Name of procedure performed
- Names of the surgeon and assistants
- Preoperative or provisional diagnosis
- A detailed description of the procedure, such as patient preparation, anesthetic, instruments and supplies used, incisions made, visualized structures, findings, alterations performed, tissue removed, estimated blood loss, closing process, and patient status
- Postoperative diagnosis

The operative report usually specifies the instruments the surgeon used (■ TABLE 56-1 and ■ FIGURE 56-2, page 1172). Instruments may carry a generic name, such as scalpel, or an eponym, such as **Mayo-Hegar** (*needle holder*) or **Metzenbaum** (*scissors*). A number indicates the size, such as a #10 blade or 5-0 Vicryl sutures.

Table 56-1 ■ **INSTRUMENTS USED BY SURGEONS**

Functional Purpose	Types
Absorption	Sponge, towel, dressing
Cutting	Knife, scalpel, scissors, electrocautery, bone saw, wire, snare, stapler
Drainage	T-tube, drain, catheter, hemovac, chest tube, water seal
Grasping, holding	Forceps, clamp, hemostat
Occlusion	Ligature (sutures), clips, clamps
Viewing	Retractor, speculum, endoscope, microscope
Wound closure	Needle holder, sutures (catgut, Vicryl, silk, nylon), stapler

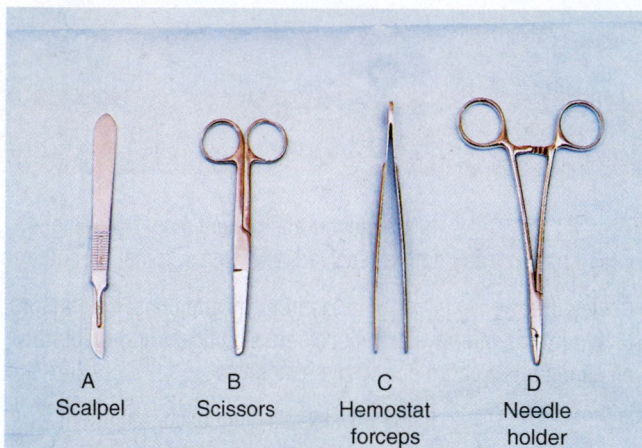

A — Scalpel B — Scissors C — Hemostat forceps D — Needle holder

Figure 56-2 ■ The operative report identifies the instruments a surgeon uses. *Source: Michal Heron/Pearson Education, Inc.*

Annotated Example of Coding from Operative Reports

To code from an operative report, apply the skills of abstracting, assigning, and arranging codes. Follow these steps and cross-reference the examples of each in ■ FIGURE 56-3 using the numbers in parentheses:

- Read the preoperative and postoperative diagnoses (1). Determine whether these are consistent with each other and/or add any details that may be required.
- Read the name of the procedure(s) performed as stated by the surgeon (2).

- Refer to the key criteria for abstracting for the body system(s) related to the diagnostic statement. Read through the entire record, noting what items support or modify the stated diagnosis.
- Identify the indications, symptoms, and signs (3). Determine whether they are consistent with the postoperative diagnosis and/or add any details that may be required by the codes (3a, 3c, 3d, 3e).
- Identify any comorbidities (3a) or complications that create an operative risk.
- Identify the code set to be used for coding procedures.
- Refer to the Key Criteria for Abstracting tables for the procedures related to the procedural description and the code set. Read through the entire record, noting what items support or modify the stated procedure.
- Refer to CPT and/or ICD-10-PCS guidelines to determine when multiple procedures should be coded.
- Identify the following for each procedure:
  - Operative approach (4) (The same operative approach may be applicable to more than one procedure.)
  - Objective of the procedure as it relates to the PCS Root Operation definition (6, 7, 8, 9)
  - Anatomic site (5, 6, 8)
  - Devices (9)
  - Other details required by the specific procedure
- Reread the entire report to confirm that all diagnoses and procedures are identified. Be certain to identify a diagnosis to support each procedure. Assign diagnosis and procedure codes according the the OGCR and coding conventions.
- Arrange (sequence) the diagnoses according to the reason for the procedure and operative findings documented by the surgeon.
- Arrange (sequence) the principal procedure followed by additional procedures (PCS OGCR).

Do not assign codes solely from the Postoperative Diagnosis or Procedure Performed sections of the operative report. You need to read the entire operative report to identify any additional details or variations.

CPT codes are assigned differently than ICD-10-PCS codes. CPT codes are assigned by physicians and outpatient services. ICD-10-PCS codes are assigned by inpatient hospitals. The code set used is determined based on who you are coding for. All entities code from the physician's operative note, but slightly different information may be required and a different number and/or type of codes might be needed for each code set. Review the abstracting criteria and guidelines for the code set being used.

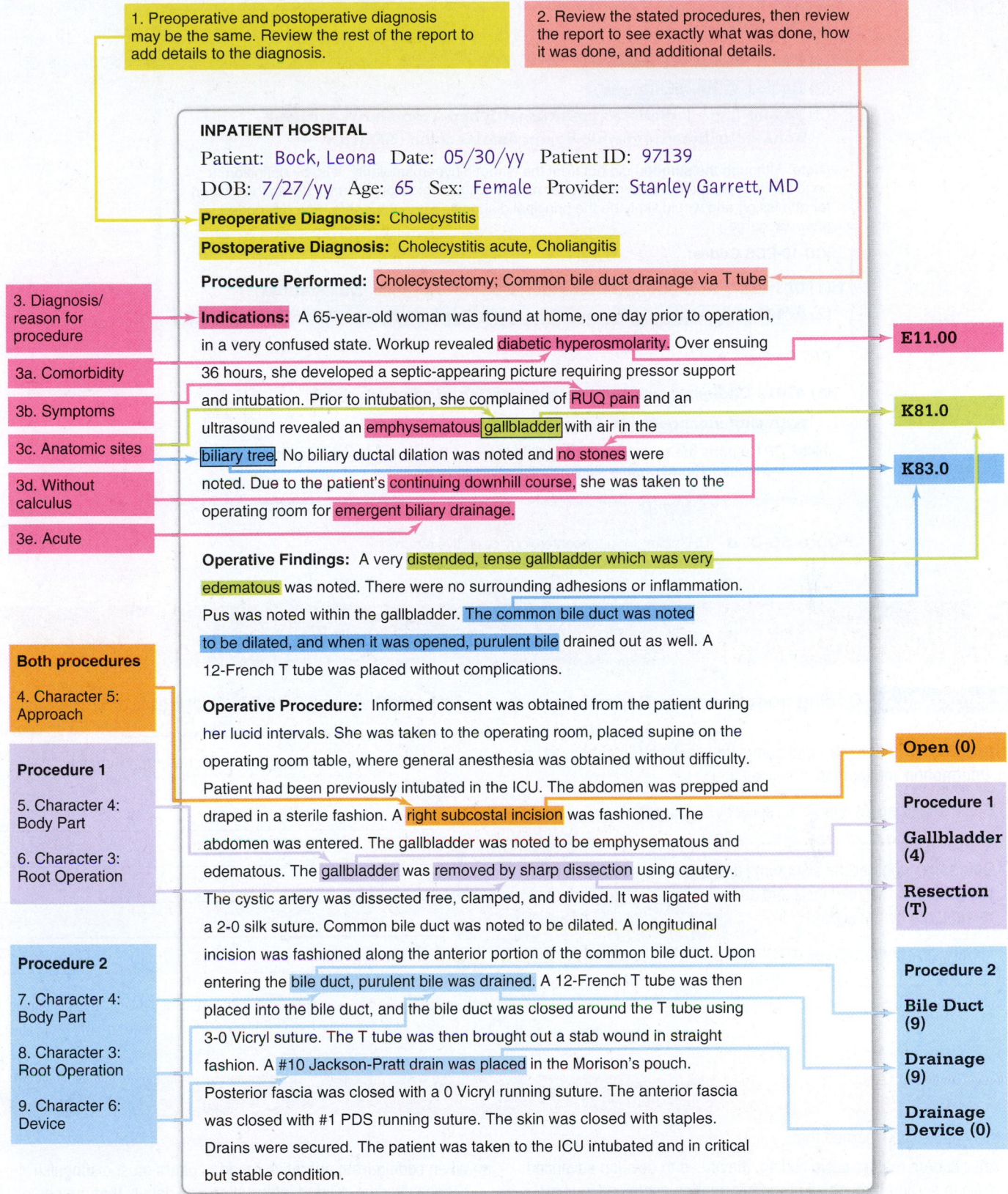

1. Preoperative and postoperative diagnosis may be the same. Review the rest of the report to add details to the diagnosis.

2. Review the stated procedures, then review the report to see exactly what was done, how it was done, and additional details.

INPATIENT HOSPITAL

Patient: Bock, Leona Date: 05/30/yy Patient ID: 97139

DOB: 7/27/yy Age: 65 Sex: Female Provider: Stanley Garrett, MD

Preoperative Diagnosis: Cholecystitis

Postoperative Diagnosis: Cholecystitis acute, Choliangitis

Procedure Performed: Cholecystectomy; Common bile duct drainage via T tube

Indications: A 65-year-old woman was found at home, one day prior to operation, in a very confused state. Workup revealed diabetic hyperosmolarity. Over ensuing 36 hours, she developed a septic-appearing picture requiring pressor support and intubation. Prior to intubation, she complained of RUQ pain and an ultrasound revealed an emphysematous gallbladder with air in the biliary tree. No biliary ductal dilation was noted and no stones were noted. Due to the patient's continuing downhill course, she was taken to the operating room for emergent biliary drainage.

Operative Findings: A very distended, tense gallbladder which was very edematous was noted. There were no surrounding adhesions or inflammation. Pus was noted within the gallbladder. The common bile duct was noted to be dilated, and when it was opened, purulent bile drained out as well. A 12-French T tube was placed without complications.

Operative Procedure: Informed consent was obtained from the patient during her lucid intervals. She was taken to the operating room, placed supine on the operating room table, where general anesthesia was obtained without difficulty. Patient had been previously intubated in the ICU. The abdomen was prepped and draped in a sterile fashion. A right subcostal incision was fashioned. The abdomen was entered. The gallbladder was noted to be emphysematous and edematous. The gallbladder was removed by sharp dissection using cautery. The cystic artery was dissected free, clamped, and divided. It was ligated with a 2-0 silk suture. Common bile duct was noted to be dilated. A longitudinal incision was fashioned along the anterior portion of the common bile duct. Upon entering the bile duct, purulent bile was drained. A 12-French T tube was then placed into the bile duct, and the bile duct was closed around the T tube using 3-0 Vicryl suture. The T tube was then brought out a stab wound in straight fashion. A #10 Jackson-Pratt drain was placed in the Morison's pouch. Posterior fascia was closed with a 0 Vicryl running suture. The anterior fascia was closed with #1 PDS running suture. The skin was closed with staples. Drains were secured. The patient was taken to the ICU intubated and in critical but stable condition.

A

3. Diagnosis/reason for procedure

3a. Comorbidity

3b. Symptoms

3c. Anatomic sites

3d. Without calculus

3e. Acute

E11.00

K81.0

K83.0

Both procedures

4. Character 5: Approach

Procedure 1

5. Character 4: Body Part

6. Character 3: Root Operation

Open (0)

Procedure 1

Gallbladder (4)

Resection (T)

Procedure 2

7. Character 4: Body Part

8. Character 3: Root Operation

9. Character 6: Device

Procedure 2

Bile Duct (9)

Drainage (9)

Drainage Device (0)

Figure 56-3 ■ (A) Example of a gastroenterology operative report. *Source: Adapted with permission from Health Professions Institute, Medical Transcription: Fundamentals and Practice, 3rd Ed., © 2007. Reprinted and electronically reproduced by permission of Pearson Education, Inc., Upper Saddle River, New Jersey.*

(continued)

ICD-10-CM Codes:

(1) K81.0 Cholecystitis, acute

(2) K83.09 Other cholangitis

(3) E11.00 Type 2 diabetes mellitus with hyperosmolarity without nonketotic hyperglycemic-hyperosmolar coma (NKHHC)

(Note: Although the surgeon did not treat the diabetic hyperosmolarity, it is, by definition, a condition that places the patient at higher risk during a surgical procedure. It was the reason for admission and would likely be the principal diagnosis when the entire record is coded after discharge.)

ICD-10-PCS Codes:

(1) 0FT40ZZ Resection, Gallbladder, Open, No Device, No Qualifier

(2) 0F9900Z Drainage, Common Bile Duct, Open, Drainage Device, No Qualifier

CPT Codes:

(1) 47612 Cholecystectomy with exploration of common duct; with choledochoenterostomy

(Note: CPT reports the resection of the gallbladder and the drainage of the common bile duct (choledochoenterostomy) with a single combination code.)

B

Figure 56-3 ■ (B) Coding for gastroenterology operative report.

CODING PRACTICE

Exercise 56.2   Coding from Operative Reports

Instructions: Write the term that completes each statement based on the information you learned in this section.

1. Begin analyzing an operative report by reading the
   _____.

2. Determine whether the symptoms and signs are consistent with the postoperative diagnosis and add any _____ that may be required by the codes.

3. Identify any comorbidities or complications that create an _____.

4. Refer to CPT and/or ICD-10-PCS Guidelines to determine when _____ should be coded.

5. Identify five pieces of information documented for each procedure.

   a. _____

   b. _____

   c. _____

   d. _____

   e. _____

CHAPTER SUMMARY

In this chapter you learned that:

- After coders master basic coding, they need to develop advanced skills in sorting through all of the information contained in chart note and operative reports.

- Continue to use the three skills of an "Ace" coder—abstract, assign, and arrange (sequence)—within the context of more detailed instructions.

- The entire chart note or operative report must be analyzed to abstract the needed information. Do not rely on a few isolated statements to arrive at the code(s).

- When coding from operative reports coders must distinguish between coding-related information and details that are not required to assign diagnosis and procedure codes, such as the anesthetic, instruments, sutures, and other supplies.

- CPT and ICD-10-PCS coding require different abstracting criteria and guidelines, so be sure to identify which code set you are working with.

- Assign and sequence codes according to the guidelines for the specific code sets being used.

CONCEPT QUIZ

Take a moment to look back at your trip through advanced coding and solidify your skills. This is your opportunity to pull together everything you have learned.

Completion

Instructions: Write the term that completes each statement based on the information you learned in this chapter. Choose from the list below. Some choices may be used more than once and some choices may not be used at all.

BP	CTA	LBP
BPH	EX	PE
CA	HTN	PMH
CC	ICD-10-PCS	postoperative diagnosis
CPT	LB	

1. _____ is the patient's stated reason for a visit.
2. _____ is a review of a patient's past conditions, which may or may not be resolved, and past surgical procedures.
3. _____ codes are assigned by inpatient hospitals.
4. Do not assign codes directly from the _____ section of an operative report.
5. _____ is the physician's examination and factual findings and results of tests performed or reviewed.
6. _____ is the abbreviation for hypertension.
7. _____ is the abbreviation for low back pain.
8. _____ is the abbreviation for blood pressure.
9. _____ is the abbreviation for clear to auscultation.
10. _____ is the abbreviation for benign prostatic hypertrophy.

Multiple Choice

Instructions: Circle the letter of the best answer to each question based on the information you learned in this chapter.

1. What condition(s) should be coded for this scenario? *A patient sees a gastroenterologist for epigastric pain and nausea and vomiting, which are due to a peptic ulcer. The patient is also seeing a urologist for BPH.*
   A. BPH and peptic ulcer
   B. Epigastric pain and nausea and vomiting
   C. BPH, peptic ulcer, epigastric pain, and nausea and vomiting
   D. Peptic ulcer

2. What condition(s) should be coded for this scenario? *A patient sees a urologist for polyuria, nocturia, and oliguria due to BPH.*
   A. Polyuria
   B. Polyuria, nocturia, and oliguria
   C. BPH, polyuria, nocturia, and oliguria
   D. BPH

3. What condition(s) should be coded for this scenario? *A patient presents with complaint of chest pain and shortness of breath. The physician diagnoses angina pectoris, rule out myocardial infarction. An EKG and blood enzyme studies are ordered to be completed ASAP.*
   A. Chest pain, shortness of breath
   B. Shortness of breath, angina pectoris, myocardial infarction
   C. Angina pectoris, myocardial infarction
   D. Angina pectoris

4. What is the meaning of *cholangitis?*
   A. Inflammation of the blood vessels
   B. Inflammation of the gallbladder
   C. Inflammation of the common bile duct
   D. Inflammation of the gallbladder and common bile duct

5. What is the functional purpose of an electrocautery?
   A. Cutting
   B. Drainage
   C. Occlusion
   D. Wound closure

6. What is the functional purpose of a retractor?
   A. Cutting
   B. Occlusion
   C. Viewing
   D. Wound closure

7. What is the functional purpose of a hemostat?
   A. Absorption
   B. Holding
   C. Drainage
   D. Viewing

8. What is the functional purpose of catgut?
   A. Cutting
   B. Wound closure
   C. Absorption
   D. Drainage

9. What is the functional purpose of wire?
   A. Cutting
   B. Wound closure
   C. Occlusion
   D. Stabilization

10. What does the eponym *Mayo-Hegar* refer to?
    A. Procedure
    B. Sutures
    C. Scissors
    D. Needle holder

CODING CHALLENGE

Instructions: Read the case, then abstract, assign, and arrange the codes indicated, using the appropriate Index and Tables. Write the code(s) on the line provided.

1. Review the annotated chart note from a gastroenterology consultation in ■ FIGURE 56-4. Abstract, assign, and arrange (sequence) the codes.

   5 ICD-10-CM Codes _____

   1 CPT (E/M) Code _____

2. Review the chart note from a urology consultation in ■ FIGURE 56-5. Abstract, assign, and arrange (sequence) the codes.

   5 ICD-10-CM Codes _____

   1 CPT (E/M) Code _____

GASTROENTEROLOGY CLINIC

Patient: Jeff Flannery   Date: 01/30/yy   DOB: 9/30/yy   Age: 56
Sex: Male   Allergies: NKDA   Provider: Stanley Garrett, MD
Referred by: Kristen Conover, MD (Family Practice Clinic)

Reason for Consultation:
[1. Reason for the referral to gastroenterologist]
Evaluation of recurrent epigastric and LUQ pain.

History of Present Illness:
[2. Symptoms]
Patient is a 56-year-old male. He reports a long history of mild dyspepsia, characterized by burning epigastric pain, especially when his stomach is empty. This pain has been relieved by OTC antacids. Approximately two weeks ago, the pain became significantly worse. He is also nauseated and has vomited several times.

Past Medical History:
[3a. Medical history]
[3b. Current problem not treated here]
[3c. Risk factor]
Patient's history is not significant for other digestive system disorders. He had a tonsillectomy at age 8. He sustained a compound fracture of the left ankle in a bicycle accident at age 11 that required surgical fixation. More recently, he has been diagnosed with an enlarged prostate gland and surgery has been recommended. However, he would like to resolve this epigastric pain before going forward with the TURP. He also has long-standing problems with alcohol dependence.

Results of Physical Examination:
[4. Examination findings and test results]
CBC indicates anemia and a fecal occult blood test is positive for blood in the feces. A blood test for *Helicobacter pylori* is positive. Erosion in the gastric lining was visualized on an upper GI. Follow-up gastroscopy found evidence of mild reflux esophagitis and an ulcerated lesion in the lining of the pyloric section of the stomach. The ulcer is 1.5 cm in diameter and deep, with evidence of bleeding. Multiple biopsies were negative for gastric CA.

Assessment:
[5. Diagnosis]
Acute peptic ulcer. Gastric cancer has been ruled out in light of negative biopsies.

Recommendations:
[6. Future treatments, prescriptions, and instructions]
A gastrectomy to remove the ulcerated portion of the stomach is indicated because the ulcer is already bleeding. Patient started on Tagamet to reduce stomach acid. Added Keflex to treat the bacterial infection and iron pills to reverse anemia. Patient was instructed to eat frequent small meals and avoid alcohol and irritating foods.

Figure 56-4 ■ Coding Challenge, Question 1, Gastroenterology chart note.
Source: FREMGEN, BONNIE F.; FRUCHT, SUZANNE S., MEDICAL TERMINOLOGY: A LIVING LANGUAGE, 4th Ed., ©2009. Reprinted and Electronically reproduced by permission of Pearson Education, Inc., **New York, NY.**

3. Review the annotated operative report from an orthopedics procedure in ■ Figure 56-6 (page 1178). Abstract, assign, and arrange (sequence) the codes.

2 ICD-10-CM Codes _____

4 ICD-10-PCS Codes (Code the four procedures identified in the figure for this exercise.) _____

3 CPT Codes: _____

_____

Procedures 1 and 2 (one CPT code) _____

Procedure 3 (one CPT code) _____

Procedure 4 (2-view x-ray) _____

4. Review the annotated operative report for a neurology procedure in ■ Figure 56-7 (page 1179). Abstract and assign the codes.

Tip: *Supratentorial* refers to the upper front portion of the brain containing the frontal and temporal lobes of the cerebrum. *Infratentorial* refers to the lower portion of the brain containing the pons and medulla.

1 ICD-10-CM Code _____

1 ICD-10-PCS Code _____

3 CPT Codes (Surgical) _____

_____

UROLOGY CLINIC

Patient: Peter Mock   Date: 03/30/yy   DOB: 7/13/yy   Age: 60   Sex: Male   Allergies: NKDA
Provider: Brent Eberhart, MD   Referred by: Kristen Conover, MD (Family Practice Clinic)

Reason for Encounter:
Has been "using the restroom a lot. I always need to go and feel like I cannot wait, but not much comes out."

History of Present Illness:
This "has been happening for awhile, but has gotten to be a problem within the last month or two." Frequency, urgency, decrease in amount and force of urinary stream.

Past Medical History:
Rotator cuff repair 20 years ago. Had physical therapy about a year ago for LBP but it is "not bothering him lately." Currently takes Lisinopril for HTN.

Results of Physical Examination:
Vital signs: T: 98.8F   P: 82   R: 20   BP: 146/89
Ht: 6´1˝   Wt: 191 lb.
General appearance: Healthy 60-year-old male. Appears uncomfortable. Hesitant in talking about symptoms.
Heart: Regular rate and rhythm. No murmurs, gallops, or rubs.
Lungs: CTA.
Abd: Bowel sounds all 4 quadrants. No masses or tenderness. No distention of bladder or renal tenderness
Prostate: DRE revealed enlarged prostate, approximately 5.5 cm, projecting 1.5 cm into the rectum. Smooth without normal central groove, no nodules or indurations, tender, firm to rubbery consistency.

Assessment: BPH

Plan: Urinalysis and PSA test. Rx finasteride 5 mg PO once a day for 6 months for BPH. FU 6 months

Figure 56-5 ■ Coding Challenge, Question 2, Urology chart note.
Source: RICE, JANE, MEDICAL TERMINOLOGY: A WORD-BUILDING APPROACH, 6th Ed., ©2008. Reprinted and Electronically reproduced by permission of Pearson Education, Inc., **New York, NY.**

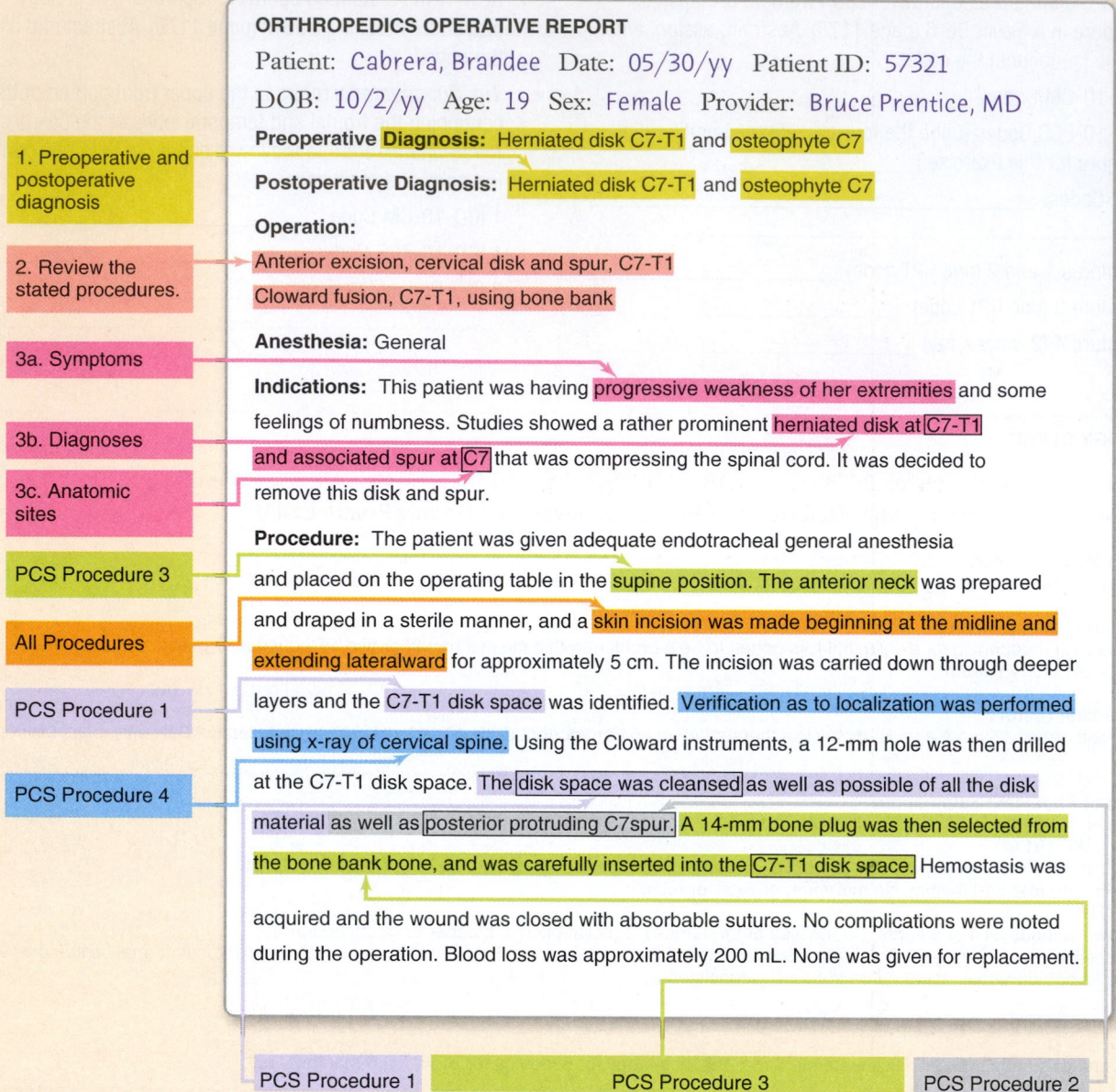

ORTHROPEDICS OPERATIVE REPORT

Patient: Cabrera, Brandee   Date: 05/30/yy   Patient ID: 57321

DOB: 10/2/yy   Age: 19   Sex: Female   Provider: Bruce Prentice, MD

Preoperative Diagnosis: Herniated disk C7-T1 and osteophyte C7

Postoperative Diagnosis: Herniated disk C7-T1 and osteophyte C7

Operation:

Anterior excision, cervical disk and spur, C7-T1

Cloward fusion, C7-T1, using bone bank

Anesthesia: General

Indications: This patient was having progressive weakness of her extremities and some feelings of numbness. Studies showed a rather prominent herniated disk at C7-T1 and associated spur at C7 that was compressing the spinal cord. It was decided to remove this disk and spur.

Procedure: The patient was given adequate endotracheal general anesthesia and placed on the operating table in the supine position. The anterior neck was prepared and draped in a sterile manner, and a skin incision was made beginning at the midline and extending lateralward for approximately 5 cm. The incision was carried down through deeper layers and the C7-T1 disk space was identified. Verification as to localization was performed using x-ray of cervical spine. Using the Cloward instruments, a 12-mm hole was then drilled at the C7-T1 disk space. The disk space was cleansed as well as possible of all the disk material as well as posterior protruding C7spur. A 14-mm bone plug was then selected from the bone bank bone, and was carefully inserted into the C7-T1 disk space. Hemostasis was acquired and the wound was closed with absorbable sutures. No complications were noted during the operation. Blood loss was approximately 200 mL. None was given for replacement.

Annotation labels (left margin):
1. Preoperative and postoperative diagnosis
2. Review the stated procedures.
3a. Symptoms
3b. Diagnoses
3c. Anatomic sites
PCS Procedure 3
All Procedures
PCS Procedure 1
PCS Procedure 4

Annotation labels (bottom): PCS Procedure 1   PCS Procedure 3   PCS Procedure 2

Figure 56-6 ■ Coding Challenge, Question 3, Orthopedics operative report.
Source: Adapted with permission from Health Professions Institute, Medical Transcription: Fundamentals and Practice, 3rd Ed., © 2007. Reprinted and electronically reproduced by permission of Pearson Education, Inc., Upper Saddle River, New Jersey.

NEUROLOGY OPERATIVE REPORT

Patient: Cassity, Janet   Date: 05/30/yy   Patient ID: 64197

DOB: 4/16/yy   Age: 61   Sex: Female   Provider: Stanley Garrett, MD

Preoperative and postoperative diagnosis →

Preoperative Diagnosis: Subacute subdural hemorrhage on the right

Postoperative Diagnosis: Subacute subdural hemorrhage on the right

Procedures →

Operation: Craniotomy and excision of subacute subdural hematoma on the right

Anesthesia: General

Symptoms →

Indications: The patient was suffering from headaches and at time had a slowed pulse. Studies showed

a rather extensive chronic or subacute subdural hematoma on the right. It was decided to excise this

Diagnosis and anatomic site →

hematoma.

Procedure: The patient was given adequate endotracheal general anesthesia and placed on the

operating table in the supine position with her head turned toward the left. The scalp was prepared and

PCS Character 5: Approach →

draped in a sterile manner, and a linear skin incision was made, beginning in front of the ear and

extending over the top of the head. The scalp was retracted and a free bone flap was turned in the right

frontoparietal region. The dura was opened, and subdural fluid was noted approximately 1 cm or so in

PCS Character 4: Body Part →

depth, which was covering the right cerebral hemisphere. This subdural was evacuated in all directions,

PCS Character 3: Root Operation →

carefully. Hemostasis was acquired, and the dura was again closed. The bone flap was plated into

position and the scalp was closed in two layers. No complications were noted during the operation.

Blood loss was approximately 100 milliliters.

Figure 56-7 ■ Coding Challenge, Question 4, Neurology operative report.
Source: Adapted with permission from Health Professions Institute, Medical Transcription: Fundamentals and Practice, 3rd Ed., © 2007. Reprinted and electronically reproduced by permission of Pearson Education, Inc., Upper Saddle River, New Jersey.

Chapter 57

Professionalism and Patient Relations

Chapter Outline

- **Professionalism Basics**
- **Professionalism and Your Employer**
- **Professional Communication**
- **Professional Workplace Relationships**
- **Professional Patient Relations**

Learning Objectives

After completing this chapter, you should have the skills to:

57.1 Spell and define the key words and abbreviations related to professionalism. (Remember)

57.2 Summarize the essential elements of professionalism. (Understand)

57.3 Describe the four areas of professionalism related to your employer. (Apply)

57.4 Identify the characteristics of verbal, nonverbal, and written communication. (Apply)

57.5 Articulate tips for working well with others. (Apply)

57.6 Assess the importance of patient relations and how to respond to distressed patients. (Evaluate)

Key Terms

at-will employment	human resources department	phone etiquette	verbal communication
clear speech	insubordination	probationary period	voice pitch
enunciate	internal customer	professionalism	written communication
external customer	nonverbal communication	slang	
extraneous	patient relations	tone of voice	

In addition to the key terms listed here, students should know the terms defined within tables in this chapter.

Source: Beth A. Rich, *Medical Coding: A Journey.* Pearson, 2013.

INTRODUCTION

You have now come to the last stop, the end of your coding journey in this text, even though your journey will continue on in the healthcare field. Regardless of how much coding you perform, you will need to possess the qualities of a professional to be successful.

You may be thinking that you already are a professional and wonder what more there is that you could possibly learn. Even the most professional people continue expanding their current knowledge of practicing professionalism, and look forward to refreshing their existing skills. Professionalism is a learned skill that people have to deliberately practice daily to become good at. It is not something that you are born with or that you "just know." Being a professional is a lifelong endeavor because successfully working with others is a lifelong endeavor.

PROFESSIONALISM BASICS

When you think of someone who is a professional, what type of person do you think about? What qualities come to mind? Would you say that this person is successful?

Can you also think of someone who you feel is unprofessional? What characteristics would you use to describe this person? Would you say that the person you thought of is unsuccessful?

Professionalism is practicing the traits necessary to be successful in the workplace, including enthusiasm, dedication, job knowledge, respect for others, and a positive attitude. The most basic traits of a professional are to show:

- *Enthusiasm* about your job, even in the midst of negative circumstances. Employer research shows that managers are more likely to hire and promote people with enthusiasm and less experience over those with more experience but who are not enthusiastic.

- *Dedication*, demonstrated by arriving for work consistently and on time, even if you do not feel like working.

- *Job knowledge*, including a thorough knowledge of your job and an understanding of how your work affects others, even when they may not understand your job.

- *Respect* for everyone, even when they are rude to you.

- A *positive attitude* and a warm smile, even if you feel bad on the inside.

Imagine a person who has one of these qualities but not the others—like someone who is very enthusiastic but does not know how to perform her job—or someone who has sound job knowledge but disrespects others. It is the combination of these skills that make a person a successful professional. These are certainly not all of the qualities that contribute to being professional. Take a few minutes to jot down a list of what *you feel* are qualities of a professional, and then answer *yes* or *no* to each of the self-assessment questions in ■ TABLE 57-1.

So, how did you do on your self-assessment? Do you feel that you have all of the traits needed to be a professional? Count how many times you answered *yes* in the left column and how many times you answered yes in the right. If you answered *yes* to most questions on the left, then you handle most situations like a professional. If you answered yes to more than two or three questions on the right, then you need to improve your professionalism and patient relations skills.

Now that you are familiar with the qualities needed to be a professional, review the following real-world workplace scenarios. Think about how you would handle each situation, drawing from your own experiences and the experiences of others you know. Check the recommendations listed after the scenarios to see how you did.

Table 57-1   ■   **PROFESSIONALISM SELF-ASSESSMENT**

A professional is someone who is …		
Honest and Trustworthy		
Do you make sure that you make up any time missed and ensure you record the missed time on your time sheet? ☐ Yes ☐ No	OR	Have you ever arrived late to work but did not make up the time or mark the time missed on your time sheet? ☐ Yes ☐ No
Do you feel that stealing is wrong, no matter what the situation is? ☐ Yes ☐ No	OR	Have you ever made personal copies at work or taken supplies, food, or materials from an employer simply because they would not miss it, they were throwing it away anyhow, or you did not receive that bonus you were promised? ☐ Yes ☐ No
Positive and Friendly		
Do you smile at people you encounter and say "hello" and ask "How are you?"? ☐ Yes ☐ No	OR	Do you feel that this is not important, so you do not bother? ☐ Yes ☐ No
Do you rise above a negative situation and work through it with a smile on your face? ☐ Yes ☐ No	OR	Do you instantly grumble when something goes wrong, once again believing it is just your bad luck? ☐ Yes ☐ No
Efficient and Accurate		
Do you double-check your work before finalizing it? ☐ Yes ☐ No	OR	Do you "wing it" because you have spent enough time on it already? ☐ Yes ☐ No
Are you organized and able to meet deadlines, keeping a to-do list and following it? ☐ Yes ☐ No	OR	Do you rely on your memory to keep all of your appointments and manage projects, sometimes or frequently missing due dates? ☐ Yes ☐ No

(continued)

Table 57-1 ■ *(continued)*

Mature and Reasonable

Are you able to keep your emotions in check, even when you are angry or upset, and think before you speak? ☐ Yes ☐ No	OR	Do your emotions get the best of you, where you easily become angry or upset, say what you think, and raise your voice to others? ☐ Yes ☐ No
Do you give others the benefit of the doubt if they are in a bad mood and try not to take their mood personally? ☐ Yes ☐ No	OR	Do you feel that it is one more time (in a long list of times) that this person has treated you this way? ☐ Yes ☐ No

Motivated and Passionate

Do you like to work, and does work give you an intrinsic (internal) satisfaction? ☐ Yes ☐ No	OR	Is work something that you do to pay the bills, and that's all? ☐ Yes ☐ No
Do you believe in what you do and feel strongly that you need to do it well? ☐ Yes ☐ No	OR	Do you watch the clock until your work is over and you can go home? ☐ Yes ☐ No

Respectful and Reliable

Can you appreciate when someone does not share your religious beliefs or personal interests or just simply disagrees with you? ☐ Yes ☐ No	OR	Do you feel that this person is simply opinionated and hard to get along with? ☐ Yes ☐ No
Do you understand that you have to take orders from your boss, or you could lose your job? ☐ Yes ☐ No	OR	Do you talk back to superiors, enforcing your opinion because you just know you are right? ☐ Yes ☐ No

Flexible and Understanding

Are you willing to perform work that you have never done before because it needs to be done? ☐ Yes ☐ No	OR	Do you say that you would rather not do the work because you are uncomfortable with it? ☐ Yes ☐ No
Can you understand that when someone else is hurting physically or emotionally, their situation can make them impatient and rude? ☐ Yes ☐ No	OR	Do you think that they are just unhappy and negative? ☐ Yes ☐ No

A professional also…

Shows Good Judgment

Can your boss/teacher/instructor/coworker rely on you to perform a task without worrying that you will waste time? ☐ Yes ☐ No	OR	Do you find that surfing the Internet, text messaging, talking on your cell phone, and using other electronic devices are absolutely necessary, even when you are at work or school? ☐ Yes ☐ No
Will you do what someone else needs you to do, regardless of how you are feeling at the moment? ☐ Yes ☐ No	OR	Would you rather do what you want, when you want, regardless of what someone else needs? ☐ Yes ☐ No

Takes Pride in His or Her Work

Do you follow up when you say you are going to, in response to someone's question or concern? ☐ Yes ☐ No	OR	Do you follow up when you think of it, even if someone has been waiting for your answer? ☐ Yes ☐ No
Do you feel good about yourself after you complete certain projects? ☐ Yes ☐ No	OR	Is it just another job done, and you are glad that it is over? ☐ Yes ☐ No

Makes Ethical Decisions

Do you understand the legalities of not discussing patient information with people who are not authorized to know it? ☐ Yes ☐ No	OR	Would you share patients' stories with friends and family members? ☐ Yes ☐ No
When you have to make a decision, do you ensure that it does not hurt someone else financially, physically, or emotionally? ☐ Yes ☐ No	OR	Do you make decisions regardless of how they affect others? ☐ Yes ☐ No

Is Fair to Others

Would you treat everyone the same because they should have to follow the same rules? ☐ Yes ☐ No	OR	Would you bend the rules according to the situation and the person involved? ☐ Yes ☐ No
Do you treat everyone the same regardless of race, ethnicity, language, religion, politics, lifestyle, and gender orientation? ☐ Yes ☐ No	OR	Do you find that you avoid or respond to people differently based on personal characteristics? ☐ Yes ☐ No

Possesses Excellent Customer Service Skills

Do you feel that every customer is as important as your family member or best friend? ☐ Yes ☐ No	OR	Are customers people whom you cannot wait to get rid of because they are in your way and wasting your time? ☐ Yes ☐ No
Do you feel that every customer is really your boss, since every customer helps to pay your salary? ☐ Yes ☐ No	OR	Do you feel that even if a customer does not come back, there will always be other customers? ☐ Yes ☐ No

Communicates Well

Do you listen to others when they speak to you, ensuring that you maintain good eye contact and concentrate on what they say? ☐ Yes ☐ No	OR	Do you find that it is easier to continue working while someone is speaking to you? ☐ Yes ☐ No
Do you double-check written correspondence that you create, including email, to ensure that there are no grammatical or spelling errors? ☐ Yes ☐ No	OR	Do you write correspondence once and check it as you go without double-checking your work when you finish? ☐ Yes ☐ No

Real-World Professionalism Scenarios

Imagine the following setting. You are working at a family practice clinic that has three physicians who specialize in primary care. Your job title is administrative coding specialist, and you perform diagnosis and procedure coding. You also assist the billing staff with appealing denied claims and help answer the phones. You report to Katie, the office manager, and you also report to the physicians.

Situations

Determine how you would handle each of the following situations, and write your answer in the space provided. Then compare your answer with the recommendation listed after the scenario.

Scenario 1: Did you ever hear the saying "Rule No. 1: The Boss Is Always Right"? Katie asks you to complete a task, and you feel that she used a rude tone of voice when she spoke to you. What should you do? _____

_____

Scenario 2: What about "Rule No. 2: If The Boss Is Wrong, See Rule No. 1"? You need to explain a situation to Katie. While you are speaking, she keeps interrupting you and tries to finish each one of your sentences. What should you do?

_____

_____

Scenario 3: The "That's Just Her" Defense. Yasmin, a billing specialist in the office, has told coworkers that she and her husband have been arguing a lot lately. Yasmin also seems to be in a bad mood frequently and is often impatient with and disrespectful to her coworkers, including you. If anyone asks Yasmin if she is all right, then she complains for what seems like forever about everything that is wrong with her husband. One day, Charise, another coworker, talks to you about Yasmin and says, "She's going through a rough time, and she always handles bad situations this way. She takes it out on others, and then later when she calms down, she's okay. You just have to tiptoe around her if you sense that she's in a bad mood because *that's just Yasmin.*" What should you do? _____

_____

Scenario 4: "I Can't Believe That You Would Suggest Such a Thing…" Katrina, a coworker, is trying to pass off her work to you. She is responsible for scheduling all appointments for patients and decides to tell you to do it today, stating that she is "way too busy with other stuff" to handle scheduling on top of everything else that she has to do for the day. She adds, "Since you told me yesterday that you finished your big project, I figured you'd be looking for work to do." Even though you finished the project, your to-do list is full of other projects and other deadlines. What should you do? _____

_____

Recommendations

There are several ways to handle these situations professionally and tactfully. A few suggestions follow and you will probably think of more.

Scenario 1 Recommendation. Ignore it. Maybe Katie is just having a bad day, and she will later apologize to you. Even though this does not excuse her behavior, you should not take offense. However, if Katie speaks rudely to you on a regular basis, then you should politely ask her if you have done something wrong because you sense that she is upset with you. If there are no problems, then Katie will hopefully realize her actions are counterproductive.

Because Katie is your boss, you should not report her to one or all of the physicians unless her behavior is abusive, in which case you may choose to find another job. Going over your manager's head, as the saying goes, could cause her to become even more upset and angry.

Scenario 2 Recommendation. Do nothing. Ignore it. Stop talking when she interrupts, and when she finishes talking, continue speaking. Some people interrupt others without realizing it. It is important to not make an issue out of it, and avoid saying something like, "Excuse me, I'd like to finish what I was saying." After all, she is the boss.

Scenario 3 Recommendation. Many people excuse their bad behavior, and others excuse it for them, by saying that it is just the way the person is. However, there are certain job requirements that everyone must meet in order to keep their jobs, including treating other people with respect, regardless of how bad their personal lives are. Imagine if everyone felt that it was acceptable to be impatient with others just because they were in a bad marriage or having a bad day!

No one should have to "tiptoe" around Yasmin because of her personal problems. It is not appropriate to carry personal problems to work to the point where they affect other employees. This is a situation that Katie should handle because Yasmin is treating everyone in the office poorly. Charise is defending the bad behavior and further encouraging it by asking you to excuse it, too. The best approach is to avoid interactions with Yasmin as much as possible, not ask questions about her personal life, and trust that Katie will step in and resolve the situation.

Scenario 4 Recommendation. Tell Katrina that you are sorry but even though you finished your project, you still have other work to do, and if she does not feel that she can keep up with her work, she should let Katrina know. Keep in mind, there will be times that you will help your coworkers with their work, and they will help you with yours. But helping is much different from being asked to complete someone else's entire job for them. It also does not mean that coworkers are permitted to delegate their work to others who do not report to them. Rather, they should *ask* for assistance instead of giving a direct order to someone else to provide it.

PROFESSIONALISM PRACTICE

Exercise 57.1 Professionalism Basics

Instructions: Read each scenario and determine the best way to handle the situation, recording your answer in the space provided.

1. *You Want Me To Do What? When?*

Today is Wednesday, and Katie gives you three assignments to complete. She tells you that they are all due next Tuesday, so you have a little less than a week to finish them. Because you have other responsibilities and are working on multiple projects, you do not feel that you will have time to finish the new assignments by next Tuesday.

What should you do?

_____

_____

2. *Would Someone Please Answer the Phone?*

For the first hour every morning, your job is answering incoming phone calls, and it is the busiest time for calls. Danielle, one of your coworkers, works beside you and helps you with the calls. For the past three mornings, Danielle has arrived at least 20 minutes late, causing you to handle a lot more phone calls because she is not there to help you.

What should you do?

_____

_____

3. *I Wish I Could Stay and Chat but ...*

Gloria is one of your coworkers and she has a tendency to talk too much. In fact, once she starts talking to you, it is very hard to break away and get back to work. She talks about what she did the night before, her son's baseball practice, her dog's recent antics, and her latest shopping trips. Today, she has you cornered again, this time in the lunch room. Your lunch ended 10 minutes ago, but you cannot seem to excuse yourself while Gloria is still talking to you.

What should you do?

_____

_____

4. *Ghostly Visits*

Dr. Svenger, one of the physicians in the practice, stops by your desk today to drop off a report. He tells you that the report contains a list of Medicare patients' demographic and insurance information and asks you to enter the patients into the computer system. He also tells you, "Once you've added them, please enter an office visit charge with code 99215." You ask Dr. Svenger where the encounter forms are for the patients, since the staff always uses them to enter charges. Dr. Svenger says, "Don't worry about it. I'll take care of the encounter forms. Just key the charges, and ask Ashley to submit their claims to Medicare." He then walks away. You check the list of patients and cannot identify that any of them as ever been a patient in the office, let alone having received a high-level office visit for an established patient.

What should you do?

_____

_____

5. *Are You Talking to Me?*

In the office this morning, one of your coworkers, Gina, raises her voice when she is speaking to you and sounds angry and mean. She questions why you performed a certain task, and she even asks you, "Don't you know anything?!" as she huffs and walks away.

What should you do?

_____

_____

PROFESSIONALISM AND YOUR EMPLOYER

Professionalism includes understanding your employer's departments, policies, and procedures. The four areas with which you should be familiar regarding your employment are:

1. Job descriptions
2. At-will employment
3. Probationary period
4. Human resources department

Job Descriptions

Every position should have a job description. The employer writes the job description and provides each employee with a copy. It is a good idea to ask for a copy of the job description before a scheduled job interview so that you will have a better idea of the job expectations. The job description includes individual job duties, and behavior expectations—such as courtesy and respect, work hours, dress code, and other criteria about the job that the employer wants to define. Being a professional means understanding and following your job description.

Job descriptions also typically state that the employee must perform "other related duties." This means that your boss can ask you to work on a project or complete a task not specifically listed on the job description but does relate to your job. This type of request is not unusual, and it is not appropriate to tell your boss, "That isn't on my job description, so I'm not doing it." Failure to perform work that your boss requests is considered **insubordination**—which means not following orders from your boss—and can cost you your job.

At-Will Employment

At-will employment means that your employment is both at your will and at your employer's will. You can legally leave your job at any time, for any reason, even without notice (although this is not recommended), and your employer can legally terminate your job at any time, for any reason, without notice.

At-will employment applies when you do not have a written or verbal contract with an employer that protects your job for a specific amount of time, such as a year. Employees who belong to labor unions usually have written contracts. Many federal and state government employees are not at-will employees. They cannot be fired unless there is a specific and well-documented reason, such as proof of engaging in an illegal activity.

At-will employment is subject to other existing laws. For example, employers cannot fire employees for reasons that violate other laws. State and federal laws prohibit employers from firing employees because of their race, color, religion, age, gender, national origin, or disability. Employers also cannot fire employees if they refuse to perform work that is illegal or if they take time off under the Family and Medical Leave Act (FMLA) of 1993. Other exceptions to at-will employment can vary by state.

Probationary Period

A **probationary period** is the amount of time that an employer allows a new employee to learn all aspects of his or her job. When you start a new job, it is common for an employer to review the probationary period with you, which typically includes one or more performance reviews to determine your progress. Employers may review new employees every 30 days or some other period of time the employer determines up until the end of the probationary period. Probationary periods can last three months to a year, or a different amount of time, depending on the employer.

An employer can legally terminate an employee at any time during the probationary period if it appears that the employee will not be successful in the new job. Employers may also reward employees who successfully complete their probationary periods by giving them raises and/or increasing their job responsibilities.

Human Resources Department

Many larger organizations have a **human resources department** whose staff are in charge of hiring and firing employees; overseeing employee benefits (medical, life, and disability insurance); processing the company payroll to ensure that employees are paid correctly and on time, and that appropriate deductions are taken from their pay; and ensuring that all employees follow employment laws, including policies for evaluating and disciplining employees. Often, when you interview for a new job, you first meet with a human resources representative whose job is to screen applicants and choose those who should return to meet with individual department managers. You should treat an interview with human resources as seriously as you would an interview with the department manager because they play a big role in determining whether you qualify for additional interviews within the organization.

PROFESSIONAL COMMUNICATION

A large part of being a professional is communicating well with others. Your boss, coworkers, patients, families, physicians, and other employees will all judge how well you communicate, and it will affect your job success and opportunities for promotion.

There are three types of communication: verbal, nonverbal, and written. You should learn how to communicate well using all three methods.

Verbal Communication

Verbal communication means speaking with others. One skill to successful communication is identifying the correct amount of information to convey so that you provide enough information, but not too much or too little.

Think about this example: You are driving along the highway looking for the nearest grocery store. You stop at a gas station, go in, and ask the clerk for directions. The clerk gives you directions, and on your way out of the station, a male customer stops you and says that he overheard you asking for directions. Before you can say that you already have them, he also gives you directions. Both sets of directions are listed next. Determine which directions you would rather receive and why.

> EXAMPLE: *The gas station clerk's directions*
> Drive out of the gas station, and turn right at the first stop light. You will be on Highway 12. Then drive about three miles and take the Glen Cove exit, and Sam's Grocery will be on your left.

> EXAMPLE: *The customer's directions*
> Drive out of the gas station, oh, I'd say for about a mile. You'll see Juan's Dairy on the right. They used to be a lot bigger, but they downsized, and now just have milk and juice. Drive for a while past a couple of farms, and you'll get to an exit; I think it's Glen Cove, but I'm not sure. [*The customer then turns to find his wife.*] Ethel, do you remember if that first exit is for Glen Cove? Oh, she's not listening. I think she's picking out some cookies to take home. I'm pretty sure it's Glen Cove, though. Take that exit, and then almost immediately, you'll see a craft store on the right. It has a big sign out front, but you don't need to worry about that …

Did you decide that you would rather have the clerk's directions? The customer obviously enjoyed talking to you, but he missed the point of the communication: You wanted directions to the grocery store. He gave too much irrelevant information that you did not need to know.

Know Your Audience

The example about asking for directions illustrates the need to *know your audience*: know who will receive your message and how much information he needs to have. This helps you identify the amount of information that you need to convey. Ask yourself if the person to whom you are speaking really needs *all* of the information that you are about to share. Do not provide unnecessary details; stay focused and communicate only what is pertinent to the listener's needs.

Phone Etiquette

Verbal communication includes face-to-face conversations and conversations over the phone. Phone etiquette means showing good manners at work while you talk on the phone. (■ FIGURE 57-1) When you work in healthcare, you talk on the phone with both internal customers—other employees of the organization, such as coworkers and superiors—and external customers, patients and others from outside organizations such

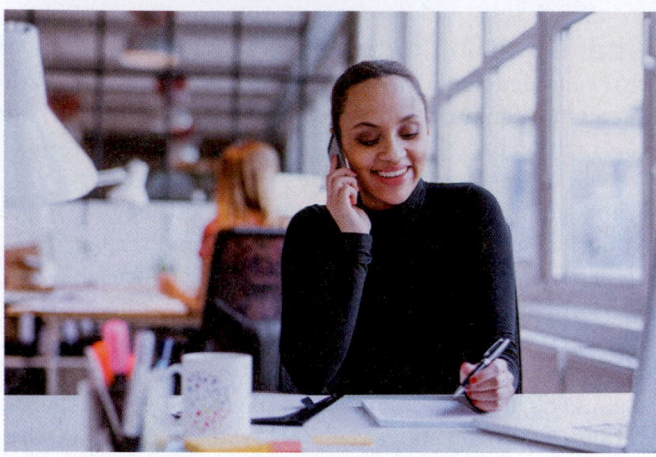

Figure 57-1 ■ All employees should know and practice good phone etiquette.

as other providers or insurance companies. Refer to ■ TABLE 57-2 to review tips for good phone etiquette.

Clear Speech

Successful verbal communication, whether it occurs in person or over the phone, includes clear speech. If you find that others often ask you to repeat what you say, then it probably means that you are not speaking clearly or loudly enough. Tips to practice clear speech are:

- Enunciate (*pronounce*) your words correctly.

- Ensure that your tone of voice (*emotion that your voice conveys when you speak*) is even-tempered, rather than upset, anxious, hurried, or mean, which can make it difficult for others to understand you and difficult for you to remain professional.

- Determine that your voice pitch (*how high or low your voice sounds*) does not interfere with your ability to communicate. If your pitch is a whisper, ranges from high to low, or is garbled, then you should improve it.

- Ensure that you do not make common mistakes, such as consistently pausing when speaking, saying "um" or "ah," swearing, or using slang. Such words and phrases are acceptable to use with friends but should not be used in a professional environment. Refer to the examples of slang

Table 57-2 ■ PHONE ETIQUETTE TIPS

Situation	Etiquette Tip
Answering the phone	Be sure to say "Good morning" or "Good afternoon," identify yourself and the organization for which you work, and ask how you may help. Example: "Good morning, Dr. Singh's office, this is Joanie, how may I help you?" rather than just saying Dr. Singh's office.
Placing a call on hold	Ask the person if you may do so instead of saying "hold, please" and hanging up. Not everyone can wait on hold and some people would rather have you call them back, or they may prefer to call back later. Ask for a call-back number in case you get disconnected.
Removing a caller from hold	Thank the caller for holding. Make sure they are still on the line.
Misunderstanding what the caller says	If you cannot hear or understand the caller, politely say, "Excuse me, can you please repeat that?" rather than saying "What?," "Huh?," or "I can't hear you!"
Taking a phone message for someone who is unavailable	Offer the caller the option to leave a message. Do not tell the caller to call back later. This is poor service and inconvenient for the caller.
	Be sure to include all necessary information, such as the caller's name, phone number, message, and best time to reach them. Many software programs and paper message pads have designated areas to list this information.
Lacking immediate information	If you do not have all the information a caller needs immediately, provide a specific day and time when you will call back. If you do not have the information by that time, then call the person back to at least tell them, and explain when you will have an answer. Not returning the call because you do not have an answer is not professional, and the other person will feel that you forgot about them.
Returning phone messages that someone leaves for you	Return calls within 24 hours or per company policy. Do not use the excuse that you are too busy because most people are busy. Returning phone calls is part of your job requirements.
Ending a call	Say "Goodbye" rather than just hanging up on the caller. You can also add "Thank you for calling" when it is appropriate for the situation.
Eating and chewing gum	Do not eat or chew gum while on the phone. It can be detected by the listener and is distracting. It can make it appear that you do not take your job seriously.
Interrupting conversations with others	Do not take a phone call in the middle of a conversation with a patient, other external customer, or another employee unless it is a true emergency.
Texting	Do not text-message while talking with a patient over the phone or in person.
Creating your voice mail greeting	Your voice mail greeting should state your name and job title. Say goodbye when you end the message. Callers should not have to guess that they have reached the correct person. Check with your supervisor if you are unsure how to set up your voice mail message.

Table 57-3   ■   SLANG WITH PROFESSIONAL TRANSLATION

Slang Word or Term	Professional Translation
Ain't	Is not or isn't
Back in the day	A long time ago
Cool	Great, wonderful, interesting, fascinating
Freak out	Become upset
Gonna	Going to
Grossed out	Become disgusted
Irregardless	Regardless
Like	Avoid using the word *like* in the following context, "It's like, a busy day at the office." Either it *is* a busy day at the office or it is *not*. It is not *like* a busy day.
Run with the big dogs	Keep up with the pace and the workload
Shoulda	Should have
Stuff your face	Eat too much
Very unique	Unique; the word *unique* means "one of a kind," so something cannot be very one of a kind. It is either one of a kind or it is not.
Wanna	Want to
Y'all or you guys	All of you

words and terms and the professional translations to say instead in ■ TABLE 57-3.

- Avoid speaking text-messaging jargon, such as LOL (laugh out loud) or OMG (oh my God!). Think about what you are going to say before you say it to ensure that you communicate clearly and professionally.

If you are not sure how you sound to others, then record your voice and determine whether you can understand what you are saying and whether you sound professional. You can also ask friends and family to critique your voice. Ask them whether they can understand you and whether they think that others could, too. This will help you to determine the areas that you need to improve. If you need to practice pronouncing words, there are many Internet websites that enable you to listen to correct word pronunciations, and you can practice pronouncing the words yourself. Then ask friends and family to listen to you as you practice to provide feedback.

Listening Skills
Successful verbal communication also depends on how well you listen. Many people appear to be listening to someone when they are really concentrating on something else. Effective listening skills will help you to hear what someone else is telling you, so be sure to concentrate when someone speaks to you to determine what they are trying to say, and you will then be able to ask them pertinent follow-up questions.

Taking notes while you are listening to someone speak is another technique that will help ensure that you capture pertinent information from the conversation. You can also repeat your notes back to the person talking to be sure you understood the message and ask if you missed anything.

Avoid interrupting a person when they are speaking or when they are finishing their sentence because it is unprofessional and does not allow the speaker to convey the entire message. It also shows that you are not listening effectively. You may think that you know what a person is going to say next, but you could be incorrect. Allow the speaker to finish talking before you respond.

Nonverbal Communication
Nonverbal communication involves communicating with others without speaking, and it can be just as important as verbal communication for successfully conveying or responding to a message. Nonverbal communication includes facial expressions, eye contact, body language, and gestures, including pointing.

Body Language
A professional uses body language appropriately when communicating with others, giving the other person his or her full attention by maintaining eye contact, sitting up straight, and showing an interested facial expression. Unprofessional body language when communicating includes rolling your eyes in disgust, making faces, slouching in your seat, ignoring the other person by working on another task, or having an uninterested facial expression.

Remember to be very aware of your body language even when you think that no one can see you. For example, let's say that Joanie, who works for a primary care physician, has a conversation with a patient whom she thinks is mean. After the patient leaves, Joanie quietly tells a coworker about the conversation and, in the process, she makes a face and rolls her eyes. Even though patients in the waiting room cannot hear Joanie's conversation, they can see her face, and they wonder if she is talking about them, another patient, or a coworker.

Joanie used poor judgment. Her unprofessional body language made the patients wonder why she felt compelled to make faces. Do you think that it would make the patients feel welcome in the office? It actually would have the opposite effect. Joanie also risked being heard by other people even though she thought she was having a private conversation. What if Joanie's office manager saw her making faces? She would then have to explain what she was doing and why. Joanie not only acted unprofessionally but also behaved immaturely.

There will always be times when another person makes you angry or upset, and you can think what you choose about that person. But conveying your thoughts through body language is a bad idea. Being professional means rising above a situation with which you do not agree and acting positively anyway, regardless of the negative thoughts you have.

Appearance and Dress
Nonverbal communication also includes taking care of your appearance and dressing appropriately for your position. It is important to follow an employer's dress code policy. Many employers allow casual dress, and clinicians can wear scrubs, but some employers require business dress. Many employers also prohibit their employees from exposing any tattoos or piercings, other than the ears. Tattoos and piercings may be an important part of an individual's self-expression, but they are not always appropriate when you are working in healthcare. Professional dress also involves maintaining good hygiene,

making sure that you are clean, and ensuring that you do not wear too much cologne or perfume. What you think smells good someone else may find offensive. Some people are also allergic to perfumes. Refer to ■ TABLE 57-4 for appearance dos and don'ts.

The Name Badge

Another form of nonverbal communication is a name badge. Many employers require employees to wear badges in a visible location that show their names, job titles, and photo. Name badges help patients and their families to know that you are an employee, so that they can ask for your assistance when needed. Wearing a name badge does not replace introducing yourself and stating your job title to a patient and their family members because not everyone will be able to read your name badge. You still need to establish a personal connection with patients.

Written Communication

Written communication means communicating with others in writing through formats such as email, business letters, memos, reports, phone messages, or notes asking others questions or to clarify information.

Successful written communication begins with knowing how to write well. Writing well does not mean that you have to be a professional writer, but it does mean that you should know the basic rules to follow for clear written communication. You can take a writing class if you need help with your writing skills, or ask someone who writes well to help you. There are also a wide variety of articles and books, as well as Internet interactive learning sites, available to assist you. Refer to ■ TABLE 57-5 for tips on successful written communications.

Email

Email is a quick and effective way to communicate with other employees, patients, and outside organizations. It is important to treat email communication the same way that you treat all other written communication, following the basic rules for clear writing. Review the following, an email that Joanie, a billing specialist, sends to her boss, Ralph. Ralph previously asked Joanie to create a financial report that he could present at the next staff meeting and asks two other employees, Babrina and Roberto, to assist.

EXAMPLE:

TO: nicotetti.ralph@medicalcenter.com
FROM: moon.joanie@medicalcenter.com
CC:
SUBJECT: report
The report is on my desk for u to pick up and bqrbna will make copies of the handouts for the meeting roberot will bring the poewr point with him when he gets their.

Believe it or not, the mistakes that Joanie made in her email are very common in the workplace, although most senders do not make all of them in the same email. Take a few minutes to see how many mistakes you can find, and then compare them with the email tips listed next for Joanie's email.

- **Be specific on the subject line**—Ralph may have several emails to review and will categorize the order to review them by their subject. He may not instantly remember what information he requested from Joanie when the subject of the email only shows "report."

- **Include a salutation**—Examples include "Hi Ralph" or "Dear Ralph." Joanie should not just start writing without acknowledging the person to whom she is addressing her message.

- **Do not use all capital letters**—Writing in all caps looks like yelling. It was unnecessary for Joanie to do this and makes the message more difficult to read.

- **Use punctuation correctly**—Notice that Joanie does not use *any* punctuation, and her sentences run together, which makes her email difficult to read.

- **Spell correctly**—Joanie used the letter *u* to replace the word *you*. Emailing is not text messaging, and Joanie should not confuse the two. She also misspelled Barb's name as BQRB and misspelled PowerPoint as POEWR POINT.

- **Use grammar correctly**—Joanie incorrectly spelled the word *there* (a place) as *their* (shows possession).

- **Do not give orders to your boss**—Joanie tells Ralph to pick up the report on her desk rather than offering to deliver it to him.

- **Ask if there is any further information needed or any more that you can do**—Asking shows courtesy and also ensures

Table 57-4 ■ APPEARANCE DOS AND DON'TS

Dos	Don'ts
❏ Wear your hair in a clean and neat style, not hanging in the face, over an eye, or big. Hair color should be believable.	❏ Do not show cleavage or wear miniskirts, tank tops, shorts, cut-off shorts, summer sandals, or clothes that are too tight. Do not go braless.
❏ Wear makeup conservatively.	❏ Do not wear brightly colored makeup or too much makeup.
❏ Be clean shaven or have neatly trimmed facial hair.	❏ Wear to work any outfit that you would wear to a club or party, the beach, to clean out your garage, on a date, or to bed. When in doubt, do not wear it.
❏ Ensure your nails are clean and neatly trimmed—for both men and women. Clinicians should keep their nails short so that they do not injure patients or harbor germs. Wear conservative nail colors—clear, light tan, or light pink tones. Avoid wearing decals and multi-colored nails.	❏ Do not wear clothes that are dirty, stained, smell bad, or wrinkled.
❏ Wear conservative and minimal jewelry. Think in terms of one—one ring, one necklace, one bracelet, and one earring in each ear. Earrings should be no longer or wider than one inch.	❏ Do not wear nose or mouth piercings. Do not wear multiple earrings in each ear or long dangling earrings.

Table 57-5 ■ **TIPS FOR SUCCESSFUL WRITTEN COMMUNICATIONS**

Spell words correctly	*Spell check* is a function in many software programs that you can use to verify your spelling to avoid mistakes such as spelling *thru* instead of *through* or *nite* instead of *night*.
Write clearly and concisely	Ensure that people can understand your writing and that you convey only necessary information. This also includes knowing when to start and end paragraphs.
Use punctuation correctly	The spell-check function can find some punctuation errors but not all of them.
Ensure that your writing is grammatically correct	Know basic rules of grammar, such as the differences among *their*, *there*, and *they're*. *Their* is a possessive pronoun. *There* refers to a place or idea. *They're* is a contraction for "they are." In choosing *loose* or *lose*, remember that *loose* means "not tight" and *lose* means "to be unable to find something or to be deprived."
Explain medical terms in common language that everyone understands	Avoid using medical terminology when you are communicating with people who may not understand it, such as patients and their family members, and those whose native language is not English.
Avoid overuse of catch phrases or buzz words that are popular at the moment	Avoid useless phrases like *at the end of the day*, *thinking outside the box*, *on the same page*, and *win–win situation*. These expressions do not convey meaningful information. Try to think of what you really mean, then say it.
Understand the appropriate amount of information to convey to the person receiving the message	Written communications should include only pertinent information, not **extraneous** information, which is irrelevant and unrelated to the subject.
Know the proper formatting for documents	Business letters, memos, and email all have standard formats that you should use when composing them. Refer to articles, books, software help functions, and Internet sites for formatting assistance.
Keyboard accurately and maintain constant speed of at least 35 words per minute (WPM)	If you do not know how to type, then it is essential to take a keyboarding course or learn through online tutorials. Successful written communication depends on having fast and accurate keyboarding skills.
Ensure that the document you create is neat and organized	Make it easy for others to read and follow the letters, email, or reports that you give to them.
Avoid sending written communication if you are upset or angry	You can easily convey your emotions in writing, and it is best to wait to calm down before writing so that you do not later regret it.

that you perform all necessary tasks related to the content of the email. Joanie's email ended abruptly without asking if her boss needed any additional information.

- **Sign your name, and provide your contact information**—A signature makes it easy for the receiver to know who sent the email without trying to decipher an email address (some addresses do not clearly identify a sender) and identify a quick way to reach her on her phone extension. Joanie failed to list any contact information in her email.

Now review Joanie's corrected email to see learn how she sounds more professional:

EXAMPLE:

TO: nicotetti.ralph@medicalcenter.com
FROM: moon.joanie@medicalcenter.com
CC:
SUBJECT: Report on unpaid claims from July to December 20XX
Hi Ralph,
I finished the unpaid claims report and will drop it off to you today. Babrina will make copies of the handouts for the meeting. Roberto will bring the PowerPoint that explains the columns of the report. Please let me know if you need anything else.
Joanie Moon
Ext. 5437

Refer to ■ TABLE 57-6 for additional tips for sending email.

Table 57-6 ■ **TIPS FOR SENDING EMAIL**

Never send an email if you are upset or angry.	Avoid writing until you calm down because you can easily convey your emotions in the email, and the receiver can forward it to anyone else at any time.
Avoid using your work email for personal purposes, including sending jokes to others and badmouthing your employer, coworkers, and boss.	Your employer can easily track your email and read what you wrote, even if you delete them. Think of email this way: Unless you would be willing to read your email on a billboard along the highway and not be embarrassed, do not send it.
Use the *Reply All* feature on email only when "all" people on the email list need to read your response.	Some people make it a habit to hit *Reply All*, even though the message may be irrelevant to all but one person. Reply only to those who need to read your message.
Respond to email within 24 hours, even if you do not have an answer to give the sender.	Send a brief message to explain why you cannot respond to them and when you expect to provide an answer.
Do not send or receive personal email while you are at work.	Avoid the use of company resources for personal purposes unless your employer occasionally permits it. Be aware that your employer has the right to read or delete all messages in their account.

SUCCESS STEP

Employees often mistakenly believe that their use of the Internet and email at the workplace is private. Your employer owns the equipment and software used in your job. They are paying you for the time you work, so it is wise not to use your employer's time and resources for personal activities. The courts have found no reasonable expectation of privacy in such use and have consistently permitted employers to monitor and review employee activity.

PROFESSIONALISM PRACTICE

Exercise 57.2 Professionalism and Your Employer; Professional Communication

Instructions: Fill in each blank with the answer discussed in this section.

1. A _____ is the amount of time that an employer allows a new employee to learn all aspects of her job.

2. _____ means speaking with others.

3. _____ means that you can leave your job at any time, for any reason, even without notice, and your employer can terminate your job at any time, as long as they do not violate public policy.

4. _____ means showing good manners at work while you talk on the phone.

5. _____ involves communicating with others without speaking.

6. List three tips for sending email.

   a. _____

   b. _____

   c. _____

PROFESSIONAL WORKPLACE RELATIONSHIPS

It is important to please your boss to be successful, but did you also know that your workplace success depends on how professionally you work with others? This is because everyone works for the same team. Coworkers rely on each other to "win the game," which can be to keep patients satisfied, stay organized, meet deadlines, perform coding and billing, and achieve many other objectives. When one team member does well, the entire team looks good. One of your jobs in healthcare is to support your own team and make each other look good. (■ FIGURE 57-2) Follow the tips outlined next for working well with others.

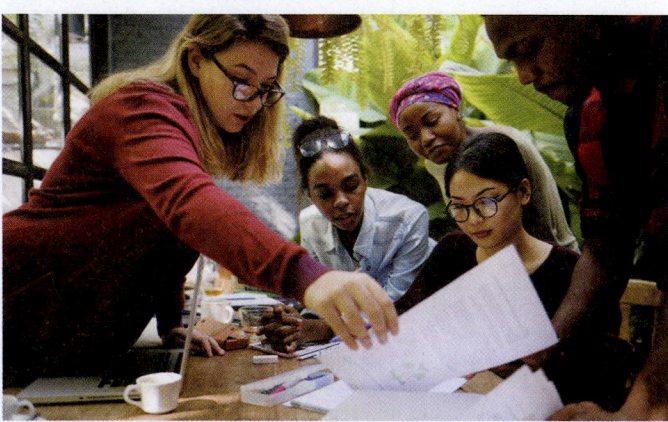

Figure 57-2 ■ Professionals must work cooperatively with a wide variety of people.

- **Support your coworkers**—Do not resent someone else if they do a good job or earn a promotion. Do not pick on a coworker for making a mistake, and do not openly criticize them in order to get a laugh from others.

- **Congratulate a team member**—Offer congratulations to someone who achieves a goal, and thank them for helping you complete a task or project. It may be easy to forget to say "please" when you are asking for someone's help and "thank you" when they help you, but using "please" and "thank you" goes a long way to ensuring that fellow teammates will support you and assist you in the future.

- **Do not give orders to coworkers**—Only give orders if it is part of your job, like if you are leading a project and have to ask coworkers to complete specific duties. It is the boss's job to delegate work and give orders. Coworkers may resent you if you give them orders and probably will not follow them. This also includes giving orders to your boss, which is inappropriate.

- **Acknowledge coworkers and other people who work in your organization**—Part of professionalism is having the manners to make eye contact, smile, and say "hello" when you encounter someone else. Not only do you have to acknowledge people whom you know; you should acknowledge everyone you encounter. A smile takes only a second and is well worth the investment. You never know whom you may encounter, including a person who may have the final say on whether you are promoted.

- **Use good manners**—Employers tend to promote mannerly, likeable people over those whom they do not like and who have poor manners. Other employees are more willing to work with people whom they like and who have good manners.

- **Embrace diversity**—Your fellow employees represent to a wide variety of ethnic and racial groups. People hold differing religious and political beliefs. Personalities range from very shy to boisterous and outgoing. Lifestyle choices and gender orientation may include practices you are personally unfamiliar or uncomfortable with. As a human being and a professional, you must be sensitive to differences such as these, accept feedback from everyone, and be willing to support and assist others without bias, regardless of these characteristics.

- **Have a sense of humor**—It is all right to laugh and joke with others at work, as long as it is not at someone else's expense and does not take up much of your day. Having a sense of humor also means not taking yourself or others so seriously that you are incapable of having occasional fun conversations. Having fun does not mean wasting time. If you enjoy what you do at work, then it is easy to make it fun.

- **Be a good observer of human nature**—You can learn a lot from others who perform their jobs well and think to yourself, "Wow, what a great way to handle that situation. I'll have to remember to do that." You can also learn from the mistakes that others make so that you do not make the same mistakes yourself. You can learn skills for working well with others by reading articles and books, taking classes, and learning from others who have more work experience and who are eager to share it with you.

Coworkers can encounter roadblocks when communicating with one another (■ TABLE 57-7). Read each roadblock and then the instructions for how the employee can navigate around the roadblock to act more professionally.

Table 57-7 ■ WORKPLACE COMMUNICATION ROADBLOCKS AND SOLUTIONS

Roadblock	Scenario and Solution
Interrupting others	*Sam walks up to Christiana's desk. She is typing on her computer, and her back is turned. Sam says, "Do you have those totals from the computer report with rejected claims that we printed last week?"*
	Solution: Sam should say, "Excuse me, Christiana, do you have time for a question?" before interrupting her in case she is in the middle of work that she cannot stop. This shows good manners and respect for another person's time and schedule. Just because it was a good time for Sam to discuss the report does not mean that it is also a good time for Christiana.
Coworker is busy	*Tobias needs to ask Nekeisha a question. When he reaches her desk, she is on the phone with a patient. He stands at her desk, waiting for her to finish.*
	Solution: If Tobias wants to wait a few minutes (not indefinitely) for Nekeisha to end the call, he should at least move away from her desk to an area nearby, rather than stand at her desk. If he does not have time to wait, then he should come back later. If it is an emergency situation, Tobias can write a quick note to Nekeisha and place it on her desk directly in front of her so she will read it. It is not polite to stand beside someone while she is on the phone. This same rule would also apply if Nekeisha were meeting with someone else at her desk.
Unnecessary email	*Mai and Rita have desks that are side by side. Rita has a question for Mai, so she sends Mai an email.*
	Solution: Rita should just ask Mai the question. She should not email someone sitting right next to her because it diminishes her ability to build rapport with a coworker.
Lack of pleasantries	*Kenyonna arrives each morning at her desk, which is situated in the middle of the department, along with eight other employees. She always removes her coat and puts her purse in her desk drawer and begins working, without speaking to anyone.*
	Solution: Kenyonna should say "good morning" to her coworkers when she arrives and "good night" when she leaves. It is courteous to speak to other people at work, rather than walking in and out without talking. If Kenyonna is consistently discourteous to those working around her, then they may not be very eager to assist her if she ever needs help. People are more apt to help those whom they like and who are positive and friendly. In addition, if Kenyonna does not have a good rapport with others, it can adversely affect her ability to succeed at work or be promoted.
Missing deadlines	*After a group project meeting on Monday morning, Jose, the project manager, asked Eugenia to prepare a report for the next team meeting on Friday morning. Now it is Thursday afternoon, and Eugenia has not had the chance to even start on the report. She tells Jose that she is sorry, but she will not have the report ready for Friday's meeting.*
	Solution: Eugenia should have started preparing the report early in the week, since Jose asked her about it on Monday morning. She did not complete the work that she was required to perform as part of her responsibilities on the team project. The group needs information for Friday's meeting. If Eugenia did not have time to work on the report, then she should have discussed it with Jose earlier in the week to explain the situation and ask for assistance. She could also have talked with her manager to determine whether she could stop working on other tasks in order to complete the report, to ensure that she finished the report on time.

PROFESSIONALISM PRACTICE

Exercise 57.3 Professional Workplace Relationships

Instructions: Read each roadblock and determine the best way to navigate around it, recording your answer in the space provided.

1. Every morning, Deborah and Likeyita say "good morning" to each other, but if Likeyita asks Deborah how she is, Deborah's only response is "good."

   - What could Deborah do differently to communicate more professionally with Likeyita? _____
   _____

2. Nathan and Filippe engage in heated debates on a regular basis when they discuss politics at their desks. Nathan's political views are very different from Filippe's views, and Nathan becomes upset when Filippe disagrees with him. One day, they debate whether abortion should be legal or illegal. The conversations disrupt other coworkers trying to complete their work.

   - What could Nathan and Filippe do differently to communicate more professionally with each other? _____
   _____

3. Jen has a tendency to be short with her coworkers when she feels that they are bothering her. The other day, when Deborah asked her a question, she told Deborah, "I'm in the middle of something and can't talk right now. You'll have to wait." Another day she told Filippe that he was "getting on her nerves."

   - What could Jen do differently to communicate more professionally with Deborah and Filippe? _____
   _____

4. When Ashley talks with others, she uses a lot of slang terms and catch phrases. She also overuses the word *like* and has a very high-pitched voice, which sounds almost childlike. Yesterday, she told Filippe about a computer problem she had to resolve, stating, "I was like, what now? I can't believe that the computer, like, failed again! But you know what, I got out the manual and was able to find the problem and, like, fix it myself! LOL!"

   - What could Ashley do differently to communicate more professionally with her coworkers? _____
   _____

PROFESSIONAL PATIENT RELATIONS

A healthcare provider is a business and needs revenue to survive. Patients, the customers, provide that revenue, and without them, there is no business. Coders do not have constant daily contact with patients as clinicians do, but you may have opportunities to talk with patients about their bill, their insurance, or other business matter on the phone or after an office visit. Treat patients well, and they will return; treat them poorly, and they will go elsewhere. To lose a patient to poor service hurts everyone: the patient, the employees, and the provider's business. Treat each patient like they are the most important patient. Only then will you ensure that the patient is satisfied with the services, you are satisfied that you've done a great job, and all the employees are satisfied that the office will continue to generate revenue. Give each patient your attention and time to make them feel important and that you truly care about their well-being. Remember that patients are not diagnoses, like "the shoulder injury," "the mole removal," or "the broken leg." Patients are people, and you should treat them that way, rather than refer to them as a diagnosis.

Patient relations involves interacting with patients and their families to ensure that they receive the best service. Many hospitals have patient relations departments whose employees address patients' questions and concerns and resolve complaints from patients and families regarding the patient's experience at the hospital. Even if you do not work in a patient relations department, you can show excellent patient relations skills because they are the same skills that you should show any customer, including courtesy, respect, sincerity, concern, and compassion. Many customer service skills are also the same as many professionalism skills, such as having excellent communication skills and follow-up abilities. The patient is a customer of healthcare, purchasing services from healthcare providers.

Your job may involve patient interactions on a daily basis, or it may involve only occasional interactions. You may talk with patients in person or over the phone. You may see them in the hallway. You may never see a patient if you have a position working from home or in a separate location where employees perform coding, billing, and collections and where there are no clinicians. But even if you do not see patients, you should still appreciate the fact that you work for them.

Just as there is wide diversity among you and coworkers, you will also come in contact a wide variety of patients. Factors such as race, language, socioeconomic status, religion, politics, lifestyle preferences, and gender orientation should never affect your interactions with patients. You should not be rude, condescending, or overly ingratiating to others because they are different than you. As a professional in the healthcare environment, you should always be aware of your tendencies and preferences and consciously work to overcome them. It takes personal insight and self-awareness to identify any subconscious judgements and biases.

Patients may not always seem cheerful or pleasant. They could be in pain, nauseated, dizzy, confused, disabled, terminally ill, or depressed, or they may have several other problems. Many times, a patient's illness also contributes to financial problems. There are patients who have gone bankrupt paying medical bills, and there are patients who cannot afford to pay anything toward their medical bills.

Not all patients are this way, but you have to be prepared for those who are. Take extra care to ensure that you treat all patients with respect, patience, courtesy, and dignity, just like you would treat your best friend or a family member. Patients pay your salary, after all, because they are the real boss!

Poor Service to Patients

Think about a time when you received poor service at a healthcare provider (physician's office, clinic, or hospital), restaurant, or store. Did you feel that the people employed there understood that you, the customer, were their boss? Would you ever go back? Review the following list of common patient complaints about bad service, and avoid repeating these errors:

- Employee failed to listen to the patient's questions, concerns, and complaints, including failing to acknowledge family members who accompanied the patient.

- Employee failed to acknowledge the patient, such as when the patient arrived for an appointment, or informed the patient of service delays (e.g., the physician is running late, the billing specialist is with another patient).

- Employee failed to greet the patient with "hello" to introduce themselves, to say "goodbye," or to thank the patient for the business.

- Employee showed a lack of interest in the patient's issue, not paying attention, ignoring the patient, or having an uninterested facial expression.

- Employee failed to follow up with a patient after promising to get back to the patient with additional information.

- Employee showed rude behavior toward the patient, including talking down to the patient as though the patient were a child, interrupting the patient when they were talking, interrupting a conversation with the patient to take personal calls, or using medical terms that the patient did not understand.

- Employee showed lack of interest in the patient's situation and lack of concern for the patient's inability to understand information.

- Employee failed to provide an interpreter for a deaf patient or a patient who speaks another language.

- Employee showed unwillingness to help the patient, failing to direct the patient to the appropriate department or area when the patient looked lost or asked for directions, or failing to help a patient or find someone to help when a patient is struggling to walk or has lost their balance.

- Employee failed to explain required forms to the patient, including patient registration forms, consent to treatment forms, and HIPAA regulations, and simply handed the patient forms to sign.

- Employee assumed that the patient knew all the provider's policies when no one ever explained them or provided the patient with written copies of them, including policies about paying for services and procedures.

Since you now know the common patient complaints about poor service, you can do something about them when you interact with patients to ensure that they are satisfied with your service. A patient's experience with a provider involves more than just one person. A patient may interact with many types of healthcare professionals from the time he or she arrives at the provider until the time he or she leaves. Everyone working for the provider must ensure that the patient's experience is as comfortable and pleasant as possible, given the patient's circumstances.

Excellent Service to Patients

You can ensure outstanding service just by smiling at and speaking to patients you see, even if you are not meeting with them. You might be walking down the hall when you see a patient arriving for an appointment. You can smile and say "Hello, how are you?" or just say "Good morning." When you see a patient leave, say "goodbye" and "thank you." Saying "Thank you" shows a patient that you appreciate his business and the fact that he or she chose to visit your provider, rather than going somewhere else. Common pleasantries like these can have a huge impact in terms of making a patient feel important and appreciated. Take the extra time, and make the effort to help patients feel important to you and the provider for whom you work. It might be the only positive interaction a patient has that day.

Assisting Distressed Patients

One of the challenges that healthcare professionals face when they are interacting with patients is responding to an angry or frustrated patient. A patient can be unhappy with the services, upset about receiving a bill, disappointed in an employee's inability to follow up on an issue, or distressed for any other reason. It is easy to be kind to others and cheerful when they are also kind to you. But it can be especially difficult when you are trying to resolve a problem for a distressed patient. It can be very upsetting when someone yells at you, criticizes you, or complains loudly. There are specific techniques that you can use to turn a negative interaction with a patient into a positive one, ensuring that you resolve the patient's problem rather than making the issue worse.

Review the following example about a frustrated patient, and then think about techniques that you could employ to calm the patient and help to resolve her situation.

EXAMPLE: You are working as a coder for Dr. Cizeron's office and covering for Judy, the front desk receptionist. Vahini, a medical assistant, is working with you. You are busy answering incoming phone calls when a patient walks up to the desk and tells you that she is upset because she received three bills for a $150 service that she says she already paid. She continues to tell you that she does not feel that the office staff is listening to her because she already called twice to say that her bill was paid, but the bills "just keep coming!" Her voice becomes louder, and her face turns red. She points a finger in your face and shouts, "You people don't know what you're doing, and you don't care how much you've inconvenienced a patient!

Why can't you make the corrections and get it right?!" There are other patients in the reception area who are witnessing her outburst. What should you do?

- What techniques did you think about?

- Would you ask Vahini to help you?

- Would you call your boss and ask her to handle the patient?

- Would you call the police because you feel threatened?

- Would you try to talk with the patient, or would you tell the patient to come back when she is calm?

- Would you insist that the patient calm down before you speak with her?

This situation is a tricky one to handle, because the patient is very upset andbecause she is in the reception area. Her reactions could easily upset other patients and risk release of her confidential information if you discuss her private details in front of others.

Tips for Responding to Patients
Review the following tips for responding to patients who might be frustrated, angry, or upset.

- Do not tell the patient, "There is nothing that I can do about it."

- Do not say, "It is our policy that …" and then say that there is nothing that you can do. Managers can review policies to determine whether they make sense and revise them or even make an exception when necessary.

- Do not give the patient orders, such as saying things like, "Your behavior is very rude, and you need to calm down," or "You are being very disrespectful to me, and I am not disrespectful to you." These comments will only make the patient more defensive, since the patient will resent you attempting to give her orders regarding her behavior, even if her behavior is inappropriate. She is upset, so allow her

the opportunity to tell you about it without policing her behavior.

- Ask for your manager's assistance if you have failed to resolve the problem yourself or with another employee's help. Then, explain the situation to your manager so that the patient does not have to repeat herself. Do not immediately call your manager every time you encounter a distressed patient.

- Call your manager, the police, or security (if your provider has a security officer) if a patient threatens you, verbally or physically, and you believe that the patient will harm you. If a patient swears at you, this does not necessarily mean that she is threatening you. It depends on what she says to you. If she is not threatening you, then you can politely ask her not to swear. If she does not stop, then you can ask for your manager's assistance because you will not be able to successfully resolve the problem if the patient does not stop swearing at you. Sometimes upset customers calm down when they know that they are talking with someone who is a higher authority.

- Avoid labeling patients after negative encounters. This means that after a patient leaves, you should not call her names when you are discussing the situation with your manager or other employees, such as calling her a "pain," "angry lady," "psycho," or "old buzzard." Even though it may feel good to complain about her, it serves no purpose and makes you look unprofessional.

- You can employ many of the same techniques for responding to patients on the phone as you in person. Apologize, listen without interrupting, introduce yourself, say that you want to help, and take notes and repeat back the information.

- You may have to meet with or handle a phone call from a family member if the patient is not present. You can use the same techniques as handling a distressed patient. Be sure that you have a signed authorization from the patient allowing you to speak with the family member.

PROFESSIONALISM PRACTICE

Exercise 57.4   **Professional Patient Relations**

Instructions: Fill in each blank with the answer discussed in this section.

1. _____ is interacting with patients and their families to ensure that they receive the best service.

2. List three examples of poor service to patients.

   a. _____

   b. _____

   c. _____

3. List three tips for responding to a distressed patient.

   a. _____

   b. _____

   c. _____

CHAPTER SUMMARY

In this chapter you learned that:

- Professionalism is practicing the traits necessary to be successful in the workplace, including enthusiasm, dedication, job knowledge, respect for others, and a positive attitude.

- Professionalism includes understanding employers' policies and procedures, including job descriptions, at-will employment, probationary period, and the human resources department.

- Successful professionals are skilled at verbal, nonverbal, and written communication.

- Workplace success includes working well with coworkers to keep patients satisfied, stay organized, meet deadlines, perform coding and billing, and achieve many other objectives.

- Patient relations involves interacting with patients and their families to ensure that they receive the best service.

CONCEPT QUIZ

Take a moment to look back at professionalism and solidify your skills. Try to answer the questions from memory first, then refer to the discussion in this chapter if you need a little extra help.

Completion

Instructions: Write the term that completes each statement based on the information you learned in this chapter. Choose from the list below. Some choices may be used more than once and some choices may not be used at all.

clear speech	phone etiquette
enunciating	probationary period
external customer	professionalism
extraneous	slang
human resources department	tone of voice
insubordination	verbal communication
internal customer	voice pitch
nonverbal communication	written communication
patient relations	

1. _____ means showing good manners at work while you talk on the phone.

2. _____ means words and phrases acceptable to use with friends, but not in a professional environment.

3. _____ means speaking clearly or loudly enough to be understood by others.

4. _____ is interacting with patients and their families to ensure that they receive the best service.

5. _____ is communicating with others without speaking.

6. _____ means pronouncing your words correctly.

7. _____ means how high or low your voice sounds.

8. _____ is a coworker or superior within your organization.

9. _____ means emotion that your voice conveys when you speak.

10. _____ is someone from outside the organization such as a patient or other provider.

Multiple Choice

Instructions: Circle the letter of the best answer to each question based on the information you learned in this chapter.

1. Which person is an example of an internal customer?
   A. A patient
   B. An insurance company representative
   C. A coworker
   D. A drug company sales representative

2. What is the professional translation of the slang expression *irregardless*?
   A. A long time ago
   B. Should have
   C. Disgusted
   D. Regardless

3. What type of communication comprises body language, appearance and dress, and the name badge?
   A. Indirect
   B. Written
   C. Nonverbal
   D. Verbal

4. What word is a contraction for *they are*?
   A. *Them*
   B. *Their*
   C. *There*
   D. *They're*

5. What is the term for information that is irrelevant and unrelated to the immediate topic?
   A. Intravenous
   B. Extraneous
   C. Redundant
   D. Repetitive

6. What document lists individual job duties and expected behavior?
   A. Time sheet
   B. Employer's policies and procedures
   C. Job description
   D. Practice management software

(continued)

(continued from page 1195)

7. What department is responsible for hiring and firing employees, overseeing employee benefits, and processing the company payroll?
   A. Honorary recruitment department
   B. Patient satisfaction team
   C. Healthcare management team
   D. Human resources department

8. What communication tip means to know who will receive your message and how much information he or she needs to have?
   A. Know your place
   B. Know your audience
   C. Know your job
   D. Know your coworkers

9. What employment rule means that you can leave your job at any time, for any reason, even without notice, and your employer can terminate your job at any time, for any reason, without notice?
   A. At-will employment
   B. Hire-at-will employment
   C. Fire-at-will employment
   D. All-risk employment

10. What are the three types of communication?
    A. Verbal, oral, and written
    B. Nonverbal, written, and email
    C. Verbal, nonverbal, and written
    D. Verbal, nonverbal, and nonspeaking

PROFESSIONALISM CHALLENGE

Instructions: Read each workplace scenario and determine the best way to handle the situation. Write your answer in the space provided.

1. You are working for Dr. Khatri's office, and a coworker, Janine, tells you during a lunch break that another coworker, Rolando, has been saying negative things about you. Janine tells you that Rolando said that you try to befriend the boss by talking with her all of the time. Janine says that Rolando is very insulting when talking about you, including criticisms of your hairstyle and clothes. What should you do? _____
_____
_____
_____

2. It is Monday, two days before an important staff meeting with all of the office staff, including your manager Chris and Dr. Khatri. Chris asks you to create sample form letters for Dr. Khatri to send to other physicians when they refer new patients to his practice and to give the letters to her before the meeting on Wednesday. You spend about two hours working on the letters. You are very proud of your work because you created a series of four letters, each with a different style, clip art, and creative details. As Chris asked, you give the letters to her before the meeting. During the meeting, Chris distributes copies of the letters in a packet to all in attendance. She then proceeds to tell everyone that she would like to begin using the letters. Dr. Khatri tells Chris that he is very impressed with the letters, and she smiles brightly and says, "Thank you." What should you do? _____
_____
_____
_____

3. You are working at the front desk at a family practice clinic, scheduling patients' appointments, answering phones, and checking in and checking out patients. You are extremely busy, and there are nine patients in the waiting room scheduled to see either Dr. Young or Dr. Snow. The phone rings, and it is Dr. Reynolds. He is on his way to the office and asks you to order him lunch from the restaurant across the street, proceeds to give you his long lunch order, and then says that after you order his lunch, he needs you to go to the dry cleaner to pick up two of his suits that his wife dropped off last week. What should you do? _____
_____
_____
_____

4. At the family practice clinic where you work, Katie calls you into her office after lunch and explains that Bernadette, the billing specialist, told her that you were rude to her this morning and acted very abruptly. Katie tells you that she will not tolerate rudeness to staff and expects you to change this behavior. You are angry because you thought that Bernadette was rude to *you* and talked down to *you*. This morning, when Bernadette stood at the front desk and began criticizing you, you ignored her and took a phone call before she huffed and walked away. What should you do? _____
_____
_____
_____

5. You are the newest employee at the family practice clinic, starting two months ago. Everyone else has worked there at least three years. It seems that your five coworkers have been giving you the cold shoulder and excluding you from their group lunches in the lunch

(continued from page 1196)

room. If they order food for pick-up, they never ask you to join them. Recently, they went out after work, talking loudly about it all day, anticipating where they would go for dinner. They did not invite you—*again*. What should you do? _____

_____

_____

6. It is 4:30 P.M. on Wednesday at the family practice clinic. Katie comes to your desk and tells you that she needs your help with a report. She says that she has been working on it all week and has a few more points to include to finish it. Katie tells you that she has to turn in the report tomorrow morning to all three physicians. You made plans after work to have dinner with family members and are supposed to meet them at 5:00 P.M. at a restaurant. What should you do? _____

_____

_____

7. For the past two weeks, you have been off, sick from a gastrointestinal infection. When you return to work, Katie speaks rudely to you, and it seems to you that she is upset that you were off. What should you do? _____

_____

_____

8. You are in charge of sending a letter to Mrs. Nunes, a patient at the family practice clinic, who requests an explanation of how much money she owes to the office. Mrs. Nunes said she wants to check the amount the office shows that she owes against her records. You check her balance owed on the computer and find that it is $580. So you write the letter to Mrs. Nunes explaining the amount she owes and why. A few days later, Mrs. Nunes calls the office and asks to speak with you manager, Katie. She is very upset and angry because she received your letter and says that according to her records she only owes $100. Katie checks the computer and finds that Mrs. Nunes is correct. She apologizes to Mrs. Nunes and explains that she will send her a corrected letter with the balance showing as $100. Katie then tells you that the amount owed in the letter was incorrect and shows you the account in the computer. You instantly see your mistake. What should you do? _____

_____

_____

9. At the family practice clinic, you work at the front desk with a medical assistant, Kierra, who constantly complains about the office and her work. She says that she does not like the hours or the physicians, and that Katie, the office manager, is too bossy. Kierra has been working at the office for six months. Each time that you see her interact with the physicians or with Katie, Kierra is very nice and gives no indication to them that she hates her job. Kierra's nonstop complaining is getting to you. What should you do? _____

_____

_____

10. At the family practice clinic, Katie asks you and two coworkers, Annalie and Lucinda, to complete a project. Each of you has to complete a lengthy section and the team needs to have regular weekly meetings to keep everyone on track. Katie asks you to be in charge of the project. You must make sure that you, Annalie, and Lucinda all have the work completed accurately and on time for each weekly meeting. You are also in charge of heading the weekly meetings and reporting the team's progress to Katie. The problem is that during your first meeting, Lucinda did not have her work completed, not even close. She told you that she had other work to complete and promised to get the work to you by the next week's meeting. You gave her the benefit of the doubt and agreed to wait until the next week. But during the second meeting, Lucinda told you the same story. You suspect that Lucinda either does not know how to complete the work required or does not want to. Annalie has completed all of her work, accurately and on time. She is now complaining to you about Lucinda. What should you do? _____

_____

_____

_____

Glossary

The glossary provides definitions for key terms, terms defined in tables, and abbreviations.

0–9

3-D ultrasound taking and combining multiple two-dimensional scans using specialized computer software to form three-dimensional images.

837I electronic equivalent of the UB-04 for; used by inpatient hospitals

837P electronic equivalent of the CMS-1500 form; used by physicians

A

AAPC a professional organization for coders founded in 1988, formerly known as the American Academy of Professional Coders

abdominal hysterectomy surgical incision into the lower portion of the uterus

abnormal finding in which the readings are not within the normal average range established for that particular test

abnormal clinical finding evidence of a disease or condition discovered through physical examination or testing

abnormal development embryonic development of a structure that occurred on schedule but took on an uncommon physical variation or development in the womb

abnormal laboratory test result of a chemistry test, blood test, or biological culture that is outside of (higher or lower than) the normal numerical range, or a microscopic specimen examination that differs from the standard visual features

abortifacient an agent that causes abortion

Abortion (ICD-10-PCS) the root operation that identifies artificially terminating a pregnancy

abortion artificially terminating a pregnancy

absence seizure a seizure characterized by muscle twitching or jerking for several seconds

abstract to read the medical record and determine which elements of the encounter require codes

abuse (financial) mistakenly accepting payment for items or services that should not be paid for by Medicare; due to improper coding and billing practices

abuse (personal) physical, emotional, or sexual mistreatment of one person by another

abuse (substance) using a substance in a quantity or frequency that creates legal, employment, social, or family problems, or places the individual at physical risk, without causing physical dependence

access location the anatomic site through which the target site for a procedure is reached

accessory organ an organ that assists an organ system in carrying out its functions but does not fulfill a major function of the system

accessory sinus an air-filled chamber, or space, inside the skull and face bones; also called paranasal sinus

Accredited Standards Committee (ASC) X12N Version 5010 the HIPAA standards for electronic transactions

Accredited Standards Committee (ASC) group that is directly responsible for setting electronic transaction standards ASC Accredited Standards Committee

acquired immunodeficiency syndrome (AIDS) a disease caused by the human immunodeficiency virus, which weakens and paralyzes the immune system

actinic keratosis a precancerous lesion

activities of daily living (ADL) daily self-care activities such as bathing, dressing, grooming, eating, and leisure activities

Activities of Daily Living Assessment (ICD-10-PCS) the root type that identifies the measurement of functional level for activities of daily living

Activities of Daily Living Treatment (ICD-10-PCS) the root type that identifies exercise or activities to facilitate functional competence for activities of daily living

activity describes what a person was doing when an injury occurred, such as running, playing sports, or preparing food

acute exacerbation a sudden increase in the intensity or type of symptoms, such as shortness of breath, wheezing, and chest tightness

acute kidney failure the rapid loss of kidney function over a period of days or weeks

acute myocardial infarction (AMI) a myocardial infarction (heart attack) that occurred within the past four weeks; also called a current myocardial infarction

acute respiratory distress syndrome (ARDS) acute respiratory failure that results in widespread injury to the endothelium in the lung caused by sepsis, massive blood transfusion, aspiration of gastric contents, or pneumonia

acute respiratory failure (ARF) insufficient oxygen passing from the lungs to the blood due to hypercapnia, hypoxemia, or both

acute rhinitis common cold

acute tubular necrosis damage to the renal tubules due to reduced blood flow or toxins in the urine

AD Alzheimer's disease; *auris dexter* (right ear)

add-on code a CPT code marked with a + in the CPT manual that must be reported with another procedure code

addiction a usage pattern that involves compulsive reliance on a substance to the extent that it is physically or psychologically difficult to stop, despite the significant problems it creates; also called dependence

additional diagnosis any diagnosis that is not the principal or first-listed diagnosis; also called secondary diagnosis

adenocarcinoma cancerous tumor of a gland

adenoma tumor of a gland

adhesiolysis use of a scalpel or electric current to destroy or cut free adhesions

adjacent tissue transfer/rearrangement (ATT/R) transfer of a section of skin or flap from that immediately next to the damaged skin, which can be moved without completely detaching it

adjustment disorder an abnormal difficulty in responding to life changes

adjuvant therapy additional treatments when more than one type of treatment is used

admitting privileges an agreement between a physician and hospital that gives the physician authority to admit a patient to the hospital

adnexa the associated anatomic structures of the eye, which includes the ocular muscles, eyelids, and conjunctiva

adrenalectomy surgical removal of all or most of an adrenal gland(s)

advanced-level job a job obtained after several years of experience that may include management of others or focus on a specialized area of technical expertise

adverse effect a negative physical reaction

aerosol therapy medication suspended in a mist that is inhaled

AHIMA American Health Information Management Association

airway obstruction a reduction in the amount of air inhaled during each breath, most commonly caused by a reduction in the diameter of the bronchioles due to inflammation

alimentary canal a continuous tube, approximately 30 feet long, that begins at the mouth; continues through the esophagus, stomach, small intestine, and large intestine; and exits the body at the rectum and anus

allergen immunotherapy treatment that exposes a patient to allergenic extracts or insect venoms to decrease his or her sensitivity to the allergen, a process called desensitization

allergenic extract a concentration of components from an allergen, such as grass or pollen

allergic rhinitis hay fever

allergy testing a skin or inhalation test to expose a patient to an allergen to determine whether it causes an allergic response

allogeneic from the same species

allograft a skin substitute, where the skin comes from another person

allopathic method of treating disease with remedies such as medicine or surgery that produce effects different from those caused by the disease

allotransplantation receiving an organ from another person

alopecia baldness

Alteration (ICD-10-PCS) the root operation that identifies modifying the anatomic structure of a body part without affecting the function of the body part

alveolus the small air sac where the bronchioles end

Alzheimer's disease (AD) a progressive degenerative brain disease that doubles in prevalence with every five years of age

ambulatory payment classification (APC) groups of CPT codes that describe similar procedures

ambulatory surgery a surgical procedure that does not require an overnight stay in the hospital

amend to add information to

American Health Information Management Association (AHIMA) a professional organization of coders founded in 1928

American National Standards Institute (ANSI) the organization with overall responsibility for setting electronic transaction standards

AMI acute myocardial infarction

amnesia condition of lack of memory

amniocentesis surgical puncture into the amniotic sac to remove fluid from the amnion

amnioinfusion introducing a substance into the amnion

amnion see *amniotic sac*

amnionitis an infection or inflammation of the amniotic sac

amnioscopy visual examination of the amnion

amniotic sac a membrane that surrounds the embryo; also called the amnion

amniotomy incision into the amnion

A-mode (amplitude) ultrasound a one-dimensional ultrasonic measurement

amyotrophic lateral sclerosis (ALS) a chronic, terminal neurological disease characterized by a progressive loss of motor neurons and muscle atrophy; also called Lou Gehrig's disease

analgesia condition of lack of pain

analyte the specific substance within a sample to be examined or tested for

anastomosis a surgical connection between two (usually tubular) structures such as the organs in the digestive tract or blood vessels

anatomic imaging captures a static image of an anatomic part

ancillary provided in addition to medical care, such as laboratory, radiology, or physical therapy services

ancillary reports narrative reports or copies of reports from additional services such as ECGs or imaging

anemia a blood disorder characterized by a reduction in the number of red blood cells, which results in less oxygen reaching the tissues

anencephaly lack of part of the brain

anesthesia a temporary state, induced by drugs, of unconsciousness, loss of memory, lack of pain, and/or muscle relaxation

anesthesia code package a group of services represented in an anesthesia code that includes preoperative visits, administration of anesthesia, and intraoperative monitoring

anesthesia conversion factor a dollar value, adjusted for geographic differences in cost, that Medicare (and other payers) assigns to one base unit of anesthesia

anesthesia time the elapsed time that begins when the anesthesia provider starts to prepare the patient for the induction of anesthesia and ends when the anesthesia provider is no longer in personal attendance and the patient can be safely placed under postoperative supervision

anesthesiologist a physician who specializes in providing perioperative care, developing anesthesia plans, and administrating anesthetics

aneurysm a bulge in the wall of an artery due to weakening, most commonly occurring in the abdominal aorta and cerebral arteries

angina intense pain and spasms

angiogram a recording of the heart vessels

angiography an x-ray taken after an opaque dye is injected into a blood vessel

angioplasty insertion into a blood vessel of an inflatable catheter that expands to compress plaque against the walls of the vessel

annulus fibrosus a fibrocartilaginous ring that comprises the outside of a disc and holds the nucleus pulposus in place

anomaly (congenital) a permanent abnormal shape of an organ or body region, resulting from arrested, delayed, or abnormal development of the embryo; also called a malformation

ANSI American National Standards Institute

antegrade the normal or forward direction of flow

antenatal see *prenatal*

antepartum see *prenatal*

anterior cruciate ligament (ACL) reconstruction replacement of the ACL with a graft

anteroposterior from front to back

antibody a protein in the blood that creates an immune response against an antigen or other invader

antigen any natural or artificial substance that produces an immune response

antrectomy a procedure in which the distal portion of the stomach is excised

anxiety disorder abnormal anxiety that interferes with normal activities

aorta the first artery leading out of the heart to the body, which then repeatedly subdivides into smaller arteries that lead to each body region and anatomic site

aortic coarctation a narrowing of the aorta

aortic valve the valve that controls blood flow from the left ventricle to the aorta

APC ambulatory payment classification

Apgar score an evaluation of a newborn's physical condition that is performed one and five minutes after birth to determine any immediate need for extra medical or emergency care

aphagia lack of ability to swallow

aphasia lack of ability to speak

aplastic anemia anemia due to loss of or lack of production of red bone marrow

appendectomy surgical removal of the appendix

appendicitis inflammation and possible rupture of the appendix

appendicular skeleton the part of the skeleton consisting of the arms, shoulders, wrists, hands, legs, hips, ankles, and feet; contains 126 bones

Appendix A (CPT) an appendix of the CPT manual that provides a full definition of all modifiers

approach (ICD-10-PCS) Character 5 in an ICD-10-PCS code; defines the surgical technique used to reach the procedure site

approach procedure (skull base) a procedure performed to access or expose a lesion

appropriate for gestational age (AGA) a fetus or newborn infant whose size is within the normal range for his or her gestational age

apraxia the inability to perform motor tasks

ARDS acute respiratory distress syndrome

area measurement the space inside a boundary; used to classify the amount of skin treated in a tissue repair or skin graft

ARF acute respiratory failure

arrange to place codes in the order dictated by the OGCR and instructional notes

arrested development embryonic development of a structure that stopped before it should have

arrhythmia an irregular heartbeat

arteriole a small artery

arteriosclerotic heart disease (ASHD) the formation of plaque in the coronary arteries; also called ischemic heart disease and coronary heart disease (CHD)

arteriotomy an incision into an artery

arteriovenous (AV) fistula creation creation of a connection between an artery and a vein

arteriovenous (AV) fistula repair closure of an abnormal connection between two vessels

arteriovenous malformation (AVM) an abnormal connection between arteries and veins, usually congenital

artery any blood vessel that carries blood from the heart to the body tissues

arthralgia a pain in a joint

arthrectomy surgical excision of a joint

arthritis damage to or inflammation of a joint

arthrocentesis aspiration of a small joint or bursa, or collection of synovial fluid from a joint with a needle

arthrodesis surgical fusion of a joint

arthrogram a record or picture of a joint

arthrography the process of recording a joint

arthrotomy cutting into a joint

AS *auris sinister* (left ear)

ASHD arteriosclerotic heart disease

aspiration of bladder the removal of urine using a needle, a trocar, or a catheter

Assessment (ICD-10-PCS) a Physical Rehabilitation and Diagnostic Audiology procedure to diagnose a condition; classified into more than 100 tests and methods

assessment a diagnostic statement; the process of a provider asking questions to arrive at a conclusion

assign to determine codes that accurately describe a patient's condition, reflect the highest level of specificity possible, and contain the correct number of characters for that code

Assistance (ICD-10-PCS) the root operation that identifies taking over a portion of a physiological function by extracorporeal means

assistance taking over a portion of a physiological function by extracorporeal means

assisted delivery a delivery of a fetus using mechanical, pharmacologic, or medical assistance

assisted vaginal delivery (AVD) birth of an infant through the vagina, with the use of drugs or techniques to induce labor and/or with forceps or vacuum extraction to aid in moving the infant through the birth canal

asthma a chronic lung disease that affects the bronchi and is characterized by inflammation of the airway, a reversible obstruction, and reshaping of the airway

astrocytoma a tumor of the brain or spinal cord that is composed of astrocytes

asymptomatic having no symptoms

ataxia a lack of coordination

atelectasis the collapse of a lung, preventing the exchange of oxygen and carbon dioxide

atherectomy a procedure in which a catheter that has a rotating shaver on its tip is threaded through the veins to cut away plaque from the artery

Atmospheric Control (ICD-10-PCS) the root operation that identifies extracorporeal control of atmospheric pressure and composition

atmospheric control extracorporeal control of atmospheric pressure and composition

atonic (seizure) a seizure characterized by a sudden loss of consciousness and falling down; affects the entire brain

atopic asthma due to allergens

atresia lack of an opening to an orifice or passage in the body

atrial fibrillation (A-fib) an irregular heartbeat in the atria characterized by an abnormal quivering of heart fibers

atrioventricular bundle (bundle of His) a group of cardiac muscle fibers that connect the atria with the ventricles

atrioventricular (AV) node an electrical relay station between the atria and the ventricles

atrioventricular (AV) valve a valve that controls the flow of blood from the atria to the ventricles

atrium two of the four chambers of the heart that receive blood from the body and the lungs

attending physician a physician who oversees and coordinates all aspects of a patient's inpatient care

ATT/R adjacent tissue transfer/rearrangement

AU *auris uterque* (each ear)

audit an investigation of a provider's billing and coding practices

auditory canal the part of the external ear that funnels sound waves

aura a sensation of hearing voices or seeing colored light

aural pertaining to the ear

auricle the visible part of the ear, which collects sound waves; also called the pinna

autograft the use of a patient's own tissue from one site to replace damaged tissue at another site

autoimmune a condition in which the body's immune system attacks and destroys healthy body tissue

autologous from the same patient

autologous islet cell transplantation a procedure in which the pancreas is surgically removed and the islet cells are isolated then injected into the portal vein

automatic adjudication a process in which a computer automatically determines which procedure codes are covered, calculates how much the insurance company is obligated to pay, then triggers the payment

autonomic nervous system the system that controls sensory impulses from the blood vessels, the heart, and organs in the chest, abdomen, and pelvis, through nerves, to the brain

AV atrioventricular

AV node atrioventricular node

AV valve atrioventricular valve

AVD assisted vaginal delivery

AVM arteriovenous malformation

avulsed ripped or torn away

avulsion forceful tearing of the nail plate

axial skeleton 80 bones that are basically stationary and make up the skull, sternum, ribs, and vertebrae

B

B-scan/gray-scale (brightness) ultrasound a two-dimensional ultrasonic scan that displays the movement of tissues and organs

BAC blood alcohol concentration

bacteria one-celled germs that multiply quickly and may release toxins that create illness

bacterial infection an infection caused by bacteria and treatable with antibiotics

BAL blood alcohol level

balloon catheter a urethral catheter with an inflatable balloon near the tip to hold the catheter in place and/or dilate the urethra

barium enema the injection of a chalky substance into the colon through the anus and viewing the organs on an x-ray; also called a lower GI series

Barlow's syndrome an eponym for mitral valve prolapse (MVP)

Bartholin's gland a gland that secretes mucus

basal cell carcinoma (BCC) a cancer appearing in the lowest layer of the epidermis; accounts for 75% of new skin cancer cases

base unit (B) a number that represents the complexity of an anesthesia, the risk to a patient, and the skills needed by an anesthesia provider to render services for each CPT Anesthesia code

basilar skull fracture a linear fracture in the anterior or middle skull base or the posterior fossa

BBB blood–brain barrier; bundle branch block

BCC basal cell carcinoma

Beam Radiation (ICD-10-PCS) the Modality that identifies aiming radiation beams at a small target area to destroy tissue

beam radiation aiming radiation beams at a small target area to destroy tissue

behavior (tumor) malignant or benign

behavioral disorder the manifestation of a mental disturbance that results in extreme or disruptive conduct, such as rage, withdrawal, or substance abuse

behavioral disturbance an action that includes aggression, wandering, depression, delusion or hallucinations, sleep disturbances, or poor eating habits

Bell's palsy the inflammation of the seventh (VII) cranial nerve, which is the facial nerve

beneficiary the recipient of services

benign not life-threatening

benign prostatic hypertrophy (BPH) the abnormal growth of epithelial cells of the prostate, causing compression or obstruction of the urethra; also called enlarged prostate (EP) or hyperplasia

Bethesda System a method of reporting findings from Pap tests that includes a statement of adequacy of the specimen; a general categorization of the specimen; a descriptive diagnosis; interpretation of abnormalities using specific nomenclature; and a statement of review and any ancillary testing

Billroth I a procedure in which the pylorus is removed and the proximal stomach is anastomosed directly to the duodenum in an end-to-end manner

Billroth II a procedure in which the greater curvature of the stomach is connected to the first part of the jejunum in a side-to-side manner

bilobectomy the surgical excision of two lobes

Biofeedback (ICD-10-PCS) the root type that identifies the provision of information from the monitoring and regulating of physiological processes in conjunction with cognitive-behavioral techniques to improve patient functioning or well-being

biopsy the scraping, punching, cutting, or removal of a small piece of body tissue or fluid sample for laboratory analysis

birth trauma any physical injury to an infant during delivery

blepharitis the inflammation and infection of hair follicles and glands at the margins of the eyelids, due to virus, bacteria, allergic response, or exposure to irritants

block (ICD-10-CM) a contiguous range of codes within a chapter

blood the bodily fluid that transports and passes nutrients, oxygen, carbon dioxide, water, proteins, and hormones to cells and transports waste products to excrete oxygen; also called the hemic system

blood alcohol concentration (BAC) see *blood alcohol level (BAL)*

blood alcohol content see *blood alcohol level (BAL)*

blood alcohol level (BAL) a measurement of the amount of alcohol present in the blood; also called blood alcohol content or blood alcohol concentration (BAC)

blood–brain barrier (BBB) a naturally occurring barrier of vessels and capillaries that filters blood flowing to the brain and prevents certain toxic substances from infiltrating brain tissue and the central nervous system

blood creatinine a blood test used to determine the amount of creatinine present; an abnormal result suggests renal dysfunction

body the main portion of a muscle

body part (ICD-10-PCS) Character 4 in an ICD-10-PCS code; defines the specific anatomic site where a physician performed a procedure

body system (ICD-10-PCS) Character 2 in an ICD-10-PCS code; defines where a procedure is performed

bone marrow connective tissue in the cavities of bones

book-based encoder an enhanced electronic coding manual that allows coders to input key words, such as the Main Term, and access hot links to potential codes

Brachytherapy (ICD-10-PCS) the Modality that identifies the insertion of radioactive implants directly into body tissue

brachytherapy insertion of radioactive implants directly into body tissue

bradycardia a slow heart rate

bradypnea slow breathing

brain the organ that governs perception of the senses, emotions, consciousness, memory, and voluntary movements

breast engorgement the temporary enlargement of breasts on female or male newborns, due to high levels of maternal hormones in the infant's blood

bronchial tree the configuration of bronchi subdividing into smaller and smaller branches

bronchiectasis the condition of a dilated bronchus

bronchiole the smallest bronchus in the bronchial tree; does not contain rings of cartilage

bronchiolitis inflammation of a bronchiole

bronchitis inflammation of the bronchus

bronchodilator a medication that relaxes muscle spasms in bronchial tubes

bronchogenic of bronchial origin

bronchogram a record or picture of the bronchus

bronchography the process of recording the bronchus

bronchoscope the instrument used to view the bronchus

bronchospasm a contraction of smooth muscle in the walls of the bronchi and bronchioles, causing narrowing of the lumen

bronchus the air tube that begins at the end of the trachea and leads to the lungs

bulbourethral gland the gland that provides a mucous secretion before ejaculation, which becomes part of the semen

bulla a blister

bundle branch a division of the bundle of His

bundle branch block (BBB) a blockage of the conduction of electrical impulses through the branches of the atrioventricular bundle

bundling edit a coding restriction frequently triggered by the words *includes* and *not separately reportable* that indicates that multiple services are included in a single code

Burch's procedure an eponym for vesicourethropexy

burn damage to the skin by heat, electricity, or radiation

bursitis the inflammation of fluid around a joint

by report based on a report submitted by a physician

Bypass (ICD-10-PCS) the root operation that identifies altering the route of passage of the contents of a tubular Body Part

bypass graft the creation of a new route around a blockage in a blood vessel using a vessel from another part of the body, another person, or a synthetic substitute

C

CA carcinoma, cancer

CA in situ cells that have begun to change but are contained within the epithelial layer

CABG coronary artery bypass graft

CAD computer-aided detection; coronary artery disease

calculi hard balls of cholesterol (fat), also called stones, that may accumulate in the kidneys, bladder, or ureters

Caldwell-Luc procedure an incision through the gum and bone to create an opening to the maxillary sinus

cancer (CA) a malignant tumor of epithelial cells, which line body cavities and organs; synonymous with carcinoma

Candida a yeast fungi

cannulation of thoracic duct the insertion of a tube (cannulation) into the thoracic duct to collect lymph

capillary the very thin-walled membrane at the end of arterioles that allows blood to diffuse into body tissues and receives waste products from the tissues to send back into the bloodstream

capsule endoscopy a technology in which patients swallow a capsule the size of a large pill that contains a video microchip, light bulb, battery, and radio transmitter

capsulectomy cutting into or the surgical excision of a joint capsule

capsulodesis the surgical fusion of a joint capsule

carbuncle a skin infection that involves a group of hair follicles

carcinoid a benign or malignant tumor arising from the mucosa of the gastrointestinal tract

carcinoid syndrome a collection of symptoms caused by carcinoid tumors, characterized by flushing, cyanosis, abdominal cramps, diarrhea, and heart valve disease; see also *carcinoid*

carcinoma (CA) a malignant tumor of epithelial cells, which line body cavities and organs

carcinoma of unknown primary (CUP) a neoplasm diagnosed at a late stage after it has metastasized and for which a physician is unable to determine the site of origin

cardiac catheterization the passage of a thin tube through a blood vessel to the heart to visualize the structure, collect blood samples, and determine the blood pressure of the heart

cardiac function test a measurement of the capacity of the heart in real time; tests include cardiac catheterization, electrocardiography, Holter monitor testing, and stress testing

cardiac scan a scan of the heart after a patient receives radioactive thallium intravenously

cardiac sphincter the valve between the esophagus and the stomach

cardiology lab a testing center used to evaluate heart problems

cardiopulmonary bypass (CPB) a heart–lung machine that takes over the function of the heart and lungs, maintaining the circulation of blood and the oxygen content of the body

cardiovascular (CV) system the body system that distributes blood throughout the body and includes the heart and blood vessels; also called the circulatory system

career path the progression of jobs and responsibilities throughout one's working life

Caregiver Training (ICD-10-PCS) the root type that identifies the training in activities to support a patient's optimal level of function

carpal tunnel release cutting of the transverse carpal ligament to release pressure on the median nerve

cartilage the fibrous tissue found at the ends of bones

case production the number of cases a coder codes each day while maintaining high accuracy

case-based a reimbursement amount (rate) determined per case, or per inpatient admission, rather than on a per diem (daily) basis or a fee-for-service basis

cataract a cloudiness of the lens of the eye that usually develops slowly over time due to aging

category (CPT) a subdivision of CPT Category I codes that shows specific methods for completing procedures

category (ICD-10-CM) three characters in length

Category I a group of permanent CPT codes, numbered 00100 to 99607, to report widely used services and procedures approved by the FDA

Category II a group of optional CPT codes used to collect and track data for performance measurement

Category III a group of temporary CPT codes for data collection and for tracking the use of emerging technology, services, and procedures

catheter a small, flexible tube inserted through a narrow opening into a body cavity to remove fluid or inject medication

catheter ablation/radiofrequency ablation the use of a fluoroscopy-guided catheter at the exact site of arrhythmia in the heart to emit radiofrequency energy that destroys heart muscle cells in a very small area (about one-fifth of an inch)

catheter procedures the implantation, revision, or repositioning of a tunneled intrathecal or epidural catheter

causal event an event or action that results in an injury

causal relationship one disease being caused by another

cause an event or action that results in an injury

CC chief complaint

CDI clinical documentation improvement

CDM charge-description master

CEHRT certified EHR technology

celiac disease an abnormal immune reaction to gluten and poor absorption of nutrients

cell type the characteristics or appearance of a cell

cellulitis inflammation under the skin

Centers for Medicare and Medicaid Services (CMS) the division of the Department of Health and Human Services (HHS) that administers Medicare

central nervous system (CNS) the control center for the nervous system, which processes information and provides short-term control over other organ systems; consists of the brain and spinal cord

cephalic version turning of a fetus so the head is oriented toward the cervix

cephalopelvic disproportion (CPD) a cause of obstructed labor due to a mismatch between the size of the fetal head and the mother's pelvic brim; also called fetopelvic disproportion

cerclage (nonobstetrical) extensive suturing around the cervix to make the opening smaller

cerclage (obstetrical) a closed cervix during pregnancy

cerebellum the portion of the brain located below and behind the cerebrum

cerebral an object located within the brain

cerebral palsy a functional disorder of the brain manifested by motor impairment

cerebrospinal fluid (CSF) shunt the creation, removal, or reprogramming of a shunt and the replacement or irrigation of a catheter that transports fluid from one area of the body to another

cerebrovascular accident (CVA) a sudden decrease in blood supplied to the brain; also called stroke

cerebrum the largest structure of the brain that controls sensory and motor activity

Certificate of Compliance (COC) a certificate issued to a laboratory that performs nonwaived (moderate and high complexity) testing

Certificate of Waiver (COW) a certificate issued to a laboratory that performs only CLIA-waived tests

certification a voluntary achievement that documents that a coder has attained a certain level of proficiency by passing a rigorous examination

certified registered nurse anesthetist (CRNA) a registered nurse with advanced education and training in the field of anesthesia

cerumen the earwax that protects and lubricates the ear

cervical pertaining to a neck (most commonly, the neck of the spine or the neck of the uterus)

cervical approach the performance of a procedure through an incision in the neck

cervical dilator insertion the transcatheter administration of a substance into the cervix to widen it

cervical dysplasia abnormal changes in the cells on the surface of the cervix that may lead to cancer if not treated

cervical intraepithelial neoplasia (CIN) cervical dysplasia seen on a cervical biopsy, classified as mild dysplasia (CIN I), moderate to marked dysplasia (CIN II), and severe dysplasia to cancer in situ (CIN III)

cervicectomy see *trachelectomy*

cesarean delivery the delivery of a fetus by making a surgical incision into the abdominal wall and uterus; also called abdominal delivery

chalazion a small, hard cyst on the eyelid caused by the blockage of a gland on the eyelid

Change (ICD-10-PCS) the root operation that identifies taking out or off a device from a body part and putting back an identical or similar device in or on the same body part, without cutting or puncturing the skin or a mucous membrane

chapter (ICD-10-CM) a subdivision of ICD-10-CM that includes codes for a body system or related conditions

character one of seven positions in an ICD-10-PCS code with an alphanumeric value; each has a distinct purpose and meaning

charge capture the process of entering nonprocedural services provided throughout a patient's stay

charge description master (CDM) a list of the nonprocedural services provided by a hospital throughout a patient's stay

CHD coronary heart disease

chemocauterization the destruction of tissue using chemicals

chemodenervation the injection of a substance into a muscle group or gland(s) to stop overactivity

chemosurgery the use of a chemical agent to destroy tissue

chemotherapy treatment using drugs

CHF congestive heart failure

chief complaint (CC) a concise statement that describes a patient's symptom(s), problem, condition, diagnosis, or history of present illness

childbirth the period of true labor and active delivery; also called parturition

Children's Health Insurance Program (CHIP) a program established in 1997 by the federal government to provide health insurance to children in families with incomes below 200% of the federal poverty level

chiropractic manipulation the use of direct manual force or an instrument to manipulate the joints of the body, most commonly the spine, to restore or enhance joint function; also called chiropractic adjustment

cholecystectomy surgical removal of the gallbladder

cholecystitis inflammation of the gallbladder

choledochocystectomy excision of the common bile duct

choledocholithiasis the condition of calculi in the common bile duct

choledochoplasty repair of the common bile duct

cholelithiasis the condition of calculi in the gallbladder

cholera an acute gastrointestinal disease

chondroplasty the reshaping and cleaning of cartilage in a joint to remove uneven surfaces and fragments

chorion the outer membrane that surrounds the amnion

chorionic villus sampling (CVS) the aspiration of fetal tissue under ultrasonic guidance,

using a catheter through the cervix or a needle through the mother's abdominal and uterine walls into the uterine cavity, for genetic analysis

choroid the opaque middle layer of the eyeball that supplies blood to the eye

choroiditis inflammation of the vascular coating of the eye

chromosomal abnormality any of a wide range of disorders in which a fetus has an abnormal number of chromosomes or a structural abnormality in one or more chromosomes

chronic bronchitis an inflammation of the bronchi with a productive cough for three months in two consecutive years

chronic kidney disease (CKD) the gradual loss of kidney function over a period of months or years

chronic obstructive pulmonary disease (COPD) the combination of chronic bronchitis and emphysema as comorbidities

chronic pain syndrome (CPS) a collection of pain conditions lasting more than six months and that are unresponsive to treatment

cineradiography the process of making radiographs of moving objects in rapid sequence and quickly projecting them back to simulate a motion picture; also called videoradiography

circulatory system the body system that distributes blood throughout the body and includes the heart and blood vessels; also called the cardiovascular (CV) system

circumstances of admission the facts, signs, and symptoms that require an admission

cirrhosis the scarring of liver tissue that blocks the normal flow of blood through the liver

cisternal puncture the withdrawal of CSF from the cisterna magna

CKD chronic kidney disease

clavicle the collar bone

clean claim a claim that passes the front-end edit checks and has no missing or invalid information

cleft lip/cleft palate a notch or division of the upper lip or roof of the mouth

cleft lip/cleft palate repair the procedure in which abnormally oriented and attached muscles are repositioned to repair the functionality of the soft palate musculature

CLIA Clinical Laboratory Improvement Amendments

click murmur syndrome see *mitral valve prolapse (MVP)*

clinical brachytherapy the application of small, encapsulated radioactive elements implanted directly into or near a tumor

clinical documentation improvement (CDI) an internal process to identify areas in which documentation does not provide all the information needed to code and educate providers regarding the details needed

Clinical Laboratory Improvement Amendments (CLIA) regulations passed by Congress in 1988 to establish quality standards for all laboratory testing to ensure the accuracy, reliability, and timeliness of patient test results regardless of where the test was performed

clinical pathology a medical specialty that is concerned with the diagnosis of disease based on the laboratory analysis of bodily fluids and tissue

clinically significant conditions those conditions defined by the Uniform Hospital Data Discharge set (UHDDS) as "all conditions that coexist at the time of admission, that develop subsequently, or that affect the treatment received and/or the length of stay. Diagnoses that relate to an earlier episode which have no bearing on the current hospital stay are to be excluded."

clitoris a small sensitive protrusion that is part of the female genital system

clitoroplasty a reduction of the size of an enlarged clitoris

clonic (seizure) a type of seizure characterized by a series of muscle contractions and relaxations on both sides of the body

closed (fracture) a type of fracture in which the bone does not break the skin

cluster headache a unilateral pain in the eye or temple

CNS central nervous system

COC Certificate of Compliance

cochlea a snail-shaped organ that makes hearing possible

cochlear device implantation the implantation of a receiver into bone, which sends signals to electrodes implanted in the cochlea

code (ICD-10-CM) the final level of subdivision

code set a distinct system of medical codes

Codes on Dental Procedures and Nomenclature (CDT®) the HIPAA-mandated code set for dental services (occupies section D of the HCPCS codes)

coding the process of accurately assigning codes to verbal descriptions of patients' conditions and the healthcare services provided to treat those conditions

coding path the sequence of Main Terms and subterms a coder must search in the Index in order to locate the code

cognitive disorder a failure to develop or the deterioration of mental comprehension

colectomy the surgical removal of all or a part of the large intestine

colloid a gelatin-like or mucous substance found in tissues

colonoscopy the use of an endoscope to view the colon

colopexy surgical fixation of the colon

colorectal cancer of the colon and rectum

colorrhaphy suturing of the colon

colostomy division of the colon, bringing the proximal end out through a stoma in the abdominal wall, bypassing the rectum and anus

colpocentesis the puncturing of the posterior vaginal wall with a needle to withdraw fluid from the peritoneal cul-de-sac

colpopexy/vaginofixation the suturing of the vagina to another structure, such as the abdominal wall

colporrhaphy the suturing of the vagina

colpotomy a procedure creating an incision into the wall of the vagina; may also include draining an abscess

Column 1 NCCI data that contain a list of all payable CPT codes

Column 2 NCCI data that contain the code that is not payable with a particular Column 1 code unless a modifier is permitted and submitted

combination code a code that describes two or more conditions in a single code

common bile duct (CBD) exploration the injection of a dye into the duct, visualization on an x-ray, removal of calculi, and introduction of a drainage bag when necessary

common descriptor the shared portion of a code before the semicolon

comorbidity two diseases occurring together

complete mastoidectomy a simple mastoidectomy with more extensive removal of the mastoid process

completeness (ICD-10-PCS) the ICD-10-PCS major attribute whereby there should be a unique code for every procedure that is significantly different in body part, approach, or method

complex partial (seizure) a seizure associated with both sides of the cerebrum; causes a change in or loss of consciousness

complex regional pain syndrome see *reflex sympathetic dystrophy (RSD)*

compliance following the rules

complication an abnormal medical reaction that results from a medical or surgical procedure

complications of care the unanticipated results of a medical or surgical procedure

complication or comorbidity (CC) a diagnosis listed in the *ICD-10-CM/PCS MS-DRG Definitions Manual* that potentially qualifies the patient for a higher-paying DRG

Compression (ICD-10-PCS) the root operation that identifies putting pressure on a body region

computed tomography (CT) the creation of a three-dimensional image of a body structure by computer, using a series of cross-sectional images

computer-aided detection (CAD) the use of pattern recognition software to help identify suspicious features on a radiological image, to decrease false-negative readings

Computerized Tomography (CT Scan) (ICD-10-PCS) the root type that identifies the computer-reformatted digital display of multiplanar images developed from the capture of multiple exposures of external ionizing radiation

computerized tomography (CT) scan the computer-reformatted digital display of multiplanar images developed from the capture of multiple exposures of external ionizing radiation

conception the fertilization of the female ova by the male sperm

concurrent care care that occurs when more than one physician treats a patient at the same time for different conditions or different aspects of the same condition

condom catheter a nonindwelling catheter consisting of a sac that fits over the penis to collect urine and drain it through a tube that leads to a collection bag; is left in place

cone a photoreceptor cell of the retina that is sensitive to bright light and color vision

confirmed a diagnostic statement that the physician is confident of

congenital a condition that appears at birth

congenital abnormality a specific type of perinatal condition that originates during pregnancy or the first 28 days of life

congestive heart failure (CHF) the inability of the heart to maintain circulation

conization of cervix the removal of a cone-shaped piece of tissue from the uterine cervix

conjunctiva the membrane that lines the eyelids

conjunctivectomy excision of the conjunctiva

conjunctivitis a viral or bacterial inflammation and infection of the conjunctiva

conjunctivoplasty repair of the conjunctiva

constant attendance modality a physical therapy treatment that requires constant one-to-one contact with the patient by the provider

consultation an evaluation of a patient requested by another physician to obtain a professional opinion on a specific problem

consulting physician the provider who receives a request from a referring physician to see a patient regarding a specific problem; also called consultant

content of service requirements guidelines that define the work done during the patient encounter; also referred to as key components

contralateral an examination on the opposite side from which catheterization was performed

contralateral lobectomy the excision of part of the opposite or second lobe in addition to a partial, subtotal, or total lobectomy of the first lobe

contrast medium a radiopaque substance that is injected or swallowed

Control (ICD-10-PCS) the root operation that identifies stopping, or attempting to stop, postprocedural bleeding

controlled hypotension a technique that lowers the mean arterial blood pressure (MAP) by 30% during surgery, with the goal of reducing intraoperative blood loss and minimizing the risk of fluid overload; also called induced hypotension or hypotensive anesthesia

contusion a bruise

convention the use of symbols, typeface, and layout features to succinctly convey interpretive information

conventional Pap test involves scraping cells from the cervix and fixing them on a slide to be evaluated by a lab

conversion factor a constant dollar value multiplied by the relative value unit to determine the price of individual services

Coordination and Maintenance Committee the group that oversees all changes, which must be consistent with WHO's ICD-10

COPD chronic obstructive pulmonary disease

cordocentesis the use of ultrasound to detect the umbilical cord and removal of a sample of fetal blood from the cord; also called percutaneous umbilical blood sampling (PUBS)

cornea the clear, hard portion of the sclera that protects the lens

coronary artery bypass graft (CABG) open-heart surgery to create a bypass around a blocked coronary artery, usually using the internal mammary artery (IMA) or a vein in the leg

coronary artery disease (CAD) an insufficient blood supply to the heart due to an obstruction of one or more coronary arteries

coronary circulation blood flow that occurs within the heart; carries blood from the aorta to the tissues of the heart to maintain the function of the heart itself

coronary heart disease (CHD) see *arteriosclerotic heart disease (ASHD)*

corrosion damage to the skin due to chemicals

cosmetic relating to aesthetics or appearance

coudé catheter a type of elbowed catheter with a slightly curved tip

Counseling (ICD-10-PCS) the root type that identifies the application of psychological methods to treat an individual with normal developmental issues and psychological problems in order to increase function, improve well-being, alleviate distress, address maladjustment, or resolve crises

covered entity a health plan, healthcare clearinghouse, or healthcare provider who electronically transmits any health information in connection with transactions for which the Department of Health and Human Services (HHS) has adopted standards

COW Certificate of Waiver

CPS chronic pain syndrome

CPT Current Procedural Terminology

CPT surgical package the services included in a procedure code in addition to the operative procedure

craniectomy excision of part of the skull

cranioplasty repair of part of the skull

craniostomy procedure in which a physician drills or cuts into the skull to drain a hematoma or abscess or to remove part of the bone of the skull to gain access to perform further surgery

craniotomy incision into the skull

Creation (ICD-10-PCS) the root operation that identifies making a new genital structure that does not take over the function of a body part

cricoid split an incision of the cricoid cartilage to open the airway

Crisis Intervention (ICD-10-PCS) the root type that identifies the treatment of a traumatized, acutely disturbed, or distressed individual for the purpose of short-term stabilization

CRNA certified registered nurse anesthetist

Crohn's disease an inflammatory bowel disease (IBD) with inflammation and ulcers in the alimentary tract characterized by a thickening of the mucous membrane

cryosurgery surgery using cold

cryotherapy the use of liquid nitrogen to destroy tissue

CSF fistula an abnormal connection between the subarachnoid space around the brain and either the sinuses or the ear that allows the passage of CSF

culture a laboratory test of secretions, such as sputum, to identify the microorganism that is causing an infection

culture and sensitivity a laboratory test of secretions to observe bacterial growth and determine antibiotic effectiveness

curettage (obstetrical) scraping-away of the uterine lining

curettement see *paring*

current MI a myocardial infarction (MI) that has occurred within the past four weeks

Current Procedural Terminology (CPT) a listing of five-character alphanumeric codes and descriptions that report outpatient medical services and procedures

cutaneous vesicostomy a temporary surgical procedure to create an opening in the umbilicus (lower abdomen), which allows urine to continuously drain from the bladder

CV system cardiovascular system

CVA cerebrovascular accident

CVS chorionic villus sampling

cyclectomy a partial excision of the ciliary body

cystectomy a partial or complete excision of the bladder; may also involve other procedures, including removing surrounding lymph nodes

cystitis a bacterial infection of the urinary bladder; also called urinary tract infection (UTI)

cystolithotomy incision of the bladder to remove calculi

cystometrography the use of a manometer (pressure-measuring device) to evaluate bladder function; the bladder is emptied using a catheter, then filled using a smaller catheter

cystoscopy visual examination of the urinary bladder

cystostomy the creation of an opening in the bladder, with possible removal of the bladder neck

cytopathology the study of abnormal cells

D

DBS deep brain stimulation

DDH developmental dysplasia of the hip

Decompression (ICD-10-PCS) the root operation that identifies extracorporeal elimination of undissolved gas from body fluids

decompression cutting into a body site to relieve pressure or provide drainage

decubitus ulcer a breakdown of the skin, usually over bony parts of the body, caused by continuous pressure, friction, moistness, and heat; also referred to as pressure ulcer or bed sore

deep brain simulation (DBS) the implantation of electrodes into a patient's brain to provide electrical stimulation to specific locations and reduce or eliminate involuntary movements

deep inferior epigastric perforator (DIEP) flap the use of blood vessels called deep inferior epigastric perforators (DIEPs), and the skin and connected fat, or skin only (but no muscle), from the wall of the lower belly to rebuild the breast

deep vein thrombosis (DVT) the formation of a thrombus within a deep vein, usually in the leg or pelvis

default code (ICD-10-CM) a code that may represent a condition most commonly associated with a Main Term, or it may represent the unspecified code for a condition

definitive drug testing a testing procedure that identifies the individual drugs present in a sample using qualitative, quantitative, or semiquantitative methods

definitive procedure (skull base) performing the repair, biopsy, resection, or excision of a lesion

definitive treatment a treatment intended to cure, eliminate, improve, or reduce the effects of a condition

deformation a change in the size or shape of a normal structure due to physical forces

degeneration the breakdown of bone or tissue

degenerative neural disease a class of diseases marked by degeneration of nerves and brain tissue, resulting in abnormalities in muscle and sensory functions

degree the depth of a burn or corrosion

delayed the status of a patient who has waited to seek care

delayed development the embryonic development of a structure that is started late or progresses slowly

delirium a state of confusion, restlessness, and incoherence

Delivery (ICD-10-PCS) the root operation that identifies assisting the passage of the products of conception from the genital canal

delivery the expulsion of the fetus and placenta from the uterus

delusion a false belief that hinders the ability to function

dementia a progressive loss of brain function that affects memory, thinking, language, judgment, and behavior

denied a claim that was processed and found to be ineligible for payment

densitometry the measurement of density

density a mass or substance

dentistry the practice of a dentist

Department of Health and Human Services (HHS) the federal government's principal agency for protecting the health and well-being of all Americans

dependence (substance) see *addiction*

dermatitis a flat or raised eruption that can be caused by irritation, allergy, or infection

dermolysis surgical loosening of the skin

dermomycosis a skin condition related to fungus

dermoplasty surgical removal or repair of the skin

Descemet's stripping endothelial keratoplasty (DSEK) the removal of only the corneal endothelium layer and replacement with a donor (cadaver) endothelial graft

Destruction (ICD-10-PCS) the root operation that identifies the physical eradication of all or a portion of a body part by the direct use of energy, force, or a destructive agent

Detachment (ICD-10-PCS) the root operation that identifies cutting off all or a portion of the upper or lower extremities

Detoxification Services (ICD-10-PCS) the root type that identifies detoxification from alcohol and/or drugs

developmental dysplasia of the hip (DDH) a disruption in the normal relationship between the head of the femur and the acetabulum (hip socket)

device Character 6 in an ICD-10-PCS code; refers to material that is intentionally left in place for a therapeutic reason at the end of a procedure

Device Fitting (ICD-10-PCS) the root type that identifies the fitting of a device designed to facilitate or support achievement of a higher level of function

DG documentation guidelines

diabetes mellitus (DM) a common disease of the endocrine system resulting in elevated glucose concentrations over an extended period of time and excess excretion of urine, usually due to malfunction of the pancreas

diabetic ketoacidosis (DKA) the condition of a high concentration of ketones that has accumulated in the blood and turns acidic

diabetic nephropathy the condition of accumulated damage to the glomerulus capillaries due to chronic high blood glucose

diabetic retinopathy the abnormal expression of blood vessels and hemorrhaging in the vessels of the retina; caused by diabetes

diagnosis a patient illness, disease, condition, injury, or other reason for seeking healthcare services

diagnosis-related group (DRG) a payment system that categorizes patients who are medically related with respect to diagnosis and treatment and statistically have similar lengths of stay

diagnostic procedure a procedure performed to obtain information needed to make a diagnosis and treatment plan

diagnostic radiology imaging services used to evaluate or diagnose a health problem

diagnostic ultrasound the use of ultrasound technology to create an image to help diagnose a condition

dialysis a treatment that filters the blood to remove waste, excess salt, and water

dialysis-related amyloidosis (DRA) a deposit of the starchy substance amyloid in the joints due to dialysis

diaphragm a muscle shaped like half of a dome that is located between the thoracic and abdominal cavities

diaphysis the long, narrow part of a long bone

diastole the time during the heart cycle when the chamber relaxes as it fills with blood

dichorionic-diamniotic (DiDi) two embryos developed from separate zygotes, resulting in each embryo having its own amnion and chorion

DiDi dichorionic-diamniotic

DIEP deep inferior epigastric perforator

digestive system the body system that receives nutrients, breaks them down, absorbs them into the blood to be used by the body, and eliminates solid waste products; also called the gastrointestinal (GI) system

Dilation (ICD-10-PCS) the root operation that identifies expanding an orifice or the lumen of a tubular body part

dilation and curettage (D&C) (nonobstetrical) the widening of the cervix and scraping of the uterine wall

direct optical observation the process of looking at results with the naked eye

discectomy the removal of all or part of an intervertebral disc

dislocation a condition in which two bones are out of place at the joint

displaced a condition in which fragments of bone move out of alignment due to a traumatic fracture

displacement therapy (Proetz type) the irrigation of sinuses with a saline solution that is then suctioned out

dissociative disorder a disruption in consciousness, memory, identity, or perception

distal epiphysis the rounded end of a bone farthest from the trunk

distributed (seizure) a seizure that is the result of abnormal activity on both sides of the brain; also called a generalized seizure

diuresis excessive urination

diverticula pouches formed when the lining of the intestine pushes through the intestinal muscle layer

diverticular disease the presence and/or inflammation of diverticula

diverticulitis a bacterial infection of diverticula

divided separated

Division (ICD-10-PCS) the root operation that identifies cutting into a body part, without draining fluids and/or gases from the body part, to separate or transect a body part

DM diabetes mellitus

DO doctor of osteopathy

doctor of osteopathy (DO) a licensed physician who has the same licensing, training, and qualifications as a doctor of medicine (MD); also called allopathic physician

document the act of recording the reason a physician saw a patient, the diagnostic techniques used, tests or treatments planned, and the overall assessment of the patient

documentation the written or electronic record of medical care and services provided

documentation guidelines (DG) criteria developed by the Centers for Medicare and Medicaid Services and the American Medical Association for Evaluation and Management (E/M) services that outline general principles of medical documentation and guidelines for documenting the history, examination, and medical decision-making components of E/M services

dominance the side of the body an individual favors, such as being left-handed or right-handed

Doppler ultrasonography/ultrasound an image created by measuring sound-wave echoes off of tissues and organs

dorsal approach the performance of a procedure through an incision in the midback

dosimetry the measurement of a dose

Down syndrome a genetic condition in which a person has 47 chromosomes instead of the usual 46; also called trisomy 21

Drainage (ICD-10-PCS) the root operation that identifies taking out or letting out fluids and/or gases from a body part

Dressing (ICD-10-PCS) the root operation that identifies putting material on a body region for protection

DRG diagnosis-related group

DRG grouper software that considers several clinical and demographic characteristics of a patient

drug withdrawal syndrome a collection of symptoms of drug withdrawal in an infant who was exposed to narcotics in the uterus; also called neonatal abstinence syndrome (NAS)

DSEK Descemet's stripping endothelial keratoplasty

dual-energy x-ray absorptiometry (DXA/DEXA) bone density study the measurement of the density or mass of a material by comparing the amounts of material absorbed from x-ray beams of two different energies

ductal (cancer) a cancer that starts in the milk ducts of the breast

duodenectomy the excision of the duodenum

duodenoscopy visual examination of the duodenum

DVT deep vein thrombosis

dysphonia difficulty speaking

dyspnea difficulty breathing

dysrhythmia an abnormal heartbeat

dystocia difficult labor

dystonia erratic jerky movements due to improperly functioning muscle tension

E

eardrum a membrane that separates the external ear from the middle ear; also called the tympanic membrane or tympanum

early onset (Alzheimer's disease) Alzheimer's disease that is diagnosed before age 65

eating disorder a serious disturbance in eating behavior

EBD endoscopic balloon dilation

ECC echocardiogram

ECG electrocardiography

echocardiogram (ECC) a recording of the sounds of the heart

echocardiography the use of noninvasive ultrasound to visualize internal cardiac structures

eclampsia convulsions occurring during pregnancy or the puerperium, associated with preeclampsia

ectopic outside of the uterus

EDD estimated date of delivery

edit a specific coding and billing criterion that is checked for accuracy based on predetermined rules

EEG electroencephalogram

EGA estimated gestational age

EGD esophagogastroduodenoscopy

EKG electrocardiography

elbowed catheter a urethral catheter with a sharp bend near the intake; used to navigate past obstructions in the urinary tract; also called prosthetic catheter

ELBW extremely low birth weight

elective surgery nonemergency surgery that is medically necessary but can be delayed at least 24 hours

electrocardiogram an electrical recording of the heart

electrocardiography (ECG, EKG) the graphical recording of the electrical activity of the heart

electrocauterization the use of a hot instrument to destroy tissue

electrocochleography the process of recording the electrical activity of the cochlea

Electroconvulsive Therapy (ICD-10-PCS) the root type that identifies the application of controlled electrical voltages to treat a mental health disorder

electroconvulsive therapy a procedure in which electric currents are deliberately passed through the brain, triggering a brief seizure; can reverse symptoms of certain mental illnesses

electrocorticography the implantation of electrodes on the brain to record electrical impulses and identify areas to surgically remove

electrodessication destruction using electrical energy

electroejaculation the insertion of an electrostimulator probe into a patient's rectum next to the prostate to transmit an electrical current and stimulate ejaculation

electroencephalogram (EEG) a recording of the electrical activity of the heart

electroencephalography the process of recording the electrical activity of the brain

electrolysis surgical destruction using electricity

electrolyte a chemical compound that separates into charged particles in a solution

Electromagnetic Therapy (ICD-10-PCS) the root operation that identifies extracorporeal treatment by electromagnetic rays

electromagnetic therapy extracorporeal treatment by electromagnetic rays

electromyogram (EMG) a recording of the electrical activity of a muscle

electrosurgery surgery using electrical energy

E/M evaluation and management

embolectomy the removal of a clot from a blood vessel

embolus an abnormal particle circulating in the blood, such as an air bubble or thrombus that has broken loose from its point of origin

emergency department an organized department of an acute care hospital that provides treatment of an injury or health problem that cannot be delayed without harm to the patient

emergency surgery surgery that must be performed immediately to save a life or prevent a disability, such as loss of a limb

emphysema the enlargement and rupture of alveolar sacs at the end of the bronchioles, causing an abnormal accumulation of air in the tissue

empyema pus in a body cavity

encephalitis a viral inflammation of the brain and meninges

encephalocele a hernia in the brain

encounter a specific interaction between a patient and a healthcare provider

endarterectomy excision of the lining of a vessel

endocarditis an inflammation in the lining of the heart or valves, due to bacteria or another disease

endocardium the smooth inner layer that reduces friction as blood flows through the heart

endocavity within a cavity

endocervical curettage scraping tissue from the endocervical canal

endocrine system the body system that produces, stores, and releases hormones

endometriosis the growth of endometrial tissue in any area other than the uterus

endoscopic balloon dilation (EBD) a procedure in which through-the-scope (TTS) balloon dilators or plastic dilators are moved over a guide wire to stretch the esophagus, pyloric valve, or duodenum

endoscopic retrograde cholangiopancreatography (ERCP) the injection of contrast medium into the bile ducts via a tube through the ampulla of Vater to visualize the entire biliary tree

endoscopic sclerotherapy a procedure in which a solution that causes inflammation and scarring is injected into a vein to close it off

endotracheal intubation placement of a tube through the mouth and glottis into the trachea to create a viable airway

endovascular aneurysm repair (EVAR) replacement of a weak section of an artery or heart wall with a patch, stent, or graft

endovascular therapy treatment that involves inserting microcatheters into blood vessels to treat aneurysms, lesions, and neoplasms, including intracranial tumors

enlarged prostate (EP) the abnormal growth of epithelial cells of the prostate, causing compression or obstruction of the urethra; also called benign prostatic hypertrophy or hyperplasia (BPH)

enteral nutrition providing nutrients to patients in the nose using a nasogastric (NG) tube, in the stomach using a gastrostomy (G) tube, or in the small intestine using a jejunostomy (J) tube

enterectomy excision of the intestine

entitlement program a health benefit plan funded by federal or state governments that pays for 47% of healthcare services

entry-level job a job performed upon graduation in order to gain basic skills, become familiar with the healthcare field, and establish excellent work habits

enucleation removal of the eyeball without removing the ocular contents of the orbit or muscles

EP enlarged prostate; established patient

epicardium the inner layer of the pericardium; also called visceral pericardium

epidermis the outer layer of the skin

epididymis spermatic duct

epididymovasostomy the removal of a portion of the vas deferens and attachment of the vas deferens to the epididymis

epikeratoplasty the transplantation of donor corneal epithelium onto a patient's cornea

epilepsy a brain disorder in which neurons signal abnormally, causing seizures and/or unconsciousness

episiotomy (obstetrical) a surgical incision into the perineum and vagina

eponym named after a person

equilibrium sense of balance

ERCP endoscopic retrograde cholangi-opancreatography

erectile dysfunction (ED) the chronic inability to achieve or maintain a penile erection until ejaculation; also called impotence

erythema redness

erythema multiforme red fluid-filled lesions that can cause layers of skin to fall off

erythremia polycythemia; a circulatory disorder

erythroblastosis fetalis a blood disorder that occurs when the blood types of a mother and baby are incompatible; also called hemolytic disease of the newborn (HDN)

erythrocyte a red blood cell

erythrocytopenia a lack of red blood cells

erythroderma red skin

erythropoiesis the process of the formation of red blood cells

Escherichia coli (E. coli) a bacterium that can cause serious food poisoning

esophageal ring an abnormal ring of tissue around the esophagus

esophagectomy a procedure in which all or part of the esophagus is surgically removed

esophagitis irritation of the esophagus caused by acid reflux and a weak cardiac sphincter

esophagogastroduodenoscopy (EGD) a procedure in which an endoscope is inserted through the mouth and moved down the throat into the esophagus, stomach, and duodenum

esophagoscopy visual examination of the esophagus

established patient (EP) a patient who has received professional services from the same physician, or another physician in the group of the same specialty and subspecialty, within the previous three years

estimated date of delivery (EDD) the anticipated due date of a pregnant woman determined by counting 40 weeks from the last menstrual period (LMP)

estimated gestational age (EGA) the number of weeks and days since the last menstrual period

ESWL extracorporeal shock wave lithotripsy

ethmoid sinus a sinus located between the eyes and nose

ethmoidectomy the process of opening the ethmoid sinus cavity

etiology cause

eustachian tube the connection between the ear and the nasopharynx

evacuation suctioning the fetus and placenta out of the uterus with a suctioning instrument placed through the vagina, into the cervix, and into the uterus

Evaluation and Management (E/M) the section of CPT codes that describe patient encounters with a physician for the evaluation and management of a health problem

EVAR endovascular aneurysm repair

evisceration removal of the ocular contents and removal of the cornea; the sclera and extraocular muscles are not removed

examination performing a visual and physical inspection, with or without the assistance of instruments, to arrive at a conclusion

exceptionally large newborn a newborn with a birth weight more than 4,500 grams (9 pounds, 15 ounces)

exchange the process of obtaining oxygen from the air and delivering it to the lungs and blood for distribution to tissue cells, and removing the gaseous waste product, carbon dioxide, from the blood and lungs and expelling it

Excision (ICD-10-PCS) the root operation that identifies cutting out or off, without replacement, a portion of a body part

excision the use of scissors, scalpel, or other sharp instrument to cut out tissue

excisional embolectomy see *thrombectomy*

Excludes2 a convention indicating the condition excluded is not part of the condition represented by the code, but the patient may have both conditions at the same time

exenteration removal of the eyeball, including the ocular contents; may include removal of bone and muscle

exfoliation falling off in scales or layers

exocrine a secretion externally via a duct

expandability (ICD-10-PCS) the major attribute of ICD-10-PCS whereby the structure of the code set allows new procedures to be easily incorporated

explanation of benefits a statement that lists all the services the provider billed, which ones were accepted for payment, how much the insurance company will pay, how much the patient owes, and how much will not be paid

External (ICD-10-PCS) the approach that identifies the entire treatment is performed on the skin or mucous membranes

external approach the performance of a procedure of the nose through the skin on the outside of the nasal structure

external cause an event such as an accident, force of nature, assault, or situation that causes an injury or adverse effect

external customer patients and others from outside organizations such as other providers or insurance companies

external ear a section of the ear that consists of the auricle or pinna, the auditory canal, and the tympanic membrane

external fixation the installation of a rigid device, external to the body, attached to the bone with pins and screws to stabilize it

external radiotherapy a treatment that directs precise doses of x-ray beams at specific sites in order to kill or shrink tumors and cancerous cells

Extirpation (ICD-10-PCS) the root operation that identifies taking out or cutting out abnormal solid matter from a body part

extracapsular cataract extraction removal of the lens of the eye while leaving the elastic capsule that covers the lens partially intact to allow implantation of an intraocular lens (IOL)

extracorporeal outside of the body

extracorporeal shock wave lithotripsy (ESWL) the use of a lithotripter to aim pulsating sound waves at a kidney stone to break it into pieces

Extraction (ICD-10-PCS) the root operation that identifies pulling or stripping out or off all or a portion of a body part by the use of force

extraluminal from outside a vessel

extremely low birth weight (ELBW) a birth weight of less than 1,000 grams (2 pounds, 3 ounces)

extrinsic (asthma) asthma due to allergens; also called atopic

F

facet the flat surface on the edge of the spinous process that forms the connection between vertebrae

facetectomy the excision of the vertebral facet

facility fee the fee charged by hospitals or other medical facilities for resources such as nursing and support staff, supplies, medication administration, social services, and the cost of space

failure to thrive (FTT) inadequate physical growth marked by child's weight for age below the fifth percentile of the standard growth chart

fallopian tube the tube through which eggs are transported for fertilization and implantation in the uterus

fallopian tube catheter introduction the insertion of a catheter through the cervix and uterus into the fallopian tube(s)

False Claims Act (FCA) a federal law that imposes penalties on individuals and companies who defraud government programs

Family Counseling (ICD-10-PCS) the root type that identifies the application of psychological methods that includes one or more family members to treat an individual with addictive behavior

family history the condition(s) that a patient's family member had in the past or currently has that causes the patient to be at higher risk of also contracting or developing the disease

Family Psychotherapy (ICD-10-PCS) the root type that identifies the treatment that includes one or more family members of an individual with a mental health disorder by behavioral, cognitive, psychoanalytic, psychodynamic, or psychophysiological means to improve functioning or well-being

family psychotherapy a method of psychotherapy whereby family members meet with a clinician to discuss the patient's condition and how to help the patient

fascia the fibrous tissue that connects muscle to muscle

fasciotomy cutting into the fascia to relieve pressure or tension

fatigue fracture a fracture of a bone that has been subjected to repeated use or impact

FBR foreign body removal

Federal Register the official daily publication for rules, proposed rules, and notices of federal agencies and organizations, as well as executive orders and other presidential documents

female catheter a short urethral catheter for passage through the female urethra

female factor infertility a problem in the female genital system that diminishes reproduction, such as scarring or obstruction of the fallopian tubes or abnormal interaction between sperm and the mucous membrane in the cervix

femur thigh bone

fenestrated endovascular aneurysm repair (FEVAR) reinforcement of a weak section of the aorta with a stent that has holes customized to accommodate arterial branches

fenestration semicircular canal the creation of an opening in the semicircular canal

fetal nonstress test (NST) testing of the fetal heartbeat and oxygenation

fetal scalp blood sampling a blood specimen from the scalp of a fetus through the dilated cervix

fetopelvic disproportion see *cephalopelvic disproportion (CPD)*

FEVAR fenestrated endovascular aneurysm repair

fibrocystic breast disease a condition of lumps of benign fibrous tissue in the breast

fimbrioplasty a procedure that obstructs a fallopian tube to save the function of the fimbriae

final rule a legally required notice of final regulations, which is published in the *Federal Register*

fine-needle aspiration (FNAB, FNA, NAB) a procedure in which a physician inserts a fine (thin), hollow needle under the skin to obtain aspirate, a small sample of cells, tissue, or fluid

first trimester the time during a pregnancy when the gestational age is less than 14 weeks, 0 days

first-listed diagnosis the diagnosis, condition, problem, or other reason for an encounter shown in the medical record to be chiefly responsible for the services provided

fistulization the creation of a passageway, or opening, in the sclera by incising the iris and allowing the aqueous humor to drain

flap a procedure whereby the blood supply remains intact, or a physician removes the skin and blood vessels and connects them to the recipient site; flaps can also involve subcutaneous tissue, muscle, fascia, and bone

flap transfer moving a section of skin and subcutaneous tissue (sometimes including muscle, fascia, and bone), with blood vessels intact, from one site to another, with anastomosis to vessels at the recipient site

flexible endoscope an instrument used for endoscopy procedures that consists of a soft tube with fiber-optic bundles that transmit an image

Fluoroscopy (ICD-10-PCS) the root type that identifies the single plane or biplane real-time display of an image developed from the capture of external ionizing radiation on a fluorescent screen; may also be stored by either digital or analog means

fluoroscopy the single plane or biplane real-time display of an image developed from the capture of external ionizing radiation on a fluorescent screen; may also be stored by either digital or analog means

focal (seizure) a type of seizure that occurs in one part of the brain

Foley catheter the most commonly used design of indwelling balloon catheter

folic acid deficiency anemia an anemia due to a lack of folic acid

folliculitis the inflammation of space around the hair root

foramen an opening in the vertebra that surrounds the spinal cord

forceps delivery the extraction of a fetus from the birth canal by grasping the head with forceps (tongs)

foreign body an object that does not belong in the body

foreign body removal (FBR) a procedure in which an object is retrieved from within the body

forequarter an extremity and all or part of the adjoining structure, such as the arm, shoulder joint, and all or part of the scapula and clavicle or the leg, hip joint, and all or part of the pelvic girdle

formed element a blood cell

four cooperating parties a federal inter-departmental committee that oversees all ICD-10 changes; comprises representatives from the Centers for Medicare and Medicaid Services (CMS), the National Center for Health Statistics (NCHS; part of the Centers for Disease Control and Prevention [CDC]), the American Hospital Association (AHA), and the American Health Information Management Association (AHIMA)

fracture broken bone

fracture reduction (manipulation) the use of force to move parts of a bone into normal alignment

fragility fracture a broken bone caused by disease rather than trauma

Fragmentation (ICD-10-PCS) the root operation that identifies breaking solid matter in a body part into pieces

fraud knowingly billing for services that were never given or billing for a service that has a higher reimbursement than the service produced

free flap a skin graft in which the blood vessels and nerves are completely disconnected from the original site and reconnected to vessels and nerves at the new site

free skin graft a skin graft in which a section of skin is replaced with skin from another area of the body, donor skin, or a synthetic substitute

front-end edit check a computerized scan of insurance claims for valid data, performed by the payer

frontal sinus a sinus located above the eyes

FTSG full-thickness skin graft

full-term pregnancy 37 weeks, 1 day of gestation to 40 weeks, 7 days of gestation

full-thickness burn a burn that causes damage to the entire depth of the dermis

full-thickness skin graft (FTSG) a skin graft consisting of the epidermis and the full depth of the dermis

function study visualizing a physiologic function in real time to observe the processes at work

functional imaging a type of radiology that allows a physician to observe organ function in real time

fungus a primitive vegetable that reproduces through spores

furuncle a skin infection involving an entire hair follicle and the surrounding skin tissue

Fusion (ICD-10-PCS) the root operation that identifies joining together portions of an articular body part, rendering the articular body part immobile

G

galactogram see *mammary ductogram*

gangrene the decay or death of tissue in the body caused by a lack of blood supply

gastrectomy excision of the stomach

gastric bypass a procedure in which the stomach is divided to create a small pouch and causes food to bypass part of the small intestine

gastritis the inflammation of the stomach lining

gastroenteritis a bacterial or viral infection of the stomach and intestines

gastroesophageal reflux disease (GERD) the backward flow of stomach contents into the esophagus

gastrointestinal (GI) system the digestive system

gastroplasty surgical repair of the stomach

gastroplication folding of the stomach

gastrorrhaphy suture of the stomach

gastroscopy visual examination of the stomach

GEMs General Equivalency Mappings

gender data mismatch an error that occurs when the patient's documented gender is inconsistent with the procedure coded

general anesthesia a type of anesthesia that affects the whole body, including the brain, and in which the patient feels nothing and has no memory of the procedure afterward

generalized (seizure) see *distributed (seizure)*

genital prolapse the downward displacement of the uterus or vagina to an abnormal position

genitourinary (GU) system the body system that includes the urinary and genital systems

geographic practice cost index (GPCI) the Medicare system of adjusting fees based on the region of the country and/or zip code in which the healthcare provider practices

GERD gastroesophageal reflux disease

gestational condition a condition that is first diagnosed during pregnancy

gestational diabetes a type of diabetes that develops during pregnancy in a woman who did not previously have diabetes

gestational diabetes mellitus (GDM) a condition in which elevated glucose concentrations are diagnosed during pregnancy in women with no history of diabetes

gestational hypertension the development of hypertension after 20 weeks' gestation in a woman who previously was not diagnosed with hypertension; also called pregnancy-induced hypertension (PIH)

gestational sac a synonym for a fetus

giant-cell bone tumor a rare, aggressive, benign tumor generally occurring in adults between the ages of 20 and 40 years

Giardia the parasite that causes giardiasis, an intestinal tract infection

Glasgow Coma Scale a standardized system for assessing the level of consciousness of patients with an acute brain injury with ratings for eye opening, verbal responsiveness, and motor responsiveness

glaucoma an increased fluid pressure within the eye that damages the optic nerve and can cause blindness

global obstetric package (CPT) the services of routine antepartum, delivery, and postpartum care provided for a single patient

global period (CPT) the number of days during which a provider must render all services related to a surgery

globin a by-product of hemoglobin

globulin a protein molecule that comprises immunoglobulins

glomerular filtration rate (GFR) a method used to measure kidney function and to determine the stage of kidney disease

glomerulonephritis inflammation of the glomerulus of the kidney, allowing protein and blood into the urine

glomerulus a cluster of capillaries that separates the urinary space from the blood

glucose tolerance test (GTT) a diagnostic measure to evaluate how the body breaks down sugar

glycouria a condition of sugar in the urine

goiter an enlargement of the thyroid gland that is not cancer

goniotomy placement of a goniolens (gonioscope) on a patient's cornea to view the iris and cornea; allows a physician to see and open the trabecular meshwork to drain aqueous humor and reduce intraocular pressure (IOP)

GPCI geographic practice cost index

grand mal (seizure) a seizure characterized by a sudden loss of consciousness and falling down; affects the entire brain

grand multipara a woman who has had five or more previous pregnancies resulting in a viable fetus

granular detailed; specific

Graves' disease overproduction of hormones by the thyroid gland due to an autoimmune condition in which autoantibodies are directed against the thyroid-stimulating hormone (TSH) receptor

gravida (G) the number of pregnancies a woman has had

gross (examination) viewing with the naked eye

Group Counseling (ICD-10-PCS) the root type that identifies the application of psychological methods to treat an individual with addictive behavior

group health plan insurance coverage offered through an employer or union

group psychotherapy a method of psychotherapy whereby a group of patients with the same disorder meets with a clinician to share information to help one another change their behaviors

Group Therapy (ICD-10-PCS) the root type that identifies the treatment of two or more individuals with a mental health disorder by behavioral, cognitive, psychoanalytic, psychodynamic, or psychophysiological means to improve functioning or well-being

GTT glucose tolerance test

guided imagery see *radiologic guidance*

guidelines (CPT) instructions that appear at the beginning of each of the six sections and apply to all codes in that section

gustatory the sense of taste

Gustilo classification system the classification of open fractures of long bones into three major categories depending on the method of injury, soft-tissue damage, and degree of skeletal involvement

H

hallucination false visual, auditory, olfactory, or tactile perception

Hb hemoglobin

HbA1c a blood test that measures the glucose attached to hemoglobin

HBW high birth weight

HCPCS Health Care Common Procedure Coding System

HCPCS Index an alphabetical listing of services and supplies organized by Main Terms and subterms

HCPCS modifier additional characters added to a code, either alphanumeric or two letters long that can be used with both HCPCS and CPT codes; provides additional information

about a service, item, or procedure and encompasses more situations than a CPT modifier does

HCPCS Table of Drugs a table that organizes HCPCS codes for generic and brand name drugs

HCPCS Tabular List the section of the HCPCS manual that arranges codes in alphanumeric order, beginning with codes that start with the letter *A*, followed by four numbers

HDN hemolytic disease of the newborn

Health Insurance Portability and Accountability Act (HIPAA) a federal law passed in 1996 that has numerous provisions relating to consumer health insurance and the privacy and security of electronic health transactions

healthcare administrator an individual in a healthcare organization who is responsible for managing the organization, including the transition to ICD-10-CM/PCS

Healthcare Common Procedure Coding System (HCPCS) the HIPAA-mandated code set for supplies, items, and services not covered by CPT, physician, and nonphysician services

Hearing Aid Assessment (ICD-10-PCS) the root type that identifies the measurement of the appropriateness and/or effectiveness of a hearing device

Hearing Aid Treatment (ICD-10-PCS) the root type that identifies the application of techniques to improve the communication abilities of individuals with cochlear implant

Hearing Assessment (ICD-10-PCS) the root type that identifies the measurement of hearing and related functions

Hearing Treatment (ICD-10-PCS) the root type that identifies the application of techniques to improve, augment, or compensate for hearing and related functional impairment

heart transplant replacement of a diseased heart with a healthy heart from a deceased donor

Helicobacter pylori (H. pylori) the bacterium that causes ulcers

Heller myotomy a procedure in which the esophageal sphincter muscle is cut

HELLP syndrome a severe form of preeclampsia with hemolysis, elevated liver enzymes, and low platelet count

helminth a plant or animal that lives in or on another living organism, or host, and often causes damage to the host; also called a parasite

hemapheresis removal of blood

hematology study of blood

hematopoiesis formation of blood

hematuria the condition of blood in the urine

hemiarthroplasty a procedure requiring only one component of a joint be replaced; also called a partial joint replacement

hemic related to blood

hemic system the method to transport and pass nutrients, oxygen, carbon dioxide, water, proteins, and hormones to cells and transport waste products to excretory oxygen; also called blood

hemilaminectomy the partial removal of the lamina; also called laminotomy

hemiplegia paralysis of one side of the body

hemispherectomy excision of one of the two cerebral hemispheres

hemodialysis (HD) a method for removing waste from the blood in which blood is processed through a machine when the kidneys cease to function

hemoglobin (Hb) the oxygen-carrying component of erythrocytes

hemolytic anemia anemia due to excessive loss of erythrocytes

hemolytic disease of the newborn (HDN) see *erythroblastosis fetalis*

hemophilia a genetic disorder in which blood takes too long to clot

hemostasis the stoppage of bleeding or hemorrhage

hepatectomy the surgical removal of all or part of the liver

hepatitis inflammation of the liver due to viruses named A, B, or C

hernia the protrusion of an organ through a weakened area in a muscle

hernia repair the surgical correction of a hernia through the use of manual manipulation, sutures, or mesh

herpes the shingles virus

HHNS hyperosmolarity hyperglycemic nonketotic syndrome

hierarchical condition category (HCC) coding a risk adjustment methodology intended to predict future costs of caring for patients with chronic, high cost illnesses

high birth weight (HBW) birth weight greater than 4,000 grams (8 pounds, 13 ounces)

histology type of tissue

history of present illness (HPI) an interview of a patient regarding symptoms related to the chief complaint and how the problem has progressed

Holter monitor a portable ECG machine worn by a patient for an extended period of hours or days to measure heart activity in a variety of situations

homeostasis the maintenance of a stable internal physical state

hordeolum the bacterial inflammation of a sebaceous gland on the edge or lining of the eyelid; also called a stye

hormones chemical messengers that regulate many body functions including growth, development, metabolism, sexual function, reproduction, and mood

hospital-acquired condition (HAC) a condition that begins during a patient's hospital stay but is considered reasonably preventable through proper patient care (evidence-based) practices

hospital laboratory a laboratory located in a hospital facility, used to perform tests needed in emergency situations, tests where STAT results are needed rapidly for patient care, and those done in high volume for both inpatients and outpatients

HPI history of present illness

HTN hypertension

human immunodeficiency virus (HIV) a virus that infects and destroys helper T cells of the immune system and causes AIDS

Huntington's disease chorea an inherited progressive, degenerative disease involving loss of muscle control and personality changes

hydrocele a fluid-filled sac in the scrotum caused by abnormal fetal development, injury, hernia, or blockages

hydrocephalus an excess of cerebrospinal fluid trapped in the brain

hydrocephaly water or fluid in the head/brain

hydronephrosis distention of the renal pelvis due to excessive urine collection in the kidney, often due to ureteral obstruction

hymenotomy incision of the hymen

hyperbaric oxygen treatment (HBOT) breathing 100% oxygen under increased atmospheric pressure

hyperbilirubinemia high concentrations of bilirubin in the blood, which causes an infant's skin and sclera to turn yellow

hypercapnia a high carbon dioxide concentration

hyperglycemia a severely elevated blood glucose concentration due to a lack or deficiency of insulin

hyperosmolarity hyperglycemic nonketotic syndrome (HHNS) an elevated glucose concentration without ketoacidosis, usually occurring in elderly type 2 diabetics with other conditions

hypertension (HTN) an abnormally high arterial blood pressure

Hyperthermia (ICD-10-PCS) the root operation that identifies extracorporeal raising of body temperature

hyperthermia extracorporeal raising of body temperature

hyperthyroidism inappropriately elevated thyroid function

Hypnosis (ICD-10-PCS) the root type that identifies the induction of a state of heightened suggestibility by auditory, visual, and tactile techniques to elicit an emotional or behavioral response

hypogammaglobulinemia a deficiency of gamma globulins and antibodies in the blood

hypoglycemia an abnormally low blood glucose concentration often due to excessive use of insulin or other glucose-lowering medications

hypospadias a congenital condition in which the opening of the urethra is on the underside, rather than the end, of the penile shaft, and may be located as far down as the scrotum or perineum

Hypothermia (ICD-10-PCS) the root operation that identifies extracorporeal lowering of body temperature

hypothermia extracorporeal lowering of body temperature

hypothyroidism a deficiency of thyroid hormone, usually due to lack of production by the thyroid or inadequate secretion of hormones by the pituitary gland or hypothalamus

hypoxemia low oxygen concentration

hysterectomy removal of the uterus and/or related structures, such as the ovaries and fallopian tubes

hysteroophorosalpingectomy excision of the uterus, ovary, and fallopian tube

hysteroplasty the repair of a malformed uterus

hysterorrhaphy (nonobstetrical) suturing of the uterus

hysterosalpingography X-ray of the uterus and fallopian tubes after injecting contrast dye

hysteroscopy visualization of the cervix and uterus using a hysteroscope that is passed through the vagina into the cervix and uterine cavity

I

IBD inflammatory bowel disease

IBS irritable bowel syndrome

ICD-10 *International Classification of Diseases*, 10th Revision

ICD-10-CM *International Classification of Diseases*, 10th Revision, Clinical Modification

ICD-10-PCS *International Classification of Diseases*, 10th Revision, Procedure Classification System (ICD-10-PCS)

ICD-10-PCS Official Guidelines for Coding and Reporting (PCS OGCR) the official rules for the use of the ICD-10-PCS coding system

idiopathic of unknown cause

ileal conduit a channel that joins the ureters to the ileum

ileostomy division of the ileum that brings the proximal end out to a stoma in the abdominal wall, bypassing the colon, rectum, and anus

ileum small intestine

ileus a condition in which the bowel does not work correctly but there is no structural problem

ilium pelvic bone

IMA internal mammary artery

imaging guidance real-time visualization of body structures during a medical or surgical procedure

imbrication of the diaphragm repair of the diaphragm to resemble normal anatomy

Immobilization (ICD-10-PCS) the root operation that identifies limiting or preventing motion of a body region by external methods and devices

immobilization limiting or preventing motion of a body region by external methods and devices

immune globulin a substance that provides passive immunity and consists of serum globulins or recombinant immune globulins

immunization administration of a vaccine (virus) or toxoid (bacteria) that provides active immunity

immunization history date and type of past vaccinations and titers (blood tests proving immunity to a specific disease)

immunodeficiency the result of a body's immune system failure or reduction in function

impairment the degree to which an individual's normal abilities are limited

impotence the chronic inability to achieve or maintain a penile erection until ejaculation

impression an effect produced on the mind by outside stimuli

impulse-control disorder an extreme difficulty in controlling impulses, despite the negative consequences

in remission (substance use) a history of past drug or alcohol dependence documented by the physician

in vitro fertilization the removal of an egg from a female patient, which is manually fertilized with sperm and then returned to the fallopian tube or implanted in the uterus

incidental appendectomy the removal of the appendix as a preventive measure during another procedure

incision site the anatomic location at which a surgeon cuts through the skin and subcutaneous tissue

incisional biopsy a tissue sample obtained with a sharp blade, other than a punch tool, to remove a full-thickness sample of tissue using a vertical incision or wedge and penetration deep into the subcutaneous tissue

inconclusive HIV a test result that means the antibody test was neither positive nor negative; also called indeterminate HIV

incontinence the inability to control bladder muscles

incubator a medical device that allows a newborn to be in an environment where the temperature, humidity, and oxygen concentration can be controlled

incus the anvil-shaped bone in the middle ear that receives vibrations from the malleus and transmits them to the stapes

indented code description indented three spaces and beginning with a lowercase letter, this description is the unique descriptor for a specific code number

independent clinical lab a Medicare-enrolled laboratory that receives a specimen and performs a test(s) for a separate, referring laboratory; also called referring lab

indeterminate HIV see *inconclusive HIV*

Individual Counseling (ICD-10-PCS) the root type that identifies the application of psychological methods to treat an individual with addictive behavior

individual health insurance a plan that people purchase directly from a health insurance company, such as those who are self-employed or do not have benefits through an employer or government program

Individual Psychotherapy (ICD-10-PCS) the root type that identifies the treatment of an individual with a mental health disorder by behavioral, cognitive, psychoanalytic, psychodynamic, or psychophysiological means to improve functioning or well-being

indwelling (catheter) a flexible, hollow tube inserted into the urinary bladder and left in short or long term to provide continuous urine flow; may be inserted through the urethra or ureters

infant of diabetic mother (IDM) an infant born to a woman who has diabetes

infection inflammation due to an infectious agent

inferior vena cava the largest veins that carry deoxygenated blood back to the right ventricle

inflammatory bowel disease (IBD) a group of disorders in which the intestines become red and swollen, probably as a result of an immune reaction of the body against its own intestinal tissue; includes Crohn's disease and ulcerative colitis

influenza an acute respiratory infection with sudden onset caused by a virus and characterized by fever, chills, headache, muscle aches, cough, and sore throat

infusion technique a slow, steady rate of release of medication over a long period of time

initial encounter (CPT) the first encounter by the admitting physician during the current admission

initial encounter (ICD-10-CM) active treatment

initial episode of care identifies that the patient received active treatment for an injury during the encounter

injection the administration of a medication using a needle

inner ear see *labyrinth*

inpatient encounter physician interaction with a patient who has been formally admitted

to a healthcare facility, such as an acute-care hospital, long-term care facility, or rehabilitation facility

Insertion (ICD-10-PCS) the root operation that identifies putting in a nonbiological appliance that monitors, assists, performs, or prevents a physiological function but does not physically take the place of a body part

insertion the position where a muscle attaches to a bone that moves

Inspection (ICD-10-PCS) the root operation that identifies visually and/or manually exploring a body part

instructional note (CPT) text that appears in parentheses after a code description; directs the user to alternative codes for closely related procedures or to codes that must or must not be used together

instructional note (ICD-10-CM) official coding directions throughout the ICD-10-CM manual

instrumentation specialized equipment, such as an endoscope or needle, used to reach an internal body part

insulin pump a small, implantable device that dispenses small doses of rapid-acting insulin

integral routine

integral component a task that is part of the intraoperative service and is not coded or billed separately

integumentary pertaining to a covering

intellectual disability the modern term for mental retardation

intent a term describing whether an event was accidental or intentional

interactive complexity a component of psychiatry services that is used when communication is challenging because of the involvement of third parties in addition to the patient

internal approach the performance of a procedure of the nose from within the nasal passage or through the mucous membrane inside the nasal passage

internal customer other employees of the organization, such as coworkers and superiors

internal fixation the use of special implants, such as plates, screws, nails, rods, and/or wires, applied directly to the bone(s)

internal mammary artery (IMA) the blood vessel located on the inside of the chest cavity, which is resistant to cholesterol buildup; often used in a coronary artery bypass graft

internal radiotherapy the use of radioactive pellets or containers within a body cavity to target a malignant area

***International Classification of Diseases*, 10th Revision (ICD-10)** a worldwide reporting system developed by the World Health Organization for classifying epidemiological and mortality data

International Classification of Diseases, 10th Revision, Clinical Modification (ICD-10-CM) a HIPAA-mandated code set for diagnosis coding

International Classification of Diseases, 10th Revision, Procedure Classification System (ICD-10-PCS) a HIPAA-mandated code set for hospital inpatient procedure coding

interspace the space between two vertebrae; identified by the vertebrae above and below

interstitial between tissues

interventional radiologist a physician who performs minimally invasive, image-guided surgeries

intervertebral disc a plate that exists between each pair of vertebrae to provide flexibility and movement to the spine; consists of the nucleus pulposus and annulus fibrosus

intestinal obstruction a physical blockage of the intestine that prevents waste from passing through

intoxication a state of impaired function that occurs when more of a substance is consumed than a person can physically tolerate, resulting in behavioral or physical abnormalities

intra-articular within a joint

intracavity within a cavity

intractable (migraine) a migraine that is resistant to treatment; may also be called pharmacoresistant or refractory

intradermal pertaining to within the skin

intralesional injection the injection of a drug, such as a corticosteroid, into a skin lesion

intraluminal from within a vessel

intraocular lens (IOL) an artificial lens inserted into the lens capsule of the eye

intraocular pressure (IOP) the pressure of fluid within the eye

intrapartum fetal hypoxia an insufficient amount of oxygen provided to the fetus during labor and delivery

intraperitoneal within the peritoneum

intrathecal into the sheath of the spinal cord

intrauterine growth restriction (IUGR) the poor growth of a baby while in the mother's womb during pregnancy; specifically, the developing baby weighs less than 90% of other babies at the same gestational age

intraventricular hemorrhage (IVH) bleeding in the brain in very-low-birth-weight premature babies that usually resolves within a few days

intravitreal injection the injection of medication into the vitreous body

intrinsic (asthma) asthma that is not due to allergens; also called nonatopic

Introduction (ICD-10-PCS) the root operation that identifies putting in or on a therapeutic, diagnostic, nutritional, physiological, or prophylactic substance except blood or blood products

introduction putting in or on a therapeutic, diagnostic, nutritional, physiological, or prophylactic substance except blood or blood products

involuntary (muscles) muscles that are controlled by a subconscious part of the brain

IOL intraocular lens

IOP intraocular pressure

ipsilateral the examination of circulation on the same side on which catheterization was performed

iridectomy excision of the iris

iridencleisis implantation of part of the iris in the cornea

iridoplasty repair of the iris

iridotasis stretching of the iris

iridotomy incision of the iris to drain aqueous humor; can include transfixion for iris bombé

iron-deficiency anemia an anemia due to insufficient iron to manufacture hemoglobin

Irrigation (ICD-10-PCS) the root operation that identifies putting in or on a cleaning substance

irrigation putting in or on a cleaning substance

irritable bowel syndrome (IBS) a combination of symptoms such as cramping, abdominal pain, bloating, constipation, and diarrhea

ischemia deficient blood supply to a local area due to obstruction of the arterial blood flow, usually due to narrowing of the arteries; also called coronary heart disease or arteriosclerotic heart disease when it affects the heart

IUGR intrauterine growth restriction

IVH intraventricular hemorrhage

J

jaundice a condition due to high bilirubin that causes the skin and parts of the eyes to turn a yellow color

joint the location where two or more bones meet

joint replacement the removal of a natural joint and insertion of an artificial ball and cup made of metal, ceramic, polyurethane, or other artificial material

K

keratectomy excision of the cornea

keratin horny tissues found in the epidermis, hair, and nails

keratitis inflammation and ulceration of the surface of the cornea

keratomileusis a form of keratoplasty in which a slice of the cornea is removed, reshaped (often with a laser), and placed back onto the cornea

keratophakia the reshaping and transplantation of donor corneal tissue onto a patient's cornea

keratoplasty repair of the cornea

keratosis overgrowth of horny tissue

key components (KCs) history, examination, and medical decision making; also referred to as content of service requirements

kidney the part of the urinary system that produces urine and regulates the level of electrolytes and body fluid

L

lab report a report that provides the results of specimen testing and other information useful to a physician in making a diagnosis

lab requisition a form that describes specimen testing to be performed

lab test/pathology results reports from lab tests; report from pathology regarding specimen testing

LABG laparoscopically adjustable gastric banding

labia major the folds of flesh that surround and protect the opening to the vagina

labia minor the fold of flesh that surrounds and protects the urethra

laboratory a department or organization that analyzes biological specimens

labyrinth a fluid-filled cavity in the temporal bone that contains the cochlea; also called the inner ear

labyrinthotomy surgical incision into the labyrinth of the ear, sometimes with the administration/injection of drugs

laceration a torn or jagged wound

lamellar keratoplasty partial-thickness transplantation involving a graft of only specific corneal layers

lamina a thin layer of bone that forms part of the vertebral arch

laminectomy the complete removal of the lamina

laminoplasty repair of the lamina

laminotomy the partial removal of the lamina; also called hemilaminectomy

laparoscopically adjustable gastric banding (LABG) a procedure in which an inflatable silicone device is placed around the top portion of the stomach to divide it into a smaller pouch and a larger pouch

laparoscopy visual examination of the abdomen

laparotomy cutting into the abdomen

large for gestational age (LGA) a fetus or newborn infant who is larger in size than normal for the baby's sex and gestational age

laryngeal reinnervation by neuromuscular pedicle the use of a neuromuscular pedicle to restore nerves

laryngectomy excision of all or part of the larynx

laryngitis inflammation of the larynx, resulting in hoarseness

laryngoscopy (direct) the use of a laryngoscope inserted through the mouth or nose to view the larynx and hypolarynx/subglottis

laryngoscopy (indirect) the use of a mirror to view the base of the tongue, larynx, and hypolarynx

larynx the voice box

last menstrual period (LMP) the last menstrual period that a woman has before becoming pregnant, which is used to determine the estimated date of delivery (EDD)

late effect a problem that occurs after active healing is completed

late onset Alzheimer's disease that is diagnosed after age 65

lateral rhinotomy the creation of an incision along the nose from the inner eyebrow to the nasolabial fold

laterality an indication of the side of the body that a condition affects, such as right, left, or bilateral sides

latissimus dorsi (LD) flap the use of a latissimus dorsi muscle flap, often combined with a tissue expander or implant, to reconstruct the breast

lavage irrigation of the maxillary or sphenoid sinus by puncturing the antrum or creating an ostium

LBW low birth weight

left atrium the upper left chamber of the heart, which receives blood from the lungs

left ventricle the lower left chamber of the heart, which ejects blood to the body

legacy system a coding system used for historical purposes

lens the clear part of the front of the eye that focuses light rays on the retina

leukemia a malignant disease of the blood-forming organs; does not produce tumors

leukocyte white blood cell

leukopenia a lack of white blood cells

level (spinal) a vertebra of the spine

Level I (HCPCS) Current Procedural Terminology (CPT) codes

Level II (HCPCS) national Healthcare Common Procedure Coding System codes

level of service in evaluation and management coding, the complexity or duration of a service provided based on the nature of the presenting problem, the history, the examination, and the medical decision making

Lewy body disease a condition in which patients have abnormal protein structures in certain areas of the brain

LGA large for gestational age

lichen an eruption of flat papules

ligament fibrous tissue that connects bones to bones

ligation closing off a vessel or tubular body part, most often done using sutures, clips, or cautery

ligature tying or binding off; or the material used to tie or bind off, such as surgical filament

ligature (skin tag) tying off a skin tag at its base with thread, eliminating blood flow to the skin tag; it eventually dies and falls off

Light Therapy (ICD-10-PCS) the root type that identifies the application of specialized light treatments to improve functioning or well-being

limited lymphadenectomy the removal of lymph nodes

linear measurement a measurement that identifies the distance between two points and is used to classify the length and the diameter of wound repairs

lipolysis surgical destruction of fat

lithoplasty surgical formation of fat

lithotripsy the use of high-frequency sound waves to break up calculus

liver biopsy the surgical removal of a small piece of the liver

liver transplant the surgical removal of a diseased liver and replacement with some or all of a healthy liver from another person

LMP last menstrual period

lobar pneumonia a bacterial pneumonia that primarily affects one lobe of the lung

lobe a segment of a lung

lobectomy the surgical excision of one lobe of an organ

lobular a breast cancer that starts in the lobules that produce milk

lobular pneumonia a pneumonia that primarily affects the bronchi and lobules; also called bronchopneumonia

local anesthesia numbs a small area of a body part; patient is awake and alert

localized an infection that primarily affects a single organ or body system, such as pneumonia or pharyngitis

localized (seizure) see *focal (seizure)*

logic-based encoder coding software that guides users through a series of questions and menu choices that ultimately lead to code choices

low birth weight (LBW) a birth weight less than 2,500 grams (5 pounds, 8 ounces)

lower respiratory tract consists of the trachea, bronchi, and lungs

lower urinary tract symptom (LUTS) a symptom relating to urine storage and voiding disturbances

Lund-Browder classification a system used by physicians to estimate the extent, depth, and percentage of burns

lung a respiratory organ composed of the spongy tissue that receives deoxygenated blood from the heart through the pulmonary artery, re-oxygenates it, and sends it back to the heart through the pulmonary vein

lymph a clear fluid containing proteins, salts, organic substances, and water

lymph chain a sequential grouping of lymph nodes in a localized area along lymph vessels, occurring in sites where the body is most vulnerable to infection

lymph node a small mass of tissue that ranges from the size of a pinhead to about one inch in diameter and is located along the lymph vessels

lymphadenectomy the surgical excision of a lymph gland

lymphangiography a radiology procedure where contrast medium is injected into a patient to visualize lymph nodes and lymph circulation

lymphangiotomy incision into a vessel of the lymphatic system

lysis of labial adhesions the destruction or freeing of adhesions between the labia minor and labia major

M

M-mode (motion) ultrasound a one-dimensional ultrasonic measurement used to display the movement of a structure

MAC monitored anesthesia care

macular degeneration the gradual loss of central vision due to aging, with no cure

magnetic resonance angiography (MRA) the use of a magnetic field and pulses of radio wave energy to visualize the heart, blood vessels, or blood flow in the circulatory system

Magnetic Resonance Imaging (MRI) (ICD-10-PCS) the root type or root operation that identifies the computer-reformatted digital display of multiplanar images developed from the capture of radiofrequency signals emitted by nuclei in a body site excited within a magnetic field

magnetic resonance imaging (MRI) the use of strong magnets and radio waves to produce computerized images of internal body tissues

Main Term the primary index entry

major complication or comorbidity (MCC) a diagnosis listed in the *ICD-10-CM/PCS MS-DRG Definitions Manual* that potentially qualifies the patient for a higher-paying DRG

male factor infertility a problem in the male genital system that diminishes reproduction, such as inability to ejaculate, lack of sperm production, or lack of live sperm

malformation (congenital) a permanent abnormal shape of an organ or body region, resulting from arrested, delayed, or abnormal development of an embryo

malignant life-threatening

Mallampati score a score that rates the potential difficulty of endotracheal intubation on a scale of I through IV

malleus the hammer-shaped bone in the middle ear that transmits vibrations to the incus

malposition of fetus any presentation of a fetus other than occipitoanterior (OA)

malunion a condition when the ends of fractured bone segments do not heal with proper alignment

mammary ductogram the use of mammography and contrast material to view the inside of a breast's milk ducts

mammography (diagnostic) X-ray imaging of the male or female breast to determine whether a problem exists or to determine the nature of a problem

mammography (screening) X-ray imaging of the breast of a woman who has no signs or symptoms of breast disease

mammoplasty the repair or reconstruction of a breast

managed care plan a company that attempts to control the cost of healthcare while providing better outcomes

manifestation a sign or symptom

manipulation the realignment of bone fragments or segments; also called reduction

manometry a procedure that evaluates muscular activity of the esophagus at rest and during swallowing to diagnose esophageal disorders involving motility or causes of heartburn; also called motility study

manual review a review done by hand instead of through an automatic process

Map (ICD-10-PCS) the root operation that identifies locating the route of passage of electrical impulses and/or locating functional areas in a body part

march fracture the fracture of a bone that has been subjected to repeated use or impact

Marfan's syndrome a genetic disorder of connective tissue characterized by elongated bones and ocular and circulatory defects

Marshall-Marchetti-Krantz (MMK) procedure an eponym for vesicourethropexy

marsupialization to incise a cyst or abscess by cutting a slit into it to drain it and then suturing the edges to surrounding tissue; the surgical formation of a pouch-like sac (marsupialization) on the Bartholin's gland

MAS meconium aspiration syndrome

mastalgia breast pain

mastitis inflammation of the breast

mastoid process the portion of the temporal bone of the skull that juts forward behind the ear

mastopexy a skin reduction with removal or reduction of underlying breast muscles to reorient the breasts into a higher position

mastostomy the incision and drainage of a breast abscess

maxillary sinus a sinus located below the eyes

maxillectomy the removal of all or part of the upper jaw bone

Mayo-Hegar an eponym for a type of surgical needle holder

maze surgery the creation of new paths for the heart's electrical signals to travel through

MBD metastatic bone disease

Measurement (ICD-10-PCS) the root operation that identifies determining the level of a physiological or physical function at a point in time

measurement the use of equipment or tools to quantify the body's response, reflex, or perception

mechanical thrombectomy a transcatheter procedure that uses a thrombolytic agent, radiological guidance, and a small blade or water jet to fragment, then suction out, a clot from an artery or vein

Meckel's diverticulum a congenital bulge in the intestine caused by a remnant of the embryonic yolk stalk

meconium aspiration syndrome (MAS) a condition in which a newborn breathes a mixture of meconium and amniotic fluid into the lungs before or during delivery

meconium peritonitis an infection of the peritoneal cavity due to perforation of the bowel and leakage of meconium

mediastinotomy incision into the mediastinum

mediastinum located in the thorax and surrounded by connective tissue, an area that separates the lungs and contains the esophagus, heart, and superior and inferior vena cava and aorta

Medicaid a program for low-income families that is funded jointly by the federal government and state governments

medical necessity establishing the medical need for services

medical payment a payment made by automobile insurance policies to pay for medical expenses incurred during an automobile accident; also called med pay

medical record the comprehensive collection of all information on a patient at a particular facility

medical review an investigation conducted by a nurse, physician, or other clinician

Medicare a federal government program that pays for healthcare services for most people age 65 and older or people of any age with end-stage renal disease (ESRD)

Medicare administrative contractor (MAC) a private company that processes Medicare Part A and Part B claims

Medicare Advantage the optional replacement of Part A and Part B that is offered by private health insurance companies

Medicare global surgical package a group, or package, of services that all relate to a single surgery and are covered by a single insurance payment, including preoperative, intraoperative, and postoperative services

Medicare Physician Fee Schedule (MPFS) a listing of CPT codes and Medicare-allowable fees published by the Centers for Medicare and Medicaid Services

Medicare Physician Fee Schedule Database (MPFSDB) a listing of CPT codes, Medicare-allowable fees, and related information published by the Centers for Medicare and Medicaid Services

Medicare severity-adjusted DRGs (MS-DRGs) a DRG system developed and used by Medicare consisting of approximately 500 DRG classifications that aggregate the thousands of diagnoses and procedures available in the coding manuals

Medication Management (ICD-10-PCS) the root type that identifies the monitoring and adjustment of the use of medications for the treatment of a mental health disorder; also, the root type that identifies the application of psychological methods that includes one or more family members to treat an individual with addictive behavior

Medigap a Medicare supplement insurance policy sold by private insurance companies to fill gaps in Part A and Part B coverage

melanoma a tumor of melanocytes

meningitis a contagious, acute inflammation of the pia mater and the arachnoid mater in the brain

meniscectomy shaving, debriding, or excising all of the meniscus

mental disorder a psychological or physical condition that disrupts an individual's personality, mind, and emotions in such a way that it affects the ability to function and interact with others

mesh prosthesis/insertion the repair of weak tissues by inserting a mesh or other prosthesis to strengthen them

metabolism the processes of digestion, elimination, breathing, blood circulation, and maintaining body temperature

metastasize to spread and invade organs other than that of origin

metastatic bone disease (MBD) the invasion of a bone by cancer that begins in another organ

method (ICD-10-PCS approach) identifies how the access location is entered to reach an internal body part

Metzenbaum an eponym for a type of surgical scissors

MI myocardial infarction

microcephaly having a small head

microscopy the visual examination of small things

middle ear a small, air-filled cavity in the temporal bone that contains the ossicles, three small bones that are critical to the hearing process

middle fossa approach through the incision and partial removal of the bone above the ear

mid-level job a job obtained after two or three years of experience

migraine headache a severe, debilitating headache caused by vasodilation

millicurie the unit of measurement for radiopharmaceutical drugs

minimally invasive (procedure) a procedure performed using only natural body openings, needles, or small incisions

misadventure an error during a medical or surgical procedure

miscellaneous code a code that allows providers to immediately bill insurances for a service or item as soon as the FDA approves its use, even though there is no permanent or temporary code that describes it

mitral valve the valve that controls blood flow from the left atrium to the left ventricle

mitral valve prolapse (MVP) a disorder in which the two leaflets that compose the valve fall backward into the left atrium, resulting in regurgitation; also called click murmur syndrome or Barlow's syndrome

mitral valve stenosis a narrowing of the valve opening, which may be caused by calcification, as often occurs with the aortic valve, or rheumatic fever, which often occurs with the mitral valve

MMR measles, mumps, and rubella vaccine

modality the method of applying a therapeutic/physical treatment

moderate (conscious) sedation use of a mild sedative to relax a patient and pain medicine to relieve pain; the patient stays awake but may not remember the procedure afterward

modified radical mastectomy a simple mastectomy plus removal of axillary lymph nodes but not the pectoralis major muscle

modified radical mastoidectomy a mastoidectomy that includes reconstruction of the eardrum and leaves a few middle ear bones intact

modifier a word that limits the meaning of another

modifier (CPT) a two-digit alphanumeric suffix appended to CPT codes to further describe circumstances

modifying term a descriptive word in the Index that appears indented under the Main Term to further describe a service or procedure; also called subterm

modifying unit (M) a value assigned to each physical status modifier and each qualifying circumstance code to represent the added difficulty of the procedure

Moh's micrographic surgery a multistage procedure in which a malignant lesion is excised in microscopic layers

monitored anesthesia care (MAC) a planned procedure during which a patient undergoes local anesthesia together with sedation and analgesia

Monitoring (ICD-10-PCS) the root operation that identifies determining the level of a physiological or physical function repetitively over a period of time

monitoring determining the level of a physiological or physical function repetitively over a period of time

monoamniotic multiple fetuses sharing the same amnion

monochorionic multiple fetuses sharing the same chorion

monoplegia paralysis of one limb

mood disorder an instability of mood; also called affective disorder

morbidity a cause of disease and illness

mortality a cause of death

motility study a study evaluating muscular activity of the esophagus at rest and during swallowing to diagnose esophageal disorders involving motility or causes of heartburn; also called manometry

Motor and/or Nerve Function Assessment (ICD-10-PCS) the root type that identifies the measurement of motor, nerve, and related functions

Motor Treatment (ICD-10-PCS) the root type that identifies the exercise or activities to increase or facilitate motor function

MPFS Medicare Physician Fee Schedule

MPFSDB Medicare Physician Fee Schedule Database

MRA magnetic resonance angiography

MRI magnetic resonance imaging

MS-DRGs Medicare Severity-adjusted DRGs

multiaxial nature (ICD-10-PCS) the major attribute of ICD-10-PCS whereby each position or character within a code has a designated meaning or purpose

multiplane fixator a fixation device that has a ring-shaped frame that surrounds the treatment site

multiple coding the use of two or more codes that are needed to fully describe a condition

multiple endoscopy rule (CPT) guidelines about how to assign endoscopy codes when more than one procedure is performed during the same session; states that when two codes from the same code family are reported, 100% is allowed on the first procedure and the allowed amount for the second procedure is the *difference* in price between the second code and the endoscopic base code

multiple-family group psychotherapy a method of psychotherapy whereby a group of families who share the same problems meets to discuss the issues they are having

multiple gestation a pregnancy that involves more than one fetus

multiple organ dysfunction the altered function of more than one organ at the same time requiring medical intervention to stabilize the patient

multiple sclerosis a chronic, progressive disorder of the CNS characterized by muscle impairment due to patches of hardened tissue in the brain or spinal cord

muscular system provides for movement of the body as well as the operation of individual organs, maintenance of body posture, and production of heat

musculocutaneous pertaining to both muscles and skin

musculoskeletal (MS) system the skeletal and muscular systems of the body that support the body, protect internal organs, produce blood cells, store minerals, provide movement to the body, maintain body posture, and produce heat

MVP mitral valve prolapse

myalgia a muscle pain

myasthenia a weakness in a muscle

myocardial infarction (MI) the death of heart tissue caused by an interruption to the blood supply; commonly known as a heart attack

myocarditis inflammation of the heart muscle

myocardium the thick, muscular inner layers that contract to pump blood

myoclonic (seizure) a seizure characterized by jerking and twitching in the upper body, arms, or legs

myomectomy removal of uterine fibroid tumors without removing healthy uterine tissue

myosarcoma a malignant tumor in a muscle

myositis inflammation of a muscle

myringectomy excision of the eardrum

myringoplasty repair of the tympanic membrane, involving the drumhead and donor area, usually with a graft of living tissue such as fat or fascia; also called tympanoplasty

myringotomy drainage of fluid or pus from the eardrum

N

narcolepsy a condition characterized by brief, sudden attacks of deep sleep

Narcosynthesis (ICD-10-PCS) the root type that identifies the administration of intravenous barbiturates in order to release suppressed or repressed thoughts

National Center for Health Statistics (NCHS) the organization that adapted ICD-10 for use in the United States

National Correct Coding Initiative (NCCI) a set of coding rules published by the Centers for Medicare and Medicaid Services that identifies pairs of codes that normally cannot be reported together; implemented to control improper coding leading to inappropriate payment

national drug codes (NDCs) a code set that identifies the manufacturer, product, and package size of all drugs and biologics recognized by the Food and Drug Administration (FDA)

National Institutes of Health Stroke Scale (NIHSS) a 15-item neurologic examination stroke scale used to evaluate the effect of acute cerebral infarction in several areas: levels of consciousness, language, neglect, visual-field loss, extraocular movement, motor strength, ataxia, dysarthria, and sensory loss

National Uniform Billing Committee (NUBC) the entity that maintains the UB-04 and is chaired by the American Hospital Association, consisting of representatives from more than 15 healthcare industry groups

native (vessel) a patient's original blood vessel

NCCI National Correct Coding Initiative

neck (of bone) area between the proximal epiphysis and the shaft

neck dissection excising lymph nodes and surrounding tissue from the neck during a thyroidectomy

neonatal intensive care unit (NICU) a section of a hospital that treats newborns with serious conditions

neonatal mortality death before 29 days of age

neonate an infant during the first 28 days of life; also called a newborn

neoplasm an abnormal growth of new tissue

neoplastic fracture a fragility fracture due to a neoplastic disease

nephrectomy the partial or complete removal of a kidney

nephritic syndrome a collection of disorders affecting the kidneys, characterized by nonpurulent inflammatory glomerular disorders that allow proteins and red blood cells to pass into the urine, resulting in proteinuria and hematuria (*blood in the urine*)

nephrolithotomy incision of the kidney to remove a calculus

nephron the functioning part of each kidney that filters waste from the blood

nephropathy disease of the kidneys

nephroplasty surgical repair of a kidney

nephroptosis downward placement of a kidney from its normal location

nephrorrhaphy suture of a kidney wound or injury

nephroscopy visual examination of a kidney with an endoscope

nephrostomy the creation of an opening in a kidney with percutaneous catheter insertion, with imaging guidance

nephrostomy catheter a catheter inserted through an existing nephrostomy

nephrotic syndrome a collection of disorders affecting the kidneys, characterized by proteinuria but not hematuria

nephrotomy incision into a kidney

nerve block the introduction or injection of an anesthetic agent

nervous system the body system that directs the body's response to internal and external stimuli and coordinates the activities of other organ systems

neurectomy the excision of a nerve

neurodevelopmental disorder a condition that results from impaired development of the nervous system during infancy or childhood

neuroendoscopy the use of an endoscope to visualize the CNS

neurofibroma a benign tumor of nerve fibers and connective tissue

neuron a cluster of nerve cells

neuropathy a disease of the nerves

neuroplasty any of a variety of surgical procedures to repair or alter a nerve

neuroplegia the paralysis of a nerve

neurostimulator procedures the implantation of electrodes under the skin; the removal or revision of spinal electrodes, plates, or paddles; the insertion, replacement, revision, or removal of a spinal pulse generator or receiver

neurotomy incision into a nerve

neutropenia a decrease in neutrophils

new patient (NP) a patient who has not previously received services from a particular physician or group of physicians in the same specialty or subspecialty

newborn see *neonate*

newborn ABO incompatibility an infant with blood type A or B affected by comingling of blood from a mother with blood type O

newborn apnea a condition in which an infant stops breathing

newborn birth status a code that identifies the location of a birth, the delivery method, and the number of multiples

newborn clinically significant condition a condition of newborns that requires clinical evaluation, therapeutic treatment, diagnostic

procedures, extended length of hospital stay (LOS), and increased nursing care or monitoring or presents implications for future healthcare needs

newborn Rh incompatibility an Rh-positive infant affected by comingling of blood with an Rh-negative mother

NF nursing facility

NIHSS National Institutes of Health Stroke Scale

Nissen fundoplication a procedure in which the upper part of the stomach is wrapped around the lower esophageal sphincter

nonatopic (asthma) asthma that is not due to allergens

nonautologous from a source other than a patient, such as a cadaver or animal

nonbiological a grafted vessel from a synthetic source

nondisplaced (fracture) a traumatic fracture in which the fragments of bone remain properly aligned

nonessential modifier (ICD-10-CM) a word included in the default description of a code and does not need to be present in the medical record in order to use the code

Nonimaging Nuclear Medicine Assay (ICD-10-PCS) the root type that identifies the introduction of radioactive materials into the body for the study of body fluids and blood elements by the detection of radioactive emissions

nonimaging nuclear medicine assay the introduction of radioactive materials into the body for the study of body fluids and blood elements by the detection of radioactive emissions

Nonimaging Nuclear Medicine Probe (ICD-10-PCS) the root type that identifies the introduction of radioactive materials into the body for the study of the distribution and fate of certain substances by the detection of radioactive emissions from an external source

nonimaging nuclear medicine probe the introduction of radioactive materials into the body for the study of the distribution and fate of certain substances by the detection of radioactive emissions from an external source

Nonimaging Nuclear Medicine Uptake (ICD-10-PCS) the root type that identifies the introduction of radioactive materials into the body for measurements of organ function, from the detection of radioactive emissions

nonimaging nuclear medicine uptake the introduction of radioactive materials into the body for measurements of organ function, from the detection of radioactive emissions

nonindwelling (catheter) includes two types of catheters that are not left in the bladder: a condom catheter placed outside the body to catch urine or a straight catheter inserted into the bladder only to drain the urine then removed; also called an external catheter

noninvasive (procedure) a procedure performed without puncturing the skin

nonmosaic Down syndrome the predominant type of Down syndrome, which occurs when there is an extra copy of chromosome 21 in every cell of the body.

nonpressure ulcer a breakdown of skin that is not the result of prolonged pressure

nonselective catheter placement the insertion of a catheter that remains in the accessed vessel or the aorta

non-ST elevation MI (NSTEMI) a myocardial infarction in which the ST segment on an EKG is not elevated, indicating that a vessel is only partially blocked

nontoxic goiter an enlargement of the thyroid that is not associated with overproduction of thyroid hormone or malignancy

nontransmural see *subendocardial (infarction)*

nonunion the failure of the ends of fractured bone segments to reunite

normal birth weight a birth weight of 2,500 grams (5 pounds, 8 ounces) to 4,000 grams (8 pounds, 13 ounces)

normal spontaneous vaginal birth (NSVB) a vaginal delivery without mechanical, pharmacologic, or medical assistance

normal spontaneous vaginal delivery the birth of an infant through the vagina, without the use of drugs or techniques to induce labor, without forceps, vacuum extraction, or cesarean delivery

novel influenza A a class of viruses that normally circulate in animals and may infect humans, such as avian flu and H1N1

NST nonstress test

NSTEMI non-ST elevation myocardial infarction

NSVB normal spontaneous vaginal birth

NUBC National Uniform Billing Committee

nuchal cord the condition of the umbilical cord becoming wrapped around the neck of a fetus

nucleus pulposus a gelatinous substance that comprises the center of a disc and provides cushioning

nursing facility (NF) a residential facility that provides professional medical and nursing care; formerly known as a skilled nursing facility (SNF)

nutritional anemia an anemia due to malabsorption or poor dietary intake of iron, folate, and/or vitamin B_{12}

O

observation extended monitoring that may require an overnight stay but does not meet the requirements for a formal inpatient admission

obstetric history prior pregnancies, complications, and their outcomes

obstructed labor a labor in which the fetus cannot progress into the birth canal, despite adequate uterine contractions, due to a physical blockage

obstructive uropathy the inability of urine to flow

occipitoanterior (OA) the presentation of a fetus in which the back of the baby's head is slightly off center in the pelvis, with the back of the head toward the mother's left thigh

Occlusion (ICD-10-PCS) the root operation that identifies completely closing an orifice or the lumen of a tubular body part

occlusion a blockage

occlusive disease a buildup of plaque or a blood clot

ocular globe the eyeball

ocular implant the insertion of a small sphere into the orbit where the natural eye used to be

OD *oculus dexter* (right eye)

Office of the Inspector General (OIG) a department within the federal government that investigates cases of fraud and imposes monetary penalties on providers who are found guilty

Official Guidelines for Coding and Reporting (OGCR) rules that provide information and direction in identifying the ICD-10-CM diagnoses and ICD-10-PCS procedures to be reported

old (healed) MI an MI more than four weeks old, as defined by ICD-10-CM

olfactory the sense of smell

olive-tip catheter a ureteral catheter with an olive-shaped end, used to dilate a constricted ureter

omental flap the removal of part of the omentum with blood vessel supply intact

omphalitis an infection of the umbilical stump in a newborn, usually presenting as superficial cellulitis

oncologist a physician who specializes in the diagnosis and treatment of tumors

oophorectomy the excision of an ovary

oophoroscopy the visual examination of an ovary

open (fracture) a fracture in which the bone breaks through the skin

Open (ICD-10-PCS) the approach that identifies an incision is made through the skin and subcutaneous tissue

open heart surgery involves exposing the heart through a 30-cm (6- to 8-inch) incision in the chest wall that requires cutting through the sternum

open wound a wound in which the underlying tissue is exposed to the air

operating endoscope a scope equipped with irrigation and suction channels, as well as channels for inserting special instruments, such as biopsy forceps, to obtain tissue samples

operating microscope a specially designed microscope used to assist in the performance of delicate microsurgical procedures, such as operations on the eye, middle ear, or nerve

operative report a detailed narrative description prepared by a physician after completing a procedure, which describes the details of what was done; also called a procedure report

opportunistic infection a disease that attacks those with weakened immune systems but does not develop in those with healthy immune systems

OPPS outpatient prospective payment system

optic nerve cranial nerve II

optional surgery a type of surgery that provides a personal benefit but provides no medical benefit, such as a cosmetic face lift or breast augmentation; rarely covered by insurance

oral pertaining to the mouth

orbital cavity the bony structure around the eye, commonly known as the eye socket

orbital implant the insertion of glass, plastic, or acrylic under an ocular implant

orbital tumor a benign or malignant tumor in the eye socket or tissues that surround the eyeball; sometimes originates from the surrounding paranasal sinuses, brain, or nasal cavity

orifice an opening

origin the point at which a muscle is attached

Original Medicare hospital insurance that covers a specific list of services for inpatient hospital care, skilled nursing facilities, hospice, and home healthcare; also called Part A

orthosis an orthopedic appliance or apparatus used to support, align, prevent, or correct deformities or to improve the function of movable parts of the body

OS *oculus sinister* (left eye)

osseointegrated implant a hearing implant that is integrated with bone

osseous pertaining to a bone

ossicles a part of the middle ear that amplifies vibrations and transmits them to the inner ear

osteoarthritis an inflammation of a bone and joint

osteoporosis the thinning of bone tissue and loss of bone density

osteoporotic fracture a fragility fracture in a person with osteoporosis

osteosarcoma a malignant tumor in a bone

ostomy an artificial opening between a hollow organ and the skin

other fracture a fragility fracture caused by a disease other than osteoporosis or neoplasm; any other type of pathological fracture

Other Procedures (ICD-10-PCS) the root operation that identifies methodologies that attempt to remediate or cure a disorder or disease

Other Radiation (ICD-10-PCS) the Modality that identifies radiation therapy modalities not otherwise identified

otitis media (OM) an infection of the middle ear

otorhinolaryngological pertaining to the ear, nose, and throat

OU *oculus uterque* (each eye)

outpatient encounter an interaction with a patient who has not been formally admitted to a healthcare institution

outpatient prospective payment system (OPPS) Medicare's payment system for outpatient hospitals, which pays a set amount for a service or procedure based on a specific classification

oval window a thin membrane that covers the opening to the inner ear and passes vibrations to the cochlea

ovary the gland in which eggs are produced in females

overcoding coding for a more complex diagnosis or procedure than is documented

overlapping lesion contiguous sites where a tumor continues from one site to an adjacent one without interruption

P

pacemaker a small electronic device that is implanted in the chest to correct arrhythmia by speeding up, slowing down, smoothing out, or coordinating the heartbeat

pacemaker insertion placement under the skin of the chest or abdomen of a small device with wires connected to the heart chambers that transmit low-energy electrical pulses to control heart rhythm

Packing (ICD-10-PCS) the root operation that identifies putting material in a body region or orifice

packing putting material in a body region or orifice

PACU postoperative anesthesia care unit

PAD peripheral artery disease

pancreatectomy the surgical removal of all or part of the pancreas

pancreaticoduodenectomy the surgical removal of parts of the pancreas, duodenum, common bile duct, and, if required, portions of the stomach

pancreatitis inflammation of the pancreas

pancytopenia an abnormal reduction in the number of all types of blood cells: red, white, and platelets

pandemic a disease outbreak that spreads to multiple continents

papilla a small vascular protrusion of connective tissue or skin

papulosquamous disorders papules and scales

para (P) the number of pregnancies resulting in a fetus of viable gestational age (20 weeks), regardless of whether the fetus was alive at birth

paracentesis a surgical puncture of a body cavity to remove ascites

paraesophageal hernia repair a procedure in which the diaphragm is repaired using sutures or mesh; part of the stomach may be wrapped around the esophagus

paranasal sinus an air-filled chamber, or space, inside the skull and face bones; also called accessory sinus

paranoia a mental condition of delusions of persecution

parasite a plant or animal that lives in or on another living organism, or host, and often causes damage to the host; also called helminth

parathyroid autotransplantation the surgical removal of the four parathyroid glands and their transplantation into a muscle in the neck or forearm

parathyroidectomy the surgical removal of all or part of the parathyroid glands

paravaginal adjacent to the vagina or part of the vagina

parent code a code whose description is left-justified and begins with a capital letter; also called standalone code

parenteral nutrition providing nutrients intravenously because the body is unable to take in nutrients orally or by other methods

parietal pericardium the outer layer of the pericardium

paring the use of a scalpel, blade, or curette to scrape away tissue; also referred to as cutting or curettement

Parkinson's disease (PD) a degenerative disease that affects muscle control and coordination, usually occurring in midlife

parkinsonian see *parkinsonism*

parkinsonism a combination of conditions in which dementia is diagnosed first, followed later by an additional diagnosis of Parkinson's disease; also called parkinsonian dementia

Part A (Medicare) hospital insurance that covers a specific list of services for inpatient hospital care, skilled nursing facilities, hospice, and home healthcare; also called Original Medicare

Part B (Medicare) the portion of Medicare that covers a specific list of physician services, outpatient hospital care, and home healthcare

Part C (Medicare) an optional replacement of Part A and Part B that is offered by private health insurance companies; also called Medicare Advantage

Part D (Medicare) prescription drug coverage offered by private insurance companies through contracts with Medicare; provides limited benefits for prescription drugs

partial (seizure) see *focal (seizure)*

partial mastectomy (lumpectomy, tylectomy) the removal of only enough breast tissue to ensure that the margins of the specimen are free of malignant cells

partial-thickness burn a burn that causes damage to the epidermis and part of the dermis

partial thyroid lobectomy the excision of less than two-thirds of one lobe of the thyroid gland

partum birth

parturition see *childbirth*

past, family, and social history (PFSH) a review of a patient's past experience with illness, injury, treatment, and operations; a review of a patient's family's medical history; and a review of a patient's social history, including current and past activities

patch testing applying an allergen to the skin to observe the reaction

patent foramen ovale an opening in the septum between the two atria of the heart

pathologic fracture a fracture caused by disease rather than trauma

pathologist a physician who studies and identifies diseases through laboratory analysis

pathology the study of the abnormal

patient type describes whether the patient is new or established

patient-controlled analgesia (PCA) a method of pain control that patients can administer in response to the level of pain experienced

payers insurance companies or public programs that pay for healthcare services

PBT proton beam treatment

PCA patient-controlled analgesia

PCS Procedure Coding System; used in this text as shorthand for ICD-10-PCS

PCS OGCR PCS Official Guidelines for Coding and Reporting

PD Parkinson's disease; peritoneal dialysis

PE physical examination

pedicle flap a skin transfer in which a flap of skin and subcutaneous is separated and moved to cover a nearby damaged area while the original blood vessels and nerves remain connected to the original site

PEG percutaneous endoscopic gastrostomy

pelvic exenteration excision of the bladder, urethra, ureters, lymph nodes, prostate/vagina, uterus, colon, and rectum; may also include a hysterectomy and resecting the rectum and colon

pelvic girdle pain (PGP) a pain at the back of the pelvis

pelvic inflammatory disease (PID) inflammation of the female reproductive tract above the cervix

pemphigus an autoimmune disease that erupts in blisters

penetrating keratoplasty (PKP) the removal of the entire cornea and transplantation of a full-thickness cornea

penetrating wound see *puncture wound*

penile in or through the penis

penis the external male organ that carries urine and semen out of the body

perceptual disturbance the misinterpretation of surroundings or events

Percutaneous (ICD-10-PCS) the approach that identifies the skin is punctured or a very small incision is made to access a site, but a full-length incision is not made

Percutaneous Endoscopic (ICD-10-PCS) the approach that identifies a surgeon makes several, usually two to four, small incisions, approximately one-half to one inch in length, and accesses the operative site with an endoscope

percutaneous endoscopic gastrostomy (PEG) a procedure in which a tube is passed into a patient's stomach through the abdominal wall

percutaneous umbilical blood sampling (PUBS) see *cordocentesis*

Pereyra procedure elevation of the bladder by attaching it to abdominal fascia

perforation the cutting or puncturing of the wall or membrane of an internal organ or structure

Performance (ICD-10-PCS) the root operation that identifies completely taking over a physiological function by extracorporeal means

performance completely taking over a physiological function by extracorporeal means

pericarditis an inflammation of the pericardial sac that surrounds the heart

pericardium a double-walled sac filled with fluid, which is the outer layer

perinatal relating to the time period before birth that continues through the 28th day following birth

perinatal condition a condition that develops before birth or during the first 28 days after birth, but excludes malformations, deformations, and chromosomal abnormalities

perinatal period the time before birth that continues through the 28th day following birth

perineal surrounding the perineum

perineoplasty repair of the tissues of the perineum

perineum the area between the anus and external genitalia

peripartum the period comprising the last month of pregnancy to five months' postpartum

peripheral artery disease the damage to arteries outside the heart resulting in decreased blood flow to the limbs

peripheral nervous system (PNS) consists of the 12 nerves that radiate out from the brain and the 31 pairs of nerves that radiate from the spinal cord to all other areas of the body

periprosthetic capsulectomy the removal of a breast implant and the entire contracture capsule surrounding the breast implant

perirenal relating to tissues surrounding the kidney

peritoneal dialysis (PD) a type of dialysis in which the peritoneal membrane is used to filter the blood

peritoneal membrane the lining of the abdomen

permanent national code a code that all U.S. providers and insurances can use for billing and statistical purposes

pernicious anemia an anemia due to insufficient absorption of vitamin B_{12}

personal history a condition a patient had in the past, was removed or resolved, and is no longer being treated, but has the potential for recurrence and therefore may require continued monitoring

personal injury protection (PIP) a payment made by automobile insurance policies to pay for medical expenses incurred during an automobile accident

personality disorder persistent, inflexible patterns of behavior that affect interpersonal relationships

pessary insertion/fitting the evaluation and placement of a rubber, silicone, or plastic device into the vagina to support surrounding structures

PET positron emission tomography

petit mal (seizure) a type of seizure characterized by muscle twitching or jerking for several seconds

petrous apicectomy excision of the petrous, including radical resection of the entire mastoid part of the posterior temporal bone

PFSH past, family, and social history

phacoemulsification destruction, usually with ultrasound, of a natural lens, which is then suctioned out of the eye

pharmacoresistant resistant to medication

Pharmacotherapy (ICD-10-PCS) the root type that identifies the use of replacement medications for the treatment of addiction

pharyngitis sore throat; inflammation of the throat

pharynx the throat

Pheresis (ICD-10-PCS) the root operation that identifies extracorporeal separation of blood products

pheresis extracorporeal separation of blood products

photochemotherapy treatment using drugs and light

photocoagulation the use of a laser to seal tears

Phototherapy (ICD-10-PCS) the root operation that identifies extracorporeal treatment by light rays

phototherapy extracorporeal treatment by light rays

physical examination (PE) a hands-on evaluation of a patient's vital signs, physical functions, and organ systems relevant to the chief complaint

physical status score a value that identifies a patient's health status at the time anesthesia begins, on a scale of 1 through 5

physical therapy noninvasive treatment to correct a musculoskeletal problem

physician office an outpatient clinic at which physicians evaluate and manage new or existing health problems and provide preventive care services

physician office laboratory (POL) a physician office that performs a limited number of laboratory tests in the office

physis the growth plate near the end of a long bone

pigmentation disorder damage to unhealthy melanin cells that give color to the skin

PIH pregnancy-induced hypertension

pinna the visible part of the ear, which collects sound waves; also called auricle

pituitary tumor an abnormal growth in the pituitary gland that is usually benign

pityriasis rough, dry scales

PKP penetrating keratoplasty

place of occurrence (ICD-10-CM) a category of external cause codes that describe where an injury occurred, such as a public street or a single-family home

place of service (POS) the location of the facility where a physician provides an evaluation and management service, such as an office, hospital, or nursing facility

placenta the organ that allows for the exchange of oxygen, nutrients, and waste between the fetus and mother

placenta previa a condition in which the placenta partially or fully covers the cervix, posing a risk that it may separate from the wall of the uterus during labor

placental infarction a scarring of the placenta due to an inadequate blood supply

Plain Radiography (ICD-10-PCS) the root type that identifies the planar (flat, single plane) display of an image developed from the capture of external ionizing radiation on a photographic or photoconductive plate

plain radiography the planar (flat, single plane) display of an image developed from the capture of external ionizing radiation on a photographic or photoconductive plate

plan the treatment that was or will be provided to address a patient's symptoms

Planar Nuclear Medicine Imaging (ICD-10-PCS) the root type that identifies the introduction of radioactive materials into the body for single-plane display of images developed from the capture of radioactive emissions

planar nuclear medicine imaging the introduction of radioactive materials into the body for single-plane display of images developed from the capture of radioactive emissions

plaque a buildup of cholesterol inside the wall of blood vessels

plasma clear fluid

plastic repair introitus restoration of the vaginal opening to its original size

plethysmography recording of volume

pleuracentesis the withdrawal of fluid from the pleural cavity/thoracic cavity

pleural effusion an abnormal amount of fluid around the lung

pleural tap the withdrawal of air or fluid from the pleural space using a needle or tube

pleurisy inflammation of the lining of the lungs and thoracic cavity with oozing of fluid or fibrinous material into the pleural cavity

pleurodesis the use of an irritant to create inflammation within the pleural space to cause the two pleura to adhere together

pleurotomy an incision into the pleural cavity/thoracic cavity

pneumocentesis the withdrawal of fluid from a lung

pneumoconiosis an abnormal condition of the lung caused by the inhalation of dust particles, such as coal dust (anthracosis), asbestos (asbestosis), iron dust (siderosis), or quartz (silicosis)

pneumonectomy the surgical excision of an entire lung

pneumonia an inflammatory condition of the lung in which the alveoli and air spaces fill with fluid; caused by a bacteria, virus, fungus, or chemical irritant

pneumonolysis the separation of the parietal pleura from the fascia of the chest wall

pneumothorax a collection of air between the chest wall and lungs, which may cause the lung to collapse

pneumotomy an incision into the lung

PNS peripheral nervous system

poisoning the improper use of a substance that causes an undesired physical response

polycystic kidney disease a condition in which numerous cysts occupy much of the kidney tissue

polycythemia an abnormal increase in the number of circulating red blood cells

polydactyly the presence of many fingers or toes

polynephritis an acute or chronic infection of the renal medulla and upper urinary tract as a result of untreated cystitis; also called pyelonephritis

polypectomy the surgical removal of a polyp(s)

polysomnography multiple recordings of sleep

POS place of service

position (patient) the position in which a patient is arranged for surgery (e.g., supine, dorsal recumbent, prone)

Positron Emission Tomography (PET) (ICD-10-PCS) the root type that identifies the introduction of radioactive materials into the body for three-dimensional display of images developed from the simultaneous capture, 180 degrees apart, of radioactive emissions

positron emission tomography (PET) the introduction of radioactive materials into the body for three-dimensional display of images developed from the simultaneous capture, 180 degrees apart, of radioactive emissions

postauricular behind the ear

posteroanterior from back to front

postnatal after birth

postoperative anesthesia care unit (PACU) an area where a patient is taken after surgery is complete to recover from the surgical procedure and the effects of anesthesia

postpartum see *puerperium*

postpartum depression a moderate to severe depression after giving birth

postpartum hemorrhage (PPH) an excessive amount of bleeding following delivery

postpartum psychosis the sudden dramatic onset of psychotic symptoms after giving birth, often occurring in patients with bipolar disorder

postpartum wound infection a bacterial infection of a cesarean delivery wound

postprocedural bleeding bleeding that occurs after a surgical procedure; also called postoperative bleeding or hemorrhage

postterm pregnancy a pregnancy with between 40 and 42 completed weeks of gestation

PPH postpartum hemorrhage

PPMP provider-performed microscopy procedure

PPS prospective payment system

Prader-Willi syndrome a genetic disorder due to a deletion of paternal chromosome 15; characterized by short stature, mental retardation, muscle weakness, abnormally small hands and feet, nonfunctioning gonads, and uncontrolled appetite, leading to extreme obesity

preauthorization prior authorization or approval of elective surgery by an insurance company

precerebral located outside of the brain

prediabetes a condition in which blood glucose concentrations are higher than normal but not yet high enough to be diagnosed as diabetes

preeclampsia a metabolic disorder of pregnancy that develops after the 20th week and involves gestational hypertension and proteinuria

preexisting diabetes diabetes that is diagnosed in a woman before she becomes pregnant

preexisting hypertension hypertension that is diagnosed in a woman before she becomes pregnant

preferred provider an exclusive network of private health insurance companies and self-insured plans

pregnancy a normal, temporary condition that occurs in the female body, beginning at the time of conception and ending with the birth of a fetus

pregnancy-induced hypertension (PIH) see *gestational hypertension*

premature rupture of membranes (PROM) the rupture of the amniotic sac and chorion more than an hour before the onset of labor; may also be called prelabor rupture of membranes

prenatal the time period from conception to the beginning of labor; also called the prepartum, antepartum, or antenatal period

prepartum see *prenatal*

prepayment edit a set of claims processing rules in which claims are electronically scanned for compliance before the payer accepts them into the claims processing system

present on admission (POA) an alphabetic indictor listed on the UC-04 or 837I claim to identify whether a particular diagnosis was present at the time of an inpatient admission

presumptive drug class screening a qualitative test that identifies the possible use or nonuse of a drug or drug class

preterm pregnancy, delivery, or labor a pregnancy with less than 37 completed weeks of gestation

primary (malignant neoplasm) a tumor in which malignant cells break through the epithelial membrane into an organ

primary intention healing wound closure performed with sutures, staples, or adhesive tape or glue

principal diagnosis as defined by the Uniform Hospital Data Discharge Set (UHDDS), the "condition established after study to be chiefly responsible for occasioning the admission of the patient to the hospital for care"

principal procedure a procedure that was performed for definitive treatment most related to the principal diagnosis, rather than one performed for diagnostic or exploratory purposes, or was necessary to take care of a complication

private health insurance coverage for healthcare services offered by private corporations

procedure a service that healthcare professionals provide to patients

procedure report a report prepared by a physician after completing a procedure that describes the details of what was done; also called an operative report

process a nodule or projection of a bone

productive cough a cough with sputum

products of conception encompasses all components of pregnancy, including the embryo, fetus, amnion, placenta, and umbilical cord

professional component part of a radiology code; covers the cost of a radiologist supervising a technician and interpreting the results

prognosis future knowledge; the expected course of the disease

progress note the record of a specific patient encounter

prolonged pregnancy a pregnancy with more than 42 completed weeks of gestation

PROM premature rupture of membranes

promoting interoperability (PI) program a program under which eligible Medicare and Medicaid providers can receive payments when they adopt, implement, or upgrade certified EHR technology (CEHRT); formerly called meaningful use

prompt pay a law that requires insurance companies to process claims within a specific period of time, such as 30 or 45 days

prophylactic prevention of the spread of disease or infection

prospective payment system (PPS) a standard payment rate is predetermined based on the average amount of staff, supplies, and other resources typically used and assigned to each DRG

prostate the part of the male genital system that secretes fluid to nourish the sperm

prostate-specific antigen (PSA) a blood test used to screen for prostate cancer

prostatectomy removal of the prostate gland, including possible biopsy or removal of the lymph nodes

prostatic intraepithelial neoplasia (PIN) neoplastic changes in the epithelial cells of the prostate ducts showing some features of cancer, but is not invasive; a potential precursor of carcinoma or adenocarcinoma

prostatomy an incision into the prostate

prosthesis an artificial substitute for a missing body part

prosthetic catheter a urethral catheter with a sharp bend near the intake; used to navigate past obstructions in the urinary tract; also called elbowed catheter

protection helps prevent invasion by pathogens, mechanical harm, and loss of fluids and electrolytes

proteinemia protein in the blood

proteinuria protein in the urine

proton beam treatment (PBT) delivery the use of noninvasive electromagnetic radiation to treat both in situ benign and malignant tumors

protozoa one-celled organisms, more complex than bacteria, that use other living things as a source of food and a place to live

provider-performed microscopy procedure (PPMP) moderate-complexity tests that require use of a microscope

proximal toward the center of the body

proximal epiphysis the rounded end of a bone that is closest to the trunk

Pseudomonas aeruginosa (P. aeruginosa) the most common Gram-negative bacterium that can cause disease in humans and animals

psoriasis round, red patches covered with white scales

psychiatric diagnostic interview an interview with a patient whereby the provider assesses the patient's mental status by reviewing the patient's medical history, asking the patient a series of questions, and communicating with family members and other providers involved in the patient's care to determine the patient's diagnosis

psychoactive substance a substance that has the ability to alter behavior, impair judgment, or create medical problems

Psychological Tests (ICD-10-PCS) the root type that identifies the administration and interpretation of standardized psychological tests and measurement instruments for the assessment of psychological function

psychometry measurement/testing of the mind

psychomotor (seizure) see *complex partial (seizure)*

psychotherapy a method of using nonphysical techniques, such as talking, interpreting, listening, rewarding, and role playing, to treat disorders

psychotic disorders delusions and hallucinations

public health lab a lab operated by state and local health departments to diagnose disease and protect the public from health threats, such as outbreaks of infectious diseases and environmental hazards

PUBS percutaneous umbilical blood sampling

puerperal see *puerperium*

puerperal mastitis the inflammation or infection of the mammary gland in the breast during the postpartum period

puerperium the six-week period following childbirth in which the female reproductive organs return to the prepregnant state; also called puerperal or postpartum

pull-through process whereby a surgeon removes the diseased portion of an organ and connects the healthy segment to the adjacent organ

pulmonary circulation occurs between the heart and the lungs; carries deoxygenated blood from the heart to the lungs, where it is replenished with oxygen, then back to the heart

pulmonary edema an abnormal accumulation of fluid in the lungs, especially the alveoli, resulting in dyspnea

pulmonary function test a diagnostic test that measures air flow into and out of the lungs, lung volumes, and gas exchange between the lungs and blood

pulmonary valve the valve that controls the blood flow from the right ventricle to the pulmonary artery

punch biopsy a tissue sample obtained with a punch tool to remove a full-thickness cylindrical tissue sample

puncture wound a wound caused by a sharply pointed object passing through the skin into the underlying tissues; also called penetrating wound

pupil the opening in the iris that dilates and constricts

Purkinje fiber the cardiac muscle that rapidly transmits impulses from the atrioventricular node to the ventricles

purpura small hemorrhages in the skin

purulent otitis media an infection of the middle ear, usually bacterial, involving the discharge of pus

push technique a one-time, rapid injection of medication into the bloodstream

pyelonephritis the acute or chronic infection of the renal medulla and upper urinary tract as a result of untreated cystitis; also called polynephritis

pyeloplasty repair of the renal pelvis

pyelotomy an incision into the renal pelvis

pyogenic arthritis an infectious arthritis in which pus is formed during the disease process

pyothorax pus in the chest

Q

quadriplegia paralysis of all limbs

qualified a diagnosis that is limited or uncertain

qualifier (ICD-10-PCS) Character 7 in an ICD-10-PCS code; describes additional information about the procedure

qualifier a word that limits the meaning of another

qualitative test a test performed to detect the presence of a substance in a specimen

query a written communication asking for clarification and/or additional details

Qui Tam a provision of the FCA that mandates a financial reward to whistleblowers, those who turn in violators

R

RAC Recovery Audit Contractor

radial keratotomy the flattening of the cornea by making a series of incisions in a radial pattern, resembling the spokes of a wheel

radiation disorders damage to the skin resulting from exposure to radiation

radiation oncologist a physician who provides cancer treatment through radiation

radical lymphadenectomy removal of lymph nodes and nearby structures

radical mastectomy removal of the breast, pectoralis major and minor muscles, axillary lymph nodes, and associated skin and subcutaneous tissue

radical mastoidectomy removal of the entire mastoid, tympanum, middle ear, and possibly the mastoid part of the posterior temporal bone

radiologic guidance use of a radiological modality to visualize access to an anatomic site in real time; also called guided imagery

radiology technician a nonphysician staff member who is trained to operate and adjust imaging equipment, explain procedures to patients and answer questions, position patients for imaging, and ensure that a patient's exposure to radiation is limited

radiolucent permits x-rays to pass into and through it, resulting in a darker, shadowy image that shows layers within a structure

radiopaque allows few x-rays to pass through; shows up as a light (white) image using plain radiography and provides a two-dimensional image of the surface

radiopharmaceutical a radioactive material used for therapeutic or diagnostic purposes

radiosurgery a form of radiation therapy that focuses high-power energy on a small area of the body (e.g., Cyberknife, Gamma Knife)

radiotherapy treatment with radiation

rapid strep test (RST) a strep test that produces results within 10–20 minutes

RBRVS resource-based relative value scale

RDS respiratory distress syndrome

real-time scan a rapid succession of B-mode images producing a moving video; a two-dimensional ultrasonic scan, with displays of both two-dimensional structures and motion with time

Reattachment (ICD-10-PCS) the root operation that identifies putting back in or on all or a portion of a separated body part to its normal location or other suitable location

recession cutting muscle from the surface of the eye and reattaching it farther back from the front of the eye to weaken or lengthen the muscle

reconcile comparison of the EOB to the original bill to verify that each service billed was paid in the amount expected

reconstruction a procedure whereby original tissue is replaced with grafted tissue to create a new structure

reconstructive relating to restoring normal function or appearance

recording creating an image of a structure or process

Recovery Audit Contractor (RAC) uses independent contractors to identify improper Medicare payments to healthcare providers and suppliers made on claims of healthcare services provided to Medicare beneficiaries

reducible a hernia that can be corrected by a physician by pushing the tissue back into place

reduction the realignment of bone fragments or segments; also called manipulation

reference lab see *independent clinical lab*

reference range numeric range of typical results in the average population and the levels considered to be high or low, determined by the statistic calculation of two standard deviations

referring physician a provider who requests a consultation for a patient with another physician

reflex sympathetic dystrophy (RSD) a chronic pain syndrome in which an extremity experiences intense burning pain and changes in skin texture and temperature

reflux nephropathy a disease of the kidneys that results from a backward flow of urine into the kidneys

refractory resistant to treatment

regional anesthesia epidural, spinal, and peripheral nerve blocks; blocks pain in an area of the body, such as an arm or leg, and patient feels nothing in that area of the body

regulation the body function that increases and decreases body temperature through constriction and dilation of blood vessels and sweat glands

regurgitation the backward leakage of blood through the opening of the left atrium

rejected claim a claim that is not accepted into an insurance company's computer system for processing due to missing or invalid data

relapse the return of disease after remission

related a symptom, finding, or sign that is connected to a disease but is not routinely associated with it

relative value unit (RVU) a value that identifies the amount of work and expense involved in providing a particular service

Release (ICD-10-PCS) the root operation that identifies freeing a body part from an abnormal physical constraint by cutting or by the use of force

release a type of soft-tissue repair/reconstruction whereby the tissue is freed from surrounding adhesions so that it can move freely within the tendon sheath

relevant as defined by UHDDS, "all conditions that coexist at the time of admission, that develop subsequently, or that affect the treatment received and/or the length of stay. Diagnoses that relate to an earlier episode which have no bearing on the current hospital stay are to be excluded."

remission blood counts return to normal and bone marrow samples show no sign of disease

remittance advice (RA) a statement that lists all the services the provider billed, which ones were accepted for payment, how much the insurance company will pay, how much the patient owes, and how much will not be paid

Removal (ICD-10-PCS) the root operation that identifies taking out or off a device from a body part

renal pertaining to the kidney

renal endoscopy endoscopy through an established nephrostomy, pyelostomy, nephrotomy, or pyelotomy

renal pelvis the portion of a kidney where urine collects

renal transplant the implantation of a cadaver or living donor kidney to take over the function of a patient's natural kidney

Repair (ICD-10-PCS) the root operation that identifies restoring, to the extent possible, a body part to its normal anatomic structure and function

repair a procedure whereby torn or damaged tissue, such as a muscle, is sewn together

repair of oval window or round window closure of an opening with soft tissue such as fat or fascia

repeat cesarean performing a cesarean delivery for a mother who had a cesarean delivery with a previous pregnancy

Replacement (ICD-10-PCS) the root operation that identifies putting in or on biological or synthetic material that physically takes the place and/or function of all or a portion of a body part

replantation the reattachment of an amputated body member

Reposition (ICD-10-PCS) the root operation that identifies moving to its normal location, or other suitable location, all or a portion of a body part

reproductive duct a part of the internal genital organs of the male reproductive system

Resection (ICD-10-PCS) the root operation that identifies cutting out or off without replacement all of a body part

resequenced code (CPT) a code that does not appear in numerical order; identified with the symbol #

reservoir/pump implantation the replacement, implantation, or removal of a subcutaneous reservoir or pump; electronic analysis of programmable implanted pump

resource-based relative value scale (RBRVS) the scale used by Medicare to establish physician reimbursement rates, which are published in the Medicare Physician Fee Schedule (MPFS)

respiratory distress syndrome (RDS) a condition in which the alveolar sacs collapse due to lack of surfactant

respiratory system the system that obtains oxygen from the air and delivers it to the lungs and blood for distribution to tissue cells and removes the gaseous waste product carbon dioxide from the blood and lungs and expels it

Restoration (ICD-10-PCS) the root operation that identifies returning, or attempting to return, a physiological function to its original state by extracorporeal means

restoration returning, or attempting to return, a physiological function to its original state by extracorporeal means

Restriction (ICD-10-PCS) the root operation that identifies partially closing an orifice or the lumen of a tubular body part

retina the innermost layer that contains sensory receptor cells

retinal pertaining to the retina

retinal detachment the separation of the retina from the choroid layer of the eye

retinopathy of prematurity (ROP) the abnormal growth of blood vessels in the eye that can lead to vision loss

retroperitoneal behind the peritoneal membrane that covers the abdominal and pelvic organs

retropubic behind the pubic bone

revascularization the restoration of flow to the coronary vessels that have been obstructed, usually due to occlusive disease

revenue code a four-digit code reported on the UB-04 that identifies a general category of service, such as accommodation, type of ancillary service, pharmacy, or supplies

review of systems (ROS) a list of questions, arranged by organ system, used by physicians to complete a system-by-system review of body functions with a patient

Revision (ICD-10-PCS) the root operation that identifies correcting, to the extent possible, a portion of a malfunctioning device or the position of a displaced device

revision mastoidectomy a total mastoidectomy following a previous mastoidectomy that failed to resolve a patient's condition

Rhesus (Rh) incompatibility a condition in which the mother is Rh negative and develops antibodies against a fetus who is Rh positive

rhinoplasty (primary) surgical repair of the nose

rhinoplasty (secondary) a second rhinoplasty that may be more complex than the primary one, including grafts of cartilage, bone, or tissue to reconstruct the nose or repair the nasal septum

rhizotomy interruption of a cranial or spinal nerve root

right atrium the right upper chamber of the heart, which receives blood from the body

right ventricle the right lower chamber of the heart, which ejects blood to the lungs

rigid endoscope an instrument used for endoscopy procedures that consists of a hard tube with a series of prisms and lenses that reflect the image

rod a light-sensitive receptor cell in the retina

root operation Character 3 of an ICD-10-PCS code; defines the objective of a procedure

ROP retinopathy of prematurity

ROS review of systems

rotational deformity an abnormal position of the femur or tibia

Roux-en-Y (RNY) a procedure in which the stomach and small bowel are joined using an end-to-side anastomosis

RSD reflex sympathetic dystrophy

RST rapid strep test

RTO return to office

Rule of Nines the division of the body into areas, each of which comprises 9% of the total body surface area

RVU relative value unit

S

SA sinoatrial

saccule a membranous pouch containing serum fluid of the inner ear

salpingectomy excision of a fallopian tube

salpingoscopy visual examination of a fallopian tube

salpingostomy the surgical creation of an opening in a fallopian tube to restore its patency

Salter-Harris classification a system that classifies epiphysis fractures to identify involvement of the growth plate and estimate the prognosis and potential for growth disturbance

sarcoidosis the formation of nodules in the lymph nodes, lungs, bone, and skin

SCC squamous cell carcinoma

schizoaffective disorder a condition characterized by an extended period in which schizophrenia is accompanied by major depressive, manic, or mixed episodes

schizoid of childhood a condition characterized by severe and sustained impairment in social interactions and restricted, repetitive patterns of behaviors, interests, and activities; also called Asperger's disease/syndrome

schizoid personality disorder a condition characterized by a persistent withdrawal from social relationships and lack of emotional responsiveness in most situations

schizophrenia a condition characterized by the inability to distinguish between thoughts and reality, think logically, and have normal emotional and social relationships

schizophreniform disorder a condition that is identical to schizophrenia except that the total duration is greater than one month but less than six months; impaired social or occupational functioning may not be apparent

schizothymia a tendency toward being severely introverted

schizotypal personality disorder a condition characterized by trouble with relationships and disturbances in thought patterns, appearance, and behavior

sclera the tough, white outer layer of the eyeball

screening procedure a procedure performed to determine whether an abnormality exists in a person showing no signs or symptoms of disease

sebaceous pertaining to oil

second trimester the time in a pregnancy when the gestational age is between 14 weeks, 0 days and 28 weeks, 0 days

secondary (malignant neoplasm) the site or metastasis where a neoplasm spreads to

secondary diabetes mellitus a condition in which glucose concentrations are elevated due to an external factor, such as medication, surgery, pancreatic disease, or other illness

secondary diagnosis any diagnosis that is not the principal or first-listed; also called additional diagnosis

secondary intention healing an extended process in which a wound is not closed with sutures but left open to granulate

secondary parkinsonism Parkinson-type abnormal movements that are caused by medication or another condition

secondary thyroidectomy a second operation to excise remaining thyroid tissue following a previous thyroidectomy; also called complete thyroidectomy

secretion the release of perspiration to control temperature and sebum to protect from dehydration and penetration by harmful substances

section (CPT) the first level of classification of CPT Category I codes

Section (ICD-10-PCS) Character 1 in an ICD-10-PCS code; defines the broad procedure category in which the code is found

segmentectomy the surgical excision of tissue from part of one lobe of a lung; also called wedge excision

selective catheter placement inserting a catheter into a vessel, moving it to the aorta, then moving it through one or more arteries that branch off the aorta to reach a specific vessel needing treatment

self-insured health plan a plan offered by large employers or unions who, rather than purchasing group health insurance, set aside money in a reserve fund and pay for employees' medical expenses from the fund

semen fluid containing sperm

semicircular canal the superior, posterior, and inferior canals in the ear that contain endolymph

semicolon (CPT) a convention used in the CPT manual to conserve space and avoid having to repeat common terminology

sensation contains sensory receptors for pain, touch, heat, cold, and pressure

sentinel lymph node the first node or group of nodes in a chain

septoplasty surgical repair of the nasal septum, with or without cartilage scoring (incising), contouring, or replacement with graft

sequela (ICD-10-CM) a late effect or problem after active healing is completed

sequela episode of care identifies an encounter at which a patient is treated for a complication after the healing phase is complete

sequence the placement of codes in the order dictated by the guidelines and instructional notes

serology a blood test used to diagnose diseases

serum assay a lab test that measures the presence and quantity of a substance in the blood

setting the location where a service is provided, such as office/outpatient, hospital, emergency department, or nursing facility; also called place of service

sexual disorder repetitive and prolonged sexual dysfunction that interferes with normal relationships or daily activities

SGA small for gestational age

shaft the long, narrow part of a bone

shaving use of a sharp instrument

Shock Wave Therapy (ICD-10-PCS) the root operation that identifies extracorporeal treatment by shock waves

shock wave therapy extracorporeal treatment by shock waves

Shone's syndrome a set of four congenital heart defects: a supravalve mitral membrane, parachute mitral valve, subaortic stenosis, and coarctation of the aorta

sialogram a record or picture of the salivary duct

sialography the process of recording the salivary duct

sialolithotomy a procedure in which calculus is removed from the salivary gland(s)

sickle cell anemia a genetic disorder in which red blood cells take on a sickle shape and lead to hemolytic anemia

sickle cell crisis pain caused because blood vessels have become blocked or defective red blood cells damage organs in the body

sign objective evidence of a disease or condition that can be observed by a physician

significant procedure a procedure that is surgical in nature, carries a procedural risk, carries an anesthetic risk, or requires specialized training

SIL squamous intraepithelial lesion

simple complete mastectomy the removal of only breast tissue, the nipple, and a small portion of the overlying skin; also called simple mastectomy and total mastectomy

simple mastoidectomy incision into the mastoid with dissection of the mastoid process; also called transmastoid antrotomy

simple partial (seizure) a seizure that affects only a small region of the brain and does not cause loss of consciousness

single-photon emission computed tomography (SPECT) the use of photons emitted by a radioactive tracer to create an image of lower quality than PET

single quantity a code for which one unit is reported for each service performed

singleton a pregnancy with one fetus

sinoatrial (SA) node the pacemaker of the heart

sinusitis sinus infection

SIRS systemic inflammatory response syndrome

site of origin the anatomic site where a growth begins

skeletal system the system that supports the body, protects internal organs, produces blood cells, stores minerals, and serves as a point of attachment for the skeletal muscles

skeletal traction placing pins and/or wires through broken bones and connecting them to stirrups, ropes, pulleys, and weights outside the body to secure bones in place until they heal

skin appendages nails, hair, sweat glands

skin replacement the use of skin from the patient's own body or a donor to replace damaged skin that cannot be repaired with sutures alone

skin substitute the use of synthetic material to replace damaged skin

skull traction applying cranial tongs or calipers to the head and attaching them to ropes and weights on the outside, which secure the spine in place

sleeping disorder an abnormal sleep problem

small-bowel transplant the surgical removal of a diseased small intestine and replacement with some or all of a small intestine from a healthy person

small for gestational age (SGA) a fetus or newborn infant who is smaller in size than normal for the baby's sex and gestational age

smallpox an infectious disease with the last known case in 1977

social history education, occupation, religious affiliation, natural support network, lifestyle

habits (e.g., tobacco use, alcohol use, illicit drug use, sexual activity)

solid matter (PCS) a non-native solid that may result from biological processes, such as calculi or a clot, or may be a nonbiological solid, such as a foreign body

somatoform a physical symptom that is not explained by a medical condition(s)

sonohysterography ultrasound of the uterus after a saline solution is infused into the uterus

special instructions (CPT) directions within each section describing specific rules and definitions for use of codes within a particular category or subcategory

specimen a sample of any bodily fluid or tissue

SPECT single-photon emission computed tomography

Speech Assessment (ICD-10-PCS) the root type that identifies the measurement of speech and related functions

Speech Treatment (ICD-10-PCS) the root type that identifies the application of techniques to improve, augment, or compensate for speech and related functional impairment

sperm washing separation of the sperm from seminal fluid and removal of chemicals that can be harmful to the uterus

spermatocele the benign cystic swelling of sperm in the ducts of the epididymis

sphenoid sinus the sinus located at the center of the base of the skull, at the back of the nose

spina bifida a congenital neural tube defect in which vertebrae do not fuse

spinal cord (seizure) see *complex partial (seizure)*

spinal tap or puncture insertion of a needle into the lumbar back to collect a sample of CSF

splenectomy the total or partial excision of the spleen

splenoplasty surgical repair of the spleen

splenorrhaphy repair of a ruptured spleen, with or without partial splenectomy

split-thickness skin graft (STSG) a skin graft consisting of the epidermis and a portion of dermis or a mucosal graft consisting of only a partial thickness of mucosa

sprain the overstretching, bruising, or tearing of a ligament

squamous cell carcinoma (SCC) cancer that occurs in flat squamous cells

squamous intraepithelial disease (SIL) cervical dysplasia seen on a Pap test, graded as low-grade (LSIL), high-grade (HSIL), and possibly cancerous or malignant

ST elevation MI (STEMI) a myocardial infarction in which the ST segment of an EKG is elevated, indicating that the MI completely occludes a vessel

stabilization immobilizing a fracture site to prevent further injury and allow for healing

stage 1 pressure ulcer skin redness due to prolonged pressure that does not go away

stage 2 pressure ulcer damage to the epidermis due to prolonged pressure that extends into the dermis

stage 3 pressure ulcer damage through the full thickness of the dermis and into the subcutaneous tissue due to prolonged pressure

stage 4 pressure ulcer skin damage extending into the muscle, tendon, or bone due to prolonged pressure

staging the process of determining how far a cancer has spread

standalone code the code whose description is left-justified and begins with a capital letter; also called parent code

standardized terminology (ICD-10-PCS) the major attribute of ICD-10-PCS whereby a code set includes definitions of the terminology it uses, with each term having only one meaning

stapedectomy excision of the stapes bone

stapedotomy incision into the footplate of the stapes; may also involve inserting a prosthesis for hearing loss

stapes the stirrup-shaped bone in the middle ear that receives vibrations from the incus

status (ICD-10-CM) the external cause code that describes a person's employment status in relation to the event that caused an injury

status asthmaticus an acute exacerbation that does not respond to the standard medical treatments with bronchodilators and steroids

status epilepticus an epileptic seizure that lasts more than 30 minutes or is a near-constant state of seizures

status migrainosus a migraine that lasts more than 72 hours

STEMI ST elevation myocardial infarction

stenosis a narrowing of a valve or vessel

stent insertion placement of a mesh tube in a blood vessel to keep it open; necessary in atherosclerosis

stereotactic imaging three-dimensional imaging to pinpoint a specific location

Stereotactic radiosurgery (ICD-10-PCS) the Modality that identifies delivery of high doses of radiation to a target area with minimal exposure to the surrounding healthy tissue

stereotactic radiosurgery the use of narrow beams of radiation with three-dimensional guidance to target lesions in difficult-to-treat areas

steroid a type of medication used to reduce inflammation

stomatitis redness, ulcers, and/or bleeding of the mouth due to bacteria, viruses, or fungi

stomatoplasty surgical repair of the mouth

stomatorrhaphy suturing of the mouth

straight catheter a nonindwelling catheter consisting of a short, rigid tube that is inserted via the urethra to allow for drainage of urine, then removed

strain the overstretching, bruising, or tearing of a bone or tendon

stress fracture a fracture of a bone that has been subjected to repeated use or impact; also called March fracture or fatigue fracture

stress testing measuring EKG and oxygen concentrations as a patient performs an increasing level of exercise on a treadmill or stationary bicycle

structural integrity (ICD-10-PCS) the major attribute of ICD-10-PCS whereby the code set can be expanded easily without disrupting the structure of the system

STSG split-thickness skin graft

subcategory (CPT) a further division of some categories of CPT Category I codes that provides more specific information about a procedure or service

subcategory (ICD-10-CM) each level of subdivision after a category and before a code; either four or five characters

subchapter (ICD-10-CM) a contiguous range of codes within a chapter

subcutaneous under the skin

subcutaneous mastectomy excision of breast tissue but not the overlying skin, nipple, and areola, making it possible for the breast form to be reconstructed

subdermal pertaining to under the skin

subdural tap withdrawal of CSF through a fontanelle

subendocardial (infarction) the death of heart tissue that affects only a small portion of the heart wall, usually due to a decreased, but not totally occluded, blood supply; also called nontransmural infarction

subheading (CPT) a division of CPT Category I codes that groups procedures by location within a body system

subluxation the partial dislocation of bones in a joint

subsection (CPT) a division of CPT Category I codes that breaks down sections by type and/or anatomic sites

subsequent encounter (CPT) the second or later encounter by the admitting provider during the current admission and to all encounters by other than the admitting physician

subsequent encounter (ICD-10-CM) treatment during the healing phase

subsequent episode of care (ICD-10-CM) treatment during the healing phase

subsequent MI an MI that occurs within four weeks of a previous AMI

substance disorder drug and alcohol use, abuse, and addiction

subterm a word indented under each Main Term that further describes the Main Term in greater detail, such as an anatomic location or other disease variation

subtotal thyroid lobectomy excision of more than two-thirds of one lobe but less than the entire lobe

sudoriferous pertaining to sweat

superficial burn a burn that causes damage to the epidermis

superficial injury an injury to the surface of the skin, such as an abrasion, blister, contusion, constriction, insect bite, or superficial foreign body

superior vena cava one of the largest veins that carry deoxygenated blood back to the right ventricle

supervised modality a physical therapy treatment that does not require continuous one-on-one contact with a patient by a provider

Supplement (ICD-10-PCS) the root operation that identifies putting in or on biological or synthetic material that physically reinforces and/or augments the function of a portion of a body part

supracervical above the cervix uteri

suprapubic catheter an indwelling catheter inserted into the bladder through a laparotomy incision a few inches below the navel; less likely to harbor infection than an indwelling urethral catheter

surgical approach the method used by a surgeon to access the operative site

surgical destruction the obliteration of tissue using electrosurgery, cryosurgery, laser, or chemical treatment; also called lysis

surgical facility the setting or location in which surgery is performed

surgical history the date and type of past operations; operative reports (a narrative of exactly how the surgeon performed the procedure)

suspended temporarily held from moving forward

symptom subjective evidence of a disease or condition, usually reported by a patient

syngenic from an identical genetic match, such as an identical twin

syndactyly the presence of webbed fingers or toes

synovectomy surgical removal of the synovial membrane

synthetic manmade; not natural

systemic a class of diseases that affect the entire body

systemic circulation the section of the circulatory system that occurs between the heart and the rest of the body

systemic inflammatory response syndrome (SIRS) a complex inflammatory state affecting the whole body

Systemic Nuclear Medicine Therapy (ICD-10-PCS) the root type that identifies the introduction of unsealed radioactive materials into the body for treatment

systemic nuclear medicine therapy the introduction of unsealed radioactive materials into the body for treatment

systole the time during the heart cycle when the chamber contracts as it ejects blood

T

T lymphocyte a white blood cell that protects against viruses and bacteria

Table (ICD-10-PCS) a reference grid used to select the body part, operative approach, and other characteristics of a procedure

tachycardia rapid heart rate

tachypnea rapid breathing

TAH total abdominal hysterectomy

tangential biopsy a tissue sample obtained with a sharp blade, oblique scalpel, or curette to remove a sample of the epidermis with or without the underlying dermis

target organ an organ receiving hormones or treatment

tattooing injection of a colored pigment into the skin

TBSA total body surface area

technical component (CPT) part of a radiology code that covers the cost of staffing and equipment

temporary national code (CPT) a code used for a service or supply that does not have a permanent code

tendon fibrous tissue that connects bones to muscles

tendon repair sewing together the damaged or torn ends of a tendon

tendonitis the inflammation of a tendon

tendonoplasty the surgical repair of a tendon

tendonorrhaphy suturing of a tendon

terrorism an event involving weapons of mass destruction or specific terrorism-related offenses

tertiary intention healing delayed primary closure; wound is initially cleaned, debrided, and left open for observation for several days before closure

testis the part of the male genital system that provides the male sex hormone testosterone

tetralogy of Fallot a congenital heart defect consisting of four malformations: pulmonary stenosis, ventricle septal defect, dextraposition of the overriding aorta, and hypertrophy of the right ventricle

thalassemia a genetic disorder that results in defective formation of hemoglobin

therapeutic drug assay testing performed to monitor a known, prescribed medication so a physician can evaluate how it is affecting a patient

therapeutic procedure a procedure performed to treat a disease or condition

therapeutic radiology treatment using radiation

therapeutic ultrasound (radiologic) the use of ultrasound technology during a procedure

thermocauterization the destruction of tissue by applying heat

therosclerosis the formation of plaque on the inner walls of arteries in the heart

third trimester the time in a pregnancy when the gestational age is between 28 weeks, 0 days and delivery

third-party administrator (TPA) a private company that processes claims for self-insured health plans

third-party payer an entity other than a patient or physician who pays for healthcare services; they reimburse physicians and hospitals for 86% of all healthcare services in the United States

thoracentesis surgical puncture of the chest wall to remove fluids

thoracoscopy the insertion of an endoscope through a small incision in the chest wall

thoracostomy creation of an opening through the chest to place a chest tube or intercostal catheter in the pleural space

thoracotomy incision into the pleural space

thrombectomy incision into a vein or artery and removal of a clot

thrombocyte a platelet

thrombophilia a tendency to create blood clots

thrombus a clot of blood formed within a blood vessel that remains attached to its point of origin

thymectomy surgical removal of all or most of the thymus gland

thyroglossal pertaining to the thyroid and the tongue

thyroidectomy surgical removal of all or most of the thyroid gland

thyroidectomy, substernal surgical removal of an enlarged thyroid that has grown behind the sternum

thyrotomy cutting into the thyroglossal duct

thyrotoxicosis an excessive quantity of circulating thyroid hormone due to over-production by the thyroid gland originating from outside the thyroid, or from loss of storage function and leakage from the gland; also referred to as thyroid storm

TIA transient ischemic attack

time units (T) the total minutes of anesthesia service provided for all procedures divided by 15

tissue expander a temporary inflatable or saline implant placed under the skin to stretch it and allow growth of new skin cells

TMR transmyocardial revascularization

tolerate the ability of a patient to absorb a substance before experiencing behavioral or physical abnormalities

Tomographic (Tomo) Nuclear Medicine Imaging (ICD-10-PCS) the root type that identifies the introduction of radioactive materials into the body for three-dimensional display of images developed from the capture of radioactive emissions

tomographic (tomo) nuclear medicine imaging the introduction of radioactive materials into the body for three-dimensional display of images developed from the capture of radioactive emissions

tongue tie a condition in which the bottom of the tongue is attached to the floor of the mouth by a band of tissue called the lingual frenulum

tonic (seizure) a seizure characterized by prolonged muscle contractions or stiffening

tonic-clonic (seizure) a seizure characterized by a sudden loss of consciousness and falling to the floor; affects the entire brain

tonsillectomy/adenoidectomy (T&A) a procedure in which the tonsils and adenoids are surgically removed

tonsillitis inflammation of the tonsils

topical anesthesia a type of anesthesia that numbs the surface area of a body part

topography the anatomic site where a growth begins

total artificial heart (TAH) implementation the insertion of a device that replaces the ventricles

total-body hypothermia a technique that lowers the core body temperature below 35°C (95°F) during surgery, with the goal of protecting neurons from injury or degeneration; also called induced hypothermia or hypothermic anesthesia

total body surface area (TBSA) the total surface area of the human body, used in a calculation when classifying burns of the skin

total/complete thyroidectomy a second operation to excise remaining thyroid tissue following a previous thyroidectomy; also called completion thyroidectomy

total thyroid lobectomy the excision of one entire lobe of the thyroid gland

Tourette's syndrome a condition that causes people to make repeated, quick movements or sounds, which they have no control over

toxic effect a harmful substance that is ingested or comes into contact with a person and causes an undesired physical response

toxoid immunization that contains bacteria that are nontoxic so that the immune system will produce antibodies but the individual will not become ill

toxoplasmosis an infection due to the parasite *Toxoplasma gondii*, usually affecting the brain, lung, heart, eyes, or liver

TPA third-party administrator

TPAL a description of parity that identifies the number of term births (T), preterm births (P), spontaneous or induced abortions (A), and living children (L)

trabeculectomy surgical excision of a small portion of the trabecular tissue lying between the anterior chamber of the eye and the canal of Schlemm

trabeculoplasty see *trabeculotomy*

trabeculotomy incision into and repair of the trabecular meshwork to improve aqueous humor outflow and reduce IOP

trachea the windpipe

tracheal cartilage the part of the body that keeps the trachea and bronchi open

trachelectomy removal of the uterine cervix; also called cervicectomy

trachelorrhaphy suture of a laceration of the uterine cervix

tracheobronchoscopy the insertion of an endoscope through an established tracheostomy incision to view the trachea and bronchi

tracheostomy the creation of an opening in the trachea through which a breathing tube is inserted

tracheostomy tube a surgical opening in the neck leading to the trachea

tracheotomy creation of a surgical incision through the neck into the trachea

Traction (ICD-10-PCS) the root operation that identifies exerting a pulling force on a body region in a distal direction

traction exerting a pulling force on a body region in a distal direction

tractotomy incision of a nerve tract in the brainstem or spinal cord

TRAM transverse rectus abdominis myocutaneous

transabdominal pertaining to across the abdomen

transabdominal approach the performance of a procedure through an incision in the abdomen

transaction standards programming specifications

transcanal through the ear canal

transcatheter through an existing catheter

transcervical through the cervix uteri

transcranial through the skull

Transfer (ICD-10-PCS) the root operation that identifies moving, without taking out, all or a portion of a body part to another location to take over the function of all or a portion of a body part

transfer of care occurs when a consulting physician assumes management of a patient's care for one or more problems or conditions

Transfusion (ICD-10-PCS) the root operation that identifies putting in blood or blood products

transfusion putting in blood or blood products

transient ischemic attack (TIA) a brief episode of cerebral ischemia

transient tachypnea of the newborn (TTN) a short-term condition of rapid breathing due to retained lung fluid that occurs shortly after birth in full-term or near-term newborns

transitory temporary

translabyrinthine through the labyrinth

transmastoid through the mastoid bone

transmastoid antrotomy see *simple mastoidectomy*

transmural MI the death of heart tissue that extends through the entire thickness of the heart muscle

transmyocardial revascularization (TMR) the use of lasers to make small channels through the heart muscle and into the left ventricle

transnasal through the nose

transoral through the oral cavity

transorbital through an incision in the orbit of the eye

transperineal through the perineum

Transplantation (ICD-10-PCS) the root operation that identifies putting in or on all or a portion of a living body part taken from another individual or animal to physically take the place and/or function of all or a portion of a similar body part

transposition a medical term that identifies moving or relocating a structure; when done without cutting it out it is mapped to the PCS root operation Reposition

transposition of the great vessels a congenital heart defect in which the aorta and pulmonary artery are switched, preventing pulmonary circulation

transpubic through the pubic bone

transthoracic approach the performance of a procedure through an incision in the chest

transurethral through the urethra

transurethral resection of prostate (TURP) the insertion of a resectoscope via the urethra and removal of a portion of the prostate; may include cystoscopy, meatotomy, and urethral dilation

transvaginal through the vagina

transverse rectus abdominis myocutaneous (TRAM) flap the use of transverse rectus abdominis myocutaneous tissue to reconstruct the breast

traumatic an acute current injury that results from an accident

traumatic amputation the accidental severing of a body part

Treatment (ICD-10-PCS) the root operation that identifies manual treatment to eliminate or alleviate somatic dysfunction and related disorders

treatment (PCS Section F) activities typically associated with rehabilitation, such as swallowing dysfunction exercises, bathing and showering techniques, wound management, and gait training

Tricare (TC) federal health insurance coverage for family members of active-duty personnel and for retired military personnel and their families

trichiasis turning inward of the eyelashes

trichinosis a disease caused by trichinae parasites

tricuspid valve the valve that controls blood flow from the right atrium to the right ventricle

trisomy a genetic disorder in which a person has three copies, rather than two, of genetic material

true labor the period during which the uterine contracts and the cervix dilates

TTN transient tachypnea of the newborn

TURP transurethral resection of prostate

tympanectomy excision of the eardrum

tympanic membrane perforation (TMP) a hole or break in the eardrum; also called ruptured tympanic membrane

tympanic membrane the eardrum; separates the external ear from the middle ear; also called tympanum

tympanolysis destruction of tympanic membrane adhesions, granulation tissue, or scar tissue

tympanometry measurement of the eardrum

tympanoplasty see *myringoplasty*

tympanostomy the creation of an opening in the eardrum to insert a plastic or metal ventilating tube to drain fluid from the middle ear

tympanotomy incision into the eardrum

tympanum the part of the external ear that separates it from the middle ear; also called tympanic membrane or eardrum

type 1 diabetes a condition in which the body's immune system attacks pancreatic beta cells so that the pancreas does not produce insulin; previously called insulin-dependent diabetes mellitus (IDDM) or juvenile-onset diabetes

type 2 diabetes a condition in which the pancreas produces insulin, but the body does not use it properly; previously called non-insulin-dependent diabetes mellitus (NIDDM) or adult-onset diabetes

U

UB-04 a standard hospital billing form; also known as the CMS-1450

UHDDS Uniform Hospital Data Discharge Set

ulcer a sore on the lining of the stomach (gastric ulcer) or duodenum (peptic ulcer)

ulcerative colitis an inflammatory bowel disease (IBD) with inflammation and sores, called ulcers, in the lining of the rectum and colon

Ultrasonography (ICD-10-PCS) the root type that identifies the real-time display of images of anatomy or flow information developed from the capture of reflected and attenuated high-frequency sound waves

ultrasonography the real-time display of images of anatomy or flow information developed from the capture of reflected and attenuated high-frequency sound waves

Ultrasound Therapy (ICD-10-PCS) the root operation that identifies extracorporeal treatment by high-frequency sound waves

ultrasound therapy extracorporeal treatment by high-frequency sound waves

ultrasound imaging the use of sound waves to capture an image of echoes bouncing off structures, showing real-time movements within the body

Ultraviolet Light Therapy (ICD-10-PCS) the root operation that identifies extracorporeal treatment by ultraviolet light

ultraviolet therapy extracorporeal treatment by ultraviolet light

uncertain diagnosis diagnoses preceded by the words *probable, possible, suspected, questionable, rule out, working diagnosis,* or a similar word

underdosing taking less of a medication than is prescribed by a provider or a manufacturer's instruction

Uniform Hospital Data Discharge Set (UHDDS) a list of data elements and definitions prepared by the Centers for Disease Control and Prevention and used by hospitals for inpatient discharge data collection

uniplane fixator a fixation device that has a single external rod that runs parallel to a long bone and is used almost exclusively on fractures of the shaft

unique definitions (ICD-10-PCS) the ICD-10-PCS attribute whereby the description of a code is based on the meaning of each value in the code, so the description is unique and cannot change

United Network for Organ Sharing (UNOS) a nonprofit organization that administers the United States' Organ Procurement and Transplantation Network, including the organ transplant waiting list

unlisted procedure (CPT) a procedure or service for which there is no specific CPT code; generally ends with the two digits 99

and appears at the end of the category or subdivision to which they apply

unrelated a symptom, sign, or abnormal finding not connected to a disease

unstable lie repeated changes in the fetal position during or after the 36th week of pregnancy

unstageable pressure ulcer an ulcer covered with dead cells, eschar, or wound exudate that cannot be visually assessed

upper respiratory tract a part of the respiratory system that consists of the nose, pharynx, and larynx

uremia a toxic blood condition due to the inability of the kidneys to remove nitrogenous substances from the blood

ureter a tube that drains each kidney

ureteral catheter an indwelling catheter inserted into the ureter, either through the urethra and bladder or posteriorly through the kidney

ureterectomy excision of the ureters

ureterolithotomy incision into a ureter

ureteroplasty repair of a ureter; may include excision of a portion of the ureter, then anastomosis of the ends that were not removed or grafting of tissue from the bladder

ureterotomy incision into the ureter; may include stent placement

urethra a tube that carries urine out of the body

urethral catheter an indwelling catheter inserted through the urethra into the urinary bladder, percutaneously or through an existing ostomy

urethroneocystostomy repair of a defect in the bladder and urethra, with reimplantation of one or both of the ureters into the bladder

urinary bladder a muscular sac that holds urine until it is expelled through the urethra

urinary tract infection (UTI) a bacterial infection of the urinary bladder; also called cystitis

urodynamic tests a variety of tests that measure the contraction of the bladder muscle as it fills and empties, ranging from simple visual observation to precise measurements using sophisticated instruments

urticaria hives

use (substance) consuming a substance in moderate amounts that do not create significant legal, social, employment, family, or medical problems

uterine suspension the shortening of the ligament that suspends the uterus by plicating and tacking it back in place; may also include presacral sympathectomy

uteroscopy visual examination of the ureters

uterus a hollow muscular organ in females that provides for the development of a fetus; also called the womb

utricle a small, saclike structure of the labyrinth of the inner ear

uvea the middle layer of the eye consisting of the iris, ciliary body, and choroid

uvula a pendant fleshy lobe, most commonly the one in the back of the mouth

V

vaccine immunization that contains antigens from a weakened strain of a virus so that the body will produce antibodies to fight it, but the person will not become ill

VAD ventricular assistive device

vagina the birth canal

vaginal birth the delivery of a fetus from the uterus through the cervix to the vagina (birth canal)

vaginal birth after cesarean (VBAC) delivery through the vagina after having a cesarean delivery in a previous pregnancy

vaginotomy making an incision into the vagina

vagotomy a procedure in which a portion of the vagus nerve in the stomach is excised

value an individual letter or number in an ICD-10-PCS code

valve repair the correction of a physical defect of the heart

valve replacement the replacement of a heart valve with a synthetic or porcine (pig) valve

valvular disorder a condition characterized by damage to or a defect in one of the four heart valves

VAP ventilator-assisted pneumonia

varicella the chickenpox virus

vascular dementia a form of dementia due to many small strokes

vascular family a network of vessels branching off the same primary vessel

vasectomy cutting out a piece of the vas deferens and cauterizing or suturing the ends closed

vasodilation enlargement of blood vessels

vasoocclusive crisis a form of sickle cell crisis in which the patient experiences severe pain due to infarctions, which may occur in nearly any location

vasotomy incision into the vas deferens

VATS video-assisted thoracoscopic surgery

VBAC vaginal birth after cesarean

vein a tube that carries blood from the capillaries back to the heart in successively larger veins leading to the superior vena cava and inferior vena cava

venography X-ray of veins by tracing the venous pulse

ventilation-perfusion scan a nuclear medicine test useful in identifying pulmonary emboli by showing whether blood is flowing to all parts of a lung

ventilator a machine that assists with breathing

ventilator-associated pneumonia (VAP) pneumonia that develops 48 hours or more after mechanical ventilation is initiated

ventricle one of the lower heart chambers that ejects blood to the lungs and the body

ventricular assist device (VAD) implantation the insertion of a mechanical pump used to support heart function and blood flow

ventricular fibrillation (V-fib) an irregular heartbeat in the ventricles characterized by an abnormal quivering of heart fibers

ventricular puncture the withdrawal of CSF from the ventricles of the brain by drilling a hole in the skull

venule a small vein

Version 5010 A1 the current version of the electronic standards for healthcare transactions

vertebra a bony segment of the spine

vertebral body the main anterior bony part of a vertebra

vertebral segment a vertebra

very low birth weight (VLBW) a birth weight less than 1,500 grams (3 pounds, 4 ounces)

vesicocentesis prenatal aspiration of fetal urine

vesicourethropexy suturing of the vaginal wall to the urethra or bladder neck, with anchoring to the pubic bone or Cooper ligament; also referred to as the Marshall-Marchetti-Krantz (MMK) procedure or Burch procedure

vesiculectomy the removal of one of the seminal vesicles

Vestibular Assessment (ICD-10-PCS) the root type that identifies the measurement of the vestibular system and related functions

Vestibular Treatment (ICD-10-PCS) the root type that identifies the application of techniques to improve, augment, or compensate for vestibular and related functional impairment

vestibulocochlear nerve cranial nerve VIII; the ear makes hearing possible by collecting sound waves from the external world and converting them into impulses that are transmitted to the brain through the vestibulocochlear nerve

Veterans Health Administration (VHA) an integrated healthcare delivery system with more than 1,400 sites of care, including hospitals, community clinics, community living centers, and various other facilities to provide health services to veterans with service-related disabilities

Via Natural or Artificial Opening (ICD-10-PCS) the approach that identifies the surgeon accesses the surgical site through a body opening that already exists, such as the mouth, nose, ear, anus, or vagina

Via Natural or Artificial Opening Endoscopic (ICD-10-PCS) the approach that identifies the surgeon inserts an endoscope through an existing natural or artificial opening

Via Natural or Artificial Opening Endoscopic with Percutaneous Endoscopic Assistance (ICD-10-PCS) the approach that identifies two endoscopes are used: one through a natural or artificial opening and the second one through percutaneous access

video-assisted thoracoscopic surgery (VATS) the use of an endoscope and video camera to perform procedures traditionally performed using a thoracotomy

videoradiography see *cineradiography*

virus a capsule that contains genetic material and uses the body's own cells to multiply

visceral pericardium see *epicardium*

vitiligo a loss of pigmentation

vitreous body the transparent jelly that fills the eyeball and is surrounded by a membrane

VLBW very low birth weight

voluntary (muscle) a muscle a person can choose to contract and relax

volvulus the twisting of a portion of the small or large intestine or stomach into a loop, which obstructs the passage of digestive material

Von Willebrand's disease a genetic disorder marked by bleeding of the mucosa

vulvectomy surgical removal of part of the vulva

vulvovaginitis inflammation of the vulva and vagina due to yeast, bacteria, viruses, parasites, or skin care products

W

wedge excision surgical excision of tissue from part of one lobe of the lung; also called segmentectomy

whistleblower someone who turns in violators

white blood cell disorder a condition that diminishes the body's immune response and increases the risk of infection

winged catheter a urethral catheter that is retained in the bladder by winglike projections on the end

workers' compensation (WC) a plan that pays for medical costs due to employment-related injuries or illnesses; each state establishes its own requirements for WC insurance but must comply with federal minimums

wound a cut or opening in the skin or mucous membrane

wound exploration the enlargement, dissection, and examination of a wound to determine the wound depth or perform a procedure

wound repair, complex a layered closure that also requires scar revision, debridement, extensive undermining, stents, or retention sutures

wound repair, intermediate the layered closure of one or more of the deeper layers of subcutaneous tissue and superficial fascia, in addition to the skin closure; also includes extensive cleaning/decontamination of wounds otherwise requiring single-layer closure

wound repair, simple a one-layer closure of epidermis, dermis, or subcutaneous tissue without significant involvement of deeper structures; includes local anesthesia and electrocauterization, when used

X

xenograft a skin substitute in which the skin comes from another species, such as a pig, or a synthetic substitute

Z

Z codes (ICD-10-CM) codes that represent reasons for encounters; may be used in any healthcare setting when the reason for the encounter is not a disease, injury, or external cause that is classified in the preceding ICD-10-CM chapters for body systems (A00 to Y99)

zooplastic from an animal

zygote a fertilized egg

References

AAPC. *About Us*. https://www.aapc.com/aboutus/

Agency for Healthcare Research and Quality (AHRQ). *Statistical Brief #113, Complicating Conditions of Pregnancy and Childbirth*, 2008. https://www.hcup-us.ahrq.gov/reports/statbriefs/sb113.jsp

Alzheimer's Association. *2016 Alzheimer's Disease Facts and Figures*, p. 84. https://www.alz.org/documents_custom/2016-facts-and-figures.pdf

Alzheimer's Association. *Younger/Early Onset Alzheimer's & Dementia*. http://www.alz.org/alzheimers_disease_early_onset.asp

American Academy of Orthopedic Surgeons. *Metastatic Bone Disease*. http://orthoinfo.aaos.org/topic.cfm?topic=A00093

American Association of Poison Control Centers. *2015 Annual Report of the American Association of Poison Control Centers' National Poison Data System (NPDS): 33rd Annual Report*, pp. 935, 936, 937, 943. https://aapcc.s3.amazonaws.com/pdfs/annual_reports/2015_AAPCC_NPDS_Annual_Report_33rd_PDF.pdf

American Board of Medical Specialties. http://www.abms.org

American Cancer Society. *About Childhood Leukemia*. https://www.cancer.org/cancer/leukemia-in-children/about/key-statistics.html

American Cancer Society. *Cancer Facts & Figures 2017*, pp. 10, 13, 21, 22, 24. https://www.cancer.org/research/cancer-facts-statistics/all-cancer-facts-figures/cancer-facts-figures-2017.html

American Cancer Society. *Key Statistics for Colorectal Cancer*. https://www.cancer.org/cancer/colon-rectal-cancer/about/key-statistics.html

American College of Allergy, Asthma, and Immunology. *Asthma Statistics*. http://www.aaaai.org/about-aaaai/newsroom/asthma-statistics

American Health Information Management Association. *Our Story*. http://www.ahima.org/about/aboutahima?tabid=story

American Hospital Association. "Diabetic Cataract," *Coding Clinic for ICD-10-CM and ICD-10-PCS*, Fourth Quarter 2016, pp. 142–143.

American Medical Association. *CPT Assistant Newsletter*. https://commerce.ama-assn.org

American Medical Association. *Current Procedural Terminology, CPT 2019*. Chicago, 2018.

American Psychiatric Association. *DSM–5: Frequently Asked Questions*. https://www.psychiatry.org/psychiatrists/practice/dsm/feedback-and-questions/frequently-asked-questions

American Society of Anesthesiologists. *CROSSWALK: A Guide for Surgery/Anesthesia CPT Codes*. Schaumburg, IL, 2018.

American Society of Clinical Oncology (ASCO). *Eye Cancer Overview*. http://www.cancer.net/cancer-types/eye-cancer/overview

American Urological Association. *About Us, Why Urology?* https://www.auanet.org/about-us/why-urology

Centers for Disease Control and Prevention. *2014 National Diabetes Statistics Report*, p. 1. https://www.cdc.gov/diabetes/data/statistics/2014statisticsreport.html

Centers for Disease Control and Prevention. *Birth Defects Homepage, Data and Statistics*. https://www.cdc.gov/ncbddd/birthdefects/data.html

Centers for Disease Control and Prevention (CDC), *National Diabetes Statistics Report*, 2017, pp. 2, 7.

Centers for Disease Control and Prevention. *Chronic Obstructive Pulmonary Disease (COPD)*. https://www.cdc.gov/nchs/fastats/copd.htm

Centers for Disease Control and Prevention. *Colorectal Cancer Statistics*. https://www.cdc.gov/cancer/colorectal/statistics/

Centers for Disease Control and Prevention. *Heart Disease Fact Sheet*. https://www.cdc.gov/dhdsp/data_statistics/fact_sheets/fs_heart_disease.htm

Centers for Disease Control and Prevention, National Center for Health Statistics. *Infant Health*. https://www.cdc.gov/nchs/fastats/infant-health.htm

Centers for Disease Control and Prevention, National Center for Health Statistics. *National Vital Statistics Reports Volume 66, Number 1 January 5, 2017, Births: Final Data for 2015*, p. 2. https://www.cdc.gov/nchs/data/nvsr/nvsr66/nvsr66_01.pdf

Centers for Disease Control and Prevention. *Second Hand Smoke (SHS) Facts*. https://www.cdc.gov/tobacco/data_statistics/fact_sheets/secondhand_smoke/general_facts/index.htm

Centers for Disease Control and Prevention. *Sepsis*. https://www.cdc.gov/sepsis/index.html

Centers for Medicare and Medicaid Services. *2019 ICD-10-PCS Official Guidelines for Coding and Reporting*. https://www.cms.gov/Medicare/Coding/ICD10/Downloads/2018-PCS-Guidelines.pdf

Centers for Medicare and Medicaid Services. *2019 International Classification of Diseases, 10th Revision, Clinical Modification (ICD-10-CM)*. https://www.cms.gov/Medicare/Coding/ICD10/2019-ICD-10-CM.html

Centers for Medicare and Medicaid Services. *2019 International Classification of Diseases, 10th Revision, Procedure Coding System (ICD-10-PCS)*. https://www.cms.gov/Medicare/Coding/ICD10/2019-ICD-10-PCS.html

Centers for Medicare and Medicaid Services. *Healthcare Common Procedure Coding System 2018*. https://www.cms.gov/Medicare/Coding/HCPCSReleaseCodeSets/Alpha-Numeric-HCPCS.html

Centers for Medicare and Medicaid Services. *ICD-10-CM Official Guidelines for Coding and Reporting FY 2019*. https://www.cms.gov/Medicare/Coding/ICD10/Downloads/2019-ICD10-Coding-Guidelines-.pdf

Centers for Medicare and Medicaid Services. *ICD-10-PCS Reference Manual 2016*, p. 39. https://www.cms.gov/Medicare/Coding/ICD10/2016-ICD-10-PCS-and-GEMs.html.

Department of Health and Human Services, Office Of Inspector General. *Improper Payments for Evaluation and Management Services Cost Medicare Billions in 2010*, pp. 11–12. https://oig.hhs.gov/oei/reports/oei-04-10-00181.pdf

Department of Health and Human Services and Department of Justice Health Care Fraud and Abuse Control Program. *Annual Report for Fiscal Year 2016*, 8.

Gabriel-Jones, and Larry, Bohn. *Medical Coding Evaluation and Management* (New York: Pearson Education, 2014), pp. 54, 160.

Institute for Safe Medication Practices (ISMP). *Error-Prone Abbreviations, Symbols, and Dose Designations*. https://www.ismp.org/Tools/errorproneabbreviations.pdf

Leukemia and Lymphoma Society. *Childhood Blood Cancer Facts and Statistics*. https://www.lls.org/http%3A/llsorg.prod.acquia-sites.com/facts-and-statistics/facts-and-statistics-overview/facts-and-statistics/childhood-blood-cancer-facts-and-statistics

Leukemia and Lymphoma Society. *Facts and Statistics*. https://www.lls.org/http%3A/llsorg.prod.acquia-sites.com/facts-and-statistics/facts-and-statistics-overview/facts-and-statistics

Medscape. *Brain Metastasis*. http://emedicine.medscape.com/article/1157902-overview

National Center for Health Statistics. *National Health Expenditures by Type of Service and Source of Funds: Calendar Years 1960 To 2015.* NHE2015.xls.

National Highway Traffic Safety Administration. *Drunk Driving.* https://www.nhtsa.gov/risky-driving/drunk-driving

National Institute of Diabetes and Digestive and Kidney Diseases. *Bladder Infection Definition and Facts.* https://www.niddk.nih.gov/health-information/urologic-diseases/bladder-infection-uti-in-adults/definition-facts

National Institute of Diabetes and Digestive and Kidney Diseases. *Chronic Kidney Disease, Causes of Chronic Kidney Disease.* https://www.niddk.nih.gov/health-information/kidney-disease/chronic-kidney-disease-ckd/causes

National Institute of Diabetes and Digestive and Kidney Diseases. *Chronic Kidney Disease, Kidney Disease Statistics for the United States.* https://www.niddk.nih.gov/health-information/health-statistics/kidney-disease

National Institute of Diabetes and Digestive and Kidney Diseases. *Digestive Diseases Statistics for the United States.* https://www.niddk.nih.gov/health-information/health-statistics/digestive-diseases

National Institute on Deafness and Other Communication Disorders. *Quick Statistics About Hearing.* https://www.nidcd.nih.gov/health/statistics/quick-statistics-hearing

National Institute on Deafness and Other Communication Disorders. *Vestibular Schwannoma (Acoustic Neuroma) and Neurofibromatosis.* https://www.nidcd.nih.gov/health/vestibular-schwannoma-acoustic-neuroma-and-neurofibromatosis

National Institutes of Health. *Any Disorder Among Children.* https://www.nimh.nih.gov/health/statistics/prevalence/any-disorder-among-children.shtml

National Institutes of Health. *Any Mental Illness (AMI) Among U.S. Adults.* https://www.nimh.nih.gov/health/statistics/prevalence/any-mental-illness-ami-among-us-adults.shtml

National Institutes of Health, "Birth Weight and Subsequent Risk of Cancer," *Cancer Epidemiology* 38, no. 5 (2014): 538–543.

National Institutes of Health, National Cancer Institute. *Cancer Stat Facts: Bladder Cancer.* https://seer.cancer.gov/statfacts/html/urinb.html

National Institutes of Health, National Institute of Neurological Disorders and Stroke. *NIH Stroke Scale.* https://stroke.nih.gov/resources/scale.htm

National Institutes of Health, "A High Birth Weight is Associated with Increased Risk of Type 2 Diabetes and Obesity," *Pediatric Obesity* 10, no. 2 (2015): 77–83.

National Institutes of Health. *Serious Mental Illness (SMI) Among U.S. Adults.* https://www.nimh.nih.gov/health/statistics/prevalence/serious-mental-illness-smi-among-us-adults.shtml

National Kidney Foundation. *End Stage Renal Disease in the United States.* https://www.kidney.org/news/newsroom/factsheets/End-Stage-Renal-Disease-in-the-US

National Uniform Billing Committee (NUBC). *Official UB-04 Data Specifications Manual*

National Uniform Claim Committee (NUCC). *1500 Health Insurance Claim Form Reference Instruction Manual.*

PB Resources, Inc. Belfair, WA.

Physicians Commitee for Responsible Medicine. *Birth Defect Statistics.* http://www.pcrm.org/research/resch/reschethics/birth-defect-statistics

Provistas, Inc. *SpeedeCoder.* Yuma, AZ.

Skin Cancer Foundation. *Basal Cell Carcinoma (BCC).* http://www.skincancer.org/skin-cancer-information/basal-cell-carcinoma

Skin Cancer Foundation. *Melanoma.* http://www.skincancer.org/skin-cancer-information/melanoma

Tammy Reynolds, C. E. Zupanick, & Mark Dombeck, 2013. *Diagnostic Criteria for Intellectual Disabilities: DSM-5 Criteria.* https://www.mentalhelp.net/articles/diagnostic-criteria-for-intellectual-disabilities-dsm-5-criteria/

The Joint Commission. *Do Not Use List.* http://www.jointcommission.org/assets/1/18/dnu_list.pdf Updated 3/5/09.

U.S. Department of Health and Human Services (HHS). *A Timeline of HIV and AIDS.* https://www.hiv.gov/hiv-basics/overview/history/hiv-and-aids-timeline

United Network for Organ Sharing. *Annual Report-2016,* https://www.unos.org/about/annual-report/2016-annual-report/

United States Bone and Joint Initiative. *The Burden of Musculoskeletal Diseases in the United States (BMUS),* 3rd edition (Rosemont, IL, 2014).

United States Preventive Services Task Force (USPSTF). *USPSTF A and B Recommendations* www.uspreventiveservicestaskforce.org. July 2018.

World Health Organization (WHO). *Smallpox.* http://www.who.int/csr/disease/smallpox/en/

Index

Coder's Index

This Coder's Index lists the specific codes discussed in the text and the pages on which they appear. Note: Page numbers followed by f, t, or g represent figures, tables, or guided examples respectively.

Key Criteria for Abstracting Tables

Abstracting is the first step in coding for every body system and every code set. These handy pull-out cards consolidate the 113 Key Criteria for Abstracting Tables presented in this text. Keep them in a notebook or folder for quick reference. The following directory identifies the original table number and the page reference in this appendix, organized by code set and body system. Refer to the corresponding chapter in the text for a full discussion of abstracting criteria.

Table 3-7 ■ KEY CRITERIA FOR ABSTRACTING DIAGNOSES (GENERAL GUIDELINES)

- ❑ What are the gender and age of the patient?
- ❑ What is the patient's chief complaint or reason for the encounter or inpatient admission?
- ❑ Is the encounter inpatient or outpatient?
- ❑ What symptoms and signs are described?
- ❑ Does the physician provide a definitive diagnosis?
- ❑ Does the physician provide a diagnosis that is uncertain, probable, possible, qualified, or rule out?
- ❑ Which symptoms and signs are integral to the definitive diagnosis?
- ❑ Which symptoms and signs are related, but not integral, to the definitive diagnosis?
- ❑ What unrelated conditions, symptoms, or signs are managed during the encounter?
- ❑ What conditions, symptoms, or signs are not managed during the encounter?
- ❑ What is the laterality, if any, of the condition?
- ❑ What is the treatment plan or procedure? Is it consistent with the diagnosis?
- ❑ Is the condition the result of an injury or external cause?

Table 4-3 ■ KEY CRITERIA FOR ABSTRACTING SYMPTOMS, SIGNS, ABNORMAL FINDINGS, AND CONFIRMED CONDITIONS

- ❑ What symptoms does the patient report?
- ❑ What signs does the physician document?
- ❑ What abnormal laboratory findings are reviewed?
- ❑ What confirmed diagnoses are documented?
- ❑ What diagnoses are identified as uncertain with words such as *possible, probable, rule out, suspected*?
- ❑ Which symptoms, signs, and abnormal findings are integral to the condition?
- ❑ Which symptoms, signs, and abnormal findings are related but not integral to the condition?
- ❑ Which symptoms, signs, and abnormal findings are unrelated to the condition?

Table 5-3 ■ KEY CRITERIA FOR ABSTRACTING NEOPLASMS

- ❑ What is the histologic description of the neoplasm or cancer?
- ❑ What is the anatomic site of the neoplasm?
- ❑ Is the neoplasm stated as malignant or benign?
- ❑ If malignant, is the neoplasm primary, secondary, in situ, or of unknown histologic origin?
- ❑ Has the malignant neoplasm metastasized? If so, to what sites?
- ❑ What complications are documented, such as anemia, dehydration, or a surgical complication?
- ❑ If anemia is present, is it due to the malignancy itself or due to a treatment such as chemotherapy, radiotherapy, or immunotherapy?
- ❑ Is the reason for the encounter or admission the malignancy or an unrelated condition?
- ❑ If the reason for the encounter is the malignancy, what is the specific purpose?
  - Treatment of the primary site
  - Treatment of a metastatic site(s)
  - Treatment of a complication
  - Chemotherapy
  - Radiotherapy
  - Immunotherapy
  - Pain management
  - Determination of the extent of malignancy
  - Aftercare
  - Follow-up care
- ❑ Is the patient in remission from leukemia, multiple myeloma, or malignant plasma neoplasm?
- ❑ If the primary malignancy was previously excised, is there any remaining evidence of primary malignancy, metastasis, or any related treatment?
- ❑ Does the patient have a personal history or family history of malignant neoplasm?

Table 6-2 ■ KEY CRITERIA FOR ABSTRACTING Z CODES

Patient Situation	Main Term
❏ Is the reason for the encounter a routine examination?	Examination
❏ Is the reason for the encounter to receive an inoculation or vaccination against a disease?	Inoculation
❏ Does the physician document a past medical condition that no longer exists and is not receiving any treatment but has the potential for recurrence?	History, personal
❏ Does the physician document that the patient has a family member(s) who has had a particular disease, which causes the patient to be at higher risk of also contracting the disease?	History, family
❏ Is the reason for the encounter testing for disease or disease precursors in seemingly well individuals so that early detection and treatment can be provided?	Screening
❏ Does the physician document a lifestyle habit that poses a risk factor?	Use
❏ Is the reason for the encounter continued care during the healing or recovery phase after initial treatment has been completed?	Aftercare
❏ Is the reason for the encounter continuing surveillance following completed treatment of a disease, condition, or injury when the condition has been fully treated and no longer exists?	Follow-up
❏ Is the reason for the encounter to receive assistance in the aftermath of an illness or injury or for support in coping with family or social problems?	Counseling
❏ Did a woman give birth during the encounter?	Outcome of delivery
❏ Is the patient a newborn who was born during the current admission?	Newborn, born
❏ Was a procedure cancelled or a surgical approach converted?	Procedure
❏ Is a newborn observed for conditions that were suspected but not found to exist?	Observation

Table 7-1 ■ KEY CRITERIA FOR ABSTRACTING EXTERNAL CAUSES

- ❏ **Diagnosis:** What physical injury(ies) or health condition did the patient sustain?
- ❏ **Intent:** What is the purpose or intent of the injury: accidental, self-harm, assault, legal intervention, military operation, or medical procedure?
- ❏ **Cause/causal event:** How did the injury or health condition happen?
- ❏ **Place:** Where did the event occur?
- ❏ **Activity:** What was the patient doing at the time of the event?
- ❏ **Status:** What was the patient's employment status at the time the event occurred: civilian employment, military, volunteer, or recreational/leisure?

Table 8-3 ■ KEY CRITERIA FOR ABSTRACTING DIGESTIVE SYSTEM CONDITIONS

- ❏ What is the condition?
- ❏ What is the anatomic site?
- ❏ What is the laterality, if any?
- ❏ Is bleeding or hemorrhaging documented?
- ❏ What other manifestations or complications are documented?
- ❏ What comorbidities are documented?
- ❏ What lifestyle habits are documented as current or with a history of, such as alcohol use or abuse and tobacco exposure, use, or abuse?

Table 9-5 ■ KEY CRITERIA FOR ABSTRACTING DIABETES MELLITUS

- ❏ What type of diabetes is documented?
- ❏ Are coexisting conditions documented as related to diabetes?
- ❏ What acute complications are documented?
- ❏ What chronic complications are documented?
- ❏ If secondary DM is documented, what is the cause?
- ❏ If either type 2 or secondary DM is documented, is insulin used on a long-term basis?
- ❏ Is a family history of DM documented?
- ❏ Which problem or complication is the reason for the encounter?

Table 9-6 ■ KEY CRITERIA FOR ABSTRACTING THYROID DISORDERS

- ❏ Is the condition hyperthyroidism or hypothyroidism?
- ❏ What is the cause of the condition?
- ❏ Is the condition congenital?
- ❏ Is goiter documented?
- ❏ Is thyrotoxicosis crisis documented?

Table 10-3 ■ KEY CRITERIA FOR ABSTRACTING CONDITIONS OF THE INTEGUMENTARY SYSTEM

- ❏ What is the type of lesion (carbuncle, abscess, urticaria, mole, corn)?
- ❏ What is the anatomic site (face, back, hand)?
- ❏ What is the laterality (right or left side)?
- ❏ Is there an underlying cause (another condition, exposure to a drug, or environmental substance)?
- ❏ What is the infectious agent, if any?
- ❏ Are there complications or manifestations (gangrene)?
- ❏ What is the depth or extent of damage?

Table 11-3 ■ KEY CRITERIA FOR ABSTRACTING MUSCULOSKELETAL CONDITIONS

- ❏ What type of condition is documented: fracture, dislocation, subluxation, sprain, infection, inflammation, or degeneration?
- ❏ What type of tissue or structure is affected: bone, joint, cartilage, muscle, tendon, or ligament?
- ❏ What is the specific subtype of condition (e.g., osteoarthritis vs. rheumatoid arthritis)?
- ❏ What is the anatomic site?
- ❏ What is the laterality?
- ❏ For osteoporosis: Does the patient have a pathologic fracture? Does the patient have a history of healed pathologic fractures?
- ❏ Is the condition acute, chronic, or a late effect?
- ❏ Is the encounter for active treatment?
- ❏ Is the encounter for aftercare during the healing phase?
- ❏ Is the encounter for follow-up after active healing is complete?

Table 11-4 ■ KEY CRITERIA FOR ABSTRACTING PATHOLOGIC FRACTURES

- ❏ Is the fracture traumatic or pathologic?
- ❏ What type of pathologic fracture is it?
- ❏ What is the underlying disease?
- ❏ What bone is fractured?
- ❏ What is the laterality?
- ❏ Were any additional bones fractured?
- ❏ Is the healing routine, delayed (*patient waited to seek care*), nonunion (*failure of the ends of the fractured bone segments to reunite*), or malunion (*ends of fractured bone segments did not heal with proper alignment*)?
- ❏ Is the encounter for active treatment?
- ❏ Is the encounter for aftercare during the healing phase?
- ❏ Is the encounter for follow-up after active healing is complete?

Table 12-5 ■ KEY CRITERIA FOR ABSTRACTING BURNS

- ❏ Is the burn due to heat or a chemical (corrosion)?
- ❏ What is the anatomic site?
- ❏ What is the laterality?
- ❏ What is the greatest depth (degree) of burn on each site?
- ❏ Are any burns nonhealing?
- ❏ Are any burns infected?
- ❏ What is the episode of care?
- ❏ What percentage of the body surface involves third-degree burns?

Table 12-6 ■ KEY CRITERIA FOR ABSTRACTING TRAUMATIC FRACTURES

- ❏ Is the fracture traumatic or pathologic?
- ❏ Does the patient have osteoporosis?
- ❏ What bone is fractured?
- ❏ What is the laterality?
- ❏ Were any additional bones fractured?
- ❏ Where on the bone is the fracture located?
- ❏ What type of fracture occurred?
- ❏ Is the fracture displaced or nondisplaced? (*Default is displaced.*)
- ❏ Is the fracture open or closed? (*Default is closed.*)
- ❏ For open fractures, what is the Gustilo classification?
- ❏ For epiphysis fractures, what is the Salter-Harris classification?
- ❏ What is the episode of care?
- ❏ Is the healing routine, delayed, nonunion, or malunion?
- ❏ Is the encounter for follow-up after active healing is complete?

Table 12-7 ■ KEY CRITERIA FOR ABSTRACTING POISONING, ADVERSE EFFECTS, AND UNDERDOSING

- ❏ What substance is involved?
- ❏ Is a diagnosis of abuse or dependence on the substance documented?
- ❏ Is the injury a poisoning/toxic effect, adverse effect, or underdosing?
- ❏ Is the injury documented as accidental, intentional self-harm, an assault, or of undetermined intent? (The default intent is *accidental.*)
- ❏ What conditions (manifestations) resulted from the injury?
- ❏ What is the episode of care?

Table 13-3 ■ KEY CRITERIA FOR ABSTRACTING CONDITIONS OF THE CIRCULATORY SYSTEM

- ❏ What part of the circulatory system is affected?
- ❏ What is the specific anatomic site?
- ❏ What type of disorder is present?
- ❏ Is the condition further specified as complete, partial, current, or old (if applicable)?
- ❏ What is the underlying cause?
- ❏ What symptoms are documented that are not integral to the condition?
- ❏ Is the condition acquired or congenital?
- ❏ Is the condition related to pregnancy?
- ❏ Does the patient have a current, subsequent, or old MI?
- ❏ Has the patient had more than one AMI in the past four weeks?
- ❏ What other cardiovascular conditions coexist?
- ❏ Does the patient have hypertension with heart or kidney involvement?
- ❏ What conditions exist in other organ systems?
- ❏ Which conditions are documented as being related to the cardiovascular condition?
- ❏ What is the patient's exposure to or use of tobacco?
- ❏ Does the patient use anticoagulants or antithrombotics on a long-term basis?
- ❏ Does the patient have a family history of cardiovascular disease?
- ❏ Does the patient wear a pacemaker?
- ❏ Has the patient had a CABG?
- ❏ If a vessel is blocked or diseased, is it an artery or vein? Is it native (*the patient's original vessel*) or a graft?
- ❏ If a grafted vessel is blocked, is the grafted vessel autologous (*from the patient*), biological nonautologous (*from a source other than the patient, such as a cadaver or animal*), or nonbiological (*synthetic*)?
- ❏ Is the patient waiting for or a recipient of a heart transplant?

Table 14-3 ■ KEY CRITERIA FOR ABSTRACTING CONDITIONS OF THE BLOOD

- ❏ What is the condition?
- ❏ What part of the hemic system does the condition involve?
- ❏ Does the condition have an underlying cause?
- ❏ Is the condition acquired or congenital?
- ❏ If anemia exists, is it due to a neoplasm or chronic disease?
- ❏ If sickle cell disease exists, what is the specific type?
- ❏ If sickle cell disease exists, is the patient in crisis?
- ❏ If sickle cell disease exists, does the patient have a fever?
- ❏ What symptoms are integral to the condition?
- ❏ What manifestations require an additional code?
- ❏ Is the condition drug induced?

Table 15-3 ■ KEY CRITERIA FOR ABSTRACTING CONDITIONS OF THE RESPIRATORY SYSTEM

- ❏ What is the specific type of condition?
- ❏ Does the record document any of the following?
  - Exposure to environmental tobacco smoke
  - Exposure to tobacco smoke in the perinatal period
  - History of tobacco use
  - Occupational exposure to environmental tobacco smoke
  - Tobacco dependence or tobacco use
- ❏ What is the lowest anatomic site affected by a respiratory infection?
- ❏ Is the condition acute or chronic?
- ❏ Does a lung abscess exist?
- ❏ What is the infectious organism? Is it a virus or bacteria?
- ❏ What are all of the respiratory-related comorbidities?
- ❏ Does influenza or asthma coexist with another respiratory condition?
- ❏ Is the condition in acute exacerbation?
- ❏ If asthma is documented, what is the level of severity?
- ❏ Is asthma in acute exacerbation or status asthmaticus?
- ❏ Is the condition the result of an external cause or procedural complication?
- ❏ If influenza is documented, what manifestations exist?
- ❏ Is the condition recurrent?
- ❏ Does the patient use supplemental oxygen or a ventilator (*a machine that assists in breathing*)?

Table 16-3 ■ KEY CRITERIA FOR ABSTRACTING CONDITIONS OF THE NERVOUS SYSTEM

- ❏ What is the condition?
- ❏ What is the subtype of the condition?
- ❏ What is the anatomic site?
- ❏ What is the underlying disease, if any?
- ❏ What is the external cause, if any?
- ❏ What is the infectious organism, if any?
- ❏ What laterality is documented?
- ❏ Is paralysis documented?

Table 16-4 ■ KEY CRITERIA FOR ABSTRACTING PAIN

- ❏ What is the site of the pain?
- ❏ What is the underlying cause of the pain?
- ❏ Is the pain due to a device, implant, graft, or trauma?
- ❏ Is the pain postoperative?
- ❏ Is it related to a specific postoperative complication?
- ❏ Is the pain related to a neoplasm?
- ❏ Is pain management the reason for the encounter?
- ❏ Is treatment of the underlying condition the reason for the encounter?
- ❏ Is the pain documented as chronic?
- ❏ Is chronic pain syndrome documented?
- ❏ Is complex regional pain syndrome documented?
- ❏ What psychological factors are associated with the pain?

Table 16-5 ■ KEY CRITERIA FOR ABSTRACTING HEADACHES

- ❏ What specific type of headache is documented?
- ❏ Is it documented as intractable?
- ❏ Is the headache documented as episodic or chronic?
- ❏ Does it affect the entire head or only one side?
- ❏ Is the headache accompanied with aura?
- ❏ Is status migrainosus or duration of 72 hours or more documented?
- ❏ Is the headache associated with another condition such as trauma, menstruation, cerebral infarction, or drug use?

Table 16-6 ■ KEY CRITERIA FOR ABSTRACTING EPILEPSY

- ❏ Is the seizure documented as epilepsy?
- ❏ Is it localized or generalized?
- ❏ Is it documented as intractable?
- ❏ Is status epilepticus or duration of 30 minutes or more documented?
- ❏ Are partial seizures documented as simple or complex?

Table 16-7 ■ KEY CRITERIA FOR ABSTRACTING PARKINSON'S DISEASE

- ❏ Is parkinsonism primary or secondary?
- ❏ Is dementia documented?
- ❏ Is dementia documented as parkinsonian dementia or Parkinson's disease with dementia?
- ❏ Is secondary parkinsonism documented?
- ❏ What is the cause?

Table 17-4 ■ KEY CRITERIA FOR ABSTRACTING GENERAL PSYCHIATRIC DISORDERS

- ❏ What is the disorder?
- ❏ What is the specific subtype of the disorder?
- ❏ Is the disorder due to an underlying physiological condition?
- ❏ Does the patient report symptoms that have no medical cause?
- ❏ What is the severity?
- ❏ Is the condition in remission?

Table 17-5 ■ KEY CRITERIA FOR ABSTRACTING MOOD DISORDERS

- ❏ What is the disorder?
- ❏ Does it have psychotic features?
- ❏ Is the condition current or in remission?
- ❏ Is the current or most recent episode manic, depressed, or mixed?
- ❏ Is the severity mild, moderate, or severe?
- ❏ Is remission partial or full?

Table 17-6 ■ KEY CRITERIA FOR ABSTRACTING PSYCHOACTIVE SUBSTANCE DISORDERS

- ❏ What is the specific substance?
- ❏ What is the class of substance (opioid, sedative, stimulant, hallucinogen, inhalant)?
- ❏ Is the disorder one of use, abuse, or dependence?
- ❏ Does the provider clearly document the relationship between the mental or behavioral disorder and the substance use?
- ❏ What is the blood alcohol level?
- ❏ Is intoxication present?
- ❏ Is withdrawal present?
- ❏ Is delirium (*state of confusion, restlessness, and incoherence*) or perceptual disturbance (*misinterpretation of surroundings or events*) present?
- ❏ Are any associated hallucinations, delusions, or other psychotic conditions present?
- ❏ Is the condition in remission?

Table 18-3 ■ KEY CRITERIA FOR ABSTRACTING CONDITIONS OF THE EYE AND OCULAR ADNEXA

- ❏ What is the condition?
- ❏ What is the subtype of the condition?
- ❏ Is a more specific subtype documented?
- ❏ What is the stage (certain types of glaucoma and macular degeneration)?
- ❏ Is laterality right, left, bilateral, or unspecified?
- ❏ For conditions affecting the eyelid, is the upper or lower lid involved?
- ❏ Is the condition acute or chronic?
- ❏ Is the eye condition secondary to diabetes or a condition from another body system?
- ❏ Do any additional eye conditions exist?
- ❏ Is the condition due to an external cause?

Table 18-4 ■ KEY CRITERIA FOR ABSTRACTING OPHTHALMIC MANIFESTATIONS OF DIABETES

- ❏ Is the diabetes type 1 or type 2?
- ❏ Is the eye condition related to diabetes (per the documentation or ICD-10-CM Index)?
- ❏ Is the condition retinopathy, cataract(s), or other?
- ❏ What is the laterality?

Retinopathy
- ❏ Is retinopathy proliferative or nonproliferative?
- ❏ Is nonproliferative retinopathy mild, moderate, or severe?
- ❏ Is retinopathy accompanied by macular edema?

Table 19-3 ■ KEY CRITERIA FOR ABSTRACTING CONDITIONS OF THE EAR AND MASTOID PROCESS

- ❏ What is the condition?
- ❏ What is the subtype of the condition?
- ❏ Is a more specific subtype documented?
- ❏ What part of the ear is affected?
- ❏ What is the laterality?
- ❏ What other conditions coexist?
- ❏ Is there an underlying disease?
- ❏ Is the condition due to a drug or external cause?
- ❏ Is there documentation of current or past use of tobacco or exposure to tobacco smoke?

Table 19-4 ■ KEY CRITERIA FOR ABSTRACTING OTITIS MEDIA

- ❏ What is the subtype of otitis media?
- ❏ Is it suppurative/purulent, nonsuppurative/serous, or another subtype?
- ❏ Is it acute, acute recurrent, or chronic?
- ❏ What is the laterality?
- ❏ Is there associated rupture of the tympanic membrane?
- ❏ What is the type or extent of the rupture?
- ❏ What is the laterality of the rupture?
- ❏ Is it a manifestation of another disease?
- ❏ Is there documentation of current or past use of tobacco or exposure to tobacco smoke?

Table 20-4 ■ KEY CRITERIA FOR ABSTRACTING INFECTIOUS AND PARASITIC DISEASES

- ❏ What is the named organism responsible for the patient's condition?
- ❏ What type of organism is it (bacteria, virus, etc.)?
- ❏ What is the subtype of the condition?
- ❏ Is a more specific subtype documented?
- ❏ Does the patient have a condition that is due to *Streptococcus*, *Staphylococcus*, or *Enterococcus*?
- ❏ Is the infection systemic or localized (organ specific)?
- ❏ Is the organism the cause of a condition that exists in a specific body system?
- ❏ Does the documentation state that the infection is resistant to antibiotics?

Table 20-5 ■ KEY CRITERIA FOR ABSTRACTING HIV AND AIDS

- ❏ Does the physician clearly document a confirmed diagnosis of HIV positive?
- ❏ Does the patient have symptoms or complications?
- ❏ Is the patient being seen (or admitted) for an HIV-related condition?
- ❏ Is the patient being seen (or admitted) for a condition *un*related to HIV?
- ❏ Has the patient been previously diagnosed with an HIV-related illness?
- ❏ Is the purpose of the encounter HIV testing?
- ❏ Did the patient receive HIV counseling?
- ❏ Is HIV serology inconclusive?

Table 20-6 ■ KEY CRITERIA FOR ABSTRACTING SEPSIS AND SEPTIC SHOCK

- ❏ What is the systemic infection underlying the sepsis?
- ❏ Is a more specific subtype documented?
- ❏ Is the sepsis documented as severe?
- ❏ Is an *associated* acute organ dysfunction documented?
- ❏ Is septic shock documented?
- ❏ Was the severe sepsis present on admission or did it develop after admission?
- ❏ Does a localized (organ-specific) infection exist in addition to sepsis?
- ❏ Is the sepsis the complication of a procedure that was performed?
- ❏ Is the sepsis associated with a wound?
- ❏ Is the sepsis associated with a noninfectious condition (such as trauma)?

Table 21-6 ■ KEY CRITERIA FOR ABSTRACTING CONDITIONS OF THE URINARY SYSTEM

- ❏ What is the condition?
- ❏ What is the subtype or anatomic site?
- ❏ What is the laterality, if any?
- ❏ Is the condition acute or chronic?
- ❏ Is an obstruction documented?
- ❏ What is the infectious organism?
- ❏ Is there a history of recurrent UTIs?
- ❏ What stage is the chronic kidney disease?
- ❏ Does the patient receive dialysis?
- ❏ Is the patient on a transplant waiting list or the recipient of a transplant?
- ❏ Do any additional conditions coexist?

Table 21-7 ■ KEY CRITERIA FOR ABSTRACTING CONDITIONS OF THE MALE REPRODUCTIVE SYSTEM

- ❏ Verify the patient's gender.
- ❏ What is the condition?
- ❏ What is the subtype or anatomic site?
- ❏ What is the laterality, if any?
- ❏ Is the condition acute or chronic?
- ❏ Is an obstruction documented?
- ❏ What is the infectious organism?
- ❏ What symptoms are associated with prostatic hypertrophy?
- ❏ Do any additional conditions coexist?

Table 21-8 ■ KEY CRITERIA FOR ABSTRACTING CONDITIONS OF THE FEMALE REPRODUCTIVE SYSTEM

- ❏ Verify the patient's gender.
- ❏ What is the condition?
- ❏ What is the subtype or anatomic site?
- ❏ What is the laterality, if any?
- ❏ Is the condition acute or chronic?
- ❏ What is the infectious organism?
- ❏ Do any additional conditions coexist?

Table 22-6 ■ KEY CRITERIA FOR ABSTRACTING CONDITIONS OF PREGNANCY

- ❏ Will the patient be under age 16 or age 35 and older at EDD?
- ❏ How many fetuses are there?
- ❏ What trimester is the pregnancy?
- ❏ How many weeks of gestation are completed?
- ❏ How many pregnancies has the patient had, including the current one?
- ❏ How many births has the patient had?
- ❏ What preexisting medical conditions exist?
- ❏ What complications exist?
- ❏ What is the current gestational age?
- ❏ For multiple gestations, how many chorions and amniotic sacs are present?
- ❏ For multiple gestations, which fetus is affected by the complication?
- ❏ What is the main reason for the encounter or the primary complication treated?

Table 22-7 ■ KEY CRITERIA FOR ABSTRACTING CONDITIONS OF CHILDBIRTH

- ❏ What is the reason for the admission?
- ❏ In what week of pregnancy did delivery occur?
- ❏ Is the delivery vaginal or cesarean?
- ❏ What is the reason a cesarean delivery was performed?
- ❏ Has the mother had a previous cesarean delivery?
- ❏ Is there a classical (vertical) or low transverse scar from any previous cesarean delivery?
- ❏ Was there a malposition of the fetus or obstructed labor?
- ❏ What other complications are present?
- ❏ How many fetuses were delivered? Were there any stillbirths?

Table 22-8 ■ KEY CRITERIA FOR ABSTRACTING CONDITIONS OF THE PUERPERIUM

- ❏ Is the encounter less than six weeks after delivery?
- ❏ What complication or condition is treated during the encounter?
- ❏ Is the condition preexisting or does it originate during the postpartum/puerperal period?

Table 23-3 ■ KEY CRITERIA FOR ABSTRACTING BIRTH ENCOUNTERS

- ❏ Was the infant born in this hospital during this admission?
- ❏ Was the infant born outside the hospital, then hospitalized?
- ❏ Was the delivery vaginal or cesarean?
- ❏ What is the birth weight?
- ❏ What is the estimated gestational age at time of delivery?
- ❏ Are any conditions documented as due to prematurity?
- ❏ Did the infant suffer any birth trauma?
- ❏ What conditions of the newborn required evaluation, treatment, extended LOS, or increased care or present implications for future healthcare needs?
- ❏ Was the newborn observed or evaluated for any suspected conditions not found?
- ❏ What maternal conditions affected the infant?

Table 23-4 ■ KEY CRITERIA FOR ABSTRACTING ENCOUNTERS AFTER THE BIRTH EPISODE

- ❏ What is the age of the patient?
- ❏ What is the reason for the encounter?
- ❏ What condition is documented?
- ❏ What is the subtype of the condition?
- ❏ What complications and comorbidities exist?
- ❏ Is the condition documented as originating in the perinatal period?

Table 24-3 ■ KEY CRITERIA FOR ABSTRACTING CONDITIONS RELATED TO CONGENITAL ABNORMALITIES

- ❏ What is the specific condition?
- ❏ What is the subtype?
- ❏ Is the condition clearly congenital?
- ❏ What manifestations are present?
- ❏ What manifestations are integral to the condition?
- ❏ What complications or comorbidities exist?
- ❏ Which condition or manifestation is the main reason for the encounter?

Table 25-7 ■ KEY CRITERIA FOR READING CPT GUIDELINES

- ❏ What is the purpose of the category and procedure(s)?
- ❏ How are anatomic sites or regions defined?
- ❏ How are the codes divided?
- ❏ What services are included in the code descriptions (not separately reportable)?
- ❏ What services can be reported separately?
- ❏ What standalone codes, indented codes, and add-on codes appear in the category?
- ❏ What instructional notes appear within the code descriptions in the Tabular List?
- ❏ What Main Term in the Index leads most directly to these codes?

Source: © PB Resources, Inc. Used with permission.

Table 25-8 ■ KEY CRITERIA FOR ABSTRACTING PROCEDURES (GENERAL GUIDELINES)

General Questions

- ❏ What service(s) were provided or procedure(s) performed at the current encounter by a physician or other qualified healthcare professional?
- ❏ What is the main service or procedure?
- ❏ What additional services or procedures were performed?
- ❏ What is the patient's age and gender?

Procedure-specific Questions

- ❏ What method, instrumentation, or approach was used?
- ❏ What anatomic site(s) were treated?
- ❏ What quantity was provided or time spent?
- ❏ What complications or unusual circumstances were encountered?
- ❏ Was more than one provider involved?
- ❏ What is the final diagnosis?

Source: © PB Resources, Inc. Used with permission.

Table 26-2 ■ KEY CRITERIA FOR ABSTRACTING HCPCS CODES

- ❏ Is the patient covered by Medicare or Medicaid?
- ❏ Does the patient's payer require/accept HCPCS codes?
- ❏ Did the patient receive durable medical equipment (DME), such as wheelchairs, crutches, hospital beds, or related accessories?
- ❏ Did the patient receive supplies to help treat or manage any of the following conditions:
  - Urinary incontinence
  - Ostomies
  - Respiratory problems
  - End-stage renal disease (ESRD)/dialysis
  - Need for parenteral and enteral nutrition
- ❏ Was radiopharmaceutical contrast administered (such as for a nuclear medicine scan)?
- ❏ Did the patient receive medication or drugs administered by a healthcare provider, including:
  - Injections
  - Chemotherapy drugs for cancer treatment
  - Immunosuppressive drugs for treatment of patients whose immune systems are compromised (including patients with AIDS)
  - Inhaled solutions
- ❏ Did the patient receive services or supplies related to orthotics or prosthetics?
- ❏ Did the patient receive preventive care services such as an immunization, mammogram, or colorectal cancer screening?

Source: © PB Resources, Inc. Used with permission.

Table 26-4 ■ KEY CRITERIA FOR ABSTRACTING AMBULANCE SERVICES

- ❏ Is the ambulance service freestanding or institution-based?
- ❏ What type of vehicle was used to transport the patient: ground (ambulance), air fixed wing (airplane), or air rotary wing (helicopter)?
- ❏ What type of services did the patient need: nonemergency, emergency, ALS, BLS, specialty care transport (SCT), or neonatal care?
- ❏ How many miles did the ambulance have to travel from its origin to its destination?
- ❏ Were extra personnel involved?
- ❏ What supplies were used?

Source: © PB Resources, Inc. Used with permission.

Table 26-3 ■ KEY CRITERIA FOR ABSTRACTING HCPCS MODIFIERS

Criteria	Modifier(s)
❏ Did the patient receive a service on a paired organ or site?	LT, RT
❏ Did the patient receive a service that treated the eyelids, fingers, toes, or coronary arteries?	E1-E4, F1-FA, TA, T1-T9, LC, LD, LM, RC, RI
❏ Was chiropractic manipulation provided?	AT
❏ Were one or more wounds dressed?	A1-A9
❏ Did the patient units of service exceed those in the medically unlikely edits (MUEs)?	GD
❏ Was a waiver of liability/Advanced Beneficiary Notice (ABN) issued or required due to the possibility of a Medicare denial for lack of medical necessity?	GA, GL, GK, GU, GZ, KB
❏ Was only the technical component of a service provided by a facility?	TC
❏ Did a dialysis patient receive dialysis-related services or non-dialysis-related services?	AX, AY, CB, CD-CF, ED-EM, G1-G6, JE, V5-V7
❏ Were psychotherapy or substance abuse services provided?	H9-HZ
❏ Did a nonphysician provider deliver the service?	AE-AJ, AS, GF, QY, SB, SD
❏ Was the service provided by a substitute or locum tenens provider?	Q5-Q6
❏ Were anesthesia services provided?	AA-AD, G8-G9, P1-P6, QX-QZ
❏ Was a screening mammogram or colonoscopy converted to a diagnostic test or done on the same day as a diagnostic version of the procedure?	GG, GH, PT
❏ Was a supply item or piece or part of equipment replaced?	FB, FC, KC, KN, KM, MS, RA, RB
❏ Were services performed that are normally bundled, but should be billed separately because of a separate encounter, separate provider, separate structure or anatomic site, or other unusual circumstances?	XE, XP, XS, XU
❏ Did the physician admit the patient to a hospital or nursing facility during the encounter?	AI

Source: © PB Resources, Inc. Used with permission.

Table 27-1 ■ KEY CRITERIA FOR ABSTRACTING CPT MODIFIERS

Criteria	Modifier(s)
Was a service provided that was more extensive than usual?	-22, -23, -47, -59
Was a service reduced or discontinued?	-52, -53
Was the service mandated (required) by a third party?	-32
Was the service bilateral (performed on both members/sides of a paired organ or site)?	-50
Was more than one surgeon involved in performing a surgical procedure?	-62, -66, -80, -81, -82
Was the service provided during the global period of a surgical procedure? Was the previous procedure performed by the physician now seeing the patient? Is the current service unrelated to the previous surgery?	-24, -25, -54, -55, -56, -79
Did the physician provide only the professional component of a service that has both technical and professional components?	-26
Was the service performed in a hospital outpatient or ambulatory surgery center?	-73, -74
Was an evaluation and management service provided on the same day or day before a surgical procedure?	-25, -57
Was the procedure repeated or a staged or unrelated procedure performed?	-58, -76, -77, -78, -79
Were surgeons other than the one who performed the surgery involved in the preoperative or postoperative care?	-54, -55, -56
Was the service habilitative or rehabilitative in nature?	-96, -97

Source: © PB Resources, Inc. Used with permission.

Table 28-1 ■ KEY CRITERIA FOR ABSTRACTING THE E/M SETTING (CATEGORY)

❏ Where (in what setting) was the service provided: office or other outpatient, inpatient hospital, or another setting (specify)?

❏ Did the service require minimal or no direct patient contact?

❏ Is the patient a neonate or child?

❏ What type of service was provided: management of a health problem, preventive care, consultation only, or other?

❏ If outpatient, is the patient new or established?

❏ If inpatient, is the encounter for the admission, continuing care, or discharge?

Source: © PB Resources, Inc. Used with permission.

Table 28-3 ■ KEY CRITERIA FOR ABSTRACTING E/M ESTABLISHED PATIENT TYPE

❏ Has the patient seen the same physician within the past three years?

• *Yes*: Patient is established.

• *No*: The next three questions must be answered *Yes* to qualify as an established patient.

❏ Did the patient see a physician of the exact same specialty as a previous physician in the same group?

❏ If previous physician was a subspecialist, did the patient see a physician of the exact same subspecialty as the previous physician in the same group?

❏ Does the visit with the same specialist or subspecialist occur within three years of the previous visit?

Source: © PB Resources, Inc. Used with permission.

Table 28-6 ■ KEY CRITERIA FOR ABSTRACTING THE E/M LEVEL OF SERVICE

❏ What are the criteria for determining the level of service: 2/3 key components, 3/3 key components, time, or other (specify)? (*You first must identify the preliminary E/M category to answer this question.*)

• What level of history was taken by the provider?

• What level of examination was performed?

• What was the complexity of medical decision making?

• How much time was spent in counseling and coordination of care?

❏ What is the patient's age?

❏ How much time was spent providing the service?

Source: © PB Resources, Inc. Used with permission.

Table 29-2 ■ KEY CRITERIA FOR ABSTRACTING MEDICINE PROCEDURES

❏ What organ system or anatomic site is involved?

❏ Is the procedure diagnostic or therapeutic?

❏ What equipment and techniques are used?

❏ What is the quantity, duration, or frequency?

❏ Is the procedure part of a more extensive procedure?

Source: © PB Resources, Inc. Used with permission.

Table 29-4 ■ KEY CRITERIA FOR ABSTRACTING IMMUNIZATIONS AND IMMUNE GLOBULINS

Immune Globulins
- ❑ Is the administration method infusion or injection?
- ❑ Is the route subcutaneous (SQ), intramuscular (IM), intravenous (IV), or intra-arterial (IA)?
- ❑ How long does the infusion last?
- ❑ How many substances or drugs are injected?
- ❑ What substance(s) or drugs(s) is given?

Immunizations
- ❑ What is the patient's age?
- ❑ Is counseling provided to the parents or family members of a child?
- ❑ How many vaccine components or combinations are administered?
- ❑ What is the route of administration of each vaccine or component?
- ❑ Is the vaccination provided in conjunction with a preventive medicine or other service?
- ❑ Is an immunization given for H1N1 influenza?

Source: © PB Resources, Inc. Used with permission.

Table 29-5 ■ KEY CRITERIA FOR ABSTRACTING PSYCHIATRY SERVICES

- ❑ What is the duration of psychotherapy services?
- ❑ Are services provided in a group or family setting?
- ❑ Is pharmacologic management provided?
- ❑ Is the service provided for crisis?
- ❑ Is interactive complexity required?
- ❑ Is testing or other services provided?
- ❑ Are separate E/M services provided?

Source: © PB Resources, Inc. Used with permission.

Table 29-6 ■ KEY CRITERIA FOR ABSTRACTING DIALYSIS PROCEDURES

- ❑ What is the patient's age?
- ❑ Where is the service provided?
- ❑ Are the services ESRD related?
- ❑ What type of dialysis is provided: hemodialysis, peritoneal dialysis, hemofiltration, or other continuous replacement therapies?
- ❑ How many days of ESRD inpatient services are provided during the month?
- ❑ How many ESRD outpatient encounters with the physician occur during the month?
- ❑ Are ESRD dialysis services provided in the hospital, a clinic, or the home?
- ❑ Are separate evaluation and management services provided, in addition to dialysis-related evaluation and management?
- ❑ For inpatient dialysis, how many evaluations are required with the hemodialysis procedure?

Source: © PB Resources, Inc. Used with permission.

Table 29-7 ■ KEY CRITERIA FOR ABSTRACTING GASTROENTEROLOGY PROCEDURES

- ❑ What site in the gastrointestinal system is involved?
- ❑ What is the nature of the test?
- ❑ Is fluoroscopy or endoscopy used?
- ❑ Which components of the service are provided: professional, technical, or both?

Source: © PB Resources, Inc. Used with permission.

Table 29-8 ■ KEY CRITERIA FOR ABSTRACTING OPHTHALMOLOGY SERVICES

- ❑ Is a diagnostic and treatment program initiated? Is the patient new or established? Is the level of service intermediate or comprehensive?
- ❑ Is contact lens service provided?
- ❑ Is spectacle service provided?
- ❑ What ophthalmic condition(s) is treated?
- ❑ Is ophthalmoscopy performed?
- ❑ What other type(s) of ophthalmic services is provided?
- ❑ Is the service bilateral or unilateral?

Source: © PB Resources, Inc. Used with permission.

Table 29-9 ■ KEY CRITERIA FOR ABSTRACTING HEARING SERVICES

- ❑ Is an evaluation and management (E/M) service provided?
- ❑ Is the service diagnostic or therapeutic?
- ❑ What anatomic site(s) is evaluated or treated?
- ❑ What specific tests are performed?
- ❑ What is the purpose of any evaluation service(s) provided?
- ❑ How much time is spent providing the evaluation?
- ❑ For speech-related services, does the service evaluate speech production and language abilities or does it evaluate the effect of residual hearing abilities on speech formation?
- ❑ What is the purpose of any therapy provided?
- ❑ What devices, tools, or equipment are used?

Source: © PB Resources, Inc. Used with permission.

Table 29-11 ■ KEY CRITERIA FOR ABSTRACTING INTERVENTIONAL CARDIOVASCULAR PROCEDURES

❏ Is the procedure diagnostic or therapeutic (interventional)?
❏ How many and which coronary arteries are treated?
❏ Which branches of each coronary artery are treated?
❏ How many grafted vessels are treated?
❏ Is contrast dye used?
❏ Is a stent or balloon used?
❏ Is intravascular Doppler velocity or coronary flow measured?

Diagnostic Angiography

❏ Is angiography performed at the same time as a coronary interventional procedure?
❏ Has the patient previously had angiography performed?
❏ Has there been a change in the patient's clinical indicators since the previous angiography?

Source: © PB Resources, Inc. Used with permission.

Table 29-12 ■ KEY CRITERIA FOR ABSTRACTING EVALUATION OF CARDIAC DEVICES

❏ What type of device is evaluated?
❏ How many leads does the device have?
❏ What type of evaluation is performed?
❏ Are programming services performed?
❏ Which components of the service are provided: professional, technical, or both?

Source: © PB Resources, Inc. Used with permission.

Table 29-13 ■ KEY CRITERIA FOR ABSTRACTING ELECTROPHYSIOLOGICAL STUDIES

❏ Which site(s) is evaluated?
❏ Is pacing performed?
❏ Is a comprehensive electrophysiologic evaluation performed?
❏ Which specific elements are evaluated?

Source: © PB Resources, Inc. Used with permission.

Table 29-14 ■ KEY CRITERIA FOR ABSTRACTING CARDIAC CATHETERIZATION

❏ Is catheterization performed for congenital heart disease?
❏ For catheterization procedures, which site(s) is catheterized: right heart, left heart, coronary arteries, bypass grafts?
❏ Is contrast dye used?
❏ Is catheterization accompanied by any of the following?
  • Transeptal or transapical puncture
  • Pharmacological study
  • Exercise study
  • Injection procedure for selective right-ventricular or left-atrial angiography; supravalvular aortography; pulmonary angiography
❏ Which components of the catheterization service are provided: professional, technical, or both?
❏ Is another procedure such as revascularization with a stent or balloon performed?

Source: © PB Resources, Inc. Used with permission.

Table 29-15 ■ KEY CRITERIA FOR ABSTRACTING NONINVASIVE VASCULAR STUDIES

❏ What body region is evaluated?
❏ Does the study involve arteries, veins, or both?
❏ What technique(s) or equipment is used?
❏ Is the study limited or complete?
❏ Is the study unilateral or bilateral?

Source: © PB Resources, Inc. Used with permission.

Table 29-16 ■ KEY CRITERIA FOR ABSTRACTING ALLERGY PROCEDURES

Allergy Testing

❏ What method(s) of testing is used: percutaneous, intracutaneous, or inhalation?
❏ What type(s) of test is performed: allergenic extracts, venoms, biologicals, or food?
❏ How many tests of each type were performed?

Immunotherapy

❏ Is the service injection only, provision of antigen and injection, or provision of antigen only?

Source: © PB Resources, Inc. Used with permission.

Table 29-17 ■ KEY CRITERIA FOR ABSTRACTING NEUROLOGY PROCEDURES

- ❑ What site(s) is treated?
- ❑ What testing method(s) is used?
- ❑ How many studies or tests are performed?
- ❑ How long does a recording last, if performed?
- ❑ Are all services—recording, interpretation, and report—provided?

Sleep Studies
- ❑ How old is the patient?
- ❑ What parameters are measured?
- ❑ Is the testing attended, unattended, or remote?
- ❑ Which components of the service are provided: professional, technical, or both?

Source: © PB Resources, Inc. Used with permission.

Table 29-18 ■ KEY CRITERIA FOR ABSTRACTING INFUSION AND INJECTION PROCEDURES

- ❑ What is the purpose of the infusion?
- ❑ What is the route of administration?
- ❑ What administration technique is used?
- ❑ How long does the administration last?

Source: © PB Resources, Inc. Used with permission.

Table 29-19 ■ KEY CRITERIA FOR ABSTRACTING PHYSICAL MEDICINE PROCEDURES

- ❑ What site(s) is treated?
- ❑ What type of evaluation or assessment is performed (if any)?
- ❑ What modality is used?
- ❑ Is the service supervised or constant attendance?
- ❑ What is the duration of treatment for each modality?
- ❑ How many spinal or body regions were treated by a chiropractor or osteopath?

Source: © PB Resources, Inc. Used with permission.

Table 30-10 ■ KEY CRITERIA FOR ABSTRACTING FINE-NEEDLE ASPIRATION

- ❑ Is the aspiration procedure specified as *fine-needle* aspiration?
- ❑ What type of imaging guidance, if any, is performed?
- ❑ Is a specimen being obtained?

Locate other codes if the answer to any of the following questions is *Yes*:
- ❑ Is the specimen being evaluated? (Use laboratory codes.)
- ❑ Does the aspirate consist of orbital contents? (Use eye codes.)
- ❑ Is the transendoscopic method used to obtain the aspirate from the esophagus, stomach, duodenum, or colon? (Use gastrointestinal system codes.)
- ❑ Is a percutaneous or core needle biopsy performed? (Use appropriate code for the anatomic site.)

Source: © PB Resources, Inc. Used with permission.

Table 31-4 ■ KEY CRITERIA FOR ABSTRACTING ANESTHESIA PROCEDURES

- ❑ What is anatomic site, type of procedure, and approach for the main procedure performed?
- ❑ What is the diagnosis(es)?
- ❑ How old is the patient?
- ❑ What type of anesthesia is provided (local, regional, general)?
- ❑ How long was anesthesia care provided?
- ❑ What is the health status of the patient?
- ❑ What type of anesthesia provider is in attendance?
- ❑ Are anesthesia services provided personally by the anesthesiologist?
- ❑ How many anesthesia providers did the physician supervise, if any?
- ❑ Did the surgeon provide anesthesia services?
- ❑ Is total-body hypothermia provided?
- ❑ Is controlled hypotension used?
- ❑ Is anesthesia complicated by emergency conditions?
- ❑ Are any unusual forms of monitoring used (intra-arterial, central venous, Swan-Ganz)?
- ❑ Is moderate sedation provided?
- ❑ Is monitored anesthesia care (MAC) provided?

Source: © PB Resources, Inc. Used with permission.

Table 32-8 ■ KEY CRITERIA FOR ABSTRACTING DIGESTIVE SYSTEM PROCEDURES

- ❑ What is the patient's age?
- ❑ What site(s) is treated?
- ❑ What primary procedure is performed?
- ❑ What other procedure(s), if any, are performed?
- ❑ Is the treatment screening, diagnostic, or therapeutic?
- ❑ What is the approach?
- ❑ What exact sites within an organ are excised or treated?
- ❑ What type of anastomosis, if any, is performed?
- ❑ What sites are joined in the anastomosis?

Endoscopy
- ❑ What approach (access) is used?
- ❑ What is the farthest site reached?
- ❑ Is the purpose of the service preventive care?
- ❑ Does a screening or diagnostic endoscopy convert to a therapeutic procedure?
- ❑ Is the endoscopy a separate procedure?
- ❑ Was more than one treatment performed during the endoscopy?
- ❑ Is moderate sedation used?
- ❑ Is the patient covered by Medicare?

Source: © PB Resources, Inc. Used with permission.

Table 33-5 ■ KEY CRITERIA FOR ABSTRACTING ENDOCRINE SYSTEM PROCEDURES

❑ What endocrine gland is treated?
❑ What is the surgical approach (e.g., open, endoscopic)?
❑ What is the anatomic approach (e.g., cervical, thoracic)?
❑ Is the procedure partial, subtotal, or total/complete?
❑ Is the procedure done to remove a malignancy?
❑ Were any adjacent tumors removed?
❑ What is the extent of lymph node excision, if any?

Source: © PB Resources, Inc. Used with permission.

Table 34-7 ■ KEY CRITERIA FOR ABSTRACTING INTEGUMENTARY SYSTEM PROCEDURES

❑ What is the procedure?
❑ What is the anatomic site?
❑ What is the depth or complexity of the repair or treatment?
❑ What is the size (length or area) of the site treated?
❑ What method is used?
❑ What is the quantity?
❑ Is a malignancy involved?

Source: © PB Resources, Inc. Used with permission.

Table 35-5 ■ KEY CRITERIA FOR ABSTRACTING SKELETAL SYSTEM PROCEDURES

❑ What is the general anatomic site?
❑ What is the specific location and/or compartment within the anatomic site?
❑ What is the laterality?
❑ What is the procedural approach (open or endoscopic)?
❑ What is the anatomic approach for spine procedures (posterior, anterior, anterolateral, or a combination)?
❑ What is the purpose of the procedure (diagnostic or therapeutic)?
❑ Is a foreign body removed?
❑ What type(s) of materials are used and/or prostheses/devices implanted?
❑ Which components of a joint are replaced (total or partial)?

Source: © PB Resources, Inc. Used with permission.

Table 35-6 ■ KEY CRITERIA FOR ABSTRACTING TREATMENT OF FRACTURES AND DISLOCATIONS

❑ What bone is fractured or dislocated?
❑ What site on the bone is fractured?
❑ What is the laterality?
❑ What type of reduction is provided (open or closed)?
❑ What general type of stabilization is provided (fixation or immobilization)?
❑ What type of fixation is provided (internal or external/percutaneous)?
❑ What type of traction is provided (skeletal or skin)?
❑ Is re-reduction of the injury required?

Application of Casts and Strapping

❑ What anatomic site is treated?
❑ Is the service an initial treatment?
❑ Is restorative treatment provided?
❑ Is restorative treatment provided by the same individual who applied the cast/strapping?
❑ Is the cast removed or repaired by the same individual who applied it?

Source: © PB Resources, Inc. Used with permission.

Table 35-7 ■ KEY CRITERIA FOR ABSTRACTING MUSCULAR SYSTEM PROCEDURES

❑ Is the procedure an excision, release, repair, transfer, or reconstruction or other type of procedure?
❑ Is the tissue a muscle, tendon, ligament, fascia, or other?
❑ What is the anatomic site?
❑ What is the laterality?
❑ What is the deepest layer of tissue treated?
❑ Is a foreign body removed?
❑ Is a malignancy involved?

Source: © PB Resources, Inc. Used with permission.

Table 36-6 ■ KEY CRITERIA FOR ABSTRACTING CARDIAC PROCEDURES

- ❏ What type of procedure is performed?
- ❏ What is the anatomic site?
- ❏ Is a device implanted or removed?
- ❏ Is imaging supervision and interpretation provided by the surgeon?
- ❏ Is moderate sedation used?

Coronary Artery Bypass Graft

- ❏ How many grafted vessels are used?
- ❏ How many and which arteries are used for grafting?
- ❏ How many and which veins are used for grafting?
- ❏ Is a venous graft obtained endoscopically?
- ❏ How many distal anastomoses are performed?
- ❏ Is cardiopulmonary bypass used?

Central Venous Access Procedures

- ❏ What type of procedure is performed (insertion, repair, partial or complete replacement, removal)?
- ❏ Is the catheter inserted centrally or peripherally?
- ❏ Is the centrally inserted catheter tunneled or nontunneled?
- ❏ Is a pump or port included?
- ❏ What is the age of the patient?

Source: © PB Resources, Inc. Used with permission.

Table 36-7 ■ KEY CRITERIA FOR ABSTRACTING PACEMAKER AND ICD PROCEDURES

- ❏ What is the type of device (pacemaker, implantable [transvenous] cardioverter-defibrillator, or subcutaneous cardioverter-defibrillator)?
- ❏ What type of procedure is performed (initial placement, removal, replacement, upgrade, or repair)?
- ❏ Which components are involved (pulse generator and/or lead)?
- ❏ How many and which chambers are involved?
- ❏ What type of leads does the pulse generator have (atrial, ventricular, dual, multiple)?
- ❏ How many leads are removed and/or inserted transvenously? How many leads are reused?
- ❏ What approach is used L (open [thoracotomy], endoscopic, or transvenous)?
- ❏ Is the device temporary or permanent?
- ❏ What other related services are provided (device evaluation, skin pocket relocation, defibrillator threshold testing)?
- ❏ Is moderate sedation used?

Source: © PB Resources, Inc. Used with permission.

Table 36-8 ■ KEY CRITERIA FOR ABSTRACTING VASCULAR PROCEDURES

- ❏ What site is treated?
- ❏ Is a catheter used?
- ❏ What type of procedure is performed?
- ❏ What is the surgical approach?
- ❏ Is a stent, filter, or other prosthesis used?
- ❏ Is moderate sedation used?

Vascular Injection Procedures

- ❏ Is the catheterization nonselective, selective, or both?
- ❏ How many access sites are used?
- ❏ What is the point(s) of access (e.g., femoral, radial, jugular, brachial)?
- ❏ Does the procedure begin at the aorta?
- ❏ Which vascular family(ies) is accessed?
- ❏ What is the first-order branch?
- ❏ Is more than one first-order branch (family) accessed?
- ❏ What is the second-order branch?
- ❏ What is the site of the examination/injection (e.g., ipsilateral or contralateral)?
- ❏ What is the most distal anatomic site to where the catheter is manipulated?
- ❏ What imaging studies are performed?

Source: © PB Resources, Inc. Used with permission.

Table 37-5 ■ KEY CRITERIA FOR ABSTRACTING HEMIC AND LYMPHATIC SYSTEMS PROCEDURES

- ❏ What is the procedure?
- ❏ What is the anatomic site?
- ❏ What is the surgical approach?
- ❏ Is the procedure performed during the same operative session as another major procedure?
- ❏ Is the harvest allogeneic or autologous?
- ❏ How many donors are used?
- ❏ What components are depleted or removed?
- ❏ Is the service a biopsy, limited removal for staging, or radical resection?
- ❏ Which specific nodes and/or chains are removed?
- ❏ Is the procedure bilateral (where applicable)?

Source: © PB Resources, Inc. Used with permission.

Table 38-5 ■ KEY CRITERIA FOR ABSTRACTING RESPIRATORY SYSTEM PROCEDURES

- ❏ What is the anatomic site?
- ❏ What is the procedure?
- ❏ What is the surgical approach (open, endoscopic, external)?
- ❏ What is the anatomic approach (transnasal, transthoracic, latero-vertical, etc.)?
- ❏ What is the purpose or variation of the procedure?
- ❏ What is the extent of the procedure (partial, total, etc.)?
- ❏ What is the laterality?
- ❏ What additional procedures were performed during the same session?

Endoscopy Procedures

- ❏ What type of endoscope is used?
- ❏ Is the procedure diagnostic, surgical, or both?
- ❏ Is moderate sedation used?
- ❏ What procedure(s) are performed during the endoscopy?
- ❏ Is the endoscopy a preoperative survey or scout?
- ❏ Is an endoscopic procedure converted to an open procedure?
- ❏ Is a decision made to perform an additional procedure during the same encounter based on the results of the endoscopy?
- ❏ What is the farthest anatomic site reached with the endoscope?

Source: © PB Resources, Inc. Used with permission.

Table 39-6 ■ KEY CRITERIA FOR ABSTRACTING NERVOUS SYSTEM PROCEDURES

- ❏ What procedure is performed?
- ❏ What is the anatomic site(s)?
- ❏ What is the surgical approach (open, closed, percutaneous, endoscopic)?
- ❏ What is the anatomic approach (anterior, posterior, epidural, subdural, etc.)?
- ❏ Is this an initial procedure or a revision/replacement?
- ❏ What other procedures are performed during the same encounter?

Vertebral Procedures (Laminectomy, Discectomy, Corpectomy)

- ❏ Which part(s) of the vertebra is treated (vertebral body, lamina, foramen, facet, disc, etc.)?
- ❏ How many and which segments or interspaces are treated?
- ❏ What is the purpose of the procedure?
- ❏ Is a facetectomy performed at the same time as another vertebral procedure?
- ❏ What is the laterality?

Source: © PB Resources, Inc. Used with permission.

Table 40-6 ■ KEY CRITERIA FOR ABSTRACTING EYE PROCEDURES

- ❏ What is the procedure?
- ❏ What part(s) of the eye is affected?
- ❏ What is the laterality?
- ❏ What is the surgical approach?
- ❏ What is the anatomic approach?
- ❏ What type of prosthesis is used?

Eyelid Procedures

- ❏ Is the upper or lower lid involved?
- ❏ Is only the skin involved, or are parts of the eye and adnexa also involved?

Keratoplasty Procedures

- ❏ How much of the cornea is removed (endothelium, epithelium, slice, partial thickness, full thickness)?
- ❏ Is the cornea reshaped?
- ❏ Is the patient's cornea reinserted or is a donor graft used?
- ❏ Is a graft secured with sutures or an air bubble?

Source: © PB Resources, Inc. Used with permission.

Table 41-6 ■ KEY CRITERIA FOR ABSTRACTING OPERATING MICROSCOPE PROCEDURES

- ❏ What is the primary procedure performed?
- ❏ Is use of the operating microscope documented?
- ❏ Do CPT guidelines or instructional notes indicate that the use of the operating microscope is included in the primary procedure?
- ❏ Does the NCCI prohibit coding for the operating microscope in conjunction with the primary procedure?

Source: © PB Resources, Inc. Used with permission.

Table 41-7 ■ KEY CRITERIA FOR ABSTRACTING AUDITORY SYSTEM PROCEDURES

- ❏ What is the procedure?
- ❏ What part(s) of the ear is affected?
- ❏ What is the laterality?
- ❏ What is the surgical approach?
- ❏ What is the anatomic approach?
- ❏ What type of anesthesia is used?
- ❏ What additional procedures are performed during the same operative session?

Source: © PB Resources, Inc. Used with permission.

Table 42-8 ■ KEY CRITERIA FOR ABSTRACTING URINARY SYSTEM PROCEDURES

- ❑ What is the procedure?
- ❑ What is the patient's gender?
- ❑ What is the anatomic site?
- ❑ What structures outside the urinary system are involved, if any?
- ❑ What is the surgical approach?
- ❑ What is the anatomic approach?
- ❑ What is the laterality?
- ❑ What type of obstruction is treated, if any?
- ❑ What structures are joined in an anastomosis, if performed?
- ❑ Is a stoma created?

Source: © PB Resources, Inc. Used with permission.

Table 42-9 ■ KEY CRITERIA FOR ABSTRACTING MALE GENITAL SYSTEM PROCEDURES

- ❑ What is the procedure?
- ❑ What is the patient's gender?
- ❑ What is the anatomic site?
- ❑ What structures outside the male genital system are involved, if any?
- ❑ What is the surgical approach?
- ❑ What is the anatomic approach?
- ❑ What is the laterality?
- ❑ What type of obstruction is treated, if any?
- ❑ What structures are joined in an anastomosis, if performed?

Source: © PB Resources, Inc. Used with permission.

Table 43-7 ■ KEY CRITERIA FOR ABSTRACTING FEMALE GENITAL SYSTEM PROCEDURES

- ❑ What is the patient's gender?
- ❑ What procedure is performed?
- ❑ What is the anatomic site?
- ❑ What additional sites are treated?
- ❑ What is the surgical approach?
- ❑ What is the anatomic approach?
- ❑ Is the procedure obstetrical or nonobstetrical?
- ❑ What is the extent of the procedure?
- ❑ What is the laterality?
- ❑ What additional procedure(s) are performed?

Source: © PB Resources, Inc. Used with permission.

Table 43-8 ■ KEY CRITERIA FOR ABSTRACTING MATERNITY CARE AND DELIVERY PROCEDURES

These criteria are specific to Maternity Care and Delivery subsection procedures. Also review the criteria for Female Genital System subsection procedures.

Delivery Procedures

- ❑ What is the trimester?
- ❑ How many weeks of gestation have been completed?
- ❑ How many infants were delivered?
- ❑ What is the method of delivery for each infant?
- ❑ Is a vaginal delivery attempted before cesarean delivery is performed?
- ❑ Has the patient had a previous cesarean delivery?
- ❑ What services are provided at the time of delivery in addition to the delivery itself?
- ❑ Is more than one physician involved in the antepartum care, delivery, and postpartum care?

  If Yes:

  - Which part of the process is provided by the current physician?
  - How many antepartum visits were provided by the same physician?

Abortions

- ❑ What is the trimester?
- ❑ How many weeks of gestation have been completed?
- ❑ Is the abortion induced?
- ❑ What method is used (evacuation, D&C, or drug administration)?
- ❑ Is the abortion complete or incomplete?

Source: © PB Resources, Inc. Used with permission.

Table 44-5 ■ KEY CRITERIA FOR ABSTRACTING RADIOLOGY PROCEDURES

- ❑ What is the patient's age?
- ❑ What is the anatomic site?
- ❑ What is the type of radiology procedure?
- ❑ Is the procedure diagnostic or therapeutic?
- ❑ How many and what views are taken?
- ❑ What body positions are used?
- ❑ What is the anatomic approach?
- ❑ What is the laterality?
- ❑ Is contrast medium used?
- ❑ Is the service technical, professional, or global?
- ❑ Is imaging guidance used to assist in another procedure?
- ❑ What additional procedures are performed?

Source: © PB Resources, Inc. Used with permission.

Table 44-6 ■ KEY CRITERIA FOR ABSTRACTING RADIATION ONCOLOGY PROCEDURES

- ❏ Is the service treatment planning or treatment delivery?
- ❏ Is treatment planning clinical or simulation?
- ❏ What is the treatment delivery modality (radiation, proton beam, brachytherapy)?
- ❏ What anatomic site(s) is treated?
- ❏ How many distinct areas are treated?
- ❏ How many and what type of ports are used?
- ❏ How many and what type of blocks are used?
- ❏ What is the total radiation dose delivered?
- ❏ How many treatments are given in the period being reported?
- ❏ Is the service technical, professional, or global?

Source: © PB Resources, Inc. Used with permission.

Table 45-4 ■ KEY CRITERIA FOR ABSTRACTING PATHOLOGY AND LABORATORY PROCEDURES

- ❏ What is the referring or ordering diagnosis?
- ❏ What specimen is tested or examined?
- ❏ How many specimens are submitted?
- ❏ How many tests or examinations are performed?
- ❏ What type of test(s) or examination(s) is performed?
- ❏ Is the test qualitative or quantitative?
- ❏ What type of equipment is used (e.g., microscope, automated, nonautomated)?
- ❏ Are any panel tests performed? Are all tests in the code description performed?
- ❏ What testing method is used?
- ❏ What constituents or analytes are tested?
- ❏ Is only the professional component provided?
- ❏ Is the physician billing on behalf of an outside laboratory?
- ❏ Is the laboratory test repeated on the same day?
- ❏ Is the service a CLIA-waived test?

Source: © PB Resources, Inc. Used with permission.

Table 47-3 ■ KEY CRITERIA FOR ABSTRACTING MEDICAL AND SURGICAL PROCEDURES (GENERAL)

- ❏ What is the stated procedure?
- ❏ What organ or body part is involved?
- ❏ How many sites are treated?
- ❏ What is the laterality (if applicable)?
- ❏ Is the procedure description what you would expect based on the name of the procedure?
- ❏ What surgical approach is used? (*Refer to Table 47-9, Key Criteria for Abstracting the Approach.*)
- ❏ Is a therapeutic device left in the patient after the procedure? (*Refer to Table 47-11, Key Criteria for Abstracting the Device.*)
- ❏ Was more than one procedure, or a combined procedure, performed?

Source: © PB Resources, Inc. Used with permission.

Table 47-4 ■ KEY CRITERIA FOR ABSTRACTING ROOT OPERATIONS

Root Operation Questions	Root Operation (Value)	Key Criteria for Abstracting (in this text)
Did the procedure take out some or all of a body part without replacement?	Destruction (5) Detachment (6) Excision (B) Extraction (D) Resection (T)	See Table 49-9
Did the procedure take out solids, fluids, or gases from a body part?	Drainage (9) Extirpation (C) Fragmentation (F)	See Table 52-8
Did the procedure involve cutting or separation only, within or around a body part?	Division (8) Release (N)	See Table 52-11
Did the procedure put in, put back, or move some or all of a body part?	Reattachment (M) Reposition (S) Transfer (X) Transplantation (Y)	See Table 50-7
Did the procedure alter the diameter or route of a tubular body part?	Bypass (1) Dilation (7) Occlusion (L) Restriction (V)	See Table 51-7
Did the procedure involve an external device left in place in, on, or in replacement of a body part?	Change (2) Insertion (H) Removal (P) Replacement (R) Revision (W) Supplement (U)	See Table 53-11
Did the procedure involve examination only?	Inspection (J) Map (K)	See Table 52-14
Operations Involving Other Repairs Did the procedure stop or attempt to stop postprocedural or other acute bleeding? Did the procedure restore a body part to its normal structure?	Control (3) Repair (Q)	See Table 53-14
Operations Involving Other Objectives Did the procedure render a joint or articular body part immobile? Was the procedure for cosmetic purposes only, without affecting the function of the body part? Did the procedure use biological or synthetic material to form a new body part to replicate a missing body part?	Fusion (G) Alteration (0) Creation (4)	See Table 53-18

Source: © PB Resources, Inc. Used with permission.

Table 47-7 ■ KEY CRITERIA FOR ABSTRACTING THE BODY PART

- ❑ What organ or body part is involved?
- ❑ What body system is the site part of?
- ❑ How many sites are treated?
- ❑ What is the laterality (if applicable)?
- ❑ Does PCS subdivide the anatomic site into multiple segments or lobes for detailed body system or body part values?
  - • If so, which segment applies to this procedure? (Refer to PCS coding manual Index, Tables, and Body Part Key.)

Table 47-9 ■ KEY CRITERIA FOR ABSTRACTING THE APPROACH

Key Criteria Questions	Method	PCS Approach
Is a full incision made?	Skin and deeper layers are cut open to reach internal organs/sites.	Open (0)
Is a needle or other puncture device used?	Skin is not cut open to expose deeper layers.	Percutaneous (3)
Is an endoscope used?	Access is made through small incisions in the skin.	Percutaneous endoscopic (4)
	Access is made thorough a natural or pre-existing artificial opening.	Via natural or artificial opening endoscopic (8)
Is a natural opening used for access to internal sites?	Direct entry access is made without endoscope.	Via natural or artificial opening (7)
	Access is made using an endoscope.	Via natural or artificial opening endoscopic (8)
Is access made through a pre-existing artificial opening?	Direct entry access is made without endoscope.	Via natural or artificial opening (7)
	Access is made using an endoscope.	Via natural or artificial opening endoscopic (8)
Is the procedure performed on the surface of the skin?	Skin is not cut open to reach deeper layers.	External (X)
Is the procedure performed in the mouth or mucous membrane?	Site can be seen without use of an endoscope.	External (X)
Is pressure applied to the skin?	Skin is not cut open. Direct or indirect force is applied, to move an internal structure.	External (X)
Are there two access sites: one through a natural or artificial opening and a second through the skin with an endoscope?	Laparoscopically assisted vaginal hysterectomy / Laparoscopically assisted anorectal pull-through procedure	Via natural or artificial opening with endoscopic assistance (F)

Source: © PB Resources, Inc. Used with permission.

Table 47-11 ■ KEY CRITERIA FOR ABSTRACTING THE DEVICE

- ❏ Was anything left in the patient to continue treating the condition?
- ❏ Was a therapeutic drain placed?
- ❏ Were clips placed around a vessel?
- ❏ Was a stent placed inside a vessel?
- ❏ Was an internal or external fixation device used to repair a fracture?
- ❏ Was a mechanical device, such as an infusion pump, placed in the patient?
- ❏ Was an electronic device, such as a pacemaker, placed in the patient?
- ❏ Was an artificial body part, such as a joint or limb, used to replace the natural part?
- ❏ Was a fusion device used?
- ❏ Was natural or artificial tissue used?
- ❏ Was an implant left in the patient?
- ❏ Was a shunt placed to move fluid from one area of the body to another?
- ❏ What material was used for the graft in a coronary artery bypass graft procedure?

Source: © PB Resources, Inc. Used with permission.

Table 47-13 ■ KEY CRITERIA FOR ABSTRACTING THE QUALIFIER

- ❏ Is the procedure a biopsy or otherwise diagnostic?

Bypass (Non-Coronary) Procedures
- ❏ What is the ending site of the bypass?

Coronary Bypass Procedures
- ❏ What vessel is bypassed from?

Amputation
- ❏ What is the exact anatomic site of the amputation?

Skin and Muscle Grafts
- ❏ To what depth is the procedure performed? Skin, subcutaneous tissue, fascia, partial thickness, full thickness
- ❏ What type of flap is created? Latissimus dorsi myocutaneous flap, transverse rectus abdominis myocutaneous flap, deep inferior epigastric artery perforator flap, superficial inferior epigastric artery flap, gluteal artery perforator flap

Spine Procedures
- ❏ What direction is the anatomic approach? Anterior (*incision/access from the front*) or posterior (*incision/access from the back*)?
- ❏ What part of the spinal column is treated? Anterior (*front side*) or posterior (*back side*)

Transplant and Replacement Procedures
- ❏ What type of tissue is used? Autologous, nonautologous, zooplastic, or synthetic

Source: © PB Resources, Inc. Used with permission.

Table 47-14 ■ KEY CRITERIA FOR ABSTRACTING MULTIPLE PROCEDURES

❏ Which components are included in the root operation (Character 3) or procedural steps?

❏ Is the same root operation (Character 3) performed on multiple body parts (Character 4)?

❏ Is the same root operation (Character 3) performed on multiple anatomic sites with the same body part (Character 4) value?

❏ Are multiple root operations (Character 3) with distinct objectives performed on the same body part (Character 4)?

❏ Is a root operation (Character 3) attempted with one approach (Character 5) then converted to a different approach?

❏ Is the initial root operation (Character 3) discontinued or otherwise not completed and a different root operation completed?

❏ Are a biopsy and a definitive procedure performed at the same operative session?

❏ Is an autograft harvested from a distinct anatomic site?

Source: © PB Resources, Inc. Used with permission.

Table 49-8 ■ KEY CRITERIA FOR ABSTRACTING ROOT OPERATIONS THAT TAKE OUT SOME OR ALL OF A BODY PART

Question	Root Operation (Value)
❏ Was a body part or abnormal tissue growth (such as a lesion or tumor) removed?	If *Yes*, continue below to root operations 5, 6, B, D, and T.
❏ Was a foreign object or abnormal material (such as calculus) removed?	If *Yes*, do not use root operations 5, 6, B, D, and T.
❏ Was the body part replaced with a natural or synthetic substitute?	If *Yes*, do not use root operations 5, 6, B, D, and T.
Answer the following questions to help distinguish Root Operations 5, 6, B, D, and T	
❏ Was removal performed by cutting?	Excision (B)
	Resection (T)
❏ Was removal performed through physical eradication, such as energy, force, or a destructive agent?	Destruction (5)
❏ Was an extremity cut off?	Detachment (6)
❏ Was removal performed through the use of force, such as pulling or stripping?	Extraction (D)

Source: © PB Resources, Inc. Used with permission.

Table 50-7 ■ KEY CRITERIA FOR ABSTRACTING ROOT OPERATIONS THAT PUT IN/PUT BACK OR MOVE SOME/ALL OF A BODY PART

Question	Root Operation (Value)
❏ Was a body part reattached, replaced, or moved? ❏ Was a body part replaced with a human or animal substitute?	If *Yes*, continue below to root operations M, S, X, and Y.
❏ Was a body part replaced with a synthetic substitute?	Do not use root operations M, S, X, or Y.
Answer *Yes* to one of the following questions to help distinguish root operations M, S, X, and Y	
❏ Was a severed or avulsed body part or extremity reattached?	Reattachment (M)
❏ Was a body part moved to a new location from an abnormal location to improve its function, with or without detaching it?	Reposition (S)
❏ Was a body part moved to a new location from its normal location where it was not functioning properly to improve its function, with or without detaching it?	
❏ Was a body part moved, without disrupting its nervous or blood supply, to serve a similar function in a new location?	Transfer (X)
❏ Was an organ or part of an organ replaced (transplanted) with a human or animal substitute?	Transplantation (Y)

Source: © PB Resources, Inc. Used with permission.

Table 51-7 ■ KEY CRITERIA FOR ABSTRACTING ROOT OPERATIONS THAT ALTER THE DIAMETER OR ROUTE OF A TUBULAR BODY PART

Question	Root Operation (Value)
❏ What tubular body part was treated?	If a tubular body part was not treated, do not use root operations 1, 7, L, or V.
Answer *Yes* to one of the following questions to help distinguish Root Operations 1, 7, L, and V	
❏ Were the contents of a tubular body part rerouted?	Bypass (1)
❏ Was an orifice or lumen expanded?	Dilation (7)
❏ Was an orifice or lumen completely closed?	Occlusion (L)
❏ Was an orifice or lumen partially closed?	Restriction (V)

Source: © PB Resources, Inc. Used with permission.

Table 52-8 ■ **KEY CRITERIA FOR ABSTRACTING ROOT OPERATIONS THAT TAKE OUT SOLIDS, FLUIDS, OR GASES FROM A BODY PART**

Question	Root Operation (Value)
❏ Did the procedure involve taking out gases, fluids, or non-native solid matter?	If *No*, do not use the root operations in this group.
Answer *Yes* to one of the following questions to help distinguish root operations 9, C, and F	
❏ Were gases or fluids let out from within a body part?	Drainage (9)
❏ Was non-native solid matter taken out of a body part?	Extirpation (C)
❏ Was non-native solid matter within a body part broken into pieces?	Fragmentation (F)

Source: © PB Resources, Inc. Used with permission.

Table 52-11 ■ **KEY CRITERIA FOR ABSTRACTING ROOT OPERATIONS INVOLVING CUTTING OR SEPARATION ONLY**

Question	Root Operation (Value)
❏ Did the procedure involve cutting or separation only, with no other objective intended?	If *No*, do not use the root operations in this group.
Answer *Yes* to one of the following questions to help distinguish root operations 8 and N	
❏ Was a body part cut into to separate or transect it, without draining fluids and/or gases?	Division (8)
❏ Was a body part freed of abnormal constraint by loosening or removing an attachment or constraint around the body part?	Release (N)

Source: © PB Resources, Inc. Used with permission.

Table 52-14 ■ **KEY CRITERIA FOR ABSTRACTING ROOT OPERATIONS INVOLVING EXAMINATION ONLY**

Question	Root Operation (Value)
❏ Was a body part examined but not treated?	If *No*, do not use the root operations in this group.
Answer *Yes* to one of the following questions to help distinguish root operations J and K	
❏ Was some or all of a body part visually or manually examined or explored?	Inspection (J)
❏ Was a brain or cardiac conduction mechanism mapped to locate electrical impulses or functional areas?	Map (K)

Source: © PB Resources, Inc. Used with permission.

Table 53-11 ■ **KEY CRITERIA FOR ABSTRACTING ROOT OPERATIONS THAT ALWAYS INVOLVE A DEVICE**

Question	Root Operation (Value)
❏ Did the procedure involve an external device left in place in, on, or in replacement of a body part?	If *No*, do not use the root operations in this group.
Answer *Yes* to one of the following questions to help distinguish root operations 2, H, P, R, U, and W	
❏ Was a device exchanged without cutting or puncturing the skin?	Change (2)
❏ Was a nonbiological device put in or on a body part?	Insertion (H)
❏ Was a device taken out and not replaced?	Removal (P)
❏ Was a device taken out by cutting or puncturing the skin?	
❏ Was a device put in to replace a body part?	Replacement (R)
❏ Was a device put in to reinforce or augment a body part?	Supplement (U)
❏ Was a malfunctioning or displaced device corrected?	Revision (W)

Source: © PB Resources, Inc. Used with permission.

Table 53-14 ■ **KEY CRITERIA FOR ABSTRACTING ROOT OPERATIONS THAT DEFINE OTHER REPAIRS**

Question	Root Operation (Value)
Answer *Yes* to one of the following questions to help distinguish root operations 3 and Q	
❏ Did the procedure stop or attempt to stop postprocedural or other acute bleeding?	Control (3)
❏ Was another root operation performed to stop postprocedural or other acute bleeding?	Assign a root operation that describes the procedure performed.
❏ Did the procedure restore a body part to its normal structure?	Repair (Q)
❏ Is the procedure more specifically identified by another root operation?	Assign a root operation other than Repair.

Source: © PB Resources, Inc. Used with permission.

Table 53-18 ■ **KEY CRITERIA FOR ABSTRACTING ROOT OPERATIONS THAT DEFINE OTHER OBJECTIVES**

Question	Root Operation (Value)
Answer *Yes* to one of the following questions to help distinguish root operations 0, 4, and G	
❏ Was the procedure for cosmetic purposes only, without affecting the function of a body part?	Alteration (0)
❏ Did the procedure create a new body part that previously did not exist?	Creation (4)
❏ Did the procedure render a joint immobile?	Fusion (G)

Source: © PB Resources, Inc. Used with permission.

Table 54-6 ■ **KEY CRITERIA FOR ABSTRACTING OBSTETRICS PROCEDURES**

Section Question	
❏ Is the procedure performed on the products of conception?	If *No*, do not use Obstetrics codes.

Root Operation Questions	Root Operation (Value)
Answer *Yes* to one of the following questions to help distinguish Root Operations in the Obstetrics (1) section	
❏ Does the procedure take a device out or off from a body part on the fetus and put back an identical or similar device in or on the same body part without cutting or puncturing the skin or a mucous membrane?	Change (2)
❏ Does the procedure take or let fluids and/or gases from a body part on the fetus?	Drainage (9)
❏ Is a pregnancy artificially terminated?	Abortion (A)
❏ Does the procedure pull or strip out or off all or a portion of a body part on the fetus by the use of force?	Extraction (D)
❏ Is a cesarean section delivery performed?	
❏ Are forceps used to assist a vaginal delivery?	
❏ Does the procedure assist a fetus, embryo, or unborn child to pass through the genital canal?	Delivery (E)
❏ Was a nonbiological appliance put in the fetus that monitors, assists, performs, or prevents a physiological function but does not physically take the place of a body part?	Insertion (H)
❏ Is all or part of a body part of the fetus visually and/or manually explored?	Inspection (J)
❏ Is a device taken off from a body part, region, or orifice on the fetus?	Removal (P)
❏ Is a body part of the fetus restored to its normal anatomic structure and function to the extent possible?	Repair (Q)
❏ Is all or a portion of a body part of the fetus moved to its normal location, or other suitable location?	Reposition (S)
❏ Is a body part of the fetus cut out or off, without replacement?	Resection (T)
❏ Does the procedure put in or on all or a portion of a living body part taken from another individual or animal to physically take the place and/or function of all or a portion of a similar body part on the fetus?	Transplantation (Y)

Source: © PB Resources, Inc. Used with permission.

Table 54-8 ■ **KEY CRITERIA FOR ABSTRACTING PLACEMENT PROCEDURES**

Section Question	
❏ Is the procedure performed on an anatomic region or natural orifice without making an incision or puncture?	If *No*, do not use Placement codes.

Root Operation Questions	Root Operation (Value)
Answer *Yes* to one of the following questions to help distinguish Root Operations in the Placement (2) section	
❏ Does the procedure take a device out or off of a body part and put back an identical or similar device in or on the same body part without cutting or puncturing the skin or a mucous membrane?	Change (0)
❏ Is pressure applied on a body region?	Compression (1)
❏ Is material put on a body region for protection?	Dressing (2)
❏ Does the procedure limit or prevent the movement of a body region?	Immobilization (3)
❏ Is material put in a body region or orifice?	Packing (4)
❏ Is a device taken off from a body part, region, or orifice?	Removal (5)
❏ Is a force pulling in a distal direction exerted on a body region?	Traction (6)

Source: © PB Resources, Inc. Used with permission.

Table 54-10 ■ **KEY CRITERIA FOR ABSTRACTING ADMINISTRATION PROCEDURES**

Section Question	
❏ Is a diagnostic or therapeutic substance given to the patient?	If *No*, do not use Administration codes.

Root Operation Questions	Root Operation (Value)
Answer *Yes* to one of the following questions to hel p distinguish Root Operations in the Administration (3) section	
❏ Is a cleansing substance put in or administered to the patient?	Irrigation (1)
❏ Is blood or blood products put in or administered to the patient?	Transfusion (2)
❏ Is a therapeutic, diagnostic, nutritional, physiological, or prophylactic substance except blood or blood products put in or administered to the patient?	Introduction (0)

Source: © PB Resources, Inc. Used with permission.

Table 54-12 ■ KEY CRITERIA FOR ABSTRACTING MEASUREMENT AND MONITORING PROCEDURES

Section Question	
❏ Does the procedure measure the level of a physiological or physical function?	If *No*, do not use Measurement and Monitoring codes.

Root Operation Questions	Root Operation (Value)
Answer *Yes* to one of the following questions to help distinguish Root Operations in the Measurement and Monitoring (4) section	
❏ Does the procedure take a single reading at a point in time?	Measurement (0)
❏ Are multiple readings of the same function taken repetitively over a period of time?	Monitoring (1)

Source: © PB Resources, Inc. Used with permission.

Table 54-15 ■ KEY CRITERIA FOR ABSTRACTING EXTRACORPOREAL OR SYSTEMIC PROCEDURES

Section Question	
❏ Does the procedure use equipment to support a physiological function?	If *No*, do not use Extracorporeal or Systemic Assistance and Performance codes.

Root Operation Questions	Root Operation (Value)
Answer *Yes* to one of the following questions to help distinguish Root Operations in the Extracorporeal or Systemic Assistance and Performance (5) section	
❏ Does the procedure take over a portion of a physiological function by extracorporeal or systemic means?	Assistance (0)
❏ Does the procedure completely take over a portion of a physiological function by extracorporeal or systemic means?	Performance (1)
❏ Does the procedure return, or attempt to return, a failed physiological function to its original state by extracorporeal or systemic means?	Restoration (2)
❏ Does the procedure use other methods, such as light, heat, cold, electromagnetic force, diffusion of fluid, or similar, to support a physiological function?	Review and select the appropriate root operation from Section 6, Extracorporeal or Systemic Therapies.

Source: © PB Resources, Inc. Used with permission.

Table 55-4 ■ KEY CRITERIA FOR ABSTRACTING ANCILLARY PROCEDURES

General Questions
❏ What is the stated procedure?
❏ What body region or body part is involved?
❏ What method is used?
❏ Is the procedure description what you would expect based on the name of the procedure?
❏ Was more than one procedure, or a combined procedure, performed?

Section Questions (Answer *Yes* to one question)	Refer to Root Types in This Section
❏ Does the procedure involve imaging/radiography?	Section B Imaging
❏ Does the procedure involve nuclear medicine?	Section C Nuclear Medicine
❏ Does the procedure involve radiation treatment for a malignancy?	Section D Radiation Therapy
❏ Does the procedure involve physical rehabilitation or diagnostic audiology?	Section F Physical Rehabilitation and Diagnostic Audiology
❏ Are mental health services provided?	Section G Mental Health
❏ Is substance abuse treatment provided?	Section 6 Substance Abuse Treatment

Source: © PB Resources, Inc. Used with permission.